Guidelines for Nursing Procedures

As you provide nursing care you want to communicate through your actions that you are a competent and caring nurse. Through developing systematic work habits you can communicate organization and efficiency that will not only save you time but are consistent with competency and help you focus on the client rather than the procedure. Plan your activities to include CDC Standard Precautions.

As you practice the procedures in this book, include the following activities in each procedure.

PRELIMINARY ACTIONS

Before you perform a procedure, always:

Confirm physician's order. When a nursing procedure is part of medical therapy or the implementation of medical therapy you need to confirm that a physician's order is written and that you are familiar with any guidelines the physician has provided.

Gather equipment. Planning the procedure and gathering the equipment will allow you to work efficiently. You want to gather all the supplies you will need to avoid repeated trips to the supply storage area. However, choose the items wisely. In the hospital setting you cannot replace supplies to a clean storage area after you have taken them to a client's room.

Confirm client's identity. Clients in an inpatient setting are identified with an armband. Check the client's armband against the chart or computer-generated worksheet. This check is especially important when the client's level of consciousness is altered or when you are working from a work station where items (especially medications) for multiple clients are stored. Asking the client to state his or her name is considered more reliable identification than asking, "Are you John Smith?"

Explain procedure to client. Form the habit of introducing yourself to the client and explaining what you are going to do. Explain in terms the client can understand. Avoid using medical or nursing jargon.

Arrange the work area. This activity may include raising the bed to a comfortable working height, clearing the over-the-bed table to provide a work surface, and placing the trash can in a convenient place.

Perform hand hygiene. You should perform hand hygiene before every procedure. Washing your hands in the client's presence adds to the client's confidence that you are providing for safety.

Provide for privacy. In a health care setting the client has the right to privacy. Close the door, pull a curtain around the bed, and drape the client if needed to avoid exposing usually private body parts.

COMPLETION ACTIONS

After you finish a procedure, always:

Make the client comfortable. Straighten the bed linens, adjust the pillow, and assist the client to a position of comfort. Lower the bed, raise one or more rails according to client need, and position the call light. Place water and personal items within easy reach.

Perform hand hygiene. You should perform hand hygiene after every procedure.

Document the care. Document the time of the procedure. Document the indication for the procedure, what was done, how it was done, supplies used, and pertinent observations made during the procedure.

OTHER CONSIDERATIONS

If you are unfamiliar with the agency policies and procedures, you should access the policy and procedure manual for guidelines specific to the agency. If you are assisting with an invasive procedure, confirm the agency's requirement for written informed consent.

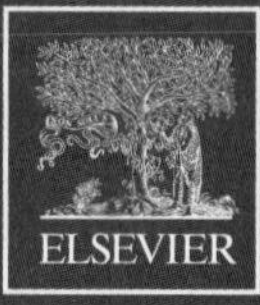

evolve

To access your Instructor Resources, visit:

http://evolve.elsevier.com/Harkreader

Evolve® Student Resources for Harkreader: ***Fundamentals of Nursing: Caring and Clinical Judgment,*** third edition, offer the following features:

Student Resources

- **Activities**
  Are an exciting, interactive way to review textbook content.
- **Review Questions**
  Test knowledge and understanding of the textbook content and include answers and rationales.
- **Video Clips**
  Demonstrate important steps in various nursing skills throughout the textbook.
- **Audio Glossary**
  Provides definitions of all key terms in addition to audio pronunciations for selected key terms.
- **WebLinks**
  Are an exciting resource that lets you link to hundreds of websites carefully chosen to supplement the content of each chapter of the text.

3rd Edition

Fundamentals *of* Nursing

Caring and Clinical Judgment

Helen Harkreader,
PhD, RN
Professor
Austin Community College
Austin, Texas

Mary Ann Hogan,
RN, MSN
Clinical Assistant Professor
University of Massachusetts–Amherst
Amherst, Massachusetts

Marshelle Thobaben,
RN, MS, APNP, FNP, PHN
Professor
Humboldt State University
Arcata, California

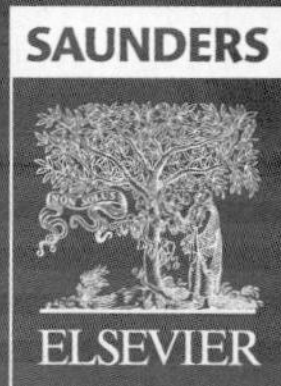

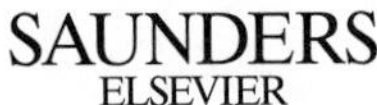

11830 Westline Industrial Drive
St. Louis, Missouri 63146

FUNDAMENTALS OF NURSING: CARING AND CLINICAL JUDGMENT ISBN: 978-14160-3436-0

Notice

Knowledge and best practice in this field are constantly changing. As new research and experience broaden our knowledge, changes in practice, treatment and drug therapy may become necessary or appropriate. Readers are advised to check the most current information provided (i) on procedures featured or (ii) by the manufacturer of each product to be administered, to verify the recommended dose or formula, the method and duration of administration, and contraindications. It is the responsibility of the practitioner, relying on their own experience and knowledge of the patient, to make diagnoses, to determine dosages and the best treatment for each individual patient, and to take all appropriate safety precautions. To the fullest extent of the law, neither the Publisher nor the Authors assume any liability for any injury and/or damage to persons or property arising out or related to any use of the material contained in this book.

The Publisher

Previous editions copyrighted 2004, 2000

ISBN: 978-14160-3436-0

Executive Editor: Susan R. Epstein
Senior Developmental Editor: Maria Broeker
Publishing Services Manager: John Rogers
Senior Project Manager: Beth Hayes
Design Direction: Jyotika Schroff

Printed in Canada

Last digit is the print number: 9 8 7 6 5 4 3 2 1

To all the people who call themselves Nurse. To those from the past who have given me a rich heritage.
To those who have accompanied me on the journey and to those who will follow.
Helen Harkreader

To my children, Michael Jr., Kathryn, Kristen, William, and Donna, who are sources of unending joy in life.
To the memory of my parents, Joseph and Marian, who taught me to pursue my dreams.
To all of my past and present students, who will help shape the future of nursing.
Mary Ann Hogan

To my current and former students who have affected my life and taught me so much.
To my husband, Kermit C. Thobaben, son, Sean C. Thobaben, daughter-in-law, Arianna M. Thobaben,
and grandson, Aidan K. Thobaben, for their love and support, and who bring joy and fulfillment to my life.
Marshelle Thobaben

About the Authors

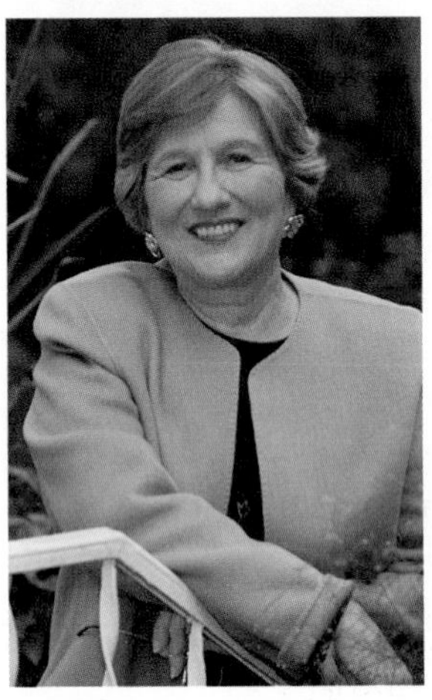

Helen Harkreader, PhD, RN, has been teaching beginning level nursing students most of her career as a nurse. Dr. Harkreader believes that her role as a teacher is to foster the individual growth of nursing students to help them develop their unique talents into professional nursing practice. Using the Myers-Briggs Type Indicator, Dr. Harkreader helps students appreciate the constructive use of differences and bring their strengths to develop an individual practice of nursing. The greatest compliment students can give her is that she has made them think. She is proud to be a nurse, bringing a background of practice in general medicine, intensive care nursing, oncology, gastrointestinal nursing, and surgical nursing to teaching in both baccalaureate and associate-degree nursing programs. Dr. Harkreader has conducted research on the effects of positioning on ventilation-perfusion ratios, caregiver burden as a factor in nursing home placement, and the utilization of vocational nurses. Dr. Harkreader received her undergraduate degree from Texas Christian University, her master's degree as a Clinical Nurse Specialist in Medical-Surgical Nursing from the University of Iowa, and her PhD in Adult Health Nursing from the University of Texas at Austin. She is a member of the American Nurses Association and NANDA International. She serves as Professor of Nursing at Austin Community College in Austin, Texas.

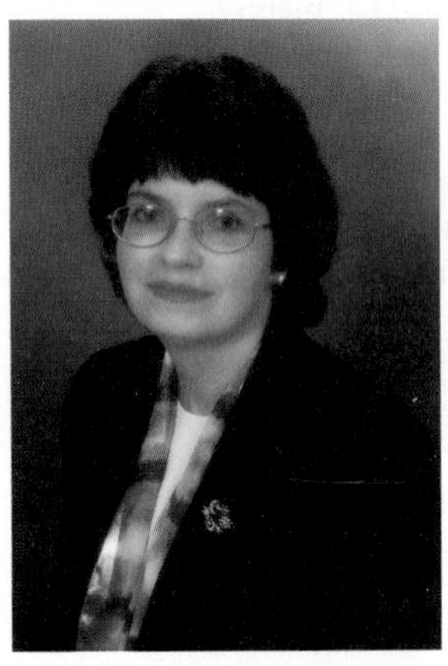

Mary Ann Hogan, RN, MSN, has practiced nursing in critical care and adult acute care units in Massachusetts and Connecticut. She began teaching in 1981 and has taught in diploma, associate-degree, and baccalaureate nursing programs. Ms. Hogan has taught fundamentals of nursing, medical-surgical nursing, and leadership and management in various nursing programs. Her ongoing interest in beginning nursing students stems from the belief that early learning has a tremendous impact on subsequent development as a nurse. Ms. Hogan's area of research interest is health-related behavior changes in older adults. She has an ongoing interest in assisting nursing students to prepare for the NCLEX-RN® licensing examination and is a former NCLEX item writer. Ms. Hogan received her Bachelor of Science degree from the University of Massachusetts–Amherst and her Master of Science Degree in Nursing from Anna Maria College in Paxton, Massachusetts. Ms. Hogan is a member of the American Nurses Association and Sigma Theta Tau International. She is a Clinical Assistant Professor at the University of Massachusetts–Amherst.

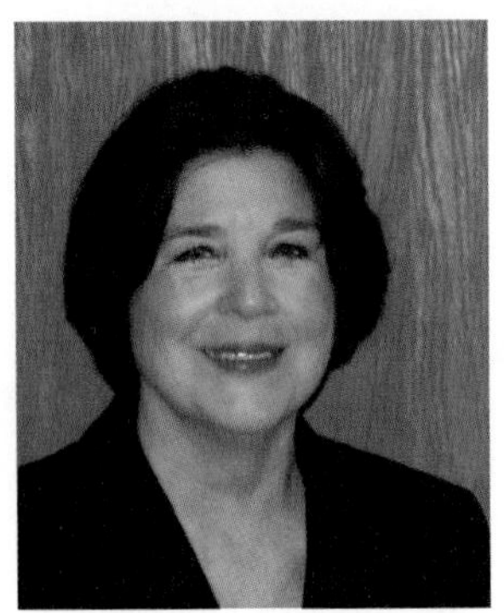

Marshelle Thobaben, RN, MS, APNP, FNP, PHN, is professor of nursing at Humboldt State University (HSU) in Arcata, California. She has taught for 30 years and been chair and director of HSU's Department of Nursing. Professor Thobaben has published more than 100 articles on international nursing education, elder abuse, and psychosocial issues affecting clients and nurses in leading nursing journals and textbooks. She has been nationally recognized for her work in elder abuse prevention and psychiatric home health. She has been a faculty leader both at Humboldt State University and at the California State University (CSU) system, and is currently the CSU Academic Senate Chair. Professor Thobaben has been honored by Humboldt State University as a Scholar of the Year for her outstanding research and received a Women of Achievement Award for her ongoing commitment to nursing education by the American Association of University Women.

Contributors

Kim B. Alten, APRN-BC, MSN, FNP
Family Nurse Practitioner
Adjunct Faculty
Azusa Pacific University
Azusa, California

Lenore L. Boris, JD, MS, RN
Associate Dean
SUNY Upstate Medical University
Clinical Campus at Binghamton
Binghamton, New York

Cynthia Bostick, PhD, APRN, CS
Lecturer
California State University–Dominguez Hills
Carson, California

Therese M. Bower, EdD, MSN, RN, CNS, CNE
Nursing Instructor
Firelands Regional Medical Center School of Nursing
Sandusky, Ohio

Karen Chang, PhD, RN
Assistant Professor
Purdue University School of Nursing
West Lafayette, Indiana

Diane E. Featherston, MSN, APRN, BC
Instructor, Clinical
Wayne State University College of Nursing
Detroit, Michigan

Janet S. Hickman, RN, EdD
Professor of Nursing and Interim Graduate Dean
West Chester University
West Chester, Pennsylvania

Janene Council Jeffery, RN, MSN, CT
Professor
Austin Community College
Associate Degree Nursing Program
Austin, Texas

Carolyn M. Kruse, BS, DC
Medical Editor
Kruisin Editorial Services
O'Fallon, Missouri

Virginia Lester, RN, BSN, MSN
Assistant Professor of Nursing
Angelo State University
San Angelo, Texas

Kristen L. Mauk, PhD, RN, CRRN-A, APRN, BC
Associate Professor of Nursing
Valparaiso University
Valparaiso, Indiana

Martha Meraviglia, RN, CNS, PhD
Assistant Professor of Clinical Nursing
School of Nursing
University of Texas
Austin, Texas

Jean Montgomery, RN, MSN
Associate Professor/Nurse Tutor
Austin Community College
Associate Degree Nursing
Austin, Texas

Kathleen Newman, MS, APRN, BC
Assistant Clinical Professor
University of Massachusetts
Amherst School of Nursing
Amherst, Massachusetts

Karen Plotkin, APRN, BC, PhD
Clinical Assistant Professor
University of Massachusetts
Amherst, Massachusetts

Donna Polverini, MS, RN
Assistant Professor of Nursing
American International College
Springfield, Massachusetts

Cecilia Prado, MSN, RN
Retired Faculty
Austin Community College
Austin, Texas

Deborah A. Roberts, RN, EdD
Assistant Professor
Humbodlt State University
Arcata, California

Heidi M. Vogtmann, MSN, BSN, RN, PHN, CPHQ
Instructor, Nursing
Ventura College School of Nursing
San Buenaventura, California

V. Doreen Wagner, RN, MSN, CNOR
Assistant Professor
North Georgia College and State University
Dahlonega, Georgia

Katherine H. West, BSN, MSEd, CIC
Infection Control Consultant
Infection Control/Emergency Concepts, Inc.
Manassas, Virginia

Mary Ellen Wilkosz, RNc, FNP, MSN, PHN
Assistant Professor
Nursing Department
Sonoma State University
Rohnert Park, California

Barbara Wroblewski, RN, MSN, MLIS
Clinical Nurse Informaticist
Cooley Dickinson Hospital
Northampton, Massachusetts

Reviewers

Barbara S. Anderson, RN, MS
Assistant Professor
William Rainey Harper College
Palatine, Illinois

Nell Ard, PhD, CNS, RNC
Director of Nursing
Collin County Community College District
McKinney, Texas

Terry Bichsel, RN, BSN
Practical Nursing Coordinator
Moberly Area Community College
Moberly, Missouri

Miriam V. Bixler, PhD, RN
Coordinator, Maternity & Mental Health Nursing
Alvin Community College
Katy, Texas

Tonya M. Broughton, MSN, RN
Assistant Professor
Ivy Tech Community College
Sellersburg, Indiana

Wanda H. Capps, RN, BSN, MSN
Associate Degree Nursing Instructor
Sampson Community College
Clinton, North Carolina

Deborah T. Castellucci, CRNP, PhD
Associate Professor
Geriatric Nurse Practitioner
Millersville University
Millersville, Pennsylvania
Center for Urologic Care
Berks Urologic Surgery Center
Wyomissing, Pennsylvania

Margaret Cole, RN, DSN
Associate Professor of Nursing
Spring Hill College
Mobile, Alabama

Lynn Marie McKenzie Derickson, APRN, P/MH
Instructor of Nursing
Wor-Wic Community College
Salisbury, Maryland

Marian T. Doyle, MSN, MS, RN
Associate Professor
Northhampton Community College
Bethlehem, Pennsylvania

Geralyn Frandsen, EdD, RN
Associate Professor of Nursing
Maryville University
St. Louis, Missouri

Sue K. Goebel, RN, MS, NP, SANE-A
Associate Professor of Nursing
Mesa State College
Grand Junction, Colorado

Christine Hobbs, BSN, AAS, RN
Assistant Professor of Nursing
Southwest Virginia Community College
Richlands, Virginia

Regina Janoski, RN, BC, MSN
Assistant Professor of Nursing
Montgomery County Community College
Blue Bell, Pennsylvania

Rosemary Kehrer, BSN, MSN, RN, CEN
Assistant Professor of Nursing
Mt. Aloysius College
Cresson, Pennsylvania

Mary Louise Kotsokalis, MSN, RN
Nursing Faculty
Central Piedmont Community College
Charlotte, North Carolina

Kay M. LaCount, BSN, MSN
Nurse Educator
Bay College
Escanaba, Michigan

Norma Lestikow, MS, BSN, RN
Nursing Faculty
Highland Community College
Freeport, Illinois

Denise Marshall, RN, BSN, EdD
Department Head Nursing
Wor-Wic Community College
Salisbury, Maryland

Patricia C. McCahan, MSN, RN
Nursing Faculty
Cabarrus College of Health Sciences
Concord, North Carolina

Pamela A. Montgomery, RN, MSN, MSEd
Instructor of Nursing
Southwestern Michigan College
Dowagiac, Michigan

Susan M. Randol, RN, MSN
Freshman/Sophomore Coordinator and Instructor
College of Nursing and Allied Health Professions
University of Louisiana at Lafayette
Lafayette, Louisiana

Terri Rebmann, PhD, RN, CIC
Associate Director of Curricular Affairs
Institute for Biosecurity
Saint Louis University School of Public Health
St. Louis, Missouri

Brenda Srof, PhD, RN
Professor and Assistant Director, Department of Nursing
Goshen College
Goshen, Indiana

Jo Ann L. St. Romain, MSN, RN, CLNC
Professor
Charity School of Nursing
Delgado Community College
New Orleans, Louisiana

Darlene Street, MSN, RN
Nursing Professor
Gardner-Webb University
Boiling Springs, North Carolina

June Tackett, MSN, RN
Associate of Science in Nursing Assistant Professor
Ivy Tech Community College
Sellersburg, Indiana

Josie Veal, MSN, RN, APRN-BC
Nursing Instructor
Milwaukee Area Technical College
Milwaukee, Wisconsin

Susan Waltz, RN, MSN
Associate Professor of Nursing
Associate of Science Program Chair
Ivy Tech Community College of Indiana
Columbus, Indiana

Kim Webb, RN, MN
Nursing Chair
Northern Oklahoma College
Tonkawa, Oklahoma

Gina Wilson, RN, MS
Fundamentals of Nursing Coordinator
Rose State College
Midwest City, Oklahoma

Linda J. Wlodyga, RN, MSN
Nursing Faculty
Century College
White Bear Lake, Minnesota

Contributors to Previous Editions

Elizabeth B. Abrahams, RN, MSN, ONC
Clinical Nurse Specialist, Materials Management
Inova Health System
Falls Church, Virginia

Kay C. Avant, PhD, RN, FAAN
Associate Professor and Chairperson
Family Health Nursing Division
School of Nursing, The University of Texas at Austin
Austin, Texas

Dee Baldwin, PhD, RN
Women's Health
Georgia State University
Atlanta, Georgia

Kathleen Barta, EdD, RN
Associate Professor
University of Arkansas
Eleanor Mann School of Nursing
Fayetteville, Arkansas

Margaret L. Bell, PhD, RN
Assistant Professor
Department of Chronic Nursing Care
The University of Texas Health Science Center
San Antonio School of Nursing,
San Antonio, Texas

Laura Bradford, PhD, RNC
Unit Director
Special Care Nursery
Rush–Presbyterian–St. Luke's Medical Center
Chicago, Illinois

Chyi-Kong Karen Chang, MSN, RN
Teaching Assistant
University of Illinois at Chicago
Chicago, Illinois
Formerly Visiting Assistant Professor and Assistant Professor
Purdue University
West Lafayette, Indiana

Carolyn Chambers Clark, EdD, ARNP, FAAN, HNC, DBFN
Adjunct Professor
Graduate Program in Nursing
Schiller International University
Dunedin, Florida
Faculty Mentor
Doctoral Program in Health Services
Walden University
Minneapolis, Minnesota

Jeannette Marie Daly, PhD, RN
Geriatric Nurse Researcher
Department of Family Medicine
University of Iowa
Iowa City, Iowa

Laura Dulski, MSN, RN
Staff Nurse
New Life Family-Centered Care Unit
Rush–Presbyterian–St. Luke's Medical Center
Chicago, Illinois

Carson A. Easley, MS, RN
Instructor of Nursing
Associate Degree Nursing Program
Antelope Valley College
Lancaster, California

Kristen L. Easton, MS, RN, CRRN-A, CS
Assistant Professor of Nursing
Valparaiso University
Valparaiso, Indiana
Community Health Education Director
Porter Memorial Hospital
Valparaiso, Indiana
Doctoral Candidate
Wayne State University
Detroit, Michigan

Shirley Eden-Kilgour, MSN, RN, FNP
Assistant Professor of Nursing
College of Nursing and Health Professions
Arkansas State University
Jonesboro, Arkansas
Retired Professor of Nursing
Loewenberg School of Nursing
University of Memphis
Memphis, Tennessee
Family Nurse Practitioner
Charter Lakeside Behavioral Health Systems
Memphis, Tennessee

Joan Engebretson, DrPH, RN HNC
Associate Professor
University of Texas Health Science Center at Houston
Houston, Texas

Kathleen A. Ennen, MS, RN
Doctoral Student
University of Illinois at Chicago
Chicago, Illinois
Part-Time Faculty
Parkland College
Champaign, Illinois

Sally Evankoe, BSN, MS, RN
Instructor
Maternal Child Nursing
College of Nursing, Rush University
Chicago, Illinois

Nancy Evans, BS
Health Science Writer/Editor,
San Francisco, California

Joanne H. Frey, PhD, RN
Assistant Professor
University of Massachusetts at Boston
Boston, Massachusetts

Richard Henker, PhD, RN
Assistant Professor
University of Pittsburgh
Pittsburgh, Pennsylvania

Karen Y. Hill, PhD, RN
Associate Professor of Nursing
Southeastern Louisiana University
School of Nursing
Hammond, Louisiana

Doris S. Holeman, PhD, RN
Associate Dean and Director, School of Nursing and Allied Health
Tuskegee University
Tuskegee, Alabama

Donna D. Ignatavicius, MS, RN, Cm
Clinical Nurse Specialist
Medical-Surgical/Gerontology Nursing
Calvert Memorial Hospital
Prince Frederick, Maryland

Susan M. Irvin, MSN, RN
Clinical Coordinator
Ambulatory Surgery Unit
Memphis Veterans Administration Medical Center
Memphis, Tennessee

Lorraine E. Kenny, MS, RN
Special Project Manager–Nursing
Governors State University
University Park, Illinois

Konnie Sue Kyle, MSN, RN, CNRN
Director
Orthopedics, General Surgery, and Neurosurgery
St. Francis Hospital and Medical Center
Topeka, Kansas

Eileen Klein, EdD, RN
Austin Community College
Austin, Texas

Kathryn Lauchner, PhD, RN
Professor of Nursing
Austin Community College
Austin, Texas

Delois Laverentz, MN, RN, CCRN
Formerly Assistant Professor
Fort Hays State University
Hays, Kansas

Jeanne Lawler-Slack, DnSc, RN
Associate Professor and Practitioner–Teacher
College of Nursing
Rush University
Chicago, Illinois

Marilyn S. Leasia, MSN, RN, FNP
Nurse Practitioner
Department of Medicine
Montefiore Medical Center
New York, New York

Janna Lesser, PhD, RN
Assistant Professor
Florida State University School of Nursing
Tallahassee, Florida

Susan J. Lewis, PhD, ARNP, CS
Advance Practice Nurse
Adult Psychiatric Mental Health Nursing
Department of Veterans Affairs Medical Center
Louisville, Kentucky

James Higgy Lerner, RN, LAc
Private Practice
Acupuncture and Oriental Medicine
Chico, California

Gwyneth Lymberis, MS, RN, ANP
Assistant Professor
Borough of Manhattan Community College
The City University of New York
New York, New York

Nancy J. MacMullen, PhD, APN/CCNS
University Professor
Governors State University
University Park, Illinois

Donna W. Markey, MSN, RN, ACNP-CS
Clinician IV, Surgical Services
University of Virginia Health System
Charlottesville, Virginia

Barbara McKinney, MSN, RN
Formerly Clinical Instructor
Ashland Community College School of Nursing
Ashland, Kentucky

Beverly M. Miller, MSN, RN
Geriatric Nurse Practitioner
Memphis Veterans Administration Medical Center
Memphis, Tennessee

Barbara S. Moffett, PhD, RN
Professor of Nursing
Southeastern Louisiana University
Hammond, Louisiana

Frances Donovan Monahan, PhD, RN
Professor and Director
Department of Nursing, SUNY Rockland
Suffern, New York
Nursing Faculty
Regents College
Albany, New York

Janet B. Moore, MS, RN, CS
Director
Robin Read Adult Day Health
West Springfield, Massachusetts
Part-Time Faculty
Elms College
Chicopee, Massachusetts

Virginia Nehring, PhD, RN
Associate Professor
College of Nursing and Health
Wright State University
Dayton, Ohio

Beatriz Nieto, MSN, RN, CNS
Assistant Professor
Department of Nursing
The University of Texas–Pan American
Edinburg, Texas

Hilario A. Pascua, MSN, CS, ARNP
Veterans Administration Medical Center
Mental Health and Behavioral Science Services
Louisville, Kentucky

Laura Roddy Redic, MA, MSN, RNC
Formerly Assistant Professor of Nursing
University of Arkansas at Pine Bluff
Pine Bluff, Arkansas

Betty Kehl Richardson, PhD, RN, CS, AANC
Professor
Austin Community College
Austin, Texas
Private Practice
Marriage and Family Counseling
Austin, Texas

Carol F. Roye, EdD, RN, CPNP
Associate Professor
Hunter-Bellevue School of Nursing
New York, New York

Barbara C. Rynerson, MS, RN, CS
Associate Professor Emerita
The University of North Carolina School of Nursing
Chapel Hill, North Carolina

Betty Samford, MSN, RN
School of Nursing
University of Texas at Austin
Austin, Texas

Katherine S. Schulz, RD, MS, LDN
Dietetic Consultant
State of Tennessee
Jackson, Tennessee

Brenda Leigh Yolles Smith, EdD, RN, CNM, ICCE
Associate Professor
College of Nursing
University of Tennessee at Memphis
Memphis, Tennessee

Carol E. Smith, PhD, RN
Professor, School of Nursing
University of Kansas
Kansas City, Kansas

Nancy Spector, DNFc, RN
Assistant Professor
Loyola University
Chicago, Illinois

Karen Stanley, MSN, RN, AOCN
Clinical Nurse Specialist
Pain and Symptom Management
Kaiser Permanente Fontana Medical Center
Fontana, California

Judy Sweeney, MSN, RN
Assistant Professor
School of Nursing
Vanderbilt University
Nashville, Tennessee

Rachel A. Taylor, PhD, RN
Formerly Assistant Professor
Department of Health Care Systems
College of Nursing
University of Tennessee at Memphis
Memphis, Tennessee

Joyce Z. Thielen, MS, RN, CS
Assistant Professor of Nursing
Elms College
Chicopee, Massachusetts

Daria Virvan, MSN, RN, CS
Nurse Psychotherapist
Town Center Psychiatric Associates
Rockville, Maryland

Phyllis Russo Wells, MSN, MEd, MPH, RNC
Women's Health Nurse Practitioner
New Horizons OB-GYN, PC
Stockbridge, Georgia

Bernie White, MSN, RN
Assistant Professor
Creighton School of Nursing
Creighton University
Omaha, Nebraska

Suzanne S. Yarbrough, PhD, RN
Assistant Professor
School of Nursing
University of Texas Health Science Center at San Antonio
San Antonio, Texas

Charlotte F. Young, PhD, RN
Retired Associate Professor
Department of Nursing
College of Nursing and Health Professions
Arkansas State University
Jonesboro, Arkansas

Deborah K. Zastocki, BSN, MA, EdM
Nursing Faculty
William Paterson University
Wayne, New Jersey
Senior Vice President
Clinical Services and Operations
Chilton Memorial Hospital
Pompton Plains, New Jersey

Sheila Rankin Zerr, BSc, MEd, RN, PHN
Visiting Faculty
School of Nursing
University of Victoria
Victoria, British Columbia
Visiting Faculty
School of Nursing
University of British Columbia
Vancouver, British Columbia

PREFACE

Thank you for choosing *Fundamentals of Nursing: Caring and Clinical Judgment,* third edition, as you begin your journey into a lifetime of learning to develop your practice of nursing. The opening chapters introduce you to the social and professional context of nursing practice, the cultural context of the people who are recipients of nursing care, and the framework to learn to "think like a nurse." Then you will use that framework as you learn about the needs and problems that nurses can help people manage. When you have completed the study of fundamentals of nursing you will be able to apply principles to provide holistic care to meet the needs of the recipients of your care. We hope your creativity is stirred and you will use this platform as a springboard to develop a richly unique nursing practice that contributes caring and clinical judgment to an ever-changing health care environment.

Plans for the third edition emerged out of a study of the current trends in health care. We cannot know what the nurse will be doing in a rapidly changing health care environment. We expect the role of the nurse to continue to evolve, with opportunities developing in long-term care, in the home and health care settings, in advanced nursing practice, and in clinical nursing research. Nurses will be increasingly relied on to meet the needs of growing populations of the elderly, the chronically ill, the poor, and the uninsured as society struggles with a right to health care for all in an environment of scarce resources. Nurses will need creativity and critical thinking to be providers of care and advocates for these populations.

There will be greater responsibility and accountability for nurses in a responsive health care system with well-informed clients, who demand more of the system as consumers of health care. We can expect the client in both the hospital and in long-term care to be sicker and have a need for more sophisticated nursing care. We can expect the public to be watching through the eyes of a highly regulated health care system.

The need for cost-effective care drives the system to employ only evidenced-based practice methodology and models of practice to prevent errors. While the current use of computers is introductory, computerized databases of the client's health record will become a means to provide the needed evidence that our practice is effective and to identify the contribution of nursing to health care.

Ethical integrity is becoming more important to nursing practice because of widespread use of alternative therapies, developments in gene therapy and use of stem cells, and emerging issues in palliative care. An increasingly multicultural society will place demands on the system for ethnically competent care.

Fundamentals of Nursing: Caring and Clinical Judgment, third edition, introduces you to a framework for practice and methodologies of practice that can be applied regardless of the setting for practice. It emphasizes the thinking skills that will help you modify your practice in a changing health care environment. Rather than learning to base nursing care needs on medical diagnoses, you will learn to assess your patient to identify needs and problems. You will use logical reasoning to plan goal-directed care.

We have added a separate chapter on the middle and older adult to place greater emphasis on the aging population. We have strengthened chapters on confusion, verbal communication, and sensory perceptual deficits because these problems are common in the elderly client. Aging content has been strengthened throughout the book.

We have added information about emerging regulations such as the use of abbreviations in documentation, increased use of lifting devices to prevent back injuries in health care workers, and reducing errors in health care.

We have restructured the chapter on nursing research to introduce evidence-based practice. Then we added Evidence-Based Practice boxes throughout the book to show you how levels of evidence can be used to justify nursing practice.

The chapter on ethical legal aspects of nursing has been restructured to focus the student on becoming first an ethically competent practitioner in a system highly regulated by law. The ethic of care has been introduced as fundamental to the nursing practice.

HOW THE BOOK IS STRUCTURED

Unit I is designed to help you understand the context of nursing practice as a profession, as a service to a multicultural society, and as part of the health care team. We practice as a member of a profession; the *profession* of nursing controls the *practice* of nursing by defining the practice of nursing, the standards for practice, and the code of ethics of nursing. Nursing is also controlled by the legal definition of nursing and legal standards for practice. We first serve the client, who is often from a culture different from our own. We work as part of a health care team to ensure that the right services are employed to best meet the client's needs.

Unit II is designed to help you develop a pattern of thinking that will give structure to your practice of nursing. Additionally, you will be introduced to the concepts of caring, critical thinking, and clinical judgment, skills that are growing in importance as health care grows in complexity. The nursing process is the method of studying how nurses think. Although the nursing process is divided into five phases that involve five types of thinking (assessment, diagnosis, planning, intervention, and evaluation), this unit shows the interrelationships among the five types of thinking. This unit concludes with content on documentation of the care that you have provided.

Unit III discusses some key "tools" used in nursing practice. Although the use of technology is paramount in health care, these "tools" of nursing are more closely related to the mental processes and human relationships nurses use in practice than to the technology of health care. Independent nursing practice often primarily uses the tool of a therapeutic relationship with the client, in which the client makes decisions about health management and learns effective methods of restoring or maintaining health. Additionally you will learn to use the tools of teaching, managing care, and research in your practice.

Unit IV describes the well client across the life span and examines some of the client's needs to maintain health. You will be introduced to growth and development and factors affecting health at each stage of life.

Units IV through XV present common client problems organized around Marjory Gordon's Functional Health Patterns. Rather than focusing on body systems and pathophysiology, these patterns focus your assessment on the client problems that are amenable to nursing care. You can use the Functional Health Patterns to systematically assess your clients, thus ensuring comprehensive assessment for any presenting problem. At the start of each chapter in these units, you will find a *Key Nursing Diagnoses* box to help serve as a focus for the chapter content, as well as a *chapter-opening case study* to enable you to study the content in the context of a real-life person. The case study is continued throughout the chapter in brief vignettes with critical thinking questions to help you reflect on the client's problems and explore solutions. A *Nursing Care Plan* and *Sample Documentation Note* for the case study client is also provided.

Unit XVI will help you integrate the information from Units V through XV to plan care for surgical clients. The client who needs surgical intervention has needs in each Functional Health Pattern.

Internally, the chapters in Units IV through XVI of the book are organized in a consistent framework revolving around the application of the nursing process to help you establish a systematic pattern of thinking.

NEW TO THIS EDITION

- Companion CD features a wide variety of student activities, NCLEX-style questions, audio glossary, and Body Spectrum, an anatomy and physiology program.
- Separate chapter on the middle and older adult.
- Evidence-based practice introduced in research chapter and boxes throughout the book
- Compliance with The Joint Commission (TJC) use of abbreviations.
- Ethic of care added to ethics chapter.
- Updated NANDA-I terminology.
- Research-based table on managing nasogastric tubes.
- New food pyramid guide (MyPyramid).
- NCLEX-style questions at the end of every chapter.
- Media Resource boxes detail what electronic resources are available to you for every chapter.
- Safety Issues added to appropriate skills to reflect TJC's increased focus on safe patient care.
- Older Adults boxes highlight important information for providing appropriate care to this growing client population.
- Case Studies now include photographs of clients to help bring these clinical situations to life for students.
- Skills in the text that are supported by Nursing Skills Online include NSO lesson numbers so students can go right to pertinent review and evaluation.
- Skills Video Clips from Mosby's Nursing Skills Videos are provided on Evolve and on the Companion CD; skills in the text are flagged to remind students to view the video.

SPECIAL FEATURES TO FACILITATE LEARNING

- Chapter-opening case studies enable you to study the content in the context of a person you will be helping. The case study is continued throughout the chapter in brief *vignettes, cross-cultural care boxes,* a *nursing care plan,* and *sample documentation note.*
- Key Nursing Diagnoses boxes help guide your thinking as you read the chapter. Almost all of these nursing diagnoses are officially approved by the North American Nursing Diagnosis Association International (NANDA-I).
- Critical thinking questions throughout chapters and at the end of chapter care plans will help you develop the habit of reflecting critically on client problems and exploring alternative solutions.
- NCLEX-style questions are included at the end of every chapter.
- Cross-Cultural Care boxes explore the implications of culture in the client whose story is introduced in the chapter-opening case study. These charts, which consist of background information, introduce you to a

wide variety of cultures and subcultures and present true-to-life examples of the impact of culture on health care. Many of these clients are based on real people encountered in a clinical setting.
- Nursing Care Plan charts based on the client in the case study demonstrate how to plan and evaluate nursing care. Each of these charts ends in a series of critical thinking questions.
- In this book, we highlight the skills and procedures most commonly taught in nursing fundamentals courses in over 70 heavily illustrated *Procedures.* Most students are more comfortable learning a small number of steps to a procedure rather than an exhaustive list; therefore we have presented each procedure with a small number of key steps, with more specific details under each step. Under each step, we have included, in *italic* type, rationales, alternative approaches, and decision-making information.
- To convey the human side of health, illness, and health care, we conducted interviews with real patients and family caregivers. The resulting charts, which we have called *A Patient's Perspective* or *A Caregiver's Perspective,* provide first-person windows into the lives of clients and caregivers. They demonstrate, in the person's own words, how health conditions, medical treatments, and nursing care have affected their lives.
- Increasingly, people are turning to complementary and alternative therapies to overcome the effects of illness or side effects of treatment. To introduce you to this topic and to give you the tools to learn more, we have provided a series of *Considering the Alternatives* boxes, written by an expert in the field of complementary and alternative medicine.
- Evidenced-based practice boxes throughout the text show the application of the concept of evidence-based practice as introduced in Chapter 15.
- In your practice of nursing you will encounter situations that require quick thinking and immediate action. Therefore throughout the text, we have included *Action Alerts,* which focus on situations that call for immediate action or immediate physician collaboration.
- We have provided two special features to help you accurately formulate nursing diagnoses: *Clustering Data to Make a Nursing Diagnosis* boxes and *Decision Trees.* These boxes show you how to apply nursing diagnoses to various client scenarios and how to differentiate between closely related diagnoses in order to select the appropriate one.
- The *Teaching for Wellness* and *Teaching for Self-Care* boxes will help you sharpen your teaching skills. *Teaching for Wellness* boxes focus on health promotion and illness prevention. *Teaching for Self-Care* boxes focus on restoration of health after illness. Both types of boxes model how to convey complex health care information in language that clients and caregivers can easily understand.
- Skills in the text that are supported by Nursing Skills Online include NSO lesson numbers so students can go right to pertinent review and evaluation.
- Skills Video Clips from Mosby's Nursing Skills Videos are provided on Evolve and on the Companion CD; skills in the text are flagged to remind students to view the video.

A MULTIMEDIA LEARNING PACKAGE

FOR STUDENTS

- *Study Guide for Fundamentals of Nursing* includes Matching, True or False, Fill in the Blanks, Exercising Your Clinical Judgment, and Test Yourself questions, along with Performance Checklists for each of the *Procedures* found in the textbook. Answers for all of the exercises are also provided.
- *Brand-new Companion CD* packaged with the textbook provides
  - Over 250 Student Activities to test your understanding of key concept and principles in each chapter
  - Nearly 600 NCLEX-style Review Questions to help you focus your study and practice for your next exam.
  - Audio Glossary
  - Body Spectrum, an anatomy and physiology program
- *Virtual Clinical Excursions.* This workbook/CD-ROM brings learning to life in a multifloor "virtual" hospital setting. Each lesson in the workbook corresponds with a textbook unit and guides you through the CD-ROM as you care for patients in the virtual hospital.
- *Evolve Learning Resources.* Be sure to visit the Evolve website at http://evolve.elsevier.com/Harkreader to access the online resources available to you. These resources include:
  - Nearly 600 NCLEX-style Review Questions to help you focus your study and practice for your next examination
  - Audio Glossary
  - Over 250 Student Activities to test your understanding of key concept and principles in each chapter
  - WebLinks for each chapter to take you to places of interest on the web

FOR INSTRUCTORS

- *Evolve Course Management System* for instructors adopting classroom quantities of *Fundamentals of Nursing: Caring and Clinical Judgment,* third edition. You can use Evolve to publish your class syllabus, outline, and lecture notes; set up "virtual office hours" and e-mail communication; share important dates and information through the online class *Calendar;* and encourage student participation through *Chat Rooms* and *Discussion Boards.* Instructors' Resources available at the Evolve website (http://evolve.elsevier.com/Harkreader) are the same as those available on the CD-ROM (listed below).

- *Instructor's Resource CD-ROM.* Consists of valuable resources including:
  - Instructor's Manual includes: Teaching/Learning Activities for the classroom, laboratory, and clinical setting; Critical Thinking Exercises; and Resources for lesson preparation and student assignments. Each chapter also includes Key Terms, Learning Objectives, Key Principles, and a chapter outline. Selected chapters include brand-new prioritization questions focusing on prioritization of nursing actions.
  - ExamView Test Bank with over 500 multiple-choice questions.
  - Electronic Image Collection with over 500 images from the textbook.
  - PowerPoint Slides with over 600 text slides to assist you with your lecture.
  - Skills Performance Checklists for each of the procedures covered in the text.

For more information about these resources, instructors may contact their Sales Representative or call Faculty Support.

A TEXT FOR THE NURSES OF TOMORROW

The third edition of *Fundamentals of Nursing: Caring and Clinical Judgment* is written for you, the nurses who will come after us to become the nursing leaders of tomorrow in a health care environment that is unpredictable and unprecedented in its complexity. It introduces the tools you need to provide the human element of care in a health care environment concerned with cost containment and efficiency; it equips you with the tools of thinking you will need to develop a practice of sound clinical judgment and continue your professional education. We are privileged to be allowed to offer *Fundamentals of Nursing: Caring and Clinical Judgment* as a forum to share our expertise in nursing with you.

Helen Harkreader, PhD, RN
Austin, Texas

Mary Ann Hogan, RN, MSN
Amherst, Massachusetts

Marshelle Thobaben, RN, MS, APNP, FNP, PHN
Arcata, California

Acknowledgments

The preparation of a fundamentals textbook is truly a team effort. We wish to thank all the people on the team for their contribution.

Susan Epstein, Executive Editor, led the team with style to ensure a uniquely sound and marketable product. Maria Broeker as Developmental Editor organized the project and ensured the team worked efficiently. The production team of John Rogers, Publishing Services Manager, and Beth Hayes, Senior Project Manager, ensured a well-coordinated and smooth production process. Beth oversaw the editing and production process, bringing greater clarity and consistency to the text, while working closely with the development team, the typesetter, and the printer to transform the manuscript into a book. Jyotika Shroff as Senior Book Designer oversaw the layout and design to give the book a fresh and sparkling new look yet in keeping with the theme of the first edition.

We do not want to forget those who contributed to and reviewed the first edition and second editions, because we relied heavily on their work for the third edition. We received many helpful suggestions from students and faculty who used the book, and we feel the book is stronger for their input. Thanks to the contributors and reviewers of the third edition. We hope all of you are as proud of the product as we are.

STUDENT PREFACE

This book was designed to help you learn. It includes the following special features.

Key Nursing Diagnoses at the beginning of each chapter help you understand how nursing actions relate to specific patient problems.

Media Resource boxes detail what electronic resources are available to you for every chapter.

Case Studies open each clinical chapter and continue with vignettes throughout.

Learning Objectives and **Key Terms** at the beginning of each chapter place focus on key information.

Decision Trees and **Clustering Data Tables** help accurately formulate nursing diagnoses by applying the diagnoses to different client scenarios and showing how to differentiate between closely related diagnoses.

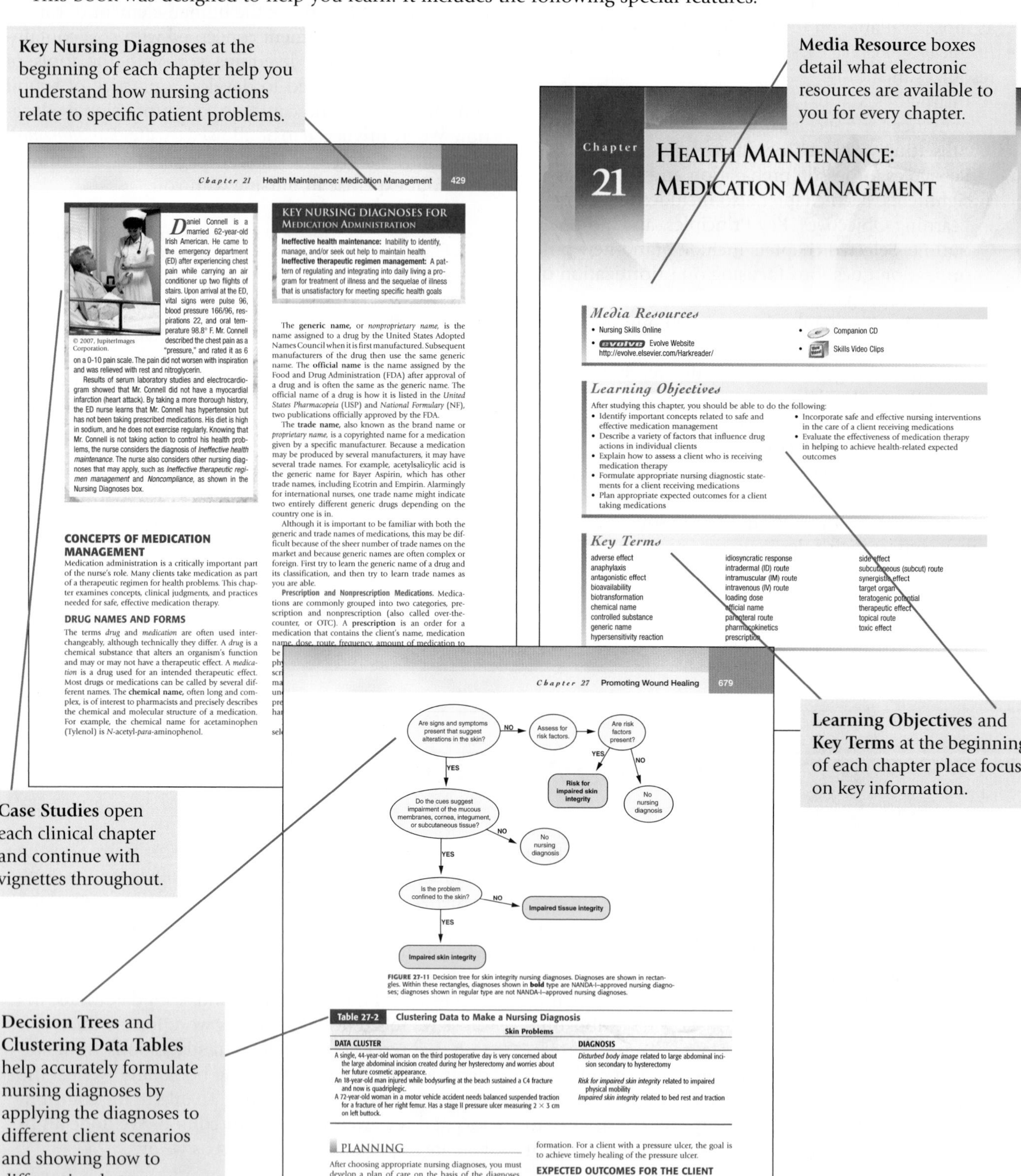

Chapter 21 Health Maintenance: Medication Management 429

Daniel Connell is a married 62-year-old Irish American. He came to the emergency department (ED) after experiencing chest pain while carrying an air conditioner up two flights of stairs. Upon arrival at the ED, vital signs were pulse 96, blood pressure 166/96, respirations 22, and oral temperature 98.8° F. Mr. Connell described the chest pain as a "pressure," and rated it as 6 on a 0-10 pain scale. The pain did not worsen with inspiration and was relieved with rest and nitroglycerin.

Results of serum laboratory studies and electrocardiogram showed that Mr. Connell did not have a myocardial infarction (heart attack). By taking a more thorough history, the ED nurse learns that Mr. Connell has hypertension but has not been taking prescribed medications. His diet is high in sodium, and he does not exercise regularly. Knowing that Mr. Connell is not taking action to control his health problems, the nurse considers the diagnosis of *Ineffective health maintenance*. The nurse also considers other nursing diagnoses that may apply, such as *Ineffective therapeutic regimen management* and *Noncompliance*, as shown in the Nursing Diagnoses box.

© 2007, JupiterImages Corporation.

KEY NURSING DIAGNOSES FOR MEDICATION ADMINISTRATION

Ineffective health maintenance: Inability to identify, manage, and/or seek out help to maintain health

Ineffective therapeutic regimen management: A pattern of regulating and integrating into daily living a program for treatment of illness and the sequelae of illness that is unsatisfactory for meeting specific health goals

CONCEPTS OF MEDICATION MANAGEMENT

Medication administration is a critically important part of the nurse's role. Many clients take medication as part of a therapeutic regimen for health problems. This chapter examines concepts, clinical judgments, and practices needed for safe, effective medication therapy.

DRUG NAMES AND FORMS

The terms *drug* and *medication* are often used interchangeably, although technically they differ. A *drug* is a chemical substance that alters an organism's function and may or may not have a therapeutic effect. A *medication* is a drug used for an intended therapeutic effect. Most drugs or medications can be called by several different names. The **chemical name**, often long and complex, is of interest to pharmacists and precisely describes the chemical and molecular structure of a medication. For example, the chemical name for acetaminophen (Tylenol) is *N*-acetyl-*para*-aminophenol.

The **generic name**, or *nonproprietary name*, is the name assigned to a drug by the United States Adopted Names Council when it is first manufactured. Subsequent manufacturers of the drug then use the same generic name. The **official name** is the name assigned by the Food and Drug Administration (FDA) after approval of a drug and is often the same as the generic name. The official name of a drug is how it is listed in the *United States Pharmacopeia* (USP) and *National Formulary* (NF), two publications officially approved by the FDA.

The **trade name**, also known as the brand name or *proprietary name*, is a copyrighted name for a medication given by a specific manufacturer. Because a medication may be produced by several manufacturers, it may have several trade names. For example, acetylsalicylic acid is the generic name for Bayer Aspirin, which has other trade names, including Ecotrin and Empirin. Alarmingly for international nurses, one trade name might indicate two entirely different generic drugs depending on the country one is in.

Although it is important to be familiar with both the generic and trade names of medications, this may be difficult because of the sheer number of trade names on the market and because generic names are often complex or foreign. First try to learn the generic name of a drug and its classification, and then try to learn trade names as you are able.

Prescription and Nonprescription Medications. Medications are commonly grouped into two categories, prescription and nonprescription (also called over-the-counter, or OTC). A **prescription** is an order for a medication that contains the client's name, medication name, dose, route, frequency, amount of medication to

Chapter 21 HEALTH MAINTENANCE: MEDICATION MANAGEMENT

Media Resources

- Nursing Skills Online
- evolve Evolve Website http://evolve.elsevier.com/Harkreader/
- Companion CD
- Skills Video Clips

Learning Objectives

After studying this chapter, you should be able to do the following:

- Identify important concepts related to safe and effective medication management
- Describe a variety of factors that influence drug actions in individual clients
- Explain how to assess a client who is receiving medication therapy
- Formulate appropriate nursing diagnostic statements for a client receiving medications
- Plan appropriate expected outcomes for a client taking medications
- Incorporate safe and effective nursing interventions in the care of a client receiving medications
- Evaluate the effectiveness of medication therapy in helping to achieve health-related expected outcomes

Key Terms

adverse effect, anaphylaxis, antagonistic effect, bioavailability, biotransformation, chemical name, controlled substance, generic name, hypersensitivity reaction, idiosyncratic response, intradermal (ID) route, intramuscular (IM) route, intravenous (IV) route, loading dose, official name, parenteral route, pharmacokinetics, prescription, side effect, subcutaneous (subcut) route, synergistic effect, target organ, teratogenic potential, therapeutic effect, topical route, toxic effect

Chapter 27 Promoting Wound Healing 679

FIGURE 27-11 Decision tree for skin integrity nursing diagnoses. Diagnoses are shown in rectangles. Within these rectangles, diagnoses shown in **bold** type are NANDA-I–approved nursing diagnoses; diagnoses shown in regular type are not NANDA-I–approved nursing diagnoses.

Table 27-2 Clustering Data to Make a Nursing Diagnosis

Skin Problems	
DATA CLUSTER	**DIAGNOSIS**
A single, 44-year-old woman on the third postoperative day is very concerned about the large abdominal incision created during her hysterectomy and worries about her future cosmetic appearance.	*Disturbed body image* related to large abdominal incision secondary to hysterectomy
An 18-year-old man injured while bodysurfing at the beach sustained a C4 fracture and now is quadriplegic.	*Risk for impaired skin integrity* related to impaired physical mobility
A 72-year-old woman in a motor vehicle accident needs balanced suspended traction for a fracture of her right femur. Has a stage II pressure ulcer measuring 2 × 3 cm on left buttock.	*Impaired skin integrity* related to bed rest and traction

PLANNING

After choosing appropriate nursing diagnoses, you must develop a plan of care on the basis of the diagnoses. When planning care, assign priorities to the nursing diagnoses, select appropriate nursing interventions to achieve expected outcomes (client-centered goals), and document the nursing diagnoses, outcomes, interventions, and evaluations on the plan of care. For a client who is bed-bound after a motor vehicle accident, the goal is to prevent skin breakdown and pressure ulcer formation. For a client with a pressure ulcer, the goal is to achieve timely healing of the pressure ulcer.

EXPECTED OUTCOMES FOR THE CLIENT WITH *IMPAIRED SKIN INTEGRITY*

The expected outcome for a client with the nursing diagnosis of *Impaired skin integrity* is to achieve wound healing without complications. General outcomes for the client may include the following:

- Maintains a normal temperature or baseline vital signs

Teaching for Wellness and **Teaching for Self-Care** boxes focus on sharpening teaching skills, health promotion and illness prevention, and restoration of health after illness.

BOX 21-2 *Teaching for Wellness*

Avoiding Common Side Effects of Medication Therapy

Purpose: To help the client remain free of the most common side effects of a variety of medications by encouraging health-promoting behaviors.
Expected Outcome: The client will remain free of common medication side effects or will have less severe side effects if they occur.

Client Instructions

Constipation. Many groups of medications, such as opioid analgesics, antispasmodics, and iron supplements, slow the action of the gastrointestinal tract. The following are helpful hints about actions you can take to decrease the risk of getting constipated while taking these medications:

- Drink increased fluids unless contraindicated by another health problem. Because foods also contain fluid, you will probably obtain a sufficient fluid intake by drinking 6 to 8 glasses of water each day in addition to the normal diet, to total 2 to 3 quarts of fluid per day.
- Walk or do some other activity that moves and stretches the abdominal muscles each day. This movement "massages" the intestines and increases peristaltic activity.
- Increase the amount of fiber in your diet. Eat plenty of fruits and vegetables, and include whole grains whenever possible instead of refined carbohydrates.

Sedation. Many medications, such as decongestants, some cough preparations, narcotics, and antianxiety agents, cause drowsiness. Although you may not be able to prevent this side effect, you can modify your activities to reduce the risk of injury while taking these medications.

Some suggestions include the following:

- Do not drive or do any other activity that requires concentration for approximately 2 to 3 hours after taking the medication. Resume these activities only after the drowsiness has worn off.
- Make sure travel paths, such as the hallway leading to the bathroom, are sufficiently lighted at night to prevent falls caused by sedation or reduced vision. Remove scatter rugs or other objects that increase the risk of falls.
- If you take the medication once a day, do so at bedtime if possible, to minimize the risks associated with sedation.
- Do not drink alcohol or take any other over-the-counter (OTC) drugs with a sedative effect while taking this medication. Consult with your physician about specific questions to obtain individualized advice.

Dizziness. Because of their effects on blood vessels, many medications taken for cardiovascular problems cause dizziness (vertigo) when you sit up or stand up. The most common ones are antihypertensives and diuretics. If you are taking one of these medications, try to do the following (especially within the first few hours after taking a dose):

- Sit or stand up slowly when rising from the bed or chair.
- Avoid extremely warm environments or hot baths because they can aggravate the problem by dilating the blood vessels.
- Do not drink alcohol while ta… alcohol dilates blood vessels … ing of blood pressure.
- If you take an antihypertensi… so at night to reduce your … If you are taking a diuretic, h… the morning. Taking it at nigh… by making you have to get u…

Action Alerts highlight situations that require important nursing actions.

such as rash, urticaria, and pruritus. Headache, rhinitis, or nausea and vomiting may also occur.

Anaphylaxis is a life-threatening allergic reaction that requires immediate intervention to prevent possible death. It is a medical emergency. Symptoms are typically cardiorespiratory in nature and include dyspnea, wheezing, stridor, tachycardia, and hypotension. They are caused by bronchoconstriction, laryngeal edema, and widespread vasodilation. Treatment includes supportive care and administration of epinephrine, bronchodilators, antihistamines, and corticosteroids to reduce the allergic response.

Action Alert! If a client begins to exhibit signs of anaphylaxis after receiving a medication, maintain the client's airway and call for help immediately.

…se allergic responses can be serious, carefully … clients about a history of drug allergy. For …mmonly known to be antigenic, such as penicillin, also inquire about a family history of drug allergy. Inquire not only about the drug but also about specific symptoms of the allergic response. This information helps determine whether the client could safely receive the drug if given with another drug (such as an antihistamine) or whether it must not be used at all. All clients with a history of drug allergy should wear or carry identification noting the drug allergy. They should also be taught to inform all future caregivers about the allergy.

Idiosyncratic Responses. An **idiosyncratic response** is an unexplained and unpredictable respon… medication. It may be a suboptimal response, … gerated response, or an abnormal type of respo… example, some medications that normally … drowsiness may cause excitability in children. … cratic responses may be listed in the drug … as rare types of adverse effects. Because these ar… predictable, skilled and conscientious nursing … ment is warranted.

Procedures include Time to Allow, Delegation Guidelines, Equipment Needed, and Rationales and **Age-Related** and **Home Care Considerations.** These streamlined procedures include key steps needed to grasp essential information.

…iew Video icons remind students …o view the video on Evolve and …n the Companion CD.

Referrals back to case studies relate chapter concepts directly to the chapter case study.

Time to Allow: Novice: 5 min. Expert: 10 min.

PROCEDURE 30-2

APPLYING A CONDOM CATHETER

Nursing Skills Online: Urinary Catheterization, Lesson 3

View Video!

The purpose of applying a condom catheter is to control incontinence in a male client without the risk for urinary tract infection and with greater comfort to the client than an indwelling catheter.

DELEGATION GUIDELINES

The application of a condom catheter is a noninvasive procedure that you may delegate to a nursing assistant who has received specific instruction in this skill. Instruction should include safety and skin care considerations.

EQUIPMENT NEEDED

- Commercially packaged condom catheter
- Soap and water
- Disposable clean gloves
- Drainage bag and tubing

1 Follow preliminary actions (see inside front cover).
2 Position the client on his back, and drape him to expose only his penis.
3 Clean his genitals with soap and water, and dry thoroughly.
4 Apply skin-protecting cream packaged with the catheter to the client's penis. Allow it to dry.
5 Wrap the adhesive spirally around the shaft of the penis (see illustration). *Be careful not to apply the adhesive too tightly. Severe edema can result if the adhesive strip constricts the shaft of the penis, and the client will develop pain and difficulty urinating.*

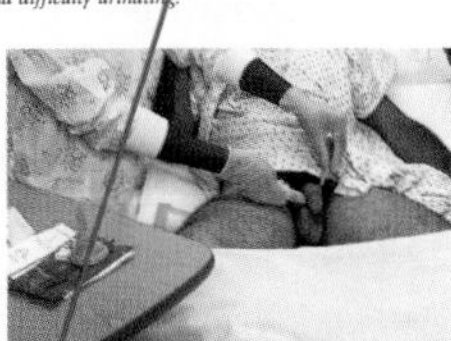

Step 5. Wrapping the adhesive spirally around the penis.

6 Place the rolled condom over the client's glans penis, and unroll the condom over the adhesive liner and the shaft of the penis (see illustration). *If the client is uncircumcised, make sure his foreskin remains in place over the glans penis as you unroll the condom. If retracted, the foreskin may be tight enough to constrict the penis and cause edema of the glans penis.*

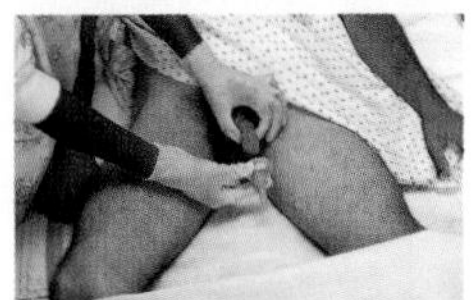

Step 6. Placing the rolled condom over the client's glans penis.

7 Attach the catheter to a collecting system and tape the tubing to the client's leg (see illustration).

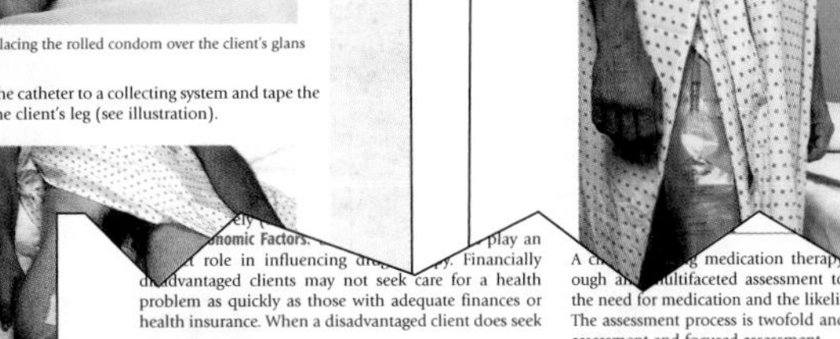

Step 7. Catheter a… to the client's leg.

8 Document date… ment of shaft of pe… client's penis after … tect such problems … in skin color.

Skills in the text that are supported by Nursing Skills Online include NSO lesson numbers so you can go right to pertinent review and evaluation.

PEDIATRIC CONSIDERATIONS

For infants and toddlers, diapers or training pants are more appropriate. Change them frequently to prevent skin irritation. Condom catheters are probably not effective until the penis reaches adult size.

GERIATRIC CONSIDERATIONS

The size of the penis may shrink with age and make it difficult to effectively use a condom catheter in some men. Skin may be more fragile.

HOME HEALTH CARE CONSIDERATIONS

Teach family caregivers to apply the catheter and care for the skin. The family should remove the condom and clean the skin daily.

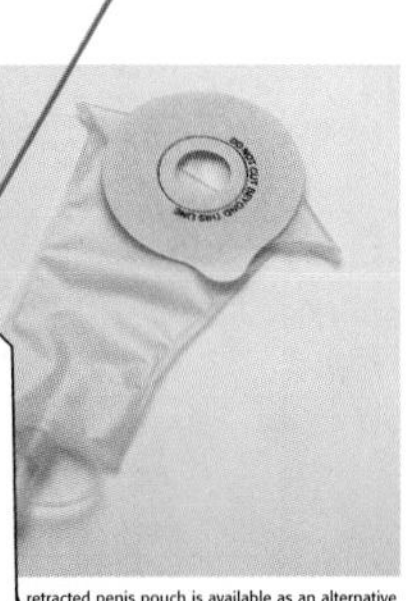

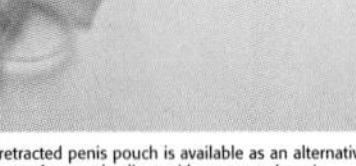

…retracted penis pouch is available as an alternative …theter for a male client with a retracted penis.

…nomic Factors. … play an … role in influencing dr… Financially disadvantaged clients may not seek care for a health problem as quickly as those with adequate finances or health insurance. When a disadvantaged client does seek

BOX 21-3 *Communicating Effectively With Clients of Other Cultures About Medication Therapy*

- Become informed about the health practices and beliefs of cultural groups in your community. Be aware that diversity may exist within subgroups of a larger cultural group.
- Encourage clients of other cultures to communicate their concerns and ask questions related to medication therapy.
- Provide printed or audiovisual medication information in the client's language if possible.
- Question the client directly about the use of remedies prescribed by a healer within the culture.
  These remedies may have an interactive effect with prescribed medication therapy.
- Watch for atypical drug responses or unexpected side effects in clients in certain cultural groups. Cultural influences such as diet, complementary therapies, or even genetic factors can precipitate unusual responses to medication therapy.

A c… medication therap… thorough an… multifaceted assessment to de… the both the need for medication and the likelihood of response. The assessment process is twofold and includes general assessment and focused assessment.

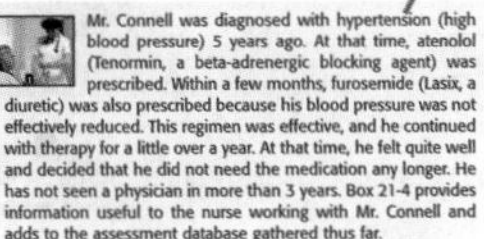

Mr. Connell was diagnosed with hypertension (high blood pressure) 5 years ago. At that time, atenolol (Tenormin, a beta-adrenergic blocking agent) was prescribed. Within a few months, furosemide (Lasix, a diuretic) was also prescribed because his blood pressure was not effectively reduced. This regimen was effective, and he continued with therapy for a little over a year. At that time, he felt quite well and decided that he did not need the medication any longer. He has not seen a physician in more than 3 years. Box 21-4 provides information useful to the nurse working with Mr. Connell and adds to the assessment database gathered thus far.

GENERAL ASSESSMENT FOR MEDICATION ADMINISTRATION

Health History. A client's health history provides information about existing health problems being managed with medications and illnesses or organ dysfunction that may increase the risk of toxicity or other adverse drug

BOX 21-4 *Cross-Cultural Care*

Caring for an Irish American Client

Daniel Connell, the client whose story we've been following through this chapter, is of Irish American descent. His family came to Boston, Massachusetts, in the late 1800s. Although there are always individual differences among clients, Irish Americans as a group tend to have the following characteristics (Wilson, 1998):

- Believe and expect that life is a difficult process.
- Understate their symptoms when ill and delay seeking health care until symptoms are severe or cannot be ignored.
- Are stoic and resist expressing emotions associated with illness or pain.
- Use facial expressions to communicate nonverbally rather than more expressive gestures, such as hand and arm movements.
- Use traditional home remedies to treat minor illnesses but seek out a traditional health care provider if these fail or if a larger health problem emerges.

Cross-Cultural Care boxes focus on the client in the case and highlight considerations for his or her cultural group.

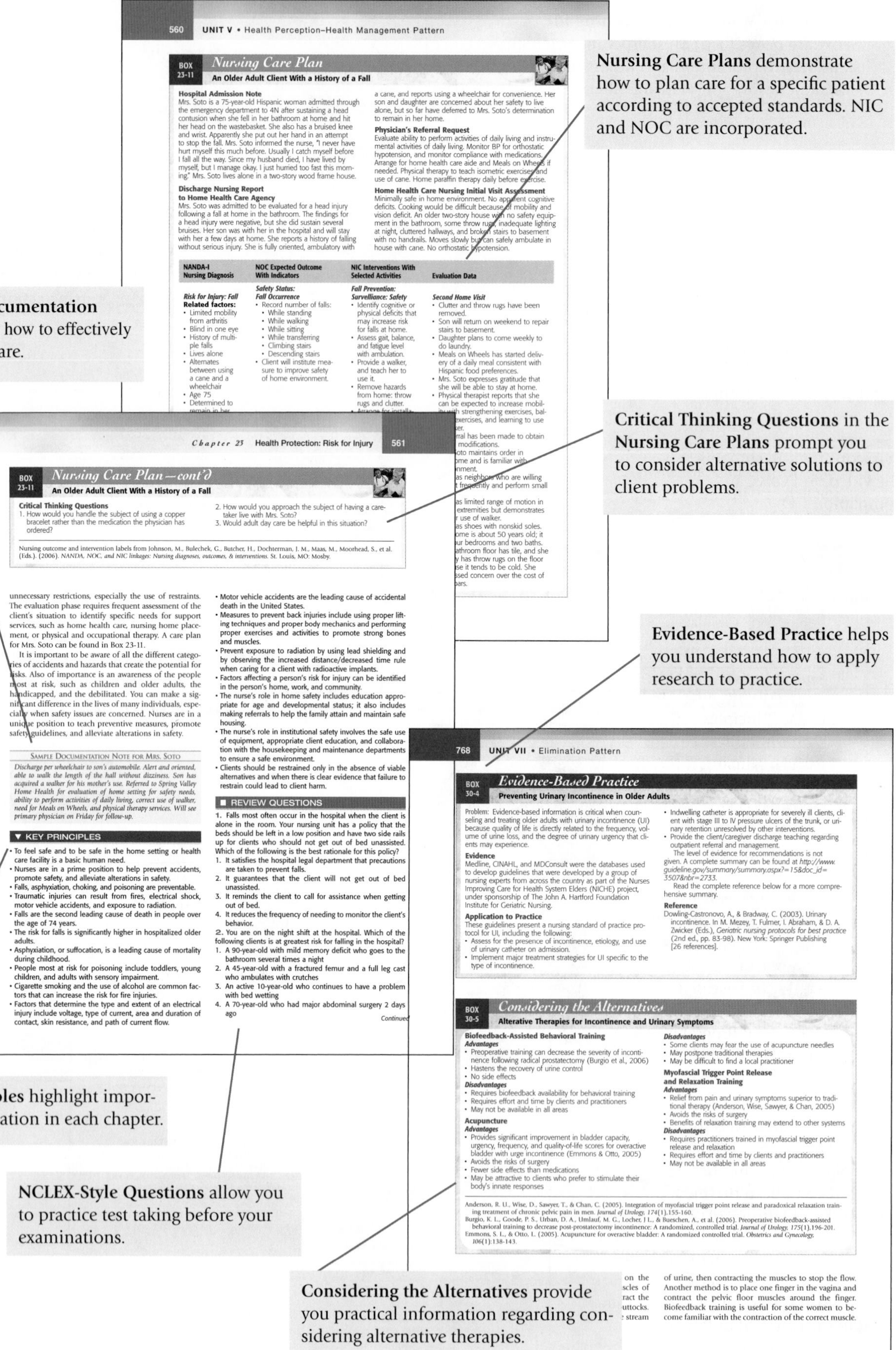

Nursing Care Plans demonstrate how to plan care for a specific patient according to accepted standards. NIC and NOC are incorporated.

Sample Documentation Notes show how to effectively document care.

Critical Thinking Questions in the **Nursing Care Plans** prompt you to consider alternative solutions to client problems.

Evidence-Based Practice helps you understand how to apply research to practice.

Key Principles highlight important information in each chapter.

NCLEX-Style Questions allow you to practice test taking before your examinations.

Considering the Alternatives provide you practical information regarding considering alternative therapies.

Contents

Unit IV The Well Client Across the Life Span

Unit VII Elimination Pattern

Unit VIII Activity–Exercise Pattern

Unit XII Role–Relationship Pattern

Unit XIII Sexuality–Reproduction Pattern

Unit XIV Coping–Stress-Tolerance Pattern

Unit XV Value–Belief Pattern

Unit XVI The Surgical Client

Chapter 1

The Nursing Profession

Media Resources

- evolve Evolve Website http://evolve.elsevier.com/Harkreader/
- Companion CD

Learning Objectives

After studying this chapter, you should be able to do the following:

- Describe various historical influences that have affected today's nurse
- Describe trends in society have influenced changes in nursing practice
- Compare the different educational programs in nursing
- Describe the influence on professional nursing practice contributed by standards of professional nursing, professional organizations, and professional nursing roles

Key Terms

autonomy
client
continuing education
health
holistic care
licensed vocational nurse (LVN) / licensed practical nurse (LPN)
National Council Licensure Examination for Registered Nurses (NCLEX-RN)
nursing
profession
registered nurse (RN)
standards of nursing practice

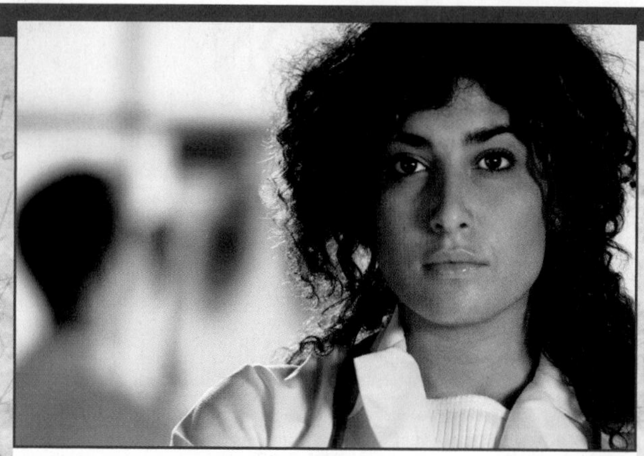

Since Diane was a small child, she always wanted to become a "nurse." She has just started her first year of nursing classes and is finally discovering what nursing is like in the "real world." She has worked hard to learn the nonnursing science classes and has gained insights about herself through the psychology classes. She expects clients to be happy to see her and wants to be professional by giving the medications and treatments in a timely and safe manner. She expects to give a great deal of time and effort to help each client get better so he or she can go home "well."

The first clinical day she was assigned to two clients to whom she was to give baths, medications, and treatments within her 5-hour clinical day. Upon arrival she was not able to finish hearing intershift report because one of her clients had a cardiac arrest and the code team was performing cardiopulmonary resuscitation (CPR). Shortly thereafter the first client died, and she was told to perform postmortem care so the family could come in to say good-bye.

She was not familiar with the postmortem care policies and had to look up the procedure before she could perform it. The research took a while, and then she had to work quickly so the family could see the client before calling the funeral home to transport the body. The family wanted someone to stay while they said goodbye and she felt responsible, so she stayed for some time before they were through.

She documented the care before the funeral home was called but had to check to make sure all forms were completed before the family could leave. By this time it was already 10:30 and she had not given her medications or checked charts for new orders on her other client. She had not fully assessed her other client since she was giving care to the client who had died. She was glad to stay with the family but felt someone else should have been there to answer their questions.

The second client had already spilled his urinal in the bed, which was being saved for a 24-hour urine test. He was also yelling in pain, and everyone in the hall could hear him. None of the regular staff was available because of another emergency at the other end of the hallway.

What will be Diane's response? Will her attitude about nursing change? What are her thoughts about her choice to make nursing her career? How does her "real" image of nursing affect her ideal description?

OVERVIEW

The nursing profession consists of the diverse group of individuals who practice nursing using a specialized and unique body of knowledge. Nursing can be considered a **profession** because it provides an essential service to society, has a theoretical body of knowledge, requires relative independence in decision making in practice, requires specialized education, and has a code of ethics for behavior of its members.

Today's practice of **nursing** is based upon the American Nurses Association's (ANA's) definition:

> Nursing is the protection, promotion, and optimization of health and abilities, prevention of illness and injury, alleviation of suffering through the diagnosis and treatment of human response, and advocacy in the care of individuals, families, communities, and populations. (ANA, 2003)

This definition reflects the activities performed by the nurse and is based upon a five-part approach to the management of clients no matter where they receive the health care services provided by nurses. This approach is called nursing process and is identified as the following phases of care: assessment, nursing diagnosis, planning, implementation, and evaluation. Nursing process is implemented in a cyclic manner that is overlapping because assessment and evaluation are ongoing. Throughout the process as new information, called data, is obtained the nurse modifies the plan and adjusts the interventions to adapt to the new changes.

The term *patient* is used to reflect the object of nursing care as a service given by the nurse. Today, the term **client** reflects more appropriately the interaction between the nurse and the recipient of nursing services. The client is expected to participate in all levels of the nursing process to help direct the expected outcomes of care provided not only by nurses but also other health care workers. This change in terminology implies that the client takes more responsibility in caring for self and helps plan the direction of care desired, which is aimed at achieving optimal **health** (physical, social, spiritual, and psychological well-being).

Today, this cooperation between the health care team and the client has resulted in a more informed public that is taking charge of their health care by using the best possible options to maximize health. Through efforts aimed at health education, health promotion, and prevention of illness, clients are increasingly receiving better health care, and this should lead to reduced health care costs in the long term. Statistically people are living longer, and by emphasizing disease prevention they will live longer and healthier lives than in previous generations.

Traditionally, the health care field was perceived as the physician and nurse working together to care for the client who has developed an illness. In contrast, today the health care team not only consists of the client,

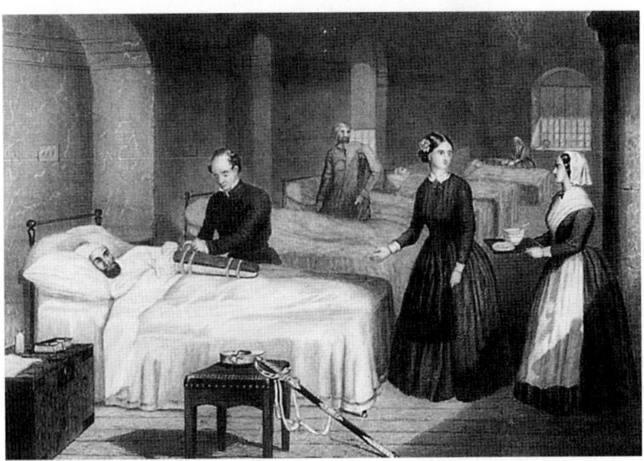

FIGURE 1-1 Florence Nightingale (1820-1910). (Courtesy the National Library of Medicine.)

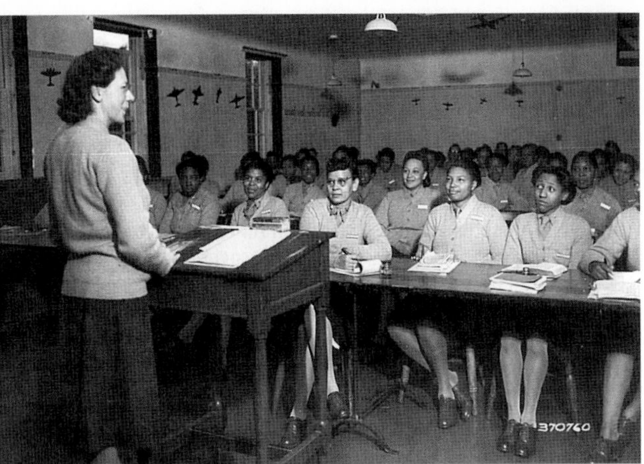

FIGURE 1-2 During World War II, training for nurses became associated with classrooms and organized curricula. (Courtesy the National Archives at College Park.)

nurse, and physician or nurse practitioner, but also includes all health care workers who contribute to the client's welfare: unit managers, nurse aides, pharmacists, therapists (physical, occupational, speech, respiratory), social workers, case managers, dieticians, environmental service workers, and engineers. These teams come together to identify and work on individual and group needs within the health care facility. Participatory management allows input and responsibility of client care to be given to all employees with the challenge to offer the best care possible in an optimum setting.

BRIEF HISTORICAL PERSPECTIVE

Traditionally, the history of nursing begins with Florence Nightingale (Figure 1-1), who became known initially from her work in the Crimean War. She was the first nurse to nurture and give care to military men during battle. Before she started her work, injured men in the Crimean War were left to die if they could not get up to fight again on their own. Florence Nightingale treated these men and believed the role of nursing was to "take charge of somebody's health" to help rid the body of disease or recover health (Nightingale, 1860). She later created principles of care based upon her observations recorded during the war and the attempts that guided her practice. These principles became the basis for the practice of "nursing" today. Her notes were written in the form of "hints" for women who were placed in charge of the health of others. She later went on to open the first hospital-based training program for nurses in London. In addition to these accomplishments, Nightingale also became the first practicing nurse epidemiologist, studying the correlation between poor sanitary conditions with diseases such as dysentery and cholera (Cohen, 1984).

Wars during the last century continued to catalyze advances in medical and nursing practice. They created greater opportunities to try new medical treatments, surgical techniques, and new chemical managements than during peace time. Wars also created new jobs for nurses (Figure 1-2).

Building upon Nightingale's foundational principles and the contributions of other early nursing leaders (Table 1-1), today's theories of practice have evolved to keep pace with the expanding role of nursing to include an interdisciplinary blending of sciences, art, and sociocultural development. There are many influences that have contributed to this evolution. With the changes based on historical progress, nursing has continued to change to meet the needs of those receiving care. Industrialization, increasing technology, and sociocultural emphasis are a few of the factors that have stimulated changes in nursing practice.

According to the International Council of Nurses (www.nursingworld.org/icn), nursing is described as follows:

> Nursing encompasses autonomous and collaborative care of individuals of all ages, families, groups and countries, sick or well and in all settings. Nursing includes the promotion of health, prevention of illness, and the care of the ill, disabled, and dying people.

Therefore, from history we have seen a change from directly caring for those that are ill to include illness prevention and health promotion based upon new technology and a better understanding of other approaches to care. By trying to prevent health problems, health care costs are reduced and clients have better overall health, which should result in a longer life span at a higher quality of life.

Industrialization has advanced the United States to offer better lifestyles to its citizens. Unfortunately, today there are still some populations who experience disparity in access to modern health care, and this remains a key issue and challenge in our society.

Table 1-1 Primary Contributions of Selected Early Nursing Leaders

NURSING LEADER	KEY DATE	CONTRIBUTION
Sojourner Truth	1827	Abolitionist, lecturer, women's rights worker. An African American nurse who made enormous contributions during the American Civil War. Worked as a nurse/counselor for the Freedman's Association after the war.
Harriet Ross Tubman	1840	An African American nurse who led more than 300 slaves to freedom during the American Civil War. Recognized for her kindness and attention to the sick and suffering.
Florence Nightingale	1854	A war nurse and founder of modern nursing education. A publisher and nurse theorist.
Mary Ann Ball	1861	"Mother Beckerdyke" was one of the greatest heroines of the American Civil War. Searched for survivors on the battlefield and organized diet kitchens and ambulance services.
Dorothea Dix	1861	Appointed Superintendent of the Women Nurses of the Army. Devoted herself to the care of the mentally ill and to improvement of jail conditions.
Linda Richards	1872	A graduate of New England Hospital for Women and Children. The first trained nurse in the United States. Later, developed and established the first nursing school in Japan.
Lavinia Lloyd Dock	1873	A well-known nurse who was actively involved in early twentieth-century women's rights issues and the suffragette movement. Wrote one of the first nursing textbooks.
Mary Eliza Mahoney	1879	Completed the 16-month training course at the New England Hospital for Women and Children to become America's first African American "trained nurse."
Clara Barton	1881	Superintendent of nurses for Union Army during the American Civil War. Developed the American Red Cross.
Mary Agnes Snively	1884	Responsible for the direction of Canadian nursing education. Director of the Toronto General Hospital Canadian Nurses Association.
Isabel Hampton Robb	1886	An outstanding nurse who was first president of the Nurses Associated Alumnae of the United States and Canada. Was first principal of Johns Hopkins School of Nursing, cofounder of the *American Journal of Nursing*.
Betty Moulder and Ada Stewart	1888	First nurses employed as occupational health nurses.
Annie Goodrich	1893	Dean of the United States Army School of Nursing in 1918. Was Professor of Nursing at Columbia Teachers College and Dean of Nursing at Yale University. Served as president of the American Nurses Association (ANA).
Lillian Wald	1893	Founded the Henry Street Settlement service, providing health care for the poor on New York's Lower East Side. Formed the National Organization of Public Health Nursing (the first specialization in nursing) in 1912.
Mary Adelaide Nutting	1894	An early nurse activist at Columbia Teachers College. Known as "the first nursing professor in the world." Influential in raising educational standards for nurses working toward undergraduate and graduate nursing degrees.
Namahyoke Curtis	1898	Employed as a contract nurse by the United States War Department during the Spanish-American War to hire black nurses to go to Cuba to care for victims of yellow fever.
Clara Maas	1898	A nurse volunteer who participated in the yellow fever research experiment in Havana, Cuba, and died from yellow fever after the Spanish-American War.
Jessie Sleet (Scales)	1900	The first African American public health nurse.
Martha Franklin	1916	Founded the National Association of Colored Graduate Nurses (NACGN).
Margaret Sanger	1916	Founded the first birth control clinic in America, the forerunner of Planned Parenthood.
Francis Reed Elliott	1918	The first African American nurse accepted by the American Red Cross Nursing Service.
Frances Payne Bolton	1923	Provided financial support that was instrumental in the development of the nursing school at Case Western Reserve University.
Isabel Maitland Stewart	1925	Conducted research to differentiate between nursing and nonnursing tasks. Successful in influencing upgraded nursing education.
Mary Breckinridge	1925	Founded the Frontier Nursing Service, which provided the first organized midwifery service in the United States.
Lucille Petry	1949	The first woman appointed to the position of Assistant Surgeon General of the United States Public Health Service.
Mildred Montag	1952	Conducted research; was instrumental in the development of the first associate degree nursing program.

CULTURAL INFLUENCES ON NURSING

Exposure to other cultures has helped nurses to understand and incorporate multicultural approaches to care that are both acceptable and necessary to meet the holistic needs of diverse clients. **Holistic care** identifies nursing care that goes beyond physical needs to include spiritual, cultural, and psychological needs to help an individual achieve health. The definition of health has evolved to include not just recovery from physical injury or disease but the balancing of the whole individual—body, mind, and spirit. To deliver care effectively and to creatively meet the individualized needs of clients, it is important to become familiar with and understand the characteristics and beliefs of other cultures. Acknowledging specific cultural influences and beliefs when planning care promotes better understanding of what the client needs from the health care team and is more likely to lead to outcomes that are congruent with those desired by the client.

According to Leininger and McFarland (2002, p. 298), the strongest past influences on the development of the nursing profession have been Anglo-Americans and the values attributed to this cultural group. Some of these values include the following:

- Individualism and self-reliance
- Independence and freedom
- Competition, assertiveness, and achievements
- Dependence on technology
- Equal gender roles and rights
- Instant time and action (doing)
- Reliance on "scientific facts" and numbers
- Generosity and helpfulness in crises

Additionally, Leininger and McFarland maintain that two prominent cultural influences have helped shape nursing today (2002). Common characteristics and beliefs of the African American and Hispanic cultures within the borders of the United States have influenced nursing practice.

Marjorie Morgan (2002) discusses three of Leininger's modes of care that were congruent with culturally specific to African American clients. African Americans' strong belief in a higher power that guides their healing is the core for accepting both good and bad news from the health care providers. Based upon a multigenerational household, family and traditional healing practices are highly valued and practiced before seeking traditional medicine. Without the influence of common African American values, today's nurse might not be as nurturing or as spiritually and family focused. Today's nurse understands and encourages family, religious practices, and incorporation of traditional healing approaches into current care to enhance recovery or the experience of death (see Chapters 45 and 48).

A second culture that has influenced today's nurse in America is that of the Mexican American and Hispanic populations from Cuba, Puerto Rico, Spain, Mexico, and Central America (Leininger & McFarland, 2002). Although they are similar, needs do vary based upon the cultural uniqueness of each. Mexico is the rising population that has the greatest influence in the southwestern United States. Surprisingly, a distinct difference is noted between cultural needs of clients who are first-generation Americans and those who are second- or third-generation Americans. Some characteristics include respecting older adults, supporting religious practices/symbols, understanding hot/cold theory as interpreted by each group, and desiring to advance education with each new generation while retaining cultural uniqueness, such as language spoken in the home. These beliefs have influenced nurses to

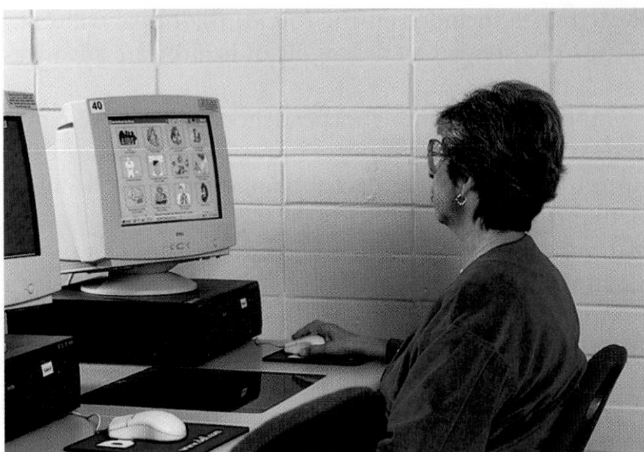

FIGURE 1-3 In the twenty-first century, nursing informatics will revolutionize nursing, and computer skills will be essential to nurses at every level of practice.

have increased respect for older adults, support kinship and family during recovery, and to possibly acquire Spanish or Tex-Mex language skills to communicate effectively with this growing population.

Despite common desires of clients, there is a need to remain unique, so remember to avoid stereotyping clients according to cultural background. As you develop experience in working with clients of various cultures, you will learn to deliver culturally appropriate care so that health care outcomes are congruent with the expectations of the client (see Chapter 3).

OTHER SOCIETAL INFLUENCES ON NURSING

Cost management, resource allocation, increased technology, new advances, and nursing shortages have lead to innovative approaches to health care delivery. These influences have also shaped the day-to-day nursing practice.

Roles and Resource Allocation. According to Saba and McCormick (2006), the newest role of the nurse is in the area of "nursing informatics." In this role, the nurse will coordinate and administer care at the bedside based upon technologic regulation (Figure 1-3). Immediate access to laboratory results, tests, and other data at the bedside using computer technology will speed the response time by the nurse, maximize health care delivery, and minimize errors

Because of nursing shortages and issues of resource allocation, procedures traditionally done by nurses have been delegated to other health care workers. Examples include the following:

- Respiratory treatments are now given by respiratory therapists.
- Ambulating of some clients may be done by physical therapists.
- Client medications are prepared by pharmacists through computerized access.

Activities included in the role of the nurse will continue to be shaped by the results of health care advances in the future.

Autonomy as relative independence and self-governance is the core of a current nurse's practice. The complexity and urgency of the decisions required by a nurse demand the expertise to make decisions quickly and autonomously to give the best possible care in a timely manner. In addition, each client must be viewed as a unique individual with needs that include not only health issues but spiritual, cultural, and mental issues that will affect the outcome of the health care delivered by the nurse.

Knowledge Explosion. While in today's classroom, tomorrow's nurse can no longer learn scientific principles and apply them to all possible circumstances in the clinical setting. Technology and theories are being discovered and developed continuously. Knowledge is based not only on facts to be learned, but on the ability to apply critical thinking and problem-solving skills to the care of clients. To participate in the advancement of knowledge in the discipline of nursing, nurses also need to be able to articulate problems amenable to nursing research. This dialogue among professionals can spur the research needed to generate new knowledge and advance the discipline of nursing as a profession engaged in evidence-based practice (see Chapter 15).

Nurses need to stay current with current research results and help bring them to the practice arena by influencing policy and procedure development in the health care facilities in which they are employed. Nurses are team contributors who participate at all levels of care, both independently and in collaboration other health care providers.

As a current nursing student, it will be important for you to learn the principles and concepts of care but not to memorize procedures in a detailed step-by-step manner. You will need to be able to analyze an individual skill and apply basic principles and guidelines, knowing that the details of performance will ultimately be adapted by tomorrow's technology. For example, you will need to learn concepts of surgical asepsis (sterile fields) and then be able apply them in all settings despite the equipment in use in the workplace.

Population. People today are technologically prepared and come to the health care setting equipped with a broader knowledge of their medical needs and available treatment options than in the past. However, if the treatment does not achieve the desired outcomes, people are increasingly likely to litigate their complaint in court. As a result, increasing insurance costs and legal fees are driving the cost of health care in an ongoing upward spiral. Some physicians and other specialized health care professionals are leaving the health care field because of these rising legal costs. Some areas of medicine are becoming scarce in various parts of the country because of increasing costs of insurance for specialization medicine.

Bomar (2004) describes today's population as "families throughout the world that are conflicted with unprecedented economical, political, social, and environmental changes that are unpredictable and complex." Bomar further explains that today's families have lost the concept of family well-being and have deteriorated into poverty and poor health status despite new medical advances. The disparity in health care confronting various racially and ethnically diverse families in the United States remains a major issue for policy makers and health care providers. In addressing these issues, nurses must understand the stressors and problems faced by these clients because they affect the plan of care and recovery after discharge from a health care facility to home. Nurses should attempt to meet as many of specialized client needs as possible to help improve health outcomes.

Another issue affecting today's population is the increased emphasis on privacy laws, which have revolutionized the way information is shared or posted. The Health Insurance Portability and Accountability Act (HIPAA) of 1996 created strict guidelines for the electronic transfer of information, including insurance agencies, clergy, friends, and family. This act was designed to minimize ability of someone to get information using computers or other technology. A great deal of time has been spent in teaching these guidelines to all health care personnel and ensuring that these guidelines are followed. A major problem can occur if the nurse does not explain clearly the permission guidelines to a client. Concerned family members may not be able to obtain information on the condition of their loved one if permission is not obtained from the client correctly. Without permission hospital staff cannot share that a client has even been admitted.

With increasing "instant" awareness of new medical advancements, the public demands instant application of research findings. With advancing research, medicine is on the cutting edge of scientific advances that require extensive moral and ethical review before using them in the clinical setting. Cost and resource management have also become the basis for guidelines that determine whether or not a procedure is done. "Can we do this?" is no longer a question; instead, the focus is "Should we be doing this and why?"

The great ethical debates of when does life begin and when does it cease have been redefined by today's technology. Decisions based on discriminating between brain death and physical death become moral dilemmas now that technology can keep a person alive almost indefinitely. Future debates will center on when an individual can end his or her own life and under what circumstances this decision can be made. Another debate is likely to be who has the legal right to decide who receives or is declined treatment. Nurses work daily with these issues and may have strong opinions based on personal beliefs, but research-based expertise must be the guide for action. Ethical review boards have been established at many facilities to create the guidelines for tomorrow's practices.

The need to provide nursing care to an increasing, large population with a decreasing number of nurses has affected nursing care delivery. Today's nurse needs to know how to prioritize care and delegate care appropriately to unlicensed assistive personnel (such as certified nursing assistants) to provide the most effective nursing care in the most efficient manner. Because the nursing shortage will grow in the coming years, these issues are likely to assume increasing importance in the health care arena.

Health Care Management. Today clients are no longer treated in the hospital until they are "well enough" to go home. The current trend is to either perform same-day surgery (with discharge the same day) or to admit surgical clients for only a day or two and then discharge them to home or another health care facility.

Rehabilitation centers, home health care, and private nursing agencies have significantly increased as hospitals have decreased the number of inpatient days to contain costs. This trend has followed the change in insurance reimbursement, which now reimburses a fixed amount per diagnosis. New guidelines in policies are giving additional funds for out-of-hospital care, which is less expensive for insurance companies and thus more attractive. Therefore services are switching to community-based organizations to decrease costs. Hospitals that have been insightful in their planning have created "new" departments that deliver home health care services and thus retain the income from those services that would be lost to other organizations.

Hospitals have become wise in their ability to cut costs by staffing changes, resource management, and redefining employees' roles. Acute care has been the basis for funding for most hospitals; specialized testing, adding different outpatient services, and subletting floor space for other hospitals to consolidate care within the same facility is becoming the norm.

Another new approach to health care management includes merging several smaller area facilities into a magnet or regional facility. Overall, these mergers tend to decrease costs by reducing expensive duplication of services and allow for greater financial stability through large-group purchasing power for equipment and supplies. In some instances, mergers have allowed smaller, financially nonviable facilities to remain open, whereas others have resulted in closure of the smaller facilities.

Interdisciplinary Collaboration. Historically, physicians led the team and directed all activities and services needed by the client. With increasing specialization and advancing knowledge bases, various health care providers now work collaboratively to maximize delivery of health care services to clients.

Examples of health care providers that collaborate in client care include medical specialists, hospitalists, clinical nurse specialists, certified nurse specialists, vocational or practical nurses, professional generalists, pharmacists, various therapists, social workers, case managers, unit managers, and technologists. With each specialized professional giving his or her expertise, the client receives the best care possible within the hospital and in the community after discharge. Nurses often help to coordinate care and refer clients for the services of various agencies in a multidisciplinary approach to care.

Other Trends. Demographically, the increase in the aging population is creating a unique problem for nurses both as workers and consumers of health care. Doctors, nurses, and a variety of health care educators are also within this aging group; the average age is in the mid-50s. Social security is stated to be declining and is estimated to be inadequate to support the larger number of people in this generation that will retire and need funding. With this decline there will be less money available to use for health care needs. A choice between food or medications may be a common problem of this age-group as funds diminish. Health care is likely to decline as well from further increases in costs and decreasing availability. An adequate health care professional staff will not be available unless we create a new generation of workers that are interested in and dedicated to providing health care.

News reports of medical advances, such as with stem cell research, genetic findings, and new drugs, seem to be almost daily events. Many people are living longer and with some degree of increased health. In contrast, the incidences of depression and suicide are increasing in older adults because of frustration and lack of resources to meet daily needs and cope with losses. Nurses will need to acknowledge and address these issues when providing care to adequately meet client needs.

Middle-age adults are referred to as the "sandwich generation," which has responsibilities of caring for their aging parents while raising the next generation. This age-group also consists of individuals who may also be grandparents raising grandchildren because their adult children cannot do so for a variety of reasons. Although this group may have increased wealth, individual clients may suffer ill effects from increasing stress and reduced leisure time because of the demands from the older and younger generations.

Although the incidence of acquired immunodeficiency syndrome (AIDS) has begun to decline in the United States, it is still a worldwide problem that has taken millions of lives and costs are staggering. Comorbidity from conditions related to AIDS is still the leading cause of death in most countries. Within the United States AIDS remains a problem for populations rendered vulnerable by "gender, race, sexual orientation, poverty, drug use, or lack of access to healthcare" (Lewis, Heitkemper, & Dirksen, 2004). Therefore nurses must continue to try to reach those that need the education and access to free health care to affect the continuing problem of AIDS.

Disparities in global health care is an increasing concern for Americans. The health of undeveloped countries could be significantly improved by use of simple low-cost treatments, administration of vitamins and medications, and health education about topics such as hand washing, use of condoms to prevent sexually transmitted infections, and principles of nutrition. Nurses are in the forefront of public efforts to address these concerns by offering their services around the world on either a short-term and long-term basis.

NURSING EDUCATORS

The nursing shortage is still present today despite an increasing number of graduates from many nursing programs. The decline is also reflected in number of prepared faculty needed to educate future nurses in all levels of nursing programs. One cause is the aging of educators who teach the nursing curriculum. The average age of nursing faculty is currently 58 years (Lenburg, 2005). This is a reflection of the aging "baby boomers" in the general population that will soon reach retirement age.

There are many challenges to establishing a sufficient pool of doctorally prepared nurse educators:

- With increased time required for education and the rising cost of doctoral programs, many nurses are choosing to specialize in practice or stop at the master's level, in contrast to continuing educational preparation at the doctoral level. There are a number of specialized fields in which to practice that have excellent pay and have the advantage of good working hours (Box 1-1).
- There are many specialty fields with various levels of educational requirements in which nurses can specialize. Although certifications are required for most at the end of a graduate program, they do not require a doctoral degree (Box 1-2).
- The immediacy of increased incomes may be the need of many students who entered nursing as a second career because of limited opportunities in other employment fields or corporate downsizing. An increasing number of today's nursing students are older with grown families, whereas in the past most had just graduated from high school. Older students are less likely to obtain advanced education than younger students because of the fewer years of employment in which to regain tuition costs and lost wages.

BOX 1-1 *American Nurses Association Certifications*

ADVANCED PRACTICE CERTIFICATION

APRN, BC (Advanced Practice Registered Nurse, Board Certified) A current registered nurse license from the U.S. or its territories and a master's or higher degree in nursing for the specialty is required. Educational program must include a minimum of 500 hours of supervised clinical practice. Criteria for specific specialties are presented in application catalogs.

Nurse Practitioners

- Acute Care Nurse Practitioner
- Adult Nurse Practitioner
- Family Nurse Practitioner
- Gerontological Nurse Practitioner
- Pediatric Nurse Practitioner
- Adult Psychiatric and Mental Health Nurse Practitioner
- Family Psychiatric and Mental Health Nurse Practitioner

Clinical Nurse Specialists

- Clinical Nurse Specialist in Community Health Nursing
- Clinical Nurse Specialist in Gerontological Nursing
- Clinical Nurse Specialist in Home Health Nursing
- Clinical Nurse Specialist in Adult Health
- Clinical Nurse Specialist in Pediatric Nursing
- Clinical Nurse Specialist in Adult Psychiatric and Mental Health Nursing
- Clinical Nurse Specialist in Child/Adolescent Psychiatric and Mental Health Nursing

NURSING ADMINISTRATION, ADVANCED

RN, CNAA, BC (Registered Nurse, Certified in Nursing Administration, Advanced, Board Certified) A master's degree is required. You must complete the equivalent of 24 months of full-time practice and 30 contact hours in the specialty.

Advanced Diabetes Management for Nurses, Dietitians, and Pharmacists A current professional license and master's degree is required. You must complete at least 500 hours of direct clinical diabetes management; however, exceptions (refer to catalog) apply depending on licensure.

- RN, BC-ADM (Masters prepared nurses who are not Nurse Practitioners or Clinical Nurse Specialists)
- APRN, BC-ADM (Clinical Nurse Specialist and Nurse Practitioner)
- RD, BC-ADM (Registered Dietitian)
- RPh, BC-ADM (Pharmacist)

BOX 1-1 *American Nurses Association Certifications—cont'd*

Diploma and Associate Degree Certification

RN, C (Registered Nurse, Certified) A current registered nurse license from the U.S. or its territories and a diploma or associate degree in nursing is required. You must have practiced the equivalent of 2 years full time as a nurse with a minimum of 2000 practice hours and 30 contact hours in the last 3 years.

- Cardiac/Vascular Nurse
- Gerontological Nurse
- Medical-Surgical Nurse
- Pediatric Nurse
- Perinatal Nurse
- Psychiatric and Mental Health Nurse

Baccalaureate and Higher Level Certification

RN, BC (Registered Nurse, Board Certified) A current registered nurse license from the U.S. or its territories and bachelor's degree in nursing is required. You must have practiced a minimum of 2 years with at least 2000 hours of practice in the specialty and 30 contact hours in the 3 years preceding application.

- Cardiac/Vascular Nurse
- Community Health Nurse
- Gerontological Nurse
- Medical-Surgical Nurse
- Nursing Professional Development
- Pediatric Nurse
- Perinatal Nurse
- Psychiatric and Mental Health Nurse

Informatics

RN, C or RN, BC (Registered Nurse, Certified or Board Certified) Credential depends on whether baccalaureate degree is in nursing. A bachelor's degree in nursing or relevant discipline is required. You must complete at least 2000 hours of practice within the last 3 years.

Nursing Administration

RN, CNA, BC (Registered Nurse, Certified in Nursing Administration, Board Certified) A bachelor's degree in nursing is required. You must complete the equivalent of 24 months of full-time practice and 30 contact hours in the specialty within the 5-year period of application.

From American Nurses Credentialing Center. (2006). Certification catalog. Washington, DC: Author. http://www.nursecredentialing.org.

BOX 1-2 *Examples of Specialty Organization Certifications**

American Association of Critical Care Nurses (AACN)
  Certified Critical Care Registered Nurse (CCRN)
American Association of Occupational Health Nurses (AAOHN)
  Certified Occupational Health Nurse (COHN)
American Association of Nurse Anesthetists (AANA)
  Certified Registered Nurse Anesthetist (CRNA)
American College of Nurse Midwives (ACNM)
  Certified Nurse Midwife (CNM)
American Society of PeriAnesthesia Nurses (ASPAN)
  Certified Post-Anesthesia Nurse (CPAN)
Association of Operating Room Nurses (AORN)
  Certified Nurse Operating Room (CNOR)
Association for Practitioners in Infection Control (APIC)
  Certified in Infection Control (CIC)
Association of Rehabilitation Nurses (ARN)
  Certified Rehabilitation Registered Nurse (CRRN)
Emergency Nurses' Association (ENA)
  Certified Emergency Nurse (CEN)
International Association for Enterostomal Therapy (AET)
  Certified Enterostomal Therapy Nurse (CETN)
National Association of Pediatric Nurse Associates/Practitioners (NAPNAP)
  Certified Pediatric Nurse Practitioner (CPNP)
National Association of School Nurses (NASN)
  Certified School Nurse (CSN)
Oncology Nursing Society (ONS)
  Oncology Certified Nurse (OCN)
The Organization for Obstetric, Gynecologic, and Neonatal Nurses (NAACOG)
  Reproductive Nurse Certified (RNC)
    Ambulatory Women's Health Care
    High-Risk Obstetric Nurse
    Inpatient Obstetric Nurse
    Low-Risk Neonatal Nurse
    Maternal Newborn Nurse
    Neonatal Intensive Care Nurse
    Reproductive Endocrinology/Infertility Nurse
  Neonatal Nurse Practitioner (NP)
  Ob/Gyn Nurse Practitioner (NP)
  Women's Health Care Nurse Practitioner (NP)

*Certificates may be awarded by closely related, but separate and independent, organizations.

Interest in nursing education must be nurtured to provide faculty to keep nursing programs in operation. Those currently teaching in nursing programs will need to continue to develop creative, nontraditional teaching approaches to attract a sufficient number of students. Currently, due to declining enrollment in nursing programs, federal legislation is being enacted to lure people back into nursing education by offering special funding, grants, discounting loans, and other benefit packages.

PROFESSIONAL NURSING EDUCATION

REGISTERED NURSE

A **registered nurse (RN)** is an individual who is granted a license to practice nursing in a particular state under that state's nurse practice act after completing the curriculum of an accredited school of nursing and passing the **National Council Licensure Examination for Registered Nurses (NCLEX-RN®)** licensing examination from the National Council of State Boards of Nursing (NCSBN) (see Chapter 2 for discussion of nurse practice acts). Nursing school graduates who receive a diploma, an associate degree of nursing, or a bachelor's degree in nursing are all eligible to take this examination (Figure 1-4). After initial licensure in one state, the registered nurse may summit a request for licensure by endorsement in another state and pay an additional fee for licensure in that state.

The NCLEX-RN examination is a computer-adapted test administered in a localized testing center, but a paper and pencil examination can be requested from the state board of nursing under special request because of learning needs.

The NCLEX-RN examination tests the graduate's ability to meet client needs in the areas of safe, effective care environment, health promotion, psychosocial integrity, and physiological integrity (NCSBN, 2003). The test reflects questions on leadership, priority setting and delegation, medical-surgical or adult health, maternal-newborn health, psychiatric mental health, and child health.

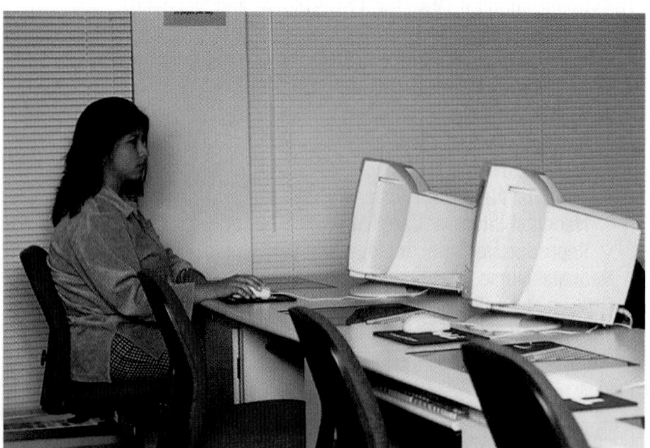

FIGURE 1-4 A graduate nurse taking the NCLEX-RN examination.

Since the first schools of nursing opened their doors in the eighteenth century, nursing education has expanded in response to ongoing changes and advances in health care. Today's nursing roles are more complex and require additional knowledge in the physical, biological, and social sciences, along with nursing practice and theory. Every three years the NCLEX-RN examination blueprint is updated to reflect the changing practice of nurses. Changes to the test plan reflect the results of research on the actual role performance expected of new graduates within the first 6 months of practice.

LICENSED VOCATIONAL NURSE/LICENSED PRACTICAL NURSE

In contrast to the registered nurse, many states recognize another health care worker known either as the **licensed vocational nurse (LVN)** or **licensed practical nurse (LPN)**. Usually this educational program is approximately 15 months in length and is primarily skills focused, although some college level preparatory courses are required. The role of the LVN/LPN as a health care team member is to assist in delivering care to clients under the supervision of an RN, who is legally responsible for the delegation of tasks to the LVN/LPN. Collaboration of all care is greatly assisted by the expertise of the LVN/LPN, who may provide much of the direct care to clients in the acute or subacute care settings.

ENTRY-LEVEL EDUCATION

Currently, four types of state-approved educational programs prepare students for entry into professional nursing practice as a registered nurse (RN). They are diploma programs, associate degree programs, baccalaureate degree programs, and graduate degree entry programs.

Diploma Programs. In the United States a diploma nursing program is a 2- or 3-year program frequently affiliated with a hospital. However, some diploma programs are associated with a junior college or university and students receive college credit for all nonnursing classes, which can lead to dual degrees. The programs retain some of the apprenticeship traditions of the past and prepare nurses for a high technical level of practice. The number of diploma programs has drastically declined over the past few decades as these programs close or become associate degree–granting programs.

Associate Degree Programs. Associate degree programs are 2-year programs offered by community colleges and universities. The program includes courses focused on scientific knowledge, nursing knowledge, and technical skills needed by nurses. Upon graduation, students receive an associate degree in nursing (ADN).

Baccalaureate Degree Programs. The basic baccalaureate nursing program is located within a university or college and requires a minimum of 4 years of study, including general education courses. The focus is on achieving a level of critical inquiry, clinical judgment, decision-making ability, and clinical knowledge imperative for professional nursing practice.

Many baccalaureate programs admit RNs with previously earned diplomas or associate degrees. Some universities offer an independent study program (external degree) without class structure. Most baccalaureate nursing programs accept student transfer credits from accredited universities and colleges. In addition, transferring students can take challenge examinations for college credit.

Graduate Degree Entry Programs. Master's and doctoral entry-level programs are offered by only a few universities. These programs prepare college graduates who have degrees in disciplines other than nursing to be entry-level nurse generalists with advanced knowledge and skills. These programs may offer tracks of specialization, such as for nurse practitioners, nurse administrators, nurse midwives, clinical nurse specialists, and nurse educators. Certification in specialty areas requires advanced testing and additional clinical practice to maintain currency of practice.

ADVANCED PRACTICE EDUCATION

Today, more nurses are earning master's and doctoral degrees to increase their nursing knowledge and expertise. These advanced degrees are also useful for those who wish to provide leadership in the policy-making arena of health care, in clinical practice and administration.

Master's Degree Programs. Master's degree programs in nursing, which usually take about 2 years to complete, prepare advanced practice nurses, such as nurse practitioners or clinical nurse specialists, nurse educators, and nurse administrators. Special emphasis is given to advanced scientific concepts and clinical practice. Theory and research in nursing form the foundation of the curriculum. As advanced practice roles increase in popularity, the addition of research will ultimately define the future role of tomorrow's nurse. Creativity and increasing application of theoretical research within the nursing field will identify advanced roles and clearer pictures of what evidence-based practice will look like in the near future. As a student you will help develop the role of the nurse tomorrow (Lenburg, 2005) (see Chapter 15).

Doctoral Degree Programs. A nurse doctorate requires in-depth inquiry and scientific research into a specific field of learning. Doctoral programs produce nurse philosophers, ethicists, theorists, and researchers. Many universities now require that nursing faculty members hold doctoral degrees. Clinical agencies are beginning to ask for nurses with doctorates to serve as nurse executives or directors of education and research. Professional organizations are also looking to nurses with doctoral degrees to represent them to those who make decisions about health policy and even to consumers.

CONTINUING EDUCATION

Continuing education (CE) is a term used to describe programs or courses that assist professional nurses in developing and maintaining the clinical expertise that promotes quality nursing care. CE is designed to enhance knowledge and skills in practice, administration, research, and education. CE for nurses is offered in workshops, institutes, short courses, conferences, telecourses, evening courses, and even supplements in professional nursing journals. The use of computers as resources for CE is growing rapidly. It is mandatory in many states to obtain a certain number of contact hours or continuing education units (CEUs) within each year or registration cycle to maintain professional licensure. A CE program may be approved to grant contact hours or CEUs if it meets certain criteria set by an approving authority. Computers have become the standard for communication and education by both local and distant continuing educational programs by various organizations (see Figure 1-3).

CE should not be confused with in-service programs, which are designed to increase knowledge and skills needed for nursing practice in a particular agency. Topics for in-service programs often relate to new policies, procedures, or equipment. CEUs are not generally given for this type of educational updates.

PROFESSIONAL NURSING PRACTICE

STANDARDS OF PROFESSIONAL NURSING

The role of the professional nurse is independent from that of the physician or other health care providers. This role derives from the discipline of nursing, which has a body of knowledge based upon theory, research, and practice. The role includes beliefs, practices, traditions, heritage, and a system of education that is applied through independent critical thinking skills of the individual practitioner (Parker 2006).

Professionalism is behavior that upholds the status, methods, character, and standards of a given profession. But what is a profession? According to Megginson, Mosley, and Pietri (1989), a profession has the following five characteristics:

- A codified body of knowledge
- A long period of education and training
- Controlled entry
- An enforced code of ethics
- Unselfish service to others

These characteristics distinguish professions from some other careers or occupations.

States and provinces regulate the professional practice of nursing through nurse practice acts, which legally define the scope of nursing practice in a given state. Even though nurse practice acts differ somewhat from state to state, they are similar in that they serve to protect the public by regulating and monitoring standards of practice and by ensuring that minimum standards for entry into the nursing profession are met. These same activities help meet the needs of the nursing profession as well.

Standards of nursing practice are a set of nursing actions constituting safe and effective client care that are generally agreed on by groups of nurses expert in their area of nursing. They establish the foundation for the professional practice of RNs. The development and implementation of these standards are major functions of nursing professional organizations. Chapter 10 further discusses standards of clinical nursing practice. Appendix A provides the American Nurses Association Standards of Clinical Nursing Practice.

PROFESSIONAL NURSING ORGANIZATIONS

According to Lenburg (2005), a professional organization is an organization of practitioners who are self-regulating, create their own standards and policies, and use political lobbyists and regulation to maximize health care delivery through policy formation and public awareness. Thus the professional organization deals with events of concern to the profession.

Nursing organizations set standards for nursing practice and education. Active involvement in nursing organizations enhances a sense of professional commitment. Clearly these organizations empower nurses through educational programs and professional publications.

In North America, there are two similar professional organizations for registered nurses. One is the American Nurses Association. Its members are state nurses' associations and individual nurses belonging to the state organization. The ANA sponsors workshops for nurses and publishes the *American Journal of Nursing*. The ANA also offers specialty certification (see Box 1-2).

The ANA is part of the International Council of Nurses (ICN), which promotes international associations of nurses and improves nursing practice standards while seeking higher status for nurses. The council provides nurses with an international power base.

The National League for Nursing (NLN) is a nursing organization that extends membership to nurses at any educational or practice level, nonnurses, and nursing agencies. The organization's main function is to promote increased development of nursing services and education in nursing.

The National Student Nurses Association (NSNA) is the preprofessional organization for student nurses in the United States. A requirement for membership in this organization is enrollment in a state-approved nursing education program.

Other organizations include the American Academy of Nursing (AAN), whose purpose is to recognize nurses who have made major contributions to the profession of nursing. The international honor society for nursing, Sigma Theta Tau, is a member of the Association of College Honor Societies. Students in baccalaureate, master's, doctoral, and postdoctoral programs are eligible ganizations support specialty practice and often provide certification in their areas (see Box 1-2). These organizations focus on specific areas of nursing practice such as oncology nursing. They strive to improve the standards of practice and welfare of nurses in that specialty.

The Nursing Organizations Alliance represents the largest number of registered nurses practicing in the United States. The organization's goal is to promote excellence in specialty nursing practice. Approximately 39 organizations are members. Membership consists of two representatives from each organization plus representatives from the ANA and the NLN.

OTHER REGULATING AGENCIES

All agencies (schools of nursing, universities, and health care facilities) are regulated by licensing organizations, accreditation boards, legislation, and public policy to achieve the maximum educational and practice standards. To continue to maintain the ability to operate, these organizations require funding and licensure (Lenburg, 2005). If an organization does not meet standards, it may be placed on warning and ultimately accreditation may be withdrawn. Funding is cut significantly or the program is closed if improvement has not occurred after warnings are given. Some nursing organizations do not regulate agencies but work through public awareness or legal influences to support the nursing practice.

PROFESSIONAL NURSING ROLES

In the past, a nurse's role consisted of providing care and comfort to clients and performing specific nursing functions. The role of modern nursing has expanded to include a heightened emphasis on illness prevention, health promotion, and concern for the client in a holistic manner, incorporating the needs of body, mind, and spirit. Today's nurse engages in eight interrelated roles: caregiver, advocate, critical thinker, teacher, communicator, manager, researcher, and rehabilitator.

Caregiver. The nurse addresses the client's holistic health care needs to promote health and the healing process. In the role of caregiver, the nurse provides treatment for specific disease processes and applies measures to restore the emotional and social well-being of the client.

Advocate. The nurse protects the client by preventing physical and/or chemical injury. In the role of client advocate, the nurse assists clients in understanding and expressing their rights whenever necessary. The nurse also works to preserve clients' legal and human rights in times of health and illness and during the process of dying. Chapter 2 discusses the legal and ethical contexts of nursing practice.

Critical Thinker. Nurses use decision-making and critical thinking skills in conjunction with the nursing process. Before actually delivering nursing care, the nurse plans the best method of care delivery for each client. Refer to Chapter 5 for additional information on critical thinking and clinical judgment.

Teacher. The nurse provides clients and family members with information about health, treatment or therapy, and lifestyle changes. As a teacher, the nurse determines if the client understands the information presented and reinforces the learning as necessary. The nurse then evaluates the client's progress toward health-related goals. The nurse uses teaching methods that are compatible with the client's knowledge, education, and literacy levels. For more in-depth information refer to Chapter 13.

Communicator. Open and consistent communication is vital for effective nursing practice. The nurse must possess excellent communication skills to provide care, rehabilitation, teaching, comfort, and protection to clients. For more in-depth information about client-nurse communication processes refer to Chapter 12.

Manager/Administrator/Executive. Today's nursing leadership role is in transition and so is the title that reflects the role performed. Nurses are responsible for coordinating, delegating, and supervising the health care team that provides the care to the client and significant others. All nurses need good management skills, whether they supervise others in the provision of nursing care or provide direct care themselves (Figure 1-5). This will become an increasingly vital role as more specialization occurs and the nurse coordinates the specialists to provide a unified goal (Lenburg, 2005). Chapter 14 further describes the role of the nurse as manager/administrator/executive.

Researcher. Nursing research provides the evolving body of knowledge and theory for the nursing profession. Research nurses may be employed in an academic area, a community agency, or an independent professional agency. The nurse researcher usually conducts studies and investigates problems to improve client health and nursing care. A graduate degree in nursing is usually the minimal educational requirement, although many nurse generalists participate in research. Chapter 15 discusses nursing research as a tool for professional practice.

Rehabilitator. Ensuring that a client returns to a maximal state of functioning requires rehabilitative activities administered by nurses along with members of other disciplines, such as physical therapy. When clients experience alterations in health, the nurse's role is to promote client adaptation and coping.

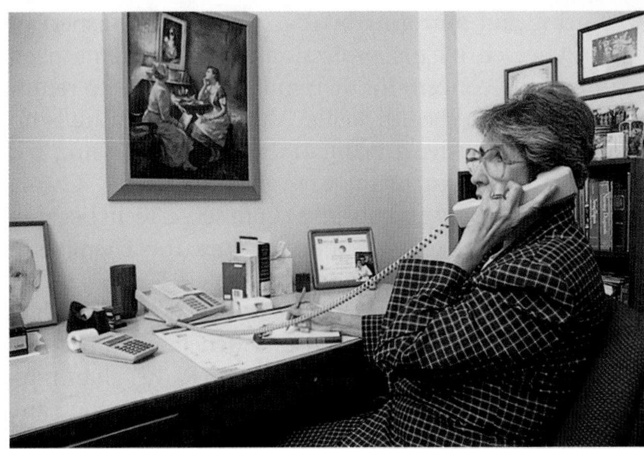

FIGURE 1-5 Whether a nurse serves as a nurse-manager or as a manager of assistive personnel, management skills are essential.

CHALLENGE

Today's nurse must know more, possess advanced skills, be able to multitask, perform a variety of roles, and maintain an even temperament while engaging in nursing practice. Treatments must be administered safely and with skill while using newer advanced technologies. Clients need education about use of and precautions with medications, treatments, after-hospitalization care, disease management, and follow-up appointments. The nurse also needs to do follow-up evaluation of this knowledge to prevent errors in home management. Often the nurse becomes a phone resource for clients after discharge to help answer any questions or problems experienced after discharge. Written directions and follow-up postdischarge checkups by nurses help to reduce errors after discharge. In sum, the nurse needs to engage in management, resource allocation, counseling, education, and client management at any given time, and this can be a complex challenge.

Another challenge is the identification of individual cultural needs during client assessment upon admission to make sure that client needs are being addressed to maximize recovery. The professional nurse should give holistic care by planning to meet the identified needs of each client. Written plans of care are documented within the legal chart to guide each nurse's approach to care based upon identified client needs and goals. Interventions, actions, and referrals are also documented to show how the goals are met or not met and the modifications needed based on client response. Evaluation of the client is an ongoing process by all staff caring for the client, but the professional nurse synthesizes client assessments and response to care into a comprehensive documentation of the client's status. Nursing documentation is a tool that aids collaboration with health care providers and other health care workers to maximize the quality of care delivered.

Caring and nurturing by the nurse is a key aspect of care delivered by the professional nurse. Clients need comfort and concern for their individual needs to return to their optimal health status. Although nurturing is no longer the exclusive domain of the professional nurse, it is still a large part of the care given to clients. Caring enhances recovery and positive client self-esteem because it demonstrates that the nurse values the client as a unique individual. Refer also to Chapters 5 and 12.

Another challenge for nurses in today's health care arena includes the effort to use evidence-based practice in planning and delivering client care. Rather than relying on tradition as a basis for delivering nursing care, health care organizations are looking to formulate policies and procedures for medical and nursing care based on what research has shown to be effective in improving client outcomes (see Chapter 15).

Today's nurse must be autonomous and self-directed in maintaining currency of practice. To do this, nurses must engage in lifelong learning to maintain a current base of nursing knowledge, by reading journals and books, attending conferences, and participating in online or face-to-face continuing education programs. Each state board of nursing dictates how many hours of continuing education credit are needed for nursing license renewal. Beyond acquiring knowledge, a final challenge to nurses in today's health care arena is to put new knowledge into practice and maintain the quest and desire to continue to learn.

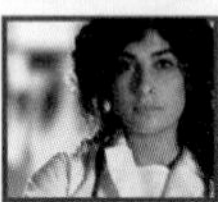

In reference to the case study presented at the beginning of the chapter, Diane stayed in school and went on to acquire her bachelor's, master's, and doctoral degrees in nursing. She became an assistant professor of nursing to assist other new and struggling students in understanding the demands on today's nurse. She continually reads and learns; many changes have occurred, but by staying current she can assist her students in using current knowledge while helping them to develop their critical thinking and clinical decision-making skills.

As a student your dedication to nursing will be evidenced by your continued study and your attempts to meet the challenges of tomorrow's clients. As a future nurse you need to feel a part of the future and remember that what you do in practice today drives tomorrow's research and role development.

▼ KEY PRINCIPLES

- Nursing is a profession in transition, and one must remain current to meet tomorrow's demands.
- Nursing is client focused.
- Nursing includes prevention of illness, promotion of health, maintenance of health, and comfort in dying.
- Nursing is team focused to give a holistic approach to management of individual clients.
- Nursing is an autonomous practice of research-based expertise that uses scientific principles to guide daily practice.
- Nurses gather data daily to contribute to research to further advance the profession.
- Nursing values the highest standard of care possible and is based upon standards that guide the profession.
- Roles of the nurse are varied, complex, and evolving with new technologies and research advances.
- The client is a multidimensional individual who has unique needs that affect health care outcomes.
- Health is the maximization of the potential improvements possible within the limitations that the individual possesses and includes a balance of spiritual, physical, and psychosocial aspects.
- All registered nurses take the same licensing examination (NCLEX-RN) regardless of the level of education used for entry into nursing practice.
- Professional organizations assist in developing and maintaining the standards of practice.
- Ongoing education is valued, expected, and required for continued licensure.

■ REVIEW QUESTIONS

1. The term *client,* when used by nurses, refers to a person who:

1. Is the passive object of nursing care as a service given by the nurse
2. Is being treated in a community setting such as a clinic
3. Participates actively in his or her own care along with health care providers
4. Purchases health care services while remaining in the home

2. The use of nursing informatics is a new role for the nurse based on which of the following influences?

1. Advances in computer technology
2. Worsening nursing shortages
3. Ongoing issues with resource allocation
4. Closing of small hospitals and greater commute for clients

3. HIPAA has positively affected the client's right to which of the following?

1. Free health care
2. Confidentiality
3. A peaceful death
4. Home health care services

4. A nursing student who attends a 2-year nursing program should expect to receive:

1. An associate's degree in nursing
2. A bachelor's degree in nursing
3. A master's degree in nursing
4. A diploma in nursing

5. The professional organization of nurses in the United States is the:

1. National League for Nursing
2. American Nurses Association
3. American Academy of Nurses
4. International Council of Nurses

Bibliography

*American Nurses Association. (1987). *The scope of nursing practice.* Kansas City, MO: Author.

*American Nurses Association. (1995). *Nursing's social policy statement.* Washington, DC: Author.

American Nurses Association. (2003). *Standards of clinical nursing practice* (3rd ed.). Washington, DC: Author.

American Nurses Credentialing Center. (2006). *Certification catalog.* Washington, DC: Author.

*Berry, A. (2002). Cultural care of Mexican American families. In M. Leininger & M. R. McFarland, *Transcultural nursing: Concepts, theories, research, and practice* (3rd ed., pp. 432-433). New York: McGraw-Hill, Medical Publisher Division.

Bomar, P. J. (2004). *Nursing in the new millennium: Promoting health in families—applying research and theory to nursing process* (3rd ed., p. 634). Philadelphia: Saunders.

*Cohen, L. B. (1984). Florence Nightingale. *Scientific American, 250*(128), 137.

*Dock, H. K., & Stewart, I. M. (1925). A short history of nursing (3rd ed.). New York: Putnam.

International Council of Nurses, The ICN definition of nursing. Retrieved October 24, 2006, from http://www.nursingworld.org/icn.

*Leininger, M. & McFarland, M. (2002). Anglo-American (United States) culture care, values, beliefs, and lifeways. In M. Leininger & M. R. McFarland, *Transcultural nursing: Concepts, theories, research, and practice* (3rd ed., pp. 298-300). New York: McGraw-Hill, Medical Publisher Division.

Lenburg, C. B. (2005). The influence of contemporary trends and issues on nursing education. In B. Cherry & S. R. Jacob, *Contemporary nursing: Issues, trends, management* (3rd ed., pp. 78-80). St. Louis, MO: Mosby.

Lewis, S. M., Heitkemper, M. M., & Dirksen, S. R.. (2004). *Medical-surgical nursing: Assessment and management of clinical problems* (6th ed., pp. 264-265). St. Louis, MO: Mosby.

*Megginson, L. C., Mosley, D. C., & Pietri, P.H. (1989). *Management concepts and applications* (3rd ed., p. 639). New York: Harper & Row.

*Morgan, M. G. (2002). African American culture care. In M. Leininger & M. R. McFarland, *Transcultural nursing: Concepts, theories, research, and practice* (3rd ed., p. 278). New York: McGraw-Hill, Medical Publisher Division.

National Council of State Boards of Nursing. (2003). *NCLEX-RN® examination. Test plan for the National Council licensure examination for registered nurses. Effective Date: April 2004.* Chicago: Author.

*Nightingale, F. (1860). *Notes on nursing: What it is and what it is not.* London: Harrison. (Reprinted in F. L. A. Bishop & S. Goldie. [1962]. *A bio-bibliography of Florence Nightingale.* London: Dawsons of Pall Mall.)

Parker, M. E. (2006). *Nursing theories and nursing practice* (2nd ed., pp. 4-11). Philadelphia: F.A. Davis.

Saba, V. K., & McCormick, K. A. (2006). *Essentials of nursing informatics* (4th ed., pp. 3-4). NY: McGraw-Hill, Medical Publisher Division.

Williams-Evans, S. A., Jacob, S. R., & Carnegie, M. E. (2005). The evolution of professional nursing. In B. Cherry & S. R. Jacob, *Contemporary nursing: Issues, trends, management* (3rd ed., p. 23). St. Louis, MO: Mosby.

---

*Asterisk indicates a classic or definitive work on this subject.

Chapter 2

ETHICAL AND LEGAL CONTEXT OF PRACTICE

Media Resources

- evolve Evolve Website http://evolve.elsevier.com/Harkreader/
- Companion CD

Learning Objectives

After studying this chapter, you should be able to do the following:

- Discuss the concepts of morals, values, and ethics as a basis for nursing practice
- Apply ethical principles to clarify values and make decisions in nursing
- Identify the elements of the codes of ethics for nursing
- Describe the application of sources and types of law in nursing practice
- Describe the professional regulation of nursing practice
- Describe the legal regulation of nursing practice
- Discuss selected client rights and their influence on nursing practice
- Describe two initiatives to improve the quality of nursing care delivered to clients
- Identify actions that can safeguard one's own nursing practice

Key Terms

accreditation
administrative law
advance directive
assault
autonomy
battery
beneficence
certification
civil law
common law
confidentiality
contract
credentialing
criminal law
defamation
defendant
durable power of attorney for health care
ethics
false imprisonment
fidelity
fraud
informed consent
invasion of privacy
justice
law
liability
license
living will
malpractice
morals
negligence
nonmaleficence
plaintiff
procedural law
professional misconduct
public law
registration
statutory law
substantive law
tort
values
values clarification
veracity

To the extent that nursing as a profession has an altruistic motivation, ethics is the foundation for nursing practice. Altruism means that nurses are motivated to act in the best interests and welfare of their clients; in other words, nurses have an ethic of care. Ethics is the system of beliefs about what is right or wrong, good or bad, in human conduct and helps us make decisions about what constitutes moral conduct and moral judgment. To be ethical is to act as an independent moral agent who accepts responsibility and accountability for one's actions.

Ethical decision making is not the same as legal decision making. Nurses have an obligation to practice within the law as written by the legislature, interpreted by the courts, and written into administrative rules of agencies given authority under the law. Law is the system of manmade rules and regulations by which a society is governed and through which people can live together. Decision making in nursing practice involves a complex interplay of a system of ethics and legal mandates. Our actions are at times determined primarily by laws, at times by ethics, and at times by a combination of the two.

Laws have the intent of promoting or protecting the members of a society and are generally in keeping with basic ethical principles. Therefore what is a legally correct action is also often a morally correct action. On the other hand, sometime a morally defensible action is not legally correct and laws are not always morally defensible.

THE ETHICAL CONTEXT OF PRACTICE

Being ethical is about having the moral character to consistently act with consideration of the consequences to the welfare of others. The development of moral character occurs from a lifetime of self-examination and study of the principles of moral behavior and the consequences of our actions.

Professional ethics is the principles that guide the practice of the members of a profession. These principles should be core or fundamental values that are embraceable by all members of the profession. Nursing ethics is the values of the profession underlying practicing in a way that achieves the best outcomes for the persons who are the objects of care.

Some of the values that guide nursing practice include the following:

- All humans have inherent dignity and worth.
- The primary commitment of nurses is to the people who receive nursing care.
- The client has the right to protection of health, safety, and human rights.
- Basic human rights include veracity, autonomy, justice, beneficence, and nonmaleficence.
- Compassionate care, the relief of suffering, and promoting the well-being of the client is central to nursing.

Nearly all nurses face ethical dilemmas. Ethical decision making is not isolationistic, egocentric, or without consequences to self and others. Health care decisions are made in the context of the values of the client, the family, the physician, the nurse, the health care institution, and society.

VALUES, MORALS, AND ETHICS

Values, morals, and *ethics* are overlapping concepts to indicate behaviors or ideas that the speaker feels are right, good, just, or proper.

Values. **Values** are ideals, beliefs, and patterns of behavior that are prized and chosen by a person, group, or society. Not all values are moral or ethical values. Nevertheless, values shape decisions in everyday life, from the clothes we wear to the movies we prefer to the food we eat to the way we behave in relationship to other people.

Values are learned behaviors that are influenced by culture, ethnicity, education, and life experiences. Values are acquired through structured and unstructured learning, experiences in our homes and communities, and interactions with family, teachers, clergy, and social organizations. As children, we are exposed to the values of adults who have influence over our lives. As we mature, we begin to develop our own values and separate fundamental moral principles from what we just happen to like. In adulthood, our behaviors reflect the values we have acquired and use in daily decision making.

Morals. **Morals** are standards of conduct that represent the ideal in human behavior that would be put forward by all rational persons as a guide to our relationships to others. Although morals are often thought of as the principles or standards of behavior derived from religious doctrine, in a broader sense morals and ethics mean the same thing. Nurses have moral agency. That is, nurses are independently responsible and accountable for their actions. Although nurses follow the physician's directives in carrying out the medical treatment plan and work within hospital policies, these duties cannot be substituted for moral responsibility.

Ethics. **Ethics** is the branch of philosophy that systematically examines behavior to determine what constitutes good, bad, right, and wrong in human behavior and provide guidance for action. In Western culture it has evolved as a process of reasoning both to examine human behavior and to prescribe action. *Bioethics* is the branch of ethics that studies moral implications of new biological discoveries and biomedical advances, as in the fields of genetic engineering and drug research. Advances in science and technology have significantly contributed to the increasing complexity of ethical decision making in health care.

ETHICAL PRINCIPLES

Principles are basic truths or laws that guide conduct and behavior. Ethical principles, also called standards, provide the framework for the practice of professional nursing. The following eight principles are considered essential to the delivery of ethical nursing care.

Ethic of Care. As an ethical position, care means to have an emotional connection that motivates both concern for the other and a desire to meet the needs of the other. It is manifest in compassion, kindness, empathy, altruism, generosity, respectfulness, trustworthiness, personal integrity, forgiveness, and courage. The ethic of care is most closely related to the theory of virtue ethics, which holds that you cannot separate the person from his or her acts. You need to know the character of the person.

Nursing's ethic of care has been criticized as lacking a rational or logical structure to give nurses a systematic way of making ethical decisions. On the other hand, proponents of an ethic of care might say that because the ethic of care is "a woman's way of decision making" from knowledge gained from "a woman's way of knowing," it cannot be described in rational, logical terms but can be understood in an intuitive way. Embracing an ethic of care can be combined with the more rational (in the sense of being logical and systematic structure) as a way to solve an ethical problem.

While the ethic of care does not solely belong to nurses, some nurses believe it is what makes nursing unique. Some of the nursing theorists who write about care are discussed in Chapter 5.

Autonomy. **Autonomy** refers to a person's right to make individual choices—that is, to self-determination. Autonomy supports respect for the client's right to make health care choices. To support autonomy, you provide detailed and realistic information to clients, who then freely choose from the available options. The principle of autonomy conflicts with "paternalism," in which an authority figure makes decisions for another person from a position of greater knowledge and intelligence.

Beneficence. **Beneficence** is the promotion of good. It requires the performance of actions that are of benefit to others. To do good implies knowledge and understanding of what is good and weighing good against any possible harm. For example, failing to turn a bedridden client who complains of pain during the turning may produce the short-term good of reduced discomfort, but it may also cause the harm of impaired skin integrity and musculoskeletal deformities.

Nonmaleficence. The word *maleficence* means to do evil or cause harm. Thus **nonmaleficence** requires the practitioner to do no harm. Nonmaleficence is the complement of beneficence. It implies that the good of your actions should outweigh any possible harm to clients. Safe, effective nursing care includes acts that cause fear, discomfort, or pain—inserting a feeding tube, for example, or giving an injection. The good of these acts (beneficence) is weighed against both the temporary pain and the potential for serious harm if the interventions are withheld.

Right to Privacy. The right to privacy is derived from the principle of autonomy and from moral rights theory. **Confidentiality** is the client's right to privacy in the health care delivery system. Confidentiality means maintaining another's privacy by safeguarding information that is entrusted to you. A further discussion of confidentiality can be found under Client Rights later in this chapter.

Fidelity. **Fidelity** means honoring agreements and keeping promises. It is derived from teleological ethics, in which a duty is owed or there is a duty to act. Establishing a nurse-client relationship implies that certain duties are owed to the client.

Justice. **Justice** is moral rightness, fairness, or equity. In the legal system it can mean that "the punishment fits the crime." In the health care system justice is generally concerned with fair and equal treatment of all clients. In applying the principle of justice, consider whether it requires that everyone be treated the same or that the same principles and standards be applied to all. Justice could be based on "to each according to his need."

The issue of justice arises in the allocation of scarce health care resources. Organ donation and transplantation is illustrative of the issues that arise in attempting to fairly allocate scarce health care resources.

Veracity. **Veracity** means adhering to the truth. It requires truth telling consistently and continually. In applying the principle of veracity, you tell the complete truth and not an altered version assumed to be in the client's best interest. Veracity also relates to the principle of autonomy because clients can make the best decisions for themselves only when given complete facts. This issue is crucial when dealing with terminally ill clients and their right to know their prognosis.

It is important to remember that respect for others guides the implementation of all ethical principles. Although respect is culturally defined, frequently it is associated with ensuring freedom of choice, promoting good, preventing harm, keeping promises, acting fairly, and being truthful.

COMMON ETHICAL PROBLEMS

Nursing care is provided in collaboration with clients, families, physicians, and other health care practitioners, thus bringing together sometimes different worldviews, personal views, and value systems (Figure 2-1). Consider the ethical principles involved in these situations:

- A client has gone into a coma overnight. You have notified the doctor, but he has not taken action or come to see the client.
- Another nurse provides care that you believe is inadequate or unsafe.

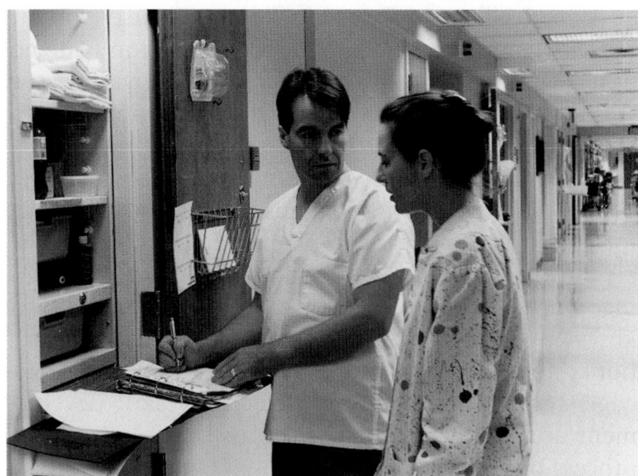

FIGURE 2-1 Nursing is not practiced in a vacuum but in collaboration with others.

- You are assigned more clients than you feel is safe. Or you are asked to perform a procedure you have not done before, but there is no one else available to do it.
- A client is being discharged from the hospital because of the limits of his medical coverage. You recognize ongoing needs that you believe the client cannot manage at home without suffering undue complications.
- A client asks you directly if his condition will lead to his death.
- A client gives you information that will result in harm to the client or others and asks you to keep this information confidential.
- A client with mild dementia is not being allowed to make decisions for herself.
- You told a client that you would return to help him to the bathroom in 15 minutes, but another client demanded your time and you were unable to return.

Issues of ethics are unavoidable in the day-to-day delivery of nursing care. Developing skills to identify when there is conflict of values or ethical principles increases your ability to be effective in care delivery. Also, being knowledgeable of the steps in the ethical decision-making process provides you with the tools to ensure that client needs are being served.

ETHICS IN NURSING

Developing professional ethics is about learning to value the principles of nursing ethics and consistently acting on those principles. Our values reflect what we hold important and what we believe when we act on them in various situations in daily life. For example, if a nurse believes that clients have a right to autonomy, the nurse demonstrates that belief by allowing the client to make choices that would not be choices the nurse would make for the client. If you understand your values and can express them clearly, you will be better prepared to handle difficult situations and make informed decisions.

A professional code of ethics is not a fully developed system of ethics. It is standards of behaviors that govern practice established by a representative body of members of a profession. It is of necessity limited because it must be acceptable to all members of a culturally diverse profession. It must be short and at the same time apply to all circumstances; therefore codes of professional ethics tend to be vague.

In the United States, the American Nurses Association (ANA) *Code of Ethics for Nurses With Interpretive Statements* (2001) is the document governing ethical nursing practice (Box 2-1). The ANA code for nurses identifies the goals and values of the profession and sets forth the philosophy of the profession. It includes interpretive statements that explain how each goal is realized in nursing practice. The code focuses on the protection of the client

BOX 2-1 *American Nurses Association Code of Ethics for Nurses*

1. The nurse, in all professional relationships, practices with compassion and respect for the inherent dignity, worth, and uniqueness of every individual, unrestricted by considerations of social or economic status, personal attributes, or the nature of health problems.
2. The nurse's primary commitment is to the patient, whether an individual, family, group, or community.
3. The nurse promotes, advocates for, and strives to protect the health, safety, and rights of the patient.
4. The nurse is responsible and accountable for individual nursing practice and determines the appropriate delegation of tasks consistent with the nurse's obligation to provide optimum patient care.
5. The nurse owes the same duties to self as to others, including the responsibility to preserve integrity and safety, to maintain competence, and to continue personal and professional growth.
6. The nurse participates in establishing, maintaining, and improving health care environments and conditions of employment conducive to the provision of quality health care and consistent with the values of the profession through individual and collective action.
7. The nurse participates in the advancement of the profession through contributions to practice, education, administration, and knowledge development.
8. The nurse collaborates with other health professionals and the public in promoting community, national, and international efforts to meet health needs.
9. The profession of nursing, as represented by associations and their members, is responsible for articulating nursing values, for maintaining the integrity of the profession and its practice, and for shaping social policy.

and the identification of standards for a nurse's interactions with clients. Because it identifies the behaviors required for ethical practice, the code can be used as a guide for evaluating nursing actions. It may also be used as a guide to ethical decision making. Although the code is not law, it is the standard by which nursing actions are judged throughout the profession.

Another code for professional nursing is the *ICN Code of Ethics for Nurses* by the International Council of Nurses (ICN) (2006) (Box 2-2). As you review, note the similarities. For example, both codes address respect for human dignity, rights, and confidentiality, and competence and responsibilities of the nurse in the delivery of health care. In addition, the codes provide a framework for ethical practice in professional nursing and can be used as a standard in legal proceedings.

Accountability and Responsibility. As a nurse, you are *responsible* and can be held accountable for your actions. That is, you are responsible for providing care within established standards of the profession. For example, you are responsible for implementing care using the nursing process. This means you assess client needs, identify nursing diagnoses, identify outcomes, formulate a plan of care, implement actions, and evaluate the effectiveness of nursing care provided. As a nursing student, you are responsible for acquiring the knowledge and skills necessary to become a safe practitioner and for acting only within your level of knowledge. Included in this knowledge and skill development are the awareness of ethical principles and the process of ethical decision making. Once you have attained licensure to practice as a registered nurse (RN),

BOX 2-2 *The International Council of Nurses Code of Ethics for Nurses*

An international code of ethics for nurses was first adopted by the International Council of Nurses (ICN) in 1953. It has been revised and reaffirmed at various times since, most recently with the review and revision completed in 2005. The ICN Code of Ethics is also available in French, Spanish, and German.

PREAMBLE

- Nurses have four fundamental responsibilities: to promote health, to prevent illness, to restore health and to alleviate suffering. The need for nursing is universal.
- Inherent in nursing is respect for human rights, including cultural rights, the right to life and choice, to dignity and to be treated with respect. Nursing care is respectful of and unrestricted by considerations of age, color, creed, culture, disability or illness, gender, nationality, politics, race or social status.
- Nurses render health services to the individual, the family, and the community and coordinate their services with those of related groups.

THE CODE

The *ICN Code of Ethics for Nurses* has four principal elements that outline the standards of ethical conduct.

ELEMENTS OF THE CODE

1. Nurses and People

- The nurse's primary professional responsibility is to people requiring nursing care.
- In providing care, the nurse promotes an environment in which the human rights, values, customs, and spiritual beliefs of the individual, family, and community are respected.
- The nurse ensures that the individual receives sufficient information on which to base consent for care and related treatment.
- The nurse holds in confidence personal information and uses judgment in sharing this information.
- The nurse shares with society the responsibility for initiating and supporting action to meet the health and social needs of the public, in particular those of vulnerable populations.
- The nurse also shares responsibility to sustain and protect the natural environment from depletion, pollution, degradation, and destruction.

2. Nurses and Practice

- The nurse carries personal responsibility and accountability for nursing practice, and for maintaining competence by continual learning.
- The nurse maintains a standard of personal health such that the ability to provide care is not compromised.
- The nurse uses judgment regarding individual competence when accepting and delegating responsibility.
- The nurse at all times maintains standards of personal conduct that reflect well on the profession and enhance public confidence.
- The nurse, in providing care, ensures that use of technology and scientific advances are compatible with the safety, dignity, and rights of people.

3. Nurses and the Profession

- The nurse assumes the major role in determining and implementing acceptable standards of clinical nursing practice, management, research, and education.
- The nurse is active in developing a core of research-based professional knowledge.
- The nurse, acting through the professional organization, participates in creating and maintaining equitable social and economic working conditions in nursing.

4. Nurses and Co-workers

- The nurse sustains a cooperative relationship with co-workers in nursing and other fields.
- The nurse takes appropriate action to safeguard individuals when their care is endangered by a co-worker or any other person.

you are responsible for maintaining competency in nursing knowledge and skills and demonstrating ethical principles in care delivery.

Being *accountable* means that you are answerable for the outcomes of actions taken. You are answerable to clients and their families, institutions, the profession, peers, and society. In addition, you are answerable to yourself to ensure that your conduct reflects ethical behavior. If you assess that a client has a high risk of injury from falls and you do not develop and implement a plan of care to protect the client from injury, you can be held accountable if the client is injured. In this instance, you are accountable to the client and his or her family. In addition, you are answerable to yourself, your employer, and the profession because the nursing care provided did not demonstrate implementation of the nursing process or provision of care within ethical principles (nonmaleficence). You are accountable for the outcomes of your nursing judgment, and this accountability cannot be alleviated by physicians' orders or institutional policies (ANA, 2001).

Advocacy. To advocate for someone means to speak for that person when the person cannot speak for himself or herself and to speak as that person perceives his or her interests. As the client's advocate, you may need to communicate the client's wishes or desires regarding health care choices to family members, physicians, or others. Advocacy can be not speaking for the client, but ensuring clients and families have effective channels of communication to express their desires/needs. It is important for you to understand your clients' values if you are to effectively represent those values to others. Nurses actively advocate for children, mentally or physically disabled persons, older adults, or other clients when they are vulnerable and unable to promote their own needs.

In a broader sense, nurses are advocates anytime they assist clients in obtaining needed help or services. Thus, providing information, helping clients explore options, and assisting clients in expressing their choices are activities integral to the advocacy role of nurses.

Making an Ethical Decision. Moral behavior is not always easy. In the complex decision-making environment of the health care system, moral principles have a way of colliding with each other and producing moral conflict. There are three situations of moral conflict:

- Moral uncertainty, when a person is unsure what values and principles are applicable or if an ethical problem really exists (some conflicts merely represent personal or cultural values that do not have anything to do with goodness, rightness, or justness)
- Moral dilemma, when moral principles are in conflict
- Moral distress, when the person understands what ought to be done but no supportive systems are available to help in reaching a decision or implementing an action

Once you recognize a moral situation, you must then be able to implement moral reasoning. Although well-developed intuitive reasoning may lead us to a correct action, rational moral reasoning is a systematic method of examination based on moral principles. Rational moral reasoning includes the following:

- Recognition of a moral situation
- Clarifying the viewpoints of the persons involved and the moral principles involved
- Examination of possible courses of action in light of moral principles and possible consequences of the actions
- Selection of an action and examination of the possible outcomes of the action
- Intention to implement morally correct behavior
- Performance of a selected behavior that resolves the dilemma

You are often called upon to make decisions that are not as easy, and the choices may conflict (Box 2-3). Not all decisions are moral decisions. A decision may be a matter of etiquette—the rules for behavior between two or more persons, for example, physician-nurse, supervisor-nurse, or nurse-nurse. The decision may be a matter of law or hospital protocol. It may be about following the orders of a superior or derived from the opinion of the majority. None of these should override ethics.

When two or more principles are in conflict or when the choices are unfavorable (i.e., no available solution is satisfactory), you have an ethical dilemma. For example, a geriatric male client is restrained because of his unsteady gait. You are concerned about his risk of injury from falling. The client is oriented and says repeatedly that he does not want to be restrained. In this situation, the principles in conflict are autonomy versus beneficence. You respect the client's right to be autonomous and make his own decisions, yet you are also bound to protect him from injury and prevent unnecessary harm.

BOX 2-3 *Ethics Discussion Scenario*

John is a 60-year-old client who fell and fractured his hip. Before this event he was physically and mentally active. On the second night after his surgery, he is on narcotics for pain and begins to hallucinate. By the next morning he is unresponsive. The physician visits and writes orders for some blood tests. He says nothing to the nurse about what he thinks. The nurse is surprised that the physician is not more aggressive in determining what is wrong with John and does not understand the physician's thinking in writing the orders he wrote.

- What do you think the nurse should do?
- What is the role of the etiquette between physicians and nurses?
- What ethical principles are involved for the nurse?
- Is this primarily an ethical situation or an etiquette situation?

You are expected to implement actions that result in good outcomes for the client yet remain in keeping with the client's wishes and desires. The following six-step ethical decision-making process will help you move beyond feelings of uncertainty and helplessness to naming and clarifying the problem and implementing solutions. Jameton (1984) provides the basis for this ethical decision-making process.

Identify the ethical dilemma. Is the situation truly an ethical dilemma, with conflicting principles or values, or is it a legal issue or a problem of faulty communication? Legal and communication issues may be present in any ethical dilemma, but in the absence of conflicting principles, legal counsel or clarification of communication may be appropriate rather than ethical analysis.

Gather pertinent data. Everyone involved in the case is a source of potentially significant data. Documents such as the health history, nurses' notes, and consent forms are also important to research. Questions to ask include the following: What are the relevant facts at issue in the dilemma? Who are the principal people involved? Are values in conflict with expected outcomes? Is there a clear therapeutic regimen for the client? Do cultural or spiritual factors need to be considered in the decision? Do institutional values and systems support the nursing decisions made? Is there a mechanism for implementing actions? Have policies, procedures, protocols, and economic factors been considered?

Examine the dilemma for the ethical principles involved. At this point it is important to have a clear understanding of the principles that are key to making an ethical decision in each case. Questions to ask include the following: With whom must the final decision be made, and is that person competent or empowered to make decisions? *(autonomy)* What is the overall good to be accomplished? (*beneficence* and *nonmaleficence*) Have the principal decision makers been given all necessary information? *(veracity)* Whose interests are being served? *(justice)* Have there been promises made or are there expectations of behaviors from caregivers? *(fidelity)* Determine which principles are applicable and which are in conflict. Does honoring one over another oppose legal requirements or institutional policies?

Examine all possible solutions. Explore all possible, reasonable actions in terms of ethical principles. In considering solutions, it is important to evaluate realistically which options you can implement within legal guidelines and agency policy. Activities such as facilitating communication, providing facts, and ensuring that participants are aware of all reasonable options are always within the purview of nursing. In addition, you must be aware of the likely outcomes of the various possible solutions. Will the consequences of actions taken be those that are intended? Will the intended good be served?

Choose solutions. After careful deliberation, choose a solution (or solutions) and take action. The chosen solutions must be consistent with ethical principles and be based on ethical analysis.

Evaluate solutions chosen. Examine solutions chosen for effectiveness. Reflect on whether expected outcomes were reached. Questions to ask include the following: Did solutions chosen resolve the ethical dilemma? What was the effect on those involved? Were additional ethical issues identified? Was the chosen solution the best one in light of the outcomes generated?

Often there is more than one possible solution. The ethical decision-making process assists you in reaching the best solution for a particular situation. The process may also help you to overcome the initial feelings of helplessness that you may experience when facing an ethical dilemma (Box 2-4). Keep in mind that a single perfect answer may not result from this process. Instead, you will search for the answer closest to the intended good for the primary parties involved in the dilemma.

Values Clarification. An understanding of personal values forms the basis for ethical decision making. The process of **values clarification** allows you to identify your personal values and develop self-awareness. This process is essential in nursing because your values provide the platform on which you will make decisions and take action. A three-step model for values clarification is described in Table 2-1, p. 24.

Guides to Ethical Decisions in Nursing

Institutional Ethics Committees. Institutional ethics committees are multidisciplinary committees of health care professionals within a facility that perform a variety of tasks related to ethical issues within that facility. Nursing is represented on such committees, but it is usually not in the majority and may be represented only at the administrative level. Ethics committees provide consultation, education, case review, decision making, and mediation when conflicts arise between health care professionals in the identification and resolution of ethical dilemmas (Figure 2-2, p. 24). They are integral to development of facility policies and procedures regarding ethics and to the implementation of such policies and procedures (Fowler & Levine-Ariff, 1987).

Nursing Ethics Forums. A nursing ethics forum can provide a mechanism for nurses to identify and address ethical issues that affect delivery of nursing care. These forums are separate from institutional ethics committees and may be hospital-wide or unit based, involving nursing rounds or case review. Nursing ethics forums focus on assisting you in developing skills in ethical analysis and decision mak-

BOX 2-4 *Case Study Using the Six-Step Ethical Decision-Making Process*

Michael R. is a 25-year-old African American client diagnosed with sickle cell disease who has undergone multiple hospital admissions in the last 2 years. He is admitted to Catherine's med-surg unit for the sixth time in the last 5 months. Catherine has cared for him on his last two admissions. She is again assigned to his care. She is aware that an ongoing issue with Michael is pain management. She is concerned when she reads the prescribed pain management regimen.

His physician prescribed the same regimen during his last two admissions, and the client frequently complained of inadequate pain relief, asking for more medication before it was time for his next dose. Because of constant pain and inadequate relief, Michael was often angry and frustrated. The nurses have labeled him hostile and difficult to manage. They expressed relief that Catherine would provide his care.

Catherine notes that the physician prescribed Demerol, 50 to 100 mg, and Vistaril, 50 mg intramuscularly every 4 to 6 hours. She knows that the nurses have a tendency to give the lower medication dose and closer to the 6-hour mark rather than the 4-hour mark. She has read recent research suggesting that morphine is a better medication for pain relief in sickle cell clients than Demerol.

Catherine also believes that patient-controlled analgesia (PCA) would probably be best for Michael. However, he is uninsured and she is afraid that the hospital would not assume the cost of PCA. She is unsure whether the physician would be willing to change the orders or listen to her ideas.

What follows is a six-step ethical decision-making process using this situation as the example.

Step 1: Identify the Ethical Dilemma

What is the situation that raises ethical problems? Is it a matter of ethics, a legal issue, or a question of communication? Are there ethical principles in conflict?

The client is not a private paying client. Some nurses have said that when he rates his pain at 10+ he doesn't appear to be in a great deal of pain. The physician in question is not noted for listening to nurses' opinions about issues that he considers to be medical practice.

Catherine has been feeling dissatisfied with the care that Michael received in the past. She is concerned that she is not protecting his rights or advocating for him. She has voiced her concern to a couple of co-workers, who did not validate her feelings. No formal action has been taken.

Step 2: Gather Pertinent Data

Review all significant data. Identify the relevant facts. Who are the people involved? Is there a conflict of values? Are there cultural influences? What are the economic and financial implications?

Is the prescribed regimen consistently implemented? Is there a mechanism for implementing action? Are there supportive nursing policies?

Catherine feels that the nursing staff is not showing care and concern. She wonders if the nurses are sensitive to cultural variations in expressing pain. She feels that adequate pain management is possible for Michael, but that the current regimen is neither effective nor implemented appropriately. She thinks that Michael should have more involvement in decision making about his pain management. Nursing policies document standards of nursing practice and nursing care that are helpful guidelines.

Step 3: Examine the Dilemma for Ethical Principles

What principles are key to making a decision here? What is the overall good to be accomplished (beneficence)? Have the principal decision makers been given all the necessary information? Whose interests are being served (justice)? What are the expectations from caregivers (fidelity)?

Catherine feels that Michael should expect pain relief. The good of the client should be the primary concern. She also feels that he can expect to be treated with respect and have his dignity maintained.

She remains unsure of the physician's response but thinks he should be approached. She feels that the nursing staff needs more information regarding pain management for clients with sickle cell disease.

Step 4: Examine All Solutions

What are all the possible and reasonable actions? What options open to Catherine are legal and within agency policy? What are the possible outcomes and consequences of actions taken? Will the intended good be served?

Catherine considers the options open to her:

- She can voice her concern to the physician and discuss nursing concerns with the unit staff.
- She can consult with the charge nurse and unit director.
- She can involve the client in decision making.
- She can consult with the unit's clinical nurse specialist and nursing education department.
- She can plan a client care conference.
- She can develop a collaborative plan of care using the nursing process.
- She can say nothing and not make waves while trying to give Michael the best care possible when she is on duty.

Step 5: Choose Solutions

After deliberation, choose solutions and act on them. Are solutions chosen consistent with ethical principles?

Catherine chooses to speak with the charge nurse and share her concerns. She shares the research information and asks for a client care conference. She involves the clinical nurse specialist in the conference. The client is involved in the decision-making process and included in the care conference. From the conference, a plan of care is developed that includes recommendation for a referral to a pain management specialist.

Catherine approaches the physician and discusses her concern. He was aware of the conference but did not choose to participate. He does not change his orders but does make a request for the pain management specialist to see the client.

Step 6: Evaluate Solutions Chosen

Was the solution effective and the expected outcome achieved? Was the ethical problem resolved, or were additional problems identified?

Consultation with the pain management specialist resulted in a change in the client's pain management regimen and client education regarding self-care. He was put in a pain management protocol study and was able to receive a PCA pump.

Catherine observed that Michael experienced effective pain relief. Other nurses said that they found him pleasant and approachable when his pain was managed. Some of the staff voiced that Catherine had gone overboard for one client.

The unit director recommended that nursing forums should be instituted on a quarterly basis to provide information on ethical principles and identify ethical issues. The nurse educator is planning seminars on the topics of pain management and cultural sensitivity.

Table 2-1 Levels/Steps in Values Clarification

LEVELS/STEPS	IMPLICATION
1. Incorporating a value begins with making a choice	To say we have chosen a value, it must be: Freely chosen, not imposed by others Chosen with knowledge of other possible choices Chosen with knowledge of consequences of our beliefs
2. Valuing our choice or intrapersonal affirmation	Owning the choice as ours Feeling positive about making the choice Sharing our choice with others
3. Behavioral affirmation	Just saying you have a value or even believing what you say is not enough, you have to: Use behavior consistent with choice Consistently act in keeping with the value Act in keeping with the value when it is not convenient or comfortable

ing. They may begin informally as discussions of issues that you have identified as ethical dilemmas.

Nursing forums can provide education in ethical theories, principles, and decision-making models. They can help you develop skills in ethical analysis and decision making by doing the following (Heitman & Robinson, 1997):

- Providing education in ethical theories, principles, and decision making
- Providing a format for nurses to exchange ideas and talk about ethical issues
- Providing a mechanism for early detection of ethical dilemmas
- Creating a format for recommendations to the institutional ethics committee

It is important that you be knowledgeable about concepts of ethical decision making and able to articulate and apply such concepts in ethical dilemmas. The services of a clinician who has expertise in ethics should be obtained to provide the needed information and instruction.

In many health care settings, you are the primary practitioner with whom clients and families interact. As such, you may be the first to obtain information regarding clients' health care choices. Your nursing skills must include the ability to recognize potential and actual ethical dilemmas. However, you do not solve ethical problems in isolation. Within a health care institution, a nursing practice committee and an institutional ethics committee are forums for resolving ethical problems. A nurse can also look outside the facility to religious leaders or medical-ethical experts to obtain support and guidance in dealing with ethical problems.

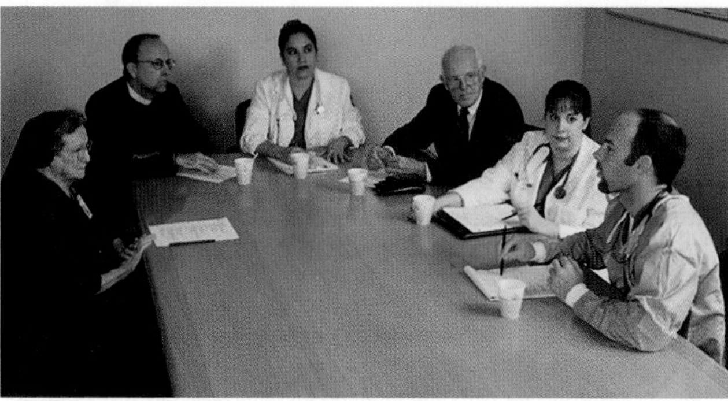

FIGURE 2-2 An ethics committee at work.

CONCEPTS OF LAW

Law is a body of rules of action or conduct prescribed by a "controlling authority," in this case the government. The Constitution of the United States created three branches of government and granted them the power to create "rules of action or conduct" governing many of the interactions between individual persons, between people and government, between people and businesses, between one business and another, and between one government and another.

A prescribed hierarchy of power exists within the levels of government, with the federal government having the highest authority. Thus local law cannot contradict or be inconsistent with state law, and state law must be congruent with federal law.

SOURCES OF LAW

Four sources of law exist at both the state and the federal level: the constitutions and the three branches of government (Figure 2-3). Laws arising from each of these sources come into being, and are modified or eliminated, through a process unique to the source. You need to understand the source of laws if you want to become involved in creating, modifying, or eliminating a law that regulates nursing practice.

The federal and state constitutions establish and outline the limits of power at different levels of government. In addition, the constitutions grant broad individual rights and responsibilities. Some of the rights particularly pertinent to nursing practice are the rights of privacy, freedom of speech, and due process. The right of privacy is embodied in your obligation to maintain client confidentiality. Freedom of speech relates to a professional registered nurse's right and obligation to share information with clients. Due process gives protection to individuals and guides execution of disciplinary proceedings.

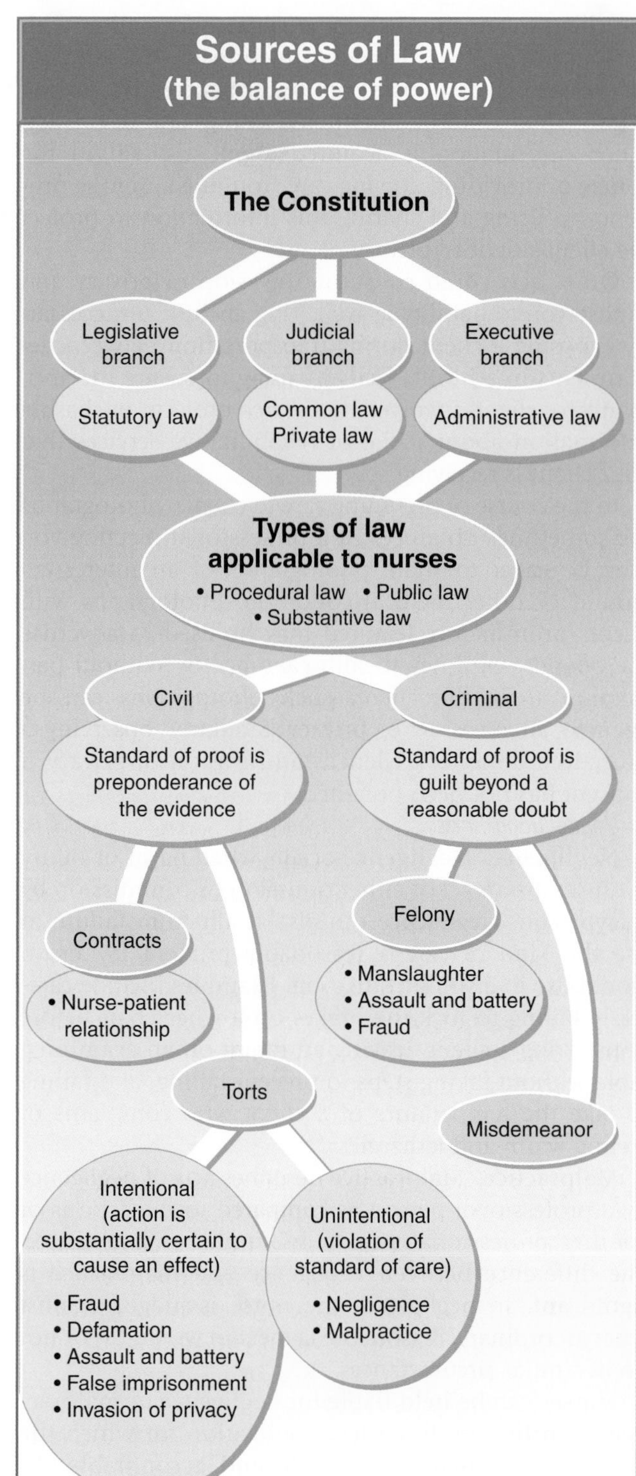

FIGURE 2-3 Sources of law for nursing practice.

The legislative branch of government is an elected body of people who are chosen to represent the interests of their constituents. The federal and state legislatures write laws, or statutes, known as **statutory law**. Examples of these laws that affect health care and nursing include nurse practice acts and the laws that created Medicare and Medicaid.

The executive branch of government has the dual responsibility of establishing the details of laws enacted by state or federal legislatures and ensuring the enforcement of laws. The executive branch works through various administrative agencies, such as the departments of health, housing, and education.

Administrative agencies, whether state or federal, are empowered to establish administrative rules and regulations through specific hearings and rule-making procedures. The resulting rules and regulations, known as **administrative law**, conform to enacted law (i.e., statutory law) and provide the detail necessary to implement them. For example, statutory laws establish the profession of nursing and the authority for administrative functions of the state boards of nursing. State boards of nursing provide the rules and regulations detailing how the profession of nursing will be practiced in each state. These rules and regulations are enforceable as law.

The judicial branch of government is responsible for resolving disputes and interpreting all types of laws. The accumulated judicial decisions have created a body of law known as *judicial, case, decisional,* or *common law.*

TYPES OF LAW

Laws differ in the topics they address, the procedures used to resolve disputes, and the remedies that are available. The types of law include administrative law, civil law, criminal law, common law, procedural law, public law, statutory law, and substantive law. These categories are not mutually exclusive. The practice of professional nursing is touched by all types of laws in some way.

Civil Law. Civil law regulates disputes between individuals and between individuals and groups. The source of much of it is judicial or common law. Civil law includes laws relating to contracts and ownership of property. A common feature is that a monetary award is provided for damages or as compensation when another person causes injury.

Torts. A **tort** is a civil wrong committed by one person against another person or that person's property. It may be intentional or unintentional. When the tort is intentional, the injury suffered by the victim was intended by the wrongdoer. Intentional torts include fraud, defamation, false imprisonment, assault and battery, and invasion of privacy. Unintentional torts include negligence and professional malpractice.

Intentional Torts

Fraud. Fraud is the false representation of some fact with the intention that it will be acted upon by another person. It would be fraud for you as a nurse to falsely represent yourself to a client as being certified in a specialty area of nursing. It is fraud to include false statements about past employment on an employment application, or about academic credentials or professional activities on a résumé, for the purpose of deceiving the potential employer.

Defamation. Defamation is either a false communication or a careless disregard for the truth that results in damage to someone's reputation. Defamation can take two forms: libel and slander. *Libel* is defamation that occurs through printing, writing, or the use of pictures. A nurse who makes false statements about a client or coworker in the client's record or the local newspaper could be guilty of libel. *Slander* is spoken defamation either by making a false statement or by making a legally unprotected statement that damages a reputation. An example of slander is telling a client that another nurse is incompetent.

Assault and battery. Assault is an attempt or a threat to touch another person unjustly. **Battery** is the actual willful touching of another person that may or may not cause harm. The terms assault and battery are distinct but are often heard together because an assault precedes a battery. A nurse who threatens a client with an injection or urinary catheterization could be found guilty of an assault. For a nurse to be guilty of battery, the touching must be wrong in some way, such as being done without permission, or done in a way that causes harm or embarrassment. The nurse who proceeds with an injection despite a client's objection could be guilty of battery.

False imprisonment. False imprisonment involves restraining a person, with or without force, against that person's wishes. Detaining clients against their wishes, such as preventing a client from leaving a health care facility, could be false imprisonment. A different analysis may be applied to clients suffering from diseases that affect judgment, such as Alzheimer's disease, before determining that a nurse's action constituted false imprisonment.

A less obvious example of false imprisonment is the use of restraints in managing clients. The use of restraints relates not only to false imprisonment but also to the issue of maintaining client rights and dignity. Concerns about the inappropriate use of restraints have been great enough that some states have issued guidelines for their use. These guidelines require a thorough assessment of the client to determine the least restrictive measures to safely accomplish the goal for which restraints are being considered.

If a client or legal representative gives permission for the restraint, there is no liability for false imprisonment. You should carefully document in the client's record the circumstances resulting in permission to restrain and undertake an ongoing assessment of the necessity for continued restraint.

Invasion of Privacy. Invasion of privacy can occur when the nurse unreasonably intrudes on the client's private affairs. Soliciting information not required for the client's care and discussing client information with persons not entitled to that information (such as employers or estranged spouses) are two examples of nursing actions that could be interpreted as invasion of privacy. Much information is acquired about a client in the course of providing nursing care. You must exercise prudence in using and sharing this information to protect the client's right to privacy.

Other acts could constitute invasion of privacy and expose you to liability as well. They include unnecessarily exposing a client during transportation between departments in a health facility, failing to ensure the anonymity of clients involved in research projects, or sharing information about social or rehabilitative services that your client is receiving.

In the course of providing care to clients, photographs are sometimes obtained. At a professional meeting you may be eager to share photographs of an interesting wound or other medical condition. Photographs with clients prominently featured may be used to advertise the opening of a new health care facility. Without permission from the client, such photographs can be deemed an invasion of privacy. Similarly, observing a procedure done to a client is an invasion of privacy if consent has not been obtained.

Unintentional Torts

Negligence. Negligence occurs when harm or injury is caused by an act of either omission or commission by a layperson. Negligence can also result from failure to use the kind of care a reasonably prudent layperson would use in a similar situation. Examples include carelessly failing to lock the brakes on a wheelchair before transferring a client, leaving an infant on an examining table without taking steps to prevent falling, and failing to take the temperature of a client who complains of feeling warm and lethargic.

Malpractice. Malpractice describes acts of negligence by a professional person as compared to the actions of another professional person in similar circumstances. The difference between negligence and malpractice is significant. In negligence, the nurse is judged against what an ordinary, reasonable layperson would do or not do in similar circumstances.

Nurses can be held liable for negligence or malpractice. **Liability** implies a legal obligation for which the nurse can be held responsible and accountable. To prove liability for negligence or malpractice, each of four elements must be proven: duty, breach of duty, causation, and damages. *Duty* involves the obligation of the nurse to use due care; that is, to exercise the kind of care a reasonably prudent nurse would use. The kind of care appropriate for a particular client is defined by standards of care. *Breach of duty* is the failure to meet the standard of care. *Causation* is demonstrated when the failure to meet the standard of care results in harm to the client. Finally, for liability to be established, the client must have suffered an actual harm or injury, called *damages.* Table 2-2 provides examples of the elements of liability for malpractice.

The standard of care is derived from professional standards, legal regulation of nursing practice, and the employer's expectations for nursing practice. Together, these sources outline the kind of care a reasonably prudent nurse would provide for a particular type of client in a particular setting. Compare the following two nurses:

- Nurse A works in a high school. This nurse's practice is guided by, among other things, a nurse practice act, standards developed by the National Association of School Nurses, and the school nurse job description. When a high school student sustains a serious injury during football practice, the position requires giving first aid, calling an ambulance, and sending the client to the nearest emergency room.
- Nurse B works in an emergency department. The nurse practice act and the employer's job description also guide this nurse's practice. However, the teenager brought from the high school now needs definitive care. Nurse B will provide that care in accordance with standards established by the Emergency Nurses Association.

Liability can ensue for almost any activity involved in the practice of nursing. Further, no practice setting is exempt from potential malpractice litigation. There are areas in which allegations of malpractice against nurses occur more frequently. Some of the common areas of concern are outlined in Table 2-3.

When clients believe they have been injured as a result of a nurse's negligence or malpractice, they may start legal proceedings. The **plaintiff**, the party bringing a lawsuit, alleges certain facts and outcomes. The **defendant** is the person against whom a lawsuit is filed. The nurse, as defendant, must show that the plaintiff is unable to prove the four elements of negligence or malpractice liability. The procedures for malpractice litigation are complex. Nurses named in a lawsuit are always advised to seek their own legal representation even if their employer is also named as a defendant.

Settlement of the legal action can occur in one of three ways. The parties may negotiate a settlement out of court. A negotiated settlement does not necessarily mean the nurse is guilty of negligence or malpractice. The cost of litigation and the potential liability may suggest settlement as the best option. If there is no settlement, the case goes to court. Both plaintiff and defendant attempt to persuade the court to rule in their favor. An expert witness may be called to testify. An expert witness is a nurse, physician, or other person qualified by education and experience who is asked to testify about the appropriate standard of care and how the care provided met or deviated from that standard. After hearing all the facts and arguments, a decision regarding liability is made. A third possible method of settling a lawsuit in some states is to present the case to a malpractice arbitration panel.

Table 2-2 Elements of Liability for Malpractice

ELEMENT	EXAMPLE
Duty	The nurse is responsible for accurate assessment and timely reporting of changes in a client's condition.
Breach of duty	The nurse fails to note that a client's thumb is warm to touch, red, swollen, and painful.
Causation	Failure to note the signs and symptoms of an infection leads to amputation of the thumb.
Damages	Loss of the thumb seriously limits the client's use of the hand.

Table 2-3 Areas of Potential Liability for Nurses

AREA	EXAMPLES
Failure to monitor and assess	• Failure to recognize significant changes in a client's condition • Failure to report significant changes in a client's condition • Failure to obtain a complete database • Failure to monitor a client as indicated by the client's condition
Failure to ensure safety	• Inadequate monitoring of a client • Improper use of restrictive devices • Failure to identify a client's risk for injury • Inappropriate use of equipment
Medication errors	• Failure to question medication orders that are unclear • Failure to adhere to established procedures in medication administration • Failure to recognize adverse drug reactions • Lack of familiarity with medication • Lack of communication in verbal or written medication orders
Improper implementation of skills or procedures	• Failure to maintain currency in clinical skills • Failure to adhere to proper techniques • Failure to follow agency policy • Performance of unfamiliar skills • Failure to initiate appropriate actions based on assessment
Documentation errors	• Failure to document nursing actions • Failure to document information relevant to a client's condition • Failure to document in accordance with agency policies

If you are named in a lawsuit, obtain legal counsel and work closely with your attorney, who probably will want to be present at all discussions of the case, including those with representatives of your health care agency. If the agency requests information, review the request with your attorney before supplying information. Avoid discussion with the plaintiff, the plaintiff's attorney, and witnesses for the plaintiff. Do not attempt to alter or enhance the client's medical record. Rather, try to put in writing everything that you can remember about the case. Your attorney will advise you of your options in each phase of the litigation.

Contracts. A **contract** is an agreement between two or more individuals that creates certain rights and obligations in exchange for goods or services. Contracts can cover the services offered by a nurse working as either an employee or an independent provider of services. Nurse entrepreneurs provide many services, including writing books, providing health teaching, consulting on breastfeeding and infant care, and monitoring high-tech venous access devices. A portion of contract law specifically addresses contracts concerning the sale of goods, which is relevant when a nurse is purchasing goods or products for a business.

Contracts come in many forms; they can be oral or written, implied or express. Several elements must be met for a valid contract to exist. All parties must be capable of entering into a contract. Examples of people who lack capacity include minors and persons declared incompetent by a court. The legal term *mutual assent* is used to describe another element. It refers to the idea that the terms of the contract must be clearly communicated and accepted. *Consideration,* a legal term for giving something of value, is also a required element. Finally, offenses that could void the agreement, such as fraud, illegality, and misrepresentation, must be absent.

Whatever the form of a contract, questions can and often do arise concerning whether the parties entered into a legally enforceable contract. The obligations incurred under a contract have value for each party. Hence, if the question arises as to whether there actually was a contract, the answer has serious consequences for both parties.

Additional questions can arise even if there is a valid and enforceable contract in place. *Can the contract be assigned?* Assignment means that one of the parties gives his or her rights under a contract to another party. For example, instead of receiving payment for services, the nurse could request that the money be donated to a charity. *Can the contract be delegated?* Delegation transfers the duty or obligation under the contract to another person. For example, the nurse may agree to teach a cardiopulmonary resuscitation class but, in the event of illness, can delegate the responsibility to another nurse. Assignment or delegation can be limited by the terms of the contract.

Finally, legal disputes can occur when one party or the other fails to perform his or her obligations under the contract. A breach of contract results from a partial or total failure to fulfill one's obligations. When a breach occurs, the nonbreaching party is entitled to damages. Remedies for a breach can include monetary payment or specific performance, which is a court-imposed requirement to perform as originally agreed.

Contract law directly or indirectly influences your practice of nursing. As nurses create new businesses, they are increasingly involved in situations that are governed by contract law. Contract law (and employment law) also governs the relationship between a nurse and an employer. A nurse who breaches contractual obligations faces monetary penalties or loss of employment but is usually not at risk of losing the license to practice nursing.

Criminal Law. Criminal law defines specific behaviors determined to be inappropriate in the orderly functioning of society. A crime is an act that violates the duties we owe to the community. Generally, statutory law creates our duties. Examples of criminal acts include larceny, homicide, manslaughter, rape, burglary, kidnapping, and arson.

Punishment for a criminal offense varies with the severity of the crime. Punishment may consist of a fine, probation, imprisonment, or death. A felony is a crime of a serious nature and is likely to be punished by imprisonment or death. A misdemeanor is a crime of a minor nature; it may be punished by a fine, a short prison term, or both.

Some actions that a nurse may take are clearly criminal matters. One example is failure to comply with the mandates of the Controlled Substance Act by engaging in activities such as diverting narcotics for personal use or selling narcotics diverted from clients. Other nursing actions that are potentially criminal in nature include participating in active euthanasia, bombing an abortion clinic, or disconnecting a life-support system. There has even been a case of alleged nursing malpractice involving a fatal overdose of medication that was considered so grievous as to warrant criminal charges.

The number of criminal actions that nurses have been involved in is quite small. When they do occur, these cases are monitored closely to determine their impact on the practice of nursing. More frequently, nurses are involved in civil lawsuits.

Common Law. Common law includes standards and rules applicable to our interactions with one another that are recognized, affirmed, and enforced through judicial decisions. This court-made law is based on the principle of *stare decisis,* or "let the decision stand." The court's decision becomes the rule (the law) to follow for subsequent cases involving similar facts. The prior court decision will be applied less rigorously or even not at all if it can be shown that the subsequent case is dissimilar and therefore that the law should not apply. With regard to nursing practice, most laws in the areas of negligence and malpractice are judicial.

Procedural Law. **Procedural law** establishes the manner of the proceeding used to enforce a specific legal right or to obtain redress. A nurse who is threatened with the potential loss of a nursing license for professional misconduct relies on procedural law to ensure a fair hearing. The procedural laws related to civil, criminal, and administrative actions vary in detail and can be quite complex. A nurse facing any kind of legal action finds that procedural laws direct the course of the legal action. A nurse who relies on procedural law without the benefit of legal representation is at a disadvantage in any legal action.

Public Law. **Public law** regulates the relationship of individuals to government agencies and may be administrative, constitutional, or statutory. The defining characteristic is that the law is applicable to a whole group of people. An example of a public law is the requirement that everyone working in a health care setting, including nurses, be tested annually for tuberculosis.

Statutory Law. **Statutory law** is law enacted by the state or federal legislative branch of government. An example of a federal statutory law relevant to nursing practice is the Americans With Disabilities Act (ADA). To illustrate, a nurse who is permanently disabled is protected by the ADA from employer discrimination. Examples of relevant statutory laws at the state level include nurse practice acts and child- or elder-abuse reporting laws.

Substantive Law. **Substantive law** is the part of law that actually stipulates one's rights and duties, in contrast to procedural law, which guides the enforcement of rights. Substantive law includes the laws of contracts, real estate, torts, and inheritance. Substantive law creates your obligations as a professional nurse. To illustrate, your obligation to assess clients and report changes in their status is a matter of substantive law.

UNDERSTANDING THE LAW

All levels of government work together to provide the legal framework for the safe practice of professional nursing. Laws are dynamic, changing with an act of legislature or interpretation by the court. Changes affecting the profession of nursing can and do occur. As a prudent nurse, you must familiarize yourself on an ongoing basis with the legal changes that affect your practice.

As our health care system and medical technology undergo dramatic changes, questions arise in the practice of nursing about whether specific situations or tasks are safe and "legal." *Is it legal to staff a 40-bed unit with only one RN or to have a staffing ratio of one RN per four intensive-care-unit clients? Is it legal for an RN to insert fetal scalp electrodes or to discontinue central lines?* Many people believe that the law provides specific answers to these and hundreds of other questions, but in many instances the law is subject to interpretation. It is uncomfortable and potentially illegal to practice in the "gray areas" of nursing (Figure 2-4). Be aware that administrative agencies offer opinions about the intent and interpretation of rules and regulations, and professional nursing organizations often attempt to clarify practice issues. Ultimately, the courts may provide an interpretation when a specific question is litigated. Understanding your legal obligations and staying abreast of legal changes is the best way to safeguard your professional nursing practice.

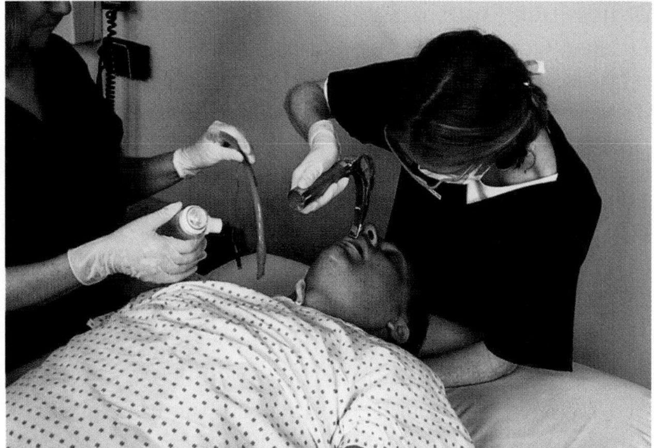

FIGURE 2-4 As professional practice changes, questions arise about the legal guidelines for practice.

UNDERSTANDING YOUR LEGAL AND PROFESSIONAL OBLIGATIONS

Failure to understand your legal and professional obligations as a nurse could jeopardize your livelihood and your ability to practice as a professional nurse. Illegal or incompetent practice could result in professional discipline, a civil lawsuit, a criminal lawsuit, or disciplinary action by your employer. It is important to note that these actions are independent; therefore more than one can be brought against you at the same time for the same incident.

Furthermore, a determination of "no wrongdoing" in one action does not mean that you will be cleared of wrongdoing in the other potential actions. The procedure used to execute each legal action, the possible outcomes, and the law on which the action is based are different.

PROFESSIONAL REGULATION OF NURSING PRACTICE

To practice nursing in a safe, efficient, competent manner, you must understand both the legal regulation of nursing practice and the voluntary professional regulation of nursing practice. There are several types of laws that direct nursing practice. Strict adherence to laws governing nursing practice may be insufficient to guide you in daily efforts to provide quality nursing care. Supplemental voluntary guidelines are provided by professional nursing organizations, the Centers for Disease Control and Prevention (CDC), employer directives, and educational programs. These guidelines do not carry the force of law, but they provide direction for your day-to-day efforts to give competent and legal nursing care.

PROFESSIONAL NURSING ORGANIZATIONS

The ANA is a professional organization for registered nurses. RNs can also join any of the professional nursing organizations that represent their area of specialization. Most of these organizations have established standards of practice that provide more specific guidance to the professional nurse than might be found in the law. Although the recommendations contained in the standards are not law, they are used to evaluate the quality of care provided by the nurse.

STANDARDS OF PRACTICE

Standards of practice provide direction for the provision of nursing care, including your role in professional activities. They reflect the nursing profession's autonomy in establishing standards of professional practice. Standards are written statements that define the acceptable level of performance in the profession. Standards also provide a set of expectations that can be consistently applied to evaluate nursing performance.

Standard of practice for nursing may delineate the process of thinking that is used by nurses. For example, the ANA's *Standards of Clinical Nursing Practice* (2003) delineates the steps of nursing care. Each step of the nursing process is identified, including descriptive behaviors. The standards can be used as guides to determine if the care you provided was in keeping with acceptable practice within the profession.

CENTERS FOR DISEASE CONTROL AND PREVENTION

The CDC is a federal agency of the U.S. Public Health Service. The CDC focuses on epidemiology, prevention, control, and treatment of communicable diseases. It offers guidance to nurses about reporting, treating, and managing communicable diseases such as sexually transmitted diseases, tuberculosis, and acquired immunodeficiency syndrome (AIDS). Isolation procedures and other infection-control recommendations come from the CDC as well.

EMPLOYER POLICIES AND PROCEDURES

Employers should not ask nursing employees to function outside the scope of nursing practice as defined by law. Employers can and do develop guidelines for the practice of nursing in a specific employment setting. Ideally, these guidelines are within the law and are consistent with established standards of practice.

An employer uses at least two methods to convey its expectations of nurses. First, the employer provides a job description to each new employee. It is important to read and understand what your employer expects of you. Although you may have expertise in starting intravenous (IV) therapy, your new community health employer may not want you to restart an IV line on your home health care client. It may seem to you to be a waste of resources to ask the client to leave the home and go elsewhere to have an IV line restarted. Nevertheless, the employer is within its rights to ask you not to perform that task. If you fail to adhere to the job expectation, you may not only lose your job but also be exposed to legal liability.

Employers also use written policies and procedures to convey their expectations about the way you will practice nursing. Occasionally, there is more than one safe and efficient way to perform a specific nursing task. Cost factors, staffing limitations, liability considerations, or other factors may direct an employer to require a specific method for performing a nursing procedure. To minimize your legal liability, it is absolutely essential to be familiar with your employer's policies and procedures, to function within your job description, and to practice consistently within established standards.

EDUCATIONAL PROGRAMS

Continuing education promotes competence in nursing practice (Figure 2-5). Some states mandate continuing education; even without this legal requirement, you have a professional obligation to maintain currency in your nursing practice.

You can obtain the newest information to keep your practice current by attending educational programs, reading professional publications, and maintaining membership in professional nursing organizations. These resources may also provide you with information about legislation that could affect your practice. Evidence of your efforts or lack thereof to keep your practice current may affect the determination of your liability in a legal action.

LEGAL REGULATION OF NURSING PRACTICE

NURSE PRACTICE ACTS

Among the powers granted to states is the ability to regulate the practice of health care providers, including RNs. Regulation of the health care professions protects the public by excluding uneducated or unlicensed persons from practicing in a health care profession and by defining the nature and scope of professional practice.

Physicians were the first health care providers to lobby for state regulation of the health care professions

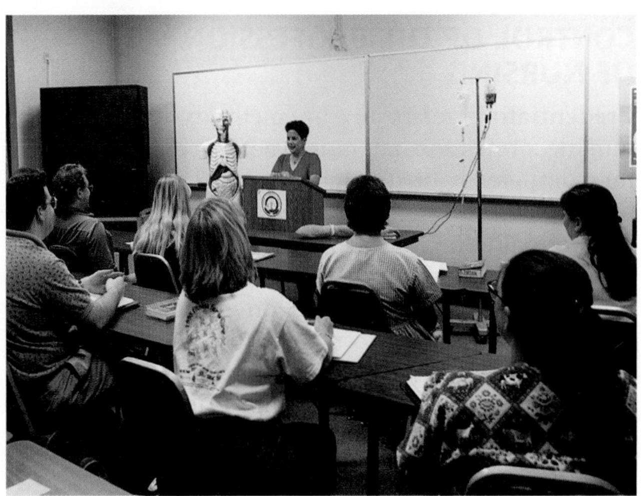

FIGURE 2-5 Continuing education promotes continued competence in nursing practice.

through licensure. The broad definition of medicine contained in legislation had a significant impact on licensure of the other health care professions. The nursing profession and others had to carefully construct practice acts that excluded responsibilities addressed in the previously adopted, well-accepted definition of medical practice. The historic dominance of medicine in defining the health care professions continues to challenge the nursing profession as nurses move into more advanced-practice roles such as nurse anesthetist, nurse midwife, and nurse practitioner.

Common Features of Nurse Practice Acts. A nurse practice act is the most important law affecting your nursing practice. Each state has a nurse practice act; therefore the definitions and descriptions of nursing differ from state to state. This has created problems for the nursing profession, particularly with regard to reimbursement for services. If the nursing profession cannot reach consensus on a definition of nursing, how can reimbursement be regulated? What services does nursing provide that should be reimbursable?

Despite the differences in the nurse practice acts of the states, they share some common topics. Nurse practice acts usually define terms found within the law, such as "treating" and "diagnosing." A nurse practice act defines the practice of nursing, both registered professional nursing and licensed practical nursing. Historically, some states attempted to list all the tasks registered nurses were legally allowed to perform. Such listings became very restrictive because of technical advances in the practice of nursing and the shifting of responsibilities from physicians to nurses. Subsequent revisions to nurse practice acts allowed flexibility by defining nursing in terms of broad categories of the services provided. These services may include assessing health responses, treating health problems, teaching on health-related topics, and providing supportive care. A nurse practice act also delineates the rules and regulations that govern nursing practice for the licensed practical nurse, the nurse practitioner, the nurse anesthetist, and the nurse midwife.

Often the relationship of the professional nurse to other health care providers is outlined in a nurse practice act. Nurses typically are obligated to implement medical regimens prescribed by physicians and dentists. The care nurses provide to clients independent of a physician's order must be consistent with the treatments ordered by the physician. There is variation from state to state about whether nurses can or must execute the orders of physician assistants, nurse practitioners, respiratory therapists, physical therapists, or other health professionals.

A nurse practice act establishes the requirements for obtaining a license to practice nursing. Completion of a basic accredited nursing educational program is a necessity. A passing score on the National Council Licensure Examination (NCLEX®) is also required. Sometimes additional requirements, such as good moral character or a minimum age must be met for licensure in a particular state.

Another common feature of a nurse practice act is the creation of a state board of nursing. The state board is created to assist in matters related to professional licensing and conduct. The specific functions and composition of a state board of nursing vary somewhat from state to state, but a board must comply with the provisions of the nurse practice act that created it. A board does have the power to create rules and regulations (administrative law) to execute its responsibilities. It can also modify these rules as the need arises.

Professional Misconduct. Finally, a nurse practice act defines **professional misconduct**, which is a violation of the act that can result in disciplinary action against a nurse. In some states, the actual language for professional misconduct, disciplinary proceedings, curricula, and other topics pertaining to the profession of nursing are not found specifically in the practice act but may be found in education law or health law. These other laws may be referenced in the nurse practice act and always work in concert to create the legal context for professional practice. Unprofessional conduct in the practice of nursing covers a wide area. Some actions viewed as professional misconduct are outlined in Box 2-5. Many states provide a nursing handbook to applicants for nursing licensure that contains the nurse practice act and other relevant law.

Disciplinary Actions. Disciplinary actions for professional misconduct are part of administrative procedure. A specific state agency, such as the Board of Nursing, the Office of Professional Discipline, or the Office of

BOX 2-5 *Examples of Professional Misconduct*

- Exercising undue influence on the client
- Moral unfitness
- Revealing personal information without the client's prior consent
- Practicing beyond the scope permitted by law
- Delegating professional responsibilities to a person not qualified to perform them
- Abandoning or neglecting a client
- Harassing, abusing, or intimidating a client physically or verbally
- Failing to maintain a record reflecting evaluation and treatment of a client
- Failing to exercise appropriate supervision over persons who can practice only under supervision of a licensed professional
- Guaranteeing satisfaction or cure from the performance of professional services
- Failing to wear an identification badge
- Failing to use scientifically accepted infection-control techniques

Regulation of the Professions is designated to review and manage allegations of professional misconduct. The state agency investigates the allegation, prosecutes or settles a disciplinary proceeding, and enforces the penalty imposed. The disciplinary proceeding may involve a hearing before an administrative officer if a settlement cannot be reached.

Penalties that a state agency can impose range from relatively mild to quite severe, and they may be temporary or permanent. The state agency may find that allegations are unfounded and take no action. An administrative warning may be issued to resolve a violation involving a minor or technical matter. The most serious penalty is revocation of the nursing license.

Other possible penalties include censure and reprimand, a fine (not to exceed a specified dollar amount), a requirement to perform community service, a requirement to complete a specified course of education or training, and an annulment of registration or license. Suspension of license is another penalty that can be imposed. A total suspension may be given for a specified period of time or until a course of therapy or treatment is completed. A partial suspension, which allows you to work in nursing but not in the area or task (e.g., giving medications) to which the suspension applies, is also possible. The suspension could last until successful completion of a course of retraining.

Penalties for professional misconduct can have a significant impact on your ability to practice nursing. Because this type of action is an administrative proceeding and not a lawsuit, nurses sometimes fail to recognize the seriousness of the proceeding and therefore do not seek legal representation. Any potential disciplinary action must be viewed very seriously. At the first notice that you are under investigation, you should seek legal representation.

CONTROL OF THE PROFESSION OF NURSING

Credentialing refers to the methods by which the nursing profession attempts to ensure and maintain the competency of its practitioners. The nursing profession uses several methods of credentialing, including accreditation, licensure, and certification. These efforts are designed to assure the public that only those persons who have met specified requirements provide nursing care.

Accreditation. **Accreditation** is a process that monitors an educational program's ability to meet predetermined standards for students' outcomes. The accreditation process examines program length, teaching methods, course objectives, clinical sites, and numerous other factors related to the structure, functioning, and stated outcomes of the educational program. A determination is then made as to whether the educational program meets the minimal standards for basic nursing education. The goals of accreditation include maintaining minimal educational standards and fostering the continuous improvement of nursing education programs.

Accreditation can be granted by a governmental agency, such as a state board of nursing, or by a voluntary organization, such as the National League for Nursing Accrediting Commission (NLNAC) or the Commission on Collegiate Nursing Education (CCNE). As a legal requirement, all nursing education programs must be accredited by the state. Accreditation by a voluntary organization is often truly voluntary, but it may be required by a state for the school to maintain state accreditation.

The NLNAC has been the major nursing education program-accrediting body for all levels of nursing education. The CCNE, an autonomous arm of the American Association of Colleges of Nursing (AACN), is another voluntary organization that accredits nursing education programs. The AACN recognizes the bachelor of science in nursing (BSN) as the minimal educational requirement for what the organization holds to be professional-level nursing practice. The AACN does not seek to deny entry of associate degree graduates into nursing. The AACN supports articulation models that move nurses with an associate degree in nursing (ADN) into higher-degree programs. However, the accreditation activities of the CCNE are restricted to ensuring quality and integrity in baccalaureate and higher-degree nursing programs. Associate degree programs are free to pursue accreditation through the NLNAC.

Licensure. A **license** grants its owner formal permission from a constituted authority to practice a particular profession. The power to grant licenses to professional health care providers is reserved for the state. The state requires the applicant to meet certain criteria to be granted a license, which indicates to the public that this person has met minimal competency standards, thus protecting the public's health and safety. All states now have mandatory licensing acts, which define the practice of nursing and the requirements for licensure.

A major exception to the requirement that you must have a license to practice nursing exists for nursing students. Students enrolled in a recognized, accredited educational program do not need to be licensed to practice nursing, provided such practice is part of the clinical and academic requirements of the educational program and occurs under the supervision and guidance of nursing faculty. Nursing students employed in health care settings in unlicensed roles as aides, client care technicians, and other positions must be cautioned to avoid applying newly acquired skills belonging solely to the domain of licensed professionals. Legal protection is not available to nursing students practicing nursing outside of their educational programs.

States require licensed professional nurses to register. **Registration** is a process by which an applicant provides specific information to the state agency administering the nursing registration process. Information may include current address and telephone number, proof of continuing education, testimonies that no legal actions have been taken against the nurse, and other information. After the initial licensing and registration of the professional nurse, registration renewal may be required every 1 to 4 years. In addition to paying a registration fee, you may need to prove that you have completed specific coursework (e.g., an infection-control update) for a particular type of registration.

In some jurisdictions, the terms *licensure* and *registration* are synonymous. Technically the terms have different meanings. Licensure is a grant to an individual to practice the profession of nursing. Registration is a method of making sure that the state agency has the most current information about a person to whom they have granted a license. Even in a state that recognizes the distinction between licensure and registration, nurses cannot practice without both a license and a current registration.

The recent dramatic changes in the health care delivery system have resulted in rising concerns about nursing licensure. Although these issues may seem theoretical and outside the experience of the beginning practitioner, potential changes in nursing licensure may at some point affect your nursing career.

Reciprocity of RN licensing between states is an issue undergoing change. A registered nurse licensed in one state who wants to practice in another state can apply for reciprocity of license. Generally this involves completion of an application and payment of a licensing fee. A nurse can hold licenses from different states but cannot practice in a given state without holding its license.

License reciprocity has limitations. Time delays, differing licensing requirements, tracking of disciplinary actions, telemedicine, and other factors have led to calls for reform of licensing regulations. Approximately eighteen states have adopted a version of multistate licensing through the Nurse Licensure Compact. This model of mutual recognition allows a nurse to have one license (in his or her state of residency) and to practice in other states, subject to each state's nurse practice law and regulation. To achieve mutual recognition, each state must enact legislation authorizing the Nurse Licensure Compact and adopt administrative rules and regulations for implementation of the compact.

State boards of nursing have not reached consensus on multistate licensure. The concept would seem to facilitate physical mobility and telehealth practices. State variations in disciplinary practices, differences in practice (e.g., delegation to unlicensed personnel), data sharing, and other issues have not been fully addressed. Thus some states are reluctant to adopt multistate licensure.

An ongoing concern within professional nursing is the concept of institutional licensure for nursing. Currently, the state issues a license to practice nursing to an individual. The boundaries of your professional practice are determined by the state. In effect, you agree to practice nursing according to the rules set forth by the state. As an outcome of this arrangement, you have flexibility to change employers with only minor variations in your professional obligations as a nurse.

In an effort to control the cost, quality, and productivity of the workforce, health care institutions have proposed changes in nurse practice acts that would give them control of nurse licensure. The health care institution would be the gatekeeper, deciding who is qualified to practice nursing within that institution. The institution would review the credentials of the applicant for a nursing position and determine suitability to practice "nursing." Or the institution could provide the education, thus creating a "nurse" tailor-made to the practice setting of the institution. Under this system, the individual nurse could lose employment mobility, leverage for pay and benefits, and control over individual practice. By decentralizing the practice of nursing, institutional licensure would seriously undermine the collective action of professional nurses to control the defining standards for the professional practice of nursing.

Another ongoing issue in professional nursing is the legal protection of the term *nurse*. Licensure of professional RNs originally came about to protect the public from uneducated persons seeking employment as nurses. The terms *licensed* and *registered* are used to notify the public that these nurses have met minimal educational and licensing requirements. In some states, however, the term *nurse* is not restricted to persons who have met the educational and licensing requirements of nursing. Thus one could advertise and gain employment as a nurse without the appropriate education and credentials. Although employers would recognize the distinction between a nurse, a licensed practical nurse, and a registered professional nurse, families seeking a nurse to provide home health care to an ailing relative might not have a sophisticated understanding of the terms. They might thus hire someone ill equipped to provide safe and competent nursing care.

A third licensing issue within the profession of nursing is agreement on the requirements for licensure of persons functioning as nurse practitioners. Nurse practitioners work mainly in primary care settings, providing assessment, teaching, and care to a given client population. It can be argued that nurse practitioners are not performing any functions that fall outside the scope of practice of a registered professional nurse and therefore do not need a separate license. Yet many nurse practitioners believe that a separate license is needed, particularly if they are prescribing medications. States have approached the licensing of nurse practitioners differently. Educational requirements, licensing, and scope of practice vary among the states.

The dramatic changes in the health care system and the creation of new roles for nurses have created new licensing concerns. Many health care organizations service clients across state lines. As a case manager or telephone "telehealth advisor," you could find yourself working with clients in states other than the one in which you are licensed, raising legal concerns you are practicing without a license. Forensic nurses apply nursing science to public or legal proceedings. They may provide direct services (e.g., to a rape victim) or assist in the investigation of abuse or homicide. Should specific education in criminal investigation and licensure as a forensic nurse be required to work in this developing area of practice?

Certification. Although not required by law, nurses often seek certification to receive recognition for their expertise in a particular area of nursing. **Certification** is a voluntary process by which a nurse can be granted recognition for meeting certain criteria established by a nongovernmental association. A nurse can become certified in many areas of nursing, including geriatrics, pediatrics, emergency nursing, community health nursing, school nursing, maternal-child health, and forensic nursing. Certification is offered through the ANA and many specialty nursing organizations. Proponents of certification believe it identifies nursing expertise. Requirements vary but typically include specific educational preparation, experience in the specialty area, evidence of continuing education, and successful completion of a certification examination.

In some states, certification can have a second meaning. In New York, for example, certificates are issued to registered professional nurses to reflect their academic preparation as a nurse practitioner. The specific requirements for education and experience for certification as a nurse practitioner are outlined in the law. This legal requirement for certification is entirely different from the certification offered by the professional nursing organizations.

OTHER LAWS AFFECTING NURSING PRACTICE

Several laws not directly focused on the practice of nursing have a significant impact on the way you must practice nursing. These laws apply to nurses and other health care providers regardless of setting. The laws include the Occupational Safety and Health Act, the Controlled Substance Acts, the Health Care Quality Improvement Act, the Americans With Disabilities Act, Good Samaritan laws, mandatory reporting laws, and the Health Insurance Portability and Accountability Act of 1996 (HIPAA).

Occupational Safety and Health Act. The Occupational Safety and Health Act of 1970 (OSHA) established legal standards that define safe and healthful working conditions. The Occupational Safety and Health Administration affects you as a nurse in two ways. First, it sets standards for your working conditions. For example, it directs the manner in which potentially toxic or flammable chemicals are handled. The use and care of electrical equipment is another area it regulates.

Second, some of the requirements of the law dictate how you manage clients. For example, The Occupational Safety and Health Administration provides standards for the management of contaminated equipment and supplies and the types of isolation techniques used for infectious clients. Promoting health and safety is both your professional obligation and your legal mandate.

Controlled Substance Acts. Several laws have been enacted that address standards for drug development and marketing. These laws affect the process by which new drugs become available to clients. Most significant for you is the Comprehensive Drug Abuse Prevention and Control Act of 1970. This law was enacted to regulate the distribution and use of drugs with the potential for abuse. These drugs include narcotics, depressants, stimulants, and hallucinogens. Your nursing obligations include proper storage and documentation of controlled substances. Failure to meet the requirements of this law is grounds for charges of professional misconduct and potential criminal action against you.

Health Care Quality Improvement Act. One of the difficult issues in attempting to protect the public from unsafe and incompetent health care providers has been the tracking of information related to adverse licensure actions, malpractice payments, and adverse professional actions. The Health Care Quality Improvement Act of 1986 was created to collect data about unsafe and incompetent practitioners. The law, which does apply to nurses, has limited the ability of health care practitioners who had adverse action taken against them in one state from moving to another state without disclosing their previous performance.

Americans With Disabilities Act. The ADA, passed in 1990, was enacted to protect persons with disabilities from discrimination in such areas as housing, employment, education, and health services. The act uses a broad definition of disability that includes persons with AIDS or infected with the human immunodeficiency virus (HIV) and persons recovering from drug or alcohol addiction. Many of your clients may be disabled. As a result, you may be assisting your clients in asserting their rights under this law, particularly if you work in an outpatient or community health setting.

Good Samaritan Laws. As a nurse, you may feel a special obligation to provide aid to people in emergency situations. In most states, there is no legal requirement for any person, including a health care provider, to provide assistance at the scene of an emergency. You (just as any other person) could choose to help or to leave the scene. However, a few states have enacted legislation specifically requiring a person trained in health care to stop and aid the injured, and it is important that you know whether your state is one of these. Even without a legal obligation, you may feel an ethical obligation to assist in such circumstances (Figure 2-6).

Good Samaritan statutes are laws enacted to encourage health care providers to respond to emergencies and to protect them from being sued when providing care to accident victims. The person must use reasonable, prudent guidelines for care within the limitations of resources available at the accident scene. Some states have specific requirements (e.g., the health professional cannot leave the victim until care is transferred to other professionals such as emergency personnel). Several conditions must be met for a health care provider to receive the protection of the Good Samaritan laws. The emergency care must be provided voluntarily and without objection from the victim. The rescuer must be offering a good faith effort to provide aid without expectation of compensation.

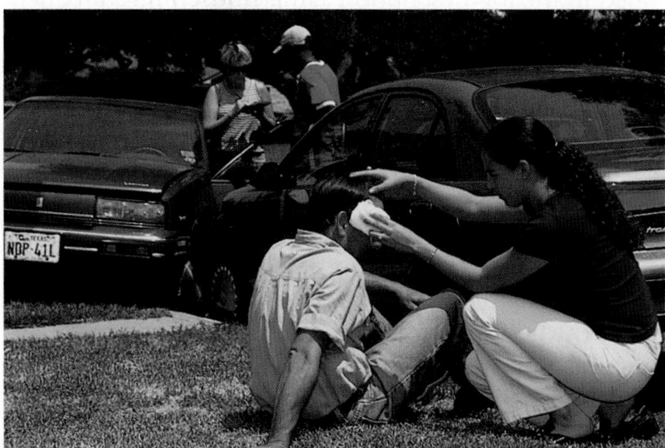

FIGURE 2-6 Good Samaritan laws offer some protection from legal liability for health care workers who stop to offer assistance at the scene of an accident.

Good Samaritan laws do not provide you with absolute immunity from legal liability. Professionals providing care to accident victims can be sued for malpractice if the care you provide can be shown to be grossly negligent or if gross professional misconduct is asserted. Nevertheless, Good Samaritan laws provide some protection against lawsuits when health care providers render aid at an accident scene.

Mandatory Reporting Laws. All 50 states have enacted some form of child abuse and neglect reporting laws. These laws identify the persons required to report suspected child abuse, including nurses and other health care providers, teachers and school personnel, social workers, law enforcement personnel, and others. The extent of knowledge that triggers the obligation to report varies. In some states a "reasonable cause to know" is all that is required. Other states set a higher knowledge standard such as "know or suspect." The failure to report can result in criminal or civil liability. Specific information about each state's mandatory reporting statutes can be accessed through the National Clearinghouse on Child Abuse and Neglect.

Health Insurance Portability and Accountability Act of 1996 (HIPAA). HIPAA is a set of federal regulations intended to protect client privacy by limiting the ways a client's personal medical information can be used. Health care providers and institutions must comply with HIPAA. Individually identifiable information, whether it is on paper, transmitted through computers, telephone, or fax, or communicated orally, is protected. HIPAA covers such areas as access to medical records, notice of privacy practices, prohibitions on marketing, and limits on the use of personal medical information. The regulations provide both civil and criminal penalties for noncompliance.

EMPLOYMENT LAW

Employment law governs employment practices and encompasses such areas as at-will employment, personal employment contracts, and collective bargaining. It also influences when and how employment may be terminated.

Most nurses work as employees rather than as independent contractors or nurse entrepreneurs. An employee is a person who works for someone else in return for a salary or wages. The agreement to work with the promise of being paid is a contract for hire and can be express or implied, oral or written. The employer has the power to control the details of the work. The employer's expectations as to the work to be done and the manner in which it is to be done are usually found in the job description and the employer's policies and procedures.

In contrast, an independent contractor agrees to provide a specific service for a fee. The independent contractor has control over the details of providing the service. The employer's control is limited to establishing the end product of the contractor's work. For example, a home health care agency can hire a nurse as an independent contractor to monitor its clients who have total parenteral nutrition. The independent contractor decides in what order to visit clients, what time of day to see them, and other particular details of monitoring this group of clients. The contract with the employer may specify details of providing the service (e.g., clients must be seen no less than once a day). The independent contractor can decide that the employer's conditions are not acceptable and refuse to provide services for that particular home health care agency.

Nurses who establish a health-related business may find themselves in the position of employer. If you are the sole employee of your business, your activities will be covered by the contracts you develop with your clients. If you employ other people in your business, your concerns about employment law will be from the perspective of an employer. Your rights and obligations as an employer are covered in a variety of employment-related laws, including the Fair Labor Standards Act, workers' compensation laws, and the National Labor Relations Act.

At-Will Employment. Most nurses work as employees of hospitals, but an increasing number work in community health, ambulatory care, long-term care, and other health care delivery settings. Regardless of the setting, the employee is usually either an at-will employee or an employee covered by a collective bargaining agreement. The at-will employment doctrine allows both the employer and the employee to terminate the employment relationship at any time and for any reason. Several exceptions to the at-will doctrine exist. Some states have modified the at-will doctrine to permit termination only for "just cause." Most nurses are at-will employees.

Collective Bargaining. About 17% of registered professional nurses are covered by *collective bargaining agreements,* which are contracts between an employer and a labor organization (i.e., a union that represents the nurses). In an employment setting covered by a collective bargaining agreement, the union represents the interests of the bargaining unit. The bargaining unit may include only registered nurses, or it may include other health care workers (e.g., licensed practical nurses, nurse's aides, physical therapists, and other workers in the facility). Excluded from the bargaining unit are persons in management positions.

The employer and the union are obligated to negotiate and reach agreement on the terms and conditions of employment for the members of the bargaining unit. The terms and conditions include pay and benefits, such as vacations, holidays, health insurance, sick leave, personal leave, and rules pertaining to such issues as lunch breaks, coffee breaks, absenteeism, tardiness, dress codes, overtime work, and safety.

Personal Employment Contracts. As an employee, you can theoretically have a personal employment contract with an employer, but the number of nurses who do is low. Typically, nurse executives, nursing faculty, nurse anesthetists, nurse midwives, and nurse practitioners have individual employment contracts. The contract is between the nurse and the employer and describes position responsibilities, terms and conditions of employment, fringe benefits, and other aspects of the employment relationship.

Employer Actions. As a registered nurse, you face three kinds of threats to your livelihood and continued practice of nursing. The first threat involves the employer's right to discipline you through a verbal or written warning, suspension, or termination of your employment. The second threat involves obligations your employer may have for reporting you to the state agency that handles allegations of professional misconduct or substance abuse. Finally, your employer may be required to provide information damaging to your career during litigation of a lawsuit brought against you. These actions are independent, and therefore more than one can be brought against you at the same time for the same incident.

An employer can discipline you for reasons unrelated to your professional practice of nursing. Employment issues common to any employee also affect nurses. Excessive absences or tardiness, failure to notify your employer when you will be absent, poor customer service skills, and poor personal hygiene are the types of issues employers regard as legitimate grounds for discipline. You may even be terminated for these reasons despite your flawless practice of nursing.

Employers also discipline nurses for reasons more closely related to the practice of nursing. A nurse who is unable to perform to the employer's expectations as outlined in the job description can face discipline. Frequent client complaints, questionable clinical skills, substandard documentation, and failure to master skills needed for the particular clinical area are examples of grounds for discipline. These deficiencies can also be justifiable causes for termination of employment even if they have not resulted in any client harm.

Usually, an employer does not terminate employment without first going through a process of notifying and advising the employee of actions needed to correct deficient performance. The process of progressive discipline is addressed in a collective bargaining agreement if a union represents the employee. Even without a collective bargaining obligation, most employers have a policy of progressive discipline as a means of avoiding a wrongful discharge lawsuit brought by a disgruntled former employee.

In some instances, nursing practice that is so substandard or that result in client harm obligates an employer to report the nurse to the state agency that investigates allegations of professional misconduct or drug violations. The state agency may impose various forms of discipline if allegations prove to be true. Types of discipline include reprimand, fines, temporary suspension, and permanent license revocation. Criminal prosecution is also a possibility if the alleged misconduct involves violation of criminal statutes. Specific state statutes vary, but allegations of client abuse, substance abuse, illegal activity, or the death of a client under certain conditions are all examples of situations that may obligate an employer to generate a report. This reporting is independent of a disciplinary action the employer may initiate.

Similarly, you may be involved in litigation arising from your employment. The employer is also usually sued. Although the situation that caused a lawsuit occurred in the place of employment, the employer will not necessarily seek to terminate the employment relationship. In this lawsuit, the employer may provide evidence damaging to your continuing practice as a nurse.

A determination of "no wrongdoing" in one action does not mean that you will be cleared of wrongdoing in the other potential actions. Suppose a postpartum client complains to your employer that you did not provide all the care she believed she should have received. The client is angry enough that she decides to report you to the state agency that addresses allegations of professional misconduct. The state agency determines that your practice met the standard of care and declines to take any disciplinary action against you. Meanwhile, your employer, concerned that this is the second time it has received complaints about your nursing care, suspends you from work for 2 days.

All potential legal actions determine the extent to which you meet or fail to meet your legal and professional nursing responsibilities. However, the procedures used to execute each legal action, the law on which the action is based, and the possible outcomes vary. Professional discipline, civil or criminal lawsuits, and employer sanctions all represent threats to your license and must be addressed appropriately.

CLIENT RIGHTS

Self-determination has long been valued in Western society, especially regarding health care choices. The American Hospital Association supports this value through the Patient's Bill of Rights in 1975 and the Patient Care Partnership: Understanding Expectations, Rights, and Responsibilities in 2003. Both these documents describe the rights of clients to have informed consent and to refuse treatment. The more recent Patient Care Partnership outlines the elements of informed consent. The American Hospital Association clearly supports clients' involvement in their treatment selections. The ethical principle of autonomy is clearly reflected in this passage. Although autonomy calls on you to respect client health care decisions, this is possible only when the client's choices are made known.

The health care client has specific rights that affect the relationship between the client and the health care provider and between the client and the health care delivery system. These rights protect each client's ability to determine the level and type of care received. Several of these rights interface with your practice of nursing. Informed consent, advance directives, do-not-resuscitate (DNR) orders, organ transplant preferences, and client confidentiality are among the client's rights that direct, in certain instances, how you must practice nursing.

INFORMED CONSENT

Informed consent involves the legal right of clients to receive adequate and accurate information about their medical condition and treatment. Such information is necessary for clients to exercise their right to select and consent to particular treatments. The presumption of the law is that all adult clients possess the decision-making capacity to make informed decisions regarding their treatment choices.

If a health care provider believes an adult client is incapable of making informed decisions, an evaluation by a specialist must take place and an opinion rendered before the client is denied the right of informed consent. When the court determines that a client is incapable of making decisions, it may appoint a personal guardian to make decisions on the client's behalf. In some states, statutes have been enacted that identify a ranked listing of who should be consulted to make decisions. The list may begin with a spouse and continue to adult children, parents, and then a sibling.

Minor children are viewed under the law as lacking decision-making capacity. Therefore the parent or legal guardian provides informed consent after receiving all the required information. In some cases, minors are able to provide their own consent for treatment, such as for a sexually transmitted disease or when the minor is married or otherwise emancipated.

Courts have established the information to be shared with a client to obtain informed consent (Box 2-6). A physician is responsible for conveying information and obtaining informed consent for medical procedures. If you are involved in obtaining informed consent for a medical procedure, in most states you are only witnessing the signature of the client on the informed consent form. You may be the person who actually ensures that the client signs the informed consent form. You should ask the client to sign a consent form only if the physician has instructed the client and you have determined that the client has reasonably understood the information.

BOX 2-6 *Elements of Informed Consent*

The client has received the following information:
- ❑ Diagnosis
- ❑ Name of procedure, test, or medication
- ❑ Explanation of procedure, test, or medication
- ❑ Reasons for recommending the procedure, test, or medication
- ❑ Anticipated benefits
- ❑ Major risks of the procedure, test, or medication
- ❑ Alternative treatments
- ❑ Prognosis if treatment is refused

The nurse has performed the following duties:
- ❑ Assessed barriers, such as hearing impediments, transcultural factors, pain, anxiety, and other factors that could influence the client's understanding of the information
- ❑ Assessed the influence of education, age, developmental level, and emotional status on the client's ability to understand the information
- ❑ Ensured that information was provided in a manner that facilitated understanding
- ❑ Determined that the client is voluntarily giving informed consent

ADVANCE DIRECTIVES

An **advance directive** is a written document that provides direction for health care in the future, when clients may be unable to make personal treatment choices. It allows clients to express their preferences for health care before an event that renders them incapable of indicating their treatment choices. Individual state laws provide for specific kinds of advance directives, including living wills and the durable power of attorney for health care.

A **living will** is a document that provides written instructions about when life-sustaining treatment should be terminated. It may indicate when and if a person may be hospitalized and what types of treatment may be implemented. Ideally, these preferences are discussed in advance with the persons who may become involved in decision making, so the client's wishes are clearly understood by all. Some living wills may contain general statements requesting that no extraordinary means be used to extend life. The more general the statements, the more open they are to interpretation.

A **durable power of attorney for health care**, also called a proxy directive, is a document that designates a person to make decisions about the client's medical treatment in the event that the client becomes unable to do so. The designated person may be a family member, an attorney, or a friend who is aware of the client's wishes. Like the living will, the durable power of attorney for health care is most effective when the client has written specific instructions. Ideally, the client will have discussed his or her preferences with the person the client appoints as his or her agent.

Often a nurse is the first health care provider to know that a client has executed an advance directive. Ensure that a copy of the advance directive becomes part of the client's record. You may also need to inform the physician and other care providers about the client's advance directive.

When working with a client's significant others, it is especially important to ensure that the decision maker is the person *legally* authorized to make the decisions. Several different family members or significant others may voice conflicting opinions about the client's care. Your obligation is to consult with the person legally authorized to make treatment decisions, even when this person is not clearly identifiable.

State laws and statutes about advance directives may vary. It is important for hospital policies and procedures to be developed and implemented in line with regulatory requirements and for you to become familiar with such policies and procedures.

Organ Transplants. As is the case for other treatments, clients have the right to decline organ transplant as a treatment option. Clients also have the right to determine whether they want to donate their organs and tissues for someone else's benefit at the time of death. The desire to donate organs can be expressed through a written document executed before death. In the absence of an express written directive providing an informed consent for donation, the Uniform Anatomical Gift Act would control the donation of any organ.

The Uniform Anatomical Gift Act is law in all states and provides a list of individuals who can provide informed consent for the donation of the deceased individual's organs. The persons on the list must be contacted in order, usually a spouse first, followed by adult children and parents of the deceased.

Do-Not-Resuscitate Orders. Implicit in the client's right to informed consent is a client's right to refuse treatment. In fact, clients have a right to refuse treatment even if that treatment is needed to sustain life.

Cardiopulmonary resuscitation (CPR) is one type of treatment refused by clients. Most health care agencies have developed policies to guide health care providers when clients choose not to be resuscitated. These policies should include a written order for a DNR status, review of the order on a regular basis, and evidence of informed consent by the client or legal representative in requesting a DNR. In addition, DNR and CPR must be specifically defined, so that the client continues to receive any desired treatment.

CONFIDENTIALITY

Confidentiality is the client's right to privacy in the health care delivery system. As a nurse, you have an ethical obligation to maintain client confidentiality. You are party to much sensitive and private information about clients and must exercise discretion in sharing that information. Sharing information about a client with people who are not involved in the client's care, such as disclosing information about one client to another client, is a violation of client confidentiality. Talking about a client in the hallways, cafeteria, grocery store, social club, or anywhere else with people who are not involved in the client's care is also a violation of client confidentiality. In addition, disclosure of confidential information could expose you to liability for invasion of your client's privacy.

Even if your conversation partner is involved in caring for the client, in public places you must guard against disclosing information within earshot of others. Some nurses mistakenly think that they have not breached client confidentiality if they talk about the client without using a specific name. If sufficient information is conveyed for another person to identify the person under discussion, client confidentiality has indeed been violated and charges of invasion of privacy could be forthcoming.

Increasingly, clients are enrolled in health care networks that offer a range of services, including ambulatory care, hospitalization, rehabilitation services, and home health care services. Planning and coordinating care is the responsibility of case managers or discharge coordinators. Such planning requires access to confidential information. In addition, third-party payers and utilization review departments access confidential information to address payment issues. This information is often transmitted by electronic means to the agencies within the network. The difficulty in maintaining client confidentiality is thus compounded by a greater number of persons accessing sensitive client information and the means by which the information is shared.

Any request for client information you receive should be evaluated very carefully. Address two questions. First, does the person requesting client information have a need to know the information requested? Suppose you work in a home health care agency. Client information might be shared with the agency's social worker for the purpose of helping the client receive social services, but the social worker may not need to know all the details of the client's medical care. Furthermore, the office administrative assistant may recognize your client as a neighbor and ask you probing questions about your client's condition. The state nurse practice act, ethical considerations, and nursing standards of care require you to protect client confidentiality.

The second question to ask yourself is whether the client has authorized the release of information. When clients consent to receive services, they usually sign a consent form for treatment that includes an authorization for information to be shared with people in the agency involved in the client's treatment. Beyond this, requests for information come from concerned family, friends, or employers. Requests also come from other health care providers, lawyers, insurance companies, and public news sources. Carefully consider whether the client has authorized release of information to these persons. When in doubt, consult with your supervisor.

Specific federal or state statutes protect the confidentiality of some client groups. Persons receiving treatment for drug and alcohol abuse, mental health care, sexual assault, HIV infection, and AIDS are among the groups whose confidentiality receives additional protection under the law. If you work with clients in these categories, you should familiarize yourself with the particulars of confidentiality requirements.

QUALITY IMPROVEMENT INITIATIVES

Quality improvement initiatives are activities that health care agencies undertake to contain costs, improve quality, and increase competitiveness. Some of the costs an agency seeks to reduce are those related to legal liability arising from adverse occurrences. *Adverse occurrence* is a term sometimes used to describe errors in practice or the injury or death of a client. Health care agencies have used several methods to manage adverse occurrences. These include incident reports, risk management committees, quality assurance committees, safety programs, and quality improvement programs.

Risk management programs and quality improvement programs are somewhat different in focus, but both can potentially reduce legal liability. Continuous quality improvement, total quality management, and quality initiatives are programs that have proliferated in recent years in health care facilities. These programs focus on improving the quality of client care or the efficient operation of the business by examining the processes used to deliver health care services. For example, a quality improvement initiative might examine how waiting time in an outpatient clinic can be reduced. In contrast, incident reports and risk management programs identify and analyze risks with the objective of taking corrective action and thus reducing legal liability. You may become involved in both types of programs.

INCIDENT OR ADVERSE OCCURRENCE REPORTS

An incident or adverse occurrence report is a tool used by health care facilities to document situations that have caused harm or have the potential to cause harm to clients, employees, or visitors. Medication errors, client falls, and accidental needlesticks are common situations documented on an incident report. The report is not part of the client's medical record and should not be referenced in the client's record. These reports are used to identify patterns of risk so that a corrective plan can be developed. The report also serves as a record of the facts surrounding the event should litigation arise at some point in the future.

The nurse who identified the potential or actual harm or who created the situation leading to actual or potential harm initiates the incident report. The incident report identifies the people involved in the event (including witnesses), describes the event, and records the date, time, location, actions taken, and other relevant information. A physician completes the report after examining the client, employee, or visitor if actual or potential injury occurred. Often, suggestions are solicited for how this event can be avoided in the future.

In some instances, incident reports can be used in a court of law. Documentation should be as factual as possible and avoid accusations. Questions of liability are for the court to decide, and therefore conclusions about who is responsible for the event should be avoided in the incident report.

RISK MANAGEMENT PROGRAMS

Risk management programs have several components. An ongoing safety program is essential to ensure the safety of clients, employees, and visitors. Periodic inspections of electrical equipment, monthly fire drills, and monitoring of the disposal of hazardous wastes are often included in safety programs. Educational programs about potential risks help reduce accidents and injuries. Identifying known risks (e.g., by putting up warning signs for construction or ice on the walkway) are also activities of a risk management program. A risk management program might examine patterns of problems, seeking to identify causes and corrective actions.

A health agency may have a designated risk manager. This person can be an invaluable resource to answer questions regarding potential risks and liabilities.

SAFEGUARDING YOUR PRACTICE

The legal threats to your continuing practice as a professional nurse are very real. Clients deserve and demand that only those persons who are able to provide safe, competent quality care should practice nursing. Administrative procedures, lawsuits, and disciplinary practices by employers help ensure that unsafe and incompetent nurses are removed from the practice of nursing. Despite the demands and complexity of nursing, you can take steps to safeguard your nursing practice and avoid having legal action taken against you.

KNOW YOUR OBLIGATIONS AND RESPONSIBILITIES

The first step in safeguarding your practice is to thoroughly understand your professional, legal, and ethical obligations and responsibilities. It is as important to be competent in the professional and legal aspects of your practice as it is to be technically competent. Read your state's nurse practice act. Read your job description and your employer's policies and procedures. Follow legislative bills that may affect your practice. Track court decisions that clarify the specifics of your practice and identify your potential legal exposure. Read the standards of practice that apply to your area of nursing, and comply with the guidance provided. These actions are important steps in making sure that your practice conforms to the expectations inherent in your license to practice nursing.

PRACTICE COMPETENTLY

The competent practice of nursing requires that, as your professional practice develops, you expand on the skills and knowledge you acquired as a nursing student. You are expected to maintain competency in three domains:

- *Technical competency:* Perform skills accurately, safely, and in a manner consistent with established procedures.
- *Cognitive competency:* Acquire knowledge and information, understand the needs of your clients, and implement appropriate nursing care.
- *Interpersonal competency:* Develop effective communication techniques for working with professional colleagues and maintaining therapeutic relationships with clients.

Clients who believe their nurse is caring and respectful are less likely to sue. Thus, the combination of technical, cognitive, and interpersonal competencies applied within the legal limits of nursing practice is an effective safeguard for your nursing practice.

KNOW YOUR STRENGTHS AND LIMITATIONS

The nursing profession is characterized by endless opportunities. The number of work settings, types of clients, specific expectations of a nursing position, conditions of employment, work hours, and any number of other factors combine to create a vast array of nursing opportunities, some of which will match your temperament, skills, knowledge, and interests. The key to finding an appropriate nursing position is an accurate assessment of your professional and personal strengths and weaknesses.

No nurse can function equally effectively in all settings. A nurse accustomed to the collegiality of an institutional setting may find the independence of community health nursing unnerving. An experienced intensive care nurse may feel that work in a physician's office is not challenging enough and may overlook critical elements of practice. A nurse who is mismatched with or overwhelmed by the demands of a particular position or type of client is inviting disciplinary or legal action.

KEEP CURRENT

A license to practice nursing signifies that you have met the minimum standards for a beginning practitioner. The expectation is that you will ultimately become a master practitioner of your chosen profession. This can occur only if you acknowledge your role as lifelong learner. Attending in-service programs, pursuing continuing education courses, reading professional publications, and attending professional meetings are evidence of your commitment to continued professional growth.

Projections made about the relevancy of the nursing information you master today suggest that much of what you know will be obsolete in 3 years. Indeed, 25 years ago, standard precautions were unheard of and gloves were worn only to keep your hands clean. At that time, AIDS, Ebola, hepatitis C, and other very serious illnesses had not yet been identified. Nursing is an evolving profession. It is incumbent upon you to keep your practice current. An outdated practice is a practice ripe for a lawsuit.

DOCUMENT YOUR CARE

Documentation of your activities while practicing nursing will not compensate for failing to render nursing care that is consistent with established standards of practice. Timely, accurate, complete, and appropriate documentation of the care you give can provide evidence that you executed your professional responsibilities in accordance with your legal and professional obligations. Client records are legal documents that may be entered as evidence in a lawsuit. In either a lawsuit or an insurance claim, documentation may be the factor upon which liability determinations are made.

There are many types of documentation formats. In all cases, the content of the documentation requires that you make decisions about the words you use, the relevance of the information you provide, the completeness of your notations, and the inclusion of certain information. Information conveyed should be an accurate, complete, objective, and relevant assessment of your client and the nursing care you provided. As in other forms of communication, excellent documentation takes practice.

The client record is a legal document that should provide a complete and accurate picture of the client's condition and the nursing care provided. Nurses are sometimes reluctant to document adverse events that happen to clients. But falls, medication errors, and other adverse incidents must be documented as completely and accurately as any other information pertinent to the client's care. Document the event in a straightforward manner, including all the steps you took to respond appropriately to the situation.

PURCHASE PROFESSIONAL LIABILITY INSURANCE

Despite competent or even expert nursing care, clients are not always satisfied with the outcomes of their health care experiences. Also, the responsibilities and complexities of practice in today's rapidly changing health care environment can create situations that expose you to greater legal risk. Although it is virtually impossible to practice flawless nursing, the cost of an error in your practice could be a lawsuit. Increasingly, nurses are being named with the agency and the physician in a lawsuit. Insurance coverage will not reduce the risk of being sued, but at least the financial impact of a lawsuit can be minimized.

In the past, plaintiffs have named in a lawsuit those persons or institutions believed to have the most money. Thus the hospital and physicians were typically sued, whereas nurses were overlooked because they lacked "deep pockets." Yet with the rise in nurses' salaries, the protection against being sued attributed to the deep-pockets theory is becoming increasingly suspect. Some people believe that a nurse who has individual liability insurance is more likely to be sued.

In a variety of employment settings, you may be told that you are covered by your employer's liability insurance and do not need to purchase individual liability insurance. Your employer's lawyers also may have an excellent record of representing their nurse employees. If you have individual insurance coverage, the approach of your insurance company to the management of a lawsuit may differ from the approach of your employer's lawyers. The resulting adversarial relationship between you and your employer could be detrimental to a mutually agreeable resolution of the lawsuit.

Despite these risks, there are several sound reasons why you should purchase your own professional liability insurance even if you are covered under an employer's insurance plan. One is to ensure that, if you are named as a defendant in a lawsuit, your best interests will be represented. An employer's first obligation is to reduce or eliminate its own liability. One way of doing that may be to shift responsibility for the incident to you by trying to demonstrate that you practiced incompetently, that you exceeded the limits of your job description, or that you did not follow agency policies and procedures. These would represent attempts to prove that you, and not the agency, should be held liable.

A second reason you should have your own professional liability insurance is to protect you when you are providing care or giving advice outside of work. An employer's insurance will cover only your professional activities while working for the employer. You may want to believe you are a nurse only while at work, but family, friends, and neighbors know otherwise. The first aid you provide at your daughter's soccer game, the health education and screening done during a health fair at the local retirement community, the advice you are asked to give to the neighbor's ailing father you meet at the grocery store, and countless other occasions may expose you to liability. You must protect yourself whether or not you are providing professional services during your employment hours.

▼ KEY PRINCIPLES

- To the extent that nursing as a profession has an altruistic motivation, ethics is the foundation for nursing practice.
- Ethics is the framework that we use to make moral decisions; that is, decisions about what is good, just, or right ways of thinking and acting.
- The ethics of nursing is centered on the client's welfare.
- Nurses have moral agency; that is, nurses are independently responsible and accountable for their actions.
- Ethical principles for nursing practice are the ethic of care, autonomy, beneficence, confidentiality, nonmaleficence, fidelity, justice, and veracity.
- In the United States, the American Nurses Association's *Code of Ethics for Nurses With Interpretive Statements* provides a guide to ethical nursing practice and can be used to evaluate nursing actions.
- In the delivery of health care, nurses are often required to make decisions, recognize ethical dilemmas, and apply ethical standards in resolving those dilemmas.
- A model for ethical decision making is systematic analysis to clarify a problem, identify possible solutions and actions, and evaluate actions taken.
- Laws include rules or standards of conduct from statutory, administrative, or judicial authority.
- The types of law affecting the practice of nursing include civil, criminal, common, private, procedural, public, statutory, and substantive law.
- Specific laws that secondarily affect the practice of nursing include the Occupational Health and Safety Act, Controlled Substance Act, Americans With Disabilities Act, and Health Care Quality Improvement Act.
- Legal liability may result from intentional torts involving assault and battery, defamation, fraud, false imprisonment, or invasion of privacy.
- Negligence and malpractice are unintentional torts. Liability is determined by proving duty, breach of duty, causation, and damages.
- Professional standards of care and practice are developed by professional nursing organizations and organizations that accredit educational programs or institutions.
- Failure to adhere to legal and professional directives regarding the practice of nursing can result in professional discipline, legal liability, or employer disciplinary actions. A nurse may simultaneously be involved in two or more of these actions.
- Employer job descriptions, policies, and procedures direct the practice of nursing in a specific employment setting. These directives should conform to professional and legal practice guidelines.
- Individual state nurse practice acts protect the public by regulating nursing practice and providing mechanisms for disciplinary action against nurses practicing in that state.
- Clients have specific rights, including confidentiality, informed consent, use of advance directives, and control over decisions about organ transplant and life-sustaining measures.
- Health care agencies undertake quality improvement initiatives to contain costs, improve quality, and increase competitiveness.
- Health care agencies try to reduce potential legal liability through the use of risk management programs and incident or adverse occurrence reporting mechanisms.
- Members of the nursing profession ensure competent and safe professional practice by reading professional publications and attending continuing education programs, professional meetings, and in-service programs.
- Legal safeguards for nurses begin with competent practice. Additional safeguards include understanding professional responsibilities and obligations, recognizing individual strengths and limitations, keeping knowledge and skills current and accurate, documenting care appropriately, and purchasing individual professional liability insurance.

■ REVIEW QUESTIONS

1. Select all of the following situations that require ethical principles as a basis for decision making:

1. Allowing a person with mild Alzheimer's disease autonomy of decision making
2. Informing a physician of a client's request to discontinue medical treatment
3. Documentation of a client's response to teaching about advanced directives
4. Informing a surgeon that a client needs further information before consenting to surgery.

2. A client is packing his belongings and preparing to leave the hospital. He has not completed the intravenous antibiotics prescribed by the physician; therefore he still has a potential serious infection. The nurse restrains him to keep him from leaving. Which tort is the most likely criminal charge to be brought against the nurse?

1. Assault and battery
2. False imprisonment
3. Malpractice
4. Invasion of privacy

3. A former client files a lawsuit against a nurse because she failed to use sterile technique when she changed the client's dressing. The nurse was not assigned to the client but was changing the dressing for the assigned nurse. The client did not have a wound infection at any time. Which element of liability is missing?

1. Duty
2. Breach of duty
3. Causation
4. Damage

4. Which would you expect to find in the nurse practice act for your state? Select all that apply.

1. Definition of nursing
2. Code of ethics
3. Standards for nursing education
4. A list of states in which you can practice
5. Standards for nursing practice

5. At-will employment means:

1. The employer can terminate the employee at any time
2. As an employee you have the right to collective bargaining
3. You are protected from lawsuits by conditions of your employment
4. Negation of your obligation to report violations of the nurse practice act

Bibliography

*American Hospital Association. (1992). *Patient's bill of rights.* Washington, DC: Author.

American Nurses Association. (2001). *Code of ethics for nurses with interpretive statements.* Washington, DC: Author.

*American Nurses Association. (2003). *Standards of clinical nursing practice.* Washington, DC: Author.

Butts, J., & Rich, K. (2005). *Nursing ethics: Across the curriculum and into practice.* Boston: Jones & Bartlett.

Eggenberger, S. K., & Nelms, T. P. (2004). Artificial hydration and nutrition in advanced Alzheimer's disease: Facilitating family decision-making. *Journal of Clinical Nursing, 13*(6), 661-667.

Ethical issue: Morality vs. ethical reasoning. (2004). *Minnesota Nursing Accent, 76*(3), 6.

Fowler, M., & Levine-Ariff, J. (1987). *Ethics at the bedside: A source book for the critical care nurse.* American Association of Critical Care Nurses. Philadelphia: Lippincott.

Garner, B.A. (2004). *Black's law dictionary* (8th ed.). St. Paul, MN: Thomson West.

Grace, P. J. (2004). Ethical issues. Patient safety and the limits of confidentiality: Do you know when you shouldn't keep patient information confidential? *American Journal of Nursing, 104*(11), 33, 35-37.

Grace, P. J., & McLaughlin, M. (2005). Ethical issues: When consent isn't informed enough- what's the nurse's role when a patient has given consent but doesn't fully understand the risks? *American Journal of Nursing, 105*(4), 79, 81-84.

Health Insurance Portability and Accountability Act of 1996. http://www.hhs.gov/ocr/hipaa.

Heitman, L., & Robinson, B. (1997). Developing a nursing ethics roundtable. *American Journal of Nursing 97*(1), 36-38.

*International Council of Nurses. (2000). Code for nurses: *Ethical concepts applied to nursing.* Geneva, Switzerland: Author.

Jacobson, J. (2005). AJN reports. When providing care is a moral issue: Is nurses' first priority protecting the patient or their own moral convictions? *American Journal of Nursing, 105*(10), 27-28.

Johnstone, M.-J. (2004). *Bioethics: A nursing perspective.* Melbourne, Australia: Saunders.

Leget, C. (2004). Avoiding evasion: Medical ethics education and emotion theory. *Journal of Medical Ethics, 30*(5), 490-493.

Liaschenko, J., & Peter, E. (2004). Nursing ethics and conceptualizations of nursing: Profession, practice and work. *Journal of Advanced Nursing, 46*(5), 488-495.

Mathes, M. (2004). Ethics, law, and policy. Ethical decision making and nursing. *Medsurg Nursing, 13*(6), 429-431.

Maze, C. D. M. (2005). Registered nurses' personal rights vs. professional responsibility in caring for members of underserved and disenfranchised populations. *Journal of Clinical Nursing, 14*(5), 546-554.

Paley, J. (2004). Commentary: The discourse of moral suffering. *Journal of Advanced Nursing, 47*(4), 364-365.

Peter, E., Lunardi, V. L., & Macfarlane, A. (2004). Nursing resistance as ethical action: Literature review. *Journal of Advanced Nursing, 46*(4), 403-416.

Peter, E. H., Macfarlane, A. V., & O'Brien-Pallas, L. L. (2004). Analysis of the moral habitability of the nursing work environment. *Journal of Advanced Nursing, 47*(4), 356-364.

Rassool, G. H. (2005). Current issues and forthcoming events. *Journal of Advanced Nursing, 51*(3), 314-315.

Rogers, B. (2003). Research & ethics corner. Nursing: An ethic of caring. AAOHN *Journal, 51*(4), 155-157.

Seedhouse, D. (2005). *Values-based decision-making for the caring professions.* Chicester, England: John Wiley & Sons.

Straunton, P., & Chiarella, M. (2003). *Nursing and the law* (5th ed.). St. Louis, MO: Elsevier.

Varcoe, C., Doane, G., Pauly, B., Rodney, P., Storch, J. L., Mahoney, K., et al. (2004). Ethical practice in nursing: Working the in-betweens. *Journal of Advanced Nursing, 45*(3), 316-325.

*Asterisk indicates a classic or definitive work on this subject.

Chapter 3

Cultural Context of Practice

Media Resources

- evolve Evolve Website http://evolve.elsevier.com/Harkreader/
- Companion CD

Learning Objectives

After studying this chapter, you should be able to do the following:

- Discuss culture and ethnicity as they relate to the delivery of nursing care
- Define humanistic care
- Outline the elements and objectives of transcultural nursing
- Describe the dangers of stereotyping
- List and explain the six concepts included in transcultural assessment
- Understand basic aspects of the European American community, African American community, Hispanic American community, the Asian American community, and the Native American community
- Anticipate the effects of cultural characteristics on the successful delivery of health care

Key Terms

cultural competence
culture
diversity
ethnic
ethnicity
ethnocentrism
humanistic care
multicultural society
stereotyping
transcultural nursing
universality

CONCEPTS OF CULTURE

Simple observation leads to the conclusion that, although people are all equal, they are not all alike. At least some of the differences among people stem from the behaviors, beliefs, and values learned from their families and other members of the society around them. Indeed, these cultural and ethnic influences can make people seem very different from one another.

As a nurse, you should transcend the differences among people. Nurses should seek to understand clients of different cultural backgrounds and to provide them with care that enhances their individual health and well-being. To do so, nurses need a basic understanding of other cultures.

CULTURE AND ETHNICITY

Culture can be defined as a patterned behavioral response that develops over time as a consequence of imprinting the mind through social and religious structures and intellectual and artistic manifestations (Giger & Davidhizar, 2003). Culture is shaped by the values, beliefs, norms, and practices held in common by members of the cultural group. It guides a person's thinking, acting, and being, and it becomes a patterned expression for that person (Giger & Davidhizar, 2003).

Madeleine Leininger, a nurse anthropologist, defines culture as "the learned, shared, and transmitted values, beliefs, norms, and lifeways of a particular group that guide thinking, decisions, and actions in a patterned way" (Leininger, 1991). Most definitions of culture imply a dynamic, ever-changing process through which a group defines itself through art, music, stories, and lifestyles.

For most people, cultural background and ethnic background are intimately related (Spector, 2004). The term **ethnic** refers to groups of people of the same race or national origin (within a larger cultural system) that are distinctive based on traditions of religion, language, or appearance. A person's **ethnicity** reflects the characteristics a group may share in some combination (Box 3-1).

BOX 3-1 *Characteristics of Ethnic Groups*

PRIMARY CHARACTERISTICS

An ethnic group shares one or more of the following:
- Race
- Color
- National or geographical origin
- Religious beliefs
- Cultural origin

SECONDARY CHARACTERISTICS

Group identity is evident in one or more of the following:
- A sense of identity as a group
- Distinctive customs, art, music, literature
- Elements of lifestyles
- Language, accent, or dialect
- Style or manner of dress
- Food preferences, spices, methods of cooking
- Attitudes derived from group identity
- Moral values
- Economic or political beliefs
- Special political interests as a group
- Health care practices

MULTICULTURAL SOCIETIES

The United States and Canada are examples of multicultural societies. A **multicultural society** is a society composed of more than one culture or subculture. It includes many groups that participate in and enjoy the larger culture. In such a society, the larger culture provides common interests and values. These shared interests and values help to create a social order that provides benefits to the society at large. In the United States, shared values include a democratic structure, equality among peoples, freedom of speech, and the right to the pursuit of happiness.

The United States contains many distinct ethnic groups that maintain some characteristics of their origins. This is largely because the United States is home to immigrants from every country in the world. Some nations—such as Germany, England, Wales, and Ireland—are well represented. Others—such as Japan, the Philippines, and Greece—have smaller populations in the United States. People from around the world continue to enter the United States, particularly from Asia, Latin America, Africa, and Caribbean nations (Spector, 2004).

In the United States, although cultures have blended to some degree, many cultural groups have remained visible and intact and function as a social force within the larger society. The social emphasis before the 1960s was on creating a "melting pot" society in which all members would blend together and create a common culture. Various cultures have blended together through marriage, membership in social organizations, and assimilation. However, a homogenized society runs the risk of losing distinctive contributions from cultural subgroups.

The multicultural societies of the United States and Canada represent all of the cultural and racial groups of the world (Figure 3-1). However, the mix of cultural and ethnic populations is shifting. Experts project that by the year 2021 the number of Asian Americans and Hispanic Americans in the United States will triple, and African Americans will double (U.S. Department of Commerce, Census Bureau, 2004).

These projections have important implications for society as a whole, and nursing in particular well into this new millennium. Recognizing the multicultural nature of society may be helpful in improving communication between

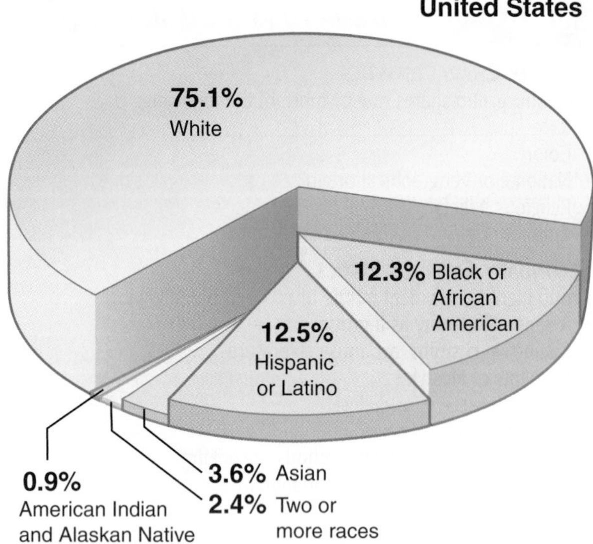

FIGURE 3-1 Racial and ethnic distribution of the populations of the United States. (Data from U.S. Department of Commerce, Bureau of the Census. [2006]. *QT-P3. Race and Hispanic or Latino: 2000.* Retrieved June 7, 2006, from http://factfinder.census.gov/servlet/QTTable?_bm=n&_lang=en&qr_name=DEC_2000_SF1_U_QTP3&ds_name=DEC_2000_SF1_U&geo_id=01000US.)

groups and increasing the likelihood that individuals will work together through common concerns and create ways to solve societal problems. Understanding the cultural context of care for multiple cultural groups will increase the nurse's ability to provide individualized care and to influence health care institutions to meet the needs of diverse groups. The challenge will be to provide culturally appropriate care to clients with widely diverse backgrounds.

TRANSCULTURAL NURSING

Nurses attempt to understand health problems from the client's unique perspective, and knowledge of the client's culture becomes a key to optimal client care. **Transcultural nursing** is culturally competent nursing care focused on differences and similarities among cultures, with respect to caring, health, and illness, based on the client's cultural values, beliefs, and practices (Leininger, 1991). To administer culturally appropriate care, nurses should avoid projecting onto the client their own cultural uniqueness and worldview. Nurses should remember that each person is a product of past experiences, beliefs, and values that have been learned and passed down from one generation to the next (Giger & Davidhizar, 2003).

Providing care within the framework of the client's culture can yield a number of benefits:

- Increased understanding of health care behavior that can be used as a basis for practice
- Improved health resulting from internally consistent health practices
- Improved compliance with the health regimen
- Increased satisfaction with services
- Creation of methods or techniques that may be useful cross-culturally

Central to the concept of transcultural nursing is the concept of care as the essence of nursing. Cultural care has many meanings, expressions, and forms. To care for another person is to take the person under your protection, using the culture's own "forms, patterns, expressions, and structures of care to know, explain, and predict well-being, health, or illness status" (Leininger, 1991).

Transcultural nursing offers a way to provide humanistic care. **Humanistic care** includes understanding and knowing a client in as natural or human a way as possible while helping or guiding the client to achieve certain goals, make improvements, reduce discomforts, or face disability or death. The goal of humanistic care is to gain full understanding of human beings and their humanity (Leininger, 1991). Three elements important to recognize when seeking to provide humanistic care are ethnocentricity, stereotyping, and cultural competence.

Ethnocentricity. Self-esteem means to hold oneself in high regard. Part of the self is produced by the cultural group with which a person identifies and from which the person has learned how to behave and what to value. **Ethnocentrism** is the belief that one's own ethnic beliefs, customs, and attitudes are correct and thus superior. Ethnocentrism includes positive regard for that part of oneself that is culturally based. However, ethnocentric behaviors in a multicultural society produce conflict between cultural groups. One way to overcome the conflict is to identify beliefs and values that are common across all cultures, even those expressed through different behaviors and customs.

All cultures have strengths and weaknesses. Strengths of a culture are those elements that enhance the life and well-being of the members of the group. For example, children who have pride in their cultural heritage have a good foundation for healthy self-esteem in adulthood (Figure 3-2). Weaknesses (such as alcohol dependency) are elements that can have detrimental effects on the group as a whole or on a significant number of people in the group. Most human characteristics can be strengths or weaknesses, depending on the circumstances and the behaviors that result.

Stereotyping. The danger of having a little knowledge about a culture is the belief that it is enough to provide culturally competent care. Instead, it may lead to stereotyping. **Stereotyping** is the assumption that an attribute present in some members of a group is present in all its members. A stereotype may be associated with a negative attribute, but not always. For example, knowing that the Chinese use acupuncture to treat many ailments might lead you to assume that a Chinese American client would be interested in or would even prefer acupuncture as anesthesia for a minor surgical procedure. In reality, both traditional and Western medicine are taught in

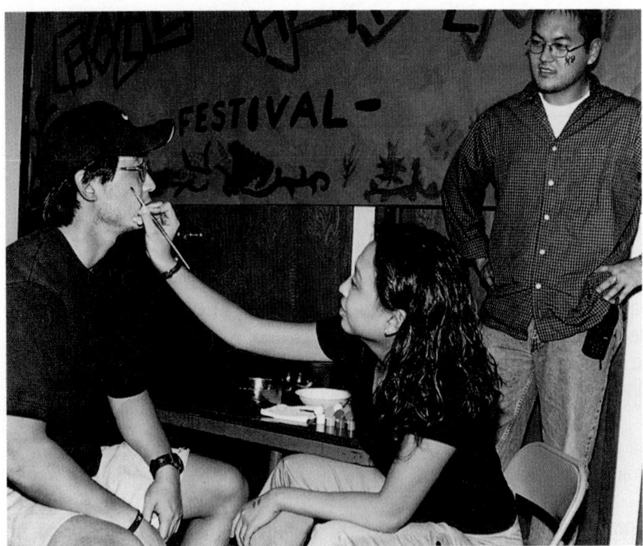

FIGURE 3-2 Healthy self-esteem in young adulthood is tied to appreciation of one's cultural heritage. These Korean Americans demonstrate pride in their cultural heritage through participation in a cultural celebration.

Chinese medical schools, and many Chinese physicians do not use acupuncture.

If nurses assume they know something about a person just because that person is Appalachian, Bostonian, Canadian, or Mexican American, they are stereotyping. This is a dangerous way of characterizing other people, even when the assumption may have some elements of truth. In trying to establish rapport, the *process* of getting to know the person may be more important than knowledge of the person.

Cultural Competence. **Cultural competence** can be described as having enough knowledge of cultural groups that are different from your own to be able to interact with a member of a group in a manner that makes the person feel respected and understood. However, knowledge alone is not enough. Nurses need an attitude that appreciates differences before they can see the strengths of a client whose values, beliefs, and behaviors differ from their own. In addition, it is important to clarify one's own values as a prerequisite to caring for clients of differing cultures (Table 3-1).

Because it is difficult to acquire enough knowledge of multiple cultures to fully understand the cultural perspective of every client you will encounter as a nurse, it is important to develop positive attitudes that are helpful to working with different clients. Culturally competent practitioners have five attributes: awareness, sensitivity, recognition, respect, and the ability to compromise.

Awareness. Awareness includes recognizing the values and beliefs of both the client and yourself. It therefore requires you to clarify your own values, as suggested earlier, and to actively seek to understand and appreciate the values of others. Thus becoming aware requires an attitude of discovery, active listening, and the desire to learn.

It is normal to filter observed behaviors through your own values and beliefs. This filtering produces bias or preconceived beliefs about the meaning of behavior or about the beliefs of another person. Bias can be favorable or unfavorable, and it is not necessarily correct.

Sensitivity. Sensitivity means recognizing the possibility of different meanings of behavior and looking objectively for cues that suggest the meaning. It requires you to validate your interpretation with the client.

Recognition. Recognizing the customs and behaviors of clients from different cultures requires knowledge. Obtaining that knowledge requires curiosity. Nurses should have the desire to explore why they are seeing, hearing, or experiencing client behaviors.

Although nurses can gain a certain amount of knowledge from books, understanding will be enhanced when nurses live among and interact with clients of different cultures. Naturally, you will not be able to live among people from all the cultures that you will encounter in nursing practice. However, learning to recognize and value the differences of even one or two other cultures will heighten your observations of other cultures.

Respect. Respect may be the most important attitude to convey when working with clients of a different culture. When nurses respect others, they recognize and acknowledge their worth and uniqueness. They also recognize and honor their rights and privileges.

Respect dictates that the nurse refrain from interfering with the beliefs and values of another. To develop respect, you must believe that there is value in diversity and then actively look for the value in lifeways that are different from your own.

Compromise. You may need a willingness to compromise when a client's values and beliefs about health care, life, family, responsibility, or medical treatment differ from yours. An attitude of compromise implies that there is more than one right way to do anything.

Diversity and Universality. Another framework for developing cultural competence is Leininger's theory of diversity and universality. It postulates that "care or caring patterns include assistive, supportive, facilitative, and enabling acts or attitudes that influence the well-being or the health status of individuals, families, groups, and institutions as well as general human conditions" (Leininger, 1991). Caring acts and attitudes can be classified into those that are universal across cultures and those that are diverse. The term **universality** describes a common mode or value of caring or a prevailing pattern of care across cultures. **Diversity** refers to the differences in modes or patterns of care between cultures and includes specific patterns of care within cultural groups.

This model assigns three major modalities to guide culturally sensitive nursing care. *Cultural care preservation/maintenance* includes helping clients to continue

Table 3-1 Values Clarification: Providing Culturally Competent Care

VALUE	RELATED ACTIONS
Make a commitment to providing culturally competent care.	• Make a commitment to providing the best nursing care possible in a manner that respects the values, beliefs, and lifeways of the person for whom you are caring. • Learn about other cultures so you can take a positive approach to their health practices and use group characteristics to improve health. You will see in other cultures what you expect to see; look for strengths. Health teaching is more successful when it builds on strengths. • Examine your own culture—not only the larger common culture but also specific subgroups to which you belong. Review your attitudes and beliefs about health, and objectively assess their origin and logic. • Examine biases, prejudices, and stereotypes that could contribute to ineffective nursing care. Plan ways to avoid the pitfalls that could harm the nurse-client relationship and lead to ineffective care. • Analyze your own communication (including facial expressions and body language) and how it may be interpreted.
Act in concert with the value of culturally competent care.	• Convey respect for the individual and respect for the individual's values, beliefs, and cultural practices. • Recognize that almost any human characteristic can be both a strength and a weakness, depending on the circumstances. • Recognize that cultural symbols and practices can bring comfort. • Support the client's practices, and incorporate them into nursing practice whenever possible.
Honor the value in differences.	• When you encounter different beliefs and values, reserve judgment until you can better understand the source of the beliefs and their meaning in the person's daily life. Do not assume that beliefs and values are wrong simply because they differ from yours. • Recognize differences in the ways clients communicate, and do not assume the meaning of a specific behavior (such as lack of eye contact) without considering the client's cultural background. • Relate your client's differing cultural beliefs to your own. In this way, you convey interest and respect for the client's beliefs.
Validate your perceptions of each client.	• Ask if a cultural practice is acceptable, desirable, or important. • Recognize individual differences. People vary within cultural groups and may make individual choices rather than follow traditional ways. • Learn how each client views health, illness, grieving, and the health care system. • Remember that clients may return to preferred cultural practices during illness; for example, the client who has learned English as a second language may revert to the primary language.

cultural practices that have importance to them. This may include using folk medicine, practicing religious rites, eating traditional cultural foods, or providing interpreters when the client's primary language is not the dominant language.

Cultural care accommodation/negotiation includes changing your behaviors or actions to be more fully understood and accepted by the client. This may include, for example, modifying your manner of addressing the client, extending visiting hours, or ensuring that the client is not interrupted during prayers or meditation.

Cultural care repatterning/restructuring includes helping the client change patterns of living that are not beneficial to healthy life patterns. An example is teaching the client different methods of food preparation, such as steaming or baking instead of frying with saturated fats.

TRANSCULTURAL ASSESSMENT MODEL

The Giger and Davidhizar (2003) transcultural assessment model considers six cultural phenomena that may vary with application, yet are present in all cultural groups. These phenomena are communication, space, social organization, time, environmental control, and biological variation (Table 3-2).

COMMUNICATION

Communication difficulties between people of different cultures involve more than speaking a different language. Misunderstanding also arises in the use of idiomatic language (language that is peculiar to a dialect, region, or social group). For example, the word *croaked* may be slang for "died," but it does not have the same meaning when translated to another language. Nor is it understood by people who have no experience in the social context in which the phrase is commonly understood.

Even nonverbal communication can lead to misunderstandings. Gestures, facial expressions, and body language may carry certain meanings commonly understood in one culture, but they would be misunderstood in another. Also, clients from different cultures may misinterpret gestures that Western nurses use to convey empathy and caring. For example, actions such as gentle touch on the hand, maintaining eye contact, or smiling and nodding may seem intrusive, disrespectful, or dismissive to clients of certain cultures.

Table 3-2 Elements of Transcultural Assessment

ELEMENT	DEFINITION
Communication	A continuous process by which one person may affect another through written or oral language, gestures, facial expressions, body language, space, or other symbols
Space	The area around a person's body that includes the individual body, surrounding environment, and objects within that environment
Social organization	The aggregate of family and other groups within a society that dictates culturally accepted role behaviors and rules of behavior. Behaviors are prescribed for such significant life events as birth, death, childbearing, and illness.
Time	A person's focus on the past, the present, or the future. Most cultures include all three time orientations, but one orientation is more likely to dominate the cultural perspective.
Environmental control	The perceived ability of an individual or persons from a particular cultural group to plan activities that control nature, such as illness causation and treatment
Biological variation	Biological differences among racial and ethnic groups may include physical characteristics, such as skin color, and physiological variations, such as lactose intolerance

From Giger, J., & Davidhizar, R. E. (2003). *Transcultural nursing: Assessment and intervention* (4th ed.). St. Louis, MO: Mosby.

SPACE

Personal space includes a person's body and the space around it. It can be used to meet the needs of security, privacy, autonomy, and self-identity. The three categories of personal space describe our physical distance from others. The intimate zone is within 18 inches of the body. The intimate zone is used when comforting, protecting, or counseling, and it is reserved for people who have a close personal bond. The personal zone is 18 inches to 3 feet from the body and is maintained with friends and some counseling sessions. The social zone is 3 to 6 feet from the body and is used for impersonal business being conducted with people who are working together. The level of discomfort generated when personal space is invaded is highly personal and is also related to culture. Generally, Americans, Canadians, and Britons require considerable personal space, whereas Latin Americans, Japanese, and Arabs need a smaller amount of personal space.

You have probably noticed that you usually begin a nurse-client relationship in the social zone and then move to the personal zone as the relationship is established. Of necessity, you enter the intimate zone when you are providing personal care and therapeutic treatments. Most clients intuitively understand and accept this level of personal space in a health care environment. However, you cannot assume that all clients would feel this way, because space varies among cultural groups.

SOCIAL ORGANIZATION

Social organization refers to family structure and organization, religious beliefs, and the group's participation in social activities. Among most cultural groups in the United States, the family is the basic unit of organization. However, there is a great deal of variety in the nature and structure of family relationships. For example, many Hispanic families have grandparents, aunts, uncles, and cousins in important roles. Similarly, Native Americans have a tribal organization of which the nuclear family is a subunit.

TIME

Time can mean many things. It typically is measured, as in the period between one sunrise and the next or the passage of years or decades. Time can refer to a duration, such as how long a person has to complete a task or how long a movie lasts. It can also refer to specific appointments, such as the time for a meeting or the time to take a medication.

Cultures vary in their awareness of time and how they use this awareness in managing their lives. Some people are more likely to focus on the task at hand as though there is nothing else to do, giving it their full attention for as long as it takes to complete. Other individuals compartmentalize time. They are more likely to set a specific amount of time for a task and work to get it done in that amount of time.

In addition, individuals may be described as oriented toward the past, present, or future (Table 3-3). Culture is only one of many factors that influence time orientation. For example, parents who have lost a child may focus on the life of the child and be unable to engage in the present or plan for the future. Poverty focuses a person's attention on the immediate. People involved in social, political, or educational activities may be focused almost exclusively on the future, neglecting their health in order to achieve a long-term goal.

ENVIRONMENTAL CONTROL

Environmental control refers both to the perception of control over the environment and to methods used to control the environment. It can be seen in a culture's attitude toward nature and in its commitment to preserving the natural environment. However, the environment can also include health care, religion, work, and governmental organizations.

Table 3-3 Selected Consequences of Time Orientation

ORIENTATION	POSSIBLE CONSEQUENCES
To past	• When traditions conflict with a prescribed treatment regimen, the person may have trouble accepting or maintaining the plan of care. • In contrast, a strong connection with the past may ground the person with others in the same culture and provide a sense of self that encourages positive health practices.
To the present	• A present-oriented person may have little concern for long-term preventive health practices and may respond better to short-term goals. • In contrast, a present-oriented person may be most able to enjoy the here-and-now and may engage fully in exercise, enjoy nutritious food, and appreciate the company of others–all attributes associated with good health.
To the future	• This person has little focus on the difficulties and inconvenience of the present, focusing instead on the future goals. • The present is important only if what is happening now will help the person realize long-term goals. • This person may have little trouble following a treatment plan as long as its benefits are clear. • However, the person may have great difficulty dealing with chronic illnesses for which no complete cure is known. • A future-oriented person naturally tends to become more of a present-oriented person with age because, as the future life becomes shorter, the present becomes more important.

The perception of being able to control the environment depends on whether the individual operates primarily from an internal locus of control or from an external locus of control. Individuals with an internal locus of control feel empowered to influence their environment. Individuals with an external locus of control are more likely to believe that events are primarily caused by chance, fate, or luck. They may feel helpless to change their environment or circumstances. These individuals may readily relinquish control to others, allowing others to make decisions for them.

BIOLOGICAL VARIATION

Biologically, humans of all races are the same, with minor variations in skin color, facial features, and body size. When a variation is shared by enough people, a group is formed. Genetic variations that produce different health problems in different races are uncommon but do exist. For example, Tay-Sachs disease is more common in people of Jewish ancestry. Thalassemia is more common among people of Mediterranean descent. Sickle cell disease is more common among African Americans.

Most illnesses that are more common in particular groups can be traced to environmental and lifestyle factors. Nevertheless, knowledge of culture is sometimes useful in identifying the lifestyle variables that contribute to disease. It is also useful to direct screening programs to groups that have a high incidence of a particular illness.

UNDERSTANDING SPECIFIC CULTURES

For the most part, a person is born into a cultural group and stays in that group. However, culture is partly a matter of choice. Individuals may choose to continue to closely identify with the group to which their parents belonged, or they may adopt the ways of the larger culture around them. This second choice may have benefits but also carries the risk of inducing a feeling of alienation from the part of the individual that came from specific cultural teachings and certain lifeways. This may require the individual to think about which group he or she most identifies with and also the degree to which the person identifies with the group into which he or she was born.

The following descriptions provide highly generalized information about certain subgroups of larger cultural groups. They do not apply to each person who belongs to a subgroup. These descriptions may include religion, social customs, health practices, and illnesses. This information may provide the first step in the goal of providing culturally competent care.

EUROPEAN AMERICAN COMMUNITY

Members of the European American community have roots in a combination of European countries—Germany, England, Italy, Ireland, and others—and therefore cannot be entirely understood through a study of the whole. Although many have integrated into the larger society and are less aware of the influence of their roots, their responses to illness and health care continue to reflect the origins of their ancestors. In addition, some pockets of European Americans have retained a specific cultural identity.

Communication. Communication patterns in the European American community may not be emotionally expressive. European Americans tend to speak directly and prefer direct eye contact with the listener. The usual distance for social conversation is 2 to 3 feet.

Time. Time is perceived as linear. Usually one topic of conversation or one individual at a time is addressed so that full attention can be given to the individual or topic. European Americans tend to be acutely aware of the pas-

Table 3-4 European American Versus Other Cultures' Values

TRADITIONAL EUROPEAN AMERICAN VALUES	OTHER CULTURES' VALUES
Personal control over environment	Fate, destiny, "God's will"
Change and variety	Tradition
Competition	Cooperation
Individualism	Group welfare
Future orientation	Past orientation
Directness	Indirectness
Informality	Formality
Time importance	Human interaction importance
Duration of life	Quality of life
Nuclear family	Extended family

sage of time and prefer to work efficiently and accomplish tasks in a timely manner.

Table 3-4 provides a general comparison of traditional European American values with values commonly found in other cultures.

AFRICAN AMERICAN COMMUNITY

The term *African American* is a descriptor that suggests pride in a cultural heritage that is a combination of African and American. It can mean the descendants of people who were brought to America as slaves or more recent immigrants from Africa. The term *black* suggests group pride and is used by some African Americans to describe their cultural group. The term African American places the emphasis on cultural heritage, whereas the term black emphasizes biological racial identity. *African American* will be used in this chapter as a means of emphasizing the cultural characteristics.

African Americans include immigrants from African countries, the West Indian Islands, the Dominican Republic, Haiti, and Jamaica. The largest importation of slaves to America from the west coast of Africa occurred during the seventeenth century, and not all African Americans are the descendants of these slaves. The first English settlers brought African slaves and servants with them. Over time other Africans immigrated to America as free persons. The history of African Americans in the northern states differs from that in the southern states. In the North, African Americans who were slaves were freed by their owners and allowed to live their own lives. In the South, most slaves were prohibited from learning to read or write and were denied access to medical care and education.

Communication. The African American dialect may be a product of the English learned by different tribes or of different languages intermingled. The syntax and grammar reflect in part the English dialect of southern white Americans. Patterns of speech have developed that are somewhat unique to African Americans. The dialect (or variation within a language) spoken by African Americans may differ from Standard English in pronunciation, grammar, and syntax. It is helpful for nurses to learn strategies for communicating (Box 3-2).

BOX 3-2 *Strategies for Communicating With Clients From Different Cultures*

- Take a little extra time to establish a level of comfort between yourself and the client.
- Ask questions in an unhurried manner. Rephrase a question and ask it again if the answer seems inconsistent with other information the client has provided.
- Observe for cultural differences in communication, and honor those differences. Use eye contact, touch, and seating arrangements that are comfortable for the client.
- Ask the client about the personal meaning of health and illness, and understanding of treatments and planned care. Investigate how the client's illness is likely to affect his or her life, relationships, and self-concept. Find out what the client considers to be the cause of his or her illness. Ask how the client prefers to manage his or her illness.
- To establish a therapeutic relationship, listen to the client's perception of his or her needs, and respect the client's perspective.
- Listen actively and attentively; try not to anticipate the client's response.
- Talk to the client in an unhurried manner that considers social and cultural amenities.
- Give the client time to answer.
- Use validation techniques to verify that the client understands. Remember that smiles and head nodding may indicate that the client is trying to please you, not necessarily that you are understood.
- Sexual concerns may be difficult for clients to discuss. Having a nurse of the same sex may facilitate communication.
- Use alternative methods of communication, such as a foreign language phrase book, an interpreter, gestures, or pictures, for clients who do not speak English.
- Learn key phrases in languages that are commonly spoken in your community.

Family/Social Structure. Historically, because of prejudice and legalized segregation, African Americans were isolated from the mainstream of society. Assimilation into mainstream society has been slow because of continued racial prejudice and a desire to build the solidarity of a strong African American community in predominantly African American neighborhoods, churches, and schools.

The family structures of African Americans in the United States include the male-headed (patriarchal) family structure and the female-headed (matriarchal) family structure. More than half of African American families have a female head of household. African American women are responsible for maintaining and protecting the health of family members, and they are assuming significant leadership roles in the community as professionals and businesswomen. Large family networks or community groups, such as churches, provide support during times of crisis and illness.

Grandmothers tend to play an active role in the lives of African American families. In fact, children may be raised by grandmothers. Grandmothers may assist with financial support. They also may be actively involved in the care of an ill child. Including a grandmother in the plan of care, therefore, can be of vital importance.

The African American community has maintained a core of strength through its churches and schools that can be expected to continue as a force in solving the problems of the community. Religion is taken very seriously, and many African Americans actively participate in church-related activities and believe strongly in the power of prayer. Some members of the African American community are practicing Muslims. Religious beliefs are an important part of the Muslim lifestyle.

Health Practices/Illnesses. The definition of health for many African Americans stems from African beliefs about life and the nature of being. Some Africans believe that life is a process rather than a state (Spector, 2004). The nature of a person is viewed in terms of energy force rather than matter. When one possesses health, one is in harmony.

Some African Americans use home remedies and folk medicine. Traditional healers are usually women who use herbs and roots to treat illness. The reliance on healers reflects the deep religious faith of African Americans. Some belief in voodoo or hoodoo is still present. Health is maintained with proper rest, diet, and a clean environment. Treating illness through prayer and laying on of hands is practiced in some religious groups.

Lack of access to health care services, low income, and the tendency to self-treat and wait until symptoms become severe tend to increase the morbidity rate among African Americans. Some perceive receiving health care as degrading or humiliating and tend to feel alienated by the system and experience a sense of powerlessness. Some clients believe they are being talked down to by the health care providers and that providers fail to listen to them. Consequently, they choose to suffer in silence. Therefore the nurse should actively ensure that a prescribed treatment or special diet is consistent with the client's needs, cultural background, income, and religious practices. The treatment plan and rationale must be shared with the client, and it is important that the client understand what is being prescribed.

Among African Americans, skin color may vary from a light, almost white color to a very dark brown. Melanin provides protection from the effects of the sun. African Americans have a lower incidence of skin cancer than light-skinned people do.

Hypertension is common among African Americans; they have a higher hypertension-related mortality rate than other groups. Sickle cell disease and lactose intolerance are genetic disorders prevalent in African Americans; other diseases and disorders common to this culture include cancer, cardiovascular disease, cirrhosis, and diabetes. African American children have a tendency to weigh less at birth.

Traditionally, the African American diet is rich in nutrients, as found in collard greens, green and yellow vegetables, legumes, beans, rice, and potatoes. Some parts of the diet, however, are low in fiber, calcium, and potassium and high in fat. The high incidence of diabetes, hypertension, heart disease, and obesity among African Americans may be related to diet.

HISPANIC AMERICAN COMMUNITY

Members of the Hispanic American community have origins in Spain, Cuba, Central and South America, Mexico, Puerto Rico, and other Spanish-speaking countries. This ethnic community is very diverse. It includes people with black skin and people with white skin. The Mexican American subgroup is one of the most prominent.

Most Mexican Americans reside in Texas, the Southwest, and California. In early U.S. history, Mexican Americans helped build many southwestern cities. Settlers learned skills such as mining, farming, and ranching. Most Mexican Americans have remained close to the region of the country that was settled by their ancestors (Giger & Davidhizar, 2003). As new immigrants arrive, they have tended to gather in these areas as well. However, they have also migrated as farm workers to other areas of the country.

Many Mexican Americans can trace their ancestry back to Indian groups such as the Incas and Mayas, who developed complex Mexican civilizations before the arrival of the Spanish explorers. Many Mexican Americans are a blend of both Indian and Spanish European cultures (Giger & Davidhizar, 2003).

Mexican Americans have been successful at retaining a unique cultural identity within the dominant culture, unlike early European immigrants, who assimilated into the overall U.S. culture. Traditional gender and family roles continue to be part of the heritage that separates Mexican Americans from other cultural groups. Some are well educated, and others are migrant workers who move around the country seeking work harvesting seasonal crops.

Communication. For many Mexican Americans, Spanish is the primary language, spoken in many dialects and differing widely between Hispanic groups. Some Mexican Americans place a high value on diplomacy and tactfulness and communicate in a manner that avoids direct confrontation and arguments, which are considered rude and disrespectful. Through the use of elaborate, often indirect communication, the Mexican American tries to accomplish the goal of communication while maintaining politeness and respect. Self-disclosure is avoided with strangers, including health care professionals. In communicating, Mexican Americans may incorporate the use of senses as well as words, and they are characterized as tactile in their relationships.

Most Mexican Americans can speak at least some English, but they may use it selectively. It is not uncommon to use English in the workplace and Spanish at home or with friends. Children of newer immigrants who have not yet mastered English may have a hard time in school. In general, Mexican American children are more likely to grow up bilingual than European American children in the same regions. In health care situations, you may observe a client speak to his or her family in Spanish, to you in English, and, when very stressed, to both the family and you in a mix of both English and Spanish.

Family/Social Structure. The strength of the nuclear family (parents and children) is the foundation of the Mexican American community. For most Mexican Americans, extended family relationships have special significance, and the family may be the most significant social organization. They take pride in family accomplishments and usually do not seek help from outsiders to meet needs or resolve problems. Men may assume the dominant role of breadwinner and decision maker. Women often work at jobs outside the home, and they are taking significant leadership roles in the community as educators, attorneys, and businesswomen.

Health Practices/Illnesses. Mexican Americans are more likely to perceive an external locus of control. They may perceive life as being under the influence of a divine will. They may also have a fatalistic belief that they are at the mercy of the environment and have little control over what happens (Giger & Davidhizar, 2003).

Some Mexican Americans may view health as purely the result of good luck or a reward from God for good behavior. Individuals are expected to maintain their equilibrium in the universe by conducting themselves in the proper way, eating the proper foods, and working the proper amount of time. The prevention of illness is an accepted practice that is accomplished with prayer, by wearing religious medals or amulets, and by keeping relics in the home. Illness may be viewed as an imbalance in the individual's body or as a punishment for wrongdoing.

Some Mexican Americans believe that an imbalance may exist between hot and cold or wet and dry. These forces are embodied in four body fluids (or humors): blood, which is hot and wet; yellow bile, which is hot and dry; phlegm, which is cold and wet; and black bile, which is cold and dry. When all four humors are balanced, the body is healthy. When an imbalance occurs, an illness is present. If an illness is categorized as hot, it is treated with a cold substance. A cold disease, in turn, must be treated with a hot substance. The classification of what is a hot disease or a cold disease varies from person to person.

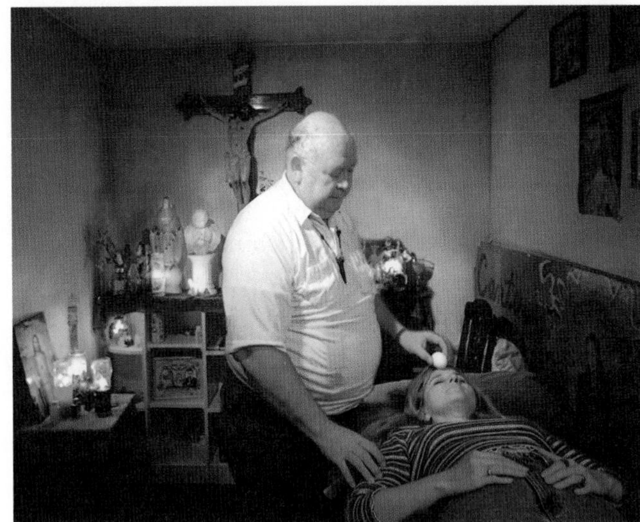

FIGURE 3-3 Within the Mexican American folk medicine system, the *curandero* is the folk healer.

Within the Mexican American folk medicine system, the *curandero* is the folk healer (Figure 3-3). The *curandero* views illness from a religious and social context rather than the scientific perspective that dominates Western society (Giger & Davidhizar, 2003). The *curandero* is a holistic healer and can be either female or male.

In the folk medicine system, illness may be caused by *susto* (fright), *mal ojo* (evil eye), *envidia* (envy), or *empacho* (gastrointestinal ailment). The most popular form of treatment by folk healers involves herbs, especially when used as teas. Treatments may also include massage, cleanings *(limpias)*, diet, rest, prayers, and supernatural rituals. Rituals include elements of both Catholic and Pentecostal rituals and artifacts: money offerings, confession, candle lighting, wooden or metal offerings in the shape of anatomical parts *(milagros)*, and laying on of hands. The *herbero* is a folk healer who specializes in the use of herbs and spices for preventive and curative purposes. *Brujos* (male witches) and *brujas* (female witches) are another level of healers. They practice black magic and may not be sought until other forms of healing have been tried.

Roman Catholicism is the predominant religion practiced by Mexican Americans. During times of crises, Mexican Americans may rely on a priest or prayers. Rituals, such as making promises, lighting candles, or visiting shrines, may be practiced when a family member is ill.

The incidence of diabetes among Mexican Americans is five times the national average, and complications are more frequent. The client with multiple health problems is a special concern in this population. Hypertension is a significant health problem. Urban, older adult Mexican

Americans are at risk for many age-related chronic health conditions associated with migrant status, lower levels of education, nutrition, and poverty. Alcoholism is also a crucial health problem among Mexican Americans (Giger & Davidhizar, 2003). Men are most often affected, because the male role may be correlated with the ability to ingest large amounts of alcohol.

The typical Mexican diet is rich in complex carbohydrates, provided by corn, beans, rice, and breads. Protein sources include fish and shellfish, eggs, beef, pork, poultry, and goat. Major changes occurred in the Mexican American diet with emigration to the United States. The intake of fats and less consumption of complex carbohydrates occurred. As a result, the incidence of obesity, cardiovascular disease, and diabetes has increased among Mexican Americans.

ASIAN AMERICAN COMMUNITY

According the Commerce Department's Census Bureau, Chinese are the largest Asian group in the United States. Chinese Americans are immigrants and their descendants, mainly from Taiwan, Hong Kong, and mainland China.

Many religions exist among Chinese Americans, such as Buddhism, Taoism, Christianity, Islam, beliefs in myths and fortunes, and worship of ancestors and deified heroes. When they are ill, Chinese Americans may practice one or more religions to help themselves get well. Respect these practices as long as the client's faith does no harm to health.

The teachings of Confucius form a primary force in Chinese culture. Confucius was a Chinese sage who established rules and codes of ethics for personal and interpersonal behaviors to maintain order and harmony in society. Lao Zi, another Chinese sage, greatly influenced Chinese medicine. Confucius encouraged people to pursue the virtues of loyalty to family, friends, and the government. He also encouraged filial piety to parents, love, faithfulness, righteousness, and peacefulness. Confucius emphasized harmonious relationships with nature and each other. He suggested accommodating rather than confronting and seeking group consensus rather than advocating individual concerns. A person is expected to demonstrate these virtues, to exert self-control, to be self-reliant, and to behave modestly. Otherwise, one brings shame to oneself, family members, and society. (Chinese call this losing face.) Consequently, Chinese Americans may be group oriented; may avoid conflicts or being different; may seem quiet, unassertive, agreeable, and pleasant; and may suppress the showing of negative emotions, such as anger, sadness, worry, and depression (Chang, 2003).

Communication. English proficiency and communication styles affect the interactions of Chinese Americans with health care providers and the health care delivery system. Once Chinese Americans are in the health care delivery system, they may experience an undue amount of stress. They may not understand their health condition and may be unable to express their concerns or needs. Even when able to express concerns, they may be misunderstood.

To reduce Chinese American clients' stress, the nurse may help them in the following ways:

- Find a translator who can speak their dialect to help them understand their health status and care. Try to not use family members if possible.
- Use plain and simple English to explain things; avoid jargon or medical terms.
- Provide written materials in addition to verbal information to clients and to family members to facilitate understanding.
- Find resources that are written in Chinese.

During the process of acculturation, some Chinese Americans may feel shame. They have low self-esteem and feel helpless, powerless, and depressed because of their limitations in English and reduced social support. Because the Chinese culture emphasizes self-control and self-reliance, they may feel shame in verbalizing emotional and social problems. They may verbalize only physical symptoms. The nurse can help them by identifying the psychosocial problems underlying physical symptoms. When they disagree with a health care provider, they may switch to another health care provider rather than confront the original one. When communicating with Chinese Americans, assess their communication style, be sensitive to nonverbal communication clues, and encourage them to verbalize any questions, concerns, or disagreements.

Family/Social Structure. Chinese Americans tend to have a hierarchy in the social and family structure. Husbands and elders have authority over wives and children. Elders and people in authoritative positions are highly respected. Chinese culture expects children to take care of their parents when they grow up. If children do not take care of their parents, the parents may feel shame and consider the children disloyal to their family.

Under the influence of democracy and American culture, Chinese Americans may challenge traditional social structure and values. They may come to value the individual more than the group. They may alter the line of authority in the family. The conflicts between traditional values and American culture may create stress. Some stress may cause physical symptoms and psychological problems. For example, elder immigrants may feel some loss of self-respect because they depend on their children for financial, physical, and psychosocial support. As a result of this dependence, the elder immigrants may experience loneliness and emotional isolation. However, they may complain only about problems with sleep or appetite because they are ashamed to admit emotional problems, or they may develop further mental illnesses and commit suicide.

When caring for Chinese Americans, assess their family structure, the line of authority, and their social support. The nurse may include family members in the plan of care. You may also involve the person who is authoritative to the client to help the client reach therapeutic goals. To identify psychosocial problems, encourage the client to express thoughts and feelings without feeling shame. For a client with limited social support, help identify available community resources to increase the client's sense of self-reliance and self-esteem (Chang, 2003).

Health Practices/Illnesses. Chinese culture does not emphasize control of the environment but rather maintenance of a harmonious relationship with nature and balance in life. To maintain health, some Chinese Americans may perform traditional Chinese exercises, such as tai chi or qi-kung, to facilitate the flow of qi and the yin-yang balance within the body. They believe that fresh air is important for quality qi. They usually exercise early in the morning in the park while the air is fresh. They may also prefer to keep windows open to allow the flow of fresh air instead of using air-conditioning.

When Chinese Americans are ill, they may take Western medicines together with Chinese herbal medicines, and both may have similar effects. Caution the client about overmedication and suggest not taking both types of medicines together. Encourage the client to work with health care providers for any problems related to medicines.

Some Chinese Americans may observe the yin-yang quality of foods and eat only foods that can balance the yin-yang quality of their diseases. For example, after giving birth (yin quality), some Chinese Americans drink only warm milk or hot water (yang quality) and will not drink or eat anything cold (yin quality). Respect this belief, and help the client obtain the preferred foods and drinks.

Some Chinese may use external Chinese medicine, such as acupuncture, moxibustion, skin scraping, or suction cupping, to promote the circulation of qi and to restore health. Acupuncture uses hair-thin needles inserted at special sites. This procedure may leave no marks and has been reported to control pain effectively.

Some of these procedures can produce skin lesions. For example, moxibustion involves placement of a burning moxa (an herb) over vital points. A crater about 1 cm in diameter on the skin may develop. Skin scraping involves scraping skin firmly at selected points with a blunt spoon or coin until bright red stripes appear. Multiple linear bruises over the neck, the bridge of the nose, along the spine, or over the chest may be observed. Suction cupping involves the use of an ignited cotton swab inside a glass cup that is quickly placed on a treatment site to create suction. When these lesions are present, do not mistake them for physical abuse. Provide care as needed to prevent infection.

Several symptoms or diseases are genetically linked to Chinese Americans. Mongolian spots (bluish pigmentation, usually at the coccygeal area) are often observed on Chinese infants. They should not be mistaken for bruises.

More than half of Chinese babies develop neonatal jaundice. Prepare Chinese American mothers before discharge to be aware of jaundice, and teach them ways to reduce or treat it.

Chinese Americans typically weigh less than whites. Their drug metabolism may also be different from that of whites. Therefore they may develop side effects or toxic effects when they take the dosages usually prescribed for whites. You need to observe if lower dosages are needed to reduce side effects.

Many Chinese adhere to a traditional Chinese diet interspersed with traditional American foods, especially breads and cereals. Usually, dairy products are not eaten in sufficient quantities. Adequate calcium is consumed through tofu and small fish. The main protein sources are fish, pork, and poultry. Vegetables and fruits make up a large part of the Chinese diet. The positive factors related to diet include low incidence of heart disease and bowel and breast cancer. Diet-related diseases are stomach cancer and lactose intolerance.

High incidences of lactose deficiency, thalassemia deficiency, and glucose-6-phosphate dehydrogenase (G6PD) deficiency have been reported among the Chinese. After drinking milk some Chinese Americans may experience abdominal cramps, diarrhea, or flatus. Thus they may avoid drinking milk. Thalassemia deficiency causes rapid destruction of red blood cells. Clients require monthly blood transfusions for life. If both parents are thalassemia carriers, infants or mothers may develop complications, such as stillbirth or preeclampsia. G6PD deficiency may result in anemia because of rapid destruction of red blood cells when some Chinese Americans take certain drugs (Chang, 2003). Screening for these deficiencies and providing information and genetic counseling are the best preventive care.

Chinese Americans are at high risk of developing hepatitis B, tuberculosis, nasopharyngeal cancer, esophageal cancer, stomach cancer, and liver cancer. The consumption of fermented, moldy, and pickled foods may contribute to the development of esophageal and liver cancers (Chang, 2003). Crowded living arrangements may be one of the contributing factors for tuberculosis. To help Chinese Americans, you may provide them information about these diseases to reduce their risk and to help them identify these diseases at an early stage.

In summary, when caring for Chinese Americans, you need to assess the impact of Chinese culture and beliefs on their health status and health care behaviors to help them cope with physical and psychosocial problems, to screen for genetic disorders, and to reduce high-risk diseases.

NATIVE AMERICAN COMMUNITY

There are about 200 Native American tribes in the United States, and they are concentrated primarily in western states as the result of forced westward migration. Oklahoma, Arizona, California, New Mexico, and Alaska have the largest numbers of Native Americans (Spector, 2004). Although many live on reservations and in rural areas, just as many live in cities, especially those on the West Coast. The term *Native American* implies tribes residing in the continental United States. One of the largest tribes is the Navajo, and elements of that culture are discussed here.

Communication. Many Navajo use English as their primary language, but many are fluent both in the Navajo language and in English. Naturally, those who do not speak English will require the assistance of an interpreter when seeking or receiving health care.

Rather than shaking hands, as is common among many Americans, Navajos tend to extend a hand and lightly touch the hand of the person being greeted. The Navajo culture holds a taboo against touching a dead person or an animal killed by lightning. Consequently, a Navajo client or family member may prefer not to touch articles associated with a dead person or animal.

The Navajo people may appear silent and reserved when first meeting strangers. Warm behavior may be demonstrated once the Navajo individual becomes familiar with you (Giger & Davidhizar, 2003). In the Navajo culture, eye contact is considered a sign of disrespect.

Family/Social Structure. The Navajo culture is very family oriented, and the definition of family may have no limits on number or on relationship. Navajo people believe that family members are responsible for each other. Therefore it is not unusual for many relatives to come to the hospital to care for a Navajo client. Decision making is mutual. The goal of the family is to help its members grow, share resources, and participate in daily activities and significant life events, such as birth, death, marriage, and sickness.

The Navajo culture is neither dead nor static but instead is a living culture, retaining its heritage and advancing with the times. Navajo members may join with other tribes and share their songs and dances to remind the people of their old ways and rich heritage. Dancers have always been a very important part of the life of the Native American (Figure 3-4). Although dance styles and content have changed, their meaning and importance have not.

Health Practices/Illnesses. The traditional Navajo belief about health is that it reflects living in total harmony with nature and having the ability to survive under exceedingly difficult circumstances. The Navajo people have practiced a holistic approach to healing for hundreds of years. This practice involves a sense of connection with place and land. Illness is viewed as a price being paid for something that happened in the past or for something that will happen in the future. Everything is the result of something else.

Native Americans do not subscribe to the germ theory of medicine. Illness is something that must be. The cause of disease or injury to a person or property, or of continued misfortune of any kind, must be traced back to an action that should not have been taken. Examples of such infractions are breaking a taboo or contacting a ghost or witch. To the Navajo, the treatment of an illness must be concerned with the external causative factors and not with the disease or injury itself (Spector, 2004).

The traditional healer of the Navajo is the medicine man. He is a person wise in the ways of land and nature. He knows the interrelationships of humans, the Earth, and the universe. He knows the ways of the plants and animals, the moon, and the stars. The medicine man takes his time to determine first the cause of the illness

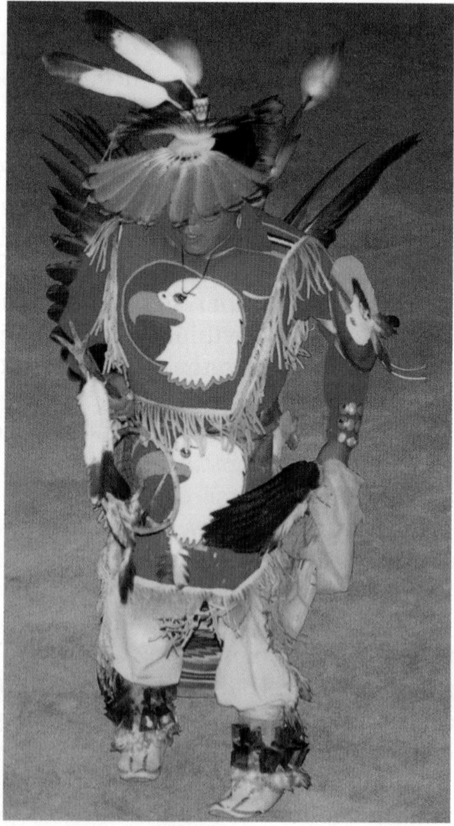

FIGURE 3-4 Dancers have always been a very important part of the life of the Native American.

and then the proper treatment. To determine the cause and treatment of an illness, he performs special ceremonies that may take several days. Navajos may rely on traditional tribal medicine, the "white man's medicine," or a combination of both. Conflicts can occur in families when there are different degrees of acceptance of scientific medical treatments.

Navajos may be suspicious of people of European descent. Initial reluctance may dissipate when a health professional respects the client's opinion and demonstrates sensitivity to the client's point of view. Nurses and caregivers must avoid "interviewing" Navajos to gain information. Often, simply listening helps the person overcome concerns about interacting with health care providers of a different culture.

The traditional diet of Native Americans was based on animal foods such as deer, elk, buffalo, goat, rabbit, fish, and shellfish. These foods were protein sources and contained small amounts of saturated fats. As processed foods became part of the Native American diet, the incidence of obesity, heart disease, and diabetes increased.

Today, Navajos are faced with a number of health problems. Health care skills inherent in the Navajo traditional ways of diagnosing and treating illness have not fully survived their migration and changing ways of life. Because of the loss of these skills and because modern health care centers are not always available, Navajos are frequently in limbo when it comes to obtaining appropriate health care. High rates of unemployment are prevalent. In addition, at least a third of Navajos live in poverty. With poverty come poor living conditions, malnutrition, tuberculosis, and high maternal and infant death rates. The leading causes of death for Navajos are tuberculosis, chronic liver disease and cirrhosis, accidents (including motor vehicle accidents), diabetes, pneumonia, suicide, and homicide (U.S. Department of Health and Human Services, 2005).

Type 2 diabetes mellitus is a major health problem for Navajos. It tends to occur early, in the teens or early twenties. As a result, complications also occur early, leading to excessive mortality in the early and middle adult years. According to the U.S. Department of Health and Human Services (2005), the age-adjusted death rate is on the rise. It is not known why diabetes is prevalent among Navajos.

LANGUAGE BARRIERS

Language may be an obstacle to providing health care. Twelve percent of the population in the United States (32 million people) speak a language other than English. Some language resources that may be available to the nurse include the following:

Bilingual staff
Staff interpreters
Volunteer staff or community interpreters
Telephone interpreter service

Use of the client's family or friend is usually not recommended because the individual may not understand medical terminology or maintain confidentiality.

IMMIGRANTS

Immigration has changed the social landscape of the United States. First-generation immigrants are those individuals born outside of the United States, its territories, or possessions. Second-generation immigrants are those born in the United States, with at least one foreign parent (Suro and Passel, 2003). First-generation immigrants confront challenges such as language barriers, socioeconomic limitations, and legal issues. Their beliefs about health and wellness are influenced by these factors. They struggle with adapting to their new environment more than second-generation immigrants. Many second-generation immigrants have assimilated into mainstream American society, have substantial differences in fluency in English and education, and more readily embrace the health care system.

▼ KEY PRINCIPLES

- In a multicultural society, distinct cultural groups retain cultural identity and contribute to the overall society the strengths and lifeways of the group.
- Stereotyping is a counterproductive tendency to assume that an attribute present in some members of a group must be present in all members of the group.
- Culture includes the values, beliefs, norms, and practices shared by a particular group that guide thinking, decisions, and actions in a patterned way.
- Six elements by which to describe cultural diversity are communication, space, social organization, time, environmental control, and biological variation.
- To communicate with persons of other cultures, you should respect each individual's values, beliefs, and cultural practices.
- Communication requires validation that all parties in the communication have been understood.
- There is perhaps as much variation within cultures as between cultures.
- Culturally competent nursing care requires understanding the health care setting from the client's point of view.

■ REVIEW QUESTIONS

1. An important step in developing cultural competence is:

1. Providing interpreter services for clients who speak a language other than English
2. Clarifying one's own values as a prerequisite to caring for clients of different cultures
3. Reviewing immigration laws as they relate to the implementation of nursing care
4. Learning about the beliefs and values of every client that you will care for as a nurse

Continued

2. Humanistic care:
1. Is the belief that one's own ethnic beliefs, customs, and attitudes are correct and superior
2. Is the assumption that an attribute present is in some members of a group is present in all its members
3. Includes understanding and knowing a client in as natural or human a way as possible
4. Includes recognizing the values and beliefs of both the client and yourself

3. Culturally competent practitioners have these attributes:
1. Awareness, sensitivity, recognition
2. Ethnocentrism, respect, sensitivity
3. Ability to compromise, diversity
4. Recognition, respect, ethnicity

4. The nurse anthropologist who defines culture as "the learned, shared, and transmitted values, beliefs, norms, and lifeways of a particular group that guide thinking, decisions, and actions in a patterned way" is:
1. Madeline Leininger
2. Mildred Montag
3. Florence Nightingale
4. Clara Barton

5. The phenomena described in Giger and Davidhizar's transcultural assessment model include:
1. Communication, space, accommodation
2. Environmental control, time, space
3. Repatterning, social organization, time
4. Biological variation, time, negotiation

Bibliography

Callister, L., C., Khalaf, I., Semenic, S., Kartchner, R., & Vehvilainen-Julkunen, K. (2003). The pain of childbirth: Perceptions of culturally diverse women. *Pain Management Nursing, 4*(4), 145-154.

Chang, K. (2003). Chinese Americans. In J. N. Giger & R. E. Davidhizar (Eds.), *Transcultural nursing: Assessment and intervention.* St. Louis, MO: Mosby.

Cioffi, J. (2004). Caring for women from culturally diverse backgrounds: Midwives' experiences. *Journal of Midwifery & Women's Health, 49*(5), 437-442.

Conti, K. M. (2006). Diabetes prevention in Indian country: Developing nutrition models to tell the story of food-system change. *Journal of Transcultural Nursing, 17,* 234-245.

Dapice, A. N. (2006). The medicine wheel. *Journal of Transcultural Nursing, 17,* 251-260.

Edwards, G. M. (2003). The health cost of soul food. *Topics in Advanced Practice Nursing eJournal, 3*(2). Retrieved from http://www.medscape.com/viewarticle/453335.

Giger, J. N., & Davidhizar, R. E. (2003). *Transcultural nursing: Assessment and intervention* (4th ed.). St. Louis, MO: Mosby.

Hoar, S. (2006). ISCOPES: *Interdisciplinary Student Community Oriented Prevention Enhancement Service—The George Washington University.* Retrieved June 7, 2006, from http://www.gwu.edu/iscopes/LearningMods_Culture.htm.

Krisberg, K. (2005). Cultural competencies needed to serve all older Americans: Cultural skills will help bridge health gaps. *The Nation's Health, 35*(5). Retrieved from http://www.medscape.com/viewarticle/507014_2.

*Leininger, M. (1991). *Culture care diversity and universality: A theory of nursing* (Publication No. 15-2402). New York: National League for Nursing Press.

Spector, R. E. (2004). *Cultural diversity in health and illness* (6th ed.). Upper Saddle River, NJ: Pearson Education.

Suro, R., & Passel, J. S. (2003). *The rise of the second generation: Changing patterns in Hispanic population growth.* Washington, DC: Pew Hispanic Center. Retrieved from http://pewhispanic.org/reports/report?ReportID=22.

U.S. Department of Commerce, Bureau of the Census. (2002). *Census 2000: Chinese largest Asian group in the United States.* Retrieved June 6, 2006, from http://www.census.gov/Press-Release/www/2002/cb02cn59.html.

U.S. Department of Commerce, Bureau of the Census. (2004). *U.S. interim projections by age, race, and Hispanic origin.* Retrieved June 7, 2006, from http://www.census.gov.

U.S. Department of Commerce, Bureau of the Census. (2006). *QT-P3. Race and Hispanic or Latino: 2000.* Retrieved June 7, 2006, from http://factfinder.census.gov/servlet/QTTable?_bm=n&_lang=en&qr_name=DEC_2000_SF1_U_QTP3&ds_name=DEC_2000_SF1_U&geo_id=01000US.

U.S. Department of Health and Human Services, Indian Health Service. (2005). *Health characteristics of the American Indian and Alaska Native adult population.* Advanced data from vital and health statistics: no. 356, Hyattsville, MD: National Center for Health Statistics.

U.S. Department of Health and Human Services, Public Health Service, National Institutes of Health. National Institute of Diabetes and Digestive and Kidney Diseases. *National diabetes fact sheet, general information and national estimates on diabetes in the United States.* Bethesda, MD: Author. (2005).

Youngblut, J. M., Brooten, D., Lobar, S. L., Hernandez, L., & McKenry, M. (2005). Child care use by low-income single mothers of preschoolers born preterm versus those of preschoolers born full term. *Journal of Pediatric Nursing,* 20(4), 246-257.

*Asterisk indicates a classic or definitive work on this subject.

Chapter 4

The Health Care Delivery System

Media Resources

- Evolve Website http://evolve.elsevier.com/Harkreader/
- Companion CD

Learning Objectives

After studying this chapter, you should be able to do the following:

- Identify the characteristics of health care as a system of delivery of services
- Compare the four types of health care services
- Identify health care personnel and describe their training, roles, and responsibilities
- Discuss inpatient, outpatient, and community settings for the delivery of health care
- Compare the types of health care financing
- Discuss current issues and opportunities in health care delivery

Key Terms

access
capitation payment system
diagnosis-related groups (DRGs)
exclusive provider organization (EPO)
health maintenance organization (HMO)
health promotion
illness prevention
managed care
Medicaid
medical model
Medicare
preferred provider organization (PPO)
prospective payment system (PPS)
rehabilitation
retrospective payment system
supportive care
unlicensed assistive personnel (UAP)

The health care delivery system in the United States is a complex array of services working together often as independent units with an interdependent relationship based on government and private systems for payment of services. The goal of these services is to provide accessible, available, affordable, quality health care focused on consumer needs. It is not truly a system in the sense of being a well-ordered, coordinated body of connected parts, but it is a system in the sense that the parts are interdependent with each affecting the work of the others.

Each person or group concerned with the system has a unique perspective on the meaning and relationship of the parts of the whole. Clients and their families, such as the parents of a child with a serious illness, seek the health care delivery system as a beneficent domain—that is, a source of nurturance and healing with solutions to their health problems. Health care providers view the system as a means to provide care to their clients. Economists on the other hand see it as a huge service industry consisting of public and private businesses providing health care services to consumers. Legislators may see it as a political agenda driven by demand from their constituents. Social theorists may claim that the system is the property of all citizens, who should be granted universal availability and coverage.

Understanding the strengths and weakness of the health care delivery system begins with knowledge of the nature of comprehensive health care services and the people and institutions that provide those services. However, full understanding takes into account the methods of health care financing, the social and economic factors affecting health care, and the framework for redesigning the system to better meet the goal of a healthy society. Indeed, these are the forces that have created the health care delivery system over the last century and that have created the opportunities and issues in health care for the twenty-first century.

SCOPE OF HEALTH CARE SERVICES

Over the last century, the medical model has largely governed the direction of health care delivery. In the **medical model** the identification and treatment of an illness or disease is the focus of care. However, four types of services have evolved as a means to provide a system of comprehensive health care: health promotion and illness prevention, diagnosis and treatment, rehabilitation, and supportive care.

HEALTH PROMOTION AND ILLNESS PREVENTION

Health promotion is a means to modify a client's knowledge, attitudes, and skills to adopt behaviors leading to a healthier lifestyle, thus achieving a higher level of wellness from any point on a continuum from health to illness. **Illness prevention** involves the use of modalities such as immunizations and medications that avert disease or detect disease in its earliest, most treatable stages.

Although the treatment of illness has made tremendous advances in the last century, the overall improvement in general health and longevity of the past few decades owes less to medical care and more to healthy behaviors and improved environmental quality. Health promotion and prevention of illness will take on new meaning as the science of gene therapy and other advances change our approach to health care.

DIAGNOSIS AND TREATMENT

The diagnosis and treatment of acute and chronic illness will continue to be a major component of the health care system. Although acute or episodic care is a major focus of the system, about 45% of noninstitutionalized Americans have chronic illnesses, and they account for 75% of personal health care spending. Although technological advances have allowed physicians to diagnose illnesses earlier and treat acute episodes of illness more effectively than in the past, the client needs to understand the medical diagnosis and treatment and assume responsibility for managing the treatment plan at home. Chronic illness requires long-term management and lifestyle changes.

REHABILITATION

Rehabilitation has the goals of restoration of function, maintenance of the remaining levels of physical and mental function, and prevention of further deterioration. Rehabilitation activities are applied to a wide range of health problems, such as cerebrovascular infarct, joint replacement, burns, or spinal cord injury, which can occur on an acute, chronic, or time-limited basis. Rehabilitation services are required by clients whose past illnesses or injuries have left them with residual physical or mental impairments that affect their ability to function normally. In addition, people with chronic illness often need rehabilitation services to optimize their level of function. Rehabilitation is discussed more thoroughly in Chapter 44.

SUPPORTIVE CARE

Supportive care includes medical, nursing, psychological, and social services aimed at helping the client manage a chronic illness, disability, or terminal illness when rehabilitation or restoration is not a realistic goal. This care can be provided in a hospital, a nursing home, a hospice, or in the client's home setting and aims to meet the physical, emotional, and spiritual needs of the client and the family. The objective is to help clients achieve or maintain the highest level of functioning possible, thus permitting the greatest degree of independence and participation in their community.

MULTIDISCIPLINARY HEALTH CARE TEAM

Multidisciplinary health care teams bring together several disciplines to work together through joint planning, decision making, and goal setting to enhance positive client outcomes in each discipline. To work effectively as a team, each discipline must understand and respect the role and contribution made by the other disciplines. The goal of the team is to provide higher-quality, better-coordinated client care than can be provided with each discipline working alone.

REGISTERED NURSES

Registered nurses (RNs) focus on health promotion and disease prevention and are major care providers for sick and injured clients. An RN is a graduate of a state-approved school of nursing and licensed by the state to practice nursing as defined by the nurse practice act in that state. Nurses are the largest single group of health care professionals in this country. Five major employment settings for RNs were identified: hospitals (59.1%), community and public health settings (18.3%), ambulatory care settings (9.5%), nursing homes and extended care facilities (6.9%), and nursing education (2.1%). There are 2,696,540 registered nurses (Division of Nursing, 2003), or 828.4 per 100,000 people in the United States (National Center for Health Statistics, 1998). The evolving health care system has created the need for nurses trained in many specialties.

ADVANCED PRACTICE NURSES

With an emphasis on holistic care, health promotion, and disease prevention, advanced practice nurses (APNs) retain their identity as nurses across multiple practice settings. This emphasis distinguishes them from physician assistants. The APN is an RN who has met advanced educational and clinical practice requirements beyond the basic nursing education required of all RNs. Advanced practice nurses generally have a master's degree as a clinical nurse specialist (CNS), nurse practitioner (NP), certified nurse midwife (CNM), or certified registered nurse anesthetist (CRNA). With the ability to provide 60% to 80% of the preventive and primary care traditionally done by physicians, the nurse practitioner contributes to the availability of primary health care in large practices and underserved areas. Clinical nurse specialists are expert clinicians in a specialized area of nursing practice. Advanced practice nursing is regulated by the various state boards of nursing, and the states vary with regard to the authority to write prescriptions and the nature of required supervision by a physician (ANA, 2006).

OTHER NURSING PERSONNEL

Nurses are extended through the use of licensed practical nurses, licensed vocational nurses, and assistive personnel. Licensed practical or vocational nurses provide nursing care under the supervision of a registered nurse or a physician. They are graduates of state board–approved nursing programs that are 12 to 18 months in length. The primary area of employment for licensed practical or vocational nurses is in nursing homes or other long-term care facilities. Hospitals vary in the practice of hiring these nurses.

The term **unlicensed assistive personnel (UAP)** refers to an unlicensed individual who is trained to function in an assistive or supportive role to the licensed nurse in the provision of direct client care or activities peripherally related to the provision of care that have been delegated by the nurse (ANA, 1997). These workers may receive only on-the-job training or a short course (a month) of training, which sometimes leads to certification for the skills taught in the course but is not a license to practice nursing. Examples of the titles given to unlicensed assistive personnel include (but are not limited to) certified nurse's aides, orderlies, nursing assistants, home health aides, attendants, and client care technicians.

PHYSICIANS

Physicians are licensed to diagnose and treat disease. A physician is a graduate of a college of medicine or osteopathy and licensed under the medical practice act by the state to diagnosis and treat disease. Education includes an undergraduate degree, a medical degree, and graduate medical education (residency). Physicians may be employed by hospitals as staff physicians, in federal or state government agencies, public health clinics, community health centers, and prisons. However, most physicians are in private practice, and increasing numbers are in group practices. The number of physicians has steadily increased from 141 per 100,000 of the population in 1950 to 262 per 100,000 in 2001 (American Medical Association, 2004).

Increasingly, physicians are specializing. Physicians trained in family medicine, general internal medicine, and general pediatrics are considered to be primary care providers or generalists. Board certification in a specialty requires additional years of training and a specialty board examination. Common medical specialties include cardiology, dermatology, family medicine, neurology, obstetrics and gynecology, ophthalmology, pediatrics, psychology, radiology, and surgery. Primary care physicians may refer clients to specialists on the basis of evaluation of the client's medical needs.

PHYSICIAN ASSISTANTS

The American Academy of Physician Assistants (2005) defines physician assistants (PAs) as "health care professionals licensed to practice medicine with physician supervision. As part of their comprehensive responsibilities, a PA conducts physical exams, diagnoses and treats illnesses, orders and interprets tests, counsels on preventive health care, assists in surgery, and in virtually all states can write prescriptions. Within the physician-PA relationship, physician assistants exercise autonomy in medical decision making and provide a broad range of diagnostic and therapeutic services. A PA's practice may also include education, research, and administrative services." Physician assistants are educated in the medical model and practice in a variety of settings, including physicians' offices, hospitals, ambulatory care centers, nursing homes, government agencies, and community health centers (American Academy of Physician Assistants, 2005).

The average PA program curriculum is approximately 26 months and grants a bachelor's or master's degree. The National Commission on Certification of Physician Assistants provides the PA with certification after completion of education and clinical experience requirements.

ALLIED HEALTH PRACTITIONERS

Allied health workers can be divided into two broad categories: therapists and technologists, and technicians and assistants in fields such as physical therapy, occupational therapy, respiratory therapy, surgery, radiology, laboratory analysis, and sonography. Generally, *technicians* and *assistants* are prepared in 2 years or less and require supervision by therapists or technologists to evaluate the treatment process. *Therapists* and *technologists* receive more advanced training to evaluate clients, diagnose problems, and develop treatment plans (Jonas, 2003). In addition, the terms *technician* and *assistant* are being used as job titles for personnel with only on-the-job training.

PHARMACISTS

A pharmacist is a graduate of an accredited program of study in pharmacology and licensed to prepare, compound, and dispense drugs when presented with a prescription from a physician, dentist, or some other licensed practitioners with prescriptive authority. A pharmacist takes an active role on behalf of clients by interpreting, evaluating, and implementing medical orders, assisting providers in making appropriate drug choices, counseling clients, and assuming direct responsibilities collaboratively with other health care professionals and with clients to achieve the desired therapeutic outcome.

MEDICAL SOCIAL WORKERS

Medical social workers help clients and families cope with problems resulting from long-term illness, injury, and rehabilitation. Medical social workers are hired by acute care hospitals, long-term care facilities, hospices, and home health care providers. They often work in clinical settings as case managers to facilitate appropriate client discharge and follow-up care and to ensure proper use of community services. Social workers may have a bachelor's, master's, or doctoral degree in social work; a graduate degree is often required for those engaged in clinical practice. Social workers' licensure and scope of practice are regulated in all 50 states.

SPIRITUAL AND RELIGIOUS PERSONNEL

Pastoral care workers provide spiritual care, which is an integral part of holistic health care. Clients and their families come from diverse religious backgrounds, ranging from Christianity to Taoism, and others practice no formal religion at all. Pastoral care assists the health care team in being receptive to clients' spiritual needs. Larger hospitals may have a department of full-time pastoral care employees to minister to their clients, families, and staff and to provide guidance in ethical decision making.

ALTERNATIVE PRACTITIONERS

Complementary and alternative medicine practitioners use many healing methods, from ancient arts such as traditional Chinese medicine and acupuncture to recently discovered food supplements (Box 4-1). Viewed by many with skepticism and sometimes even labeled as quackery, the use of alternative therapies is growing in typical health care settings. Some think these methods could reduce the need for physicians and therefore the cost of health care. Proponents believe that some forms of alternative medicine may prove to be superior to traditional Western medicine. Nontraditional or alternative therapies include homeopathy, herbal formulas, acupuncture, therapeutic touch, and biofeedback. Even meditation, imagery, massage, spiritual guidance, and prayer are often included in discussions of nonconventional and alternative therapy options. Dietary changes and vitamin supplements have become popular for preventing or treating health problems for several reasons: dissatisfaction with traditional medicine, a desire to manage symptoms not well understood by traditional medicine, and the expectation that we can live longer and better. The lack of definitive research does not seem to deter the marketing of these therapies.

HEALTH CARE SETTINGS

Health care delivery occurs within a continuum of health care settings and services from outpatient to inpatient and from acute care to long-term care. *Inpatient* denotes care given in the context of an overnight stay in a hospital or other facility. Inpatient treatment is provided in long-term care facilities such as nursing homes, psychiatric hospitals, and rehabilitation centers. *Outpatient* services

BOX 4-1

Considering the Alternatives

Complementary, Alternative, and Integrative Therapies in Health Care

Description and History

Complementary and alternative medicine (CAM) is a major industry in the United States, Europe, and other English-speaking countries. CAM incorporates a wide range of products, practices, and health-related activities that are not part of conventional medical treatment. Many of these therapies originated in healing systems from historically or geographically different cultures. *Complementary* means in conjunction with, *alternative* means in place of, and *integrative* means together with; each represents a different viewpoint on the use of nonconventional therapy.

Both the nursing and the medical professions have organizations related to holistic health: the American Holistic Nurses Association (AHNA) and the American Holistic Medical Association (AHMA). This shift in health care on the part of professionals and the lay public coincides with the increasing emphasis on health and with the expansion of health care to include concerns about quality of life and prevention of diseases and disability. Over two thirds of the medical schools in the United States now have courses on CAM.

The National Institutes of Health (NIH), following a mandate by Congress, established the Office of Alternative and Complementary Medicine in the early 1990s. This was upgraded to the National Center for Complementary and Alternative Medicine (NCCAM) in 1998 with the mission of supporting research and disseminating knowledge to the public. In 2002, the White House Commission presented its report recommending continued research, education, and dissemination of information as well as an office to address concerns related to regulating safety, efficacy, and preparation of providers. Some health care organizations are offering CAM to their clients, and some insurance companies now cover select modalities.

1. *Alternative medical systems* are systems of healing, such as traditional Chinese medicine (TCM), Ayurvedic medicine, and homeopathy.
2. *Mind-body interventions* facilitate relaxation and other modalities that might enhance health through the psychoneuroimmunological framework.
3. *Biologically based therapies* include diet modifications, diet supplements, and other biologically based modalities.
4. *Manipulative and body-based methods* include bodywork, massage, and other structural manipulations.
5. *Energy therapies* include magnets, touch therapies, and other modalities known as biofield therapies.

Potential Benefits

Because many complementary therapies act to bolster the body's natural health-promoting capacity, their beneficial effects may be more generalized and more effective. Some may be effective in the early stages of a disease. Others have efficacy in symptom control, such as in reducing pain or side effects of treatments or reducing anxiety and stress. The relationship between a CAM provider and the client may be more engaging, which may explain some of the positive benefits of CAM modalities. NCCAM is currently studying the placebo effect.

Concerns

The first area of concern is lack of proven efficacy and regulation. Much of the evidence for efficacy is antidotal. Some CAM practitioners may exploit or actually harm clients. Others, although well intentioned, have no medical knowledge and thus may inadvertently harm vulnerable clients by giving inappropriate advice. In addition, practitioners may not embrace health care ethics and may violate confidentiality, informed consent, or professional accountability.

A second major concern is that of replacing or delaying effective biomedical treatment. Clients may spend valuable time and resources pursuing CAM treatments and thus fail to get an effective biomedical treatment.

A third area of concern is about the interaction of a CAM therapy with biomedical treatments. Dietary supplements, herbs, and other substances may have a synergistic, cumulative, or counteractive effect with medications. Assessment must include herbs, diet supplements, or over-the-counter medications.

The fourth concern is about the interaction of the CAM treatment and the disease process. For example, using very vigorous bodywork with a client with a clotting disorder could lead to injury.

Resources

Books

Dossey, B., Keegan, L., & Guzzetta, C. (Eds.). (2005). *Holistic nursing: A handbook for practice* (3rd ed.). Boston: Jones & Bartlett.

Micozzi, M. (Ed.). (2006). Fundamentals of complementary and integrative medicine. St. Louis, MO: Elsevier.

Snyder, M., & Lindquist, R. (Eds.). (2006). Complementary/alternative therapies in nursing (5th ed.). New York: Springer.

Journals

Advances in Mind Body Medicine
Alternative and Complementary Therapies
Alternative Therapies in Health and Medicine
HerbalGram
Holistic Nursing Practice
Journal of Holistic Nursing

Websites

Center for Mind Body Medicine, http://www.cmbm.org/
Commonweal, http://www.commonweal.org/
Fetzer Foundation, http://www.fetzer.org
National Center for Complementary and Alternative Medicine (NCCAM), http://www.nccam.nih.gov

do not require an overnight inpatient stay in a hospital or long-term care facility. Outpatient services, also called ambulatory care, include a wide range of services, from routine tests and treatments to complex procedures and therapies. The managed care environment has made outpatient settings increasingly important in the delivery of health care services.

Services based in the community are provided through voluntary, public, or proprietary organizations and include adult day care, respite care, congregate meals, transportation, and case management programs. A variety of funding sources include Medicare, Medicaid, Title II of the Older Americans Act established in 1965, and other federal, state, and local social services programs. The extent of services provided and the eligibility requirements vary by service, funding source, and locality.

HOSPITALS

A hospital is an institution for the medical treatment of ill and injured persons needing a combination of complex services with a high risk of complications and nursing care. Hospital services are appropriate when intensive monitoring is required for the early detection or prevention of complications or deterioration of the client's condition. The need for hospitalization may be based on the risks associated with a medical or surgical treatment. Hospitals offer a variety of inpatient and outpatient services for management of acute and subacute conditions. Services may also include emergency, rehabilitative, and skilled nursing care.

Although some hospitals serve multiple purposes in a community, in general there are three levels of hospitals. The first tier of the hospital system includes the general hospital, the community hospital, and the rural community hospital. The general hospital offers a range of medical, surgical, obstetrical, pediatric, and emergency services. A community hospital serves a specific location (an area of a city, a rural community) or population (women, children, heart patients). Rural hospitals are often more limited in the scope of their services than urban hospitals. Poor economic conditions, isolated rural areas, weather conditions, limited availability of transportation, and long distances affect rural residents' access to health care. Rural hospitals also have difficulty recruiting health care providers such as pediatricians, obstetricians, internists, dentists, and nurses.

The second tier is a larger, usually urban, general hospital with a full range of services, including up-to-date, high-level technical care by specialists. The third tier or tertiary care hospitals are large medical centers that provide the most sophisticated, advanced care and maintain extensive research and teaching programs. Tertiary care centers draw clients from a larger geographical region.

Hospitals are also classified as public or private. Public hospitals are owned by agencies of federal, state, or local government. Federal hospitals are maintained for special groups of federal beneficiaries, such as military and governmental personnel, veterans, and Native Americans. State governments generally limit themselves to operating hospitals intended to safeguard public health by treating mental illness and contagious diseases such as tuberculosis.

Private hospitals are owned and operated by corporations or charitable organizations. As health care grew to be one of the largest industries in the United States, multihospital chains developed in response. The change in reimbursement methods and a need to constrain costs while still providing a variety of health care services forced cost constraints that allowed large corporations to have an advantage over smaller, single-hospital systems.

EMERGENCY AND RESCUE CARE

Ambulance service and first aid treatment to victims of acute illness, accidents, and disasters by trained paramedics and emergency medical technicians (EMTs) are the most common mobile medical services. Paramedics are the highest level of prehospital providers; EMTs are the basic level personnel. Paramedics and EMTs are often the first medical people at the scene of an accident or sudden illness; they give immediate care to heart attack victims, car crash victims, gunshot victims, and poisoning victims. They even assist in childbirth. The sick or injured are then transported to health care facilities in specially equipped emergency vehicles. Most urban centers have developed formal emergency medical systems to provide a quick response to emergencies. Rural areas access medical centers through ambulance services and helicopter medical transport units. Specialized ambulance services, such as cardiac care units and shock/trauma units, initiate complex care at the scene and during transport.

Most hospitals provide some level of emergency services. The hospital emergency department provides services around the clock for clients with emergent problems, as well as services after office hours for other clients. A trauma center has a full range of services for complex trauma victims.

PSYCHIATRIC CARE

In both public and private psychiatric facilities, the number of beds devoted to inpatient psychiatric services has decreased over the past two decades. New treatment techniques, consumer protection laws, and issues of cost are responsible for the shift from inpatient care to community care. However, the result of the shift to community care and the client's right to refuse treatment has been an increased number of homeless people who are not managing their mental illness well.

REHABILITATIVE CARE

Rehabilitation services specialize in providing restorative services to optimize the level of function in chronically ill and disabled clients (Figure 4-1). Clients who are dis-

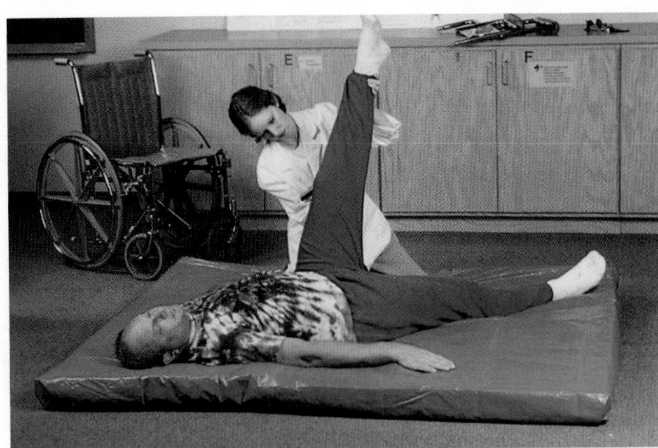

FIGURE 4-1. Rehabilitation hospitals specialize in providing restorative services to rehabilitate chronically ill and disabled people.

charged from a short-term inpatient stay may transfer to a freestanding rehabilitation hospital, a rehabilitation unit in a general hospital, or an outpatient rehabilitation service. Most rehabilitation hospitals offer nursing, physical therapy, occupational therapy, psychological services, social services, and vocational services.

LONG-TERM CARE

Long-term care describes a range of health and housing services provided to people unable to care for themselves independently or in need of assistance to maintain their independence. In addition to traditional nursing home care, options include assisted living facilities, residential care facilities, and retirement centers. Assisted living provides services associated with a resident's activities of daily living. Residential care, also known as sheltered care or board and care, offers some services, such as meals and assistance with taking medicine. Retirement centers offer residents the opportunity to maintain their own lifestyle while having some services available for those who need them.

More than half of the financial support for long-term care comes from public funds such as Medicaid and Medicare. Long-term care is heavily regulated through licensure and certification requirements. The growing industry of long-term care insurance generally provides assistance when the insured needs assistance with one or more activities of daily living on a long-term basis and after a predesignated period.

After a client's hospital stay, Medicare will pay for care for a short period of time when the care can be expected to assist the client in returning to independent living. The care has to include medically necessary services requiring professional nursing skills. Skilled care, as a Medicare level of care, is offered on special hospital units, in nursing homes, and in subacute care hospitals. Subacute care addresses the needs of clients who have recovered from the acute phase of an illness or injury but have ongoing medical needs.

For clients who are unable to care for themselves and have no expectation of improvement, the only source of public funding for long-term care is Medicaid. To receive Medicaid funding for long-term care, the client has to demonstrate financial need. As a result, clients must spend almost all of their resources before qualifying for Medicaid.

HOSPICE

Hospice is a concept that includes a cluster of special services to address the special needs of dying people and their families. It blends medical, spiritual, legal, financial, and family-support services. Hospice is a model of care that regards the client together with the family as the unit of care. It is a concept, not a location. The venue of care can vary from a specialized facility to a nursing home to the client's own home. Services can be organized out of a hospital, a nursing home, a freestanding hospice facility, or a home health care agency. Hospice care is available through Medicare when the client is expected to die within 6 months.

PHYSICIANS' OFFICES

Private physicians working solo, in partnerships, or in private group practices are the dominant providers of outpatient care. The physician's office is the usual setting for most basic outpatient services, such as physical examinations, diagnostic and screening services, minor illness care, medication administration, counseling and advice, and routine treatment follow-up. Today this office is most likely to be part of a group practice or medical clinic complex.

AMBULATORY CARE CENTERS

The ambulatory care center provides health services on an outpatient basis to those who visit a hospital or other health care facility and depart after treatment on the same day. This category covers managed care programs and hospital-based ambulatory services, including clinics, walk-in and emergency services, mobile units, and health promotion centers. Freestanding "surgi-centers" and "urgi- or emergi-centers," health department clinics, neighborhood and community health centers, organized home health care, community mental health centers, school and workplace health services, and prison health services are additional examples of ambulatory care settings.

Mobile medical services take advanced diagnostic services to clients in rural communities in a convenient and cost-effective manner. For example, mobile eye care and dental care units can be brought to a nursing home site or to a workplace, where they can efficiently serve a large number of clients. Mobile diagnostic services include mammography, magnetic resonance imaging, and cardiac assessment and health screening services such as blood sugar, blood pressure, and cholesterol checks.

ADULT DAY CARE CENTERS

Adult day care (ADC) is a daytime program for frail (usually older) adults who require supervision and care while members of the family or other informal caregivers are away at work. ADC is generally a structured, comprehensive weekday program that provides personal care, midday meals, social services, and transportation in a protective setting. It complements informal care given in the home by family members and helps delay or prevent institutionalization. ADC may also work as respite to help reduce caregiver stress. Many ADC programs provide a mix of medical, maintenance, and social-psychological services. Group socialization and recreational activities are important as well.

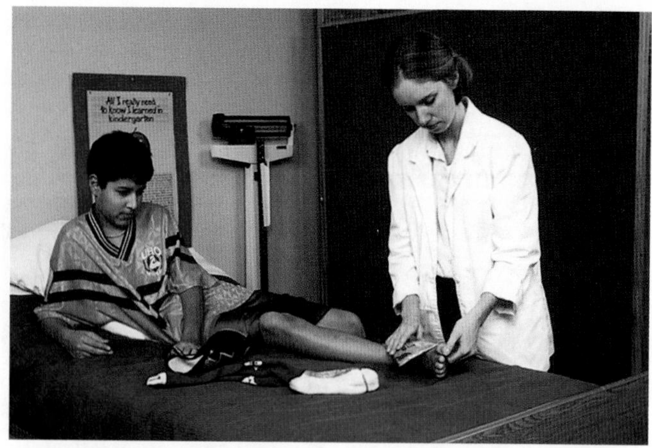

FIGURE 4-2. The work of most school-based health programs is carried out by a registered nurse and is confined to basic first aid, case finding, and prevention of certain chronic or epidemic diseases.

RESPITE CARE SERVICES

Respite care is defined as a service that provides temporary relief to informal caregivers such as family members. Respite care is the most frequently suggested intervention to address family caregivers' feelings of stress and burden. ADC, home health care, and temporary stays in nursing homes, hospitals, group homes, or foster care homes are examples of respite care services or programs. In-home respite care provides temporary homemaker, chore, or home health care services. The focus of respite care, regardless of how it is provided, is to give the client's informal caregiver time off while meeting the assistance needs of frail, older, or disabled chronically ill clients.

SCHOOL HEALTH CLINICS

Almost all educational institutions provide some form of ambulatory health services to students. Services are provided by local health departments or by school boards in conjunction with the local health department.

The work of most school-based health programs is supervised by a registered nurse and confined to basic first aid, case finding, and prevention of certain chronic or epidemic diseases (Figure 4-2). Very little disease treatment is done in the health program of a public school (kindergarten to twelfth grade). Vision and hearing screenings and various immunizations are commonly offered. When indicated, referrals for diagnosis and treatment are made to the student's parents and physician. Colleges and universities provide a broader set of services, including many basic diagnostic and treatment services. In some school settings there are programs to help students deal with mental, physical, and substance abuse problems.

OCCUPATIONAL HEALTH SERVICES

Industrial or occupational health services are provided in most large businesses and factories. The actual number of these "in-plant" health units in the United States is unknown. In smaller firms it may be simply a first aid box; larger firms may provide systematic health services staffed by industrial nurses and part-time physicians. In a few firms the health services are comprehensive, with complete care for all health disorders, whether or not the disorders are work related.

Optimal health accomplished through changes in lifestyle improves the overall health of America's workforce. Work-site health promotion or wellness programs create awareness of health factors, help employees make lifestyle changes, and develop workplace environments that are conducive to health.

HOME HEALTH CARE SERVICES

Home health care services, such as nursing, therapy, and health-related homemaker or social services, are brought to clients in their own homes because these clients are unable to leave their homes safely to get the care they need. Home health care is provided to clients and their families at their place of residence to promote, maintain, or restore health and minimize effects of disability and illness. Home health care services are provided mainly to older adult clients. Seventy-five percent of home health care clients are age 65 or over.

COMMUNITY HEALTH CENTERS

Community health centers concentrate on the delivery of primary health care services to the community as a whole and to individuals. They serve as a primary care safety net for our nation's poor and underserved in both inner-city and rural areas. Community health centers have become expert in managing the health care needs of these special populations. Long-standing outreach programs, case management, transportation, translation services, alcohol and drug abuse screening and treatment, mental health services, health education, and social services are provided to roughly 30% of the country's indigent population served by these centers nationwide.

HEALTH CARE FINANCING

Over the past few decades a complex blend of private and public mechanisms has arisen to affect how Americans pay for health care. Since the early 1980s the basic approach for reimbursing hospitals, physicians, and long-term providers of services has been restructured.

After Medicare, private health insurance has been the most prevalent source of financing for the United States health care system. Insurance is a mechanism created to help protect against risk, and it protects against potential substantial financial loss from a low-probability event. A person protected by insurance against a specific risk is called the insured, and the insuring agency that assumes the risk is the insurer.

However, the term *health insurance* is often used to mean a wide array of health care financing mechanisms, including the "social insurance" of Medicare and the public assistance of Medicaid, the self-insurance plans used by employers, and the managed care programs of health maintenance organizations (HMOs) and preferred provider organizations (PPOs). Clients pay for some of their health care themselves. Persons not covered by either private or government-sponsored health care financing programs are called uninsured. Medicare and private health insurance play an important role in influencing the direction and structure of our nation's health care system.

The American health care system is the most expensive and unique system in the developed world. U.S. citizens spent $5,267 per capita for health care in 2002—53% more than any other country (Anderson, Hussey, Frogner, & Waters, 2005). However, over the years public outlays for health care financing have increased, and private financing has shrunk proportionately. In 2002 the number of people without health insurance was 43.6 million, or 16% of the population (U.S. Census Bureau, 2003). The figures for children show that 11.6% had no health insurance in 2002 (U.S. Census Bureau, 2003); 31% of people in poverty do not have health insurance. The government's share of the nation's health care bill includes 20% of the national budget for Medicare and Medicaid (Congressional Budget Office, 2006). Private resources financed 54% of personal health services, $585 billion in 1997, down from 60% in 1990 (Levit et al., 1998). All of the money to pay for health care services ultimately comes from the American people.

PRIVATE HEALTH INSURANCE

Private health insurance may be purchased by an individual or a group. Group insurance measures the risk for the insured group, resulting in lower premiums for each member. Indemnity (commercial) health insurance reimburses health care providers on the basis of a fee for each health service provided to the insured person. The traditional method of reimbursement was the **retrospective payment system**—that is, the amount of insurance paid was based on the service received. This type of insurance was considered to be catastrophic coverage, thus paying only for major medical events like an automobile accident or major surgery.

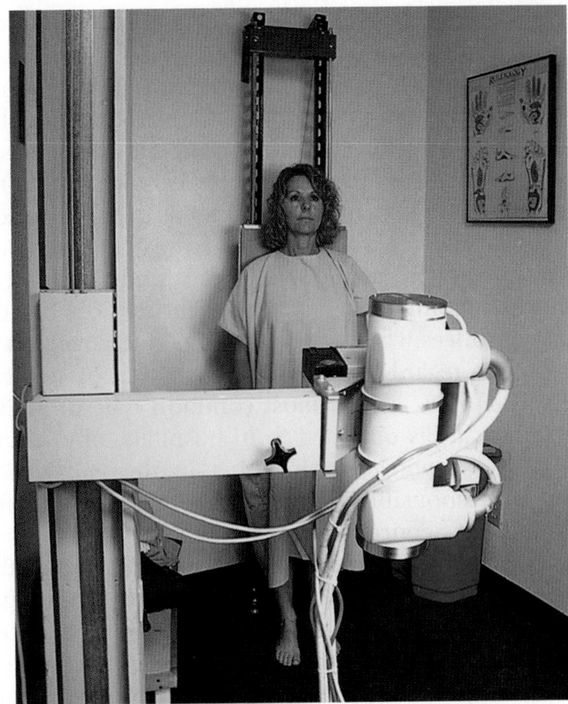

FIGURE 4-3. Under managed care the primary care physician serves as a "gatekeeper" for referral for diagnostic procedures and specialty care.

MANAGED CARE ORGANIZATIONS

Currently, health care coverage is more likely to be administered by a managed care organization (MCO). MCOs were the most significant development in America's system of health care delivery in the twentieth century. **Managed care** is a system that combines the functions of health insurance and the actual delivery of care in a way that controls utilization and costs of services by limiting unnecessary treatment (Shi & Singh, 1998).

Health care delivery under MCOs is designed to affect the operation and structure of the health care system and thus to affect the use of services by the consumer. Managed care attempts to control cost by controlling access to unnecessary care. The opponents of managed care say it limits consumer choice and access, and it involves insurers in the client-provider relationship.

The primary care physician is the "gatekeeper" in the managed care systems. This provider has the coordinating role for the client's health care needs through being responsible for all primary care for the client and determining when referral to specialists is necessary (Figure 4-3). The gatekeeper concept manages the client's use of resources, reduces the self-initiated use of specialty services, and ensures overall coordination without duplication of care.

A **health maintenance organization (HMO)** is a prepaid health plan that delivers comprehensive health care to members through designated providers, has a fixed monthly payment for health care services, and requires members to be in a plan for a specified period of time (usually 1 year). HMOs are a type of group health care practice that provides basic and supplemental health maintenance and treatment services to voluntary enrollees who prepay a fixed periodic fee that is set without regard to the amount or kind of services received. HMOs are the most common type of MCO. All health care is obtained from hospitals, physicians, and other providers participating in the HMO. The HMO is responsible for establishing standards for the quality of services provided.

The **preferred provider organization (PPO)**, the most common type of MCO after the HMO, is an organization of physicians, hospitals, and pharmacists whose members discount their health care services to subscribers (clients). A PPO may be organized by a group of physicians, an outside entrepreneur, an insurance company, or a company with a self-insurance plan. The PPO is the insurance industry's response to the growth of HMOs. PPOs negotiate contracts with companies to lock in the business of treating their employees. The PPO makes contractual arrangements with providers for the delivery of health care services on a discounted fee schedule (Shi & Singh, 1998).

An **exclusive provider organization (EPO)** is similar to a PPO in its organization and purpose, but enrollees are restricted to the EPO's list of providers of health care, called exclusive providers. Like HMOs, EPOs use a gatekeeping approach to health care service delivery as a means of decreasing cost.

GOVERNMENT INSURANCE PLANS

Public financing of health care services accounts for roughly 46% of the total expenditures on health care in the United States. Governmental spending supports *categorical programs* designed to provide benefits to certain groups of people. The most well-known examples are Medicare and Medicaid. Like Social Security, Medicare is an *entitlement program*. Because people have contributed toward Medicare through taxes, they are "entitled" to the benefits regardless of their income and assets. In contrast, Medicaid is a welfare program, in which the level of benefits depends on a person's income and assets. Medicare and Medicaid purchase government-funded services from the private sector.

Medicare is a federally funded national health insurance program in the United States for people over 65 years of age and for some chronically ill persons. Medicare is the first national social insurance program in the United States to finance medical care. Medicare was enacted in 1965 as Title XVIII of the Social Security Act. Health care services are provided for those disabled persons who are eligible for Social Security benefits and for those who have end-stage renal disease. Although there is no monthly fee for Medicare Part A, which pays for hospitalization and some skilled care afterward, the recipient must pay the first $764, and the number of days is limited. For part B coverage, there is a monthly premium and Medicare pays only 80% of the allowable charges. Most people need supplemental insurance. Medicare recipients can participate in an MCO.

Medicaid is the largest health insurer in the United States, covering medical services and long-term care for nearly 40 million people (Centers for Medicare and Medicaid Services [CMS], 2002). It was established along with Medicare in 1965 under Title XIX of the Social Security Act. **Medicaid** is a grant program providing partial health care services for indigent people. Federal and state governments support it jointly. The federal government provides matching funds to the states on the basis of the per-capita income in each state. By law the federal matching dollars cannot be less than 50% or more than 83% of the total state Medicaid program costs.

A **prospective payment system (PPS)** is a payment system in which the amount paid for a specific service is predetermined. This system was implemented for short-stay inpatient hospitalizations (Medicare Part A) in the mid 1980s under the Social Security Act of 1983. The predetermined reimbursement amount is set according to **diagnosis-related groups (DRGs)**, a system of classification or grouping of clients according to medical diagnosis for purposes of paying hospitalization costs. Payment is based on diagnosis and date of discharge rather than length of stay (per diem). Payment is at a rate set for "bundled services." It involves approximately 500 DRGs corresponding to the most prevalent diagnoses found in clients using inpatient services. The PPS has helped Medicare to control the per-case rate of increase for Part A hospital expenditure reimbursement. In the older *retrospective payment system*, payment was determined after the provision of care and was based completely on the costs incurred by the facility.

Another form of prospective payment is a **capitation payment system.** In this system, payment for health care services is an arrangement between the purchaser of care and the provider, and the provider receives a flat fee to provide a defined level of care. The enrollee (insured person) may or may not need the services being covered. Thus the provider theoretically has an investment in keeping the enrollee healthy.

In the United States, health care is not administered or controlled by a central department or agency of the government. However, many other industrialized countries maintain central control of health care delivery. Three types of basic systems are in use.

In the Canadian system, the government finances health care through general taxes, but private providers deliver health care services. Canada's system demonstrates that the use of a national health care budget can be effective in controlling the growth of health care expenditures.

In Great Britain, the government's National Health Service not only finances the program but also manages the infrastructure for the delivery of medical care. Under this system the government operates most of the medical institutions, and physicians in this type of system are employees of the government.

In Germany's system of socialized health insurance, employers and employees finance health care through government-mandated contributions. Private providers deliver health care. Private, not-for-profit insurance companies, called sickness funds, are responsible for collecting the contributions and paying physicians and hospitals.

Generally, the three national health care systems described have common features: (1) every citizen is entitled to a defined set of health care services, (2) national budgets determine total health care expenditures and allocate resources, and (3) the budget limits determine the availability of services and the payments to providers. The governments control the proliferation of health care services, especially those that involve high technology. Resource allocation determines the extent to which the governments can offer citizens health care services (Shi & Singh, 1998).

The United States has long resisted the idea of moving from a private practice model for delivery of health care to a national health plan. However, the issue continues to be discussed. Oregon has led the way in developing a model for a state-administered health care system that guarantees certain basic services to all its citizens. In 1989, the Oregon state legislature passed the Basic Health Services Act, creating the Oregon Health Services Commission (OHSC) (1991). The OHSC defined basic health care as a bottom-line standard for the services to be available to all people. The OHSC created three levels of health care benefits: "essential," "very important," and "valuable to certain individuals." It also developed a priority list of 709 health services (Hadorn, 1991).

Oregon's health plan was originally seen as extreme, but rationing of health care is no longer seen as radical. Every state is struggling to keep Medicaid costs under control. So far, the Medicaid portion of the Oregon plan has been successful, signing up about 126,000 new members since 1994 (Bodenheimer, 1997; Montague, 1997).

Although many people resist the idea of rationing health care, the current system of delivery does in essence ration health care. Instead of being rationed by the state, it is rationed by the HMOs.

ISSUES AND OPPORTUNITIES IN HEALTH CARE DELIVERY

In the last few decades, the United States has experienced significant changes in its demographics, family structures, communities, and lifestyles. Unemployment and poverty clash with rising health care costs, raising many legal and ethical issues related to the distribution and availability of health care services. Nurses support a health care system that assures access, quality, and services at affordable costs (American Nurses Association, 2005).

ISSUES AFFECTING HEALTH CARE DELIVERY

Health Care Disparities. The elimination of disparities in health is a goal of *Healthy People 2010*. For people who live in the right geographical region of the United States, have the right health care coverage, and have a disease on which the health care professionals have chosen to focus, the American health care system is the best in the world. However, the distribution of and access to health care services for the American people is significantly uneven.

Race. There is significant variation in the rates of medical procedures by race, even when insurance status, income, age, and severity of conditions are comparable. Racial and ethnic minorities are less likely to receive even routine medical procedures and experience a lower quality of health services (Institute of Medicine [IOM], 2003). Health care disparities are costly. When care is ineffectively managed or illness is underdiagnosed, avoidable complications increase the cost to the system. Racial and ethnic minorities are less likely to receive high-quality care (IOM, 2003).

Poverty. The uneven distribution of wealth is a contributing factor to the uneven distribution of health care. American workers' wages have stagnated or declined in recent decades. In addition, the wealth and income in the United States are becoming increasingly concentrated in the hands of just a few people, producing a large gap between those who have and those who do not. Over 12% (12.7%) of Americans live below the poverty level. Sixteen percent of children age 5 to 17 years and 20% of children under 5 years are living in poverty. Two of every five Hispanic children and one of every two African American children are poor (U.S. Census Bureau, 2003).

Many Americans living in poverty are the victims of social and environmental ills such as drug addiction, acquired immunodeficiency syndrome (AIDS), crime, and prostitution. Their children likewise suffer from addiction, low birth weight, and resultant mental and physical problems. Women, African Americans, and Hispanics experience poverty at a higher rate than other Americans. Although the socioeconomic status of our nation's older adults (older than 65 years) varies dramatically on the basis of their sources of income and assets, the poverty rate for people age 65 to 74 is 8.4% and 75 or older is 11.1%.

The need for health services for vulnerable populations is closely tied to the economic conditions often produced by their health conditions. Homelessness may result from health problems or staggering medical bills. The treatment of AIDS is an economic hardship even with health insurance. Substance and alcohol abuse are costly experiences crossing all economic and social levels in our country. Women, children, and older adults who are chronically ill, disabled, mentally ill, cognitively impaired, neglected, or abused make up the high-risk categories of vulnerable populations that make increasing demands on society as a whole and on the health care system in particular.

Access to Health Care. Access to health care is an important prerequisite to obtaining quality care. Some access barriers, whether perceived or actual, can result in adverse health outcomes. Clients may perceive barriers to delay seeking needed care, resulting in presentation of illness at a later, less treatable stage of illness. Health care in this country is neither universally available nor universally accessible. There are wide variations depending on residence (urban or rural), health care insurance, economic status, and skill in negotiating the system.

Access to health care is a complex construct representing the personal use of health care services and the structures or processes that facilitate or impede that use. *Realized access* is the actual use of health care providers and services. Whether access is equitable or inequitable depends on what determines realized access. For example, to the extent that they are precursors of need, age, gender, and ethnicity are indicators of equitable access or inequitable access when they determine who obtains access to health care.

Effective access is the link between utilization of health care services (realized access) and health outcomes that include enhanced health status and consumer satisfaction. Evaluating the effectiveness of access involves assessment of health care utilization within the context of predisposing, enabling, need, and health behavior variables. Predisposing variables are factors (such as age, gender, and social support) that could influence a person's health status after treatment. The presence of enabling resources such as health insurance and income can lead to expeditious medical treatment that takes advantage of state-of-the-art technology. Its absence can lead to delays in seeking medical care and result in episodic, fragmented treatment with the potential for a negative impact on outcomes and on satisfaction with the care received.

To help formulate public policy that works to enhance access to health services, consumers need to get involved in the political process. For example, older adults have had a major impact in influencing the political process in our country. As a group they are better educated than ever; organizations such as the American Association of Retired Persons (AARP) have a legislative agenda and their own lobbyists in Washington, D.C., to advance their causes. Their ability to influence legislation and policy relating to specific issues of concern lies in numbers—their voting power. In contrast, the change in work patterns from a blue-collar manufacturing workforce with dwindling union membership to a white-collar, services-based workforce has affected organized labor's ability to influence politicians and has allowed businesses to receive more support for their issues.

Demographic Changes. Changes in the composition of a population are important for the planning of health care services. The age of the population, the contribution of family support systems, and health problems of specific groups affect the need for specific services.

The health care system can expect an increase in the need for services to older adults. The U.S. Census Bureau (2004) estimates that people age 65 and over represented 12.4% of the population in 2000. In the year 2020, it is predicted that approximately 16.3% of Americans will be age 65 years or older, with about 7.3 million age 85 years and older. People in the 85 or older category are the fastest-growing group of the U.S. population. Older adults consume more health care services than the younger population. A growing older adult population will have a serious impact on health care expenditures in the future. By 2020, it is estimated that the proportion of children (age 19 and under) in the population will be reduced from 28.5% in 2000 to 26.6% (U.S. Census Bureau, 2004). The median age of the population in the year 2003 was 36 years (U.S. Census Bureau, 2000). However, subgroups such as Hispanics have a lower median age than the general population.

Families make up 67% of the households in the United States. This figure includes both married-couple families (50%) and other families (17%). Most of the nonfamily households are people living alone, but some were composed of people living in households in which no one was related to the householder. The average household size is 2.61 people (U.S. Census Bureau, 2003b).

Family support systems have declined as America has evolved from a rural economy with large families to a nation of city dwellers with small families often a long distance from their family of origin. The last U.S. Census showed a trend toward increasing urbanization and persistent rural losses. In 2000, 79% of the population lived in urban areas, up from 63% in 1960.

One-parent families continue to increase, contributing to the small average family size. Only 26% of American households with children under the age of 18 years include a married couple. Women living alone head 11.7% of all households in the United States and are likely to be part of the 89% of all households receiving at least one noncash benefit such as Medicaid or food stamps (World Almanac, 1995).

At the same time, there are 25.8 million family caregivers providing $200 billion worth of health care services per year, almost double the annual amount the United States spends on nursing home and home health care. Cutting costs in the health care delivery system will shift the burden of caregiving to an already strained family system (Gordon, 2001).

The changing ethnic composition of the United States is creating a demand for a health care system more responsive to minority population needs. In the United States 11.1% of the people are foreign born, and 17.9% speak a language other than English at home (U.S. Census Bureau, 2003b). Less than 7% of U.S. residents fail to report a specific ancestry. Hispanics, Asians, and Muslims are among the minority groups whose presence is visibly increasing in the United States. There will be a growing demand for health care providers who speak languages other than English and understand the health needs of a multiethnic society. Health care providers currently encounter over 190 different languages.

Lifestyle. The nature of common health problems has changed from primarily acute disease to chronic or "lifestyle" diseases. The major causes of death in the United States are from chronic diseases such as heart disease, stroke, cancer, and chronic obstructive pulmonary disease. One in six deaths in this country is attributable to smoking. Dietary practices have a direct role in 5 of the top 10 causes of death and contribute to 3 more through alcohol abuse. Lifestyle diseases are the result of human behaviors.

In addition, Americans are more vulnerable to health problems from our interactions with other countries. Diseases like Ebola and food-borne illness are easily imported from distant lands. Through global telecommunications and expanding travel, we live in a world of people who continuously exchange ideas and influence each other's national cultures, languages, and lifestyles.

OPPORTUNITY FOR RESTRUCTURING THE SYSTEM

The American health care system will continue to face the challenge of balancing three competing goals—containing costs, improving access to health care services, and enhancing the quality of care. The dehumanization of the reformed and reengineered health care system of the 1990s led to consumer activism in the areas of clients' rights and client safety. Tumultuous change in the health care delivery system requires health care providers, including nurses, to be vigilant to ensure that the level of quality achieved not be left to chance.

For their part, consumers must insist that an adequate mechanism for assessing value and effectiveness of care and services be in place to monitor and report to federal, state, and private sector providers. Consumers must be willing to respond to lack of satisfaction in their health care and health services in the same way they would for any other product or service, if necessary by lobbying for legislation, by legal action, and with media campaigns. Today's consumers are better educated, more aggressive, and not limited to thinking that "the doctor knows best" or that illness prevention is the only way to improve their health and overall quality of life (Box 4-2).

COST OF CARE

The most visible problem in the health care delivery system is how to pay for the increasingly staggering cost of services. In 2003, health care spending in the United States reached $1.7 trillion and was projected to reach $1.8 trillion in 2004, representing 15.3% of the gross national product (CMS, 2003). Major areas of growth in cost include prescription drugs and health insurance. Prescription drugs for older adults and others with certain diseases can be devastating. Although managed care has been effective in decreasing the cost of care, it may have reached the limits of cost savings that can be accomplished with reduction in hospitalization days.

Savings could come through better coordination of care (especially for clients with complex, expensive, or chronic conditions). Case management has the potential to improve coordination for those with continuing health care needs by reducing the fragmentation of the system, promoting consumers' active participation in decisions about their health, and creating an advocate on their behalf.

Savings could come from a wider use of a range of qualified health professionals to increase access to care, especially in primary health care and in underserved urban and rural areas. Consumers could have the option of selecting the most cost-effective provider, such as using advanced practice nurses for primary health care.

Other savings can result from controlling the cost of prescription drugs, controlling the profits of MCOs, controlling expensive litigation, giving individuals and families more power in the system, decreasing the amount of time spent complying with regulations, reducing overhead cost, and reducing the incidence of errors.

To participate in positive changes in the system, nurses must understand the economic forces driving change, the needed evolution to meet the needs of society, and how nursing should respond to fulfill the profession's responsibility to meet the health care needs of society.

Economic constraints and cost-cutting measures exacerbate ethical problems in the delivery of health care. The ever-increasing availability of technology is creating situations that require decision making about who receives what services. These decisions are often made under complex and stressful circumstances (Figure 4-4). Competition pushes health care executives to walk a

BOX 4-2

A Patient's Perspective

"Sad to Say, This May Be as Good as It Gets in Today's Health Care System."

If every pregnancy and childbirth were like my first experience, people would never have big families. As a health science editor, I considered myself well prepared to deal with the health care system, especially during what should be a normal physiological process. Never in my worst nightmares had I imagined what actually happened.

Five months into my pregnancy, I realized I was in the wrong place to get the right kind of care. There was little or no personal interaction or education. If I had a problem or a question, I had to tell it to an answering machine. I decided it was time to take charge and make a change.

On the basis of advice from three different people, I went to a practice associated with the university medical center. They made me feel better instantly. There were five physicians, two nurse midwives, four nurse practitioners, and one maternity triage nurse—what I now know was an ideal situation. Whenever I called with a question or a problem, I talked with a person, not a machine. The triage nurse was always available, either immediately or through her beeper.

At 27 weeks, after being really sick all week, I became dehydrated and went into preterm labor. I was hospitalized and spent 2 days in labor and delivery, terrified that I would lose the baby. At 31 and 32 weeks, it happened again—2 more days in labor and delivery.

When I began having preterm labor every week, my doctor intervened and advised my employer that I needed some flexibility in my work life. Easing my schedule helped a lot; the last month was much easier. In my fortieth week, I went into labor on my way to the office.

During the next 38 hours, I saw every doctor in the practice but only two nurses. One of them stayed with me for the entire last day; she was a saint. I was given epidural anesthesia twice—the first one wore off, and the second was given too close to the time when I needed to push, so I felt like I had no legs; I couldn't push. The baby was stuck, and they had to use forceps. Then whoosh—there she was—the beautiful, perfect baby we had hoped for.

In the first hour after delivery, things began to get confusing. I got very brief instruction in breastfeeding, and then they had to take the baby away because I was in an older, unsecured section of the hospital. Next morning, two different nurses gave me two different sets of instructions for breastfeeding. Finally, the discharge nurse gave me yet another set of instructions about breastfeeding. Baby and I went home Christmas day, a Thursday, and had no success with breastfeeding because all the various recommendations were so conflicting. I was exhausted, confused, and frustrated. The baby was hungry. My breasts were engorged, and a terrible pain was beginning to build in my abdomen.

By Monday the abdominal pain was excruciating, so I went to the clinic and was examined by my least-favorite physician, who diagnosed the problem as constipation or gas and recommended milk of magnesia. Two days later, on New Year's Eve, my temperature was 102.5° F, and I was immobilized by the pain. This time the doctor told me to drink plenty of fluids. Finally, on Friday, I was doubled over in pain, ghostly white, feverish, too weak even to hold my daughter. The doctor said to meet him in the emergency department, which I did at 2 PM. After poking and prodding my tender abdomen, he did an ultrasound but was still baffled. Around midnight he concluded that it might be appendicitis and decided to operate.

Surgery solved the mystery. A fibroid tumor on my uterus had caused the preterm labor; fueled by the pregnancy hormones, my uterus began shrinking, causing the tumor to pull at the appendix until it burst.

I was in the hospital for 5 days after the appendectomy. The surgeon thought it was too soon after delivery to remove the tumor. Each doctor from the obstetric clinic came in to apologize for not diagnosing my problem sooner. During those 5 days, I tried valiantly to maintain my milk supply by using a breast pump (the one they brought in was industrial size!), and it was a real disaster. Not a single medical-surgical nurse could remember how to operate the pump.

Later I made two more trips to the emergency department because the pain just wouldn't stop. The surgeon said the fibroid would have to come out, but I disagreed. Enough was enough. It took a month just to be able to walk again, and 9 months later I still don't have any feeling in my abdomen.

I did go back to breastfeeding for a time, but it was a struggle. After 4 months, I gave up.

I'm an educated health care consumer. I was in one of the best medical centers in the country—certainly the best in the region—but my care left a lot to be desired. Yet I would recommend that hospital and that ob-gyn group because I believe, sad to say, this may be as good as it gets in today's health care system.

fine line between what is good for the business and what is ethical.

ACCESS TO CARE

The American Nurses Association (ANA) advocates for universal coverage at least at the level of a standardized package of essential health care services to be provided and financed through an integration of public and private plans and sources. Furthermore, the ANA says insurance reforms are needed to ensure improved access to coverage, including affordable premiums, reinsurance pools for catastrophic coverage, and other steps to protect both insurers and individuals against excessive costs (ANA, 2005).

The standard package of essential health care services for insurance coverage advocated by the ANA would include the following:

- Primary health care services, hospital care, emergency treatment, inpatient and outpatient professional services, and home health care services
- Prevention services, including prenatal and perinatal care; infant and well-child care; school-based disease prevention programs; speech therapy, hearing, dental, and eye care for children up to age 18; screening

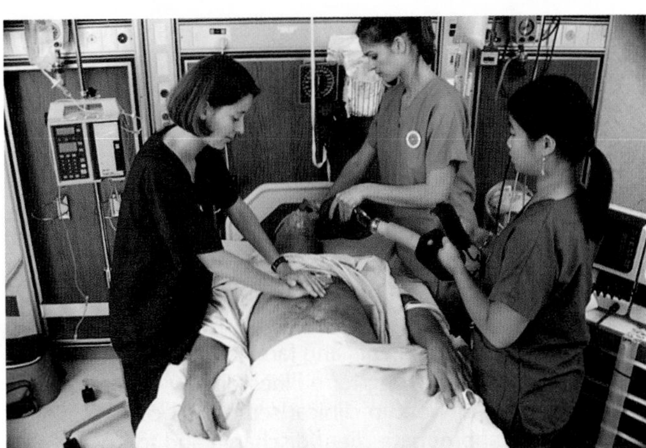

FIGURE 4-4. Modern technology leads daily to situations that require decision making under complex and stressful circumstances.

procedures; and other preventive services with proven effectiveness

- Prescription drugs, medical supplies and equipment, and laboratory and radiology services
- Mental health services and substance abuse treatment and rehabilitation
- Hospice care
- Long-term care services of relatively short duration
- Restorative services determined to be essential to the prevention of long-term institutionalization

The ANA also advocates that the system should be restructured with a direct focus on consumers. Access should include the provision of care in community settings where the consumers live and work. In addition, consumers will be encouraged to assume more responsibility for their own health. Health professionals will work in partnership with consumers to evaluate the full range of their needs and available services. Together, the consumer and the health professional will determine a course of action that is based on an understanding of the effectiveness of treatment.

QUALITY OF CARE

The U.S. health care system is a patchwork of many subsystems loosely connected to provide medical care rather than health care to those who are insured. Although the system is undergoing major changes, most of these are focused on improving delivery of and payment for illness care rather than providing better health care. Reform should look to systems that would integrate services and activities to minimize risks and provide early detection and treatment of emerging diseases. These systems must also place a greater emphasis on wellness and public health for the health care system reform to eventually affect the overall health of the American population.

Technological Progress. The technological advances of recent decades have significantly affected the delivery of health care and its outcomes. Selected developments include computerized clinical laboratory and diagnostic equipment, multiple organ transplants, improved invasive and noninvasive surgical techniques, genetic engineering, and the use of lasers. These advances have allowed the health professions to treat certain conditions more quickly, more safely, and more effectively, with less pain and fewer complications.

In spite of the benefits of "high-tech" equipment and procedures, many fear that they will increase the use of machines and decrease human interaction. It is this fear of depersonalization of health care that is fueling the demand for more humane or "high-touch" care systems, such as hospice care, birthing rooms, and neighborhood clinics. Some high-tech equipment, notably computers, can also be used to increase human contact. For example, electronic mail and Internet services can be used to help people communicate and share information with each other. The use of computers in health care institutions and agencies is likely to intensify. They have become critical to various functions within a health care organization, such as client records, billing and accounting, information processing and retrieval, hiring and staffing, and ordering and tracking supplies.

Unquestionably, computers have helped to improve the delivery of health care services in our country. Integrated computerized systems within health care agencies link a client's care with every department within the facility. Outside the hospital, computer-assisted communication techniques are making speedy transmission of health information and new knowledge a powerful influence in molding public opinion.

Quality Improvement. The growth of managed care with its emphasis on cost containment has prompted the concern that containing costs will diminish and disrupt quality. Differing definitions of quality by clients, providers, and payers translate into different expectations of the health care delivery system and evaluations of its quality. Quality can mean improved health in populations, client satisfaction with the level of care received, reduction in complications that result from errors, reduced death rates, prolonged life, or access to multiple options in care.

The basic goal of the health care system in the United States is to provide those services that will optimize the overall health of the resident population. The key to achieving this goal is the commitment to quality—its assurance, monitoring, evaluation, and improvement. The Joint Commission (TJC) has published standards to help health care organizations continuously improve and meet this basic goal.

The future of our health care delivery system and the quality of its services will depend on the ability of health care professionals to work with consumers, policy makers, and payers. The ethical dilemmas surrounding access, impact of technology, cost versus quality versus amount of service, business orientation of the delivery system, provider turf battles, and availability of alternative health and illness care treatments will challenge everyone to be partners. Professionals, policy makers, providers, payers, and consumers must act in concert with each other to ensure that basic health care services are delivered by a system that acknowledges the ties between quality and the caring interaction.

Environmental Health Challenges. In addition to the behavioral and biological factors that determine health, a complex array of environmental influences must also be considered. Environmental determinants of health can be divided into three components: physical, social, and psychological. In a health context, the physical environment includes hazards such as air, noise, and water pollution, with the potential consequences of hearing loss, infectious diseases, gastroenteritis, cancer, emphysema, and bronchitis. The social environment produces child abuse, homelessness, and drug abuse. The psychological environment produces diseases related to stress.

Social and psychological components of environmental health can be combined to address the major issues of behavior modification, perceptual problems, and interpersonal relationships. Crowded living spaces, physical or social isolation, rapid and persistent change, and increased social interchange may all contribute to homicide, suicide, stress, and environmental overstimulation, which negatively affect the overall health of the individual and the community. Professional nursing must be involved in policy-making decisions that set standards for and controls on responsible agencies and industries. These decisions should be directed toward the control of potential threats to health and safety in our physical environment.

▼ KEY PRINCIPLES

- Until recent decades, the diagnosis and treatment of identifiable disease or illness has largely governed health care delivery in the United States (biomedical model).
- *Health promotion,* aimed at modifying a client's knowledge, attitudes, and skills to adopt behaviors leading to healthier lifestyles, may contribute more to longevity than medical care.
- *Illness prevention* that relies on strategies described as primary prevention, such as immunizations, health screenings, and medications that avert disease, may be more cost-effective than treatment of illness.
- Registered nurses focus on health promotion and disease prevention and are also the major care providers of sick and injured clients.
- Physicians, the major providers of health services, play a central role in the diagnosis and treatment of diseases, illnesses, and injuries.
- The American Academy of Physician Assistants (1996) defines a *physician assistant* as "a member of the health care team who works in a dependent relationship with a supervising physician to provide comprehensive care."
- Allied health workers can be divided into two broad categories: therapists and technologists, and technicians and assistants.
- The role of the pharmacist includes instructing clients about medications, as well as advising physicians and other health care providers about new and complex pharmaceutical management regimens.
- Social workers help clients and families cope with the problems resulting from long-term illness, injury, and rehabilitation. They often work in clinical settings as case managers to facilitate appropriate client discharge and follow-up care and to ensure proper use of community services.
- The term *inpatient* is used in conjunction with an overnight stay in a hospital or other facility. Inpatient treatment is provided in long-term care facilities such as nursing homes, psychiatric hospitals, and rehabilitation centers.
- Outpatient services do not require an overnight inpatient stay in a hospital or long-term care facility, although these institutions may offer these services.
- Managed care is a system that combines the functions of health insurance and the actual delivery of care, where costs and utilization of services are controlled.
- Changes in the composition of a population are important for the planning of health care services.
- Economic markets exist for allocating scarce resources to pay for the provisions of goods and services.
- The U.S. health care system will continue to face the challenge of balancing three competing goals—containing costs, improving access to health care services, and enhancing the quality of the delivered health care services.

■ REVIEW QUESTIONS

1. Your 30-year-old client has come to a clinic for health screening. He has no health problems. You teach him about the importance of a healthy diet and regular exercise. Which health service are you providing?
1. Health promotion
2. Prevention
3. Diagnosis and treatment
4. Supportive care

2. A client is being discharged from the hospital and will need to manage an open wound at home. Which health care worker would be most qualified to provide the teaching?
1. Social worker
2. Nurse
3. Unlicensed assistive personnel
4. Physician's assistant

3. A client has a terminal condition but is not expected to die within the next 6 months. He remains active and can manage his activities of daily living but needs to manage his condition with occasional infusions of intravenous medications. Which type of setting is most appropriate for his care?
1. Home with visits to outpatient clinic for infusions
2. Long-term care
3. Hospice
4. Hospital

4. A client is hospitalized for an appendectomy. He experiences severe hypoglycemia and dehydration postoperatively and has to stay 3 days longer than expected. The hospital is most likely to be paid in keeping with the actual care provided if the payment system is:

1. Capitation
2. Prospective
3. Retrospective
4. By diagnosis-related groups

5. Which of these situations is a measure of realized access to health care services?

1. Fifty percent of persons in a given population who are at risk for heart attacks see a cardiologist once a year.
2. A cardiology clinic performs 500 angioplasties in 1 year.
3. The incidence of heart attacks in a clinic's population is reduced by 10% in 1 year.
4. A cardiology clinic implements a program to increase the use of a preventive medication by 20%.

Bibliography

Alliance for Health Reform. (2004) *Covering health issues: A Source book for journalists.*. Health care costs (Chapter 8). Retrieved from http://www.allhealth.org/sourcebook2004/pdfs/chapter8.pdf.

American Academy of Physician Assistants. (2005). *General information.* Alexandria, VA: Author. Retrieved from http://www.aapa.org.

American Medical Association. (2004). *Physician characteristics and distribution in the U.S.: 2004-2005 edition.* Chicago: Author.

American Nurses Association. (1997). *Position statement: Registered nurse utilization of unlicensed assistive personnel.* Retrieved from http://www.nursingworld.org/readroom/position/uap/uapuse.htm.

American Nurses Association. (2005). *Nursing's agenda for health care reform.* Washington, DC: Author. Retrieved from http://www. nursingworld.org/readroom/rnagenda.htm.

American Nurses Association. (2006). Advanced practice nursing: A new age in health care. Retrieved from http://www.nursingworld.org/readroom/.

Anderson, G. F., Hussey, P. S., Frogner, B. K., & Waters, H. R. (2005). Health spending in the United States and the rest of the industrialized world. *Health Affairs, 24*(4), 903-914. Project HOPE DOI: 10.1377/hlthaff.24.4.903. Retrieved from http://content.healthaffairs.org/cgi/content/abstract/24/4/903.

*Bodenheimer, T. (1997). The Oregon health plan: Lessons for the nation. *New England Journal of Medicine, 337* (9), 651-655.

Centers for Medicare and Medicaid Services. (2004). *The official U.S. government site for people with Medicare.* Retrieved from http://www.medicare.gov/basics/overview.asp.

Congress of the United States Congressional Budget Office. (2006). The budget and economic outlook: An update. Retrieved from http://www.cbo.gov/ftpdocs/74xy/doc/7492/08-17-budgetupdate.pdf.

Division of Nursing. (2003). *Seventh national sample survey of registered nurses.* Washington, DC: Health Resources and Services Administration, Department of Health and Human Services. Retrieved from http://bhpr.hrsa.gov/healthworkforce/reports/rnsurvey/default.htm.

Enthoven, A. C., & Tollen, L. A. (2005). Competition in health care: It takes systems to pursue quality and efficiency. *Health Affairs.* Retrieved from http://content.healthaffairs.org/cgi/content/full/hlthaff.w5.420/DC1.

Gordon, S. (2001). Families on call. *The American Prospect, 12*(1). Retrieved from http://www.prospect.org/print/V12/1/gordon-s.html.

*Hadorn, D. C. (1991). The Oregon priority-setting exercise: Quality of life and public policy. *Hastings Center Report, 21*(3), 11-16.

Hecker, D. C. (2001). *Monthly labor review.* Washington, DC: Bureau of Labor Statistics. Retrieved from http://stats.bls.gov/opub/mlr/2001/11/art4full.pdf.

Institute of Medicine. (2003). Unequal treatment: *Confronting racial and ethnic disparities in healthcare.* Washington, DC: National Academies Press.

Jonas, S. (2003). *An introduction to the U.S. health care system* (5th ed.). New York: Springer.

Leininger, M. M. (2006). *Culture care diversity and universality: A theory of nursing.* Boston: Jones & Bartlett.

Levit, K., Cowan, C., Braden D., Stiller, J., Sensenig, A., & Lazenby, H. (1998). National health expenditures in 1997: More slow growth. *Health Affairs, 17*(6), 99-110.

*Montague, J. (1997). Why rationing was right for Oregon. *Hospitals & Health Networks, 71*(3), 64-65.

National Center for Health Statistics. (1998). *Health United States,* 1995 (Public Health Service Publication No. 96-1236). Hyattsville, MD: Department of Health and Human Services.

Office of Management and Budget (2004).

*Oregon Health Services Commission. (1991). *Prioritization of health services: A report to the governor and legislature.* Salem, OR: Author.

Shu, L., & Singh, D. A. (1998). *Delivering healthcare in America: A systems approach.* Gaithersburg, MD: Aspen.

*Steinbrook, R., & Lo, B. (1992). The Oregon Medicaid demonstration project: Will it provide adequate medical care? New England Journal of Medicine, 326, 340-344.

The world almanac and book of facts. (1994). Mahwah, NJ: Funk and Wagnall.

U.S. Census Bureau. (2000). Fact finder: Profiles of general demographic characteristics: 2000. Washington, DC: U.S. Government Printing Office. Retrieved from http://factfinder.census.gov.

U.S. Census Bureau. (2003a). *Current population reports: Health insurance coverage in the United States: 2002.* Washington, DC: U.S. Government Printing Office. Retrieved from http://www.census.gov/prod/2003pubs/p60-223.pdf.

U.S. Census Bureau. (2003b). *2003 American community survey.* Washington, DC: U.S. Government Printing Office. Retrieved from http://factfinder.census.gov/.

U.S. Census Bureau. (2004). *U.S. interim projections by age, sex, and race, Summary files.* Retrieved from http://www.census.gov/ipc/www/usinterimproj/natprojtab02a.pdf.

U.S. Department of Health and Human Services. *Healthy People 2010.* (2001). pp. 11-16. Retrieved from http://www.healthypeople.gov/About/goals.htm.

U.S. Department of Health and Human Services Centers for Medicare and Medicaid Services (2003). *Centers for Medicare and Medicaid Services.* Retrieved from http://www.cms.hhs.gov/statistics/nhe/projections-2003/t2.asp.

*Asterisk indicates a classic or definitive work on this subject.

Chapter 5 CARING AND CLINICAL JUDGMENT

Media Resources

- Evolve Website http://evolve.elsevier.com/Harkreader/
- Companion CD

Learning Objectives

After studying this chapter, you should be able to do the following:

- Discuss the importance of theory in nursing practice
- Compare and contrast nursing theories about caring
- Differentiate between critical thinking, problem solving, decision making, diagnostic reasoning, and clinical judgment
- Describe the elements of the T.H.I.N.K. model of critical thinking
- Discuss Benner's stages of skill proficiency in nursing practice
- Recognize obstacles to critical thinking
- Describe the five interwoven phases of the nursing process
- Apply the T.H.I.N.K. model to the nursing process

Key Terms

abstract
Benner's stages of skill acquisition
caring
clinical judgment
concept
critical thinking
decision making
diagnostic reasoning
empirical
nursing process
problem solving
theory
T.H.I.N.K. model

This chapter will provide the reader with a beginning understanding of the theories that support the science and the practice of nursing. This content represents the content or the *"what"* of nursing. Discussion of nursing theory is followed by information about critical thinking and clinical judgment and their application in practice. This represents the *"how"* of nursing practice.

THINKING ABOUT NURSING

When we think about the profession of nursing, a set of words and images come to mind: caring, tender loving care, compassion, and an expectation of clinical competence. We might have a historical mental picture of a female nurse dressed in white, wearing a white cap and a flowing navy blue cape with a red cross on it. Although multicolored scrubs and lab coats have replaced the starched white uniforms and caps, the qualities of the nursing profession represented by these historical symbols continue. To understand the source of this mental image, we can try to understand what has guided the development of today's practice of nursing.

In 1859, Florence Nightingale published *Notes on Nursing, What It Is and What It Is Not.* This small but incredibly important volume established nursing as a profession, a profession that provides a kind of caring often equated with motherhood but that is in fact more than and different from that kind of nurturing. Furthermore, nursing has developed as both an art and a science. To explain the relationship between the art and the science of nursing, Parse (1992) defines nursing as a basic science, the practice of which is a performing art. She states that the knowledge base of the discipline is the science of the art, and the performance is the art creatively lived. When you think about how you apply theory—what you have learned in the laboratory and classroom—to a real clinical situation, you as the nurse *perform* the practice of nursing. You do this *creatively,* using both your assessment data and your knowledge base to individualize care for each of your clients and their families. Libster (2001) suggests that how nurses demonstrate caring is the art of nursing.

The science of nursing continues to be a topic of significant debate in the current nursing literature. Simply stated, nursing science focuses on *phenomena* related to human health, such as facts, behaviors, problems, and events that describe a reality. From the description of the phenomena, the concepts present in nursing practice can be named and their relationships described.

A **concept** is an idea, thought, or notion conceived in the mind. It may be *empirical* or *abstract.* **Empirical** concepts can be observed or experienced through the senses. A stethoscope is an example of an empirical concept; it can be seen and touched. **Abstract** concepts are those that are not observable, such as caring and hope. All concepts become abstract in the absence of the object. For example, once you have become familiar with a stethoscope, you are able to see the concept of a stethoscope in your mind without having one physically present. Abstractions such as hope or caring are more difficult to mentally visualize.

Chinn and Kramer (1999) define a **theory** as "a creative and rigorous structuring of ideas that project a tentative, purposeful, and systematic view of phenomena." From their view, theories are *tentative* and therefore open to revision as new information emerges. More simply stated, theories suggest a direction or structure of how to view facts and events. Think about how your view changes when you put on a pair of sunglasses. Nursing theories can be thought of as different colored lenses, each color both affecting and structuring how you perceive your professional practice.

Theories cannot be equated with scientific laws, which predict a given outcome every single time. Laws compose the basis of the natural sciences such as chemistry. However, because nursing is a human science, the rigor and objectivity of the chemistry laboratory are both inappropriate and impossible to duplicate in nursing practice. As the research base from which nursing theories are developed is tested, the predictability of nursing theories will become more reliable.

Theories are composed of concepts and their definitions and of propositions that explain the relationships between the concepts. For example, when Nightingale proposed a beneficial relationship between sunlight and health, she had the beginning of a nursing theory. A complete theory is one that contains context, content, process, and goal (Barnum, 1998). Context is the environment in which the nursing act takes place, content is the subject matter of a theory, process is the method the nurse uses to apply the theory, and the goal is the intended aim of the theory—what the nurse hopes to achieve.

Two major and opposing schools of thought exist in nursing science today. The *received view* is the scientific position, which requires that all truths be confirmed by sensory experiences. It is objective and value free and requires study of the smallest parts of phenomena using the scientific method. In this view, the whole is equal to the sum of its parts. Nursing theories that view human beings as biopsychosocial-spiritual entities are reflective of the *received view* and are considered to be the majority view in nursing practice today.

The *perceived view,* on the other hand, views human beings as irreducible wholes in constant interrelationship with the universe. Nursing theorists of the received view define health as a state of well-being as measured against norms, whereas perceived view theorists view health as something that the client determines it to be. Although the perceived view is currently considered the minority view in nursing practice, it is gaining ground in practice circles and it is widely used in current nursing research.

Nursing theories interpret and explain the reality of nursing, thus guiding practice, education, and research activities for nursing as a profession. When nurses have a theoretical base of knowledge, they have professional autonomy. That is, nurses make decisions on the basis of nursing theory as opposed to always taking direction from another profession. Theory is useful for demonstrating that although nursing is a practice discipline, it is also a profession with a unique body of knowledge. This knowledge base is needed and trusted by society to (1) help individuals, families, groups, and communities retain and promote health and (2) intervene when there is illness and disease. Thus theory underlies both the science and art of nursing.

The concepts of person, environment, health, and nursing are the most recognized organizing realities of nursing theory. These concepts have provided the boundaries and the shared viewpoint that have helped nurses focus their practice over the last half century. Recently, nurse scientists have added caring to this group of concepts. Clarification of caring may broaden the boundaries of nursing and reaffirm our long-standing social directive. **Caring** is to be attentive to or watch over the needs of another person, thus implying responsibility in the context of a human relationship (Figure 5-1).

Nursing theory and research can be viewed as interdependent components of the scientific process. When constructing a theory, the theorist must be knowledgeable about the empirical findings and formalize the available knowledge by validating or verifying knowledge through research activities. A theory is accepted when the consensus of the nursing profession is that the theory provides an adequate description of reality. In the broadest sense, nursing research and theory development are necessary for the continued evolution of nursing as a science.

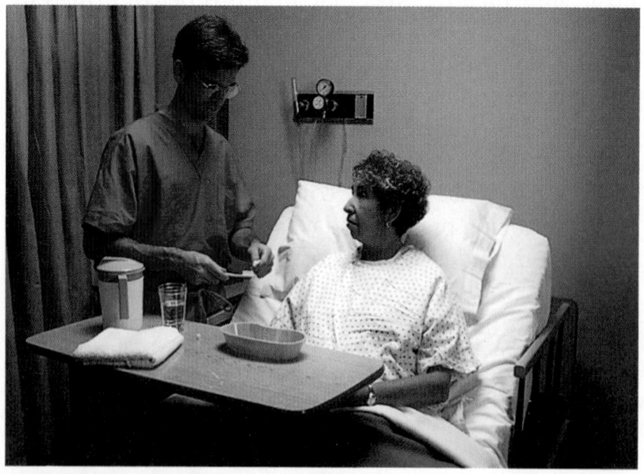

FIGURE 5-1 In entering into relationships with clients, nurses use the self to establish a caring relationship.

HISTORICAL PERSPECTIVE

The following historical perspective gives an overview of the nursing theorists. Although no one of these theorists is recognized as having provided a complete theoretical basis for nursing practice, each has added to our understanding of nursing through explanations of the phenomena of nursing practice. Table 5-1 summarizes the work of selected nurse theorists.

Nightingale. *Florence Nightingale* wrote extensively on what she and other nurses were attempting to do during the Crimean War. She gathered statistics on the death rate in the hospital before and after nurses intervened. She was our first researcher, using statistics to show the effect of nursing care. She was our first theorist, recognizing the importance of the environment and basing her theory of nursing on it. She believed environment included all external conditions and influences that affect life, including ventilation, food, warmth, odors, noise, and light (Nightingale, 1859). Through being supportive and physically present, nurses also enhanced a sense of well-being in suffering clients.

Nightingale created the first formal nursing education curriculum based on her writings. This approach guided nursing education in Great Britain and in America until the mid–twentieth century.

The 1950s. During the 1950s, nursing education was in the early stages of moving into college and university settings, and the scientific basis for nursing practice was developing. There was a need to prepare nurses at the graduate level for positions in nursing administration and education. Columbia University's Teachers College developed graduate education programs to meet these needs, and the first wave of nursing theorists were graduates of these programs. These theorists include Peplau (1988), Harmer and Henderson (1955), Hall (1959), and Abdellah (Abdellah, Beland, Martin, & Matheney, 1960).

The nurse theorists of this era operated from a biomedical model and nursing research. This model focused primarily on what nurses do—that is, their functional roles, and most theorists considered patient problems and needs to be the focus of nursing practice.

However, *Hildegarde E. Peplau* focused on the nurse-patient relationship. She introduced her interpersonal concepts in 1952 and departed from the biomedical model by basing them on several psychosocial theories. Peplau is known as the first to borrow from other scientific fields and to relate the data to nursing theory. Her ideas and theory development are the basis for psychiatric nursing practice and have contributed to all nursing practice. Peplau believed that in the nurse-patient relationship, the nurse assumes many roles: stranger, teacher, resource person, surrogate, leader, and counselor. She also identified four phases of the nurse-patient relationship: orientation, identification, exploration, and resolution.

Virginia Henderson (1966) defined nursing as doing for patients what they would do for themselves if they had the necessary knowledge, will, or strength. Her definition of nursing was adopted by the International Council of Nursing and later by the World Health Organization. Henderson also identified 14 basic patient needs that define the components of nursing care. From Henderson's perspective, nursing has the basis for a comprehensive and systematic approach to care. Henderson's basic needs have evolved into nursing diagnoses as we use them today.

However, Henderson's model did not seem to adequately include the "caring" component of nursing. *Lydia E. Hall* (1959) presented her theory of nursing by drawing three interlocking circles, each circle representing a distinct aspect of nursing: care, core, and cure. This is the first theoretical model that speaks specifically to the concept of caring. Hall defined the care circle as representing the nurturing component of nursing. She further defined nurturing as the care and comfort of the person and the provision of the person's teaching and learning activities.

Faye G. Abdellah and her colleagues (1960) laid the foundation for a process of critical thinking in nursing practice when they developed a problem-solving approach to deal with the 21 nursing problems they had identified in clinical practice. Nursing practice changed when her book, *Patient Centered Approaches to Nursing,* was published in 1960. Its list of nursing problems outlined everything nurses did, from improving nutrition to increasing comfort. This approach built on Henderson's model and formed the basis for the nursing process as a way of approaching nursing care problems.

The 1960s. In the 1960s, theories of nursing roles moved from a focus on problems (or needs) and function, to a focus on the relationship between the nurse and the patient. In these theories the process (between nurse and patient) of nursing is as important as the procedures and practices. Here the interest is not only how nurses practice but also how patients perceive their situation and the effects of nursing on that perception. Theorists representative of this era include Henderson (1960, 1966), Orlando (1961/1990), and Levine (1967, 1996).

In 1961, *Ida Jean Orlando* suggested that all nurses use interpersonal relationships to meet the needs of the patient as defined by that patient, not as defined by the nurse. Orlando also introduced the nursing process as a tool for nursing practice. She delineated automatic actions and deliberate actions from the three elements of a nursing situation: patient behavior, nurse reaction, and nursing actions. The patient became more important as a member of the health care team.

Building on work of earlier theorists, *Myra E. Levine* (1967) further developed the idea of a comprehensive approach to patient care and hypothesized the mechanism of the relationship of nursing actions to improved patient health. She suggested that the focus of all nursing actions is to conserve the patient's energy, structural or physiological integrity, personal integrity, and social integrity. Based on Levine's nursing activity analysis, these four components became *four conservation principles* used by nurses to help patients adapt to the environment. She presented the patient holistically and as the center of nursing activities.

The 1970s. In the 1970s, new theories were developed to explain the unique nature of nursing and to provide holistic caring for clients (as opposed to patients) of all backgrounds. These theories elaborated on previous ones to provide increasingly complex explanations of the practice of nursing. Theorists included Rogers (1970), King (1971), Orem (1971), Neuman (1974), Roy (1976), Paterson and Zderad (1976), and Newman (1979).

The theories presented in this decade were diverse. One group furthered the holistic approach to nursing

Table 5-1 Overview of Selected Nursing Theory

THEORIST	KEY DATE	CONCEPTUAL FOCUS OF THEORY
†Nightingale	1859	Environmental manipulation crucial to health and the client's ability to regain health
†Peplau	1952	Nurse-client therapeutic relationship; the basis for interpersonal psychiatric nursing
†Henderson	1955	Known for her definition of nursing and for the identification of 14 basic needs of clients
†Hall	1959	Nursing represented as core, care, and cure
Orlando	1961	Emphasizes the reciprocal relationship between client and nurse using nursing process
†Rogers	1970	First perceived-view theorist; the science of unitary humans continuously exchanging energy with the universe
King	1971	Nursing as a system; decision-making process and outcomes of mutual goal attainment are specified for nurse-client interactions
Orem	1971	Delineation of the need for nursing care that comes from a client's self-care deficit
Neuman	1970	Nursing as a system, with the client seen as a system functioning in relation to environmental influences
Roy	1976	Clients exist through adaptation to a changing environment, with the nurse as a regulatory mechanism in situations of health and illness
Parse	1981	Man-living-health theory, perceived-view theory that became the theory of human becoming in 1992

†Deceased

practice. Rogers and Newman introduced the concept of human beings as irreducible energy fields, the first of the perceived-view theorists. King, Roy, and Neuman based their theories on general systems theory.

Other groups expanded on the importance of the nurse-client relationship. Paterson and Zderad based their theory on existential philosophy, and Watson addressed the nurse's role of caring and healing as it pertains to sustaining humanity and wholeness.

Martha E. Rogers (1970) saw human beings as dynamic energy fields integral to or interwoven with environmental fields, both identified and recognized by their pattern, existing in a multidimensional universe. Rogers's theory of unitary human beings focuses on integration of humans with environment and the interrelationships of energy fields. Her theory is well known for capturing the complexities of interactions between nurse, client, and environment. She emphasized that nursing was not something a person does but a body of abstract knowledge, a learned profession that is both science and art. Rogers's theory was revolutionary and provided the foundation for a large body of research.

Betty Neuman (1974) introduced a comprehensive conceptual model for nursing that is based on a "systems" point of view to evaluate nursing problems. She views the client as a system functioning harmoniously in relation to environmental influences. The focus of this model is the stability of the client system as it encounters stressors in the environment. The goal of keeping the client system stable is achieved through nursing actions derived from prevention measures.

The work of *Imogene M. King* (1971) can be categorized as a systems model derived from three dynamic interacting systems: personal systems or individuals, interpersonal systems or groups, and social systems or society. King defines nursing as a human interaction process between nurse and client, who communicate to set goals, explore actions for reaching the goals, and then agree on which actions are to be used. Her theory of goal attainment highlights the importance of the decision-making process and the outcomes of nursing care.

Dorothea E. Orem (1971, 2001) defines nursing as a human service and theorizes that the special concern of nursing is assisting people in achieving self-care. Orem's focus is primarily on the needs of the client and the actions of nursing to meet those needs. Her theory of self-care maintains that nursing care is needed when people are affected by limitations that do not allow them to meet their self-care needs. According to Orem, the need for nursing care stems from a client's self-care deficit.

The adaptation model of *Sister Callista Roy* (1976) views humans as biopsychosocial beings who exist through adaptation within an environment. Her model combines divergent thinking, such as systems, stress, and adaptation, into a convergent view of a client interacting with the environment. Roy's model differentiates nursing from medicine by focusing its activity on client adaptation as opposed to health or illness alone.

Josephine G. Paterson and *Loretta T. Zderad* (1976) introduced the theory of humanistic nursing. This theory relates to nursing practice that is developed from the lived experiences of the nurse and the person receiving care. It is based on existential thought.

Margaret Newman (1979) describes health as expanding consciousness. She views health as a fusion of disease and nondisease. She defines nursing as caring in the human health experience and believes that caring is a moral imperative for nursing.

The 1980s. As it now had a solid theoretical base, nursing knowledge was able to grow rapidly in the 1980s. Many nursing theories were revised on the basis of research findings that refined and expanded them, and new theories were developed. The works of Johnson (1980), Leininger (1980), Parse (1981), Erickson, Tomlin, and Swain (1983), Benner (1984), and Eriksson (1987) developed from the perspective of previous nursing theory and began the process of connecting theory to practice.

In fact, by 1988, the theory of nursing was sufficiently advanced to warrant its own scientific publication, and *Nursing Science Quarterly* debuted. This journal, edited by Rosemarie Rizzo Parse, is devoted exclusively to the presentation of nursing theory and research based on nursing theory.

Building on the systems theory approach, *Dorothy E. Johnson* (1980) presented a behavioral system model in which the various parts of the system strive to achieve balance. She believes that each individual has patterned, purposeful, repetitive ways of acting that compose that person's behavioral system. She identified seven subsystems. The role of the nurse in this model is to foster balance, or equilibrium, in the individual.

Madeleine M. Leininger (1980) expanded on the theme of the importance of care in the nurse-client relationship. She believes that caring is the central theme in nursing knowledge and practice. Educated in cultural and social anthropology, Leininger states that caring varies among cultures in its processes and patterns, is largely culturally derived, and is culturally expressed. Her theory of transcultural care focuses on culture-specific and culture-universal nursing practices. She identifies culture as the broadest and most holistic way to view, understand, and be effective with people.

In 1981, *Rosemarie Rizzo Parse* presented her theory of man-living-health. This theory is based on existential-phenomenological philosophy and the work of Rogers (1970). Parse's theory is an example of the perceived view, in which the whole person is in constant and dynamic interaction with the universe. The goal of nursing is quality of life from the client's perspective. In 1992, Parse changed the title of her theory to the "human becoming" (Parse, 1992), and in 1998 she stated that her theory has evolved into the human becoming school of thought.

Helen C. Erickson, Evelyn M. Tomlin, and *Mary Ann P. Swain* (1983) explained the role of the nurse. Their theory of modeling and role modeling requires the nurse to assess (model), plan (role model), and intervene on the basis of the client's perspective of the world. At all times the nurse respects the client's self-care knowledge and assists the client in accessing and using self-care resources.

The phenomenological theory of *Patricia Benner* describes caring as a common bond between people situated in a meaningful relationship. This situation is essential to nursing. Skill and skilled practice, as defined by Benner (1984), refer to skilled nursing interventions and clinical judgment skills in actual clinical situations. She sees clinical nursing practice in terms of nurses making a positive difference by being in the situation in a caring way. Further development of this research led to an interpretive theory of nursing practice that she (together with Wrubel) explained in *The Primacy of Caring: Stress and Coping in Health and Illness* (1989). The primacy of caring is concerned with helping clients cope with the stress of illness. Benner is credited with helping us understand the decision-making process in nursing. Table 5-2 summarizes the work of those theorists who focus on caring.

Jean Watson (1988), in her philosophy and science of caring, wrote that caring must be central to nursing practice to preserve human dignity and humanity. As a moral ideal, nursing practice is based on humanistic or altruistic values in the development of a helping-trust relationship between the nurse and the client. Watson's theory includes 10 *carative factors* that represent both feelings and actions pertaining to the nurse and the client and that include elements to be felt, experienced, expressed, and promoted by every nurse. Examples of carative factors include developing a helping-trusting, human caring relationship with the client and the instillation of faith-hope. Her theory contributes to nursing by sensitizing nurses to humanistic aspects and caring.

Katie Eriksson is the author of the theory of caring science. Eriksson belongs to the Finland-Swedish minority in Finland, and her native language is Swedish (Lindstrom, Lindholm, & Zetterlund, 2006). The emphasis of caring science is the phenomenon of caring, and the aim has been to create a humanistically oriented caring science. Eriksson's theory of caring science integrates both religion and spirituality. Her theoretical assumptions (Box 5-1) demonstrate this integration. The leading idea of caring science is to alleviate human suffering and to preserve and safeguard life and health. Eriksson clearly states, however, that the core of caring is not primarily tied to a specific discipline (2002).

Table 5-2 Caring-in-Nursing Theorists

THEORIST	DESCRIPTION OF THEORY
Nightingale, 1859	Caring provided by trained nurses is more than and different from the nurturing provided by mothering. Nursing care involves the environment to the benefit of the client's health.
Leininger, 1978-present	Caring is the central theme in nursing knowledge and in culture-specific and culture-universal nursing practice (now known as the theory of culture care diversity and universality).
Watson, 1979-present	Theory of transpersonal caring seeks to connect with and embrace the spirit of the client through processes of caring and healing. From the original 10 carative factors have emerged 10 caritas processes that guide nursing practice. Watson ties the future of nursing to Nightingale's sense of "calling," a sense of deep commitment to human service (Watson, 2001).
Benner, 1984-present	Describes caring as a common bond between people in a meaningful situation, which is essential to nursing.
Eriksson, 1987-present	Caring science focuses on the phenomenon of caring, not on the profession. Caring implies alleviating suffering in charity, love, faith, and hope. Natural, basic caring is expressed through tending, playing, and teaching in a caring relationship (Eriksson, 2002).
Swanson, 1991-present	Caring is defined as a nurturing way of relating to a valued 'other' toward whom one feels a personal sense of commitment and responsibility. Caring consists of five processes: knowing, being with, doing for, enabling, and maintaining belief (1991).
Boykin and Schoenhofer, 1993-present	Caring nursing is living in caring and growing in caring. "The intention of nursing as a practice discipline is nurturing persons living in caring and growing in caring" (Boykin & Schoenhofer, 2001, p. 393).

The 1990s. In the 1990s research studies that tested and expanded nursing theory were numerous. In addition to those discussed below, eleven nurse-theorists refined and republished their theories.

Kristen Swanson conducted extensive research on the nature of caring in nursing and has derived a middle-range theory of caring. Swanson defines caring as "a nurturing way of relating to a valued other toward whom one has a personal sense of commitment and responsibility." She describes five processes that are essential to caring for another person:

1. *Maintaining belief:* Conveying to another person that there is a personal meaning to be found in his or her current situation. It includes a commitment to "stick with" the person, conveying hope and optimism.

BOX 5-1 *Basic Assumptions of Eriksson's Theory*

1. The human being is an entity of body, soul, and spirit.
2. The human being is fundamentally a religious being, but all human beings have not recognized this dimension.
3. The human being is fundamentally holy. Human dignity means accepting the human obligation of serving with love, of existing for the sake of others.
4. Health means a movement in becoming, being and doing, and striving for integrity and holiness which is compatible with bearable suffering.
5. The basic category of caring is suffering.
6. The basic motive of caring is the *caritas* motive.
7. Caring implies alleviating suffering in charity, love, and hope. Natural basic caring is expressed through tending, playing, and teaching in a sustained caring relationship.
8. Caring relationship forms the meaningful context of caring and derives its origin from the ethos of love, responsibility, and sacrifice, that is a caritative ethic.

From Eriksson, K. (2002). Caring science in a new key. *Nursing Science Quarterly, 15*(1), p.62

2. *Knowing:* Striving to understand a person's situation, seeking information and cues. It involves avoiding assumptions and establishing a partnership.
3. *Being with:* Being present and actively listening to another person without quickly jumping to conclusions. It conveys the belief that what happens to another matters.
4. *Doing for:* Doing for others what they would do for themselves if they were able. It consists of setting up opportunities for people to problem solve or perform well.
5. *Enabling:* Enabling others to practice self-care. It includes informing, coaching, assisting, and supporting another person.

Ann Boykin and *Savina Schoenhofer* (1993) proposed their theory in their book, *Nursing as Caring.* They view caring as a process of daily becoming, not a goal to be attained. The basic premise of this theory is that all persons are caring. Caring is living in the context of relational responsibilities—for self and others. At the heart of the caring relationship is the importance of the person-to-person connection. The focus of nursing is "nurturing persons living in caring and growing in caring" (1993). Nursing is the response to the human need to be recognized as a caring person.

ADVANTAGES OF MULTIPLE THEORIES

There were alternative viewpoints as nursing evolved as a profession. Some believed that nursing used only borrowed theory—that is, borrowed from other disciplines. Other nurses demanded that the profession create its own research methods and knowledge so that nursing concepts would be unique. Today we recognize that no discipline owns knowledge. Therefore nursing uses knowledge from other fields and shares knowledge with other disciplines.

What you as a nurse observe, document, choose as an intervention, and evaluate depends on the theoretical perspective that guides your nursing practice. Having more than one theoretical perspective increases your options and choices. The more ways you can analyze the needs of a particular client, the more potential there is for seeing different needs.

A FEW THOUGHTS ON CARING

For centuries, caring has been synonymous with the profession of nursing. In 2002, Johnson & Johnson launched a media campaign designed to attract more people into the nursing profession using the slogan "Dare to Care." The campaign's central theme is that nurses have opportunities to touch lives in special ways by offering care and caring. Johnson & Johnson has continued this effort; see http://www.discovernursing.com.

Barnum (1998) eloquently discusses caring as an ideology for nursing. She states that there is general agreement that nurses are caring people, but the fact that most nurses act in a caring way is different from asserting that the *act of caring* is at the heart of nursing practice. Barnum goes on to explain that nurses disagree on just what *caring* means. It is an ambiguous term, having at least three different meanings. The first meaning is *taking care of* in the sense of tending to the needs of another. Taking care of is expressed in nursing actions to meet client needs. This meaning is reflective of motor activity, of doing something for.

The second definition that Barnum (1998) discusses is the notion of *caring* as an emotion or attitude that occurs in the nurse in relation to the client. The nurse who "cares" is one who is emotionally invested in the client's welfare, who has a positive concern for the client. This meaning is affective in nature in contrast to the first meaning, which was labeled as motor activity. Libster (2001) expands on this theme by stating that demonstrating care to another human being involves effective communication. She states that although some people really appreciate a comforting word, others need to feel and see the demonstration of caring feelings. They perceive caring through gesture, posture, and body language more than through words.

Barnum (1998) states the definition of caring involves *caution,* of *being careful* to do something correctly. This meaning contains a sense of guarding against harm or injury. In this sense caring has to do with safety and precision in one's acts. This meaning is cognitive; it speaks to the nurse's having the knowledge base to provide clinically competent care to a client.

Barnum (1998) contends that a nurse may take care of a client, with a caring attitude, while being careful to ensure that things are done correctly and competently. Thus all three senses of caring may occur simultaneously. She later describes a personal experience as a client where the caring attitude of her nurse did not in any way compensate for clinical incompetence. One might consider that ideally *all* three senses of caring *should* occur simultaneously in professional nursing practice.

Kyle (1995) presented of a review of quantitative and qualitative literature on caring and concluded that caring is complex phenomenon involving more than a set of caring behaviors. It is a process including moral, cognitive, and emotional components that is culturally derived. She reports that the studies on caring highlight a marked difference between clients' and nurses' perceptions of caring. She concludes that although caring has been most often studied from a quantitative approach, a qualitative approach is the preferred method to study the concept of caring.

Swanson (1999) conducted a meta-analysis of literature about caring in nursing science and created a hierarchical structure of five levels of studies: capacity of caring, concerns and commitments underlying caring, conditions inhibiting or enhancing caring, caring actions, and consequences of caring. She suggested that future discussion and research about caring be oriented around these five theoretical themes.

In a concept analysis of caring, Brilowski and Wendler (2005) continue to report that the concept of caring remains ambiguous. Their findings suggest that the core attributes of caring are: *relationship, action, attitude, acceptance,* and *variability.* Factors such as trust, rapport, understanding of self and other, and commitment were identified as antecedents and need to be present for caring to occur. The consequences of caring include an increased ability to heal for clients and an increased sense of personal and professional satisfaction for nurses. These are important and significant consequences!

Fahrenwald et al. (2005) state that caring is a multidimensional concept that is best demonstrated by a nurse's ability to embody the five core values of professional nursing. Core nursing values that are essential to nursing education include human dignity, integrity, autonomy, altruism, and social justice (American Association of Colleges of Nursing [AACN], 1998).

CRITICAL THINKING AND CLINICAL JUDGMENT

The theoretical basis of nursing practice affects how we think about nursing situations. The extent to which your critical thinking and clinical judgment is derived from nursing theories determines the unique contribution you make to health care. As health care becomes more complex, nurses must exercise increasingly complex thinking skills. Indeed, the body of knowledge that nurses need is increasing at such a rate that it is impossible to succeed in nursing simply by applying standardized responses. Even clients who have common needs express those needs in highly individualized ways. Consequently, critical thinking is an important and integral part of nursing practice.

Because critical thinking is an abstract concept rather than something you can observe and measure, defining it can be somewhat difficult. In fact, a number of respected scholars have created different definitions of the critical thinking process. However, all of these definitions include thinking skills that you can learn, practice, and integrate into your nursing care. Using these critical thinking skills will result in sound decisions, safe practice, and creativity in addition to promoting the well-being of your clients.

THE LANGUAGE OF CRITICAL THINKING

Critical thinking is defined as purposeful, self-regulatory judgment that gives reasoned and reflective consideration to evidence, contexts, conceptualizations, methods, and criteria (Facione, 1990). Richard Paul for the Center of Critical Thinking defines critical thinking as "Thinking about your thinking while you are thinking, in order to improve your thinking" (Paul & Heaslip, 1995). Consistent themes in definitions of critical thinking include the following:

- The importance of a good foundation of knowledge, including formal and informal logic
- The willingness to ask questions
- The ability to recognize new answers, even when they are not the norm and not in agreement with preexisting attitudes (Jackson, Ignatavicius, & Case, 2006).

Snyder (1993) differentiates critical thinking from regular thinking by defining critical thinking as "the ability to solve problems by making sense of information using creative, intuitive, logical, and analytical mental processes . . . (and the process is continual)." This definition defines critical thinking as a whole brain operation, using both the right (creative and intuitive) and the left side (logical and analytical) as well as a continuous process.

Critical thinkers examine all elements of a situation and think through alternative strategies to achieve an end. The goal of critical thinking is not to devise a single solution but rather to envision a number of scenarios that could occur depending on actions taken or not taken. Rather than one right answer, critical thinkers determine a number of possible outcomes. They use creativity to overcome barriers (Figure 5-2). Built on the nurse's knowledge, clinical experience, and intuition, critical thinking takes a holistic approach to the client.

Embedded in the broad concept of critical thinking are several more specific thinking skills, including

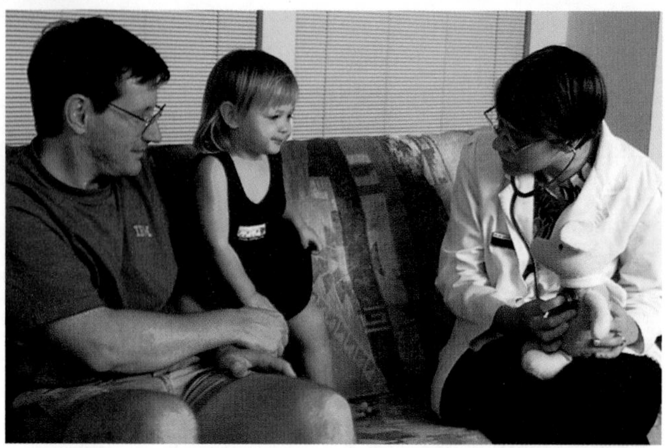

FIGURE 5-2 A nurse adept at critical thinking uses creativity to overcome barriers to quality nursing care.

problem solving, decision making, diagnostic reasoning, and clinical judgment. Typically, all of these processes take place within the framework of the nursing process.

Problem solving is defining a problem, selecting information pertinent to its conclusion (recognizing stated and unstated assumptions), formulating alternative solutions, drawing a conclusion, and judging the validity of the conclusion (Watson & Glaser, 1964). Problem solving is a process used to arrive at an answer or a solution. There is an implied gap of information or action that must be bridged to arrive at the solution. There is also the expectation that the solution be "right" according to a particular standard of measure.

Decision making involves choosing between two or more options as a means to achieve a desired result. Typically, the decision is goal directed, in which case the goal or goals direct the outcome. For example, if you were to plan a dinner party, your menu (goal) would direct your decisions in grocery shopping and food preparation. Decision making in the clinical setting yields approaches for nursing care selected from a variety of possible nursing interventions. You must decide which intervention(s) will be most likely to achieve the desired client outcomes.

Diagnostic reasoning is the process of clustering assessment data into meaningful sets and generating hypotheses about the client's human responses. Diagnostic reasoning can be carried out as a deliberate, conscious activity, or it may occur intuitively with little conscious awareness.

Clinical judgment is a conclusion or an opinion that a problem or situation requires nursing care. It includes determining the cause of the problem, distinguishing between similar problems, and discriminating between two or more courses of action.

The **nursing process** is a critical-thinking framework in which you will exercise decision making, diagnostic reasoning, problem solving, and clinical judgment. It is composed of five interwoven phases: assessment, diagnosis, planning, intervention, and evaluation. Although the nursing process is sometimes criticized as being linear or unidirectional, it is more appropriately thought of as a dynamic, constantly interactive process, where new client data and feedback continuously affect each phase. The nursing process provides a framework to guide you to thinking critically in the clinical setting.

THINKING ABOUT THINKING

To improve your ability to think critically, you need to examine how you think. Thinking about thinking means bringing your mental activities to conscious awareness. It means recognizing the thinking patterns that you use in different situations and evaluating the effectiveness of those patterns in achieving desired results. It means understanding yourself and the elements included in your thinking.

Thinking involves multiple mental functions grouped into two broad categories:

- Taking in information
- Using information to make decisions

Information is perceived through the five senses and stored in the brain. Storing information requires that the information be processed into meaningful patterns so that it can be retrieved or used in some way. The ways in which you process and understand information form your basic functions of thinking.

People have different preferences for processing information, and they seem to create meaning from information more efficiently when they receive it in the manner that most closely matches their preference. For example, some people process information best when they see it (visual learners), whereas others process information best when they hear it (auditory learners). Think about how you learn best. You may find that you learn better if you have both visual and auditory cues.

Thinking is ever changing. Before beginning to read this chapter you may have *thought* about the other choices you have for this period of time. You also may have *thought* about whether you would sit at your desk to read or sit in a comfortable chair. You might have *recalled* that a study-skills teacher told you that concentration improves when you study in one place consistently. Making a decision about each of the options requires thinking. Likewise, every action you will take in nursing practice requires thinking. Clearly, understanding your thinking process will enhance that thinking.

Thinking occurs on more than one level of awareness. Sometimes we consciously think by saying to ourselves that a problem must be solved, a decision must be made, or simply that we will pay attention to a symphony. In any event, cognitive activity is occurring in the brain. Appreciating a symphony is a more passive activity than decision making. However, even when you are making a decision consciously, adaptive unconscious activity is also going on in your brain to influence the decision. Gladwell (2006) states that the study of the adaptive unconscious is one of the important new fields in psychology. In this field, the adaptive unconscious is thought of as a kind of giant computer that quickly and quietly processes a lot of data. Gladwell suggests that when you walk out into a street and suddenly realize that a car is bearing down on you, you do not think through your options, you just act. In this sense the brain is able to make very quick judgments based on very little information.

New ideas about exercising the brain can be found at www.keepyourbrainalive.com. At this site, two behavioral psychologists suggest over 83 exercises for "neurobics." They suggest doing habitual tasks in different ways to form new brain pathways. An example would be taking a shower with your eyes closed. Try this site!

THE T.H.I.N.K. MODEL

Nursing educators Rubenfeld and Scheffer (1999) propose a critical thinking model, the **T.H.I.N.K. model**, that incorporates five modes or processes of thinking that occur in combination or simultaneously. Whereas some situations may seem to require only one mode of thinking, the authors emphasize the importance of effectively using all of the thinking modes. Together, the five modes constitute a broad definition of critical thinking. You can use the mnemonic device T.H.I.N.K. to help remember them (Box 5-2).

BOX 5-2 *The T.H.I.N.K. Model*

T = Total Recall
H = Habits
I = Inquiry
N = New Ideas and Creativity
K = Knowing How You Think

From Rubenfeld, M. G., & Scheffer, B. K. (1999). *Critical thinking in nursing: An interactive approach.* Sudbury, MA: Jones and Bartlett. Retrieved from http://www.jbpub.com. Reprinted with permission.

Total Recall. Total recall involves remembering facts, such as names, dates, normal values, and telephone numbers. Thinking based on total recall is useful when you want to dial a phone number, drive to work, perform a nursing procedure, or obtain complete information during a client interview.

How total your recall is depends on your memory and how you process information into memory. One way to increase recall is to put information into patterns of similar or related items. Telephone numbers in the United States—a three-digit area code, a three-digit prefix, and a four-digit number—use a pattern that is easier to remember than a string of 10 numbers. Similarly, grouping clinical data into patterns can help you remember the data.

Another way to aid total recall is to attach significance to a fact by relating that fact to an experience (Rubenfeld & Scheffer, 1999). You may remember how to give an injection to a client at your clinical setting because you practiced injection techniques in the learning laboratory. One of the most important aspects of nursing education occurs in the clinical setting where students actualize what they have read in texts and heard in lectures. It is much easier to recall how a client looked and behaved while in respiratory distress than it is to memorize the signs and symptoms of pulmonary edema. Putting real people's faces into one's memory in the context of the clinical learning setting helps you learn about clinical practice.

Having total recall of essential facts is crucial to thinking. It allows you to sort information in different ways to solve problems, to make decisions, or to create scenarios. (Remember, however, that the way you sort or cluster information affects the way you interpret that information.) Ready recall of information also frees your mind to engage in other modes of thinking.

Habits. Habits are accepted ways of doing things that work, save time, or are necessary. Habits are behaviors that have been repeated so many times that they become second nature. When a behavior is habitual, you need not think through the individual steps involved. Knowing how to drive a car and knowing how to swim are examples of habitual activities. Most of the activities that you learn in the nursing skills laboratory will become professional habits as you gain experience in nursing practice.

Forming habits allows you to do one thing while thinking about another. Much as you can drive a car while having a conversation, you can change a dressing while considering whether the wound has become infected. Naturally, habitual behaviors can be unsafe if unsafe steps become incorporated into the pattern.

Inquiry. Inquiry means examining issues in depth and questioning things that may seem obvious on the surface. It is the primary kind of thinking by which you reach conclusions. Inquiry involves analyzing information to confirm your hunch about a situation. Through feedback and further analysis, you can validate a conclusion. Nurses use this process to verify that the best interpretation is made of the client's clinical situation. Typically, the client provides the main source of information, as well as validation for your perception of reality.

Inquiry also includes the quality of being curious or wondering about the meaning of information. It is a spirit of wanting to know more, to understand, or to be able to explain facts that arise. Having a spirit of inquiry means never being satisfied with an interpretation of facts until you are sure that it is complete and accurate.

New Ideas and Creativity. New ideas and creativity occupy the opposite end of the spectrum from total recall and habit. They emphasize new and different ways of looking at information, and they form the basis for individualized client care. No two clients have identical values, life situations, preferences, and concerns. If you need to teach a person to care for a wound after discharge from the hospital, you need to consider how the client learns, whether the level of anxiety will permit learning to occur at this time, what supplies are available in the home, and the complexity of terminology the client can understand. A creative plan considers all of these variables.

Knowing How You Think. Knowing how you think is called metacognition, which literally means "in the midst of knowing." Knowing how you think means that you recognize when you are using logical reasoning to reach a conclusion. It leads you to ask yourself questions about how you think. Did I get all the facts before making a decision? Am I making assumptions that may not be true? In the example of teaching a client to manage a wound, you recognize that you have made an assumption that all clients want to learn wound care, so you seek validation that the assumption is true. Another question might be, Do I spend so much time making sure I have all the facts that I am blocked from making a decision? Box 5-3 lists strategies you can use to gain understanding about how you think.

CRITICAL THINKING AS CLINICAL JUDGMENT

In making a clinical judgment, you form an opinion using critical thinking to identify problems, solve problems, or make decisions. Sound clinical judgments stem from knowledge, clinical experience, and a holistic approach to the client's needs. As you learn to recognize patterns of behavior, the process also begins to include your powers of intuition.

Kataoka-Yahiro and Saylor (1994) have proposed a model of critical thinking that helps nurses make the clinical judgments needed for effective nursing care. The first component of the model is a *specific knowledge base.* Thinking depends on the knowledge base that each individual brings to the thinking process. The nurse's knowledge base includes sciences, liberal arts, and the nursing content needed to provide nursing care. Physical sciences help you understand the functions of the body and how humans think and respond to health care situations. The liberal arts provide a basis for understanding human values and cultural variations. Nursing knowledge incorporates these elements, contributes understanding of what it means to be ill, and provides methods of increasing the client's level of wellness.

The second component of the model is *experience.* As a nursing student, you bring a unique set of individual experiences to the nursing education. Material presented as part of that education will be understood and applied within your experience. During nursing education, you gain additional experiences through the practice of nursing in the clinical setting. Classmates share clinical experiences in formal clinical conferences. Each of these experiences adds to your knowledge. As your clinical experience increases, so does your ability to think critically in the setting.

The third component of the model is called *competencies* and refers to the cognitive processes used to make clinical judgments. Competencies that you need as a nurse include the following:

- The ability to identify problems caused by illness
- The ability to recognize health needs
- The ability to make decisions about how to improve a client's health
- The ability to recognize when and why nursing care has improved the client's condition

The fourth and fifth components of the model are *attitudes* and *standards* of critical thinking. Attitudes associated with critical thinking include a spirit of inquiry, the desire to understand a situation from more than one perspective, and valuing or seeking the truth. Paul's (1993) work, discussed shortly, expands on the attitudes and standards of critical thinking.

BOX 5-3 *Strategies for Gaining Understanding About How You Think*

- Keep a journal of how you use thinking skills. If you find a principle that works for you, jot it down! If something helps to make a thinking connection for you, jot it down!
- Share your journal with classmates in clinical conference. Compare how different thinking styles work for each of you.
- Discuss with classmates the thinking connections that you find difficult. Share problems and solutions.
- Always consider multiple solutions to any problem.
- Keep at it! Remember that critical thinking is the key to good nursing care and the foundation of accountability.

CHARACTERISTICS OF CRITICAL THINKING

In critical thinking, the most fundamental concern is excellence of thought. The idea that the study of critical thinking is important is based on two assumptions: first, that the quality of our thinking affects the quality of our lives, and second, that all of us can learn how to continually improve the quality of our thinking. The idea is to systematically form and shape our thinking to function purposefully to exacting standards. Critical thinking is disciplined, comprehensive, and based on intellectual ideals. As a result of the process of examining critical thinking, well-reasoned thinking develops (Paul, 1993).

Comprehensive critical thinking has the following characteristics (Paul, 1993):

- It is thinking that is responsive to and guided by such intellectual standards as relevance, accuracy, precision, clarity, depth, and breadth. Without standards to guide it, thinking cannot achieve excellence.

- It is thinking that deliberately supports the development of intellectual traits in the thinker, such as humility, integrity, perseverance, empathy, and self-discipline.
- It is in thinking that the thinker can identify the elements of thought present in the process. For example, the thinker can make logical connections between the elements and the problem at hand. Paul states that the critical thinker will routinely ask probing questions such as these: What is the purpose of my thinking? What question am I trying to answer? What information am I using? How am I interpreting it? What conclusions am I coming to? What assumptions am I making? If I accept the conclusion, what are the implications and the consequences? Table 5-3 applies these elements to nursing.
- It is thinking that is routinely self-assessing, self-examining, and self-improving. Paul stresses that if students are not assessing their own thinking, they are not thinking critically.
- It is thinking in which there is integrity to the whole system.
- It is thinking that yields a predictable, well-reasoned answer from the comprehensive and demanding process that the thinker pursues.
- It is thinking that is responsive to the social and moral imperative to argue from alternative and opposing points of view and to seek and identify the weaknesses and limitations of one's own position.

Critical Thinking and Nursing. Scheffer and Rubenfeld (2000) conducted a Delphi study to arrive at a consensus statement on the definition of critical thinking in nursing. Fifty-one nurses representing practice, education, and research served on the international panel of experts. After five rounds of data analysis, the following consensus statement was reached:

> Critical thinking in nursing is an essential component of professional accountability and quality nursing care. Critical thinkers in nursing exhibit these habits of the mind: confidence, contextual perspective, creativity, flexibility, inquisitiveness, intellectual integrity, intuition, open-mindedness, perseverance, and reflection. Critical thinkers in nursing practice the cognitive skills of analyzing, applying standards, discriminating, information seeking, logical reasoning, predicting, and transforming knowledge (p. 357).

Box 5-4 provides descriptions of the habits of the mind and the cognitive skills that nurse–critical thinkers exhibit.

Table 5-3 Paul's Elements of Critical Thinking Applied to Nursing

ELEMENT	APPLICATION EXAMPLES
Assumptions	• The nurse-client relationship is a helping relationship. • Clients have a right to make decisions about their health care.
Information	• Data, facts, and observations about the client • Knowledge about the pathophysiology and etiology of disease • Knowledge about human behavior
Concepts	• Theories, definitions, principles, and laws that give meaning to information and that are used to interpret clinical data and make decisions about effective management of the client's problems
Purpose of thinking	• To make decisions about data to be collected • To diagnose problems and make clinical judgments • To determine client goals or outcomes • To determine the nature of the client's presenting problem
Question of an issue	• To identify ethical and legal issues in practice
Points of view	• The nurse's and client's perception of the clinical situation • Perspective of health team members
Interpretation and inference	• Diagnostic reasoning that results in nursing diagnoses, plans, and interventions
Implications and consequences	• Client outcomes and modifications of care

BOX 5-4 ***Definitions of Habits of the Mind and Skills of Critical Thinking***

HABITS OF THE MIND

- **Confidence:** Assurance of one's reasoning abilities
- **Contextual perspective:** Considering everything relevant to the whole situation, including relationships, background, and environment
- **Creativity:** Intellectual inventiveness, used to generate, discover, or restructure ideas; imaging alternatives
- **Flexibility:** Capacity to adapt, accommodate, modify, or change thoughts, ideas, and behaviors
- **Inquisitiveness:** Eagerness to know by seeking knowledge and understanding through observation and thoughtful questioning to explore possibilities and alternatives
- **Intellectual integrity:** Seeking the truth through science and honest processes, even if the results are contrary to prior assumptions and beliefs
- **Intuition:** Insightful sense of knowing without conscious use of reason
- **Open-mindedness:** A viewpoint characterized by being receptive to divergent views and sensitive to one's biases
- **Perseverance:** Pursuit of a course with determination to overcome obstacles
- **Reflection:** Contemplation on a subject, especially assumptions and thought processes, for the purposes of deeper understanding and self-evaluation

Scheffer, B. K., & Rubenfeld, M. G. (2000). A consensus statement on critical thinking in nursing. *Journal of Nursing Education, 39,* 358.

Continued

BOX 5-4 Definitions of Habits of the Mind and Skills of Critical Thinking—cont'd

SKILLS

- **Analyzing:** Separating or breaking a whole into parts to discover their nature, function, and relationships
- **Applying standards:** Judging according to established personal, professional, or social rules or criteria
- **Discriminating:** Recognizing differences and similarities among things or situations and distinguishing carefully as to category or rank
- **Information seeking:** Searching for evidence, facts, or knowledge by identifying relevant sources and gathering objective, subjective, historical, and current data from those sources
- **Logical reasoning:** Drawing inferences or conclusions that are supported or justified by evidence
- **Predicting:** Envisioning a plan and its consequences
- **Transforming knowledge:** Changing or converting the condition, nature, form, or function of concepts among contexts

From Scheffer, B. K., & Rubenfeld, M. G. (2000). A consensus statement on critical thinking in nursing. *Journal of Nursing Education, 39,* 358.

CRITICAL THINKING AND EVIDENCED-BASED PRACTICE

Evidence-based practice (EBP) in nursing means using the best evidence available to make clinical decisions, instead of making decisions based on tradition. The Institute of Medicine (2003) envisioned EBP as "the integrations of best research evidence, clinical expertise, and patient values in making decisions about the care of individual patients." In EBP, one must decide when it is necessary to search for evidence, what constitutes evidence, where and how it can be found, the quality of the evidence, how best to translate that evidence into practice, the potential consequences of using approaches advocated by the evidence, and after using it, how to determine if it was "best" (Centre for Health Evidence, 2001; "Evidence-based clinical. . ,"n.d.). Rubenfeld and Scheffer (2006) contend that this statement implies the use of critical thinking skills of analyzing, applying standards, discriminating, information seeking, logical reasoning, predicting, and transforming knowledge. It also implies the habits of the mind such as contextual perspective, inquisitiveness, intellectual integrity, and open-mindedness. They believe a clear connection exists between all dimensions of critical thinking and EBP. These connections are diagrammed in Figure 5-3.

DEVELOPMENT OF CRITICAL THINKING

Critical thinking is a skill that develops over time and with conscious application of total recall, habits, inquiry, new ideas and creativity, and knowing how you think. As you gain more experience in nursing, your thinking will evolve and advance.

STAGES OF SKILL ACQUISITION

In *From Novice to Expert,* Patricia Benner (1984) applies the Dreyfus model of skill acquisition to nursing practice. The Dreyfus model suggests that a person passes through five levels of proficiency in acquiring and developing a skill. Applying this model to professional nursing practice, Benner identifies these stages as novice, advanced beginner, competent, proficient, and expert (Figure 5-4). Each of these stages requires that the nurse be able to think critically; however, the depth and breadth of the nurse's ability to think critically evolve with each stage. One can also hypothesize that as the nurse progresses through the levels of proficiency, the adaptive unconscious provide the basis for intuitive actions.

Benner's stages of skill acquisition in professional nursing practice reflect changes in three general aspects. The first change is from reliance on abstract principles stored in memory to the use of past concrete experiences to guide actions. The second change is the individual's perception of the situation; it is seen as a whole in which only certain elements are relevant. The third change is from being a detached observer to being an involved performer.

Novice. Benner describes the behavior of the *novice* nurse as being rule-governed, limited, and inflexible. Critical thinking operates in the total recall mode. Because the novice has no experience of the situation at hand, rules are used to guide performance. The student nurse follows rules because they are "correct." But, Benner cautions, rules legislate against ultimately successful performance because rules do not specify the most relevant tasks in actual situations.

Advanced Beginner. According to Benner, the *advanced beginner* (or new graduate) has experienced enough real situations to note the recurring meaningful aspects and attributes in a situation. The advanced beginner can formulate guidelines on the basis of experience but may miss their differential importance, thereby treating them equally. Benner states that the advanced beginner benefits from assistance, given by an instructor or a preceptor, in setting priorities. This stage demonstrates the very beginning of the development of professional habits, part of the T.H.I.N.K. process.

Competent. Benner reports that the third stage of proficiency—*competence*—is typified by the nurse who has been in the same or a similar position for 2 to 3 years. In this setting, the nurse begins to interpret actions in light of long-range goals or plans with conscious awareness. The plan dictates which aspects of the current and future situation are most important and which can be ignored. Therefore the competent nurse can develop a plan on the basis of considerable conscious, abstract, and analytical contemplation of the

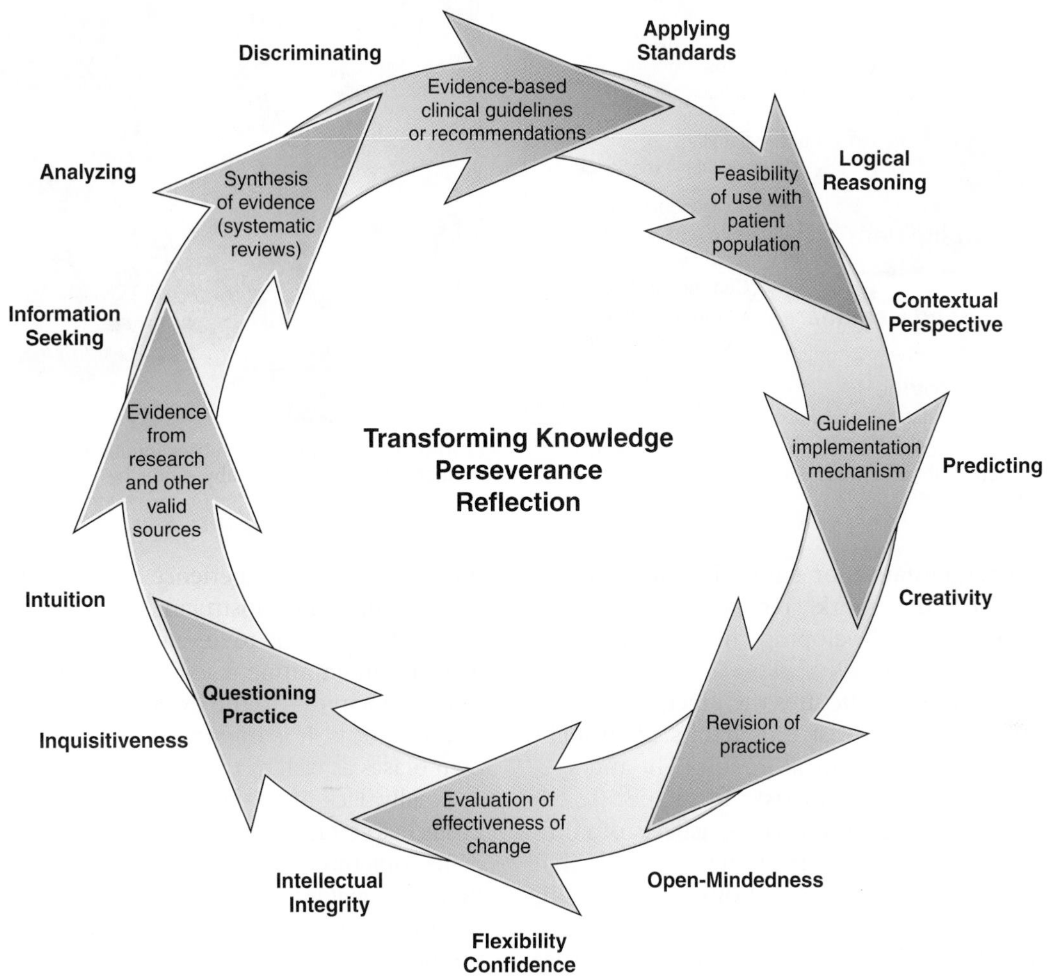

FIGURE 5-3 Use of critical thinking skills is closely related to the development of evidence-based practice as depicted in the inner circle of arrows. (From Rubenfeld, M.G., & Scheffer, B. K. [2006]. *Critical thinking tactics for nurses*, p. 146. Sudbury, MA: Jones & Bartlett Publishers. Used with permission.)

problem. The competent nurse lacks the speed and flexibility of the proficient nurse but does have a feeling of mastery and the ability to manage the required nursing care. In this stage, the nurse relies on all modes of the critical thinking process.

Proficient. Benner describes the *proficient* nurse as one who perceives each situation as a whole, rather than its individual aspects. She states that the nurse's perception is the key element in this stage. The perspective is not consciously thought out; instead, it "presents itself" on the basis of experience and recent events. Proficient nurses understand a situation as a whole because they perceive its meaning in terms of long-term goals. They operate in a holistic mode where, on the basis of their clinical experience, they can clearly understand nuances in clinical situations. It typically takes 3 to 5 years in one setting to become proficient. This is an advanced level of critical thinking, possibly involving highly complex clinical situations.

Expert. Benner states that the *expert* nurse no longer relies on an analytical principle to connect the understanding of a situation with an appropriate action. The expert nurse has an intuitive grasp of each situation and zeroes in on the accurate region of the problem without wasteful consideration of alternative actions (Figure 5-5). It takes 5 to 15 years in a setting for a nurse to become expert. Practice at this stage demonstrates the highest level of critical thinking in that the expert nurse knows holistically what to do without consciously thinking through all the data.

Advanced Clinical Judgment. Benner, Hooper-Kyriakidis, and Stannard (1999) studied the nursing practice of critical care nurses. They identified two pervasive habits of thought and action that provide a rich description of clinical judgment—*clinical grasp* and *clinical forethought.* Clinical grasp describes clinical inquiry in action and includes problem identification and clinical judgment across time. It has four compo-

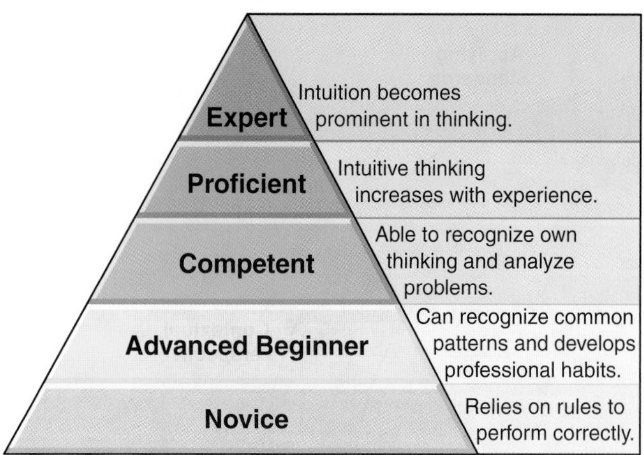

FIGURE 5-4 Growth in critical thinking from novice to expert. Advancing to expert is not automatic. It requires commitment to continued growth.

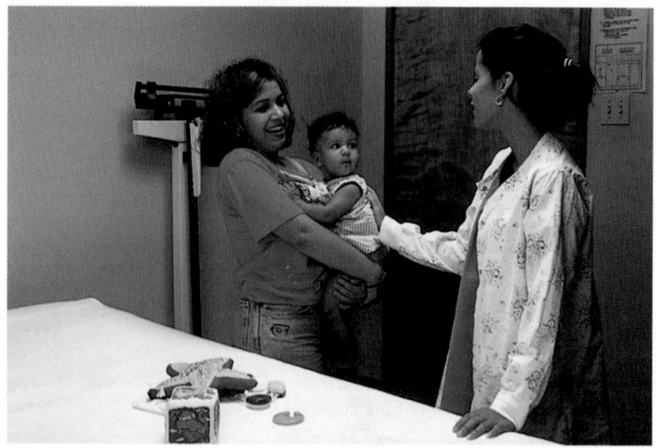

FIGURE 5-5 An expert nurse uses intuition to ascertain that this mother is happy and the baby is healthy.

nents: making qualitative or subjective distinctions, engaging in detective work, recognizing changing clinical relevance, and developing clinical knowledge in specific client situations.

Clinical forethought structures the practical logic of clinicians. It refers to at least four habits of thought and action: future-think, clinical forethought and specific diagnosis, anticipation of risks for a specific client, and seeing the unexpected. These aspects of clinical judgment are advanced nursing practice skills that the novice nurse can watch for and observe in experienced nurses.

Obstacles to Critical Thinking. A number of obstacles impede the developing and exercising of your critical thinking skills. By being aware of them, you can ensure that your thinking remains sound.

One of the most common obstacles involves overuse of the habit mode. Nurses tend to develop routines and habits to make sure that work gets done efficiently. However, habits can narrow the focus of your thinking. Unquestioned habits may cause you to miss important cues and could be dangerous to your clients. Every person for whom you provide care is unique. By assuming that habitual behaviors will be correct for all clients, you leave yourself open to mistakes.

Another obstacle to good thinking is anxiety, especially severe anxiety, which can render even the most prepared person unable to perform. Dealing with anxiety requires you to focus on yourself, thus reducing the focus and energy available to your clients.

Working under deadlines may affect your ability to think critically because you simply may not have enough time to think through all available information before arriving at a solution. You may make decisions prematurely, without all the facts or before the client is ready. Clearly, clinical practice often takes place under real time pressures, depending on the setting. One way to overcome this obstacle is to prepare as thoroughly as possible for the clinical experience at hand. Also, make good use of your clinical instructor.

Another obstacle to developing critical thinking skills is an overcommitment to ideological, religious, or political principles—to the extent that your mind is closed to other ideas. It is important that you understand your own biases as well as those that your client might have.

Finally, lack of confidence in your thinking can be an obstacle to critical thinking (see Figure 5-3). Nursing students sometimes lack the confidence to stand up for what they believe; it may feel safer to defer to an authority figure (staff nurse, instructor, or physician) than to defend your position. However, if you think clearly, logically, and with consideration for the values of others, then you can always have confidence in your thinking.

CRITICAL THINKING AND THE NURSING PROCESS

In clinical practice, the nursing process provides the structure in which critical thinking, diagnostic reasoning, and clinical judgment take place. It is a continuous process composed of five interrelated phases: assessment, nursing diagnosis, planning, intervention, and evaluation (Figure 5-6).

ASSESSMENT

In the first phase of the process, *assessment,* you collect data that you then can use to identify client needs that can be managed or treated with nursing care. The focus of your assessment may be narrow or broad and may generate a large amount or a relatively small amount of data, depending on the setting and the client's condition. A specific nursing theory may be chosen to direct the structure of your assessment.

A comprehensive assessment is holistic and includes a physical examination, a health history, and a psychosocial-cultural assessment. Client-centered data are usually col-

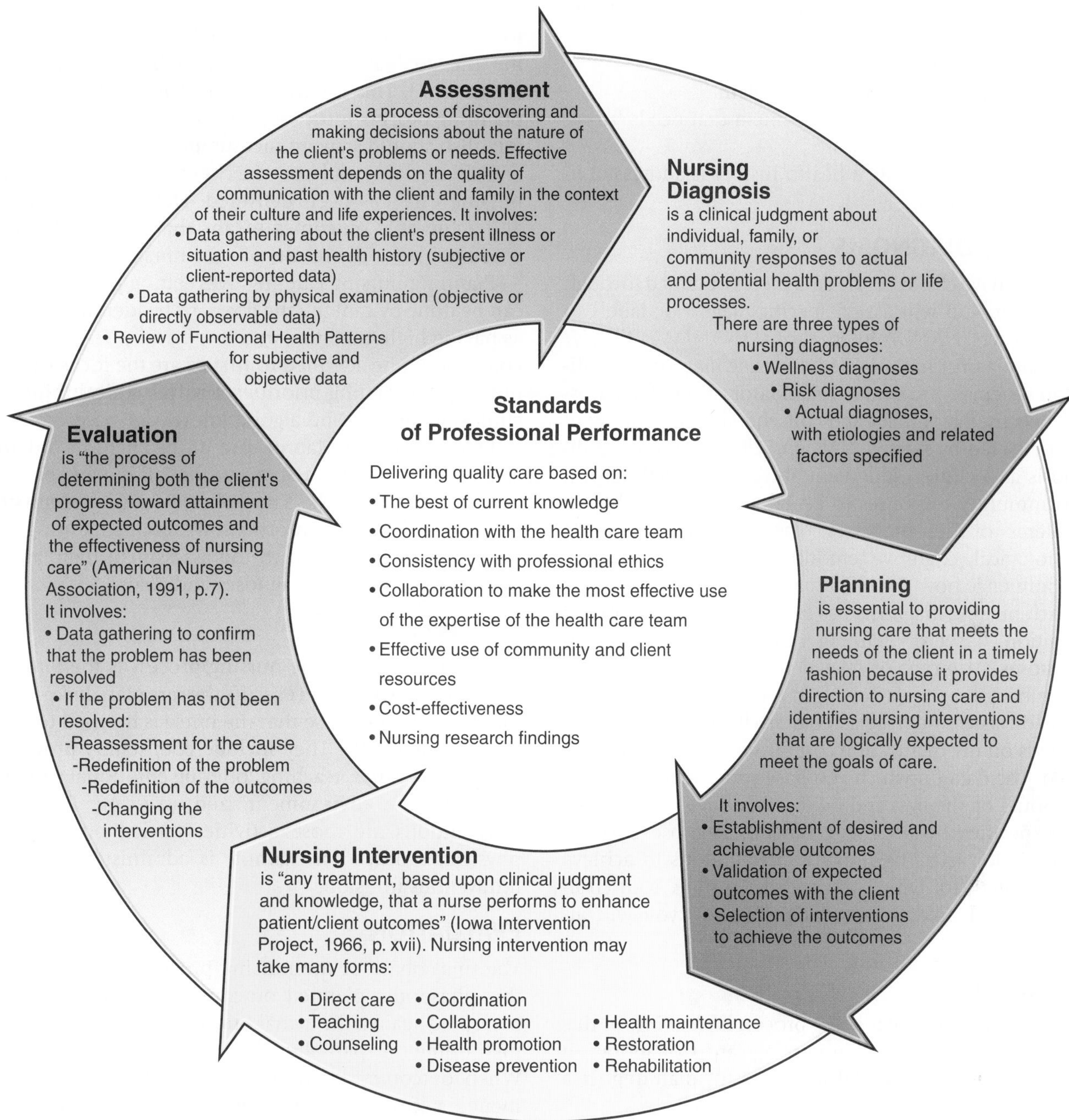

FIGURE 5-6 The nursing process and standards of professional performance.

lected to understand the client's history in the areas of health needs. This health history is organized in a framework that is most pertinent to identifying the care needs of the client. Most health care agencies have a form for collecting a health history. Proceeding though scripted questions, you listen for cues that suggest a problem or a need. These cues direct you to explore those areas of concern in more depth. Critical thinking directs this exploration.

The nursing assessment is performed in all nursing specialties and settings. You may encounter clients in the hospital setting where a presenting problem or illness becomes the starting point of the assessment. In contrast, in a community setting you may screen healthy clients for risk factors for a particular disease.

As you collect assessment data, you will engage in critical thinking, mentally grouping data into clusters for specific meaning related to the client's situation. You will listen actively and make observations about the client. As the pieces of data form meaningful patterns or information clusters, you will critically analyze them. This is the process of diagnostic reasoning. Diagnostic reasoning is not innate; it is a skill that you can learn and improve with practice, experience, and an ever-increasing knowledge base.

As a result of your assessment, you will arrive at one of the following outcomes:

- You will identify no problem.
- You will identify a potential problem.
- You will identify an actual problem that needs further assessment.

The process of taking a health history is addressed in detail in Chapter 6.

NURSING DIAGNOSIS

Once you have clustered the data pieces obtained through assessment, you will assign specific diagnostic labels to those clusters. NANDA International (NANDA-I) (http://www.nanda.org) has adopted a *nursing diagnosis* classification system to promote the standardization of diagnostic labels used by nurses and consequently the quality of care delivered by nurses. NANDA-I defines a nursing diagnosis as a clinical judgment about individual, family, or community responses to actual and potential health problems or life processes. These responses include physiological, cognitive, emotional, and social changes that influence how an individual functions.

Each nursing diagnosis has five components: a label, a definition, a set of defining characteristics (signs and symptoms), a group of related factors, and risk factors. The nursing diagnoses you choose for each client will be based on assessment data for that client; their accuracy depends on the quality and completeness of the data collected. The data on which you base your nursing diagnoses should be the best and most reliable available to you.

As specified by NANDA-I, nursing diagnoses provide the basis for selecting nursing interventions to achieve the outcomes for which you are responsible. Your clinical judgment determines which diagnosis you will attend to first.

PLANNING

The third phase of the nursing process is *planning.* In this step you set goals and plan nursing care. Collaboration with the client is essential to successful planning. If a goal that you create on your own holds no importance for the client, the client will have little interest in pursuing the goal and no incentive to become interested (Figure 5-7). This is why the goals (or outcomes) of the planning process must be client oriented. The goals you establish should state, in measurable terms, what the client will be doing and how the client will be doing it after nursing care has been delivered. Determining realistic and achievable outcomes means that you can be held accountable for the results of your nursing care.

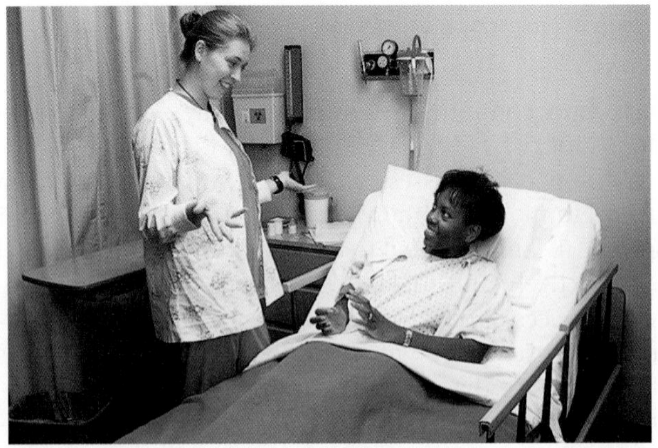

FIGURE 5-7 Planning for interventions that are acceptable to the client requires the nurse to use creativity to engage the client in the process.

Planning nursing care involves setting priorities. This can be done by ranking the goals, or by identifying goals as having high, medium, and low priority. High-priority goals should be attended to first or are the focus of your nursing care. Setting priorities involves critical thinking, clinical judgment, and a good knowledge base.

Document your plan of care in the client record and also on the nursing care plan so that all nursing personnel can work from the same plan. Because the nursing process is dynamic, information obtained during the planning stage is added to the assessment data, and it may alter the nursing diagnoses and goals.

INTERVENTION

The fourth phase of the nursing process is the *intervention* phase, in which you execute the care plan. *Independent* interventions are those that the nurse is licensed to carry out independently. They include counseling, providing comfort measures, teaching, offering emotional support, managing the environment, and assessing. *Dependent* interventions are those activities carried out under a physician's order. An example is administration of an intravenous infusion.

EVALUATION

The final phase of the nursing process is *evaluation.* In this phase, the planned outcomes of nursing care are measured against the actual outcomes. Outcomes can be met, unmet, or partially met and are recorded as such. When outcomes are unmet or partially met, reassessment is necessary to determine why this result occurred. The care plan is then revised accordingly.

Clinical pathways and case maps are evaluation tools that can help nurses monitor client progress. They show the average path that a client with a certain diagnosis is likely to take. These evaluation tools provide you with a daily measure of the client's progress on the clinical path. They are examples of building quality assurance measures into nursing care.

APPLYING T.H.I.N.K. TO THE NURSING PROCESS

You will use each of the five modes of critical thinking outlined in the T.H.I.N.K. model while carrying out the nursing process. Doing so will help you to more accurately and completely provide for each client's needs.

USING T.H.I.N.K. IN ASSESSMENT

Total recall is used in assessment when you follow a specific list of questions, or a guide, to collect assessment data. An assessment guide ensures that your assessment covers all essential elements of data collection. *Habits* come into play when you develop consistent patterns of behavior that you use in the assessment process. You use *inquiry* when you explore abnormal findings and form additional questions to obtain more information that may improve your understanding of the problem—and perhaps reveal the cause of the problem. You use *new ideas and creativity* by listening to what is not said as well as to what is said and by formulating questions that help the client express sensitive feelings or describe embarrassing symptoms. You use *knowing how you think* by asking yourself such questions as, Have I been thorough? Have I identified all the necessary cues? Is there sufficient evidence to support my conclusions?

USING T.H.I.N.K. IN DIAGNOSIS

You use *total recall* and *habits* to cluster assessment data into meaningful patterns. *Inquiry* is used as you ask yourself how the data patterns affect the client's health. *New ideas and creativity* are used in the process of diagnostic reasoning to arrive at nursing diagnoses. *Knowing how you think* assists you in the analytical process of diagnosing.

USING T.H.I.N.K. IN PLANNING

You use *total recall* to remember the usual goal for the problems that you have identified. *Habits* help you to develop goals and outcomes that are measurable and achievable. *Inquiry* is used to validate goals with the client, thus making sure that you and the client agree. *New ideas and creativity* may be needed when the client denies that a problem exists or is unwilling to engage in behaviors that improve health. *Knowing how you think* leads to questions about the logic used in connecting the expected outcomes to solving the problems that have been identified.

USING T.H.I.N.K. IN INTERVENTION

Total recall is used to remember the steps of a procedure and the principles or elements that are critical to safe and effective intervention. You rely on *habits* to achieve a well-organized, smooth procedure. *Inquiry* helps you to determine if the methods of intervention are the best for the particular client situation. *New ideas and creativity* modify the intervention for client preferences or situational variables. *Knowing how you think* helps you to evaluate the methods of intervention by asking such questions as, Was the client comfortable? Was the intervention successful?

USING T.H.I.N.K. IN EVALUATION

Total recall and *habits* are used to compare the goals of care with the outcomes of care. *Inquiry* helps you to determine client satisfaction (or dissatisfaction) with the achieved outcomes. *New ideas and creativity* may be necessary to modify the plan of care. *Knowing how you think* helps you to assess an outcome objectively.

▼ KEY PRINCIPLES

- The basis of any discipline is theoretical. Theories identify important concepts and the relationships between them.
- Theories help the nurse learn, organize knowledge, apply knowledge, seek new knowledge, and communicate quickly and effectively with other nurses.
- Nursing theory provides a basis for clinical practice.
- More than any other single component, nursing theory helps the nurse to engage in thoughtful, experienced, skillful care of clients, whether that client is an individual, family, or community.
- T.H.I.N.K. is a mnemonic device for a model that reflects the key elements of critical thinking: total recall, habits, inquiry, new ideas and creativity, and knowing how you think.
- Nurses typically develop skill proficiency in the following order: novice, advanced beginner, competent, proficient, and expert.
- Obstacles to critical thinking include an inadequate knowledge base, an overreliance on habits, anxiety, too little time to make reasoned decisions, zealous adherence to circumscribed sets of beliefs, and lack of confidence in thinking ability.
- The nursing process is composed of five interrelated phases: assessment, diagnosis, planning, intervention, and evaluation. It provides a framework in which to exercise critical thinking.

■ REVIEW QUESTIONS

1. Nurse theorists who define health as a state of well-being as measured against norms are representative of the following view:

1. Received
2. Perceived
3. Elemental
4. Irreducible

2. The nurse theorist who focuses on manipulating the environment to provide the most positive client outcomes is:

1. Roy
2. Orem
3. Nightingale
4. Watson

3. The nurse theorist who authored the theory of caring science is:

1. Peplau
2. Eriksson
3. Rogers
4. Parse

4. The goal of critical thinking is to:

1. Determine the safest nursing action to take
2. Use creativity to solve client problems
3. Consider possible outcomes based on actions taken
4. Guide client-centered nursing practice

5. A critical thinking model created by nurse educators is called:

1. Adaptive unconscious
2. T.H.I.N.K.
3. Clinical judgment
4. Outcomes assessment

Bibliography

*Abdellah, F., Beland, I. L., Martin, A., & Matheney, R. V. (1960). *Patient centered approaches to nursing.* New York: Macmillan.

American Association of Colleges of Nursing. (1998). *Essentials of baccalaureate education for professional practice.* Washington, DC: Author.

Barnum, B. S. (1998). *Nursing theory: Analysis, application, and evaluation* (5th ed.). Philadelphia: Lippincott.

*Benner, P. (1984). *From novice to expert: Excellence and power in clinical nursing practice*. Menlo Park, CA: Addison-Wesley.

Benner, P., Hooper-Kyriakidis, P., & Stannard, D. (1999). *Clinical wisdom and interventions in critical care: A thinking-in-action approach*. Philadelphia: Saunders.

*Benner, P., & Wrubel, J. (1989). *The primacy of caring*. Menlo Park, CA: Addison-Wesley.

Boykin, A., & Schoenhofer, S. O. (1993). *Nursing as caring: A model for transforming practice*. New York: NLN Press.

Brilowski, G. A., & Wendler, M.C. (2005). An evolutionary concept analysis of caring. *Journal of Advanced Nursing, 50*(6), 641-650.

Centre for Health Evidence. (2001). *User's guides to evidence-based practice*. Available at http://www.cche.net/users-guides/guideline.asp.

Chinn, P., & Kramer, M. K. (1999). *Theory and nursing: A systematic approach* (5th ed.). St. Louis, MO: Mosby.

Erickson, H. C., Tomlin, E. M., & Swain, M. A. P. (1983). *Modeling and role modeling*. Lexington, KY: Pine Press.

Eriksson, K. (1987). *Pausen: En beskrivning av vardvetenskapens kunskapsobjekt* [The pause: A description of the knowledge of caring science]. Stockholm, Sweden: Almqvist & Wiksell.

Eriksson, K. (2002). Caring science in a new key. *Nursing Science Quarterly, 15*(1), 61-65.

*Facione, P. A. (1990). *Executive summary: Critical thinking—A statement of expert consensus for purposes of educational assessment and instruction*. Millbre, CA: California Academic Press.

Fahrenwald, N. L., Basset, S. D., Tschetter, L., Carson, P. P., White, L., & Winterboer, V. J. (2005). Teaching core nursing values. *Journal of Professional Nursing, 21*(1), 46-51.

Gladwell, M. (2006). *Blink: The power of thinking without thinking*. New York: Little, Brown.

*Hall, L. E. (1964). *Nursing: What is it? Canadian Nurse 60:*150-154.

*Harmer, B., & Henderson, V. (1955). *Textbook of the principles and practice of nursing*. New York: Macmillan.

Henderson, V. (1960). *Basic principles of nursing care*. Geneva: International Council of Nurses.

Henderson, V. (1966). *The nature of nursing*. New York: Macmillan.

Jackson, M., Ignatavicius, D. D., & Case, B. (2006). *Conversations in critical thinking and clinical judgment*. Sudbury, MA ; Jones & Bartlett.

*Johnson, D. E. (1980). The behavioral system model for nursing. In J. P. Riehl & C. Roy (Eds.), *Conceptual models for nursing practice* (2nd ed., pp. 207-216). New York: Appleton-Century-Crofts.

*Kataoka-Yahiro, M., & Saylor, C. (1994). A critical thinking model for nursing judgment. *Journal of Nursing Education, 33*, 351-355.

*King, I. (1971). *Toward a theory for nursing: General concepts of human behavior*. New York: Wiley.

Kyle, T.V. (1995). The concept of caring: A review of the literature. *Journal of Advanced Nursing, 21*, 506-514.

Leininger, M. M. (1978). *Transcultural nursing: Concepts, theories, and practice*. New York: Wiley.

Leininger, M. M. (1980). Caring: A central focus of nursing and health care services. *Nursing and Health Care, 6*, 209-212.

Levine, M. (1967). The four conservation principles of nursing. *Nursing Forum, 69*(10), 93-98.

*Levine, M. (1996). The conservation principles: A retrospective. *Nursing Science Quarterly, 9*, 38-41.

Libster, M. (2001). *Demonstrating caring: The art of integrative nursing*. Albany, NY: Delmar Thomson Learning.

Lindstrom, U. A., Lindholm, L., & Zetterland, J. E. (2006). Theory of caritative caring. In A. Marriner-Tomey & M. R. Alligood, *Nursing theorists and their work* (6th ed.). St. Louis, MO: Mosby.

*Neuman, B. (1974). The Betty Neuman health care systems model: A total person approach to patient problems. In J. P. Riehl & C. Roy (Eds.), *Conceptual models for nursing practice* (pp. 99-114). New York: Appleton-Century-Crofts.

Newman, M. A. (1979). *Theory development in nursing*. Philadelphia: Davis.

*Nightingale, F. (1859, 1992). *Notes on nursing* (Com ed.). Philadelphia: Lippincott.

*Orem, D. E. (1971, 2001). *Nursing: Concepts of practice*. New York: McGraw-Hill.

*Orlando, I. J. (1990). *The dynamic nurse-patient relationship*. New York: Putnam. (Original work published 1961.)

Parse, R. R. (1981). *Man-living-health: A theory of nursing*. New York: Wiley.

Parse, R. R. (1992). The performing art of nursing [Editorial]. *Nursing Science Quarterly, 5*, 147.

*Parse, R. R. (1998). The human becoming school of thought. Thousand Oaks, CA: Sage.

Paterson, J. G., & Zderad, L. T. (1976). *Humanistic nursing*. New York: Wiley.

*Paul, R. W. (1993). *Critical thinking: What every person needs to know in a rapidly changing world* (3rd ed.). Rohnert Park, CA: Center for Critical Thinking.

Paul, R. W., & Heaslip, P. (1995). Critical thinking and intuitive nursing practice. *Journal of Advanced Nursing, 22*, 40-47.

*Peplau, H. E. (1988). *Interpersonal relations in nursing*. New York: Putnam. (Original work published 1952.)

*Rogers, M. E. (1970). *An introduction to the theoretical basis of nursing*. Philadelphia: F. A. Davis.

*Roy, C. (1976). *Introduction to nursing: An adaptation model*. Englewood Cliffs, NJ: Prentice-Hall.

*Rubenfeld, M. G., & Scheffer, B. K. (1999). *Critical thinking in nursing: An interactive approach* (2nd ed.). Philadelphia: Lippincott.

Rubenfeld, M. G., & Scheffer, B. K. (2006) *Critical thinking tactics for nurses*. Sudbury, MA: Jones & Bartlett.

*Scheffer, B. K., & Rubenfeld, M. G. (2000). A consensus statement on critical thinking in nursing. *Journal of Nursing Education, 39*, 352-359.

Snyder, M. (1995). Critical thinking: A foundation for consumer-focused care. *The Journal of Continuing Education in Nursing, 24*(5), 206-210.

Swanson, K. M. (1991). Empirical development of a middle range theory of caring. *Nurse Researcher, 40*(3), 161-166.

Swanson, K. M. (1999). What's known about caring in nursing science: A literary meta-analysis. In A. S. Hinshaw, S. Feetham, & J. Shaver (Eds.), *Handbook of clinical nursing research* (pp. 31-60). Thousand Oaks, CA: Sage

Watson, G., & Glaser, E. M. (1964). *Watson-Glaser critical thinking appraisal*. New York: Harcourt, Brace World.

Watson, J. (1988). *Nursing: Human science, human care*. New York: National League for Nursing.

*Asterisk indicates a classic or definitive work on this subject.

Chapter 6

CLIENT ASSESSMENT: NURSING HISTORY

Media Resources

- evolve Evolve Website http://evolve.elsevier.com/Harkreader/
- Companion CD

Learning Objectives

After studying this chapter, you should be able to do the following:

- Make preliminary decisions in preparation for data collection
- Understand data collection as a critical thinking process
- Employ interviewing techniques in taking a health history
- Develop a systematic framework for organizing data
- Document the assessment in the client's health record

Key Terms

active listening
active processing
assessment
biographical data
cardinal signs and symptoms
chief complaint
closed question
cue
data
database
demographic data
functional health patterns
inference
interview
intuition
leading question
minimum data set
nursing history
objective data
open-ended question
orientation phase
signs
subjective data
symptoms
termination
validation
working phase

Assessment is the process of gathering information about a client's health status to identify concerns and needs that can be treated or managed by nursing care (Figure 6-1). The **data** gathered consist of subjective and objective information about the client, such as signs and symptoms of disease, results of diagnostic tests, and the client's health practices. Data collection marks the beginning of the nursing process and continues throughout the process. As you gather data, you organize the information into groups or meaningful clusters that describe the problems to be treated. Thus assessment also involves analyzing data to identify a client's problems and arrive at appropriate nursing diagnoses.

Assessment begins before the actual collection of data; that is, assessment begins with thinking about the data you will need and the best method of obtaining the data (Figure 6-2). Assessment is an active mental process requiring critical thinking about the data to be collected rather than merely obtaining answers to a specific list of questions. To gather information wisely, you need well-developed skills in observing and listening. At the same time, the mental skills of translating, reasoning, intuiting, and validating will make the data meaningful.

The assessment process is organized in a framework that helps you to identify the nature of data to be collected and classify it into common problem areas. As you collect data in each category prescribed by the framework, you will produce an initial clustering of information about the client. The framework for data collection affects which problems are distinguished or emphasized. For example, if you studied colors by examining red, blue, and yellow, all colors could be put into one of those categories. However, you would not be able to identify or classify the uniqueness of purple, green, and orange, much less the millions of subtle shades in between. In the same fashion, data about a client can be classified by physiological systems, but you might fail to identify social, psychological, and spiritual problems that influence the client's health. In this chapter you will learn to organize data using functional health patterns.

Rarely will you perform assessment as a single isolated step in the nursing process. Rather, as you elicit information about a client, you will begin to consider nursing diagnoses and formulate plans. In some cases, during the assessment you will include interventions such as giving information to the client. In other words, assessment is often combined with teaching. In other cases, assessment and implementation take place almost simultaneously, as when the person has a compromised airway or needs emergency surgery. In all cases, assessment serves to establish priorities for care.

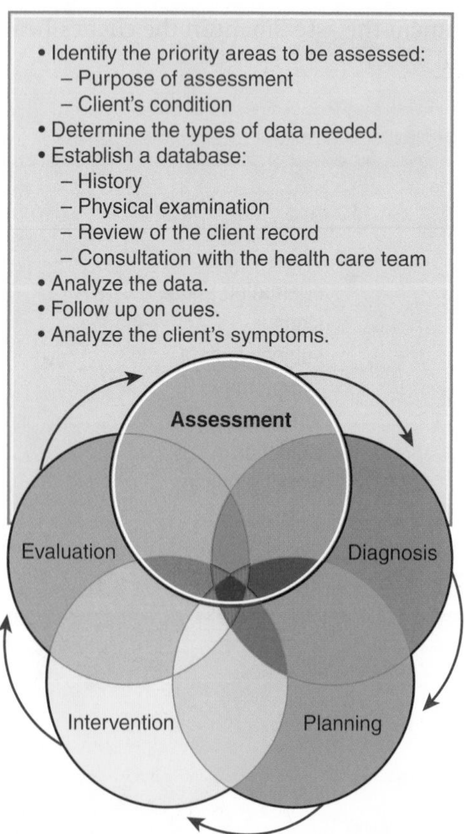

FIGURE 6-1 Assessment is the process of gathering information about a client's health status to identify concerns and needs that can be treated or managed by nursing care.

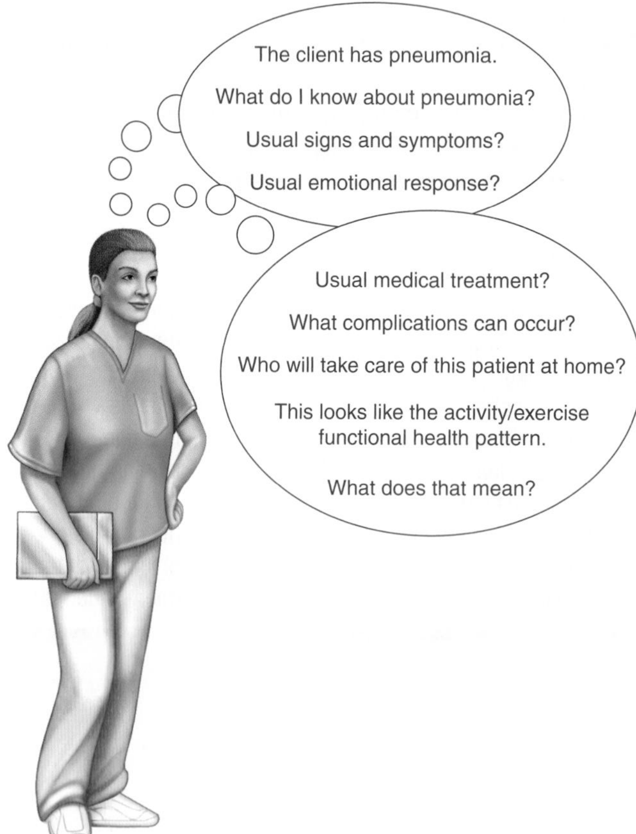

FIGURE 6-2 Assessment begins with thinking.

PRELIMINARY DECISION MAKING

Any time you interact with a client, for virtually any reason, you will assess the person's problems, needs, and concerns. To efficiently and effectively collect data, you must make decisions about the type of assessment required, the sources of data to be consulted, how to structure and focus the assessment, and how much information to collect before developing a plan of action.

PURPOSE OF ASSESSMENT

An assessment may have a comprehensive focus or a specific, narrow focus. Depending on the purpose, assessment may involve asking two or three specific questions, or it may involve spending an hour in an in-depth conversation with the client. The purpose of the assessment may be to do any of the following:

- Establish a database with which to plan and evaluate comprehensive care
- Identify actual and potential problems to make nursing diagnoses
- Focus on a specific problem
- Determine immediate needs to establish priorities
- Determine the cause (etiology) of a problem
- Determine related or contributing factors
- Identify strengths as a basis for changing behavior
- Identify the risk for complications
- Recognize complications

TYPES OF ASSESSMENT

To help you begin to identify the purpose of your assessment, consider four major types of assessment: initial, focused, emergency, and ongoing. The initial assessment is made at the first contact with the client. A focused assessment is a detailed examination of a specific problem. An emergency assessment identifies or rules out life-threatening problems and those problems that need immediate treatment to prevent complications. Ongoing assessment refers to the data collection that takes place during every contact with the client throughout the client's association with the health care agency.

Initial Assessment. Assessment on initial contact with the client is typically more comprehensive than subsequent assessments. It begins with the problems that prompted the client to seek nursing services, and it obtains a holistic overview of the client's level of functioning. The objective is to rule out as well as to identify problems.

The nature of the client's problems—and therefore of the services to be provided—dictate the course and depth of the assessment. The client entering the hospital for surgery or for treatment of a medical condition has a specific problem and needs nursing care aimed at managing the treatment for the problem. The client entering a long-term care facility needs a general evaluation of health status to ensure that medical problems are stabilized and to identify the scope of anticipated nursing care. Wellness services typically take place in community settings, such as schools or clinics, where the nurse may screen for health problems in addition to helping clients manage specific concerns. In any setting, the focus of the nursing assessment is to identify how the nurse can help the client.

The focus of the initial assessment relates directly to the goals of prevention, maintenance, restoration, or rehabilitation. As a screening procedure, assessment is an overview designed to detect risk factors and evidence of certain problems. When prevention is the focus, assessment examines risk and lifestyle factors. A health maintenance assessment examines health and health behaviors. When the goal is restoration, assessment focuses on the need for support of body functions and the detection and prevention of complications. Rehabilitation considers the potential for restoring function and the resources needed to modify the lifestyle.

Not every initial assessment is comprehensive. In general, the thoroughness of an assessment is directly proportional to the length of expected care. If the client has an acute, short-term problem, such as a need for sutures in an accidentally inflicted minor wound, you will gather only minimal lifestyle information. However, when caring for clients with serious injuries resulting in admission to a rehabilitation unit, you are able to provide better long-term care by knowing the client's complete health history.

Focused Assessment. Once the client's general problems have been identified, you may perform a focused assessment on each problem or problem area. The focused assessment examines the evidence in detail, considers possible etiologies, looks for contributing factors, and considers client characteristics that will help solve the problems. Imagine, for example, that you have identified a diagnosis of *Ineffective coping (use of alcohol as primary coping mechanism)* for a client. You then can focus on this diagnosis to gather information about the person's pattern of drinking, defense mechanisms that maintain the behavior, effects on the family, and other information helpful in developing an appropriate plan of care.

Focused assessment also takes place when the client has a complaint or describes a new problem. Common complaints include pain, shortness of breath, difficulty urinating, and visual changes. You must be prepared to assess the severity of the problem, determine a possible cause, evaluate effects on the client's health, and decide on an appropriate course of action.

Emergency Assessment. When the client's situation is life threatening or time is an important factor in preventing complications, assessment will include only key data directly related to the immediate problem. The initial information you collect will vary, depending on the urgency of the situation. Additional data can be collected after the client's condition is stable. Emergency assessment uses ABC—airway, breathing, and circulation—to prioritize the client's needs.

Vital needs are for an open airway to take in oxygen-laden air, respiratory effort to breathe, and the circulation of blood to transport oxygen to body tissues.

Ongoing Assessment. Continuous or episodic assessment occurs throughout the client's health care experience. Episodic assessment may occur monthly, weekly, daily, or hourly, depending on the client's condition and the nature of the services being offered, but you continuously assess with each encounter with the client. Continuous assessment takes place in critical care or during anesthesia via electronic monitoring equipment. Weekly assessment may be appropriate for a client on a weight-loss program. Clients in a nursing home may have a formal assessment only once a month.

Nurses routinely make decisions about the frequency, the depth, and the breadth of client assessment. To make these decisions effectively, you must anticipate the potential for a client's condition to change, the speed at which it could change, and the evidence that would indicate a change. For example, when a client takes a new medication, assessment decisions are based on the expected effects of the medication, how rapidly those effects occur, and potential adverse effects.

TYPES OF DATA

As you interact with a client, you will gather information that is directly observable and that is only available by listening to the client's experience. Either type of information can provide a **cue**, an indicator of the presence or existence of a problem or condition that represents a client's underlying health status. The data of greatest significance in diagnosing a particular illness, disease, or health problem are called **cardinal signs and symptoms**.

Subjective Data. Information that is provided by the client and that you cannot observe directly is called **subjective data.** When subjective data supplied by the client describe characteristics of disease or dysfunction, those characteristics are known as **symptoms.** Pain, nausea, cramps, dizziness, and ringing in the ears are examples of symptoms because you cannot observe them directly. The client must inform you of their presence.

You may be able to directly observe evidence related to the client's symptom. For example, you may notice grimacing, an increased heart rate, and a doubled-over posture in a client who complains of pain. However, these observations could apply to pain, nausea, or cramps and can be confirmed only by asking the client to name the complaint. You may help the client describe or quantify subjective findings, but you should not make judgments about whether or not the symptom exists. The client is the best—indeed, the only—source of information about subjective findings.

Objective Data. Characteristics about the client that you can observe directly are called **objective data**. When these data indicate characteristics of disease or dysfunction, they are known as **signs.** Objective data can be observed through your senses of sight, hearing, taste, touch, and smell. These data can be measured (or quantified), and they can be reliably replicated from one examiner to the next, a concept called *interrater reliability.*

For example, you can measure the size of a wound and the amount of drainage it produces. The number of red blood cells in a sample of blood can be counted. Because they are factual, objective data have a high degree of certainty. However, objective information is not necessarily superior to subjective information.

SOURCES OF DATA

When assessing a client, you will need to make decisions about the most effective use of multiple sources of data, possibly including the client, the client's significant others, your colleagues, and the client's records. You will need to confirm that each data source is appropriate, reliable, and valid for each assessment. *Appropriate* means that the source is suitable for a particular purpose, person, or occasion. *Reliable* means that you can trust the information to be accurate and honestly reported. *Valid* means that the information can be substantiated or confirmed.

Client. Usually, the client is in the best position to provide accurate, reliable, and valid information about subjective data that describe health problems. In fact, some symptoms can be validated and accurately described *only* by the client. Always start by considering the client as the primary source of assessment data. However, sometimes a client may be too ill to provide information, may be confused, or may suffer from memory loss or otherwise not be able to provide accurate information.

Significant Others. You may ask the family for information when the client is unable to give reliable information or simply prefers to have a family member help describe events. Family members may be able to contribute significant details, provide a different perspective, or clarify the information. In addition, it is often important to help the family feel included in the process.

Before discussing the client's problems with family members or significant others, however, you must consider the client's right to confidentiality. Although many times an ill person relies on a family member to help remember details and ask important questions, that client may prefer to maintain some privacy from the family. Making an accurate determination of the client's wishes requires you to respond sensitively to subtle cues that may suggest the client's willingness, even preference, to have a family member remain in the room while you conduct the interview. Remember that you are in a position to ask family members to leave during the interview unless the client expresses the desire to have them stay.

Colleagues. All members of the health care team who have worked with the client can be important sources of data. Each team member will have a unique perspective on the client's problems, and therefore team members may make different observations. For example, the physical therapist may recognize that pain is preventing the client from walking or getting adequate exercise; the dietitian may suggest that pain is interfering with the client's ability to learn important information about a newly prescribed diet.

In contrast to nurses in hospitals, nurses who work in the home setting may have fewer opportunities to confer face-to-face with other members of the health care team. Consequently, other forms of communication may become more important in ensuring complete assessment and continuity of care. Usually, the client's record provides the primary method of communication to ensure continuity of care among various health care team members.

Client Records. The client has a right to expect members of the health care team to communicate adequately with each other. Likewise, the client has a right to expect you to be informed about the reason for admission or care. If the client has a medical or nursing record in the agency, you will usually begin by reviewing that record.

For the admission assessment of a hospitalized client, the record will indicate the reason for admission and the physician's admitting orders. In a home health care agency, the initial record may show the reason for the referral and a brief history of the current problem. At a follow-up visit in a clinic setting, reviewing the record will help you detect any ongoing problems as well as any new problems. Naturally, clients will feel more confidence in the health care team if you and other members take time to review the record before beginning an assessment and if you can avoid collecting data that are already in the record.

STANDARDS OF PRACTICE FOR ASSESSMENT

One characteristic of a profession is that it has the means to regulate and control its practice. As the official voice of nurses in the United States, the American Nurses Association (ANA) develops and disseminates standards for clinical practice (ANA, 2004) (see Appendix A). These standards are broad guidelines that require clinical judgment. They may be used in a court of law when determining what a reasonable and prudent nurse would do in a similar situation.

COLLECTING THE DATA

Assessment requires more than obtaining the answers to an established list of questions; it is a process of discovery, of gathering information in a manner that reveals the client's needs. The health assessment forms used by many health care facilities provide plausible and reasonable guides to data collection; however, forms are not a substitute for critical thinking skills (ANA, 2001). Whether or not you use a health assessment form, you will gather data using active listening and active processing.

ACTIVE LISTENING AND ACTIVE PROCESSING

When assessing a client, you will be (1) observing and listening to the client and (2) processing information through translating, reasoning, intuiting, and validating. To accomplish these goals effectively, you will use **active listening**. In other words, you will attend to what the client says and help the client clarify and elaborate and give additional pertinent information.

In addition, you will use **active processing**, which involves a systematic series of mental actions to analyze and interpret the information about the client. When you process information actively, you help yourself form mental impressions by thinking through such questions as "How does this information fit with what I know about a certain disease or health problem?" and "What questions do I need to ask to see how well it fits the pattern?"

Active listening and active processing are closely related concepts that occur simultaneously. Together they require you to use all your senses, to make judgments about the meaning of information, and to validate that meaning. For example, you may see that a client is exhibiting a particular symptom, hear the client describe an alteration in health, and then make a judgment about the meaning of these cues for this client. Finally, you may think about other experiences involving these cues and ask further questions.

As you assess a client, your mind continually shifts back and forth from general or global scanning to focusing on a specific problem. An initial assessment often follows a standardized format that directs your mental activity toward the global scan. Proceeding through specified questions, you listen for cues that suggest a problem or a need, or for other cues relevant to the present circumstances. Then you ask questions to follow up any cues that arise so you can determine whether a problem exists.

After categorizing this specific information in the context of the global assessment, you continue scanning for problems. Assessment of a specific cue may lead to one of three conclusions: no problem exists, a potential problem exists, or an actual problem exists and needs further assessment. Some potential problems may need

BOX 6-1 *Active Processing*

The line on the simple assessment checklist reads *Recent weight gain/loss?* Rather than simply placing a check mark on the form to confirm that the client has lost weight recently, the nurse follows up with the following conversation:

Nurse: How much weight have you lost?

Client: About 30 pounds in the past 2 months.

Nurse: How do you account for losing so much weight?

(The nurse knows weight loss can be associated with cancer. This question is looking for any other possible cause.)

Client: I don't know. I guess I just haven't had much appetite.

Nurse: Have you had any nausea or vomiting?

(The nurse is still exploring for other possible causes.)

Client: No.

Nurse: Have you had any blood in your stool? Or had black, tarry stools?

(Not finding any explanation for the weight loss, the nurse moves to other warning signs of cancer.)

Client: I haven't seen any blood, but I have sometimes had really dark, sticky bowel movements. Does that mean something?

Nurse: Well, it could be blood. I don't really know what it means. Have you discussed it with your doctor?

(The nurse has begun to explore a plan with the client.)

Client: I know I need to. I guess I don't want to know. My father died of cancer.

(The client has revealed a need for teaching.)

Nurse: Blood can mean several things, only one of which is cancer. How long ago did your father die?

(The nurse is looking for further information before being satisfied with the teaching.)

Client: Oh, it's been 30 years. They didn't know how to treat cancer then. I guess I really should see about it.

Nurse: We can do a screening test for blood in your stool. However, even if it is negative at this time, I want you to make an appointment with your doctor. If there is blood in your stool, it is best to make sure it is not from cancer. Will you do it?

Client: Yes.

Nurse: Remember that cancer is only one of the possibilities. If it turns out to be cancer, you know that there are many new treatments that were not available when your father died. However, whatever the cause, you need to see the doctor.

(The nurse then gives the client a Hemoccult test slide and instructions to collect the specimen.)

From American Nurses Credentialing Center. (January 2003). Certification brochure. Washington, DC: Author. Retrieved from http://www.nursecredentialing.org.

further assessment; others may need to be noted only for future reference. Box 6-1 illustrates a conversation with a client in which the nurse is actively processing information to guide assessment questions.

Observing. Assessment involves using all of your senses to observe the client for physical and behavioral cues. Observable physical cues could be difficult breathing, pale skin, odors, noisy respiration, or feeling a lump in the abdomen. Behavioral responses include verbal and nonverbal responses: a clinched fist, a tense expression, or a loud cry. Observe for consistency or discrepancy between nonverbal and verbal responses. Interpret eye contact, body language, and facial expressions in the context of what the client says in response to your questions.

Listening. Listening is an active process that involves hearing what the client says as well as the meaning behind it. Active listening involves validating what you think you understood. When you listen actively, you formulate questions that help the client describe a problem completely by providing all pertinent information. For example, if the client has difficulty describing the intensity of nausea, you may suggest using a scale from 0 to 10, with 10 being the worst nausea imaginable. And it may be helpful to know if eating makes the nausea better or worse.

Failing to listen attentively to both what a client says and does not say can keep you from identifying a problem or understanding it completely. Denying the possible seriousness of a problem can cause the client to withhold information. The client may leave out important details, believing that the problem is not important or that certain symptoms are not relevant and that seeking help was not appropriate.

Naturally, most clients describe their problems from a layman's point of view. Consequently, they often include extraneous information. You must decide how long to listen before refocusing the client to more pertinent data. If you interrupt the client too soon or too abruptly, the client may feel misunderstood and will probably feel that you have little interest in helping to identify the problem.

Translating. Assessment further involves translating information into clear, succinct, meaningful statements that will be understood by other health care personnel. The client may express concerns in slang terms or lengthy descriptions. You will then translate and document these descriptions in medical terminology, which has the advantage of abbreviating the description and conveying meanings that are commonly understood by other health care team professionals. However, if you feel that a medical term or interpretation could be misinterpreted, choose instead to document the client's own words.

Grouping data into meaningful patterns is also part of translation. For example, you would group cyanotic skin color, restlessness, and rapid respirations together because they all relate to tissue oxygenation.

Reasoning. Assessment includes actively processing information to make mental connections of the data to diseases, health patterns, or the current situation. Nurses who have a wide knowledge base are more likely to make appropriate mental connections. For example, the nurse who understands pathophysiology can determine

BOX 6-2 *Understanding Inferential Reasoning*

CORRECT INFERENTIAL REASONING

Fact: *Mr. Smith has a bowel movement every 3 days, and the stool is soft and easily passed.*

Premise: *Constipation is the presence of hard, dry stool that is difficult to pass.*

Conclusion: *Mr. Smith is not constipated.*

Explanation: *Asking whether information included in the premise is sufficient to establish the presence of constipation can corroborate this correct conclusion. Because the premise includes a standard definition of constipation, the conclusion is based on sufficient evidence.*

INCORRECT INFERENTIAL REASONING

Fact: *Mr. Smith has swelling in his ankles and feet.*

Premise: *Persons with right-sided heart failure have swelling in their ankles and feet.*

Conclusion: *Mr. Smith has congestive heart failure.*

Explanation: *Although the premise is correct, the information in both the fact and the premise are insufficient to support the conclusion. Because ankle swelling can result from other problems besides heart failure, more evidence is needed to determine that heart failure has caused Mr. Smith's swollen ankles.*

whether the client's signs and symptoms are consistent with normal progression of an illness or whether a complication may be developing. Knowing the problems or complications that can occur with an illness, medical treatment, or surgical procedure can help you determine the meaning of the data you collect.

Reasoning also includes recognizing and understanding psychological and social responses to a health problem. These responses must be distinguished from the signs and symptoms of the illness itself.

Reasoning includes making **inferences** from the data, which means that you attach meaning to the data or reach a conclusion about the data. Inferential reasoning is based on a premise or proposition that supports or helps to support a conclusion. Correct inferential reasoning is based on knowing that the facts are correct, that the premise is correct, and that the known information is sufficient to reach the conclusion. Box 6-2 illustrates examples of correct and incorrect inferential reasoning.

You will routinely make inferences about the meaning of information as you collect it. However, reaching a conclusion too rapidly can result in errors. Always validate the data and explore the problem further. Look for evidence that you can use to judge the extent of the problem, and look for logical relationships between the data and the probable causes.

Using Intuition. **Intuition** is an ability to understand the whole without having to systematically examine the parts. It is knowing without always knowing why you know. The knowing comes in a flash of understanding, or a gestalt, without being aware of the thinking that has preceded the understanding. This kind of thinking starts with the whole and then examines the parts to validate that the thinking is correct.

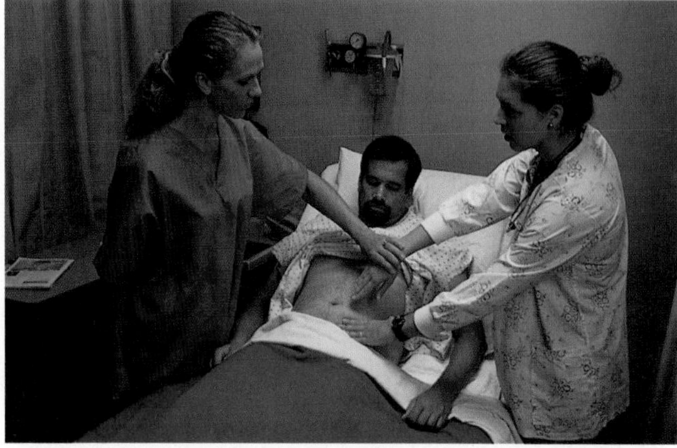

FIGURE 6-3 Well-developed intuitive reasoning distinguishes the expert nurse from the novice. Here, an expert nurse guides a novice nurse through a systematic physical examination guided by intuitive reasoning.

Some people appear to be naturally intuitive thinkers, having developed a preference for intuitive reasoning from early childhood. However, poorly developed or untrained intuition skills can lead to faulty reasoning, and an excessive reliance on intuitive reasoning raises the danger of accepting a conclusion without verifying that the facts support the conclusion. A novice should never rely on intuition alone.

Intuition can be developed through repeated systematic examination of data to arrive at an appropriate conclusion. After multiple experiences with similar situations and similar correct conclusions, you will begin to develop intuitive reasoning as a valid basis for nursing actions.

Well-developed intuitive reasoning distinguishes the expert nurse from the novice (Figure 6-3). With intuition the nurse acts correctly, seemingly without thinking, and cannot always explain the basis for the action. Intuition is efficient reasoning that allows the nurse to act quickly to save a life or prevent a complication. It allows the nurse to recognize a client's feelings or sense a level of understanding and respond appropriately (Benner, 1999; Benner, Tanner, & Chesla, 1996).

Validating. **Validation** means substantiating or confirming the accuracy of information using another source or another method. Cross-validation of both objective and subjective data increases the accuracy of all the data. For example, you can validate your interpretation of nonverbal behavior by asking the client about it. When the client reports symptoms (subjective data), you can try to validate them with objective findings. Imagine that a client has reported being constipated; you can look for such objective evidence as lack of a bowel movement, a hard and dry stool, or a distended abdomen.

Sometimes family members or significant others can be used to validate information given by the client. The family can be especially helpful when the client has developed symptoms too gradually to be aware of their onset.

When the client and a family member provide conflicting reports, you must make a clinical judgment about which information to accept. Sometimes you can validate the most accurate account by using other sources, such as the medical or health record, objective observations, other family members, or the judgments of other team members. For example, suppose a client reports having an occasional alcoholic beverage, whereas a family member reports that the client is a heavy drinker. You check the medical or health record and find that the client's blood alcohol level on admission indicates heavy drinking. This information does not confirm that the client continually drinks large amounts of alcohol, but it does provide evidence that supports the family member's position.

INTERVIEWING

An **interview** is a planned series of questions designed to elicit information for a particular purpose. Whether you enter a client's room to assess a complication or a complaint, make a phone call to a home health care client, or take an initial history, the interview has a definite purpose. You know in advance exactly what information is needed. An interview can be formal or informal; the following principles can be applied to either.

A well-conducted interview helps the client explain his or her own interpretation and understanding of the condition or reason that prompted the visit. The interview usually begins with an open approach that allows the client to talk until you develop an understanding of the client's perspective. Next, you will ask a series of questions while continuing to give the client some control of the interview. The client should feel like your partner in explaining and defining health problems.

The initial assessment interview begins with information about the client's **chief complaint,** which is the problem that caused the client to seek health services, call the physician, or request a visit with a nurse; it is the client's description of the problem. The initial assessment typically includes both nursing and medical emphases. The **nursing history** is a narrative of the client's past health and health practices that focuses on information needed to plan nursing care. The medical history focuses on illness and the treatment of disease. The medical and nursing histories have some elements in common. Both types are collected through interviewing the client, and they use an assessment framework to ensure thoroughness. The physical examination follows the assessment interview.

PHASES OF THE ASSESSMENT INTERVIEW

A successful interview depends on preparation that anticipates the client's needs and sets the stage for the interview. Additional skills are engaged to ensure that the assessment is comprehensive and that the time with the client is productive. Interviewing skills are engaged in each of four phases of the interview process: preparation, orientation, the working phase, and termination.

Preparation. You need to prepare for each assessment both mentally and physically to assess each client systematically and thoroughly. The extent of your preparation depends on the purpose of the assessment. It may be as brief as asking a colleague to provide pertinent data before entering a room to assess a client's report of pain. A comprehensive health assessment requires more extensive preparation.

As part of your preparation, you will set the stage for the assessment interview. Ideally, a comprehensive health history should take place in a private setting because some of the conversation may be sensitive or embarrassing to the client.

Of course, all client information is confidential. Assure the client that the information you solicit will be shared only with the health care team and only for purposes related to providing care. Do not suggest that any information will be kept confidential from the health care team. In some cases, you may need to inform the client of your obligation to share information with legal authorities; as needed, do so before asking for information that may be incriminating.

In addition, the client should be comfortable and have any immediate needs met before the interview begins. Immediate needs may be as simple as going to the bathroom, or they may require you to treat pain or reposition the client to ease difficult breathing. The client's condition always determines how much information can be collected in one sitting. Before beginning the interview, assess the client's probable reliability in providing or reporting health information.

Orientation. The **orientation phase** is a brief exchange to establish the interview's purpose, the examination procedures, and the nurse's role in the interview process. The orientation phase in the initial interview is important because it establishes the nurse-client relationship as a legally binding contract. The nurse should be seen as a person who can be trusted with confidential information, trusted to provide competent care, and trusted in some cases with the client's life. The relationship will benefit from establishing an atmosphere that communicates care for the client.

Therefore the first step in client assessment is establishing a nurse-client relationship based on mutual trust and understanding. In other words, you must build rapport with the client. *Rapport* means that there is a sense of understanding and trust between the nurse and client, suggesting that each of you has a vested interest in the client's well-being. When rapport is present, the client is more likely to reveal personal information.

Your demeanor can help establish rapport and trust to the extent that you portray yourself as a professional, knowledgeable person who is interested in the client.

In a social relationship, flirting, giggling, joking, exchanging personal stories, or talking about sports events are expected forms of interchange. In a professional relationship, however, the conversation focuses on the reason for the relationship: the client. The client is the most important person in the relationship. A small amount of social interchange can help some clients be more comfortable with you, but you must avoid using a client relationship to meet your own personal or social needs.

Begin the assessment by identifying the client's immediate concerns and addressing them. A mother admitted to the hospital for elective surgery may need to know how to use the telephone to call her children before she will be interested in talking about the upcoming surgery. One client who is admitted for open-heart surgery may be worried about the surgery itself, whereas another may have questions about the postoperative diet and smoking cessation plan. Allow the client's questions and concerns to shape and focus the assessment, but do not limit the interview to these areas. Box 6-3 lists key points for the orientation phase.

Working Phase. The **working phase** is the phase of the interview process in which the client and nurse work together to review the client's health history and establish potential and actual problems that will be addressed as part of the care plan. The nurse gains insight about the client's concerns and expectations. The client feels assured these concerns will be addressed.

Termination. Skillfully ending the interview leaves both the nurse and the client feeling satisfied that the purpose has been accomplished, the client has been understood, and there is no unfinished business. The nurse prepares the client for **termination** of the interview by announcing in advance the approximate length of time the interview will take. The client will know how much time the nurse expects to devote to the process. As the interview nears an end, it may be helpful to state that you have just a few more questions. The last phase of the interview allows time for the client to ask questions and address any additional concerns that have not been covered in the interview.

BOX 6-3 *Key Points for the Orientation Phase*

- Establishing rapport with the client is essential. Rapport implies understanding and trust between the nurse and the client.
- The initial contact with the client sets the tone for the interview.
- The client who feels acceptance and positive regard is more likely to discuss feelings, thoughts, and values.
- Your tone of voice, body language, choice of words, and dress all give direct messages to the client.
- The psychosocial interview can involve discussing sensitive personal information; privacy is important.
- The interview should have a basic structure and a quality of professionalism.
- Begin by introducing yourself, and then describe your credentials, your role in the person's care, and the purpose of the interview.

TYPES OF INTERVIEWS

You will need to choose the method of conducting an interview on the basis of the type of information you need to collect, the purpose of the interview, and the client's skill in describing problems. Interviews can be primarily directed or nondirected. Most interviews will make use of a combination of approaches.

Directed. In a directed interview, you maintain control over the interview by asking a list of questions that call for specific information from the client. The directed interview is used to elicit specific information and to ensure that the interview covers all relevant areas of assessment. One advantage of the directed interview is its ability to focus the client on information that is pertinent to the immediate concern, avoiding extraneous information. The directed interview is an efficient way to collect data in a short time.

The directed interview makes use of **closed questions**, questions that call for a specific, short response from the client. For example, to assess pain the nurse asks, "Do you have pain? Where is the pain? Describe the pain? How severe is the pain?" The directed interview may also use **leading questions,** questions that suggest a possible appropriate response. An example of a leading question is, "Are you frightened that the diagnosis will be cancer?" Using closed questions can help you collect the most pertinent information in the shortest time.

The directed interview has the disadvantage of not providing the opportunity for clients to freely express their concerns, fears, or feelings. You can obtain the most basic and necessary information, but the client may be left feeling that you are not concerned enough. Clients need to express their feelings and describe their symptoms from their own point of view to feel understood.

Nondirected. The nondirected interview gives more control to the client, thus allowing freer expression of concerns and feelings. Many clients try to "make sense" of their symptoms and may have associated meanings and antecedents to events surrounding the onset of symptoms that may or may not be relevant. The nondirected interview offers the client the opportunity to discuss and seek clarification about these meanings and events.

The nondirected interview uses primarily **open-ended questions** that ask for longer, interpretive responses. Open-ended questions do not call for a specific answer and may be phrased as a request rather than a question, such as "Tell me about the events that brought you to the hospital" or "Describe your symptoms." Open-ended questions are more useful for eliciting information from the client's point of view. A disadvantage of the nondirected interview is the client can become involved in discussing tangential information that is not pertinent.

ORGANIZING THE DATA

A **database** is all of the information that has been collected about the client and recorded in the health record as a baseline for the initial plan of care. It typically includes the data from the physician's client history and physical examination, the nurse's assessment, laboratory and diagnostic test results, and input from other members of the health care team. The database is used for comparing the client's response to treatment with the client's baseline condition.

A health care agency establishes a **minimum data set** that specifies information that must be collected from every client entering or being admitted to an institution. There is usually some commonality among clients in a particular setting that directs the decision about what to include in the minimum data set. Many institutions have assessment forms designed to ensure the collection of the minimum data set. Box 6-4 illustrates a typical minimum data set for a hospitalized client.

BOX 6-4 *Typical Minimum Data Set for Admission of a Hospitalized Client*

At Admission
- Admitted from *(home, physician's office, emergency medical service, or emergency department)*
- Mode of arrival *(ambulatory, wheelchair, or stretcher)*
- I.D. band on *(yes/no)*

Present Illness
- Vital signs
- Height and weight
- Time and type of last oral intake
- Chief complaint
- Observations

Allergies
- List drugs, food, other
- Describe reaction
- Allergy band on *(yes/no)*

Prostheses
- Dentures
- Glasses
- Contact lenses
- Hearing aid
- Artificial limb
- Artificial eye
- Other

Equipment: Adaptive Devices Used
- Safety rails
- Pickup extension
- Ramp
- Chairlift

Medication History
- List dose, frequency, date and time of last dose
- Medications brought to hospital
- Disposition (list medications)
- Valuables (to safe [policy explained], to home [with whom])

Medical Health History
- Previous illness or hospitalization
- Bleeding tendencies
- Circulatory problems
- Previous transfusion
- Hypertension
- Asthma
- Hay fever
- Arthritis
- Heart problems
- Kidney problems
- Cancer
- Diabetes
- Epilepsy

Functional Status (Activities of Daily Living)
- Primary language spoken
- Diet
- Hygiene (bathing, dressing, grooming)
- Sleeping patterns
- Communication/speaking
- Comprehension
- Seeing/hearing

Mobility (Describe Limitations)
- No limitations
- Unable to sit
- Unable to stand
- Requires walker/cane
- Requires wheelchair
- Requires partial/complete assistance

Admission Instructions Given
- Bathroom emergency light
- Visitor policy
- Meals/guest meals
- Smoking
- Room: Bed control, phone, call light, TV control, side rails
- Electric appliances OK. *or* maintenance notified of non-U.L. equipment

Social Assessment/Discharge Planning
- Religion
- Culture
- Apparent family support system
- Are any persons in your home dependent on you?
- Obvious family conflicts that may impair health care in the future
- Able to administer all medications
- Indications of possible neglect or abuse
- Do you anticipate any problems after discharge?
- Able to return to previous living situation
- Will you need help when you go home?
- Independence in the home setting?
- Are you being seen by any health service/agency?
- Do you have any suggestions that will help us with your care here?
- Identified client/family education needs
- Person to notify in emergency
- Respondent *(if other than client)*

BEGINNING THE HEALTH HISTORY

Health care agencies generally use a standardized assessment tool or form on which to record your health history interview. This tool may vary, depending on the goals for care and the type of services offered by the agency. Acute care agencies with short-term stays will need only the information necessary to manage the short-term experience. Some information is gathered for the purpose of helping clients plan their care after discharge. If a client appears to need extensive assistance with discharge planning, additional information may be gathered.

Some agencies use a form organized as a review of body systems, whereas functional ability or other nursing assessment schemata organize other forms. In all cases, the goal is to achieve a systematic, comprehensive assessment appropriate to the services of the agency. No matter what organizational framework you use, your assessments will be more efficient when you use a consistent, thorough pattern.

In an effort to reduce the time spent documenting, ensure comprehensive assessment, and meet the legal requirements for documentation, assessment forms have been developed that allow you to complete a checklist and possibly write brief notes. Computerized charting systems take the idea one step further, and you may choose from a list to record your findings. You may need to add a narrative nursing note to be sure you have completely documented the assessment.

Usually, a systematic assessment begins with an exploration of the client's biographical data, expectations and goals, reason for the visit, and medical and family histories. It then can expand into a holistic approach on the basis of an assessment framework (functional health patterns or body systems) that addresses all aspects of the client's health.

Biographical Data. **Biographical data** consist of information that identifies and describes the person, such as name, address, age, gender, religious affiliation, race, occupation, other people residing in the household, and the number of dependent children. This kind of information is also referred to as **demographic data** because it is factual information that can be aggregated to describe populations of clients. Biographical information helps the health provider anticipate problems common to a particular group. For example, the probable causes of difficulty in urinating would be different in a 55-year-old man and in a 16-year-old boy. Biographical data may also be collected by having the client complete an admission form or by reviewing the client's record.

Expectations and Goals. In describing their symptoms or concerns, clients may provide cues to their feelings about their illness, expectations of the health care encounter, or health care goals. You should listen for information that suggests that the client fears a serious or life-threatening problem. Sometimes you can provide information that calms those fears or helps the client gain a realistic perspective.

The client's goals and expectations are affected by the setting. In home health care, the client may be seeking information to decide whether to call a physician or information to determine whether the family has the resources to manage a problem. The family may expect you to give them information or help them manage the problem. The hospitalized client may be expecting a short hospital stay, full recovery, and immediate return to usual activities. Other expectations of the hospitalized client include being free from pain, being treated with respect, being safe, and receiving appropriate treatment for the presenting problem. The nurse needs to know if the client's expectations and goals match those of the health care team.

Social and cultural history provides cues to the person's values and experience with health care (Figure 6-4). It may also suggest the need to investigate problems that are more likely to occur within a particular group. Care can be planned that is consistent with the client's values.

Reason for the Visit. The health care provider usually begins by finding out the reason for the encounter from the client's point of view. The physician often writes only brief descriptions of the client's problems in the medical record; therefore you may need a more complete description from the client. Most clients appreciate the opportunity to review the details of the experience that has led them to seek health care.

While listening to the client's account of the reason for the visit, you are gathering information about the client's knowledge level and feelings about the problem and areas for teaching. Using active listening techniques, you may discover that the client has misunderstandings about the medical treatment plan. If you cannot remedy these misunderstandings, you will need to share this information with the physician.

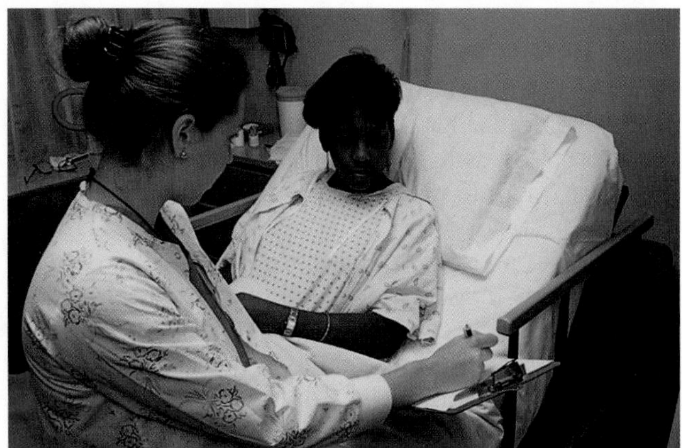

FIGURE 6-4 The social and cultural history provides important clues to the client's health-related values and to the client's experience with the health care system.

History of Present Illness. Information about the history of the present illness helps to anticipate problems the client may have and to understand the illness from the client's point of view. Having described the reason for the visit, the client may have given a complete account of the history of the present illness. If not, you can help the client fill in missing information. It is helpful to know when the symptoms began, the severity of the symptoms, and what actions were taken to control them. The client who enters the hospital may have been managing an illness for a long time through outpatient services, or the symptoms may have had a sudden onset. The following questions may be helpful: Have you been seeing a physician for this problem? What did the doctor tell you about the problem? What medications have you been taking? Did the medication help? Have you received other treatment?

Assessing the Chief Complaint. You can encourage the client to describe the chief complaint by asking questions such as these: How can I help you? What brought you to the hospital? or Tell me about your problem. Told in the client's own words, the chief complaint establishes the purpose of the contact, provides direction for the assessment, and establishes the nurse-client relationship.

Then you will gather information to fully describe the client's problem. Ask questions that help the client describe the specific signs and symptoms associated with the problem and provide a history of the present illness. The following seven variables provide a core description of most problems. Although all the variables may not apply to every symptom, using this general pattern of assessment will help you to be thorough.

Location. Symptoms are often associated with a particular body part. Ask the client to be specific about the location of pain, numbness, or other sensation. For example, you might ask, "Can you point to the exact location of the pain in your abdomen?" or "Where does it hurt?" The location of a rash or other lesion may help identify the cause.

Quality. You are seeking the client's description of how the symptoms feel. Avoid giving the client words to describe the symptom but, if the client cannot find any words, you can offer choices. People will often describe a symptom by using an analogy, such as "pins pricking my skin," "a knife stabbing me," "something very heavy on my chest," or "something tearing." Clients' choices of analogies are fairly consistent for particular diseases and therefore may provide a definitive cue to the medical diagnosis.

Quantity. Measuring quantity is an attempt to determine the intensity or severity of the symptom. Quantity can be elicited as frequency, volume, number, effects on activity, and extent. You might ask, "How severe is your symptom?" or "How often does it occur?" To get more objective data about pain, it may be useful to have the client rate the pain or other symptom on a scale of 0 to 10, with 10 being the most severe pain imaginable.

Chronology. It may be helpful to know how long the client has had the symptom. Was the onset insidious (slow, gradual) or acute (sudden)? Is the symptom constant, or does it come in episodes? Does the intensity vary with time? Does the symptom disturb the client's sleep?

Setting. Where was the client, and what was happening when the symptoms first occurred? The setting may suggest that stress, activity, or environmental pollution is affecting the symptom. For example, the onset of asthma when the person goes to a park may suggest an environmental trigger for the attack.

Aggravating or alleviating factors. Ask what the client has found to be helpful in relieving the symptom. What attempts has the client made to relieve the symptom? Is there any activity that makes it worse? Does eating make it worse or better? Does resting help? Was aspirin used to reduce a fever?

Associated factors. Look for anything else that might have been missed. Associated factors will vary according to the nature of the problem. You may ask about common associations. For example, for a client with diarrhea and abdominal cramps, ask if that person has recently traveled to a foreign country or eaten a food that might have produced the problem. The client may have an idea about what brought on the problem.

Medical History. A medical history is a review of problems or diseases that required or continues to require treatment by a physician. You are looking for any past medical problems that might influence the present illness by contributing to the problem or that might require altering the care for the current problem. A medical history may be elicited through a written checklist of common chronic problems, filled out by either the client or the nurse. Specific questions are asked about each illness in the client's history. By using a checklist, the client is encouraged to be thorough, and the focus of the interview is narrowed to pertinent information.

The medical history also includes a history of allergies to medications, pollutants, foods, and pollens. When the planned treatment includes the administration of medications, it is most important to ask about allergies to medications. If the client reports an allergy, obtain information about the type of reaction and how the reaction has been managed in the past.

Family History. As you ask about the client's medical history, you will also ask about the family history of any illnesses that are genetic or familial. As the name implies, genetic illnesses are passed through genes. Familial illnesses tend to be more prevalent in families, but the cause of the increased incidence in a family may be unknown. Familial illness may have a basis in lifestyle, diet, stress, or environmental factors.

REVIEW OF FUNCTIONAL HEALTH PATTERNS

One method of holistic assessment that provides information from a nursing rather than a medical perspective uses **functional health patterns,** a concept that refers to the positive and negative behaviors a person uses to interact with the environment and maintain health. During assessment you will examine the client's behaviors to determine whether each pattern is functional or dysfunctional. Assessment includes the usual pattern of behavior, complaints, limitations, problems associated with the pattern of behavior, behaviors used to manage the problem, and the client's coping skills. Each pattern is examined for biological, social, psychological, cultural, developmental, and spiritual factors influencing behavior. Box 6-5 lists categories of information to be assessed in each health pattern.

A few key questions in each category may be sufficient to determine that the person does or does not have a problem (Box 6-6). If a problem is suggested, you will ask further questions. However, assessment of functional patterns includes the client's strengths as well as weaknesses, problems, and limitations. Information about methods of health maintenance can be combined with indicators of physical function to develop possible causal relationships between the two. Additional questions are asked not to identify problems but to elicit the client's usual pattern of function. You need this information to more effectively support the client's usual pattern of functioning while providing care.

Clustering of data by functional health patterns also helps you identify problems that are responsive to nursing intervention and helps you assign appropriate nurs-

BOX 6-5 *Assessment of Health Patterns*

For each pattern, assess the following categories:

FUNCTIONAL PATTERN
- Present function
- Personal habits
- Culture and lifestyle factors
- Age-related factors

DYSFUNCTIONAL PATTERN
- History of dysfunction
- Diagnostic tests
- Risk factors associated with medical treatment plan
- Types of adaptations used

WHEN A PROBLEM IS IDENTIFIED IN A FUNCTIONAL PATTERN
- Relationship to other functional patterns

BOX 6-6 *Nursing History Questions Arranged by Functional Health Pattern*

HEALTH PERCEPTION–HEALTH MAINTENANCE PATTERN
- Client's description of general health
- Health practices; may include those related to managing a specific chronic illness
- Use of alcohol, tobacco, and other substances
- Home, school, and occupational safety
- Client's description of the cause of the illness (if present) and actions taken to manage it

NUTRITIONAL–METABOLIC PATTERN
- Does the client seem well nourished and well developed in general appearance?
- Is the client overweight or underweight for the age and height? Weight changes over last 6 months?
- What is the client's usual dietary pattern? Describe typical daily food and fluid intake.
- Does the client adhere to a special diet?
- How does the client's skin look? Are there lesions? Is the skin dry?
- What is the client's body temperature?
- What was the client's recent cholesterol level?
- Does the client have diabetes or a family history of diabetes?
- Does the client have dental problems? Swallowing problems?
- History of gastrointestinal or endocrine problems?

ELIMINATION PATTERN
- What are your usual bowel and bladder habits?
- What are the frequency, consistency, and color of your stool?
- Do you have difficulty with urination?
- Do you experience incontinence?
- How would you describe your use of laxatives or other aids to elimination?
- Do you have a history of bowel or bladder problems?

ACTIVITY–EXERCISE PATTERN
- What are your usual daily activities?
- What is your general level of physical fitness?
- Do you have a history of cardiac or respiratory problems?
- What activities give you the most pleasure?
- Do you need help with home maintenance?
- What is your activity tolerance?
- What is your usual pattern of exercise?
- Do you lead a sedentary lifestyle?
- Are you satisfied with your level of activity?
- Do you smoke? How many packs per day? For how many years?
- Are you able to feed yourself, bathe, go to the toilet, groom yourself, and move about in bed?
- Can you do the shopping and cooking, maintain your home, and achieve general mobility?
- Do you use a cane or walker or need help for walking?

SLEEP–REST PATTERN
- What is your usual pattern of sleep? Rituals? Reading, teeth brushing, stretching, meditation, watching TV?
- Do you feel rested in the morning?
- Do you use sleep aids?
- Are you able to sleep through the night?
- Do you have trouble falling asleep?

COGNITIVE–PERCEPTUAL PATTERN
- Do you have any difficulty with vision? Do you need glasses for reading or distance vision?
- Do you have any difficulty with hearing? Do you use a hearing aid?
- What is your name? Where do you live? What brought you to the hospital? What day is it?
- How long have you been here? Pain/discomfort? Heat/cold intolerance?

Continued

BOX 6-6 *Nursing History Questions Arranged by Functional Health Pattern—cont'd*

SELF-PERCEPTION–SELF-CONCEPT PATTERN
- What can you tell me about yourself?
- How will this hospitalization affect your life?
- How would you describe your support systems?
- Who relies on you?
- Where do you go for moral support?
- What do you do to "take care of yourself?"
- How do you feel about being ill? In the hospital?
- Do you have anxiety? How does it affect you?
- Do you have a history of anxiety disorders? Have you used psychotropic drugs? Alcohol? Street drugs?

ROLE–RELATIONSHIP PATTERN
- Who are the members of your household?
- How would you characterize the strength of your marriage?
- Is your family dependent on you? How are they managing during your hospitalization or illness?
- What are the ages of your children? Where do they live?
- Do close family ties characterize your family?
- When someone is ill, how does your family offer support?
- Do you have trouble sharing your problems and concerns with others?
- Do you have concerns that this illness will affect your ability to perform in your occupation?
- If you are unable to continue in your present occupation, are you in a position to retire?
- Do you have problems with your children that are difficult for you to manage?

SEXUALITY–REPRODUCTIVE PATTERN
- How would you characterize your satisfaction with your sexual relationship?
- Would disruption of your sexual relationship with your spouse be a factor in making a decision about having this surgery (taking this medication)?
- What was the date of your last menstrual period?
- At what age did you start menstruation? Are your menstrual periods regular?
- Do you use birth control? What method do you use?
- How many times have you been pregnant? How many live births?

COPING–STRESS TOLERANCE
- How are you managing (name the current problem or situation)?
- Have you talked to your (significant other) about (the current situation)?
- Have you informed your family and friends of your (current situation)?
- How would you characterize the level of stress in your life over the past year?
- Do you have someone with whom you are comfortable talking about problems or changes in your life?
- Do you use alcohol or other drugs to relieve stress?

VALUE–BELIEF PATTERN
- Is your life satisfying? Is your life good?
- What are your plans for the future?
- Do you have a religious affiliation?
- Do you actively practice a religion?
- Is spirituality important in your daily life?
- Will this hospitalization interfere with any religious practices?

ing diagnoses to dysfunctional patterns. Nursing care is more concerned with helping the person manage or function with a health problem than with diagnosing and treating illnesses. Therefore the focus of functional health patterns is on nursing diagnoses rather than on medical diagnoses.

Marjorie Gordon (2002) introduced a formal framework for assessing functional health patterns in 1982. She identified patterns of human function in 11 categories that address physical, psychological, spiritual, and social needs. Rather than treating the illness, nursing care is aimed at maintaining or improving the client's functional status in each of the 11 areas.

HEALTH PERCEPTION–HEALTH MAINTENANCE PATTERN

The health perception–health maintenance pattern describes the client's personal view of health and behaviors associated with the quest to be healthy. The client's risk factors for altered health and altered health maintenance should be explored. Although health maintenance is inherent in the other 10 patterns of functioning, exploring the health perception–health maintenance pattern separately gives you the opportunity to focus on health behaviors and risk factors. Important components of this pattern of behavior include the beliefs held by a person about control over health and the actions taken to change the state of health.

Assessment of the client's lifestyle can reveal areas where health can be improved. Knowledge of the client's health-seeking behaviors will provide you with cues to help the client plan care that will improve health. Assessment would include health-related activities in each of the functional patterns.

Assessment of health perceptions may begin by asking the client to describe any current health problems. Information about health perceptions and beliefs may be inherent in the response.

Another way to elicit information about health perceptions is to ask, "Have you had a similar experience in the past?" You may get information about previous illnesses or hospitalizations, including the client's perceptions of these experiences. In eliciting information about the current illness, ask the client to describe it, including the onset and the cause. Ask about previous treatment, whether the client complied with the treatment regimen, and whether the client anticipates having any problems in self-care as a result of the illness. When assessing health perception–health maintenance, you are looking for evidence of a healthy lifestyle.

Asking about the use of caffeine, herbs, supplements, prescription medications, over-the-counter drugs, tobacco products, alcohol, and illegal drugs should be a routine part of a health assessment. A nonjudgmental manner is essential to getting truthful information. Accurate information is particularly important if the hospitalized client is expected to have anesthesia or to be confined long enough for withdrawal symptoms to occur.

You also need to know whether the client has sufficient information to understand and manage the presenting health problems. Allow time to address the client's concerns, and frequently ask whether the client has any questions. By having the client describe problems and review information received from a physician, you can often detect whether the person has any misunderstandings.

NUTRITIONAL–METABOLIC PATTERN

The nutritional–metabolic pattern includes the client's dietary habits in relationship to metabolic need, and indicators of metabolic function, such as the skin, mucous membranes, and body temperature. Nutritional patterns are learned from early childhood; they may be modified by lifestyle changes, new knowledge, economics, or health problems. General health is affected by nutritional intake (Figure 6-5).

You will assess the dietary pattern to ascertain the feasibility of improving the client's general health in relationship to the health problems or potential health problems of obesity, undernourishment, uncontrolled diabetes, or high cholesterol. Metabolism is related to the gastrointestinal system and the endocrine system; therefore gastrointestinal, thyroid, and pancreatic functions are included.

ELIMINATION PATTERN

The elimination pattern overlaps with the effects of the nutritional pattern. Nutritional intake and fluid intake are important determinants of the pattern by which a person eliminates wastes from the body. This pattern includes bowel and bladder habits, the effect of activity on elimination, and the use of laxatives and other aids to elimination. Fluid loss through the skin must also be considered. The elimination pattern describes the function of the gastrointestinal tract, kidneys, and bladder.

ACTIVITY–EXERCISE PATTERN

The activity–exercise pattern includes the person's ability to be active and the level of activity the person chooses. Energy is expended in exercise, daily routines, leisure, and recreation. The person's ability to engage in activity affects both productivity and the quality of life. The activity–exercise pattern includes the person's physical capability for self-care, an attribute that also depends on

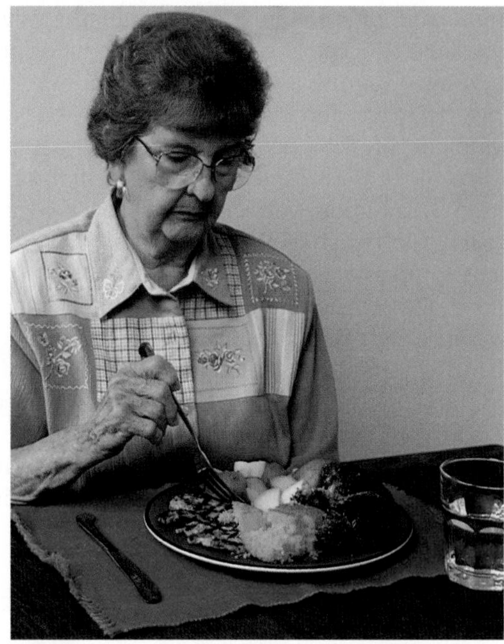

FIGURE 6-5 General health is affected by nutritional intake. This woman understands the importance of maintaining a well-balanced diet in older adulthood, even though it is difficult on a retiree's fixed income.

cognitive function, mobility, resources, knowledge, and motivation.

Assessment includes obtaining information about limitations of mobility, type of exercise, duration of exercise, ability to perform activities of daily living, and satisfaction with level of activity. The person's ability to perform activities is related to the musculoskeletal system, the neurological system, the cardiovascular system, and the respiratory system. You may need to assess each of these areas in depth, or simple observation may be sufficient to recognize, for example, that the client is or is not capable of adequate self-care.

SLEEP–REST PATTERN

All persons need sleep and rest, but the amount they need is variable. Assessment of the sleep–rest pattern includes the usual pattern of sleep and rest, aids to sleep, the person's satisfaction or feeling of being rested, and routines associated with sleep and rest. Problems related to the sleep–rest pattern may form the presenting complaint, or they may be secondary to the chief complaint.

COGNITIVE–PERCEPTUAL PATTERN

The cognitive–perceptual pattern includes sensation, perception, and cognition. Sensation is the reception of stimulation through receptors of the nervous system. Sensory functions include vision, hearing, touch, taste, smell, and proprioception (sense of body movement and position). Pain is a sensation and therefore included in this functional pattern. Perception is the ability to receive input from the senses, interpret the information in the brain, and interpret it in a meaningful way. The closely related concept of cognition is the act or process of knowing. Cognitive functions include memory, thoughts, language, and reasoning.

Assessment of the cognitive–perceptual pattern includes neurological assessment and the mental status examination. In addition, you will assess how a cognitive–perceptual problem alters the client's daily life and how the client compensates for the deficit.

Begin your assessment of the cognitive–perceptual pattern by spending a few minutes getting acquainted and conversing with the client. Listen for cues that the client is hearing and understanding you; is oriented to time, place, and person; and has memory of recent and past events. Evaluate the client's language for unusual speech patterns and reasoning. You may perform this assessment without asking any questions specific to the pattern.

SELF-PERCEPTION–SELF-CONCEPT PATTERN

The self-perception–self-concept pattern includes how the person views the self. Self-concept is an attitude, a feeling about self, or an evaluation of self; self-esteem is the affective component of self-concept that describes an attitude, feeling, or evaluation of self-worth. To understand a client's self-concept, you will need information about the person's perception of cognitive, affective, and physical abilities as well as the perception of body image and identity, the general sense of worth, and the general emotional pattern.

When assessing this pattern, you would like to know if the client has mental problems or emotional needs that must be addressed to provide the best care. It is particularly important for the home health care nurse to recognize depression, because this condition has a high potential for interfering with the client's ability to comply with the therapeutic regimen. The home health care client may have anxiety about managing at home and getting help when it is needed. The hospitalized client is at high risk for anxiety because of the potentially serious nature of problems that require hospitalization.

You will assess this pattern through active listening rather than by asking specific questions. Listen for negative self-talk, lack of confidence, and beliefs about how others regard the client. Also consider body posture, eye contact, voice tone, speech patterns, and general appearance.

ROLE–RELATIONSHIP PATTERN

Roles are the parts one plays in one's own life. Typically, they relate closely to relationships with children, spouse, friends, and co-workers. For example, a person may have the roles of mother, teacher, friend, and colleague. Roles and relationships are the means through which the need for love and belonging is met and self-esteem is developed.

Examining living arrangements, support systems, and family life assesses the role–relationship pattern. Complaints may include isolation, loneliness, abuse, and marital problems.

SEXUALITY–REPRODUCTIVE PATTERN

Sexuality is present from birth to the end of a person's life. The expression of sexuality varies among individuals by age, culture, beliefs, health, life circumstances, and social norms. Assessment of the sexuality–reproductive pattern must include the person's satisfaction and perceptions of appropriate sexual and reproductive behavior. Many of the external indicators of sexual patterns may be misleading or lead to stereotypical assumptions that may not be valid.

Generally, the sexuality–reproductive pattern is not assessed explicitly unless you have a reason to do so. For example, the client may indicate that a potential problem exists or that a potential problem is secondary to the problem for which the client is seeking treatment. Possible indicators include the strength of the client's relationship with a spouse, flirting behavior, an overtly sexy way of dressing, a single parent, children with different fathers, discomfort with persons of the opposite sex, and adults who remain unmarried beyond the usual age for marriage.

COPING–STRESS TOLERANCE PATTERN

Stress is a part of life that results from both positive and negative experiences, from hardships and joys, and from internal and external forces. A person's experience of stress varies with the perception of stress-producing events and the person's skills in managing both the events and the responses to them. During assessment, you would consider the client's evaluation of the current situation and experience with similar situations. In addition, how the client managed stressful situations in the past may provide useful information.

You may not assess this pattern directly, although hospital nurses commonly ask about previous reactions to hospitalization. In the process of describing the previous experience, the client often provides cues to how he or she coped with the experience. One client may say, "I don't know how I could have managed without my wife," whereas another may suggest that a warm, friendly relationship with the nurses helped in managing the experience. The home health care nurse may get cues from the home environment. A well-ordered, well-planned living environment may suggest that order and planning are a possible coping strategy.

VALUE–BELIEF PATTERN

The value–belief pattern describes the philosophical position that guides a person's choices or decisions in life. The spiritual self is a major component of this pattern. It also reflects what the individual perceives as important

Table 6-1 Data Illustrating Functional Health Patterns

A 50-year-old man is admitted to the hospital for abdominal pain. He is being evaluated for a bowel obstruction. Although pain applies specifically to the cognitive/perceptual pattern, it has the potential to affect all other functional patterns as well. Assessing its relationship to other functional patterns might reveal findings such as those listed here.

PATTERN	POSSIBLE FINDINGS
Self-Perception–Self-Concept	Client has never been hospitalized and denies that anything could be seriously wrong. "I must have food poisoning. The doctor will probably give me an antibiotic and send me home. One of the guys at work had the same thing." Well-developed muscles emphasized by tight-fitting shirt with rolled-up short sleeves. Attempts to flirt with the nurses.
Value–Belief	Lists Christian as religious preference. Wife says she will call the minister if he has to go to surgery, but her husband does not attend church very often.
Role–Relationship	States he is angry at his wife because she insisted that he come to the hospital. Is employed as a lineman for the city utility company and is concerned because a recent electrical storm has left a number of power lines down. Has a 30-year-old son who is married and works with his father as a lineman. A 33-year-old daughter is unmarried and lives in another city.
Elimination	Usually has a daily bowel movement after breakfast. Has not had a bowel movement in 5 days. Abdomen hard and distended. Bowel sounds absent. Voids without difficulty. Urine dark and concentrated. Results of abdominal computed tomography (CT) scan pending. Father and one uncle died of cancer of colon.
Activity–Exercise	Usually engages in daily weight lifting but has not exercised since the onset of pain 3 days ago. No history of cardiovascular problems. Has never had cholesterol checked. Vital signs: blood pressure 100/70, pulse 108, respiration 34, temperature 101.2° F. Skin is pale, cool, and clammy. Became dizzy after getting out of bed to go to the bathroom. Hemoglobin and hematocrit levels slightly elevated. Skin turgor sluggish. Eyes sunken. Breath sounds diminished in lung bases.
Cognitive–Perceptual	Complains of severe, diffuse abdominal pain; a 7 on a scale of 0 to 10. Agrees to take pain medication to make his wife happy. Alert and oriented.
Nutritional–Metabolic	Has not eaten much for 3 days and nothing for 24 hours. Last meal caused severe nausea followed by vomiting. Appetite is generally good. Often eats in fast-food places for lunch. Coffee, eggs, and toast for breakfast. Wife prepares a balanced meal for supper. No family history of diabetes. Intravenous infusion of D5/NS started in left forearm at 125 mL/hr. Nasogastric tube to low intermittent suction. Serum sodium and potassium levels slightly high.
Sexuality–Reproductive	Appears to have a close relationship with wife.

to quality of life. Often values and beliefs are derived from a religious or other formal philosophical base. Family strongly influences the formation of values and beliefs as well. Health care that is consistent with and supportive of the person's value system is most likely to result in positive health outcomes. Table 6-1 illustrates assessment data obtained for a client and grouped by functional health patterns.

DOCUMENTING THE DATA

The assessment data that you collect must be documented in the client's medical record so that the entire health care team has access to it. Thus the record serves as a means of communication and sharing information for the health care team. The database includes the information contributed by all members of the health care team.

Clearly, it is crucial that data recorded about the client be accurate, complete, clear, and concise. The data will be used to make treatment decisions not just for nursing care but for medical care, respiratory care, physical therapy, diet therapy, and others. The record should contain all information pertinent to the client's condition. Statements should be succinct, using the least number of words needed to convey meaning accurately. Often, potential or actual problems identified on an assessment form will need to be described in more detail in your nurse's notes.

Only factual information should be documented. Clear documentation differentiates between objective and subjective data. When the data come from the client, always indicate that the client has stated the information. Avoid including your opinions. Almost always, it is better to chart the facts that caused you to develop an opinion rather than the opinion itself. More information on documentation appears in Chapter 11.

▼ KEY PRINCIPLES

- Assessment does not exist in isolation from the other steps of the nursing process; making diagnoses, planning, and establishing outcomes take place simultaneously with assessment.
- Critical thinking is a necessary part of assessment to know what questions to ask, what the answers mean, how to follow up, and how to recognize the etiology of the problem.
- The most appropriate format for assessment depends on the purpose and type of the assessment.
- Using multiple sources of data increases the accuracy of the database.

Continued

- Prudent health assessment requires that you collect data about sensitive subject matter in a private setting.
- Assessment requires active listening and active mental processing, not merely asking a list of questions.
- During assessment, the client's immediate concerns should occupy your focus of attention.
- Assessment begins with the chief complaint, proceeds to health history, and ends with a physical examination.
- When a symptom is revealed, it should be followed with symptom analysis that helps the client describe the symptom.
- A systematic method of data collection can help ensure a comprehensive, holistic assessment.
- The collected data are documented in the health record to aid continuity of care and communication with the health care team.

REVIEW QUESTIONS

1. Your client has put on the call light and reported that he is in pain. Which assessment type is most appropriate to this situation?

1. Holistic assessment
2. Establishing ABC priorities
3. Analysis of a symptom
4. Ongoing assessment

2. Your client has just returned to the surgical nursing unit from the recovery room. His surgery ended 3 hours ago. Which assessment type is most appropriate to this situation?

1. Ongoing assessment
2. Analysis of a symptom
3. Focused assessment
4. Comprehensive assessment

3. Your client has moderate Alzheimer's disease. You are trying to determine if he needs an as-needed (prn) laxative. Without any hesitation, he tells you that he cannot be constipated because he has a daily bowel movement. Which is the best action?

1. Accept his assessment, and hold the laxative.
2. Validate the information with his daughter.
3. Examine his abdomen for bowel sounds and distention.
4. Tell him the doctor wants him to have the medication, and give it.

4. Which is the best method of terminating an initial assessment interview?

1. When you are almost done, say, "I just have a few more questions."
2. When you are finished, say, "That's all I need to know."
3. After the last question, close your notebook and stand up.
4. After the last question, say, "If you have any further questions, your doctor will be here is a couple of hours."

5. You have gathered information about how the client manages his diabetes. In which functional health pattern would you group this data?

1. Activity–exercise
2. Nutritional–metabolic
3. Cognitive–perceptual
4. Coping–stress tolerance

Bibliography

*American Nurses Association. (2001). Don't just simply "follow the form." *Same-Day Surgery, 25*(6), 66.

American Nurses Association. (2004). *Nursing: Scope and standards of practice* (3rd ed.) (Publication No. 9801ST). Washington, DC: Author.

*Benner, P. (1999). Nursing leadership for the new millennium: Claiming the wisdom and worth of clinical practice. *Nursing and Health Care Perspectives, 20*(6), 312-319.

*Benner, P. A., Tanner, C. A., & Chesla, C. A. (1996). *Expertise in nursing practice: Caring, clinical judgment, and ethics.* New York: Springer.

Casper, G. R., & Kenron, D. A. (2005). Information technology and the clinical nurse specialist: A framework for technology assessment—approaches for the selection of a home technology device. *Clinical Nurse Specialist, 19*(4), 170-174.

Consider patient use of OTC medications. (2005). *ED Nursing, 8*(4), 46.

Cutilli C. C. (2005). Do your patients understand? Determining your patients' health literacy skills. *Orthopaedic Nursing, 24*(5), 372-379.

Dulak, S. B. (2004). A practical guide to a thorough history. *RN Travel Nursing Today, 67, TNT 14-21.*

Gordon, M. (2002). *Manual of nursing diagnosis* (10th ed.). St. Louis, MO: Elsevier Health Sciences.

Graf, C. (2006). Functional decline in hospitalized older adults: It's often a consequence of hospitalization, but it doesn't have to be. *American Journal of Nursing, 106*(1), 58-68.

Jarvis, C. (2004). *Physical examination and health assessment* (4th ed.). Philadelphia: Saunders.

Klymko, K. W. (2005). Assessment: Cognitive assessment in elderly African American adults with hypertension. *Journal of Gerontological Nursing, 31*(11), 15-20.

Madsen D., Sebolt, T., Cullen, L., Folkedahl, B., Mueller, T., Richardson, C., et al. (2005). Listening to bowel sounds: An evidence-based practice project. *American Journal of Nursing, 105*(12), 40-49.

Magnan, M. A., Reynolds, K. E., & Galvin, E. A. (2005). Barriers to addressing patient sexuality in nursing practice. *Medsurg Nursing, 14*(5), 282-290.

Manias, E., Aitken, R., & Dunning, T. (2004). Decision-making models used by "graduate nurses" managing patients' medications. *Journal of Advanced Nursing, 47*(3), 270-278.

Narayan, S. M., Corcoran-Perry, S., Drew, D., Hoyman, K., & Lewis, M. (2003). Decision analysis as a tool to support an analytical pattern-of-reasoning. *Nursing & Health Sciences, 5*(3), 229-243.

Protocol designed to identify often-overlooked problems in the elderly. (2005). *Senior Care Management, 8*(7), 82-83.

Robichaux C., Dittmar, V., & Clark, A. P. (2005). Are we providing culturally competent care? *Clinical Nurse Specialist, 19*(1), 11-14.

Ryan, B. A. (2005). Advice of counsel: Can a nurse adequately assess what she didn't see? *RN, 68*(11), 70.

Saunders, C. S. (2002). Tips for better history-taking. *Patient Care, 36*(8), 58-60, 65, 69.

Scanlan, B. C. (2005). The value of comprehensive geriatric assessment. *Care Management Journals: Journal of Case Management; The Journal of Long Term Home Health Care, 6*(1), 2-8.

Velez-McEvoy, M. (2004). Occupational health: Spanish. Nursing assessment: Taking the history. *AAOHN Journal, 52*(1), 8-9.

*Asterisk indicates a classic or definitive work on this subject.

Chapter 7

Assessing Vital Signs

Media Resources

- Nursing Skills Online
- evolve Evolve Website http://evolve.elsevier.com/Harkreader/
- 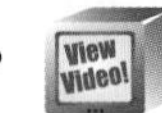 Companion CD
- View Video! Skills Video Clips

Learning Objectives

After studying this chapter, you should be able to do the following:

- Identify the rationale for the assessment of vital signs
- Interpret deviations from the normal ranges of each vital sign according to the client's age
- Describe the normal physiological features of each vital sign
- List factors that influence temperature, pulse, respirations, oxygen saturation, and blood pressure
- Safely and accurately measure axillary, oral, rectal, and tympanic temperatures; apical and radial pulses; respirations and oxygen saturation; and blood pressure
- Measure vital signs in an organized, accurate manner
- Document and report vital sign measurements correctly

Key Terms

apical pulse
auscultatory gap
basal metabolic rate (BMR)
bradycardia
bradypnea
diastolic blood pressure
eupnea
Korotkoff's sounds
orthostatic hypotension
oxygen saturation
peripheral vascular resistance
pulse deficit
pulse oximeter
pulse pressure
systolic blood pressure
tachycardia
tachypnea
thermogenesis
thermolysis
tidal volume

Vital signs are a basic component of assessment of the physiological and psychological health of a client. Body temperature, pulse, respiration, oxygen saturation, and blood pressure are the signs of life, and their assessment allows you to (1) identify specific life-threatening clinical problems and select nursing interventions and (2) detect changes in the client's health status. There are many situations in which you may assess a client's vital signs:

- As part of a physical examination
- To establish a baseline on admission to a health care facility
- For routine monitoring during the client's stay in a hospital
- To make a nursing diagnosis of ineffective thermoregulation
- To determine the effects of surgery or other invasive procedure
- To determine the effects of medications on temperature or the cardiovascular or respiratory systems
- To evaluate the effectiveness of the medical treatment plan
- To evaluate the effectiveness of nursing interventions, such as ambulation
- To detect improvement or deterioration in the client's condition
- To validate health status on discharge from a nursing unit

As in any scientific measurement, accuracy depends on precision of measurement. A careless assessment can result in inaccurate planning, interventions, and evaluation. Perform the procedures methodically to ensure accurate readings and maintain your client's safety.

INTERPRETING VITAL SIGNS

To interpret the significance of vital sign measurements, you need to analyze the data in relationship to other findings in the assessment. The significance of vital signs does not stem from a single value but from the *relationship* of the vital signs to each other and to other assessment findings. In addition, the *trend* of changes in vital signs is highly important and should guide your conclusions about the client's condition.

First, compare the client's readings with the average normal parameters. Normal values are different for children, adults, and older adults (Table 7-1). For example, 30 respirations per minute is normal for an infant but abnormally high for an adult.

Next, compare the data with the client's baseline and previous readings to consider what is normal for the specific client. Have any vital signs increased or decreased since the previous measurement? If the previous measurements were recent, is the client's condition changing quickly? If the condition is changing for the worse, how soon will you need to assess the vital signs again to verify the continuing trend? This may be as soon as 5 or 10 minutes. Do you need an emergency plan to prevent serious or fatal consequences?

Next, compare your data with the client's complete health history and condition. In a client with a history of hypertension, you may note a blood pressure that is higher than normal. In a client who just underwent surgery, pain may cause an increased pulse and blood pressure. Perhaps the client is taking a drug that adversely affects vital signs. For example, some medications, such as digitalis, may slow the heart rate. Others, such as aminophylline, may raise the heart rate. Be sure to review any over-the-counter medications or herbal supplements the client may have taken recently. Overall, the goal is to consider whether the client's vital signs are consistent with the history and current clinical status. If not, measure the vital signs again to make sure your readings are correct. If changes in the client's vital signs stem from a medication, consult the physician, who may change the dose.

In addition, consider the effects of the environment, activity level, and mental status on your results. Generally

Table 7-1 Average Range for Vital Signs According to Age-Group

AGE-GROUP	TEMPERATURE (ORAL) IN °F (°C)	PULSE PER MINUTE	RESPIRATIONS PER MINUTE	*Blood Pressure (in mm Hg)* SYSTOLIC	DIASTOLIC
Newborn	98.2 (axillary) (36.8)	100-180 (Mean, 125)	35-40	60-90	20-60
Infant up to age 1	99.4 (axillary) (37.4)	100-160 (Mean, 120)	30-40	85-105	50-65
Toddler ages 1 to 3	99.0-99.7 (37.2-37.6)	80-120 (Mean, 110)	25-40	95-105	50-65
Preschooler ages 3 to 6	98.6 (37)	70-110 (Mean, 100)	22-35	95-100	55-60
Child ages 6 to 12	98.6 (37)	65-100 (Mean, 90)	20-30	100-110	60-70
Adolescent ages 12 to 18	97.8-98.6 (36.6-37)	60-90 (Mean, 80)	16-20	110-120	60-65
Adult	98.6 ± 1 (37 ± 0.5)	60-100 (Mean, 75)	12-20	110-130	60-80
Older adult	97.6 ± (36 ± 0.5)	60-100 (Mean, 75)	12-20	120-140	70-90

vital signs should be assessed in quiet, comfortable, resting conditions. Is the room hot or cold? Does the client appear anxious, angry, or stressed? Has the client been exercising? Is the client a child who is upset and crying?

Action Alert! Reassess elevated blood pressure, pulse, and respiratory rate after the client has sat quietly for 10 to 15 minutes.

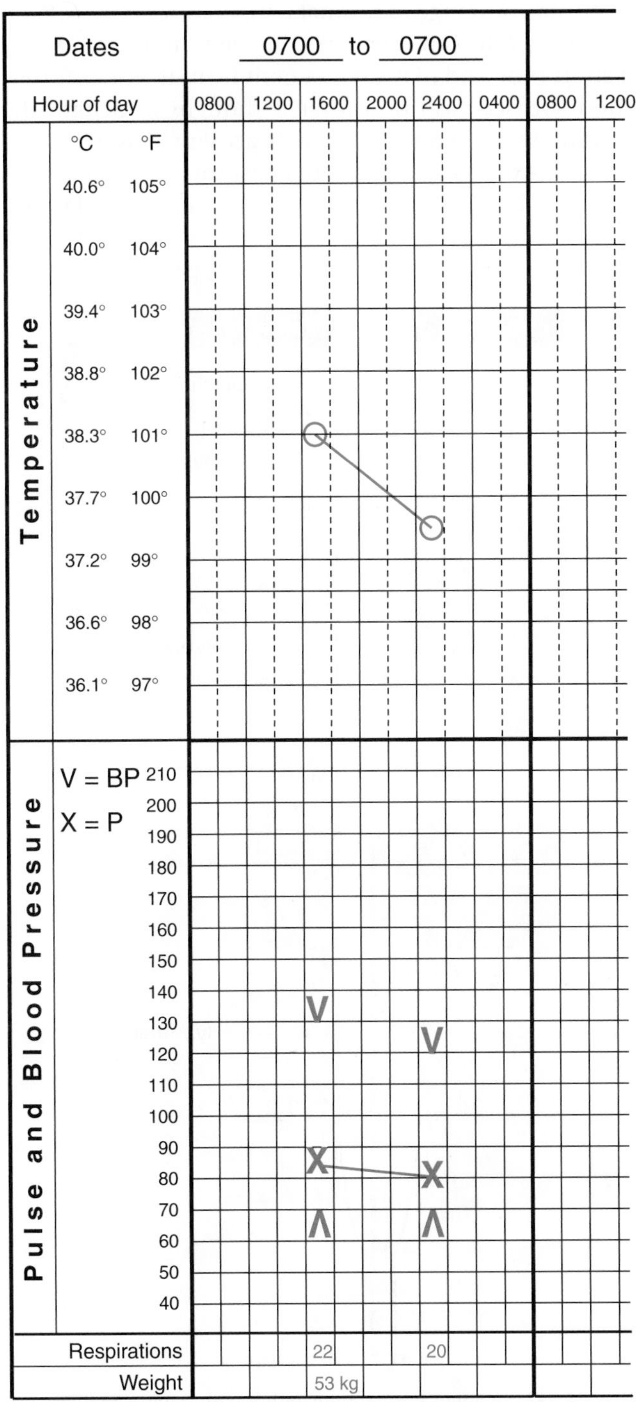

FIGURE 7-1 An example of how to chart vital signs.

Through interpretation of vital signs, nurses make decisions about the frequency of vital sign assessment. Although a physician's order or nursing unit policy typically specifies the minimum frequency for measuring vital signs, you are responsible for assessing vital signs any time a need arises. For example, if the client's temperature rises above 100.4° Fahrenheit (F) or 38° Celsius (C), you may decide to measure the temperature again in 60 minutes, even though the physician may have ordered temperature assessment every 4 hours.

Action Alert Increase the frequency of vital sign assessment if the client is at risk for a complication or a change in condition. Frequent assessment is indicated for fever, infection, recent surgery, chest pain, or shortness of breath.

As a nurse, you will also delegate vital sign assessment to unlicensed assistive personnel. You will be responsible for ensuring they know proper technique, and you will also need to specify what values or changes in values should be reported to you. Remember that you are ultimately responsible for awareness of vital signs as part of the client's overall clinical picture.

Pain has been referred to in the literature by some as the fifth vital sign. The reason is that, despite the many methods available to treat pain, nurses continue to inadequately assess and incompletely manage it. Pain and its management are discussed in depth in Chapter 37.

COMMUNICATING VITAL SIGNS

Whether your client's vital signs are normal or abnormal, you must communicate the findings to other health care providers. Document the vital signs on the appropriate form in the client's record immediately. A typical graphic record is easily read and shows trends in vital signs, and it may be used even where records are computerized (Figure 7-1).

Action Alert! Verbally report significantly abnormal vital signs or changes to the nurse in charge or to the physician/nurse practitioner. Changes in vital signs are key parameters for making changes in the treatment plan.

In addition, the client and family may request information about vital signs. Be prepared to provide health teaching about how to measure and interpret vital signs. Many clients must track vital signs as part of their ongoing health maintenance. For example, a client who takes an antihypertensive medication may need to routinely self-monitor blood pressure.

TEMPERATURE

Body temperature is measured to monitor for signs of inflammation or infection, but it may also reflect problems in thermoregulation. It reflects the balance between heat production and heat loss from the body. A healthy body effectively maintains a balance between heat production and heat loss. **Thermogenesis** is the generation of heat from chemical reactions that take place during cellular activity. In the presence of inflammation or infection these chemical reactions accelerate, causing a rise in body temperature. Heat is dispersed from the body through radiation, conduction, convection, and evaporation, a process called **thermolysis** (see Chapter 28).

Although the average normal body temperature is 98.6° F or 37° C, heat production varies with the **basal metabolic rate (BMR),** which represents the energy needed to maintain essential basic body functions, expressed as calories per hour per square meter of body surface. Heat production increases with muscular activity, sympathetic nervous system stimulation (which produces epinephrine and norepinephrine), and thyroid gland stimulation (which produces thyroxine). Thus normal body temperature varies by approximately plus or minus 1° F or 0.5° C.

UNDERSTANDING THERMOREGULATION

Thermoregulation balances heat production and heat loss to maintain a constant body temperature in a range between 96.8° F and 99.4° F (36° C and 37.4° C). The body temperature has a rhythmic biological variation throughout each 24-hour period, which is called *circadian rhythm*. For most people, temperature is lowest in the morning because the BMR slows during the inactivity of sleep. In the afternoon the increased activity of the day may raise the temperature by about 1° F. Stress, strong emotions, and exercise can increase cellular activity and thus also raise temperature within a normal pattern of variation.

Other factors can alter temperature as well. For example, estrogen causes women to have a slightly higher average temperature than men. Newborns, children, and older adults have a reduced capacity for thermoregulation. A cold environment speeds up heat loss, and a warm environment slows heat loss. Internally, infection and inflammation can raise body temperature through their pyrogenic influence on the medulla of the brain.

Physiological compensatory mechanisms are involuntary and help maintain a normal core temperature in the body. The autonomic nervous system helps to keep the core body temperature at 98.6° F (37° C) through receptors in the skin, abdomen, and spinal cord. These receptors sense internal and external temperature changes and send this information through the nervous system to the hypothalamic region of the brain. The data are integrated, and the appropriate effector mechanisms (such as blood vessels, sweat glands, and skeletal muscles) are activated.

The cardiovascular system plays an important role in maintaining body temperature through its vast network of blood vessels. An increase in body temperature causes blood vessels near the skin surface to dilate, called vasodilation. By bringing an increased volume of warmed blood to the skin surface, vasodilation enhances heat loss. In contrast, a decrease in body temperature causes vasoconstriction, which keeps warmed blood closer to the center of the body, thus maintaining its core temperature. By insulating the body, fat also helps to control heat loss. The act of shivering generates heat and helps to control heat loss as well.

Keep in mind that body cells function within a relatively narrow range of normal temperatures (Figure 7-2). However, cells can tolerate a change in temperature for a short time and may even benefit from it. For example, the increased heat of a fever is thought to benefit the immune system and increase its activity. However, prolonged, extreme temperature elevation (hyperthermia) or reduction (hypothermia) can lead to tissue damage

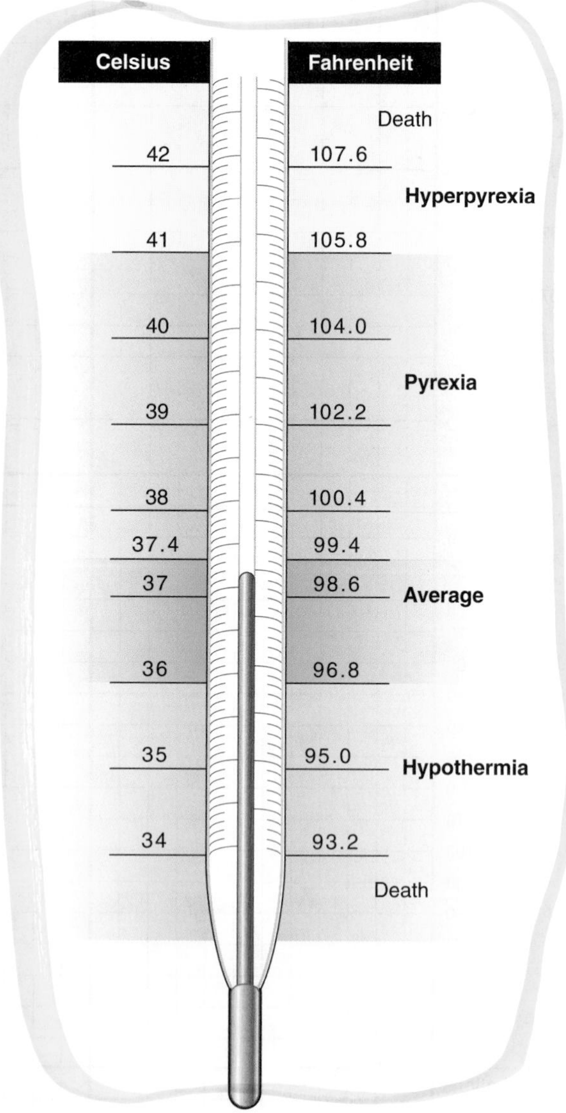

FIGURE 7-2 Range of normal body temperature and alterations in body temperature on the Celsius and Fahrenheit scales.

and death. High temperatures damage cells by inactivating proteins and enzymes. Low temperatures damage cells when ice crystals form and puncture the cell membranes.

We assist the body in maintaining a normal temperature by changing our behavior; for example, we may move to the shade, regulate the thermostat, or remove extra clothes. When attempting to lose heat, we may maintain an open posture with arms away from the body and possibly swing them (to enhance heat loss by convection). To conserve heat, we may have a closed the body posture with arms encircling the body.

Naturally, if a client cannot alter his or her temperature, is unconscious, or is unaware of the environment, you may need to intervene and help with temperature regulation. Even when clients can regulate temperature normally, your assessment of temperature offers vital information about their condition.

MEASURING TEMPERATURE

Temperature can be measured using either the Fahrenheit or the centigrade (or Celsius) scale (see Figure 7-2). The Fahrenheit scale has long been the standard in English-speaking countries and continues to be commonly used despite the movement of the scientific community to the centigrade scale. A hospital may use the centigrade scale, and you may need to discuss this with clients who use the more commonly understood Fahrenheit scale. Any reading can be converted from one scale to the other by completing a simple calculation (Box 7-1). Depending on client needs, you may use a glass thermometer, an electronic thermometer, a tympanic thermometer, chemical dots, or an intravenous catheter to measure temperature.

Glass Thermometer. Most glass thermometers are calibrated hollow cylinders with a liquid-filled bulb at the base. When heated, the liquid expands and rises in the hollow tube. Temperature is measured by the height of the column of liquid. The most common liquids are mercury and alcohol.

BOX 7-1 *Conversion Formulas for Fahrenheit and Celsius Scales*

CONVERTING FROM FAHRENHEIT TO CELSIUS

- Subtract 32 from the Fahrenheit reading.
- Multiply the resulting number by $5/9$.

For example, the following formula shows the conversion of 98.6° F to Celsius:

$$98.6° \text{ F} - 32 = 66.6 \times \{5/9\} = 37° \text{ C}$$

CONVERTING FROM CELSIUS TO FAHRENHEIT

- Multiply the Celsius reading by $\{9/5\}$(or 1.8).
- Add 32 to the resulting number.

For example, the following formula shows the conversion of 37° C to Fahrenheit:

$$37° \text{ C} \times \{9/5\} = 66.6 + 32 = 98.6° \text{ F}$$

For infection-control purposes, glass thermometers are color coded to signify rectal or oral use (Figure 7-3, *A*). The rectal thermometer is always red tipped and has a blunt tip to avoid trauma to delicate membranes.

Glass thermometers containing mercury, a poisonous substance, are no longer used in health care settings. Although they are inexpensive, easy to use, easily disinfected, and can be used multiple times for the same client, they cannot be shared between clients, have small calibrations that can be difficult to read, and take 5 to 7 minutes to get an accurate reading. The readings are recorded to the nearest 0.2° F.

The use of medical devices that contain mercury, such as thermometers and sphygmomanometers, is being systematically eliminated. Mercury-filled thermometers are being removed from retail stores. All forms of mercury are toxic to humans, but organic forms (i.e., methylated mercury) are much more toxic than the inorganic forms used in medical devices. However, if improperly disposed of, the inorganic form changes to an organic form. Disposal of mercury from medical facilities accounts for about 10% of the mercury contamination in the environment. Short-term exposure to high levels of mercury can produce severe respiratory irritation, digestive disturbances, and marked renal damage. With long-term exposure, mercury is a neurotoxin.

Action Alert! Do not attempt to clean up a mercury spill yourself. Call the hazardous waste disposal team at your agency, because the mercury must be recovered according to strict guidelines established by the Occupational Safety and Health Administration (OSHA).

Electronic Thermometer. You are more likely to use an electronic thermometer that has a heat-sensitive probe attached by a thin wire to a battery-powered control unit (Figure 7-3, *B*). It offers a convenient, safe, accurate, and fast method for measuring temperature. The reading is quickly displayed on the unit and is easy to read. Typically, the unit beeps when the measurement is complete. Readings can be measured to the nearest 0.1°.

An electronic thermometer can be used for oral, axillary, or rectal temperature measurements, and it can be used with multiple clients. The use of disposable probe covers (also called sheaths) prevents the transmission of microorganisms between clients. For visually impaired clients, electronic thermometers are available that give auditory temperature readings. The disadvantages of electronic thermometers are their high cost and the need for regular maintenance.

Tympanic Thermometer. The tympanic thermometer was designed to measure temperature quickly and easily in clients who cannot easily hold a thermometer in the mouth. A heat-sensitive probe is placed into the ear canal to measure the temperature of the blood in the tympanic membrane (Figure 7-3, *C*). Readily visible measurements are displayed on the unit and reflect temperature to the nearest 0.1°. The unit can be used for multiple clients because the disposable probe covers avoid the transmission of microorganisms. Tympanic thermometers are more costly than glass thermometers and must be regularly checked for accuracy.

Temperature Strip and Chemical Dot. A temperature strip or chemical dot is an inexpensive, disposable product for measuring temperature. Although the strip or dot lacks precision, it can ensure infection control for a client in an isolation unit, and it is easy to use at home (Figure 7-3, *D*). As the client's temperature rises or falls, the strip or dot changes color.

The disadvantage of the strip or dot is that it gives less accurate and variable temperature readings. In addition, sweating can alter the contact between the device and the client's skin, and this change may alter the reading.

Core Body Temperature. Core body temperature can be directly measured using a urinary bladder probe or a central venous catheter. The central venous catheter uses a thermistor attached to the central line. It is more accurate and reliable for measuring core temperature, but it is used only for clients in intensive care units because of the potential complications of infection and air emboli. Both methods require expertise in using the device.

ROUTES FOR MEASURING TEMPERATURE

The oral, rectal, axillary, and tympanic sites for measuring body temperature have been chosen because these sites approximate the core body temperature (Procedure 7-1) and provide reasonably consistent readings for most clinical purposes. Core body temperature is the

A

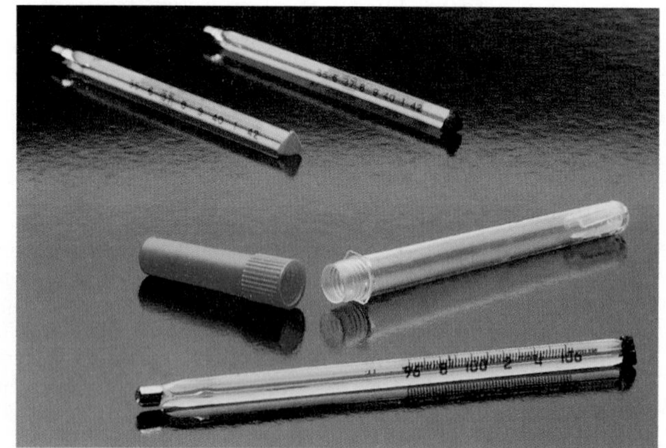

B

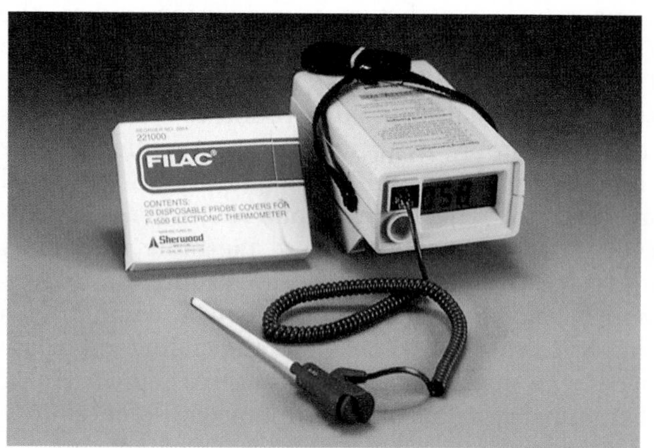

C

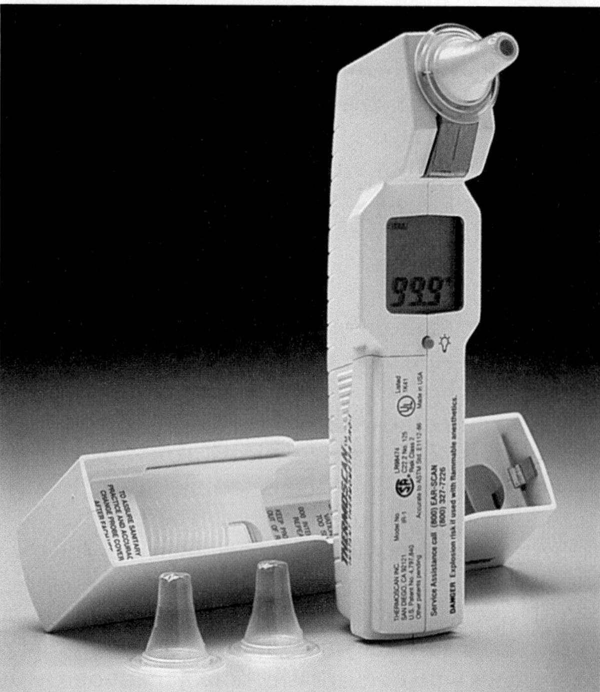

D

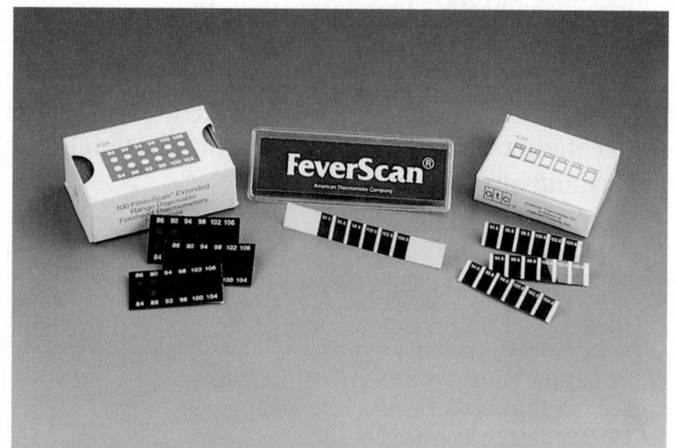

FIGURE 7-3 Types of thermometers. **A,** Glass thermometers. **B,** Electronic thermometer. **C,** Tympanic thermometer. **D,** Disposable temperature strips. (**A** courtesy American Diagnostic Corporation, Smithtown, NY; **B** through **D** courtesy Medline Industries, Mundelein, IL.)

temperature at the center of the body or in deep tissues (e.g., in the cranium and thoracic, abdominal, and pelvic cavities). It is more constant than skin temperature. The traditional method for temperature measurement in adults is to place the thermometer (glass or electronic) under the tongue in the pocket created by the frenulum linguae.

To accurately reflect the core body temperature by the oral route, you must consider factors that affect the temperature of the mucous membranes. The client must be able to follow directions and breathe with the mouth closed. Nasal oxygen cannulae and nasogastric tubes do not seem to affect the reading adversely. However, if the client has just eaten, ingested fluids, or

TIME TO ALLOW: **NOVICE:** 2 min. **EXPERT:** 2 min.

PROCEDURE 7-1 ASSESSING TEMPERATURE

Nursing Skills Online: Vital Sign, Lesson 1 and 2

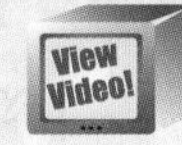

We measure body temperature primarily to detect inflammation and infection, and it can be an independent or a dependent nursing action. However, because some disorders and medications can have an effect on body temperature, its measurement can give important information about a client's health.

DELEGATION GUIDELINES

The measurement and recording of body temperature is a simple, low-risk procedure that you may delegate to a nursing assistant. Be sure the assistant indicates the route by which to take the temperature. You remain responsible for your knowledge of the temperature measurement and your assessment of changes in the client's temperature.

EQUIPMENT NEEDED

- Thermometer (oral, rectal, electronic, tympanic)
- Water-soluble lubricant
- Disposable probe covers
- Clean gloves and tissues
- Watch with a sweep second hand

1 Perform preliminary actions (see inside front cover).

2 Select an appropriate route, and obtain a corresponding thermometer. You may choose the oral, rectal, axillary, or tympanic route, whichever is safest and most convenient for the client. For consistency of results, use the same route for succeeding temperature measurements.

3 Prepare the thermometer.

GLASS THERMOMETER

a. Ensure that the glass thermometer (see Figure 7-3, *A*) is clean and free of defects. Follow agency policy for storage and cleaning. A common practice is to provide each client with an individual thermometer. Cleanse the thermometer with an alcohol wipe between uses, wiping from the stem to the bulb using a rotating motion. Thoroughly rinse away any disinfectant in cool water before use. *Hot water will expand the liquid and can break the glass. Consider covering the thermometer with a disposable sheath to protect both you and the client, and use a clean sheath for each measurement. A well-designed sheath inverts on itself as it is removed, thus preventing you from contact with oral mucus. The sheath also helps contain the glass if the thermometer breaks.*

b. Ensure that the liquid is confined to the bulb (i.e., the thermometer registers 96° F or 35.6° C). Hold the thermometer firmly by the tip. Using a flicking wrist motion, shake the thermometer. This action forces the liquid into the bulb. Check the reading on the thermometer to ensure that it is below body temperature. *Hold the thermometer with the numbers positioned to be read from left to right. Slightly rotate the thermometer toward you until the column of liquid is visible. Most thermometers have a white or yellow background to increase visibility of the liquid. You should be viewing the liquid against the background*

ELECTRONIC OR TYMPANIC THERMOMETER

a. If using an electronic thermometer (see Figure 7-3, *B*), turn on the device by removing the probe. If using a tympanic thermometer (see Figure 7-3, *C*), turn on the unit.

b. Place a disposable sheath or cover over the probe (see illustration). *A probe cover prevents transmission of microorganisms between clients.*

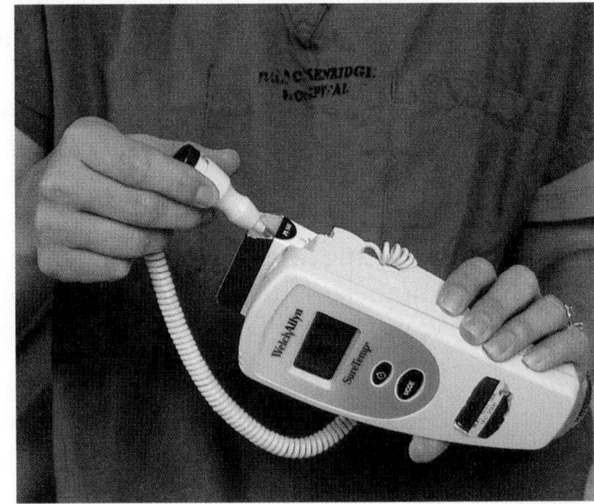

Step 3b. **Electronic or Tympanic.** Placing a disposable sheath, or cover, on the probe.

4 Measure the temperature.

Continued

ORAL ROUTE

a. Place the thermometer or electronic probe under the client's tongue, in the sublingual pocket next to the frenulum linguae, for 2 to 4 minutes or according to your facility's policy (glass thermometer) or until unit beeps (electronic thermometer). *Although most glass thermometers are calibrated to register in 1 minute, waiting at least 2 minutes results in a more reliable measurement.*
b. Have the client close his or her mouth and hold the thermometer in place with the lips (see illustration). Make sure the bulb remains in direct contact with the sublingual tissue. *Warn the client not to bite on the thermometer, especially a glass one, because the glass could break.*

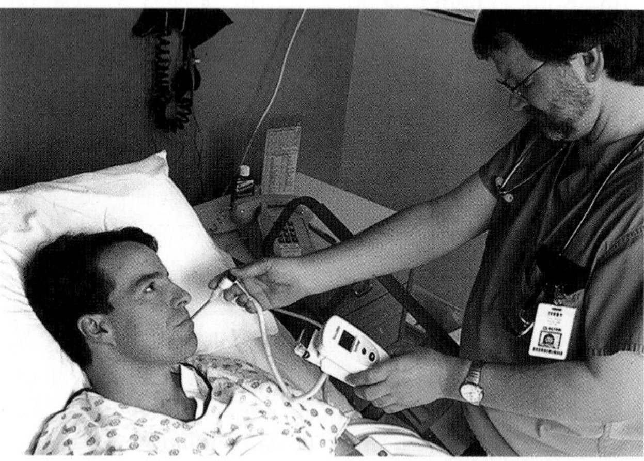

Step 4b. **Oral Route.** Holding the probe in place for oral temperature assessment.

RECTAL ROUTE

a. Position the client in the side-lying (left Sims') position, and drape for privacy. The left Sims' position allows easy access to the client's anus. Appropriate draping helps to minimize the client's discomfort.
b. Put on clean gloves. Taking a rectal temperature has a higher risk of contact with fluid from mucous membranes.
c. Lubricate the bulb of the thermometer with water-soluble jelly. Lubrication prevents rectal trauma.
d. Gently insert the thermometer about 1.5 inches into the rectum. Angle the thermometer toward the client's umbilicus during insertion.
e. Hold the thermometer in place for 2 to 4 minutes or according to your facility's policy (see illustration).

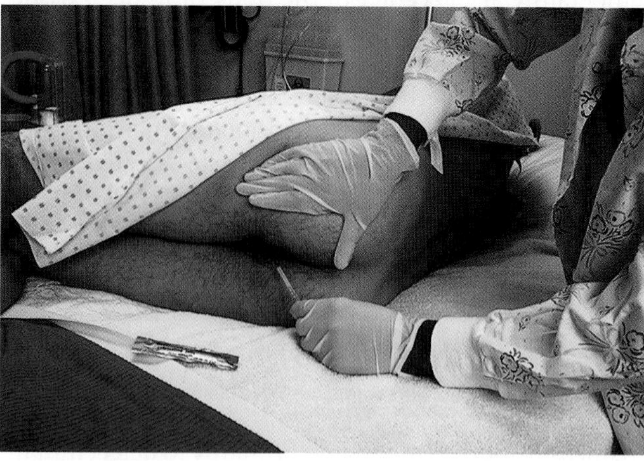

Step 4e. **Rectal Route.** Holding the probe in place for rectal temperature assessment.

AXILLARY ROUTE

a. Place the thermometer in the center of the client's axilla, and leave it in place for 8 to 10 minutes or according to your facility's policy (see illustration). *To secure the thermometer and make sure the bulb of the thermometer remains in contact with the axillary skin, have the client cross his or her arm across the chest.*

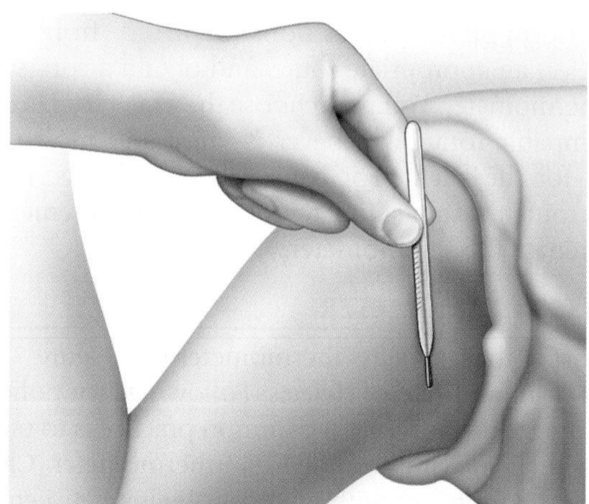

Step 4a. **Axillary Route.** Placing the probe for axillary temperature assessment.

TYMPANIC ROUTE

a. Pull the client's auricle back, and then gently obtain the temperature measurement (see illustration). For a child, pull the auricle down and back. For an adult, pull the auricle up and back. Doing so straightens the ear canal and helps to direct the probe toward the tympanic membrane.

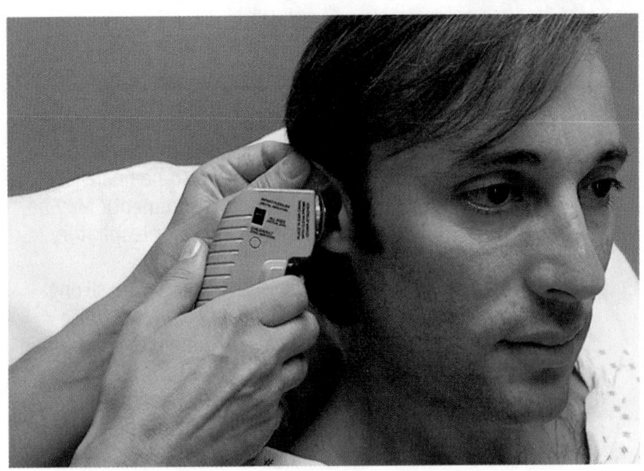

Step 4a. **Tympanic Route.** Inserting the tympanic probe into the ear canal.

b. Place the probe into the ear canal, pointing the tip of the probe toward the client's nose. The probe must be directed toward the tympanic membrane. Errors in measurement occur when it is directed toward the wall of the ear canal.
c. Holding the probe steady, quickly press the activation button.
d. A buzzer will sound when the temperature has been measured. A tympanic reading usually takes only 2 or 3 seconds.

5 Read the temperature measurement.

a. After an appropriate time or after the electronic thermometer beeps, remove the thermometer from the client's mouth, axilla, ear canal, or anus.
b. After removing a glass rectal thermometer, wipe it with a tissue, using a rotating motion from stem to bulb. Discard the tissue, or remove the disposable sheath. *This cleaning pattern moves from clean to contaminated areas of the thermometer and prevents transmission of microorganisms.*
c. Read the temperature measurement indicated on the thermometer. If using an electronic thermometer, obtain the measurement, and then discard the probe cover directly into the trash by pressing the release button. *This prevents transmission of microorganisms.*

6 Document the client's temperature in the medical record as soon as you obtain the reading. *Note whether the reading was oral, rectal, or axillary by writing oral, R, or Ax next to the measurement. Report an abnormal temperature to a charge nurse or physician. A normal oral temperature for an adult is 98.6° F (37° C), a normal rectal temperature is 99.6° F (37.5° C), and a normal axillary temperature is 97.6° F (36.5° C).*

PEDIATRIC CONSIDERATIONS

Rectal temperatures are taken only when there is no other feasible route. Rectal temperatures can cause rectal perforation in young infants and are especially contraindicated in the neonate, the immunosuppressed child, or the child with rectal surgery, diarrhea, or a bleeding disorder. If it is necessary to take a rectal temperature, insert a well-lubricated thermometer no more than the length of the bulb.

GERIATRIC CONSIDERATIONS

Rectal temperatures can also cause bleeding in older adults who have hemorrhoids; use caution and use gentle technique. Also consider that older adults may have limited mobility and they may need assistance in positioning before taking a rectal temperature.

smoked a cigarette, wait 20 to 30 minutes before obtaining the temperature reading. Avoid using this method for any client who could be injured by the thermometer, who cannot breathe with a closed mouth, or who cannot follow simple instructions.

The rectal or axillary route is sometimes used for infants and for small children who cannot hold a thermometer safely in their mouths. It is also used for adults who are unconscious or confused, have respiratory difficulty, or have had recent oral surgery. However, this route should be used with caution, especially with uncooperative or combative clients. The rectal route is contraindicated for clients who have had rectal or perineal surgery or injury, and for clients who have severe hemorrhoids. It is also not used in clients with cardiac disease because the thermometer can stimulate the vagus nerve, slowing the heart rate. The axillary route is less invasive than the rectal route but offers less accurate readings because it measures only surface body heat. It is contraindicated if the client is uncooperative or combative.

The tympanic membrane thermometer is a fast, safe, easy, and noninvasive method that can be used for children and adults. It is reliable and accurate when used properly. However, it is contraindicated for clients who have had a recent ear infection or ear surgery.

After obtaining a client's temperature, document the reading in the client's medical record. Temperature readings are usually charted on a graph with connecting lines to illustrate trends over time (see Figure 7-1). Rectal and axillary temperatures are charted with the designations *R* and *Ax*, respectively. Document other factors associated with temperature, such as diaphoresis or chills, in the nurse's progress notes section of the medical record.

PULSE

A pulse wave is created throughout the arterial system with each contraction of the ventricles of the heart (systole). It is best felt with the tip of a finger at a point where the artery is close to the surface and rests against a bone. Thus the pulse is a rhythmic fluctuation of fluid pressure against the arterial wall created by the pumping action of the heart muscle. Between contractions the heart muscle rests (diastole), and the pulse wave disappears.

UNDERSTANDING PULSE CHARACTERISTICS

The characteristics of the pulse are described as rate, rhythm, and strength. Examining these characteristics provides information about the strength of the myocardial contraction, its rhythm, the volume of blood in the vascular system, and the patency and resiliency of blood vessels. Abnormal pulse patterns are described on the basis of changes in the client's heart rate, rhythm, and strength (Table 7-2).

Table 7-2 Pulse Patterns

PATTERN	DESCRIPTION
Pulsus paradoxus	A regular rhythm of an increase and then a decrease in the pulse amplitude associated with respirations (may also be heard on the blood pressure measurement). May be a sign of a serious cardiac or respiratory condition.
Pulsus alternans	A regular rhythm with a pattern of a strong normal pulse followed by a weak pulse (every other beat is strong). One of a group of signs that indicate a failing heart.
Pulse bigeminy	Cardiac arrhythmia results in an irregular rhythm with a pattern of a strong normal pulse (beat originating in the sinus node) followed quickly by an early, weak pulse (beat originating elsewhere in the heart). May progress to ventricular fibrillation and death.
Sinus rhythm	The electrical impulse is generated in the normal pacemaker (sinus node). Usually a regular rhythm with a rate between 60 and 100 beats per minute for an adult.
Tachycardia	Regular rhythm with a rate greater than 100 beats per minute for an adult. Decreases cardiac output by decreasing ventricular filling time. If prolonged, may lead to shock.
Bradycardia	Regular rhythm with a rate less than 60 beats per minute for an adult. Rate is insufficient to meet the demands for oxygen. May lead to cardiac standstill.
Sinus arrhythmia	Slightly irregular rhythm that speeds up and slows down with respirations. Originates in the sinus node. Does not usually affect cardiac output or vital signs

Rate. The pulse rate of a normal adult varies from 60 to 100 beats per minute. A heart rate less than 60 beats per minute is called **bradycardia.** A heart rate greater than 100 is termed **tachycardia.** Rate cannot be viewed as the sole criterion for normal, however; instead, it must be considered together with any signs and symptoms that might produce, or be produced by, an abnormal rate. The heart rate is primarily controlled by the two opposing parts of the autonomic nervous system. The sympathetic nervous system (SNS) increases the heart rate, whereas the parasympathetic system decreases it. Both changes stem largely from the body's response to the cells' need for oxygen.

Any psychological stressor (producing anxiety, fear, or anger) or physiological stressor (such as exercise, pain, or blood loss) causes the body's compensatory mechanisms to launch a fight-or-flight response. Information is relayed to the cardiac center in the medulla, and the SNS is stimulated to produce an increase in the pulse.

Other factors can influence the pulse rate as well (Table 7-3). For example, infants and children have a higher BMR and thus a slightly higher pulse rate than adults. Some medications (such as digitalis and beta-adrenergic blockers) slow the heart rate, and others (such as amphetamines) increase it. Low blood pressure, dehydration, fever, and pain can stimulate the SNS. In contrast, rest and relaxation can stimulate the parasympathetic nervous system.

Rhythm. Normally myocardial contraction is initiated in the sinus node in the atrium and produces a normal rate and regular rhythm. However, chemical disturbances, such as inadequate oxygen in the heart muscle and electrolyte imbalance, may cause the heart to beat irregularly. Some children, and even some adults, have a normal variation in rhythm in which the heart rate increases with inhalation and decreases with exhalation. Even if normal, report all irregular rhythms to the nurse in charge or to a physician.

Strength. The quality of the pulse reflects the strength of cardiac contraction and the volume of blood available in the vascular system. A normal contraction of the heart muscle combined with an adequate blood volume will create a strong pulse wave. A weak heart contraction combined with a low blood volume will create a weak, thready pulse wave. An increased heart contraction combined with a large blood volume will create a full, bounding pulse wave.

A number of conditions can alter the strength of a client's pulse. For example, heart failure can cause the strength of the heart's contraction to vary on alternating beats while the rhythm remains regular, a condition called pulsus alternans.

You also may detect an abnormality (in adults) in which the strength of the client's pulse wave increases

Table 7-3 Factors That Influence Pulse Rate

FACTOR	INFLUENCE
Age	Infants and children have a slightly higher heart rate than adolescents and adults. As the client ages, the pulse rate gradually decreases.
Emotions and stress	Anxiety, fear, anger, and pain stimulate the sympathetic nervous system and cause the pulse rate to increase. Relaxation stimulates the parasympathetic nervous system and decreases the rate.
Exercise	Exercise increases the oxygen demand, and the rate increases. A conditioned athlete can have a slow but effective resting heart rate.
Rest and sleep	During rest and sleep, oxygen needs decline, and the rate decreases.
Temperature	Hyperthermia and fever increase the heart rate. Hypothermia decreases the heart rate.
Dehydration, shock, and hemorrhage	Decreases in blood volume or cardiac output result in an increased pulse rate because of sympathetic stimulation.
Hypoxia and hypoxemia	When oxygen levels in the blood decrease, the heart rate increases in an attempt to compensate.
Vomiting	Vomiting stimulates the vagus nerve and causes the pulse rate to drop.
Head injury and increased intracranial pressure	Head injuries cause the pulse to decrease as a compensatory mechanism as intracranial pressure rises.
Electrolyte balance	Changes in potassium and calcium affect the pulse rate and rhythm.
Medications	Certain medications cause the heart rate to increase, such as adrenalin and atropine, and others decrease the pulse, such as digitalis and beta-adrenergic blockers

during inhalation and decreases back to normal during exhalation, a condition called pulsus paradoxus. This can also be heard when measuring blood pressure. Finally, the nervous system can alter the strength of the client's pulse. Stimulation of the SNS increases the force of myocardial contraction, increasing the amount of blood ejected from the heart with each beat (stroke volume) and creating a stronger pulse. Stimulation of the parasympathetic nervous system decreases the force of contraction, thus decreasing stroke volume and creating a weaker pulse.

MEASURING PULSE

Significant clinical decisions, such as medication administration, are based on pulse values. To facilitate accurate pulse measurement, apply light pressure over the client's artery with the pads of the two middle fingers. Press firmly enough to detect the pulse wave without occluding the artery. If you use your thumb or index finger, you may feel your own pulse rather than the client's (Procedure 7-2).

Peripheral Pulses. Peripheral pulse sites are located where arteries lie over bony surfaces. Nine sites are available to assess peripheral pulses: the carotid artery in the neck; the brachial, radial, and ulnar arteries in the arms; and the femoral, popliteal, dorsalis pedis, and posterior tibial arteries in the legs and feet (Figure 7-4). The temporal artery can also be used, but it is not easily palpated in all people.

The most common site for assessing the quality, rate, and rhythm of the pulse is the radial artery. The radial artery, on the inner surface of the wrist on the thumb side, is easily accessed and palpated. Other sites (e.g., at the cardiac apex and the carotid and femoral arteries) are used for special purposes. In an emergency or during

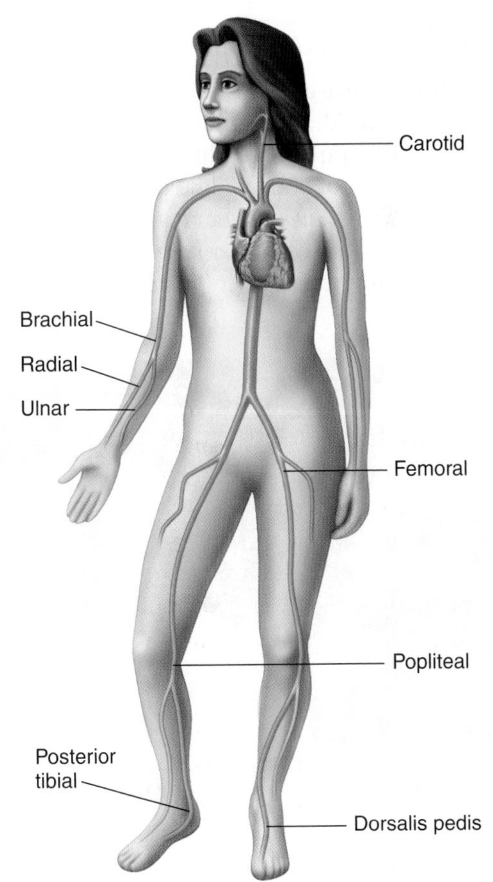

FIGURE 7-4 The eight sites commonly used to assess peripheral pulses.

TIME TO ALLOW: NOVICE: 1 min. EXPERT: 1 min.

PROCEDURE 7-2 ASSESSING RADIAL AND APICAL PULSES

Nursing Skills Online: Vital Signs, Lesson 3

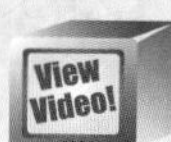

A person's pulse reflects the function of the person's heart and the condition of his or her arterial system. Usually, we measure a client's radial pulse in his or her wrist. In some cases, however, we need to measure the apical pulse instead of or in addition to the radial pulse.

DELEGATION GUIDELINES

The measurement and recording of the radial pulse rate is a simple procedure that you may delegate to a nursing assistant who has received training in this technique. Training should include careful instructions about specific findings that necessitate your immediate notification. You remain responsible for knowledge of the pulse rate and your assessment of a client with any reported irregularities. Measurement of apical pulse rate may also be delegated but is more likely to be completed by the nurse based on a need for specific cardiac assessment.

EQUIPMENT NEEDED

- Stethoscope
- Watch with sweep second hand

1 Perform preliminary actions (see inside front cover).

2 Prepare the client for pulse measurement.

a. Place the client in a comfortable position. Have the client relax. *If the client is not relaxed, wait 10 or 15 minutes before obtaining the pulse reading. This will enhance accuracy by preventing false elevations caused by stress or anxiety.*

3 Measure the pulse.

RADIAL PULSE MEASUREMENT

a. Place the client's arm across his or her abdomen or in another relaxed, comfortable position. Locate the client's radial pulse (see illustration).

b. Place the pads of your middle fingers on the inside of the client's wrist. *Do not use your thumb or first finger to palpate the pulse because they have pulses of their own.*

c. Compress the radial artery firmly against the underlying bone.

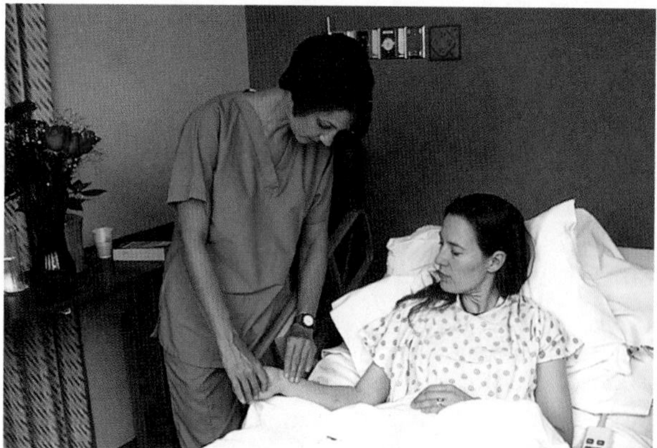

Step 3a. **Radial Pulse.** Locating the radial pulse.

d. Occlude the pulse, and then gradually release pressure until the pulse becomes palpable. *Occluding and then restoring the pulse verifies its presence.*

e. Assess the quality and rhythm of the client's radial pulse as you count the pulse. *If the radial pulse is irregular or weak, assess the client's apical pulse. If the radial pulse is regular and of normal strength, count the number of beats for 30 seconds and multiply by 2. If it is irregular, count for a full minute. For rapid approximation, you can count for 6 (×10), 10 (×6) or 15 (×4) seconds. The most accurate count requires counting for a full minute.*

APICAL PULSE MEASUREMENT

a. Place the client in the supine position, and locate the apical pulse at the fifth intercostal space to the left of the midclavicular line on the anterior thorax (see illustration). *If you have difficulty hearing, a left-lying position or a forward-leaning position (with the client seated) enhances transmission of heart sounds through the chest wall.*

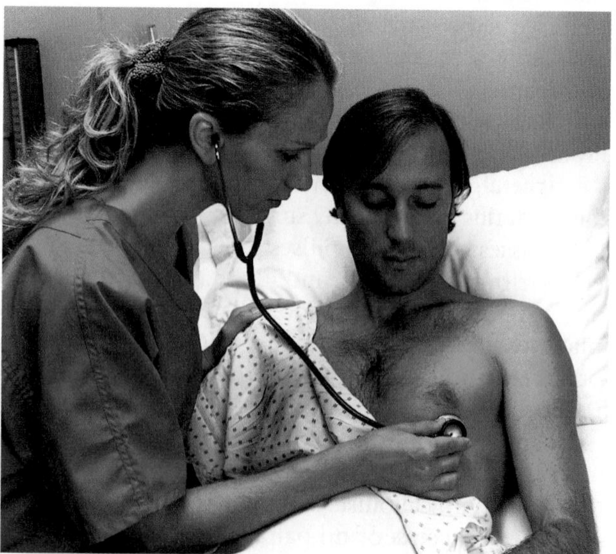

Step 3a. **Apical Pulse.** Locating the apical pulse.

b. Keep the client covered appropriately, exposing the chest only as needed.
c. If necessary, lift a female client's breast to find her apical pulse. *Finding the correct anatomical location of the apex increases the accuracy of the apical pulse measurement.*
d. Place the earpieces of the stethoscope in your ears and the diaphragm firmly against the client's chest. Avoid rubbing it against clothing or linens. *The diaphragm is used for high-pitched sounds, such as heart tones. Firm skin contact enhances sound transmission. Clothing may cause interfering noises.*
e. Assess the rate and rhythm of the client's apical pulse, which is heard as a "lubb-dupp" (S_1 and S_2) and corresponds with one cardiac contraction. *The apical pulse is the most likely to reveal irregularities of heart rhythm. Count the apical pulse for 1 full minute. This will increase the accuracy of your reading.*

4 Document the rate and any abnormality of rhythm or strength as soon as you obtain the reading. Report an abnormal pulse to a charge nurse or physician.

PEDIATRIC CONSIDERATIONS

An apical pulse is recommended for an infant or a child younger than 2 years.

GERIATRIC CONSIDERATIONS

Because many older adults take medications that require apical pulse measurement, check the medication list to ensure you know when to measure an apical pulse instead of a radial pulse. Also, if a client has an enlarged heart or heart failure, the location of the apex of the heart may be displaced downward and further to the left. Note on the client's history and physical the location of the point of maximal impulse (PMI), which corresponds to where you want to measure the apical pulse.

cardiopulmonary resuscitation (CPR), you may assess the client's heart rate or monitor the effectiveness of cardiac compressions using the carotid or femoral pulse in an adult or the brachial pulse in an infant.

Other pulses also have specific uses. The brachial artery, located in the antecubital fossa (the inner aspect of the elbow), is used to measure blood pressure (BP). The popliteal artery, located behind the knee, can also be used for BP measurement. The dorsalis pedis and posterior tibial arteries are used to assess the status of the peripheral vascular system but not to assess heart rate and rhythm.

No matter how you measure a client's pulse, always document your findings immediately in the medical record (see Figure 7-1). If you obtained an apical pulse, note it with an A. Place other information about the client's pulse in the nurse's notes or progress report section of the chart.

Apical Pulse. The **apical pulse** is the heart rate counted at the apex of the heart on the anterior chest. If a client has weak or ineffective heart contractions, cardiac disease, an irregular heart rhythm, or a history of taking cardiac medications that affect the heart's action, you may not be able to palpate all cardiac contractions at the radial pulse site. For these clients, apical pulse measurement provides a more accurate assessment. The apical pulse is preferred for infants and children because it can be difficult to palpate their peripheral pulses. You may choose to perform an apical pulse measurement instead of a radial pulse measurement on any client for whom you think it would be helpful.

To take an apical pulse you will need a stethoscope. A stethoscope consists of earpieces connected to two stiff tubes that join with a single flexible tube that ends in a sound-transmitting device that has a diaphragm on one side and a bell on the other (Figure 7-5). Place the earpieces into your ear canals with the ends pointing slightly toward your nose, not the back of your head. Use the bell to assess low-frequency sounds and the diaphragm to assess high-frequency sounds. Remember that a stethoscope does not magnify heart sounds. It simply focuses them into the end piece and eliminates outside sounds. To decrease the transmission of microorganisms, wipe the diaphragm and bell with alcohol between clients.

When you listen to the client's anterior chest, you will hear two sounds produced by a normal heart. The first heart sound, called S_1, results when the mitral and tricuspid valves close during systole. This creates the "lubb" of the "lubb-dupp" heart sound. It can be heard best at the apex of the heart, near the fifth intercostal space, just left of the midclavicular line. The second heart sound, called S_2, results when the aortic and pulmonic valves close during diastole. This creates the "dupp" of the "lubb-dupp" heart sound. It can be heard best at the base of the heart, by the second intercostal space, right or left of the sternal border. When assessing a client's apical pulse rate, count S_1 and S_2 together ("lubb-dupp") as one beat.

Apical-Radial Pulse. To gain further information about the heart's effectiveness as a pump in the event of dysrhythmias and cardiac disease, take an apical-radial pulse to assess for a pulse deficit. When the apical pulse rate exceeds the radial pulse rate, the difference is described as a **pulse deficit**. To be accurate, both pulses must be counted simultaneously. Because it is difficult to count both pulses at the same time, work together with a colleague so that one auscultates the apical rate while the other palpates the radial pulse. Both of you must start

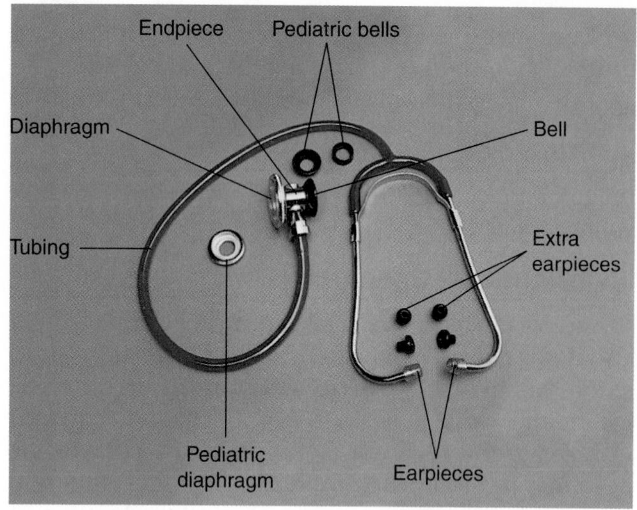

FIGURE 7-5 Components of a stethoscope.

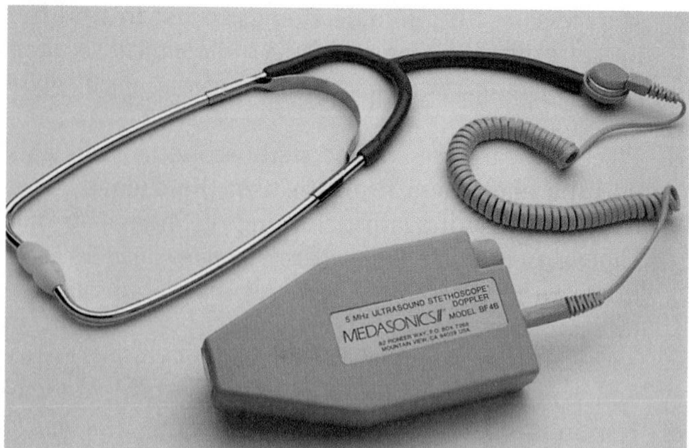

FIGURE 7-6 A Doppler ultrasound stethoscope. (Courtesy Medasonics, Inc., Newark, CA.)

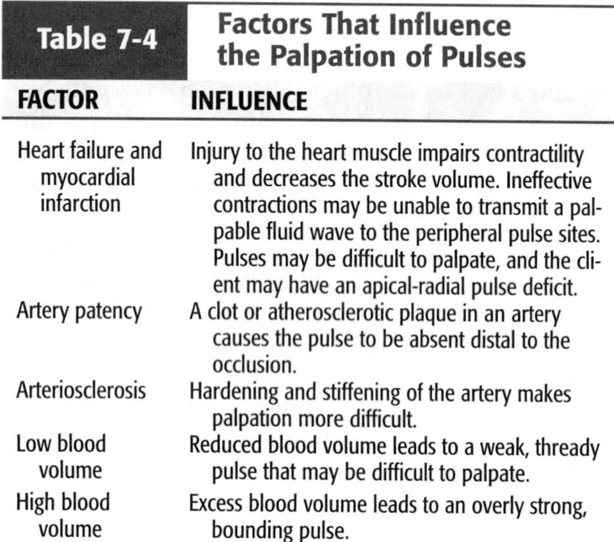

Table 7-4 Factors That Influence the Palpation of Pulses

FACTOR	INFLUENCE
Heart failure and myocardial infarction	Injury to the heart muscle impairs contractility and decreases the stroke volume. Ineffective contractions may be unable to transmit a palpable fluid wave to the peripheral pulse sites. Pulses may be difficult to palpate, and the client may have an apical-radial pulse deficit.
Artery patency	A clot or atherosclerotic plaque in an artery causes the pulse to be absent distal to the occlusion.
Arteriosclerosis	Hardening and stiffening of the artery makes palpation more difficult.
Low blood volume	Reduced blood volume leads to a weak, thready pulse that may be difficult to palpate.
High blood volume	Excess blood volume leads to an overly strong, bounding pulse.

counting at the same time, count for a full minute, and compare your findings. The difference is documented as a pulse deficit.

Pulse Quality. Quality refers to the strength or weakness of the pulse. A weak pulse is caused by any condition that slows or restricts the blood flow, such as decreased blood volume, weak heart contractions, or partial obstruction of arteries (Table 7-4). For example, vasoconstriction can cause the artery to become so narrowed that the pulse wave is difficult to feel. Likewise, in shock, the blood volume may be reduced to a point at which you can no longer feel the pulse wave. In contrast, in vasodilation and overhydration, the extra blood volume can make the pulses pronounced.

In addition, to produce a palpable pulse, the wall of an artery must have enough elasticity to respond to the pulse wave. The harder and stiffer the wall of the artery, the less the pulse wave can distend it. The result is a weak pulse that is difficult to palpate.

If you have trouble palpating a pulse wave, you may need to use a Doppler ultrasound stethoscope to assess the weakened pulse (Figure 7-6). By enhancing pulse sounds, it can also improve the accuracy of your assessment. The Doppler stethoscope can help detect a pulse when you cannot palpate one. It may be especially helpful for a client who has total occlusion of an artery. To use the device, place the transducer over the artery while listening through the earpieces. A sensor picks up the arterial pulse wave and magnifies the sound, giving it a "whooshing" sound. Like any device used on multiple clients, the transducer should be cleaned between clients, following the manufacturer's directions.

RESPIRATION

To survive, the cells of the body must receive enough oxygen to meet metabolic needs. They must also release carbon dioxide, the major byproduct of metabolism. As you know, breathing—also known as respiration—accomplishes these purposes.

UNDERSTANDING RESPIRATION

A person's respiratory rate and depth vary with the cellular demand for oxygen and with levels of carbon dioxide and hydrogen ions (pH) in the blood (see Chapter 34). Receptors throughout the body feed to the brain information about the level of oxygen available to cells. The brain, in turn, regulates the person's respiratory rate. For example, peripheral chemoreceptors located in the aorta and the carotid arteries are especially sensitive to low blood levels of oxygen (hypoxemia). Central chemoreceptors in the medulla are especially sensitive to high levels of carbon dioxide (hypercapnia) and changes in pH. When these receptors sense a change in oxygen, carbon dioxide, and hydrogen ions, they communicate via the autonomic nervous system to the respiratory center in the medulla for integration. As a result, the rate, depth, rhythm, or effort of respiration may change. During rest and sleep, cells need less oxygen, and respirations become shallow, quiet, and slow.

MEASURING RESPIRATIONS

The act of breathing is primarily involuntary. In fact, people usually are not aware of their breathing. When you measure respirations, you are assessing this natural, involuntary function. However, breathing can come under voluntary control as well. When a person concentrates on breathing, the rate may change. Consequently, when you assess a client's respirations, try to do so when the client is not aware of your actions. This ensures that you will be assessing the client's natural respirations. To keep the client unaware of your assessment, try counting respirations just after you take the client's pulse, while still holding the wrist (Procedure 7-3). Count one cycle of inspiration and expiration as one breath. Make sure to assess the client's complete breathing pattern, including rate, rhythm, depth, and effort.

A quiet, easy respiration, with a rate between 12 and 20 breaths per minute in an adult at rest, is known as **eupnea**. A rate of more than 20 breaths per minute is called **tachypnea**, and a rate less than 12 breaths per minute is called **bradypnea**. Children normally have slightly higher respiratory rates than adults.

Normally, breathing has a regular rhythm with periodic sighing. Irregular breathing in an adult is often accompanied by dyspnea and can result from head injury, increased intracranial pressure, or cardiovascular dysfunction (Table 7-5). Document and report irregular breathing to the charge nurse or physician immediately, being sure to describe the pattern. Infants and children normally have a slightly irregular pattern of breathing.

The normal rhythmic volume of ventilation, called **tidal volume**, indicates the volume of air exchanged with each breath (about 500 mL). Because you cannot measure this volume as part of vital signs, you will need to estimate whether there is an adequate volume of air exchange with each breath. With normal depth, you will see a moderate amount of chest movement. With deep breathing, the chest expands fully. With shallow breathing, you may see little chest movement at all. Fast, deep breathing is known as hyperventilation or hyperpnea. Slow, shallow breathing is known as hypoventilation (see Chapter 34). Normal respiration includes periodic deep breaths known as sighing. Sighing is a protective mechanism that periodically expands unused alveoli and prevents their collapse.

Normal ventilation is effortless and quiet. It results from movements of the intercostal muscles and diaphragm. Accessory muscles are not used. Exercise, shortness of breath (dyspnea), or respiratory diseases can lead to an exaggerated respiratory effort to breathe. Infants and children often flare their nostrils if they are having difficulty breathing.

On occasion, you may use a stethoscope to count a client's respirations, especially if they are shallow and slow. You also may use palpation to assess slow, shallow respirations. Place your hand on the client's lower chest or abdomen and feel for a slight rise and fall with each breath. Document the client's respirations immediately after obtaining the reading (see Figure 7-1). Other information about the client's respirations can be documented in the nurse's notes or progress report. For example, you would document other indicators of respiratory status, such as pulse oximetry readings, a blue tinge to the client's skin or mucous membranes, or restlessness.

TIME TO ALLOW: NOVICE: 1 min. EXPERT: 1 min.

PROCEDURE 7-3

ASSESSING RESPIRATIONS

Nursing Skills Online: Vital Signs, Lesson 4

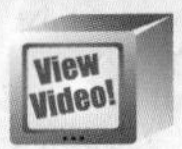

Respiration is a largely involuntary process, but it may come under voluntary control at times. By assessing respirations without the client's knowledge, you can gain important information about the client's respiratory and cardiovascular systems.

DELEGATION GUIDELINES

The measurement and recording of the client's respiratory rate is a simple procedure that you may delegate to a nursing assistant who has received training in this technique. Training should include specific instructions about findings that necessitate your immediate notification. You must complete the full respiratory assessment if one is indicated (see Chapter 34).

EQUIPMENT NEEDED

- Watch with a sweep second hand

Continued

1 Perform preliminary actions (see inside front cover).

2 Make sure the client is relaxed and quiet and either sitting or lying down. Make sure that the client's anterior thorax is easily visible and that the lungs can complete the full excursion of respiratory movement without hindrance. *If necessary, wait 10 or 15 minutes before counting respirations. Anxiety, discomfort, and exercise increase the rate and depth of respirations and may result in a false reading.*

3 Make sure the client does not know you are counting the respirations. *If aware, the client may alter the respirations or concentrate on them, which can alter the natural count. Many nurses simply continue holding a client's wrist after taking a pulse measurement. The client thinks the pulse measurement is still continuing while the nurse has begun counting respirations.*

4 Watch the rise and fall of the client's chest. Count each cycle of inhalation and exhalation as one breath. *If necessary, you may place your hand on the client's lower thorax or abdomen and palpate the movement.*

5 Count the client's respirations. *For an adult with a regular rhythm, count for 30 seconds, and multiply your result by 2. For an infant, a child, or an adult with an irregular rhythm, count for a full minute to obtain the most accurate reading. Infants and children normally have a slightly irregular rhythm.*

6 Document the respirations as soon as you obtain the reading. *Normal adult respirations are 12 to 20 per minute, regular, of moderate depth, and effortless.*

7 Report abnormal respirations to a charge nurse or physician.

PEDIATRIC CONSIDERATIONS

For very small children or infants who have small tidal volumes (breaths), you may need to place your hand lightly on the chest to measure respirations.

GERIATRIC CONSIDERATIONS

Clients who are confused may try to talk or be uncooperative when measuring respirations. Try to be as inconspicuous as possible, as noted in the text of this chapter.

Table 7-5 Breathing Patterns

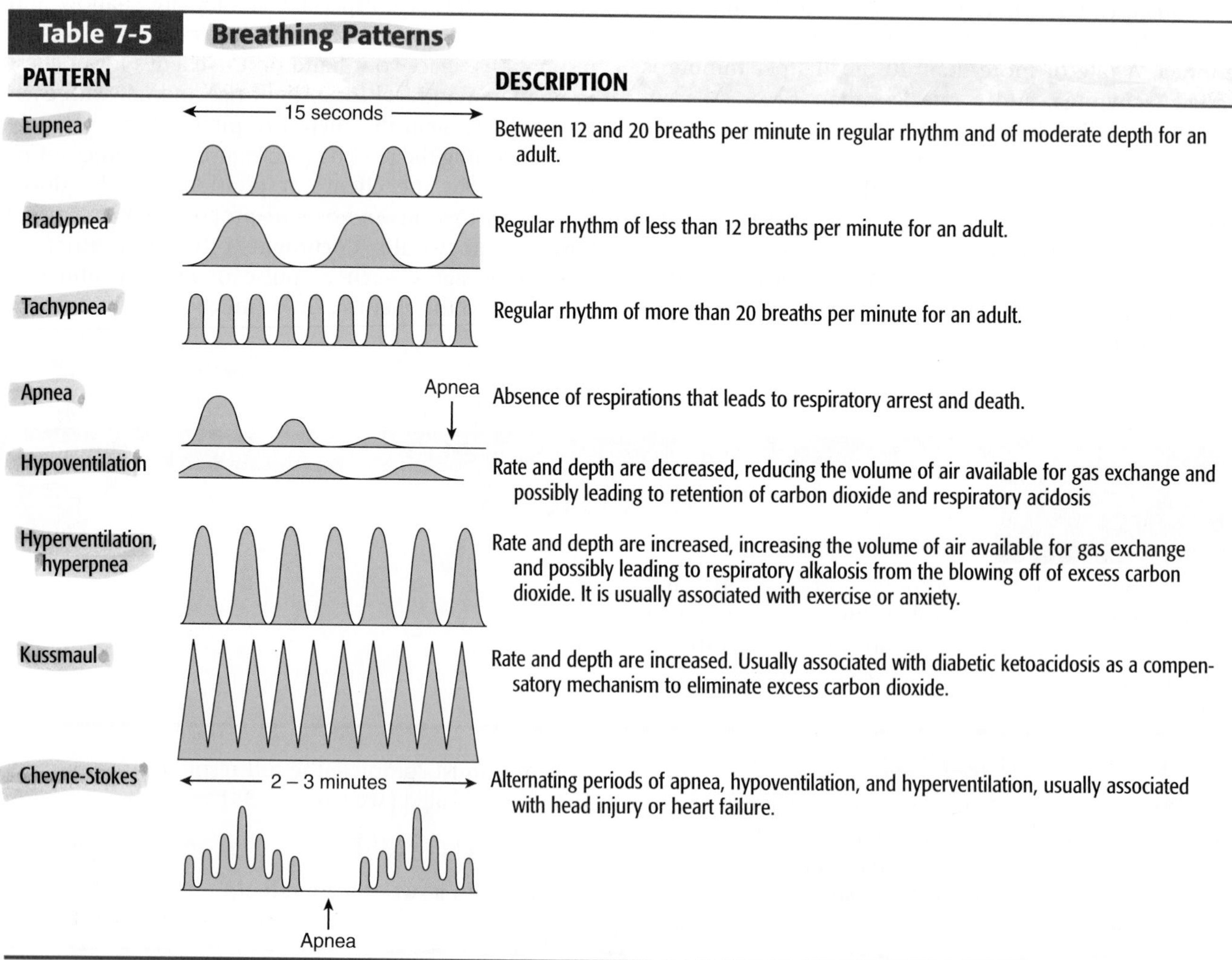

PATTERN	DESCRIPTION
Eupnea	Between 12 and 20 breaths per minute in regular rhythm and of moderate depth for an adult.
Bradypnea	Regular rhythm of less than 12 breaths per minute for an adult.
Tachypnea	Regular rhythm of more than 20 breaths per minute for an adult.
Apnea	Absence of respirations that leads to respiratory arrest and death.
Hypoventilation	Rate and depth are decreased, reducing the volume of air available for gas exchange and possibly leading to retention of carbon dioxide and respiratory acidosis
Hyperventilation, hyperpnea	Rate and depth are increased, increasing the volume of air available for gas exchange and possibly leading to respiratory alkalosis from the blowing off of excess carbon dioxide. It is usually associated with exercise or anxiety.
Kussmaul	Rate and depth are increased. Usually associated with diabetic ketoacidosis as a compensatory mechanism to eliminate excess carbon dioxide.
Cheyne-Stokes	Alternating periods of apnea, hypoventilation, and hyperventilation, usually associated with head injury or heart failure.

OXYGEN SATURATION

Although measurement of respirations provides an indication that sufficient oxygen is brought into the lungs, it does not provide an indication of how much oxygen actually enters the bloodstream. The use of a **pulse oximeter** can provide information about the saturation of the client's arterial blood with oxygen (called **oxygen saturation** or SaO_2).

UNDERSTANDING OXYGEN SATURATION

As oxygen enters the lungs, it diffuses across alveolar membranes into the pulmonary capillaries and attaches to hemoglobin on the red blood cells (RBCs). The RBCs carry oxygen through the left side of the heart and arterial blood vessels to body tissues, where oxygen is released according to local tissue needs. Normally, between 95% and 100% of hemoglobin in arterial blood is saturated with oxygen. Because body tissues extract oxygen from the RBCs, the oxygen saturation in the venous system (SvO_2) is lower, approximately 70%. When measuring oxygen saturation via pulse oximetry in the clinical setting, you are measuring arterial saturation, not venous, and the value of 95% to 100% is the expected normal value. This is a useful clinical tool because the SaO_2 level will drop before other signs of hypoxemia occur, such as dusky skin color or dusky nail beds.

Various factors can affect the SaO_2. These include lung disease and decreased circulation (from disease or cool temperatures), which can lower the value. Excessive movement at the site, shivering, and some types of nail polish can lead to an inaccurate reading. Interestingly, anemia (low hemoglobin level) may not lower the reading. This is because the hemoglobin that is present is fully saturated, even if the body does not have a sufficient amount of hemoglobin. As with any other vital sign measurement, you should know not only the current reading, but also how it compares to previous readings. Report an oxygen saturation below 90%.

MEASURING OXYGEN SATURATION

The pulse oximeter unit has two parts: the oximeter unit and the sensor unit. The oximeter unit contains electronics, an inlet connection for the sensor cable, and a faceplate that displays both SaO_2 and pulse rate. The unit also has alarms that can be set during continuous SaO_2 monitoring if the client's reading drops below a predetermined level. The sensor unit or probe attaches to a fingertip, toes, nose, earlobe or forehead, or the hand or foot of a newborn (Figure 7-7). The sensor emits light (red and infrared) through light-emitting diodes (LEDs) from one side of the probe. A photodetector on the other side of the probe measures the amount of red and infrared light absorbed by oxygenated and deoxygenated hemoglobin and reports it as the SaO_2. Procedure 7-4 (p. 130) describes how to measure oxygen saturation.

BLOOD PRESSURE

The BP reflects information about the person's cardiovascular system. Blood pressure is the pressure (measured in millimeters of mercury or mm Hg) of the blood against the inner walls of the arteries. It is recorded at the highest and lowest points of pressure.

During myocardial contraction (systole), when blood is ejected from the heart and into the arteries, BP reaches its height. During diastole, when the heart rests, BP falls to its baseline level. These values are known as **systolic blood pressure** and **diastolic blood pressure.** The difference between these is the amount of pressure that produces the palpable pulse, and it is known as the **pulse pressure.** For an adult, systolic BP normally varies from 100 to 130 mm Hg. Diastolic BP normally varies from 60 to 80 mm Hg. Blood pressure is usually expressed and documented as a ratio of systolic over diastolic. Hypertension is defined as a BP that is greater than 140/90 mm Hg. Pulse pressure is normally about 30 to 50 mm Hg. By correlating a client's blood pressure readings with the history and other signs and symptoms, you can draw important conclusions about health changes.

UNDERSTANDING BLOOD PRESSURE

Several factors combine to form the reading reported as the BP (Figure 7-8). An important factor is the volume of blood in the vascular system. Less blood yields a lower BP; more blood yields a higher BP. A second factor is the action of the heart. An increased cardiac output raises BP, whereas a decreased cardiac output lowers it. A third factor is the impediment to blood flow through the vascular

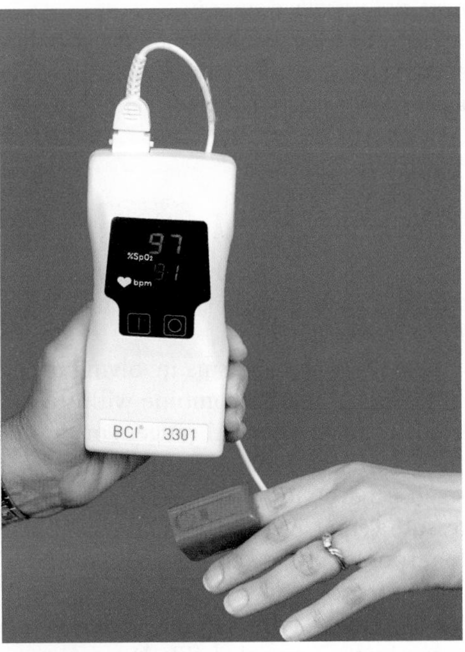

FIGURE 7-7 Placement of fingertip sensor/probe for oxygen saturation measurement.

PROCEDURE 7-4

TIME TO ALLOW: NOVICE: 1 min. EXPERT: 1 min.

ASSESSING OXYGEN SATURATION

Nursing Skills Online: Vital Signs, Lesson 6

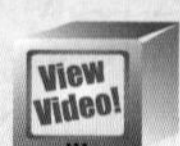

Measuring oxygen saturation detects hypoxemia before other clinical signs may be apparent. For selected clients, oxygen saturation is measured routinely with vital signs. Some hospitals purchase electronic vital sign monitoring equipment that provides automatic oxygen saturation readings along with pulse and blood pressure.

DELEGATION GUIDELINES

The measurement and recording of the client's oxygen saturation is a simple procedure that you may delegate to a nursing assistant who has received training in this technique. Training should include specific instructions about findings that necessitate your immediate notification. You must complete a full respiratory assessment if one is indicated (see Chapter 34).

EQUIPMENT NEEDED

- Pulse oximeter
- Alcohol wipe
- Nail polish remover (acetone) if indicated

1 Perform preliminary actions (see inside front cover).

2 Choose a site that has adequate capillary refill. *Use the nose or forehead if fingers, toes, and earlobes are not suitable.*

3 Choose proper sensor according to location and client's size and weight. *Weight limits of sensors overlap, so an adult sensor may be used for a very large child. Use a sensor without adhesive if the client is allergic to adhesive tape.*

4 Cleanse the site with alcohol, and remove nail polish that is dark or contains blue pigments. *This improves the likelihood of obtaining accurate readings.*

5 Attach sensor probe to site, and attach to pulse oximeter unit if not already connected. *Explain that fingertip probe looks like a clothespin but does not pinch or hurt.*

6 Turn on power to activate unit. Observe pulse waveform on screen, and listen to audible beep. *Waveforms and beeps should correlate with each other; if not, check probe placement and possibly change it.*

7 Wait for machine to display a fairly constant reading and record value. *This may take 10 to 30 seconds, depending on machine, probe placement, and client.*

8 Shut off machine and remove probe if single reading is obtained, or leave in place if continuous monitoring will be done. *Explain to client that alarm will beep if probe is removed or otherwise displaced from site, or if value changes beyond preset parameters on machine.*

9 Report abnormal respirations to a charge nurse or physician.

PEDIATRIC CONSIDERATIONS

Site selection is often based on the size of the client and the ability to cooperate. Explain that the probe will not hurt or "pinch."

GERIATRIC CONSIDERATIONS

Because cardiovascular disease is widespread in older adults, be sure to assess the area to be used for adequate local circulation before applying the probe.

system, known as **peripheral vascular resistance.** The diameter of the vessel and the viscosity of the blood create resistance. When vascular resistance increases, BP rises, and vice versa.

Compensatory mechanisms involving the brain, kidneys, and adrenal glands combine with these factors to help keep BP in the normal range. For example, when nervous system receptors (baroreceptors) in the great vessels sense a drop in BP, they relay that information to the pressure center in the medulla, which activates the SNS. In response, blood vessels constrict, and blood volume rises in response to sodium retention by the kidney and catecholamine (epinephrine and norepinephrine) production by the adrenal glands. When the parasympathetic nervous system is activated, a series of events occurs to cause the BP to decrease.

Other factors that help to regulate BP to some degree include atherosclerotic plaque, viscosity of blood; velocity of blood flow; levels of oxygen and carbon dioxide in the blood; the client's age, emotions, pain, and exercise; time of day; stressors; and medication use (Table 7-6). Finally, hemorrhage, shock, dehydration, and blood loss reduce BP by lowering the circulating blood volume. Renal failure and other causes of fluid overload can raise BP. Head injuries can raise BP as well, by interfering with regulatory mechanisms in the medulla.

MEASURING BLOOD PRESSURE

To measure a person's BP, you will use a sphygmomanometer and a stethoscope to listen to a series of sounds, usually in the client's brachial artery. A sphyg-

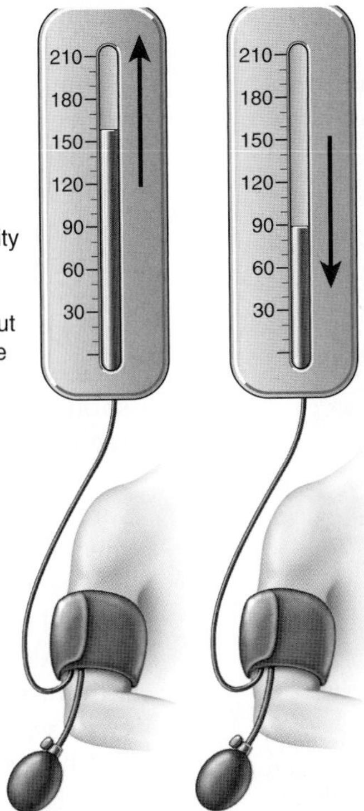

FIGURE 7-8 Physiological factors affecting blood pressure.

Table 7-6 Factors That Influence Blood Pressure

FACTOR	INFLUENCE
Age	Newborns and infants have the lowest blood pressure. Blood pressure increases as age increases. It is highest in older adults because of a decrease in the elasticity of vessels, which causes an increase in resistance to blood flow. However, even in older adults a blood pressure above 140/90 mm Hg should not be considered normal.
Stress and emotions	Anxiety, pain, tension, worry, and stress raise blood pressure by stimulating the sympathetic nervous system, which causes vasoconstriction and a resulting increased heart rate.
Medication	Medications that lower blood pressure include narcotics, tranquilizers, hypnotics, diuretics, antihypertensives, and certain cardiac medications (particularly vasodilators). Medications that raise blood pressure include antihistamines, estrogen, and corticosteroids (glucocorticoids and mineralocorticoids).
Diurnal variation	Blood pressure is typically lowest in the early morning, with decreased activity, and highest in the afternoon or evening, with increased activity.
Sex	After puberty, males tend to have higher blood pressure than females. After menopause, women tend to have higher blood pressure than men of the same age.
Environment	A hot environment can lower blood pressure by causing vasodilation. A cold environment can raise it by causing vasoconstriction.
Exercise	Blood pressure increases with activity and exercise because the sympathetic nervous system responds to the body's increased need for oxygen.
Body position	Blood pressure is lowest in the recumbent position. It is slightly higher in the standing position because of sympathetic nervous system stimulation.
Right versus left arm	About one fourth of the population has a difference of 10 ($\pm$5) mm Hg between the right and left arms.
Arm versus leg	There is a difference of 10 to 40 mm Hg in systolic blood pressure between measurements taken using the arm and measurements taken using the leg.
Vasodilation	Parasympathetic nervous system stimulation causes blood vessels to increase in lumen diameter, thus lowering blood pressure. This may happen in response to warm temperatures, fever, and relaxation, for example.
Vasoconstriction	Sympathetic nervous system stimulation causes blood vessels to decrease in lumen diameter, thus raising blood pressure. This may happen in response to cold temperatures, for example.
Head injury	Injuries to the head and increased intracranial pressure result in increased blood pressure.
Reduced blood volume	Blood pressure decreases if the circulatory system contains an inadequate volume of blood, as from low cardiac output, hemorrhage, or shock.
Increased blood volume	Too much fluid in the cardiovascular system increases blood pressure.

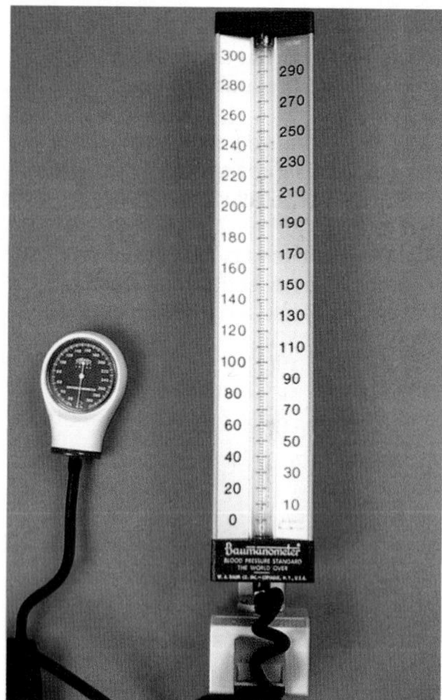

FIGURE 7-9 Manometers: aneroid *(left)* and mercury *(right)*. (From Polaski, A. L., & Warner, J. P. [1994]. *Saunders' fundamentals for nursing assistants: Slide package.* Philadelphia: Saunders.)

momanometer includes a pressure manometer (Figure 7-9), an inflatable cuff, and a pressure bulb. The manometer can function either with air (aneroid) or with mercury. In addition, a variety of automatic BP cuffs are available ranging from inexpensive over-the-counter models to high-tech programmable models that can inflate the cuff and check the BP at preset intervals. Mercury-filled manometers are being phased out in many health care settings because of the mercury hazard. All devices record BP standardized to millimeters of mercury (mm Hg). Before taking a person's BP, you should calibrate the manometer to zero to avoid a false high reading.

To most accurately detect significant changes, measure BP under constant conditions. The site for measurement (usually the upper arm) should be level with the left ventricle. The person should be in a comfortable, relaxed position without crossing the legs or constricting the abdomen. Do not allow the client to hold up the arm during the measurement, because this isometric exercise will raise the pressure (Pickering et al., 2005).

Choose a BP cuff of appropriate size for your client (Procedure 7-5). Cuffs come in newborn, infant, child, and adult sizes for both arm and leg measurements. The

PROCEDURE 7-5

TIME TO ALLOW: NOVICE: 2 min. EXPERT: 2 min.

ASSESSING BLOOD PRESSURE

Nursing Skills Online: Vital Signs, Lesson 5

View Video!

Blood pressure is the pressure exerted by blood against the inner walls of the arteries. Measuring a client's BP gives you information about the health of the cardiovascular, circulatory, and renal systems.

DELEGATION GUIDELINES

Measuring and recording a client's BP is a simple, low-risk procedure that you may delegate to a nursing assistant who has received training in this technique. Training should include specific instructions about findings that require your immediate notification. You remain responsible for assessing any variance or irregularities in the client's BP.

EQUIPMENT NEEDED

- Sphygmomanometer with cuff of correct size
- Stethoscope

1 Perform preliminary actions (see inside front cover).

2 Select a cuff of correct size for the client and the limb you intend to use.

a. Select a bladder that fits almost completely around the client's arm.
b. Select a cuff width that is about two-thirds the length of the client's upper arm. *A cuff that is too wide will result in a false low reading. A cuff that is too narrow will result in a false high reading.*

3 Choose the arm on which you will take the BP reading. *Avoid taking a BP measurement on an arm used for hemodialysis or that has a shunt, burn, cast, intravenous line, or traumatic injury. Also avoid using an arm contiguous with the site of breast or axillary surgery. If you cannot use one of the client's arms to take a BP reading, use a leg and measure BP at the popliteal artery.*

4 Position the client's arm so it is level with the heart, palm up, in a relaxed and comfortable fashion. If the client is supine, you may place the arm on the bed. If the client is sitting or standing, position the arm on the table over the bed, or hold it with your elbow. *Positioning the arm below heart level will result in a false high reading. Positioning it above heart level will result in a false low reading. Positioning it with palm up exposes the brachial artery.*

5 If the client is changing from a lying to a sitting position, wait at least 2 minutes before taking the BP measurement. *This time allows the body's compensatory mechanisms to stabilize the BP.*

6 Affix the cuff onto the client's arm.

a. Do not place the cuff over the client's clothing and do not push clothing up so it constricts the brachial artery.
b. Place the bottom edge of the cuff 1 inch above the client's antecubital fossa (see illustration).

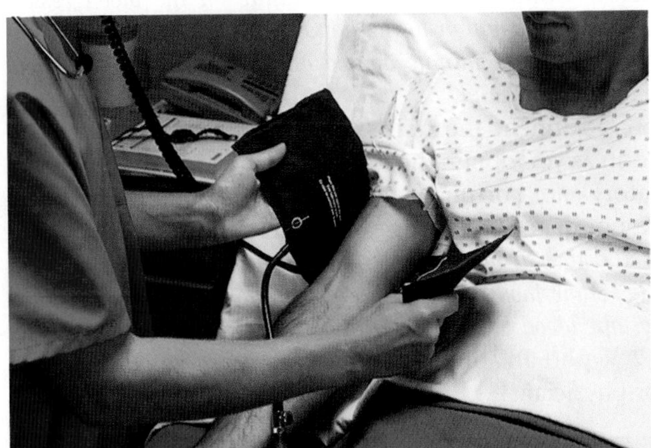

Step 6b. Placing the cuff 1 inch above the antecubital fossa.

c. Place the center of the cuff directly over the brachial artery.
d. Wrap the cuff snugly around the client's arm while allowing space to place the stethoscope over the brachial artery. *This ensures uniform and complete compression of the brachial artery. A cuff that is too loose will result in a false high reading.*

7 Position the sphygmomanometer at eye level. The liquid in a manometer or the needle of an aneroid gauge should be at zero (see illustration). *Positioning the manometer above eye level results in a false high reading. Positioning it below eye level results in a false low reading.*

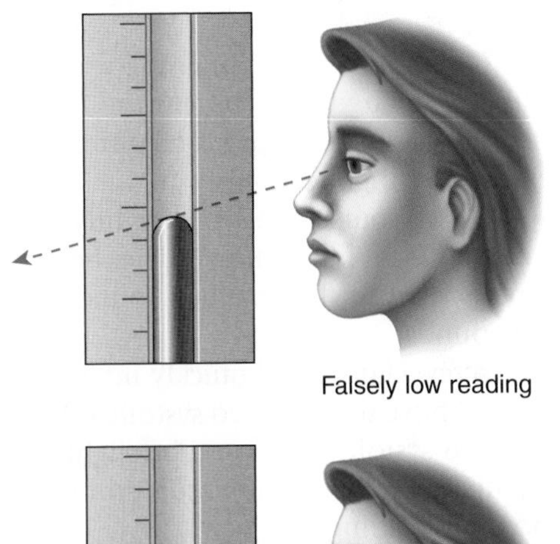

Falsely low reading

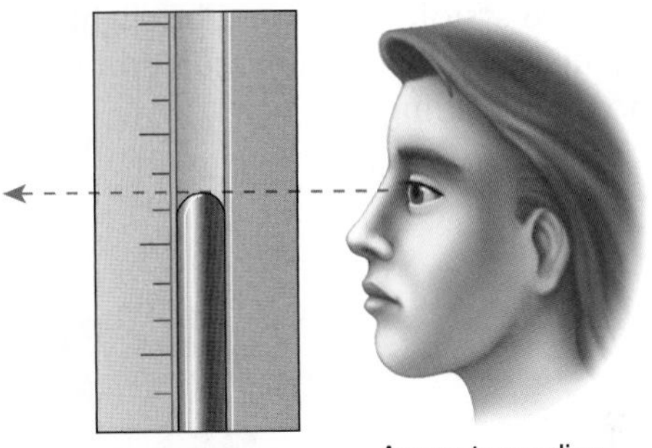

Accurate reading

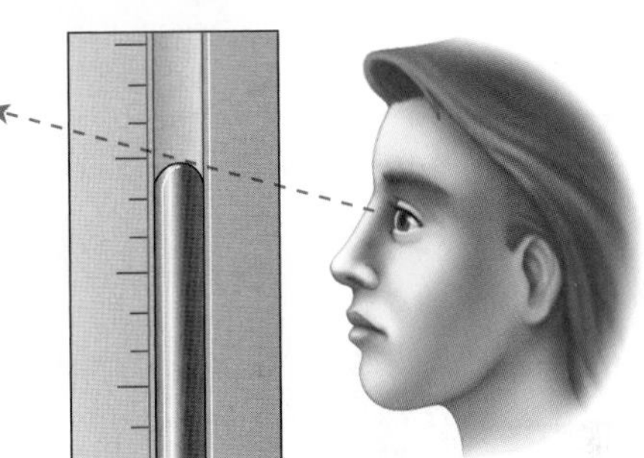

Falsely high reading

Step 7. Effect of viewing the meniscus at different levels. Viewing at eye level gives the most accurate reading.

8 Obtain a palpated systolic blood pressure. Palpated blood pressure measurement should be performed on any client whose BP is being read for the first time. It ensures that the cuff is sufficiently inflated to give an accurate systolic reading by auscultation. It also provides information about an auscultatory gap. Failure to identify such a gap results in a false low systolic reading.

a. Palpate the brachial or radial pulse.
b. Inflate the cuff until the pulse disappears.
c. Release the pressure slowly until the pulse returns, and note this reading.
d. Quickly release the cuff.

Continued

9 Obtain the BP reading without talking during the measurement.

a. Wait 30 to 60 seconds after obtaining the palpated systolic BP. *If you attempt to obtain the BP reading too soon after obtaining the palpated systolic BP, you will receive a false high reading.*

b. Place the bell of your stethoscope lightly over the brachial artery (see illustration). *The bell of the stethoscope is used for low-pitched sounds, such as extra heart sounds.*

c. Tighten the screw clamp, and quickly inflate the cuff to 30 mm Hg above the palpated systolic BP reading. *The auscultated systolic BP should be slightly higher than the palpated reading. Slow inflation can result in an inaccurate reading.*

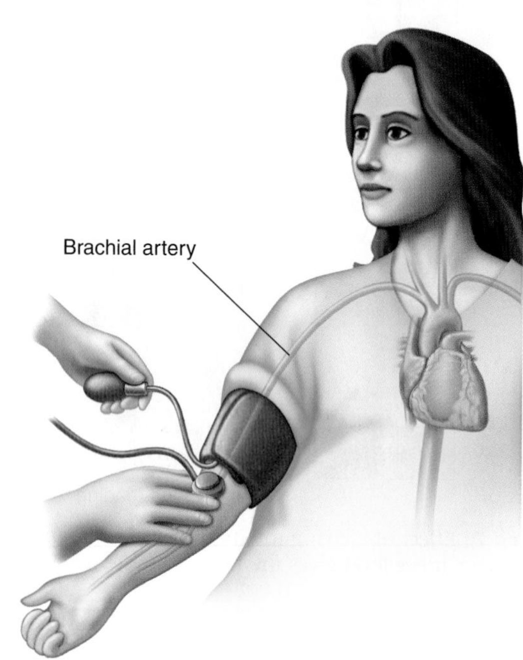

Step 9b. Positioning the stethoscope over the brachial artery.

d. Deflate the cuff slowly and steadily at 2 to 3 mm Hg per second until you hear a soft, tapping sound. This is the first Korotkoff sound and indicates the client's systolic BP. *Deflating the cuff too rapidly results in a false low systolic reading. Deflating the cuff too slowly results in a false high diastolic reading.*

e. Continue deflating the cuff slowly. Listen for a murmur or swishing sound (Korotkoff II), a clear tapping (Korotkoff III), and a muffling of sound (Korotkoff IV). *Muffling of sound correlates with the beginning of diastole and is the best indicator of diastolic BP in children.*

f. Continue deflating the cuff slowly, listening for the sounds to stop. *Cessation of sounds correlates with the end of diastole (Korotkoff V) and is the best indicator of diastolic BP in adults. In children and athletes, the sounds of phase V may continue all the way to zero.*

10 Deflate the cuff at a moderate rate and completely. If you must take another BP reading, wait 1 to 2 minutes before doing so. *Continued pressure on the blood vessels decreases circulation to the hand, causing the client discomfort. Waiting a minute or two allows normal circulation to return to the hand.*

11 Document the client's BP in the medical record as soon as you obtain the reading. If you identify an auscultatory gap, document the reading (in mm Hg) that corresponds to the length of the silence. *Normal systolic BP is 100 to 130 mm Hg. Normal diastolic BP is 60 to 80 mm Hg. Some facilities require that you document three sounds: systolic blood pressure, muffling, and diastolic blood pressure.*

12 Report an abnormal blood pressure to a charge nurse or physician.

PEDIATRIC CONSIDERATIONS

Select the proper cuff size for accurate measurement. Explain to the child that the arm will not hurt, but will feel like it is being "hugged" or "squeezed."

GERIATRIC CONSIDERATIONS

Select the proper cuff size for accurate measurement. Explain the procedure to a confused client to gain cooperation.

inflatable bladder inside the cuff should be long enough to encircle 80% of the client's limb, and the bladder width should be 40% of the client's limb circumference. A too-narrow cuff will produce a false high reading. A too-large cuff will produce a false low reading. Place the cuff directly over the client's brachial artery to ensure complete and equal compression.

To hear the sounds on which to base BP measurement, you will need to know how to use a stethoscope correctly. Some sounds are very faint, and the possibility of error is considerable (Table 7-7). To improve the sound, place the diaphragm of the stethoscope directly over the brachial artery. Insert the stethoscope earpieces so the tips point toward your nose, not the back of your head. Turn the television or radio down or off and, if necessary, ask people in the room to be quiet. You will need to practice and refine your technique for measuring BP to make sure you can do it accurately.

Table 7-7 Blood Pressure Measurement: Sources of Error and the Effect on Results

SOURCE OF ERROR	EFFECT ON BLOOD PRESSURE READING
Cuff size too wide	False low
Cuff size too narrow	False high
Cuff wrapped too loosely	False high
Arm below heart level	False high
Arm above heart level	False low
Manometer below eye level	False low
Manometer above eye level	False high
Cuff deflated too rapidly	False low systolic
Cuff deflated too slowly	False high diastolic
Failure to wait 30 to 60 seconds between successive blood pressure readings	False high
Failure to identify an auscultatory gap with a palpatory systolic blood pressure measurement	False low systolic
Defective equipment, poorly calibrated manometers, hearing impairment, or improper use of stethoscope	Inaccurate readings

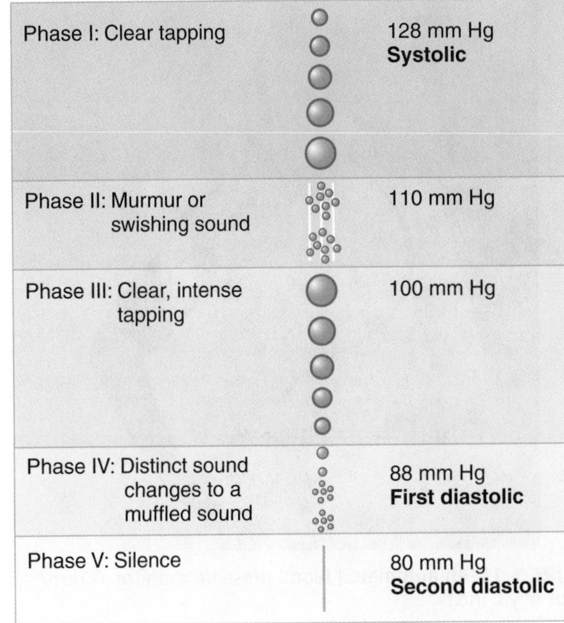

FIGURE 7-10 The Korotkoff sounds (also called phases).

The five distinct sounds you will listen for when measuring BP are called **Korotkoff's sounds** or Korotkoff's phases. When blood is flowing freely through an artery or the artery is totally obstructed, no sound can be detected even with a stethoscope. However, if you partially constrict the artery, turbulent blood flow vibrates the walls of the artery and produces sound. Thus the BP cuff is used to temporarily obstruct the artery. As you slowly release pressure from the cuff, the obstruction is gradually reduced, and the sounds change. When the blood flows freely again, the sound disappears.

The first sound you will hear as turbulent blood begins flowing through the partially compressed artery is Korotkoff I, a clear tapping sound (Figure 7-10). As you continue to release pressure, the other sounds follow. Korotkoff II is a murmur or swishing sound. Korotkoff III is a clear, intense tapping. Korotkoff IV is a distinct change to a muffled sound and indicates the first diastolic blood pressure. Korotkoff V is the disappearance sound caused by freely flowing blood; it indicates the second diastolic blood pressure.

To assess a client's cardiovascular function fully, you may need to check for **orthostatic hypotension,** in which BP drops by 20 mm Hg or more with position changes (see Chapter 33). To do so, measure the BP when the client is lying, sitting, and standing. Wait about 2 minutes between position changes to allow the client's compensatory mechanisms to stabilize the BP before taking the next reading. Orthostatic hypotension may result from a reduced blood volume or from certain medications.

Action Alert! Ensure the safety of clients with orthostatic hypotension by sitting them up and getting them out of bed slowly.

If the client has hypertension, you may not hear Korotkoff II. This absence is called an **auscultatory gap.** You will hear a faint first Korotkoff sound, then silence until the third Korotkoff sound comes in loud and crisp. The cause of this gap is unknown. However, recognizing it is crucial. If you fail to recognize it, you could mistake the third Korotkoff sound (instead of the first) as the client's systolic pressure. Doing so produces a false low systolic reading.

If the normal tapping sounds disappear on inspiration and return on expiration, the client has pulsus paradoxus. Slowly decrease the cuff pressure, and listen for the paradoxical pulse to cease. If it is present for more than 10 mm Hg, it may be a sign of serious cardiovascular problems.

If you cannot use the client's arm to measure blood pressure, you may need to use the popliteal artery behind the knee. Use an appropriate thigh-sized cuff. Systolic pressures in the leg can differ by 10 to 40 mm Hg from pressures in the arm. When documenting your findings, make sure to note that the reading is from the client's leg.

Finally, if you have trouble hearing the Korotkoff sounds, you may need to use Doppler ultrasound to measure the client's BP. This problem may result from severe hypotension, shock, or circulatory instability. The Doppler transducer picks up and amplifies blood

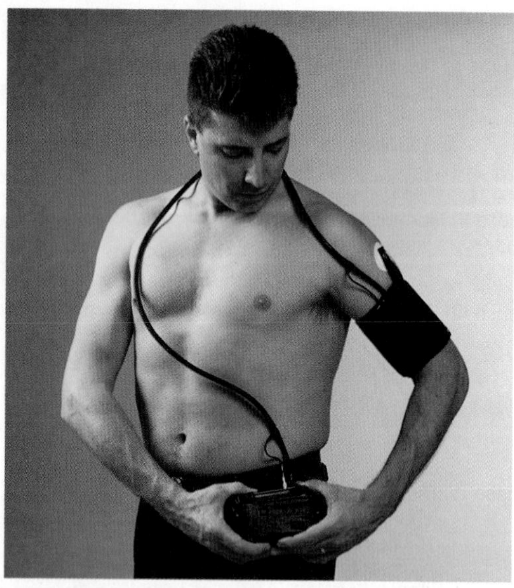

FIGURE 7-11 An automated blood pressure monitor. (Courtesy Welch Allyn, Inc.)

pressure sounds so you can hear them. However, you will be able to determine only a systolic pressure measurement with this device. If you need to take frequent BP readings, you may want to use an automated BP machine to obtain quick, accurate measurements (Figure 7-11).

In all cases, document your client's BP as soon as you obtain the reading. If you are documenting BP for the first time, measure it in both arms as a baseline. When there is a difference in the measurements obtained between arms, record both BP readings and note the location from which they were obtained. Thereafter the same arm (the one with the higher pressure) should be used for consistency in readings and accurate interpretation of trends (Pickering et al., 2005; Schell et al., 2005). Follow your health care facility's policy when documenting pressures. Most continue to use the two-part measurement that lists systolic and diastolic levels. However, a growing number of facilities require a three-part documentation. If yours does, you will need to chart systolic, muffling, and diastolic readings. Along with the numerical readings, you should also document the location from which you took the reading and the client's position.

▼ KEY PRINCIPLES

- Assessment of vital signs provides you with crucial information about a client's psychological and physical state of health.
- Body temperature is a balance between heat production and heat loss.
- Body temperature is affected by the client's health, age, stress, and time of day.
- Common types of thermometers are glass, electronic, and tympanic.
- Routes for temperature measurement are oral, axillary, rectal, and tympanic.
- The pulse is a wave of blood in the arteries created by the pumping action of the heart.
- Assessment of the radial and apical pulses includes the rate, rhythm, and strength.
- The rate and depth of respirations change according to the body's need for oxygen, the release of carbon dioxide, and the person's emotions.
- Oxygen saturation provides an indication of the amount of oxygen that is available for use by tissues of the body and is being increasingly used as one of the standard vital signs.
- Blood pressure is largely a reflection of blood volume, cardiac output, and vascular resistance.
- Blood pressure measurements record the highest pressure (systolic) and the lowest resting pressure (diastolic) of the fluid in the vessels.
- Accurate documentation is essential for communication of vital sign data to other health care providers.

■ REVIEW QUESTIONS

1. The nursing assistant reports to the nurse that the temperature of a first-day postoperative client is 100.6° F. Which of the following actions should the nurse take first?

1. Instruct the nursing assistant to recheck the temperature using a different thermometer.
2. Instruct the nursing assistant to recheck the temperature in 30 minutes.
3. Compare this temperature to previously documented temperatures.
4. Notify the physician of the rise in temperature.

2. The nurse is checking routine vital signs on four assigned clients. For which client would the nurse measure an apical pulse instead of a radial pulse?

1. A client receiving digitalis, a cardiac medication
2. A client who will be going to surgery the next morning
3. A client who will be discharged to home later in the day
4. A client who is reporting pain

3. The nurse measures a respiratory rate of 16 respirations per minute for a newly admitted adult client. Which of the following actions should the nurse take next?

1. Recheck the measurement in 15 minutes
2. Document the measurement on the flow sheet
3. Ask another nurse to measure the respiratory rate
4. Check the client's medical record for history of respiratory disease

4. The nurse determines that which of the following clients has the greatest need to have an oxygen saturation measurement done with vital signs?

1. A client who smokes a pipe
2. A client who has a broken ankle
3. A client who is 25 pounds overweight
4. A client who has lung disease

5. The physician's order reads, "Take orthostatic blood pressure measurements once daily." The nurse would measure the blood pressure in which of the following positions?

1. Lying, standing, and then sitting
2. Lying, sitting, and then standing
3. Sitting, standing, and then lying
4. Standing, sitting, and then lying

Bibliography

Ayers, D. M., & Lappin, J. S. (2004). Act fast when your patient has dyspnea. *Nursing, 34*(7), 36-42.

*Bayne, C. G. (1997). Technology assessment: Vital signs: Are we monitoring the right parameters? *Nursing Management, 28*(5), 74-76.

Carroll, P. (2003). Pulse oximetry in context. *RN, 66*(9), *Acute Care Decisions,* (30, ac 1-7).

Considine, J. (2005). Consult stat. Taking vitals on a patient with orthostatic hypotension. *RN, 68*(1), 50.

Considine, J. (2005). The reliability of clinical indicators of oxygenation: A literature review. *Contemporary Nurse, 18*(3), 258-267.

*Erickson, R. S., Meyer, L. T., & Woo, T. M. (1996). Accuracy of chemical dot thermometers in critically ill adults and young children. *Image Journal of Nursing Scholarship, 28*(1), 23-28.

*Flo, G., & Brown, M. (1995). Comparing three methods of temperature taking. *Nursing Research, 44*(2), 120-122.

Giuliano, K. K., & Higgins, T. L. (2005). New-generation pulse oximetry in the care of critically ill patients. *American Journal of Critical Care, 14*(1), 26-39.

Hakemi, A., & Bender, J. A. (2005). Understanding pulse oximetry, advantages, and limitations. *Home Health Care Management & Practice, 17*(5), 416-418.

Harper, J. P. (2004). Post-anesthesia care unit nurses' knowledge of pulse oximetry. *Journal for Nurses in Staff Development, 20*(4), 177-180.

*Henker, R., & Coyne, C. (1995). Comparison of peripheral temperature measurements with core temperature. *AACN Clinical Issues, 6*(1), 21-30.

Khorshid, L., Eser, I., Zaybak, A., & Yapucu Ü. (2005). Comparing mercury-in-glass, tympanic and disposable thermometers in measuring body temperature in healthy young people. *Journal of Clinical Nursing, 14*(4), 496-500.

Molony, S. L., Kobayashi, M., Holleran, E. A., & Mezey, M. (2005). Assessing pain as a fifth vital sign in long-term care facilities: recommendations from the field. *Journal of Gerontological Nursing, 31*(3), 16-24.

Occupational Safety and Health Administration, U.S. Department of Labor. (Revised April 1999). *Occupational safety and health guideline for mercury vapor.* Retrieved January 20, 2006, from http://www.osha.gov/SLTC/healthguidelines/mercuryvapor/recognition.html.

Occupational Safety and Health Administration, U.S. Department of Labor. (2004). Pediatric corner. Don't get a sick child's temperature wrong: Inaccurate readings can impact care. *ED Nursing, 7*(6), 64-65.

Pickering, T. G., Hall, J. E., Appel, L. J., Falkner, B. E., Graves, J., Hill, M. N., et al. (2005). Hypertension. *Circulation, 45,* 142-161.

Popovich, D. M., Richiuso, N., & Danek, G. (2004). Pediatric health care providers' knowledge of pulse oximetry. *Pediatric Nursing, 30*(1), 14-22.

Pullen, R. L. (2003). Caring for a patient on pulse oximetry. *Nursing, 33*(9), 31.

Pullen, R. L. (2003). Using an ear thermometer. *Nursing, 33*(5), 24.

Schell, K., Bradley, E., Bucher, L., Seckel, M., Lyons, D., Wakai, S., et al. (2003). The unvarnished truth about nail polish. *Nursing, 33*(9), 33.

Schell, K., Bradley, E., Bucher, L., Seckel, M., Lyons, D., Wakai, S., et al. (2005). Clinical comparison of automatic, noninvasive measurements of blood pressure in the forearm and upper arm. *American Journal of Critical Care, 14*(3), 232-241.

Sund-Levander, M., Grodzinsky, E., Loyd, D., Wahren, L. (2004). Errors in body temperature assessment related to individual variation, measuring technique and equipment. *International Journal of Nursing Practice, 10*(5), 216-223.

Thomas, J., & Feliciano, C. (2003). Measuring BP with a Doppler device: Learn how this ultrasound tool can amplify a faint pulse sound. *Nursing, 33* (7), 52-53.

Viverais-Dresler, G., & Bakker, D. A. (2004). Blood pressure monitoring: Older adults' perceptions. *Journal of Gerontological Nursing, 30*(1), 44-52.

*Winslow, E. H. (1995). Research for practice: Are 60-second pulse counts necessary? *American Journal of Nursing, 95* (1), 53.

*Winslow, E. H., Jacobson, A. F., & Beazlie, M. A. (1997). Research for practice: Tympanic thermometers—Accuracy is questionable. *American Journal of Nursing, 97*(5), 71.

Yucha, C. B., Yang, M. C. K., Tsai, P., & Calderon, K. S. (2003). Comparison of blood pressure measurement consistency using tonometric and automated oscillometric instruments. *Journal of Nursing Measurement, 11*(1), 73-86.

*Asterisk indicates a classic or definitive work on this subject.

Chapter 8

Physical Assessment

Media Resources

- evolve Evolve Website http://evolve.elsevier.com/Harkreader/
- Companion CD

Learning Objectives

After studying this chapter, you should be able to do the following:

- Describe the four techniques used in physical examination: inspection, palpation, percussion, and auscultation
- Identify the purpose of the primary instruments used in physical assessment
- Acquire nonthreatening techniques for physical examination to ensure client comfort and prepare the client for each regionally focused area of a complete physical examination
- Perform a complete physical examination on a client using a head-to-toe approach
- Recognize normal physical findings
- Recognize when physical findings deviate from normal

Key Terms

accommodation
auscultation
bronchial
bronchovesicular
ecchymosis
inspection
lesion
ophthalmoscope
otoscope
palpation
percussion
point of maximal impulse (PMI)
precordium
respiratory excursion
tactile fremitus
turgor
vesicular

The physical examination is a systematic means of collecting objective assessment data. Objective data may be used to verify findings from the history or to determine the meaning of the findings. Although the history and the physical examination are often conducted separately, the information is synthesized to identify and explain the client's problems.

As you collected the nursing history, you identified problems and possible problems in the client. In doing a physical examination, you are now looking for objective evidence commonly associated with these problems. The findings may confirm the problems you suspected or at least add evidence to substantiate the hypotheses.

Physical assessments can be either *comprehensive* or *focused*. A comprehensive physical assessment is often limited to the first time that a client sees a specific health care provider or enters a health care agency. Subsequently, assessment is focused on the reason for the visit and the client's current needs. When a client presents in acute distress with need of immediate intervention for a specific problem, assessment is focused on the most important data for the immediate problem. How quickly you narrow the focus may depend on the client's needs and your knowledge level. A focused assessment assumes you have the knowledge to rule out the need for examination of particular body parts or functions.

Regardless of the purpose, all physical assessment is aimed at detecting problems related to altered function, establishing baseline data against which subsequent data can be compared to judge whether the client's condition is improving or worsening, and identifying factors that place the client at risk for additional health problems. To learn to perform physical assessment, you must first learn to recognize normal findings. As you continue to study each health pattern, you will add knowledge of some common abnormal findings.

PREPARATION FOR PHYSICAL EXAMINATION

TECHNIQUES OF PHYSICAL EXAMINATION

The four basic techniques used in physical examination are inspection, palpation, percussion, and auscultation, and they are generally performed in that order. Inspection is always done first. Palpation follows, except during examination of the abdomen, when it is done last so that it does not alter bowel sounds and change the findings on percussion and auscultation.

Inspection. **Inspection** is the systematic visual examination of the client. It involves observation of color, shape, size, symmetry, position, and movement, using the sense of smell to detect odors, and using hearing to detect sounds. For inspection to yield accurate findings, the area to be inspected must be fully exposed and the environmental light must be good. Use natural light when it is important to avoid distortion of color. Use tangential lighting (lighting that shines from one side and casts shadows) to increase your ability to detect variations in body surface such as changes in abdominal contour (Figure 8-1).

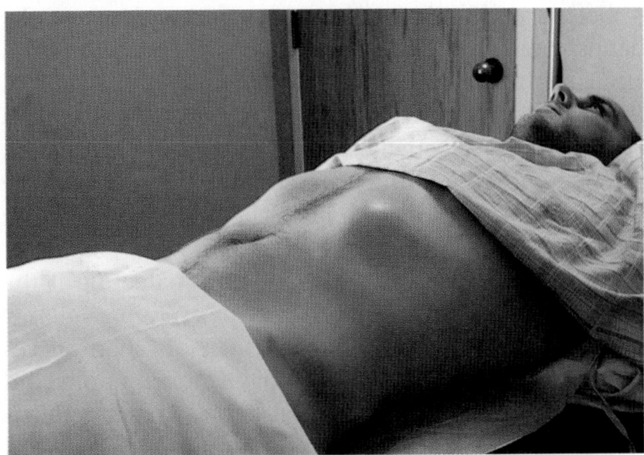

FIGURE 8-1 Tangential lighting (lighting that shines from one side and casts shadows) increases your ability to detect variations in body surface, such as changes in abdominal contour.

Palpation. **Palpation** is examination of the body through the use of touch. It is used to obtain information regarding temperature, moisture, texture, consistency, size, shape, position, and mobility. You palpate to assess pulses as well as to check for tenderness, guarding, abdominal distention (enlarged or swollen abdomen), masses, and edema.

When checking temperature, use the back (dorsal surface) of the hand, because it is usually more sensitive than the palm. When assessing texture, shape, size, muscle tone, movement, or tenderness, use the pads of the fingers. When assessing vibration, use the ulnar aspect of the hand.

Palpation may be either light or deep. Use light palpation to examine lesions or masses on the surface of the skin or lying immediately under the skin. A light touch helps you avoid changing the shape of the lesion or mass. For light palpation, place the hand, with fingers together, flat on the area to be palpated. Press the finger pads into the area to a depth of 1 to 2 cm ($^1/_2$ to $^3/_4$ inch). Repeat this action in ever-widening circles until you have palpated the entire area to be examined. Use light palpation to check muscle tone and to check for tenderness. Light palpation is always done before performing deep palpation.

Use deep palpation to identify abdominal organs and abdominal masses. With deep palpation, hold the hand at a 60-degree angle, fingers together, and use the finger pads and fingertips to press inward to a depth of 4 cm (2 inches). For two-handed deep palpation, place one hand on top of the other and palpate as just described. Two-handed palpation may help you keep the lower hand relaxed and thus more sensitive to underlying structures.

Before performing palpation, wash and warm the hands. Make sure the fingernails are short to avoid scratching the client's skin. If the client is ticklish, spread the fingers and add the client's fingers between yours until the hypersensitivity is lessened and the client's hand can be removed. During palpation, tell the client to take slow deep breaths through his or her mouth to decrease muscle tension, which can interfere with palpation. Palpate any tender areas last, and stop palpating if the client has pain at any point during the examination.

Percussion. **Percussion** is the use of short, sharp strikes to the body surface to produce palpable vibrations and characteristic sounds. Percussion is performed to determine the size, shape, density, and location of a body organ, and to elicit pain and tenderness. In addition, it can be used to detect whether tissue or a body cavity is fluid filled, air filled, or solid. With the exception of costal vertebral tenderness, percussion is an advanced skill.

Generally, as the amount of air present in the area being percussed increases, the sounds produced become louder, longer, and deeper. Softer, higher-pitched, shorter sounds are produced from more solid areas. The five types of percussion sounds are *resonance* (hollow sound), *hyperresonance* (booming sound), *tympany* (musical or drum sound), *dullness* (thud), and *flatness* (extremely dull sound). Resonance is heard over the normal lung, hyperresonance is heard over an emphysematous lung, tympany is the sound produced by air-filled bowel, dullness is heard over dense structures such as the liver and heart, and flatness is heard over very dense structures such as skeletal muscle and bone.

The two types of percussion are direct and indirect. For direct percussion, you use a sharp, rapid movement of the wrist so that the pad of the middle finger strikes the area of the client's body to be percussed (Figure 8-2, *A*). Direct percussion is used primarily to assess the sinuses in adult clients.

Indirect percussion involves two hands. Place the middle finger of the nondominant hand in contact with the client's body, then use the dominant hand fingertip, not the finger pad, to strike the first joint of the nondominant finger (Figure 8-2, *B*). Hyperextend the middle finger, and avoid touching the client with the palm or other fingers because this will also damp the vibrations. Strike at a right angle, then withdraw immediately to avoid damping the resulting vibrations. Strike each area twice, and then move to a new area. In general, the thicker the body wall is in the area being percussed, the greater the force of the strike needed to produce a clear tone.

Percussion that uses either the ulnar surface of the hand or the fist to strike the surface to be percussed is called blunt percussion. If the area to be percussed is struck directly, it is direct blunt percussion. It is indirect blunt percussion when the palm of the nondominant hand is placed flat on the area to be percussed and the back of the hand is struck.

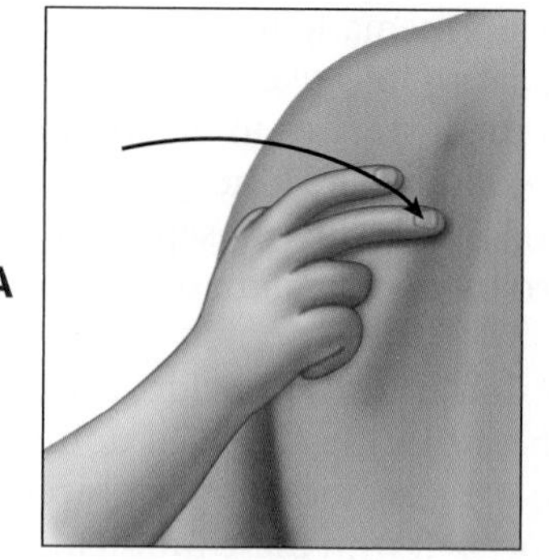

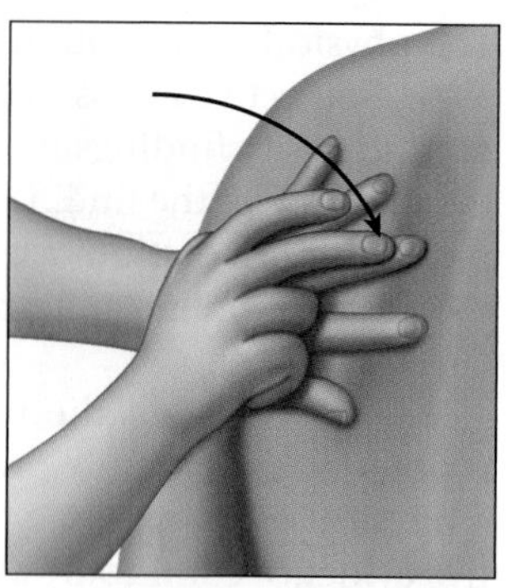

FIGURE 8-2 Techniques for direct percussion **(A)** and indirect percussion **(B)**.

Auscultation. **Auscultation** is the process of listening to sounds generated within the body. Examples of such sounds are those produced by the passage of air in and out of the lungs (breath sounds), those produced by the flow of blood through the heart and blood vessels (heart and vascular sounds), and those produced by the movement of fluid and gases through the intestinal tract (bowel sounds). Each sound is described in terms of intensity (loudness), pitch, quality, frequency, and duration. Sounds can be judged abnormal on the basis of where they are located or because changes are noted in one or more of these characteristics.

Auscultation is most often done using a stethoscope. However, you may also listen without a stethoscope to detect breath sounds, clicking or popping sounds from joint movements, and other sounds of body functions.

EQUIPMENT FOR PHYSICAL EXAMINATION

To perform a physical examination, you will rely heavily on the use of the five senses, particularly the ability to observe (inspect). Much of the examination is a mental activity rather than something you actually do. However, some equipment is used for specific aspects of the basic physical examination, and additional equipment may be used for special parts of the examination (Figure 8-3).

For most purposes, you will need a stethoscope, sphygmomanometer, and thermometer to take vital signs. A tongue blade and penlight are useful to examine the oral cavity and throat. The tuning fork, cotton-tipped swabs, Snellen chart, paper clip, and safety pins are needed only for the neurological examination.

For safety and accuracy, conduct the examination in a manner that is both time-efficient and conducive to client comfort and satisfaction. It is essential that all equipment be clean, accessible, in working order, and warmed if it will touch the client. Most nurses carry a stethoscope and a penlight, because they are most commonly used.

As you listen with a stethoscope, visualize the underlying anatomy and physiology. To use a stethoscope you will need to limit extraneous sounds. The room should be quiet. If this involves turning off suction devices that are being used on the client, first ascertain the safety of doing

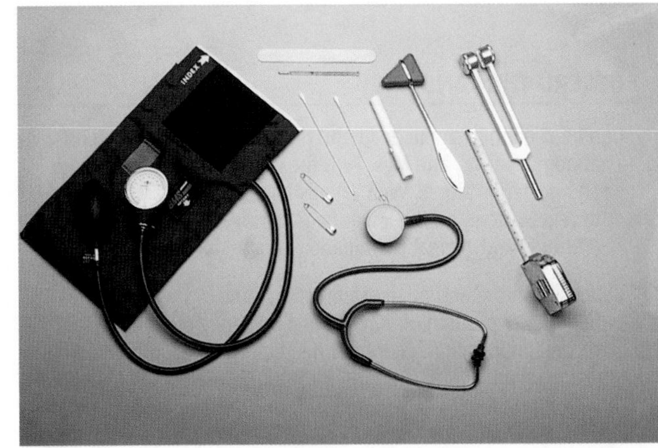

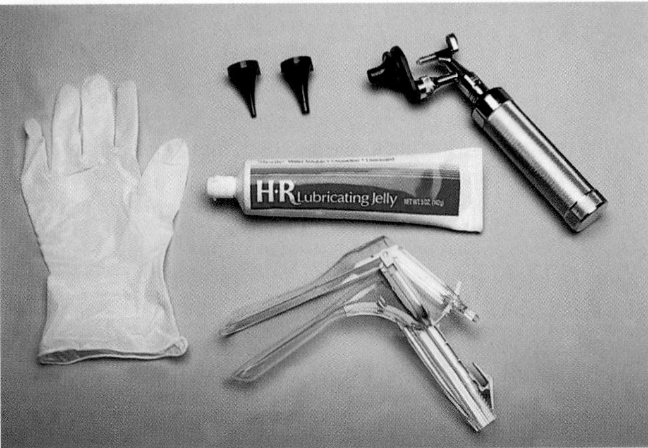

FIGURE 8-3 **A,** Equipment used for a basic physical examination: sphygmomanometer, stethoscope, tongue blade, thermometer, safety pins, cotton-tipped applicators, penlight, percussion hammer, tape measure, and tuning fork. **B,** Equipment used for specialized aspects of the physical examination: clean gloves and water-soluble lubricant, otoscope, and vaginal speculum.

so. In addition, the room should be warm. Shivering may distort the sound. Listening through clothes can create extraneous noise and damp the sounds. Hair on the chest can mimic abnormal lung sounds.

Place the diaphragm of the stethoscope firmly, but not pressing, on the client's skin, and keep the tubing still. Place the bell lightly on the skin. Practice until you can hear very quiet, soft sounds. As you listen to normal body sounds, imagine the normal function that is occurring and associate the sound with the function. You should mentally "see" what is happening in the body.

CONDUCTING THE PHYSICAL EXAMINATION

It is critical that the physical examination be conducted in a manner that will promote the collection of complete, accurate assessment data. This means that you should follow a regular pattern of examination, position the client for the most accurate collection of data, and describe the findings in a manner that can be understood by other health care providers.

There is no one correct pattern for physical examination; the importance of the pattern is to ensure a comprehensive assessment through systematic data collection. You may choose, for example, a head-to-toe approach, or you may proceed from one body system to the next. The pattern may be modified as appropriate for the physical condition of the client and the information needed. The approach you choose should become second nature to you, thus helping to ensure that no aspect of the assessment is overlooked and that the data are organized in a meaningful fashion. The head-to-toe approach helps you proceed from clean to dirty. Thus you are not examining the mouth with a hand that has touched a foot.

To prepare the client, introduce yourself and describe what the examination will involve. Be sensitive to the client's personal or cultural need for privacy, touch, and communication. Reassure the client about the confidentiality of the examination. Ask the client to immediately report any fatigue or discomfort.

Before starting the examination, provide the client with the opportunity to use the bathroom and to assume a comfortable position. Throughout the examination, drape the client for privacy. Repositioning will be necessary as the different parts of the body are examined (Table 8-1).

For the ambulatory client, the physical examination usually starts with the sitting position or walking into the room, at which time you can assess gait, posture, effort, assistance, and clothing. For the hospitalized client, the examination is often started with the client lying in bed. You need to plan the examination to avoid having the client change positions any more than necessary while still allowing you to obtain all needed data.

To accurately describe the findings of a physical examination, you need to use terms that have a common meaning to other health care providers. To describe the location of the area you are examining, imagine that the body is divided by three planes that divide it into anterior-posterior, inferior-superior, and medial-lateral aspects (Figure 8-4).

The frontal plane divides the body into anterior and posterior surfaces. The anterior surface is called the *ventral surface,* and the posterior surface is *the dorsal surface.*

The transverse plane divides the body into inferior and superior aspects. The terms *inferior* and *superior* are also used in relation to a point of reference, usually the heart or the thorax. For example, the knee is inferior to the thigh and superior to the foot. Similarly, the terms *distal* and *proximal* are used in relation to a reference point, or the point of origin of the body part. Distal means away from, with reference to a point of origin such as the arm. In other words, the hand is distal to the elbow. Proximal means nearer to a point of origin. The elbow is proximal to the hand.

Table 8-1 Client Positions for Physical Examination

POSITION		DESCRIPTION AND USE
Dorsal recumbent		Can be used to examine head and neck, anterior thorax, breasts, abdomen, arms, and legs. Turn the client to examine the back and posterior thorax. With client's knees flexed, can be used to relieve strain on the lower back during the examination. (Perineal and vaginal examination can be done in this position.)
Sitting		Client sits on the end of an examination table or the side of a bed. Better position of anterior and posterior chest than dorsal recumbent position. Client will need to lie down for abdominal examination.
Lithotomy		The feet and legs are put in stirrups. Used for vaginal and rectal examination in a female.
Genupectoral (knee-chest)		Used for a rectal examination.
Prone	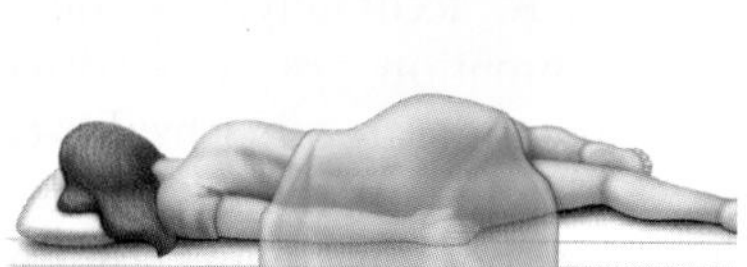	Can be used to examine the posterior thorax in this position. Most common use is for range of motion (extension) in hip.
Sims'		Can be used to examine the posterior thorax. Used as an alternative position for vaginal and rectal examination when lithotomy position is contraindicated.

The sagittal plane divides the body into right and left halves. The sagittal plane is described as the midline. Although *medial* refers to the center of the body and *lateral* to the sides, the terms medial and lateral are also used in relation to a point of reference. For example, you might describe a lesion as on the lateral aspect of the right thigh, 2 inches superior to the patella.

GENERAL SURVEY

The general survey is the first step in physical assessment. It provides information on the overall state of the client. It begins on first meeting the client, continues through the health history interview, and includes the measurement of height, weight, and vital signs. The general survey provides a basic impression of the client derived from overall physical appearance relative to age, body development, height, weight, movement, behavior, and vital signs, and it helps guide both the health history and the detailed physical examination.

Inspection of body posture may reveal significant information about the client's emotional and physical status. Assess it as the client enters the examination room or sits on the examination table, on the bed, or in a chair. Observe posture frontally, laterally, and posteriorly.

Record the client's height, weight, and body mass index (BMI) as parameters of general health status (Figure 8-5).

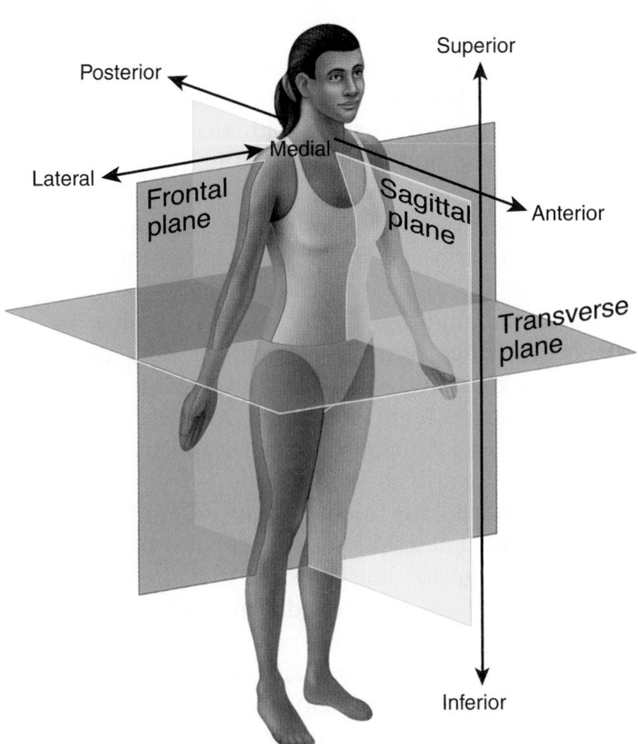

FIGURE 8-4 The body is divided by three planes. The frontal plane separates the body into anterior and posterior aspects. The transverse plane separates the body into inferior and superior aspects. The sagittal plane runs through the midline and separates the body into left and right halves and lateral and medial aspects.

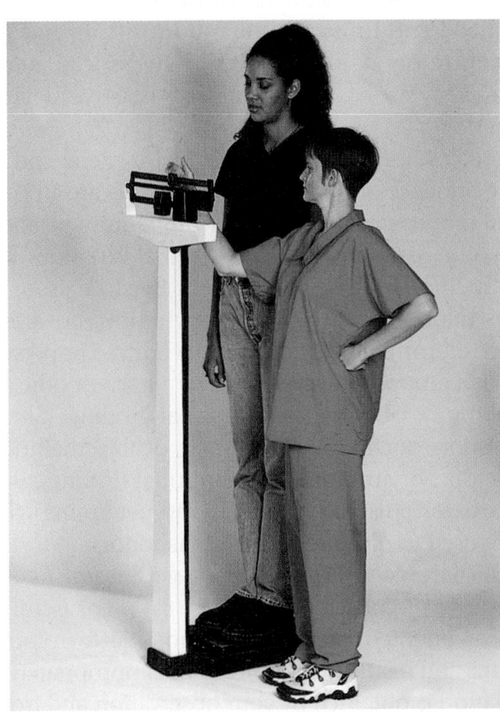

FIGURE 8-5 For both children and adults, compare height and weight to determine whether the person is overweight or underweight. This is one indicator of general health status and nutrition.

Measure the height and weight rather than relying on the client's report. However, if it is not possible to weigh and measure the client, record the client's report and note that it is approximate. Because medication doses may be calculated based on the recorded height and weight, actual measurements are important to obtain.

A standardized balance scale is preferable to a spring-loaded scale. This scale can easily be checked for balance at the zero mark each time a client is weighed, and more accurate and consistent weights are obtained. Ideally, in successive assessments a person is weighed at the same time of the day, wearing the same clothes, on the same scale, and immediately before eating. To measure a client, be sure the client is standing erect and looking straight ahead. No shoes should be worn for the most accurate measurement.

Scales are available to suspend a bedridden client in a sling, to lay an infant on a platform, to roll a wheelchair on a platform, or even as part of high-tech hospital beds. If sheets, clothes, wheelchairs, or items are weighed with the client, weigh the item separately and subtract to obtain the person's actual weight.

Height, weight, and head circumference up to age 2 are important measurements in children to determine that growth and development are proceeding at a normal rate. For both children and adults, compare the height and weight to determine if they are overweight or underweight. This is one indicator of general health and nutrition.

Signs of Acute Distress. The general survey begins with observing the client for obvious signs of distress. These include posture, cyanosis, labored breathing, bleeding, diaphoresis, writhing, moaning, crying, vocalizations, or guarding of a body part. If any of these signs is present, determine whether immediate intervention is needed. If no sign of distress requiring immediate intervention is present, the general survey continues.

Age, Physical Development, and Nutritional Status. Assess the client in terms of apparent age versus reported age. This assessment is based on signs of aging such as skin changes, gait, posture, muscle strength, and mental alertness. It answers the question, "Does the client look older or younger than the actual chronological age?" Note general body shape, muscular development, and fat distribution. Draw an impression regarding apparent nutritional status (see Chapter 24). Does the client seem to be well nourished, malnourished, obese, thin, emaciated?

The general survey includes an assessment of sexual development. Note the client's secondary sexual characteristics, such as facial hair, breast size, and voice quality. Are they appropriate for the client's age and sex?

Observe for normal body proportions, the size and symmetry of facial features, facial mobility, length of limbs, and symmetry of body parts. Also observe the symmetry, smoothness, and coordination of movement, as well as the absence of involuntary movement of the head and limbs; posture, both sitting and standing; balance on standing and walking; speed, smoothness, and style of gait; and use of assistive devices or prosthetic limbs.

Skin color and condition, personal hygiene and dress, and the presence of body and breath odors are all components of the general survey. On encountering a person with a body odor, you must consider cultural variation. Typical values in the United States dictate freedom from body odor as the norm. In many other cultures, however, the presence of normal body odor is the norm. For persons of all cultural groups, however, a fecal, urinary, or other-than-normal body odor is an abnormal finding. Similarly, breath odors, such as a sweet smell, or the smell of alcohol, acetone, or ammonia are abnormal findings. Be alert to the excessive use of perfumes, and determine whether they are used to disguise an abnormal odor.

Orientation, Mood, Manner, Affect, and Speech. Assess the client's level of consciousness (Box 8-1). For example, is the client oriented, alert, aware, and able to respond to questions and instructions quickly and appropriately? This information is obtained by your observation and from the responses to routine questions in the health history.

Observation of the client's mood, manner, affect, and speech is also a part of the general survey. Mild anxiety with a cooperative, attentive attitude, and with mood and affect appropriate to the situation, are normal findings. Abnormal findings include marked nervousness; restlessness; agitation; combative or uncooperative behavior; bizarre mannerisms; apathetic, depressed, or euphoric attitude; and stooped posture. In observing the client's speech, note the speech pattern, pace of speech, use of words, thought pattern, and sentence structure. Also note the tone, clarity, and strength of the voice and whether the client has any speech defects.

Abnormal findings include excessively slow or fast speech; halting, slurred, garbled, or very deliberate speech; an excessively soft or loud voice; or a voice that is weak, hoarse, high pitched, or monotone. Aphasia, dysphasia, use of inappropriate vocabulary, stuttering, and lisping are also abnormal findings.

Mental Status. The mental status examination provides a detailed description of the client's cognitive functioning at a given time (Box 8-2). You can ascertain whether the client understands what is happening and how well the client can cooperate with the treatment plan. The depth of the mental status examination depends on the reason the client is being seen, the relevant medical problems, and the expected goals for treatment. If mental status is part of the chief complaint or related to the chief complaint, then a thorough mental status examination should be conducted. For example, for the confused client, consider evaluating the elements in the following paragraphs.

General *appearance* may provide a clue to the client's level of functioning. Poor hygiene and grooming can suggest depression, schizophrenia, organic brain disease, or lack of sufficient cognitive functioning for self-care. Bizarre dressing and makeup may be seen in manic-depressive (bipolar) illness.

Assess whether or not the *behavior* is appropriate for the client's reference group, age, and social may indicate a mental disturbance. Assess whether or not the client is able and willing to *cooperate with the interviewer.*

Affect refers to the external expression of emotion attached to ideas or mental representation of ideas. Affect is normally an expression of the internal mood of the

BOX 8-1 *Describing a Client's Level of Consciousness*

Awake and Alert: The client is aware of the surroundings and can respond appropriately to internal and external stimuli. Awake means not asleep and should not be confused with alert.

Lethargic or Somnolent: Easily drifts off to sleep or is not fully alert even though awake. This person may appear to be asleep but can be aroused with difficulty.

Obtunded: More difficult to arouse than lethargic. Technically refers to someone who is heavily dosed with narcotics and not only may be difficult to arouse but also may not be breathing adequately.

Stupor, Semicoma, Comatose: A state of almost complete unconsciousness. May respond to strong stimuli such as loud noise, shaking, or pain. These terms may represent a continuum, with stupor being the most arousable; however, they are difficult to distinguish. For this reason, record precisely the observations you make, such as spontaneous movement, opening eyes, attempts to speak, or level/type of stimulus that elicits a response.

Coma: A state of unconsciousness from which the client cannot be aroused even by painful stimulus. Painful stimulus is applied by rubbing deeply on the sternum. If there is no response, the coma is deep. **Caution:** Sternal rubbing can cause bruising and should be used only if absolutely necessary.

Orientation: If the mental status is not certain, ask the client to identify person (state his or her name), place (where he or she is), and time (what day it is).

BOX 8-2 *Brief Mental Status Examination*

Ask the client to respond to the following instructions and questions:

- State your full name.
- Where are we? Hospital? City? State?
- What is the date today? Month? Year?
- What day of the week is it?
- I am going to name three objects, and I want you to repeat them back to me when I ask you.
- Where do you live? Address? City? State?
- How old are you?
- Name the three objects I listed for you.
- Count backward from 100.

person. Assess whether the affect is appropriate for the topic of conversation or situation. Inappropriate affect is inconsistent with content of the client's speech or ideas, such as laughing at a sad story. A flat affect is a lack of emotional expression and is associated with depression, Parkinson's disease, and other disorders.

Assess *speech* for clarity, choice of words, rate, and any unusual patterns. Speech may be slowed in depression or rapid in manic-depressive illness. The person with organic brain damage may have difficulty speaking.

Orientation is the most basic assessment. Ask direct questions to determine whether the client knows who he or she is, where he or she is, and whether he or she has some orientation to time (see Box 8-2). Orientation to time should take into consideration the normal tendency to lose track of time without the usual cues to the time of day. Most people normally can convey some frame of reference, such as "after lunch" or "nighttime." However, not knowing the day of the week may simply be a function of a lifestyle in which keeping up with the day of the week is not important.

Cognitive functioning refers to the client's patterns of thinking. Assess for logic, relevance, organization, and coherence of the pattern of thinking.

Ask clients if they have any problems with *memory* or concentration, or if they have noticed any changes in memory. Assess recent and remote memory. Assess recent memory by asking about recent events, such as what was eaten for the evening meal or what occurred in today's news. Remote memory is generally considered to deal with events that occurred 6 months or more in the past. The client's birth date, names of children, and names of past presidents may serve as reference points.

Intellectual functioning includes abstract thinking, concentration, content and process of thinking, perceptions, social judgment, and insight.

- *Abstract thinking* is frequently assessed by giving the person a proverb and asking what it means. The client who can think abstractly will give the nonliteral meaning. Useful proverbs include these: "a rolling stone gathers no moss," "as the twig is bent so grows the tree," "a stitch in time saves nine," "a penny saved is a penny earned."
- *Concentration* is tested by asking the person to remember a series of numbers or unconnected words and asking him or her to repeat them later in the examination.
- *Thought* is examined for content and process Abnormality in content includes delusions. Abnormality of process means that associations between thoughts are vague, lack sequence, coherence or relevance; thoughts are loosely connected, poorly organized, or illogical.
- *Perception* is the ability to see the environment as it is; assessment includes asking about illusions and hallucinations. Illusion is misinterpreting external sensory stimuli. Hallucinations are false perceptions of any of the five senses: vision, hearing, taste, touch, or smell.
- *Social judgment* is whether or not the client can compare and evaluate alternatives, make and carry out reasonable decisions, and behave in an appropriate manner for a given social situation.
- *Insight* refers to the client's ability to evaluate and understand the events and behavior that resulted in the present situation; or to recognize that his or her disturbed behavior is abnormal.

Vital Signs. The final component of the general survey is vital signs: temperature, pulse, respiratory rate, blood pressure, and a scale for the fifth vital sign (pain). Vital signs are an important determinant of the person's overall health. Assessment of vital signs is discussed in Chapter 7.

ASSESSMENT OF THE SKIN, HAIR, AND NAILS

Assessment of the skin requires that you be able to recognize a vast array of normal variations in skin color, tone, distribution of pigmentation, effects of the sun, hair growth, and distribution of hair. Physical assessment of the skin, hair, and nails involves the following:

- Inspecting the skin for color, cleanliness, hair distribution, and presence of lesions
- Palpating the skin to determine moisture, temperature, texture, mobility, and turgor
- Inspecting the hair for quantity, distribution, color, and cleanliness
- Feeling the texture of the hair
- Inspecting the scalp for cleanliness, parasites, and lesions
- Inspecting the fingernails and toenails for color, shape, contour, smoothness, uniformity of thickness, and presence of lesions

Skin

Appearance. To inspect and palpate the skin, expose and cleanse areas as needed. Use good, preferably natural, light to avoid distortion of color. Make the room temperature comfortable to prevent color or other changes that might be caused by excessive heat or cold. In assessing skin color, note general color as well as local or patchy variations.

Normally skin is intact, free of lesions, and pink toned in light-skinned persons or an underlying healthy glow in dark brown or olive-skinned persons. In dark-skinned persons, the lips, palms, nail beds, and soles are commonly light toned. Normal variations in dark-skinned persons include blue-black areas over the sacrum and pigmented spots on the nail beds and in the sclera.

Abnormalities of skin color include pallor, cyanosis, flushing, and yellowing. Pallor, which appears as a loss of rosy tones in dark skin, is best seen in the nail beds, lips, oral mucous membranes, and palpebral conjunctiva (inner lining of eyelid). Cyanosis, or blueness, in light skin is seen as ash gray in dark skin. Central cyanosis is best seen in lips, buccal mucosa, and the tongue. Peripheral cyanosis is best observed in the nail beds and in the skin of the arms and legs. Jaundice (yellow skin from liver disease) is seen in the bulbar conjunctiva (lining over the surface of eye), lips, and hard palate as well as the skin.

Lesions. Many different types of lesions occur in the skin. A **lesion** is a wound, injury, or pathological change in the body. A thorough description of a lesion is useful in determining whether the lesion is primary or secondary and whether it is benign or malignant. A *primary lesion* is the most significant or one that arises from the original source, condition, or set of symptoms in a disease process. A secondary lesion occurs secondary to or arises as a result of changes or complications from the primary condition.

The characteristics of a lesion may help determine the nature of an injury or of the disease process. Observe characteristics of the lesion. Then palpate to determine whether it is hard, soft, freely mobile with the skin, or attached to underlying structures. Also palpate for temperature and sensation. Various types of lesions are illustrated in Figure 8-6 and further described in Chapter 27.

Descriptions of skin lesions should include size, color, shape, borders, distribution, and arrangement of the lesions. The size descriptors may include the area of redness, size of a raised area, or depth of the lesion. The color descriptor usually includes redness and blue discoloration and uniformity. A bruise, or **ecchymosis,** is a hemorrhagic infiltration of the skin producing a bluish discoloration that changes to yellow as the blood cells are broken and reabsorbed. Erythema is redness of the skin caused by congestion of capillaries close to the surface of the skin.

The shape can be round, oval, irregular, ringlike (or annular), or annular with a center target. The distribution can be regional, generalized, scattered, on exposed body surfaces, at pressure sites, or on intertriginous areas (where skin surfaces touch). The arrangement of skin lesions can be described as linear (in a line), discrete (separate), confluent (running together), arciform (in an arch), or clustered. Additional terms used to describe lesions include the following:

- *Rash:* A skin eruption characterized by macules (flat spots), papules (superficial, circumscribed, solid elevations of the skin less than 0.5 to 1 cm in diameter), vesicles (serous fluid-filled elevations of epidermis—blisters), or erythema
- *Excoriation, abrasion:* Removal of surface skin by scraping or rubbing
- *Fissure:* A thin, linear crack in the epidermis
- *Ulcer:* An open lesion extending deeper than the dermis

Moisture, Texture, and Temperature. Assess the moistness and texture of the skin using the pads of the fingers. Normally the skin is dry, soft, smooth, and even. Excessively dry, damp, sweaty, oily, rough, thick, or uneven skin is an abnormal finding. Check skin temperature with the back of the hand. It is normally warm or cool, not hot or cold. General skin temperature, as well as temperature of any reddened areas, should be checked bilaterally. Assess for purulent discharge, exudates, or transudate from any lesion. Purulent discharge, which contains dead cells and leukocytes, indicates infection. Exudate is fluid with protein and cells that have escaped from blood vessels, usually as the result of inflammation. Transudate is similar but is mostly fluid.

Turgor and Mobility. Skin **turgor** is a reflection of the skin's elasticity, measured as the time it takes for the skin to return to normal after being pinched lightly between the thumb and forefinger. To check skin turgor and mobility, pinch and lift a fold of skin on the hand or forearm, over the sternum, or over the clavicle. Observe the ease of moving the skin and the speed with which it returns to its original position (Figure 8-7, p. 149). If mobility is normal, the skin moves easily. If turgor is normal, the pinched-up skinfold immediately returns to normal position. Turgor is abnormal if the skinfold remains tented (elevated) for more than 3 seconds. In older adults who have lost subcutaneous adipose tissue and skin elasticity, use the skin over the sternum. In an infant, use the abdomen.

Hair and Scalp. To assess the hair and scalp, ask the client to remove any wig, hairpiece, or other head covering. Observe the quantity, distribution, and color of the hair, then palpate the hair to determine its texture. Abnormal findings include patchy or sudden hair loss and brittle hair. Next, part the hair in several areas and inspect the scalp. It should be smooth, clean, and intact. Look for discolorations, lumps, scales, or open areas. Inspect the base of the hair shaft for nits, which are tiny, white, opaque eggs of head lice found attached to the hair shafts. Palpate the skull for lumps or tender areas.

Nails. Inspect the fingernails and toenails to determine their color, shape, contour, smoothness, thickness, and cleanliness. Abnormal findings are described by comparing the nail to a normal nail. Normal nails are clean, curved, and hard, with a pink to light brown nail bed. The angle between the nail and its base is 160 degrees. Abnormal findings include soft or brittle nails, inflammation, and pale or cyanotic nail beds. Cleanliness and grooming of nails are a cue to hygienic practices. Examples of abnormal changes in nails include spoon-shaped nails, Beau's lines, splinter hemorrhages, paronychia, and clubbed nails (Figure 8-8, p. 149).

ASSESSMENT OF THE HEAD AND NECK

Head and Face. Physical assessment of the head and face involves the following:

- Observing the size, symmetry, position, and movement of the head as a whole and of the facial features

PRIMARY LESIONS

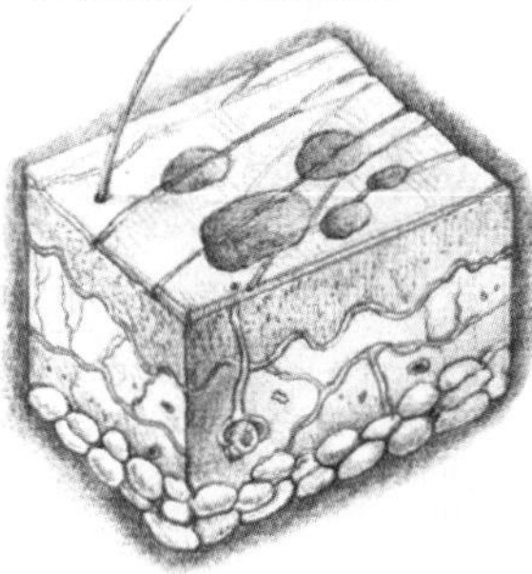

Macules (such as *freckles, flat moles,* or *rubella*) are flat lesions of less than 1 cm in diameter. Their color is different from that of the surrounding skin—most often white, red, or brown.

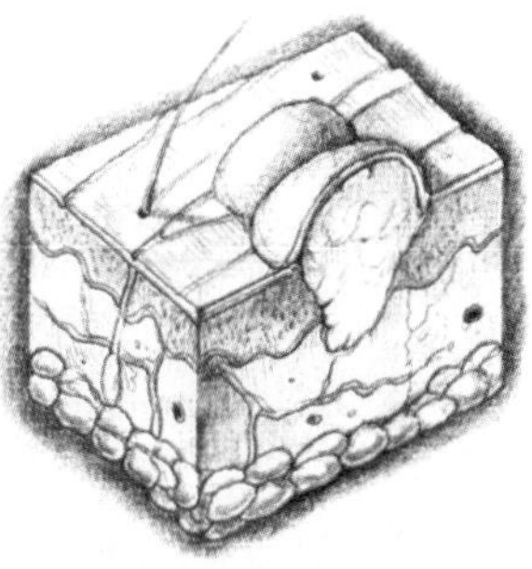

Nodules (such as *lipomas*) are elevated, marble-like lesions more than 1 cm wide and deep.

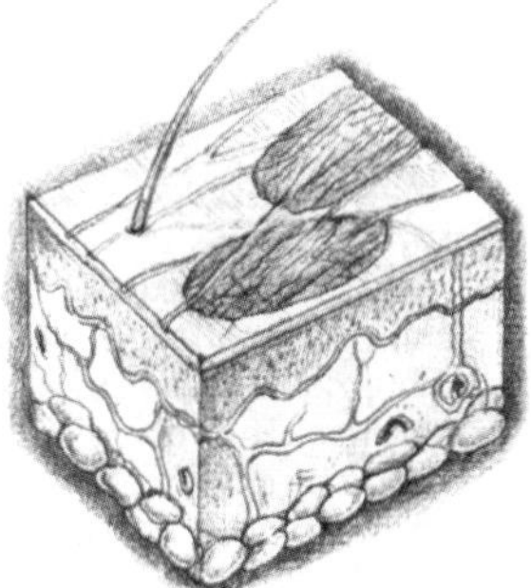

Patches (such as *vitiligo* or *café au lait spots*) are macules that are larger than 1 cm in diameter. They may or may not have some surface changes—either slight scale or fine wrinkles.

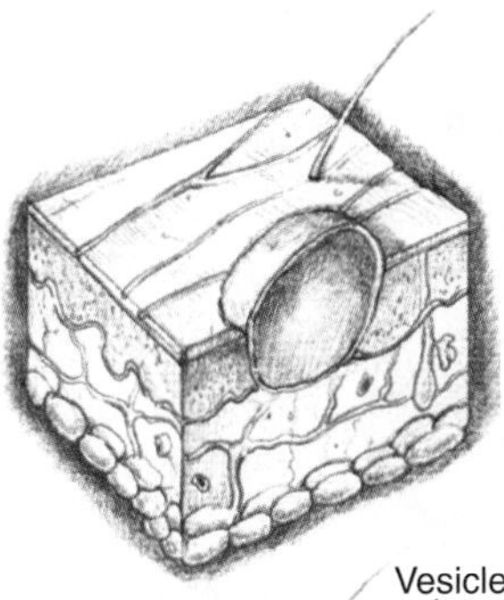

Cysts (such as *sebaceous cysts*) are nodules filled with either liquid or semisolid material that can be expressed.

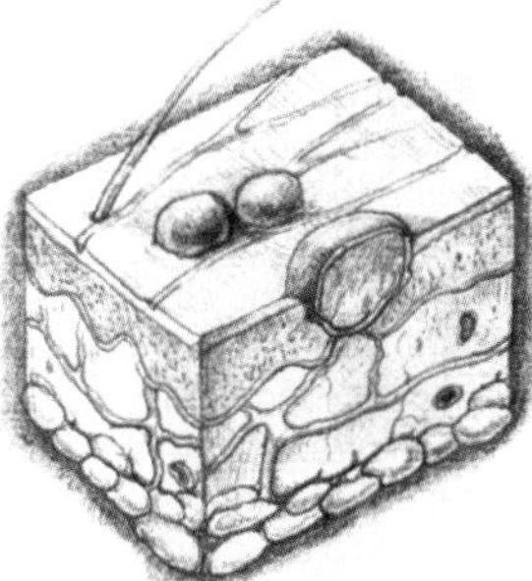

Papules (such as *warts* or *elevated moles*) are small, firm, elevated lesions less than 1 cm in diameter.

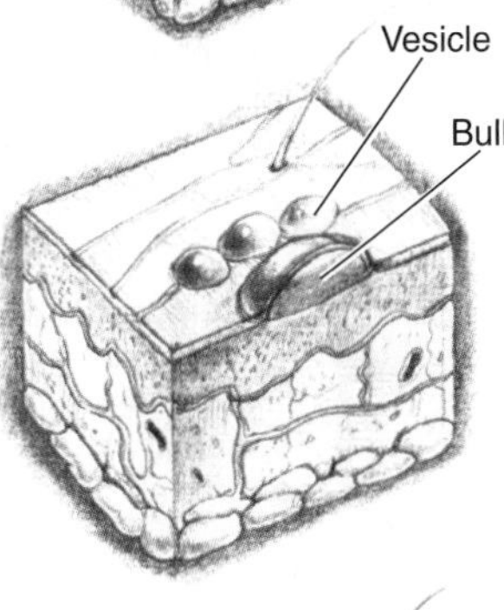

Vesicles (such as in *acute dermatitis*) and **bullae** (such as *second-degree burns*) are blisters filled with clear fluid. Vesicles are less than 1 cm in diameter, and bullae are more than 1 cm in diameter.

A

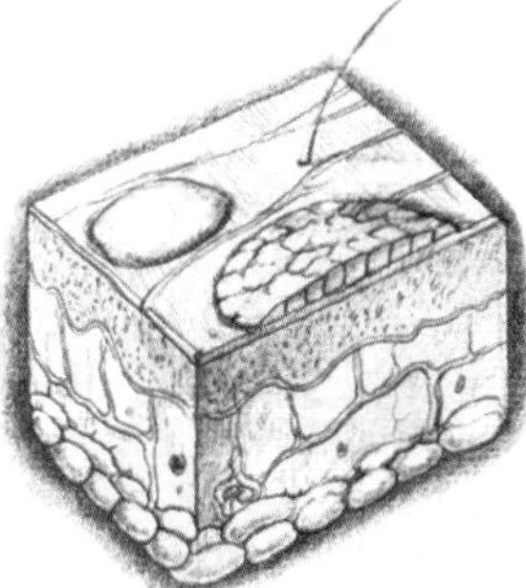

Plaques (such as in *psoriasis* or *seborrheic keratosis*) are elevated, plateau-like patches more than 1 cm in diameter that do not extend into the lower skin layers.

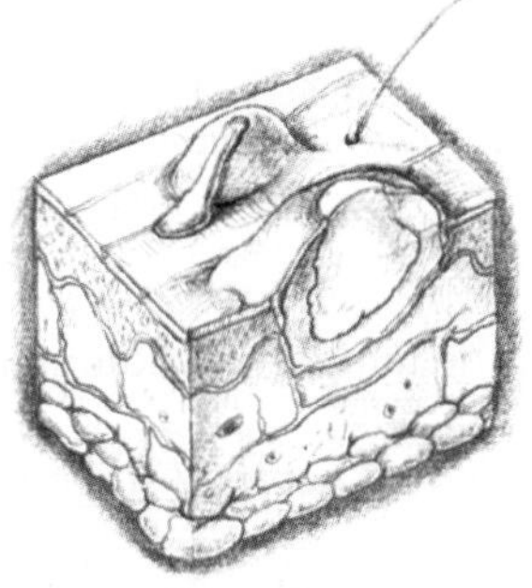

Pustules (such as in *acne* and *acute impetigo*) are vesicles filled with cloudy or purulent fluid.

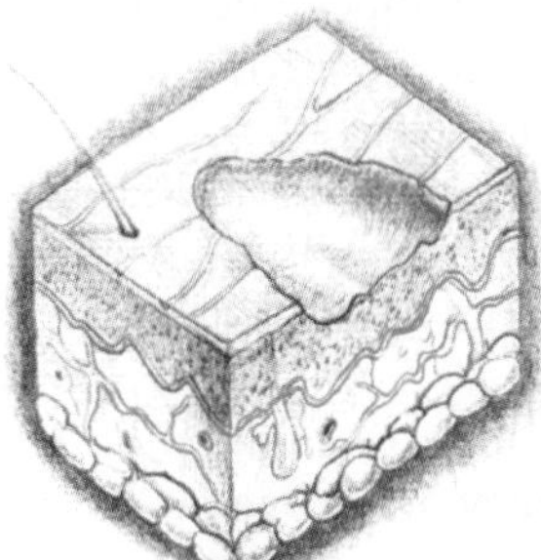

Wheals (such as *urticaria* and *insect bites*) are elevated, irregularly shaped, transient areas of dermal edema.

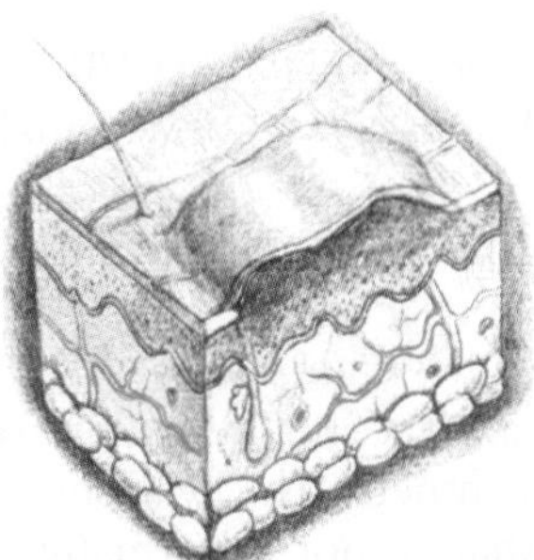

Erosions (such as in *varicella*) are wider than fissures but involve only the epidermis. They are often associated with vesicles, bullae, or pustules.

FIGURE 8-6 A, Primary skin lesions. (From Ignatavicius, D., & Workman, M. L. [2006]. *Medical-surgical nursing: Critical thinking for collaborative care* [5th ed.]. Philadelphia: Saunders.)

Continued

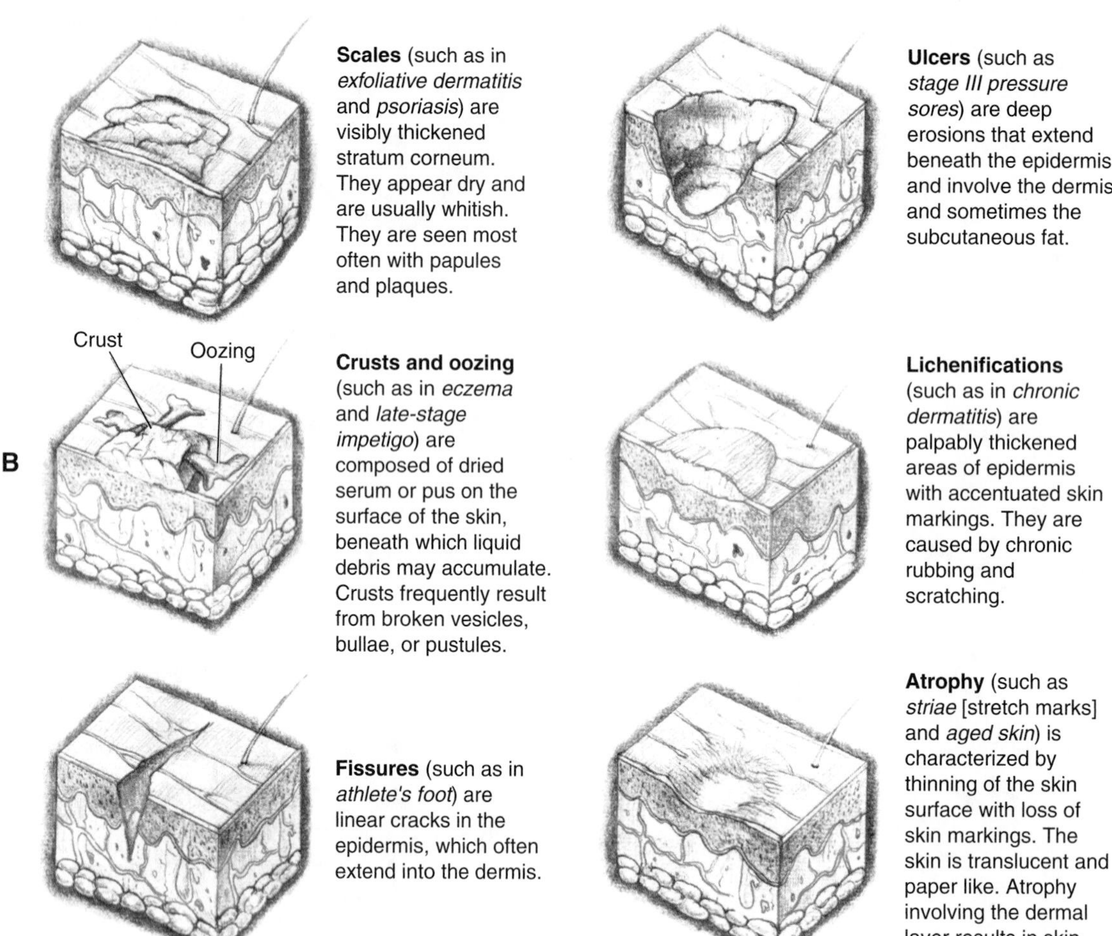

FIGURE 8-6, cont'd B, Secondary skin lesions. (From Ignatavicius, D., & Workman, M. L. [2006]. *Medical-surgical nursing: Critical thinking for collaborative care* [5th ed.]. Philadelphia: Saunders.)

- Checking the temporal artery
- Checking the function of the temporomandibular joint
- Checking the function of cranial nerves V (trigeminal) and VII (facial)
- Examining the eyes (includes cranial nerves II, III, IV, and VI)
- Examining the ears (includes cranial nerve VIII)
- Examining the nose and sinuses (includes cranial nerve I)
- Examining the lips, mouth, and throat (includes cranial nerves X and XII)
- Examining the neck (includes cranial nerve XI)

Assessment of the head and face begins with observation of size, position, and symmetry. The head should be normal in size (normocephalic), not abnormally small (microcephalic) or large for the person's age. In older adults the nose and brows are often prominent and the lower face may appear small, with the mouth shrunken if the person is edentulous (without teeth).

The head should be in a normal upright position, not tilted backward, forward, or to the left or right side. It should also be symmetrical in shape—that is, the same on the right and left sides. The eyebrows, palpebral fissures, and nasolabial folds should be equal (on the right and left) in size, shape, and position. The sides of the mouth should be similar in appearance and free of any abnormal one-sided droop or sag. Facial movements and expressions should be free, variable, and symmetrical. Distorted, absent, or asymmetrical movement or expression is abnormal. Involuntary movement is also abnormal, although in older adults mild rhythmic tremors are common.

Temporal Artery. Although the temporal artery is not routinely assessed, you may do so by palpating the temporal artery, located superior to the temporalis muscle. The pulsation can be felt in front of the ear. Normally it is nontender, smooth, and pliable. Tenderness or hardness is abnormal. The temporal arteries are often prominent and tortuous in older adults.

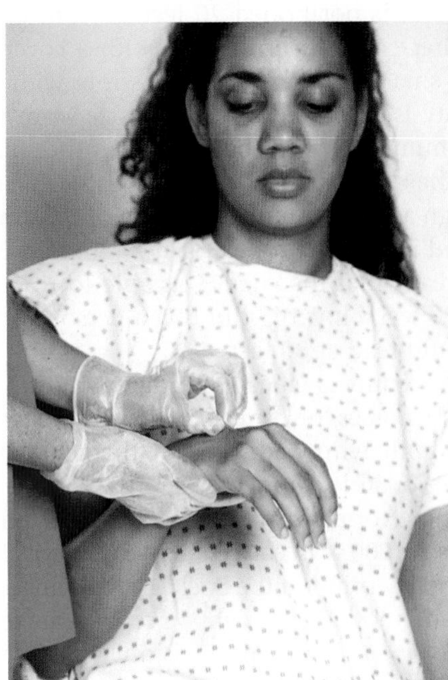

FIGURE 8-7 Checking skin turgor and mobility in a young person.

Temporomandibular Joint. Examine the temporomandibular joint (TMJ) to determine its range of motion (ROM) and to check for any swelling or tenderness. To do this, place the tips of the index fingers on the sides of the client's face just in front of the tragi of the ears. Ask the client to open the mouth while the fingertips slide into the joint space when the mouth opens.

Normally the mouth will open 3 to 6 cm and the lower jaw can move laterally 1 to 2 cm. Snapping or popping sounds when the mouth is opened are common and not pathological. Restricted motion, deviation of the lower jaw to one side when the mouth is opened, pain, or crepitus (crackling or rubbing sound) are abnormal findings.

Cranial Nerve VII. Cranial nerve VII (the facial nerve) is routinely tested. It is a mixed nerve, which means it has both motor and sensory components, but only the motor component, which innervates the facial muscles and is responsible for closing the eyes and for movement of the lips, is routinely tested. To test motor function of cranial nerve VII, ask the client to smile, frown, raise the eyebrows, show the upper and lower teeth, and keep the eyes tightly closed while you attempt to open them (Figure 8-9). As the client performs these actions, observe for symmetrical strength and movement. Ask the client to puff out the cheeks. Then use the finger pads to press the puffed cheeks in. Air should escape equally from both cheeks with this maneuver.

Cranial Nerve V. Cranial nerve V (the trigeminal nerve) is also a mixed nerve. Its motor component innervates the muscles of mastication, and its sensory component is responsible for sensation in the face, scalp, cornea, and the mucous membranes of the

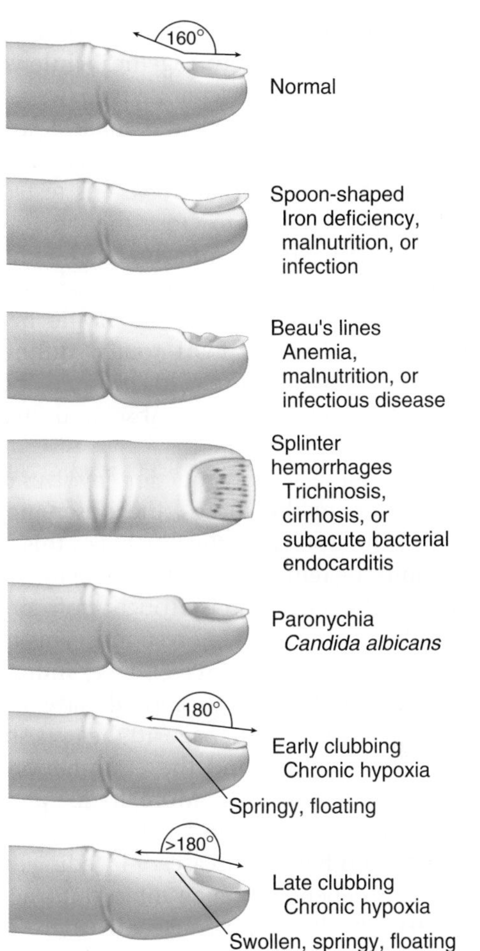

FIGURE 8-8 Comparing normal nails with examples of abnormalities. Some possible causes are listed.

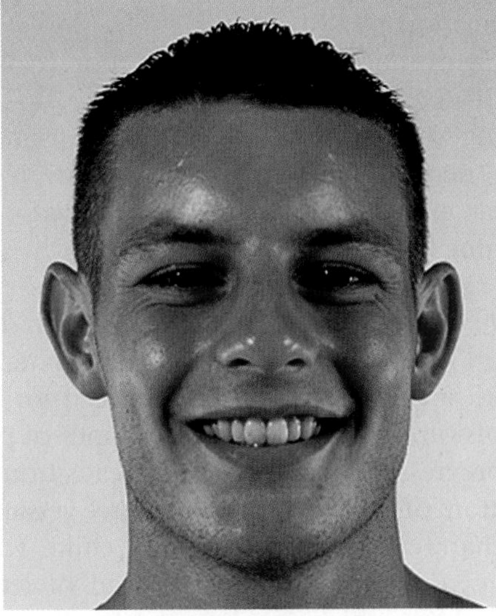

FIGURE 8-9 Assessing cranial nerve VII function. (From Jarvis, C. [2004]. *Health assessment and physical examination* [4th ed.]. Philadelphia: Saunders.)

mouth and nose. Its motor function is tested by asking the client to clench the teeth together while you push down on the chin to try to separate the jaws. Normally the jaw cannot be separated and muscle strength is equal on both sides.

Sensory function of cranial nerve V is tested in two ways. First, ask the client to close the eyes, and then you touch the chin, cheeks, and forehead with a sterile pin or cotton ball. Ask the client to describe what is felt and where it is felt. The client should be able to distinguish sensations of light touch, dullness, and sharpness and identify their location as being on the forehead, cheeks, or chin. Absent, decreased, or unequal sensation is abnormal.

The second test of sensory function involves touching a wisp of cotton to the cornea and observing for the normal blink in response to the touch. For this test, contact lenses must be removed, and the client looks straight ahead while the cotton wisp is brought in from the side to prevent the natural blinking response. This test is often omitted during a normal screening examination.

Eyes. People under age 40 should have their eyes tested every 3 to 5 years. After age 40 the eyes should be examined every 2 years, and the examination should include glaucoma screening. More frequent examinations are needed if the person has hypertension, diabetes, glaucoma or other eye disease, or bleeding disorders. Visual acuity is dependent on an intact optic nerve (cranial nerve II), a healthy retina, a clear lens, movement of the eye, and focusing light. Physical assessment of the eye involves the following activities:

- Testing visual acuity for distance vision, near vision, and peripheral vision
- Inspecting the outer eye structures, including lids, lashes, sclera, conjunctiva, cornea, iris, and pupil
- Testing pupillary response to light and accommodation (pupils equal, round, reactive to light and accommodation [PERRLA])
- Checking extraocular muscular function (cranial nerve III—oculomotor)
- Checking visual fields and conjugate movements (cranial nerve III—oculomotor, cranial nerve IV—trochlear, and cranial nerve VI—abducens)
- Examining the ocular fundus

Distance Vision. Visual acuity is the clearness of the visual image or the degree of detail the eye can discern in an image, which allows the eye to discriminate between forms. The Snellen chart is used to screen for acuity of distance vision. This chart consists of lines of print that become progressively smaller as one reads from the top to the bottom of the chart. There are three versions of the Snellen chart: one for the preschool child, which has commonly recognized symbols instead of letters; the Snellen E chart, which can be used for the preschool child or others who cannot read; and the standard Snellen chart, which consists of random letters.

The client is positioned 20 feet in front of the chart and is directed to cover one eye with a cover card and read the smallest line of print possible with the other eye. Acuity is recorded as 20 (distance from the chart) over the number printed by the side of the smallest line of print the client can read with at least 50% accuracy. A minus sign and the number of letters of this line that the client read incorrectly follows. An example is 20/80 −1, which means that the client was able to read with one error at 20 feet a line of print that a person with normal vision could read at 80 feet.

This procedure is repeated for the other eye. If corrective lenses, glasses, or contacts are worn, distance vision is tested both with and without them and CC (with correction) or SC (without correction) is recorded after the acuity ratio. Normal acuity is 20/20. Legal blindness is defined as 20/200 with correction in either eye. If the client cannot see any print on the Snellen chart, finger counting ability, hand motion, and light perception are tested.

Near Vision. Acuity of near vision is tested in adults over age 40 and in those who present with a complaint of difficulty reading. This is done by asking the client to read lines of print of different sizes on a Jaeger chart, which the client holds 14 inches in front of the face. A Jaeger card is similar to a Snellen chart, but the print size is scaled to be equivalent to the print size at 20 feet when read at 14 inches. Results, which indicate the smallest line the client can read, are recorded as J1 (smallest letters) through J12 (largest letters). A person with normal near vision acuity can read J1 with each eye without hesitation and without moving the card. Near vision acuity can also be checked by having the client hold and read any printed materials at a comfortable distance from the face. If this type of test is used, the type of material and the distance it is held from the face is recorded.

Outer Eye Structures. To examine the structures of the eye, begin with the outer structures and work your way inward. Begin inspection of the outer eye structures by noting the position of the eyelids in relationship to the globe. Normally no sclera (white) is visible between the upper lid and the iris. The lids are also observed for the presence of abnormalities such as ptosis (drooping of the upper lid), incomplete closure, redness, swelling, and presence of discharge or other lesions. The eyelashes are observed for even distribution and outward curve. Uneven distribution, inward growth touching the globe, crusting, or lesions are abnormal findings.

The globe, conjunctiva, sclera, iris, and pupil are also inspected. The right and left globes should be aligned and neither sunken nor protruding. To inspect the sclera and conjunctiva, separate the lids using the index finger and the thumb and ask the client to look up, down, and to each side. The palpebral (eyelid) conjunctiva is inspected by everting the lower lid with the thumb while asking the client to look up. The sclera should be smooth, moist, and glossy, and the conjunctiva should be clear, pale pink, and glistening, often with small blood vessels visible. The irises should be similar in shape, color, clarity, and markings. The pupils should be 3 to 5 mm in diameter, round, and equal in size in both eyes. Excessively dilated or constricted pupils as well as irregular or unequal pupils are abnormal. Shining a light from the side onto each eye and observing for cloudiness or opacities checks the clarity of the cornea.

Pupillary Response to Light and Accommodation. PERRLA stands for pupils equal, round, reactive to light and accommodation. With the client looking straight ahead into the distance, bring a bright light in from the side (one side at a time) to the front of the pupil to test pupillary response to light. The illuminated pupil (direct response) and the nonilluminated pupil (indirect response) should constrict. Bringing the light in from the side elicits a direct response and consensual response; however, it may eliminate an accommodation response. Speed and degree of constriction should be equal in both pupils and should be followed by equal dilation. Absence of constriction or an asymmetrical response is abnormal. Degree of constriction is recorded as millimeters before and after exposure to the light, and speed is described as brisk or sluggish.

Accommodation is adjustment of the eye for seeing objects at various distances. To test accommodation, hold a finger or an object such as a pen 10 to 15 cm (4 to 5 inches) in front of the client's nose. Tell the client to look ahead into the distance and then to quickly look at the finger or other object. If accommodation is normal, the pupils constrict. The irises of both eyes also converge or move toward midline as the finger moves toward the nose. Normal pupillary findings are recorded with the acronym PERRLA.

Extraocular Muscle Function. The function of the extraocular muscles (cranial nerves III, IV, and VI) is tested for parallel gaze (corneal light reflex) and coordinated eye movement (direction of gaze). To test the corneal light reflex, shine a light straight into the client's eyes from a distance of 31 cm (12 inches) while the client looks straight ahead. Normally the light is reflected on or just medial to the pupil in both eyes. Reflection of the light in a different location in each eye is abnormal and requires further evaluation.

Coordinated eye movement through the six cardinal directions of gaze is checked by holding a finger 31 cm (12 inches) in front of the client and moving it from the center to one of the six locations, holding a moment, and then returning it to center (Figure 8-10, *A*). This action is repeated for each of the six locations while the eyes are observed for normal parallel movement. As the gaze moves up and down, the upper lid is observed and should be seen to overlap the iris at all times. Both eyes should remain parallel as the finger is tracked through the six locations. Weakness of extraocular muscles or cranial nerve dysfunction results in nonparallel tracking. In addition, you should look for nystagmus, which is involuntary, rapid, rhythmic movement of the eyeball when the eye is gazing laterally within the field of binocular gaze. A few beats of nystagmus is normal with extreme lateral gaze or in the first few hours after birth.

Visual Fields. The visual field (the range of peripheral vision) is the entire area seen by the eye when looking at a central point (Figure 8-10, *B*). Position yourself 2 to 3 feet in front of the client so that your faces are at the same level. Cover your left eye, and have the client cover the right eye. Hold your right hand at arm's length, equidistant between you and the client. Wiggle your fingers and bring your hand into the field of vision. Have the client say "stop" when he or she sees your fingers, and compare with your own peripheral vision. Repeat from four directions. Normal results are about 90 degrees from the temporal side, 50 degrees from above, 70 degrees from below, and 60 degrees from the nasal side.

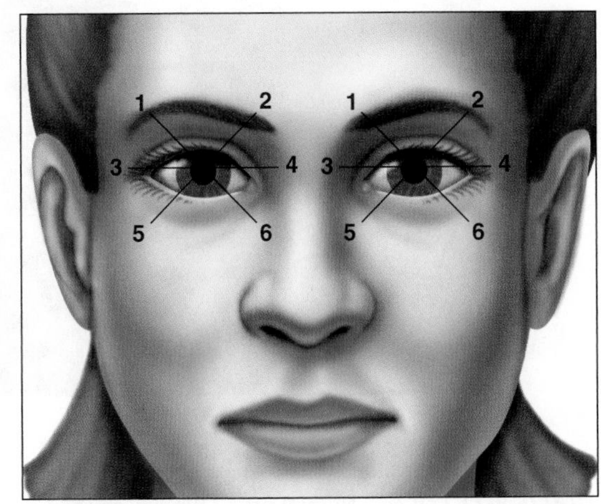

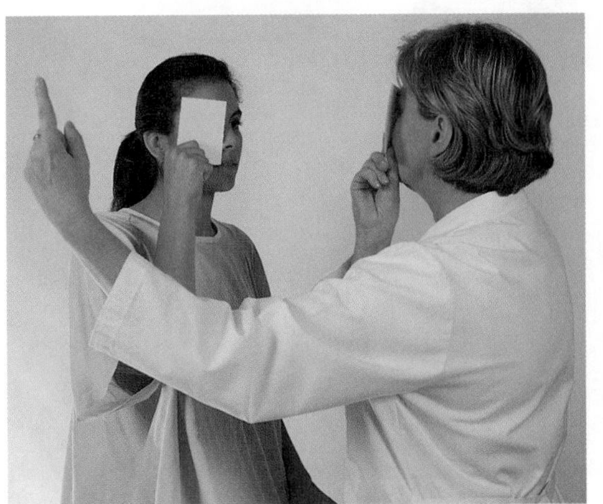

FIGURE 8-10 A, The six cardinal directions of gaze used in checking for coordinated eye movement. **B,** The visual fields or confrontational test assesses for peripheral vision by comparing the client's peripheral vision to your own.

Normal findings are recorded as "Visual fields full." This gross check of visual fields is repeated for the other eye. Loss of visual fields could result from a cerebrovascular event, glaucoma, or retinal detachment.

Ocular Fundus. You can examine the inner eye using an **ophthalmoscope** to direct a light through the window of the pupil to view the lens, anterior chamber, vitreous, and ocular fundus, or retina (including the optic disc, macula, and retinal blood vessels). Change the aperture of the ophthalmoscope until you have found the small round, white light to examine undilated pupils.

The client must be able to cooperate and hold the eyes still by looking at a distant object to dilate the pupils. The examiner holds the ophthalmoscope in the right hand while using the right eye to examine the client's right eye (Figure 8-11). The ophthalmoscope is used as an appendage to the examiner's own eye. To prevent losing sight of the fundus during the examination, stabilize the ophthalmoscope on the eyebrow or nose and move the head and the instrument as one unit. The index finger rests on the lens wheel to focus easily during the examination, and the thumb rests on the lower jaw to stabilize the hand. The light should be adjusted to maximum if tolerated by the client.

The ophthalmoscope contains a set of lenses to control the units of measurement (dioptrics), thus focusing for vision from near to far. The black numbers are positive dioptrics for focusing on nearer objects, and the red numbers are negative dioptrics for focusing on objects farther away.

The examination is done in a darkened room and begins with the examiner positioned about 8 to 12 inches away and 15 degrees to the side of the client's line of vision. As the light beam from the ophthalmoscope is directed toward the pupil of the eye being examined, an orange-red glow called the red reflex appears in the pupil. This glow should be uninterrupted and fill the pupil. Dark shadows or black dots interrupting the glow are abnormal. When you have found the red glow (the reflection of the light off the inner retina), move closer to the client until your heads are almost touching. If you lose the red glow, move back, relocate the glow, and move forward again.

As you advance, adjust the lens to +6 and note any opacity in the lens. Opacities appear as black areas or dark shadows interrupting the red reflex. Continuing to move forward, adjust the lens setting (diopter) to bring the fundus into focus. When both you and the client have normal vision, this should be at 0. Adjust to red dioptrics for nearsighted eyes and to black for farsighted eyes.

Begin the examination of the optic fundus by finding the optic disc (Figure 8-12). The optic disc is an area on the nasal side of each retina. The blood vessels of the retina converge at the optic disc. If the optic disc is not visualized, track a blood vessel as it grows larger toward the disc. Outside the optic disc, the retina is light red to dark brown-red, with the shade varying in accord with skin color.

Assess the structures in the ocular fundus: optic disc, retinal vessels, general background, and macula. The optic disc is normally yellow orange to creamy pink in color, with distinct margins except at the nasal edge. Pallor, hyperemia, irregular shape, or blurred margins are abnormal findings. Visualized retinal vessels should consist of one artery and one vein passing to each quadrant of the retina, with a progressive decrease in the diameter of both veins

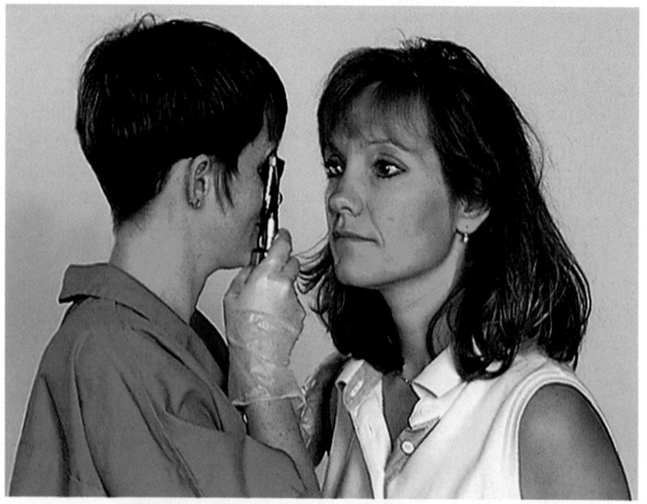

FIGURE 8-11 Ophthalmoscopic examination.

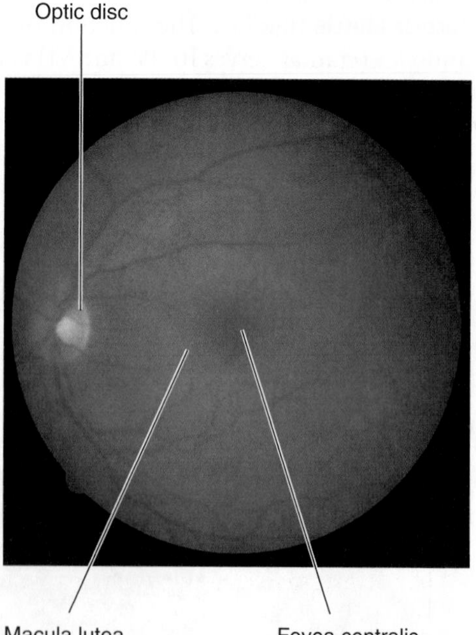

FIGURE 8-12 Left eye. Normal ocular fundus, as seen on ophthalmoscopic examination. Note the location of the optic disc. (Courtesy Dr. Harry Kaplan and Dr. Lawrence P. Roach, Philadelphia.)

and arteries as they extend toward the periphery. Arteries are brighter red than veins. Abnormal findings include the absence of major arteries, constricted arteries, dilated veins, and extreme tortuousness. The general background should be free of lesions such as hemorrhage or exudate. The macula lutea is the yellow oval spot at the center of the retina responsible for sharp, detailed vision (also called visual acuity). It receives and analyzes light only from the center of the visual field. At the macula, which is about 1 DD (one disc diameter—i.e., the size of the diameter of the optic disc), the color may be darker than that of the rest of the retina, but all areas should be free of clumped pigment, which occurs with aging, trauma, or retinal detachment. Hemorrhage or exudate may represent macular degeneration. For further details on examination of the ocular fundus, a specialty text on physical assessment should be consulted.

Ear. Physical assessment of the ear involves the following activities:

- Inspecting and palpating the external ear
- Inspecting the external auditory meatus
- Using an otoscope to examine the external auditory canal and the tympanic membrane (eardrum)
- Testing the acuity of hearing (cranial nerve VIII)

External Ear. Inspection of the external ears involves noting their placement on the sides of the head, their alignment with each other, and their size, shape, symmetry, and skin color. The top of the pinna (the projecting part of the ear, also called the auricle or helix) is normally level with the outer corner of the eye, and the whole ear is normally angled less than 10 degrees toward the occiput (the back of the head). The skin of the external ear should be the same color as the face and should be intact, smooth, and free of drainage or lesions. In older adults, earlobes may be pendulous and coarse, and stiff hairs may be present on the external ear.

Next, the external ear is palpated to identify nodules or other irregularities. The pinna is moved up and down, the tragus (the cartilaginous projection anterior to the ear canal) is palpated, and the area behind the ear (mastoid bone) is palpated, with normal findings being no pain or tenderness on manipulation. The external auditory meatus is inspected for redness, swelling, discharge, or the presence of a foreign body. The size of the opening is noted and should be unobstructed.

External Auditory Canal. The external auditory canal is examined using an otoscope fitted with the largest speculum that can be inserted comfortably into the auditory canal. An **otoscope** is a handheld instrument used to examine the external ear, the tympanic membrane, and, through the tympanic membrane, the ossicles of the middle ear. It consists of a light, a magnifying lens, a speculum, and sometimes a device for insufflations.

With the client in a sitting position, move to the side and slightly to the back of the ear to be examined. Ask the client to tip the head toward the shoulder on the opposite side (Figure 8-13). Grasp the top of the pinna and pull it up and slightly away from the head with the nondominant hand to straighten the ear canal in the adult, and maintain throughout the examination. In the infant or child, the pinna is pulled downward because the canal is directed downward.

The otoscope is commonly held in an upside-down position in the dominant hand, which is kept firmly braced against the side of the client's head; thus if the head moves, so does the otoscope, preventing accidental trauma to the auditory canal. The speculum is slowly inserted at a slightly downward and forward angle approximately 1/2 inch into the auditory canal. Because of its sensitivity to pain, avoid touching the medial wall of the canal. The examiner carefully positions the otoscope and then positions the eye to the otoscope.

Once the speculum is inserted, the canal can be observed. If you cannot see anything but the wall of the ear canal, angle the otoscope slightly toward the client's nose. You may need to rotate the otoscope to see the entire tympanic membrane.

Normally the walls are pink and uniform, with small to moderate amounts of cerumen present. Cerumen, or earwax, is moist and honey colored to dark brown or black in most white or African American individuals and dry, gray, and flaky in most Asians and Native Americans. Large amounts of earwax, swelling, redness, discharge, foreign bodies, or other lesions are abnormal, as are marked pain on insertion of the speculum and foul odor. Sometimes you will have to remove earwax for good visualization. Ear irrigations are discussed in Chapter 38.

Tympanic Membrane. Following inspection of the external auditory canal, the tympanic membrane is also inspected with the otoscope, and the positions of the

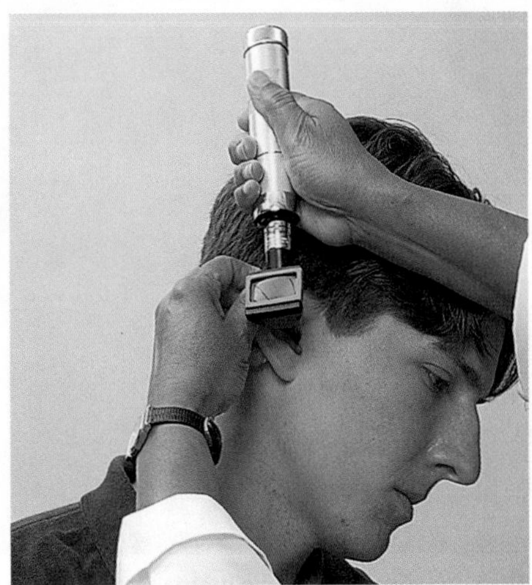

FIGURE 8-13 Otoscopic examination. (From Wilson, S. F., & Giddens, J. F. [2005]. *Health assessment for nursing practice* [3rd ed.]. St. Louis, MO: Mosby.)

handle of the malleus, the umbo, the short process, and the cone of light are noted. The tympanic membrane separates the external and middle ear and is tilted obliquely toward the ear canal. Normally the tympanic membrane is intact, pearly gray, shiny, translucent, and conical, although in older adults it may be whiter, duller, and thicker than in younger adults.

Assess for landmarks. The cone of light seen at the 4 to 5 o'clock position in the right ear and at the 7 to 8 o'clock position in the left ear is a reflection of the otoscope light. The malleus is the primary landmark. The short process of the malleus stands out as a knob. The manubrium, or the handle of the malleus, extends downward from the short process to the umbo (Figure 8-14). Having the client hold the nose and swallow assesses mobility of the tympanic membrane; the membrane should be seen to flutter. Abnormal findings include perforations, scarring, dullness, blue, red, or amber coloring, retraction with accentuated landmarks, bulging with partially occluded landmarks, and a fluid level in the middle ear.

Hearing Acuity. Hearing is mediated by the acoustic (formerly vestibulocochlear) nerve, which is cranial nerve VIII. Testing of hearing acuity involves checking gross acuity, checking ability to lateralize sound, and comparing air and bone conduction of sound.

Gross hearing is evaluated during the course of normal conversation. The voice test is a more specific measure of gross hearing acuity. For this test, press on the tragus of one of the client's ears with the index finger to occlude the auditory canal. Stand 1 to 2 feet in front of the client. With the client's eyes closed or your mouth covered to prevent lip reading, exhale and whisper words of two equally accented syllables toward the ear being tested. The same procedure is used for the other ear. Normally the client can repeat the whispered words accurately. Repeat with spoken words. Whispered words are higher tones, which are more commonly lost than the lower tones of spoken words.

Lateralization of sound is evaluated by means of the Weber test. For this test, set a 512- or 1024-Hz tuning fork to vibrate lightly by tapping the tines against your hand. The base of the tuning fork is then placed in the middle of the top of the client's head or in the middle of the forehead. Ask whether the client hears the tone only in the right ear, only in the left ear, equally in both, or more in one ear than in the other (specify). Normally the tone is heard equally in both ears. If a *conductive* hearing loss exists, the tone is lateralized to the affected ear because the normal ear is more likely to be distracted by room noises. In the case of *sensorineural* hearing loss, the sound is lateralized to the unaffected ear.

Air and bone conduction are compared by means of the Rinne test. In this test, a lightly vibrating tuning fork is placed on the client's mastoid process (bone conduction) and the client is asked to indicate when the tone is no longer heard (Figure 8-15). When the client so indicates, quickly move the tuning fork so that the tines are in front of the auditory meatus (air conduction). Then ask the client if a tone is heard; if the answer is Yes, have the client indicate when it ends. Air conduction is heard twice as long as bone conduction. Then repeat the procedure for the other ear.

Normally, air conduction lasts twice as long as bone conduction, so the client is able to hear the tone when the tines are placed in front of the auditory meatus for as long as the tone was heard when the tuning fork was on the mastoid process. In sensorineural hearing loss, air conduction lasts longer than bone conduction but not twice as long. It is equal to or shorter than bone conduction in conductive hearing loss.

Nose and Sinuses. Physical assessment of the nose and sinuses involves the following activities:
- Checking patency of the nares (nostrils)
- Inspecting the outside and the inside of the nose

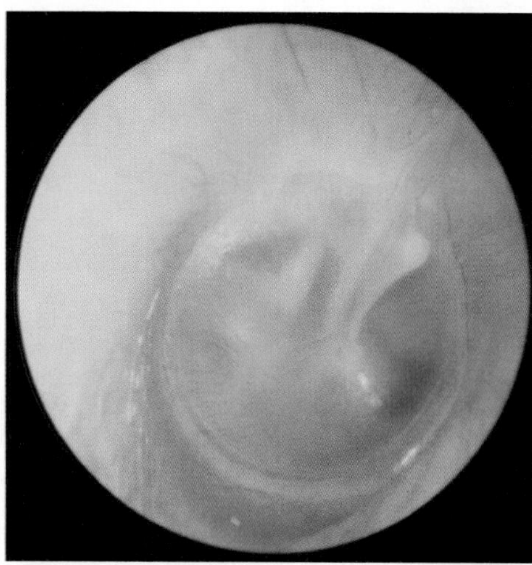

FIGURE 8-14 Normal right tympanic membrane as seen on otoscopic examination. (From Swartz, M. H. [1994]. *Textbook of physical diagnosis: History and examination* [2nd ed.]. Philadelphia: Saunders.)

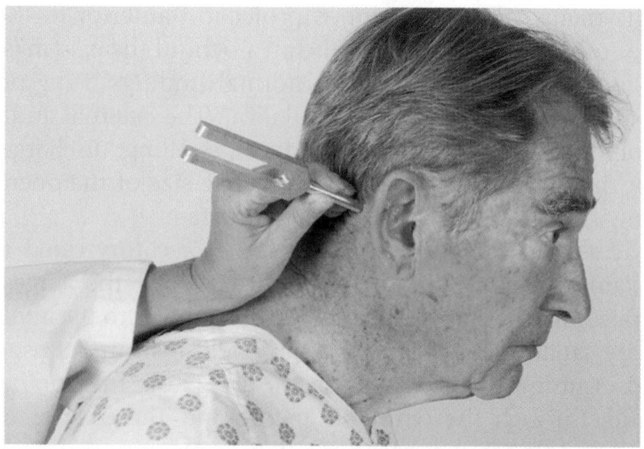

FIGURE 8-15 Place the stem of the vibrating tuning fork on the mastoid process, and ask the client to signal when the sound goes away.

- Palpating the sinuses for tenderness
- Testing the function of cranial nerve I

Nose. Observe the external aspect of the nose for abnormalities such as asymmetry, lesions, or signs of inflammation. Check the patency of the nares by asking the client to close his or her mouth; then occlude each naris in turn while you feel for exhaled air from the nonoccluded naris. Next, inspect the inside of the nose using an otoscope fitted with a short, wide nasal speculum and magnifying lens. With the client's head tilted back and the handle of the otoscope held to the side, insert the speculum 1 cm into each naris without touching the nasal septum. Direct it back and somewhat upward to allow both the upper and lower nose to be seen.

Normally the mucosal lining of the nose is intact, smooth, and deep pink; the nasal septum is straight, and the turbinates are smooth and of the same color as the rest of the mucosa. The nasal mucosa is redder than the oral mucosa. The septum is somewhat deviated in most adults. The lateral wall of the nose consists of inferior, middle, and superior turbinates. The inferior turbinate is the largest and lies like a finger along the lower lateral wall of the nose.

Pale, bright red, or gray mucosa is abnormal. Bogginess, exudate, swelling, bleeding, ulcers or fissures, polyps, or a perforation or deviation of the septum are other abnormal findings.

Sinuses. The paranasal sinuses are pockets within the cranium that lighten the weight of the skull. They are lined with a ciliated mucous membrane and communicate with the nasal cavity. The frontal and maxillary sinuses are within the frontal and maxillary bones (Figure 8-16). The sphenoid sinuses are deep within the skull in the sphenoid bone, and the ethmoid sinuses are between the orbits of the eyes.

Examination of the sinuses is performed by indirect methods of inspection and palpation of the overlying soft tissues (frontal and maxillary sinuses) and by noting secretions that may drain from the nose. Use the pads of your thumbs to palpate the frontal and maxillary sinuses. Palpate the frontal sinuses by pressing up from under the medial aspect of the brow ridges. Palpate the maxillary sinuses by pressing up and in under the zygomatic arch. Normally the sinuses are nontender on palpation.

Cranial Nerve I. To test cranial nerve I, the olfactory nerve, the client closes his or her eyes while you occlude one naris and hold a substance with a familiar odor under the other. Ask the client if he or she smells anything and, if so, to identify it. The procedure is then repeated for the other naris. Normally, familiar odors such as coffee or vanilla can be distinguished. The sense of smell is often decreased in older adults.

Lips, Mouth, and Throat. Physical assessment of the mouth and throat involves the following activities:

- Inspecting the lips, gums, teeth, buccal mucosa, roof and floor of the mouth, top, bottom, and sides of the tongue, throat, tonsils, and uvula
- Checking motor function of the palate, pharynx, and larynx (cranial nerve X)
- Testing the client's ability to move the tongue (cranial nerve XII)

Lips. Observe the color and moistness of the client's lips. Also inspect them for cracking, ulcers, and lumps. Normally the lips are smooth, pink, moist, intact, and free of lesions. A blue tinge to the pink coloration due to the presence of melanin pigment is a normal finding in some dark-skinned people. Abnormal findings include

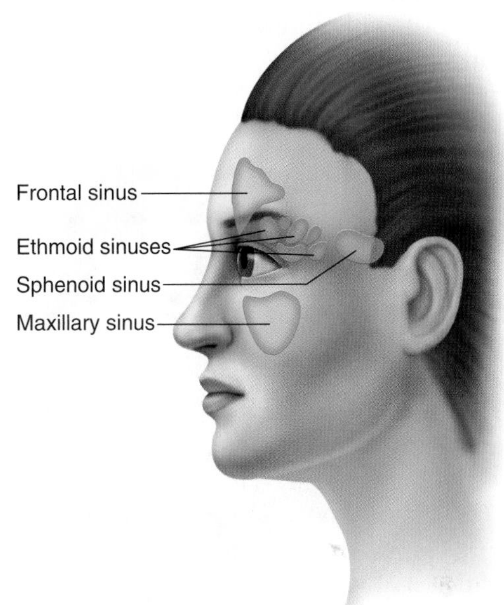

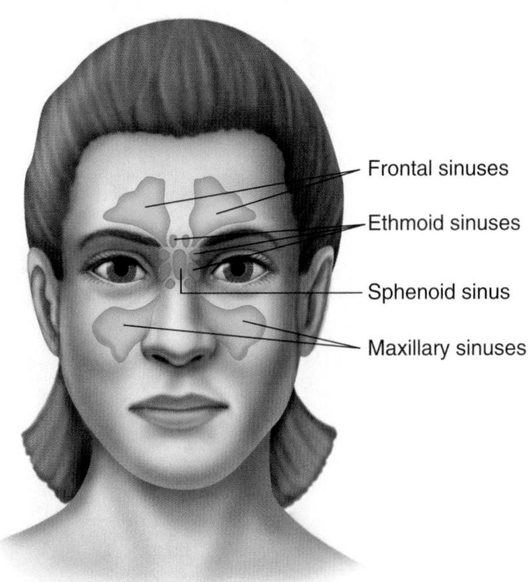

FIGURE 8-16 The paranasal sinuses.

dryness, cracks, fissures, pallor, cyanosis, drooping, and involuntary movements. Inspect the oral mucosa of the lower lip for color and lesions by everting the lip (Figure 8-17, *A*).

Mouth and Throat. Ask the client to remove any dentures and open his or her mouth. Inspect the buccal mucosa, gums, teeth, roof of the mouth, top, bottom, and sides of the tongue, and floor of the mouth. To allow good visibility of the buccal cavity, good light and a tongue blade are essential (Figure 8-17, *B*). Use the tongue blade to expose the buccal mucosa, which can then be inspected for color, intactness, and presence of lesions.

Like the lips, the buccal mucosa is normally intact, smooth, moist, and pink, with areas of dark pigmentation in dark-skinned clients. The tongue should be shiny, pink, and moist, with an even distribution of papillae arranged in an inverted V.

Inspect the teeth for dental caries (cavities) and periodontal disease (pyorrhea). The enamel should be smooth, white, and shiny. Brown or black discoloration of the enamel may indicate staining or the presence of caries. Gingivitis (red, swollen gums, bleeding, receding gum lines, and the formation of pockets between the teeth and gums) is characteristic of periodontal disease. In advanced disease, the teeth may be loose and pus may be present.

You should also assess for other inflammatory conditions of the mouth. Glossitis is inflammation of the tongue. Stomatitis is inflammation of the oral mucosa. Fungal infection or oral candidiasis is a common cause of stomatitis. Parotitis is inflammation of the parotid gland (the largest of the salivary glands) and results in obvious swelling of the lower cheek. The most well-known infection of the parotid gland is mumps.

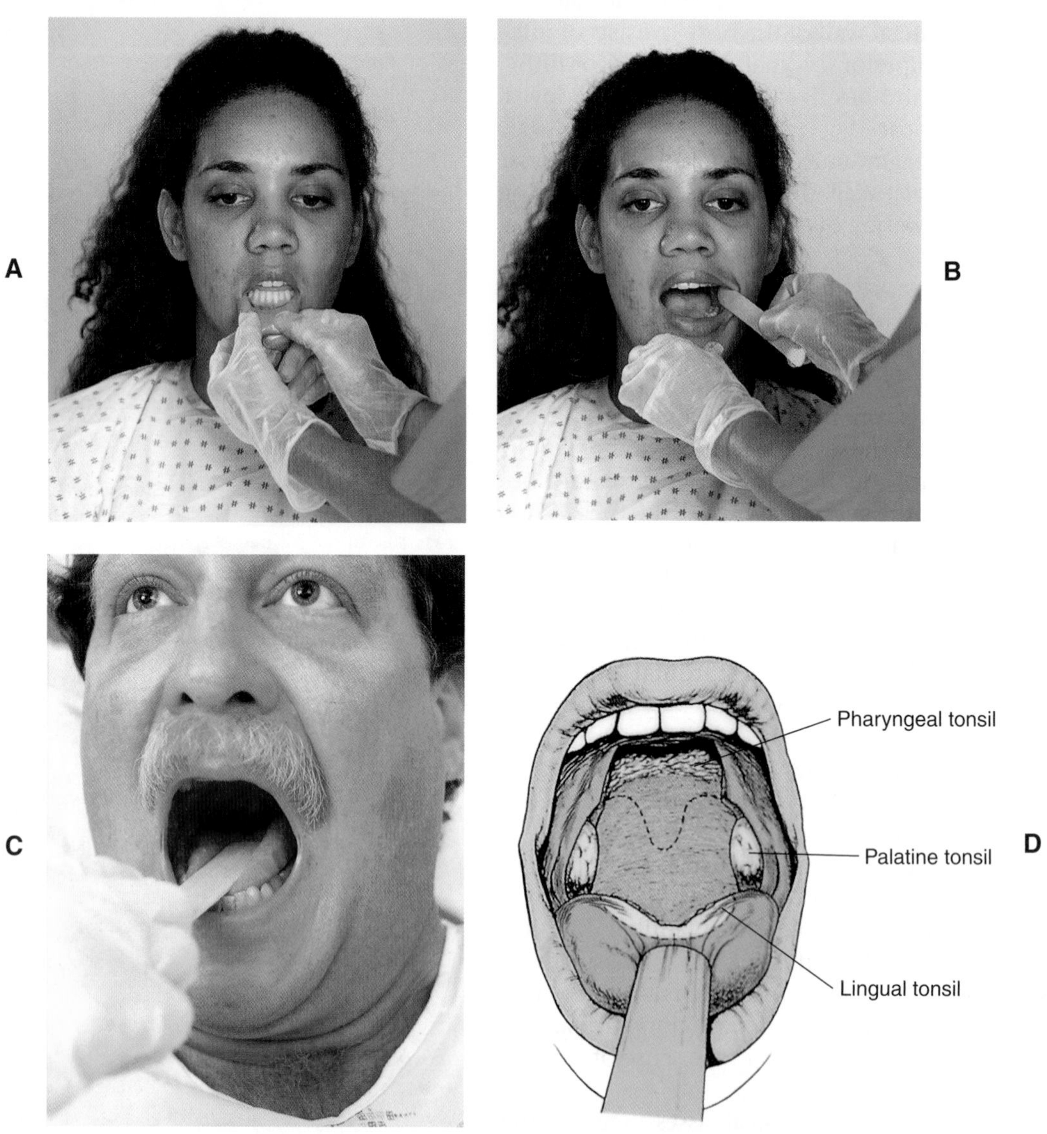

FIGURE 8-17 Examination of the oral cavity. Inspecting the mucosa of the lower lip **(A)** and the buccal cavity **(B).** Assessing the oropharynx **(C)** and the tonsils **(D).**

To assess the oropharynx, have the client tilt his or her head back and open his or her mouth. Use the tongue blade to depress the tongue about halfway back, and shine a penlight on the throat (Figure 8-17, C). Depress one side at a time to avoid eliciting the gag reflex. In the oropharynx, or throat, the uvula should be at the midline. The lingual tonsils lie on either side of the dorsal surface of the tongue. These tonsils normally do not protrude beyond the tonsillar pillar and are of the same color as the rest of the oropharynx. The tonsils may have crypts with exfoliated epithelium that gives a white appearance. Examine the throat for redness, swelling, and the presence of lesions, plaque, or exudate. The tonsils are graded from 1 to 4 (often charted as +1 +2 +3 +4). Grade 1 is normal. In grade 2, the tonsils are between the pillars and the uvula. In grade 3, the tonsils touch the uvula. In grade 4, one or both tonsils extend to the midline of the oropharynx.

Neck. The neck contains a number of important structures (Figure 8-18). The major blood vessels supplying the head are the carotid arteries and jugular veins. The neck is also highly lymphatic, receiving lymph drainage from the head. The esophagus and the trachea course through the neck supported by the cervical spine. Strong muscles support the head and assist with multidirectional ROM. Physical assessment of the neck involves the following activities:

- Observing the shape, symmetry, position, and motion of the neck
- Inspecting the carotid arteries and jugular veins
- Inspecting and palpating the trachea
- Inspecting and palpating the thyroid gland
- Palpating cervical lymph nodes

Appearance and Motion. With the client in an upright position, begin assessment of the neck by observing for symmetry and proportion to the head and shoulders. To assess for normal movement, direct the client to put his or her head back to check extension, put the chin on the chest to check flexion, touch the chin to each shoulder to check rotation, and bend the right ear to the right shoulder and the left ear to the left shoulder without raising the shoulder to test lateral abduction.

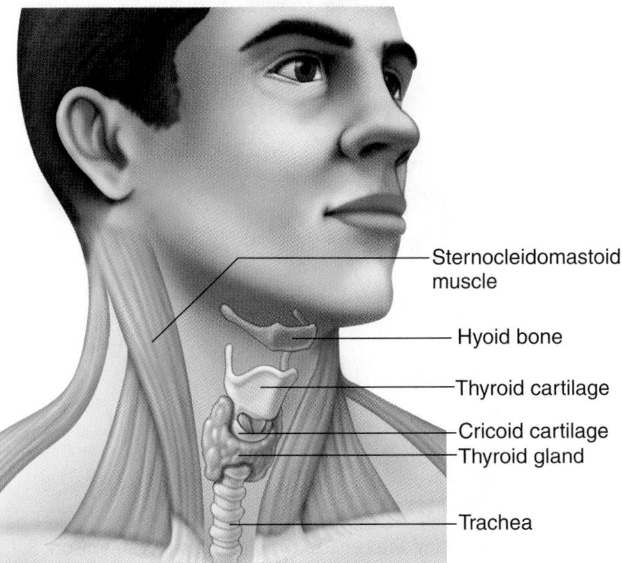

FIGURE 8-18 Major structures of the neck.

Normally the neck flexes 45 degrees, extends 55 degrees, laterally flexes 40 degrees, and rotates 70 degrees (and is free of uncoordinated, uncontrolled movements). This check of ROM must be performed slowly in geriatric clients, because they may become dizzy with the lateral movements.

Assess for muscle strength by having the client turn his or her head to one side against the resistance of your hand. Ask the client to shrug his or her shoulders against the resistance of your hands. The strength should be equal on both sides.

Abnormal findings include unusual shortness of the neck, lack of symmetry, fullness, edema, masses, and scars. In older adults, the neck may appear shortened. This is a normal finding that occurs as a result of muscle atrophy, compression of vertebrae, and loss of fat.

Jugular Veins and Carotid Arteries. Observe the side of the neck over the jugular vein and the carotid artery. Normally the jugular vein is not distended and only a mild pulsation of the carotid artery can be seen. A distended jugular vein or marked pulsations of the carotid are abnormal.

Trachea. Observe the middle front of the neck and then palpate for any sign of tracheal deviation from the midline. To palpate for tracheal deviation, place the index finger along one side of the trachea and note the distance between the side of the trachea and the sternocleidomastoid muscle. Repeat this action on the other side, and compare the two distances. Normally the distances should be equal, and the trachea should be nontender with distinct rings palpable. Soreness or swelling indicated by nonpalpable rings is abnormal.

Thyroid. The thyroid gland has two lobes, one on each side and slightly in front of the trachea, and each lobe is about the size of a thumb pad. The thin isthmus that connects the lobes lies over the trachea just below the cricoid cartilage.

To assess the thyroid gland, ask the client to lift his or her chin so you can observe the neck for a visible thyroid. You may also ask the client to take a sip of water, lift his or her chin, and then swallow while you watch the movement of the thyroid in the neck. Normally the thyroid is not visible with this inspection.

Next, palpate the size, shape, and consistency of the thyroid. This is done by standing behind the client and asking him or her to tilt the head back slightly. Place the fingers of both hands on the sides of the client's neck with the index fingers just below the cricoid cartilage (Figure 8-19). Then ask the client to swallow while you feel for the thyroid isthmus to rise. Then move the fingers downward and laterally to identify any palpable parts of the lateral lobes. Generally the thyroid is not palpable; if it is, the normal thyroid feels smooth and rubbery. If palpable, the lobes should be symmetrical and painless.

Cervical Lymph Nodes. Lymph nodes in the neck collect lymph from the head and neck (Figure 8-20). There are 10 major groups of superficial cervical lymph nodes:

- Preauricular (in front of the ear)
- Posterior auricular (behind the ear, over the mastoid process)
- Parotid
- Submaxillary
- Submental (midline, beneath the tip of the mandible)
- Anterior or deep cervical chain
- Supraclavicular (between the sternocleidomastoid muscle and the trapezius muscle at the base of the neck)
- Occipital (at the base of the skull)
- Tonsillar
- Posterior cervical (posterior to the sternocleidomastoid muscle and along the edge of the trapezius muscle in the posterior triangle of the neck)

Cervical lymph nodes are assessed by palpating both sides of the neck simultaneously using the pads of the index and middle fingers. Bend the client's head slightly forward or to the side to relax the soft tissues and muscles around the area being examined.

To examine the submental and submandibular nodes, place the fingertips under the mandible and move the skin over the nodes. To assess the supraclavicular nodes, have the client flex his or her neck forward. Exert light to moderate pressure, and move the skin over the underlying tissues beginning in front of the ear and progressing systematically over the areas of the neck where the groups of cervical lymph nodes are located. There is no one right order for palpation of cervical nodes (Figure 8-21). It is simply important that you select an order and use it consistently so that no area is accidentally missed.

Normally, cervical lymph nodes either are not palpable or are smooth, firm, less than 1 cm in diameter (with definite margins), mobile, and nontender. In older adults, submandibular salivary glands commonly prolapse and may be felt as soft masses in the upper neck, below the jaw.

Enlargement of the lymph nodes is called lymphadenopathy. Describe the location, size, consistency, pres-

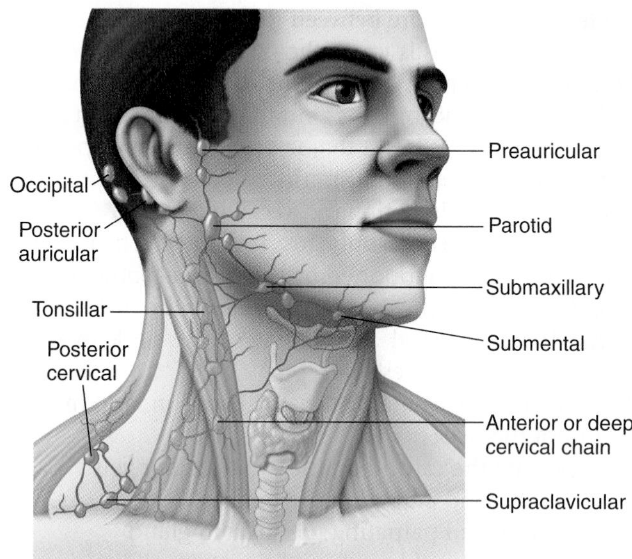

FIGURE 8-20 The cervical lymph nodes.

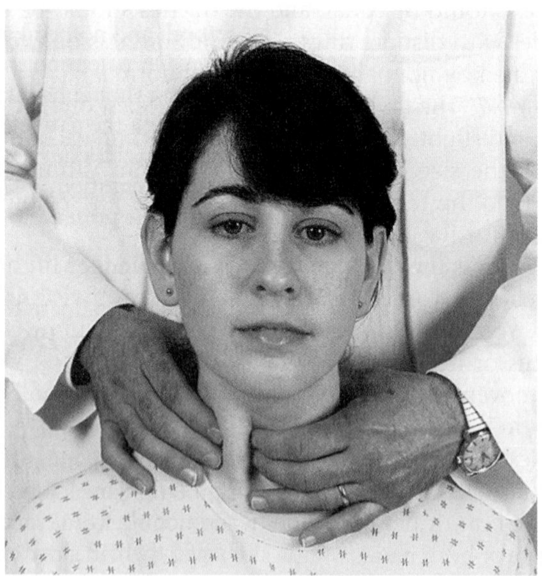

FIGURE 8-19 Palpating the thyroid gland. (From Seidel, H. M., Ball, J. W., Dains, J. E., & Benedict, G. W. [2006]. *Mosby's guide to physical examination* [6th ed.]. St. Louis, MO: Mosby.)

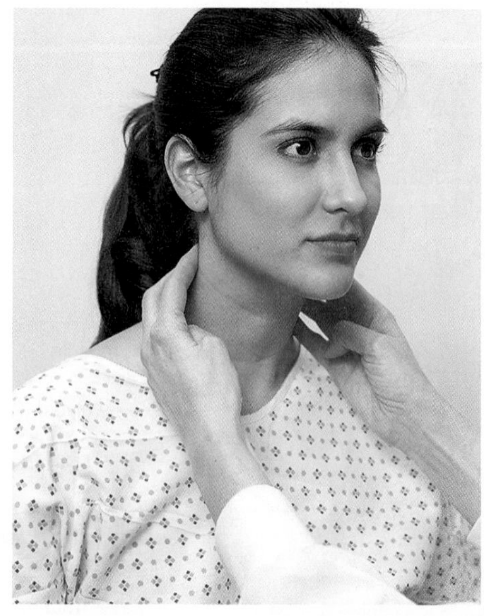

FIGURE 8-21 Palpating the cervical lymph nodes. (From Wilson, S. F., & Giddens, J. F. [2005]. *Health assessment for nursing practice* [3rd ed.]. St. Louis, MO: Mosby.)

ence of tenderness, inflammation, and whether they are freely moveable. Enlargement can result from infections or neoplasms of the oral pharynx or nasopharynx, from systemic diseases, or from infections such as mononucleosis or measles. Infection of the mouth or oropharynx is the most common cause.

ASSESSMENT OF THE BREASTS AND AXILLAE

Breasts. The breasts of both men and women are composed of glandular, fibrous, and adipose tissue. Adult women have more adipose tissue and fully developed (mature) glandular tissue, whereas it is rudimentary in men. However, the breasts in both sexes should be inspected and palpated for malignancy. Breast cancer is rare in men, but one of nine women will acquire breast cancer at some point in life. Therefore, women should be taught breast self-examination (see Chapter 46).

The glandular tissue in the female breast is concentrated in the upper outer quadrant, where a tail of breast tissue projects into the axilla and is known as the tail of Spence. The breast is drained by four groups of axillary lymph nodes: central axillary nodes high in the midaxilla; pectoral nodes, along the outer edge of the pectoral muscle at the anterior axillary line; subscapular nodes, along the posterior axillary line at the lateral edge of the scapula; and lateral nodes, inside the upper arm along the upper humerus.

Physical assessment of the breasts involves the following activities:

- Observing the size, contour, symmetry, skin color and appearance, and vascularity of the breasts
- Observing the areolae for shape, color, and hair
- Observing the size, shape, symmetry, and direction of point of the nipples
- Palpating each breast for consistency, tenderness, and presence of masses or palpable lymph nodes
- Checking for nipple discharge

Size, Shape, and Skin Appearance. To inspect the breasts, begin with the client sitting with her arms at her sides and then ask her to raise her arms over her head, lower them, and press her hands against her hips. If she has pendulous breasts, ask her to lean forward. As the client performs these actions, observe the size, symmetry, contour, vascular pattern, and skin appearance of the breasts.

Normal breasts are symmetrical, although one may be larger than the other. They are conical to pendulous in shape, their contour is even, and the skin is similar to normal skin on the trunk, with a faint, symmetrical vascular pattern evident.

Abnormal findings include asymmetrical breasts; breasts markedly different in size; areas of retraction, dimpling, or flattening; erythematous or peau d'orange (orange peel appearance) skin; and asymmetrical vascular dilation.

Palpation. First, palpate the breasts with the client sitting with her hands at her sides. Then have her lie on her back with the arm on the side being examined raised and positioned so that the hand is behind her head; place a pillow under the shoulder on the side being examined. This position allows the breast tissue to flatten evenly over the chest wall. In palpating the breasts, move the pads of the fingers in small, firm circular motions to slide the skin over the breast tissue. The examination pattern should be systematic and include the tail of Spence (Figure 8-22). Start at the axilla in the midaxillary line, and cover the breast by palpating in parallel lines to the sternum (Figure 8-23). Palpate from the clavicle to the lower border of the breast and from the axillary line to midsternum. Examination of the

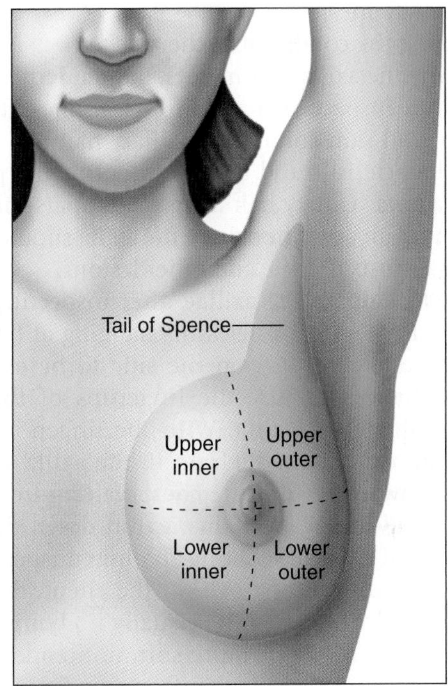

FIGURE 8-22 The four breast quadrants and the axillary tail of Spence.

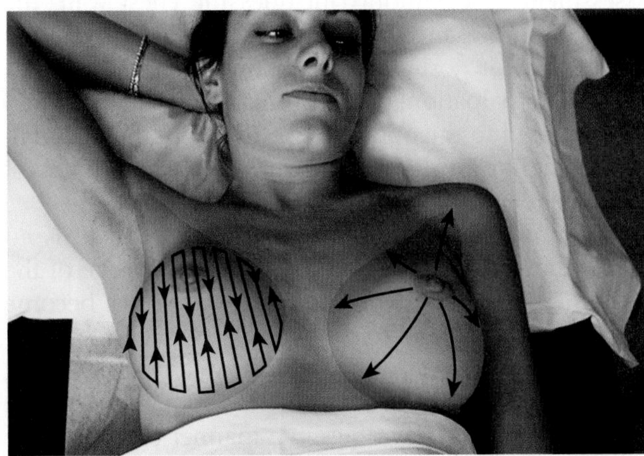

FIGURE 8-23 Client position and assessment patterns for breast palpation.

axillae for lymph nodes should follow breast examination. Examination along the chest wall is especially important. The position and size of any nodes should be recorded. In judging the findings, one breast must be compared with the other.

Normally, breast tissue feels uniformly loose or dense, smooth, and either firm or soft. The finding of areas of thickening, palpable masses, or tenderness or pain on palpation (except in the premenstrual female) is abnormal. Following palpation, the nipple of each breast is gently compressed between the thumb and forefinger to check for nipple discharge. With the exception of lactating women, the appearance of discharge with or without nipple compression is abnormal, as is retraction, deviation, or recent inversion of a nipple.

Axillae. Physical assessment of the axillae involves the following activities:

- Inspecting the condition of the axillae
- Palpating the axillae for masses and tenderness

Inspection. Inspect each axilla for cleanliness, hair distribution, and skin condition. Axillary hair is a secondary sex characteristic and thus is absent before puberty. In older adults, axillary hair is normally sparse and gray. In persons of all ages, the skin of the axilla should be free of redness, crusts, rashes, and other lesions.

Palpation. Palpate the axillae after inspecting them. Have the client sit with her arms hanging at her sides. Support the client's arm on the side to be examined with one hand, and use the fingertips of the other hand to palpate the axilla. With the fingers together, slightly cupped, and as high up in the axilla as possible, press inward toward the chest wall and move the fingers downward. Repeat this action down the anterior border of the axilla, along the inner aspect of the upper arm and, standing behind the client, down the posterior border of the axilla. Usually no lymph nodes are felt; however, one or more soft, nontender central nodes are an occasional insignificant finding.

ASSESSMENT OF THE THORAX

Assessment of the thorax includes the chest wall, the lungs, the heart, and the great vessels. Begin with either the anterior or posterior chest, using the techniques of inspection, palpation, percussion, and auscultation, and then proceed to the opposite chest wall. In the hospitalized client, it is common to begin with the anterior chest for convenience when the client is lying in bed.

Examining the organs within the chest cavity is an indirect examination that is based on knowledge of the location of the underlying structures. You must become familiar with the landmarks on the chest wall to associate your findings with the underlying structures. Using imaginary reference lines, you will be able to describe the location of your findings in a manner that will have the same meaning to anyone reading your description. Useful landmarks include the ribs, the sternal notch, the angle of Louis, the *xiphoid process*, the vertebra prominens, and the scapula.

As you begin learning to identify key locations on the chest wall, it is useful to count the ribs. Once you are comfortable with the locations, you will no longer need to count. The first rib is hidden beneath the clavicle; therefore, the first space is the first intercostal space, and the first rib to be felt is the second rib. The angle of Louis separates the manubrium from the body of the sternum. The second intercostal space is at the same level as the angle of Louis. In addition, the trachea bifurcates at the angle of Louis. All 12 ribs articulate with the thoracic spine.

The right lung has three lobes, and the left lung has two lobes. Figure 8-24, *A*, helps you locate the lobes of the lungs using landmarks on the anterior surface of the chest wall. On the right, the horizontal fissure that divides the upper lobe from the middle lobe follows the fourth rib. The fissure between the middle and lower lobes starts at the midclavicular line under the sixth rib and angles diagonally to the midaxillary line in the axilla. On the left, the heart occupies the space that would otherwise be the middle lobe. Only small portions of the lower lobes are accessible anteriorly on either the right or the left side.

The best access to the lower lobes is posteriorly. With the client's arms raised over the head, the division between the upper and lower lobes starts at the third thoracic vertebra and runs obliquely, following the edges of the scapulae (Figure 8-24, *B*).

On the lateral left side, the upper and lower lobes are divided obliquely from the midclavicular line at the sixth rib to the axilla at the level of the third thoracic vertebra (Figure 8-24, *C*). The same line on the right side divides the upper and middle lobes from the lower lobe. A horizontal line from the fourth or fifth rib at the midclavicular line divides the upper and middle lobes (Figure 8-24, *D*). The right side provides the best access to the right middle lobe.

Chest Wall and Lungs. Physical assessment of the chest wall and lungs should include the following:

- Inspection and palpation of the chest for shape, contour, and symmetry
- Inspection of the pattern of breathing
- Palpation of tactile fremitus
- Palpation of respiratory excursion
- Percussion of the posterior, anterior, and lateral thorax
- Auscultation of the posterior, anterior, and lateral thorax

Inspection and Palpation. To assess the thorax and lungs, evaluate the anterior, posterior, and lateral areas of the thorax, using the techniques of inspection, palpation, *percussion*, and *auscultation*.

Anterior landmarks. The anterior chest is divided into sections by imaginary vertical lines, that serve as anatomical landmarks (Figure 8-25, p. 162):

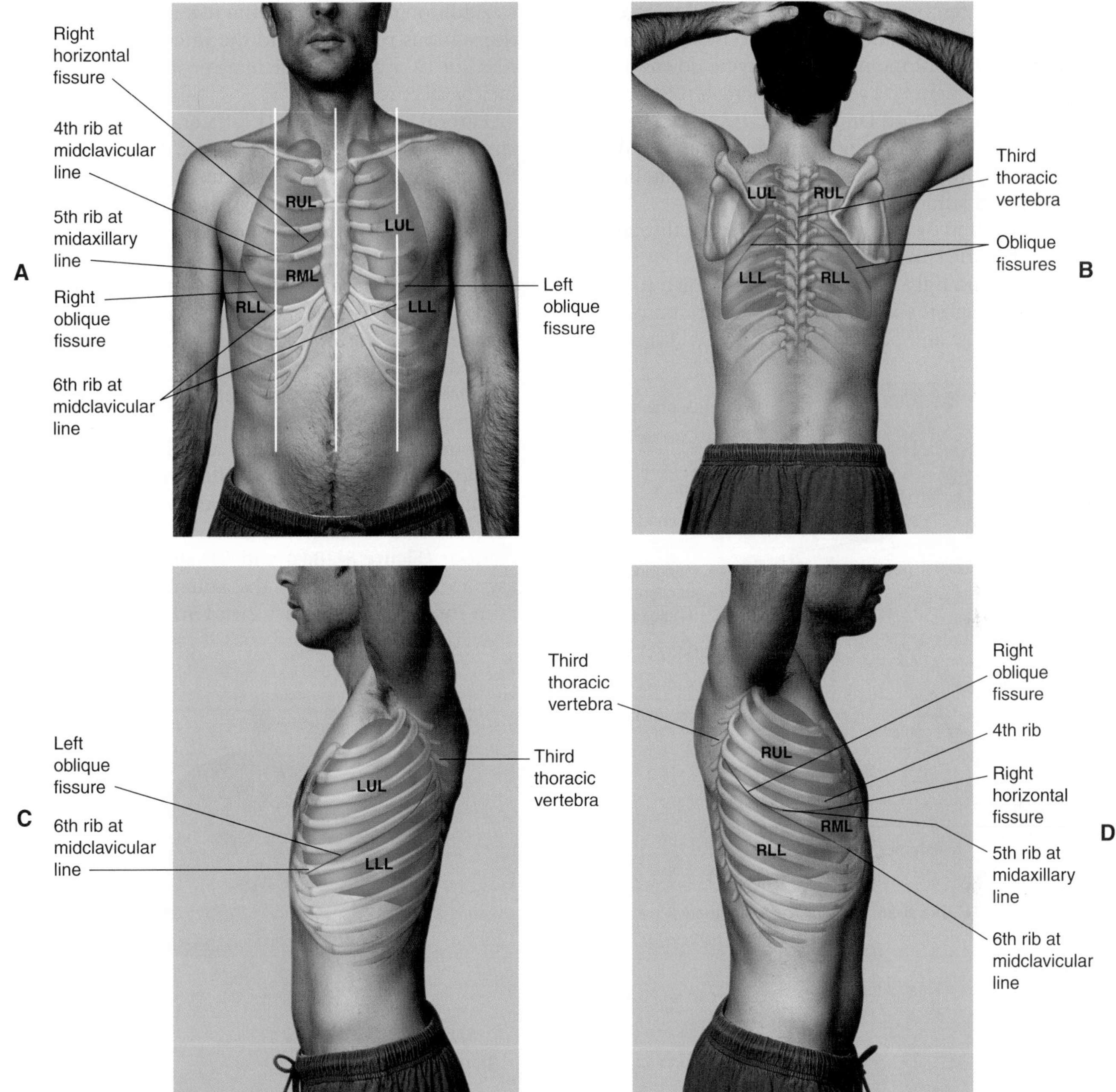

FIGURE 8-24 Chest landmarks. **A,** Anterior chest landmarks and underlying lungs. **B,** Posterior chest landmarks and underlying lungs. **C,** Left lateral chest landmarks and underlying lungs. **D,** Right lateral chest landmarks and underlying lungs.

- The midsternal line, drawn vertically through the center of the sternum
- The left and right midclavicular lines, drawn vertically through the midpoint of the left and right clavicles and running parallel to the midsternal line
- The left and right anterior axillary lines, drawn vertically through the anterior axillary folds and running parallel to the midsternal line

Additional anterior anatomical landmarks include the manubriosternal junction, the suprasternal notch, the costal angle, the clavicles, and the ribs. Anteriorly, the ribs articulate with the manubrium and the sternum. Posteriorly, they articulate with the vertebral processes. The first seven ribs articulate with the manubrium and the body of the sternum, and the last five ribs are fused into a bony and cartilaginous costal angle anteriorly. This angle should be less than 90 degrees. They are supported and connected by the intercostal muscles and attached to each other by costal cartilage. The exceptions are the eleventh and twelfth ribs, which remain unattached (or floating) anteriorly. The palpable spaces between the ribs are called intercostal spaces (ICSs) and are numbered in ascending order beginning at the base of the neck and moving downward (i.e., the first left or right ICS, second left or right ICS, etc.). They are used as anatomical landmarks.

Posterior landmarks. The posterior chest is divided similarly by three imaginary vertical and parallel lines that serve as landmarks (Figure 8-26):

- The vertebral or midspinal line, running through the center of the spinous processes
- The left and right midscapular lines, which run vertically through the midpoint of the inferior angle of the scapulae and parallel to the vertebral line

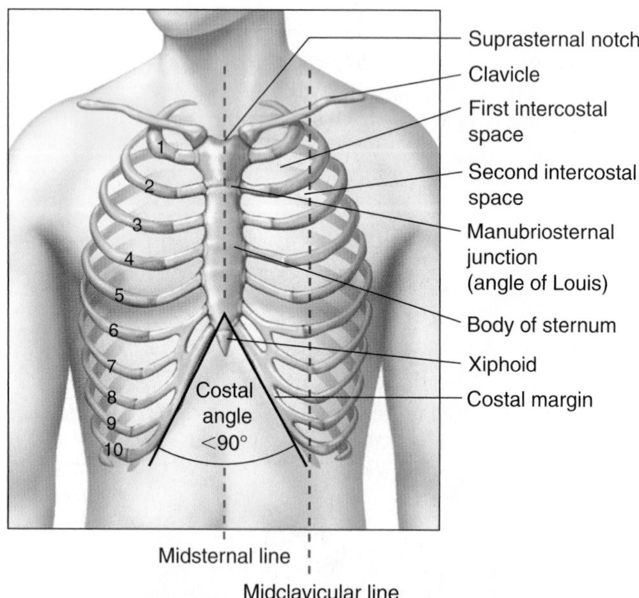

FIGURE 8-25 Anterior chest landmarks.

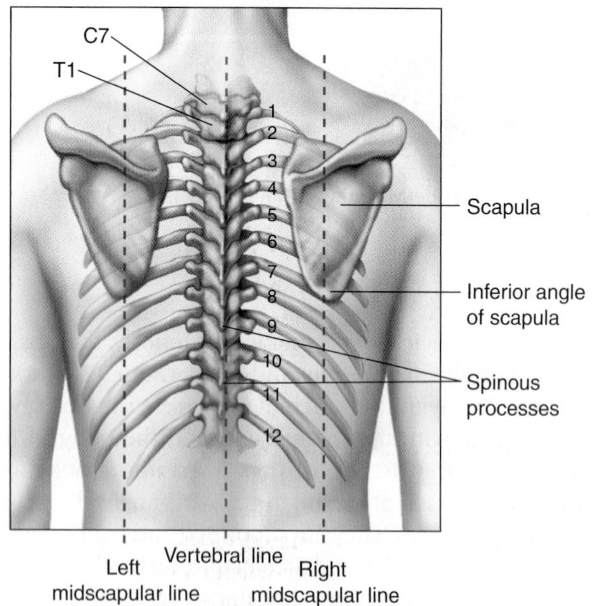

FIGURE 8-26 Posterior chest landmarks.

Additional posterior landmarks include the scapulae, the spinous processes, and the intercostal spaces of the ribs. All 12 of the ribs articulate posteriorly with the thoracic vertebrae.

Lateral landmarks. The lateral chest is divided similarly by three imaginary lines: the anterior axillary line, the midaxillary line, and the posterior axillary line (Figure 8-27). The midaxillary line is drawn vertically through the midpoint of the left and right axillae. The anterior axillary line is drawn vertically through the anterior axillary folds and parallel to the midaxillary line. Finally, the posterior axillary line is drawn through the posterior axillary folds parallel to the midaxillary line.

Shape, Contour, and Symmetry. Begin the assessment of the chest and lungs with the client undressed from the waist up and sitting up on the examining table. Observe the posterior thorax from a midline position behind the client. Observe the anterior thorax with the client lying supine. Note whether the chest is of normal size and contour (Figure 8-28, *A* and *B*). Does the chest appear asymmetrical? Normally the anteroposterior to lateral ratio should be between 1:2 and 5:7.

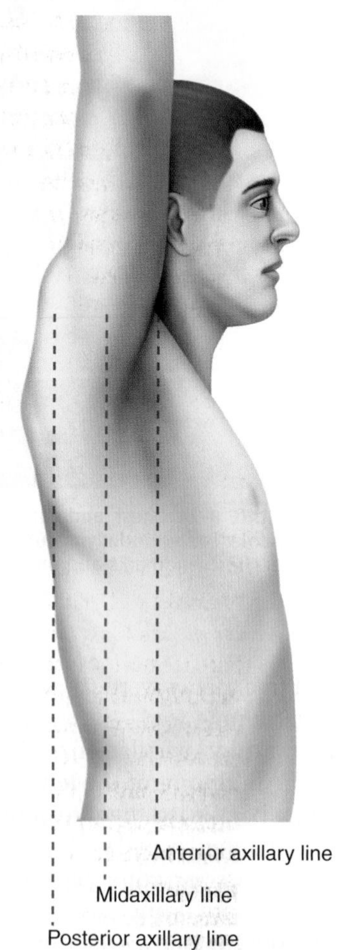

FIGURE 8-27 Lateral chest landmarks.

Note whether there are congenital anomalies, past traumatic injuries, disfigurements, or surgical alterations. Inspect and palpate the thorax, clavicles, scapulae, ribs, and spine for contour and abnormalities. Note any congenital abnormalities, traumatic injuries, postsurgical alterations, masses, lesions, tenderness, or abnormal slopes or contours. Ask the client to bend over at the waist to further inspect the curvature of the spine.

Figure 8-28, *C* through *F*, illustrates normal variations and abnormalities of chest configuration. Pigeon chest (Figure 8-28, *C*) and funnel chest (Figure 8-28, *D*) are considered normal congenital variations and are not corrected unless the deformity interferes with cardiopulmonary function or the client desires correction for cosmetic reasons. Barrel chest (Figure 8-28, *E*) is associated with chronic obstructive pulmonary disease (COPD). Kyphosis (Figure 8-28, *F*) and scoliosis (see Figure 32-5) can be severe enough to interfere with breathing.

Pattern of Breathing. Inspect the client's breathing pattern. Attempt to observe the respirations without making the client aware that you are doing so. A commonly used technique is to pretend you are taking the pulse while you are actually observing the respiratory pattern. Note any abnormalities of breathing rate or rhythm. A rate of 12 to 20 breaths per minute is considered normal for an adult. Inspiration time is slightly shorter than expiration time.

Any variations in rate and rhythm, such as tachypnea (rapid breathing), bradypnea (slow breathing), hyperpnea (sighing), hyperventilation (rapid deep breathing), apnea (periods of cessation of breathing), Cheyne-Stokes respirations (irregular breathing with long pauses), Kussmaul's respirations (rapid, deep breathing seen in

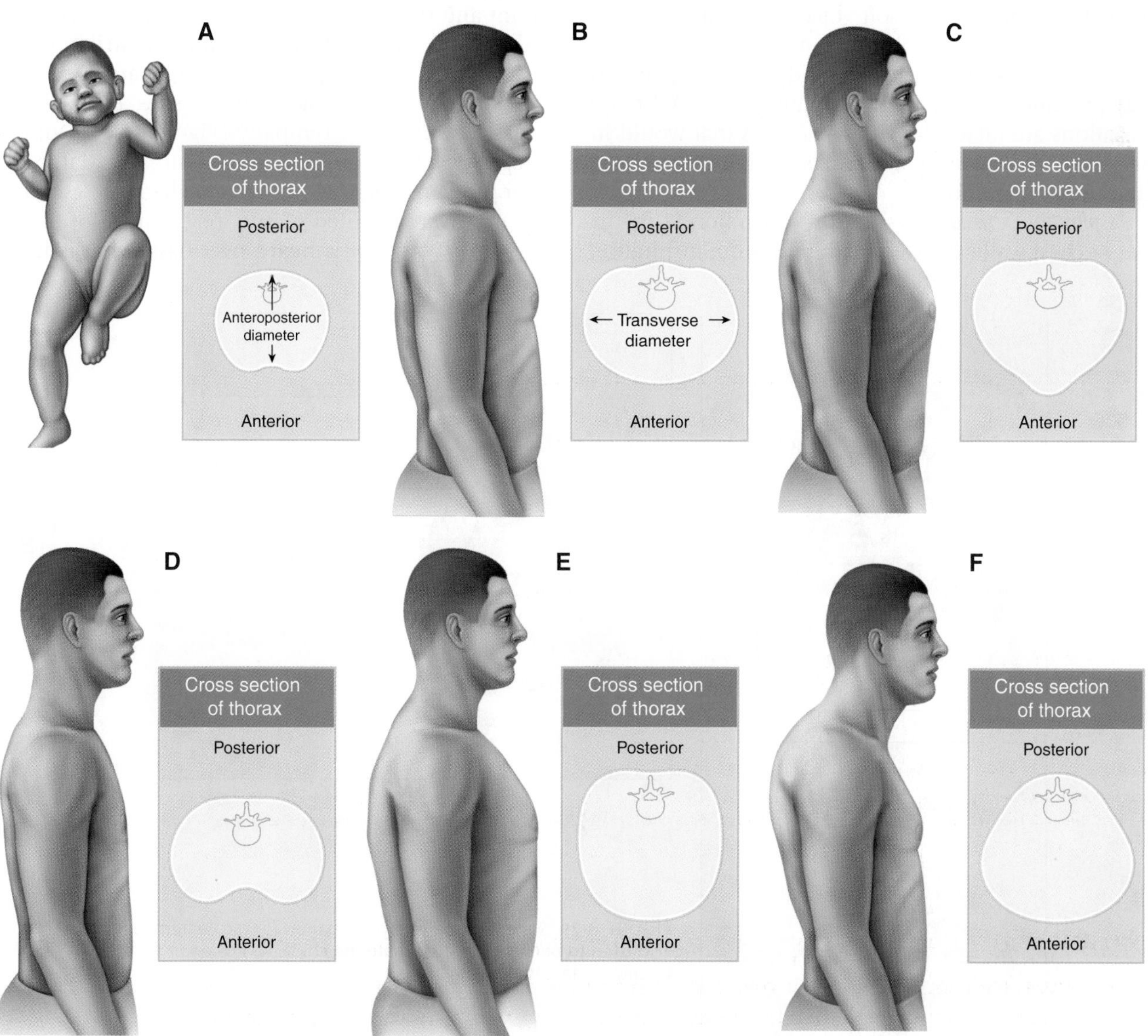

FIGURE 8-28 Normal configuration of the thorax in an infant **(A)** and an adult **(B)**. Normal variations and abnormalities of chest configuration include pigeon chest **(C)**, funnel chest **(D)**, barrel chest **(E)**, and kyphosis **(F)**.

diabetic ketoacidosis), wheezing (squeaking or whistling), pauses, prolonged expiration, bulging of the intercostal spaces, or use of accessory muscles to breathe should be clearly noted.

Tactile Fremitus. Palpate for tactile fremitus (also called vocal fremitus). **Tactile fremitus** is a vibration in the chest wall that is felt on the thorax while the client is speaking. It occurs over an abnormal area, such as an area where secretions have collected. Ask the client to repeatedly say "ninety-nine" as you place the ball of the hand (the posterior palm near the proximal finger joints) on each of the target areas diagrammed in Figure 8-29. The pattern shown for palpating for tactile fremitus will later be repeated for percussion and auscultation.

Compare the transmission of the client's voice through the chest wall in opposite symmetrical areas of the chest. The vibratory transmission of the voice should be equivalent in symmetrical areas. Vibratory sensations are decreased in clients with a soft voice, laryngeal disease or obstruction, bronchial obstruction, chronic obstructive pulmonary disease, effusions (fluid), fibrosis (thickening), pneumothorax (air), or infiltrating tumor. Vibratory sensations are increased with conditions that would increase the transmission of sound, such as a consolidated lung (lobar pneumonia).

Respiratory Excursion. **Respiratory excursion** is the extent of chest wall expansion with maximum inspiration; it should be bilaterally equal. Place your hands lightly over the lower rib cage as shown in Figure 8-30, and ask the client to take a deep breath. Allow your hands to move with the expansion of the chest wall. Observe the movement of the thumbs, and note the expanded distance between them. Normal respiratory excursion will separate the thumbs by 2 to 4 cm. Limited respiratory excursion may occur with chronic fibrotic disease of the lungs, COPD, emphysema, pulmonary tumors, an abdominal mass, or pain. Unilateral excursion would occur when one lung is unable to expand, such as a collapsed lung.

Percussion. Percuss the posterior and anterior thorax to reveal the nature of underlying tissue. To obtain a percussion "note," press the middle finger of the nondominant hand firmly on the surface. Cock the middle finger of the dominant hand, and strike the middle finger of the nondominant hand between the distal joint and the fingernail. Work your way down the posterior and then the anterior thorax, striking at least twice in each of the percussion target areas in intercostal spaces, and compare side to side. Listen for dullness, resonance, or tympany (Figure 8-31). Dullness is heard over solid or fluid-filled tissue (e.g., large underlying organs such as the liver or heart). Resonance is heard over air-filled tissue (e.g., most of the lung spaces). Tympany is heard over tissue that is hyperin-

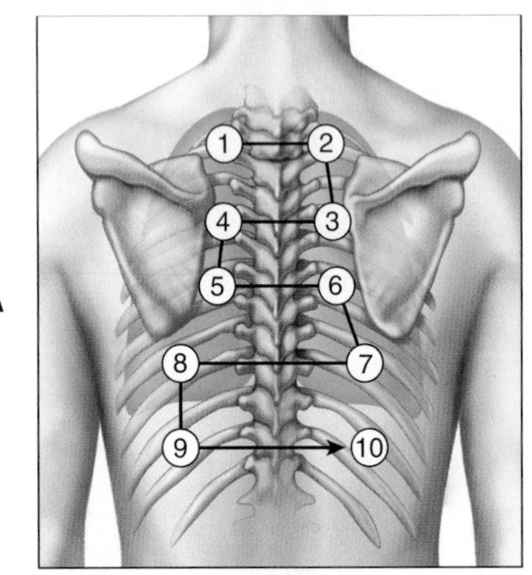

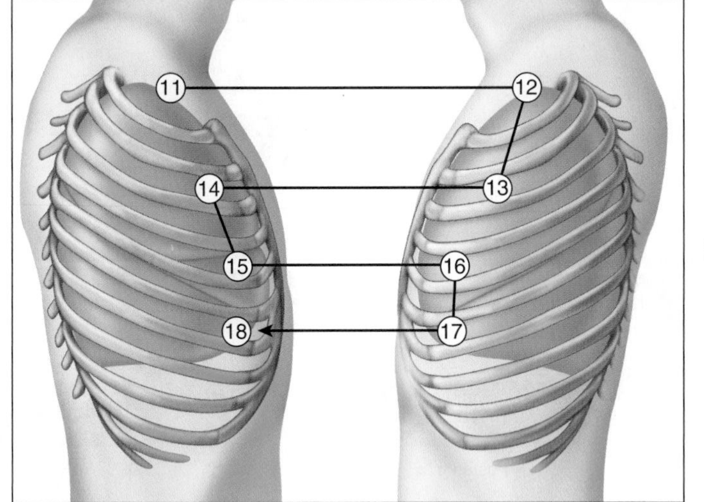

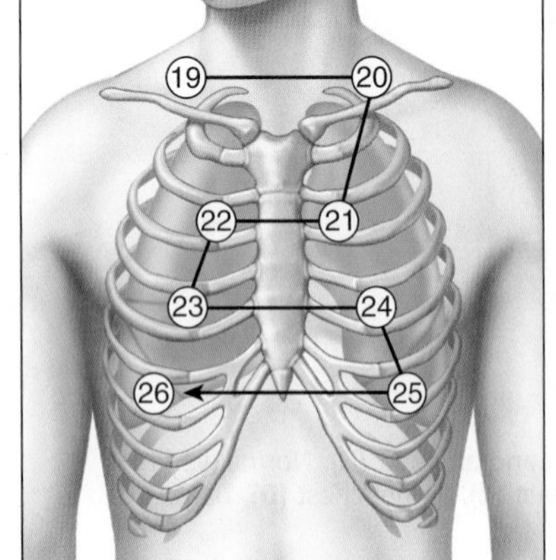

FIGURE 8-29 Systematic pattern of palpation for tactile fremitus, also used to percuss and auscultate the chest. **A,** Posterior; **B,** lateral; **C,** anterior target areas.

flated with air or where a large amount of air is common, such as the gastric air bubble.

On the posterior chest wall, percuss for diaphragmatic excursion or the ability of the lungs to expand as evidenced by the movement of the diaphragm. Ask the client to exhale and hold it. Percuss downward from a point of resonance toward the diaphragm. Mark the point where dullness is initially heard. Ask the client to exhale, then inhale and hold it. Again percuss downward from a point of resonance to the area where diaphragmatic dullness is initially heard. Mark this point and measure the distance between the two points. Normally the diaphragm will descend 3 to 6 cm. Excursion of the diaphragm is decreased in COPD.

Auscultation. Auscultate the posterior and then the anterior thorax in the pattern diagrammed for palpation (see Figure 8-29). Have the client (undressed from the waist up) sit up for both posterior and anterior chest auscultations, because abnormal findings may be masked in a supine client. With the diaphragm of the stethoscope on bare skin, listen to the client breathing. Move across and down the posterior and then the anterior chest comparing left side to right side. Be alert for artifacts, and eliminate them before proceeding. Artifacts are sounds made inadvertently from clothing, chest hair, muscle contractions, paper, scratching, or from the fingers resting on the stethoscope or the client's chest.

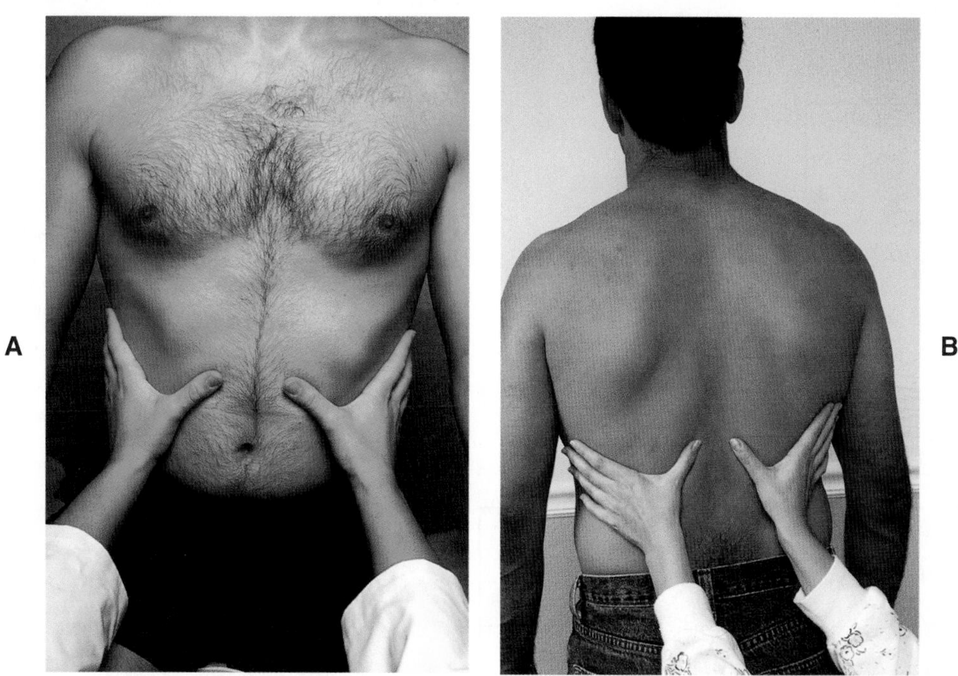

FIGURE 8-30 Position of the hands for assessing respiratory excursion on the anterior **(A)** and posterior thorax **(B)**.

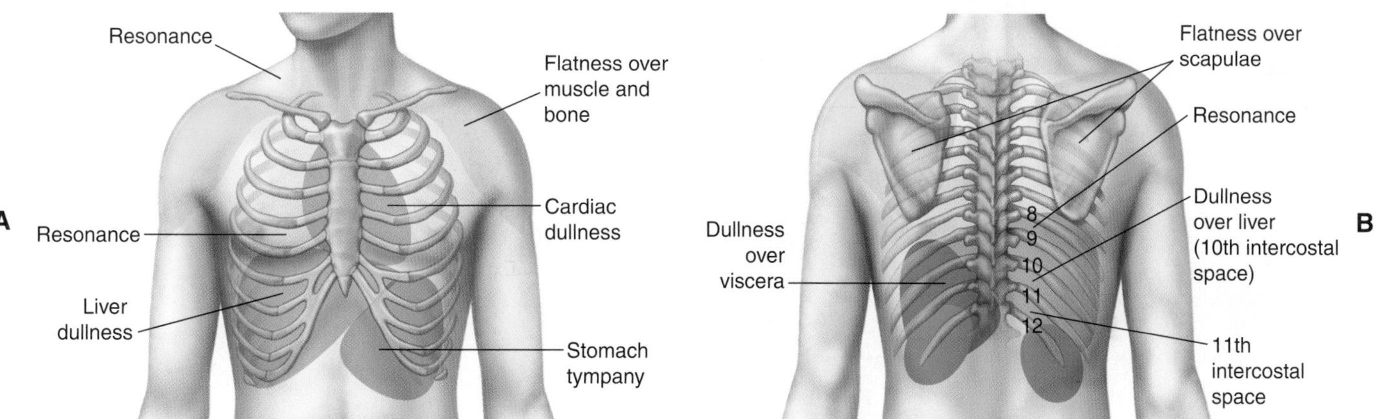

FIGURE 8-31 Normal percussion notes over the anterior **(A)** and posterior **(B)** chest and upper abdomen.

Identify the bronchial, bronchovesicular, and vesicular breath sounds (Figure 8-32), and distinguish these sounds from artifactual and abnormal breath sounds. **Bronchial** breath sounds are normal sounds heard over the main bronchus; tracheal sounds are those heard over the trachea. Inspiration is shorter than expiration. **Bronchovesicular** breath sounds are normal breath sounds heard over the right and left bronchi; these sounds are a combination of the sounds from the bronchi and the alveoli. Expiration and inspiration are of equal duration and sound like blowing through a hollow tube. **Vesicular** breath sounds are a soft, rustling sound heard over the peripheral lung fields, characteristically higher pitched during inspiration and falling rapidly during expiration. Inspiration is longer than expiration.

Adventitious is derived from a Latin word meaning from an outside source. Thus, adventitious breath sounds are produced by a source other than normal lungs. There are basically three types of adventitious breath sounds: discontinuous, coarse and fine crackles that indicate the presence of fluid in the airways; continuous, including high- and low-pitched wheezes that indicate narrowing or partial obstruction of the airways from inflammation, mucus, edema, a foreign body, or a mass; and rubs, grating sounds heard on end-inspiration and beginning-expiration and caused by the rubbing together of inflamed pleural surfaces. Note the timing (inspiratory or expiratory), location, and whether the adventitious sound clears with coughing, deep breathing, or position changes. Adventitious sounds are further discussed in Chapter 34.

A

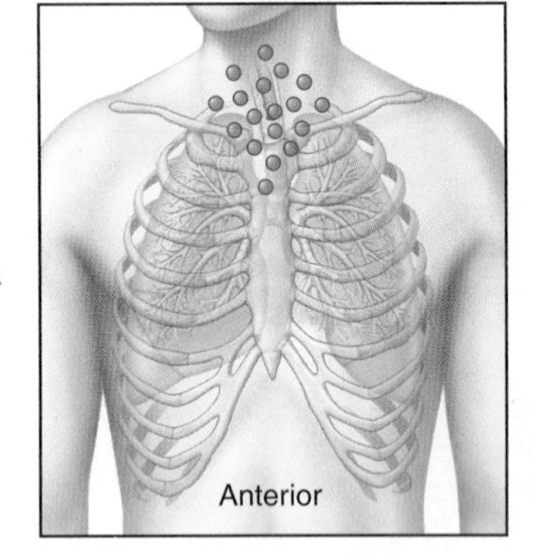

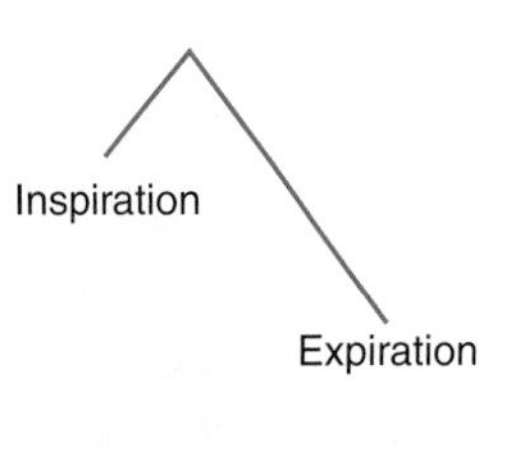

FIGURE 8-32 Normal breath sounds. **A,** Bronchial: hollow, blowing sounds over the trachea and main bronchus. **B,** Bronchovesicular: blowing sounds of medium pitch and intensity over the right and left bronchi. **C,** Vesicular: soft, low-pitched sounds over the periphery of the lungs.

B

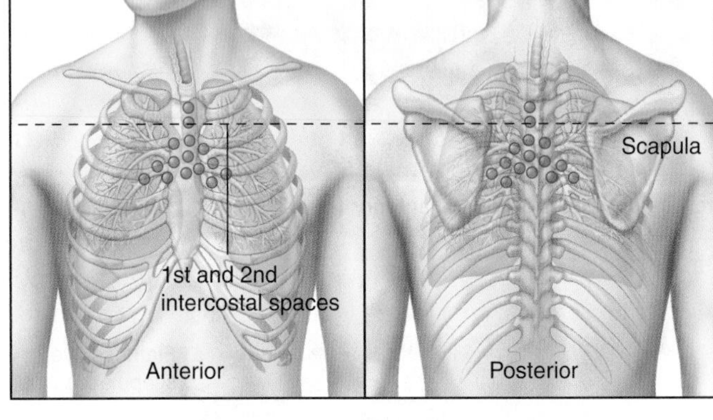

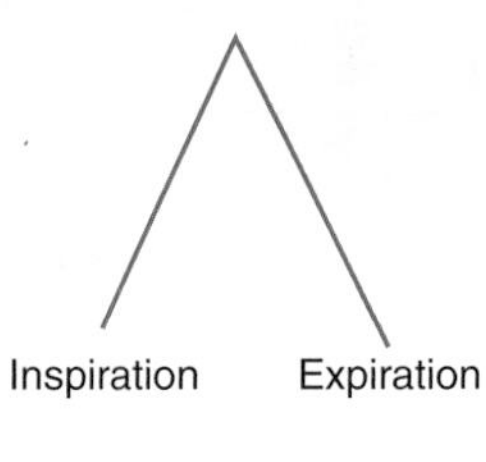

C

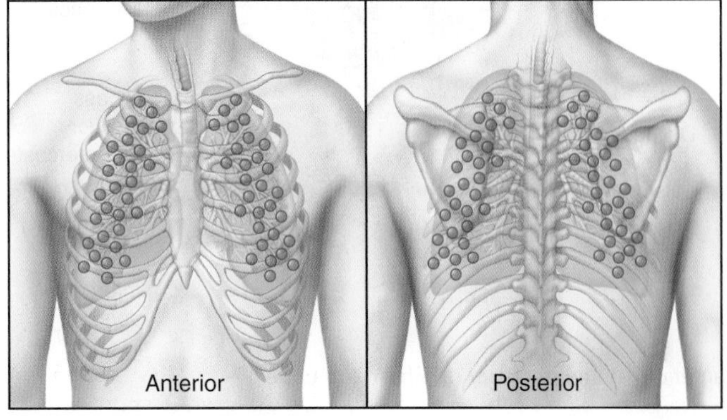

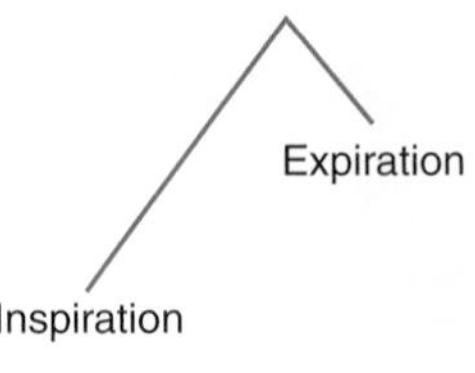

Heart. Examination of the heart should include the following steps:

- Inspect and palpate the anterior and posterior chest.
- Palpate the apical impulse or point of maximal impulse.
- Palpate the carotid pulse.
- Percuss the cardiac border to assess the size of the heart.
- Auscultate the heart for rate and rhythm.
- Compare the apical and radial pulses if the rhythm of the heart is found to be irregular.
- Auscultate the heart at each of the five anatomical landmarks.
- Auscultate S_1 and S_2.
- Auscultate for extra heart sounds.
- Auscultate for and evaluate any heart murmurs.

Anatomical Landmarks. The location of the heart in the anterior chest begins with identification of the anatomical landmarks that identify the precordium. The **precordium** is the area on the anterior chest overlying the heart and great vessels. The heart extends from the right border of the sternum to the left midclavicular line and from the second intercostal space to the fifth intercostal space. The heart can be thought of as an inverted isosceles triangle in the chest with the base at the top and the apex pointing down and to the left. It is slightly rotated with the right side anterior and the left side posterior.

There are six anatomical landmarks for listening to heart sounds. Four are associated with the heart valves: aortic, pulmonic, mitral, and tricuspid. The areas to listen to for the sounds are not directly over the valves but over the area to which the sound produced by the valve is transmitted (Figure 8-33). Sound is transmitted in the direction of blood flow. Although these areas are depicted as a single spot on the precordium, the valve sounds are heard in a larger area that overlaps with other areas. The area associated with the pulmonic valve is the second intercostal space to the left of the sternum. The area associated with the aortic valve is the second intercostal space to the right of the sternum. The area associated with the tricuspid valve is the fifth intercostal space at the left sternal border. The area associated with the mitral valve is the fifth intercostal space at the left midclavicular line. Erb's point is the fifth area, located in the third intercostal space on the left sternal border, and it is here that some murmurs are best heard. The **point of maximal impulse (PMI)** is the area of the chest wall where the apex of the heart comes closest to the chest wall; the heartbeat can be felt in approximately 75% of adults and may even be seen in a thin chest wall. In a healthy adult, the PMI is the mitral area.

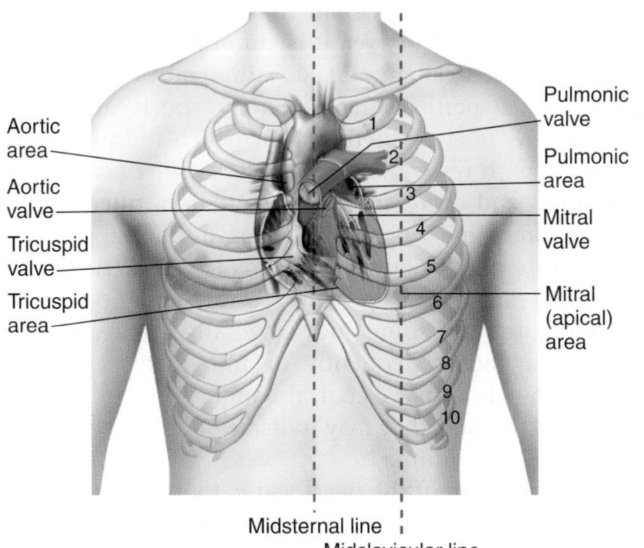

FIGURE 8-33 Anatomical sites for assessment of the precordium.

Events of the Cardiac Cycle. The heart is evaluated in relationship to the events of the cardiac cycle. The cardiac cycle is the time from the beginning of the contraction of the ventricles to the beginning of the next contraction. Systole is the contraction phase, and diastole is the relaxation phase. When the ventricles contract, pressure immediately increases in the ventricles, causing the mitral and tricuspid valves to close and the aortic and pulmonic valves to open. When the ventricles relax, the pressure drops to below that of the aorta and the pulmonary artery, causing the aortic and pulmonic valves to close. The greater pressure in the atria opens the mitral and tricuspid valves.

Two heart sounds are produced by the events of the cardiac cycle. The first heart sound, S_1, is the heart sound caused by the closure of the mitral and tricuspid valves. S_2, the second heart sound, is caused by the closure of the aortic and pulmonic valves. Thus, S_1 is associated with the beginning of systole, and S_2 is associated with the beginning of diastole. The heart sounds are often described as a "lubb-dupp" sound with the "lubb" being S_1 and the "dupp" being S_2.

Inspection and Palpation. Begin the assessment of the heart with inspection and palpation of the anterior thorax. Have the client undress to the waist, and examine the client first sitting up, then lying down, under adequate lighting. Be sure to inspect the client from the side and at an angle to take full advantage of lighting.

Inspect and palpate the aortic area, the pulmonic area, Erb's point, the tricuspid area, and the apical area. Palpate using the ball of the hand and the posterior side of the proximal finger joints placed lightly on the chest surface in each area. No pulsations should be visible. No pulsations, heaves, or thrills should be palpable. Heaves are forceful pulsations that bound up against the hand. Thrills are vibrations.

Apical pulse. As defined in Chapter 7, the *apical pulse* is the heart rate counted at the apex (the PMI) of the heart on the anterior chest. Palpate the apical impulse by placing the hand over the fifth intercostal space at the midclavicular line. Usually you will feel a light tapping sensation occurring in the apical area at the left fifth intercostal space at the midclavicular line. Normally the area of the tapping sensation is limited to 1 to 2 cm in diameter and confined to one intercostal space. Displacement of the apical impulse or an impulse felt in an area that is larger than 2 cm in diameter may be a result of abnormal curvatures of the spine, cardiomegaly, emphysema, obesity, increased musculature, or enlarged breasts. A faint or barely perceptible PMI may also be related to any condition that increases tissue mass or fluid between the heart and the chest wall, such as pericardial effusions (inflammatory fluid in the pericardium), pulmonary effusions (inflammatory fluid in the pleural space), or tumors.

Carotid pulses. Palpate and evaluate the carotid pulses. The carotid arteries are located in the groove between the trachea and the sternocleidomastoid muscle and can usually be easily felt anywhere along this groove. To locate the most prominent pulse, ask the client to turn his or her head away from the side chosen for palpation. Observe the neck for pulsations. Figure 8-34 shows the major arteries and veins of the right side of the neck. Place the tips of two fingers held together (usually the index and second finger) lightly over the pulsations. The right and left carotid are palpated separately and compared for strength. If the pulse is palpated while auscultating the heart, the carotid pulse will coincide with S_1.

Percussion. Rarely is the technique of percussion employed to determine cardiac size in current practice because chest radiographs now provide a much more reliable assessment of cardiac size and contour. However, when chest radiographs are not readily available, this may be a useful technique to know.

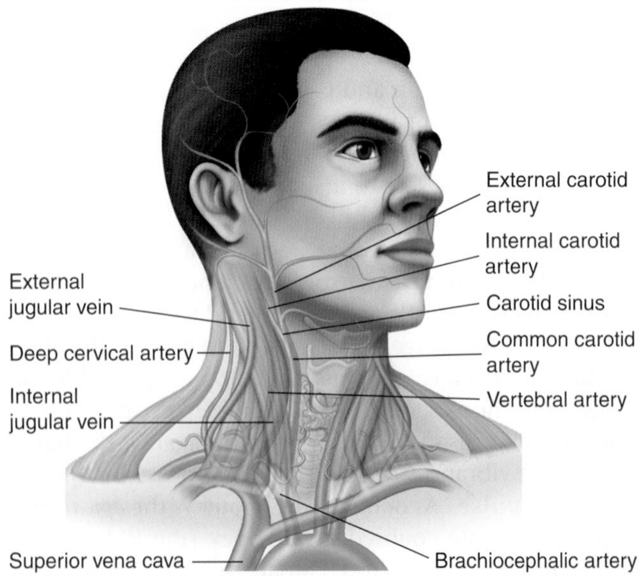

FIGURE 8-34 Arteries and veins of the right side of the neck.

Using the percussion technique described previously, percuss the borders of cardiac dullness and assess the size of the heart. The heart tissue is dull to percussion amid surrounding resonant lung tissue. The left border of cardiac dullness is usually at the fifth intercostal space at the midclavicular line and at the second intercostal space at the sternum. The right border of cardiac dullness is usually at the sternum.

A number of conditions, such as cardiomegaly (enlarged heart), left ventricular hypertrophy (enlarged left ventricle), pericardial effusions, or a cardiac mass, may account for increased heart size. A small number of clients may have congenital anomalies such as dextrocardia (abnormally rotated or positioned heart) or situs inversus (organs located on the side opposite of normal), which will result in markedly abnormal findings.

Auscultation. Auscultate the heart for rate and rhythm. Using the diaphragm of the stethoscope, auscultate the apical area of the heart for the rate and rhythm, counting the first heart sound (S_1) and the second heart sound (S_2) in combination as one beat, "lubb-dupp."

Assess the apical heart rate by counting the number of beats in 1 full minute. Assess the cardiac rhythm. Listen to several full cycles, paying particular attention to the length of the systolic pauses between S_1 and S_2. The length of both the systolic and the diastolic pause should be consistent in all cycles. Any variation in length of systolic or diastolic pauses, an abnormally long pause, or a sudden increase in heart rate over 100 cycles constitutes an irregular rhythm.

The average heart rate for adults is between 60 and 100 beats per minute (bpm). The average heart rate for children varies depending on age. Sinus bradycardia, or heart rate less than 60 bpm, may be normal in well-conditioned athletes but is abnormal when associated with hypothermia, hypothyroidism, and drug overdoses (narcotics and digoxin). Sinus tachycardia, or a heart rate greater than 100 bpm, may be normal with increased exercise; however, it is abnormal in association with increased caffeine intake, stimulant overdoses, fever, pain, hyperthyroidism, anxiety, shock, and heart disease. A sinus dysrhythmia, in which the pulse rate changes with respirations, increasing at the peak of inspiration and decreasing with expiration, often occurs in children and young adults as a normal variant. Premature ventricular contractions (PVCs) result in irregular heart rhythms perceived as beats that occur out of sequence and sometimes singularly or in couplets. They may occur frequently or infrequently and are caused by abnormal electrical conduction through the ventricular tissue; they may indicate or be a precursor to a serious dysrhythmia.

If the rhythm of the heartbeat is found to be irregular, compare the apical and radial pulses. Compare the rate (per full minute) between the apical and radial pulses. Usually the apical and radial pulses will be equivalent in rhythm. If a pulse deficit occurs, the lost beats were not strong enough to send a pulse wave to the radial artery; the peripheral circulation may be compromised by the deficit.

Auscultate the heart in each of the six anatomical landmarks using first the diaphragm of the stethoscope and then the bell. Apply firm pressure when using the diaphragm and light pressure when using the bell. At each site, listen for the rate and rhythm, S_1, S_2, systole and diastole, extra heart sounds, and murmurs.

Heart sounds. Identify and carefully auscultate S_1 and S_2. The first heart sound (S_1) occurs at the same time as the carotid pulse. It is heard best at the apex of the heart and is louder than the second heart sound (S_2) at the apical and tricuspid areas. It is softer than S_2 at the pulmonic and aortic areas. The second heart sound (S_2) is heard best in the aortic area. It is louder than S_1 in the aortic and pulmonic areas.

Listen to S_1 and S_2 carefully and separately. S_1 is associated with the systolic or contraction phase; S_2 is associated with diastole or the relaxation phase. Usually systole and diastole are silent. Figure 8-35 will help you compare the heart sounds to the events of the cardiac cycle and the electrocardiogram.

Once you have identified S_1 and S_2, note whether the heart sounds are normal, accentuated (loud), or split. A split sound means you can distinguish more than one sound in S_1 or S_2. A physiological split of S_2 can occur with respiration. The change in intrapulmonary pressure causes blood to sequester in the lungs with inspiration, resulting in late closure of the pulmonic valve. Hence, closure of the aortic and pulmonic valves is heard separately. A physiological split of S_2 is easily identified because it varies with respiration.

Extra heart sounds. Auscultate for extra heart sounds. Note whether there are third (S_3) and fourth (S_4) heart

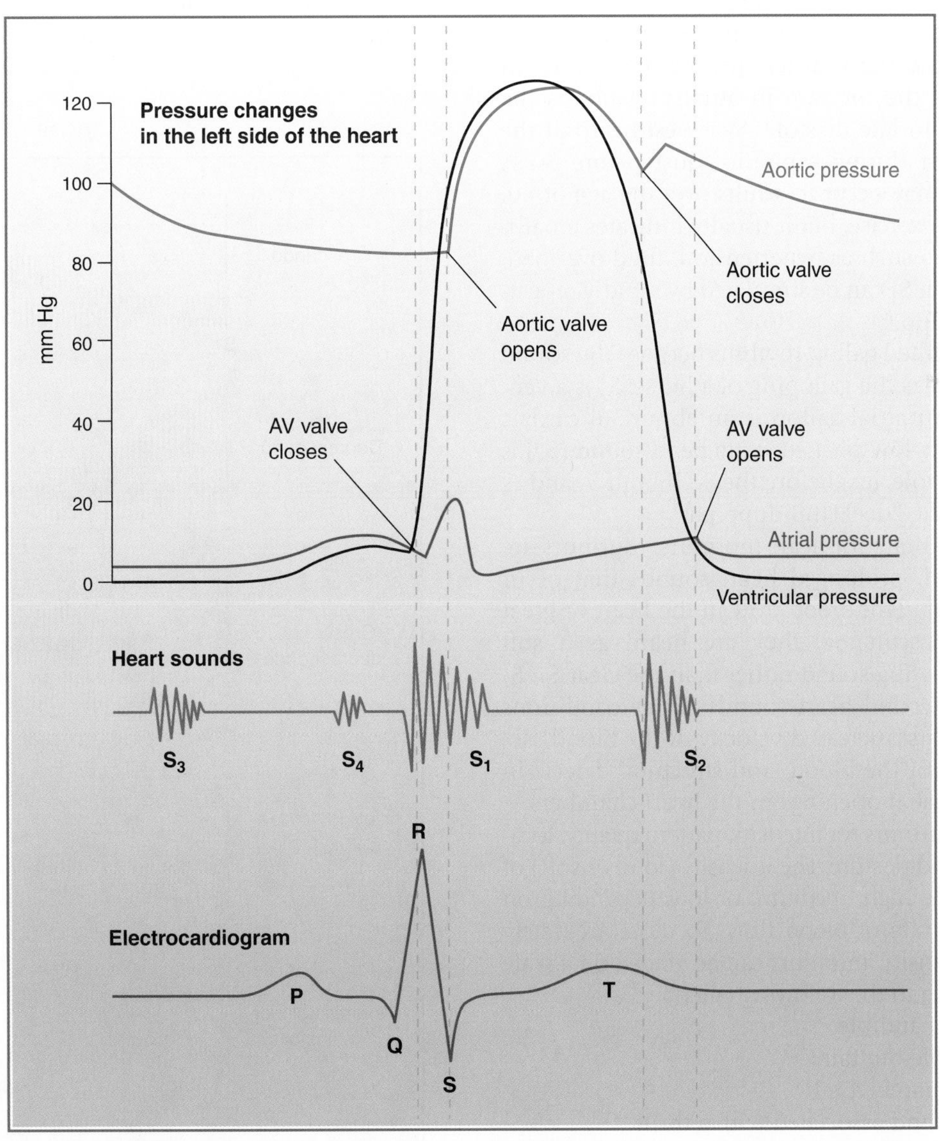

FIGURE 8-35 Relationship of heart sounds to the events of the cardiac cycle and the electrocardiogram.

sounds, split sounds, or audible clicks. S_3 and S_4 are sounds produced by rapid ventricular filling. Split sounds are the result of one valve closing before the other. Clicks are the result of diseased valves being forced open or incompletely closing. S_3 and S_4 are a good introduction to extra heart sounds.

S_3 is heard most clearly at the apex of the heart just after S_2 in early diastole. As the atrioventricular valves open, ventricular filling occurs with a rush of blood into the ventricles, which creates vibration that produces sound. It occurs when the ventricles are resistant to filling during the early rapid filling phase of diastole. S_3 is best heard at the apex in the lateral position or lower left sternal border with the client in the left side-lying position or leaning forward. S_3 is normal in children and in young adults, but after age 40 it is usually considered to be a sign of heart failure. The sound of an S_3 can be simulated by rapidly repeating "LUBB-dupp-pa."

The cause of S_4 is vibrations of the ventricular walls when they are suddenly distended by blood from the atria at the end of diastole. As the atria contracts, it forces the last blood into the ventricle just before systole. In Figure 8-35 note the increase in atrial pressure as the atrium contracts in late diastole. S_4 is best heard at the apex of the heart during expiration just before S_1. A physiological S_4 may occur in adults over the age of 40, particularly after exercise, but it usually indicates a pathological condition such as hypertension, fluid overload, or heart failure. An S_4 can be simulated by rapidly repeating "deeLUBB-dupp."

S_3 and S_4 are called gallop rhythms because the sound produced resembles the galloping of a horse. S_3 is a ventricular gallop. An atrial gallop is an abnormal cardiac rhythm in which a low-pitched, extra heart sound (S_4) is heard late in diastole, just before the S_1. If both S_3 and S_4 exist, it sounds like "deeLUBB-dupp-pa."

Murmurs. Auscultate for heart murmurs. Murmurs are muffled, softened, prolonged heart sounds that occur when there is turbulent blood flow in the heart or great vessels. When auscultated, they are heard as a soft swooshing or blowing sound rather than the clear S_1, S_2 of the first and second heart sounds. Three conditions can cause murmurs: increased velocity of the blood, decreased viscosity of the blood, and structural defects in the valves or unusual openings in the heart chambers.

Evaluate all murmurs for intensity, pattern quality, location, radiation, and posture. The intensity (loud or soft) of a murmur may be high, medium, or low, depending on the pressure and rate of blood flow. To more accurately describe their intensity, murmurs can be graded on a scale of 1 to 6 according to the following criteria:

Grade 1: Barely audible
Grade 2: Audible but faint
Grade 3: Moderately loud
Grade 4: Loud and associated with a thrill
Grade 5: Loud and heard with the edge of the stethoscope lifted off the chest wall
Grade 6: Loudest and heard easily without a stethoscope or with a stethoscope held just above the chest wall

Murmurs may also vary in their pattern of intensity (Figure 8-36). They may grow louder in intensity (crescendo), taper off in intensity (decrescendo), or increase in intensity to a peak and then taper off all within one systolic or diastolic pause (a crescendo-decrescendo or diamond-shaped pattern). The murmur may be pansystolic or holosystolic (or pandiastolic or holodiastolic); that is, it occurs throughout the entire length of the systolic (or diastolic) pause. It may occur only in the early, middle, or late part of systole or diastole. Whatever pattern the murmur exhibits, it should be carefully and accurately described to help differentiate the possible underlying causes. Although some patterns of intensity are introduced here, it is beyond the scope of this chapter to provide more detailed explanations of the characteristic murmurs associated with each cardiac abnormality.

The location of a murmur refers to its position within the cardiac cycle. A murmur heard during the S_1, or sys-

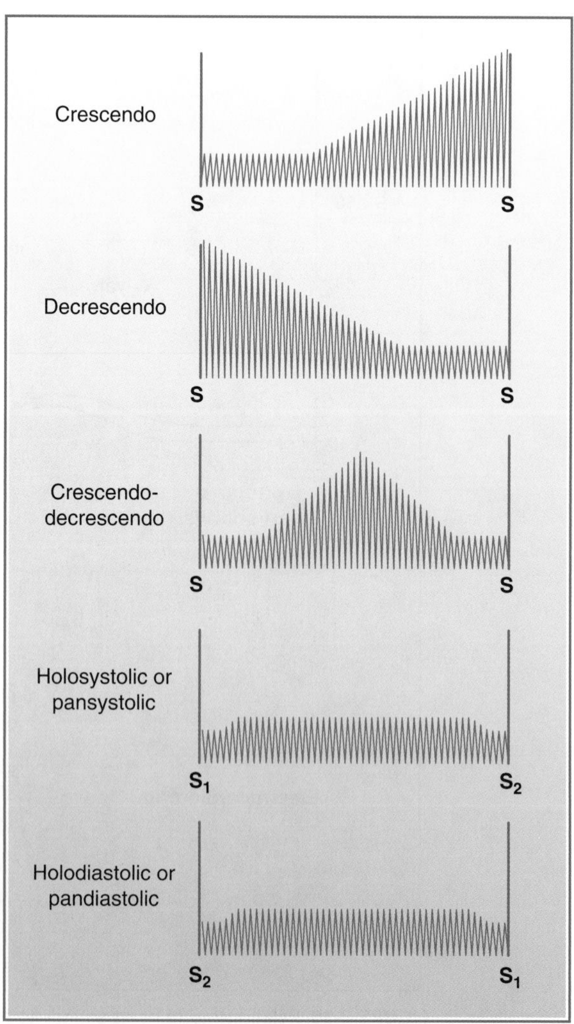

FIGURE 8-36 Characteristics of heart murmurs.

tolic phase, is a systolic murmur; one heard during the S_2, or diastolic phase, is a diastolic murmur.

A murmur can radiate downstream of the blood flow and be heard in a different area of the precordium. The degree to which a murmur can be heard can vary with posture. Therefore, a thorough examination of the heart includes listening with the client in the supine, forward-sitting, and left side-lying positions (Figure 8-37).

ASSESSMENT OF THE PERIPHERAL VASCULAR SYSTEM

Include the following in the assessment of the peripheral vascular system:

- Assessment of the client's blood pressure
- Inspection and palpation of the carotid arteries
- Assessment of the jugular venous pulsations
- Assessment of the peripheral venous circulation
- Assessment of the peripheral arterial circulation

Ask the client to undress to underwear and to don an examination gown. The examination of the peripheral vascular system will require that the client sit, stand, or lie down as necessary.

Blood Pressure. Using the stethoscope and sphygmomanometer, assess blood pressure while the client is relaxed and sitting and again just after standing. Blood pressure normally varies in an individual. In general, systolic pressure in the adult varies from 95 to 140 mm Hg and diastolic pressure varies from 60 to 90 mm Hg. Compare the blood pressures in each arm. A difference of 10 to 15 mm Hg or less systolic is considered normal. Assess whether there are orthostatic changes in blood pressure; orthostatic hypotension is usually defined as a drop in systolic pressure greater than 20 mm Hg when changing to the upright position. Sometimes you may want to take the blood pressure with the client lying, sitting, and standing. Refer to Chapter 7 for a more thorough discussion of blood pressure and vital signs.

Carotid Arteries. Inspect and palpate the carotid arteries. With the client sitting, inspect and palpate the pulsations of the carotid arteries. Use the index and middle

A

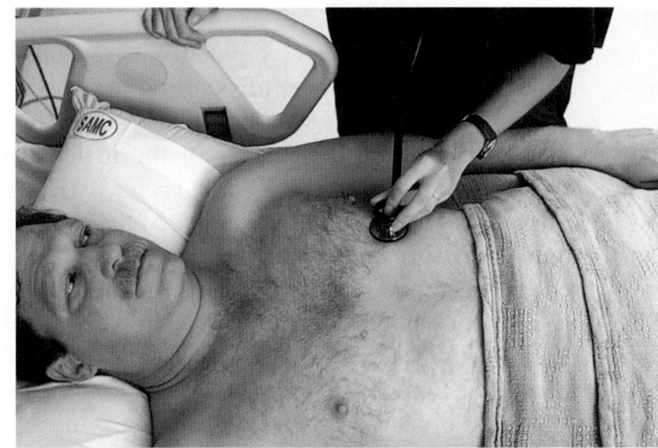

B

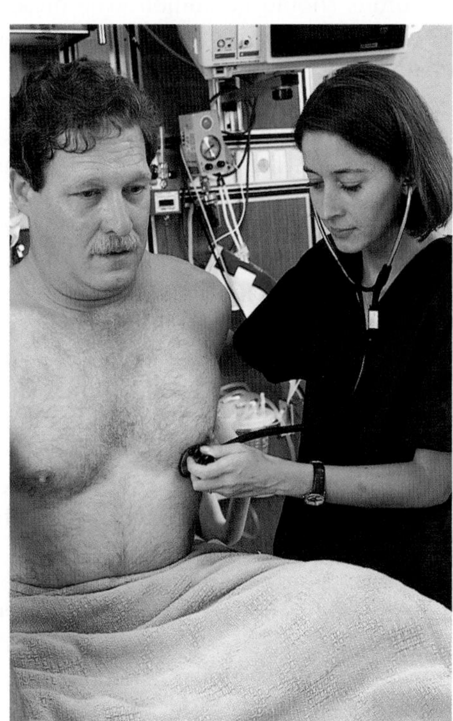

C

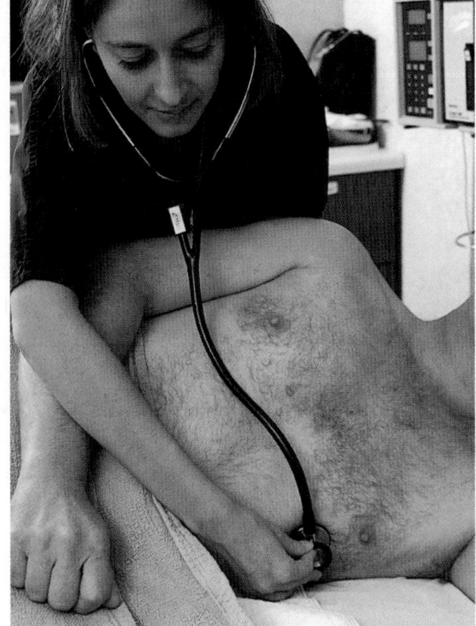

FIGURE 8-37 Positions for auscultation of the heart. **A,** Supine. **B,** Forward-sitting. **C,** Left side-lying.

fingers together to gently palpate the carotid arteries on either side of the neck near the medial edge of the sternocleidomastoid muscle.

Examine one artery at a time. It may help to turn the client's head slightly away from you for inspection and then back toward you for palpation. Compare and note the rate, rhythm, and strength of pulsations of both carotid arteries. A normal rate varies between 60 and 90 bpm bilaterally. The carotid pulsations should feel strong, elastic, and regular. Note whether the rate is synchronous with the client's heartbeat and whether the rate changes with inspiration or expiration.

Use the bell to listen for a bruit. A bruit is an abnormal blowing, swishing, or murmurlike sound heard while auscultating a carotid artery, organ, or gland, such as the liver or thyroid. Ask the client to hold his or her breath (to prevent artifact from the tracheal breath sounds) while you auscultate each carotid artery for bruits (Figure 8-38). Assess at the angle of the jaw, middle third of the neck, and just above the clavicle. Use light pressure because compressing the artery can create an artificial bruit. Normally no bruits should be audible. The presence of bruits may indicate thrombosis or severe thickening of the lumen from atherosclerosis.

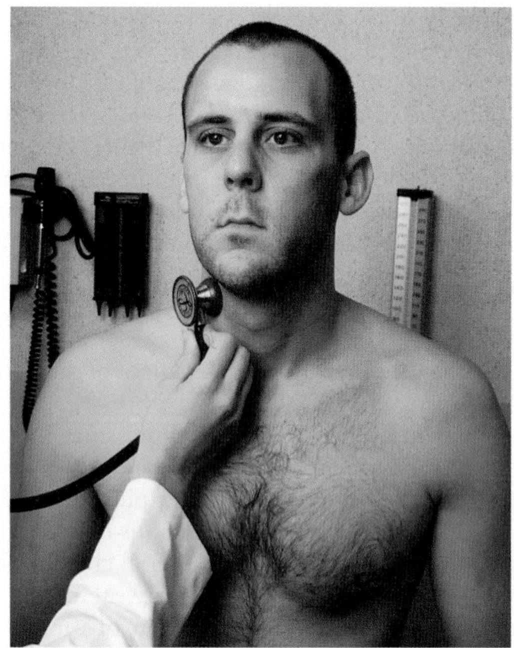

FIGURE 8-38 Assessing for a carotid bruit.

Neck Veins. Inspect for distention of the jugular veins with the client lying down with the head raised slightly at a 30- to 45-degree angle. The pressure in the jugular vein reflects the pressure where the vena cava enters the right side of the heart. The height of the pulsation on the neck is related to the central venous pressure. Jugular vein distention to more than 3 cm above the sternal angle is associated with increased blood volume or congestive heart failure. Assess the jugular venous pulsations in the internal jugular vein. A jugular pulsation results from a backward wave associated with contraction of the right atrium. The level of pulsations of the internal jugular vein may be more definitive for increased central venous pressure than the level of distention of the external jugular vein. Chapter 35 further discusses jugular vein distention.

Peripheral Veins. Assess the lower extremities for changes in peripheral venous circulation. Inspect and palpate for signs of peripheral venous insufficiency (changes in the skin, changes in temperature, presence of edema, varicosities, phlebitis, and thrombosis). Note signs of pallor, cyanosis, dermatitis, ulcers, necrosis, edema, or cellulitis. Note whether there is clubbing of the client's fingers or toes. Bilateral comparison is useful to distinguish normal from abnormal in one individual.

If edema is present, assess the extent or height of involvement on the leg and whether it is pitting or nonpitting. The edema of peripheral vascular disease is usually ascending. It may begin in the ankles and ascend up the legs, depending on the severity of the vascular compromise. Chapter 35 discusses edema in greater detail.

Inspect and palpate the lower extremities for varicosities. Varicose veins are swollen, distended, and knotted veins resulting from incompetent valves that allow the blood to back-flow, thus distending and stretching the veins. They appear as swollen, thick, tortuous veins seen or palpated along the surface of the lower extremities. Inspect and palpate the superficial veins for signs of phlebitis or inflammation. Look for reddened, thickened, or tender veins. If varicosities are present, palpate the vessel with one hand while pressing down on the vessel with the second hand at a point just above the first hand. Palpate for the impulse of blood flow. Normally there should be none. If any varicosities occur in the lower legs, assess for phlebitis (inflammation of a vein).

To check for the presence of phlebitis, *gently* compress the calf muscle against the tibia and note the presence of any tenderness. You also can perform a maneuver to elicit Homans' sign. With the client's knee flexed, sharply dorsiflex the foot. A positive Homans' sign is a characteristic, sharp calf pain (Figure 8-39). However, Homans' sign is nonspecific; a positive Homans' sign is present in only 20% of cases of deep vein thrombosis (DVT) and may be present without DVT.

Peripheral Arteries. Assess the peripheral arterial circulation. Inspect and palpate for signs of peripheral arterial insufficiency. Inspect the skin and nails. Note the presence of thin shiny skin, scaly skin, decreased hair growth, or thickened nails. Note whether the extremities are cool to the touch. Note whether the client demonstrates any sensory deficits. Test the client's ability to perceive soft, dull, sharp, and vibratory sensations with the eyes closed.

Check each of the peripheral pulses (temporal, radial, ulnar, brachial, femoral, popliteal, dorsalis pedis, and posterior tibial). See Chapter 7 for more information about pulses. Because each person's anatomy varies

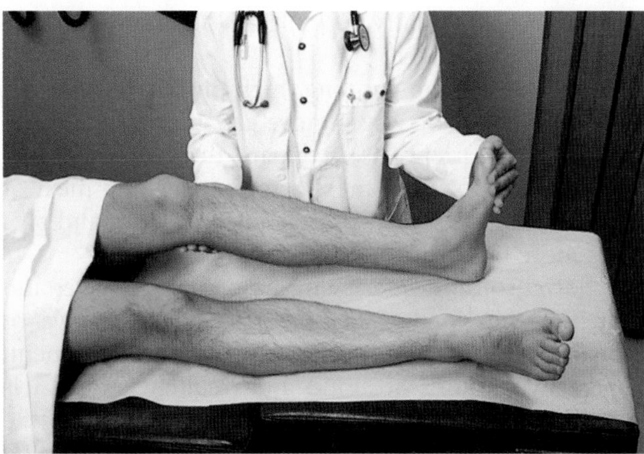

FIGURE 8-39 Assessing for Homans' sign.

slightly, pulses are located primarily by touch. Exert light pressure with the index and middle fingertips held together, and palpate the arterial pulses. Compare pulses side to side for rhythm, strength, and equality. If the pulse is not palpable, you may need to use a Doppler or ultrasound stethoscope to amplify the sound of the arterial pulsations (see Chapter 7).

ASSESSMENT OF THE ABDOMEN

The abdomen is a large oval cavity extending from the diaphragm to the floor of the pelvis. It is lined with the parietal peritoneal membrane that covers the wall of the abdomen and is continuous with the visceral peritoneal membrane that covers the organs of the abdomen. To assess the abdomen, you must know the precise location of the visceral organs underlying the skin and abdominal muscles. A routine nursing examination generally includes inspection, auscultation, and light palpation. Deep palpation and most percussion are more likely to be part of a diagnostic medical examination.

The abdomen can be divided into four or nine sections. Commonly the abdomen is divided into four quadrants by vertical and horizontal lines at the umbilicus (Figure 8-40, *A*). However, the older nine-section method is sometimes useful to describe findings more precisely (Figure 8-40, *B*).

The lower ribs on the right protect the liver and gallbladder, and thus only the lower border of the liver is normally palpable, if at all. The lower ribs on the left protect the spleen. The organs of the abdominal cavity are not normally palpable. The lower left colon may be palpable if filled with feces, and the bladder if filled with urine. The uterus and ovaries are palpable with a bimanual vaginal examination.

The following should be included in assessment of the abdomen:

- Inspection of the abdomen
- Auscultation for bowel sounds and vascular sounds
- Percussion of the abdomen
- Percussion of the size and span of the liver
- Percussion of the gastric air bubble
- Percussion of the kidneys
- Percussion of the spleen
- Palpation of the abdomen in all four quadrants using light and deep palpation techniques
- Palpation of the umbilicus
- Palpation of the liver
- Palpation of the gallbladder
- Palpation of the spleen
- Palpation of the aorta
- Palpation for ascites in the distended abdomen
- Ballottement of a suspected mass

Inspection. To prepare for an examination of the abdomen, ask the client to undress to the waist and don an examination gown. Cover the legs and genitalia with a sheet, and have the client lie supine with knees slightly flexed and arms at the side or folded across the chest. You may need to provide pillows for the head and knees to make the client more comfortable. Ask the client to locate any tender areas before proceeding, and examine these areas last. Examine the client with warm hands and a warm stethoscope. Try to distract the client with conversation throughout the examination, and watch facial expressions for any grimaces or confirmations of pain.

Observe the client's posture. Note whether the client is guarding or splinting the abdomen, lying perfectly still, constantly changing positions, frequently leaning forward, or favoring one side or position.

Inspect the skin of the abdomen (refer to Assessment of the Skin, Hair, and Nails, earlier). Note its color, its turgor, and the presence of erythema, ecchymosis, lesions, masses, striae (stretch marks), old scars, or venous abnormalities. Note whether the client has markedly diminished or excessive adipose tissue.

Note the symmetry, the contour (flat, convex, or concave), the presence of surface movements (breathing, peristalsis, aortic pulsations), bulging (hernias, cysts, tumors), obesity, and distention (obstruction, ascites). Asymmetry above the umbilicus may indicate gastric dilation, a pancreatic cyst, or malignancy. Asymmetry below the umbilicus may indicate pregnancy, fibroid uterus, ovarian cancer, bowel or bladder obstruction, hernias, tumors, or cysts. It is normal to see the pulsation of the aorta and waves of peristalsis in thin persons.

Assess for abdominal distention. Inspect the abdomen from all angles while the client is lying supine and again while the client holds a deep breath. Mild distention of the abdomen below the umbilicus may be the normal result of a full bladder or stool in the colon. Abnormal distention of the abdomen occurs with the accumulation of fluid, feces, or gas in the intestine, often from bowel obstruction or absent peristalsis. It may also be secondary to infection or inflammation, such as in appendicitis or after surgery. The cause might also be inflammation, infection, or free fluid in the peritoneal cavity. If the appendix ruptures, the entire peritoneal cavity becomes inflamed (peritonitis). A glistening, taut abdomen might indicate the presence of ascites, the abnormal accumulation of lymphatic fluid within the peritoneal cavity secondary to liver disease.

Auscultation. Because percussion and palpation can change the bowel sounds, auscultate before you palpate and percuss. Place the diaphragm of the stethoscope lightly on the abdomen to auscultate for bowel sounds. Auscultate the abdomen by beginning in the left lower quadrant (LLQ) or right lower quadrant (RLQ) and following the bowel until you have listened in all four quadrants; listen for up to $1^1/_2$ minutes in each quadrant. Usually 10 to 15 seconds provides the information you need.

Bowel sounds are gurgling, high-pitched sounds occurring as peristaltic waves move gas through the intestine. Their occurrence is irregular—there may be anywhere from 5 to 20 or more a minute. After a meal or other stimulus to peristalsis, the bowel is active and produces more frequent sounds.

If bowel sounds are present, note their character and frequency and whether they are normal, hyperactive, or hypoactive. Hypoactive sounds are quiet and infrequent. Hyperactive sounds are loud and frequent. Normal is somewhere in between. The loud, audible sound of the stomach "growling" or the loud, gurgling, tinkling

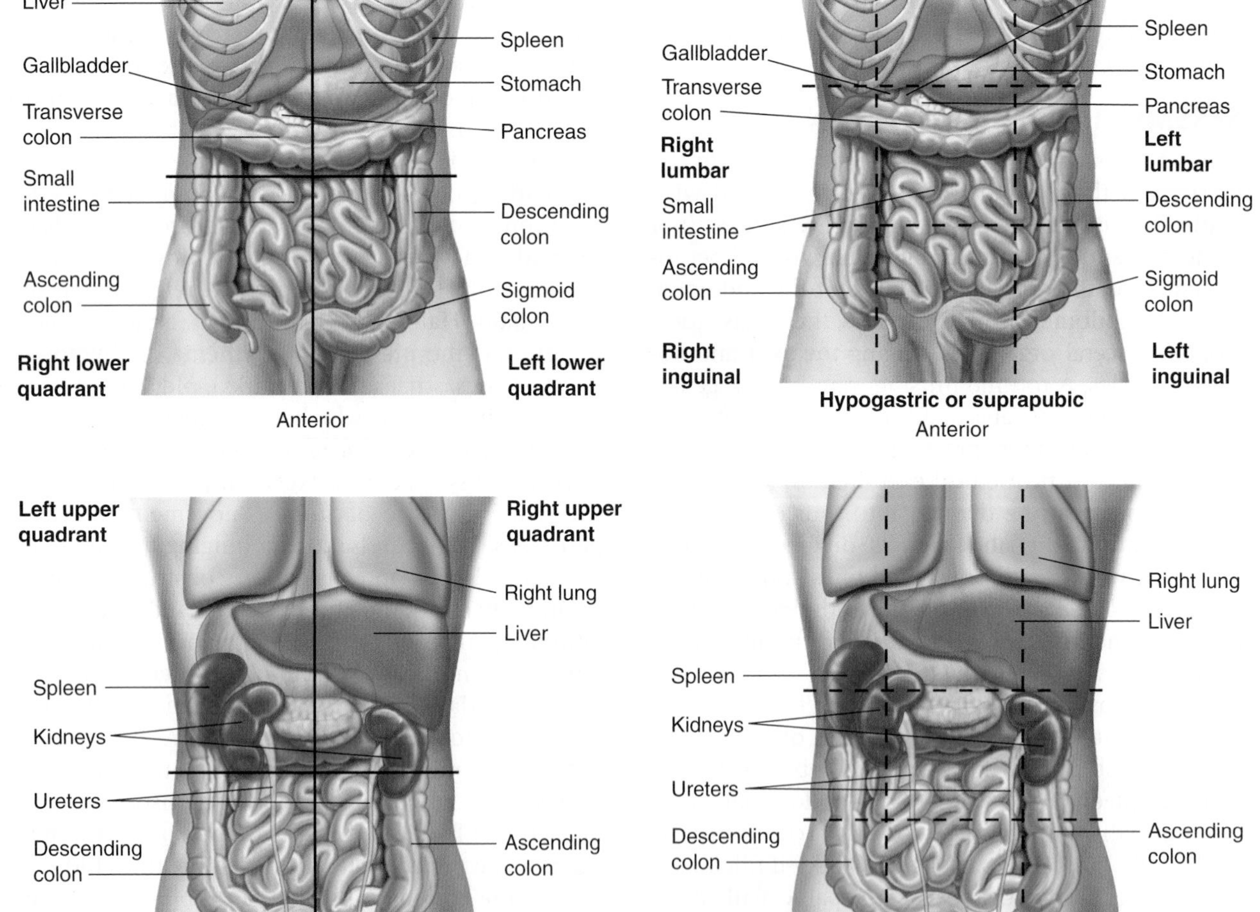

FIGURE 8-40. A, The four abdominal quadrants and their underlying organs. **B,** The nine regions of the abdomen and their underlying organs.

sound of the hyperactive bowel is termed borborygmus. The complete absence of bowel sounds indicates a nonfunctional intestine. You would need to listen for as much as 5 minutes before deciding absolutely that bowel sounds are absent.

Bowel sounds do not necessarily occur in all four quadrants but should occur in at least one, most frequently the RLQ at the ileocecal valve. However, hyperactive bowel sounds may occur in response to inflammation of the bowel, laxative abuse or overuse, and certain spicy foods. Hypoactive bowel sounds or the complete cessation of bowel sounds may occur in response to conditions that decrease the gastric motility, such as pancreatitis with peritonitis, paralytic ileus (absence of peristalsis), or an intestinal obstruction.

Bowel sounds are described as present, absent, increased, decreased, high pitched, tinkling, gurgling, and rushing. The bowel sounds are higher pitched, with rushing and tinkling sounds, when there is increased tension in the bowel such as occurs in intestinal obstruction.

Auscultate for abdominal bruits. Using the bell of the stethoscope, auscultate for vascular sounds. Listen carefully for bruits, hums, and friction rubs in the epigastric area and in all four quadrants over the aortic, renal, iliac, and femoral arteries. Bruits may occur normally in healthy young adults. However, the presence of bruits, venous hums, or friction rubs may indicate an underlying stricture, thrombosis, or aneurysm. If bruits are present, notify the physician and do not further palpate the abdomen, as this may damage an existing aneurysm.

Percussion. Percuss the abdomen using the percussion techniques previously described. Percuss all four quadrants of the abdomen to determine the nature of underlying tissue. Hollow organs, such as the gastric air bubble in the left upper quadrant (LUQ), produce tympanic sounds, and solid or fluid-filled tissue, such as the liver, kidneys, spleen, pancreas, and distended bladder, produce a dull sound. Percussion for the tympanic sound of excess flatus may be useful to the nurse in general practice.

If you need to assess for urinary retention, percussion may be a more useful tool than palpation. Percuss the lower abdominal area, just above the symphysis pubis. A distended bladder may sometimes extend almost to the umbilicus and may deviate to one side; however, it is usually just above the symphysis pubis. Percussion of the bladder produces a dull sound when compared to the sound heard in the surrounding gut.

When you have had more experience and training, you may add the technique to percuss the size and span of the liver. The liver is normally dull to percussion. Begin at a point just below the umbilicus on the right midclavicular line and percuss upward to the lower edge of the liver. Mark the area where the dullness of the lower liver border begins. Next, percuss downward from an area of resonant lung to the upper liver edge. Mark the area where the dullness of the upper liver edge begins. Measure between the two marks with a ruler or tape measure. Record this measure as the liver span. The normal liver span should be from 6 to 12 cm ($2^1/_2$ to 5 inches) in width. An enlarged liver (span greater than 12 cm) may indicate cirrhosis, hepatitis, hepatoma, cyst, abscess (localized collection of pus), or other extrinsic mass or malignancy that impinges on the liver.

Percussion of the kidney is used to detect pain or tenderness. Ask the client to sit or stand, and percuss the posterior costovertebral angle at the scapular line. The kidneys should be dull and painless to percussion. Tenderness of the costovertebral angle may indicate acute pyelonephritis or glomerulonephritis.

Percuss the spleen in the area of the left tenth rib just posterior to the midaxillary line to determine its size by identifying the small oval area of splenic dullness. You may also assess for splenic enlargement by percussing the normally tympanic area in the lowest left interspace on the left anterior axillary line. If this area grows dull when the client takes a deep breath, the spleen may be enlarged.

Palpation. Palpate the abdomen in all four quadrants using the technique of light palpation, compressing the skin to a depth of 1 cm (Figure 8-41). The client should be supine with knees slightly bent to facilitate assessment. Use the finger pads or palmar surface of three or four fingers held together. Move methodically through each quadrant, depressing the abdomen not more than 1 to 2 cm, while using dipping or circular motions. Identify and note the size and location of any abnormalities and areas of increased resistance or tenderness. While distracting the client, return to and further evaluate areas of increased resistance and tenderness to determine whether the resistance is voluntary or involuntary. With the client relaxed, palpate for any abnormal rigidity of the rectus muscles.

Palpate the abdomen in all four quadrants using the technique of deep palpation to a depth of 5 to 8 cm. Use

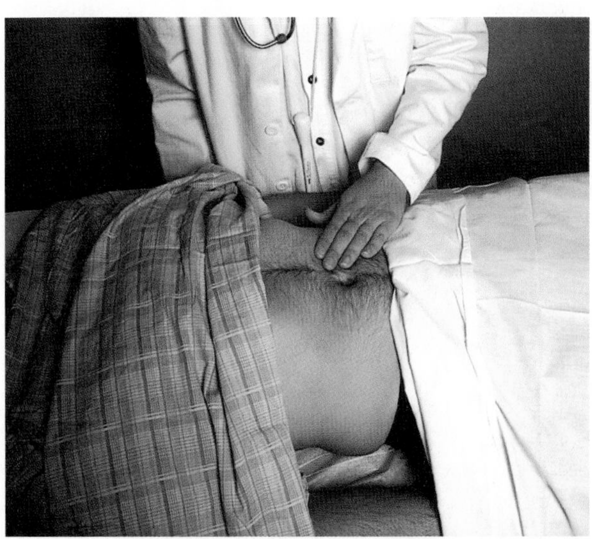

FIGURE 8-41 Light palpation of the abdomen.

bimanual palpation if necessary to overcome the resistance of a large abdomen (Figure 8-42). Using the palmar surface or finger pads of three or four fingers held together, deeply palpate the abdomen, depressing underlying tissue as you move methodically through each quadrant. Move the fingers back and forth over underlying tissue to delineate organs and detect less obvious masses. Deeply palpate for rebound tenderness, which occurs after the sudden release of deep pressure on the abdomen if an acute inflammatory process is present. Proceed cautiously, and avoid deeply palpating any areas of known severe tenderness, pulsating masses, or recent surgical incisions.

Palpate the umbilicus for tenderness, masses, bulges, hernias, lesions, and discharge.

Palpate the liver. Place the left hand under the client's right posterior thorax parallel to and at the level of the eleventh and twelfth ribs. Place the right hand on the client's right upper quadrant (RUQ) over the midclavicular line with fingers pointing toward the head and positioned below the lower edge of liver dullness. Ask the client to take a deep breath while you press inward and upward with the fingers of the right hand. With inspiration, the liver descends lower in the abdomen. Attempt to feel the edge of the liver as it descends (Figure 8-43). Normally the liver edge is not palpable. When palpable, the liver edge should feel smooth, firm, and nontender and have a regular contour. If you can feel the liver edge extending from under the ribs, the liver is enlarged. Abnormalities may indicate the presence of cirrhosis, hepatitis, hepatoma, cyst, abscess, malignancy, or other extrinsic mass compromising the integrity of the liver.

Palpation of the gallbladder is usually not performed on routine physical examinations. Ask the client to take a deep breath, and palpate deep below the liver margin for enlargement of the gallbladder. Because the gallbladder is usually not palpable, a palpable gallbladder is more than likely enlarged. An enlarged, palpable, tender gallbladder may indicate cholelithiasis (gallstones), cholecystitis (infection), malignancy, abscess, or obstruction by an extrinsic mass or malignancy. A positive Murphy's sign (abrupt cessation of inspiration during deep palpation of the gallbladder) is further indication of an acute process.

Palpate the spleen. Place the left hand under the client's left costovertebral angle and the right hand on the abdomen below the left costal margin. Ask the client to take a deep breath while you press the fingertips of the right hand inward. Palpate the edge of the spleen as it descends with inspiration. The spleen is often not palpable; if it is palpable, it may be enlarged.

Palpate the aorta. Use the thumb and forefinger to palpate the aorta by pressing deeply just to the left of the vertical midline of the abdomen. Unless the client is morbidly obese, the aorta will be palpable with strong and regular pulsations. Faint or irregular pulsations may indicate cardiovascular disease. A distinct pulsating mass indicates an aneurysm and should not be further palpated, to avoid possible inadvertent rupture.

Palpate the bladder. Palpate the area above the pubic symphysis if the client's history indicates possible urinary retention. Use only gentle palpation, as pressing on a full bladder is uncomfortable. It may be sufficient to ask if the client experiences the urge to urinate as you gently press on the lower abdomen. You may be able to feel the top of a full bladder because it rises above the symphysis pubis. Sometimes it will deviate to one side or the other. The alert client will be able to describe the sensation of the urge to urinate when you press on a full bladder.

If the abdomen appears distended, palpate for ascites below the right costal margin. Ask the client to lie supine. Have a colleague assist you by pressing his or her hand and forearm firmly along the vertical midline of the abdomen. Place the hands on either side of the client's abdomen. Strike one side of the client's abdomen forcefully with the fingertips and, with the other hand, feel for the rebounding impulse of a fluid wave. Another

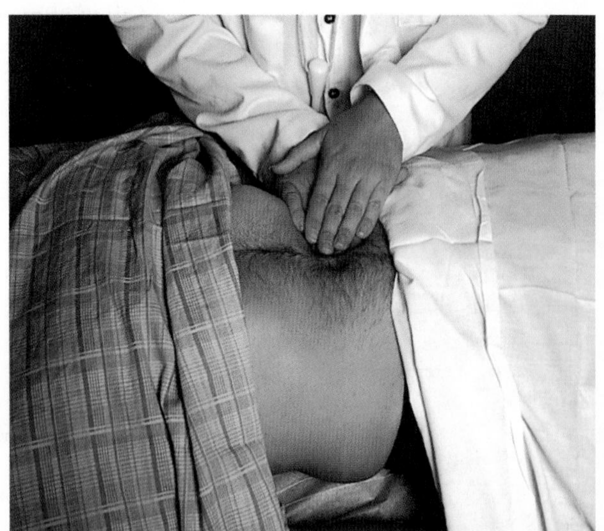

FIGURE 8-42 Deep palpation of the abdomen.

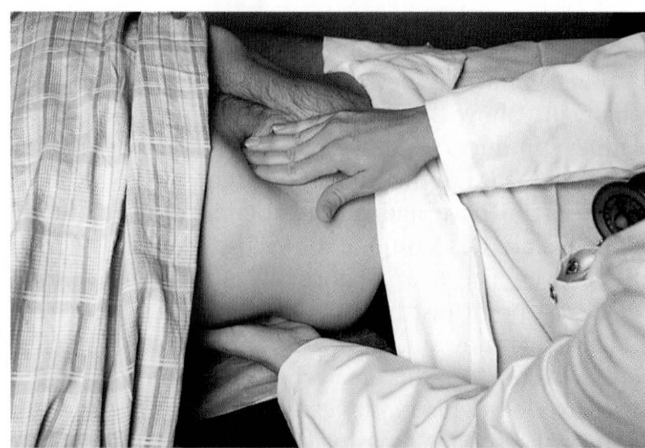

FIGURE 8-43 Palpating the liver.

technique for determining the presence of ascites is to percuss for "shifting dullness" in the abdomen. With the client lying supine, percuss from the midline of the abdomen to the flank. Mark the level of dullness. Ask the client to lie on one side and percuss again over the same area, this time from the flank to the vertical midline of the abdomen (Figure 8-44). Note any change in the level of dullness. If ascites is present, the level of dullness will be slightly higher with the client lying on one side. The presence of ascites may result from a number of medical problems, primarily liver disease, congestive heart failure, or ovarian cancer.

Perform ballottement for any suspected masses. It may be difficult to palpate a suspected mass in a person with marked ascites. In this situation, ballottement may prove helpful in determining the presence of a mass. To perform ballottement for a suspected mass, thrust the fingers of the right hand quickly and firmly into the area of the suspected mass. If the mass is freely mobile, it will initially retreat into the abdomen and then immediately rebound back against the fingers.

ASSESSMENT OF THE MUSCULOSKELETAL SYSTEM

Include the following in your assessment of the musculoskeletal system:

- Assessment of the client's posture, stance, and gait
- Inspection for gross abnormalities
- Inspection of the skin and surrounding tissues of all the bones, joints, and muscle groups
- Inspection of the temporomandibular joint and jaw and assessment of their range of motion
- Inspection of the neck and spine and assessment of their range of motion
- Inspection of the upper extremities and assessment of their range of motion
- Inspection of the lower extremities and assessment of their range of motion

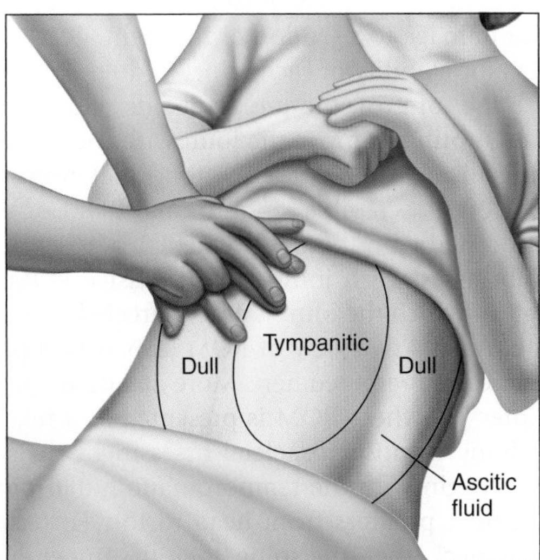

FIGURE 8-44 Assessing for ascites.

Posture, Stance, and Gait. Assess the client's posture, stance, and gait by observing inconspicuously as the client enters the examining room. The client should be able to stand erect with head up, face forward, arms hanging straight at the sides, shoulders and hips parallel, and legs straight with both knees and feet side by side and a few inches apart.

The client's paired extremities should appear grossly symmetrical, and equal in size, shape, and length. Note whether the client appears unable to stand erect or exhibits a hunched, bent, or stooped posture. Note any apparent abnormal curvature of the spine as in kyphosis (humpback) or scoliosis (a lateral bending of the spine). Also note any contractures or deformities of the extremities. Note whether the client is able to stand on both feet comfortably without assistance or support and without any swaying or loss of balance. Note whether the client is able to stand on one foot at a time without difficulty. Note any evidence of uneven distribution of weight, swaying, stumbling, or loss of balance, favoring one foot, standing on the heels, toes, or edges of the feet, uneven depth of footprints, or toes pointing laterally or medially rather than straight ahead.

Assess gait by asking the client to walk across the room. The client should be able to walk with strides that are equal and symmetrical with respect to timing, weight bearing, and distance. The client's steps should consist of a rhythmic planting of first the heel and then the toe of the foot, and the toes should point forward. While walking, the client may sway slightly as he or she shifts weight from foot to foot but should not demonstrate an unsteady gait, loss of balance, shuffling, limping, propulsive walking, veering off in one direction, footdrop, foot lag, or any irregularity in the timing of the stride.

Gross Abnormalities. Inspect for any gross or obvious abnormalities that are easily noticed on an initial head-to-toe inspection (such as amputation, congenital deformities, contractures, paralysis, and so on). Inspect and palpate the skin and surrounding tissues of all the bones, joints, and muscle groups (refer to Assessment of the Skin, Hair, and Nails, earlier). Inspect for color, temperature, swelling, edema, skinfolds, and lesions. Note any abnormalities.

Muscle Tone and Strength. Assess all muscle groups for bilateral symmetry, tone, and strength. Bilateral muscle groups, or those muscles identically paired, as in the left and right biceps, should be symmetrical in size, shape, contour, position, and alignment of like joints. Note any variances.

Assess all muscle groups for muscle tone. You can assess muscle tone and strength at the same time as ROM by noting the degree of resistance felt on passive ROM (Figure 8-45). Normally a slight resistance is felt.

Assess muscle strength by asking the client to pull away from or push against an opposing force that you impose. Repeat these same maneuvers with the contralateral joint,

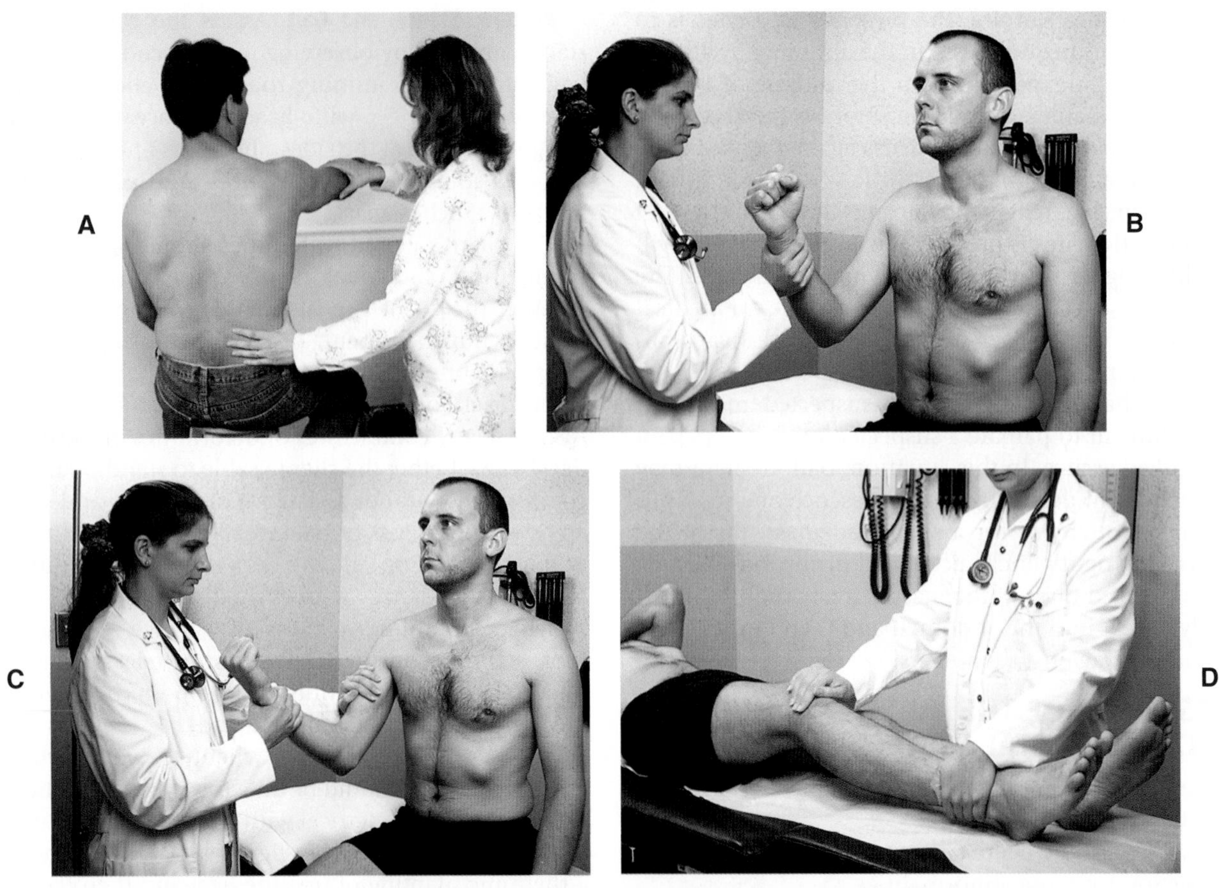

FIGURE 8-45 Assessing for muscle tone and strength. **A,** Ask the client to flex his shoulder muscle against your hand as you apply resistance. **B,** Ask the client to extend his elbow as you apply resistance. **C,** Ask the client to flex his elbow as you apply resistance. **D,** Ask the client to raise his knee as you apply resistance.

and assess bilateral muscle strength. Usually a particular muscle group has normal tone if slight resistance is demonstrated against passive ROM exercises. A hypertonic muscle exhibits increased resistance to passive ROM exercises. A hypotonic muscle presents as a boggy, flat, flabby, or flaccid muscle that offers little or no resistance against passive ROM exercises.

Assess the strength of all muscle groups. Each muscle group should be relatively equal to the contralateral muscle group. The dominant hand or arm may normally be slightly stronger. Measure (preferably with a tape measure) the size (diameter) of any muscle or muscle group that demonstrates weakness. A smaller size of a particular muscle or muscle group may indicate atrophy, and an unusually large muscle may indicate hypertrophy.

Bilateral Bones and Joints. Assess bones and joints bilaterally for symmetry with respect to size, shape, position, alignment, stability, and ROM. Asymmetry may be the result of congenital anomalies, arthritis, bony tumors, fractures, dislocations, adhesions, or surgery. Malalignment may be secondary to fracture dislocation, congenital anomalies, or surgical procedures. The joints should be able to be moved passively in all directions and degrees expected for the specific groups. There should be no abnormal movements or sounds produced by movement or manipulation of the joints. Any pain or stiffness elicited upon movement of a joint that has no associated fracture or dislocation usually indicates arthritis or damage to a tendon or ligament.

Assess the stability of each joint. To do this, grasp and stabilize the joint on the proximal side with one hand while attempting to move the joint with the other hand from the distal end. Note any abnormal movements, unusual sounds, crepitus, or abnormal ROM or tenderness associated with these movements.

Finally, assess each joint for full passive ROM. Note the angle at which the joint is able to freely bend in each position. A brief overview of ROM as part of a physical examination is presented here. More details are provided in Chapter 32, where ROM is presented as a treatment. When doing a musculoskeletal assessment, it is often easiest to begin with the temporomandibular joint and jaw and then progress from head to toe. For example: assess the neck, then the spine, then the upper extremities, and then the lower extremities.

Jaw and Temporomandibular Joint. Inspect and palpate the jaw and the TMJ. Simultaneously place two or three fingertips of each hand in the depression over the two TMJs. Ask the client to open widely and close his or her mouth two or three times while your fingertips are in place. Palpate for any unusual clicking sounds, sliding, or "catching" of the joint. With the client's mouth as wide open as possible, the normal distance between the top and bottom front teeth is 3 to 6 cm. Ask the client to slide the lower jaw forward and from side to side. The lower teeth should be able to be moved beyond and overlap the upper teeth. Normal side- to-side movement is 1 to 2 cm. Note any misalignment of the upper jaw and lower jaw, inability to move the lower jaw sideways or forward, inability to open or close the jaw, or pain on mastication or movement of the jaw.

Neck, Cervical Spine, Thoracic Spine, and Lumbar Spine. Inspect and palpate the neck, cervical spine, thoracic spine, and lumbar spine, with the client first standing erect and then bending over at the waist. Inspect from directly behind the client and again from the side. Normally the cervical spine is concave, the thoracic spine convex, and the lumbar spine concave. Note any abnormal curvatures, palpable masses, compression fractures, lesions, or pain along the spine. An abnormal curvature of the spine may be a result of kyphosis (an accentuated posterior curvature of the thoracic spine), sway back or lordosis (an accentuated lumbar curvature), scoliosis (a lateral curvature of the spine), ankylosing spondylitis (evidenced by persistence of the lumbar concavity and failure of the spinous processes to separate when the client bends over at the waist), or spondylolisthesis (a forward slipping and fusing of the vertebrae).

Assess the ROM of the neck and spine. Assess flexion by asking the client to touch the chin to the chest. Assess hyperextension by asking the client to bend the head backward with the chin pointing up toward the ceiling. Assess rotation by asking the client to turn the head as far as possible to the left and then to the right with the ears facing the front and back. Assess lateral bending by asking the client to bend the head laterally, attempting to touch the ear to the shoulder. The normal ROM for flexion is 70 to 90 degrees; for hyperextension, 55 degrees; for rotation, 70 degrees; and for lateral bending, 35 degrees.

Assess the ROM of the spine. To assess flexion, ask the client to bend forward at the waist; to assess extension, ask the client to bend backward at the waist. To assess rotation, ask the client to stand with feet planted and toes pointed forward and attempt to rotate the upper torso so that the shoulders attempt to face backward. To assess lateral bending, ask the client to bend laterally at the waist with shoulders pointing toward the floor or feet. Normal ROM for flexion is 75 degrees; for extension, 30 degrees; for rotation, 30 degrees; and for lateral bending, 35 degrees.

Upper and Lower Extremities. After the assessment of the neck and spine, assess the upper and then the lower extremities. Work your way down from top to bottom, assessing first the right side and then the left side. For example, assess the right and then the left shoulder, then move to the elbows, then the wrists, then the fingers, then the hips, then the knees, then the ankles, and then the toes. After inspection and palpation of each joint and muscle group, assess each for ROM and muscle strength.

Shoulders. Assess the shoulders for ROM and muscle strength, starting from the anatomical position with the arms at the side. Assess flexion by asking the client to lift the arm forward and above the head until the arm is straight and horizontal to the floor, then move the arm backward toward the spine. Assess extension from the anatomical position by moving the arm backward with the arm straight. Assess horizontal extension by asking the client to abduct the arm to a point horizontal to the floor and then bring the arm back to the anatomical position and across the chest.

To assess abduction, lift the arm away from the body straight up above the head. To assess adduction, adduct the arm toward the midline of the trunk. Note any pain, which may be secondary to arthritis, inflammation, infection, bursitis, tendinitis, bony spurs, calcific deposits, masses, fractures, and dislocations. A frozen shoulder, evidenced by the inability of the client to abduct the arm without characteristic "shrugging" suggests a rupture of the supraspinal tendon or rotator cuff injury. Normal ROM for the shoulders can be expected to be 180 degrees for flexion, 130 degrees for horizontal flexion, 60 degrees for extension, 45 degrees for horizontal extension, 180 degrees for abduction, and 45 degrees for adduction.

Elbows. Assess the ROM for the elbows. Assess flexion by asking the client to bend the lower arm up toward the biceps. Assess extension by asking the client to open his or her arm to a fully extended resting position. Assess hyperextension by asking the client to extend his or her arm beyond the normal resting position. Assess supination by asking the client to turn the lower arm so that the front faces upward. Assess pronation by asking the client to turn the lower arm so that the front faces downward. Normal ROM for the elbows is expected to be 150 degrees for flexion, 150 degrees for extension, 0 to 10 degrees for hyperextension, 90 degrees for supination, and 90 degrees for pronation.

Wrists. Assess the ROM for the wrists. Assess flexion by asking the client to flex the wrist toward the lower arm. Assess extension by asking the client to extend the wrist backward. Assess radial deviation by asking the client to deviate the wrist toward the radius. Assess ulnar deviation by asking the client to deviate the wrist toward the ulna. Normal ROM for the wrists is expected to be 80 to 90 degrees for flexion, 70 degrees for extension, 20 degrees for radial deviation, and 30 to 50 degrees for ulnar deviation.

Fingers. Assess the ROM for the fingers. Assess flexion by asking the client to close his or her fingers into a fist. Assess extension by asking the client to fully open his or her fingers. Assess abduction by asking the client to spread his or her fingers apart. Assess adduction by asking the client to cross the fingers together so that they touch and overlap. Assess opposition by asking the client to touch each finger with the thumb of the same hand. Normal ROM for the fingers is expected to be 80 to 100 degrees for flexion, 0 to 45 degrees for extension, and 20 degrees for abduction. Normal adduction is demonstrated if the client is able to cross his or her fingers. Normal opposition is demonstrated if the client is able to touch each finger to the thumb of the same hand.

Hips. Assess the ROM of the hips. Assess flexion with both a straight knee and a bent knee. Ask the client to first raise his or her leg straight up without bending the knee and then to raise it again with the knee bent. Assess extension by asking the client to lie prone and then extend the leg backward. Assess abduction by asking the client to abduct a partially flexed leg outward. Assess adduction by asking the client to adduct a partially flexed leg inward. Assess internal rotation by asking the client to flex the knee and swing the foot toward the midline. Assess external rotation by asking the client to flex the knee and swing the foot away from the midline. Normal ROM for the hips is expected to be 90 degrees for straight-knee flexion, 110 to 120 degrees for bent-knee flexion, 30 degrees for extension, 45 to 50 degrees for abduction, 20 to 30 degrees for adduction, 35 to 40 degrees for internal rotation, and 45 degrees for external rotation.

Knees. Assess the ROM of the knees. Assess flexion by asking the client to fully bend the knee so that the posterior calf and posterior thigh are nearly touching. Assess hyperextension by asking the client to extend the knee beyond the normal point of extension. Assess internal rotation of the hip by asking the client to rotate the knee and lower leg toward the midline. Assess external rotation of the hip by asking the client to rotate the knee and lower leg away from the midline. Normal ROM is expected to be 130 degrees for flexion, 15 degrees for hyperextension, and 10 degrees for internal rotation.

Ankles. Assess the ROM of the ankles. Assess dorsiflexion by asking the client to bend the ankle of the foot so that the toes point toward the head. Assess plantar flexion by asking the client to bend the foot downward with the toes pointing downward. Assess eversion by asking the client to turn the foot away from the midline. Assess inversion by asking the client to turn the foot toward the midline. Normal ROM is expected to be 20 degrees for dorsiflexion, 45 degrees for plantar flexion, 20 degrees for eversion, and 30 degrees for inversion.

Toes. Assess the ROM of the toes. Assess flexion by asking the client to curl the toes under the foot. Assess extension by asking the client to lift the toes to point upward. Assess abduction by asking the client to spread the toes apart. Normal ROM is expected to be 35 to 60 degrees for flexion, 0 to 90 degrees for extension (depending on the specific joint), variable capability for abduction, and inability to adduct the toes.

Reflexes. A muscular reflex is an involuntary response to a stimulus in which the sensory nerve carries the message to the spinal cord and directly back to cause a contraction in a muscle. All muscles contract reflexively when stimulated. However, only a few reflexes are tested clinically as indicators of motor function (Figure 8-46).

Reflexes are classified as superficial and deep tendon reflexes. Superficial reflexes are elicited by stroking or stimulating the skin. Deep tendon reflexes are elicited by stretching a tendon by tapping with a percussion hammer. Testing reflexes requires sensitivity to slight contractions of muscles. Reflexes are classified as 0, no response; 1+, slightly diminished; 2+, normal; 3+, brisker than normal; and 4+, hyperactive. This scale is subjective, and the ratings may vary between examiners and with experience.

The biceps, triceps, and brachioradialis reflexes provide information about the function of the nerves of the cervical spine (C5 to C8). All three are deep tendon reflexes. To test the biceps reflex, have the client partially flex the elbow and rest the arm on his or her own thigh or on your forearm. Place your thumb in the antecubital space over the biceps tendon. Tap your thumb with the percussion hammer. A positive response is slight movement of the forearm with contraction of the biceps muscle.

To test the triceps reflex, flex the client's arm at the elbow and hold it suspended at a right angle to the shoulder. The arm should be relaxed with the forearm hanging freely. Directly tap the triceps tendon just above the elbow. The forearm should extend slightly. Alternatively, you may have the client hold the forearm across the chest, flexed 90 degrees at the elbow.

To test the brachioradialis reflex, have the client rest the forearm on his or her thigh. Grasp the thumb to suspend the forearm in a relaxed position. Tap the forearm directly on the lateral aspect of the radial bone 2 to 3 cm above the joint. The forearm should flex slightly, turning toward the supinated position.

In the lower extremity, the knee jerk, Achilles, and plantar reflexes are tested. The knee jerk or patellar reflex tests function of L1, L2, and L3 nerves. The Achilles reflex tests function of S1 and S2 nerves. These are deep tendon reflexes. To test the patellar reflex, have the client sit on a table or bed from which the foot and lower leg can hang freely. Strike the tendon directly below the patella (kneecap). The lower leg should extend.

To test the Achilles reflex, position the person supine with the hip externally rotated and the knee flexed. Hold the foot in a relaxed dorsiflexed position and strike the Achilles tendon with the percussion hammer. You should feel the foot plantar flex against your hand.

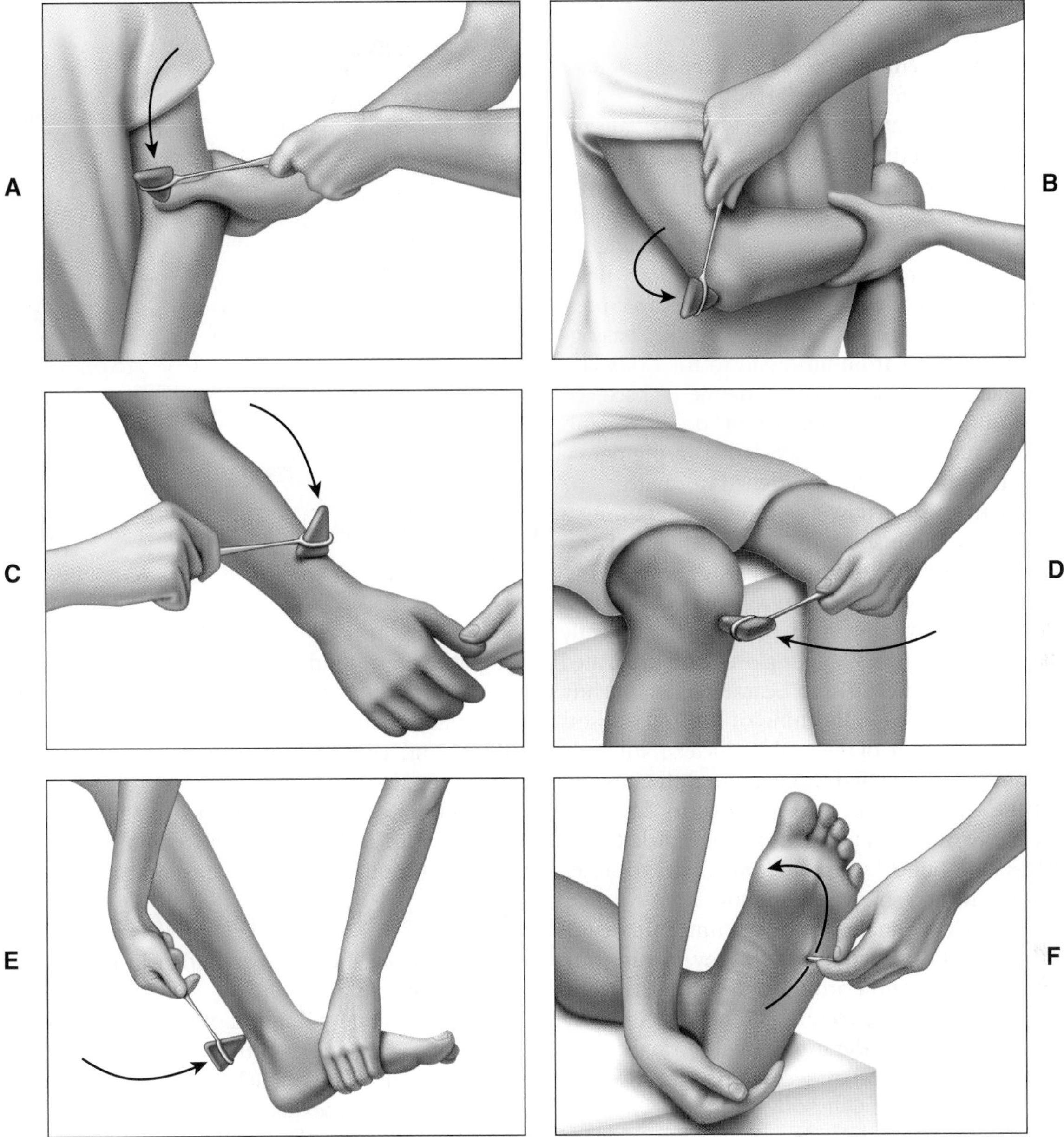

FIGURE 8-46 Assessing reflexes: biceps reflex **(A)**, triceps reflex **(B)**, brachioradialis reflex **(C)**, patellar reflex **(D)**, Achilles reflex **(E)**, and plantar (Babinski) reflex **(F)**.

The plantar, or Babinski, reflex is a superficial reflex that is present in the first 8 to 10 months of life, then disappears and should be absent in adults. This reflex should be tested with the client in a relaxed supine position. With a blunt instrument, apply firm pressure and draw a line from the heel along the lateral aspect of the sole of the foot and across the footpad under the toes. With a positive response (the Babinski sign), the toes spread outward and the big toe moves upward. This finding in an adult indicates upper motor neuron disease of the pyramidal tract. In a normal adult, the toes curl toward the sole of the feet. A positive response is normal in an infant until neurologically ready to begin walking.

ASSESSMENT OF THE ANUS, RECTUM, AND PROSTATE

The following should be included in the assessment of the anus, rectum, and prostate:

- Inspection and palpation of perianal tissue and perineum
- Inspection for the appearance of protrusions of masses with straining
- Digital examination to palpate the anus, rectum, and prostate
- Assessment of the tone and musculature of the anal sphincter
- Palpation of the muscular anal ring and rectum

- Palpation for high masses
- Palpation of the prostate in men
- Palpation of the uterus and cervix in women
- Examination of the fecal material

Perianal Tissue and Perineum. Inspect and palpate the perianal tissue and perineum. Position the client (male or female) on his or her side in the *Sims'* position with knees slightly flexed. Gently retract the buttocks with your gloved hand, and inspect the anal and perianal tissue. Note color, texture, lesions, masses, prolapse, hemorrhoids, erythema, ecchymosis, skin breakdown, pressure ulcers, fistulas (an abnormal, tubelike passage between two organs or from an organ to the body surface), sinus tracts (a recess, cavity, or channel), abscesses, masses, lesions, and any evidence of poor hygiene. Perianal tissue may appear slightly darker in pigmentation, and anal tissue is slightly reddened normally.

Ask the client to bear down as though attempting a bowel movement, and inspect for the appearance of protrusions, masses, hemorrhoids, prolapse, or polyps.

Digital Rectal Examination. Perform a digital examination to palpate the anus, rectum, and prostate. Press gently against the anal sphincter with your gloved and lubricated index finger pad. Ask the client to bear down, and gently press your fingertip into the opening of the anus. Assess the tone and musculature of the anal sphincter. (Normally the anal sphincter will tighten firmly around the inserted finger and the client may express the urge to defecate.) Palpate the entire surface of the anal sphincter. Ask the client to tighten the buttocks around your finger to allow assessment of tone and strength of the sphincter.

Palpate the musculoanal ring and rectum. Palpate the entire surface of the musculoanal ring by turning the finger in a circular motion around its own axis. Then, move further inward to the rectum and repeat. Note any palpable lesions, masses, lacerations, or abnormalities or a palpable rectal shelf (often secondary to peritoneal metastatic disease).

Palpate for high masses. With a gloved finger as far into the rectum as possible, ask the client to bear down and palpate for any descending masses. Note the presence of any high mass descending against the inserted fingertip when the client bears down.

Palpate the prostate in men (only after the onset of puberty). Turn the finger to palpate the anterior rectal wall. Gently palpate the prostate (Figure 8-47). Try to identify the two lateral lobes and the median sulcus. Normally the prostate feels rubbery and smooth to palpation, and less than 1 cm of the prostate tissue is palpable protruding into the rectal wall. Note any enlargement, irregularity in shape, palpable mass, tenderness, or softening (bogginess).

Palpate the uterus and cervix in women. Turn the finger to palpate the anterior rectal wall. Gently palpate the uterus and cervix. Normally they feel rubbery and smooth. Note any enlargement, irregularity in shape, palpable mass, tenderness, or softening (bogginess).

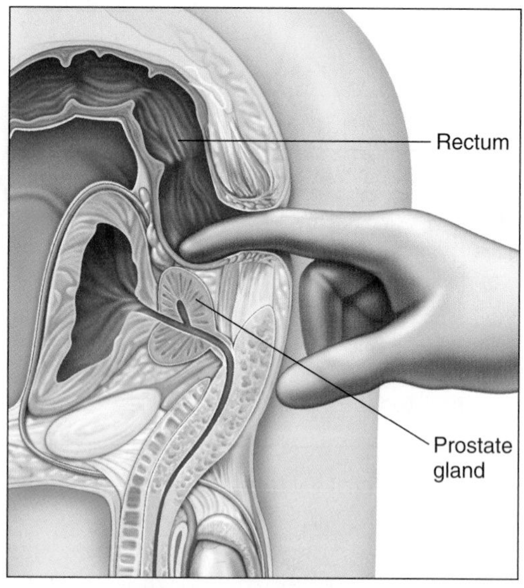

FIGURE 8-47 Palpating the prostate gland through the anterior wall of the rectum.

Withdraw the gloved finger, and examine the fecal material on the glove for color (brown, gray, yellow, black) and consistency (watery, loose, greasy, formed, hard, impacted). Using a Hemoccult card, test the fecal material for occult blood. Normally the stool should appear brown, feel formed, and contain no evidence of frank or occult blood.

ASSESSMENT OF THE FEMALE GENITALIA

The following should be included in the assessment of the female genitalia:

- Inspection and palpation of the vulva for lesions, masses, and abnormalities
- Inspection of the pubic hair for infestations, density of growth, and sexual maturity
- Inspection and palpation of the labia majora for lesions, masses, inflammation, swelling, and abnormalities
- Inspection of the labia minora
- Inspection of the clitoris
- Inspection of the urethral meatus and Skene's glands
- Inspection of the hymen and vaginal introitus
- Inspection of Bartholin's glands
- Inspection of the cervix
- Inspection of the vaginal wall
- Palpation of the cervix
- Palpation of the ovaries and fallopian tubes
- Palpation of the uterus

External Genitalia. Prepare the client for the examination. Ask the client to urinate and empty her bladder. Have her undress from the waist down and assume a semirecumbent position on the examining table with her knees and thighs draped and her feet in the stirrups. Ask the client to rest her hands on her waist and to relax her knees and let them fall to the side as far as possible.

Wear gloves to inspect and palpate the vulva for lesions, masses, and abnormalities. Inform the client before touching, and touch the client's thigh initially to avoid startling her, then proceed with the examination, parting the pubic hair as necessary to facilitate thorough examination. Palpate any noticeable masses, lesions, swelling, or abnormalities. Normally the skin is smooth, warm, and pink in light-skinned people and olive to brown in dark-skinned people, and it may be lighter in color than the rest of the body because of lack of exposure to sun. Note any hematomas, ecchymosis, irregular pigment, macules, papules, wheals, vesicles, ulcers, or other rashes.

Inspect the pubic hair for density of growth and sexual maturity (Tanner staging). Part the pubic hair to look for infestations of pubic lice often found at the base or root of the pubic hair. Also inspect for nits (tiny teardrop-shaped white or gray eggs) adhering to the hair stalks. Assess the sexual maturity of the client.

Inspect and palpate the labia majora and labia minora for lesions, masses, inflammation, swelling, and abnormalities. It may be necessary to grasp the labia majora between two fingers to accomplish a thorough examination. Part the labia majora with gloved fingers to inspect the labia minora. Note and thoroughly palpate any observed lesions or abnormalities.

Inspect the clitoris for position, size, lesions, masses, and abnormalities. The clitoris can be found between the anterior junction of the labia majora and the labia minora. Normally the clitoris is a small pink nodular form that does not exceed 0.5 cm in width and 2 cm in length. Separate the labia minora, and locate the urethral meatus, a small orifice just below the anterior junction of the labia minora. Inspect for lesions, prolapse, polyps, fistulas, edema or tenderness, masses, or discharge. If there is inflammation or if urethritis is suspected, milk the urethra gently by inserting a gloved finger into the vagina and stroking its anterior wall in a downward motion toward you. Culture any discharge for gonorrhea, chlamydia, and bacteria. Perform a potassium hydroxide and wet preparation to discern the presence of yeast and *Trichomonas,* respectively.

Inspect the hymen and vaginal introitus. The hymen is usually intact in children and sexually inexperienced women; however, usually only remnants of the hymen remain in sexually active women. If the hymen is edematous, torn, or absent in small children, sexual abuse must be considered as a possible cause.

With the labia separated by gloved fingers, inspect the vaginal introitus or vaginal opening. Ask the client to bear down to allow the support of the vaginal outlet to be evaluated. Observe and note any abnormal swelling or bulging. The introitus is usually open and unobstructed, but in older, multiparous women it is not uncommon to observe a cystocele (a bulging mass arising from the anterior wall of the vagina) or a rectocele (a bulging mass arising from the posterior vaginal floor). Cystoceles and rectoceles are caused by inadequate support of the vaginal outlet. A large, smooth, pink, protruding mass may actually be a uterine prolapse with the cervix visible in the vaginal canal. Uterine prolapse can be staged as first degree, second degree, or third degree depending on the severity of drop in the vaginal vault. In first-degree prolapse, the cervix is palpated slightly lower than usual in the vaginal vault; in second-degree prolapse, the cervix can be palpated halfway down the vaginal vault; and in third-degree prolapse, the cervix is at the introitus or sometimes even visibly protruding from the vaginal opening.

Inspect the Bartholin's glands located bilaterally at the base of the vaginal opening. The Bartholin's glands are normally not visible other than as a small pinpoint duct opening inside the labia. Palpate the glands between a gloved index finger and thumb by placing one finger inside the vaginal opening and one on the outside of the labia majora. Normally the Bartholin's glands are nontender and not palpable. Note any pain, swelling, masses, or discharge. A large, nontender, unilateral mass may be a Bartholin's cyst. A large, tender, fluctuant, unilateral or bilateral mass may be a Bartholin's abscess. The abscess may have spontaneously ruptured, or remained exquisitely tender and fluctuant. Gently compress the glands between two gloved fingers and culture any discharge exuding from the duct openings for gonorrhea, chlamydia, and bacteria.

Internal Genitalia. After you have completed the examination of the external genitalia, prepare to perform the speculum examination of the internal genitalia. Figure 8-48 illustrates a vaginal speculum used to hold the vagina open to visualize the cervix. Lubricate your gloved fingers and speculum with warm water. Water is used as the lubricant to prevent contamination when a smear for cytology is part of the examination. Insert one or two fingers into the vaginal opening and press downward on the posterior aspect to further open the introitus and facilitate the insertion of the speculum. Insert the closed speculum, holding it so that the blade width is in a vertical position. Gently push in a downward and sloping fashion, while at the same time rotating the blade so that the width is now in a horizontal position. Follow the vaginal canal to the cervix. Open the speculum, and manipulate the cervix into position. Observe the cervix, obtain specimens for cytology, and culture any discharge.

The cervical os appears as a small rounded opening within a central depression on the cervix in nulliparous women. It takes on a more "fish-mouthed" appearance in multiparous women. There are usually no lesions, masses, erythema, or cervical motion tenderness. Usually

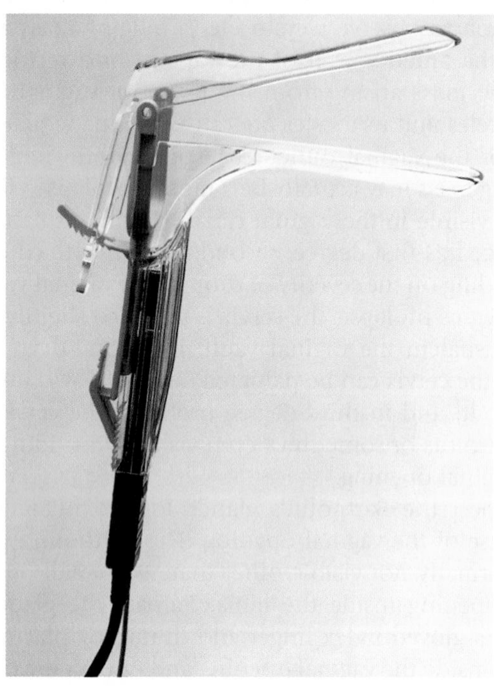

FIGURE 8-48 A vaginal speculum. (Courtesy Welch Allyn, Inc., Skaneateles Falls, NY.)

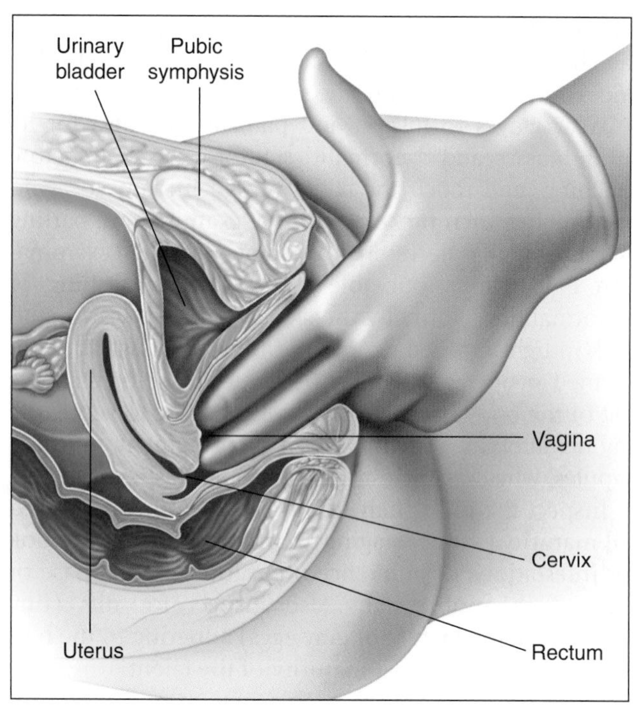

FIGURE 8-49 Palpating the uterus and cervix.

the cervix appears as a smooth, rounded, pink, moist, sometimes glistening, and firm mass. Although the cervix usually remains about 1 inch in diameter, it enlarges, softens, and becomes bluish-tinged normally in pregnancy and may appear pale during menopause.

The Papanicolaou smear, or Pap smear, is a cytology test to screen for cervical cancer. The method of collecting the specimen is dependent on the product used for testing. A Pap smear often is not performed during the menstrual period or if the client has infectious discharge. Ideally the woman should not have intercourse, douche, or use vaginal products 24 hours before the test.

Unclamp the speculum, and hold it open as you withdraw it slowly from the vaginal canal. As you withdraw the speculum, inspect the walls of the vaginal canal. Use a gooseneck lamp or penlight to better illuminate the canal.

Normally you will see rugae with thin, clear or cloudy, odorless secretions. Note any abnormal findings of masses, lesions, vesicles, papules, warts, or thick, foul-smelling discharge. Palpate the vaginal wall by inserting the lubricated and gloved middle and index finger of the right hand into the vagina (Figure 8-49). Palpate the anterior, posterior, and lateral walls of the vaginal canal.

Palpate the cervix with the tips of your fingers. Note the position, shape, consistency, and mobility of the cervix. Gently move the cervix from side to side and test for cervical motion tenderness, which can be a telltale sign of a pelvic inflammatory disease or other acute pelvic process. Attempt to admit one fingertip into the cervical os to determine its patency. Usually the cervical os remains closed and offers tight resistance. If the os admits one fingertip, or offers no resistance, it is considered open and may indicate a threatened or inevitable abortion or incompetent cervix.

Palpate the ovaries and fallopian tubes. Place the left hand on the client's abdomen about halfway between the umbilicus and the symphysis pubis. Push inward and downward toward the symphysis pubis while at the same time pushing upward on the vaginal mucosa lateral to the cervix with the fingers of the right hand. Try to palpate the small almond-shaped ovary on each side.

Palpate the uterus with your hands positioned as just described. Push downward toward the symphysis pubis with the left hand while pushing upward on the cervix with the fingers of the right hand. Attempt to grasp the uterus between the fingers of your two hands. Note the position, size, shape, consistency, and mobility of the uterus. Note also whether the uterus is tender. The fundus will not be palpable above the symphysis pubis. If it is enlarged, soft, or tender, it may indicate pregnancy, fibroids, hydatidiform mole, or the presence of a mass.

ASSESSMENT OF THE MALE GENITALIA

The following should be included in the assessment of male genitalia:

- Assessment of sexual maturity
- Assessment of the prepuce or foreskin
- Assessment of the glans penis
- Assessment of the urethral meatus

- Assessment of the penile shaft
- Assessment of the scrotum and testes
- Assessment of the presence of hernias

Sexual Maturity. Assess the external genitalia for sexual maturity (see Chapter 46). Note the distribution and quantity of pubic hair. Pubic hair is absent in infants and children and is thick, extending onto the thighs, in adults. The density of growth and distribution of hair should be consistent with that expected for the client's age-group. An abnormal quantity or distribution may indicate hormonal imbalances, chronic disease, dermatitis, or a response to medications. Hair loss may be symmetrical and nonscarring, or asymmetrical and scarring.

Penis. Note the shape and size of the penis. The penis attains adult size and shape after puberty. Note the size, color, and texture of the scrotum. The scrotum darkens and develops rugae after puberty. Assess the sexual maturity using Tanner's Sexual Maturity Rating (SMR) (see Chapter 46).

Part the pubic hair as necessary to facilitate thorough examination of the skin. Inspect and palpate the skin for color, temperature, lesions, rashes, masses, excoriations, lacerations, abnormalities, infestations, or lack of hygiene. Gently move and manipulate the penis and scrotum to allow visualization of their posterior sides. Palpate thoroughly and note the type and location of any lesions, macules, papules, ulcers, vesicles, rashes, lacerations, excoriations, or masses. Hot, red skin may indicate cellulitis, infection, or inflammation. The presence of lesions may indicate dermatitis or sexually transmitted disease.

Inspect and palpate the prepuce and foreskin in uncircumcised males. Note any lesions, swelling, edema, lacerations, erythema, or ecchymosis. Gently retract the foreskin and inspect. Smegma, a whitish, pasty exudate, may be present normally. Pay particular attention to the junction between the prepuce and the glans, because this is a common site for lesions of sexually transmitted diseases. Any difficulty in retracting or inability to retract the foreskin (phimosis) or difficulty in replacing or inability to replace a retracted foreskin (paraphimosis) is abnormal and should be noted and further evaluated.

Inspect and palpate the full surface of the glans. The glans normally appears moist and pink in uncircumcised males. Note the presence and exact location of any lesions, masses, swelling, edema, abnormalities, erythema, ecchymosis, or balanitis (inflammation of the glans with marked erythema and edema).

Note the location of the urinary meatus. It normally appears as a pink slitlike opening located in the center of the glans. Check for hypospadias, congenital displacement of the urethral meatus (usually found on the posterior side of the glans or penile shaft). Note the location and type of any lesions or abnormalities. Inspect for urethral prolapse, a perceivable small rosette of prolapsed membranes protruding from the meatus. Inspect also for fissures and fistulas. Open the meatus slightly by gently compressing the glans between your thumb and finger (or allow the client to do this). Inspect the color of the lining of the meatus and culture and describe any obvious discharge (e.g., yellow, white, clear, blood tinged), which may well indicate the presence of a urethritis. Discharge should be cultured for gonorrhea, chlamydia, and bacteria, and a potassium hydroxide and wet preparation should be performed at this time to assess for the presence of yeast and *Trichomonas,* respectively. If the client has complained of discharge and none is seen, you may need to gently "milk" the shaft of the penis to produce a bead of discharge for culture.

Inspect and palpate the shaft of the penis. Gently manipulate and lift the penis to allow inspection and palpation of the entire surface area. Note the exact location and type of lesions, masses, or abnormalities. Palpate for induration (hardness) and tenderness along the ventral surface of the penis. In infants and children, this may be omitted. Tenderness or induration along the ventral surface may indicate urethral stricture and periurethral inflammation, or carcinoma.

Scrotum and Testes. Inspect and palpate the scrotum and testes. Gently palpate the testicles by grasping them between your thumb and forefinger. Palpate the epididymis, spermatic cord, and vas deferens. Note any lesions, masses, tenderness, or enlargement. Transilluminate the scrotum and testicle if a mass is suspected or an enlargement is observed. A fluid-filled mass will illuminate well, whereas a mass filled with blood, pus, or solid tissue will not.

Normally the scrotum consists of coarse, loose, rugate skin of slightly darker pigmentation than the rest of the body. The left testicle is normally lower than the right. When compressed gently between your two fingers, the testes are sensitive but not painful and should not feel much greater than 1 inch in diameter. Check for undescended testicles (cryptorchidism) and a poorly developed scrotum on one or both sides. Note any nontender swelling or masses such as hydrocele or spermatocele (fluid-filled cysts of the tunica vaginalis and epididymis, respectively). Both hydroceles and spermatoceles transilluminate when a penlight is held up against the scrotal sac.

Palpate for testicular cancer, a hard, palpable, nontender nodule usually favoring the anterior side of the testes. Note any tender swelling or mass. This may be caused by scrotal edema (from congestive heart failure, chronic renal failure, or nephrotic syndrome), epididymitis (an acute bacterial infection of the epididymis), or testicular torsion (a painful swelling caused by torsion or twisting of the spermatic cord).

Palpate the vas deferens and spermatic cord. Note any thickening, which may occur with chronic infections and tuberculosis. Note the presence of a varicocele, a

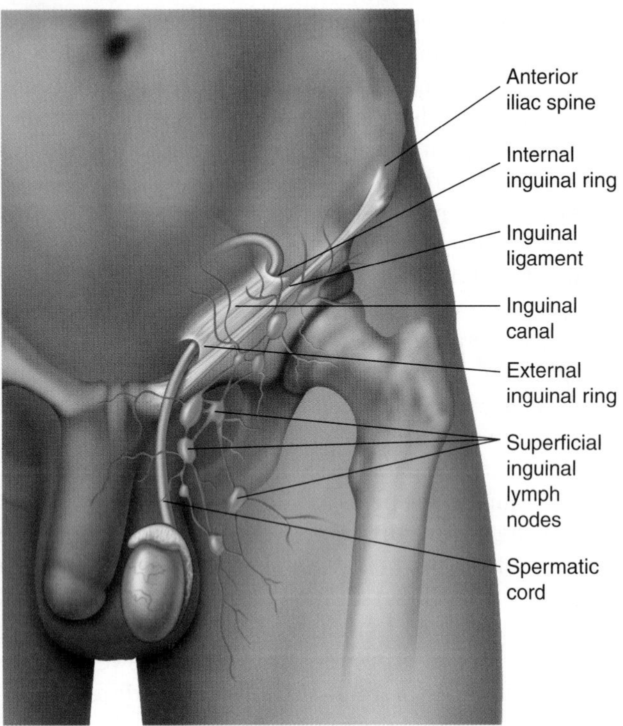

FIGURE 8-50 Structures of the inguinal area.

string of beadlike nodules or varicosities (which feel characteristically like a "bag of worms"), palpated usually on the left side.

Inguinal Canal. Inspect and palpate the inguinal canal for hernias. Figure 8-50 illustrates the structures of the inguinal area. Ask the client to stand and bear down as though having a bowel movement. Inspect the inguinal areas and scrotum for any bulging or masses. With one finger, press inward on the loose skin at a low point on the scrotum. Follow the spermatic cord upward by invaginating loose scrotal skin until you can palpate the external inguinal ring. If possible, follow the inguinal canal to the internal inguinal ring.

Ask the client to bear down and again feel for any bulging or masses. If a hernia is palpable, apply gentle pressure and note whether it is reducible. Never force your finger into the inguinal canal. If you meet with resistance or the client complains of pain, discontinue the examination.

Identify any existing hernias. A direct inguinal hernia is palpated above the inguinal ring, bulges anteriorly, does not travel down the inguinal canal, and may, but rarely does, invade the scrotum. An indirect inguinal hernia is palpated above the inguinal ligament close to the internal inguinal ring; it travels down the inguinal canal and often invades the scrotum. A femoral hernia is palpated below the inguinal ligament and appears more lateral than an inguinal hernia and is often difficult to distinguish from an enlarged inguinal lymph node. All hernias may become painful if strangulation occurs either by torsion of the bowel or by compression by surrounding tissues.

▼ KEY PRINCIPLES

- The physical examination is a systematic means of collecting objective assessment data.
- The four basic techniques used in physical examination are inspection, palpation, percussion, and auscultation, and they are performed in that order, except for abdominal assessment.
- In performing a physical examination, you rely heavily on the use of the five senses, particularly your ability to observe.
- Physical examination should be conducted following a regular pattern of examination and with the client positioned for the most accurate collection of data.
- The general survey provides information on the overall state of the client.
- The mental status examination provides a detailed description of the client's cognitive functioning at a given time.
- Good, preferably natural, light should be used to avoid distortion of color when inspecting the skin.
- A thorough description of a lesion is useful in determining if the lesion is a primary or secondary lesion and whether it is benign or malignant.
- Specific tests for hearing are performed only if gross hearing testing suggests a problem.
- Assessment of the heart provides cues to its structure and function.
- Assessment of the peripheral vascular system focuses on the blood pressure and the pulses (and other signs of peripheral circulation) in relationship to cardiac function.
- Assessing the function of the veins is part of assessing venous return to the heart.
- Abdominal assessment determines function of the bowel and detects abnormalities of other organs and structures in the abdomen.
- Assessment of the musculoskeletal system detects abnormalities of the structure and function of bones, muscles, and joints.
- The physical assessment is focused on the areas and techniques used to detect problems as appropriate to the client's history and reason for seeking care.

■ REVIEW QUESTIONS

1. Which of the following is a correct description of the relationship of one body part to another?

1. The forearm is proximal to the elbow.
2. The knee is inferior to the foot.
3. The hand is distal to the forearm.
4. The sternum is lateral to the chest wall.

2. For which of these clients would an assessment of the hair and scalp be the most important?

1. A newly admitted client following a motor vehicle accident
2. A client who is 1 day following abdominal surgery
3. A client who is mentally confused
4. A client with poison ivy on the arms and hands

3. Testing visual field means you are trying to determine the client's:

1. Extraocular eye movements
2. Peripheral vision
3. Distance vision
4. Visual acuity

4. Which would be a normal finding in the Rinne test?
1. Air conduction is half as long as bone conduction.
2. Bone conduction is equal to air conduction.
3. Air conduction is twice as long as bone conduction.
4. Only bone conduction is present.

5. Which of the following is within the limit of normal for the palpation of cervical lymph nodes?
1. Irregular, slightly tender, 1 cm in diameter, and immobile
2. Hard, mobile, nontender, 2 cm in diameter, and smooth
3. Clustered, irregular, 0.5 cm in diameter, and soft
4. Smooth, firm, less than 1 cm in diameter, mobile, and nontender

6. Which of the following correctly describes the location of the lower lobes of the lungs on the anterior surface?
1. Comprises the chest wall from the fourth intercostal space to the lower border of the ribs
2. Small triangles on the lateral chest wall, in the fifth and sixth intercostal spaces
3. Only exists on the right side between the fifth and sixth intercostal spaces
4. Small triangles on the lateral chest wall, in the seventh and eighth intercostal spaces

7. Which of the following is the most likely meaning of a carotid bruit?
1. A heart murmur being referred to the neck
2. Atherosclerotic plaque narrowing the carotid artery
3. High blood pressure
4. A rapid heart rate

Bibliography

Barkauskas, V., Baumann, L., & Darling-Fisher, C. S. (2002). *Health and physical assessment* (3rd ed.). St. Louis, MO: Mosby.

Beckow J., & Dickinson, E. T. (2005). The truth about capillary refill. *JEMS: Journal of Emergency Medical Services, 30*(1), 14.

Bickley, L. S., & Szilagyi, P. G. (2004). *Bates' guide to physical examination and history taking.* Philadelphia: J.B. Lippincott.

Bledsoe, B. E., Porter, R. S., & Cherry, R. A. (2005). 25 physical examination pearls: Important tips to help you polish your hands-on patient assessment skills. *JEMS: Journal of Emergency Medical Services, 30*(3), 58-60, [62-63], 64-74 passim.

Csokasy, J. (1999). Assessment of acute confusion: Use of the NEECHAM confusion scale. *Applied Nursing Research, 12*(1), 51-55.

Danter, J. H. (2003). Put a realistic spin on geriatric assessment. *Nursing, 33*(12), 52-55.

Hines, S. E. (2000). Performing a focused physical examination. *Patient Care, 34*(23), 76.

Jarvis, C. (2004). *Physical examination and health assessment* (4th ed.). Philadelphia: Saunders.

Leasia, M. S. (2002). *A practical guide to health assessment.* Philadelphia: Saunders.

Peate, I. (2005). Nursing assessment. Examining adult male genitalia: providing a guide for the nurse. *British Journal of Nursing, 14*(1), 36-40.

Physical assessment of the oral cavity. (2004). *Health Care Food & Nutrition Focus, 21*(7), 8-9.

Protopapas M. G., & Cymet, T. C. (2005). Musculoskeletal examination: A complete review. *Comprehensive Therapy, 31*(1), 12-20.

Reddish, S. (2004). Assessment of women in midlife. *Australian Family Physician, 33*(11), 883-887, 933-934.

Rushing, J. (2005). Clinical do's & don'ts. Assessing for ascites. *Nursing, 35*(2), 68.

Seidel, H. M., Ball, J. W., Dains, J. E., & Benedict, G. W. (2006). *Mosby's guide to physical examination* (6th ed.). St. Louis, MO: Mosby.

Wheeldon, A. (2005). Respiratory assessment. Exploring nursing roles: Using physical assessment in the respiratory unit. *British Journal of Nursing, 14*(10), 571-574.

Chapter 9

Nursing Diagnosis

Media Resources

- evolve Evolve Website http://evolve.elsevier.com/Harkreader/
- Companion CD

Learning Objectives

After studying this chapter, you will be able to do the following:

- Discuss the concept of standardized nursing diagnosis language.
- Describe the five components of a NANDA International (NANDA-I) nursing diagnosis
- Compare three types of nursing diagnoses on NANDA-I's health axis and collaborative problems
- Describe the process of diagnostic reasoning and stating a nursing diagnosis
- Discuss ways to avoid sources of diagnostic error

Key Terms

clinical judgment
collaborative problem
cue
defining characteristic
descriptor
diagnostic label
diagnostic reasoning
differential diagnosis
nursing diagnosis
related factors
risk factors
"risk for" nursing diagnosis
taxonomy
wellness nursing diagnosis

In the second phase of the nursing process, nursing diagnosis, you make conclusions about the meaning of the assessment data (Figure 9-1). As you gathered assessment data through the nursing history and physical examination, you recognized interrelationships among pieces of data and began to form clusters to identify problems or needs. The nursing diagnosis is a decision or judgment about the nature of a client's problems or needs. It is the result of the analysis and synthesis of your assessment data.

The process of nursing diagnosis is naming the client problems or needs that are amenable to treatment with nursing care. Nurses treat human responses to illness or health needs rather than diagnosing and treating the illness or condition that created the response. Thus nurses may manage symptoms, response to treatment, attitudes, feelings, or changes in lifestyle associated with an illness. Nursing diagnoses focus on the client's problems rather than on the nurse's problems in providing the care.

In their strictest sense, nursing diagnoses are problems or needs for which you are accountable and that you are capable of diagnosing and treating *independently.* However, many client problems in a health care setting require collaboration with a multidisciplinary health care team. A **collaborative problem** is a clinical problem that cannot be solved independently by the nurse but requires substantial nursing judgment to assist the client in managing or to implement the physician's orders.

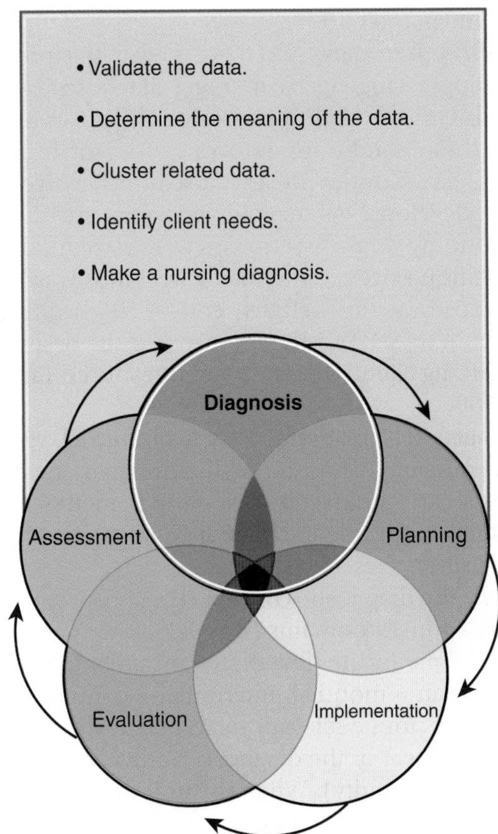

FIGURE 9-1 Nursing diagnosis is the second phase of the nursing process.

Nursing diagnosis is an ongoing part of the nursing process requiring changes as the client's condition changes. The phases of the nursing process are interlinked and function as a whole to help you make sound clinical judgments. Making a nursing diagnosis establishes a link between assessment and planning interventions. With accurate diagnoses, you will be able to select or design interventions to meet the client's individual needs or solve problems.

Making nursing diagnoses helps you think critically in nursing practice. One of the most important skills that you must possess as a nurse is the ability to analyze problems and make sound clinical judgments about the needs of clients under your care. Making a nursing diagnosis may be as simple as giving a name to an obvious problem or client need. At other times, complex thinking skills may be required to correctly identify the problem, its cause, and the factors that contribute to it. In a constantly changing health care environment driven by economic constraints, providing quality care requires that you be skilled in critical thinking (see Chapter 5). Nurses who can think critically about all aspects of nursing care increase their ability to be safe practitioners.

CONCEPT OF STANDARDIZED NURSING DIAGNOSIS LANGUAGE

A standardized language for nursing diagnoses means that all nurses are using the same words to describe the phenomena treated or managed by nurses. All sciences have a standardized language—when a microbiologist writes about *Staphylococcus,* all microbiologists understand what is meant. Nursing has borrowed language from medicine, physiology, and psychology but is only beginning to develop language for the human conditions that are uniquely responsive to nursing care.

NANDA International (NANDA-I) is the organization officially sanctioned by the American Nurses Association as the body responsible for developing a system of naming and classifying nursing diagnoses. NANDA-I defines a **nursing diagnosis** as a clinical judgment about individual, family, or community responses to actual or potential health problems/life processes that provides the basis for definitive therapy toward achievement of outcomes for which a nurse is accountable (NANDA-I, 2005).

EVOLUTION

Making nursing diagnoses is a trend in nursing practice that developed in the second half of the twentieth century. However, if nursing diagnosis is a technique for describing areas of human concern that nurses are qualified to help clients manage, then nurses have been making diagnoses since nursing practice began. Until the 1950s, nurses were reluctant to use the term *diagnosis* because it created confusion between medical practice and nursing practice. Virginia Henderson and Faye Abdellah are credited with advancing nursing as a profession by providing the beginnings of a language that encouraged nurses to identify *client-centered problems* instead of nursing tasks as the focus of nursing practice. In Chapter 5 you learned about the human needs identified by these theorists.

Many other nurses then began writing about client problems, and some began calling them nursing diagnoses. By 1971, the American Nurses Association included nursing diagnosis in its standards for nursing practice, and the term began to appear in nurse practice acts. Believing that the profession of nursing would benefit from the use of a common language, the faculty at Saint Louis University organized the first national conference for the classification of nursing diagnosis in 1973. As a result of this conference, the North American Nursing Diagnosis Association (NANDA) was established in 1982. This group, now known as NANDA International (NANDA-I), continues to meet every other year to accomplish its ongoing work. Its purpose is to increase the visibility of nurses' contribution to patient care by continuing to develop, refine, and classify phenomena of concern to nurses (NANDA-I, 2006).

RATIONALES FOR USING A STANDARDIZED NURSING LANGUAGE

A language of nursing diagnoses communicates the role of the nurse and the problems or conditions that are treated by nurses. Nurses, clients, and other members of the health care team benefit from clear communication about the phenomena treated by nurses and thus about the contribution of nursing to the client's welfare. Some of the benefits of a shared diagnostic language include the following:

- Provides a common language for nurses to communicate with one another and the health care team
- Defines the nursing scope of practice and body of knowledge
- Contributes to the autonomy and self-regulatory capacity of nursing
- Fosters critical thinking by placing the emphasis on the client's problem rather than on nursing problems
- Provides a method for identifying the focus or goal of nursing activity
- Increases the likelihood of using creative approaches to solve client problems
- Ensures documentation that is recognizable and retrievable for quality improvement studies of nursing care
- Facilitates nursing research through retrieval of nursing data from a computerized medical record
- Paves the way for third-party reimbursement for nursing care that can be proven to be beneficial and cost-effective.

The advent of computerized medical and health record systems has increased the need for a standardized nursing language that reflects nursing practice in the client's record. In agencies, such as home health care, where nursing is the primary service offered, client record systems need to clearly document client problems treated by nurses. On the other hand, in hospital records, practitioners from multiple disciplines document in the same record. A multidisciplinary approach to documentation often subsumes nursing care into the care of other practitioners, particularly physicians, and as a result the contribution of nursing care is virtually invisible.

The NANDA-I nomenclature is a systematic means of reflecting nursing practice in the client's record. When the system of naming problems does not reflect any options specific to nursing, the nurse is challenged to enter data into the system that shows the benefit of nursing care to the client.

TAXONOMIES

A **taxonomy** is a system of identifying, naming, and classifying phenomena. In nursing, the phenomena are human responses for which nursing care can be beneficial. A taxonomy is useful to nursing scientists in distinguishing various client problems and improving methods of nursing practice. There are three major taxonomies for nursing diagnoses. Taxonomies for nursing interventions and nursing outcomes are discussed in Chapter 10.

NANDA-I Taxonomy. NANDA-I began the process of developing a language of nursing diagnoses by listing the problems or conditions treated by nurses and classifying these conditions into categories of human responses. Taxonomies in any discipline evolve as the science develops. As new diagnoses were added to the taxonomy, some weaknesses were recognized in the classification system. One major weakness was the lack of diagnoses at the wellness end of the health-illness continuum. NANDA-I then researched the best method of classifying client problems and introduced Taxonomy II in 2000.

Taxonomy II. Taxonomy II is a multiaxial system of naming nursing diagnoses. With more than one axis, the diagnosis can capture up to seven parameters to make the diagnosis specific to the individual needs of the client. The seven axes are as follows:

- *Axis 1:* The diagnostic concept. These concepts are classified in 13 domains (Box 9-1).
- *Axis 2:* Time (acute [less than 6 months] to chronic [more than 6 months], intermittent, continuous). Time may not be relevant to all diagnostic situations.
- *Axis 3:* Subject of the diagnosis (individual, family, group, community). When the unit of care is the individual, it need not be specified.
- *Axis 4:* Age (fetus, infant, toddler, child, adolescent, young adult, middle adult, older adult).

BOX 9-1 *Domains of the Diagnostic Concepts*

DOMAIN 1: HEALTH PROMOTION. The awareness of well-being or normality of function and the strategies used to maintain control of and enhance that well-being or normality of function
Health awareness–Recognition of normal function and well-being
Health management–Identifying, controlling, performing, and integrating activities to maintain health and well-being

DOMAIN 2: NUTRITION. The activities of taking in, assimilating, and using nutrients for the purpose of tissues maintenance, tissue repair, and the production of energy
Ingestion–Taking food or nutrients into the body
Digestion–The physical and chemical activities that convert foodstuffs into substances suitable for absorption and assimilation
Absorption–The act of taking up nutrients through body tissue
Metabolism–The chemical and physical processes occurring in living organisms and cells for the development and use of protoplasm, production of waste and energy, with the release of energy for all vital processes
Hydration–The taking in and absorption of fluids and electrolytes

DOMAIN 3: ELIMINATION. Secretion and excretion of waste products from the body
Urinary system–The process of secretion and excretion of urine
Gastrointestinal system–Excretion and expulsion of waste products from the bowel
Integumentary system–Process of secretion and excretion through the skin
Pulmonary system–Removal of by-products or metabolic products, secretions, and foreign material from the lungs or bronchi

DOMAIN 4: REST/ACTIVITY. The production, conservation, expenditure, or balance of energy resources
Sleep/rest–Slumber, repose, ease, or inactivity
Activity/exercise–Moving parts of the body (mobility), doing work, or performing actions, often (but not always) against resistance
Energy balance–A dynamic state of harmony between intake and expenditure of resources
Cardiovascular/pulmonary–Cardiopulmonary mechanisms that support activity/rest

DOMAIN 5: PERCEPTION/COGNITION. The human information-processing system including attention, orientation, sensation/perception, cognition, and communication
Attention–Mental readiness to notice or observe
Orientation–Awareness of time, place, and person
Sensation/perception–Receiving information through the senses of touch, taste, smell, vision, hearing, and kinesthesia, and the comprehension of sense data resulting in naming, associating, and/or pattern recognition
Cognition–Use of memory, learning, thinking, problem solving, abstraction, judgment, insight, intellectual capacity, calculation, and language
Communication–Sending and receiving verbal and nonverbal information

DOMAIN 6: SELF-PERCEPTION. Awareness about the self
Self-concept–The perception(s) about the total self
Self-esteem–Assessment of one's own worth, capability, significance, and success
Body image–A mental image of one's own body

DOMAIN 7: ROLE RELATIONSHIPS. The positive and negative connections or associations between persons/groups of persons and the means by which those connections are demonstrated
Caregiving roles–Socially expected behavior patterns by care-providing persons who are not health care professionals
Family relationships–Associations of people who are biologically related or related by choice
Role performance–Quality of functioning in socially expected behavior patterns

DOMAIN 8: SEXUALITY. Sexual identity, sexual function, and reproduction
Sexual identity–The state of being a specific person in regard to sexuality and/or gender
Sexual function–The capacity or ability to participate in sexual activities
Reproduction–Any process by which new individuals (people) are produced

DOMAIN 9: COPING/STRESS TOLERANCE. Contending with life events/life processes
Post-trauma responses–Reactions occurring after physical or psychological trauma
Coping responses–The process of managing environmental stress
Neurobehavioral response–Behavioral responses reflecting nerve and brain function

DOMAIN 10: LIFE PRINCIPLES. Principles underlying conduct, thought, and behavior about acts, customs, or institutions viewed as being true or having intrinsic worth
Values–The identification and ranking of preferred modes of conduct and status
Beliefs–Opinions, expectations, or judgments about acts, customs, or institutions viewed as being true or having intrinsic worth
Value/belief/action congruence–The correspondence or balance achieved between values, beliefs, and actions

DOMAIN 11: SAFETY AND PROTECTION. Freedom from danger, physical injury, or immune system damage; preservation from loss; and protection of safety and security
Infection–Host response following pathogenic invasion
Physical injury–Bodily harm or hurt
Violence–The exertion of excessive force or power so as to cause injury or abuse
Environmental hazards–Sources of danger in the surroundings
Defensive processes–The processes by which the self protects itself from the nonself
Thermoregulation–The physiologic process of regulating heat and energy within the body for purposes of protecting the organism

DOMAIN 12: COMFORT. Sense of mental, physical, or social well-being or ease
Physical comfort–Sense of well-being or ease
Environmental comfort–Sense of well-being or ease in/with one's environment
Social comfort–Sense of well-being or ease with one's social situations

DOMAIN 13: GROWTH/DEVELOPMENT. Age-appropriate increases in physical dimensions, organ systems, and/or attainment of developmental milestones
Growth–Increase in physical dimensions or maturity of organ systems
Development–Attainment, lack of attainment, or loss of developmental milestones

NANDA-I. (2005). *Nursing diagnoses: Definitions & classification, 2005-2006.* Philadelphia: Author.

- *Axis 5:* Health status (wellness, risk, actual). This axis indicates the health status as the position on the health-illness continuum.
- *Axis 6:* Descriptor (limits or specifies the meaning of the diagnostic concept). Examples include compromised, delayed, ineffective, effective, readiness, desires.
- *Axis 7:* Topology (parts or regions of the body).

You first choose the diagnostic concept or the human response that explains the individual's situation and the descriptor from the descriptor axis. Then you have five more axes to help make the diagnosis specific.

Diagnoses have not been developed or approved for testing with all possible combinations of axes, and some combinations would not make sense. For example you could add *risk for* to any diagnosis. As you begin to use NANDA-I nursing diagnoses, you should start with the list of approved diagnoses (Box 9-2). Although you are free to create diagnoses using the axes in any combination, you should carefully consider the logic of your decision and whether or not your diagnosis clearly communicates the client's problem.

Omaha System. The Omaha System is a classification system developed by the staff of the Visiting Nurse Association (VNA) of Omaha, Nebraska, as a documentation and data management system that conveys the autonomy of community health nursing practice. The project to develop the system represents 15 years of research. The system includes a problem classification scheme or taxonomy of nursing diagnoses valuable to community health nurses. Thus the domains within the scheme reflect the home and community practice setting. For example, diagnoses within the environmental domain address material resources, physical surroundings, and the client's community. This system has the advantage of having been developed from what visiting or home health care nurses actually do within the framework of reimbursable nursing practice (Martin, 2005).

Saba System. The Saba Nursing Diagnoses for Home Health Care: Classification and Coding Scheme was developed through a project that reviewed 8961 clients of home health care agencies. The system consists of nursing diagnoses and interventions that serve as a framework for home health care nursing practice. Like the Omaha System, the Saba system is closely linked to services that can be provided under Medicare. The Saba system also has the advantage of communicating the actual work of home health care nurses. Many of the Saba nursing diagnoses are identical to those of NANDA-I.

Psychiatric Nursing Diagnoses. Because psychiatric nurses thought that the list of NANDA-I diagnoses did not capture the client problems managed by psychiatric nurses, a task force was formed in 1984 under the American Nurses Association to develop psychiatric nursing diagnoses. In 1994, this group turned its work over to NANDA-I for further refinement and development. Because psychiatric nurses find the *Diagnostic and Statistical Manual of Mental Disorders* useful, the psychiatric group has proposed that some of the diagnoses from this manual be recognized as nursing diagnoses. That

BOX 9-2 *Nursing Diagnoses by Functional Health Patterns**

HEALTH PERCEPTION–HEALTH MANAGEMENT PATTERN

Disturbed **E**nergy field
Ineffective **H**ealth maintenance
***H**ealth-management deficit*†
Health-seeking behaviors
Risk for **I**nfection
Risk for **I**njury
Noncompliance
Risk for **P**oisoning
Ineffective **P**rotection
Risk for **S**uffocation
Therapeutic regimen management

NUTRITIONAL–METABOLIC PATTERN

Latex **A**llergy response
Risk for **A**spiration
Risk for imbalanced **B**ody temperature
Impaired **D**entition
Adult **F**ailure to thrive
Readiness for enhanced **F**luid balance
Deficient **F**luid volume
Excess **F**luid volume
Hyperthermia
Hypothermia
Ineffective **I**nfant feeding pattern
Nausea
Readiness for enhanced **N**utrition
Imbalanced **N**utrition: less than body requirements
Imbalanced **N**utrition: more than body requirements
Impaired **O**ral mucous membrane
***P**ressure ulcer*
Impaired **S**kin integrity
Risk for impaired **S**kin integrity
Impaired **S**wallowing
Ineffective **T**hermoregulation
Impaired **T**issue integrity

ELIMINATION PATTERN

Bowel incontinence
Constipation
Diarrhea
Functional urinary **I**ncontinence
Reflex urinary **I**ncontinence
Overflow urinary **I**ncontinence
Stress urinary **I**ncontinence
Urge urinary **I**ncontinence
Total urinary **I**ncontinence
Impaired **U**rinary elimination
Readiness for enhanced **U**rinary elimination
Urinary retention

*For a complete list of NANDA I diagnoses, see NANDA-I. (2005). *Nursing diagnoses: definitions & classification, 2005-2006.* Philadelphia: Author.
†Italicized diagnoses are not currently accepted by NANDA-I but are found useful in clinical practice.

BOX 9-2 *Nursing Diagnoses by Functional Health Patterns*—cont'd*

Activity–Exercise Pattern
Activity intolerance
Risk for **A**ctivity intolerance
Ineffective **A**irway clearance
Autonomic dysreflexia
Risk for **A**utonomic dysreflexia
Ineffective **B**reathing pattern
Decreased **C**ardiac output
Risk for delayed **D**evelopment
***D**evelopmental delay: self-care skills*
Risk for **D**isuse syndrome
Deficient **D**iversional activity
Fatigue
Impaired **G**as exchange
Risk for disproportionate **G**rowth
Delayed **G**rowth and development
Impaired **H**ome maintenance
Disorganized **I**nfant behavior
Readiness for enhanced organized **I**nfant behavior
Risk for disorganized **I**nfant behavior
*Risk for **J**oint contractures*
Impaired bed **M**obility
Impaired physical **M**obility
Impaired transfer **M**obility
Impaired wheelchair **M**obility
Risk for **P**eripheral neurovascular dysfunction
Bathing/hygiene **S**elf-care deficit
Dressing/grooming **S**elf-care deficit
Feeding **S**elf-care deficit
Toileting **S**elf-care deficit
Total **S**elf-care deficit
Delayed **S**urgical recovery
Ineffective **T**issue perfusion
Impaired **W**alking

Sleep–Rest Pattern
Sleep deprivation
Delayed **S**leep onset
Disturbed **S**leep pattern
Sleep-pattern reversal
Readiness for enhanced **S**leep

Cognitive–Perceptual Pattern
Attention-concentration deficit
Risk for **C**ognitive impairment
Impaired verbal **C**ommunication
Readiness for enhanced **C**ommunication
Decisional **C**onflict
Acute **C**onfusion
Risk for acute **C**onfusion
Chronic **C**onfusion
Impaired **E**nvironmental interpretation syndrome
Deficient **K**nowledge
Readiness for enhanced **K**nowledge of (specify)
Impaired **M**emory
Uncompensated **M**emory loss
Unilateral **N**eglect
Pain (acute, chronic)
***P**ain self-management deficit*
***S**ensory deprivation*
***S**ensory overload*
***S**ensory perception*
*Disturbed **T**hought process*

Self-perception–Self-Concept Pattern
Anxiety (mild, moderate, severe)
Anticipatory **A**nxiety (mild, moderate, severe)
Death **A**nxiety
Disturbed **B**ody image
Fear
Hopelessness
Disturbed personal **I**dentity
Risk for **L**oneliness
Powerlessness
Readiness for enhanced **S**elf-concept
Chronic low **S**elf-esteem
Risk for situational low **S**elf-esteem
Situational low **S**elf-esteem

Role–Relationship Pattern
Risk for impaired parent/infant/child **A**ttachment
Weak parent/infant **A**ttachment
Caregiver role strain
Risk for **C**aregiver role strain
Parental role **C**onflict
***D**evelopmental delay*
***D**evelopmental delay: communication skills*
Dysfunctional **F**amily processes: alcoholism
Interrupted **F**amily processes
Readiness for enhanced **F**amily processes
Grieving
Complicated **G**rieving
Unresolved **I**ndependence-dependence conflict
Impaired **P**arenting
Readiness for enhanced **P**arenting
Risk for impaired **P**arenting
Ineffective **R**ole performance
*Parent/infant **S**eparation*
Social isolation
Impaired **S**ocial interaction
Chronic **S**orrow
Relocation **S**tress syndrome
Risk for **V**iolence (self-directed/other-directed)

Sexuality–Reproduction Pattern
Rape-trauma syndrome (compound/silent reaction)
Sexual dysfunction
Ineffective **S**exuality patterns

Coping–Stress-Tolerance Pattern
Risk prone Health behavior
Compromised family **C**oping
Coping (defensive, ineffective, *avoidance*)
Disabled family **C**oping
Ineffective community **C**oping
Readiness for enhanced community **C**oping
Readiness for enhanced **C**oping
Readiness for enhanced family **C**oping
Ineffective **D**enial
Post-trauma syndrome
***S**upport system deficit*
Stress overload

Value–Belief Pattern
Spiritual distress
Readiness for enhanced **S**piritual well-being
Moral **D**istress

Modified from Gordon, M. (2006). *Manual of nursing diagnoses* (10th ed.). St. Louis, MO: Mosby; and NANDA-I. (2005). *Nursing diagnoses: Definitions & classifications, 2005-2006.* Author.

group of nursing diagnostic labels is listed in the 1999-2000 NANDA-I manual as undergoing development (NANDA-I, 1999).

COMPONENTS OF A NURSING DIAGNOSIS

A NANDA-I nursing diagnosis has five components: a label, a definition, a set of defining characteristics, a group of related factors, and risk factors (Box 9-3). The label and related factors are documented in the client's plan of care. Applicable defining characteristics are documented as assessment findings.

LABEL

The **diagnostic label** is the name of the nursing diagnosis. *The label or stem is used to develop the goal of nursing care.* It is a concise term or phrase that represents a pattern of related cues that are characteristics, signs, or symptoms. It may include a **descriptor**, or a judgment that modifies, limits, or specifies the meaning of a nursing diagnosis, such as *decreased, deficient, excessive,* or *readiness* (NANDA-I, 2005).

DEFINITION

The *definition* of the diagnosis provides a description of the pattern of signs and symptoms, delineates the meaning of the label, and helps to differentiate it from similar or related diagnoses.

DEFINING CHARACTERISTICS

Defining characteristics are descriptions of a client's behavior that determine whether a nursing diagnosis is present and whether a particular diagnosis is appropriate or accurate. Defining characteristics are either directly or indirectly observable clinical cues. **Cues** are the indicators of the presence or existence of a problem or condition that represents a client's underlying health status. Subjective and objective data (symptoms and signs) of a problem provide the clinical cues that a problem is present.

RELATED FACTORS

Related factors show some type of patterned relationship to the nursing diagnosis. The related factor may be antecedent (prior) to, associated with, contributing to, or abetting the nursing diagnosis. These specific related factors help direct how the problem should be managed. The related factors may be an etiology or causative factor; therefore the treatment is to remove the cause. However, the etiologies of nursing diagnoses are often medical diagnoses that a nurse cannot treat. The nurse can help the client manage the medical treatment or manage the symptoms until the medical treatment becomes effective. The nurse can also manage factors that contribute to the problem. By identifying a related factor, nursing management focuses on treating responses and thus supporting the medical treatment. Writing the "related to" part of the nursing diagnostic statement is often a creative process based on understanding of the medical condition and the client's patterns of behavior (Box 9-4).

RISK FACTORS

Risk factors are factors in the internal or external environment that increase the vulnerability of a person, family, or community to an unhealthful state or event. A significant part of nursing practice is preventive, thus nursing language must be able to express client problems that require prevention.

BOX 9-3 *Components of a Sample NANDA-I Nursing Diagnosis*

Diagnostic Statement
Urge urinary incontinence

Definition
Involuntary passage of urine occurring soon after a strong sense of urgency to void.

Defining Characteristics
Urinary urgency
Bladder contracture/spasm
Frequency (voiding more often than every 2 hours)
Nocturia (more than two times per night)
Voiding in small amounts (less than 100 mL) or in large amounts (more than 550 mL)
Inability to reach toilet in time

Related Factors
Alcohol, caffeine, decreased bladder capacity (e.g., history of pelvic inflammatory disease, abdominal surgeries, indwelling urinary catheter), increased fluids, increased urine concentration, irritation of bladder stretch receptors causing spasm (e.g., bladder infection), overdistention of bladder.

BOX 9-4 *Questions to Consider When Identifying Related Factors*

Etiology
- What is the cause of the problem?
- Can nursing care remove or change the cause?
- Do the related factors allow me to understand the etiology?
- Is the cause of the problem clear?
- Will removing or ameliorating the cause solve the problem?

Contributing Factors
- What client behaviors contribute to the problem?
- Are there client behaviors that can be changed to reduce or eliminate the problem? Examples: health habits, knowledge.

Providing Direction to Nursing Care
- Do the related factors help me decide which interventions are most appropriate?
- Can nursing care change the related factors?
- If so, which factors can be changed by nursing care?
- Will changing the related factors solve the problem, manage the problem, or help the client tolerate the problem until a definitive solution can be found?

THE HEALTH AXIS

The health axis helps you identify the client's position on a continuum from health to illness. Because nursing care focuses on prevention, restoration of health, and maintaining wellness, nursing diagnoses can be described as actual, risk, or wellness diagnoses that represent these different spheres of nursing care. Nurses also help to manage problems where collaboration with the physician is necessary.

ACTUAL NURSING DIAGNOSES

Actual nursing diagnoses describe human responses to health conditions/life processes that exist at the present time (NANDA-I, 2005). Thus they describe a client's current problem. When a client has an actual diagnosis, you can identify the signs and symptoms (defining characteristics) that indicate the presence of the diagnosis. For example, if your client is unable to completely empty urine from the bladder, you would make an actual diagnosis of *Urinary retention.*

"RISK FOR" NURSING DIAGNOSES

A **"risk for" nursing diagnosis** describes human responses that *may* develop in a vulnerable person, family, or community. Risk-for diagnoses are supported by risk factors that contribute to increased vulnerability (NANDA-I, 2005). These nursing diagnoses are used when the client does not have a sufficient number of defining characteristics present to justify making the actual nursing diagnosis. Thus risk-for diagnoses are used to help you plan nursing care aimed at *preventing* the problem.

For instance, an older adult woman in a nursing home might have a risk for impaired skin integrity. The client does not actually have any broken skin or abraded areas visible. Nonetheless, she is thin, eats poorly, is confined to bed, is not using pressure-relieving devices, and sometimes wets the bed at night. All of these factors predispose her to skin breakdown. The nursing diagnosis *Risk for impaired skin integrity* alerts the nursing home staff that preventive measures should be taken to reduce the risk of skin breakdown.

Although the current NANDA-I taxonomy lists individual risk-for nursing diagnoses, risk is an element of Axis 5 and may be used with any nursing diagnosis for a client who does not actually have the problem but is at risk. Making diagnoses that define the client's risk communicates this important information to clients and suggests a plan of preventive care. Some agencies prefer that nursing diagnoses be made only when actual problems exist, and thus they make the assumption that preventive nursing care is provided.

WELLNESS NURSING DIAGNOSES

A **wellness nursing diagnosis** is a human response to a state or level of wellness in an individual, family, or community that has the desire to move toward a higher state of being healthy; it is usually the result of deliberate action (Carpenito-Moyet, 2006; NANDA-I, 2005). The client is functioning effectively but desires a higher level of wellness.

For example, the nursing diagnosis *Health-seeking behavior* related to a request for information about birth control might be used with a young woman who is engaged to be married. This diagnosis reflects that the woman desires information to maintain health in the future.

COLLABORATIVE PROBLEMS

In some client situations, the problems to be resolved require the interventions of more than one member of the health care team. In such cases, health team members share the responsibilities associated with solving those problems. There is overlap between medical and nursing diagnoses and problems identified by such others as physical therapists, nutritionists, and social workers. Carpenito-Moyet (2006) calls these *collaborative problems,* because the solutions require interventions from several members of the team (Figure 9-2). However, many nursing diagnoses represent problems treated or managed by both the physician and the nurse. Some aspects of the care are independent nursing interventions, and other aspects are dependent nursing interventions.

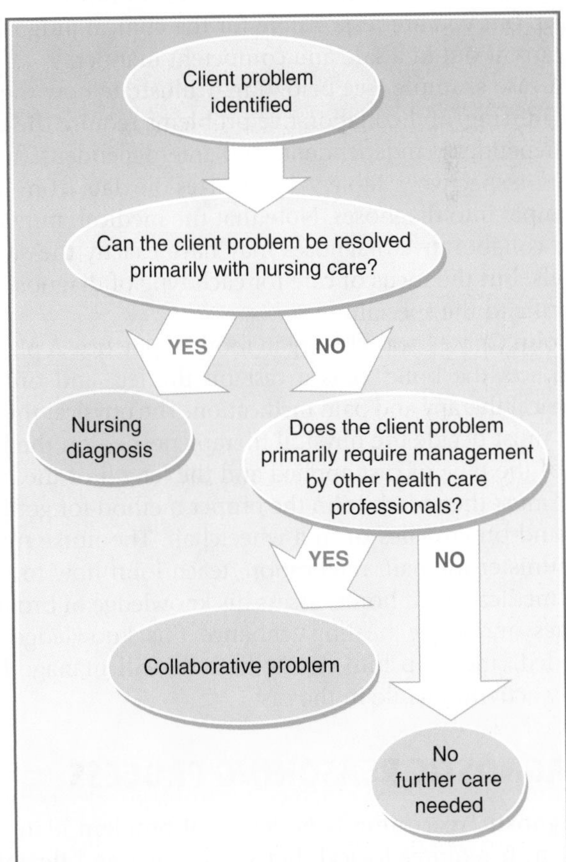

FIGURE 9-2 Differentiating between nursing diagnoses and collaborative problems.

Table 9-1 Examples of the Relationships Between Medical, Collaborative, and Nursing Problems and the Functions of the Health Care Team Members

COLLABORATIVE MEDICAL PROBLEM/ DEPENDENT FUNCTION	PROBLEM/INTERDEPENDENT FUNCTION	NURSING PROBLEM/INDEPENDENT FUNCTION
Pain: Physician orders pain medication. Nurse administers medication safely.	*Pain:* Physician orders pain medication. Nurse teaches client how to use medication at home.	*Pain:* Nurse teaches relaxation techniques and positioning methods to reduce the need for pain medication.
Impaired physical mobility: Physician orders physical therapy. Physical therapist carries out orders.	*Impaired physical mobility:* Physical therapist determines types of therapy needed and initiates a treatment plan. Nurse helps client understand how to do exercises at home.	*Impaired physical mobility:* Nurse helps client decide how client will manage daily activities at home and in school while the cast is on.
	Deficient knowledge: Physical therapist teaches client how to ambulate on crutches. Nurse encourages client to practice crutch walking in the corridor before going home.	*Deficient knowledge:* Nurse assesses client's knowledge about bone healing and provides information about the relationship between diet and bone growth.

A collaborative problem suggests that you are working interdependently and cooperatively with all health team members needed to solve the problem. This is in contrast to your independent functioning, when you work alone or with other nursing colleagues to solve the problem, and to your dependent functioning, when you follow someone else's orders (usually those of a physician). In the dependent function, you do not write the order, but you are responsible for the clinical judgment to carry it out in a safe and competent manner.

A case example (see below) may illustrate how medical, nursing, and collaborative problems require the use of dependent, independent, and interdependent functions, respectively. Table 9-1 organizes the data from this example into diagnoses. Note that the medical, nursing, and collaborative diagnoses may have exactly the same labels, but the focus of care for each type of diagnosis is specific to the specialty.

John Chase breaks his leg in football practice. A physician sets the bone, puts a cast on the leg, and orders physical therapy and pain medication. The physical therapist must decide the physical therapy needed on the basis of the type of cast applied and the length of the cast and must then teach John the proper method for getting around on crutches or in a wheelchair. The nurse must administer the pain medication, teach John how to use the medication at home, assess his knowledge of broken bones and bone healing, enhance this knowledge as needed, and help him decide how he will manage his daily activities while in the cast.

DIAGNOSTIC REASONING PROCESS

Diagnostic reasoning is professional problem identification. It requires logical, but value-laden and flexible, thinking to identify problems and related factors that both accounts for individual client needs and uses the strengths of client and nurse to the fullest extent possible. Diagnostic reasoning in nursing is somewhat different from diagnostic reasoning in medicine. Although the steps are similar for both, the contexts and the factors under consideration are different. The task of medical diagnosis is one of assessing, identifying, and labeling disease states. The physician generates hypotheses on the basis of signs and symptoms that are part of a well-defined and widely shared vocabulary. The steps in medical diagnostic reasoning include the following:

- Assess the signs and symptoms present.
- Generate several hypotheses about what the disease state might be.
- Form a mental set of descriptors, evaluate and differentiate potential diseases.
- Select the disease that best describes the client's set of signs and symptoms.
- Select the best treatment for the disease on the basis of the underlying cause(s) of the disease.

Even though experienced nurses can often identify specific disease states in some clients, the nurse's function is not to diagnose disease. However, the process of diagnostic reasoning in nursing requires the same clear, logical steps in thinking that are required for medical diagnosis. The difference, however, is that nurses diagnose the *human responses* to actual and potential health problems that *result from* or have *an impact on* disease, lifestyle, and life situations. Human responses include physiological, cognitive, emotional, and social changes that have to do with the meaning of health and illness to the person, as well as how the person is able to function.

Because you must take into account the psychosocial and life circumstances of the client (in addition to the medical diagnosis) when making any nursing diagnoses, nursing diagnosis often requires both complex and creative critical thinking. In contrast to medicine, making a nursing diagnosis does not necessarily limit the possibilities for treatment to a narrow choice of known protocols. Diagnostic reasoning in nursing takes into account both the assets and the deficits of each client, and it occurs in cycles that are repeated until the problem is resolved.

CRITICAL THINKING

Critical thinking links the idea of rationality, reasonableness, and reflection to the practical decision making necessary in nursing. In addition, critical thinking in nursing must be done within the context of the nurse-client interaction, the client's value system, and the interdisciplinary health care system.

The level of critical thinking needed to make nursing diagnoses about a client's life and health requires that you have a high level of ability in diagnostic reasoning and clinical judgment. You will use steps similar to those used for diagnostic reasoning in medicine.

- Assess the client, and analyze the data.
- Cluster logically related cues to identify patterns of responses.
- Form hypotheses about the meaning of the client's responses.
- Review potential nursing diagnostic labels.
- Select the labels that best describe the client's human responses.
- Determine the causes or related factors for each diagnosis chosen.
- Plan interventions on the basis of the related factors to treat the diagnosis.

The challenge for the beginning nurse is clustering client assessment data into meaningful sets and generating hypotheses about the client's human responses. The ability to cluster cues develops with clinical experience and knowledge of illness and medical treatments. As you study the health patterns in this textbook, learn about specific diseases, and practice making nursing diagnoses on the basis of your assessment of clients, you will learn to identify common response patterns.

Nursing diagnoses, then, are the labels you apply to the cue clusters generated from your assessment of the client. All of the defining characteristics do not need to be present for you to make a diagnosis. However, there should be a good match, or "fit," between the actual client data and the defining characteristics of the diagnosis. The diagnoses are then linked to the factors that caused or are related to the diagnoses. Nursing interventions are planned on the basis of those causal or related factors.

Action Alert! Write related factors that will give direction to nursing care.

Sometimes one cue is sufficient to make a diagnosis, but generally a diagnosis is made from a cluster of cues. Recognizing the complete cluster of cues will help you plan care. Once you can recognize common patterns of cue clusters, your diagnostic reasoning ability will improve rapidly.

When you make a diagnosis, you are making a clinical judgment. A **clinical judgment** is a conclusion or an opinion that a problem or situation requires nursing care and that determines the cause of the problem, distinguishes between similar problems, or discriminates between two or more courses of action. In addition, clinical judgments involve making decisions about what to observe, how to observe, prioritizing problems, and deciding what to do in a clinical situation. Clinical judgment encompasses both critical thinking and diagnostic reasoning.

As a novice, you cannot expect to have the same clinical judgment abilities as an experienced nurse; however, even a novice is capable of quite sophisticated judgments given practice, time, and good supervision. The more experience you have with a particular client population, the more sensitive, specific, and expert your clinical judgments will be about the clients under your care.

STEPS IN THE DIAGNOSTIC PROCESS

The process of arriving at a nursing diagnosis involves several interrelated steps; no step exists in isolation from the whole. The process is also ongoing: each step is repeated until you are satisfied that the plan of care is the best one possible on the basis of the data available.

In the initial contact with the client, often on admission to a facility or service, the emphasis is on gathering assessment data and generating tentative diagnoses. Making the first set of nursing diagnoses for a client takes more time and effort than updating and changing the care plan. A carefully constructed initial care plan will ultimately save you time. Box 9-5 illustrates an example of how to use the diagnostic reasoning process described here.

Review the Assessment Data. The first step in making a nursing diagnosis is to review the assessment data, including the client and family information, medical history and physical examination, diagnostic tests and medical treatment plan, as well as data obtained from the current nursing assessment. As you review the data, you will learn to make distinctions between relevant and irrelevant data by asking two questions: What is the significance of these data for nursing care? What problems could the client have on the basis of this information?

Cluster the Data. A single cue often alerts you to a problem. However, it is almost never enough to make a definitive diagnosis, and it is certainly not enough to associate the diagnosis with a related factor. Thus the next step in generating nursing diagnoses is to mentally organize the data into clusters of cues that seem to fit logically together and lead to insights or inferences about the client's condition. For example, a cough could

BOX 9-5 *Making a Nursing Diagnosis: A Case Example*

Mrs. Brown is a 45-year-old woman who was admitted to the hospital with a medical diagnosis of "moderately severe vaginal bleeding secondary to fibroadenoma." She was sent directly to the operating room (OR), where she underwent an abdominal hysterectomy. She was transferred to the surgical nursing unit from the postanesthesia care unit (PACU). She had an intravenous (IV) infusion of D_5 lactated Ringer's solution running in her left arm, a surgical dressing on her abdomen that was clean and dry, and an indwelling catheter in her bladder. She responded to verbal commands but was still sedated when she arrived on the nursing unit. Her color was pale. Her vital signs were as follows: blood pressure, 126/78; pulse, 88; temperature, 97.8° F.

STEP 1: REVIEW THE ASSESSMENT

When the nurse, Janine Cole, comes on duty 2 hours later, she reviews Mrs. Brown's chart. She finds that Mrs. Brown began bleeding suddenly and heavily the night before and was driven to the hospital by her husband. Her estimated blood loss before surgery was 500 mL. Blood loss during surgery was estimated at 750 mL. In the PACU her hemoglobin was 9.0 and hematocrit, 32%. She received one unit of blood.

When Janine enters Mrs. Brown's room, she finds Mrs. Brown awake but drowsy. Her husband is in the room with her. He looks tired and worried. The client's vital signs are as follows: blood pressure, 110/76; pulse, 78; and temperature, 98.6° F. Her color is pink. Her capillary refill rate is less than 3 seconds. The dressing has a 5-cm circle of pink drainage but is otherwise dry. Her urine output was 50 mL in the last hour.

Mrs. Brown is restless and complains of discomfort. She is reluctant to move or to have Janine touch her or the bed because she says it hurts when the bed is jostled. Aside from her discomfort, she seems to be primarily worried about her husband. She keeps asking him if he is all right and encouraging him to go home and rest. She tells Janine that he has been up all night and has had no sleep.

STEP 2: CLUSTER THE DATA

Janine clusters data under the appropriate functional health patterns. She does not have data on some of the health patterns, so she uses only the ones that are appropriate at this time.

- *Health perception–health management:* 4 hours postoperative (abdominal hysterectomy)
- *Nutritional–metabolic:* Nothing by mouth (NPO) last night and until 9 AM this morning, IV 5% LR at 20 gtt/min, now taking small sips of clear liquids. Temperature is 98.6° F, abdominal wound present, dressing slightly pink in one 5-cm spot but otherwise dry.
- *Elimination:* In the last hour indwelling catheter drainage is 50 mL and intake from IV was 120 mL, no bowel sounds on auscultation.
- *Activity–exercise:* Has been immobile in OR, still recumbent and inactive as a result of sedation. Pulse is 78, blood pressure is 110/76.
- *Cognitive–perceptual:* Drowsy but alert to surroundings. Restless, complains of discomfort, reluctant to move or have bed touched.
- *Self-perception–self-concept:* No data on how she feels about hysterectomy and impact this will have on her sense of self as woman.
- *Role–relationship:* Husband is present and concerned. She is more concerned about him than about her own discomfort.

STEP 3: SELECT POSSIBLE NURSING DIAGNOSES

Janine considers the data clusters and makes the following list of possible nursing diagnoses: *Impaired skin integrity, Risk for infection, Acute pain, Impaired urinary elimination, Impaired physical mobility, Bathing/hygiene self-care deficit,* and *Anxiety.* Some of these diagnoses may be ruled out when Janine compares the actual data about Mrs. Brown with the defining characteristics of the diagnoses initially selected (see Table 9-2, p. 200).

STEP 4: DIFFERENTIATE AMONG POSSIBLE DIAGNOSES

Janine then compares the defining characteristics of the possible diagnoses with the actual data she has about Mrs. Brown.

STEP 5: IDENTIFY APPROPRIATE DIAGNOSES

Janine compiles the final list of nursing diagnoses and arranges them by priority:

- *Acute pain*
- *Risk for infection*
- *Impaired physical mobility*
- *Impaired skin integrity*
- *Bathing/hygiene self-care deficit*
- *Risk for impaired urinary elimination*

Anxiety was removed from the list as not valid. The highest priority is to help Mrs. Brown get comfortable and become free of pain. When she is no longer uncomfortable, it will be easier to help her groom herself and get out of bed.

STEP 6: DETERMINE RELATED FACTORS

Janine now links the nursing diagnoses with their "related to" factors or etiologies and comes up with the following final list of diagnoses:

- *Acute pain related to inflammatory response in abdominal incision*
- *Impaired skin integrity related to abdominal surgical incision 4 hours post op*
- *Impaired physical mobility related to pain from abdominal incision, sedation, IV in arm*
- *Risk for infection related to impaired skin integrity, history of blood loss, and presence of indwelling catheter and IV site*
- *Bathing/hygiene self-care deficit related to presence of IV in one arm, indwelling catheter in bladder, pain, and sedation due to recent operative procedure*
- *Risk for impaired urinary elimination related to edema secondary to pelvic surgery*

STEP 7: DISCUSS THE DIAGNOSES WITH THE CLIENT

Janine returns to Mrs. Brown's room to administer her pain medication and to verify the other nursing diagnoses she has made. Although the diagnoses of *Impaired skin integrity, Risk for infection,* and *Bathing/hygiene self-care deficit* are based on objective evidence and might not require validation from the client, Janine discusses them with Mrs. Brown to establish mutual goals. Mrs. Brown recognizes the need to manage her wound, prevent infection, accept assistance with bathing, and walk to prevent postoperative complications. Mrs. Brown says that she is not anxious about anything, just worried that her husband has been up all night and has not had any sleep. Once Mrs. Brown has validated the nursing diagnoses, Janine enters them into the nursing care plan.

STEP 8: PLAN THE NURSING CARE

Janine plans her nursing care for Mrs. Brown on the basis of the etiologies of the nursing diagnoses. Because the highest priority was Mrs. Brown's pain, Janine gave the prescribed pain medication and repositioned her for comfort. The diagnoses *Impaired skin integrity* and *Risk for infection* share "related to" factors: the abdominal wound and the catheter. In addition to maintaining strict asepsis with dressing changes and catheter care, Janine plans to urge Mrs. Brown to deep-breathe frequently to reduce the risk of postoperative pneumonia. A third intervention she plans will be to ambulate Mrs. Brown as soon as possible to increase bowel peristalsis, reduce the risk of paralytic ileus, and prevent pneumonia.

Janine also plans to assist Mrs. Brown with her bath today to alleviate the *Bathing/hygiene self-care deficit* diagnosis; the presence of an IV in one arm, a painful abdominal wound, and a catheter significantly reduce Mrs. Brown's ability to manage her own hygiene. Finally, Janine will help Mrs. Brown get out of bed and move around several times during the day to help her increase her physical mobility.

Janine will continue to monitor Mrs. Brown's progress and will alter, delete, or add to the list of nursing diagnoses as needed throughout Mrs. Brown's hospital stay. Reviewing the nursing process steps frequently (at least once a shift, and more often if needed) during a client's stay is crucial to maintaining an accurate picture of the client's needs and giving the best possible care on the basis of those needs.

be a cue to a number of nursing diagnoses. However, the cluster of wheezing, dyspnea, cyanosis, and a history of asthma forms a pattern that suggests the nursing diagnosis *Impaired gas exchange related to airway obstruction secondary to asthma.*

Remember that not all data are useful as cues and fit into any meaningful clusters. On the other hand, some important cues may not be available. Thus you may have to reassess the client or review the database to obtain the missing information.

Before moving on to the next step, review the clusters you have generated. Do they make sense conceptually and logically? Do they provide insights into the client's condition? Do the clusters indicate probable nursing diagnoses?

Select Possible Nursing Diagnoses. After answering these questions, review each potential problem represented in a data cluster. Analyze the nursing diagnoses that might be relevant to the situation. Remember that diagnoses cannot be selected in isolation from the goals of care. When you understand the client's reason for seeking service, goals for health, preferences in managing care, and lifestyle, you will be more likely to choose a diagnosis that is appropriate for the individual client and that is realistically manageable within the care setting. For example, the hospital nurse probably does not often use the diagnosis of *Impaired home maintenance,* and the school nurse may have little use for *Decreased cardiac output.*

Differentiate Among Possible Diagnoses. Finding the most useful nursing diagnosis involves ruling out several possible diagnoses. Once you have identified possible nursing diagnoses for your client, you will need to narrow the possibilities until you identify the most appropriate diagnosis for each problem. **Differential diagnosis** is the process of deciding among several possible diagnoses to most accurately describe the client's problem. This process involves comparing the client's assessment data with the defining characteristics of possible diagnoses to determine which one has the best fit. The following steps are useful in differentiating among diagnoses:

- Determine if the cluster of cues matches one of the diagnoses better than the others.
- If the data are insufficient, collect the information you need to make a decision.
- Review the defining characteristics and data to find the best match. Perhaps there is now a high probability of two or more diagnoses being correct.
- If there is insufficient data to make a decision, you can keep both diagnoses in the care plan until the situation becomes clearer, and you can consult with the client about which diagnosis is correct.

Identify Appropriate Diagnoses. After selecting possible diagnoses and undertaking the process of differentiating between them, you will identify the most appropriate nursing diagnoses for your client. You will need to exercise clinical judgment to determine which nursing diagnoses are amenable to intervention at this time. Also exercise your judgment to prioritize diagnoses.

Determine Related Factors. Next, complete the diagnosis by determining what the "related to," or etiologic (causal), factors are for the diagnoses you have selected. The related-to or etiologic statement is important because it *gives direction to nursing care,* guiding your choice of nursing interventions to alleviate the client's health concern.

When selecting a related factor, it might be helpful to ask yourself, "Does this information help me decide which interventions are most appropriate?" For example, selecting the diagnosis *Risk for infection related to postoperative care* is neither desirable nor useful. It focuses on nursing actions, not the client's problem. A better choice would be *Risk for infection related to shallow breathing, use of indwelling catheter, and surgical incision.* Selecting the more specific and client-focused factors makes determining interventions more efficient.

A second question to ask yourself is, "Does this information make a difference in the interventions that will be performed for this client?" For example, for a client who has had a total joint replacement and must learn to walk again, you would select the diagnosis *Impaired physical mobility related to pain.* This diagnosis reflects your knowledge that pain management will be a major factor in helping the client begin to walk. It therefore focuses nursing care on pain management. The diagnosis *Impaired physical mobility related to a total hip replacement* fails to reflect your knowledge that the hip is stable and that the client *can* walk but does not want to because of the pain.

In some cases, nursing interventions are methods of implementing medical therapy for a specific medical diagnosis and it is tempting to make the medical diagnosis the related factor. For example, given the diagnosis *Disturbed thought processes related to stage 3 Alzheimer's disease,* you must recognize that neither you nor the physician can change the client's advanced Alzheimer's disease. It could have been written to focus on nursing: *Disturbed thought processes related to irreversible cognitive changes secondary to stage 3 Alzheimer's disease.* This diagnosis tells you that the change in thinking is irreversible, so the plan of care focuses on helping the client manage within the limitations imposed by the illness. Now consider the same label with a different etiology: *Impaired thought processes related to reversible cognitive changes secondary to lithium toxicity.* This diagnosis reveals that the client has a reversible problem. The nursing interventions, therefore, focus on the client following the physician's treatment plan for hydration, helping the client cope, reducing anxiety, and maintaining safety.

Validate Nursing Diagnoses With the Client. Finally, discuss your nursing diagnoses with the client and family

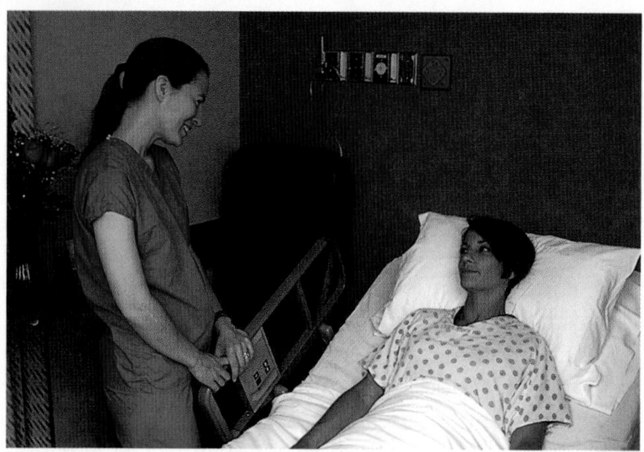

FIGURE 9-3 Discussing nursing diagnoses with client and family ensures that diagnoses match the needs of the client and family.

(Figure 9-3). Does the client agree with your inferences? Validation of your nursing diagnoses ensures that your goals and those of the client match. Table 9-2 summarizes the diagnostic reasoning process.

WRITING THE NURSING DIAGNOSTIC STATEMENT

Writing a useful nursing diagnosis means identifying the client's problem clearly so that all nurses who use the nursing care plan have the same understanding of the client's problems. How a problem is stated focuses nursing care and provides a basis for evaluating the effectiveness of the chosen care. As noted earlier, the related factor is especially important in providing needed clarity. The following paragraphs provide some useful tips for writing diagnostic statements that are meaningful and useful.

Identify the Client's Needs. The diagnosis should identify client needs or problems rather than nursing problems. One of the advantages of using NANDA-I diagnoses is that they focus on client problems and human responses. You may be tempted to write the related-to statement in terms of services or procedures; however, stating the need for services as a nursing diagnosis will not help you make decisions about how to provide those services.

You may also be tempted to write the related-to statement in terms of the technology being used. Again, the management of technology is your problem, not the client's. Asking yourself why the technology is being used may help you identify the client's problem. Likewise the medical diagnosis may be part of the cue cluster, but it should not be the related factor because a nurse is not licensed to treat it. Instead, focus on the factors associated with the medical diagnosis that affect the client's ability to function.

Avoid Legally Inadvisable Statements. State all of your nursing diagnoses in a manner that meets the legal guidelines for entries into the health record. Your related factors should not place a value judgment on the client's behavior or make a judgment that could be construed as libel in a court of law. Also avoid statements suggesting that nursing care has been or is potentially negligent. Table 9-3 gives examples of legally inadvisable nursing diagnostic statements.

Table 9-2 Applying the Diagnostic Reasoning Process*

ACTUAL CLIENT DATA	POSSIBLE NURSING DIAGNOSIS	DEFINING CHARACTERISTICS	NURSING DECISION
Client has broken skin and traumatized tissue due to abdominal surgery. Indwelling catheter is inserted in bladder.	*Impaired skin integrity*	*Present:* Disruption of skin surface; invasion of body structures *Not present:* Destruction of skin layers	This is a valid diagnosis. Two out of three of the defining characteristics are present.
Client has broken skin and traumatized tissue due to abdominal surgery. Indwelling catheter is inserted in bladder. Altered bowel peristalsis due to general anesthesia and abdominal surgery; hemoglobin is decreased, surgery is an invasive procedure, and no antibiotics ordered at present.	*Risk for infection*	*Present:* Inadequate primary defenses (broken skin, traumatized tissue), inadequate secondary defenses (decreased hemoglobin, altered peristalsis), tissue destruction, and increased environmental exposure (invasive procedure) *Not present:* Inadequate primary defenses (decrease in ciliary action, stasis of body fluids, change in pH secretions); inadequate secondary defenses (leukopenia, suppressed inflammatory response) and immunosuppression; chronic disease; malnutrition; pharmaceutical agents; trauma; rupture of amniotic membranes; insufficient knowledge to avoid exposure to pathogens	This is a valid diagnosis for most postoperative clients for at least the first few days, especially for those who are not receiving antibiotics. The client is at risk for wound infection, respiratory infection (because abdominal surgery may decrease ability to breathe deeply), paralytic ileus (intestinal paralysis caused by handling of the bowel during surgery), and urinary tract infection because of a urinary catheter.

Table 9-2 Applying the Diagnostic Reasoning Process*—cont'd

ACTUAL CLIENT DATA	POSSIBLE NURSING DIAGNOSIS	DEFINING CHARACTERISTICS	NURSING DECISION
Verbalized discomfort, expressed concern about movement causing pain, reluctance to let anyone touch the bed, and restless behavior.	*Acute pain*	*Present:* Verbal or coded reports; protective behavior; expressive behavior, such as restlessness *Not present:* Observed evidence; antalgic position and gestures; guarding behavior; facial mask; sleep disturbance. Self-focus; narrowed focus; distraction behavior, autonomic alteration in muscle tone; autonomic responses; changes in appetite and eating	This is a valid nursing diagnosis. There are several defining characteristics present.
A hysterectomy results in edema in the pelvic region, which may result in difficulty in passing urine. Preventive measure (an indwelling catheter) is in place.	*Impaired urinary elimination*	*Present:* Retention; risk for inability to pass urine without Foley catheter	The diagnosis is valid. Write the diagnosis as *Risk for urinary retention,* and institute preventive measures when indwelling catheter is discontinued.
Client is reluctant to move, intravenous catheter in arm, indwelling urinary catheter in bladder, abdominal incision, pain.	*Impaired physical mobility*	*Present:* Inability to purposefully move within the physical environment, including bed mobility, transfer, and ambulation; reluctance to move; imposed restriction of movement *Not present:* Limited range of motion; decreased muscle strength, control, or mass	This is a valid diagnosis. The client will very likely need help to get out of bed and to ambulate the first time or two. However, this diagnosis will very likely be valid only for a short time because the client will be encouraged to be out of bed as soon as possible.

*This table shows a comparison between actual client data, possible diagnoses, defining characteristics of possible diagnoses, and nursing decisions about the validity of choosing the diagnoses.

Table 9-3 Examples of Legally Inadvisable Nursing Diagnostic Statements

INADVISABLE DIAGNOSIS	PROBLEM	APPROPRIATE DIAGNOSIS
Ineffective airway clearance related to infrequent suctioning	Suggests negligence	*Ineffective airway clearance* related to diminished cough reflex
Risk for infection related to improper aseptic technique	Implies lapse in standards of care	*Risk for infection* related to operative incision in abdomen
Ineffective infant feeding pattern related to poor mothering	Judgmental and derogatory	*Ineffective infant feeding* pattern related to poor suck/swallow rhythm
Bathing/hygiene self-care deficit related to poverty	Judgmental	*Bathing/hygiene self-care deficit* related to lack of running water in home
Ineffective breastfeeding related to maternal self-absorption	Implies mother is neglectful	*Ineffective breastfeeding* related to maternal uncertainty and anxiety

SOURCES OF DIAGNOSTIC ERROR

Naturally, it is possible to make errors during the process of making a nursing diagnosis. Errors can occur during data collection, clustering, or interpretation. It is also possible to overdiagnose or underdiagnose the client's problems.

ERRORS IN DATA COLLECTING

You can begin with a medical diagnosis and anticipate a client's possible problems on the basis of problems that commonly occur with that diagnosis. However, additional comprehensive assessment is always needed to determine that the client actually has the problems and to identify additional problems unrelated to the medical diagnosis.

A second error in data collection occurs if you make your diagnoses without comprehensive data. One problem is making an inferential leap to the wrong diagnosis on the basis of insufficient data (Table 9-4). A second problem is that you may fail to make a needed diagnosis because you lack the necessary clinical cues. Except in an emergency situation, always take the time to do a thorough assessment.

ERRORS IN CUE CLUSTERING

Errors in cue clustering often result from inadequate data, poor critical thinking, or lack of familiarity with either the clinical population or the nursing diagnosis language. If cues from assessment data are incorrectly clustered, you may name the cluster incorrectly and choose the wrong nursing diagnosis. The wrong diagnosis results in ineffective interventions, and the client's problem does not get resolved. The nurse's time and energy are wasted on ineffective nursing care.

Another error in cue clustering made frequently by novices is making a nursing diagnosis on the basis of a single cue. Only rarely are accurate diagnoses based on a single cue. Almost always, more data are needed before inferences can be drawn. Validate or confirm your diagnoses with the client as one means of avoiding cue clustering errors.

ERRORS IN INTERPRETATION

A frequent source of error is interpreting cues inappropriately. In some cases, assessment data may be ambiguous and difficult to interpret, or the data may lead you to infer two or more equally possible diagnoses. The best solution is to verify the possible diagnoses with the client or the client's family.

Failure to identify and include client health strengths in your analysis of cues is another source of inappropriate interpretation. Clients have strengths and resources that nurses may not know about. These strengths can have a significant impact on their health status and their ability to cope with health problems and life processes.

Table 9-4 Selected Sources of Diagnostic Error

CUES USED TO FORM DIAGNOSIS	INCORRECT DIAGNOSIS	DIAGNOSTIC ERROR	CUES IGNORED IN FORMING DIAGNOSIS	CORRECT DIAGNOSIS
Heart rate 50 beats per minute.	*Decreased cardiac output*	Inferential leap; failure to consider all significant cues	Skin warm and dry, blood pressure 125/80, color pink, usual heart rate 52.	None needed; cue reflects normal function
Client asks to be left alone.	*Social isolation*	Inappropriate interpretation of cues	Client did not sleep last night and needs a nap.	*Fatigue*
Urine output is 30 mL per hour.	*Deficient fluid volume*	Insufficient cues	Client has a history of renal failure and is developing edema.	*Excess fluid volume*
Client appears uncomfortable and is restless after surgery for a fractured hip.	*Acute pain*	Inaccurate cue grouping	Further assessment reveals that the bladder is full and the client needs a bedpan.	*Self-care deficit (toileting)*
The client has not had a bowel movement in 3 days.	*Constipation*	Use of a single cue as the basis of the diagnosis	The client normally has a bowel movement every 3 days.	None needed; cue reflects normal function
Client has not monitored blood glucose levels for last 10 days and expresses frustration and anger with managing diet and insulin.	*Ineffective therapeutic regimen management*	Inconsistent or ambivalent cues	Client has been well controlled and able to manage in the past. Client separated from spouse last week.	*Ineffective individual coping*
Client is immobilized from a fractured leg and has a long-leg cast in place.	*Impaired home maintenance*	Inferential leap from insufficient data	Family has housekeeper, but all bedrooms are located upstairs.	*Impaired physical mobility*

Failure to assess for strengths as well as problems often leads to misinterpretation.

UNDERDIAGNOSIS AND OVERDIAGNOSIS

Overdiagnosis and underdiagnosis lead to ineffective and/or inefficient care. An underdiagnosis can occur because of failure to do a comprehensive assessment. You need a systematic method of assessing and documenting the client's health status. If the documentation method lacks a sufficient number of categories, important areas may be subsumed in a larger category and be overlooked. Broad categories should have subcategories. For example, if one category is physiological, the body systems can be used as subcategories to make sure the physical assessment is complete. Underdiagnosis also results from an insufficient knowledge base, causing you miss the significance of important cues. The more you know about the client's medical problem and responses to that problem, the more specific and sensitive your nursing diagnoses will be.

Overdiagnosis occurs when you anticipate possible problems, write a diagnosis, and fail to validate its actual existence. This approach suggests inadequate assessment. A second kind of overdiagnosis occurs when you attempt to diagnose every problem the client has now, may have soon, and could have at any time in the future. This practice results in a long list of diagnoses, many of which are irrelevant to the client's immediate problem or the setting for care. Determine which problems have priority, represent the immediate concerns, or are important to the client. Again, always validate nursing diagnoses and goals with the client.

▼ KEY PRINCIPLES

- As the second phase of the nursing process, nursing diagnosis is the end product of collection and analysis of data.
- A nursing diagnosis is a clinical judgment about individual, family, or community response to actual or potential health problems or life processes and provides the basis for selecting interventions to achieve outcomes for which nurses are accountable.
- Nursing diagnoses are human responses—the way clients respond to health conditions. Nursing diagnoses are not problems that nurses have but that clients have.
- Nursing diagnosis is the link between assessment and planning interventions. Without clear and accurate diagnoses, you cannot determine effective interventions.
- Nursing diagnoses identify problems for which nurses can be held accountable.
- Components of a NANDA-I nursing diagnosis are a label, a definition, a set of defining characteristics, a group of related factors, and risk factors.
- Diagnostic reasoning consists of collecting and reviewing client assessment data, generating clusters of cues and forming hypotheses about what the client's human responses might be, evaluating probable nursing diagnosis labels that reflect the cue clusters generated, selecting the best diagnosis to describe the client's human responses, determining the related factors, and planning interventions on the basis of each diagnosis and its related factors.
- Common errors in nursing diagnosis occur when data are incorrectly collected, clustered, or interpreted.
- Underdiagnosing or overdiagnosing the client's condition is an impediment to effective and efficient care.

■ REVIEW QUESTIONS

1. Select the statement that is the best description of a nursing diagnosis:
1. A clinical problem that is solved in collaboration with the physician
2. An actual problem the client has resulting from the medical diagnosis
3. A response to an actual or potential health problem
4. A problem a nurse has in providing nursing care

2. Select the most important reason for nursing to develop a standardized language.
1. It will make it easier to document nursing care in a computerized record.
2. It increases logical reasoning and focuses nursing care on the client's problems.
3. It makes it easier for a computer programmer to write a documentation system.
4. It makes it easier to retrieve nursing care from the computerized medical record.

3. A postsurgical client has an intravenous line, a Foley catheter, and a cast on his leg. This is the first day after surgery. You write a nursing diagnosis of *Self-care deficit.* Which is the correct classification of this diagnosis?
1. Actual nursing diagnosis
2. Risk-for nursing diagnosis
3. Wellness nursing diagnosis
4. Collaborative problem

4. A postsurgical client has an intravenous line, a Foley catheter, and a cast on his leg. This is the third day after surgery. The physician writes orders to remove the Foley and ambulate the client with crutches. He also writes no weight bearing on affected limb. Select the most helpful nursing diagnosis:
1. *Impaired physical mobility related to cast on leg*
2. *Impaired physical mobility related to lack of knowledge of crutch walking*
3. *Impaired physical mobility related to Foley catheter and intravenous line*
4. *Impaired physical mobility related to fractured leg*

5. A postsurgical client has an intravenous line and a cast on his leg. This is the fourth day after surgery, and the physician has written an order for discharge. You plan to validate that the client can safely walk with crutches and care for his cast and to provide the client with instructions for pain management and a follow-up visit with the physician before discharging him. Select the best nursing diagnosis:
1. *Impaired physical mobility related to lack of knowledge of crutch walking*
2. *Ineffective health maintenance related to need to manage postdischarge care*
3. *Ineffective individual coping related to managing ambulation with a cast*
4. *Acute pain related to bearing weight on a fractured leg*

Bibliography

Benner, P. (2004) Using the Dreyfus model of skill acquisition to describe and interpret skill acquisition. *Bulletin of Science Technology Society, 24,* 188-199.

Benner P. (2004). Using the Dreyfus Model of Skill Acquisition to describe and interpret skill acquisition and clinical judgement in nursing practice and education, *Bulletin of Science Technology Society 24,* 188-199.

Carpenito-Moyet, L. J. (2006). *Nursing diagnosis: Application to clinical practice* (10th ed.). Philadelphia: Lippincott Williams & Wilkins.

Florin, J., Ehrenberg, A., & Ehnfors, M. (2005). Quality of nursing diagnoses: Evaluation of an educational intervention. *International Journal of Nursing Terminologies and Classifications, 16*(2), 33-43.

Gordon, M. (2006). *Manual of nursing diagnosis.* St. Louis, MO: Elsevier Health Sciences.

*Kim, M. J., McFarland, G. K., & McLane, A. M. (1984). *Classifications of nursing diagnoses: Proceedings of the second national conference.* Philadelphia: North American Nursing Diagnosis Association.

Lunney, M., Delaney, C., Duffy, M., Moorhead, S., & Welton, J. (2005). Technology: Advocating for standardized nursing languages in electronic health records. *Journal of Nursing Administration, 35*(1), 1-3.

Lyon, B. Getting back on track: Nursing's autonomous scope of practice. (2005). *Clinical Nurse Specialist, 19*(1), 28-33.

*Martin, K. S. (2005). *The Omaha System: A key to practice, documentation, and information management* (2nd ed.). Philadelphia: Saunders.

Mrayyan, M. T. (2005). The influence of standardized languages on nurses' autonomy. *Journal of Nursing Management, 13*(3), 238-241.

NANDA-I (2005). *Nursing diagnoses: Definitions & Classification 2005-2006,* Philadelphia, Author.

NANDA International. (2006). *About NANDA International.* Retrieved from http://www.NANDA.org/html/about.html.

North American Nursing Diagnosis Association. (1999). *Nursing diagnoses: Definitions and classification.* 1999-2000. Philadelphia: Author.

Top drawer: Sabacare announces new version of Home Health Care Classification System. (2005). *CIN: Computers, Informatics, Nursing, 23*(1), 2-3.

Wing, R. R., Phelan, S., & Tate, O. (2002). The role of adherence in mediating the relationship between depression and health outcomes. *Journal of Psychosomatic Research, 53*(4), 877-881.

*Asterisk indicates a classic or definitive work on this subject.

Chapter 10

PLANNING, INTERVENING, AND EVALUATION

Media Resources

- Evolve Website http://evolve.elsevier.com/Harkreader/
- Companion CD

Learning Objectives

After studying this chapter, you should be able to:

- Describe types of planning for individual clients
- Describe the process of planning for individual client care, including nursing diagnoses, priorities, expected outcomes, and interventions
- Discuss the skills and types of interventions to individualize care for each client
- Describe the process of evaluating expected outcomes and nursing interventions

Key Terms

Care plan conference
Case management
Clinical pathway
Collaboration
Computerized care plan
Consultation
Discharge planning
Evaluation
Expected outcomes
Goals
Individualized care plan
Long-term goal
Nurse-initiated intervention
Nursing care plan (NCP)
Nursing interventions
Nursing Interventions Classification (NIC)
Nursing Outcomes Classification (NOC)
Nursing-sensitive client outcome
Physician-initiated intervention
Short-term goal
Standardized care plan
Standards of practice

After the nurse performs a thorough and holistic assessment of the client and identifies the client's problems, the nurse needs to address these problems in the planning phase. During this phase, the nurse will identify expected outcomes and devise interventions to achieve expected outcomes for each problem (Figure 10-1). The client problem is stated as a nursing diagnosis. The nursing diagnostic label establishes a global goal for the problem. Related factors provide directions to plan for expected outcomes and nursing interventions. **Expected outcomes** are specific, measurable, and realistic goals to achieve related to the specific problem. **Nursing interventions** are treatments initiated by nurses, physicians, or other health care providers, based upon clinical judgment, clinical practice guidelines, and scientific knowledge, to meet expected outcomes of each problem (Dochterman & Bulechek, 2004). In collaboration with the client and the other health care providers, expected outcomes and nursing interventions are formulated (American Nurses Association [ANA], 2004). The result of the assessment and planning process is a **nursing care plan (NCP)**. The NCP serves as a tool to communicate the plan of care to all members of the health care team when it is recorded in the client's health record.

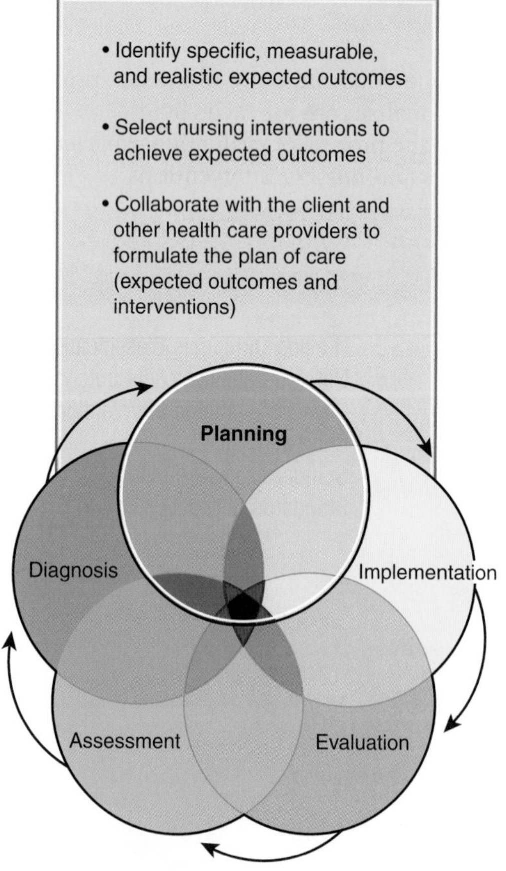

FIGURE 10-1 During the planning phase of the nursing process, you will set goals with the client, identify expected outcomes, select interventions to achieve the desired outcomes, and confirm the plan with the client.

Planning is essential for determining and providing optimal nursing care. As health care resources become more limited, planning becomes even more important. Systematic planning allows the nurse to make the best use of the resources available while avoiding use of ineffective—and therefore wasted—resources.

Although planning is the third phase of the nursing process, planning is interwoven with all phases of the nursing process (see Figure 10-1). The nurse needs to modify plans when new assessment or evaluation findings are obtained or new client problems are identified.

PLANNING FOR INDIVIDUALS

Planning for an individual client involves identifying the person's health problems and developing a plan of care to address them. The nurse plans care both independently and collaboratively with the client and other health care providers. The nurse begins to plan for nursing care at or before the initial contact with each client. The nurse modifies and updates the client's plan of care throughout the client's stay in the hospital or other health care facility. The nurse also may plan for home or community care after the client's discharge.

As the client's condition changes, plans must be reviewed and modified, sometimes together with other members of the health care team. *Planning* for discharge begins during the initial contact with the client by establishing the expected outcomes and anticipating follow-up care that may be needed.

INITIAL PLANNING

The nurse begins to assess the client at the first contact. The nurse completes a thorough history and performs a physical examination to gather data to identify actual and potential problems. While collecting data, the nurse begins to form impressions about the client's most acute, immediate, or important problems. After the problems are identified, the nurse needs to decide the priority of the problems. Problems with high priority will need intervention first.

The nurse also assesses the client's perception of his or her health problems. If the client and the nurse have different perspectives regarding these problems, the nurse needs to work with the client to identify the problems that they agree to work together on.

After problems are identified, the nurse will develop the plan of care for the client that spans the length of stay or duration of services. The nursing plan includes steps needed to support the client during medical care and to help the client become independent in self-care.

Although the plan primarily addresses the reason for seeking health care, it should also include strategies to manage other problems that could influence the resolution of the client's primary problem. Consequently, the plan may need to include interventions from other health care providers and referrals to other settings for additional services.

As an example, consider an older adult client admitted to the hospital with fractured ribs and difficulty breathing after falling at home. When assessing her, the nurse immediately notices rapid respirations and shortness of breath. The client complains of severe pain. In this case, the nursing care plan would include oxygen therapy and pain medication. The nurse calls a respiratory therapist to begin oxygen therapy while giving the client prescribed pain medication. At the same time, the nurse begins to formulate a plan to assess reasons for the fall and needs for a skilled nursing care facility after discharge—in other words, discharge planning is initiated.

All initial plans should be documented in the client's record to ensure coordination of care among members of the health care team. In the example given, the nurse would record the interventions applied and results attained rather than the plan to treat pain and administer oxygen, because the interventions were begun immediately. However, the plan to assess reasons for the fall and needs for a skilled nursing care facility after discharge would be recorded.

ONGOING PLANNING

During a client's stay in a health care facility, planning is ongoing because the client's health condition may change. These changes may lead to new problems, or some problems may be resolved. Thus, the priorities of the problems may be changed. Planning for the updated problem list also needs to be revised.

In an acute care setting, a client's condition may change rapidly, thus altering the initial plan. For example, you may plan to check a client's vital signs twice daily, only to find that the client has become weak and dizzy in the interim. If you determine that the vital signs must be checked more often than originally planned, you will need to revise the care plan in the client's record so other members of the health care team are aware of the change.

In a long-term care setting, where changes are often gradual and sometime subtle, ongoing planning may be more formal. If a client's functional abilities decline in two areas, a change-of-status assessment and a revised care plan must be initiated. For example, if your client's mental function declines and his or her ambulation changes from steady to unsteady, you would need to create a new plan of care. Prompt revisions to the client's plan of care not only ensure the correct care but also help maintain funding for the client's care, especially from Medicare.

DISCHARGE PLANNING

At the moment a client enters the health care system, the nurse begins discharge planning for the client. **Discharge planning** is to prepare the client to move from one level of care to another level of care, which may occur within or outside the current health care facility (Dochterman & Bulechek, 2004). Although discharge planning is an independent nursing activity, the nurse may need to collaborate with other health care team members to address the client's needs after discharge. Discharge planning may include arranging for home health care to help the client recover fully after hospital discharge. It may include rehabilitation services for a client recovering from a stroke, being fitted for an artificial leg, or learning to walk on an implanted hip joint. Box 10-1 presents a list of discharge planning activities.

In addition to specifying which services a client will need, discharge planning also addresses the setting in which those services should be delivered. Typical settings include inpatient facilities, outpatient facilities, skilled nursing facilities, and the client's home. The client's support system, home environment, and transportation options are all important considerations in planning for safe ongoing care after discharge.

BOX 10-1 *Discharge Planning Activities*

- Prepare the client, family, and significant others for discharge.
- Collaborate with client, family, significant others, and other health care providers in planning for continuity of health care.
- Coordinate efforts of different health care providers to ensure a timely discharge.
- Identify the client's and the primary caregiver's understanding of knowledge or skills required after discharge.
- Identify what the client should be taught for care after discharge.
- Monitor readiness for discharge.
- Communicate the client's discharge plans.
- Document the client's discharge plans in the chart.
- Formulate a maintenance plan for follow-up after discharge.
- Assist the client, family, and significant others in planning for the supportive environment necessary to provide the client's care after leaving the hospital.
- Develop a plan that considers the client's health, social, and financial needs.
- Arrange for evaluation after discharge.
- Encourage self-care.
- Arrange discharge to the next level of care.
- Arrange for caregiver support.
- Discuss financial resources if the client needs health care after discharge.
- Coordinate referrals relevant to linkages among health care providers.

Modified from Dochterman, J. M., & Bulechek, G. M. (2004). *Nursing interventions classification (NIC)*. St. Louis, MO: Mosby.

COLLABORATIVE PLANNING

Some clients' problems may need collaborative planning. **Collaboration** is a team effort that may involve clients, family members, nurses, physicians, dietitians, social workers, and other health care providers to achieve a common goal. The team works in partnership to identify the plan of care regarding the client's problems. In the collaborative planning meetings, each member contributes ideas based on personal and professional knowledge and experiences in regard to the client's problems. Authority in a collaborative situation is derived from professional knowledge, sphere of activity, and responsibility rather than from a hierarchical relationship. Collaborative planning facilitates the continuity and coordination of care among the team members.

CONSULTATION

Consultation is the act of two or more health care professionals, one of whom is an expert or specialist solicited to offer an opinion, deliberating for the purpose of making decisions. When the nurse lacks the knowledge or expertise to solve a problem or determines that a plan of care is not effective, the nurse should consult with a person who has more experience in the problem area. Nurses working in institutional settings have multiple nursing resources available for consultation. Head nurses, charge nurses, supervisors, and clinical nurse specialists all can provide consultation in the planning process. Consultation may occur during all phases of the nursing process, but it is very important in the planning process.

Consulting with specialists and experts can help the nurse provide optimal care for each client. Each consultant brings a different viewpoint and area of expertise to the development of the care plan. For example, an enterostomal therapist could provide information on a special paste that facilitates adhesion of a stomal wafer to the skin for bag attachment. A physical therapist could discuss the benefits of using a transfer board instead of a lift for moving a client from bed to chair.

Successful consultation has five important elements. First, the nurse identifies an appropriate person with expertise in the problem area. Second, the nurse provides the consultant with factual information about the client and the nature of the problem. Third, the nurse allows the consultant to make an independent judgment about the nature of the problem and possible solution. Fourth, after the consultant has made a judgment, the nurse and the consultant discuss recommended solutions. Fifth, the nurse and consultant decide who should implement the recommended care.

CARE PLAN CONFERENCES

Care plan conferences may be organized for collaborative planning. A **care plan conference** is the action of a group conferring or consulting together to plan care for the client (Figure 10-2). Various members of the health care team may organize a care plan conference to review the client's problem list and to plan interventions to achieve the outcomes established for the client. Typically, the client, family members or significant others, and any team members involved in the client's recovery are invited to the care plan conference.

The frequency and attendees of care plan conferences vary with the setting and the client's situation. A conference may occur spontaneously, which may include a nurse, a physician, and a family member to discuss the client's care in a private area on the unit. A conference may be planned ahead where all persons involved in the client's care agree to meet at a specific place and time.

In long-term care, formal care plan conferences are held when the client is admitted to the facility, at 3-month intervals, and when the client's condition changes. Health care professionals who usually attend these meetings include the nurse, activity director, social worker, dietitian, and other therapists, such as a physical therapist or speech therapist. The client is included in the conference or may be represented by a family member. The physician may also be involved.

In the hospital setting, formal conferences are less common but may occur in special situations. For example, in some hospitals, interdisciplinary teams work together to plan for the treatment of child abuse and neglect. The composition of these teams varies but may include nurses, social workers, psychiatrists, abuse counselors, physicians, and teachers.

Teamwork is necessary for effective care plan conferences. The group leader can facilitate the interdisciplinary team meeting by keeping the group focused on important issues and concluding the meeting in a reasonable amount of time. During the meeting team members are consulted to ensure that the plans of the entire team are consistent with expected outcomes.

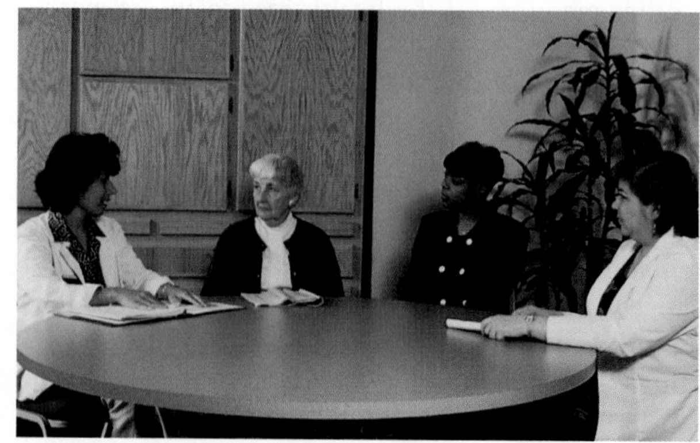

FIGURE 10-2 A care plan conference allows members of the health care team to discuss and revise the client's care plan as needed. Often, the client or a family member is invited to attend.

THE PLANNING PROCESS

Planning for individual client care includes establishing priorities, making decisions about the desired outcomes, and selecting the interventions most likely to achieve those outcomes. The client's care must be organized on the basis of the priority of activities essential for life and recovery. It also must consider the client's perceptions and self-care abilities.

ESTABLISHING PRIORITIES

During the planning process, the nurse must decide the priorities of nursing diagnoses. Establishing priorities means that nursing diagnoses are ranked in the order of importance. Some diagnoses need immediate attention, some can be safely postponed, and some can be treated in another setting. The meaning of *importance* varies with the setting, the client's condition, and the client's needs. The nurse should treat the diagnoses with high priority *(high importance)* first.

Maslow's hierarchy is a helpful tool for thinking about priorities (Figure 10-3). Abraham Maslow is credited with being one of the founders of the humanistic psychology movement. He hypothesized that human needs motivate behavior on the basis of a hierarchy of the potency of these needs. He arranged human needs in a pyramid that suggests both the order in which we satisfy the needs and the order in which these needs contribute to development over a lifetime. Albeit imperfect as a framework for establishing nursing priorities, Maslow's hierarchy of needs is useful in giving general guidance.

Threats to Physiological Integrity. When a client has a threat to physiological integrity, physical needs demand highest priority. The degree of the threat may influence how completely the client screens out other needs. Basic human needs include air, water, and food. Related to these basic needs, the first priority is any threat to the vital functions of breathing, heartbeat, and blood pressure. A person having difficulty breathing will not want a nurse to discuss the person's sense of self-worth. The immediate need is to relieve the difficult breathing.

Imagine a client with lung cancer, who is struggling to breathe, nauseated from chemotherapy, too weak to rise from bed unassisted, and aware that she will die in a short time. The following is a prioritized list of diagnoses for this client:

- *Ineffective breathing pattern related to obstructed airway*
- *Imbalanced nutrition: less than body requirements, related to nausea and vomiting*
- *Impaired physical mobility related to generalized weakness*
- *Bathing/hygiene self-care deficit related to generalized weakness*
- *Hopelessness related to coping with the diagnosis of a terminal illness*

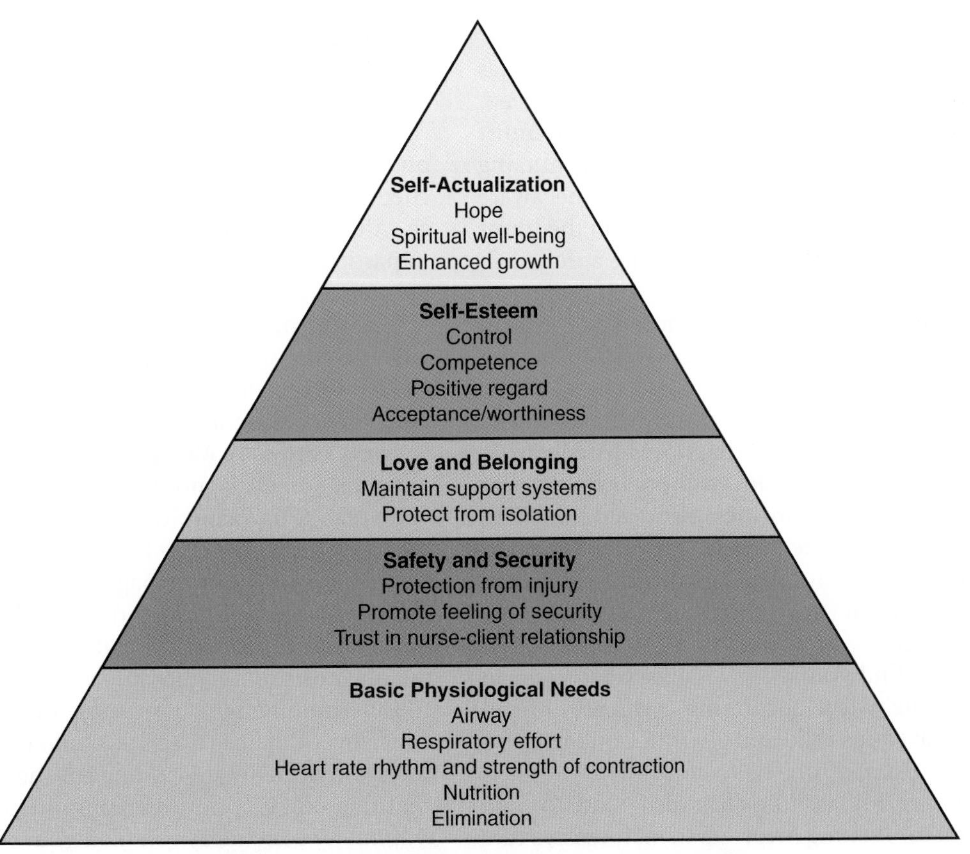

FIGURE 10-3 Using Maslow's hierarchy to establish priorities.

All of the problems listed are important, but breathing is basic to life. If the breathing pattern is life threatening, this diagnosis will have the highest priority. Getting enough to eat is secondary in importance at that moment. When vital functions are stable, attention can be turned to the other physiological systems.

Action Alert! Give top priority to basic survival needs when your client has a threat to physiological integrity.

Ensuring safety and security is the second level of need. Although you might forego safety for physiological integrity on a rare occasion, the principle that safety is a priority second only to physiological integrity is apparent from Maslow's hierarchy. Making the client feel secure through a trusting nurse-client relationship is also important.

Another nursing goal is to help clients satisfy their need for love and belonging through their relationships with significant others. In Chapter 48 you will learn about the concept of the family as a client. In addition, clients' relationships with the health care team can be valuable in helping them meet the need for belonging. The nurse should strive to help the client feel like an important member of the team.

Self-esteem develops when the need for love and belonging is met; it develops out of successful relationships or interactions with others. On the other hand, clients with low self-esteem are prone to develop depression, which affects clients' adherence to medical regimens (Wing, Phelan, & Tate, 2002).

When planning care, be prepared to adjust priorities as the client's condition and needs change. Indeed, only rarely are priorities clear and stable. You must consider the strong interrelationships among nursing diagnoses when establishing priorities, and be aware that higher-level needs can drive the needs on the lower levels of the pyramid. For example, feeling a deficit in love and belonging, a person may seek self-esteem in other ways. Then, it may be that finding self-esteem separate from others is the force that drives this person to self-actualization.

The interrelationships may also have effects in the other direction. In the nursing diagnoses listed earlier for the client with lung cancer, hopelessness was placed low on the list of priorities. However, hopelessness may need to be treated before the client is interested in food. Recognizing that one diagnosis has priority does not mean the remaining diagnoses are ignored or delayed.

You will often find yourself meeting several needs at once. For example, while suctioning a client, you can monitor an intravenous fluid and give hope and comfort through your touch and tone of voice.

The Health Care Setting. Priorities also tend to vary with the health care setting involved. In an intensive care unit, for example, the nursing diagnosis *Ineffective breathing pattern* may be the top priority of nurses working to sustain the client's life. After discharge, the client may have the same diagnosis. However, the diagnosis *Deficient knowledge related to inexperience with managing a medical condition* may become the higher priority because the client's breathing pattern has stabilized and the focus of home health care shifts to health education.

In the hospital setting, priorities are more likely to involve physiological diagnoses, and care typically addresses physical needs. The priorities in the care plan can change daily or even hourly as the person's condition improves or worsens. As physical needs are stabilized, other problems can be managed.

In a long-term care setting, where the client's physical needs are stable, quality-of-life issues may take on greater importance than physical care. Consider the following nursing diagnoses in a long-term care setting:

- *Disturbed thought processes*
- *Bathing/hygiene self-care deficit*
- *Dressing/grooming self-care deficit*
- *Impaired physical mobility*

The top priority for care is to increase the client's independence. Being well groomed may not be as important as the client's being able to manage self-care. Thus, the plan of care for *Disturbed thought processes* and *Impaired physical mobility* would be a higher priority than the plan of care for *Bathing/hygiene self-care deficit* or *Dressing/grooming self-care deficit.*

Client's Perception of Need. Another consideration in planning priorities for nursing diagnoses is the client's perception of the situation. If a client has just come to a nursing unit after an emergency appendectomy and complains of pain, the nurse would place a high priority on the client's physical safety and would respond to the client's concern by establishing *Pain* as a priority diagnosis. Alternatively, a long-term care client who prefers not to participate in social activities would not choose *Social isolation* as a diagnosis to receive high priority.

Clearly, considering a client's input helps you to provide care that is individualized and satisfying to the client. However, the planning process also allows you to help clients recognize problems and accept help.

Client's Self-Care Ability. For the client able to provide self-care, some diagnoses will have a lower priority in your plan. For example, *Bathing/hygiene self-care deficit* may have a high priority for a postsurgical client but not for a client who can manage self-care independently. If surgery involved the arms or shoulders, the client may not have adequate self-care abilities, which would raise the diagnosis to a higher priority.

Determining which nursing diagnoses take precedence over others is a decision-making process that may change repeatedly depending on the client's condition. Learning to set priorities appropriately, however, will reap many benefits as you plan your client's care.

ESTABLISHING OUTCOMES

As part of the planning process, the nurse needs to establish expected outcomes—desirable end results—of nursing care for each client problem (nursing diagnosis). By devising expected outcomes, the nurse states reasonable expectations that can be achieved as a result of nursing care. The nurse can be held accountable for the results of the care planned.

Expected outcomes should be *realistic, measurable, acceptable to the client,* and include a *time-frame* to reach expected outcomes. *Realistic* expectations are established when the nurse has a thorough assessment of the client, carefully evaluates the client's disabilities, resources, and unique life circumstances, and uses logical reasoning to verify whether nursing care can achieve expected results.

Measurable terms should be used to describe expected outcomes so that outcomes can be directly observed. Any member of the health care team reading the statement of expected outcomes should have the same concept of expected results as the nurse who develops expected outcomes. The nurse should use verbs that are measurable to describe cognitive, affective, and psychomotor actions (Box 10-2). For example, if the nursing diagnosis is *Deficient knowledge related to lack of experience in giving insulin,* you would expect your nursing care to result in the client knowing how to self-administer insulin. However, if you phrase the expected outcome as "The client knows the steps needed to self-administer insulin," you have no way to measure how the client "knows." Therefore, you should use a measurable action verb. In cognitive terms, you can describe the outcome as "The client will state the steps to follow in self-administering insulin." In terms of psychomotor performance, you can state the outcome as "The client will correctly administer insulin to himself."

The expected results should be *acceptable to the client.* Always remember that planning is done not only *for* the client but also *with* the client (Figure 10-4). When the client can collaborate, you should work with the client to establish expected results, which could lead to favorable results and client satisfaction. You can help the client set realistic expectations and encourage the client to be a full partner in care. You can listen to client's concerns, talk frankly, negotiate, and sometimes compromise to elicit a client's participation in the planning process. Many people welcome the opportunity to be more actively involved in decision making. Including the client's family and friends in setting goals and outcomes may be helpful as well. Significant others are often responsible for carrying out the care plan after discharge. They may be more willing to continue the therapeutic regimen at home if they understand its rationale and have had input into the decision-making process.

Finally, planning should include a *time frame* to achieve the intended results. The time frame may reflect short-term goals or long-term goals. A **short-term goal** suggests that the resolution of the nursing diagnosis can be accomplished in an hour, a day, or a week, and it is sometimes an intermediary goal that shows progress toward the longer-term goal. A **long-term goal** suggests that the expectation for resolution of the nursing diagnosis will take place in small measurable steps but may take a few weeks or months. Especially in a rehabilitative or long-term care setting, a long-term goal may be ongoing.

BOX 10-2 *Verbs for Writing Measurable Outcome Statements*

COGNITIVE DOMAIN

Knowledge: choose, circle, define, identify, label, list, match, name, outline, recall, report, select, state

Comprehension: describe, discuss, distinguish, estimate, explain, generalize, give example, locate, recognize, summarize

Application: apply, demonstrate, illustrate, implement, interpret, modify, order, revise, solve, use

Analysis: analyze, arrange, calculate, classify, compare, conclude, contrast, determine, differentiate, discriminate

Synthesis: categorize, combine, compile, correlate, design, devise, generate, integrate, reorganize, revise, summarize

Evaluation: appraise, assess, conclude, criticize, debate, defend, judge, justify

AFFECTIVE DOMAIN

Receiving: accept, admit, ask, attend, focus, listen, observe, pay attention

Responding: agree, answer, conform, discuss, express, participate, recall, relate, report, state willingness, try, verbalize

Valuing: assert, assist, attempt, choose, complete, disagree, follow, help, initiate, join, propose, volunteer

Organization: adhere, alter, arrange, combine, defend, explain, express, generalize, integrate, resolve

Characterization: assert, commit, discriminate, display, influence, propose, qualify, solve, verify

PSYCHOMOTOR DOMAIN

Perception: attend, choose, detect, differentiate, distinguish, identify, isolate, perceive, relate, select, separate

Set: attempt, begin, develop, display, position, prepare, proceed, reach, respond, show, start, try

Guided response mechanism and complex overt response: align, arrange, assemble, attach, build, change, choose, clean, compile, complete, construct, demonstrate, discriminate, dismantle, dissect, examine, find, grasp, hold, insert, lift, locate, maintain, manipulate, measure, mix, open, operate, organize, perform, pour, practice, reassemble, remove, repair, replace, separate, shake, suction, turn, transfer, walk, wash, wipe

Adaptation: adapt, alter, change, convert, correct, rearrange, reorganize, replace, revise, shift, substitute, switch

Origination: arrange, combine, compose, construct, create, design, exchange, reformulate

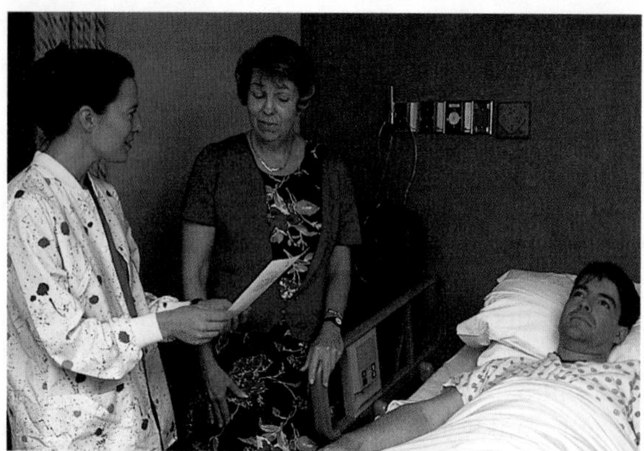

FIGURE 10-4 Planning is done not only *for* the client and family but *with* the client and family. Mutual goal setting ensures that the nurse, client, and family are working together.

It is essential that you be able to determine realistic time frames for attaining expected outcomes. Specifying the date for achieving an expected outcome reflects your best judgment about the time needed. This judgment is based on knowledge about the problem, the person's condition, the support systems available, and the necessary nursing interventions. For example, consider the expected outcome that the client will no longer have hard, dry stools. If the client takes a cathartic medication, the time frame for evaluation of the expected outcome could be 3 days. If the client prefers to resolve the problem by a diet change and activity increase rather than medication, the time frame may be 2 weeks.

In a general sense, setting appropriate time frames can provide benefits beyond those inherent in achieving an expected outcome. For example, setting time frames can accomplish the following:

- Motivate the client to strive toward resolution of the problem
- Provide the client (and nurse) with a sense of accomplishment
- "Pace" nursing care and encourage focus on continued progress
- Prompt the nurse to evaluate the achievement of the outcome

If an expected outcome is unmet, you may need to reconsider the time frame, modify the expected outcome, or devise new interventions. Of course, expected outcomes must be revised as the client's health status changes.

Defining Outcomes. The term *outcome* has come into popular use from the idea that nurses should be able to demonstrate the results of care in specific, measurable terms. The best of nursing care may not be worthwhile if it fails to result in measurable changes in the client's behavior or condition.

A *goal* describes something that you expect to happen or that you desire as a result of nursing care. Commonly, however, **goals** are broad, general statements about the desired results of nursing care; *expected outcomes* offer specific criteria for measuring results. The stem of the diagnosis provides direction for the goal. For example, the goal of the nursing diagnosis *Activity intolerance related to ineffective breathing secondary to emphysema* is to increase the client's activity tolerance. To meet the goal of activity tolerance, you would devise a set of expected outcomes to measure the progress of activity tolerance. You would use the goal (activity tolerance) and methods to modify the factors (related to ineffective breathing) to develop expected outcomes. Expected outcomes for the problem of activity intolerance might include the following:

- The client will take bronchodilator on a regular schedule.
- The client will correctly use inhaler before attempting exercise.
- The client will walk one block without shortness of breath.

The expected outcomes in this case illustrate specific ways to accomplish—and measure the accomplishment of—that goal.

Regional and institutional differences in the use of terminology and documentation systems may determine your use of goals, outcomes, and other terms. The important idea that remains, however, is that concrete descriptions of client behaviors are used to demonstrate when the plan of care has been successful. The outcomes or goals that you devise should be linked to your nursing diagnoses and direct interventions to achieve the desired changes.

Types of Outcomes. Ways to measure health care outcomes have developed over time. Early in the twentieth century, common outcome measurements included morbidity, mortality, length of client stay, and infection rate. However, as the health care industry has become more sophisticated and the consumer more knowledgeable, these measures have been deemed inadequate to capture the complexity of health care and to measure specific outcomes.

Now, client satisfaction forms an important outcome measure as well. Global multidisciplinary measures describe the client's satisfaction with care, the hospital stay, activities of daily living, and cognitive function. Other outcome measurements may include structural or process characteristics that judge the effectiveness and efficiency of a health care setting. Such outcomes in this situation may be cost, profit, unscheduled readmissions, unscheduled repeat surgeries, and unnecessary procedures. Global measurements are adequate for assessing the effectiveness of a health care system but are not specific for measuring the results of nursing care or specific outcomes for individual clients.

Discipline-specific outcomes can be influenced and changed by the discipline involved. A **nursing-sensitive client outcome** is the state, behavior, or perception of an individual, family, or community that is measured along

Table 10-1 An Example of NOC-Vital Signs

Definition: Extent to which temperature, pulse, respiration, and blood pressure are within normal range
Outcome target rating: Maintain at ________ Increase to ________

INDICATOR	SEVERE DEVIATION FROM NORMAL RANGE	SUBSTANTIAL DEVIATION FROM NORMAL RANGE	MODERATE DEVIATION FROM NORMAL RANGE	MILD DEVIATION FROM NORMAL RANGE	NO DEVIATION FROM NORMAL RANGE
Body temperature	1	2	3	4	5
Apical heart rate	1	2	3	4	5
Radial pulse rate	1	2	3	4	5
Respiration rate	1	2	3	4	5
Systolic blood pressure	1	2	3	4	5
Diastolic blood pressure	1	2	3	4	5
Pulse pressure	1	2	3	4	5

Moorhead, S., Johnson, M., & Maas, M. (Eds.). (2004). *Nursing outcomes classification (NOC)/ Iowa outcomes project* (3rd ed.). St. Louis, MO: Mosby.

a continuum in response to a nursing intervention(s) (Moorhead, Johnson, & Maas, 2004). The American Nurses Association (1996) identifies the following client outcomes as nursing-sensitive quality indicators for acute care settings: pressure ulcers, client falls, client satisfaction with pain management, client satisfaction with educational information, client satisfaction with overall care, client satisfaction with nursing care, and nosocomial infection rate. In planning and implementing nursing care, the nurse should strive to reach these outcomes (i.e., to prevent nosocomial infection and client injury, to increase client satisfaction with nursing care, pain management, and educational information).

Nursing Outcomes Classification System. The **Nursing Outcomes Classification (NOC)** is a standardized terminology and measures to evaluate effects of nursing interventions (Moorhead, Johnson, & Maas, 2004). It is developed by the University of Iowa outcomes research team. The current NOC system has 330 outcome labels. The complete list of 330 NOC labels can be found at http://www.nursing.uiowa.edu/centers/cncce/noc/noclabels.htm.

Each outcome label has a definition, a target outcome rating, a list of indicators, and a five-point Likert scale to measure changes (positive, negative, or lack of) resulting from nursing interventions. In the facility using the NOC system, the nurse selects outcomes and indicators relevant to nursing diagnoses to establish outcomes for client problems. For example, "Activity Tolerance" is the outcome for "Activity Intolerance." The nurse selects indicators pertinent to client status to measure activity tolerance. Table 10-1 provides an example of NOC-Vital Signs.

The language used in the NOC system is common to all health care professionals. Increasingly, nurses and facilities are recognizing the benefits of using a standardized outcome classification system. The National Library of Medicine has included NOC in the Unified Medical Language System.

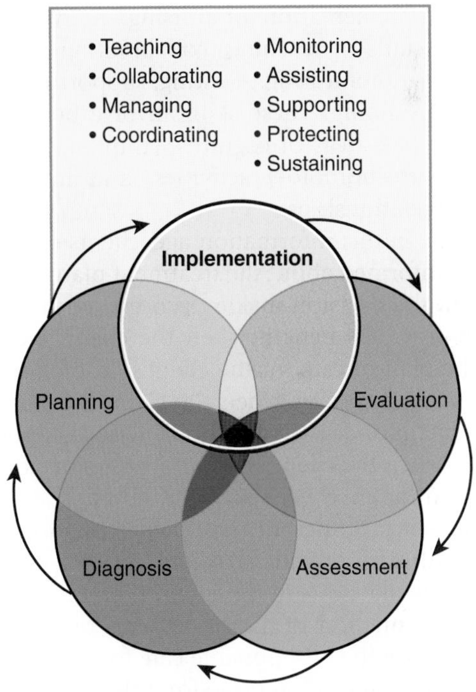

FIGURE 10-5 Implementation is the action phase of the nursing process. During the implementation phase, you provide the services identified during the planning process to support and protect your client. Implementation involves teaching, collaborating, managing, coordinating, monitoring, assisting, supporting, protecting, and sustaining.

IMPLEMENTATION

Implementation is the action phase of the nursing process—the phase in which you implement the plans developed in the planning phase (Figure 10-5). In the planning phase, nursing diagnoses are identified, individualized interventions are selected or designed to reach expected outcomes and to resolve factors identified in "related to" in nursing diagnoses. These interventions may be called nursing orders, nursing activities, or nursing approaches. When communicated to the nursing team, nursing interventions should contain elements that clearly explain the action to be performed by all nursing staff.

Having recognized actual or potential client's problems and established care plans, you implement nursing interventions to change the client's level of physical, psychosocial, or spiritual functioning in the context of the client's support system. You may help the client make lifestyle changes, support physical function, support homeostasis, support psychosocial well-being, support the family unit, and make effective use of the health care delivery system to solve problems.

SKILLS OF IMPLEMENTING INTERVENTIONS

Effective implementation of nursing interventions requires the skills of teaching, collaborating, managing, coordinating, monitoring, assisting, supporting, protecting, and sustaining. These skills involve being able to function in the areas of cognitive (thinking) processes, technical (psychomotor) activities, and interpersonal (affective) relationships.

Teaching. In this information age, clients expect to be kept well informed about the treatment plan and to participate in the decision-making process. Both the client and the providers benefit when the client is educated about the plan of care for the client's problems. For example, safety improves when the client has knowledge of the benefits and risks of care. Likewise, complications are fewer when the client knows how to manage a disorder or monitor a recovery period at home.

Collaborating. Sometimes you will collaborate with other health care providers to identify and implement the most adequate care to the client. Collaboration is the professional method of asking for and receiving assistance to ensure the best possible care for your client.

Managing. You can intervene for a client by managing care provided by others, and parts of your nursing care plan can be delegated to other health care workers. For example, a nursing assistant may provide personal hygiene care to the client. Although the intervention is delegated, you are still accountable for the activity. You need to know that the intervention was completed; the nursing assistant needs to report any abnormal findings observed while implementing the intervention.

Coordinating. When multiple health team members are involved in the client's care, coordination of the client's care is vital to meeting the client's needs. Commonly, a nurse takes charge of that coordination. Nurses have broad general knowledge of the roles and functions of the health care team and are in the best position to coordinate the various services that might be needed by the client.

Monitoring. Surveillance or monitoring is a primary nursing intervention, particularly in acute care settings. Monitoring the client's status and reporting changes to the physician is a major component of nursing. It ensures that the physician receives the information necessary to accomplish the client's health goals and to prevent complications. The purposes of monitoring are to detect complications, to evaluate the effectiveness of the interventions, and to ensure that the interventions are carried out correctly.

Assisting. Assisting is providing direct physical care when the client is unable to perform self-care. Interventions may involve assisting a client who is partially or fully unable to care for himself or herself. The client may be disabled and need assistance to perform the basic activities of daily living or may lack the manual dexterity to perform medical treatments. You would provide assistance when the client needs help to take medications, seek health-related services, or plan for the management of a health problem.

Supporting. Interventions may be supportive when the client has the ability and the knowledge but lacks willpower, resilience, or the motivation for self-care. Supportive care makes the client feel able to face adverse circumstances, find inner strength, and believe in self-efficacy. To give supportive care you do not necessarily change your client's methods of self-care; rather, you strengthen the client to get needs met.

Care is also classified as supportive when a client's physiological processes are marginally functional, and care is needed to maintain life functions. Physiological support involves implementing the physician's plan. You may give intravenous fluid or blood to maintain blood pressure or medications to strengthen the heart or control arrhythmias.

Protecting. Nurses play a major role in protecting clients from harm. The health care facilities (such as hospitals, rehabilitation centers, clinics, and skilled care facilities) should be the safest environment possible, whether the client is critically ill, having surgery, learning to walk after a stroke, learning to cope with blindness, or needs protected living in old age. However, medical treatment always involves some degree of risk, which means that clients need constant surveillance and intervention to prevent harm. For example, the nurse monitors and provides interventions to prevent the complications of bed rest, adverse effects of medications, and injuries.

Sustaining. Nursing interventions sustain life and physical function when the client's condition is critical. The most obvious example is the implementation of cardiopulmonary resuscitation when the heartbeat or respiration has stopped. Critical care, recovery room, and emergency room nurses are involved in life-sustaining interventions.

TYPES OF INTERVENTIONS

Nursing interventions can be direct or indirect and may originate with a nurse, a physician, or other health care providers.

Direct Care Nursing Interventions. A direct care intervention "is a treatment performed through interaction with the client(s)" (Dochterman & Bulechek, 2004, p. xxiii). Direct care interventions include both physiological and psychosocial nursing actions to improve the client's health or modify the environment in a way that is conducive to health or that prevents disease.

Examples of physiological direct care nursing interventions include bowel training, cast care, cardiac precautions, constipation/impaction management, ambulation, eye care, and self-care assistance (toileting, for example). Examples of psychosocial direct care nursing interventions include counseling, emotional support, hope instillation, humor, and presence. Figure 10-6 shows a nurse performing a direct care intervention.

Indirect Care Nursing Interventions. Nursing includes many activities intended to maintain a safe environment and to coordinate the client's care. Even though these activities are not at the client's bedside and may not be specific to an individual, they are necessary for client welfare. "An *indirect care intervention* is a treatment performed away from the client but on behalf of a client or group of clients. Indirect care interventions include nursing actions aimed at management of the client care environment and interdisciplinary collaboration. These actions support the effectiveness of the direct care intervention" (Dochterman & Bulechek, 2004, p. xxiii). Examples of indirect care nursing interventions include delegation, emergency cart checking, shift report, and telephone consultation. Box 10-3 shows an example of an indirect care intervention needed for continuity of care in an acute care facility.

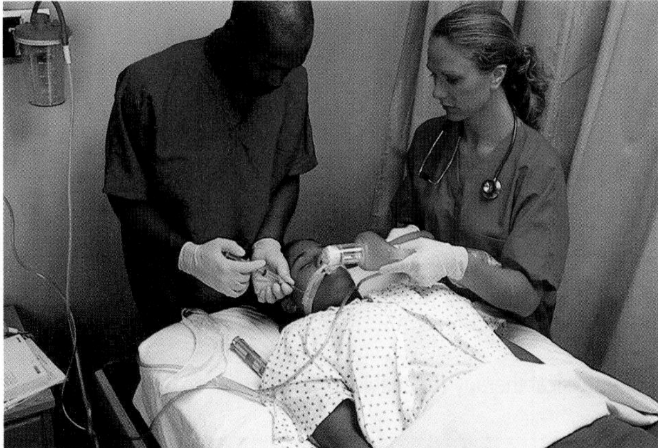

FIGURE 10-6 In today's health care environment, nurses must be prepared to accomplish highly technical direct care interventions. Remember, however, that a highly technical setting makes sensitive psychosocial interventions more important than ever.

Nurse-Initiated and Physician-Initiated Interventions. Nurses provide two types of care for their clients. Independent nursing care is within the scope of nursing practice and does not require a physician's order. Interdependent nursing care is within the scope of nursing practice but is carried out only as part of a physician's treatment plan. Both types of actions are correctly described as nursing care because these actions require a nurse's expertise to ensure the client's safety.

A **nurse-initiated intervention** is "an intervention initiated by the nurse in response to a nursing diagnosis. It is an autonomous action based on scientific rationale that is executed to benefit the client in a predicted way related to the nursing diagnosis and projected outcome" (Dochterman & Bulechek, 2004). Helping the client to dress is an example of a nurse-initiated intervention or independent action (Box 10-4).

A **physician-initiated intervention** is "a treatment initiated by a physician in response to a medical diagnosis but carried out by a nurse in response to a 'doctor's order.' Nurses may also carry out treatments initiated by other providers, such as pharmacists, respiratory therapists, or physician assistants" (Dochterman & Bulechek, 2004). An example of a physician-initiated intervention

BOX 10-3 *Example of an Indirect Care Nursing Intervention*

SHIFT REPORT

Definition: Exchanging essential client care information with other nursing staff at change of shift

Activities

- Review pertinent demographic data, including name, age, and room number.
- Identify chief complaint and reason for admission, as appropriate.
- Summarize significant health history, as necessary.
- Identify key medical and nursing diagnoses, as appropriate.
- Identify resolved medical and nursing diagnoses, as appropriate.
- Present information succinctly, focusing on recent and significant data needed by nursing staff assuming responsibility for care.
- Describe treatment regimen, including diet, fluid therapy, medications, and exercise.
- Identify laboratory and diagnostic tests to be completed during the next 24 hours.
- Review recent pertinent laboratory and diagnostic test results, as appropriate.
- Describe health status data, including vital signs and signs and symptoms present during the shift.
- Describe nursing interventions being implemented.
- Describe client and family responses to nursing interventions.
- Summarize progress toward goals.
- Summarize discharge plans, as appropriate.

Modified from Dochterman, J. M., & Bulechek, G. M. (2004). *Nursing interventions classification (NIC).* St. Louis, MO: Mosby.

is management of the client's diet when the client is recovering from an illness that has caused a medical need for dietary limitations (Box 10-5).

ELEMENTS OF AN INTERVENTION

Nursing interventions should be individualized and written clearly on the client's medical record so that all nurses involved in the client's care can provide the same care. Planning involves making decisions about the *who, what, where, when, why, and how* of client care (Table 10-2). *Who* refers to the person who provides the care, such as a physical therapist, a nurse, a nursing assistant, a family member, the client, or another practitioner. *What* refers to the care that will most effectively meet the client's needs. *Where* could be the client's home, a clinic, or a hospital. *When* refers to the time that the care is delivered or to the priorities of events to be carried out. The time may be before the client is admitted to a hospital, during a hospital stay, after discharge, during a clinic visit, or at a particular time of day. *Why* provides the rationale for care and includes evidence that the care is important, will work, or will meet individual client needs. *How* defines the methods of intervention required and may specify measures needed to individualize a client's care.

BOX 10-4 *Example of a Nurse-Initiated Nursing Intervention*

DRESSING

Definition: Choosing, putting on, and removing clothes for a person who cannot do this for self

Activities

- Identify areas where client needs assistance in dressing.
- Monitor client's ability to dress self.
- Dress client after personal hygiene is completed.
- Encourage participation in selection of clothing.
- Encourage use of self-care devices, as appropriate.
- Dress affected extremity first, as appropriate.
- Dress in nonrestrictive clothing, as appropriate.
- Dress in personal clothing, as appropriate.
- Change client's clothing at bedtime.
- Select shoes or slippers conducive to ambulation.
- Offer to launder clothing, as necessary.
- Continue giving assistance until the client can assume full responsibility for dressing self.

Modified from Dochterman, J. M., & Bulechek, G. M. (2004). *Nursing interventions classification (NIC).* St. Louis, MO: Mosby.

BOX 10-5 *Example of a Physician-Initiated Nursing Intervention*

DIET STAGING

Definition: Instituting required diet restrictions with subsequent progression of diet as tolerated

Activities

- Determine presence of bowel sounds.
- Institute NPO, as needed.
- Clamp nasogastric tube and monitor tolerance, as appropriate.
- Monitor for alertness and presence of gag reflex, as appropriate.
- Monitor tolerance to ingestion of ice chips and water.
- Determine if client is passing flatus.
- Collaborate with other health care team members to progress diet as rapidly as possible without complications.
- Progress diet from clear liquid, full liquid, soft, to regular or special diet, as tolerated, for adults and children.
- Progress from glucose water or oral electrolyte solution, half-strength formula, to full-strength formula for babies.
- Monitor tolerance to diet progression.
- Offer six small feedings, rather than three meals, as appropriate.
- Post the diet restrictions at bedside, on chart, and in care plan.

Modified from Dochterman, J. M., & Bulechek, G. M. (2004). *Nursing interventions classification (NIC).* St. Louis, MO: Mosby.

Table 10-2 Individualized Nursing Interventions: Specify Who, What, When, Where, How, Why*

PHYSICIAN'S ORDER	NURSING INTERVENTION
Ambulate tid	Encourage client to walk at 0900, 1300, 1800; 20 steps in the room with a walker.
	ALTERNATIVE Encourage client to walk 4 lengths of the hall morning, afternoon, and evening, before discharge.
	ALTERNATIVE Walk with physical therapy tid using gait belt, progressing from standing at bedside to walking the length of the hall before discharge. Give Vicodin on request at the onset of pain (to prevent severe pain).
Vicodin DS, 1 tablet by mouth q4-6h prn	**ALTERNATIVE** Give Vicodin 30 minutes before ambulating with physical therapy (to enable to walk).
	ALTERNATIVE Give Vicodin q4h until pain is controlled.

*NOTE: "Client will" is assumed; the "why" is in parentheses because it is not necessarily stated in writing interventions.

Nursing Interventions Classification System. For nurses to communicate with each other and to describe nursing to the health care team, the language of nursing needs to be standardized so that it has a common meaning among nurses. A standardized language can facilitate communication for care-plan development, research, staff education, or curriculum development, for example.

The **Nursing Interventions Classification (NIC)** system is a standardized language to describe nursing activities (Dochterman & Bulechek, 2004). It is developed by a researcher team at the University of Iowa. The NIC system has been recognized by the American Nurses Association and the National Library of Medicine.

The NIC system consists of 514 nursing intervention labels. Each label is provided with a definition and a list of nursing activities. The nurse can use the NIC system to develop a care plan by selecting nursing intervention labels and nursing activities pertinent to nursing diagnoses and expected outcomes. The nurse may select several nursing intervention labels for one nursing diagnosis. By using the NIC system, the nurse does not need to describe an array of nursing activities and needs to write only a few words when necessary. The NIC system can be used in a computerized system or a paper-based system to document nursing interventions. Most of the NIC interventions are appropriate to use in any health care setting or specialty area.

THE NURSING CARE PLAN

The nursing care plan consists of three components of the nursing process: client problems (nursing diagnoses), expected outcomes, and interventions. Client problems may be presented as a common problem list for the health care team to use or may be described as nursing diagnoses for nurses. The common problem list facilitates a multidisciplinary team approach. The problem list of nursing diagnoses delineates the contribution of nursing to client care.

The nurse may use the traditional approach to develop a care plan by writing client problems list, expected outcomes, and intervention statements. The nurse may also use the NANDA International (NANDA-I) (2005) approved nursing diagnoses to describe the client's problems, the NOC system to identify outcomes and specific indicators, and the NIC system to select pertinent nursing interventions. The standardized language systems can help the nurse develop a nursing care plan in a timely manner. The use of the NANDA-I, NIC, and NOC systems is rapidly growing in computerized record-keeping systems and may become the standard for documentation.

For public health nursing care, two standardized language systems may be used to plan and document nursing care: the Omaha System and the Clinical Care Classification (CCC) system, previously known as the Home Healthcare Classification (HHCC) system. Both systems are also recognized by the American Nurses Association and the National Library of Medicine.

The Omaha System (Martin, 2005) is developed for multidisciplinary health care providers to document health care related to public health. It consists of three components: assessment (Problem Classification), intervention (Intervention Scheme), and outcomes (Problem Rating Scale for Outcomes). Case studies of using the Omaha System to plan and document public health nursing care can be found at http://www.omahasystem.org/.

The CCC system was developed originally for home health care and is now expanded to ambulatory care and other health care settings (Saba, 2002, 2006). The CCC consists of two taxonomies: CCC of Nursing Diagnoses and Outcomes and CCC of Nursing Interventions and Actions. It is used to assess, document, classify, and evaluate outcomes of home health care. Further information about the updated CCC system can be found at http://www.sabacare.com/.

GUIDELINES FOR DEVELOPING CARE PLANS

The plan of care establishes priorities and guides the efforts of the client, the nurses, and other members of the health care team for individualized client care. As these decisions are made, the care plan is written to provide documentation for all health care personnel who will be caring for the client.

The traditional nursing care plan is formatted in three columns (problems, outcomes, and interventions), with additional columns for the date and signature of the person who developed the plan and for the dates when outcomes are achieved. Evaluation information is charted in nursing progress notes. The student care plan may consist of five components: nursing diagnoses, goals and measurable outcomes, nursing interventions, scientific rationale for the interventions, and evaluation. The student care plan is designed to help students apply and document the nursing process (assessment, diagnosis, planning [expected outcomes and interventions], implementation, and evaluation) for each client problem.

PURPOSES OF A WRITTEN CARE PLAN

The written care plan has evolved as a tool for providing current information for client care. The purpose of a nursing care plan is to communicate the planned care to the health care team, thus ensuring continuity of care. A written plan should be concise to communicate information efficiently. It should also provide specific information to ensure that everyone providing the care will provide the same care. The purposes of a care plan can also include the following:

- Identify all problems being treated
- Provide a detailed guide for nursing care
- Individualize the care provided
- Set priorities

- Coordinate care among all health care workers
- Guide evaluation of care
- Provide for individual and family participation in planning
- Document current nursing practice

TYPES OF CARE PLANS

There are different types of care plans in practice today, each with advantages and disadvantages. These types of care plans have varying degrees of individualization and standardization.

Individualized Care Plans. An **individualized care plan** is one written specifically for each client who enters a health care facility (Box 10-6). This type of care plan is developed from the admission history, physical and functional assessment, and problems anticipated on the basis of the physician's treatment plan.

Individualized care plans allow you to identify the unique problems of each client, to decide on the outcomes to be achieved, and to identify which nursing interventions will be appropriate to achieve those outcomes. These plans contain only the applicable nursing diagnoses, outcomes, and interventions. The disadvantage of individualized care plans is the time required to write them.

Standardized Care Plans. **Standardized care plans** are typically written by a group of nurses who use their collective expertise to produce a plan to direct nursing care for clients with specific medical diagnoses (such as myocardial infarction) or nursing diagnoses (such as *Pain* or

BOX 10-6 *Nursing Care Plan*

Sample Nursing Care Plan Using Standardized Language

Mrs. Worden tripped over her space heater at home and fell. She burned her left anterior thigh on the space heater and fractured her right hip. Her frail older adult husband called the emergency number (911), and an ambulance responded. Mrs. Worden was admitted to the local hospital, where she underwent an open reduction and internal fixation to repair the fractured right hip. Treatment was also started for the second-degree burn on her left thigh. After 4 days on the inpatient surgical unit, she was ready for discharge but not independent enough in mobility or activities of daily living to return home. She was discharged to a skilled unit in a local nursing home.

Admission data included the following:

- White female, age 84. Height 5 ft. 3 in. Weight 128 pounds.
- BP 148/72, T 97.6, RP 68 and regular, R 18.
- Wound anterior thigh measured 4 cm × 3.3 cm with a depth of 0.5 cm.
- Incision right hip measured 9 cm in length with 13 sutures intact. Skin was pink with no signs of infection. Skin edges approximated.
- Range of motion: all extremities within normal limits except right hip abduction was only 20 degrees and right knee flexion was only 45 degrees. Pain noted on movement of right leg during range of motion.
- Ambulated 4 yards with pain and fatigue.
- Is continent of bladder and bowel.
- Oral intake has been a regular diet with intake of 75% to 100% at each meal.
- Last known bowel movement was 2 days before with a usual routine of daily defecation.
- Oriented to time, person, and place.
- Very upset that she could not go home for physical and occupational therapy rather than going to the nursing home.

NANDA-I Nursing Diagnosis	NOC Expected Outcomes With Indicators	NIC Interventions With Selected Activites	Evaluation
Acute Pain **Related Factors:** • Second-degree burn on left thigh from contact with space heater As manifested by: • Reports pain 6/10 during dressing change • Appears tense and jerks away from nurse when dressing removed	***Pain Level:*** • Report of pain will decrease to moderate (3-4/10). • Physiological signs of pain will be slight to moderate.	***Analgesic Administration:*** • Check medical order for drug, dose, and frequency of analgesic prescribed. • Check for history of drug allergy. • Administer analgesic (oxycodone with acetaminophen [Percocet] one tablet every 6 hours, in this case) 30 minutes before dressing change. • Advise that drowsiness can occur. Put side rails up and call light within reach. • Document response.	***24 Hours After Administration:*** • Percocet one tablet PO was given 30 minutes before dressing change. • Reported pain of 2/10 during dressing change. • Appeared to sleep through most of dressing change. No change in facial expression, restlessness, or muscle tension with dressing change. • Side rails up and call light within reach.

Nursing outcome and intervention labels from Johnson, M., Bulechek, G., Butcher, H., Dochterman, J. M., Maas, M., Moorhead, S., et al. (Eds.). (2006). *NANDA, NOC, and NIC linkages: Nursing diagnoses, outcomes, & interventions.* St. Louis, MO: Mosby.

Anxiety). They are also developed for clients undergoing special procedures (such as cardiac catheterization).

These care plans are duplicated and made available to the appropriate units in the health care facility. The format is designed with extra space so you can individualize the plan by filling in specific client characteristics, related factors associated with the nursing diagnosis, deadlines for the outcomes, and additional details in the interventions. For example, you can individualize interventions by adding frequencies, amounts, times, and client preferences.

Standardized care plans have the advantage of saving you time by reducing the amount of writing required. They are also particularly helpful to nurses working in unfamiliar areas. The main disadvantage of standardized care plans is the lack of individualization. Not all of the nursing diagnoses, outcomes, and interventions listed on the standardized care plan pertain to every client. Using a standardized care plan requires you to critically analyze its applicability to an individual.

Computerized Care Plans. A **computerized care plan** is a care plan created by a computer program. Many software vendors have developed computerized care plans written by expert clinicians.

A computerized care plan has nursing diagnoses, client outcomes, and nursing interventions, and it also allows for the relevant dates to be inserted. You choose the appropriate nursing diagnoses, outcomes, and interventions for the individual client. Advantages of computerized care plans include their legibility and the ease with which they can be changed or updated. They also allow nurse researchers to collect data about groups of clients. The disadvantage is that, like standardized care plans, they lack individualization. However, computerized care plans can be simpler to individualize than standardized forms.

The NANDA-I, NIC, NOC, Omaha, and CCC systems are recognized as standardized nursing languages and are integrated into computerized client records in some health care settings. Nurses working in these settings can develop nursing care plans promptly by selecting problems, outcomes, and interventions pertinent to the client with a few clicks and typing a few notes in the computer to individualize client outcomes and interventions.

Case Management Plans. **Case management** is "a collaborative process of assessment, planning, facilitation and advocacy for options and services to meet an individual's health needs through communication and available resources to promote quality cost-effective outcomes" (retrieved May 4, 2006, from http://www.cmsa.org/ABOUTUS/DefinitionofCaseManagement/tabid/104/Default.aspx). Case management is used across the health care continuum from home health care to long-term care to hospitals. In most settings, case management is performed by nurses (Cohen, 2005).

Case management involves health assessment and planning for services to meet the comprehensive needs of the client. The standards of care management plans or clinical pathways are used to plan for client care. The case manager works with the client, family, health care team, and payers to develop client goals and plans to reach those goals. Once a plan is formulated, the case manager carries out the plan, revises the plan if it is ineffective, and coordinates all care. The case manager ensures that the client's care is well coordinated, with no gaps or overlaps in service during the course of an illness.

The goals of case management are to do the following:

- Coordinate needed care and services across disciplines to reduce fragmented or duplicated care
- Achieve satisfactory clinical outcomes
- Reduce cost per case
- Reduce the length of hospital stay and use resources effectively
- Reduce readmission rates (Cohen, 2005)

Case management models exist on a continuum from working with an individual client to managing a system of service delivery. At the client end, a hospital nurse case manager may be responsible for client care from before admission to after discharge, such as in perinatal case management. In another model, the case manager may focus on services provided to groups of clients, and on planning a system that controls costs and reduces the length of hospital stay, such as in heart failure case management. At the extreme business end of the spectrum is outcome management. An outcome manager's function is similar to that of a case manager but is more focused on researching and analyzing cost-effective ways to produce desired outcomes among large groups of clients.

Nurses who are case managers use both nursing terminology and the terminology of other disciplines to develop plans of care for clients in multiple settings over a period of time. For example, a client with chronic obstructive pulmonary disease may have home health care services, be admitted for an acute exacerbation of the disease, and be discharged to long-term care before being able to go home again. The case manager would plan this entire span of services.

Clinical Pathways. A **clinical pathway** is a standardized multidisciplinary care plan that projects the expected course of the client's treatment and progress over the hospital stay. It is a method for describing the plan of care by predicting the course of the client's hospital stay and prescribing the care and outcomes on a day-by-day basis. It provides clinical practice guidelines for health professionals in hospitals, home health care, and long-term care.

Clinical pathways are also called care maps, clinical paths, critical paths, critical pathways, collaborative care plans, and multidisciplinary care plans. All have the commonality of containing all the critical elements of the client's care. No matter which name is applied to it, a clinical pathway is a plan of care with a predictable timetable for the client to achieve the goals. This type of plan is seen by many as a way to maintain quality care and coordinate services while controlling costs.

Most clinical pathways are written on a grid that lists the client's problems, outcomes, and interventions by multidisciplinary staff along a specified time line. Figure 10-7 shows an example of a clinical pathway. Usually, the facility's pathway is developed by a group of multidisciplinary clinicians who care for clients with specific illnesses. In fact, the pathway's primary value lies in its multidisciplinary approach. Ideally, the clinical pathway should include each discipline's standardized language.

Clinical pathways are available for procedures, conditions, illnesses, and diagnosis-related groups. Time lines can range from a few hours or days to a period covering weeks or months, depending on the condition or procedure for which the pathway was developed. For example, a clinical pathway for a client having a sigmoidoscopy would cover just a few hours. A clinical pathway for a client having a total hip replacement may include a 3- to 4-day acute care phase after surgery, followed by another 4 days of skilled nursing care before discharge.

EVALUATION

Evaluation is a systematic and ongoing process of examining whether expected outcomes have been achieved and whether nursing interventions have been effective (Figure 10-8, p. 224). However, evaluation must also examine the quality of nursing care delivery and link positive client outcomes to quality care.

To evaluate the client's progress toward attaining expected outcomes, you will first need to review the expected outcomes for each diagnosis. The purposes of expected outcomes are to direct nursing interventions, to maintain continuity of nursing care, and to measure the effectiveness of nursing interventions. Keep in mind that accurate, meaningful evaluation relies on expected outcomes that are measurable, realistic, and attainable in relation to a client's capabilities and available resources.

Standards are established to evaluate the quality of care and to guide nursing practice. Nurses must agree on the standards and consistently practice according to the standards if nursing care is to be identified as the cause of positive outcomes. This chapter introduces evaluation by outcomes and by standards of practice.

EVALUATING CLIENT OUTCOMES

The process of evaluating nursing care reconsiders each phase of the nursing process. Was assessment accurate and thorough? Was the nursing diagnosis derived correctly from the data, and did it accurately identify the problem? Were the expected outcomes measurable, realistic, and appropriate? Were the interventions appropriate and appropriately implemented? During the evaluation phase, ask yourself the following key questions:

- What are the client's responses to interventions in relation to expected outcomes? Are the responses desirable or undesirable?
- Are the interventions effective in meeting expected outcomes? If not, why are the interventions ineffective? Is it necessary to revise outcomes or interventions?
- Is the nursing diagnosis still active? Is it necessary to revise it or to add new nursing diagnoses?

Examining the Client's Responses to Interventions. As you are intervening, you should evaluate the client's physical and psychosocial responses and document desirable or undesirable responses. Desirable responses indicate that the purposes of interventions are achieved and the client is progressing toward expected outcomes. Undesirable responses indicate poor progress toward expected outcomes or the occurrence of complications or side effects. Your evaluation may include responses to both medical and nursing interventions.

To assess physical and psychosocial responses to medications or treatments, you evaluate whether the purposes of medications or treatments are being achieved, the occurrence of complications or side effects, and the client's understanding of the medications or treatments. Through the process of continuous evaluation, you may identify problems that need additional attention. For example, some clients stop taking antibiotics or antihypertensives when their symptoms have subsided. When you evaluate the client's psychosocial responses to medications, you identify the problem of lack of understanding of medications.

Evaluating responses to diagnostic tests or procedures is another important aspect of nursing care. Throughout tests or procedures, the client may have many questions or concerns and may develop complications. Care can then be provided to ease the client's anxiety, increase the client's understanding, or detect complications or side effects at an early stage.

After providing nursing interventions, you should evaluate responses of the client and family members. You need to evaluate their understanding of the teaching. They may not understand the information completely or may have some misunderstanding. Some families may need further information. Others may need reinforcement to perform appropriate health behaviors.

Evaluating the client's and family members' perceptions of care provided is also important. You may perceive that good nursing care has been provided, but the client or family members may think otherwise. The client's perceptions of nursing care influence the satisfaction with nursing care, which is often used as a quality indicator of care by health care agencies. Therefore, you need to seek feedback from the client or family members to understand their perceptions of the care received and

Text continued on p. 224

VALLEY BAPTIST MEDICAL CENTER
Harlingen, Texas

ADMISSION ORDERS - PNEUMONIA

1. ☐ Admit to medical floor. ☐ Other ____________
2. ☐ Admit to the service of Dr. ____________
3. Diagnosis ____________
4. ☐ Initiate Pneumonia Restorative Care Path.
5. LAB: ☐ ER Profile (CBC w/diff, Chem 14)
   ☐ Blood cultures X 2, 15 minutes apart - separate sticks
   ☐ Aminophylline Level, if patient taking.
   ☐ Sputum C&S / Induction p.r.n. by RT.
   ☐ UA
   ☐ If SpO_2 <92%, collect ABG
   ☐ ____________
6. ☐ Chest X-ray
7. ☐ O_2 at ____________ LPM via ____________ ☐ Follow O_2 Protocol
8. ☐ Respiratory Treatment: ____________
   ☐ Bronchodilator Protocol ☐ Suction p.r.n.
9. ☐ Diet: ____________
10. ☐ IV: ____________
11. ☐ Antibiotic Therapy: ____________
    ☐ Initial Dose NOW
12. ☐ Acetaminophen gr X, 1 suppository or 650 mg P.O. for Temp >100.6F° q 4 hrs p.r.n.
13. ☐ Old charts to the floor.
14. ☐ Vital signs q 4 hours until stable, then routine.
15. Activity: ☐ Ambulate at least BID ☐ Bathroom with assistance ☐ Bed rest
16. ☐ Social Service to evaluate.
17. ____________

Date ____________ Time ____________ ____________ M.D.
Physician Signature

VBMC 1965-129-0396

FIGURE 10-7 An example of a clinical pathway for a client with pneumonia. (Courtesy Valley Baptist Medical Center, Harlingen, Texas.)

Continued

VALLEY BAPTIST MEDICAL CENTER
Harlingen, Texas

RESTORATIVE CARE PATH

PNEUMONIA > 17 Years of Age

KEY: Initials=Completed; N/A = Not Applicable; 0 - Variance

Page 1 of 2 VBMC 1620-005-0196

Initial	Signature/Status	Initial	Signature/Status

DRG: 79 and 89 Special Considerations: Case Manager

	Date: ☐ ER ☐ PATT ☐ Direct Adm RN Review	Date: Day 1: RN Review	Date: Day 2: RN Review	Date: Day 3: RN Review	Date: Day 4: RN Review	Date: Day 5: RN Review	EXPECTED OUTCOMES
Consults	_______Call Internal Medicine or primary MD to admit.		_______If not improved 48 hrs after admission, consider pulmonary consult.	-------> _______All consults notified	-------> ------->	-------> ------->	All consults notified
Tests	_______ER Profile _______Blood Culture X 2 (separate sticks) 15 min. apart _______Aminophylline Level (if taking) _______UA _______Sputum C&S / Induction p.r.n. by RT _______CXR _______If O_2Sat <92, collect ABG	_______Call MD for abnormal labs _______ABGs p.r.n. _______Swab for MRSA for nursing home patients or transfers _______If sputum not collected, in 4 hrs, notify MD	_______Call MD for abnormal labs _______In 48 hrs, if no clinical improvement, consider CBC, CXR, alternate means of sputum collection	------->	------->	------->	All labs WNL or stable for patient.
Assessment & Evaluation	_______Initiate Database _______Vital signs q 1 hr or as indicated _______F/C if unable to void _______I&O _______Assess for TB risk factors	_______Vital signs q 4 hrs _______Check voiding ------->	-------> -------> ------->	-------> -------> ------->	_______If pt afebrile X 24 hrs, consider disch -------> ------->	-------> -------> ------->	Pt afebrile, consider disch Voiding adequate I&O WNL
Activity / Safety	_______Assess PPI Level _______Raise HOB 30°	_______Bed rest with BRP ------->	-------> Activity as tolerated ------->	-------> ------->	-------> ------->	-------> ------->	Return to previous activity level
Treatments	_______O_2 ___________ L/min (NC / Mask / Trach) _______Resp.Tx: ___________ _______O_2 Sat Monitor _______Suction p.r.n.	_______O_2 protocol -------> -------> ------->	-------> -------> -------> ------->	-------> -------> -------> ------->	-------> -------> -------> ------->	-------> -------> -------> ------->	Respiratory status stable
Diet		_______Assess nutritional status Dietitian? ☐ Yes ☐ No	Diet: ___________	Diet: ___________	Diet: ___________	Diet: ___________	Patient tolerates prescribed diet

FIGURE 10-7 An example of a clinical pathway for a client with pneumonia. (Courtesy Valley Baptist Medical Center, Harlingen, Texas.)

VALLEY BAPTIST MEDICAL CENTER
Harlingen, Texas
RESTORATIVE CARE PATH
PNEUMONIA > 17 Years of Age

Page 2 of 2 VBMC 1620-005-0196

	Date: ☐ ER ☐ PATT ☐ Direct Adm RN Review	Date: Day 1: RN Review	Date: Day 2: RN Review	Date: Day 3: RN Review	Date: Day 4: RN Review	Date: Day 5: RN Review	EXPECTED OUTCOMES
Meds / IV Fluids	______Start IV ______Start Antibiotic Protocol ______________ ______________ ______List Home meds ______ER Fever Protocol	______ IV __________ @ ______ hr ______Continue IV antibiotics ______Adjust antibiotics per culture results.	______Reevaluate antibiotic therapy if no clinical improvement ------->	______Consider Saline lock ______Consider P.O. antibiotics	-------> ------->	-------> ------->	D.C. with P.O. antibiotics
Pain Management	______Medicate as ordered; document effect.	------->	------->	------->	------->	------->	Prescription for pain meds as needed.
Patient/Family Education	______Explain procedures, meds & equipment. ______Provide opportunity for questions. ______ Provide patient pathway	______Provide educational materials ______Reinforce teaching ______Return demo & document progress	-------> ------->	-------> ------->	-------> ------->	-------> ------->	Pt/family verbalize understanding of D/C instructions, follow-up appointment/classes.
Psychosocial	______Allow verbalization of feelings ______Consider referral to Pastoral Services.	-------> ------->	-------> ------->	-------> ------->	-------> ------->	______No anxiety ------->	No anxiety noted
Discharge Planning / Continuum of Care	______ Obtain old chart & send to floor with patient. ______ Discharge Planning Assessment ______ Discharge home ______ Admit (consider STO)	______Social Service Consult	------->	------->	-------> ______Consider discharge	------->	Discharge: ☐ Home ☐ NHP ☐ Home Health ☐ Transfer ☐ Rehab ☐ Other ________ ☐ Records faxed ☐ Report called ☐ D.C. instructions given.
Signatures 7 - 3							
Signatures 3 - 11							
Signatures 11 - 7							

FIGURE 10-7 An example of a clinical pathway for a client with pneumonia. (Courtesy Valley Baptist Medical Center, Harlingen, Texas.)

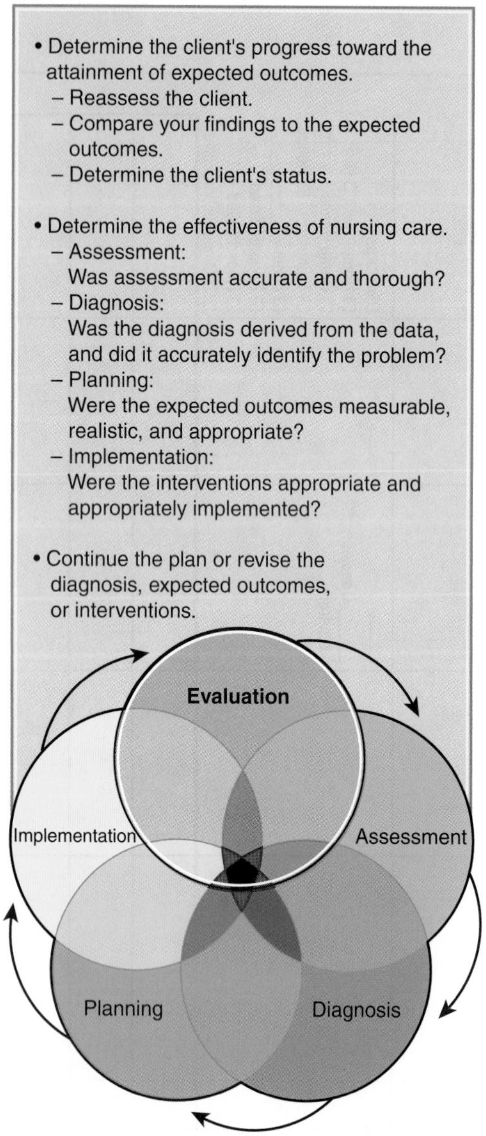

- Determine the client's progress toward the attainment of expected outcomes.
  - Reassess the client.
  - Compare your findings to the expected outcomes.
  - Determine the client's status.
- Determine the effectiveness of nursing care.
  - Assessment:
    Was assessment accurate and thorough?
  - Diagnosis:
    Was the diagnosis derived from the data, and did it accurately identify the problem?
  - Planning:
    Were the expected outcomes measurable, realistic, and appropriate?
  - Implementation:
    Were the interventions appropriate and appropriately implemented?
- Continue the plan or revise the diagnosis, expected outcomes, or interventions.

Evaluation
Implementation
Assessment
Planning
Diagnosis

FIGURE 10-8 The process of evaluation.

to help improve client satisfaction with nursing care. If a client or family member is dissatisfied with the care, you need to identify the causes of this dissatisfaction and seek ways to reduce or alleviate it.

Appraising the Success of Interventions. After evaluating the client's responses to interventions, you must judge the success of the interventions in achieving expected outcomes. Continue effective interventions, and try to determine why others are ineffective. Interventions that are inappropriate or insufficient to meet the goals need to be discontinued or revised.

Outcomes may be completely met, partially met, or not met. When the client responds as expected, outcomes are completely met. When the client's responses indicate some progress toward the goals, outcomes are partially met. When the client's responses do not show any progress toward expected outcomes, none of the outcomes are met. If the expected outcomes were not appropriately customized to the client's health status, for example, they may need to be revised.

Continuing, Revising, or Resolving the Care Plan. After evaluating the success of interventions in achieving the outcomes, you will need to decide whether the nursing care plan should be continued or revised (Figure 10-9). If the client attained the expected outcomes, the nursing diagnosis is said to be resolved. If the expected outcomes were only partially attained, you may need to revise interventions, add new ones, or discontinue others (Box 10-7, p. 226). However, there may be justification for continuing interventions when the problem is not resolved. For example, you may determine that more time is needed and thus continue the interventions.

When your evaluation identifies new problems, you will need to revise the client's existing care plan to address those problems. For example, acute pain is a common problem after surgery, and narcotics usually control surgical pain. However, because these clients commonly develop constipation, your care plan needs to address reducing or preventing constipation.

FACTORS AFFECTING OUTCOMES ATTAINMENT

Many factors affect the attainment of client outcomes. Evaluate yourself frequently to see if you are enhancing or impeding outcome attainment.

Facilitators. Stated clearly, realistic outcomes facilitate evaluations. A clear understanding of the client's illness and treatments will help you to select reasonable expected outcomes. After thoroughly identifying the client's problems and gathering adequate supporting data, you will be able to establish individualized and realistic outcomes.

Evaluation is a continuous process (Figure 10-10, p. 227). It requires frequent monitoring to gauge the client's progress in attaining expected outcomes. Observe for signs that progress is being made or that the client's condition is conducive to progress.

Maintaining continuity of care facilitates outcome attainment. Because all of a client's health problems may not be resolved with one episode of care, document all pertinent information about the client's problems, care plans, and progress toward expected outcomes. That way, the client's care plan can be continued, and the progress toward attaining the expected outcomes can be continuously assessed.

Collaborating with other health care professionals is also crucial for facilitating outcome attainment. You should not only work closely with physicians but also recognize the client's need for other health professionals. Using an interdisciplinary approach to meet the client's needs will expedite recovery.

Client participation facilitates attaining outcomes. Clients who understand what you seek to accomplish through the interventions applied are more motivated to

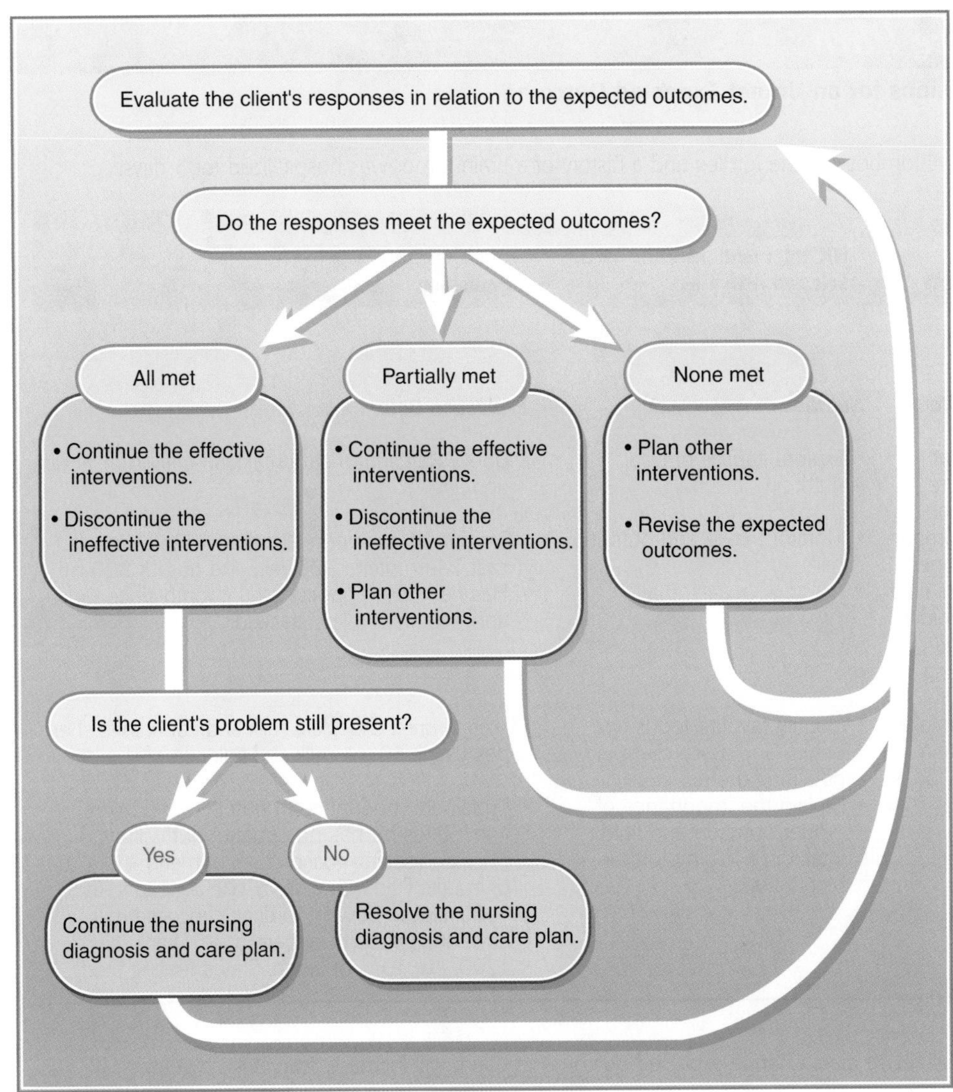

FIGURE 10-9 The process of evaluating a care plan.

reach the goals. Box 10-8 (p. 227) summarizes factors that facilitate outcome attainment.

Barriers. Barriers that impede the attainment of expected outcomes need to be evaluated as well. Barriers involve you and your colleagues more than the client and his or her condition. For example, a lack of critical thinking can leave you unaware of the client's problems and uncertain about why the goals are not being attained. Avoid focusing on routine tasks, such as taking vital signs or giving medications and treatments. Instead, think critically as you work through the nursing process to identify and solve the client's problems. Ask yourself wide-ranging questions as you evaluate the success of the nursing process in your client's care (Box 10-9, p. 227).

Lack of knowledge about client care, diseases, and treatments is another barrier that affects outcome attainment. To think critically, you need to equip yourself continuously with knowledge relevant to client care. You can use many methods to keep your knowledge current and comprehensive.

Fragmented nursing care is another factor that hinders outcome attainment. In today's fast-paced clinical settings, interventions may not be consistently implemented, documented, and reassessed from shift to shift. Consequently, client problems may take longer than necessary to be resolved (Figure 10-11, p. 228).

To avoid fragmented care, you need to improve the team's working relationship and to maintain continuity of care. Strive to develop a system to facilitate verbal and written communication among the staff regarding each client's care. Some health care institutions use clinical care guidelines and computerized client records to facilitate continuity of care.

Lack of communication among professionals in different disciplines can also deter outcome attainment. When health professionals fail to communicate or to make adequate referrals, the client's problem may not resolve appropriately.

Lack of involvement by the client himself or herself is another barrier to outcome attainment (Box 10-10, p. 228). Usually, that lack of involvement stems from a lack of adequate information. Most clients want to be informed about their condition, their treatment, and what

BOX 10-7

Nursing Care Plan

An Example of Revisions for an Unmet Expected Outcome

Client Data

A 72-year-old man with deep vein thrombosis in the left leg and a history of a brain tumor was hospitalized for 3 days.

NANDA-I Nursing Diagnosis	NOC Expected Outcomes With Indicators	NIC Interventions With Selected Activities	Evaluation
Imbalanced Nutrition: Less Than Body Requirements	***Nutritional Status:***	***Nutrition Management:***	***Evaluation Data:***
Related Factors:			
• Poor appetite	• Client will eat 75% or more of each meal.	• Explore causes of poor nutrition.	• 0800. Refuses to eat breakfast; has no appetite.
• Decreased oral intake	• Explain the importance of proper nutrition and fluid intake in avoiding further blood clots and facilitating recovery.	• Monitor intake and output daily.	• Oral intake has been less than 25% of meals. Last 24-hr intake 900 mL, and output 800 mL. Has had poor appetite for 1 month since radiation. Mouth dry, lips cracked.
	• Encourage intake of high-protein, high-calorie foods.	• Identify favorite foods and drinks, and assist client in obtaining them.	• Likes to drink chocolate milk and eat orange sherbet. Drank 50 mL milk and half cup of sherbet.
		• Explain the importance of proper nutrition and fluid intake in avoiding further blood clots.	• Explained importance of nutrition and hydration. States he has no appetite but will try. • Discussed setting goal of 25% of meals and a cup of favorite fluid q2h while awake. Agreed to try. • 1000. Does not want to drink chocolate milk anymore. Offered cranberry juice. Drank 20 mL. • 1200. Ate 10% of lunch. States feeling tired.

Revisions

Continues to have poor nutrition; will revise plan. Change expected outcome to Client will increase oral intake by eating 25% of meals.

Add Nursing Diagnosis

Impaired oral mucous membrane	***Oral Hygiene:***		
• Dryness, dehydration	• Client will have moist, pink mucous membranes.	• Contact physician about dehydration and adding protein drink to diet. • Assess oral membranes daily. • Provide oral baking soda and saline mouth rinse before each meal.	

Nursing outcome and intervention labels from Johnson, M., Bulechek, G., Butcher, H., Dochterman, J. M., Maas, M., Moorhead, S., et al. (Eds.). (2006). *NANDA, NOC, and NIC linkages: Nursing diagnoses, outcomes, & interventions.* St. Louis, MO: Mosby.

they can do to improve their health or prevent problems. Most clients also want to be involved in making decisions about their care. To help a client reach the expected outcomes, explain the plan of care and encourage the client to participate in it. Encourage questions and clarify anything that is confusing to the client.

STANDARDS FOR EVALUATION

Standards are authoritative statements that define the nursing profession's accountability to the public and the outcomes that nurses are responsible for (ANA, 2004). They are used to evaluate nursing practice. Professional standards are not legally binding; how-

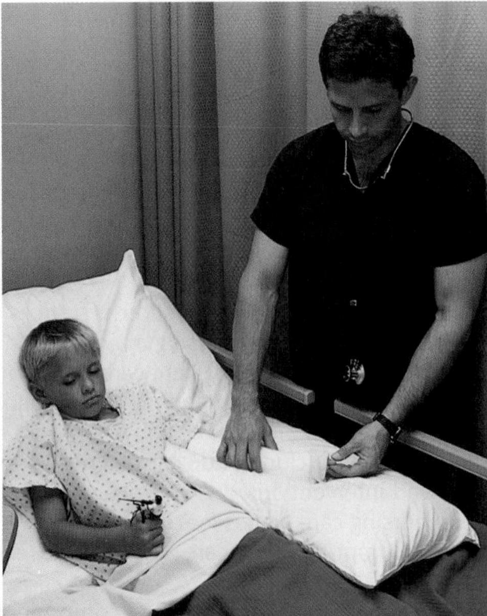

FIGURE 10-10 Evaluation is a continuous process. This nurse evaluates the circulation in a child's casted arm in an ongoing, regular manner.

BOX 10-8 *Factors Facilitating Outcome Attainment*

- Understand clearly the expected outcomes for each problem.
- Understand the client's disease and treatments.
- Assess the client accurately and thoroughly.
- Identify all pertinent problems.
- Formulate realistic and individualized outcomes.
- Revise outcomes and interventions when necessary.
- Maintain the continuity of care.
- Work as a team with other health care professionals.
- Encourage the client's participation in identifying problems and setting goals.

ever, the Nurse Practice Act and regulations adopted by each state do have the power to be legally binding.

The standards of nursing practice established by the American Nurses Association include standards of practice and standards of professional performance. The **standards of practice** for registered nurses include assessment, diagnosis, outcome identification, planning, implementation (coordination of care, health teaching and health promotion, consultation), and evaluation. Standards of professional performance include quality of practice, education, professional practice evaluation, collegiality, collaboration, ethics, research, resource utilization, and leadership. Criteria to measure these standards are also delineated (see Appendix A). Nurses are expected to use the nursing process to provide nursing care and to participate in activities related to professional performance standards to demonstrate competent nursing practice.

Standards of care (internal and external) are used in court cases to evaluate the quality of care delivered and the competence of the nurses delivering it. When the evidence indicates that nurses failed to meet these standards, the duty of care has been breached. The nurse is vulnerable to a malpractice claim. Thus nurses are responsible for performing—and documenting—competent care that meets all internal and external standards.

BOX 10-9 *Evaluating the Success of the Nursing Process*

ASSESSMENT

- What is the pathophysiology of the client's medical diagnoses?
- What are the results of diagnostic or laboratory tests? What are the relationships between abnormal results, the client's responses, and treatments?
- What are the client's physical and psychosocial responses to the present illness, diagnoses, and treatments?
- What are the client's treatments (e.g., diet, routine and prn medications, activity, and so on)? Why are these prescribed? What is the relationship between the client's diagnoses and treatments?

DIAGNOSIS

- What actual and potential problems can I identify from assessment data?
- What is the priority of these problems?
- How do I describe these problems with nursing diagnoses approved by the NANDA International?
- Do I have sufficient evidence (contributing factors, signs, symptoms) to confirm the diagnoses?
- Do I need to seek further data from current or past medical records, other health team members, family members, or other references to confirm or to rule out the nursing diagnoses?

PLANNING

- Are these outcomes client focused? Is my client aware of the expected outcomes? Is my client ready to participate in setting specific goals (outcome criteria)?
- Are these outcomes measurable and achievable in the short term or the long term?
- Are these outcomes aimed to restore, maintain, or promote my client's health?

INTERVENTION

- What interventions can be implemented to achieve expected outcomes?
- Do these interventions conform to professional standards and organizational standards and protocols?
- How should I implement these interventions safely and effectively?
- What can I do to maintain the continuity of care?

EVALUATION

- What are the client's responses to interventions in relationship to the expected outcomes?
- Are outcomes all met, partially met, or not met? Is it necessary to revise some outcomes to make them attainable?
- Are these interventions effective toward achieving the expected outcomes? Are there problems with interventions? Are there better ways to implement these interventions?
- Are there alternative approaches to reach the goals?
- Should I continue, revise, or discontinue these interventions?
- Should I continue or resolve the nursing diagnoses?
- Has evaluation identified any new problems that require a nursing response?

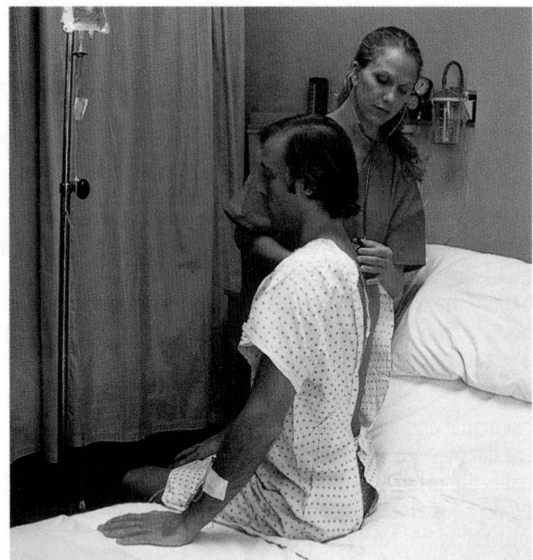

FIGURE 10-11 Avoidance of fragmented nursing care is critical to the achievement of expected outcomes. This nurse continuously reassesses and documents her client's respiratory status.

BOX 10-10 *Barriers to the Attainment of Expected Outcomes*

- Lack of critical thinking to understand the client's problems
- Lack of logical reasoning in connecting diagnoses, expected outcomes, and interventions
- Lack of adequate validation with client
- Inadequate assessment of the client's responses to interventions
- Fragmented care, in nursing or across the health care team
- Lack of collaborative work with other health care professionals
- Lack of client's involvement

▼ KEY PRINCIPLES

- The planning phase of the nursing process involves setting priorities, establishing expected outcomes and the time frame to reach outcomes, and identify nursing interventions for each nursing diagnosis.
- Planning for individuals is initiated with entry into the health care system, continues throughout the time of service, and ensures ongoing care through discharge planning.
- Planning for individuals is a team effort through collaboration, consultation, and/or care plan conferences.
- Planning for groups of clients with a common set of needs involves designing services for the population being served, determining the level of staffing, and designing the environment of care.
- The planning process involves setting priorities on the basis of the client's physical needs, the services expected in the setting, the client's perception of need, and the client's ability to provide self-care.
- Predicting the outcomes of nursing care implies that nursing can be held responsible for nursing-sensitive outcomes, not just for the provision of nursing care.
- The Nursing Outcomes Classification system is a standardized language for stating nursing-sensitive outcomes.
- The skills required for successful intervention are cognitive, technical, interpersonal, and ethical/legal.
- Implementation always includes reassessment and the continuation of the planning phase.
- Intervention is not complete until the care is documented.
- Nurse-initiated and physician-initiated interventions treat the related factors to resolve the signs and symptoms that define the nursing diagnosis.
- The Nursing Interventions Classification system is a standardized language for stating nursing interventions.
- A nursing care plan is a guide to client care that coordinates the actions of the nursing team and improves continuity of care over the course of an illness.
- A nursing care plan includes nursing diagnoses, expected outcomes, and interventions.
- The type of nursing care plan is less important than the goal of providing comprehensive care designed to meet the needs of the individual client.
- Evaluation is a systematic and ongoing component of the nursing process to determine if the client's progress toward expected outcomes is achieved, if interventions provided are effective in meeting expected outcomes, and if nursing care is provided according to standards of practice.
- Expected outcomes should be established before evaluation. Outcomes should be measurable and individualized and have an estimated time frame.
- After interventions are implemented, the client's physical and psychosocial responses to the interventions are evaluated. Desirable and undesirable responses are noted, and interventions for undesirable responses are made.
- The success of interventions should be appraised and a determination made to continue, revise, or resolve care plans.
- Nurses should evaluate themselves frequently to ensure that they are facilitators of, and not barriers to, outcome attainment.
- ANA standards consist of standards of care and standards of professional performance. Standards of care describe competent practice of nursing process. Standards of professional performance depict competent professional behaviors.

■ REVIEW QUESTIONS

1. A client is newly diagnosed with adult-onset diabetes and before discharge needs to learn how to give himself an insulin injection daily. Which one of the following is the most appropriate expected outcome? The client will:

1. Understand the mechanics of the injection technique
2. Demonstrate the correct injection technique before discharge
3. Develop a procedure for injection suitable to his lifestyle
4. Know how to give insulin injection

2. A client is admitted with a wound infection. There is an order to give vancomycin 500 mg intravenously every 6 hours. Which one of the following interventions clearly reflects a direct and nurse-initiated intervention?

1. Administer the diluted vancomycin intravenously over at least 30 minutes.
2. Establish the schedule to administer vancomycin.
3. Discuss side effects of vancomycin with a pharmacist.
4. Teach the client about the purpose and side effects.

3. A 70-year-old male client had a left total knee replacement 2 days ago and was receiving adequate doses of morphine through a patient-controlled analgesia (PCA) pump. He is weaned off PCA and is receiving an oral analgesic medication for pain control. Which one of the following statements is the best way to evaluate the extent of pain relief with the oral medication?

1. "Are you as comfortable now as you were on the PCA pump?"
2. "It has been 30 minutes since you took the pain medication. On a 0 to 10 scale, could you rate your pain?"
3. "Which type of medication works better for you? The PCA pump or the oral medication?"
4. "What do you think about this new oral medication? Is it better in controlling your pain?"

4. The nurse cares for an adult male client who had an abdominal surgery 3 days ago and recognizes that this client has a nursing diagnosis of *Acute pain.* The outcome criteria for this problem are the client will verbalize that pain is reduced or controlled and the client will use noninvasive pain relief measures effectively. He states that music helps him to relax and feel less pain. The nurse notices that he fell asleep and took a 90-minute nap after he put on earphones to listen to a portable CD player. What one of the following adequately reflects the evaluation of the outcomes?

1. Being met
2. Being partially met
3. Not being met
4. Irrelevant to the care of the client

5. What should the nurse do when evaluating whether the client has reached expected outcomes?

1. Have a general idea about the client's plan of care
2. Assess the client thoroughly and accurately
3. Not be overly concerned with revising the plan of care
4. Consult with the family, but not the client, about expected outcomes

Bibliography

*American Nurses Association. (1985). *Code for nurses with interpretive statements.* Kansas City, MO: Author.

*American Nurses Association. (1994). *Guidelines on reporting incompetent, unethical, or illegal practices.* Washington, DC: Author.

*American Nurses Association. (1996). *Nursing quality indicators: Definitions and implications.* Washington, DC: American Nurses Publishing.

American Nurses Association. (2004). *Nursing: Scope and standards of practice.* Washington, DC: Nursesbooks.org—The Publishing Program of ANA.

*Case Management Society of America. (1995). *Standards of practice for case management.* Little Rock, AR: Case Management Society of America.

Cohen, E. L. (2005). *Nursing case management: From essentials to advanced practice application.* St. Louis, MO: Mosby.

Dochterman, J. M., & Bulechek, G. M. (2004). *Nursing interventions classification (NIC).* St. Louis, MO: Mosby.

Florin, J., Ehrenberg, A., & Ehnfors, M. (2005). Quality of nursing diagnoses: Evaluation of an educational intervention. *International Journal of Nursing Terminologies and Classifications, 16*(2): 33-43.

*Gronlund, N. E. (1985). *Stating objectives for classroom instruction* (3rd ed.). New York: Macmillan.

Johnson, M., Bulechek, G., Butcher, H., Dochterman, J. M., Maas, M., Moorhead, S., et al. (Eds.). (2006). *NANDA, NOC, and NIC linkages: Nursing diagnoses, outcomes, & interventions.* St. Louis, MO: Mosby.

Lee, T. (2005). Nursing diagnoses: Factors affecting their use in charting standardized care plans. *Journal of Clinical Nursing, 14*(5): 640-647.

Lunney, M. (2006). Helping nurses use NANDA, NOC, and NIC: Novice to expert. *Nurse Educator, 31*(1): 40-46.

Martin, K. S. (2005). *The Omaha System: A key to practice, documentation, and information management.* St. Louis, MO: Elsevier Saunders.

*Maslow, A. (1954). *Motivation and personality.* New York: Harper & Row.

Moorhead, S., Johnson, M., & Maas, M. (Eds.). (2004). *Nursing outcomes classification (NOC)/ Iowa outcomes project* (3rd ed.). St. Louis, MO: Mosby.

NANDA International. (2005). *Nursing diagnoses: Definitions and classification, 2005-2006.* Philadelphia: Author.

Saba, V. (2002, August). Nursing classifications: Home Healthcare Classification system (HHCC): An overview. *Online Journal of Issues in Nursing.* Available at http://nursingworld.org/ojin/tpc7/tpc7_7.htm.

Saba, V. (2006). *Clinical care classification system.* New York: Springer.

Sims, C. (2003). Increasing clinical, satisfaction, and financial performance through nurse-driven process improvement, *Journal of Nursing Administration, 33*(2), 68-75.

Walsh, S. (2004). Formulation of a plan of care for culturally diverse patients. *International Journal of Nursing Terminologies and Classifications, 15*(1), 17-26.

Wing, R. R., Phelan, S., & Tate, D. (2002). The role of adherence in mediating the relationship between depression and health outcomes. *Journal of Psychosomatic Research 53*(4), 877-881.

Wingard, R. (2005). Patient education and the nursing process: meeting the patient's needs. *Nephrology Nursing Journal, 32*(2): 211-215.

*Asterisk indicates a classic or definitive work on this subject.

Chapter 11

Documenting Care

Media Resources

- Evolve Website http://evolve.elsevier.com/Harkreader/
- Companion CD

Learning Objectives

After studying this chapter, you should be able to do the following:

- Understand the purposes of documentation
- Identify the methods of implementation of the principles of documentation
- Identify content pertinent to various types of nursing entries, special populations, and facilities
- Differentiate among documentation formats and the usefulness of various types of flow sheets
- Apply the principles of documentation to electronic documentation systems

Key Terms

admit note (admission note)
APIE (PIE) charting
charting by exception
computerized provider order entry (CPOE)
critical or clinical pathways (care maps)
discharge note
documentation
electronic health record (EHR)
electronic medical record (EMR)
electronic medication administration record (eMAR)
flow sheet
focus charting
interval or progress note
narrative charting
problem-oriented medical records
SOAP charting
transfer note

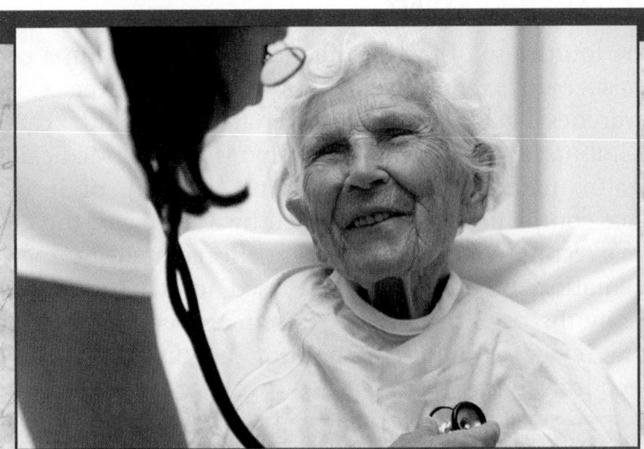

Geraldine Peters, age 88, lives alone and was working in her garden when she fell and fractured her left hip. She was taken to the emergency department of a hospital nearby, where she was evaluated. She was admitted to an orthopedic nursing unit and placed in traction until she could be prepared for surgery. The next morning she was transferred to the operating room for an open reduction and internal fixation (ORIF) of her left hip. From the recovery room she went to the intensive care unit (ICU) for an overnight stay to monitor her heart, and then she was transferred back to the orthopedic unit. Ms. Peters's care and her responses to that care are documented in each department to ensure communication among the members of the health care team and coordination of care across multiple services. This chapter addresses the purposes, principles, and methods of documenting client care.

Documentation is the recording of information relevant to assessment, planning, implementation, and evaluation (client response); it is a legal record that is permanent and retrievable for future purposes. Record-keeping systems are either handwritten or electronic, and the format varies among health care agencies. Although the primary purpose continues to be creating a record of the client's health problems, treatments, and results, documentation systems have evolved in an effort to adjust to changes in health care delivery, to reflect changes in nursing practice, and to incorporate requirements of regulatory agencies.

PURPOSES OF DOCUMENTATION

As you saw in the case study of Ms. Peters, a health record is used to communicate to multiple members of the health care team. If Ms. Peters is admitted to the same hospital next year, the record may be retrieved to review her history. If an untoward event occurs, and she decides to sue the hospital, her record will be used in court. The hospital may use her record to review the quality of care given on the orthopedic unit. The Joint Commission (TJC) may retrieve her record to examine compliance with standards of care. The Centers for Medicare and Medicaid Services (CMS) or other insurers may review the record to confirm the reimbursement of her care. Effective documentation will meet the requirements of all these uses of the client's record.

COMMUNICATION

The primary purpose of documentation of a client's care is communication among health care team members to promote continuity of care among departments, throughout 24 hours of care, and during the entire hospital stay. It is essential that all personnel provide documentation of anything they have observed or done with a client to ensure coordination of activities and continuity of care. Proper documentation informs appropriate personnel about a client's condition and response to illness, the care that has been given, and the results of care.

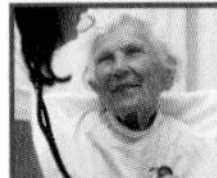

For example, the operating room personnel would examine Ms. Peters's chart for information relevant to surgery. Among other things, they need to know that she is allergic to penicillin, has a history of heart disease, and fell after becoming dizzy.

QUALITY ASSURANCE

A second purpose of documentation is to provide substantiation of quality of care. As part of a quality assurance program, health care agencies periodically conduct chart audits to determine whether or not the care provided meets established standards for care. In addition, health care accrediting agencies, such as TJC, require regular quality assurance audits of client care.

The client record must show evidence of compliance with standards of care. Standards of care are guidelines that represent generally accepted practice and are derived from a variety of sources including the American Nurses Association (ANA), the nurse practice act, TJC, national quality initiatives, and agency policy or procedure. For example, the ANA *Nursing: Scope and Standards of Practice* (2004) requires the use of the nursing process in providing care to clients. Communication of the use of this process is primarily through documentation in the client's medical record. ANA standards of care relevant to documentation are summarized in Appendix A.

Good documentation serves as the basis for collecting this quality assurance data. The record provides evidence that professional and agency standards have been incorporated into the client's care. The record should reflect initial and ongoing assessment, the problems identified through assessment, expected outcomes of care, interventions, and evaluation of progress toward expected outcomes. Data that evaluate care are critical in monitoring for quality assurance in client care and are necessary to ensure that standards of care are met. Currently in quality assurance auditing, an emphasis is placed on client outcomes as the measure of quality, and these are monitored through complete and accurate documentation.

LEGAL ACCOUNTABILITY

The third purpose of documentation of care is to provide legal evidence through which nurses are held accountable for their actions. Legally, nurses can be held accountable for failure to practice within the applicable standards of care. Documentation should, therefore, verify the need for interventions, verify the type of care given, and allow examination of progress toward expected outcomes.

Common liability issues for nurses include protection from avoidable injury, monitoring and reporting changes in condition, and performing interventions correctly. The record should document assessment of clients at risk and safety measures implemented. The use of restraints is a safety factor that requires a physician's order (including a time limit). Specific agency policy should be followed for documentation.

In the event of an injury or potential for harm to a client, visitor, or staff member or for a deviation from established policy or procedure for any reason, it is important to complete an *incident* or *safety report*. These reports document the date, time, and location of the occurrence or discovery, who was notified, facts relevant to the occurrence without conjecture, blame, opinion, or conclusions, and your assessment of the client with any follow-up care (Sullivan, 2003). An example of documentation of a medication error in the client progress notes is as follows:

SAMPLE CHARTING

7/16/07	4:30 P.M.	Awake, alert, and oriented X3. Resp. 18, BP 110/72. Dr. Johnson notified of administration of morphine sulfate 10 mg IM. C. Larsen, RN
	5:00 P.M.	Awake, alert, and oriented X3. Resp. 16, BP 112/76. C. Larsen, RN

Safety reports are not part of the legal client record; rather these forms are used to track incidents for the purpose of discovering methods of prevention and determining the root cause of the incident. Documenting in the legal record that an error was made and that a safety report was completed is not necessary and is never recommended. Safety reports are confidential and sent directly to your nursing leadership or the risk manager for follow-up.

> ***Action Alert!*** Remember that the chart is a legal record and protects the client, the nurse, and the health care agency.

REIMBURSEMENT

The fourth use of the information documented in a client's record is reimbursement by third-party payers. Cost awareness has become important in health care. Reimbursement for client care by Medicare, Medicaid, health maintenance organizations (HMOs), or insurance companies is often decided by a review of the client's record. As cost-containment efforts intensify, documentation of nursing care is used to determine and justify the need for services. Case managers and utilization review committees monitor lengths of stay and need for services.

> ***Action Alert!*** Document the client's condition, nursing activities, and treatments and procedures completely. Reimbursement may be decreased or denied if the care delivered is coded at a lower level due to inadequate documentation.

Cost awareness has increased the emphasis on what care is necessary and how care is to be implemented. Clear, concise, and accurate documentation is essential for capturing scarce resources for client care. Complete data related to admission, supplies used, monitoring activities, follow-up, education, and discharge planning are necessary for appropriate reimbursement.

RESEARCH

Finally, documentation is used to provide data for nursing research. Nursing research results in new approaches to client care, and it increases professional knowledge. The value of this research depends on complete and accurate documentation of client data. Research has led to development of standardized formats for collecting and recording data and allows researchers to detect trends that predict health care needs of the individual and the community. In addition, research questions are often generated through review of data trends obtained from health care records.

PRINCIPLES OF DOCUMENTATION

Whether documentation is electronic or handwritten, the principles are the same. These principles imply rules for legibility, terminology, brevity, sequence, corrections, omissions, completeness, signing, and confidentiality. Proper charting should follow the principles of effective documentation, and it uses correct terminology as well as abbreviations. Charting too quickly may lead to incomplete entries or statements that do not communicate the intended meaning.

The client's chart is a legal record and therefore must conform to certain legal standards. Because the record is a permanent legal record, ink is used in handwritten records. Black ink allows the chart to be duplicated with adequate readability for long-term storage. Documentation that is clear, accurate, timely, and legally sound follows certain rules of charting (Box 11-1).

BOX 11-1 *Do's and Don'ts of Charting*

- DO be sure to know the agency policies and procedures about documentation.
- DO check the name on the chart before making an entry.
- DO chart brief, concise, and complete entries. Eliminate all unnecessary words.
- DO sign each entry or follow agency policy for initialing entries.
- DO use objective, measurable terms.
- DO use black ink.
- DO write neatly and legibly.
- DO use standard abbreviations only when necessary and avoid the use of error-prone ones.
- DO use quotes whenever appropriate to relate what the client actually said.
- DO write entries logically and sequentially, date and time each entry.
- DO make addenda as needed.
- DO make entries about nursing care as close to the time of delivery as possible.
- DO report failure of client to follow treatment regimens and to take medications or receive treatments, and the rationale given by the client.
- DON'T sign anyone else's entry or document for someone else.
- DON'T skip lines or spaces.
- DON'T use the word *client* or *patient* throughout the document.
- DON'T write opinions or biased statements.
- DON'T make entries suggesting an error or unsafe practice.
- DON'T repeat narratively if flow sheets and other forms are used for the same information.

TERMINOLOGY

Terminology should be commonly understood by the health care team and should communicate clearly and concisely. Entries in clients' records include standard medical and nursing terminology and commonly recognized abbreviations to facilitate communication. Standard abbreviations and certain symbols are consistently used in the health professions to communicate in an abridged format. Consistency in their use saves time and space without interrupting communication. Health care facilities also enforce lists of error-prone abbreviations and symbols not to be used in documentation from TJC and the Institute for Safe Medical Practices (ISMP) to enhance client safety. It is your responsibility to become acquainted with accepted and unapproved abbreviations in a particular agency. (See Appendix B.)

What may be an acceptable medical abbreviation in one geographical or specialty area may be unknown or used differently in another area. For example, PAT is a fairly common abbreviation for paroxysmal atrial tachycardia, but this term may also be used on obstetrical units to abbreviate pregnancy at term or on other units to indicate preadmission testing.

Action Alert! Never use abbreviations from TJC do-not-use list.

Symbols and medical terms that represent root words, prefixes, and suffixes are used to condense charting entries. When you break down words into root words and understand prefixes and suffixes added to root words, it helps you to decipher what unfamiliar words mean. Knowledge of these word parts will assist you in building a good medical vocabulary, and they should be committed to memory (Table 11-1).

LEGIBILITY

Legibility is essential when documenting in the health care record. Entries may be made in script or print—whichever is more legible. Proper use of terms and correct spelling are extremely important. Poor handwriting and spelling reflect negatively on you and could be translated by a jury as inadequate nursing care.

Action Alert! Consider the consequences of trying to interpret charting that is not readable. Recalling information from illegible entries may be difficult or even impossible if the record is requested in a court of law several years after the entries were made.

BREVITY

Charting entries should be as brief as possible. Sentences are stripped to essential components, eliminating all words that can be stripped without changing the intended meaning of the entry. This includes articles such as "a" and "the," as well as the subject of the sentence.

SAMPLE CHARTING

7/16/07 0700 Dentures removed/cleaned with Polident. Oral mucous membranes smooth, pink, lesions. Assisted bed bath, linens changed.
C. Lott, RN

Note that neither the client's name nor the word *client* or *patient* was charted because *all* entries are about the client. If necessary, the name of the person notified when the client is admitted, results of laboratory work, or any important detail that is to be reported by orders of the physician may be used in the charting. Using an actual name should be followed by the title or position of the person. This is not absolutely necessary, but it does eliminate confusion if the physician did not receive the information requested. An example would be the following:

SAMPLE CHARTING

7/16/07 0940 Report of stat CBC called to Jane Doe, RN, at Dr. Smith's office.
C. Lott, RN

Table 11-1 Symbols, Root Words, Prefixes, and Suffixes Used in Documentation

TERM	MEANING	TERM	MEANING
SYMBOLS		**PREFIXES**	
↑	increase	a- or an-	without
↓	decrease	anti-	against
Δ	change	bi	twice, two
~	approximately	bio-	life
+	positive	brady-	slow
−	negative	chole-	bile; gall
c/o	complains of	di-	double
✓	check on	dys-	difficult, painful
		ecto-	outside
ROOT WORDS		endo-	within
adeno	gland	hemi-	half
angio	vessel	hyper-	above; excessive
arterio	artery	hypo-	decreased
arthro	joint	leuko-	white
cardio	heart	noct-	night
cerebro	brain	olig-	deficiency
cyst	bladder	para-	beside
cyto	cell	peri-	around
derma	skin	poly-	many; multiple
hemo	blood	retro-	backward
hepato	liver	supra-	above
hystero	uterus	tachy-	fast
lith	stone; calculus	trans-	across
meningo	meninges	uni-	one
myelo	bone marrow, spinal cord		
myo	muscle	**SUFFIXES**	
nephro	kidney	-cele	swelling, protrusion
neuro	nerves	-ectomy	removal
-oma	tumor	-emesis	vomiting
ophtha	eye	-emia	blood
ortho	straight	-graph, -gram	tracing
osteo	bone	-itis	inflammation
oto	ear	-ostomy	artificial opening
-oxia	oxygen	-otomy	incision of; cutting into
patho	disease	-penia	deficiency; lack of
phlebo	vein	-plasty	repair of
pnea, pneum	breathing; lungs	-rhea	discharge
pyelo	renal pelvis	-uria	urine
pyo	pus		
pyro	heat		
reno	kidney		
thrombo	blood clot		
thora	chest		
uro	urine		
vaso	vessel		
veno	vein		

COMPLETENESS

Although brevity is essential, you should document all information necessary to explain the events of a shift. Anyone reading the documentation should have a clear picture of what took place or is being described. If necessary, direct quotes can be used to describe what a client said. The need for complete entries is critical when a record is used in a court of law. Medical records may be called into court or peer review for several years after an admission and in the case of a minor, until the age of consent as determined by each state's legislature.

Action Alert! Always chart each significant event with the time it occurred. Entries do not have to be made on the hour but when they occur. From a legal perspective, entries not made in a client's record imply actions not taken or treatments not given. It may be helpful to remember the saying, "If you didn't chart it, you didn't do it."

SEQUENCE AND TIMELINESS

Recording of information on the client's record must be sequential. Noting the time and date is important for evaluating client care and for legal purposes. Every charting format has a single place for the year, month, and date to be recorded, thus eliminating the need for documenting the date with every entry. However, the exact time for every event must be included with each entry and should include AM or PM unless military time is used. Electronic medical records (EMRs) automatically enter a time and date for each entry, as well as capturing the recorder's identity.

The exact time events occur during the shift and the amount of time between events becomes critically important when special medication is given, follow-up care is necessary, a client's condition changes, or vital procedures, such as organ transplants, are being planned. Inaccurate times or prolonged time between entries may indicate poor implementation of standards of care.

Charting statements should be logically organized according to time (0800, 0840, 0915, 0935, and so on) and content. Just as you must use an organized sequence so that you do not omit any information when assessing a client, documentation of data collection should also be organized and logical in sequence. The statement is also more easily read when written in a logical pattern. Entries should be logical according to the format of charting being used (e.g., head-to-toe approach, body systems).

CORRECTIONS

The two types of corrections commonly made to a record are correcting a written entry and adding an entry later. Individual agency policies may vary for the correct format to use when correcting an entry. Common policies include drawing a single line through the entry alone or drawing a single line and writing the word *void* or *error* in the space above the incorrect entry, followed by the initials of the writer. The word *error* may still be used by some agencies, but it is no longer recommended because it implies a wrong. A single line instead of multiple lines is required to keep the incorrect entry legible.

> ***Action Alert!*** Never attempt to obscure original entries. Erasing, whiting out, or blackening the entry is not permitted because of the implication of covering up an error or mistake.

In the event an entry needs to be made on the client's record for 0830, but another nurse has already made a notation for 0915, making the entry out of sequence, an addendum must be written. It would be incorrect to avoid entering the note on the chart. This information must be noted as an addendum. Consider the following example:

SAMPLE CHARTING

7/16/07	0910	Abdominal dressing changed per Dr. Jones. Suture line intact with small amt. pink drainage noted at proximal edge. C. Lott, RN
7/16/07	0910	Bulb drain intact, compressed, & draining 400 mL pink fluid. Reports no discomfort. Foley draining clear, yellow urine with 300 mL output. C. Lott, RN
	0935	Addendum 0830 Assisted to chair per P.T. assistance X2 and use of walker. c/o weakness and instructed not to weight bear on left leg. C. Lott, RN

Note that in the previous example, the time of each entry remains sequential (0910, then 0935). The event time of the late entry (0830), however, is made after the word *addendum*. The time 0830 is when the nursing action actually occurred. Addenda should be avoided as much as possible. Charting in real time or near real time throughout the shift instead of once or twice toward the end of the shift usually prevents entries from being out of sequence. Real-time documentation is essential for optimizing the safety benefits of clinical decision support alerts and reminders in an EMR. Timely documentation also promotes adequate detail and helps with overall time management of the shift in the event of emergent transfer of a client.

If information that is omitted is recalled a day or several days later, it should be noted in the current notes with the current date and time, followed by "addendum to nurse's notes of [month, day, and year]," followed by the entry. Agency policy will specify if the term *late entry* rather than *addendum* should be used.

In rereading an entry, you often discover that certain words needed to clarify an entry have been accidentally omitted. An omitted word or phrase must not be squeezed between words in small letters or inserted above or below a written line. An addendum would need to be made to clarify the entry with the necessary description.

OMISSIONS

Blank spaces are not to be left on the chart. As much as possible, you should write to the end of a line instead of leaving the space blank. Avoid writing outside of the lines (in the margin) of the charting form. A horizontal line is drawn through any empty space to the right margin to prevent later entries from being made in front of a signature.

If a part of a page is blank at the end of the 24-hour time period, an X should be drawn through the remainder of the page. Notes should flow from shift to shift, and a new set of notes should be started after 24 hours.

If it is necessary to recopy a page of the chart, the person copying the page should date and time the entry and write "Copied by . . ." followed by his or her signature.

Copying a chart usually requires written consent by the client or responsible party.

SIGNATURES

The correct way to sign a notation in the client's record is using the first initial and full last name, followed by the abbreviation of the health care worker's position title (RN, LPN, SN). Some agencies require the full first and last names followed by an abbreviation of the individual's current position. You usually sign to the far right of the entry once it is complete.

Traditionally, SN has been the accepted abbreviation for student nurse. Even if the student has another title such as LPN (licensed practical nurse), he or she is to use the abbreviation for student nurse when functioning in that capacity. The student nurse may also be required to write the initials of the school affiliation along with the title SN. A written signature must follow every entry into a client's record. In this way, institutions provide a guarantee that the right person gave the care. It is also how an agency would determine who gave the care, if a record is reviewed at a later date.

The correct format would be as follows:

SAMPLE CHARTING

7/16/07	1530	Awake & oriented to time, place,
		& person. Skin warm and dry.
		C. Lott, RN
	1600	CBC drawn per lab. C. Lott, RN
	1645	To radiology via wheelchair for CXR.
		C. Lott, RN

When a form has only enough space for initials, there will always be a signature key for the professional to sign, to identify the initials.

CONFIDENTIALITY

All client records are confidential files that require written permission of the client to be copied. Information within the chart is often of a personal matter as well as legal evidence of the care provided and should be available to the necessary health care team members only. Client records are not accessible to insurance companies, significant others, research teams, or third parties (including payers) without the written permission of the client. Clients themselves must sign and submit a request for the information from their medical file.

> ***Action Alert!*** Safeguard all client information. It is the responsibility of the nurse and other health care team members to maintain confidentiality concerning medical records within any medical facility. This includes being sure that no documents are left unattended in public areas and that no client-specific data is viewable to the public on computer screens.

CONTENT OF DOCUMENTATION

Although agencies vary in their specific requirements about what needs to be charted, you should develop a systematic approach to documentation of client care. The system may be a head-to-toe, body systems, problem oriented, human needs, functional health patterns, or any other organized approach for deriving significant data to be documented. Regardless of your choice of organizational method, there are guidelines that should be followed. All significant client care should be documented either in narrative (progress) notes or on **flow sheets** (forms used to document data that can be more easily followed in graphic or tabular form).

On admission to a facility, most health care agencies require a health history or screening to be completed, followed by a current needs assessment or problem list. These may be combined or on separate forms. The format and degree of detail will vary according to the health care agency. The registered nurse on the unit usually completes these initial admission forms, which then become a permanent part of the chart and guide the interdisciplinary care for this admission. Some forms for this process are more structured, such as a checklist format with which you can easily check or circle observations. Other forms are unstructured but usually list areas to be assessed, with room for you to write narrative observations. If no specific form is used by the agency for this purpose, write narrative notes. After completing these forms, document the client's arrival and subsequent care needs, including consults identified.

TYPES OF ENTRIES

Various types of entries may be made in a chart. Among these are admit notes for a newly admitted client, change-of-shift notes, assessment findings, interval or progress notes, transfer and discharge notes, client teaching notes, and descriptions of observations.

Admit Notes. On assuming responsibility for a new client who just entered the facility, you usually record an admit note. An **admit note** (or admission note) is the first nurse's note acknowledging the arrival of a new client. Following the admit note, a narrative entry noting the complete assessment is made, and this is followed by notes describing the client's current status at appropriate intervals, with notations of any changes in the client's condition. On arrival, documentation of the client's orientation to the facility should be made. If the admission history or assessment form provides a place for this information, an additional narrative note is not necessary.

The admit note usually includes the following: time of arrival, age, sex, how the client arrived, where the client came from, medical diagnosis, chief complaint, general appearance, treatments in progress, allergies, vital signs (if required by the agency or if abnormal), notification of physician, and stat (from the Latin *statim*, meaning immediately) laboratory work or orders that have been completed (Figure 11-1).

Change-of-Shift Notes. At the change of shift, you do not need to document an admit note for a client who has been in the facility for a period of time. Instead, you usually begin each shift with documentation of the client assessment made on rounds. Any format is acceptable, but the documentation should include a thorough assessment of the client's current status, followed by interval notes describing any change in the client's status related to expected outcomes. It may be a requirement of the facility to note that a report was received or given and by whom.

SAMPLE CHARTING

7/16/07	0834	Shift report received from S. Smith, RN. Awake & alert on rounds. [continue note with current assessment data]

Assessment Notes. After an admit note or a beginning shift note, a complete assessment of the current status of the client should follow. Documentation of the complete assessment may be entered using different formats: narrative, flow chart, charting by exception, or a combination of various formats. Various methods for charting any entry narratively are acceptable: head-to-toe assessment, body systems, functional health patterns, or nursing diagnosis (Figure 11-2).

Interval or Progress Notes. After the complete assessment is made, interval notes should be entered. Agencies use one of the following terms: *interval notes, progress notes*, or *daily notes*. **Interval notes** or **progress notes** are interdisciplinary notes entered at various times during a shift; they reflect any aspect of change in client condition or anything affecting the client such as tests, stat or prn (as needed) medications, and procedures. Content to include in an interval note is determined by you and by the condition of the client, but it may include the following: treatments, medications, new orders, ambulation, periods of rest, presence of visitors, special tests, and client symptoms.

When you make rounds on clients, the status of their condition is noted. Documentation at intervals usually means every 2 to 4 hours. This will vary depending on the agency policy and perhaps the policy on a unit within the agency. In more critical situations, or whenever a client's

7/14/03	1400	68-year-old female admitted to room 268A via stretcher from ER with dx. Fx. Ⓛ hip. P 92, BP 142/89, R 21, T 98.8. c/o pain to Ⓛ hip from mid-thigh to greater trochanter area, marked bruising noted in same area s̄ edema at present. Stated fell while gardening and unable to "get up again," lives alone, neighbor called 911. IV of D5W infusing at TKO rate to Ⓡ upper arm s̄ signs of infiltration or inflammation c̄ 950 ml TBA. Nursing history and assessment noted, NKA, Dr. Parker notified of admit, new orders noted. ——— C. Lott, RN

FIGURE 11-1 Example of an admit note.

7/14/03	1430	Awake, alert, oriented x3. PERRLA. Stated feels "tired and exhausted from experience." Resp. even, non-labored. Lungs clear in all lobes. Heart sounds normal S_2 and S_2, regular rhythm. Radial pulses equal, regular, and palpable + 2/3. IV to Ⓡ upper arm of D_5W infusing at TKO rate c̄ 900 mL TBA s̄ signs of infiltration or phlebitis. Finger capillary refill less than 3 sec. bilaterally. Abdomen soft c̄ active bowel sounds in all 4 quadrants. Denies difficulty c̄ bowel or bladder. Ⓛ hip bruised, non-edematous, painful to touch. Trochanter roll in place to keep leg aligned. Peripheral pulses palpable, +2/3, equal. No edema to extremities. Feet warm and dry c̄ toe capillary refill less than 3 sec. SR up x2, neighbor at bedside.——— C. Lott, RN

FIGURE 11-2 Example of an assessment note.

7/18/03	0900	Transfer arrangements to Heritage skilled facility for services of Dr. Warren complete. Hospital chart copied, to be sent with client. ——— C. Lott, RN
	1110	Transferred to Heritage skilled facility by stretcher per AST Ambulance Service. Neighbor, Sandy, present, copy of hospital chart given to ambulance attendant, J. Wild. No treatments in progress. No acute distress, skin warm and dry. Color flesh-toned. Ⓛ hip incision clean and dry s̄ irritation or redness. Denies pain at present. Peripheral pulses palpable, + 2/4, and equal. T 98.9, P 76, R 18, BP 132/78. ——— C. Lott, RN

FIGURE 11-3 Example of a transfer note.

condition warrants, entries may be required more often than every 2 hours and they should include who was notified and if orders were obtained. Charting more frequently than the agency requires is a nursing judgment as long as the agency guidelines are followed for the minimal amount of documentation needed.

If the interval is too long between notations or there is lack of sufficient explanation leading up to a serious change in status, the documentation is not acceptable. The status of the client may remain unchanged on rounds and can be noted as such by you.

Transfer and Discharge Notes. When a client is transferred to another facility or to another unit, whether temporarily or permanently, you should write a transfer note. A **transfer note** is a nursing note that reflects the movement of a client from one unit to another within the agency, or to another agency. Policies should exist in the facility for specific content to include in a transfer note. Generally, the notation includes the reason for transfer, method of transportation, person giving and receiving the report, notification of physicians or family members, and the condition of the client, including vital signs and treatments in progress (Figure 11-3).

A similar notation should be made when a client is sent for a test within the same facility, but less information is usually required. Information to be included depends on the client's condition and may include place (e.g., laboratory, x-ray), method of transfer (e.g., wheelchair, stretcher), persons accompanying the client, attachments (e.g., drainage tubes), level of consciousness, and vital signs.

When the client returns to a unit, a note should be made that includes appropriate assessment of the client's condition, time of arrival, method of transfer, and attachments. Depending on the reason for the absence from the unit, specific assessment findings may be required in this entry, such as vital signs, level of consciousness, and ability to swallow.

When a client is discharged from the hospital, a discharge note should be made to close the chart. A **discharge note** is an interdisciplinary note that reflects the circumstances around the release of a client from a facility. This entry should not be made until all other necessary entries have been completed. The specific information needed for a discharge note may vary according to the type of facility. Some agencies require a summary of the client's stay showing improvement or reason for discharge, client teaching, and a note addressing the client's understanding of the self-care needed. Like the transfer note, a discharge summary should generally include preparations for the discharge, the time of departure, method of transportation, family members present, condition of the client, vital signs, community resources to assist the client, client teaching, prescriptions, and any other necessary paperwork given to the client (Figure 11-4).

Client Teaching Notes. Instructions given to a client need careful documentation in a narrative note, on an interdisciplinary client teaching form or plan of care. If the client is unable to understand or prefers, a family member or significant other should be taught. An assessment should be conducted to determine the learning method preferred by the client or family member.

Client teaching may include knowledge of the disease state, medications, wound care, diabetic care, activity restrictions or progression, or diet. The method of teaching may include videos, discussion, reading, demonstration, and return demonstration. The content that is taught needs to be documented, as does the method of teaching. In addition, the time frame, person responsible for teaching, client's readiness to learn, and the results of the teaching need to be charted. If more than just the client is involved, noting who attended the teaching session is important. If pamphlets or booklets are given to the client for further reading, they (along with title and date of publication) should be noted.

How the client responds to the teaching must be documented. To evaluate the teaching, it is essential to determine whether clients or family members can

7/30/03	1320	Dr. Warren visited c̄ orders to discontinue current meds. Home health nurse S. Beil, RN, notified of discharge and arrangements for first visit made. PT notified of discharge and need for education. —— K. Smith, RN
	1400	PT visited concerning walker and reinforced proper use. —— K. Smith, RN
	1430	Neighbor notified and on her way. —— K. Smith, RN
	1500	Neighbor present. HL in Ⓡ upper arm discontinued. Site s̄ redness or warmth. T 98⁶, P 68, R 22, BP 110/72. No complaints. Skin warm and dry. Ⓛ hip incision healing, intact s̄ inflammation or irritation. Pedal pulses + 2/3, equal, feet warm and dry. Discharge instructions given c̄ prescription for Lasix and Lanoxin. Neighbor stated she would pick up her prescriptions on the way home. —— K. Smith, RN
	1525	Discharged per wc s̄ distress. —— K. Smith, RN

FIGURE 11-4 Example of a discharge note.

return-demonstrate a skill such as wound care or explain the information in their own words.

All teaching that occurs should be noted, including reinforcement of information already taught. Special teaching forms may be required in an agency by staff assigned to this responsibility. When client educators teach the client or family, you should note that in the narrative.

Descriptions of Observations. Nurse's notes should be recorded objectively. State observations rather than opinions. Furthermore, if you believe that a client is less alert today than yesterday, you should describe the client's state of awareness today rather than stating "not as alert today."

Subjective data presented by the client are included in the nurse's notes and should be clearly labeled as such. Precede the subjective data by "States," indicating that the client is relating the information, or by using quotation marks around the client's exact words.

Vague documentation should be avoided at all times. Words such as "seems to be" or "apparently" should not be used. It is more descriptive to document the behavior that led to a conclusion. Similarly, adjectives such as *good, some, a little, bad,* and *better* should be avoided, because these terms are relative and may have different meanings for people using them.

Although the term *normal* may be used to describe some physical assessment, it is usually not the best choice for most entries. Of course, unflattering adjectives that characterize the client's behavior (e.g., obnoxious, ignorant) should never be used.

Action Alert! Write nurse's notes to convey an accurate, objective picture of the client or the facts pertaining to a client situation.

Symptoms and Complaints. Any symptom or complaint should be documented in detail. Documentation may include subjective or objective data and should be specific in terms of location, duration, intensity, amount, size, and frequency. With any complaint noted, there should be evidence of care given and the client's response to the care.

Dressings, Tubes, or Attached Devices. Observations of tubes should be documented in the initial entry of each shift and at least every 2 hours thereafter. Documentation should be more frequent when the condition requires it. Notations about dressings should include the location of the dressing, the nature of the secure attachment of the dressing to client, and the amount as well as a description of any drainage observed. If a dressing is removed, the condition of the skin and wound under it should be described, including size, shape, stage, tunneling, undermining, exudate, color, edema, drainage, edges, sutures, or staples (Baranoski & Ayello, 2005) (Figure 11-5).

Tubes providing intravenous (IV), nasogastric, or gastrostomy feeding should be observed for the fluid being administered, the rate of flow, and correct placement, and to ensure that devices are secured with tape or holder. In addition, the infusion site should be noted for any tenderness, redness, edema, or warmth. An IV site is usually assessed at least every 2 hours. Notation of the IV site may be included on a flow sheet. The type and condition of any feeding or gastrostomy tube (e.g., Levin, Keo-feed, percutaneous endoscopic gastrostomy [PEG]) should also be recorded, along with documentation of patency and proper placement. Use of an infusion pump and the reason for it must be noted (see Figure 11-5). If an agency policy requires the use of a pump for certain age-groups or for clients with specific conditions, this can be noted as "IV D_5W 50 mL to right arm per pump."

Notations concerning any drainage tubes should include the location and patency of the tube, attachment to any drainage or suction system, and a description of any drainage. The description of drainage should include color, character, odor, and amount. Specific amounts are recorded on the intake and output (I&O) flow sheet at specified intervals (see Figure 11-5). Agencies may use

Dressing	7/15/03	2030	Dressing on Ⓛ hip c̄ red 2 cm area of drainage. Dressing changed. Staples present, incision c̄ 2 cm area of redness noted at lateral end. —— S. Richards, RN
Tubes	7/15/03	2030	IV D5W in Ⓡ antecubital space infusing at 50 cc/hr c̄ 300 cc TBA. Site free of redness or edema. Hemovac to Ⓛ hip intact, depressed c̄ 50 cc red drainage. —— S. Richards, RN
Attached Devices	7/15/03	2030	Foley catheter to GU bag patent and draining 300 cc clear, amber urine. —— S. Richards, RN
Medication and Treatment	7/15/03	2030	Holding Ⓛ leg and C/O constant throbbing pain at incision area. Tylox tabs ii given PO. SR up x4, instructed not to get OOB s̄ assistance, call bell in reach. —— S. Richards, RN 7/10 scale. Oral med given.
		2245	States "feels much better." No nonverbal expression of discomfort noted. —— S. Richards, RN
		2130	PT reports pain at 2/10 scale with relief acceptable below goal of 3/10.
Valuables	7/14/03	1430	Jewelry and keys placed in folder #2396, sent to admit office c̄ J. Zimmerman, clerk. Client provided receipt. —— S. Richards, RN

FIGURE 11-5 Descriptions of observations.

flow sheets rather than narrative notes for documenting all data related to attachments.

Medications and Treatments. Most agencies maintain a medication administration record (MAR) or **electronic medication administration record (eMAR)** for the purpose of documenting all medications and treatments. Sometimes a medication or treatment is directed to be given stat (immediately). When the direction is to give the medication or treatment prn (as needed), with the decision based on your judgment, a statement should be charted in the progress notes about the events that led to your decision. For example, if you give a client a medication that has been ordered prn for pain, you should document when you gave it by entering the time you gave it and your initials on the MAR. In the progress notes or flow sheet write why you gave it, and include an adequate description of the pain (e.g., location, type, intensity). A follow-up note must be recorded at an appropriate interval to evaluate the effectiveness of the medication or treatment. When documenting the effects of a medication or treatment, take care to record all the information objectively (see Figure 11-5).

> ***Action Alert!*** Documentation should include a follow-up note related to the client's response to prn medications at appropriate time intervals, to show an acceptable standard of care.

There are times when a medication or treatment is not given as ordered. This may be because, in your judgment, it would be harmful for the client at that time, or because the client refuses the treatment or is off the floor when it should be done. In any case, the withholding of the treatment should be documented, along with the explanation for the action. It is also appropriate to notify the physician if any routine medication is withheld, and this too should be documented. An example for Ms. Peters might be as follows:

SAMPLE CHARTING

7/16/07	0910	C/O sharp, constant pain in left hip 5/10 scale, requesting pain medication. BP 98/50, P 62, RR 10. Oriented X3. Responds to verbal stimuli but easily returns to sleep. Explained the need to wait for pain medicine due to low BP & resp. and length of time since last injection 3 hours (order is for q4 hrs). Repositioned, will reassess in 15 minutes. ______ C. Lott, RN
	0920	Continues to c/o pain in left hip. Pain a level 7 on 0-10 scale with 10 being most severe. VS unchanged. Pain medication not lasting between ordered frequency. Dr. Smith notified of complaint of pain. New orders noted. ______ C. Lott, RN

Observations of Psychosocial Status. In addition to physical needs, you should document significant data related to psychosocial status. Assess the client's sensorium in relation to level of consciousness and orientation to time, place, and person. Any confusion or change in consciousness is significant and should be documented specifically.

The safety and security needs of clients seeking health care are frequently threatened, resulting in anxiety. Any evidence of fear or anxiety should be documented in the client's record. If a client decides to leave the facility against the advice of the physician (unless ordered by law to be admitted), note the same information as a routine discharge but chart "left AMA" (i.e., against medical advice). If the client states a reason for leaving, this should be included in the narrative. The physician should be notified of any AMA situation and an entry made in the chart as to this no-

Table 11-2 Necessary Charting Entries for Safety Concerns

Medication administration	Side rails placed up if sedating, instructions given not to get OOB without assistance.
Transporting client	Side rails placed up, attendant with client at all times.
Admit	Instructions given on using call light and the difference in regular and emergency light.
Restraints	Notation according to agency policy; offered water, meal, bathroom privileges; ROM and skin condition checked.
Ambulation	Assistance required, use of house shoes, use of assistive devices such as walker, cane.
Change in LOC or sensorium from a recent major event such as surgery	Instructions given not to get up the first time without health care assistance. VS taken if dizziness experienced or change in LOC. Side rails up if disoriented, notification of doctor if status changes, presence of sitter or family member.
Falls	Actual facts as reported by client, family, and health care workers should be included. Actual assessment findings on first discovering the accident, including the position client was in when found; notification of physician, family, or house supervisor. Also specific accounts leading up to the event. Report what was done, such as x-rays and notification of physician. Note the history of falls during last hospitalization or at home when admitting the client.

LOC, Level of consciousness; *OOB,* out of bed; *ROM,* range of motion; *VS,* vital signs.

tification. Any additional agency policies should also be followed.

Activities of Daily Living. Activities of daily living (ADLs) are often documented primarily on flow sheets and should be recorded by the person administering care. If a flow sheet is not available, ADLs should be noted in narrative format. Information recorded related to ADLs includes type of bath, oral hygiene, change of linen, and type of assistance needed. The type of assistance and the number of health care workers needed to move a client from place to place should also be included. Examples of ways to note transfer needs include independent, minimal supervision and/or assistance, continuous supervision and/or assistance of one person, continuous assistance of two persons, or total care. ADLs can also be charted using terminology that indicates the client's degree of independence.

Valuables. When a client enters a facility with jewelry or valuables that need to be secured during the stay, an entry should be made that these items were sent to the appropriate department. The detailed description of specific items such as jewelry, and the amount of money in the wallet, should be included with the belongings, usually on the outside of the folder in which they are placed, rather than charted (see Figure 11-5). Describe any valuables such as jewelry in general terms. Instead of "solid gold, 1-carat diamond ring," a better description is "yellow ring with clear stone." Agencies may require the signature of two health care professionals on any documentation of valuables, with a copy placed in the client's chart. If valuables are sent home with a family member, it is important to document the name of the person who took the valuables and the relationship to the client.

Spiritual Care. Spiritual care is often neglected in documentation, but it is an important entry for complete documentation of client care. Entries may need to be included that describe signs and symptoms of spiritual distress, symbols or articles of spiritual meaning, rituals practiced, source of hope, expressions of grief, and notification of chaplain or spiritual advisor.

Safety Concerns. A significant area needing detailed and complete documentation is that of safety issues for the client, particularly the older adult or immobile client. Although flow sheets now include many of these safety concerns, narrative charting may still be needed. Regardless of where the information is written, documenting safety measures taken for each client while in a facility is essential. Examples of important safety concerns include side rails, unsteady gait, assistance needed with ambulation, past medication or surgery, ability to use call lights, knowledge of emergency call lights, use of restraints, offering toiletry if immobile, history of falls, mental status changes (especially confusion), and transporting clients. Equipment and monitor alarms should be on, audible, and set to individual client limits whenever possible. Client teaching about safety should be adequately documented.

Many facilities have special guidelines for including safety concerns, and these are usually required for every client. However, you have the right and responsibility to note safety issues in a factual manner as often as needed (Table 11-2).

SIGNIFICANT NOTATIONS FOR SPECIAL POPULATIONS

Documentation entries need to be made for special groups, such as older adults, children, and culturally diverse clients. Life span considerations in older adults as well as in children are a part of the charting that may not be as necessary for other clients. Issues specific to a client, such as language barriers or dietary customs of a specific culture, should be noted.

Older Adult Clients. Special care should be taken to include accurate and complete descriptions of the skin, ADLs, mobility, mental status, and the behavior of older

7/14/03	0800	Remains alert, oriented x3. Assist c̄ AM care on a daily basis, dresses self. Attends activity 1 or 2x per month, joins in c̄ other residents. Likes to visit Mrs. Brown in room 112-A. Family visited 3x this month and took her on pass for a day. Seemed to enjoy the visit. Eating in the dining room and assists others c̄ their trays. No change in overall condition. Ⓛ hip incision healed, uses Ⓛ hip c̄ assist of walker. Physical therapy visits 2x per week, tolerates P.T. s̄ any problems. Continent of bowel and bladder. Sleeps uninterrupted for 6–8 hours per night.
		———————— S. Richards, RN

FIGURE 11-6 Example of an entry in a long-term care facility.

BOX 11-2 *Guidelines for Extended and Long-Term Care*

- Know the requirements of the regulating body of the agency; read quarterly reviews, know when to document.
- Know policies and procedures of the facility.
- Note phone calls, visits by relatives, interactions with other clients.
- Verify how nurses spend their time with the client on a visit; be aware of issues concerning reimbursement.
- Be specific in indicating progress or lack thereof (e.g., ambulated 10 feet on 7/21/07, progressed to 15 feet on 7/22/07).
- Record supplies used.
- Note activities performed by nurses for other departments on the weekends: continuous passive motion machines, physical therapy, electrocardiography, and so on.
- Describe a clear picture that includes fine details: could not open milk carton or use utensils; after meat cut and packages opened, self-fed without problems.
- Include entries that reflect progress or lack of progress toward the goals and objectives on the client's plan of care.
- Include the client's response to drug therapies.

adult clients. Accurate and descriptive documentation of the physical assessment of these clients on admission is crucial, especially if abuse is suspected or if they experienced confusion in a previous hospitalization. Notes should include how prepared older adults are to go home, the type of assistance needed at home (or, if they are unable to go to their own home, discharge planning—beginning on the day of admittance), and any emotional needs. Throughout older clients' stay in a health care facility, it is essential to document progress in their ability to carry out ADLs so that, if possible, it can be shown on discharge that they are sufficiently able to perform self-care.

Pediatric Clients. Special attention should be paid to documenting observations about the relationship between parents and child, dependence of the child on the parent, developmental level of the child (related to age), ability of the child to play, language used by child and parents, and any additional emotional needs for children. Examples might include the following: mother rocks child and reads a book; child speaks in complete, simple sentences; or child able to stack blocks, play hide-and-seek, and self-entertain with colors. Accurate and descriptive documentation of the physical assessment of children on admission is crucial, especially if abuse is suspected.

Clients From Varied Cultures. Suggested areas for documentation for culturally diverse clients include native language, fluency of English, ability to read and write, beliefs about cause of illness, dietary differences (foods excluded or preferred), special concerns related to religious beliefs, and individual needs, such as for uninterrupted time for meditation.

EXTENDED AND LONG-TERM CARE

Extended-care facilities may have additional forms that are used for documentation. The use of a classification system to show acuity and specifications of the amount or type of equipment or supplies is often included in documentation for extended-care and long-term care facilities. Group sessions with family members, planning a home visit in preparation for discharge, or visits with social workers to discuss discharge options are also included. Long-term care facilities may require weekly or monthly charting in a summary manner as opposed to daily or shift notations. Narrative entries are usually made about such items as the client's abilities, progress, or degenerative changes (Figure 11-6). Box 11-2 is a list of guidelines for documentation in these types of facilities.

HOME HEALTH CARE GUIDELINES

Documentation in a home health care setting is often different from documenting in an acute care facility because of the need to justify the visit by a professional nurse. Home health care nurses usually document an initial assessment with a complete database. Visits thereafter are usually progress notes for each visit and include direct care, teaching or instructions given, performance of skills, and evaluation of homebound status. Home health care nurses use progress notes written in narrative format that should be consistent with other disciplines charting on the same client. With each visit, the need for the help of a professional health care worker must be noted. Reimbursement for the visit is directly related to the accuracy and wording of the documentation showing a need for professional assistance. General guidelines are offered for beginning nurses in a home health care setting (Table 11-3).

Additional suggestions for effective charting in a home health care situation include the following:

- Leave out extraneous information that could affect reimbursement.
- Record all equipment and supplies used at the visit. Know which medical equipment can be provided, and document why.
- Avoid vague statements like "doing better" or "no acute distress."
- Monitor new procedures to ensure that all personnel are doing the same thing.
- Note safety concerns such as "throw rugs removed from path to BR."

Key terms in home health care include *assessment, instructions,* and *skilled care.* Home health care nurses must be especially confident in knowing definitions and in medication administration. All charting should be made with the assumption that the documents will probably be audited. Following is an example of home health care charting:

SAMPLE CHARTING

7/16/07	0905	Wound area remains open, wound edges irregular; sacral wound area intact, stage 2 has decreased in size: 2 cm L X 2 cm W X 0.5 cm D without undermining or tunneling. No change in size of left heel pressure ulcer stage 2. Family turning client q 2 hours and keeping heels clear of mattress as directed. Family still unable to perform wound care. ________ K. Hobson, RN

Problem areas frequently identified in charting for home health care clients include the following:

- Lack of a clear picture of what is going on with the client
- Discrepancies between what went on with the client and what appeared in the chart
- Difficulty in determining the client's status, functional limitations, current level of activity, or homebound status
- Why the nurse is seeing and needs to continue seeing the client
- Failure to document for Medicare reimbursement

SPECIAL ENTRIES

Finally, several situations require special notations in which you should make complete and accurate explanations. First, notification of physicians should include the time they were notified, how they were notified (e.g., direct call, beeper), and why. When the physician responds, note the time and the action taken as a result of the phone call. Failure on the part of the physician to respond should be noted as well. Second, any follow-up entry should emphasize what actions were taken, why, and the client's response.

Third, charting results of specific laboratory tests or nursing actions when administering certain classifications of medications is generally expected (Table 11-4). For example, adjusting a heparin drip according to a sliding scale order would include noting the partial thromboplastin time (PTT) value and the adjusted rate of the heparin. Documentation of a blood pressure or pulse is required for many classes of cardiac medications such as digoxin (Lanoxin) or antihypertensives.

Table 11-3 Guidelines for Beginning Nurses in a Home Health Care Setting

DIRECT SKILLED CARE Diverse and involved care that can be provided only by trained professionals	• Catheter changes, catheter care • Wound care • Treatments/administering medications • Injections/administering medications • Ostomy care • Aseptic technique • Heat treatments • Tube feedings
CLIENT TEACHING A part of any skill done	• Inclusion of client and family • Response to information • Ability to perform activity independently • Verbalizes understanding of the instruction • Booklets or educational material left for client or family
HOMEBOUND STATUS Inability to leave home to obtain similar health care services at a clinic, doctor's office, or outpatient clinic	• Reason for status on admit, and weekly thereafter • Support of other disciplines • Evaluation

DOCUMENTATION FORMATS

TYPES OF RECORDS

JCAHO has encouraged the use of health care records that are organized in an interdisciplinary problem-oriented manner to better reflect collaboration and a client-centered focus. The emergence of case management has introduced critical/clinical pathways as another method of organizing client care information.

Problem-oriented medical records are a form of documentation originally designed to organize information

Table 11-4 Examples of Charting Entries for Medications

Irritating medications such as hydroxyzine (Vistaril) or iron	Must chart IM "Z-track"
Antiarrhythmics	Change in the cardiac rhythm
Pain medication	Client rating of the pain, scale used, client goal, safety measure after administered, VS, relief obtained
Antianginals/antihypertensives	VS, may need orthostatic BP checks
Insulin administration	Glucose value before administration, condition of client during peak times
Diuretics	Recent electrolyte values, signs or symptoms of electrolyte loss, I&O
Heparin or anticoagulants	Coagulation laboratory tests; PT, PTT, INR
Allergies	What specific response the client has

BP, Blood pressure; *IM,* intramuscular; *INR,* international normalized ratio; *I&O,* intake and output; *PT,* prothrombin time; *PTT,* partial thromboplastin time; *VS,* vital signs.

according to identified client problems, with all health care team members documenting information sequentially. Problem-oriented records have four components: the database, the problem list, initial plans for each problem, and progress notes for each problem. All members of the health care team make entries on the same record using the same problem list. Problems are added to the list using the language appropriate for the health care provider making the entry. For example, physicians would add medical diagnoses, whereas nurses would use nursing diagnoses. The primary advantages of this system are the inclusion of a common problem list and the ease with which all members of a health care team can monitor progress related to each problem.

DOCUMENTATION FORMAT

Regardless of the organization of the medical record itself, health care agencies may choose from a variety of formats for documentation. The format chosen depends on the type of agency, the primary purposes of documentation, and the types of health care workers involved. Regardless of the format, the principles, the mechanics, and generally even the content remain the same. How the content is recorded, however, depends on the format chosen. This discussion addresses several formats currently used, including the use of flow sheets for documenting relevant data.

The format for documentation may be a free-style narrative, a problem-focused or process-focused format, or a combination of these. Source-oriented records that separate parts of the chart by discipline might still use a problem-oriented approach to documenting nursing care. In addition, flow sheets are used to document routine daily care.

Narrative Charting. **Narrative charting** is a method of charting that provides information in the form of statements that describe events surrounding client care. It is often relatively unstructured, providing flexibility in determining how information is recorded, or the format may be structured and problem focused. Free-style narrative charting allows anyone reading the record to easily follow a sequence of events. Medical as well as nursing interventions may be included and may relate to more than one identified problem at the same time. This style also allows inclusion of significant events related to the client that might not be directly related to an identified client problem.

The method is, however, time consuming and makes it difficult to retrieve information and track client progress and outcomes. In addition, the lack of specific prompting of notations (such as by time or identified problems) often leads to entries that fail to sufficiently address client problems. Entries may also include unnecessary or meaningless notations simply because the nurse feels compelled to write *something* at periodic time intervals. Avoid duplication of content already included on the record to reduce discrepancies in data.

Narrative documentation can easily be combined with flow sheets to retain the advantage of complete descriptions when desirable, together with the brevity of the flow sheet when descriptive data is not needed. Examples of narrative charting have been used throughout this chapter.

Problem-Focused Charting. APIE (PIE), focus, and SOAP formats for charting allow documentation using the nursing process. Advantages of problem-focused formats include easy reference to specific problems and use of the nursing process. One disadvantage cited by nurses is that all entries must relate to a specific problem on the problem list, making it difficult to document events unrelated to an identified problem. Most systems require charting about problems periodically, even if unchanged. Therefore, this format may not be the most efficient for some settings, particularly long-term care. If several problems are included on the problem list, documentation may be lengthy. Regardless of the format used, the problem list must remain current and accurate.

APIE (PIE) Charting. In **APIE (PIE) charting** the acronym APIE stands for the following:

A Assessment
P Problem identification
I Interventions
E Evaluation

The process begins with an admission assessment that is usually completed on a separate form, and the initiation of a problem list (using either nursing diagnoses or problem statements) that is based on the initial assessment. An example of a problem list for Ms. Peters is found in Figure 11-7, and Figure 11-8 shows examples of data entries using the APIE format.

Date/Initials	Problem #	Nursing Diagnosis	Date Resolved/Initials
7/15/03 BSM	#1	Pain related to surgical incision.	
7/15/03 BSM	#2	Risk for infection related to surgical incision.	
7/15/03 CRT	#3	Impaired home maintenance related to impaired mobility.	

FIGURE 11-7 Example of an APIE problem list.

Date	Time	Problem #	Remarks
7/16/03	1600	#1	I = Oral analgesic given for c/o incisional pain 4/10 scale. — S. Richards, RN
	1630	#1	E = Sitting in chair at bedside. States pain relieved. — S. Richards, RN
			States pain relieved now at 1/10 scale.
		Assessment	States she feels constipated. Last BM 7/12. Abdomen firm.
		P#4	Constipation related to decreased activity and change in diet. —
		I#4	Dr. Alvarez notified. Stool softener adm. as ordered. Encouraged to ↑ fluid intake. Nutrition consult for foods with fiber. — S. Richards, RN

OR

Date	Time	Problem #	Remarks
7/16/03	1600	IP#1	Oral analgesic given for c/o incisional pain 4/10 scale. — S. Richards, RN
	1630	EP#1	Sitting in chair at bedside. States pain relieved. — S. Richards, RN
			States pain relieved now at 1/10 scale.
		Assessment	States she feels constipated. Last BM 7/12. Abdomen firm. —
		P#4	Constipation related to decreased activity and change in diet. —
		IP#4	Dr. Alvarez notified. Stool softener adm. as ordered. Encouraged to ↑ fluid intake. — S. Richards, RN

FIGURE 11-8 Example of APIE data entries.

Some agencies include data to support the problem identified, by adding AEB (as evidenced by) to the diagnosis. For example, *Acute pain related to surgical incision AEB guarding of incision and verbal complaints of pain.* Some problem lists may also include goals or expected outcomes for each problem.

Documentation of client care is focused on interventions and evaluation related to problems listed. Each entry in the progress notes is preceded by the date, time, and problem number, and it indicates whether the entry relates to implementation or evaluation (see Figure 11-8).

Each problem should be evaluated at least once per shift (some agencies may require more frequent entries). Only information related to implementation or evaluation of problems on the problem list is included in the progress notes. Once the initial or admission assessment is complete, routine assessment is recorded each shift on a flow sheet. An "assessment" entry is not required in the progress notes unless there is a change in the client's status. For example, if the client introduced earlier with the nursing diagnosis of *Acute pain related to surgical incision* complains later of constipation, this would be noted as in Figure 11-8. Problem number 4 would also be added to the problem list. As problems are resolved, the date is indicated on the problem list.

Focus Charting. **Focus charting** addresses client problems or needs and includes a column that summarizes the focus of the entry. It may or may not utilize nursing diagnosis (some agencies use nursing diagnoses for the focus; others do not). This focus can include a nursing diagnosis, activities or concerns of the client, or other incidents. The format requires using the acronym DAR or the acronym DAE:

DAR	DAE
Data	Data
Action	Action
Response	Evaluation

Data should include all subjective and objective observations, whereas *action* indicates any interventions resulting from the observations. *Response* or *evaluation* entries document the effect of the intervention on the client and may be recorded immediately or at a later time if appropriate. For example, if medication is given for pain, the response will not likely be assessed until sufficient time has been allowed for the medication to be effective. This

Date	Time	Focus	Notes
7/16/03	1600	Pain	D = c/o pain at incision site Ⓛ hip. Pain 4/10 scale. Requests pain medication. — S. Richards, RN A = Oral analgesic given PO. — S. Richards, RN
	1600	Dressing	D = Abd. dressing c̄ mod. amt. serous drainage. — S. Richards, RN A = Dsg. reinforced. — S. Richards, RN
	1630	Pain	R = States pain relieved 1/10 scale. — S. Richards, RN
		Dressing	R = Dsg. dry and intact. — S. Richards, RN

FIGURE 11-9 Example of focus charting.

Date/Time	Problem	Progress Notes
7/16/03 1600	#1 Pain related to surgical incision	S = States discomfort in Ⓛ hip at 4/10 scale. O = Grimaces c̄ movement to Ⓛ side. Requests pain medication q3h. A = No change. P = Continue pain meds prn. S. Richards, RN

FIGURE 11-10 Example of a progress note in SOAP charting.

format also employs flow sheets for documentation of routine observations and interventions. Figure 11-9 provides an example of focus charting.

Advantages of focus charting include flexibility, easy data retrieval, and close alignment with the nursing process. One disadvantage is the possibility of inconsistency in the labeling of problems.

Soap Charting. **SOAP charting** is used to record progress notes with problem-focused charting. The progress notes include narrative notes as well as flow sheets, and they are used by all members of the health care team. The narrative notes specifically relate to a problem list and are numbered and titled accordingly. For example, a reference made to a client's surgical incision would be preceded by the problem number (from the problem list) and/or the name of the problem (e.g., No. 1, Open reduction and internal fixation).

The format contains four parts, remembered by the acronym SOAP, which stands for

Subjective data
Objective data
Assessment
Plan

Subjective data describe the client's problem as the client sees it; neither measurable nor observable, subjective data must be reported to the health care provider by the client. *Objective data* are measurable or observable by another person—for example, laboratory or physical assessment findings. In the *assessment* component of the note, conclusions are summarized on the basis of the data presented, whereas the *plan* outlines actions to address the identified problem. For example, the plan may include further diagnostic tests, therapeutic medical or nursing interventions, or client education. Often the plan is simply to continue the previously outlined plan.

Sometimes, not all SOAP elements are present or appropriate. For example, if there are no objective data to support a problem, "none" is written by the "O" in the SOAP note. One example of a progress note in the SOAP format is found in Figure 11-10. Advantages of the SOAP format include a uniform problem list used by all personnel and easy reference to data related to specific problems. Disadvantages include lack of flexibility (as seen in the APIE method), because all documentation is directed toward a specific problem.

Charting by Exception. **Charting by exception** provides documentation only if the data are significant or abnormal. This format reduces lengthy and repetitive charting and allows client progress to be followed more easily. This system provides comprehensive flow sheets for documentation of both medical and nursing orders. If assessment is within normal limits or unchanged from the previous assessment, no narrative progress notes are necessary. Charting by exception is predicated on establishment of norms for assessment, with forms varying by agency. For example, the 24-hour assessment example included in Figure 11-11 and the entry made in Figure 11-12 are examples of charting by exception.

The flow sheet provides a column for each hour in a 24-hour period. Simply place a check mark (✓) or initials in each block to indicate findings at a given time. If assessment findings are normal, no other documentation is needed. Specific notations can be included in the block that indicate specific observations. In Figure 11-11, the notation of 100% is included under diet to indicate the proportion of food consumed at each meal or snack. A letter is placed in the block indicating client position for supine, right or left lateral. If the nurse initials findings that are considered abnormal, a detailed description is then required in the progress notes.

Although charting by exception is time efficient and reduces duplication, it is more difficult to identify omissions in care, details are often limited, and it is more difficult to follow the nursing process. Charting by exception is well suited to the electronic medical record, where the clinical information system is built to help fill in both the normal assessment data and the selection of the exceptions specific to the unit and facility.

Text continued on p. 251

Cooley Dickinson Hospital

Medical/Surgical Flowsheet

Form 195 7/14/06

Date:________ Precautions: □ Contact □ Aspiration □ Airborne □ Droplet □ Latex
Protocols: □ CIWA □ Falls □ Suicide □ Seizure □ Chemo □ PrU Other: ___________

	Time:															
	Initials:															
Vital Signs	Temp															
	Pulse															
	Resp															
	BP	/	/	/	/	/	/	/	/	/	/	/	/	/	/	/
Oxygen	SpO_2															
	O_2Mode															
	O_2 Amt															
Pain	Location															
□ Faces	Intensity															
□ 0/10	Quality															
□ Words	Intervention															
□ Behav	Reassess & Time done	/	/	/	/	/	/	/	/	/	/	/	/	/	/	/
Pt Goal: ____	Acceptable															

Continued

TREATMENTS / ACTIVITY

Time:															
Initials:															
Bedside Blood Glucose Ref. range 70– 110mg/dL															
Oral / Denture Care √															
Peri / Foley Care √															
Toileted √															
Reposition in Bed(R,L,S)															
Chair / Dangle (C / D)															
Ambulated (I, A1, A2)															
Distance ambulated															
Device (G, CN, CR, W)															
AROM / PROM (A,P)															
Sleeping √															
Incentive Spirometry **Vt**															
Cough/Deep Breathe √															
Call bell in reach √															
# of Side Rails up															
Bed Position low															
Equipment Alarms on √															
NGT/GT Placement verified															
Residual checked___ml															

Hygiene □ Bath □ Shower □ Refused □ Self □ Assist □ Total Care Initials: ____ Time: ______

FIGURE 11-11 Nursing 24-hour assessment. (Courtesy Cooley Dickinson Hospital, Northampton, MA.)

Cooley Dickinson Hospital

Medical/Surgical Flowsheet

Form 195 7/14/06

Date:______________ * focus note with changes

Assessment for WNL	**Nights** Initials: ____ Time: _____	**Days** Initials: ____ Time: _____	**Evenings** Initials: ____ Time: _____
Neurological Alert & Oriented to person, place time. Follows commands. Speech clear and understandable. Able to swallow secretions.	□ **WNL** □ Unable to follow commands **Disoriented:** □ Person □ Place □ Time **LOC:** □ Unresponsive □ Confused □ Agitated □ Sleeping □ Lethargic **Pupils:** □ Equal, responsive □ Unequal (describe): __________ **Speech:**□Slurred □Dysphasic □Aphasic □ Artificial airway:__________	□ **WNL** □ Unable to follow commands **Disoriented:** □ Person □ Place □ Time **LOC:** □ Unresponsive □ Confused □ Agitated □ Sleeping □ Lethargic **Pupils:** □ Equal, responsive □ Unequal (describe): __________ **Speech:**□Slurred □Dysphasic □Aphasic □ Artificial airway:__________	□ **WNL** □ Unable to follow commands **Disoriented:**□ Person □ Place □ Time **LOC:** □ Unresponsive □ Confused □ Agitated □ Sleeping □ Lethargic **Pupils:** □ Equal, responsive □ Unequal (describe): __________ **Speech:**□Slurred □Dysphasic □Aphasic □ Artificial airway:__________
Musculoskeletal Equal strength all 4 extremities bilaterally. No muscle weakness. AROM and Sensation intact all 4 extremities.	□ **WNL** **Motion:** Ltd/Absent **Strength:** Weak RUE □ □ RUE □ LUE □ □ LUE □ RLE □ □ RLE □ LLE □ □ LLE □ **Sensation** abnormal: □ RUE □ LUE □ RLE □ LLE Other: __________	□ **WNL** **Motion:** Ltd/Absent **Strength:** Weak RUE □ □ RUE □ LUE □ □ LUE □ RLE □ □ RLE □ LLE □ □ LLE □ **Sensation** abnormal: □ RUE □ LUE □ RLE □ LLE Other: __________	□ **WNL** **Motion:** Ltd/Absent **Strength:** Weak RUE □ □ RUE □ LUE □ □ LUE □ RLE □ □ RLE □ LLE □ □ LLE □ **Sensation** abnormal: □ RUE □ LUE □ RLE □ LLE Other: __________
Cardiovascular Apical pulse regular rate/rhythm. No peripheral edema. Pedal pulses palpable bilaterally. Nailbeds and mucosa pink. Capillary refill within 2 seconds.	□ **WNL** □ Edema: __________ **Heart Rate:** □ Irregular **Heart Sounds:** □ Abnormal □_____ **Pulses:** 0 = Absent 1+ = Weak Radial Right __ Left __ Pedal Right __ Left __ Carotid Right __ Left __ Other: ____ Right __ Left __ **Color** abnormal: __________ Other: __________	□ **WNL** □ Edema: __________ **Heart Rate:** □ Irregular **Heart Sounds:** □ Abnormal □ _____ **Pulsesl:** 0 = Absent 1+ = Weak Radial Right __ Left __ Pedal Right __ Left __ Carotid Right __ Left __ Other: ____ Right __ Left __ **Color** abnormal: __________ Other: __________	□ **WNL** □ Edema: __________ **Heart Rate:** □ Irregular **Heart Sounds:** □ Abnormal □ _____ **Pulsesl:** 0 = Absent 1+ = Weak Radial Right __ Left __ Pedal Right __ Left __ Carotid Right __ Left __ Other: ____ Right __ Left __ **Color** abnormal: __________ Other: __________
Respiratory Breath sounds clear, equal throughout. Respirations symmetrical, unlabored. No cough or sputum production.	□ **WNL** **Respirations:** □ Diminished □ Shallow □ Labored □ Accessory muscles used Other: __________ **Breath Sounds:** Crackles □RUL □RML □RLL □LUL □LLL Wheezes □RUL □RML □RLL □LUL □LLL **Chest Tube:** □ Right □ Left___ cm SX **Secretions:** __________ Other: __________	□ **WNL** **Respirations:** □ Diminished □ Shallow □ Labored □ Accessory muscles used Other: __________ **Breath Sounds:** Crackles □RUL □RML □RLL □LUL □LLL Wheezes □RUL □RML □RLL □LUL □LLL **Chest Tube:** □ Right □ Left___ cm SX **Secretions:** __________ Other: __________	□ **WNL** **Respirations:** □ Diminished □ Shallow □ Labored □ Accessory muscles used Other: __________ **Breath Sounds:** Crackles □RUL □RML □RLL □LUL □LLL Wheezes □RUL □RML □RLL □LUL □LLL **Chest Tube:** □ Right □ Left___ cm SX **Secretions:** __________ Other: __________
Gastrointestinal Bowel sounds present. Abdomen soft, non-tender. Tolerating diet. Last BM: ________	□ **WNL** **Bowel Sounds:** □ Absent **Abdomen:** □Tender □Firm □Distended **Nausea:**□Yes □ No **Flatus:**□Yes □ No **Tubes:** □ NGT □ GT □ JT □ Colostomy □ Ileostomy Other: __________	□ **WNL** **Bowel Sounds:** □ Absent **Abdomen:** □Tender □Firm □Distended **Nausea:** □Yes □No **Flatus:** □Yes □No **Tubes:** □ NGT □ GT □ JT □ Colostomy □ Ileostomy Other: __________	□ **WNL** **Bowel Sounds:** □ Absent **Abdomen:** □Tender □Firm □Distended **Nausea:** □Yes □No **Flatus:** □Yes □No **Tubes:** □ NGT □ GT □ JT □ Colostomy □ Ileostomy Other: __________
Genitourinary Urine clear yellow in adequate amounts (at least 30ml / hr if on I/O). DTV:_________	□ **WNL** □ Urostomy **Voiding:** □ Incontinent □ Frequently □ Painful □ Retention □ Foley □ CBI □ Hemodialysis, access patent Other: __________ **Color:** ________	□ **WNL** □ Urostomy **Voiding:** □ Incontinent □ Frequently □ Painful □ Retention □ Foley □ CBI □ Hemodialysis, access patent Other: __________ **Color:** ________	□ **WNL** □ Urostomy **Voiding:** □ Incontinent □ Frequently □ Painful □ Retention □ Foley □ CBI □ Hemodialysis, access patent Other: __________ **Color:** ________
Integumentary Skin warm, dry & intact; Mucosa moist; Turgor rebound 3 sec or less	□ **WNL** □ Moist □ Cool □ Clammy □ Ecchymotic □ Rash __________ □ Open Areas- See Wound/Skin Record □ Dressing dry/intact □ Incision clean/dry	□ **WNL** □ Moist □ Cool □ Clammy □ Ecchymotic □ Rash __________ □ Open Areas- See Wound/Skin Record □ Dressing dry/intact □ Incision clean/dry	□ **WNL** □ Moist □ Cool □ Clammy □ Ecchymotic □ Rash __________ □ Open Areas- See Wound/Skin Record □ Dressing dry/intact □ Incision clean/dry
Psychosocial Mood, affect, behavior & interactions are appropriate for age.	□ **WNL** **Behavior** abnormal: □ Depressed □ Anxious □ Irritable □ Distracted □ Withdrawn Threat to □ Self □ Others	□ **WNL** **Behavior** abnormal: □ Depressed □ Anxious □ Irritable □ Distracted □ Withdrawn Threat to □ Self □ Others	□ **WNL** **Behavior** abnormal: □ Depressed □ Anxious □ Irritable □ Distracted □ Withdrawn Threat to □ Self □ Others

FIGURE 11-11, cont'd Nursing 24-hour assessment. (Courtesy Cooley Dickinson Hospital, Northampton, MA.)

Cooley Dickinson Hospital

Medical/Surgical Flowsheet

Form 195 7/14/06

Date: ____________________

FALL RISK ASSESSMENT – Done on admission and every shift				
Mobility	**Score**	**N**	**D**	**E**
Amb w/no gait disturbance	**0**			
Amb or transfers w/devices or assist	**1**			
Amb w/unsteady gait and no assistance (**PT consult)**	**1**			
Unable to ambulate or transfer	**0**			
Mentation: Alert, oriented x3	**0**			
Periodic confusion	**1**			
Confusion at all times	**1**			
Comatose/unresponsive	**0**			
Elimination: Independent in elimination	**0**			
Independent, w/frequency or diarrhea	**1**			
Needs assistance w/toileting	**1**			
Incontinent	**1**			
Prior Fall History: Yes, before admit **(PT consult)**	**1**			
Yes – during this admission. Date:	**2**			
No known history	**0**			
Current Medications: *Score 1 if receiving meds in any class or more than 4 meds.* Cardiac/Antihypertensives IV infusing Opioid Analgesics Diuretics Laxatives Antidepressants Muscle Relaxants Antiemetics Anxiolytics Antipsychotics	**1**			
Implement Falls protocol if score is 3 or more. Score:				
Initials :				

PRESSURE ULCER Precautions(√)	**N**	**D**	**E**
Sign and stickers posted			
Turn every 2 hours			
Incontinent Care every 2 hours			
Air pump on bed & checked			
Ointment to prominences **bid**			
Heel boots on / Heels elevated			
Waffle chair cushion			
Head to toe skin check daily			
Initials:			

FALLS Protocol (√)	**N**	**D**	**E**
Explain Protocol to patient and family.			
Falling star sign above bed / CCU door			
Chair alarm on when out of bed.			
Bed alarm on when patient is in bed.			
Stickers on Kardex, chart, door binder			
Toileting schedule; stay with patient prn			
Consult PT where noted on risk score			
Initials:			

BRADEN SCALE done on Admission and Daily		
Sensory Perception:	**Moisture:**	**Activity**
□ 1 Complete limited	□ 1 Constantly moist	□ 1 Bedfast
□ 2 Very limited	□ 2 Moist	□ 2 Chairfast
□ 3 Slightly limited	□ 3 Occasionally moist	□ 3 Walks occasionally
□ 4 No impairment	□ 4 Rarely moist	□ 4 Walks frequently
Mobility:	**Nutrition:**	**Friction & shear:**
□ 1 Complete immobile	□ 1 Very poor	□ 1 Significant problem
□ 2 Very limited	□ 2 Inadequate	□ 2 Problem
□ 3 Slightly limited	□ 3 Adequate	□ 3 Potential problem
□ 4 No limitations	□ 4 Excellent	□ 4 No problem
Implement Pressure Ulcer (PrU) Precautions for: Score 18 or less age 65+; Score 16 or less under 65yr; or a Score of 2 or less in any category		**Score:**
		Initials: **Time:**

FIGURE 11-11, cont'd Nursing 24-hour assessment. (Courtesy Cooley Dickinson Hospital, Northampton, MA.)

Continued

Cooley Dickinson Hospital

Medical/Surgical Flowsheet

Form 195 7/14/06

Date: _______ Today's weight: _____ Kg Previous weight: _____ Kg Date ________

Diet: _________________ Scale used: □ Bed □ Standing Admit weight: _____ Kg

INTAKE								OUTPUT					
Meals: B %___ S%___ L %___ S%___ D%___ S%___													
	Oral	**Tube**	**IV**	**IV**	**IV**	**IVPB**	**Colloid**	**Urine**	**Stool**				**Hourly's**
0000													
0100													
0200													
0300													
0400													
0500													
0600													
0700													
Total													
0800													
0900													
1000													
1100													
1200													
1300													
1400													
1500													
Total													
1600													
1700													
1800													
1900													
2000													
2100													
2200													
2300													
Total													
24 Hr Totals													

Intake Grand Total:	Output Grand Total:	24 Hr Balance (I – O) =
Cumulative Balance this admission (Todays 24 hr balance + Yesterdays) =		Positive Negative fluid balance

IV site check WNL = within normal limits – dressing dry/intact, no pain, no edema, no redness *focus note for deviations

Location / Size	Nights	Days	Eves	Inserted	Removed	Dsg Chg	Tubing Chg
IV:							
IV:							
IV:							

Signature:______________________ Shift:___ Initials:___ Signature:______________________ Shift: ___ Initials:___

Signature:______________________ Shift:___ Initials:___ Signature:______________________ Shift: ___ Initials:___

Signature:______________________ Shift:___ Initials:___ Signature:______________________ Shift: ___ Initials:___

FIGURE 11-11, cont'd Nursing 24-hour assessment. (Courtesy Cooley Dickinson Hospital, Northampton, MA.)

7/15/03	1610	c/o pain in Ⓛ hip. States 8 on a scale of 1–10. Instructed to use PCA as needed. Dressing to Ⓛ hip c̄ mod. amt. serous drainage (6-cm diameter). Dressing reinforced. IV D5W @ 100 ml/hr c̄ 450 ml TBA. —— S. Richards, RN
	1630	States mild discomfort. Pain rated 4 on a scale of 1–10. Reinforcement to dsg. clean and dry. —— S. Richards, RN

FIGURE 11-12 Example of charting by exception.

Flow Sheets. Regardless of the format, flow sheets are often used to document data that can be more easily followed in graphic or tabular form. They are used in many agencies to document routine assessment data and nursing interventions in checklist format. Trends related to ADLs, body systems review, and other nursing observations and activities can be easily followed using flow sheets. Flow sheets not only are often more legible, but also facilitate consistent documentation of assessment and interventions. All flow sheets require the date and the signature of the person who is making the observation. Some observations will require further description in narrative progress notes.

Graphic Records. The graphic records used to record vital signs in many agencies have largely been replaced by electronic medical records, which can graph vital signs and laboratory data and create custom graphs of selected data. Clinical information systems can also capture vital signs from client monitors for direct entry into the medical record at set intervals or as selected by the nurse. Some agencies use tabular forms for recording *all* vital signs, and some use such forms only when vital signs are recorded at frequent intervals.

Other Types of Flow Sheets. Other flow (Figure 11-13) sheets commonly used for recording data include the following:

- I&O
- Wound assessment
- Medication administration records
- Intensive vital signs
- Neurological checks
- Peritoneal dialysis
- Fetal monitoring

Clinical Pathways. **Clinical pathways,** also called **critical pathways** or **care maps,** may be recorded using an interdisciplinary approach or organized by health care discipline. Outcomes of care and planned interventions are derived collaboratively by all members of the health care team and reviewed and updated regularly. Any exceptions (variations) are documented, along with suspected causes for the variance and actions taken in response.

ELECTRONIC DOCUMENTATION

An **electronic medical record (EMR)** is used in many health care settings to record client care for a specific episode of care, as an admission. An **electronic health record (EHR)** is a comprehensive record of a client's care across different facilities and/or admissions. Electronic records contain information that is identical to that found in traditional records, but they eliminate repetitive entries by entering data once and having it sent to many different forms that require it and allow more timely access to the client data repository (Box 11-3).

Confidentiality and security of the computer system are major concerns. To keep the client's record confidential, the person who enters data into a computer logs on to the system using a secure password, which should be changed monthly to maintain security. The Health Insurance Portability and Accountability Act (HIPAA) of 1996 is administered by the U.S. Department of Health and Human Services to protect the privacy of clients' health information. These regulations protect individually identifiable health information in any format while enabling health care agencies and insurers to aggregate data and manage their business needs. Health care agencies have a privacy officer to ensure compliance with HIPAA regulations and respond to client concerns about privacy. Their networks are protected by a firewall and individually recognizable data is further protected by the use of encryption and authentication software whenever it is transmitted outside the agency.

A second issue is the clinical information system's impact on work flow. Studies have shown that computerized systems can enhance time efficiency, direct client care time, user satisfaction, accuracy of data, and completeness of the record (Poissant, Pereira, Tamblyn, & Kawasumi, 2005). Nurses' attitudes and acceptance of documenting with a computer have also affected the adoption of EMRs (Smith, Smith, Krugman, & Oman, 2005). The use of **computerized provider order entry (CPOE)** has had a significant impact on work flow because as orders are entered into the computer they are automatically routed to the appropriate clinical area for action. Orders can be added to work lists, diagnostic testing can be readily scheduled, and medications are added to eMARs.

A third issue is the vocabulary used to name the nursing problems, the lists of data for assessment, and anything else that is entered by picking from a list. The Systematized Nomenclature of Medicine Clinical Terms (SNOMED CT) is one reference vocabulary that enables terms to be mapped across the different nursing vocabularies included in it such as Nursing Interventions Classification (NIC) and Nursing Outcomes Classification (NOC). This is a key element of evidence-based practice. It enables nursing leaders and researchers to understand relationships in the data to predict trends and

NORTHOAKS

Attachment D: Skin Injury/Wound Assessment Flowsheet

R L L R

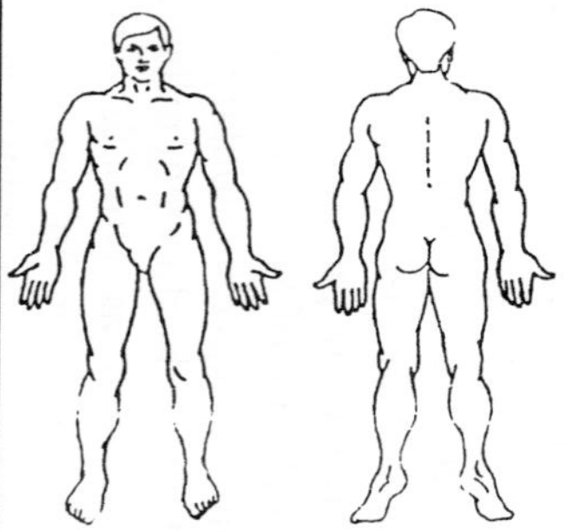

STAGE 1: Nonblanchable erythema of intact skin.

STAGE 2: Partial thickness skin loss involving epidermis and/or dermis.

STAGE 3: Full thickness skin loss involving damage or necrosis of subcutaneous tissue that may extend down to, but not through, underlying fascia.

STAGE 4: Full thickness skin loss with extensive destruction tissue necrosis or damage to muscle, bone or supporting structures.

Unable to stage due to eschar covering wound.

(Addressograph)

Number each injury/wound on the diagram. Complete a full row of information for each injury/wound.

Injury/Wound Types		Drainage	Odor	Color
Stasis Ulcer	Bruises	Serous	Mild	Pink
Pressure Ulcer	Skin Tear	Purulent	Foul	Red
Arterial Ulcer	Rash	None	None	Black
Surgical Wound	Hematoma	Other: Specify.	Other: Specify.	Eschar
Laceration	Other: Specify.			Other: Specify.

Date	Site#	Injury/Wound Type (Specify)	Stage	Length Width cm	Depth cm	Tunneling Yes/No	Color	Drainage Amt/Type	Odor	Culture Date	Treatments & Comments	Signature & Title

IS#128 JOB#2841.4+(2/18/98)

FIGURE 11-13 Example of a skin injury/wound assessment flow sheet. (Courtesy North Oaks Health System, Hammond, LA.)

BOX 11-3 *Characteristics of Computerized Records*

- Meet the legal criterion of legibility
- Automatically enter the time of the entry; the time of care must be added
- Recorder is identified by password-protected entry, rather than by a signature
- Entered data cannot be changed; incorrect entries must be noted by entering a correction entry
- Require keyboarding and mouse skills
- Employ security systems to protect confidentiality
- Can force charting to address problem list, the nursing process, or other specific needs of the agency
- Allow reduction of keyboarding required by using a menu option list, forced choice system, or technologies such as touch screen.
- May limit the ability to adequately convey meaning if the forced choices are not well constructed
- Allow for late data entries
- Allow retrieval of information for specific problems across multiple records

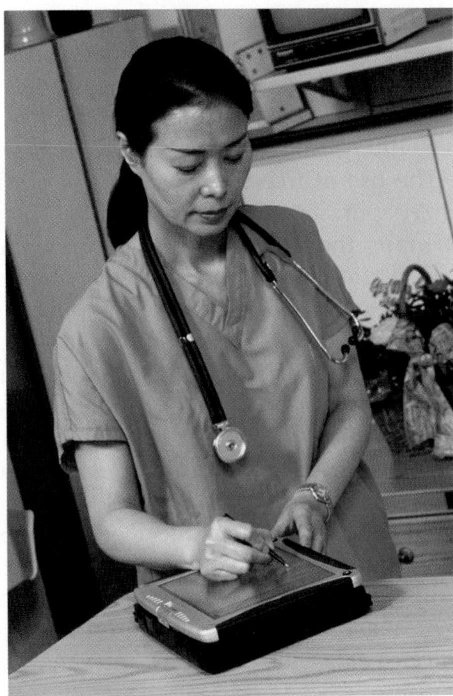

FIGURE 11-14 A tablet computer solution. (Courtesy Panasonic Corporation, Toughbook CF-18.)

consequences of care in an interdisciplinary model (Lunney, Delaney, & Duffy, 2005).

The use of computer systems for documentation in health care agencies varies in scope depending on the agency. Most health care agencies have incorporated information systems for management of admissions; billing; communication of orders for diet, pharmacy, and diagnostic tests; and reporting the results of laboratory and radiology studies. Use of these systems allows departments within an institution to interact, and it provides a database for research and quality assurance. In addition, clinical information systems are more efficient at simplifying and standardizing documentation with less reliance on memory through the use of automated reminders, alerts, checklists, protocols, clinical pathways, and reference databases as point-of-care knowledge resources. Many agencies have incorporated software for documentation of client care. Systems may include options for generating individualized care plans, automated Kardex, and acuity levels, as well as providing a mechanism for recording ongoing assessment data.

Bedside charting systems, also referred to as point-of-care (POC) systems, include handheld systems such as a personal digital assistant (PDA), notebook computers, tablet computers (Figure 11-14), and mobile computers on wheels (COWs). These technologies are evolving through the growth of secure wireless networks large enough to handle client data and images such as radiology studies sent over picture-archiving communication systems (PACS). They also improve work flow through the use of touch screens and handwriting and voice recognition software to reduce the amount of keystrokes or mouse clicks needed to input client data. In addition, automated documentation helps to reduce duplication of questions asked of the client by sending the information to all documents in which it is needed at once, provides quick responses to key questions by exception charting, builds safety by automated alerts, enables documentation in real time, sends referrals automatically based on client responses, and develops an audit trail for performance monitoring and quality review (Ligon & Das, 2004). Legibility of information is an added benefit from computer documentation systems.

Although charting by computer is an efficient method of documentation, concern about protecting client rights with regard to the security of the information has increased. Major concerns include confidentiality, access to information, and inappropriate alterations in client records. Documentation on the client's computerized record requires the individual charting to have a log-in and password for entering the computer record system. It is imperative that this password not be shared with anyone. Anything entered will be credited to the person to whom the password or signature is assigned. In addition, you should log off the computer before leaving the terminal to ensure that information about a client is not displayed on the monitor for others to view. Computer-generated printouts should also be protected so that information about clients is not indiscriminately duplicated or distributed. Most agencies using computer charting incorporate a system for logging and tracking computer printouts.

Charting procedures for computer records systems vary by agency. Data are often recorded in flow-sheet format for easy storage and retrieval. Systems can also be designed to record standard phrases such as nursing diagnoses, interventions, or outcomes classification systems. The use of free-text narratives in addition to standardized phrases, allows for specific documentation but limits the incorporation of this data into a controlled medical vocabulary for data mapping and therefore is discouraged until better mapping technologies evolve. The ANA's Nursing Information and Data Set Evaluation Center (NIDSEC) developed guidelines for nursing information systems. The standards provide a framework for evaluation of nomenclature, clinical content, storage and retrieval of data, and confidentiality and security components (ANA, 2005).

Nursing Informatics. Nursing informatics (NI) began in the early 1980s and was recognized by the ANA as a specialty in 1992. It incorporates nursing science, computer science, and information science to manage and communicate data, information, and knowledge in nursing practice (Saba & McCormick, 2005). It is concerned with providing an economical, efficient data management system that is beneficial to all users of the system to support the health of clients. To design nursing informatics systems, information specialists are concerned with the development of a common vocabulary for nursing assessment, diagnosis, outcomes, interventions and evaluations.

Nursing informatics has an important role in ensuring that nursing's data and knowledge are structured in such a way that they can be understood and used by other members of the health care team. However, because nursing utilizes information for purposes different from those of other clinical disciplines, it may require programs and information management tools that are tailored to the unique goals of clinical nursing.

Thus the practice of nursing informatics includes the following:

- The development and evaluation of applications, tools, processes, and structures that assist nurses with the management of data required to take care of clients and to support the practice of nursing
- Adapting or customizing existing informatics technology to the requirements of nurses
- Collaboration with other health care and informatics professionals to develop informatics products and standards for nursing and health care informatics

The Future. Nursing informatics does not involve just storing data; it involves storing data in a way that is clinically useful. Examples of possible clinical uses include the following:

- Nursing care planning: You enter the client's signs and symptoms, and the computer generates a list of possible nursing diagnoses, outcomes, and interventions. The accuracy of this list would of course depend on your accuracy in entering the data and on the program used to transform that data into a care plan.
- Access to knowledge: Your client is having a possible drug reaction. You enter data about the reaction. The computer already knows what medications the client is taking and is connected to a database of medication information. It generates a list of possible medications that could have caused the reaction.
- Promoting continuity of care: You access your client's chart and are alerted to pertinent information—for example, the client has received pain medication every 4 hours for the past 24 hours, has not had a bowel movement in 4 days, or is due for an IV site change.

Building a computer program to automate or even support such transformations requires an understanding of the nature and structure of the information to be processed, the transformations that will be uniquely useful in nursing, and the algorithms (decision trees) and heuristics (rules of thumb) used by expert nurses for decision making.

Current research is identifying the best way to implement these tools in the clinical environment and to make them fit naturally into the clinician's work flow. Client safety concerns are paramount in designing intuitive and robust clinical information systems. Work-flow studies are being conducted to identify areas where automation can have significant impact and to identify where poor work flow needs to be corrected before automation is begun. Nursing informaticists are adding significant findings to impact care delivery and quality of care now and into the future.

▼ KEY PRINCIPLES

- The purposes of charting are communication, quality assurance, legal accountability, reimbursement, and research.
- All documentation entries should include standard medical terminology and approved abbreviations.
- Common principles of good documentation include legibility, brevity, logical sequence, making corrections appropriately, omitting blank spaces, completeness, signing properly, and using black ink.
- All medical records are confidential.
- Content can be documented using several types of entries: admit note, change-of-shift note, assessment findings, interval notes, and discharge note.
- Special notations should be made when a client is transferred or discharged or when client teaching is conducted.
- All objective and subjective observations should be documented completely, accurately, and specifically.
- Significant data concerning psychosocial status, ADLs, valuables, spiritual care, and safety concerns should be documented as directed by agency policy.
- Older adults, children, and culturally diverse clients require specific documentation particular to their population.
- Documentation for extended-care, long-term, and home health care agencies should include life span issues, support for reimbursement, and key terms specific to the various types of agencies.

- Entries can be made using various formats for documentation.
- Flow sheets, used to document data in an abbreviated form, allow quick reference for specific data.
- Electronic records allow systematic data entry and retrieval and facilitate consistency for purposes of client safety, quality assurance, and research.

▼ REVIEW QUESTIONS

1. The nurse would use guidelines from which of the following agencies while documenting client care in the medical record?

1. State Department of Public Health (DPH)
2. Joint Commission on Accreditation of Healthcare Organizations (JCAHO)
3. American Hospital Association
4. American Nurses Association

2. The nurse would complete an incident report for which of the following situations?

1. The wife of a client is reluctant to leave the hospital when visiting hours end.
2. A client's meal tray does not contain the food items requested.
3. The laundry cart routinely has insufficient towels for the needs of the unit.
4. A client's eyeglasses could not be found after changing the bed linens.

3. The nurse forgot until 2:00 PM to write a client's response to pain medication administered at 10:00 AM. Which action should the nurse take at this time?

1. Write an incident report
2. Wait and report the data in intershift report
3. Document the finding in the record
4. Reassess the client for current pain level

4. The nurse has made an error while writing a note in the client's medical record. What should the nurse do to correct the error?

1. Draw a single line through the entry and write "void" above it.
2. Erase the entry as much as possible.
3. Blacken out the entry so it is illegible.
4. Use a paper liquid product to "white out" the entry.

5. The nurse has emptied the urinal for a male client. After noting the amount of the voiding, the nurse records the amount on which of the following most appropriate forms?

1. The progress notes
2. The vital signs sheet
3. The care plan
4. The intake and output record

Bibliography

*American Nurses Association. (2004). Nursing: *Scope and standards of practice.* Silver Spring, MD: Author.

American Nurses Association. (2005). *NIDSEC standards and scoring guidelines.* Silver Spring, MD: Author.

Baranoski, S., & Ayello, E. A. (2005). Using a wound assessment form. *Nursing, 35*(3), 14-15.

Institute of Medicine of the National Academies. (2004). Work and workspace design to prevent and mitigate errors. In A. Page (Ed.), *Keeping patients safe: Transforming the work environment of nurses* (pp. 225-284). Washington, DC: The National Academies Press.

Ligon, K., & Das, E. (2004). The benefits of automated nursing documentation. *Nurse Leader, 2*(5), 29-31.

Lunney, M., Delaney, C., & Duffy, M. (2005). Advocating for standardized nursing languages in electronic health records. *Journal of Nursing Administration, 35*(1), 1-3.

Poissant, L., Pereira, J., Tamblyn, R., & Kawasumi, Y. (2005). The impact of electronic health records on time efficiency of physicians and nurses: A systematic review. *Journal of the American Medical Informatics Association, 12*(5), 505-516.

Saba, V. K., & McCormick, K. A. (2005). *Essentials of nursing informatics* (4th ed.). New York: McGraw-Hill.

Smith, K., Smith, V., Krugman, M., & Oman, K. (2005). Evaluating the impact of computerized clinical documentation. CIN: *Computers, Informatics, Nursing, 23*(3), 132-138.

Sullivan, G. H. (2003). Incident reports are a must. *RN, 66*(11), 71-72, 74.

*Asterisk indicates a classic or definitive work on this subject.

Chapter 12

THE NURSE-CLIENT RELATIONSHIP

Media Resources

- Evolve Website http://evolve.elsevier.com/Harkreader/
- Companion CD

Learning Objectives

After studying this chapter, you should be able to do the following:

- Describe the nature of a therapeutic relationship based on the nursing theories, the communication process, and verbal and nonverbal behaviors that affect communication
- Identify nursing attitudes that promote therapeutic communication
- Describe phases of the nurse-client relationship
- Discuss effective therapeutic communication techniques
- Discuss nontherapeutic communication techniques

Key Terms

acting-out behaviors
active listening
attending behaviors
body language
communication
context
decoder (receiver)
empathy
encoder (sender)
feedback
language
message
nonverbal communication
paralanguage
personal space
sensory channel
therapeutic rapport
therapeutic relationship
unconditional positive regard
verbal communication

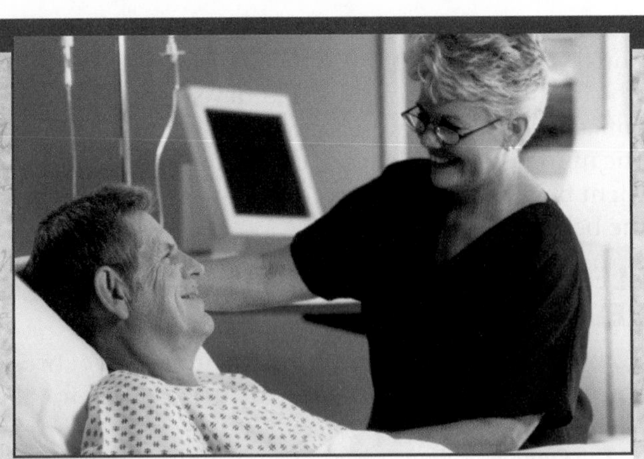

Jane Smith, RN, was dispensing bedtime medications in a busy medical-surgical unit. As Mr. Lewis took his pills, he quietly commented, "I feel pretty scared about my operation tomorrow." Ms. Smith looked at him condescendingly. "That surgery is a piece of cake," she said. "You have nothing to be afraid of." Mr. Lewis did not respond, but when Ms. Smith came to work the next day she learned that her client had had a sleepless night. "We all tried to talk to him about what was bothering him," reported the day nurse, "but he said nobody at this hospital cared enough to talk to him." What went wrong?

Had Ms. Smith been more aware of therapeutic communication techniques, she might have avoided upsetting her client. What could she have done better? What did she do that she should not have done? How might she have responded in a more sensitive and empathetic manner? The answers to these questions lie in an understanding of therapeutic communication

This chapter will orient you to beginning theories, principles, and techniques of therapeutic communication related to the nurse-client interaction. It is vital that you learn therapeutic communication techniques early in your student experience because you will be expected to use these techniques throughout your professional career. You will continue to develop competence and gain mastery of these techniques as you use them in the clinical setting. In addition, the more you practice the techniques, the more confident you will be, and the better the outcomes will be.

NATURE OF A THERAPEUTIC RELATIONSHIP

THEORIES ABOUT THE NURSE-CLIENT RELATIONSHIP

Several nursing theorists have provided us with a better understanding of the nurse, the client, and communication and of the interaction among these elements in a therapeutic relationship. Selected examples follow:

Peplau's Theory. Hildegard Peplau, a psychiatric nurse and one of the first nurse theorists, identified six roles that are assumed by the nurse in a therapeutic relationship with a client (Peplau, 1952):

- *The stranger:* This role is shared by both the nurse and the client entering the therapeutic relationship. The nurse offers the client respect, interest, and acceptance in a nonpersonal manner. The client is assumed to be emotionally intact unless conflicting evidence arises.
- *The resource:* The nurse assumes the role of a resource person, helping the consumer-client to negotiate the health care system by providing care and offering answers to specific questions.
- *The teacher:* The nurse assumes the role of teacher to help educate the client and to help the client understand and use experiences within the health care system to attain health goals.
- *The leader:* The nurse assumes the leadership role to help the client-follower contribute to and participate in a democratic nursing process.
- *The surrogate:* The nurse assumes the role of surrogate parent to help the client resolve interpersonal problems that need to be safely worked out in the presence of an understanding other and to give the client a corrective interpersonal experience.
- *The counselor:* The nurse assumes the counselor role to help integrate reality and the client's emotional responses to illness into the total life experience.

Peplau believed that nurses who related with clients in a healthy way could provide corrective interpersonal experiences for them; that is, if clients had positive relationships with nurses, they could then have healthier relationships with others. She encouraged nurses to promote trust in their relationships by relating to their clients in an authentic manner. For Peplau, relating in an authentic manner meant sharing feelings and thoughts appropriately. For example, note how Mrs. Lyons, a renal nurse, shares her feelings with Mr. Little when he learns his second kidney transplant is failing. His eyes are red and he is clenching his fists, but he is unable to verbalize his feelings.

> Mrs. Lyons *(making eye contact with Mr. Little):* "This is a hard piece of news for you."
>
> Mr. Little *(silent, but starts to cry)*
>
> Mrs. Lyons: "I feel sad too, Mr. Little. Having two transplants fail is very hard."

Peplau noted that closeness in a therapeutic relationship builds trust, increases the client's self-esteem, and leads to new personal growth for the client.

Travelbee's Theory. Joyce Travelbee pointed out that the nurse is a human being who is vulnerable to stereotypes, labels, and generalizations (Travelbee, 1966). Travelbee noted that it is not possible for a stereotype (of a nurse) to relate to another stereotype (of a client) in a human way. In the following example, Miss Lane is a nurse working with paralyzed adults. In Miss Lane's stereotyped view, paralyzed clients have enough problems and should not be overly challenged. She also believes she is overworked and underpaid and that her clients should be grateful for the care she gives. Miss Lane is assigned to work with Lisa Simmons, a 28-year-old woman recovering from a devastating car crash. Lisa is alert, bright, and highly motivated.

Miss Lane: "Good morning Lisa. Let me cut up your breakfast for you."
Lisa: "My arms are fine, it's my legs that don't work."
Miss Lane *(to herself)*: You poor thing, you need all the help you can get. You're lucky I'm your nurse today. *(to Lisa)* "No, darling, let's do it my way. I don't have all day for this."

Not only has Miss Lane not related to Lisa as another human being who is deserving of respect and consideration, but she has also given Lisa a reason to view nurses as callous, rude, and insensitive.

Travelbee noted that one nursing goal is to change the distorted beliefs others have about nurses and nursing. The client is the help-seeker whose overt and covert needs are the focus of the therapeutic relationship. She proposed that understanding the individual client's experience is paramount and that people cannot be known if their uniqueness is not appreciated. Your task, then, is to see the individual "with fresh eyes" and without labeling or stereotyping.

An important component of Travelbee's theory concerns the process of *human reduction*. This term, a synonym for dehumanization, refers to viewing the client as other than a human being. Viewing the client as an illness ("the heart attack in room 210"), a task ("the bed-bath-and-dressing-change on Team B"), or a stereotype ("all amputees") are three examples of human reduction. It is only in overcoming assigned labels that you and the client can relate on a human level and establish a therapeutic relationship.

Like Peplau, Travelbee conceptualized the communication process as a means of fostering the development of human relationships. She believed that the human-to-human relationship allows the nurse to help clients and their families cope with illness and find meaning in the experience. She believed communication to be reciprocal, dynamic, and influential. Each interaction has differences and similarities, which prohibits the forming of rigid rules of action but does permit the nurse to develop skill as a communicator.

King's Theory. Imogene King (1981) developed a nursing theory based on interacting personal, interpersonal, and social systems. Individuals involved in an interactive process mutually identify goals and the means by which to achieve them. In the nurse-client relationship, it is the nurse's responsibility to establish an interpersonal relationship, with the interaction focused on meeting the client's needs. Communication is verbal, nonverbal, situational, perceptual, transactional, and irreversible. It is viewed as the vehicle by which human relationships are developed and maintained, and it requires an atmosphere of mutual respect. The nurse uses knowledge of communication to observe client behavior and accurately interpret the meaning of the behavior (King, 1981).

ELEMENTS OF THE THERAPEUTIC RELATIONSHIP

Communication is the meaningful interaction between you and the client that leads to such growth for the client.

The Communication Process. **Communication** is a complex process in which information is exchanged between two or more individuals, called senders and receivers. It is the basic element of human interactions, and it includes both verbal and nonverbal messages. Each message consists of several components. A widely accepted model for the communication process consists of the following six elements (Figure 12-1):

- **Encoder (sender):** This person initiates a transaction to exchange information, convey thoughts and feelings, or engage another person.
- **Message:** This is the content a sender wishes to transmit to another person (the receiver) in the process of communication. The message must be encoded in a language of symbols or cues that are understandable to both sender and receiver.

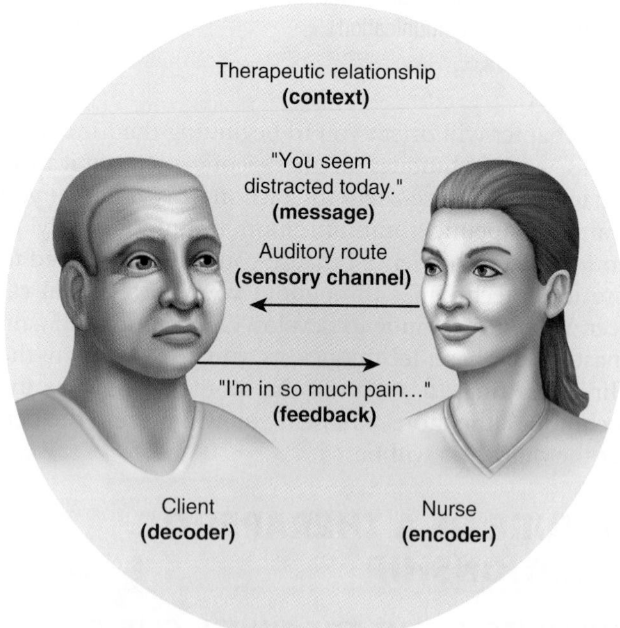

FIGURE 12-1 This diagram shows the six elements of communication within the therapeutic relationship: the encoder (sender), the message, the sensory channel, the decoder (receiver), feedback, and context.

- **Sensory channel:** This is the means by which a message is sent. The three primary channels are visual, auditory, and kinesthetic. Using these three channels, a wink, a tone of voice, and a hand gesture can all effectively convey a message without benefit of words.
- **Decoder (receiver):** This is the person to whom a message is aimed. This person must be able to decode the message sent to understand it clearly. If the message that the sender transmits is what the receiver understands, then clear and effective communication has occurred.
- **Context:** This is the condition under which a communication occurs.
- **Feedback:** This is the process by which effectiveness of communication is determined.

The feedback process is an extremely important element of communication. There are four types of feedback: internal, external, positive, and negative.

Internal feedback is a mechanism of self-perception. When you communicate, you automatically assess what you have said or done. For example, if you make a verbal blunder, you react self-consciously after realizing your mistake. If, however, you feel you have communicated clearly what you meant, you are pleased and satisfied with the effort.

External feedback is received from another or others in the form of visual, auditory, or kinesthetic information. The response to the message sent gives information about how effectively you transmitted the message.

Positive feedback affirms your efforts to communicate by rewarding and reinforcing successful communication. If your messages are met with a smile or exclamation of relief, you feel good and continue to use those communication behaviors.

Negative feedback is a response that tells you your original message was poorly transmitted or received and needs to be modified. It may also be judgmental and indicate that the receiver disagreed with your message.

It is important to note that both sender and receiver can seek feedback and clarify and qualify the message as needed. For example, consider the following interaction between Mrs. Herbert and Rick Jones, RN, after Mr. Jones completes Mrs. Herbert's diabetic teaching:

> Mrs. Herbert: "I think I understood the procedure better yesterday."
> Rick Jones, RN *(insulted by an unfavorable comparison to another nurse and seeking clarification)*: "Are you thinking that I have confused you with today's teaching?"
> Mrs. Herbert *(realizing that Mr. Jones misunderstood)*: "I wasn't saying it was your fault. I was just more with it yesterday."

Had Mr. Jones not clarified what Mrs. Herbert meant, he might have left the interaction with negative feelings about Mrs. Herbert and about his own ability to do diabetic teaching.

With this example, you can see how disruptive it could be to an interaction, and even to a relationship, if an unclear message is not clarified by seeking and receiving feedback or correction. It is unfortunate in this situation that the client had to be the one to seek feedback and to clarify, because the nurse should have done this. A more helpful question by Mr. Jones might have been, "Can you tell me more about why you feel more confused today?" This would have allowed Mrs. Herbert to clarify her statement without having to be burdened by considering the effect of her statement on Mr. Jones.

Action Alert! Clarify the understanding of a message to ensure communication is both clear and therapeutic.

TYPES OF COMMUNICATION

There are generally two types of communication: verbal and nonverbal. Each type has several components.

VERBAL COMMUNICATION

Verbal communication involves the use of words to convey messages. This type of communication is achieved by speaking or writing in a code that is mutually understood by sender and receiver. The tool of verbal communication is language. **Language** is a set of words that have meanings that are comprehensible within a group. Because a word has a definition, however, does not guarantee that its meaning will be interpreted in the same way by all group members. For example, in the English language, the word *hot* could refer to something very warm, something stolen, or something sexually attractive. It is important, therefore, to validate meaning between you and the client.

Talking. Talking is the act of verbalizing symbols to convey thoughts, feelings, or ideas. It is a skill so taken for granted that it is almost impossible to communicate without it. Clients often feel a sense of helplessness when they are intubated, do not speak the dominant language, or are rendered speechless by surgery or a neurological disorder. It is important that you use clear language, appropriate vocabulary, and speak at the client's level of understanding.

Writing. Written communication transfers a thought or spoken symbol into printed form. Being able to communicate accurately and clearly in writing is critical for you when documenting nursing care and communicating with clients who have sensory impairments. Refer to Chapter 38 for more in-depth information. You need to write as clearly as you speak.

When communicating with clients in writing, you should write at a level and in a language understood by the client, spell correctly, and print large and dark enough to be legible. You need to make sure that the client's room lighting is conducive to reading, and that the client is wearing reading glasses, if needed.

NONVERBAL COMMUNICATION

Nonverbal communication is a set of behaviors that conveys messages either without words or by supplementing verbal communication. It consists of body language, paralanguage, and any other means by which one communicates with others without the use of words. As a health care professional, you are very concerned with body language and paralanguage.

Body language refers to nonverbal communication behaviors that are accomplished by the movement of our bodies or body parts, by the presentation of ourselves to the world, and by the use of our personal space (see later). Common body language behaviors include personal appearance, conscious and unconscious changes in facial expressions, body posture and gestures, the distance maintained from others, and how we touch others. **Paralanguage** refers to nonverbal components of spoken language. These components give speech its rhythm and humanness and include stress, accent, pitch, pause, intonation, rate, volume, and quality.

> ***Action Alert!*** Astutely assess a client's nonverbal behavior. It often provides a more reliable indication of the person's true message because it is unconscious.

Body Language. Clients communicate a great deal using body language, which is important in the overall assessment of the client (Figure 12-2). A few examples of the general areas you may assess in this way follow.

Personal Appearance. A rapid assessment of the client's general appearance gives an initial impression of factors as varied as self-esteem, emotional status, and social standing. Because most persons are aware of being judged by their general appearance, they usually take steps to alter their appearance to create a more favorable impression, even in a health care setting.

You can obtain useful information about a client's condition by observing whether the client has attended to good grooming. A client's neglected personal appearance may be caused by a variety of reasons, including lack of bathing facilities, physical handicap, lack of appropriate socialization, lack of energy (resulting from severe depression, physical weakness or handicap, or disease), or lack of time. You must be careful not to make judgments about a client on the basis of personal appearance.

> ***Action Alert!*** Avoid hasty judgments about client's personal appearance. Validate initial impressions with additional client data.

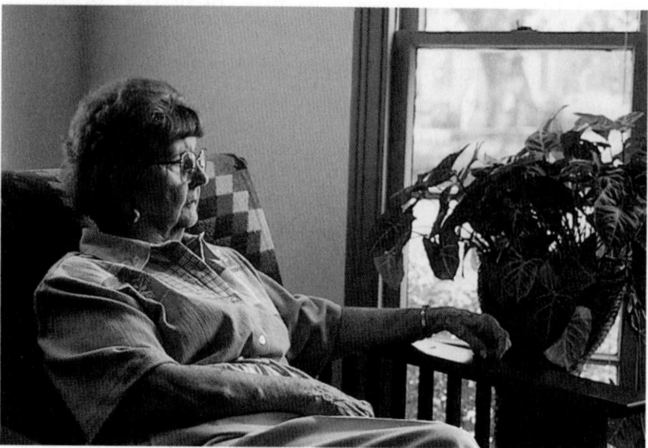

FIGURE 12-2 Body language is one important form of nonverbal communication. What might this woman's body language be saying?

Facial Expressions. Assessing a client's eyes and facial movements can also yield valuable information. Assess whether the movements are voluntary or involuntary (winks or smiles versus tics or twitches) and whether the client can focus and maintain eye contact. Observe the eyes for redness, clarity, and tearing, and the face for the raising and lowering of eyebrows or the presence of a smirk, smile, or frown.

A client can communicate pain, fear, anger, sadness, happiness, contentment, or excitement with the eyes and with facial muscular activity. Do not be too quick to assign meaning to facial expressions alone, however, because reading body language is not an exact science. For example, if you note a client's eyes are red rimmed and teary and that he has difficulty making eye contact with you, further investigation is warranted. It may be that the client is embarrassed that he has been crying, or he may be a bashful person who is suffering from a seasonal allergy. Use your observations of facial expressions as cues to alert you to instances in which further assessment might be needed.

Body Posture. As is true of facial movement, body posture and stance can also provide cues to a person's physical and emotional state. To assess body posture, note whether the person is standing straight, is slumped, or is hunched over. An erect posture usually signifies a feeling of fitness and confidence. Slumping often occurs in persons who are physically exhausted, weak or emotionally depressed. Hunching can signal a desire to be left alone. A client who is hunching with forearms crossed over the abdomen may be guarding a painful abdomen. A more severely hunched posture, with head down, forearms brought up across the chest, and knees brought up to guard the abdomen (a fetal position), may indicate extreme fear or depression.

Gestures. Observe the types of gestures used by clients. Some clients talk with their hands by gesturing while they speak. Emphatic gestures often convey messages of urgency accompanied by distress, great happiness, or excitement. They may represent the conversion of pent-up emotional energy into physical energy that can be released when a client has strong needs to be heard (and perhaps assisted), or they may be used as a means of coping when the person is unable to adequately convey urgent messages verbally. It is also important to understand what gestures mean within different cultures to avoid misunderstanding when communicating with clients from diverse backgrounds.

Personal Distance. We all have a **personal space,** a private zone or "bubble," around our body that we believe is an extension of ourselves and belongs to us. We carry this personal space around with us at all times. A select number of people are allowed to enter this space, at various distances and at certain times. We tend to be uncomfortable if others enter our personal space and behave in ways to prevent this from happening.

People within each culture respect others' personal spaces and use culturally determined body language signals to help maintain appropriate distances from each other. The size of this space appears to be culturally determined, at least in part, and it can vary considerably from culture to culture. In Western culture, the four zones of interpersonal space are as follows (Munoz & Luckmann, 2005):

- *Intimate space:* From contact to 18 inches. When you bathe clients or take their vital signs, you occupy this space, which is normally reserved for people in close relationships.
- *Personal space:* From 18 inches to 3 feet. When you talk with clients about their illnesses or when you are teaching clients, you generally occupy this space. It is the usual space of interaction with friends.
- *Social space:* From 3 to 6 feet. This is the space of normal business. When you make nursing rounds with a nursing supervisor, you normally occupy this space.
- *Public space:* Greater than 6 feet. When your professors are lecturing, they use this space. The communication is formal.

Touching. Nurse-client touching is an issue that requires great sensitivity. Assess the client's feelings about touch before using it. A rule of thumb is to ask permission before touching. Because nursing is a hands-on profession, it is daily practice to touch clients often and intimately. It is easy to ask, "May I touch your arm?" Asking can help avoid possible problems. Most clients feel neutral about a casual touch such as a pat on the arm during the course of normal conversation. Many clients are hungry for a handclasp or other form of human touch and will demonstrate this by reaching out to you (Figure 12-3).

You need to be constantly aware that touch conveys many meanings to clients. It may indicate agreement, caring, loving, or even sexual desire. However, clients who have been physically or sexually abused tend to see uninvited touch as a boundary violation. It is accepted more or less readily in different situations and cultures. For example, a hug may be greeted with relief by a family member in a hospice when support is needed most, but it would probably be perceived as a violation of personal space in an initial meeting with a client in a clinic. Touching can soothe or disturb people to their very depths. Therefore, it must be used judiciously, on the basis of an assessment of the client's needs and wishes.

Paralanguage. A more comprehensive understanding of communication occurs when you understand not only the verbal, but the nonverbal components of speech, or paralanguage. It helps you understand the content of the client's message and become attuned to the emotional component of the message—the client's mood.

Stress. Stress refers to the part of a word, phrase, or sentence that is highlighted by changing pitch or elongating the syllable. Words that are stressed are generally the more important words. For example, the following statements have slightly different meanings because of the way stress is used:

"Nice to meet you." (with no particular stress)
"*Nice* to meet you."
"Nice to *meet* you."
"Nice to meet *you.*"

Accent. Accent refers to the different pronunciation of syllables used by nonnative speakers of a language. Accent alone can cause a loss of clarity that can result in a breakdown in communication. Do not pretend that you understand what someone has said when you do not. Seek to clarify what has been said by asking the person to repeat what was said, to use different words, or to write out the troublesome phrase.

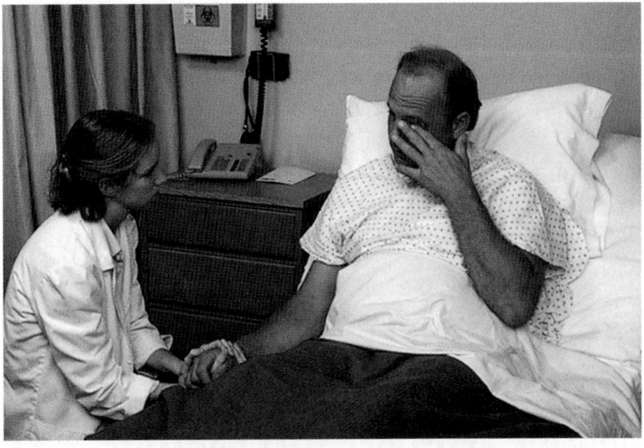

FIGURE 12-3 Many clients are hungry for a handclasp or another form of human touch. By touching the client when appropriate, you can convey warmth and empathy. However, if the client feels touch is inappropriate, draw back and respect the person's feelings. Otherwise, you risk undermining your attempt to communicate.

Pitch. Pitch refers to whether the voice is high or low. Pitch results from the speed of vocal cord vibrations. Pitch is related to gender in that most men's voices are pitched lower than most women's voices. It is also related to age in that children's voices are usually pitched higher than adults' voices. In any individual, changes in pitch can alter the meaning of the content of a message. For example, pitch rises at the end of a question (interrogative sentence) and stays the same or becomes lower in making a statement (declarative sentence). Thus, the meaning of the interrogative "You have tuberculosis?" is very different from the meaning of the declarative "You have tuberculosis."

Pause. Pauses punctuate speech with periods of silence or nonword sounds, such as "Let me see . . ." or "Hmm, I believe you are right." A pause indicates that the person is still considering something, is considering whether to share something, or is searching for the words to encode properly what is to be told. Pauses are used for effect as part of varying intonation. The pause should be respected and the person given adequate time to complete the communication interrupted by a pause.

Intonation. Intonation is the variety of stress and pause patterns within a phrase or sentence. For example, people often use one intonation when giving a formal speech and other intonations when communicating with a superior at work or with a close friend.

Rate. The *rate* of speech refers to how many syllables are spoken per unit of time. Rate also takes into account the number of pauses made. Increased rate of speech may indicate nervousness or agitation. It is sometimes possible to control anxiety by focusing on a rapid speech rate and slowing it.

Volume. Volume comprises the loudness and intensity associated with the speaking voice. Intensity is a measure of forcefulness and can convey a message about the speaker's emotions. Generally, a loud voice indicates anger or frustration, and the speaker uses it as if loudness could somehow increase the power of the words to control the listener or others. Changes in volume (either up or down) may also occur in anxiety.

Quality. Voice *quality* is a measure of clarity, hoarseness, or nasality in the speaker's voice. Physical and emotional conditions can cause a change in voice quality. For example, the voice often becomes husky with deeply felt emotions, harsher with anger, and more nasal with a cold.

FACILITATING EFFECTIVE THERAPEUTIC COMMUNICATION

NURSING ATTITUDES THAT PROMOTE THERAPEUTIC COMMUNICATION

Therapeutic communication is enhanced when you adopt helpful attitudes to indicate interest in and regard for the client. These nursing attitudes are sometimes referred to as *responsive attitudes.*

Awareness. In showing awareness, you acknowledge the presence of the client. **Attending behaviors** show that you are paying attention and listening to what the client is saying. Examples of attending behaviors that can be used to facilitate communication include facing the client, leaning toward the client, using appropriate eye contact, keeping your eyes open with eyebrows raised, and maintaining an *open body posture,* a body position in which the arms and legs are uncrossed.

Acceptance, Respect, and Unconditional Positive Regard. Acceptance is openness to the unique qualities and attributes of individual clients. It means accepting clients for who they are, even if their behavior is undesirable. It does not mean condoning inappropriate client behaviors.

Respect is more than an attitude of acceptance. It also includes valuing, highly regarding, or esteeming clients for who they are. **Unconditional positive regard,** a term coined by the psychologist Carl Rogers (1951), describes respect for the client that does not depend on the client's behavior. You learn to value and care for clients simply because their humanity warrants your care.

You avoid being critical, derogatory, or judgmental. You understand that the client's imperfections are part of the total picture; the imperfections may be undesirable behaviors, but they are coping mechanisms the client needs at the time. Many clients struggle with the dehumanizing aspects of illness and dependency. You empower clients by showing respect and by appreciating their humanness without ridiculing or demeaning them.

Another reason to avoid judging clients is that they should not view you as a judge. When this type of relationship occurs, clients may seek to please you, which diverts attention from the goal of focusing on the clients' needs.

Empathy. **Empathy** is the accurate perception of the client's feelings. It is the ability to "be in the other person's shoes" without taking on the client's feelings or thoughts. Empathy is not sympathy, wherein you feel pity or compassion for the client. Rather, it is a sense of understanding or "being with" the client. During your nursing career, you will experience both empathy with and sympathy for clients, but empathy will help you build important bridges in communicating with clients.

Relatedness. Relatedness is the recognition of similarities between you and the client and the forging of emotional connections based on those similarities. Relating to clients helps to establish human-to-human ties that make communication possible. Common experiences enable you and the client to be more readily known to each other.

Caring. Caring is taking an emotional risk to feel a personal interest in the client's welfare. By investing yourself in the client, you consciously decide to take emotional risks and give of your skills, compassion, and experience. Such concern can be draining, and you must continually assess personal psychic energy and emotional resources to prevent exhaustion and burnout.

Objectivity. Objectivity is an unbiased, reality-based stance that allows you to assess the facts of a client's situation without being emotionally pulled into the client's difficulties. You can be objective and still have caring feelings for the client and attend to the client's thoughts and feelings. Thinking about the client objectively allows you to understand client experiences and to identify areas of difficulty in order to guide the client toward developing appropriate problem-solving skills.

Protectiveness. Protectiveness leads you to shield the fragile and vulnerable client during the person's recovery from illness. There is a fine line between protectiveness and fostering dependence. Protectiveness is a caring attitude that should be used judiciously while you continue to evaluate the client's capacity to defend the self.

Genuineness. Genuineness is your ability to be honest, open, and sincere in self-presentation. The phrase "what you see is what you get" describes the demeanor of a genuine person. It is important not to confuse being genuine with being totally self-disclosing or casually spontaneous, as one would be with friends or family. For example, you may share a family's joy on the birth of a baby and demonstrate it with warm congratulations for the parents and admiration for the baby. For a client with a new baby, a warm, encouraging smile might be sufficient.

Openness. Being open with a client reflects your ability and willingness to be real, genuine, and emotionally accessible. Openness does not mean that boundaries are violated. It means that you choose what to share with the client and share it in an authentic manner. When you are open with a client, the client tends to lower defenses and to relate more honestly to you.

Professional Closeness or Distance. The nurse-client relationship is characterized by professional boundaries. In this relationship, there is a delicate balance between maintaining objectivity and professional distance, and the warmth, openness, and availability associated with professional closeness. You should be accessible to the client while maintaining awareness that the therapeutic relationship is not a friendship or other social relationship. At the same time, be careful not to be impersonal and not to treat clients with indifference.

Professional closeness and stance vary throughout the relationship as you and the client come together as strangers, work on mutual goals, and proceed to termination. New nurses may feel uncomfortable with attempts at maintaining professional closeness and stance. A good rule to follow is to become invested without being engulfed. This means that you care about clients and allow yourself to know their concerns, but it does not mean taking their thoughts, feelings, or attitudes as your own.

Sense of Humor. An appreciation of the humorous side of life can be a desirable attitude in nurses. You must be able to laugh at yourself and at humorous situations that can arise. Being a role model of this openness and demonstrating the appropriate use of humor can be therapeutic for clients just as it is for you.

The ability to use humor therapeutically is a talent that not all nurses possess. When you are comfortable with the sensitive use of humor, you can sometimes use it to put clients at ease, defuse emotionally loaded situations, or simply inject a light note into an otherwise difficult day. You must assess each client's readiness for humor. If the client is likely to perceive any levity as a put-down, it is much better to maintain a more serious demeanor. Although clients can appreciate wit as much as anyone, they must first feel that you are trustworthy, dependable, and invested in their well-being. Certain types of humor must be avoided, such as morbid humor, humor based on sarcasm, or humor that degrades anyone. These are inappropriate and unprofessional.

RESPECTING DIFFERENCES

You must develop effective communication skills to enhance your work with clients of different groups, of different cultures, and at different stages of health.

Developmental Differences. Communication techniques must be appropriate for the client's stage of development; otherwise, communication can be diminished. Examples of how to apply therapeutic techniques to children, adolescents, and adults of all ages have been provided in the tables appearing later in this chapter. Refer to Chapters 16-18 for a more in-depth understanding of developmental differences among age-groups.

Cultural Differences. Whether or not clients from different cultures speak your language, they often have different customs, values, mores, and social structures, such as who is the decision maker for the family, all of which can affect communication. Clearly, the more you understand about your client's culture, the better you will be able to communicate. It is helpful to learn crucial words and sentences in the client's language or to have a translator write out cards with commonly used bilingual sentences. Understanding the nonnative client requires more than just learning a few new phrases. You must be aware of any personal biases to avoid stereotyping and labeling these clients. Respect for the client's experience and acceptance of the differences that exist between you can help establish a safe, therapeutic environment in which maximal communication can occur.

Gender Differences. Men and women communicate differently, and understanding these differences enhances therapeutic relationships. A number of experts have studied differences in communication styles between men and women. Torppa (2002) reported that studies indicate that women, to a greater extent than men, are sensitive to the interpersonal meanings that lie "between the lines" in the messages, and men are more sensitive to "between the lines meanings" about status. These differences in emphasis on interpersonal versus status implications of messages typically lead women to expect relationships to be based on interdependence (mutual dependence) and cooperation and for men to expect relationships to be based on independence and competition.

THE THERAPEUTIC RELATIONSHIP

A **therapeutic relationship** is a helping relationship. Nurses are helpers, clients are those seeking help, and both are active participants. It is personal, focused on the client, and aimed at realizing mutually determined goals that are to be met within a desired timeframe that has been established by both participants.

Three elements are present in all phases of the therapeutic relationship: you, the client, and the communication between the two of you. You are a helper educated in skills that facilitate client growth, whereas the client is seeking help with personal growth in the areas of health promotion or adaptation to or recovery from illness. Clients bring their own life experiences, intelligence, achievements, values, beliefs, feelings, and motivations for change to the relationship. You bring experience, understanding, and skills. You work with clients to promote their health and solve their health care problems. You and your client can be viewed as unique systems that intersect on a common ground: the therapeutic nurse-client relationship.

People often help each other in social relationships, but it is more reciprocal, with both persons sharing personal beliefs, feelings, and opinions with each other. Social relationships involve an infinite range of nonspecific helping activities, such as walking the neighbor's dog or helping a person who is using a walker to cross the street safely. The interaction involved in helping may give the helper more satisfaction than the person being helped. In contrast, the help provided in the therapeutic relationship is the main reason for the relationship; it is focused on the client and has a specific purpose. You share your feelings with the client only when such sharing is appropriate for the benefit of the client.

PHASES OF THE THERAPEUTIC RELATIONSHIP

At any time in the relationship, you may begin to feel a bond with your client. **Therapeutic rapport** is a special bond that exists between a nurse and a client who have established a sense of trust and a mutual understanding of what will occur in their relationship. Therapeutic relationships develop and evolve over time, which may be brief, extend over weeks, months, or even years. Regardless of the length of time, there are three distinct phases to the relationship: the orientation phase, the working phase, and the termination phase. Because relationships are fluid, the phases flow into each other; nevertheless, each phase may be recognized by the tasks associated with it.

Orientation Phase. During the orientation phase of the therapeutic relationship, you and the client are introduced and make a verbal agreement regarding mutual roles and responsibilities to solve one or more of the client's problems. This forms the basis for the work you will accomplish together. A primary goal of the orientation phase is the establishment of trust (Figure 12-4). It is helpful to be aware of your personal feelings, such as feeling anxious, uncomfortable, or inadequate.

Trust is enhanced when you connect with the client in a respectful and nonintrusive manner that conveys personal consideration and concern. The client may feel unsure about you and may need to know that you are willing and able to help. Honesty and enthusiasm help to establish trust. You can convey these two traits in such responses such as "I don't know the answer right now, but I will find out and let you know in an hour," or "I cannot promise I can help solve your problem, but I can listen."

> ***Action Alert!*** Do not pretend to know an answer to a client's question if you do not. Your deception will erode the client's trust. Your candor is necessary to promote client confidence.

Trust is also promoted when you establish confidentiality as a ground rule for the relationship. Confidentiality is an ethical obligation to share a client's health care information only with those who have a professional need to know it. It is unrealistic to promise a client absolute confidentiality about the communications between you. You may safely promise your clients that you will respect their privacy and will share information only when there is a medical need to do so. It is important to tell your clients that you cannot maintain confidentiality if doing so would endanger their health and well-being or that of others.

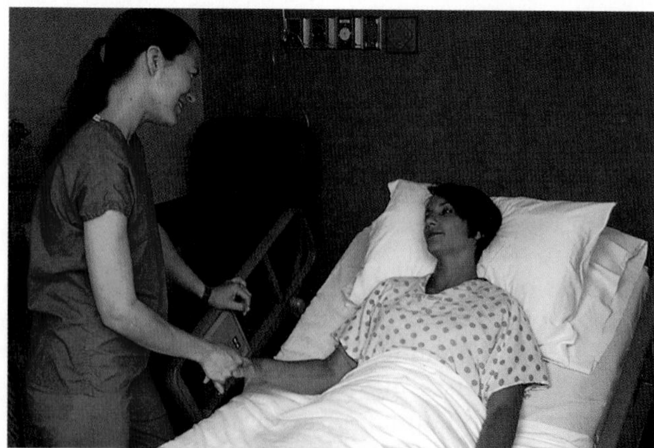

FIGURE 12-4 Establishing trust with the client is a key goal of the orientation phase of a therapeutic relationship. You can do this by conveying respect, personal consideration, and concern for the client's needs.

Unrealistic promises could create an ethical dilemma for you if the client confides something that must be revealed to others for the client's protection or for the protection of others. Consider the following example. A client confides in you that he has active tuberculosis and works with clients with acquired immunodeficiency syndrome (AIDS). He is afraid he will lose his job if his boss finds out. If you do not report this information to your supervisor, you risk the possibility of an infectious disease catastrophe. If you reveal it, you have broken your word and violated the client's trust. Maintaining appropriate levels of confidentiality should make clients feel that you will protect them and will not allow them to hurt themselves or others. If clients feel safe, they will feel a sense of trust, and the therapeutic relationship will be reinforced.

Besides establishing trust, you should establish other ground rules for the relationship. If you will be meeting with a client frequently, be sure to specify clearly where, when, and for how long each meeting will be. For example, a primary nurse might say, "I will be teaching you how to care for your Hickman catheter so you will know how to care for it when you are discharged. We will meet here for an hour tomorrow at 10:00 AM so that I can assess your current knowledge. After tomorrow, we will work together 30 minutes a day for 5 days while you are hospitalized until you can comfortably and safely take care of your catheter." As you establish meeting times and places, honesty and achievability are paramount. Do not promise what you may not be able to do. For example, if you can only meet the client for 15 minutes each day, do not promise 30-minute sessions.

Working Phase. Once trust has been established and the relationship has been structured, the working phase (middle phase) of the therapeutic relationship begins. This is a time for completing nursing interventions that address expected nursing outcomes. You work with the client to meet the client's physical and psychosocial needs and achieve mutually acceptable goals.

You respond to clients mainly by presenting information and by validating and clarifying their understandings. Rather than directing clients, you attempt to help them become self-directed. It is a time when clients can formulate and test solutions to their problems.

You perform additional client assessment and analyze the resulting data, and initial nursing diagnoses are corrected, or additional nursing diagnoses are formulated. The client's feelings, values, beliefs, and attitudes are sought out and examined. Evaluation also occurs in this phase of the relationship and, when necessary, the care plan is revised.

> ***Action Alert!*** Focus on assessing the client's feelings, thoughts, and values, and center on achieving the client's goals.

Termination Phase. The termination phase of the therapeutic relationship occurs near the end of the relationship, when the work of the client and nurse is coming to a close. The termination itself should not be abrupt or unexpected and should be acknowledged from the beginning of the relationship by both you and the client.

Recall the example given earlier, in the discussion of the orientation phase of the therapeutic relationship. The primary nurse clearly stated she would work with the client on catheter care for a certain amount of time each day for a specified number of days. The client should not have interpreted the nurse's offer to meet as extending beyond the hospital stay. The nurse was saying, in effect, "I will be meeting with you only until you are discharged." Clear communication helps to clarify expectations from the start of the relationship.

Even when the termination is thoughtfully planned, it may still be difficult to end a meaningful interaction. You and the client are aware that this phase precedes a permanent separation, and you both may feel anxiety, sadness, and a sense of loss.

How the client reacts to the termination depends on the meaning assigned to it, the length of the relationship, and the extent to which outcomes were achieved. Many relationships terminate with mutual satisfaction; however, some clients may display denial and regret and may engage in acting-out behaviors.

Acting-out behaviors are inappropriate or unexpected client behaviors that communicate the client's true or subconscious feelings and concerns. A client who is acting out during termination may refuse to talk when meeting with you, fail to keep appointments, and become more forgetful. You can help clients by acknowledging their feelings, offering support, emphasizing positive changes that have occurred during the relationship, and expressing optimism for the future while being clear about terminating the relationship. Although this process can be uncomfortable for you, it provides clients with clear boundaries and expectations.

TECHNIQUES THAT ENHANCE THERAPEUTIC COMMUNICATION

To maximize therapeutic communication it is important to use techniques that encourage clients to open up and speak more freely. A number of techniques of therapeutic communication that are generally considered helpful to use are listed in Table 12-1. Like any other tools, if they are used inappropriately, they can impede communication instead of enhancing it. It is helpful to know what to do and what not to do when using them. Here are some guidelines:

- Individualize each technique to the client's level of understanding. For example, you might tell a 40-year-old man, "I will demonstrate the correct technique for injecting your insulin," but to a 6-year-old girl you might say, "I will show you how to give your doll a shot."

- Vary the communication technique. Avoid using a single technique repeatedly. For example, saying "Tell me more" shows interest in what the client is saying and is therapeutic. But if you say "Tell me more" after everything the client says, it demonstrates that you are not giving a thoughtful response to each of the client's answers. Too many repetitions of the same response can be counterproductive.
- Use paralanguage appropriately to convey your intended meaning. For example, you may say something generally considered to be therapeutic, such as "I see," and say it sarcastically, icily, or in some other tone that is nontherapeutic. Another nurse may say something generally considered to be nontherapeutic but say it so warmly and with such caring that it is actually therapeutic for the client. Two nurses may say the same words, and one will be seen as helpful and the other as condescending. In such cases, paralanguage may make the difference.
- If you are using therapeutic techniques correctly, your client will be doing most of the talking as you listen and guide the interaction. If you find you are doing most of the talking, something is wrong, and you need to pause and reflect about how to get back on track.
- You will probably make mistakes in talking with clients, and you will say some things that are not the best possible responses. There may be times that you will be angry with yourself because you said something nontherapeutic. If you have a genuinely therapeutic relationship with the client, the relationship will survive.
- As you enter the clinical area to talk with a client for the first time, relax and realize that most clients want to talk with you.
- Any specific techniques of communication might be used at any time, according to the client and the situation, but some techniques tend to be more helpful at the beginning of an interaction, and some tend to be more helpful in the middle or at the end of an interaction.

BEGINNING THE INTERACTION

Offering Self. Offering self is a technique in which you offer to stay with the client and either talk or just sit quietly. In offering self, you need to clearly establish parameters for the amount of time offered. For example, "I have 30 minutes available to talk with you at 10 o'clock today" or "I will stay with you while you wait for your family." Additional examples are found in Table 12-1.

In some cases, it is therapeutic to give the client a choice about your offer. Say, for example, "Would you

Table 12-1 Therapeutic Communication Techniques

TECHNIQUE	DESCRIPTION/DEFINITION	EXAMPLE
Offering self	The nurse offers to stay with the client and either talk or just sit quietly.	*Nurse with child:* "Let's sit in the playroom together and play for 10 minutes." *Nurse with adolescent:* "Let's have juice or soda together." *Nurse with adult:* "I'll be back in 15 minutes to sit with you."
Providing broad openings	The nurse invites the client to select a topic.	*Nurse with child:* "What will we talk about today?" *Nurse with adolescent:* "Tell me what I can teach you about your dialysis." *Nurse with adult:* "What shall we cover next?"
Providing silence	The nurse allows the verbal conversation to stop to provide a time for quiet contemplation of what has been discussed, for formulation of thoughts about how to proceed, or to reduce tension.	(Silence)
Focusing	The nurse selects one topic for exploration from among several possible topics presented by the client.	*Nurse with child:* "Tell me your favorite food for breakfast before you tell me about lunch." *Nurse with adolescent:* "You mentioned several things you like about school. What do you like best?" *Nurse with adult:* "You mentioned several advantages to your hip surgery. What is the single greatest improvement you have noticed?"
Asking for clarification	The nurse lets the client know that what was said was unclear. If necessary, the nurse asks for clarification or suggests ways to make the message clearer.	*Nurse with child:* "I did not understand what you said. Would you say it again for me?" *Nurse with adolescent:* "Maybe you would explain more about what you mean so I can be more helpful." *Nurse with adult:* "Let me tell you what I heard you say to me."

Table 12-1 Therapeutic Communication Techniques—cont'd

TECHNIQUE	DESCRIPTION/DEFINITION	EXAMPLE
Reflecting	The client asks a question, and the nurse turns the question around and reflects it back to the client, or the client makes a statement, and the nurse selects one or more words to reflect back to the client for consideration. This technique strengthens the client's confidence.	*Nurse with child:* Child: "Should I wear blue or green?" *Nurse:* "Which would you like to wear?" *Nurse with adolescent:* Adolescent: "My mom won't let me pierce my tongue." Nurse: "What would it be like to have a pierced tongue?" *Nurse with adult:* Nurse: "What should I tell the doctor?" Nurse: "What would you like to tell the doctor?"
Placing events in time or sequence	The nurse asks the client to explain more about when an event occurred (placing the event in time) or to explain the sequence of events (placing events in the order in which they occurred) to clarify for the nurse.	*Nurse with child:* "Did you get sick before or after you ate?" *Nurse with adolescent:* "Tell me the steps you followed in changing your dressing." *Nurse with adult:* "Did your blood sugar go up after breakfast today or yesterday?"
Restating	The nurse paraphrases what the client has said. This paraphrased message may be fed back to the client in the form of a statement or a question to provide the client the opportunity to agree or disagree and clarify further.	*Nurse with child:* Child: "I want my blankie." Nurse: "You would like your blankie." *Nurse with adolescent:* Adolescent: "I just puked." Nurse: "You were sick to your stomach." *Nurse with adult:* Adult: "It's no use." Nurse: "You are pretty discouraged."
Seeking consensual validation	The nurse attempts to verify with the client that a certain term means the same thing to both parties.	*Nurse with child:* "You want Baby Lisa? Is she your doll?" *Nurse with adolescent:* "When you say you were high, did you mean you had just taken some drugs?" *Nurse with adult:* "Tell me if I understand your meaning correctly."
Encouraging descriptions of perceptions	The nurse asks the client to describe perceptions and associated emotions. This is particularly useful in understanding a client's experiences during hallucinations.	*Nurse with child:* "Tell me what you saw when I turned off the light." *Nurse with adolescent:* "How do you think the other kids feel about you?" *Nurse with adult:* "Describe what it is like when you hear the messages from God."
Presenting reality	When a client has had an unrealistic perception of reality, the nurse accepts the fact that the client has misperceived something but indicates that the nurse did not have a similar perception. When something in the environment is stimulating the misperception, the nurse attempts to point this out.	*Nurse with child:* "I think that shadow on the wall might look like a monster to you." *Nurse with adolescent:* "The other kids tell me they worry that you don't seem to like them." *Nurse with adult:* "I have heard that God usually speaks to our hearts instead of our ears."
Summarizing	The nurse briefly states, in an orderly manner, what has been discussed. The purpose is to help ensure that client and nurse are in agreement about what went on, what decisions were made to help ensure that nothing was omitted, and to bring the relationship to a close.	*Nurse with child:* "Tomorrow we will do your bath before breakfast and cartoons." *Nurse with adolescent:* "Let me review the steps for coughing and deep-breathing exercises." *Nurse with adult:* "You have told me all the appropriate things to do to take care of that wound. I think you are ready to do it by yourself from now on."

like to meet with me for 20 minutes at 1 o'clock today?" However, some clients, such as those who are depressed, need to have you with them but will tend to reject your offer. Others should not be asked to make decisions about anything, because it raises their anxiety level. As you learn more about your clients and their individual needs, you will learn who can be asked and who should be told that you are there for them. Until you do know, or if you are ever in doubt, it is always safe to offer self without allowing a choice.

Offering self can be very helpful when you are talking with those clients who seem unable to express their thoughts or who do not want to talk at the moment. You can say something like, "It is okay if you don't feel like talking right now. I'll just stay here with you for 20 minutes." If you make this time commitment, be sure to honor it for as long as you indicated. This helps establish that you are someone who can be trusted.

Providing Broad Openings. Early in a meeting with a client, it may be useful to provide a broad opening. You invite the client to select a topic for discussion. Here, too, it is therapeutic to set some parameters concerning what you are willing to discuss. For example, in most instances, it would not be helpful for the client to discuss your personal information or for you to engage in social-level small talk with the client. It is not always appropriate to say, "We can talk about anything you like." It is better to say, "We can discuss the issues that are bothering you." The latter is a very broad, client-focused opening.

Making Observations. In making observations, you acknowledge that something or someone exists or has changed in some way. Make observations without appearing to judge either positively or negatively. For example, you may observe that your client is distracted and pacing nervously. Sharing your observation by commenting "You seem distracted and nervous" may provide the opportunity for the client to discuss what has led to this behavior.

Suggesting Collaboration. Suggesting collaboration is a technique in which you offer to work together with the client. This technique is useful at the beginning of a relationship because it establishes that you and the client will work together as a team. Initially, the work may involve discussing some of the issues of concern to the client. Later, as problems are identified and nursing diagnoses are made, the work may shift to establishing and meeting client outcomes. At all times, the work focuses on the client.

Action Alert! Begin any therapeutic interaction with clarity, and focus on the client.

CONTINUING THE INTERACTION

Providing Silence. Providing silence in a therapeutic manner allows the verbal conversation to stop and provides a time for quiet contemplation of what has been discussed or for formulating thoughts about how to proceed. The silence can also provide an opportunity for reducing tension when the interaction has been concerned with powerful issues and when emotions have been particularly deep.

Many people (nurses as well as clients) are uncomfortable with silence and will talk continuously about nothing in particular just to avoid it. This is clearly not a therapeutic approach to take. If you find that you are uncomfortable with silence, think about what has been going on during the silence, and use it constructively to think about what you will say next. You will find that, with practice, you can become more and more comfortable with silence.

Accepting Messages. Accepting messages is a way of providing feedback to acknowledge to the client that you have heard and understood what the client said. The acknowledgment is done in a manner that is neutral in tone, without agreeing, disagreeing, or providing any judgments about the message. The accepting may be done verbally or nonverbally. Your method of accepting messages should be brief and should allow the client to continue on with a train of thought without any real interruption.

Providing General Leads. In ordinary social communications, people take turns communicating. After your clients have spoken for a while, they may hesitate because they are uncertain about whether it is appropriate to continue or whether they should try to draw you into the conversation. It is your task to keep clients focused on their own issues and to ensure that they continue to feel comfortable discussing them. To do this, you may use the technique of providing general leads. General leads are brief interjections ("Yes, I see" or "And then what happened?") that let clients know that they are on the right track and should continue. The leads provided should not cause real interruptions in the train of thought as they urge clients forward.

Exploring. As clients talk, they may mention something that you believe is significant enough to warrant further attention. If they have introduced the subject and have not indicated that further discussion is undesirable, it is appropriate to attempt to delve into the matter in greater detail. To do this, you use the technique of *exploring*. To explore, ask the client to describe something in more detail or to discuss it more fully. However, be careful not to use the nontherapeutic technique of *probing*. If your client gives an indication that further discussion is off limits, honor this, and use another technique, such as providing a general lead to get the client to continue with what he was saying. For example, if your client says, "I won't discuss what that doctor told me," it is counterproductive and disrespectful to ask further questions about that subject.

Focusing. When clients are talking with you, they may bring up many different topics or concerns at once. These may all be worth exploring further, but you cannot explore them simultaneously. When this happens, it is best to select one subject to explore further while keeping others in mind for future discussion. Selecting one subject for exploration from among several is termed *focusing*.

For example, an adult client may say, "Things really fell apart after my second heart attack. I knew if I didn't control my diabetes that I would wind up near dead. You know, diabetics can lose their kidneys if they are not careful. I have two uncles who went bad from too much sugar. I think I'm a goner." How do you decide which point to explore? You may choose to focus on how the client feels about being diabetic, about the possible effects of diabetes, about having had two heart attacks, or about mortality.

If you focus on one point, you can always return to other issues later on. You might prepare the client for this by making an observation, focusing, and then requesting further exploration in the future. For example, you might say, "You have given me a great deal to think about, and much of it seems worth talking about *(making an observation)*. For now, I would like to know more about your most recent heart attack *(focusing)*, and later on, perhaps we can discuss your other concerns *(requesting further exploration in the future)*."

Action Alert! Keep your interaction client centered, and clarify without speaking for the client.

Active Listening. Listening is the process in which spoken and other auditory information is received. It is an integral part of therapeutic communication. **Active listening** is participation in a conversation with a client in which you attend to what the client says and have a part in helping the client communicate thoughts, feelings, and beliefs and clarify, elaborate, and give additional pertinent information. You take an active part in listening by eliciting details from the client and by inviting the client to think more about what is being said. You build trust with the client and show respect.

Active listening is a means of "being with" the client and indicating acceptance and agreement, using verbal and nonverbal cues. It is an art and the key to therapeutic interaction. To use active listening, you must understand and be able to use all of the other therapeutic techniques of communication. Compare the following examples:

Passive listening:
Client: "I just learned I have cancer."
Nurse: "I see."
Client: "I'm afraid I will die."
Nurse: "Hmm."
Active listening:
Client: "I just learned I have cancer."
Nurse *(with concern in voice and turning to face client)*: "I wonder how you're feeling about this."
Client: "I'm afraid I will die."
Nurse: "Dying feels like a real possibility to you."
Client: "My mother died of cancer when I was 8, and I have an 8-year-old."
Nurse: "This really hits close to you."

Note how active listening brought out information not available to the passive listener. This is the basis for therapeutic interaction.

Action Alert! Actively listening to what the client says and responding to it in a considered way demonstrates that you care and have concern for the client and the client's message.

Keeping Communication Clear

Asking for Clarification. Sometimes clients say things that are unclear, that have more than one specific meaning, or that are simply vague. These garbled messages can impede communication. When this occurs, you can use several techniques to help clarify the message for both you and the client. The most straightforward technique is asking for clarification. Simply let the client know that you are not certain about what was said and, if necessary, request that the client clarify anything that is obscure. If you are unsure of the meaning, you could say, "I'm not sure I follow what you mean." If the client does not understand what was unclear, you may have to tell the client how it could be clarified for you.

Restating. Another way to clarify is to use the therapeutic technique of *restating*, or paraphrasing, what the client has said. To do this, you alter the client's words to express your understanding of the client's meaning. You send this back to the client in the form of a statement or question, and you provide the client the opportunity to agree or disagree that this was the intended message and, if necessary, to clarify further.

Seeking Consensual Validation. Sometimes, when a certain term used by a client has been unclear, you can use the technique of seeking consensual validation to help ensure that both you and the client agree on the meaning of the term. For example, at the end of a lesson about insulin injection, a client might say, "I'm through."

You may interpret this in one of three ways:

- The client has learned the information well enough to self-inject insulin.
- The client is feeling tired after intense teaching.
- The client is feeling discouraged and needs extra support.

Focus on one of these three, and seek to verify whether or not that is what the client meant. You might ask, "When you say you are through, I understand that you are tired. Is that correct?" This gives the client the opportunity to agree or disagree and clarify further.

Placing Events in Time or Sequence. Often in describing an event or a series of events, clients fail to relate the story in strict chronological order. This can make the client's message about the occurrence difficult to follow. When this happens, you can ask the client to explain more about when the event occurred (placing the event in time) or to explain the sequence of a series of events (placing events in sequence).

Helping the Client Increase Self-Awareness

Verbalizing the Implied. With the technique of *verbalizing the implied*, you understand the words the client has said but believe the words have an underlying meaning that was hinted at but not voiced specifically. You may need to verbalize this underlying message. The client may then verify that the message you received was indeed true. This frees the client to discuss with you some underlying feelings that were not voiced before. On the other hand, it is possible that the client did not mean to imply anything more than the actual words expressed. In this case, verbalizing the implied allows the client to verify that you have an inaccurate perception of the message.

Encouraging Assessment of Emotions. It is important for people to be in touch with their own feelings. Too often, to cope with overwhelming feelings, clients wall themselves off from all emotions. This can be very unhealthy. To help clients get back in touch with their feelings, use the technique of encouraging assessment of emotions. To do this, ask clients to focus on their feelings, and ask them how they feel.

Translating Into Feelings. Sometimes clients find it difficult or impossible to express their feelings verbally by using appropriate terms for common emotions. You can help clients by translating their messages into verbal expressions of feelings. You should always be open to correction if the client finds the translation in accurate.

Reflecting. In this technique, you reflect questions and statements back to the client to help the client to think about them and come to a conclusion. This helps the client gain confidence in making assessments and decisions and encourages the client's self-reliance.

There are two forms of reflection. One form is used when clients ask a question and the question is turned around and reflected back to them. For example, the client might ask, "How am I doing with my physical therapy?" and you might reflect back with, "How do you think you're doing?" This demonstrates that you value the client's opinion.

The second form reflects back to clients some of their own words and is referred to as selective reflection. This should not be confused with *parroting,* in which all of the client's words are directed back without thought on your part. With reflection, however, you think about the message and select the word or words that are important for the client to think about. This requires active involvement by both you and the client. For example, the client might say, "I'm scared about my surgery tomorrow." With reflection, you might ask, "Scared?" and suggest that the client consider and further discuss the feeling of being scared.

Encouraging Comparison. To help clients integrate new experiences into what they know of life and to help them learn, you can encourage comparison. To do this, you may ask the client to compare or contrast a certain life experience with another.

Helping the Client Maintain Contact With Reality

Encouraging Descriptions of Perceptions. Sometimes clients perceive things that others do not. It can be helpful for the client to describe such perceptions and the emotions attached to them. This technique of encouraging descriptions of perceptions is suitable when working with clients who have hallucinations of various types. It is not recommended that you attempt to communicate with a client who is actively hallucinating. If you know this is happening, wait until the hallucination has ended before attempting to elicit the client's perceptions and emotions.

Presenting Reality. If you are with clients when a misperception of reality occurs, you can help them identify what is real and what is not. This technique, called *presenting reality,* can be very reassuring to some clients. This is different from voicing doubt, because you accept the fact that the client has perceived something that you have not perceived, but you let the client know that you did not have a similar perception. You might say, for example, "It must be very frightening for you to hear sirens wailing, but I don't hear anything."

CONCLUDING THE INTERACTION

Encouraging Formulation of a Plan of Action. The technique, encouraging the client to formulate the plan, occurs once you enter the working phase of the relationship, and you and the client have identified problems, diagnoses, and desired outcomes, and you encourage formulation of a plan of action. It is more therapeutic and more likely to be successfully carried out if the plan comes from the client rather than from you.

To encourage formulation of a plan of action, ask the client to consider what might be the best thing to do in a future situation. This future situation might be one that the client has never experienced or has experienced but was not able to handle successfully. This allows the client to think things out in advance and to be prepared.

This technique may also be used near the end of a relationship in which the client has had an opportunity to try out a plan and has not been successful. After evaluating with the client what went wrong, you might suggest formulation of a new plan of action. This helps the client to see that new approaches can always be tried.

Summarizing. One therapeutic technique that might be done at intervals is summarizing. You summarize by briefly stating, in an orderly manner, what you and the client have discussed to that point in the interaction. If a client presents a great deal of data to you, it is often helpful to stop and summarize briefly at opportune times. Summarizing is usually thought of as a final activity, because it ensures that you and the client have agreement about the decisions that were made and helps to ensure that you covered all of the information you both wanted to discuss. It can help bring closure in the termination phase of a therapeutic relationship.

TECHNIQUES THAT IMPAIR THERAPEUTIC COMMUNICATION

Just as there are techniques that facilitate communication, there are also barriers to therapeutic communication. Nontherapeutic communication techniques impair the flow of communication in what would otherwise be a progressive movement toward client growth. Some nontherapeutic techniques thwart communication by undermining you, such as by calling into question your honesty or diminishing the client's trust in you. Other nontherapeutic techniques thwart communication by undermining the client.

Nontherapeutic techniques that undermine the client are those that are demeaning, those that reinforce or strengthen irrational ideas or beliefs, those that tend to raise client anxiety levels, and those that tend to make the client dependent on you. Still other nontherapeutic techniques block the flow of ideas between the client and you. For example, if you exclude the client and make the interaction incomprehensible by using nursing jargon (the specialized language used by a group), you are talking down to the client. It can confuse the client and can distance the client from you. Some nontherapeutic techniques block communication in more than one way. Table 12-2 describes many nontherapeutic communication techniques along with selected examples that might be used with pediatric, adolescent, and adult clients.

Table 12-2 Comparison of Systematic Nontherapeutic Communication Techniques

TECHNIQUE	DESCRIPTION/DEFINITION	EXAMPLE
Belittling feelings expressed	The nurse minimizes the degree of the client's distress or discomfort, thereby implying that the client's feelings are insignificant.	*Nurse with child:* Child: "I hate shots." Nurse: "You are not the only one." *Nurse with adolescent:* Adolescent: "There is no reason to go on." Nurse: "Aren't you being a little dramatic?" *Nurse with adult:* Adult: "My life means nothing." Nurse: "If you take a walk, you will feel better."
False reassurance	The nurse implies that the anxious client has no cause for worry or concern.	*Nurse with child:* "No need to fuss over such a small needle." *Nurse with adolescent:* "One day you will look back at this and laugh." *Nurse with adult:* "Your chest pain isn't a heart attack."
Parroting	The nurse mechanically repeats the client's words without evaluating what has been said and without helping the client to think things through. It indicates a lack of interest, respect, and relatedness on the nurse's part.	*Nurse with child:* Child: "My mommy left." Nurse: "Your mommy left." *Nurse with adolescent:* Adolescent: "I am not going for dialysis." Nurse: "You are not going for dialysis." *Nurse with adult:* Adult: "I do not see any options for treatment" Nurse: "You do not see any options for treatment."
Disapproving	The nurse makes a negative value judgment about the client's behavior or thinking.	*Nurse with child:* "Shame on you!" *Nurse with adolescent:* "I cannot believe you did that." *Nurse with adult:* "Why don't you stop all this foolishness?"
Disagreeing	The nurse opposes the client's thinking. The nurse's disagreement implies the client is wrong and must defend the position.	*Nurse with child:* "I think you are wrong about this." *Nurse with adolescent:* "You can say what you like, but it does not make it right." *Nurse with adult:* "I definitely disagree with you.
Rationalizing feelings expressed	The nurse provides a seemingly rational (but untrue) excuse for the client's expression of emotions to avoid an emotional reaction to the client's feelings or to avoid having to respond appropriately to the client. This rationalization of feelings robs affective material shared by the client of its power.	*Nurse with child:* Child: "I'm mad." Nurse: "Maybe you are just tired." *Nurse with adolescent:* "Jack, crying because you hurt will only make it worse." *Nurse with adult:* Adult: "Now I am just a heart patient." Nurse: "Wouldn't you be worse off if you had AIDS?"
Interpreting	The nurse attempts to tell the client the meaning of the client's experience by seeking to make conscious that which is unconscious.	*Nurse with child:* "What you really mean is . . . ." *Nurse with adolescent:* "Your true feelings are . . . ." *Nurse with adult:* "On a deeper level, you believe . . . ."

Continued

Table 12-2 Comparison of Systematic Nontherapeutic Communication Techniques—cont'd

TECHNIQUE	DESCRIPTION/DEFINITION	EXAMPLE
Advising	The nurse literally tells the client what to do. This implies that the nurse knows best and the client is incapable of independent problem solving.	*Nurse with child:* "Tell the doctor how much better you feel today." *Nurse with adolescent:* "Stop eating sweets, and you will lose weight." *Nurse with adult:* "I would choose option A."
Blaming	The nurse inappropriately expresses feelings of anger or impatience with the client as a means of faulting the client because the nurse-client relationship is not progressing well. This is a therapeutic dead end that negates the nurse's role as a client advocate, destroys trust, and takes away client motivation to work with the nurse to identify and explore sensitive topics.	*Nurse with child:* "Well, you can't expect a sticker when you cry every time I come near you." *Nurse with adolescent:* "Get your act together, and things will go better for you." *Nurse with adult:* "Nobody told you to pull your back out, did they?"
Patronizing	The nurse treats the client in a condescending manner, thereby demeaning the client. This makes acceptance, respect, and mutual decision making impossible.	*Nurse with child:* "Just go play somewhere now." *Nurse with adolescent:* "Of course your ideas are important to me, sweetie." *Nurse with adult:* "Let's put on our slippers before we fall."
Making stereotypical comments	The nurse makes empty conversation using trite phrases and clichés, thereby encouraging the client to do the same rather than honestly exploring issues.	*Nurse with child:* "You will thank me later." *Nurse with adolescent:* "Pretty is as pretty does." *Nurse with adult:* "Let a smile be your umbrella."
Introducing an unrelated topic	The nurse changes the subject when the client brings up material the nurse prefers not to discuss.	*Nurse with child:* Child: "What is sex?" Nurse: "Finish your lunch before it gets cold." *Nurse with adolescent:* Adolescent: "What is my diagnosis?" Nurse: "Did you see the game last night?" *Nurse with adult:* Adult: "The doctor says that I am dying." Nurse: "Time for a bath."
Using jargon	The nurse excludes the client and makes the interaction incomprehensible by using nursing jargon (the specialized language used by a group).	*Nurse with child:* "Do not regurgitate your nutritional supplement." *Nurse with adolescent:* "Your increased sexual preoccupation indicates progression toward full maturation." *Nurse with adult:* "Coronary abnormalities are indicated on the angiogram."
Giving literal responses	The nurse responds to the client's figurative statement as though it were factual. The nurse misses a chance to explore material with the client.	*Nurse with child:* Child: "My insides are exploding." Nurse: "That sounds messy." *Nurse with adolescent:* Adolescent: "I am losing my mind." Nurse: "Find it." *Nurse with adult:* Adult: "My world is ending" Nurse: "The world is not ending."
Requesting an explanation	The nurse asks "why" of the client, thereby asking for a reason for feelings and behaviors when the client may not know the reason.	*Nurse with child:* "Why don't you stop crying?" *Nurse with adolescent:* "Why are you upset?" *Nurse with adult:* "Why can't you fall asleep?"
Probing	The nurse digs for information or persistently questions the client even after the client indicates unwillingness to discuss the issues.	*Nurse with child:* Nurse: "Tell me about the test." Child: "I do not want to." Nurse: "Tell me anyway." *Nurse with adolescent:* "Tell me more about that terrible event." *Nurse with adult:* "I cannot help you if you do not give me all the information about your drug habit."

▼ KEY PRINCIPLES

- The three phases of the therapeutic relationship are the orientation phase, the working phase, and the termination phase. Each phase has certain tasks associated with it.
- The six elements of communication are encoder, message, sensory channel, decoder, feedback, and context.
- Two types of communication are verbal and nonverbal.
- Verbal communication includes using words through talking or writing.
- Body language is a form of nonverbal communication that consists of human communication by alterations in personal appearance, changes in facial expressions, changes in body posture, use of gestures, maintenance of personal distances, and use of touching.
- Paralanguage is a form of nonverbal communication that consists of the elements of stress, accent, pitch, pause, intonation, rate, volume, and quality.
- Nursing attitudes that facilitate effective therapeutic communication include awareness, acceptance, respect, unconditional positive regard, empathy, relatedness, caring, objectivity, protectiveness, genuineness, openness, appropriate professional closeness or distance, and a sense of humor.
- It is vital to recognize nontherapeutic communication techniques in order to avoid using them.
- Inappropriate use of therapeutic communication techniques can change them from therapeutic techniques into nontherapeutic techniques.
- Although any specific therapeutic technique might be used at any time, some techniques tend to be more helpful at the beginning, the middle, or at the end of an interaction.

■ REVIEW QUESTIONS

1. The three phases of the therapeutic relationship are the orientation phase, the working phase, and the termination phase. During the orientation phase of a therapeutic relationship:
1. The nurse and client make a verbal agreement to work together to solve one or more of the client's problems
2. The work of the client and nurse is coming to a close
3. The nurse seeks out the client's feelings, values, beliefs, and attitudes and examines them
4. The nurse establishes additional nursing diagnoses

2. A widely accepted model for the communication process consists of six elements. The decoder element is:
1. The person who initiates a transaction to exchange information
2. The content of the message
3. The person to whom a message is aimed
4. The means by which a message is sent

3. The nurse was discussing her concerns about the client with her supervisor. The nurse mentioned the stress, intonation, rate, and volume of the client's speech. The nurse was referring to the following nonverbal component of spoken language:
1. Body language
2. Personal appearance
3. Personal space
4. Paralanguage

4. The nurse said: "You mentioned several advantages to your hip surgery. What is the single greatest improvement you have noticed?" This nurse is using which therapeutic technique?
1. Offering self
2. Encouraging descriptions of perceptions
3. Focusing
4. Asking for clarification

5. A pediatric client says to the nurse, "My mommy left." The nurse responds to the child, "Your mommy left." This is an example of which nontherapeutic communication technique?
1. Advising
2. Parroting
3. Blaming
4. Probing

Bibliography

Arnold, E., & Boggs, K. U. (2003). *Interpersonal relationships: Professional communication skills for nurses* (3rd ed.). Philadelphia: Saunders.

Dieruf, T. (2005). Mini-rounds: A team communication tool. *Rehabilitation Nursing, 30*(4), 128, 131.

Kesselman, S. K. (2005). What Ruth knew. *Nursing, 35*(7), 43.

*King, I. M. (1981). *A theory for nursing: Systems, concepts, process.* New York: Delmar.

Munoz, C., & Luckmann, J. (2005). In *Transcultural communication in nursing* (2nd ed). New York: Thomson Delmar Learning.

*Peplau, H. (1952). *Interpersonal relations in nursing.* New York: McGraw-Hill.

Philpin, S. M., Jordan, S. E., & Warring, J. (2005). Giving people a voice: Reflections on conducting interviews with participants experiencing communication impairment. *Journal of Advanced Nursing, 50*(3), 299-306.

Riley, J. B. (2004). *Communication in nursing* (5th ed.). St. Louis, MO: Mosby.

*Rogers, C. R. (1951). *Client-centered therapy.* Boston: Houghton Mifflin.

Salladay, S. A. (2005). Ethical problems: Asking the hard questions. *Nursing, 35*(3), 22.

Salladay, S. A. (2005). Ethical problems: Breach of confidence. *Nursing, 35*(6), 20.

Sully, P., & Dallas, J. (2005). *Essential communication skills for nursing.* St. Louis, MO: Elsevier Mosby.

Torppa, C. B. (2002). *Gender issues: Communication differences in interpersonal relationships.* Ohio State University Extension, The Ohio State University. Retrieved September 18, 2005, from http://ohioline.osu.edu/flm02/FS04.html.

*Travelbee, J. (1966). *Interpersonal aspects of nursing.* Philadelphia: Davis.

Ufem J. (2004). Insights on death and dying: Three keys to communication. *Nursing, 34*(10), 12.

*Asterisk indicates a classic or definitive work on this subject.

Chapter 13

CLIENT TEACHING

Media Resources

- evolve Evolve Website http://evolve.elsevier.com/Harkreader/
- Companion CD

Learning Objectives

After studying this chapter, you should be able to do the following:

- Explain the rationale for client teaching, including its purpose and benefits
- Describe the teaching and learning process, including domains of learning and principles of effective teaching
- Describe factors that affect client teaching
- Discuss the nursing diagnosis *Deficient knowledge*
- Develop a teaching plan for a client
- Explore strategies for effectively implementing client teaching
- Discuss methods for evaluating teaching and learning

Key Terms

affective learning domain
cognitive learning domain
learning
learning contract
learning objectives
psychomotor learning domain
teaching
teaching plan

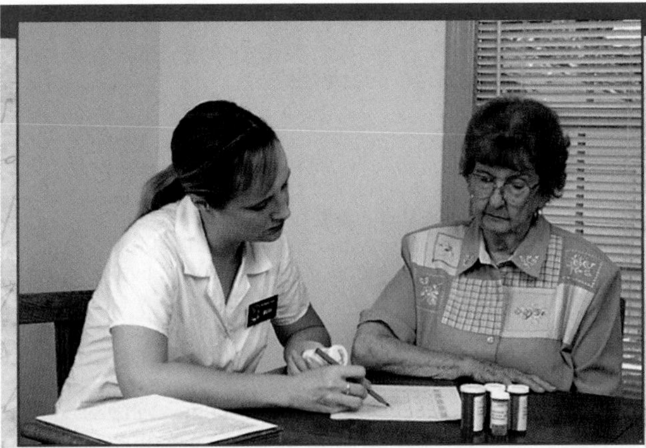

Charlotte Avery is an 82-year-old who lives in Boca Raton, Florida. Mrs. Avery is a retired restaurant manager. She lives alone in the home she shared with her third husband, Charles, who passed away 2 years ago. Mrs. Avery was recently diagnosed with type 1 diabetes mellitus, which requires insulin therapy. She needs information about her condition and self-care regarding diet, exercise, and medication therapy. The nurse makes the diagnosis of *Deficient knowledge* (see key nursing diagnosis box).

KEY NURSING DIAGNOSIS FOR TEACHING AND LEARNING

Deficient knowledge (specify): State in which a person lacks skills or information to successfully manage his or her own health care

CONCEPTS OF CLIENT TEACHING

Public access to health care information has never been greater. Self-help books and medical reference texts are available in bookstores. New medical research findings are published in newspapers and magazines and even reported on the evening news. Pharmaceutical companies advertise prescription drugs in television commercials. Via the Internet, consumers can retrieve information from around the world on any health topic within minutes.

Although access to health information has risen, so has the public's need. Because length of stay in hospitals continues to decline, nurses must ensure that clients and their families learn the information necessary to manage their health conditions post discharge. Nurses are uniquely well suited to do client teaching. Nurses understand and can explain complicated topics in simple terms, filtering less significant material. They can also evaluate the effectives of client education and are accountable for outcomes of client education as part of overall nursing care.

CLIENT RIGHTS AND NURSING STANDARDS

Although health-related client education is an integral part of nursing practice, it is also legally mandated through the nurse practice act in each state (Bastable, 2003). The Joint Commission (TJC), which accredits hospitals, also has client education standards (Chai, 2004). These include the following:

- Clients are provided with education to enhance their knowledge, skills, and behavior related to their health conditions after assessing their needs, capabilities, and readiness to learn.
- Hospitals support and provide resources for client teaching.
- There is interdisciplinary participation in client teaching as appropriate.
- Documentation includes information about client understanding of the information.

The American Hospital Association (AHA) (1975, 2003) published the *Patient's Bill of Rights* and the *Patient Care Partnership: Understanding Expectations, Rights, and Responsibilities*. These documents support the rights of clients to receive complete and current information concerning diagnosis, treatment, and prognosis in terms they can understand. In addition, the U.S. Department of Health and Human Services (2006) has published *Healthy People 2010*, which outlines national objectives for health promotion and disease prevention. These objectives call for public education programs to reduce risk behaviors and promote positive health practices.

BENEFITS OF CLIENT TEACHING

The benefits of teaching are well documented and include positive client outcomes and decreased readmissions to the hospital (Box 13-1). Client teaching also helps to control costs and maintain quality care.

Cost Control. Client teaching is an important factor in controlling costs within health care systems because it may do the following:

- Prevent illnesses that may require expensive care
- Enable the client to manage a prescribed treatment regimen after discharge from an acute care facility
- Promote client safety to decrease or prevent complications and ultimately reduce costs
- Prepare the client to anticipate and recognize complications and to seek help early to prevent hospital readmission
- Increase the care that can be given at home, including high-technology care and diagnostic testing
- Increase compliance with the treatment regimen, thus reducing the need for more costly medical procedures

Quality Control. Client teaching is also a critical component of maintaining quality of care because it does the following:

- Encourages the client and family to be active partners in the delivery of health care, thus improving the outcome

BOX 13-1

A Patient's Perspective

"The Clinic Nurses Have Taught Me So Much About How to Manage Diabetes"

When I was 48, I began to feel like my body was shutting down. I was tired all the time, I had no energy, and I was losing weight. But my doctor didn't seem concerned, so I just chalked it up to stress. And there was plenty of that. My dad was dying of a brain tumor, my mother had been diagnosed with Alzheimer's, and, as the oldest daughter, I was the primary caregiver.

After Dad died in 1991, I took my mother to Vermont to visit my brother and his family. One afternoon as we were walking through the woods, I slipped and grabbed onto a nearby tree branch to keep from falling. Unfortunately, a thorn on the branch pierced my hand. It wasn't terribly painful, so I just put some ointment and a bandage on it and thought nothing more about it. The next morning, my arm was twice its normal size! A local doctor gave me a shot of antibiotics and a prescription and told me to check in with my regular doctor when I got home, which I did. He couldn't explain why I had such an extreme reaction but thought that maybe I had multiple sclerosis. A few months after that, however, he came up with the real diagnosis: diabetes.

As soon as my doctor diagnosed the problem, he put me on 130 units of insulin a day.* Almost immediately, I began to gain weight, even though I was walking 3 to 5 miles a day. Eventually, I gained a hundred pounds. My vision began to deteriorate, because the blood vessels in my eyes were hemorrhaging. So the doctor sent me to a specialist for laser treatments to stop the hemorrhaging, at a cost of $1500 per treatment. My vision loss made it impossible for me to work, so it wasn't long before I ran out of money and was forced to go to a public clinic for all my medical care. Ironically, that turned out to be the best thing that could have happened to me.

The clinic is run by nurses, and it is wonderful. I can't say enough good things about the way they treat you. Everyone there is friendly. They always call you by name. They take time to listen. They make sure that you're scheduled for routine screenings, such as Pap smears, mammograms, and so on. They recognize that people's circumstances change, and they don't punish you because you don't have money. What's more, I get better care now than when I did have money!

The doctors who work at my clinic are all volunteers, and they are excellent. My endocrinologist is a woman, and she keeps up on all the latest research. My former doctor was not good at controlling my diabetes. Over a period of time, my clinic doctor has gotten me totally off insulin and onto oral medications. My diet was pretty good, but she fine-tuned it. She also suggested that I find an additional caregiver for my mother. Those changes have made a huge difference in my life, in my weight, and in my blood sugar.

The clinic nurses have taught me so much about how to manage diabetes. And every 3 months I have tests for long-term blood sugar control and liver function because of the oral medications I'm taking. So far, my diabetes is under really good control.

*Author note: This is an unusually high dose of insulin.

- Increases client satisfaction by helping the client understand what can reasonably be expected from the health care system
- Increases the client's sense of control, which is derived from knowledge
- Ensures that clients have the knowledge they need to provide self-care
- Increases communication between the client and provider
- Increases client satisfaction through a mutually respectful relationship

THE TEACHING AND LEARNING PROCESS

Teaching and learning are mutually dependent aspects of a dynamic, interactive process. **Teaching** is a set of planned activities performed to influence knowledge, behavior, or skill. To teach effectively, you must understand the subject to be taught, accurately assess the client's learning needs, control the learning environment, and use methods appropriate for the client's needs.

Learning is the acquisition of knowledge, behavior, or skill through experience, practice, study, or instruction. Learning may cause people to change their attitudes, perceptions, habits, and methods of problem solving.

There are many theories about how people learn, and an understanding of well-known learning theories can increase your effectiveness in client education. Table 13-1 briefly outlines major learning theories.

CORRELATION WITH THE NURSING PROCESS

The teaching and learning process correlates with the nursing process (Table 13-2). However, the teaching-learning process is focused on only one aspect of care, which is meeting clients' learning needs about self-managing their health condition.

DOMAINS OF LEARNING

Learning theorists have identified the following three primary domains of learning:

- Cognitive domain: the ability to make sense of and use information
- Affective domain: the feelings and values associated with information
- Psychomotor domain: manipulative and motor skills

In a classic work, Bloom (1956) defined a taxonomy that categorizes behaviors according to complexity within each domain, which is useful in developing learning objectives. Although described separately, cognitive, affective, and psychomotor behaviors do not occur in isolation but are interdependent processes that

Table 13-1 Overview of Major Learning Theories

LEARNING THEORIST	KEY ELEMENTS OF THEORY
Albert Bandura	Behavior is influenced and regulated by internal means, such as self-efficacy.
Jerome Bruner	The learner actively participates in the learning process. Culture and value systems influence learning.
John Dewey	Education should support and promote independence of the learner. The learner needs to have an understanding of learning goals.
Robert Gagne	There is an orderly process to learning. Learning proceeds from simple to complex and from concrete to abstract.
Ivan Pavlov	An individual as a learner is passive and is controlled by the environment.
B. F. Skinner	Teaching involves deliberate manipulation of the environment.
Edward Thorndike	Learning can be transferred from one situation to another; assessment of learner behavior is necessary.
John Watson	Learning is a combined result of conditioning and experiences. A change in the environment may encourage learning.

Table 13-2 Comparison of the Nursing Process and the Teaching Process

STEP	NURSING PROCESS	TEACHING PROCESS
1	• Collect and analyze data. • Assess client needs.	• Collect and analyze data about client's knowledge. • Identify learning needs.
2	• Label needs with nursing diagnoses.	• Make an educational diagnosis, such as *Deficient knowledge, Ineffective health maintenance,* or *Health-seeking behaviors.*
3	• Identify desired outcomes. • Plan nursing interventions.	• Prepare a teaching plan by writing objectives, content, time frame, teaching format, and methods to teach content, such as by using audiovisual equipment.
4	• Implement nursing care.	• Implement the teaching plan and delivery of content.
5	• Evaluate client's outcomes. • Reassess as needed.	• Evaluate client learning on basis of objectives. • Reassess as needed.

occur simultaneously. By integrating these domains into client teaching plans, you will improve the quality of teaching and promote client learning. We will now briefly explore each domain in more detail.

Cognitive Domain. The **cognitive learning domain** is considered the "thinking" domain. It includes acquiring knowledge, comprehending, and using critical thinking skills (Figure 13-1). Learning takes place at several levels in the cognitive domain (Bloom, 1956), and the lower levels are especially pertinent to clients learning new health information:

- **Acquisition:** To acquire knowledge, the client obtains information, commonly by memorizing terms, facts, principles, and procedures. An example would be a client who memorizes that digoxin (Lanoxin) is a cardiac glycoside that helps the heart pump more effectively.
- **Comprehension:** The client understands new information, repeats the content back in his or her own words, relates the information to something already known, or attaches meaning to the information. An example is that the client states that digoxin will help reduce the symptoms of heart failure that occurred following a myocardial infarction (heart attack).
- **Application:** The client has the intellectual ability to use acquired information in similar but different situations. An example is that a client taking digoxin (Lanoxin) calls the health care provider after recognizing early signs of digoxin toxicity.

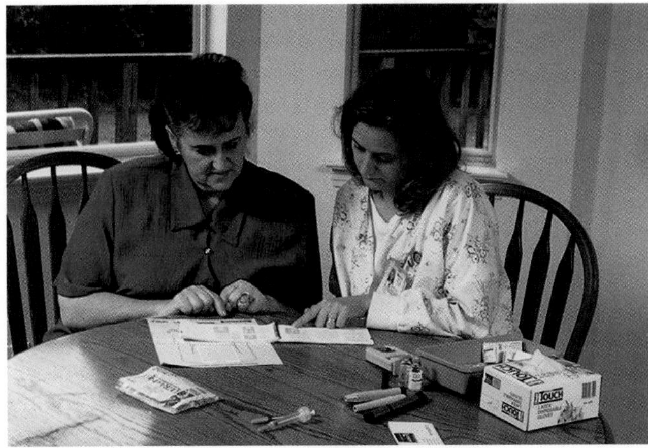

FIGURE 13-1 In the *cognitive* domain, the client is able to discuss the signs and symptoms of low blood glucose.

- **Analysis:** The client can separate information into components of the whole.
- **Synthesis:** Synthesis is reassembling parts to identify a new whole. The client uses the information that you provide and communicates a creative and unique use of the information.
- **Evaluation:** The client makes judgments about the effects of the treatment.

Synthesis and evaluation are the highest levels of cognitive ability. Although nurses routinely synthesize and evaluate information at these levels, clients—especially

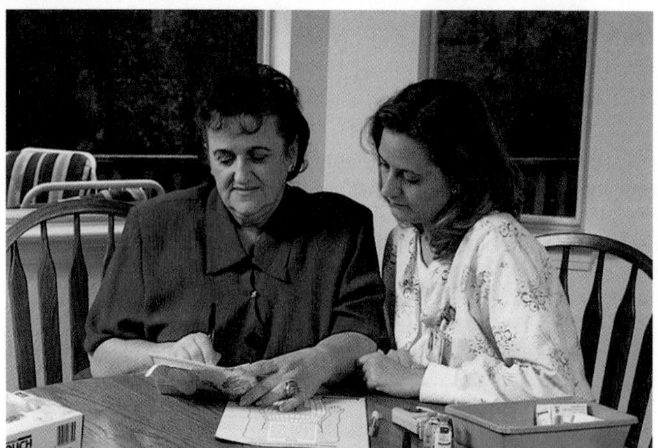

FIGURE 13-2 In the *affective* domain, the client commits to performing daily self-injections.

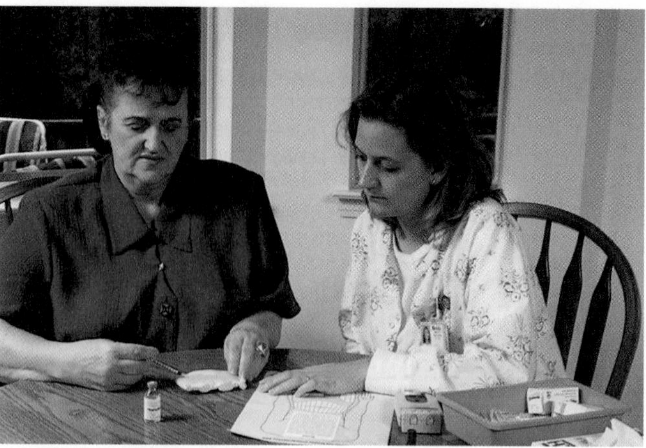

FIGURE 13-3 In the *psychomotor* domain, the client manipulates the equipment to perform self-injection.

sick clients—are not always able to attain this level. Clients may be only able to comprehend the steps of a carefully prescribed routine; they may not be able to analyze or modify that routine. When teaching such a client, limit yourself to essential information, such as the cause of an illness, lifestyle changes needed to prevent complications, basic symptom management, and specific skills as needed, such as how to irrigate a colostomy. Usually, the client can function when given this amount of information; in-depth explanations can be added as the client asks questions or later during postdischarge follow-up care.

Affective Domain. The **affective learning domain** includes values, beliefs, feelings, and attitudes (Figure 13-2). Thus teaching in the affective domain can address a client's health-seeking behaviors and choices at a deep and powerful level.

Emotions are also addressed in the affective domain. Anger, frustration, relief, and joy are often experienced as part of obtaining health care, being diagnosed with an illness, or even receiving a clean bill of health. Helping a client understand and manage feelings is essential to integrating new learning into activities of daily living.

You can promote a client's health and well-being by facilitating high-level learning in the affective domain. To do so, you must accomplish the following three personal goals:

- Understand your own value system, and provide information to clients in a manner that minimizes your own biases.
- Respect the validity and uniqueness of each individual's personal, cultural, and religious value system, even when it differs from yours.
- Provide accurate and complete information about health and illness, thereby setting the stage for affective learning.

Learning in the affective domain can be difficult to evaluate and typically is an ongoing process. Some clients may take years to internalize feelings and values fully enough to change their behavior.

Psychomotor Domain. The **psychomotor learning domain** includes physical and motor skills, such as giving injections (Figure 13-3). These skills may require varying levels of dexterity, coordination, and the ability to manipulate equipment and objects. Development of psychomotor skills involves integration of the other two domains as well. Psychomotor learning also includes perceptual processes that some theorists consider a separate domain.

A clear understanding of the interdependence of cognitive, affective, and psychomotor domains of learning enables you to assess learning needs with confidence. Once these are identified, you can negotiate learning objectives with clients and teaching in all domains.

FACTORS AFFECTING CLIENT TEACHING

Many factors can influence your teaching effectiveness, including you, the client, the family or significant others, and the situation. In addition, time to teach is a factor. Because you will have limited interaction with clients, you must maximize your teaching effectiveness to compensate for the short teaching time available. You will also need to document for continuity of care (if other nurses are teaching the client also) and advocate for referrals until learning is complete.

CLIENT CHARACTERISTICS

Many characteristics can influence a client's approach to learning, such as age, race, gender, medical diagnosis, and clinical progress. Likewise, religious beliefs and cultural background may alter the client's learning needs and therefore affect the methods by which you present materials in particular content areas. Other important assessment factors include literacy, education, developmental level, and learning style.

Literacy Level. The 2003 National Assessment of Adult Literacy found that a total of 18% of adults had below basic elementary level literacy skills (13%), were nonliterate in English (3%), or could not be tested because of language barriers (2%) (National Center for Education Statistics, 2005). Because of this, you are likely to encounter clients who cannot read or who cannot read English. Those who can read will have varying abilities, from very basic to very advanced. Often, clients are embarrassed to admit inadequate literacy, and thus you must assess their ability to read and understand health-related information. Do not rely solely on the number of years in school as a guide, because it is often an inaccurate measure of literacy. It is more useful to observe client behavior for clues of illiteracy, including confusion, nervousness, making excuses, or irrelevant statements that indicate lack of communication. You may have a client read aloud printed health information as an indicator of reading ability or check comprehension of material by having the client explain it back to you. Be prepared to provide privacy and use educational methods that complement each client's learning ability.

Level of Knowledge. Before teaching a client, assess general health knowledge, perception of current illness, and the type of teaching that will be most helpful and easily understood. You are likely to consider the client's level of formal education, but do not assume that a well-educated person is a well-informed person when it comes to health education. Determine how much a client knows or how well the client can perform a skill before initiating a teaching plan.

In addition to assessing a client's knowledge level, determine the following:

- What the client has been told by a physician or has learned from media sources
- What the client knows about his or her illness
- What the client's previous experience is with illness, the health care system, or hospitalization

These factors may influence the client's knowledge level and readiness to learn.

Developmental Level. Learning can also be influenced by whether the client is a child, an adolescent, an adult, or an older adult. In addition, a client who is developmentally delayed will need particular attention so that teaching, if appropriate, is done at an optimal level. Before beginning client teaching, assess the client's developmental level.

Children. For children, the teaching and learning process can be fundamentally different than that used by adults. Adjust the complexity and volume of information taught to each child's age and cognitive level, and include the caregiver whenever possible. Carefully choose terms and examples to keep them appropriate for the child's age level.

Young children may learn best by playing games, drawing, or watching video-modeling of behavior. Using dolls, stuffed animals, or other toys may be helpful. For older children, actual medical supplies, such as dressing materials, are useful aids when teaching about medical procedures. Many children are receptive to instruction that involves role-playing, which can be therapeutic as well as educational. Children and their parents may require specialized teaching approaches (Box 13-2). Note that parents may need affective domain assessment for their emotional reactions to their children's problems.

BOX 13-2 *Tips for Teaching Children*

- Trust is essential to a therapeutic relationship with a child.
- In general, the younger the child, the shorter the attention span.
- Children are exposed to various levels of information about health care. Be sure to assess the child's knowledge.
- Children form misconceptions easily. A child's imagination may create greater fear than the truth, told directly and simply.
- Parents can often provide cues to the child's emotional response and capacity for understanding information. However, some parents may underestimate or overestimate their child's capacity.
- Children may regress developmentally in a situation of illness.
- Children may better manage uncomfortable information through role-playing with dolls and models.

Adolescents. Developmental influences are highly important when teaching adolescents. They are able to conceptualize at a higher level than children and generally have more advanced reading skills and comprehension. In addition, they are highly influenced by peers, including pressures regarding behavior and appearance. Role-playing and group teaching sessions with other adolescents are often effective teaching strategies with this age-group.

Adolescents expect honesty, openness, and the truth about their illness. Assist them in developing independent and informed decision making about health matters by asking their opinions and engaging them in problem-solving activities.

Adults. Knowles (1980) identified four characteristics that characterize adult learning (Table 13-3). Of course, people differ, and not all of the characteristics may apply to any one client, but by sensibly integrating the principles into the learning process, you can create a successful and supportive learning environment.

Older Adults. Although intelligence may actually increase as a person ages, the capacity to learn is affected by functional changes. These changes may not appreciably affect performance until a person's 80s or 90s. However, chronic and debilitating diseases often alter intellectual abilities.

Reaction time (amount of time required for a response to a stimulus) slows with age. An older person needs more time to process information, perform psychomotor skills, and make decisions that involve thinking about multiple aspects of a problem. Keep instructions free of unnecessary detail and explanations, which could lead to confusion from paying too much attention to irrelevant detail. If this occurs, redirect the client to the main learning points.

Table 13-3 Characteristics of Adult Learning

CHARACTERISTIC	DESCRIPTION
Self-directed	Adults identify their own learning needs and take action to acquire knowledge when they need it. This stems from their independence and fully developed self-concept.
Builds on previous knowledge	Adults bring a lifetime of accumulated learning to each new learning experience. To facilitate adult learning, make use of previous learning and experiences as resources to enhance present learning.
Practical	Adults are more likely to learn there is an opportunity to immediately apply what is learned. For this reason, health education tends to be more effective during times of illness.
Purposeful	Adults tend to learn better when information is seen as useful or necessary. Adult learning is often problem based (arising from real-life problems, such as preventing an illness or retaining health), and it is most effective when immediate results are obtained.

Although memory may not be severely impaired, an older person is often slower in acquiring, storing, and recalling new information. To compensate, the person uses selective attention to screen out extraneous information and thus could sometimes miss important information. By slowing the pace of teaching new information, you can help older persons compensate for their changes in memory.

The capacity to learn is affected by stress and fatigue. The older person often fatigues more easily and thus has more difficulty paying attention to new information. In addition, stress is associated with multiple stimuli or trying to think about a number of things at the same time. If the older adult becomes overwhelmed by the information provided, prioritize the key or "survival" points as a lesson summary. This will enhance client safety by identifying what is necessary to promote health.

Age-related physical changes could impair psychomotor learning. Manual dexterity for manipulating equipment, such as syringes, may be decreased. Visual impairment could require the use of large-print teaching materials. Carefully assess these needs before beginning a teaching session.

Remember also that changes with aging are highly variable. Older adults have written a first novel, taken up painting, and otherwise developed new skills. Do not globally underestimate their learning ability.

Learning Styles. Every client has a preferred learning style, a way of processing information that works best. You can enhance teaching effectiveness by discovering this style for each client early in the course of teaching. Unfortunately, many nurses use the teaching strategy that is most comfortable for themselves, rather than accommodating the client's style of learning.

One way of classifying learning styles is to describe them as auditory, visual, or kinesthetic. Some clients prefer to hear you talk about a topic. Others prefer to read a pamphlet or handout independently, or to view a videotape, and then ask questions. Some clients need to practice a skill repeatedly until learning takes place. Ask your clients how they most enjoy learning new information; then adapt your teaching strategy to their preference (Bastable, 2003). When the spouse, significant other, or family is the actual target of health teaching, these principles still apply.

FACTORS THAT FACILITATE LEARNING

To teach effectively, you must understand and use factors that facilitate learning. These factors—readiness and motivation—can guide your decisions about teaching children, adults, families, groups, and communities.

Readiness. The client should be both physically and emotionally ready to learn. Health status may adversely affect readiness to learn if an illness diminishes cognitive ability and energy level. Readiness to learn often depends on the concern generated by illness or the threat of illness. Clients who are acutely ill are generally focused on short-term needs. As recovery progresses, more attention can be devoted to prevention. Because of shortened lengths of hospital stay, health teaching sometimes proceeds even if the client is not in an ideal state of readiness to learn. Continued learning can then occur as part of outpatient or follow-up care.

People also differ in the amount and type of health information they can tolerate. Some people become anxious if they feel uninformed about their illness, including its cause, prevention, and treatment. Others become anxious if you try to talk about their disorder. When anxious clients resist instruction, try to wait until they begin asking questions or show other signs of readiness. When anxiety has lessened, they may be more receptive to new information.

Motivation. Clients learn more if they have a genuine desire or motivation to learn. Motivation is greatest in clients who recognize their learning needs and perceive the available teaching as meaningful. Motivation depends on acceptance of self-responsibility for health. As clients become more independent, learning becomes more self-directed.

Because motivation can be difficult to measure and influence, ask questions or engage the client in a conversation about the health topic to gauge interest. An unmotivated client will become distracted, change the subject, or otherwise show signs of not paying attention.

Some clients will suggest that you give the information to their spouse or significant other.

Motivation to learn increases in an atmosphere of acceptance, in which clients feel that you are genuinely interested in helping them learn. They also need time to assimilate ideas and develop new skills. They have the right to make mistakes and even to fail at a task without "losing face." You can increase their motivation by acting as a facilitator, not as a judge.

FACTORS THAT INHIBIT LEARNING

Barriers to learning may include physiological, psychological, cultural, environmental, and socioeconomic factors.

Physiological Factors. Clients who are critically ill, in severe pain, restless, oxygen deprived, fatigued, weak, or hearing or vision impaired face physical obstacles to learning. These obstacles interfere with learning because they reduce the person's ability to concentrate, deplete energy, or impair the senses. Postpone all but the simplest information until the client is able to attend to learning, and repeat any information provided during a serious illness as the client recovers. If the client has a vision or hearing sensory deficit, consider this when selecting visual aids or teaching strategies.

Psychological Factors. Psychological barriers relate to motivation. Attitude often changes throughout the course of a serious illness and also when a person moves from being well to being ill. Understanding what the client's personality and self-image were like before the onset of the present illness is helpful because clients sometimes experience a personality change from a real or perceived threat to their self-esteem or present lifestyle.

Psychological stressors also interfere with concentration. People who feel anxious, fearful, and angry about their illness may have difficulty learning. Those who have trouble adjusting to a new diagnosis may experience denial, which postpones their readiness to learn.

Teaching content may be altered by the medical or nursing prognosis. A client who is terminally ill may have different learning needs and capabilities than those of a client not facing death.

Cultural Factors. Teaching and learning can be complicated when a client's language, cultural or ethnic background, or values are different from yours. In all cases, you and your clients will benefit from your awareness of cultural differences and your willingness to obtain assistance with teaching when needed.

Some ethnic groups follow unique beliefs and practices, many of which involve diet, nutrition, health and illness, and family roles. Certain foods may be forbidden, while certain health rituals may be required. Consider a client's cultural and religious values when assessing overall learning needs; however, avoid stereotyping a client based on ethnic or cultural background. Lack of cultural sensitivity on your part may distance those clients who most need health teaching and result in ineffective or wasted teaching time.

Also recognize that your values will vary from those of your clients at least some of the time. For example, you may value self-care and independence; the client may not. You may have trouble identifying with a client who says, "Just tell my wife. She gives me all my pills." Yet you must regard each client as a unique individual with valid wishes about teaching and learning.

Environmental Factors. Learning is facilitated in a pleasant, quiet environment, free from distractions. The teaching area should be well lit, comfortably warm, and (if possible) away from the hub of activity. When the room is too hot or cold, the client may be too uncomfortable to concentrate.

Noise, interruptions, and lack of privacy can seriously disrupt teaching sessions and can occur in any setting. In group teaching sessions, some clients may be distracted by the movements and noises of others in the room. Imagine the possible distractions in a homeless shelter or in a client's cluttered home, with barking dogs, small children, or a loud television. Even a hospital room does not always offer the privacy and quiet needed for teaching, because visitors, physicians, and other nurses enter the room to complete their roles. Reducing stimuli to gain your client's full attention may challenge you to be creative for teaching and learning sessions.

Socioeconomic Factors. When teaching clients about their illness and the care required, it helps to consider their home situation, living arrangements, and usual activities. Evaluate their relationships with significant others to determine the strength of their personal support system. Assess their type of work and their level of stress. Knowing their financial situation enables you to plan cost-effective health and maintenance care when possible. Keep in mind, however, that some clients are very private about financial matters. Be prepared to explain your need to know about their financial condition.

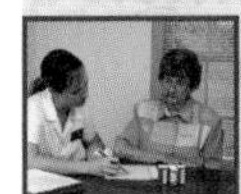

What factors might affect Mrs. Avery's ability to learn?

IMPLEMENTING THE TEACHING-LEARNING PROCESS

Health teaching involves assessment of client learning needs, determining learning objectives, planning appropriate teaching strategies, implementing the teaching plan, and evaluating the outcomes of the instruction. The process closely parallels the nursing process.

ASSESSMENT

For a client with learning needs, follow the phases of the nursing process just as you would for a client with physiological needs. Assess client characteristics, as well as current factors that facilitate or inhibit learning. Several nursing diagnoses can be applied to clients with learning needs, but *Deficient knowledge* is the most common. In certain client situations, a related diagnosis—such as *Noncompliance, Ineffective health maintenance,* or *Self-care deficit*—may be more appropriate. *Deficient knowledge* is defined as "the absence or deficiency of cognitive information related to [a] specific topic" (NANDA International [NANDA-I], 2007).

Focused Assessment for *Deficient Knowledge*. Any client can have a need for health-related knowledge; however, several factors may increase the risk of *Deficient knowledge.* Clients at greatest risk include those with chronic illnesses that require complex treatment regimens, those needing special procedures, and those for whom preventive measures are important, such as pregnant clients, older adult clients with respiratory disease, and clients with impaired immunity.

Generally, uneducated clients are thought to be at greater risk, but highly educated clients often do not understand or have experience with medical or health problems. Family members, including children, also need information, as does anyone who acts as the client's caregiver.

Defining Characteristics. Verbalization that a client has no knowledge, incomplete knowledge, or incorrect knowledge is a defining characteristic for the nursing diagnosis *Deficient knowledge.* Clients may tell you directly that they need knowledge, or they may ask questions that indicate the specific knowledge sought. Look for objective clues that they do not have appropriate knowledge or understanding. The evidence may be indirect, as when they fail to follow instructions accurately or perform poorly on tests or return demonstrations.

Related Factors. Related factors may give direction to your choice of interventions. These factors may require you to modify your teaching to minimize the factor or to remove it before implementing the teaching plan. Related factors for *Deficient knowledge* include the following:

- Cognitive limitation
- Information misinterpretation
- Lack of interest in learning
- Lack of motivation
- Lack of readiness to learn
- Lack of recall
- Limited exposure to information (specify)
- Limited practice of skill
- Unfamiliarity with information resources

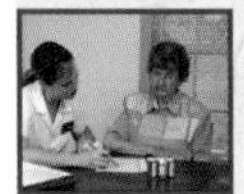

Think again about Mrs. Avery. What questions would you ask her to elicit information about her teaching-learning needs?

DIAGNOSIS

Although teaching is an appropriate intervention for many nursing diagnoses, *Deficient knowledge* is the nursing diagnosis identified most often for clients with learning needs. You must consider the goal of client teaching before selecting the diagnosis. If the goal of teaching is to maintain health, the diagnosis should be *Ineffective health maintenance.* If the goal of teaching is to ensure compliance with the treatment regimen, the diagnosis should be *Ineffective therapeutic regimen management.* If the goal of teaching is to remove barriers to complying with treatment regimen, the diagnosis is *Noncompliance.*

The diagnosis *Deficient knowledge* can be used when there is a barrier to learning that needs to be removed—for example, limited vision that interferes with reading labels, or situational depression that interferes with desire to learn about illness. When the goal of care is to help the client learn, it is appropriate to identify the diagnosis as *Deficient knowledge.*

Action Alert! Determine the highest-priority nursing diagnosis before developing the plan for meeting learning needs.

Related Nursing Diagnoses. *Ineffective health maintenance* is closely related to *Deficient knowledge.* Assess the client's ability to identify an adaptive behavior, manage a health-related behavior, or seek assistance (NANDA-I, 2007). Client teaching is a pertinent intervention when the related factor is a lack of material resources, a lack of (or significant alteration in) communication ability, or a lack of effective individual coping. All affect the teaching and learning process.

Assess the client for *Health-seeking behaviors.* Determine if the client needs assistance to actively seek ways to alter personal health habits and/or the environment to move toward a higher level of health (NANDA-I, 2007). Assess the client's knowledge of ways to achieve his or her health goals or change unhealthy behaviors.

Assess for *Ineffective coping.* Identify adaptive behaviors and abilities of the client to meet life's demands and roles (NANDA-I, 2007). Teaching may be needed to develop good nutrition habits, to manage stress, or to develop coping strategies.

PLANNING

After selecting the appropriate nursing diagnosis, you must decide what the client is expected to accomplish. Expected outcomes depend on the individual assessment, and examples might include that the client can do the following:

- Express interest in learning new information
- Repeat the key facts or principles to be learned
- Apply the information in a novel situation
- Demonstrate correct use of the information by selecting foods correctly, performing a psychomotor skill, or other action

Goals and *objectives* provide a framework for reaching desired outcomes. Goals are broad, multidimensional, long-term expectations. They are derived by identifying what the client wants to achieve, and they take into consideration the resources available to attain the expected outcomes.

Learning Objectives. Learning objectives are specific tasks to be accomplished in order to achieve broader goals. A **learning objective** is a statement that describes the intended results of learning rather than the process of instruction. It documents in a clear, realistic, and measurable manner how a client will demonstrate competency in a certain area. It must be client centered and stated in behavioral terms to allow measurement and evaluation of the client's progress. A well-written learning objective includes the following elements:

- The expected performance
- Conditions in which the behavior will be performed
- Criteria by which the performance will be evaluated

Compare the following learning objectives:

- *Objective 1:* Mrs. Avery will understand diabetes mellitus before discharge from the health care facility.
- *Objective 2:* By the end of the second teaching session, Mrs. Avery will be able to state the signs and symptoms of hyperglycemia (high blood glucose) with 100% accuracy.

The first objective is vague and ambiguous and therefore difficult to evaluate. The second objective is specific and measurable and has a clearer statement of the desired outcome, because it contains the following elements:

- *Performance:* State the signs and symptoms of hyperglycemia
- *Condition(s):* By the end of the second teaching session
- *Criterion:* 100% accuracy

A clear objective that includes measurable terminology allows you to evaluate whether the desired learning has occurred. In addition, Mrs. Avery will know the goals of your teaching sessions, and she will be able to focus her efforts on meeting those goals. Because the management of diabetes mellitus requires a number of procedures, you may need several learning objectives (in a variety of domains) to help Mrs. Avery learn to assume the responsibility for self-care. Such objectives might include the following:

- By the end of the first teaching session, Mrs. Avery will correctly explain the pathophysiology of diabetes in terms appropriate to her level (cognitive domain).
- By the end of the first teaching session, Mrs. Avery will verbalize the importance of adhering to her prescribed diet (affective domain).
- Each morning before breakfast, Mrs. Avery will correctly measure her blood glucose level, using the fingerstick method, aseptic technique, the proper equipment, accurate interpretation of the results, and correct documentation of the findings (psychomotor domain).
- On the day before discharge, Mrs. Avery will use a list provided to her to choose appropriate foods and plan a sample breakfast, lunch, and dinner menu with 100% accuracy (cognitive domain).

What to Teach. After determining expected learning outcomes, you must decide what to teach the client, when to teach it, and how to teach it. Together with the client, develop a specific teaching plan that (1) builds on the client's present knowledge base, (2) provides new information, and (3) increases the client's level of understanding about health status. Topics selected should be based on the client's learning needs and specific, measurable learning objectives. Learning needs may vary according to client location. For example, the hospitalized client might have learning needs related to an unfamiliar environment, whereas a client at home might have learning needs related to self-care and available resources.

> ***Action Alert!*** Continually assess clients' learning needs and identify other areas of interest unique to each client. Ask clients for input into the teaching plan to ensure that the content is interesting and relevant to their needs.

Teaching Plan. A **teaching plan** is an organized, individualized, written presentation of what the client must learn and how the instructions and information will be provided. It should be outcome oriented, with individualized goals set by the nurse and the client. Like a nursing care plan, it follows the steps of the nursing process. A standardized teaching plan may be designed for groups of clients, such as clients newly diagnosed with diabetes or clients who have had coronary bypass surgery; however, *each plan should be individualized for the specific client.* A sample teaching plan is prepared for Mrs. Avery, who is beginning insulin therapy for her diabetes (Box 13-3). Sources of teaching plans include nursing

BOX 13-3 *Nursing Care Plan*

Teaching Plan for a Diabetic Client Beginning Insulin Therapy

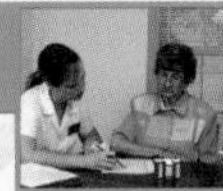

Admission Data

Charlotte Avery is an 82-year-old woman who lives in Boca Raton, Florida. After Mrs. Avery's parents died, she became the proprietor of her family's restaurant business. Mrs. Avery retired 7 years ago. Her son now runs the restaurant, and she cares for two great-grandchildren. When Mrs. Avery fainted in her home 3 days ago, her 9-year-old great-grandchild called 911. It was later found that Mrs. Avery's diabetes was out of control. Her physician told her that she would no longer be able to control her diabetes with diet and oral medications alone. She must now learn to monitor her blood glucose and self-administer insulin. The nurse developed the following teaching plan for Mrs. Avery.

Continued

BOX 13-3

Nursing Care Plan—cont'd

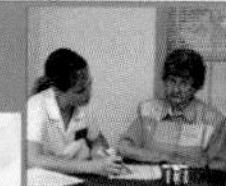

Teaching Plan for a Diabetic Client Beginning Insulin Therapy

NANDA-I Nursing Diagnosis	NOC Expected Outcomes With Indicators	NIC Interventions With Selected Activities	Evaluation Data
Deficient Knowledge: Diabetes Management (Affective)	***Knowledge: Diabetes Management***	***Teaching: Individual***	***After 1 Month of Care***
Related Factor: • Readiness to learn	• Client will discuss her feelings about taking insulin.	• Provide a quiet environment that supports discussion of feelings.	• States has survived birth of five children, death of three husbands, and loss of first restaurant by fire. This seems like minor problem in comparison.
	• Client will accept the need for insulin and dietary change.	• Assess client's desire to self-administer injections.	• States need to remain healthy to care for two great-grandchildren so has been willing to try to modify diet and take insulin.
	• Client will articulate confidence in her ability self-administer insulin injections.	• Provide constructive and positive feedback. in the learning process	• States she knows she can learn but the information is confusing.
	• Client will make a commitment to keep daily records of glucose monitoring and insulin injections and reactions.	• Provide a record book for recording.	• Records sample data accurately in record book.
	Knowledge: Medication	***Teaching: Prescribed Medication***	
Related Factor: • Seeking knowledge	• Client will complete a multiple choice test of knowledge of insulin and its effects.	• Provide video explaining effects of insulin and mechanism of action.	• Observed video twice and asked appropriate questions.
	• Client will list the differences between regular and intermediate-acting insulin.	• Provide multiple choice test, and provide instructions.	• Correctly answered 90% of questions. Indicated understanding after discussion of incorrect items.
		• Describe differences in types of insulin, and provide handout.	• Listened and read information about insulin. • Stated, "NPH will last all day. Regular is only good for one meal."
	Knowledge: Treatment Procedures	***Teaching: Psychomotor Skill***	
Related Factor: • Lack of experience with injectable medications	• Client will inject accurate dosage of insulin using correct technique.	• Demonstrate correct procedure for drawing medication and subcutaneous injection. Observe return demonstration.	• Withdrew amount accurately. Hesitant to inject self. Injected correctly on second attempt.
	• Client will demonstrate correct procedure for monitoring blood glucose.	• Demonstrate procedure for fingerstick and use of Glucometer. Observe return demonstration.	• Used appropriate technique for fingerstick. Initially confused about use of Glucometer. Completed procedure with coaching.

Critical Thinking Questions

1. The following is documented during a follow-up visit to the clinic: Verbalized that she had an episode of low blood glucose last weekend. Action taken was to check her blood glucose level (which was 42), drink a glass of orange juice, eat two peanut butter crackers, and rest. Repeated her blood glucose 30 minutes later; reading was 96. Stated she felt better and continued her housework. From this documentation, how would you evaluate the effectiveness of the teaching plan for Mrs. Avery?
2. Considering the change in learning ability that can occur with aging, how many teaching sessions would you need before Mrs. Avery self-injects her insulin? Can Mrs. Avery be expected to administer her insulin independently? How would you explain the pathological changes associated with diabetic complications?

textbooks, client teaching guides, pharmaceutical or medical equipment company literature, and computerized teaching plans that can be retrieved from a hospital information system.

In general, clients will be more successful in remembering and assimilating information if you begin with simple information and proceed to complex. In a well-developed teaching plan, each concept presented is based on a broader and more fundamental concept. Clearly, a person cannot understand abnormalities of function without first understanding normal function. Likewise, a client will not comprehend treatment and prevention of a disease without first learning about its cause. Thus, when teaching about illness and therapy, begin with a broad discussion of the normal anatomy and physiology of the diseased organ or system. Then proceed to describe factors that cause the disease, and end the discussion by describing how the client can take part in the treatment and rehabilitation program.

When to Teach. Keep in mind that teaching can take place at any time and can be scheduled or unscheduled. For example, instruction can be given at specific designated times that are spaced throughout the day or informally when a person asks questions or encounters new experiences. Environment and timing help determine success in the teaching-learning process. If possible, the client should choose the best time and place for teaching, and the environment should be quiet, with good lighting, and relatively stress free. In general, try to avoid noisy, hectic times or other times when the client is distracted (such as during meals or immediately after administration of pain medication). Involve the family and significant others when able, because their support will be helpful in achieving outcomes.

How to Teach. Many avenues are available for making the best use of your teaching time. Depending on the client's needs and the resources available, you can use one-to-one instruction, group lectures, printed materials, programmed instruction, computerized teaching, other teaching aids, and other expert teachers. Sometimes clients will benefit from more than one mode of instruction. Table 13-4 lists common learning needs across the life span, along with suggested teaching strategies.

Individual or Group Instruction. One-to-one instruction, whether formal or informal, allows you to pace and customize your teaching to the client's learning rate. It also allows more flexibility in considering the client's comfort level and ability to absorb content.

Group instruction requires a meeting place, handout materials, a meeting agenda and lesson plan, and seating that facilitates group interaction (chairs placed in a circle, for example). You must deliver a prepared lecture on the chosen topic, lead a discussion, review major points covered in the discussion, and arrange for the next meeting.

The three major advantages of group meetings are the economy of teaching time, the possibility of delivering a large amount of factual information, and the opportunity for clients with similar problems to share experiences, viewpoints, opinions, and questions with each other. Two disadvantages are the lack of ability to pace your teaching to individual learning rates and the possibility that some clients will be too intimidated to ask questions in front of the group.

Printed Materials. Printed materials—such as pamphlets and brochures—allow clients to read and study at their own pace. They are affordable, portable, and can be used to teach or reinforce a learning experience. Also, clients can share the materials with family and significant others so that all have similar information. Remember to follow up with the client to answer questions if printed materials are used in teaching.

Action Alert! Be sure to assess reading level before distributing printed materials.

Programmed or Computer-Assisted Instruction. Programmed instruction involves a prepared program of study that lists learning objectives and provides activities to meet those objectives. It may include a pretest and posttest for self-evaluation. Computer-assisted instruction (CAI) is similar to programmed instruction, except that the learner uses a computer program and there may be an interactive component that printed materials do not have. Computerized learning packages are being increasingly used at all educational levels, and client education software is becoming more common. This teaching method requires client self-direction and therefore tends to be more effective with highly motivated and computer-literate clients.

Audio and Visual Instructional Aids. Teaching can be enhanced by the proper use of aids, such as drawings, models of organs, charts, graphs, audiotapes, a bulletin board, a blackboard, posters, pictures, an overhead projector, slide shows, films, videotapes, closed-circuit television, flash cards, programmed instruction, and games (Weston-Eborn & Sitzman, 2005). Increasing numbers of websites are also available for on-line instruction. Clients should be cautioned to establish credibility by determining the source of the information.

Human Resources. The use of a specialized resource person can be extremely helpful to a client's learning process. For example, when teaching about a special diet, you could have a dietitian attend your session and share information as needed. Physicians, physical therapists, and occupational therapists all make significant contributions to teaching and learning.

Other experienced clients can help as well, especially those who have successfully changed behaviors or managed a similar condition. For example, a person who successfully managed lifestyle changes after cardiac bypass surgery might be called to talk with a client preparing for the surgery.

Table 13-4 Common Learning Needs and Teaching Strategies Across the Life Span

COMMON AGE-RELATED LEARNING NEEDS	SUGGESTED TEACHING STRATEGIES
INFANTS	
Infant care and nutrition Sleep patterns Preventing diaper rash Maintaining infant safety Growth and development	Teach the parents or other primary caregivers. Consistently role-model appropriate behavior, including nurturing the infant. Use demonstration and return demonstration for infant care skills.
TODDLERS AND PRESCHOOLERS	
Nutrition Dental hygiene Child safety Immunizations	Use age-appropriate language, but do not "talk down" to the child. Give simple instructions. Include the parents to reduce anxiety in the child. Continue to foster parenting skills as needed. Avoid teaching when the child is tired, irritable, or already excessively stimulated. Use teaching aids such as puppets, dolls, picture or coloring books, audiotapes, and appropriate medical supplies. Allow the child to hold favorite toy if possible. Use play as a teaching strategy for preschoolers, recalling that they express feelings through actions and may not fully comprehend the meaning of words. Give the child immediate rewards (such as stickers or toy) for appropriate behavior.
SCHOOL-AGE CHILD	
Nutrition Safety Hygiene Peer socialization	Recall that children at this age understand the use of symbols and can follow simple directions. Assess reading ability before providing written materials. Effective teaching strategies include use of toys, books, and games. Demonstration and role play are other useful strategies, especially because school-age children may seek to do the "right thing" to secure approval.
ADOLESCENTS	
Physiological changes Self-esteem Sexuality and birth control Safety education (automobile, sports) Preventing substance abuse	Recall that peer groups are important, so group teaching sessions are effective unless topic is threatening or could affect self-esteem or the esteem of others. Provide printed materials at appropriate literacy level. Explain benefits of using new information, and correct previously learned misinformation. Understand that this age-group tends to feel invulnerable and may not appreciate that negative health consequences could happen to them.
YOUNG AND MIDDLE ADULTS	
Nutrition and exercise Stress management Sexuality and parenting (young adults) Signs of illness (middle adults)	Use principles of adult learning when conducting teaching. Assess literacy level before providing written materials. Discussion, demonstration, and role play are effective teaching strategies. Recall that young adults have a strong need for independence, whereas middle adults gradually become aware of personal vulnerability.
OLDER ADULTS	
Disease-specific information Maintaining activities of daily living Stress management Loss and grief	Recall that aging does not reduce intelligence but learning may be slower. Principles of adult learning still apply. Teaching aids may be selected to compensate for physical limitations (large-print pamphlets, aids to dexterity). Use discussion and demonstration of skills needed to maintain health (such as blood glucose monitoring); allow opportunities for repeated practice of skills.

INTERVENTION

To implement teaching, you will need to use effective strategies and appropriate learning activities. Teaching content and methodology is documented in the health record as a nursing intervention.

Strategies for Effective Teaching Intervention. As the teacher, your behaviors have a profound influence on the client's ability to learn. By employing the following strategies for effective teaching intervention, you can maximize the learning process.

Select Appropriate Teaching Methods. The teaching method depends on the subject matter and the client's background, personality, and needs. Teaching may involve formal lectures and demonstration, but informal individual or group discussions are more appropriate for most clients in a health care setting.

When using adjunct methods, it is imperative to be available afterward to ask and answer questions and evaluate what clients have learned. Before using print or video teaching aids, verify their content and assess the comprehension level of your audience. For general audiences, a reading level between grade 4 and grade 6 is best. For each client, do your best to provide accurate, current, and relevant information at the level and in the style most likely to meet the person's unique learning needs.

Reward Positive Behaviors. Rewards for correct behaviors reinforce learning. Behaviors that are rewarded are more likely to be repeated, and immediate rewards are better than delayed rewards. For ill clients, rewards tend to involve the following:

- Reduced pain or other symptoms
- Return of a normal or near-normal lifestyle
- Avoidance of complications
- Positive regard from a nurse or physician

> ***Action Alert!*** Compliment immediately when a client asks a thoughtful question, demonstrates something learned, or performs a procedure satisfactorily.

Encourage Active Participation. People learn more effectively when they participate in their health education program. Active participation generates interest; lack of participation generates boredom.

Encourage participation in a number of ways. For instance, when presenting written materials, make sure the client understands by discussing them. Clients who are merely handed a list of instructions may not understand their importance and may or may not follow them. After demonstrating a procedure, ask the client to work through each step with you rather than waiting for a full return demonstration.

Repeat Key Facts and Concepts. Repetition of key facts and concepts reinforces learning. Likewise, practice reinforces new skills. Reviewing materials presented earlier prepares the client for receiving new materials. Encourage your clients to repeat, practice, and review.

Encourage Immediate Practice. Clients retain new information and skills longer when they put them into practice right away. For example, in many obstetric units, it is common practice for new mothers to begin caring for their infants almost immediately. Under supervision, mothers learn how to bathe, feed, and diaper. New mothers are encouraged to practice skills right away, under supervision, instead of being sent home to flounder alone. In contrast, when clients cannot use their knowledge right way, they tend to forget what they have learned.

> ***Action Alert!*** If a client does not have an opportunity to use newly acquired information or skills soon after learning, provide written information for the client to refer to later.

Help the Client Surmount Learning Plateaus. Clients occasionally reach learning plateaus, where it may appear that they have lost interest or even seem discouraged. Remember, however, that learning plateaus are normal. To surmount them, use visual aids, movies, or other stimulating methods of presentation, which give the client a break from structured learning until the previous level of enthusiasm returns.

Negotiate. By actively involving clients in the decision-making process, nurses stimulate clients' motivation to learn. Clients are more apt to be enthusiastic about learning information that they have identified as important to them. Combining client interests with content necessary to reach health care goals makes the teaching and learning process mutually gratifying.

Some clients resist learning. Perhaps they are in denial about the disease process or feel angry at the adjustments needed in their lifestyle. They may also resist for other reasons: they "don't have time," are presently asymptomatic, or lack family support, as examples. For these individuals, contracting may be an effective way to elicit their participation. In a **learning contract,** much like any business contract, each party (nurse and client) agrees to contribute certain things to the contract. The nurse provides information, and the client agrees to use that information.

Mager (1975) states that instruction is effective to the degree that it succeeds in changing behavior in the desired direction. The learning contract helps the client commit to goals to achieve the desired outcomes in the learning situation. The nurse prioritizes the most essential aspects of care within the contract. As times goes by, the contract helps the client experience the satisfaction or reward of accomplishment in learning, and the contract can be changed to include other learning needs.

Learning Activities. Clearly, teaching and learning can take place in many settings. Three of the most important activities for any form of learning are discussion, demonstration, and role-playing.

Discussion. Discussion encourages clients to participate actively in the health education program. You can draw clients into a discussion by asking for a response to something you just taught. For example, you might ask clients to share ways in which the information applies to their life, such as examples of personal experiences or related opinions. In a class for clients receiving radiation treatment, for example, you might ask how they coped with hair loss.

Demonstration. Demonstrations provide the best method for teaching motor skills, such as how to give a self-injection or transfer safely from a bed to a wheelchair. To prepare for a demonstration, complete the following steps:

- Make notes and organize your thoughts so you can narrate your demonstration clearly.

- Obtain the needed equipment, and make sure it works.
- Outline the procedure on a handout so your client can follow along with you.
- Practice the demonstration until you can do it skillfully.

When giving the demonstration, make sure clients can see it clearly. Proceed slowly, allowing questions as you go. Afterward, immediately reinforce learning by having the clients return the demonstration to the best of their ability.

Role-Playing. Role-playing is a creative learning activity in which a person can act as different people (physician, nurse, spouse, employer) in a variety of real-life situations to help clients learn new behaviors or solve problems. Initially, some people may feel shy or embarrassed about role-playing. As they become comfortable, however, they discover that it can be a very effective strategy for gaining new insights in a safe environment. Role-playing can be effective in teaching parenting and other interpersonal skills.

General Teaching Tips. The following helpful teaching strategies can enhance a well-planned teaching session:

- Teach basic information first, and add variations or details later.
- Use a combination of senses (vision, hearing, touch) to enhance learning.
- Consider the client's time orientation.
- Be cautious when using humor.
- Ensure that sensitive or potentially embarrassing procedures (such as self-catheterization of bladder) for adolescents and young adults are taught by a nurse of the same gender.
- Carefully evaluate client nonverbal behavior (smiling, nodding, looking away, as examples).
- Avoid the use of medical jargon.
- Recommend changes that can be implemented at home (do not recommend taking oatmeal baths at home for skin itching if client only has a shower, as an example).

Documentation of Teaching. Use documentation to record progress when teaching is done in multiple sessions. In addition, documentation records the cost-effectiveness of your teaching for quality evaluation, confirms the outcomes of the teaching and learning process, and provides legal material that could be considered in a court of law. As in other areas of nursing, accurate and complete documentation of your teaching is crucial.

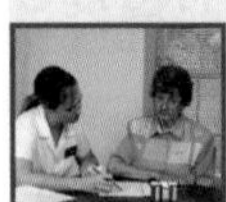

When Mrs. Avery is discharged from the hospital, the nurse writes the following discharge note shown at the top of this page.

SAMPLE DOCUMENTATION NOTE FOR MRS. AVERY

Discharged per wheelchair with granddaughter to automobile. Able to walk in the hall. Has given self insulin correctly with supervision. Referred to home health care agency for follow-up teaching. Has appointment with physician in 1 week.

EVALUATION

Evaluating how well the nurse and the client have met teaching and learning goals is an important part of the teaching and learning process. Remember that it is important to develop learning objectives in terms of behaviors and measurable outcomes *before* beginning the teaching and learning process. Then, after the program, you can evaluate its success by determining how well the client has made positive life changes. Ideally, evaluation should determine that *learning has occurred* and that you were effective as a teacher. If discrepancies exist between the desired and actual outcomes, systematic problem solving can help to rectify them and strengthen the teaching and learning process even more (see Box 13-3).

Action Alert! Be aware that, to ensure the client's learning needs are met, you may need to modify the original teaching plan on the basis of the evaluation results.

Evaluation of Teaching. Evaluation of the teaching process measures whether the short-term learning goals have been met and whether the knowledge results in long-term behavioral changes. Evaluation also examines the effects of the change in behavior on health status and whether resources used to produce the change in health status are the most cost-effective method of treatment.

Short-Term Goals. Ask yourself a variety of questions to determine whether short-term learning has occurred and is being acted on. These may include the following:

- Has the client been given the necessary information for a safe discharge?
- Has the client accomplished the learning objectives?
- Can the client demonstrate proficiency in the skills needed for self-care?
- Is there a measurable difference in the client's attitude about the highest level of health attainable?
- Can the client cope with limitations imposed by the illness?
- Does the client show a willingness to make necessary lifestyle changes?
- Do the client's significant others understand the client's problems and demonstrate readiness to provide appropriate support?

Long-Term Goals. If you focus only on evaluation of short-term learning (i.e., what a client learns before discharge), you will neglect the importance of long-term changes in behavior. The client, the facility staff, the outpatient nurse, and the physician all share responsibility for reinforcing long-term learning and evaluating its success over time.

Long-term evaluation may involve follow-up questionnaires or telephone calls at selected intervals after discharge. This method allows clients to demonstrate the success of learning in a real-life situation. Many times, when clients are in a health care facility and away from the demands of everyday living, they assume that a behavioral change will be easy to implement. However, the ideal is seldom encountered at home or in the workplace. Additional learning, problem solving, and creativity may be necessary to integrate the desired change at home. In contrast, in the relaxed and familiar home environment, the person may discover a readiness to learn that was not present during the stress of the institutional environment. For these reasons, the primary nurse seeks to understand the "big picture" when encountering the client post discharge. Questions that may be helpful include, "How have you been managing with. . . since you came home?" or "What has been the most challenging part of coming home from the hospital?"

Realize that short-term outcomes may differ from the long-term reality. Clients may "know" what is needed at discharge but forget or neglect that need over time, especially if they lack support or reinforcement. Long-term follow-up can renew information learned in the hospital. By reinforcing what was previously learned, the primary care nurse in the community provides continuity and promotes retention of learning.

Evaluation of Learning. Helpful methods to evaluate a client's learning include discussion, oral tests, written tests, and return demonstration. Testing should be fun, easy, and nonthreatening. It should give the client positive reinforcement that learning has occurred, rather than focusing on what needs to be learned. In client education, testing can be as much a teaching tool as an evaluation process.

Discussion. The discussion method is used to review what has been learned. Review three or four main points. Ask the client questions to evaluate whether learning has occurred. Observe the client's comfort level with the information, and evaluate the client's ability to apply the information to the health care concern and, as a result, change the behavior.

Oral Tests. Oral testing requires preparation on your part and can be quite time consuming because it is accomplished one-to-one with the client. Large-group oral testing may be ineffective because not all clients are able to answer. If a client has trouble articulating answers, outcomes are difficult to evaluate.

Oral testing can be beneficial when a reading level cannot be matched to a written test or the client has visual deficits. The desired outcome is for the client to verbalize the key points and to apply the knowledge.

Written Tests. Written tests prepared for individuals or groups require that clients be able to read. They can be in the form of multiple choice, true-or-false, matching, or essay questions. They require a space that is quiet, comfortable, and conducive to thinking, because they ask the client to recall teaching. The goal of written testing is to reflect what the client has learned and give the client a sense of satisfaction. Written test items should be piloted and analyzed for clarity and relevance before administration to the client. This reduces the likelihood of confusion and frustration for the client and increases the validity of test results.

Return Demonstration. Return demonstration is an excellent means of evaluating a skill or task. After you demonstrate the skill or task, ask the client to return, or mirror, the skill. Giving the client written steps or instructions along with the demonstration enhances recall when the demonstration is finished. The desired outcome is for the client to perform all the steps independently without error.

▼ KEY PRINCIPLES

- Nursing standards for practice and agency accreditation standards include client education. They assume that clients have a right to information and that nurses have a legal mandate to provide it.
- In addition to the client's right to information, client education benefits health care through cost control and quality control.
- The purposes of client education are to promote health, prevent illness, restore health, and help clients cope with illness.
- Learning theorists have identified three primary domains of learning: cognitive, affective, and psychomotor.
- Client characteristics affecting teaching are literacy, level of education, developmental level, and learning style.
- Readiness to learn and motivation facilitate learning.
- The client must be physically and psychologically able to learn.
- Cultural and environmental factors can affect learning.
- The ability of the nurse as an educator affects learning positively or negatively.
- *Deficient knowledge* is diagnosed when the client lacks knowledge of health management practices that are necessary to achieve or maintain health.
- Other nursing diagnoses commonly used for client education are *Ineffective health maintenance, Health-seeking behaviors,* and *Ineffective coping*.
- Planning to teach includes selecting topics, developing a teaching plan, and writing learning objectives.
- Although most client teaching is one-to-one instruction, many teaching methods are available to maximize efficiency and effectiveness.
- Strategies for effective implementation include selecting appropriate teaching methods, rewarding positive behaviors, encouraging active participation, repeating key facts and concepts, encouraging immediate feedback, helping the client surmount learning plateaus, and negotiating.

Continued

- Evaluation of learning requires evaluating both the short-term goal of acquiring knowledge and the long-term goal of changing behavior.
- The method of evaluation should reinforce learning.

■ REVIEW QUESTIONS

1. When preparing a teaching plan for a client with heart disease, the nurse would complete which of the following as the first step?
1. Develop a teaching plan
2. Write learning outcomes
3. Formulate a nursing diagnosis
4. Assess the client's learning needs

2. When a client needs to learn information to manage a newly diagnosed health problem, the most common nursing diagnosis for the nurse to consider is which of the following?
1. Ineffective health maintenance
2. Deficient knowledge
3. Noncompliance
4. Ineffective therapeutic regimen management

3. Which of the following learning objectives is the most appropriate for a client who needs to learn how to use a walker for assistance with ambulation?
1. Asks for assistance before ambulating with a walker
2. Asks questions about how to use a walker by end of shift
3. Ambulates 25 feet with walker independently by end of shift
4. Ambulates length of hall with walker without falling

4. The nurse would choose individual instruction over group teaching under which of the following circumstances?
1. A need to pace the flow of information according to learning needs
2. A need to be economical with teaching time
3. When there is a need to deliver large amounts of factual information
4. When teaching would be aided by sharing with clients who have similar problems

5. The nurse has just taught a 50-year-old client newly diagnosed with diabetes mellitus how to check blood glucose. The nurse would optimally evaluate the client's learning through which of the following methods?
1. Posttest
2. Oral quiz
3. Return demonstration
4. Discussion

Bibliography

*American Hospital Association. (1975). *A patient's bill of rights.* Chicago: Author.

American Hospital Association. (2003). *Patient care partnership: Understanding expectations, rights, and responsibilities.* Chicago: Author.

Bass, L. (2005). Health literacy: Implications for teaching the adult patient. *Journal of Infusion Nursing, 28*(1), 15-22, 68-71.

Bastable, S. B. (2003). *Nurse as educator* (2nd ed.). Boston: Jones & Bartlett.

*Bloom, B. J. (1956). *Taxonomy of educational objectives, Book 1. Cognitive domain.* New York: Longman.

*Bloom, B. J., Englehart, M. S., Furst, E. J., Hill, W. H., & Krathwohl, D. R. (1956). *Taxonomy of educational objectives: The classification of educational goals, Handbook 1. Cognitive domain.* New York: David McKay.

Boswell, C., Cannon, S., Aung, K., & Eldridge, J. (2004). An application of health literacy research. *Applied Nursing Research, 17*(1), 61-64.

Boyington, A.R., Dougherty, M.C., & Phetrasuwan, S. (2005). Effectiveness of a computer-based system to deliver a continence health promotion intervention. *Journal of Wound and Ostomy Care Nursing, 32*(4), 246-254.

Chai, K. (2004). *JCAHO patient education requirements: 2004 and beyond.* Glendale, CA: CINAHL Information Systems.

Forrest, S. (2004). Learning and teaching: the reciprocal link. *Journal of Continuing Education in Nursing, 35*(2), 74-79.

*Johnson, M., Bulechek, G., McCloskey, Dochterman, J., Mass, M., & Moorhead, S. (2006). *Nursing diagnoses, outcomes, & interventions: NANDA, NOC, and NIC linkages.* St. Louis, MO: Mosby.

*Knowles, M. (1980). *The adult learner: A neglected species* (2nd ed.). Houston: Gulf.

Leino-Kilpi, H., Johansson, K., Heikkinen, K., Kaljonen, A., Virtanen, H., & Salanterä, S. (2005). Patient education and health-related quality of life: Surgical hospital patients as a case in point. *Journal of Nursing Care Quality, 20*(4), 307-318.

*Mager, R. F. (1975). *Preparing instructional objectives* (2nd ed.). Belmont, CA: Fearon-Pitman.

NANDA International. (2007). *Nursing diagnoses: Definitions and classification 2006-2007.* Philadelphia: Author.

NANDA International (NANDA-I). (2007). *Nursing diagnoses: Definitions & Classification, 2006-2007.* Philadelphia: NANDA-I.

National Center for Educational Statistics. (2005). *NAAL: A first look at the literacy of America's adults in the 21st century.* Retrieved from http://www.nifl.gov/.

Nettles, A.T. (2005). Patient education in the hospital. *Diabetes Spectrum, 18*(1), 44-48.

Oermann, M. H. (2003). Using health web sites for patient education. *Journal of Wound and Ostomy Care Nursing, 30*(4), 217-223.

Olinzock, B. J. (2004). A model for assessing learning readiness for self-direction of care in individuals with spinal cord injuries: A qualitative study. *Spinal Cord Injury Nursing, 21*(2), 69-74.

Piredda, M. (2004). Patient education: A concept analysis. *International Nursing Perspectives, 4*(2), 63-71.

Smith, C. E., Koehler, J., Moore, J. M., Blanchard, E., & Ellerbeck, E. (2005). Testing videotape education for heart failure. *Clinical Nursing Research, 14*(2), 191-205.

*U.S. Department of Health and Human Services. (2006). *Healthy people 2010.* Retrieved October 13, 2006 from http://www.healthypeople.gov.

Valente, S. M. (2005). Evaluation of innovative research-based fact sheets. *Journal for Nurses in Staff Development, 21*(4), 171-176.

Weston-Eborn, R., & Sitzman, K. (2005). The teaching corner. Creating teaching plans for the adult learner. *Home Healthcare Nurse, 23*(3), 192-194.

Weston-Eborn, R., & Sitzman, K. (2005). The teaching corner. Selecting effective instructional resources. *Home Healthcare Nurse, 23*(6), 402-403.

*Asterisk indicates a classic or definitive work on this subject.

Chapter 14

MANAGING CLIENT CARE

Media Resources

- evolve Evolve Website http://evolve.elsevier.com/Harkreader/
- Companion CD

Learning Objectives

After studying this chapter, you should be able to do the following:

- Describe the impact of organizational philosophy on the structure and methods of communication in nursing practice in a complex health care agency
- Distinguish between nursing as a leadership role and as a management role in a health care agency
- Describe the organization of nursing service as a means to providing quality client care
- Describe the impact of change management, risk management, and conflict management on client care
- Identify the role of the nurse in a collaborative health care team

Key Terms

accountability
authority
change-of-shift report
concurrent audit
continuous quality improvement (CQI)
delegation
for-profit
leadership
management
non-profit
not-for-profit
nurse manager
peer review
performance appraisal
policy
primary nursing
procedure
protocol
quality assurance
responsibility
retrospective audit
risk management
standards of practice
standards of professional performance
team nursing
total client care
transactional leadership
transformational leadership

Because approximately 60% of nurses are employed in acute care hospitals, a major setting for nursing practice is a complex, business-oriented health care organization. In this setting, nursing is challenged to fulfill the professional values associated with caring for people. Nursing is a service profession that gives care through providing one-on-one practical help and meeting the unique and holistic health needs of the client. To be effective in providing quality nursing care in a health care organization, nurses need to understand the system and use it effectively to provide leadership in meeting the needs of the clients.

Nursing is a leadership role in a health care agency whether the nurse manages care by working one-to-one with the client, by coordinating the care with other providers, by delegating aspects of the care to others, or by providing leadership to a team of providers. Nursing leadership derives its power from nurses' unique role in the health care setting: nurses have a 24-hour relationship with the client and are concerned with the client's comprehensive needs. They have overall **responsibility** for care (the obligation to act or direct actions of others to accomplish a goal). In addition, nursing leadership includes the role of an advocate for clients and families.

The leadership role of nursing in the health care organization is perhaps most visibly identified with the role of the nurse manager. **Nurse manager** usually refers to a nurse's role in organizational management as nurse executive, middle manager, and first-line manager of nursing services (Table 14-1). First-line managers are identified with the direct delivery of care (Figure 14-1). However, all nurse management roles share the goal of providing quality service to meet the client's needs. Nurse managers have **accountability** for their respective units; that is, they are answerable for personal actions and the actions of other nursing staff.

Management can be thought of as the implementation of strategies that promote effective and efficient use of resources to meet goals. The goal at all levels of nursing service is to provide high-quality nursing care in a cost-effective manner. This definition of management can also be applied to managers of direct client care—for example, the staff nurse.

The leadership and management roles involved in a staff nurse position are evident when the nurse is working with a nursing team, coordinating with other departments, delegating to team members, collaborating with

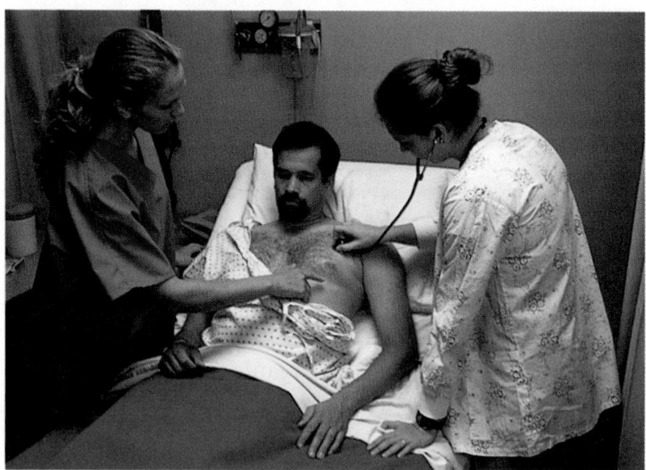

FIGURE 14-1 First-line managers are identified with the actual delivery of care. Here, a first-line manager works side-by-side with a staff nurse, giving direct care to a client.

Table 14-1 Characteristics of Nurse Managers at Different Levels

LEVEL	TITLE	PREPARATION/EXPERIENCE	TASKS
First-line manager	• Team leader • Case manager • Charge nurse	• RN • 1 to 2 years of nursing experience	• Manage client care • Supervise team members • Know status of all clients • Know all team members' roles
Middle manager	• Unit manager • Supervisor	• RN • BSN or MSN preferred • 1 to 5 years of nursing experience	• Supervise nurses and ancillary staff • 24-hour accountability • Manage resources • Motivate others • Act as change agent • Manage quality • Manage budgets • Manage risk
Nurse executive	• Director of nursing • Vice president for nursing • Nursing CEO	• RN • MSN or PhD in allied health preferred • Management experience	• Operationalize nursing • Provide resources • Facilitate quality care • Facilitate efficiency • Manage financial aspects of nursing care

RN, Registered nurse; *BSN,* bachelor of science in nursing; *MSN,* master of science in nursing; *PhD,* doctor of philosophy; *CEO,* chief executive officer.

the physician and other health care providers, and being an advocate for the client. The staff nurse is the person who most directly influences the quality of care received by the client.

Therefore you need to understand the context of the health care organization, what it means to be a leader, the qualities needed by nurses who manage client care, the role of the nurse manager at the organizational level, and the organizational patterns of nursing units.

THE HEALTH CARE ORGANIZATION

Nursing care is usually delivered within a health care agency that has an organizational structure for the delivery of health services. In addition to nursing services, the health care agency provides pharmacy services, diagnostic services, medical services, food services, and housekeeping services. A complex organizational structure, or social system, exists for the purpose of coordinating these departments to ensure that the client receives needed services in a timely manner. The organizational structure varies with the services provided and the size of the organization. Whether the agency is a hospital, nursing home, clinic, or home health care agency, a nurse plans and delivers care within an organizational framework designed to effectively and efficiently meet the needs of its clients.

Therefore, the delivery of nursing care must be understood within the context of the philosophy of the institution; how the philosophy is translated into goals, policies, and procedures; and the management style of its leaders. Also, the health care organization's definition of itself and the product it intends to deliver guides development of the parameters for quality care within the agency.

PHILOSOPHY AND MISSION

The philosophy of an organization states the values and beliefs that underlie the delivery of services. When a philosophy is effectively implemented, it is reflected in the services provided and the methods of providing services; it permeates the organization from the top down and from the bottom up. The philosophy may be communicated through a mission statement that clarifies the agency's commitment to the public. A philosophy may be developed from the rationale for establishing an agency. Therefore it may be concerned with providing access to care, providing quality care, meeting community needs, or making a profit (cost-effectiveness).

A philosophy of providing access to care means ensuring that services are readily available and easily accessible to the clients to be served. A hospital may be established to provide access to health care in a town where the residents would otherwise have to travel a long distance to receive services, or to provide services for an indigent population. For example, a small rural hospital may decide that its role is to provide basic services, but it provides links to larger metropolitan hospitals for more advanced levels of care.

Providing quality care can mean the latest technology, personalized care, well-coordinated services, or high standards for care. For example, a heart hospital may be established to provide all cardiac care services at one location, thus improving the quality of cardiac care in the community. On the other hand, the mission statement of a home health care agency may define quality through expression of the value of maintaining independence and functional ability of older adult residents in the community.

The philosophy of a health care organization may be to meet a community need. For example, a hospital may be established to provide for the specific needs of women. Or a community with a problem of overcrowded emergency departments might establish minor emergency or urgent care facilities to serve clients who do not need full emergency department services.

Regardless of the values that underlie a health care agency's philosophy, in today's environment of managed care, both cost and quality care are driving forces. An institution may include in its philosophy that health care is a business and that cost-efficiency is an important component. Some hospitals are **for-profit,** meaning that the agency exists to make a profit. In a competitive marketplace, a for-profit institution can be expected to provide quality care. A **not-for-profit** hospital may make a profit but does not exist for that purpose. The profit is often returned to the institution to maintain or upgrade equipment or to meet other needs. A **nonprofit** hospital does not make a profit and may be supported by charitable donations or taxes. However, any of these types of agencies is concerned with cost control.

The philosophy of a department of nursing reflects the values of the institution and further defines the values of nursing in that institution. These values direct nursing behavior and serve as the basis for determining the means to accomplish nursing services. When nursing values are apparent in the institutional philosophy, the organization is more likely to have a commitment to professional values and the development of nursing.

GOALS AND OBJECTIVES

Goals are the means to ensuring that the values expressed in the philosophy are upheld in the delivery of services. In other words, goals express the philosophy in more specific terms. For example, the home health care agency designed to maintain independent living for older adults may have a goal of increasing the independence of its clients. A goal for a major medical center is to provide state-of-the-art technology to improve the survival of certain client populations. Objectives are more specific plans to implement goals. A specific objective would be to obtain or develop the technology to improve the survival of burn victims.

POLICIES AND PROCEDURES

Objectives become the guidelines for establishing policies and procedures. Organizations develop policies and procedures on the basis of standards of practice and standards of client care. A **policy** is a set of rules and regulations that govern nursing practice and nursing care. Policies may pertain to clients, such as the client's bill of rights, or to the nursing staff, such as the staff's employment, duties, and assignments. Staff policies include staffing patterns, staff mix (the relative number of registered nurses [RNs], licensed practical nurses [LPNs] or licensed vocational nurses [LVNs], and nursing assistants), attendance, sick leave, chemical dependency, incident reports, and floating to other units.

A **procedure** is a detailed description of a specific method of accomplishing a task or performing nursing care. Procedural guidelines, such as medication administration, insertion of nasogastric tubes or urinary catheters, and isolation, are published in a procedure manual. The procedure manual describes who is responsible for performing the procedures, what equipment or supplies are necessary, and what information should be assessed and documented, as well as guidelines for how to perform the procedure.

A **protocol** contains detailed guidelines for nursing care for clients with specific conditions or medical treatment. For example, protocols may be developed for alcohol withdrawal, cardiac catheterization, fall risk, skin risk, restraints, surgical client management, and chest pain. Protocols are also developed to allow nurses to perform procedures beyond the usual scope of nursing practice. For example, the critical care unit may develop a protocol that specifies how the nurse can treat life-threatening arrhythmias before the physician arrives. This protocol defines life-threatening arrhythmia, the dosage and frequency of medications or treatments to be used, the staff responsible for administering the medication or treatment, and the assessment and documentation to be done.

Nurse managers with input from staff nurses have an important role in developing and implementing policies, procedures, and protocols, as well as in monitoring and measuring the success of carrying out the institutional mission. Nurses must monitor nursing's role in the provision of health care to demonstrate that nursing care is appropriate, safe, effective, and efficient.

EXTERNAL STANDARDS

In addition to the organization's philosophy and mission, the policies and procedures of a health care organization are also influenced by external standards. Two major examples are The Joint Commission (TJC) and the American Nurses Association (ANA).

TJC Standards. Policies and procedures are often derived from the standards of TJC. TJC accredits health care organizations, which is not only prestigious but also necessary for them to continue to receive federal funds, for example. Although TJC is a voluntary accreditation organization, federal and state regulatory agencies and insurance carriers require that health care organizations be accredited by TJC to be certified, to be licensed, or to receive reimbursement.

TJC evaluates each health care organization every 3 years. The extent of an organization's compliance with TJC standards determines the organization's accreditation status. In the past, accreditation indicated that an organization had the capability to provide quality care. However, the public demands the evaluation of actual performance, or outcome information, instead of potential capability. Thus TJC continuously improves and revises its standards so that an organization's accreditation reflects its actual performance of quality care (TJC, 2006).

During the accreditation process TJC examines the organization's performance in *doing the right thing* and *doing the right thing well.* The characteristics of doing the right thing are efficacy and appropriateness. The characteristics of doing the right thing *well* are availability, effectiveness, timeliness, safety, efficiency, continuity, respect, and caring. TJC believes that the organization demonstrating these characteristics is more likely to provide high-quality care with optimal client outcomes and efficient resource use.

ANA Standards. The ANA published the first standards of practice for the nursing profession in 1973. These standards defined the nursing professional's accountability to the public and described the nursing professional's responsibilities. To clarify the nature and scope of nursing practice, the ANA revised and elaborated on the original standards in 1991, 1998, 2004 (see Appendix A). The revisions addressed two dimensions: standards of practice and standards of professional performance.

Standards of practice describe a "competent level of nursing care as demonstrated by the critical thinking model known as the nursing process" (ANA, 2004). The elements of the nursing process are crucial to a systematic decision-making process intended to result in logical, reasonable, and client-centered decisions.

Standards of professional performance are defined as "authoritative statements that describe a competent level of behavior in the professional role, including activities related to quality of care, performance appraisal, education, collegiality, ethics, collaboration, research, and resource utilization" (ANA, 2004). Appendix A lists behaviors that demonstrate the standards of professional performance (ANA, 2004).

NURSES AS LEADERS AND MANAGERS

All nurses should strive to be leaders in the health care setting. However, only a few nurses are interested in a management role in the organization.

LEADERSHIP ROLE

Leadership is a means of shaping the future through influencing others to change direction in thinking or acting. Leadership differs from management in that leadership empowers the followers with a vision and the desire to achieve high goals. It includes activities or interactions that provide a sense of direction toward goal achievement, coaching and mentoring, and demonstrating proactive behaviors. A leader on a nursing unit will listen to the concerns of colleagues and provide feedback to help the person manage stressful situations or improve nursing care. Role modeling as a leadership strategy can involve dress, language, and social skills as well as excellence in nursing techniques and communication with clients. You do not have to be a nurse manager to be a leader in providing quality care.

Successful nurse managers employ leadership skills to increase their effectiveness as managers. Managers incorporate leadership strategies to further an organization's objectives by using interpersonal interactions that inspire others to work toward those goals. Whereas management involves implementing strategies to accomplish organizational goals, leadership involves showing others the way, directing others in a course of action, going ahead of others, or going with and inspiring others.

Theories of leadership incorporate communication skills, understanding of group process, and a vision for health care as the means to effect group movement in a specific direction. Leaders use open, honest, clear, and concise communication. They listen actively and use group process to build consensus and stimulate enthusiasm for projects. Nurse leaders understand the importance of their work, and they incorporate the values of the profession in all aspects of it.

Because the position of a nurse manager involves inspiring others to work, all nurse managers should be leaders. However, leaders can do the work of inspiring others from any position. A nurse may be a leader among a group of peers, influencing the way the group goes about the daily activities of providing for clients. Leaders work to create change that benefits clients throughout the health care industry. Leadership qualities are an essential component of the effective nurse's storehouse of strategies for promoting health. Leadership style can be either transactional or transformational (Table 14-2).

Transactional leadership seeks to motivate others through a cost-benefit, economic exchange in which followers' material and psychic needs are met in return for services rendered by the follower. Transactional leaders use a contingent reward for a desired behavior approach to management. Workers are given clear expectations of the desired behaviors and the rewards for those behaviors.

Transformational leadership seeks to motivate others by inspiration, arousing and satisfying higher needs, thus engaging the full person of the follower and stimulating intellectual growth while considering individual needs for support, encouragement, and developmental experiences. In transformational leadership, the leader shares a vision and a sense of mission and shows respect and confidence by trusting the employee to act in a way consistent with the mission (Figure 14-2). Although the transformational

Table 14-2 Styles of Leadership Communication

TRANSFORMATIONAL	TRANSACTIONAL
Empowers, values, and trusts employees; lets go of things others can do	Views giving reward for expected behaviors as motivation
Focuses on goal attainment, both individual and corporate	Focuses on expected behaviors
Shares responsibility and accountability	May be authoritarian
Facilitates participation; encourages initiative, ideas, and risk taking	Demands or coerces
Encourages discussion	Tells
Encourages staff input	Makes rules and rewards compliance
Uses data to solve problems	May punish; does not always mention the punishment, but it is inherent
Delegates to challenge, develop, and empower	Talks; creates clear structures whereby it is clear what is required of subordinates and the rewards that they get for following orders
Listens	Monitors and watches
Observes; coaches to ensure success	Imposes rules
Communicates beliefs	Demands results
Communicates expectations; shares information, knowledge, and skills	Dictates; expects actions even without full knowledge of the situation
Gives factual messages	
Encourages dependency	
Has positive attitude	
Rewards contributions; positive reinforcement for a job well done	
Builds consensus	Expects consensus

leader may recognize and respond to the transactional needs of followers, the transformational model appeals to the need for self-actualization.

Empowerment is one of the most important influences transformational leaders have on followers. Retention rates for nurses (Bethune, Sherrod, & Youngblood, 2005) are higher when there is shared leadership or shared governance. Shared leadership is a form of stewardship based on trust. Shared **authority,** control, decision making, and accountability increase the staff nurse's investment in quality of care and point-of-care decisions, as well as job satisfaction, compared to traditional leadership. Nursing staff are more likely to assume responsibility for developing work processes to enable delivery of quality client care (Shiparski, 2005).

Transformational nurse managers actively seek employee input about policies and procedures rather than imposing rules without regard for their applicability. They maintain a positive attitude toward work and try to create a satisfying work environment. Responsibilities are shared rather than imposed. They trust that others are motivated to produce and capable of achieving a quality product. And they can risk their sense of control, or authority, in the interest of promoting a cohesive work unit.

ROLES OF MANAGERS

The roles filled by a nurse manager result largely from the responsibilities incurred at various levels of the organization's hierarchy. In general, however, those roles involve managing quality of care, budgets, and personnel.

Managing Quality. **Quality assurance** refers to the process of achieving excellence in the service rendered to every client. A quality assurance program is based on a clear definition of quality and the reliable and valid outcomes used to measure it. Although the current trend in health care is toward cost containment, the goal is to achieve this without reducing the quality of client services. Managing quality means accentuating positive outcomes as well as avoiding negative outcomes.

Three main steps are involved in quality assurance activities. First, each nursing unit selects aspects of care to represent the standards for care, criteria for achievement of the standards, and methods of monitoring. Second, the nursing unit collects and analyzes data to determine compliance with the criteria. Third, the unit seeks ways to improve compliance with the criteria.

Retrospective audits and concurrent audits are used to conduct quality assurance activities. The **retrospective audit** is an evaluation method that uses an after-the-fact review of the medical record for documented evidence of compliance with the standards. This method requires less time than a concurrent audit and thus is used most often by the health care organization. The **concurrent audit** is an evaluation method to inspect the nursing staff's compliance with predetermined standards and criteria while the nurses are providing care. The auditor compares the performance against other nurses' performance and over time.

Generally, each organization designates responsibilities for conducting an audit to the quality assurance staff, the head nurse, the charge nurse, or the nurse educator. However, a peer review approach in which every member of the nursing staff is involved in auditing for quality of care is a growing trend (Figure 14-3).

As an example of the retrospective audit method, suppose a nursing unit has established a criterion that 90% of clients in restraints will be checked every hour. Every member of the nursing staff randomly selects and examines three charts per month to determine if the documentation complies with the criterion. Thus, if less than 90% of the charts comply with the standard, the unit will analyze the causes of substandard performance. Reasons for not performing according to the standards, and ways to improve compliance, will be identified.

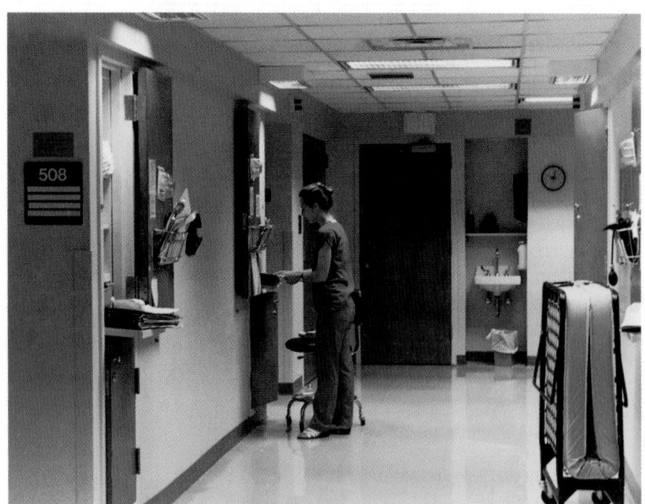

FIGURE 14-2 Employees who feel trusted will behave more responsibly. This nurse is working independently to help accomplish the organization's mission.

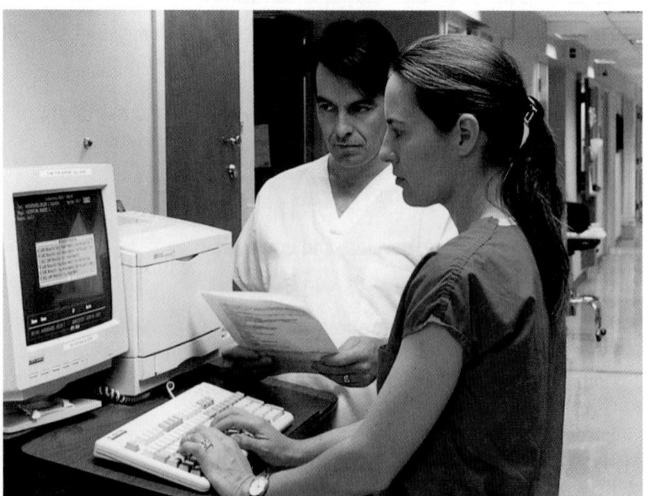

FIGURE 14-3 Recently, nursing staff members have become involved in auditing the performance of other staff members through the review of client records.

The concurrent audit method is often used to evaluate nursing staff during their orientation period. When new nurses are performing intravenous therapy, for example, they are expected to find the nurse educator or a mentor nurse who can observe their performance and ensure that it meets the standard of intravenous therapy.

Because quality assurance activities require tedious, comprehensive evaluation of documentation to show compliance with standards, there may be a delayed impact on quality of care. Thus quality assurance activities have been gradually replaced with continuous quality improvement activities. **Continuous quality improvement (CQI)** is a systematic approach to control and improve quality from the perspective of both professionals and clients. It is also called *total quality improvement* or *total quality management.* It incorporates professionals' and clients' perspectives of quality to set desirable outcomes and uses statistical methods to measure processes of care and outcomes. And it requires the relevant health care personnel to continuously improve processes of care to achieve predetermined outcomes. CQI is based on two main assumptions: (1) quality can always be improved, and (2) the health care delivery system often prevents health care providers from providing quality care. Thus CQI works on the system to improve the quality of care. When predetermined outcomes are not achieved, all relevant health care personnel work together to identify the problems and to seek ways to improve the system until desirable outcomes are achieved.

Managing Budgets. Cost containment is a major goal in health care today and affects all health care practitioners. The challenge for nurses is to balance the value of nursing and the quality of care with the cost of providing care, while continuing to fulfill our obligation to be client advocates.

Nurse managers strive to ensure the highest quality care at the lowest possible cost. As health care costs have risen, third-party payers have become more vigilant about requiring justification for expenditures. In addition, private, for-profit health care agencies are in business to make a profit and must answer to investors when they do not realize that profit. Therefore, they are extremely cautious about the expenditures that they are willing to incur while providing care.

Agencies that pay for health care (such as managed care organizations) expect health care providers, including nurses, to document evidence of the necessity of all services provided to a client. Nurse managers also must justify the number and types of staff, the supplies, and the equipment needed to produce quality health care. In short, they must provide a reasoned argument that quality nursing care is being delivered in the most efficient way possible.

Managing Personnel. Nurse managers are responsible for hiring and evaluating performance of the nursing staff. Managing personnel includes coaching, counseling, staff development, and education to assist the personnel in developing their skills.

A **performance appraisal** is an organized and uniform method of evaluation of a nurse's job contribution, quality of work, and potential for advancement, made by the nurse's supervisor. Performance appraisals focus on each staff member's consistent compliance with standards. They may be used formally or informally to identify performance strengths and areas for improvement. Often the results of a performance appraisal are used to determine promotion, selection, termination, or a pay raise. When appraisals indicate that a nurse consistently fails to comply with standards, the nurse's performance is deficient; counseling and more frequent evaluation may be needed.

The process of performance appraisal varies with each organization. The organization defines a job description for its staff on the basis of institutional standards, and then it conducts regular reviews of employees based on the job description. The process of performance appraisal must be described in the policy and procedure manual (JCAHO, 2006).

Each organization determines how each staff member should be evaluated. In general, nurses are expected to perform self-evaluation according to the institution's performance appraisal form. The nursing supervisor uses the same form to evaluate nurses' performance. Some organizations may also require each nurse to perform peer reviews. A **peer review** is the evaluation of the performance of one staff member by another staff member to judge the quality of care provided.

Managing Communication. Communication is a key element of an empowering leadership style; it facilitates all other management activities. It is a process of giving and receiving messages for the purpose of transmitting or exchanging information. An empowering nurse manager can communicate goals, delegate responsibilities and authority, coach, and inspire others through words and actions. Table 14-3 provides examples of empowering communication.

An empowering manager can also obtain information by being an active listener and an acute observer to understand behavior from the perspective of the employee. Rather than accusing, empowering nurse managers state an observation and discuss alternatives. They listen to concerns and discuss alternative solutions without creating a defensive posture.

An empowering communicator uses messages that indicate personal ownership of beliefs, values, and needs. For example, the person says, "I want" or "I need" rather than "you must" or "you didn't." An empowering manager also communicates beliefs and expectations about values and goals. This approach promotes group participation rather than imposing values and coercing work.

An empowering communicator structures messages to make them more understandable and to facilitate clear communication. Jargon and abbreviations, especially when communicating with people from other disciplines, can lead to misinterpretation or confusion. Factual messages, using appropriate details rather than

Table 14-3 Empowering Communication Techniques

EFFECTIVE MESSAGES	LESS EFFECTIVE MESSAGES
"I observed that you were able to manage your clients' care today, but that you have to stay past work hours to complete your nurse's notes most days. I believe that work assignments should be set up in a way that lets us complete all of our duties within the scheduled work time. Is there something that we can do to help you accomplish that goal?"	"You never get your nurse's notes written during your shift. You need to get organized so you can get them done on time. I won't pay you overtime for notes anymore." OR "I'll have Mary Jane change your assignment since you always have to stay overtime to finish your nurse's notes."
"Our client census is at a peak right now with some acutely ill clients. We are going to need one more nurse than usual for the next three shifts. These are the options available to us. . . ."	"I need three nurses to work overtime with the way the census is running. This is the new staffing schedule." OR "Can anybody work an extra shift to cover the increased census? My husband told me that he won't tolerate my covering all of the extra shifts for the unit any more."
"The team worked well together on this project. Through your efforts, we accomplished the changes in client outcomes that we needed."	"Lucky for you guys we met our goals somehow."

global emotion-laden metaphors empower the listener to interpret the meaning of the facts. Emotional messages will get an emotional response rather than constructive analysis of the information.

Managing Conflict. Conflict in the work place occurs when two or more values, perspectives, and opinions are present in a work group. Conflict is inevitable and often a productive route to getting the most out of diverse values, perspectives, and opinions. It is healthy when it helps to analyze problems, energizes work on the most appropriate issues, motivates people to participate, and helps people learn how to recognize and benefit from their differences. Conflict is a problem when it is used to attain power over others, gets in the way of productivity, damages self-esteem, or leads to inappropriate behaviors.

When effectively managed, conflict leads to new ideas and growth. The five steps in conflict management are analyzing the conflict, determining management strategy, prenegotiation, negotiation, and postnegotiation.

Analysis is an information-gathering process to determine the factors in the conflict. Choice of a management strategy depends on this analysis. In the collaborative management strategy the objective is to reach consensus resulting in a win-win situation for everyone. In the compromise strategy the outcome is "win some/lose some." Compromise may be best in the interest of time or avoiding power struggles as long as important values and long-term objectives are not compromised. Competition is often destructive because the outcome is "win/lose." Accommodation is appealing when the stakes are high for some, but not for others. This "lose/win" strategy may result in failure to consider important issues. In avoidance the outcome is "lose/lose" because the conflict is ignored because it seems trivial or other matters seems more important.

In the prenegotiation stage the process is initiated and assessment is done through joint fact finding. Ground rules should be established and the group organized. During negotiation all the interests, needs, concerns and motivations should be heard by concentrating on inventing options for satisfying interests without judgment of ideas. The options should not be discussed until multiple options are laid out. By documenting areas of agreement and disagreement the group can ensure common understanding of the problem. The group should discuss and agree upon methods to ensure partners understand and will honor their commitments. The last phase—postnegotiation—is often neglected, which renders the process ineffective. The change should be monitored while continuing to ensure communication and collaboration as the agreement is carried out.

ORGANIZATION OF NURSING UNITS

When you start to work on a nursing unit, you need to understand the pattern of organizing the work of the unit. Each unit has its own method of organizing and working together as a team. The best method is the one that is efficient and produces the outcomes of quality client care as defined by the nurses on that unit. Basic methods of organizing exist: functional, team, total client care, and primary nursing assignments. All methods are some variation on these forms.

PATTERNS OF WORK

Perhaps the most efficient form of nursing unit organization is also the oldest method—functional nursing. It focuses on getting the work done in a timely manner. Using this method, tasks are assigned to the individual members of the team who possess the knowledge and skill to accomplish them. One nurse may give medication; another may change dressings and administer treatments. Usually, giving baths and making beds is assigned to the least skilled member of the team. Although this method of making assignments is efficient in terms of getting the tasks done, it has fallen into disfavor because it tends to fragment care: no one person assumes responsibility for total client care.

Team nursing overcomes some of the disadvantages of functional nursing while retaining the ability to effectively use multiple levels of personnel. **Team nursing** is more a concept than a specific pattern for organizing a work group. In a team every team member feels responsible for the care of all the clients assigned to the team. A team is created when a group of clients is assigned to a group of nursing personnel, which often consists of a combination of registered nurses, vocational or practical nurses, student nurses, and nursing assistants who work together and share responsibility for the care of the clients. A registered nurse is the team leader and makes assignments to team members on the basis of the abilities of the team members. A team results in a small group, which facilitates communication.

A **total client care** assignment avoids the possibility of care being fragmented. One nurse is assigned to provide comprehensive care to a small group of clients. A nurse is assigned to a client by matching the nurse's expertise to the client's needs. In this system, it becomes difficult to make assignments when personnel have widely different levels of skill.

Using **primary nursing** enhances comprehensive care and continuity of care across the client's hospital stay. Primary nursing gives the client a nurse who is at the bedside and responsible for the client's care over a 24-hour period from admission to discharge. When the primary nurse is "off duty" a co-nurse is responsible for implementing the care plan of the primary nurse. Primary nursing is more likely to be used in hospitals staffed entirely by registered nurses. However, some institutions use vocational or practical nurses as primary nurses when the client's care is within the knowledge and scope of practice for these nurses.

With the increased use of unlicensed assistive personnel, many hospitals are returning to the concept of team nursing. However, the size of the team has been reexamined. Using a work pattern of only two or three people working together is expected to improve communication and reduce the time it takes to keep the team working together. The dyad could be a registered nurse and an unlicensed assistive person. The triad could be two nurses with one nursing assistant or some other combination depending on the skills required to meet the client's needs. The registered nurse will spend more time at the bedside than when a larger team is used, but an assistant will do tasks that do not require the registered nurse's skill.

There are two ways of working on a team. In one method, the work is divided and all members work independently to accomplish the tasks. In the other method, nurses are physically next to each other, accomplishing the same goal together. In the second method, the team members do not feel alone. Each member of the team is sharing the work with the others, and each makes a unique contribution to accomplishing the work. Each member is more likely to be attuned to the thinking of the others, and thus they are all more likely to coordinate their actions to accomplish the shared goal. The nursing assistant learns in direct contact with the professional nurse, is more likely to continue to work within the same plan of care when working alone, and is more likely to communicate appropriate information to the professional nurse.

However, team nursing does not simply mean professional nurses working with personnel who have less training or education; it also means professional nurses working with other professional nurses to improve nursing care. Team nursing improves the quality of nursing care by allowing all levels of personnel to learn from the more experienced and knowledgeable members of the team. Team nursing provides the opportunity to see alternatives and discover new solutions to old problems. It causes nurses to look at themselves and one another both critically and supportively.

COMMUNICATION

Communication is a key element of well-coordinated care when multiple caregivers are involved in that care. Because nursing care in a hospital setting is provided 24 hours a day and 7 days a week, many people must be involved in the care of any single client. Many methods and levels of communication are necessary to ensure that all personnel have the information necessary to provide care that is comprehensive and coordinated.

Physicians and sometimes physician's assistants or nurse practitioners are the members of the team who admit clients to a hospital. The client is admitted for a medical or surgical problem that requires nursing care to manage. The physician communicates the medical treatment plan by writing orders.

Nurses are responsible for implementing the physician's orders and for providing nursing care the client needs both in connection with the medical treatment plan and otherwise. The nurse writes a nursing care plan to communicate the needed nursing care to all nursing personnel over a 24-hour period and to ensure that the care is a well-coordinated effort.

Nursing care is then documented in the client's chart or record. Changes in the client's condition are also documented in the record. Through written communication, any nurse can review the chart to know what has been done for the client, whether the client's condition has changed, and whether the nursing care has been effective. In addition, the chart serves as a permanent legal record of the client's hospital stay.

In addition to the written record, communication occurs through oral reports. When a nurse gives an oral

Table 14-4 Change-of-Shift Report

INFORMATION TO BE EXCHANGED	RATIONALE/HINTS
Name, room number, physician, date of admission or date of surgery.	Orient the listener to who and what you are talking about. For example, if the client is 1 day after surgery, the nurse will listen with a different mind-set than if the client is 5 days after surgery.
Medical diagnosis or surgery performed. A *brief* medical history of the current problem may be useful.	Experienced nurses will form a mental picture of what problems to anticipate and will begin to ask themselves questions about what needs to be done.
Surgery, tests, or procedures scheduled for the next 24 hours.	Give this information early in the report. It is usually the priority and helps plan the day.
Vital signs, abnormal findings, information to report to physician.	Identifies client's current status.
Tubes and equipment; include status (e.g., IV rate, amount left in bag, I&O, amount of drainage).	Identifies essential nursing activities.
Treatments.	Identifies essential nursing activities.
General information: bath, activity, physical and mental impairments, assistance needed.	Describes client's personal needs.
New orders, special problems, needed teaching, client-family dynamics.	Describes client's personal needs

I&O, Intake and output; *IV,* intravenous.

report at the end of a shift to the next nurse who will assume responsibility for care of the client, it is called a **change-of-shift report.** The nurse's work is not done until responsibility for the care of a client is passed to another nurse. This form of passing responsibility also occurs when a client is transferred from one unit to another. For example, the client may be moved to a more intensive care nursing unit or to a lower level of care.

Reporting in a manner that very quickly and efficiently provides another nurse with an overview of the client's condition, treatment plan, and needs in a manner that can be stored in an easily retrievable fashion in the mind of another person is an art. The reporter can err on the side of not supplying enough information, thus leaving out an element that is essential to the client's safety and well-being. On the other hand, too much detail overwhelms the listener, and important information is lost amid the deluge of sometimes interesting but insignificant facts.

A good report always begins by orienting the listener to what is to come, proceeds in a systematic manner, and highlights essential events and findings. When reports are given in a consistent order, it is easier for the listener to mentally store and manage the information. Table 14-4 summarizes information to be provided in a report.

Nurses also provide verbal reports to the physician and to nursing supervisors. The same principles apply to these reports. When giving a report to a physician, anticipate the questions you might be asked and have the information readily available. For example, if the client becomes suddenly short of breath, before calling the physician you should take the vital signs, assess the lungs, and gather information about the onset of the shortness of breath. When you assess the client at the beginning of the shift, you are gathering information that may need to be reported to the physician.

ORGANIZING YOUR DAY

Nurses employ organizational skills to implement processes that lead to quality outcomes. They do so because nurses must manage multiple tasks to accomplish their mission. Thus they must use time effectively and maximize productivity. Time management requires organization and judicious delegation of tasks (Box 14-1).

Organization requires the nurse to identify tasks, obligations, and activities that must be accomplished in a given period of time. Then the nurse must estimate the time required by each task and rank the tasks, obligations, and activities in priority order. Establishing priorities involves asking questions such as what clients have immediate threats to safety and well-being, what procedures/surgeries are scheduled, for which medications is timing essential, and which needs can wait. Once the nurse has identified times and priorities, the next step is to establish a plan for accomplishing the tasks and activities.

A nurse's workday is both a series of anticipated events and a chaotic environment of constant change. Any shift has certain events that recur on a regular basis, such as meals, visiting hours, bedtime, and medication schedules. Other events are scheduled on a daily basis and thus can be anticipated. Diagnostic testing by other departments, surgery, and special procedures are often scheduled in advance. However, many events cannot be anticipated: the client's condition changes, the physician writes new orders, family arrives from out of town, or a nursing assistant is called to cover another unit, leaving you without help. Use a work sheet to make a general plan for the day. Box 14-2 shows a typical pattern of work for a day shift (7 AM to 3 PM).

BOX 14-1 *Time Management Tips*

- Identify tasks, obligations, and activities.
- Write a list of tasks using a work management sheet, make a tentative schedule, and mark off as they have been accomplished. List tasks by clients and by time.
- Add notes to your work management sheet as needed throughout the day.
- Focus on the task at hand; complete each task before moving on to the next one.
- Control interruptions.
- Identify which tasks must be completed in specified time frames. Work ahead, not behind.
- Prioritize according to importance. Work on the most important first.
- Delegate tasks that do not require your expertise. Remember to give specific directions and to follow up on progress regularly.
- Do not accept assignments that you are not capable of completing.
- Avoid the need to be perfect.

BOX 14-2 *Typical Structure of the 8-Hour Day Shift*

0645	Receive report from the night shift; nursing assistant takes vital signs
0700	Make rounds and assess assigned clients; nursing assistant starts baths
0730	Administer medications scheduled before meals; help nursing assistant serve trays; nursing assistant feeds clients if needed
0830	Prepare and administer medications due at 0900; baths by nursing assistant; physicians are making rounds (from 0600 to 1000); check for new orders; update physicians on clients' status
0930	Break
0945	Dressing changes, other treatments, 1000 medications; catch up on physician orders, charting; nursing assistant has a break, then does more baths
1130	Lunch; nursing assistant takes noon vital signs
1200	Noon medications; help nursing assistant with lunch trays
1230	Charting, 1300 medications; nursing assistant has lunch
1400	Intake and output calculations, charting, make rounds for final assessment, prepare for report to next shift
1445	Give report to next shift

DELEGATION

Some tasks need not be done specifically by the nurse and can be delegated. **Delegation** involves assigning responsibility for certain tasks to other people, thereby allowing the manager to concentrate on higher-level activities—tasks that can be accomplished only by a registered nurse. Box 14-3 lists strategies for effective delegation.

When a nurse delegates a task to another member of the health care team, the nurse must communicate all aspects of that task to the person charged with accomplishing it. A clear understanding of the nurse's expectations will help the person accomplish the task independently and successfully. The person to whom the task was delegated should have the freedom to decide on a course of action for accomplishing the task.

BOX 14-3 *Steps in Effective Delegation*

- **Identify the task.** Know whether the task can be legally delegated. You retain responsibility for assessment of the client's nursing care needs.
- **Analyze the skill and knowledge needed to accomplish the task.** Consider whether the task is within the scope of the assignee's education and ability, whether the circumstances are appropriate to delegate the specific task, whether directions and other communications have been sufficient, and how much direct supervision is needed. Know whether the person can properly and safely perform the task without jeopardizing the client's welfare and whether the task requires professional nursing judgment. Instruct the unlicensed person in the delegated task, or verify the competency to perform the nursing task through knowledge of individual characteristics, education, or training. Validate the person's understanding.
- **Assign the task.** Provide clear and concise details about the task, including the time frame and expected outcome, the purpose of the task, and any limitations in responsibility or authority for accomplishing the task.
- **Periodically evaluate the delegation of tasks.** Let the assignee complete the task with occasional follow-up and feedback. Adequately supervise the performance of the delegated nursing task. DO NOT delegate a task if you feel uncomfortable about someone else having control over how it will be completed.

Therefore that person should have ability, knowledge, and motivation to accomplish the delegated task.

The nurse must know each employee's capabilities and the constraints dictated by licensure and education level. No nurse should delegate responsibility to ancillary personnel who lack the ability, education, or licensure to make appropriate nursing decisions. If the task requires nursing judgment, the task should not be delegated.

For example, a nurse may ask a personal care assistant—a nurse's aide—to take morning vital signs for all clients. However, although the assistant may be able to take and record blood pressures, this person does not have the ability to make judgments about the values obtained. Therefore the delegating nurse must devise a specific mechanism for the assistant to report all morning vital signs to an identified nurse before delegating the task. The ultimate responsibility for a task lies with the person who delegated it.

In a general sense, work does flow more easily when shared with others. Consequently, nurses who use their knowledge of others, the work to be accomplished, and tasks appropriate for delegation will work more effectively and efficiently. In addition, they can accept responsibility and accountability for the work of others because tasks will have been delegated appropriately.

MANAGEMENT ISSUES

A major issue for nurse managers is managing change. The one constant in today's health care delivery system is change. Quality management programs are based on the ideal of continuously improving processes to continuously improve outcomes. To achieve that ideal, policies and procedures must be continuously evaluated and revised so institutions will function more effectively and efficiently. Deficiencies identified in quality indicators are viewed as opportunities for improvement and the impetus for change.

A second major issue is risk management. The public is highly aware of the possibility of injury or other untoward events in the health care environment and of the possibility of seeking reparation for damages through a lawsuit. The nurse manager has a responsibility for evaluating the risk and reducing it.

MANAGING CHANGE

Nurse managers, acting as change agents, are obligated to influence the direction of change and maintain professional nursing standards. Change occurs more readily when it is planned and managed. Changes that happen without planning result in chaos. Consequently, effective nurse managers use steps similar to those in the nursing process to plan and accomplish changes in policies and procedures for their work units. Box 14-4 lists steps in the change process.

The Change Process. First, the manager identifies the need for change through assessment. Quality indicators, usually client outcome data, are assessed to detect trends that suggest a need for improvement.

In most cases, the nurse manager acts as a member of a process-improvement team. Staff nurses also participate in these teams in the interest of promoting democratic change. The planning phase of the process includes formulating how the policy or procedure should be rewritten, in keeping with professional standards, and how the rewritten version should be implemented. If the team decides that one more nurse is needed to cover a certain number of calls, the process must also involve budget analysis to justify the expense of hiring another nurse, plans for advertising and hiring a new nurse, instituting policies and procedures for orienting the new nurse once hired, and staffing patterns for the entire team once the new nurse is oriented.

Once the plans are made, the next step is to implement them. In this example, the new nurse is hired. The change process does not end with implementation of the new policy or procedure, however. The next step entails evaluating the effectiveness of the planned change. And in the final step, further evaluation reveals either the need for more planning, if the new process fails to improve the outcome, or the means to incorporate successful new behaviors into practice. Theoretically, when employees see the value of a planned change, they are more likely to accept it and incorporate the new behaviors it represents.

Controlling Anxiety. Nurse managers understand that change, even when planned carefully, causes anxiety, Indeed, the natural response of employees—virtually everyone, in fact—is to resist change. As the change agent, the nurse manager can initiate changes successfully by soliciting input from staff affected by the change, implementing the plan in stages, and demonstrating the effectiveness of the change through evaluation, thereby decreasing anxiety related to the change.

Several theories have been proposed to address resistance to change and ways to overcome that resistance. Change is effectively brought about in systems or organizations when the need for a change is recognized and accepted by those affected by the change: the employees. The first steps of the change process (assessment and analysis) help the manager raise the employees' awareness of a need for change. This starts the process of overcoming resistance.

Once employees have begun to recognize and accept the need for change, the nurse manager seeks input from them about how to implement the change. By facilitating employee involvement in the process, the nurse manager allows resistance to be addressed directly. People involved in the change process are more likely to become invested in the new process and accept the change when their concerns are heard and addressed as part of the planned change. Instituting changes in a stepwise manner also makes the process less threatening and therefore more acceptable. Finally, changes are most likely to be accepted and incorporated into new behaviors when evaluation shows the new plan to be effective.

The nurse manager is responsible for implementing the change, but the change itself requires the cooperation of everyone involved. It also requires the understanding that change is continuous. To help accomplish changes peacefully, the nurse manager needs leadership skills, communication skills, and education to influence acceptance of the change. Trusting relationships that result from an empowering leadership style and a consensus-building outlook form the basis for effective change.

BOX 14-4 *Steps for Managing a Planned Change*

- Identify the need for change (assess).
- Identify the potential causes of a problem, or opportunity for improvement (analyze structures and processes).
- Identify potential actions (plan).
- Implement actions (implement).
- Evaluate outcomes (evaluate).
- Incorporate new behaviors into new structures or processes (evaluate).

MANAGING RISK

Risk management is the process of identifying, evaluating, and reducing or financing the cost of predictable losses. These losses include losses from litigation (lawsuits). Although risk management can be performed at the individual level to prevent personal lawsuits, the nurse manager implements risk management strategies at the institutional level.

The nurse manager must be keenly aware of competing professional, legal, and ethical claims. Nurse managers must evaluate all new programs, policies, and procedures in terms of their potential for doing good, causing harm, or both (Figure 14-4).

Malpractice and Negligence. The major legal issues faced by bedside nurses involve avoiding malpractice or negligence claims. Nurse managers are responsible for overseeing the legal practices of the health care providers they manage. They also must consider the legal implications of client care decisions and management practices when delegating care to other providers. Box 14-5 lists steps taken by nurse managers to minimize legal risk. The best protection comes from following professional standards of safe care when instituting policies and procedures used to guide nursing practice. Managing the legal risks in client care is closely tied to quality management activities.

Litigation can result from problems in performing technical skills or from problems in interpersonal communication. Therefore the nurse manager is responsible for creating an environment in which clients perceive both technical competence and an ethic of caring. Nurse managers have to assume a proactive stance in monitoring, evaluating, and correcting the services provided by other health care providers. They must ensure that providers have the tools (education, supplies, policies, and procedures) that enable them to provide the best possible care, technically and emotionally.

Discrimination and Safety. In their agency advocacy role, nurse managers also must act to avoid litigation brought by employees. Indeed, they are obligated to abide by federal, state, and local laws governing health care. The Equal Employment Opportunity Act, Americans With Disabilities Act, and Family Leave Act all provide guidelines that help to ensure fair and impartial treatment to all employees.

Most institutions have human resource departments that help nurse managers resolve issues related to gender, race, age, or disability discrimination. Nurse managers who are proactive about maintaining quality health care and who use empowering communication styles to manage employees will be more effective in avoiding legal problems related to infringement of an employee's rights.

Nurse managers must know and abide by Occupational Safety and Health Administration (OSHA) regulations regarding maintenance of a safe work environment. That includes implementing policies about infection control, the use of chemical and biological agents, and the use of special equipment.

Institutional Licensure and Certification. It is often easy to think of potential good and harm only in terms of the effect on clients. However, nurse managers must also protect the institution when implementing policies and procedures. Loss of revenue is only one type of harm that could befall the institution. Other issues can affect the longevity of any health care agency. For example, governmental rules and regulations must be followed to maintain licensure or certification.

Nurse managers are obligated to abide by regulations imposed by those who pay for health care, such as the Centers for Medicare and Medicaid Services (CMS) of the federal government (formerly Health Care Financing Administration [HCFA]). CMS regulates Medicare and Medicaid, and as payment for services provided under those programs. Each insurance program, health maintenance organization, preferred provider service, and so on also imposes rules regarding allowed services and how they are provided.

Agencies such as TJC also impose stringent guidelines regarding the provision of client care services. Nurse managers must know all of these regulations and the influence they have on practice in each environment. Any health care agency found to be out of compliance

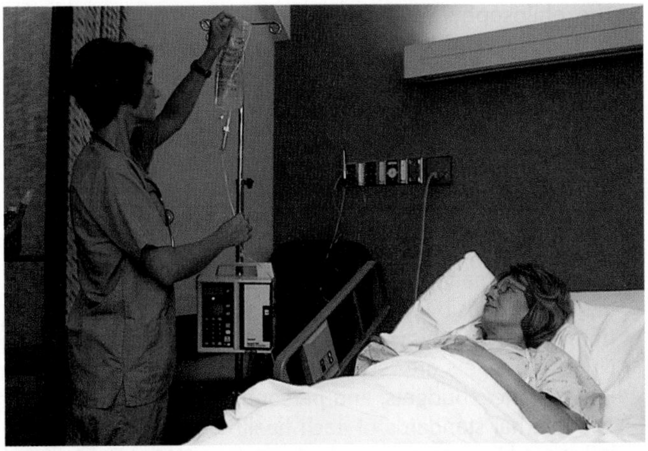

FIGURE 14-4 This nurse manager is evaluating a client's intravenous therapy to validate the effectiveness of her institution's policy for intravenous therapy.

BOX 14-5 *Risk Management/Quality Assurance Strategies*

- Determine quality indicators essential to client care in this institution.
- Determine methods for measuring those indicators.
- Implement measurement strategies (measuring indicators and mapping trends).
- Assess and analyze variations from expected norms.
- Plan and implement strategies for improving performance.
- Gather data related to occurrences (indicators of potential problems, such as medication errors or employee injuries) and follow procedures to assess, analyze, plan, and implement strategies to alter the causes of the unusual occurrences.

with these regulations could lose the license or certification that is required to do business.

Therefore nurse managers utilize leadership strategies to help other health care providers understand the rules and regulations and incorporate strategies to promote compliance. In an overall sense, they must use their knowledge of professional standards, legal implications of nursing practice and management, and ethical models to balance their obligation to act as client advocates with their obligation to promote the health care agency.

COLLABORATIVE HEALTH CARE TEAMS

Regardless of the type of health care facility involved, nurses are expected to participate in collaborative (multidisciplinary or interdisciplinary) health care teams as managers and as leaders. Client care is no longer the domain of one or two health care disciplines. Today, more people are living with chronic health conditions than ever before, and they require more assistance than that provided by physicians and nurses.

BOX 14-6 *Multidisciplinary Health Care Teams*

Goal—To facilitate client's achievement of therapeutic goals, to improve client services, and to avoid overlap of client care services.

Membership—Those participating in the care of a single client or a group of clients being served by an institution or by a unit within an institution.

Purpose—Planning client care. Each discipline shares data of their care plan: client's progress toward therapeutic goals, response to individualized interventions. The entire team evaluates progress and plans future interventions.

Roles—Team members have a clear knowledge of their professional roles and the standards that guide their practice, which they share with the other team members in planning client care.

Nursing role—Nurses share nursing processes, nursing theories, and nursing research that influence their choice of interventions. They offer input regarding the standards and regulations that affect their practice in each unique client care setting.

ESSENTIAL COMPONENTS FOR A SUCCESSFUL TEAM EFFORT

- Shared goals
- Shared commitment to client care
- Shared accountability for client outcomes
- Open communication about interventions (care plans)

COMMON MEMBERS OF A MULTIDISCIPLINARY TEAM

- Nurse
- Physical therapist
- Occupational therapist
- Speech therapist
- Social worker
- Pastoral care provider
- Dietitian
- Physician
- Client
- Client's family

Collaborative health care teams have evolved as the means to ensure coordination of services and successful outcomes for clients. Box 14-6 lists the essentials of a multidisciplinary health care team. Each discipline is responsible and accountable for the outcomes of its specific interventions. No one discipline has the power or right to negatively influence work being done with a client by another. Therefore it is extremely important that all providers work together to avoid overlapping services. They need a shared goal to produce the best client outcome efficiently and effectively.

Health care organizations have adopted collaborative team models that promote and protect professional autonomy for each discipline. In these models, all disciplines meet and confer about client care. Each member has an equal part but a different role in the client's care. No member of a team is more important than another, although, depending on the client's problem, one team member may be more involved at a given time. Members of collaborative health care teams share their expertise with other group members to plan, implement, and evaluate care strategies. Clients are involved as equal participants in the process.

Nurses have the opportunity to function as health care leaders in collaborative teams. Nurse managers, in the facilitator role, can provide education and guidance. They can model the behaviors that enhance communication and group cohesiveness. And they can evaluate the performance of nurses on these teams and coach them in improving communication and group participation. Nurse managers may also provide expert views on reimbursement, legal issues, professional standards, and organizational issues that affect team activities. Nurse managers make use of all the elements of management—quality, budgets, people, change, and risk—as tools to facilitate nurse participation and leadership in collaborative teams and all areas of practice.

▼ KEY PRINCIPLES

- The philosophy and mission of an institution affects the performance of the organization; the goals, objectives, policies, and procedures flow from the philosophy.
- Leadership is a quality of nursing practice regardless of the nurse's role within the organizational structure of a health care agency.
- Accomplishing multiple complex functions in a transformational management environment is a leadership style that empowers others and encourages their participation.
- Both nurse managers and staff nurses have the characteristics of responsibility, accountability, leadership, and commitment to quality.
- Nurse managers are responsible and accountable for quality assurance, budgets, and personnel.
- The internal standards of each health care organization are influenced by external standards, such as ANA standards and standards of federal, state, and private regulatory agencies.

- TJC surveys health care organizations to assess certain dimensions of the organization's performance. The demonstration of these characteristics indicates that the organization is likely to provide high-quality care.
- An organization develops internal standards to guide nursing practice, in the form of policies, procedures, and protocols.
- Change theories direct nurse managers through processes in which they recognize the need for change, plan for change, implement strategies for change, motivate employees to embrace change, and evaluate the effects of change.
- Nurse managers know and use ethical and legal models as they implement nursing care within the limitations of professional practice standards.
- In collaborative health care teams, client care is never exclusively the domain of any single health care discipline.

REVIEW QUESTIONS

1. A hospital has been chartered as a community hospital servicing the southeastern part of a major city. Its philosophy includes optimal access to care for the citizens of this part of town. Select the policy that is most supportive of this philosophy.

1. Provides transportation to the city hospital for indigent women in labor
2. Offers after-hours primary care for minor emergencies in the emergency department
3. Refuses ambulance admissions for major neurological trauma cases
4. Provides limited cardiac care, excludes open heart surgery

2. Select the charge nurse who is displaying a quality of leadership.

1. Tells a staff nurse that she will be fired if she does not comply with the rules for documentation
2. Solicits input from the nursing staff about the most important principles of documentation
3. Monitors the documentation on the unit by reviewing the documentation of all staff nurses
4. Posts guidelines for documentation in the medications room and in the charting areas

3. Which of the following is most accurately described as a concurrent audit?

1. A staff nurse is assigned to review a sample of charts from the month of May and look for evidence of perineal care on clients who had a Foley catheter.
2. The clients with pressure ulcers on a medical unit are monitored during a 3-day period to determine the treatment of pressure ulcers.
3. Follow-up phone calls are made within 48 hours after discharge to determine satisfaction with client's contact with RNs.
4. A questionnaire is sent to surgical clients 2 weeks after surgery to identify if they have symptoms of a wound infection at that time.

4. Which method of organizing a nursing unit is expected to provide the client with identification of a nurse who is responsible for his or her care?

1. A dyad of a nurse and a client care technician are assigned to provide care to 7 clients.
2. A nurse writes the care plan and monitors the care from admission to discharge.
3. A charge nurse is responsible for all the clients on the unit and assigns duties to the other nurses, who provide direct care to the clients.
4. A team of an RN, an LPN, and a nursing assistant are assigned to provide care to 15 clients.

5. Which best describes the goal of a collaborative health care team?

1. To use the expertise of each member of the team
2. To facilitate the client's achievement of the therapeutic goals
3. To make sure the standards of practice for each discipline are followed
4. To ensure separation of the duties of each member of the team

Bibliography

Alexis, O. (2005). Applied leadership. Managing change: Cultural diversity in the NHS workforce. *Nursing Management (London), 11*(10), 28-30.

American Nurses Association. (2004). *Scope and standards of practice.* Washington, DC: American Nursing Publishers.

Bethune, G., Sherrod, D., & Youngblood, L. (2005). 101 tips to retain a happy, healthy staff. *Nursing Management, 36*(4), 24-30.

Ferrario, C. G. (2004). Developing clinical reasoning strategies: Cognitive shortcuts. *Journal for Nurses in Staff Development, 20*(5), 229-235.

Gingerich, B. S. (2005). Leadership styles and communications. *Home Health Care Management & Practice, 17*(2), 128-129.

Hawkins, A. (2002). Self-awareness a key skill in influencing and leading others. *AACN News, 19*(1), 14.

Huffman, M. H., & Cowan, J. A. (2004). Redefine care delivery and documentation. *Nursing Management, 35*(2), 34-38.

Joint Commission on Accreditation of Healthcare Organizations (JCAHO). (2006). *2006 Comprehensive accreditation manual for hospitals: The official handbook (CAMH).* Oakbrook Terrace, IL:. Author.

Manion, J. (2005). Supporting nurse managers in creating a culture of retention. *Nurse Leader, 3*(2), 52-56.

Murphy, L. (2005). Transformational leadership: A cascading chain reaction. *Journal of Nursing Management, 13*(2), 128-136.

Pulce, R. (2005). Hints in human resources. Manager, coach, or both? *Nurse Leader, 3*(1), 6-7.

Scott, L., & Caress, A. (2005). Shared governance and shared leadership: Meeting the challenges of implementation. *Journal of Nursing Management, 13*(1), 4-12.

Shiparski, L. A.(2005). Engaging in shared decision making: Leveraging staff and management expertise. *Nurse Leader, 3*(1), 36-41.

Chapter 15

Evidence-Based Practice and Nursing Research

Media Resources

- Evolve Website http://evolve.elsevier.com/Harkreader/
- Companion CD

Learning Objectives

After studying this chapter, you should be able to do the following:

- Describe the importance of nursing research
- Identify the types of ethical dilemmas in nursing research and the mechanisms for the protection of human subjects
- Describe the types of research personnel, types of studies, and the parts of a typical research study
- Explain the steps of the research process
- Describe how evidence-based practice uses the results of nursing research to improve client care

Key Terms

abstract
data
data collection
dependent variable
evidence-based practice
experimental research
hypothesis
independent variable
informed consent
institutional review board (IRB)
instruments
nonexperimental research
operational definition
qualitative research
quantitative research
quasi-experimental research
research design
research problem
sampling
theoretical framework

Imagine that you are in the library, and you take a break from studying your fundamentals text. You notice a nursing research journal on the table, and, as you flip through the journal, you come upon the following text:

> The purpose of this study was to determine the accuracy and reliability of three types of thermometers: IVAC (IVAC Corp., San Diego, CA), TempraDOT (PyMaH Corp., Somerville, NJ), and an off-the-shelf mercury thermometer used to take oral temperatures. Roy's adaptation model provided the theoretical basis for the study. The convenience sample consisted of 35 adults who volunteered for the study. Information was collected by two registered nurses following the manufacturers' recommendations required for an accurate reading. Interrater reliability was established as well as content validity. Results indicated no statistically significant differences among the measurements obtained by the three types of thermometers.

Just then, your instructor stops by and says, "I see you're reading the study about thermometers." She asks you the following questions:

- Do you think a sample of 35 adults is large enough that you could use this research with all adult clients?
- If you were working in pediatrics, could you use this study to guide your practice with children?
- Do other factors besides the recommendations made by the manufacturer affect the accuracy of temperature measurement?
- How would you know which temperature reading was correct if the readings varied from one thermometer to another?
- If you were going to take rectal or axillary temperatures, would an IVAC and a mercury thermometer be equally accurate?

How would you answer?

Welcome to the world of nursing research. It shapes your daily practice in ways you never imagined. Indeed, it forms the basis for most of the nursing knowledge you will use in your nursing career and for many of the facts and concepts presented in your nursing courses.

Research improves nursing practice. However, before you can begin to incorporate research successfully into practice, you must be able to evaluate it. Questions such as those just asked and many others need to be answered before you can accept any research study as a valid basis to change your practice. The purpose of this chapter is to help you ask the right questions and evaluate the answers before you use nursing research results in your practice.

IMPORTANCE OF NURSING RESEARCH

Nursing research is the method used to develop knowledge about issues important to current and future nursing practice. More than ever before, nurses are being asked to determine their role in the delivery of health care and to document the effectiveness of that role. To define a distinct nursing role in health care delivery, nurses need a body of knowledge that separates nursing from other health professions. The body of knowledge developed through nursing research helps nurses articulate what they do and how their actions improve the health of their clients.

In addition, research can provide a guide for decision making in nursing practice. Research can help you answer important questions, such as the following: What should I assess? Which clients can reach the goal of self-care? Which interventions produce the best client outcomes? When should evaluation take place? Nursing research has the potential to answer these and other questions to help achieve the outcome of a healthier society.

The National Institutes of Health recognizes the importance of nursing research. To support nursing research, the National Institute of Nursing Research (NINR), a division of the National Institutes of Health, was established. The NINR mission is to establish a scientific basis for the care of individuals across their life span, to promote healthy lifestyles, to promote quality of life in those with chronic illness, and to care for individuals at the end of life (NINR, 2005). This mission is accomplished by supporting grants to universities and organizations and by research conducted at laboratories in Bethesda, Maryland. The NINR website, http://www.nih.gov/ninr/research/diversity/mission.html, lists specific goals and objectives as well as strategic plans for the twenty-first century.

CONTRIBUTIONS TO SOCIETY

Nursing research has improved the quality of life for many people. Through nursing research, new knowledge has been developed to improve nursing care for clients of all ages and cultures. For example, neonatal research has provided nurses with new methods for stimulating respiration in low-birth-weight infants and knowledge about the effects of parental touch and environmental lighting for preterm infants. Children and adolescents have benefited from studies about the psychosocial stress of being hospitalized or isolated because of a chronic illness. Adults have benefited from studies about spousal and elder abuse and about adaptation to pain.

Nurse researchers have addressed topics of concern to our clients. A rapidly growing body of nursing research knowledge exists to improve the physical and psychosocial well-being of clients with many types of illnesses or conditions. Many client teaching pamphlets and videos are based on the findings from nursing research studies.

ADVANCEMENT OF THE NURSING PROFESSION

In addition to contributing to society, nursing research also advances the profession of nursing by expanding the body of nursing knowledge. Expansion of the knowledge base is essential for the continued growth of the profession and for ongoing improvement of nursing care. Through nursing research, nurses learn new ways to solve old problems and address current professional issues. Examples of research in this area include the nursing shortage, the aging of nurses, staff ratios and effects on nursing care, the nursing faculty shortage, and teaching/learning methodologies and evaluation tools in nursing education.

Nursing research contributes to the profession by expanding the scientific basis for nursing practice. For example, through research, nurses have discovered personal characteristics related to compliance with therapeutic regimens, identified groups at risk for specific health problems, designed effective nursing interventions for particular types of clients, and demonstrated how cultural beliefs influence health care. Solutions to clinical problems are commonly found in nursing research.

Finally, nursing research contributes to the profession by developing theories of nursing practice. Although accumulating facts is important, organizing facts into theories increases our understanding of these facts. Nursing theory generates a view of the world of nursing and its influence on client care. There are diverse theories promulgated by a variety of nurse theorists that incorporate a framework and define metaparadigm concepts.

ETHICS OF NURSING RESEARCH

Ethical standards are especially important in nursing research because studies of health patterns involve the use of human subjects whose rights must be protected. To protect research subjects from ethical violations, many professions have established their own codes of ethics for research. A code of ethics serves to guide researchers in protecting the rights of human subjects. Various professions and government agencies have published codes of ethics that address the principles of ethical human research and include particular concerns of the individual professions.

In addition to professional codes of ethics, the National Commission for the Protection of Human Subjects of Biomedical and Behavioral Research (1978) issued a code of ethics that formed the basis of regulations for research sponsored by the federal government. Known as the Belmont Report, this document identified the ethical principles of human subject research and required informed consent and institutional review.

RISK/BENEFIT RATIO

Conducting ethical research involving human subjects requires analyzing the risk/benefit ratio. This ratio measures whether the risks to research subjects outweigh the possible benefits. Nursing research is completed to accomplish the following:

- Improve client care
- Expand the body of nursing knowledge
- Explore and describe new phenomena to enhance understanding of a concept and/or generate a theory
- Provide sound rationales for nursing interventions

All research involves risk to the subjects. In most cases the risks are minimal, but researchers should always try to reduce even minimal risks. The most common types of potential risks to subjects include the following:

- Psychological factors, such as fatigue or anxiety caused by self-disclosure or the loss of privacy, despite assurances of confidentiality
- Physical factors, such as physical harm, discomfort, or adverse effects
- Sociological factors, including the loss of time and financial costs for extra laboratory tests or transportation

In addition to the benefits to society and the nursing profession, the subjects themselves may benefit from participation in the study. These benefits may include increased knowledge about themselves, knowledge that they may be helping others, enhanced self-esteem, access to an intervention that may be available only through research, comfort in disclosing their concerns to a nonjudgmental researcher, and direct monetary or material gains. (Some researchers give study participants a small honorarium or other token rewards for their time.)

REVIEW BOARDS

Hospitals, universities, and other institutions where research is frequently conducted have a review board to protect the rights of subjects. These review boards, sometimes called *human subjects committees*, are formal committees with protocols for reviewing research proposals and plans.

Research supported by federal funds is subject to strict guidelines concerning the use of human or animal subjects. An **institutional review board (IRB)** is a committee whose duties include making sure that proposed research meets the federal requirements for ethical research. The federal government requires a committee structure be in place if the institution is receiving federal funds for research (Code of Federal Regulations, 1983).

Because not all research receives federal support or is conducted in institutions with review boards, some studies may not undergo review by an IRB. Regardless of the lack of a formal review process, all researchers have a responsibility to ensure that their research plans adhere to ethical guidelines. Many solicit an external review even when not required to do so.

When publishing research, most authors acknowledge that an IRB or human subjects committee has reviewed the study. When the author identifies a formal review by a committee, you can assume that the study was reviewed for ethical considerations.

INFORMED CONSENT

Informed consent means that subjects have been given sufficient information about the research to enable them to consent voluntarily to participate or to decline to participate with no repercussions or denial of care (Box 15-1). Subjects must be able to comprehend the information they are given about the study. Violations of the informed consent rule exist when there is no consent or when a consenting client is either not fully informed of the details of a research study or not continually informed of study changes or results (Karigan, 2001).

Most researchers provide subjects with a written consent form, which the researcher will ask the subject to sign before joining the study. The researcher keeps this document, and the subject retains a copy. A sample research consent form is shown in Figure 15-1.

The procedure as described protects the rights of most subjects, but sometimes researchers are interested in studying special, vulnerable groups of subjects who may be incapable of giving fully informed consent. Vulnerable groups typically include infants, children, pregnant women, the terminally ill, institutionalized or hospitalized clients, and mentally, emotionally, or physically disabled individuals. With these vulnerable subjects, the researcher may be required to undertake additional procedures and be especially sensitive about protecting subjects' rights. The researcher should make sure that risks are minimal and possible benefits are pronounced.

BOX 15-1 *Elements of Informed Consent to Participate in a Research Study*

A participant in a research study has a right to the following information. This information should be included in the consent form to be signed by the participant, and the participant should be given a copy of the form.

1. What the researcher hopes to learn
2. The type of information to be collected
3. How the information will be used in the study
4. The requirements of the participant (e.g., time, travel, invasive procedures)
5. How the information will be collected (e.g., drawing blood, answering a questionnaire, interview)
6. How participants are selected
7. Potential physical or emotional harm or discomfort
8. Potential benefits to the subject (e.g., better health, monetary payment for participation)
9. Potential benefit to others, individual, or society
10. Names of researchers, institutional affiliation, whom to contact with questions or concerns about the study
11. Information about the right to withdraw at any time without penalty
12. Information about the methods to ensure confidentiality of participants

ETHICAL DILEMMAS IN NURSING RESEARCH

Nurse researchers rarely decide purposely to violate the ethical principles of research. However, enthusiasm for conducting research may pose ethical dilemmas for the nurse researcher who comes to believe that the knowledge gained from research is more important and beneficial than the rights of subjects or ethical principles. Following are some examples of research questions and associated ethical dilemmas.

Research question: Do maternity clients discharged 24 hours after childbirth experience fewer complications when visited by a home health care nurse? *Ethical dilemma:* If a home health care nurse visits only some clients, other clients are not visited. If one group is receiving treatment, and the other group is not receiving treatment, are there potentially hazardous consequences to the group not receiving treatment? If the answer to this question is yes, the researcher is endangering the group not receiving treatment. How can this problem be resolved?

Research question: How do clients cope with the new diagnosis of an impending terminal illness? *Ethical dilemma:* Clients diagnosed with a terminal illness are very vulnerable. To answer the question, the researcher may need to ask intrusive questions. By asking these questions, the researcher may cause psychological trauma and increase the client's anxiety level. However, the results of this study may give nurses valuable insight into the coping mechanisms used by newly diagnosed terminally ill clients. Is this study fair to the subjects?

As these examples illustrate, nurse researchers frequently encounter ethical dilemmas. Ethical codes and IRBs help guide researchers in resolving these dilemmas and protecting subjects' rights.

THE RESEARCH STUDY

The research project itself is usually called a study or an investigation. The tools used by a researcher to conduct a study are called **instruments.** Instruments can be thermometers, laboratory tests, a list of questions, or a checklist. The term **data** designates the information the researcher is interested in collecting. Data may take the form of words or may have numeric value.

The people being studied are called subjects, study participants, or informants. Subjects are enlisted from *populations,* the groups of individuals that the researcher is interested in studying. For example, if a researcher wants to determine which wound dressing is most effective in aiding wound healing, clients could be placed randomly in control or experimental groups to test the dressing materials, the frequency of dressing changes, or a combination of these (depending on the actual

CONSENT TO PARTICIPATE IN A RESEARCH STUDY

In signing this consent form, I understand that I will be part of a research study that will focus on the effects of exercise on weight loss. I understand that I am agreeing to participate in the study for a total of six weeks, during which I will be asked to consume only prepackaged meals and snacks totaling 2000 calories per day. The foods and snacks will be provided for me free of charge, and I will be able to select the foods from a list that will be provided. I understand that I will keep a record of all foods and fluids consumed by me and will present this record weekly. I also understand that I will need to be present at the Tomlinson Health Sciences Center each Monday morning during the length of the study between 6:00 a.m. and 6:30 a.m., where I will be weighed without clothes, after emptying my bladder, and before I have consumed any food or liquids. I understand that I may or may not be asked to walk continuously for 30 minutes on Mondays, Wednesdays, and Fridays.

I have been informed that participation in the study is entirely voluntary, and that even after the study begins I can terminate my participation at any time. I have been told that my weight and records will not be given to anyone else and that no reports of this study will ever identify me in any way.

This study will help to develop a better understanding of the relationship between weight loss and exercise. I understand that the results of this research will be given to me if I ask for them and that Dr. Kathy Lauchner is the person to contact if I have any questions about the study or about my rights as a study participant. Dr. Lauchner can be reached by collect call at 1-800-555-1212.

Date: ________ Participant's Signature ____________________

Researcher's Signature ____________________

FIGURE 15-1 A sample research consent form.

research question). If the sample truly represents the population of clients with wound dressings, the researcher can derive conclusions about the whole population from the sample.

PERSONNEL

The person who undertakes a research project is usually called a researcher but is sometimes called an *investigator.* When a team of people undertakes a research project, the person directing the study is called the *principal investigator* or *project director.* Other personnel involved include data collectors or observers, who actually collect data for the study.

TYPES OF STUDIES

The type of research depends on the questions asked by the researcher and the topic under study. Some research questions may be asked in different ways, which influences the type of research.

Research studies range from experimental to nonexperimental. **Experimental research** is a study in which the researcher manipulates a treatment or intervention,

Table 15-1 Types of Nonexperimental Research

TYPES OF DESIGN	CHARACTERISTICS
Correlational	Examines the relationship between two or more variables to see if, when one variable changes, the other variable also changes without any active intervention
Descriptive	Accurately identifies and describes the characteristics of individuals, situations, or groups
Case study	Involves the detailed investigation of an individual, group, or institution to understand which variables are important to the subjects' history, care, or development
Historical	Examines events that have occurred in the past through systematic collection of data and critical evaluation
Needs assessment	Involves the collection of data to estimate the needs of a community or an organization so that decisions can be made
Survey	Collection of data from a sample of subjects who resemble the population in terms of variables being studied; studies to examine opinions, attributes, behavior, or characteristics of a population

randomly assigns subjects to either a control or an experimental group, and has control over the research situation. Because nurse researchers study human subjects, often in health care situations, a true experimental design is difficult. Consequently, nursing research is most commonly quasi-experimental or nonexperimental research. **Quasi-experimental research** is a type of study in which the researcher manipulates a treatment or intervention but is unable to randomize subjects into groups or lacks a control group. **Nonexperimental research** is a type of study in which the researcher collects data without the introduction of a treatment or intervention. The major types of nonexperimental research appear in Table 15-1.

STEPS IN THE RESEARCH PROCESS

As you read nursing research, you will find that the research process follows a series of unique and essential steps. Although these steps may vary with the type of research conducted, a typical research study follows this order:

- Statement of the research problem
- Review of the literature (also clarifies concepts or constructs)
- Development of a theoretical construct or framework
- Identification of variables
- Clarification of operational definitions
- Formulation of the research question(s) or hypothesis
- Selection of a research methodology (design, data, statistical analyses)
- Collection of data
- Analysis of data to obtain results
- Interpretation of findings

These steps help the researcher address a problem in an orderly way. They also help consumers of research to understand and evaluate the study. Most research articles are organized and written according to these steps. The steps are common to all research, not only nursing research.

STATEMENT OF THE PROBLEM

A **research problem** is an observation, situation, occurrence, or even a hunch that an investigator chooses to research. Initially, it may simply be an area of interest that the researcher then further defines. Most problems begin with something the researcher has observed in practice. For example, if in clinical practice a nurse observes that some clients with diabetes are better able to control their blood glucose levels than others, the researcher might question the reason for this difference.

In addition to the significance of the study, researchers must consider whether it is possible to design a study to research the problem. Not all problems are amenable to all research methods. For example, issues that are of a moral or ethical nature are not easily researchable.

Another consideration that researchers must address is the feasibility of conducting the research. All researchers face limitations, such as time, availability of subjects and resources (such as equipment), cooperation of institutions, financial support, and the facilities needed to conduct the research. Many researchers must change or limit their research problems based on availability of resources.

The research problem or purpose of the research should be stated early in the research report. In the problem or purpose statement, the researcher should clearly identify what the study is about, any suspected relationships, and the population of interest. For example, a purpose statement might be, *The purpose of this study is to compare the effects of grief on the physiological health of women who experienced the death of a spouse within the preceding 12 months and the effects of grief on the physiological health of women who experienced the death of a child within the preceding 12 months.*

The researcher's use of verbs in the purpose statement often identifies the state of the knowledge about the subject or the manner in which the researcher sought to solve the problem. The verbs *explore* or *describe* usually indicate a topic about which little is known, whereas *test* or *compare* suggests a more thoroughly developed knowledge base. Verbs such as *show, prove,* or *demonstrate* indicate possible researcher bias and should not be used.

REVIEW OF THE LITERATURE

The researcher begins by reviewing current information about the problem. A literature review is essential to all types of research and serves as the foundation for the research study. The researcher conducts this review by thoroughly examining all available literature related to the research problem. The purposes of the literature review are to help the researcher identify or refine the research problem, strengthen the rationale for the research, develop a conceptual framework, and provide a useful approach for the study.

The researcher typically conducts the literature review using a computer search. Computer searches are used to reach bibliographic information stored in databases. A computer search may be completed at any computer that has access to the database. Library computers usually have access to databases, or the librarian can help you find access to the desired database. Table 15-2 identifies databases of interest to nurses. These are the same databases you would use to look for information about any nursing topic of interest.

Table 15-2 Computer Search Database Resources

DATABASE	TYPES OF LISTINGS
CINAHL	Corresponds with the information in *Cumulative Index to Nursing and Allied Health Literature* from 1983 to present
MEDLARS/ MEDLINE	Corresponds with the information in *Index Medicus, International Nursing Index,* and *Index to Dental Literature* from 1966 to present
EMBASE	Corresponds with the information in *Excerpta Medica* from 1974 to present
HEALTH	Corresponds with the information in *Hospital Literature Index* from 1975 to present
ERIC	Corresponds with the information in *Resources in Education* and *Current Index to Journal in Education* from 1966 to present
SOCIAL SCISEARCH	Corresponds with the information in *Science Citation Index* from 1965 to present
PsycINFO	Corresponds with the information in *Psychological Abstracts* from 1967 to present
Sociological Abstracts	Corresponds with the information in *Sociological Abstracts* from 1963 to present
Dissertation Abstracts Online	Corresponds with the information in *Dissertation Abstracts International* from 1961 to the present
BIOETHICSLINE	Includes citations from 1973 to present concerning ethical questions in health care; housed at the National Library of Medicine and the Kennedy Institute of Ethics
CANCERLIT	Includes all cancer-related literature from 1963 to present

In addition, many nursing journals can be accessed at www.nursingcenter.com from any computer with an Internet connection. This site provides full-text access to many articles and has its own search engine. There are other websites that provide free access to nursing journals worldwide. The major difficulty when using journal websites is that web addresses change.

Researchers and nurses frequently read abstracts to determine the potential usefulness of an article. To fully evaluate the research, however, the entire article must be examined. At the end of the article, the reference list can be used to obtain further articles about the topic of interest.

DEVELOPMENT OF A THEORETICAL FRAMEWORK

A **theoretical framework** is a logical but abstract structure that suggests the relationships among the variables in a research study. The framework allows for the organization and explanation of all the information included in the study. Working within a framework enables the researcher to tie the research to the body of nursing knowledge. All frameworks are based on key concepts and the relationships among those concepts.

For example, a researcher who wants to examine the effect of poor health on life satisfaction must recognize that both poor health and life satisfaction are abstract concepts. Such concepts are frequently organized into theories. In this example, the researcher might want to use the Roy adaptation model (Roy & Andrews, 1999) as the theoretical basis for the study. In this model, poor health would be viewed as a focal stimulus to trigger adaptation and lead to either life satisfaction or lack of satisfaction. Without the model, it might be tempting to look only at the negative effects of poor health. Using a theory helps researchers clarify relationships and explain relationships. In addition, theory use contributes to the testing of that theory, which increases nursing knowledge.

IDENTIFICATION OF VARIABLES

The concepts under investigation in research studies are called variables because they are expected to change or differ from one person to another or from one time to another. The researcher is often trying to study how variation in one concept produces change in another concept. Almost anything in people and their environments may vary and thus be considered a variable. If all humans were 5 feet tall and weighed 100 pounds, then height and weight would not be variables. Disease conditions are variables because not all people have the disease; those who do may have varying degrees of severity. Other examples of variables include temperature, weight, knowledge, nursing interventions received, self-concept, health, and grief.

Researchers talk about independent and dependent variables rather than about cause and effect because, even though a relationship may exist between two variables, the relationship does not prove cause and effect. An **independent variable** may change during the study, but the change is expected to remain constant or to cause change in another variable. A **dependent variable** is expected to change with the treatment—that is, it is expected to result from (or be caused by) an independent variable. Following are three easy ways to distinguish between dependent and independent variables:

- The independent variable is the cause, and the dependent variable is the effect.
- The independent variable is what the researcher will manipulate, and the dependent variable is the outcome of that manipulation.
- Changes in the dependent variable depend on changes in the independent variable.

Now apply these criteria to a research problem: Do clients who receive home nursing care after discharge experience fewer complications? *Home health care nursing* is the independent variable, because home health care nursing may be the cause of fewer complications, and it is what the researcher will manipulate. The dependent variable is *complications* or the effect. *Complications* depend on changes in the independent variable *(home health care nursing)*. For more practice in determining independent and dependent variables, see Table 15-3.

CLARIFICATION OF OPERATIONAL DEFINITIONS

Research requires precision in measurement of the concepts. An **operational definition** is the precise meaning of the concept as it is being used in the study, defined in a manner that specifies how the concept will be measured. For example, if the researcher has identified height as a study variable, the operational definition may be the distance from the bottom of the feet to the top of the head as measured in inches using a specified measuring device. This definition specifies that information will be collected in inches, not centimeters. Also, this definition specifies to other researchers and readers exactly how this term is used in this study, allowing the replication of the study in the future.

Operational definitions are even more important when researchers are studying variables that are not as easily defined as height. Variables such as self-concept, pain, grief, stress, and adaptation may be very difficult to operationalize.

FORMULATION OF A HYPOTHESIS

A **hypothesis** is a tentative prediction of the relationship between two or more variables being studied. It includes independent and dependent variables. In a previous example, the research problem was to compare the effects of grief on the physiological health of women who had experienced the death of a spouse versus a child during the preceding 12 months. The hypothesis for this problem could be as follows: *Women who have experienced the death of a child in the past 12 months will report less grief and better physiological health than women who have experienced the death of a spouse in the past 12 months.* If the hypothesis fails to propose a relationship between two or more variables, it cannot be tested.

A hypothesis should be based on a thorough review of the literature or on previous research, or it could be deduced from a theory. The researcher should present a sound, justifiable, logical rationale for the study hypothesis.

SELECTION OF A RESEARCH DESIGN

A **research design** is a researcher's strategy for testing a hypothesis. The hypothesis should guide the design, but the researcher must decide what design is best for the study. Research designs are categorized as either quantitative or qualitative. **Quantitative research** is a type of study that uses variables analyzed as numbers, and **qualitative research** is a type of study that uses ideas that are analyzed as words. Quantitative designs usually are best suited to studies that focus on determining

Table 15-3 Examples of Independent and Dependent Variables

RESEARCH QUESTION	INDEPENDENT VARIABLE	DEPENDENT VARIABLE
Does involvement in health promotion activities increase the level of adaptation?	Involvement in health promotion activities	Adaptation
How does the client's culture affect the request for pain medication?	Client's culture	Request for pain medication
Do clients who receive pain medication frequently after surgery experience fewer postoperative complications?	Receiving pain medications	Experience fewer complications
Does cigarette smoking cause lung cancer?	Cigarette smoking	Lung cancer
Do mothers experiencing the birth of their second child feel less anxiety than mothers experiencing the birth of their first child?	Birth of the first or second child	Anxiety

relationships, whereas qualitative designs are best suited to studies that focus on discovery or exploration. Quantitative studies are considered to be more rigorous research, but qualitative studies are often more suited to the kinds of value-laden phenomena of interest to nurses.

COLLECTION OF DATA

After acquiring the subjects of the study via sampling, **data collection** is the process by which the researcher collects the information needed to answer the research question. It is the actual measurement of the study variables. Researchers use various instruments or tools—such as questionnaires, interviews, scales, observations, and physiological measurements—to collect data.

Any instrument used in research should be reliable and valid. *Reliability* is the degree of consistency with which an instrument measures a variable. For example, if an instrument is used to measure temperature, that instrument (in this case a thermometer) should measure the temperature accurately each time it is used. With physiological measures, instruments are usually straightforward. Concepts, such as health or stress, can be difficult to measure. *Validity* is the ability of an instrument to measure what it is designed to measure. For example, a valid measure of self-concept must measure a person's perception of the self, not another person's assessment of the study subject's beliefs about self. One method of addressing validity is to ask experts to evaluate the instruments. To evaluate an instrument's validity, the reader of the research must decide if the experts are in fact experts, if the number of experts was sufficient, and if the author revised the instrument on the basis of input by the experts.

Sampling is the process of selecting subjects from the population being studied. It is an economical and efficient means of collecting data when using an entire population is not feasible. Sampling techniques and the criteria used to define the population affect whether the findings can be *generalized* as being true of the whole population. The sample should reflect the same variations as those of the population. Generally, the largest sample size possible is the best.

There are two basic sampling techniques used in nursing research: random (or probability) sampling, and nonrandom (or nonprobability) sampling. *Random sampling* is the only method of obtaining a representative sample. In a randomly selected sample, each member of the population has an equal chance of appearing in the sample. It reduces the possibility of researcher bias. *Nonrandom sampling* involves the selection of subjects using nonrandom techniques—for example, using clients who volunteer to participate in the study. It is less rigorous and results in a less representative sample. The major disadvantage of nonrandom samples is that they limit the researcher's ability to generalize from the study results.

ANALYSIS OF DATA

The primary purpose of data analysis is to impose order on the quantity of data so that conclusions can be made and communicated. The researcher's choice of research design determines how the data should be analyzed. Quantitative research uses statistical computation to summarize the collected data, compare and contrast the data, test theoretical relationships, generalize about the population on the basis of sample findings, and evaluate possible cause-and-effect relationships. Most researchers use computers to help with statistical analysis.

Qualitative research should be analyzed through words and logic. It depends on intuitive and analytical reasoning to guide the organization, clustering, and reduction of data. *Reduction* is the organization of volumes of narrative data into concepts that allow the researcher to deduce meanings. After the data are reduced, they may be displayed using tables, graphs, and matrices. From the data display, the researcher draws conclusions and attaches meaning to the findings.

INTERPRETATION OF FINDINGS

To interpret research findings, the researcher examines, organizes, and attaches meaning to the results obtained from the data analysis. Study findings should be drawn from the data analysis and related back to the theoretical framework.

The researcher forms conclusions from the current study coupled with information learned from previous research studies. When forming conclusions, the researcher must clearly state that the research *supports* or *does not support* a position; the researcher must not state that the research *proves* a position. No single study ever proves a hypothesis. Also, conclusions should result from a logical reduction of the data and not extend to include variables not addressed in the study. When formulating conclusions, the researcher should provide practical suggestions for implementing the findings in nursing, including the areas of nursing in which they can be implemented. Finally the researcher should address implications for nursing education and further nursing research.

READING A RESEARCH REPORT

The reading of a research report begins with an **abstract,** which is a short summary that contains brief information about the purpose of the study, the number of subjects, the methodology used to select subjects, the type of study conducted, and the major results obtained from the study. The reader uses the abstract to decide whether the study contains information of interest. Some nursing journals print only the abstract of a study along with a reference that readers use to locate the full study report. An example of an abstract and a brief research article appear in Figure 15-2.

Effects of Exercise on Weight Loss

ABSTRACT: The purpose of this 6-week study was to determine the effects of 30 minutes of walking, three times a week, on weight loss. A random sample of 100 adult males and females, enrolled in a structured weight loss program, participated in the study. All of the subjects continued their normal activity levels, while one-half of the subjects agreed to increase their exercise level by walking three times a week. The Roy adaptation model served as the theoretical framework. Results indicated that those subjects who walked three times a week had a significantly greater weight loss than those subjects who maintained their normal activity.

Americans are increasingly striving to lose weight. The majority of the population is overweight, and Americans spend approximately $30 million each year on weight loss medications and dietary aids (Sampson, 1997). Obesity is a major health problem in the United States and one that influences the physical and mental health of the population. The purpose of this study was to determine the effects of 30 minutes of walking, three times a week, on subjects enrolled in a weight-loss program consisting of a 2000-kcal/day diet. The hypothesis was that people who walked 30 minutes three times a week would lose more weight than people who did not.

Several researchers have studied the effects of exercise on weight loss. Johnson (1995) studied 400 adults over the age of 65 who attended a 30-minute exercise class a minimum of once a week for a 6-month period. The results of that study indicated that subjects who attended the exercise class a minimum of three times a week lost weight, while those who attended less than three times a week did not lose weight. Likewise, Smith (1997) found that children who played baseball three times a week also lost weight, while children who played baseball less than three times a week did not lose weight.

The theoretical framework for the current study is the Roy adaptation model. According to Roy (Roy & Andrews, 1996), focal, contextual, and residual stimuli influence adaptation in the physiological, self-concept, role function, and interdependence modes. This study examined the need for nutrition and activity and rest in the physiological mode. The researchers viewed weight loss as an adaptation in the physiological mode, diet as a focal stimulus, and exercise as a contextual stimulus.

Methods

During the 6 weeks of the study, all 100 participants consumed prepackaged meals and snacks totaling 2000 kcal/day. On a flowsheet designed for this study, each subject was required to record all food and fluid intake immediately upon consumption. In addition, the subjects assigned to an exercise group were required to walk for 30 minutes on Mondays, Wednesdays, and Fridays for the 6 weeks of the study. Each participant in the exercise group was given a stopwatch to time the length of the walking. All participants were weighed using the same scale each Monday morning between 6:00 a.m. and 6:30 a.m. without clothes, after emptying their bladders and before consuming any foods or fluids.

Approval of the institutional review board was obtained for this study. All research data were collected by the researcher, who explained the study to each participant and procured informed consent.

Subjects for the study were solicited from an advertisement in a local newspaper. Of the 400 adults who responded to the advertisement, 150 met the criteria established by the researcher. These criteria included willingness to follow the study protocol, absence of physical or mental illnesses, and ability to pass a physical examination conducted by the researcher. Of the 150 respondents who met the criteria, 100 were randomly selected for inclusion in the study and randomly assigned to either the exercise or nonexercise groups. All of the subjects completed the study.

Subjects ranged in age from 22 to 64 and included 56 females and 44 males. The majority of the subjects, 82%, were employed outside the home, and education levels ranged from completion of the sophomore year of high school to a master's degree.

Instrumentation used to gather data included a Brice-Jones scale and Olympic stopwatches. The scale was calibrated by a technician from the state Bureau of Weights and Measurements each Monday morning prior to collecting the weight data. Between each subject the scale was reset at the 0 level. During the time of the study, the scale was not moved. New stopwatches were used for the study. Prior to the beginning and at the end of the study, each stopwatch was tested by a computer timing device to ensure accuracy.

Data Analysis

The data were analyzed using a t-test. The mean weight loss for the nonexercise group was 6 lb, while the mean weight loss for the exercise group was 9 lb. These results were significant ($p < .05$).

Results

The results of this study indicate that exercising three times a week for 30 minutes contributed to weight loss. The weight loss for the exercise group was

FIGURE 15-2 Example of a brief research article.

Continued

approximately one-third greater than for the nonexercise group. The flowsheets for both groups indicated that study participants adhered to the study protocol and consumed only the prepackaged meals. The amount of fluids consumed by the subjects varied from 1400 mL to 3200 mL, with the mean consumption being 2200 mL. One subject in the exercise group was unable to exercise on the specified day, but did exercise the following day.

Discussion of the Results

The findings from this study suggest that exercise does influence weight loss. These findings support the previous studies conducted by Johnson (1995) and Smith (1997). Exercise seems to increase weight loss in adults, as well as in children and older adults. These three studies may represent a beginning body of knowledge about the effects of exercise on weight loss.

The amount of fluids consumed by the subjects varied greatly, and may have influenced weight loss. The effect of fluid consumption on weight loss is an area for further study. In addition, the ability of the subjects to adhere to the diet deserves further consideration. The researcher acknowledges that in most studies, the subjects do not report such strict adherence to the diet. The adherence in this study may be due to the limited time frame of the study or to the prepackaged meals. This too is an area for further research.

This study supports the Roy model. The exercising subjects lost weight, and the researcher viewed this weight loss as a physiological adaptation to the focal stimulus of diet and the contextual stimulus of exercise.

References

Johnson, K. N. (1995). Exercise and weight loss in children. *Journal of Pediatric Conditions, 65*(5), 332–336.

Roy, C., & Andrews, H. A. (1996). *The Roy adaptation model* (2nd Ed.). Norwalk, CT: Appleton & Lange.

Sampson, T. R. (1997). *American weight loss statistics.* Bluffs, MT: Sanderson.

Smith, P. T. (1997). Weight loss in older adults. *Journal of Gerontological Physiology, 6*(4), 11–28.

FIGURE 15-2, cont'd Example of a brief research article.

If the entire study is included in the journal, you will typically find the following parts:

- *Introduction:* Usually, this section describes the research problem, presents the purpose of the study, reviews current literature, outlines the theoretical background or conceptual framework, and explains the research questions or hypotheses.
- *Methods:* This section describes how the researchers sought to answer the research questions. This section also includes the sample size, how the sample was selected, how the data were collected, and the instruments used to collect data.
- *Data analysis:* Here the researcher describes how the data were analyzed and which statistical tests were used to analyze the data. This section frequently includes tables, charts, or graphs.
- *Results:* This section describes the results obtained by the study, usually by addressing each research question individually.
- *Discussion:* This section includes the researchers' interpretation of the results, any conclusions drawn from the study, the relationship of the study findings to the theoretical background, and suggestions for future research.
- *References:* Here you will find all the other studies and journal articles referred to in the study.

Many research reports found in current nursing literature are primary sources. A *primary source* is the original research report written by the researchers. A *secondary source* is any other published material that reports on the study. When a research report or textbook cites a study, it becomes a secondary source. A secondary source is an adaptation of the primary source and may contain another person's interpretation of the research.

RESEARCH IN NURSING PRACTICE

The goal of nursing research is to improve nursing practice. Consequently, nursing research findings are intended to be incorporated into nursing practice. Nursing practice identifies areas for research, and nursing research helps solve clinical practice problems. This reciprocal relationship improves practice and provides new professional knowledge.

RESEARCH FUNCTIONS ACCORDING TO LEVEL OF PRACTICE

All nurses, including nursing students, share the responsibility for improving practice, and all can contribute to nursing research. Because students and practicing nurses may be unsure of their role in nursing research, the American Nurses Association (ANA) has identified the investigative functions of nurses at various educational levels (Table 15-4).

Nurses at all educational levels can contribute to nursing research by collecting data for an ongoing research study. It is important for all nurses to understand

Table 15-4 Educational Preparation for Participation in Nursing Research

EDUCATIONAL PREPARATION	INVESTIGATIVE FUNCTIONS
Associate Degree in Nursing	• Helping to identify clinical problems in nursing practice • Assisting in the collection of data within a structured format • In conjunction with nurses holding more advanced credentials, appropriately using research findings in clinical practice
Baccalaureate Degree in Nursing	• Identifying clinical problems requiring investigation • Assisting experienced investigators to gain access to clinical sites • Collecting data and implementing nursing research findings
Master's Degree in Nursing	• Being active members of the research team • Assuming the role of clinical expert • Collaborating with experienced investigators in proposal development, data collection, data analysis, and interpretation • Appraising the clinical relevance of research findings • Providing leadership for integrating findings in clinical practice
Doctoral Education	• Contributing to nursing knowledge through the conduct of research aimed at theory generation or theory testing • Designing studies independently or in collaboration with other researchers or clinicians • Acquiring funding for research • Disseminating research findings to the scientific community, to clinicians, and, as appropriate, to policy makers and the lay public

From the American Nurses Association Council. *Position statement on education preparation for participation in nursing research.* Reprinted with permission. Available at http://www.nursingworld.org/readroom/position/research/rseducate.htm.

factors that can affect research results and to make sure that the data collected is as accurate as possible.

When assisting with research data collection, it is critical to follow the research protocol. Slight differences in protocol may make significant changes in study results. If, for example, the research protocol states to draw blood 30 minutes after administration of a medication, and you draw blood 60 minutes afterward, the study results may be invalid. If the study protocol cannot be followed, contact the principal investigator to determine what to do with the data. Never just assume that the 30 minutes (for example) makes no difference. The value of research depends on accurate, precise data collection.

IDENTIFYING NURSING RESEARCH PROBLEMS

Nursing research problems begin as questions to be answered or problems to be solved. The nurse's everyday experience provides a rich supply of problems for investigation. Student nurses and practicing nurses alike encounter occurrences or situations that are puzzling or problematic. As a student, you may have asked such questions as, "Why is this procedure done this way?" "Is there a better way?" "Why did this happen?" "What would happen if . . . ?" These questions are frequently the beginning of research problems.

Research problems may also come from nursing literature. Most research articles include recommendations for further research, in which the author discusses areas of related research that, if conducted, would build on current knowledge. Also, inconsistent findings among reported research studies often provide ideas for further study. Similar studies may yield conflicting results, possibly because of the different samples or different situations. Nursing knowledge benefits from the replication of studies with different samples and in different situations to establish the validity and generalizability of previous findings.

A third source of research problems comes from nursing theory. To be useful in practice, theories must be tested through research. When theory is used as a basis for research, deductions from the theory must be developed. The researcher would ask such questions as, "If I use this theory, what behavior would I expect in this situation under this condition?" "Can I predict what would happen using this theory?" "What study findings would provide support or nonsupport for this theory?"

External sources also identify nursing research problems. Some organizations or government agencies sponsor funded research and may identify topics for research on the basis of current social concerns or problems. For example, in recent years many government agencies have requested a variety of research projects affecting minority populations (NINR, 2003). In addition, many nursing specialty practice groups fund research related to the specialty area.

EVALUATING RESEARCH FINDINGS

Research in a practice profession, such as nursing, provides information to improve practice based on study problems identified by practicing nurses. The practicing nurse should have the skill to evaluate research findings and develop interventions that make appropriate use of the information. Nursing research has relevance for all nurses, not just the minority of nurses who are nurse researchers. The following sections offer an introduction to the evaluation of nursing research.

Tentative Nature of Research Findings. The results of research never prove that a hypothesis or theory is true.

Rather, all research results are tentative. A hypothesis tests only one small part of a theory, and researchers cannot even state that the small part of the theory tested by the hypothesis is true. The hypothesis may be faulty, the sample may be too small, the sample may not be representative of the population, or there may be another serious flaw in the study. Instead of indications of proof, watch for phrases such as *the data support* or *the data indicate* as you read studies. Research results are always tentative and are based on the sample and study involved.

Research Bias. Bias is a factor that can change or distort the results of a study. In a good research study, you can feel confident that a change in the dependent variable occurs because of the independent variable. However, when a researcher does not attempt to control for bias, this relationship may not be true. Bias may result from the researcher's conscious or unconscious desire to demonstrate a relationship between variables. Bias is commonly introduced when studies are designed to elicit specific results.

Another source of bias is the difference among subjects in groups that are being compared. When groups are formed on a nonrandom basis, the risk of bias is always present. For example, in a study in which blood cholesterol level is the dependent variable and diet and exercise are the independent variables, a major concern is that individuals with high cholesterol may differ from those with low cholesterol in ways not connected with the independent variables. Other differences, such as metabolism and family history, may cause high or low cholesterol. Unless these other differences, called extraneous variables, are controlled, the resulting biases make it difficult for the researcher to conclude that lower cholesterol levels are related to diet and exercise.

When study data are collected by observation, the researcher's beliefs may unconsciously bias objective collection. To prevent bias from occurring, a *double-blind* technique is often used. The double-blind technique removes observer bias because both the subject and the person collecting the data are "blind" to the research objective, for instance. If this technique cannot be used, many researchers use two or more independent observers to reduce or eliminate observer bias.

Threats to Validity. If a study has validity, it actually measures what it was designed to measure. When evaluating research, you should examine factors within the design and factors external to the study that could affect the results, called internal and external validity.

Internal validity depends on the extent to which a change in the dependent variable can be attributed to the independent variable. True experiments possess a high degree of internal validity because they use control groups and randomization to control for extraneous variables. This helps to rule out most alternative explanations for the study results.

Other research designs always have alternative explanations for the study results because extraneous variables, in addition to the independent variable, could cause a change in the dependent variable. These alternative explanations are called threats to internal validity and have been grouped into several classifications:

- *History:* Have any extraneous variables occurred during the time of the study? Were there any changes in the environment that could have influenced the study findings?
- *Maturation:* Has the passage of time since the beginning of the study affected the results? Are there any internal changes in subjects—such as aging, growth and development, or wound healing—that would affect the study results?
- *Mortality:* Did the loss of subjects from different groups during the study affect the results? Was the loss of subjects from each group approximately equal?
- *Selection:* If the subjects were not randomly assigned to groups, were there preexisting differences between groups?
- *Testing:* Were the pretests and posttests identical? Could the subjects remember the material from the pretest to the posttest?
- *Instrumentation:* If the pretest and the posttest were not identical, were they equal? If different observers were collecting data, how were these people trained to ensure that each used the same technique and scored the data in the same manner?

External validity refers to the extent to which findings can be generalized to other populations, samples, or situations. Researchers almost never conduct studies to use the findings with only one group of subjects; rather, they hope other nurses in similar situations can also use the findings. There are several threats to external validity, two of which will be discussed here.

- *Sample inadequacy:* Does the sample represent the population? Is the sample large enough for the researcher to draw conclusions?
- *Hawthorne effect:* Did the study cause the subjects to act in a way that was different from how they usually acted because they were being observed?

Faulty Statistics. Statistical analysis allows the researcher to make quantitative data meaningful. It allows the researcher to summarize, organize, compare, evaluate, and communicate numerical data. Without statistics, data would be a mass of numbers with little or no meaning.

Statistics are classified as either descriptive or inferential. Descriptive statistics are used to describe data. Examples of descriptive statistics include averages and percentages. Researchers use inferential statistics, on the other hand, to make inferences or draw conclusions about a population. The difference between the two is that descriptive statistics are concerned only with characteristics of the data obtained by the researcher, whereas inferential statistics are concerned with generalizations to a population.

When researchers use inferential statistics to generalize findings to a population, the statistical tests used have assumptions that should be met in order to use the test. If these assumptions are violated, then the test results may be questionable. If the researcher uses an inappropriate measurement level (nominal, ordinal, interval, ratio) or violates major statistical assumptions, then the study results may be invalid.

IMPLEMENTING RESEARCH FINDINGS

The responsibility for implementing research findings is shared by all nurses (Figure 15-3). In fact, nurses' behaviors and attitudes are critical to the success of any efforts to base nursing practice on research findings (Estabrooks, 1998). Individual nurses can contribute to implementing research findings by doing the following:

- Read and evaluate nursing research articles.
- Attend professional research conferences.
- Support nursing research projects.
- Participate in institutional research projects.
- Share research findings with other nurses.

Expanding Professional Knowledge Base. Nursing students and staff nurses who read research reports and look for opportunities to apply sound research findings improve their own clinical skills and improve client outcomes. When research findings are incorporated into individual clinical practice, nursing knowledge expands.

Every nurse has an important role to play in making use of nursing research. Nurses have not only the right but the responsibility to ask for evidence that care practices and procedures are effective. Clinical decisions must be based on sound rationales. Practices and procedures must be challenged and changed on the basis of current knowledge rather than simply accepted because "it's always been that way."

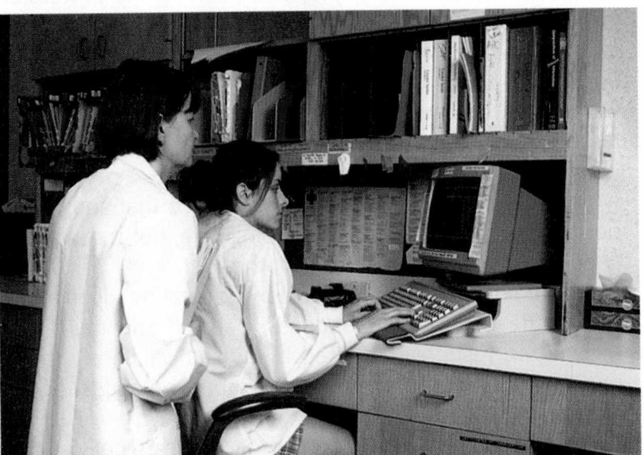

FIGURE 15-3 All nurses share the responsibility for implementing the findings of nursing research.

The use of research evidence to guide nursing practice has evolved into evidence-based nursing practice. Although the terms *evidenced-based nursing practice* and *nursing research* are frequently used interchangeably, evidence-based nursing practice may include nursing research, but it may also include the consensus of expert clinicians. Nursing research, on the other hand, is based on the steps of the research process. The outcome of nursing research is the generation of new knowledge, whereas the outcome of evidence-based practice is usually clinical guidelines for practice (see also section that follows).

Making Clinical Decisions. There is tremendous potential for using nursing research to make clinical decisions. The nursing process requires nurses to make many decisions. What will be assessed? What are the priority nursing diagnoses? What plan of care will produce the best outcomes? What interventions are necessary? How and when will the results be evaluated? Nursing research plays an important role at each phase of the nursing process by helping nurses make informed decisions.

Improving Quality of Care. The best way for you, as a student, to use nursing research to improve the quality of your practice is to identify where you have unanswered questions. Go online or to your library, and conduct a literature search using manual or computer techniques, using a librarian's assistance as needed. Once you have located several research articles of interest, consult the listing of periodicals for your library or access journal websites to select one or two journal articles. If your library does not have research journals or if you cannot access journal websites, the reference librarian may be able to help you obtain them through an interlibrary loan. After you have obtained the articles, it is helpful to photocopy or print them so that you can make notations in the margins.

As you read the articles, try to identify the positive and negative aspects of the articles and any flaws in the research. Pay particular attention to the implications for clinical practice. Then identify how you can use the research to improve the quality of care you provide to your clients. Incorporating nursing research into your clinical practice provides constant renewal of your nursing knowledge and that of the profession at large.

EVIDENCE-BASED PRACTICE

Evidence-based practice (EBP) is a conscientious integration of the best research evidence into clinical practice and decisions about client care and takes into account also the clinical expertise of the health care provider and the client's preferences and values (Sackett, Straus, Richardson, Rosenberg, & Haynes, 2000). Originating in medicine, today the movement toward EBP, sometimes referred to as "best practice," extends into nursing and allied health disciplines.

Background of Evidence-Based Practice. Dr. Arnie Cochrane, a British epidemiologist and medical researcher, pioneered a movement in England in the mid-1980s to use research rather than tradition as a basis for medical care to improve client outcomes. He also advocated the need for a comprehensive literature analysis to systematically review the amount and level of research evidence available on any given clinical topic. These reviews could then provide the basis for determining the most effective practices to use in providing health care to clients. Today, the Cochrane Centers for Systematic Reviews updates and disseminates current research evidence on many clinical topics.

In the United States, the Agency for Health Care Policy and Research (AHCPR) developed and published many clinical practice guidelines that were available for use by nurses and other health care providers. In 2002, this agency was renamed the Agency for Healthcare Research and Quality (AHRQ), and it has an expanded mission to support nursing research, to publish updated reviews of evidence for many health-related topics, and to continue to publish clinical practice guidelines. This federal agency, in concert with the American Medical Association and American Association of Health Plans Foundation, provides free access to current evidence-based clinical guidelines for nurses via the National Guideline Clearinghouse (http://www.guideline.gov).

Evidence-based nursing practice has been promoted internationally by nursing organizations as well. Sigma Theta Tau, the International Honor Society for Nursing, provides systematic reviews to guide nursing practice through the journal *Worldviews on Evidence-Based Nursing* (http://www.nursingsociety.org). The Australia-based Joanna Briggs Institute for Evidence-Based Nursing and Midwifery provides information on a wide variety of topics, from managing infant colic to reducing medication errors in older adults through their Best Practices Information Sheets (http://www.joannabriggs.edu.au/pubs/best_practice.php#).

Many evidence-based practice centers are forming at schools of nursing in various universities in the United States, such as those at Case Western Reserve University, Arizona State University, and University of Texas at San Antonio. There is likely to be an increase in the number of these centers over time.

LEVELS OF EVIDENCE

The Joanna Briggs Institute has outlined four levels of evidence for research studies based on the strength of the evidence they provided. Evidence is ranked according to feasibility, appropriateness, meaningfulness, and effectiveness. The rating system is simple and easy to understand and consists of the following:

- Level 1: Evidence obtained from a systematic review of all relevant randomized controlled trials (RCTs)
- Level 2: Evidence obtained from at least one properly designed RCT
- Level 3A: Evidence obtained from well-designed controlled trials without randomization
- Level 3B: Evidence obtained from well-designed cohort or case control analytic studies, preferably from more than one center or research group
- Level 3C: Evidence obtained from multiple time series with or without the intervention; dramatic results in uncontrolled experiments
- Level 4: Opinion of respected authorities, based on clinical experience, descriptive studies, or reports of expert committees (Joanna Briggs Institute, 2000).

Future Directions. During your nursing career, evidence-based practice as derived from nursing research and the research of other disciplines will increasingly play a key role in how you deliver care. Hospitals and other health care agencies are using research results not only to develop protocols for delivering care, but also to formulate and revise clinical policies and procedures that are implemented at the bedside. As a nurse, you can best contribute to the profession by being an active reader of nursing research, becoming active in agency committees that develop clinical policies and procedures, and participating in research studies being implemented in your health care agency.

▼ KEY PRINCIPLES

- Nursing research is important because it serves the public through improved health care, and it establishes a scientific basis for nursing practice.
- Ethical research protects study participants by rigidly following protocols that maintain the rights of subjects.
- Because of the nature of the issues studied and how the sample is obtained, nursing research is often quasi-experimental rather than experimental.
- The steps of the research process follow a standard format that reflects the scientific method and produces rigorous, disciplined study that can be replicated.
- Every nurse has a role to play in advancing the profession of nursing through research, either by conducting research or by using interventions that are based on the research findings.
- Research problems ideally come from problems encountered in a clinical practice setting, the resolution of which would improve the outcomes of client care.
- A single research study can offer evidence that supports a position, fact, or belief about nursing care, but it cannot be used to prove the truth of a hypothesis.
- Research contributes to practice by generating ideas about the nature of human responses, naming and describing the human responses treated by nurses, validating methods of intervention, and demonstrating nursing-sensitive outcomes.
- Evidence-based practice is an approach to care delivery that systematically incorporates the use of research to ultimately improve client outcomes.

▼ REVIEW QUESTIONS

1. A nurse wonders why some surgical wounds heal better than others, especially in clients who are of comparable age and have the same surgical procedures. This is an example of which of the following?
1. A hypothesis
2. A variable
3. An operational definition
4. A research problem

2. A nursing student has volunteered to be a participant in a research study. Which of the following information would not be given to the student participant as part of informed consent?
1. How participants are selected
2. Assignment to a control group or an experimental group
3. What the researcher hopes to learn
4. Methods used to ensure confidentiality

3. The degree to which a research instrument is able to measure what it is supposed to measure would be discussed under what topic in a nursing research study?
1. Data collection
2. Sampling
3. Validity
4. Reliability

4. The behavior of a group of pregnant women attending a childbirth education class changes when a nurse researcher observes the group. The researcher then needs to include which of the following threats to external validity of the study when writing the report?
1. Selection
2. Testing
3. Sample inadequacy
4. Hawthorne effect

5. A nursing student has read a nursing research study that provided evidence obtained from a systematic review of all relevant randomized controlled trials (RCTs). Using the Briggs Institute levels of evidence for a research report, the student concludes that this study represents which of the following levels of evidence?
1. Level 1
2. Level 2
3. Level 3A
4. Level 4

Bibliography

*Agency for Healthcare Research and Quality (AHRQ). (2002). *Systems to rate the strength of scientific evidence.* Fact Sheet (AHRQ Publication No. 02-P0022). Rockville, MD: Author. Available at www.ahrq.gov/clinic/epcsums/strenfact.htm.

*American Nurses Association. (1975). *Human rights guidelines for nurses in clinical and other research.* Kansas City, MO: Author.

*American Nurses Association. (1997). *Education for participation in nursing research.* Retrieved January 24, 2002, from http://www.nursingworld.org/readroom/position/research/rseducat.html.

The Cochrane Collaboration. (2006). *Cochrane brochure.* Retrieved March 2, 2006, from http://www.cochrane.org/cochrane.

*Code of Federal Regulations. (1999). Protection of human subjects. 45 C.F.R 46 (revised as of March 8, 1983). Washington, DC: U.S. Government Printing Office.

Dufalt, M. A., & Willey-Lessne, C. (1999). Using a collaborative research utilization model to develop and test the effects of clinical pathways for pain management. *Journal of Nursing Quality Care, 13*(4), 19-33.

*Estabrooks, C. A. (1998). Will evidence-based nursing practice make practice perfect? *Canadian Journal of Nursing Research, 30*(1), 15-36.

*Joanna Briggs Institute. (2000). Appraising systematic reviews. *Changing Practice: Evidence Based Information Sheets for Health Professionals, 2000* (Suppl. 1), 1-5. Available at http://www.joannabriggs.edu.au/pdf/CP1.pdf.

*Karigan, M. (2001). Ethics in clinical research: The nursing perspective. *American Journal of Nursing, 101*(9), 26-31.

Kittson, A. (2004). The state of the art and science of evidence-based nursing in UK and Europe. *Worldviews on Evidence-Based Nursing, 1*(1), 6-8. Available at www.blackwellpublishing.com/wvn.

*National Commission for the Protection of Human Subjects of Biomedical and Behavioral Research. (1978). *Belmont report: Ethical principles and guidelines for research involving human subjects.* Washington, DC: U.S. Government Printing Office.

National Institute of Nursing Research. (2003). *Research themes for the future.* Retrieved April 2, 2006, from http://www.nih.gov/ninr.

*National Institute of Nursing Research. (2005). About NINR. *Mission statement.* Retrieved May 20, 2006, from http://www.nih.gov/ninr/ research/diversity/mission.html.

*Omery, A., & Williams, R. P. (1999). An appraisal of research utilization across the United States. *Journal of Nursing Administration, 29*(12), 50-56.

Polit, D. F., Hungler, B. P., Beck, C., & West, J. D. (2004). *Nursing research: Principles and methods* (7th ed.). Philadelphia: Lippincott Williams & Wilkins.

Roy, C., & Andrews, H. (1999). *The Roy adaptation model* (2nd ed.). Norwalk, CT: Appleton & Lange.

Rycroft-Malone, J., Bucknall, T., & Melnyk, B. M. (2004). Editorial. *Worldviews on Evidence-Based Nursing, 1*(1), 1-2. Available at www.blackwellpublishing.com/wvn.

Sachett, D. L., Straus, S. E., Richardson, W. S., Rosenberg, W., & Haynes, R. B. (2000). *Evidence-based medicine: How to practice and teach EBM* (2nd ed.). Edinburgh: Churchill Livingstone.

*Asterisk indicates a classic or definitive work on this subject.

Chapter 16

Infancy Through School-Age Development

Media Resources

- Evolve Website http://evolve.elsevier.com/Harkreader/
- Companion CD

Learning Objectives

After studying this chapter, you should be able to do the following:

- Compare and contrast significant theories of growth and development
- Identify developmental milestones from infancy through school-age
- Describe environmental, socioeconomic, nutritional, and physiological factors affecting growth and development for the child from infancy through school-age
- Describe the assessment of growth and development and health maintenance from infancy through school-age
- Discuss assessment strategies to detect delayed growth and development and to promote health maintenance
- Select an appropriate related nursing diagnosis for the well infant, toddler, and school-age child with problems in growth and development and health maintenance
- Plan interventions to promote growth and development and health maintenance from infancy through school-age
- Evaluate outcomes from infancy through school-age for *Delayed growth and development* and for *Ineffective health maintenance*
- Assess, plan, and intervene with parents who exhibit alterations in parenting

Key Terms

attachment
cephalocaudal
concrete operations
conservation
critical periods
development
differentiated development
growth
object permanence
proximodistal
sensory stimulation
symbolic play

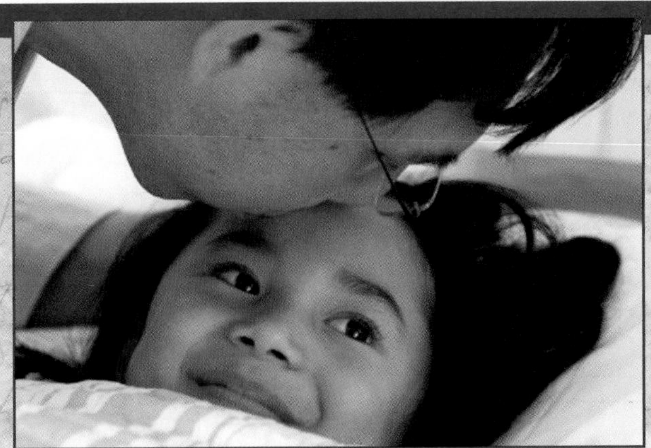

Yung Hi is a 33-month-old Korean girl who has been in the United States for only 6 months. She and her mother, maternal grandmother, and brother joined her father, who has been employed as a physics professor at the local state university for more than a year. Dr. Kim speaks fluent English, but the rest of the family understands more English than they can speak.

Yung Hi fell while playing in the parking lot of their apartment complex. Her older brother tripped and fell on her outstretched leg as it extended over the curb. Yung Hi's mother witnessed the accident. When Dr. Kim attempted to move her and was unable to, he called for an ambulance.

Yung Hi is admitted to the hospital with a diagnosis of a greenstick fracture of the right femur. She has been scheduled for placement of a spica cast. Because of this immobilization, there is concern that Yung Hi's normal developmental activities will be interrupted. Therefore the nurse considers the nursing diagnoses *Risk for delayed growth and development* and *Ineffective health maintenance.*

KEY NURSING DIAGNOSES FOR GROWTH AND DEVELOPMENT

Delayed growth and development: The state in which an individual demonstrates deviations from the norms for his or her age-group

Ineffective health maintenance: Inability to identify, manage, or seek out help to maintain health

Risk for impaired parenting: Risk for inability of the primary caregiver to create, maintain, or regain an environment that promotes the optimal growth and development of the child

Every nurse should be aware of growth parameters and developmental milestones in clients. Knowledge of growth and development will help you in assessing whether or not the client is developing and growing normally. Assessment leads to planning and to implementing interventions to enhance these processes. You need to recognize when there are abnormalities of growth and development and to provide nursing care accordingly.

CONCEPTS OF GROWTH AND DEVELOPMENT

The words *growth* and *development* have separate and distinct definitions even though they are often used together. Human growth and development is a dynamic process and continues through the life span. **Growth** is the physiological development of a living being and is the quantitative (measurable) change seen in the body. It refers to an increase in specific parameters, such as height and weight. Variations in growth occur with each person. Growth is often sporadic, with rapid spurts occurring at several points, such as the prenatal, neonatal, infant, and school-age stages.

Development is a progression of behavioral changes that involve the acquisition of appropriate cognitive, linguistic, and psychosocial skills. Development is a qualitative change and refers to increasing competence in behavioral functioning. During each developmental stage, certain goals should be achieved. Attainment of these hallmarks of development indicates whether a child is progressing normally. The following principles about the basic processes of growth and development are important for you to know:

- Human growth and development follows predictable, continuous, and expected sequential patterns that are influenced by genes, environment, and positive and negative factors that are present or absent in a person's life.
- Each stage of development depends on adequate completion of the previous stage and is itself the foundation for the development of new skills.
- Neuromuscular growth and development starts at the head and moves toward the feet, a pattern called **cephalocaudal.** For example, infants first achieve head control and then shoulder and trunk control before learning to sit or walk.
- Skill development starts at the midline of the body and moves outward, a pattern called **proximodistal.** Infants begin to move their arms and then to use their hands together before using each arm separately or beginning to use the fingers to manipulate objects.
- Periods of time when a person has an increased vulnerability to physical, chemical, psychological, or environmental influences are called **critical periods.** Growth or development may stop temporarily or regress during stressful life events.
- Development becomes increasingly differentiated over time, starting with a generalized response and progressing to a skilled specific response. This is called **differentiated development.** For example, a newborn's initial response to a playful stimulus involves the total body, whereas a 3-year-old can respond more specifically with laughter.

THEORIES OF GROWTH AND DEVELOPMENT

Stages of physical growth usually correspond to certain developmental changes. A variety of theories have been proposed to explain how a person develops. Developmental theories related to specific age-groups include the psychosocial, the cognitive, and the developmental task theories.

PSYCHOSOCIAL THEORY

Psychosocial development involves subjective feelings and interpersonal relationships. Erik Erikson described a series of psychosocial stages to outline the emotional and social development of the personality. Each stage defines a task that must be achieved. The resolution of the task may be successful, partial, or unsuccessful. Successful completion or mastery of each stage is built on the satisfactory completion of the previous stage. Erikson believed that the greater the task achievement, the healthier the personality of the individual; failure to achieve a task influences the person's ability to achieve the next task (Erikson, 1968). Erikson's theory is useful to nurses, because it describes expected emotional behaviors from birth through later adulthood.

Erikson describes eight major psychosocial crises experienced by people as they progress in their development. The stages reflect both positive and negative aspects of the critical periods every person goes through. Resolution of the conflicts at each stage enables the person to function effectively in society. Newborns to children 3 years of age experience the first two stages, trust versus mistrust, and autonomy versus shame and doubt. Preschool and school-age children experience the second two stages of initiative versus guilt and industry versus inferiority.

COGNITIVE THEORY

The intellectual process of knowing characterizes cognition, which includes perception, judgment, use of language, and memory. Cognitive development represents a progression of mental abilities from illogical thinking to logical thinking, from simple to complex problem solving, and from understanding concrete ideas to understanding abstract ideas.

The theorist best known for exploring cognitive development is a Swiss psychologist, Jean Piaget. He described cognitive development as involving the increasing ability to think and reason in a logical manner. Piaget believed that intellectual development is an adaptive process that occurs as a regulatory function of both physiological and intellectual growth.

According to Piaget, a person uses three abilities during cognitive development: assimilation, accommodation, and adaptation. Assimilation is the process of learning from new experiences. People acquire knowledge and skills, as well as insight into the world around them. Accommodation is a process of change, or modifying old ways of thinking to fit new situations. This adjustment is possible because new knowledge has been assimilated. Adaptation, or coping behavior, is the change that occurs as a result of assimilation and accommodation.

BOX 16-1 *Havighurst's Developmental Tasks of Infancy and Early Childhood*

- Learning to take solid foods
- Learning to walk
- Learning to talk
- Learning to control elimination of body wastes
- Learning gender differences and sexual modesty
- Achieving psychological stability
- Forming concepts of social and physical reality
- Learning to relate emotionally to others
- Learning to distinguish right from wrong and developing a conscience

DEVELOPMENTAL TASK THEORY

Robert Havighurst believed that living and growing are based on learning and that people must continuously learn to adjust to the changing society around them. He described these learned behaviors as developmental tasks. A developmental task is an important activity that arises at a certain period in life (Box 16-1). Successful achievement of these tasks leads to happiness and success in later tasks, whereas failure leads to unhappiness, societal disapproval, and difficulty with later tasks (Havighurst, 1972).

People progress from birth to death by working their way from one stage of development to the next while solving problems encountered at each stage. Tasks arise mainly from the biological nature of the human, but they can be derived from cultural patterns as well. Thus lists of developmental tasks will not be the same for all cultures. Infancy and early childhood represent the first of six life stages, each associated with essential developmental tasks. Havighurst's remaining five life stages include middle childhood, preadolescence and adolescence, early adulthood, middle age, and later life.

DEVELOPMENTAL MILESTONES

Growth and development are evaluated by comparing an individual's characteristics with the range of growth and developmental characteristics expected for a person in the same age-group. *Developmental milestones* are the predictable patterns of normal development according to age. Table 16-1 lists developmental milestones for newborns, infants, and toddlers. The following sections

Table 16-1 Comparison of Systematic Developmental Milestones for Newborns, Infants, and Toddlers

AGE	DEVELOPMENTAL MILESTONE
0 to 1 month	• Differentiates between light and dark • Turns toward direction of sound • Responds to touch
1 to 3 months	• Supports upper body with arms when prone • Raises head and chest • Brings hand to mouth • Opens and shuts hands • Begins hand-eye coordination
4 to 7 months	• Begins babbling and cooing • Rolls from stomach to back • Sits with support and then sits independently • Finds hidden object • Babbles, laughs, and squeals • Performs social play (such as peek-a-boo)
8 to 12 months	• Rocks • Moves from sitting or crawling to a prone position • Makes initial walking effort • Uses pincer grasp • Mimics gestures • Shakes, throws, and drops objects • Drinks from cup • Responds to verbal cues
1 to 2 years	• Walks alone • Climbs • Scribbles • Sorts objects • Shows return of separation anxiety • Imitates others
2 to 3 years	• Runs • Peddles tricycle • Screws and unscrews jar lids or objects • Holds writing instrument • Begins to make circular and horizontal strokes

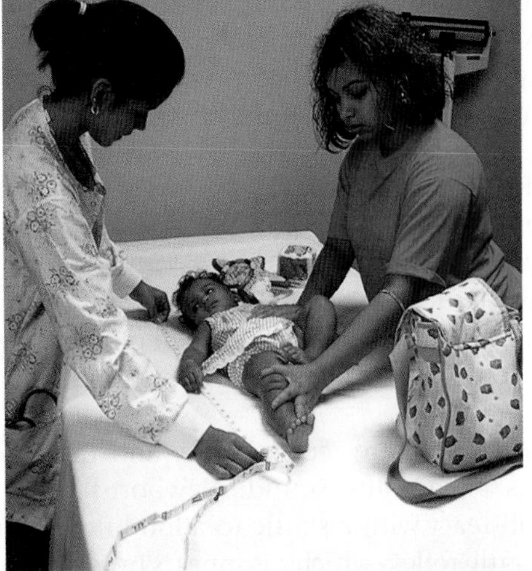

A

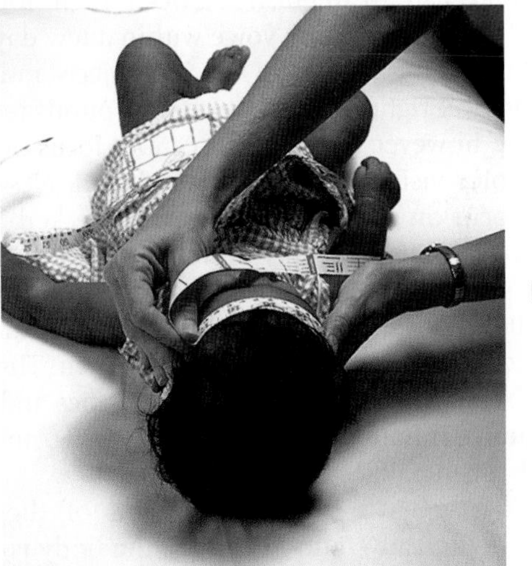

B

FIGURE 16-1 Measuring growth. **A,** Body length. **B,** Head circumference.

discuss growth and development characteristics from infancy through school-age.

NEWBORNS

A newborn is an infant from birth to 28 days. The child's parents usually follow growth and development of the newborn intensely and enthusiastically. They may have many questions about the "normalcy" of their baby's behavior. Even so, they are often able to provide you with significant cues to the progression of the child's development.

Growth Parameters. At birth, the average weight for a European American female is 7.5 pounds (3.4 kg), and for a male, 7.7 pounds (3.5 kg). Normal weights may range, however, from 5.5 pounds (2.5 kg) to 8.5 pounds (4 kg). Newborns of Asian and Native American descent are somewhat smaller, approximately 0.5 pound less. Because most (70% to 75%) of a newborn's weight is from water, the typical newborn loses 5% to 10% of the birth weight in the first few days after birth. This weight loss is normal, and newborns usually regain that weight in about 1 week (Behrman, Kliegman, & Jenson, 2004).

A newborn's length is measured from head to heel (Figure 16-1, *A*). Average normal lengths range from 19 to 21 inches (48 to 53 cm). Female babies are, on average, smaller than male babies. For the most accurate measurement of length, newborns should be placed flat on their backs with at least one leg extended.

At birth, a newborn's head is about one-third the size of an adult's head. Measurement of head circumference is of particular importance in babies to determine the growth rate of the skull and the brain (see Figure 16-1, *B*). The usual newborn head circumference ranges from 12.5 to 14.5 inches (32 to 37 cm). The head circumference should be about 1 inch (2.5 cm) greater than the chest circumference. A newborn who deviates from this normal range may have central nervous system anomalies and conditions casing smaller circumference, or microcephaly, or larger, as with hydrocephalus. Microcephaly may be caused by chromosomal abnormalities, trauma, metabolic disorders, or hypoxia, whereas hydrocephalus involves disturbances in the cerebral spinal fluid dynamics (Behrman et al., 2004).

Sensory Development. A newborn can smell at birth, as soon as the nose is cleared of mucus and other fluids. Newborns can recognize the smell of their mother's milk and respond to this smell by turning toward the mother.

Familiar sounds are recognizable, and the newborn often turns toward the sound. Newborns with intact hearing will react with a startle to a loud noise, referred to as the startle reflex, which disappears by age 4 months. Usually they can distinguish between their mother's voice and another woman's voice within a few days.

Newborns can follow large moving objects and blink in response to bright lights. A newborn's pupils respond very slowly, however, and the eyes cannot focus on close objects. Color vision is not fully developed. Newborns prefer to focus on geometric shapes and checkerboards.

A newborn's sense of touch is well developed at birth. The baby's positive response to the warmth and security of swaddling, holding, and touching demonstrates the importance of touch for healthy development. The newborn is also sensitive to temperature extremes and pain. Babies cannot isolate the discomfort, however, and they react with a generalized response.

Motor Development. The development of the newborn's ability to move and to control the body is called motor development. Initially, the newborn has uncoordinated body movement. A newborn's normal motor activity includes involuntary reflexes and turning the head from side to side when in a prone or supine position. Infants are unable to hold their head erect and will continue to have a head lag for 4 months. As the baby obtains more muscle control, body movements become smoother and more purposeful.

> ***Action Alert!*** Instruct parents to always place babies on their backs to sleep. Research has demonstrated a significant decrease in sudden infant death syndrome (SIDS) deaths since the introduction of the "Back to Sleep" campaign.

Reflexes. Reflexes in the newborn are involuntary responses. The presence of these specific reflexes indicates normal nervous system development in the newborn. The natural progression of neural development is cephalocaudal, proximodistal, and general to specific. Also present at birth are the abilities to yawn, stretch, sneeze, burp, and hiccup.

Psychosocial Development. Erikson's stage of trust versus mistrust occurs from birth to age 1 year. The most important person for the infant at this stage is the mother or primary caretaker, and the quality of this relationship and the degree to which the infant's needs are met are extremely important to the development of trust. While building this relationship, an infant receives information through all the senses. **Sensory stimulation** is the activation and exhilaration of the senses. An appropriate amount of sensory stimulation enables the infant to develop trust. If the infant's needs are not met, either through overstimulation or neglect, then some degree of mistrust develops.

Psychosocial development in the newborn is initiated with the process of attachment. **Attachment** is the development of strong ties of affection of an infant with a significant other (mother, father, sibling, caretaker). Recognizing that attachment occurs both from infant to parent and from parent to infant, researchers developed the concept of mutual bonding through observation of premature infants. Bonding is a process of forming an attachment between parent and newborn. Although bonding was initially studied as occurring during the first hours after birth, it continues to develop during the first year and possibly beyond.

The emotional bond between mother and newborn is developed and sustained through cyclical cues and communication from one to the other (Figure 16-2). Even at this early stage, newborns attempt to communicate and are consoled by gentle human touch. Crying is the primary means by which newborns make their needs and wants known. Parents are often able to distinguish between different types of cries, such as those of hunger and those of discomfort. The process of parent-child attachment is not instantaneous. Most parents require several months before they feel they know their newborn.

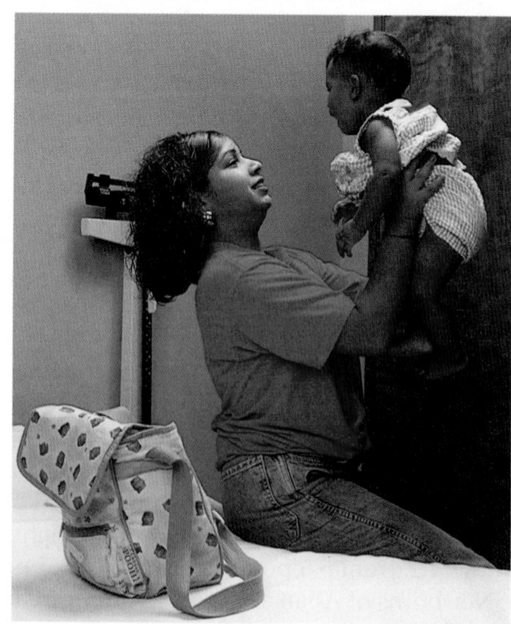

FIGURE 16-2 The emotional bond between mother and infant is developed and sustained through cyclical cues and communication from one to the other.

Cognitive Development. Cognitive development in the newborn is primarily reflexive. However, the newborn reacts socially to caregivers by paying attention to the face or voice and by cuddling when held. The baby is able to interact with the environment by responding to various stimuli, such as touch and sound. The newborn displays displeasure by crying and shows satisfaction by quieting and making soft vocalizations. According to Piaget (1950), a Swiss psychologist, newborns are active participants in learning through their senses. In addition, as motor function progresses from reflexes to purposeful activities, the child rapidly increases interactions with the environment.

INFANTS

Infant is the term given to a child from the age of 1 month to the end of 12 months. Infancy is a time of continuous and rapid growth and development. Most parents of infants carefully monitor their baby's height and weight throughout the first year and celebrate the achievements of numerous developmental milestones.

Growth Parameters. Height and weight are predictable along a growth curve. An infant usually gains 5 to 7 ounces weekly for about the first 4 to 6 months. By 4 to 7 months the birth weight doubles (Hockenberry, Wilson, Winkelstein, & Kline, 2003). By 1 year of age, the normal infant weighs about three times its birth weight. The average male baby weighs 22 pounds (10 kg), and the average female baby weighs 21 pounds (9.5 kg) by the first birthday (Behrman et al., 2004).

The rate of increase in height is largely influenced by the baby's size at birth and by nutrition. By the end of the infant's first year, recumbent length has increased 50% since birth, and the average range is 28 to 32 inches. Head growth begins to slow down between 8 and 12 months of age. By 10 months, head and chest circumferences are about the same. Head circumference is usually 18 inches (47 cm) by the end of infancy (Behrman et al., 2004). Because the rate of growth for each child differs, these measurements should be compared with the percentile curves on a growth chart.

Sensory Development. The senses of smell and taste continue to develop throughout the first year. Many new smells and tastes are introduced with the taking of solid foods at 4 to 6 months of age. With each new food experience, the infant begins to show discrimination toward favorite tastes and smells.

Eyes begin to focus and fixate at 4 months. The infant can recognize familiar objects and follow moving ones. Most 5-month-old babies can recognize facial characteristics and often smile in response to a familiar face. By the end of the first year, depth perception has developed, and the infant will be able to recognize a change in level, such as the start and finish of a step or the edge of a bed.

At about 5 months, the infant will pause while feeding to listen to the mother's voice. A 9-month-old baby will locate the source of sounds and be able to recognize familiar sounds or voices. By 1 year of age, the infant listens to sounds, begins to distinguish words, and can respond to simple commands.

Touch remains important. Infants continue to demonstrate positive responses to the security of being held and cuddled. Touching different-textured fabrics and object shapes also positively stimulates babies. Exploration through touching and placing items in the mouth to further explore them begins at 3 months of age and may last through toddlerhood.

Motor Development. From 1 to 3 months of age, the infant attains additional physical skills and becomes more neurologically sophisticated. In the prone position, infants can raise their head and chest and support their upper body with their arms. By 4 to 7 months, the infant can roll from stomach to back and vice versa. By 5 months, an infant can sit with support. By the end of 7 months, most infants can sit without support.

From 8 to 12 months of age, infants make great developmental strides. They can get up on their hands and knees and rock back and forth on both knees. Crawling begins by the tenth month. Infants of this age can move from a sitting to a crawling to a prone position. The infant makes first efforts toward walking, such as pulling to stand, standing briefly with support, cruising along furniture, and walking two to three steps unassisted. The pincer grasp is developed, and the infant takes great pleasure in manipulating objects (Figure 16-3). Parents can encourage the development of this skill by offering items that promote grasping, such as cereal bits and containers to put them in.

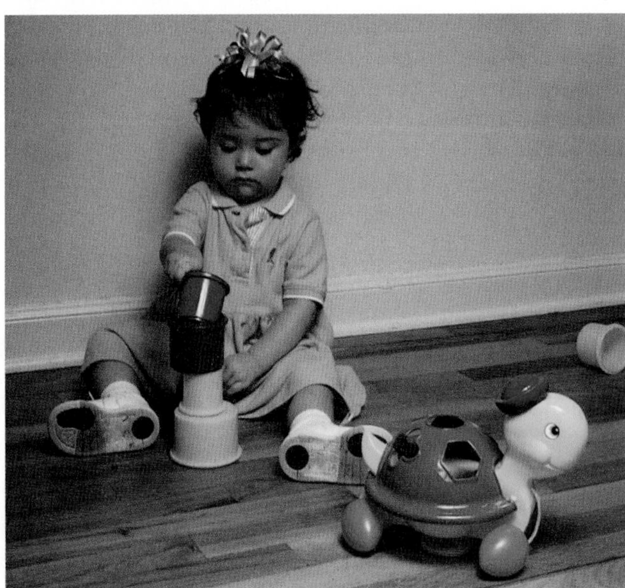

FIGURE 16-3 With development of the pincer grasp, the infant takes great pleasure in stacking objects and putting objects into containers and removing them.

Reflexes. As the infant develops neurologically, the primitive or neonatal reflexes begin to disappear. Later infant reflexes develop at 3 months of age, beginning with the Landau reflex (lifts both head and legs when suspended prone with support under abdomen).

Psychosocial Development. Psychologically, the infant begins to communicate through body language. There are attempts to imitate some facial expressions and movements, such as a social smile, by the end of the second month. The 4-month-old infant enjoys interacting with people and will vocalize displeasure when left alone. Infants mimic gestures, babble with inflection, say "mama" and "dada," and try to imitate other words by about 6 months of age. The infant responds to simple verbal cues and uses simple gestures, such as shaking the head "no" and waving "bye-bye." Smiling, laughing, waving, and reaching out to others are examples of purposeful interactive social behavior.

Self-esteem develops through trust and increasing control of the body. Trust develops when the parent or caregiver can be counted on to provide essential needs. However, by 6 to 9 months the infant begins to have a greater awareness of self as separate from mother or father. Separation anxiety emerges as crying when the infant is separated from parents or approached by strangers.

Cognitive Development. Infants learn about their world through their activities. They anticipate feeding times and "going bye-bye." They become excited when they see their parents. They have an increasing ability to concentrate and to recognize and respond to a familiar environment or a friend of the family.

Rudimentary language skills are developing. Babies begin to coo and make sounds soon after birth, and by 12 months they can convey their wishes through several key words. Use of syllable repetition (ma-ma, da-da), early phonetic expression (babbling), and imitation of intonations and sounds are characteristic of the language development of infants.

Piaget's first stage of cognitive development, the sensorimotor stage, has six substages, four of which are related to infancy (Edelman and Mandle, 2006). The first substage is reflexive, the emergence of directed behavior (birth to 1 month). The second substage is scheme coordination and early goal directions (1½ to 4 months). During this time, the infant discovers enjoyment of random behaviors, such as sucking a thumb, and repeats them. Piaget's third substage, intention, beginning independence of action and thought (4 to 6 months), is when infants relate their own behavior to change in the environment, such as intentionally shaking a rattle to hear the sound.

By 6 to 12 months, an infant can coordinate more than one thought pattern at a time to reach a goal, such as repeatedly throwing an object on the floor. Infants in this substage are also beginning to develop a sense of object permanence. **Object permanence,** the awareness that unseen objects do not disappear, is evidenced when the infant searches for an object that has been moved out of sight. This behavior is the first sign of object permanence.

TODDLERS

Toddler is the term for a child from 1 to 3 years of age. The term is derived from the pattern of locomotion of children in this age-group. Toddlers walk with their feet several inches apart and their arms held out to maintain balance. The ability to walk is an important developmental milestone as toddlers move toward the increasing independence of childhood, leaving the dependency of infancy behind.

Growth Parameters. The most noticeable physical change during the toddler years occurs as head growth slows and the relatively short legs and trunk of an infant begin to lengthen. Baby fat begins to decrease. Physiological growth and development continues steadily, but the pace of the gains is considerably slower than during infancy. Weight gain is about 4 pounds (2 kg) yearly, with height increases averaging 2.2 inches (6 cm) yearly. By age 2, the female toddler is about 34 inches (86.4 cm) tall and weighs 27 pounds (12.2 kg). Boys average 34 inches (86.4 cm) and almost 28 pounds (12.7 kg) by age 2. Head circumference increases about 2 cm by age 2 as compared to 12 cm during the first year. By age 2 the child's chest circumference has grown larger than the head (Behrman et al., 2004).

Sensory Development. All the senses continue to develop and become more associated with each other during the toddler stage. Toddlers use all their senses to explore their environment. Walking enhances their ability to explore without relying on others. Vision is fairly well established by ages 1 and 2. Visual acuity is about 20/40. The ability to focus on near and far objects is fairly well developed by 18 months and continues to develop with age. Hearing is at adult levels by age 3.

The toddler's taste buds are sensitive to the natural flavors of food, and taste preferences begin to emerge. Toddlers are less likely to try a new food if the food has an unfamiliar appearance, smell, texture, or taste. Touch is also a very important sense to the toddler. A distressed toddler often uses tactile sensations as a self-comforting technique, such as stroking the satin ribbon on a favorite stuffed animal.

Motor Development. Fine muscle (fine motor) coordination and large muscle (gross motor) activity improve during toddlerhood. At 18 months of age, a toddler can pick up beads and put them in a cup. The toddler can also hold a spoon and a cup and walk up stairs with assistance. By age 3, fine motor skills have continued to improve and include turning the page of a book one at a time, screwing and unscrewing objects, turning handles, and making vertical, circular, and horizontal strokes with a writing instrument. Gross motor skills of the 3-year-old include climbing, walking up and down stairs unassisted, running easily, bending over without falling, peddling a tricycle, and kicking a ball.

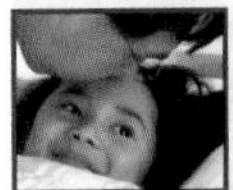

Remember that Yung Hi is in the toddler stage of her growth and development. She had been running and playing with her brother when the accident occurred. What types of activities will Yung be able to accomplish while in a spica cast? How can you help her maintain the developmental milestones she has already achieved?

Reflexes. Neural growth continues during the toddler years, with additional myelinization and cortical brain development. Neurological growth and musculoskeletal development allow the toddler to perform more complex physical tasks. The primitive reflexes of infancy must disappear before voluntary behaviors appear. By age 3, deep tendon reflexes (biceps, triceps, patellar, and Achilles) are well developed.

Psychosocial Development. Erickson's second stage, autonomy versus shame and doubt, applies to children from age 2 to 3. This stage is influenced by toddlers' maturing muscle systems, which gives them a sense of control over their body. This mastery enables the toddler to experience a sense of power and, thus, autonomy.

According to Erikson, toddlers enter the stage of autonomy versus shame and doubt. Independence increases and is demonstrated by the toddler's self-feeding, walking, talking, and toileting. A major developmental gain for this age is the achievement of a sense of independence and autonomy. The struggle between choosing independence over dependence is a frustrating decision for the toddler. Toddlers tolerate their parents being out of sight in a comfortable setting and revel in their independence, but the return of separation anxiety can be a significant problem if the settings or people are unfamiliar. The fear of abandonment is great during early toddler years. Separation anxiety can be very traumatic for both parents and children and is frequently seen during these years.

Toddlers also begin to develop their sense of autonomy by asserting themselves with frequent use of the word "no." It may be used to refuse a request, to demonstrate lack of understanding, or to practice a word that the child notices has a dramatic effect on others. They can become very negative, practicing the power of "no" every day for months.

Temper tantrums usually make their appearance at about age 2. Tantrums stem from the child's striving for power and control and the sudden loss of both. There are so many activities toddlers want and struggle to do but that they are not developmentally ready to perform.

Toddlers enjoy playing near others, but they frequently do not share objects or engage in close interactive activities with other children. In parallel play, toddlers play beside but not with their friends. The types of play that appeal to toddlers are those that allow them to use large muscles, those that include repetitive and rhythmic motions, and those involving language. Play is a natural way to enhance the toddler's physical and psychosocial development.

Self-concept and body image are also part of psychosocial development. Toddlers develop their sense of self-esteem not only through others' responses to them but also through pleasure in their accomplishments. Mastering toilet training, gaining motor skills, and making choices all enhance a toddler's self-confidence. Sexuality is another aspect of toddler development. Toddlers begin to develop some gender-based expectations, can describe themselves as a girl or a boy, and can accurately apply gender labels to those around them. Havighurst's developmental task during toddlerhood shows the child learning to control the elimination of urine and feces (toilet training), learning gender differences, forming concepts, learning language, and distinguishing right from wrong.

Cognitive Development. According to Piaget, substage 5 is the search for knowledge through trial and error. In this substage (12 to 18 months) the toddler demonstrates solving problems by trial and error. Substage 6—mental combinations of symbolic schemes (15 months to 2 years)—is a culmination of sensorimotor stages and a transition to the next stage. For example, a toddler will not handle a toy immediately to see how it works but will look at it carefully to think about how it works. Toddlers are becoming more differentiated from the environment. They will search for a hidden object where they last saw it, showing increasingly thorough understanding of object permanence.

By the end of the second year, the toddler enters the first part of the preoperational stage with preconceptual thinking. This stage is characterized by the beginning use of symbols, mental imagery, and increased language skills. A toddler continues to be very concrete and self-centered in thinking, which is the source of many miscommunications between parent and child.

During this time, language skills increase tremendously. Toddlers engage in collective monologues by themselves or in groups of children. The understanding of language increases. Toddlers can follow a two- or three-word command and can understand many sentences. The understanding of physical relationships begins with concepts, such as "on," "in," and "under." A 3-year-old can say name, age, and gender and use four- to five-word sentences. Strangers are beginning to understand what the toddler is trying to say. The child at this age can recognize all common objects and pictures.

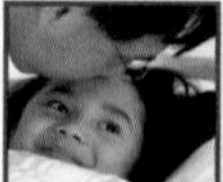

Yung Hi cries occasionally and remains nonverbal with the nurses. She speaks Korean with her parents and clings to her mother. Yung Hi's father has been attempting to explain the placement of the cast and hospital room to his wife and child. This may be a good time to have the father translate and assess for developmental data that will help you determine how to make Yung Hi's long stay less traumatic.

PRESCHOOLERS

Developmental Theory. A preschooler is a child between the ages of 3 and 5 years. Certain developmental changes take place throughout this time, particularly in the area of cognition, which is the act or process of knowing. Piaget's stages pertinent to the preschool- and school-age child are the preoperational stage (2 to 7 years), discussed here, and the concrete operational stage (7 to 11 years), discussed under School-Age Children later.

The preoperational stage is divided into two phases: the preoperational phase, ages 2 to 4, and the phase of intuitive thought, ages 4 to 7. During the preoperational phase, children shift from totally egocentric thought to social awareness and the ability to consider others' viewpoints. They acquire language and learn that they can use thought to deal with the world symbolically. They use words to describe actions and mentally and symbolically accomplish actions through the use of words. They develop the ability to imagine an action without performing the act. For example, they can imagine pulling a toy even if they do not actually have the toy to pull.

As the phase of intuitive thought begins, at about age 4, preschoolers first begin to think about the future and start to plan what they will be doing later in the day or in a few days, instead of concentrating on the here and now. This reflects their increasing ability to think. Around age 5 they show an increasing ability to use language to describe their emotions. An important requirement for preschoolers' mental development is that they be reared in an intellectually stimulating environment.

Action Alert! Counsel parents to give their children age-appropriate materials and to encourage them to explore their environment. Maximum mental growth takes place when they are stimulated mentally, year after year.

Physical Development. During the preschool period, a significant change in body contour occurs. The prominent lordosis and protuberant abdomen characteristic of the toddler change to slimmer, taller, and more childlike proportions. The child's future body type becomes more apparent. Body types may be *ectomorphic* (lanky body build), *mesomorphic* (medium muscular body), or *endomorphic* (large build). Weight, height, and growth differentials depend on genetic factors (e.g., tall parents generally have tall children), cultural and ethnic characteristics, dietary habits, and the general health of the child. In the United States, Asian children often plot low on the growth charts for both height and weight compared to European American children. African American children plot taller than both of the above groups (Pillitteri, in press).

Growth Parameters. The average preschool child gains weight slowly, only 4.5 pounds (2 kg) a year. It is not unusual for parents to perceive that the child is losing weight during this developmental period, whereas they are actually seeing age-appropriate changes in body contours. Preschoolers also grow slowly, gaining only 2 inches (51 mm) to 3.5 inches (89 mm) in an average year.

Physiological Changes. Preschool-age children undergo many physiological changes. Increased growth of lymphatic tissue increases the levels of antibodies in the child, so illnesses become more localized, as in a runny nose, with diminished systemic reaction such as fever. Heart murmurs may be heard on auscultation; this is because the heart changes its size in relation to the thorax, and murmurs at this stage are not normally a cause for concern. The heart rate decreases to about 85 beats per minute, and blood pressure stabilizes at about 100/60 mm Hg. The bladder is still quite small, so voiding occurs about eight to ten times daily; this explains why preschool children forget to use the toilet when they become absorbed in an activity and instead wet their clothes.

Dentition. Preschoolers generally have all 20 of their deciduous teeth by age 3 years. Rarely do new teeth erupt during this period. The American Academy of Pediatric Dentistry (2005) recommends initiating dental care when the first tooth erupts, with checkups twice a year thereafter.

Motor Development. Preschoolers experience tremendous improvement in large and fine muscle coordination. They can run well, walk up and down stairs, and learn to hop. By age 5 years, they can usually skip and throw and catch balls (Table 16-2). Improving fine motor skills and hand-eye coordination enables them to copy circles, squares, and triangles and to print letters and numbers. Their motor development depends primarily on overall physical maturation and is influenced by their opportunities for exercise and practice of activities such as skipping and hopping.

Language Development. By age 5, preschoolers have a vocabulary of more than 2000 words. They can use all parts of speech correctly. They tend to use more verbs than nouns. Their sentences average four to five words in length. They can define familiar objects, identify colors, and express their feelings. They understand the concepts of "under," "over," "up," and "down" and of opposites, such as "open" versus "closed." The pattern of asking questions is at its peak, and they will repeat a question until they receive an answer.

Psychosocial Development. The psychosocial development of preschoolers is marked by an increasing sense of personal identity and willingness to work with others. Erikson identifies this third of his eight psychological stages as the tasks of sense of initiative over guilt.

Peer Relationships. The development of peer relationships is one of the most important aspects of a child's social development. Four-year-olds continue to play in groups but may become involved in more arguments as they begin testing their roles in the group. The increasing conflict may cause parents to worry that their child is regressing, but it is really a forward movement. Five-year-olds begin selecting their "best" friends. They depend less on parents and more on peers for social interaction. They tend to offer approval, make demands on one another, and demonstrate the ability to show empathy when others are distressed (Sugarman, 2001).

Gender-Role Development. At ages 4 to 5, preschoolers develop gender-role identification and begin to assume the roles of persons of their own sex. Kohlberg (1966), a psychologist credited with identifying the reasoning ability of children, states that the child's self-categorization as a boy or girl is the basic organizer of the gender-role attitudes that develop. Children act consistently in accordance with gender expectations communicated to them by family members and society. Boys and girls are socialized differently from birth. In the United States, boys are often expected to be more active and aggressive, whereas girls are expected to be polite and less aggressive. However, these behavioral tendencies are at least partially biological, thus they will not entirely be suppressed by changes in socialization.

Play. Play promotes physical, social, and mental development of preschoolers. Five-year-olds continue to enjoy the rough-and-tumble play that they participated in at age 4, but they become more interested in group games, such as board games or sports such as soccer. This helps them learn to take turns and to be able to accept losing or winning and to cooperate with other children in a group. Active play is important for physical growth, refinement of motor skills, and releasing pent-up energy; the use of tricycles, wagons, sports equipment, and water play can help develop muscles and coordination. Playtime also helps them to learn to control their impulses and feelings and to express them in socially acceptable ways. Imaginative play is a healthy outlet for ill children because it allows them to think of creative solutions to their illness experiences and to develop problem-solving skills.

Action Alert! Inform parents that playtime is especially significant for the child who is ill. Through play, children can express and work out fears, anger, and misunderstandings about their illness.

Symbolic play is pretend or imaginative play that enables preschool children to recreate experiences and to try out roles (Figure 16-4). They create imaginary companions with whom they talk and play and who become a regular part of their daily routines. Reassure parents that it is normal for their preschoolers to create imaginary playmates and that it helps the child differentiate between fantasy and reality.

Fears. Common fears that develop at this time include fear of the dark, separation from parents, and, in some cases, fear of bodily harm.

Table 16-2 Motor Skills of the Child 4 to 11 Years Old

AGE	MOTOR SKILL
4 years	• Walks on tiptoes • Alternates feet when descending stairs • Hops or jumps forward • Holds a pencil with control • Can cut and paste
5 years	• Skips • Throws overhand with some accuracy • Can catch a bounced ball • Handles scissors with skill • Rides a tricycle
6 years	• Ties own shoes • Runs, jumps, climbs • Skips • Rides a bike with training wheels • Learns to swim
7 to 8 years	• Can use in-line skates • Rides a bicycle • Swimming improves • Continues to refine small muscle control • Is more graceful • Can throw and hit a baseball
9 to 11 years	• Can participate in most sports • Has good hand-eye coordination • Refines gross and fine motor skills • Can do craft projects • Can catch a ball in one hand

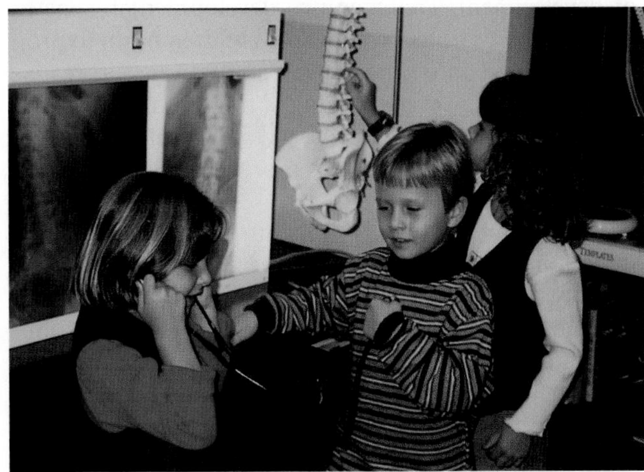

FIGURE 16-4 Symbolic play enables preschool children to recreate experiences and try out various adult roles.

- *Fear of the dark:* The vivid imagination of the preschool-age child can turn a stuffed toy by day into a threatening monster in the dark. Parents must be prepared for this fear and understand that it is a normal phase of growth. They may need to reassure their child who is reluctant to go to sleep unless a light is on or who wakes up screaming from a nightmare.
- *Fear of separation or abandonment:* Fear of separation continues to be a concern for preschoolers because they do not have a sense of time. They are not comforted by mother's reassurances that she will return to preschool in 2 hours.
- *Fear of mutilation:* Some preschoolers have a fear of bodily harm that may make it difficult for them to cooperate with medical personnel and treatments, such as needlesticks or an otoscopic examination. They cry out not only from the pain but also from the sight of injury.

Moral Development. Piaget (1997) describes the development of moral judgment as a gradual cognitive process enhanced by the increasing social relationships of children. Early in their moral development, children are constrained by the "rules of the game." As children develop, they learn that rules are not absolute but can be altered by social consensus and that adult rules are no longer sacred.

Preschoolers begin to have an elemental concept of God if they have been provided some exposure to religion. This belief in an outside force aids the development of conscience (Kohlberg, 1981), but preschoolers tend to do good out of self-interest rather than because of spiritual motivation. They enjoy the security of religious rituals, such as grace said before meals. Praying to God and observing religious traditions can help children through stressful periods such as hospitalization.

SCHOOL-AGE CHILDREN

Developmental Theory. According to Piaget (1980), school-age children are in the concrete operational stage of development. The cognitive developmental stage of **concrete operations** occurs when children begin to project themselves into other people's situations and realize that their own way of thinking is not the only way. Decentering accommodation is a child's ability to adapt thought processes to perceive more than one reason for a person's actions.

At this time, children's thoughts become increasingly logical and coherent, and they are able to classify, sort, and organize facts. However, they still lack the capacity to generalize or deal in abstract ideas. School-age children are able to increase their understanding of many concepts associated with objects. Class inclusion is a child's ability to understand that objects can belong to more than one group. The ability to group things into categories enables the child to expand knowledge through category-based indicators, which enables them to solve problems. **Conservation** is a child's ability to understand that changing the shape of a substance does not change its volume. Preschool-age children lack this perception (Figure 16-5). Understanding this concept helps limit sibling arguments over who has more milk when two different-shaped glasses of equal volume are presented.

> ***Action Alert!*** Teach parents to understand that their school-age child may demonstrate varying abilities to handle problems and can most effectively handle one major problem at a time.

Language Development. At age 6, the child's vocabulary is quite large, about 10,000 words, and it reaches about 40,000 by adolescence. School-age children enlarge their vocabularies by analyzing the structure of complex words and thinking about them and using them more precisely. They appreciate the multiple meanings of words. Their conversational strategies become more refined, and they can speak in full sentences. Children have generally mastered most of the grammar of their language when they enter school, and a 12-year-old can easily converse with an adult (Behrman et al., 2004).

Psychosocial Theory. According to Erikson's stages of development, the developmental task of the school years is the establishment of a sense of industry, in which the child is motivated to expend effort in a purposeful activity. During this stage, a child masters social and cognitive skills. However, there is a risk that the child will not gain competency at a chosen task and will develop a sense of inferiority rather than of industry. Successful completion of this stage of development

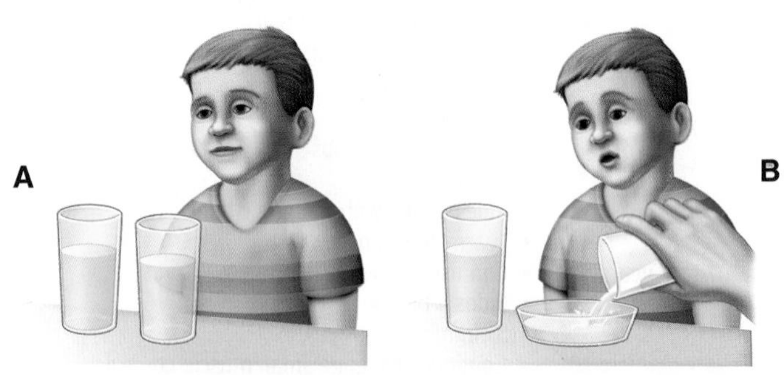

FIGURE 16-5 The preschool child does not yet understand the principle of conservation. **A,** The preschooler is able to understand that two glasses of the same size contain equal amounts of liquid. **B,** However, when the contents of one of the glasses is poured into a dish of equal volume, the child becomes perplexed because he does not understand that changing the shape of a substance does not change its volume.

enables children to recognize their abilities as well as their liabilities and to develop a sense of competence. Competition is also important; by comparing themselves to their peers, children can understand their own personal strengths and weaknesses.

Physical Development. A school-age child is a child between 6 and 11 years old. Although some girls begin puberty during the end of this period, most researchers consider these girls developmentally preadolescent despite their physical changes. During the school years, children's rate of physical growth is steady but slower than at any time since birth; however, their motor, cognitive, and psychosocial development progresses rapidly.

Growth Parameters. On average, school-age children grow 1 to 2 inches (25 to 51 mm) and gain 3 to 5 pounds (1.36 to 2.27 kg) per year. Boys are slightly taller and heavier than girls during the early school years, but by age 9, girls experience acceleration in skeletal growth and begin to be taller and heavier than boys to the acute discomfort of both. Boys experience acceleration in growth around 12 years of age (Hockenberry et al., 2003).

Physiological Changes. Cardiovascular function is usually stable in school-age children. Growth of the brain is complete around age 10, and this results in the refinement of fine motor coordination. Maturation of the respiratory system leads to increased oxygen–carbon dioxide exchange, increasing exertion ability and stamina. The frontal sinuses are developed, and sinus-caused headaches become a possibility.

Dentition. During the school-age years, all primary teeth are lost and the majority of permanent teeth have erupted. The timing is somewhat variable, depending on both heredity and nutrition (Figure 16-6). Children need to brush and floss daily to maintain healthy teeth and gums. A dentist needs to be consulted about jaw malformations or misaligned teeth.

Action Alert! Remind parents that children should have a dental examination and teeth cleaning every 6 months.

Sexual Maturation. The hypothalamus transmits an enzyme to the anterior pituitary gland to begin production of gonadotropic hormones, which activate changes in testes and ovaries at about 10 years of age (Edelman and Mandle, 2006). Timing of sexual maturity varies widely between 10 and 14 years of age. Puberty is occurring increasingly earlier, and it would not be unusual to find school-age girls already menstruating at age 11 or earlier.

Action Alert! Encourage parents to discuss sexual responsibility with the child. Children at this age should also be reminded that their body is their own to be used only in the way they choose.

Motor Development. As musculature increases in size, coordination continues to improve. Most 6- to 11-year-olds can learn to in-line skate; play baseball, soccer, or tennis; and do gymnastics. Fine motor skills continue to develop as well. School-age children can sew, learn to use garden tools, handle a hammer and a saw, draw in proportion, and master penmanship in writing. Reaction time depends on brain maturation, which is why so many children ages 5 to 7 have trouble catching a ball. Any sport that requires quick reactions, distance judgment, and hand-eye coordination may be difficult for younger school-age children.

Peer Relationships. Learning to understand and get along with children who are different from them are important developmental tasks; generally, school-age children prefer same-sex friends. Their acceptance by their peers is very important and influences their adjustment during adolescence (Box 16-2).

Gender-Role Development. Gender stereotypes are learned through parents, teachers, peers, and the media. Children's understanding of gender roles broadens, and their gender role identities change as they think more about people as personalities.

Play. During the school years, group activities dominate playtime. Through group dynamics, school-age children learn to work cooperatively toward a common goal. Success in physical and cognitive play is important.

Fears. As children explore the world around them, having new experiences and confronting new challenges, fears and anxieties are an unavoidable part of growing up. Children between the ages of 6 and 11 have many fears and concerns, such as fear of darkness, animals, high places, or thunderstorms. The death of a close friend or family member may cause them much anxiety about the health of those around them. Children want to be reassured that these terrible things will not happen to them. It is important to let children talk about a frightening situation and to share what is on their minds.

Action Alert! Children may be concerned about what they see on TV or read in the newspaper. Encourage parents to reassure their children and provide them the perspective they need to understand what they are viewing. To handle terrifying and confusing situations, children take their emotional cues from the adults around them.

Moral Development. At age 6 or 7, children know the rules and behaviors that are expected of them, but they do not understand the reasons behind them. Rewards and punishments guide their judgments. Older school-age children are able to understand what prompts an action and therefore do not judge an action only on its consequences.

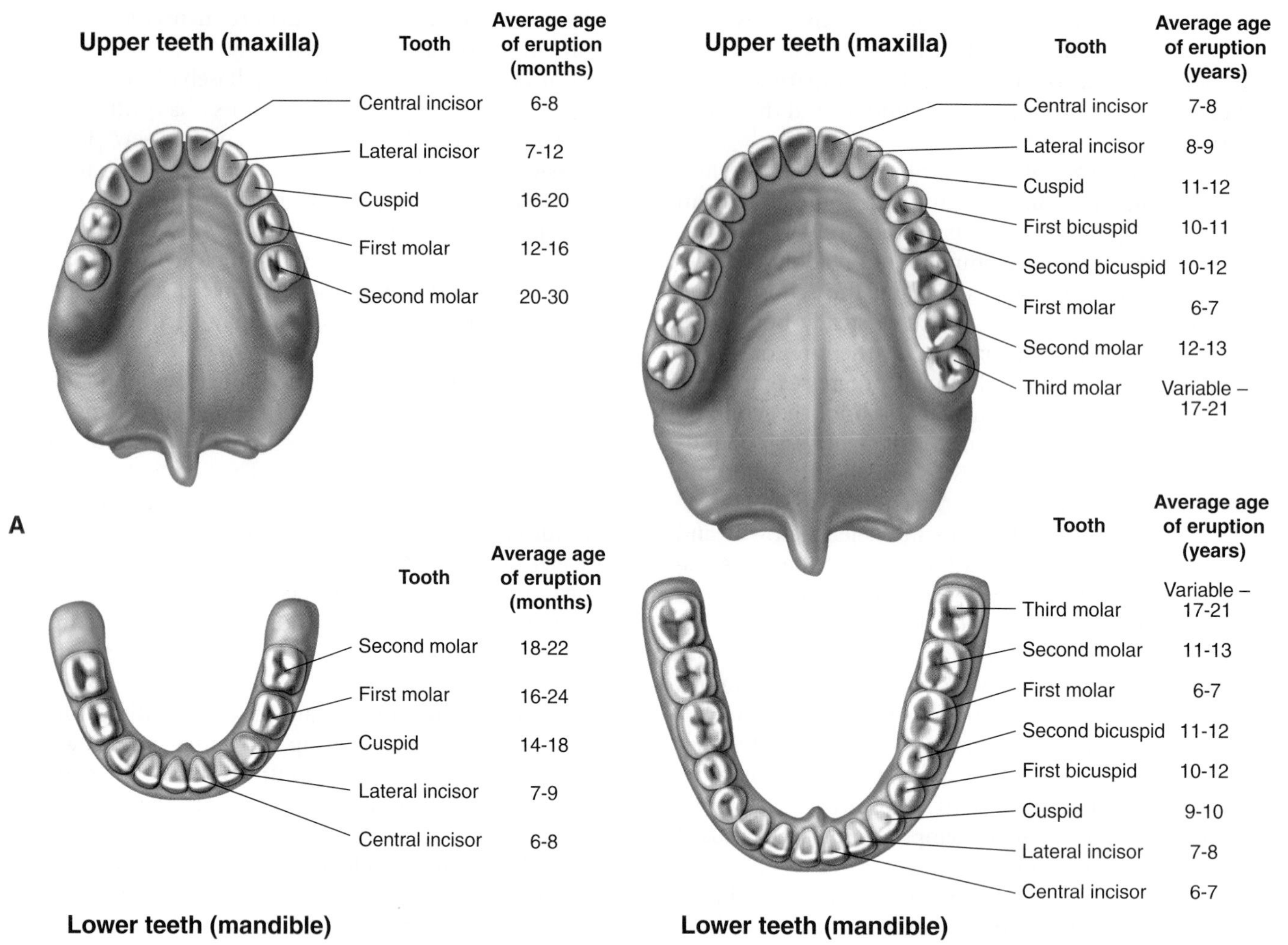

FIGURE 16-6 Sequence of eruption of primary **(A)** and secondary **(B)** teeth.

BOX 16-2 *Behavioral Characteristics That Promote Peer Acceptance*

- Being outgoing, socially interactive
- Being physically attractive (girls); having athletic ability (boys)
- Having a high level of energy
- Participating early in social events
- Having a good sense of humor and being good natured
- Accepting others even when they are different from oneself
- Performing well in school
- Having the ability to communicate effectively

FACTORS AFFECTING GROWTH AND DEVELOPMENT

Many factors, such as environment, socioeconomic status, nutrition, and physiological status, influence growth and development. In all stages of development, lifestyle and psychological factors influence health behaviors. The interaction of these factors greatly affects response to everyday situations. These factors also influence the choices caregivers make regarding health care behaviors.

RISK FACTORS/NEEDS ACROSS THE LIFE SPAN

Family Dynamics. Family dynamics is the pattern of interpersonal relationships within a family. This pattern is affected by the structure, size, and composition of the family. A child's ability to feel secure about self and relate to others depends on how well identity is established and how supportive the family members are of the child. Parents who are nurturing, supportive, and consistent in enforcing rules will help to foster childhood development.

Family Structure. Each individual has a position in the family structure and plays a defined role in interactions within the family group. Structure includes traditions

BOX 16-3 *Cross-Cultural Care*

Caring for a Korean Toddler

Yung Hi, the young client presented in this chapter, and her family are Korean and new to the United States. Koreans, like many Asian peoples, are of Mongolian-Tungus descent. Although each person is unique, Korean people are generally characterized as being generous, kind, and resourceful. The following behaviors also have been identified as culturally characteristic and valued by Korean people:

- Putting the family's welfare ahead of the individual's
- Viewing infants and young children as passive and dependent
- Having a strong sense of self-respect and self-control
- Maintaining a stoic demeanor and offering few complaints
- Being polite by giving a person the response he or she is expecting
- Avoiding physical contact
- Upholding men as authorities, with women expected to be obedient
- Believing that education is important
- Viewing health as a balance between positive and negative energy forces (yin and yang)

and values that set standards for interaction within and outside the group. Family size and composition also influence child development. Parents treat children differently, and sibling interactions vary depending on the child's position within the family. Age differences between siblings affect the childhood environment. The arrival of a baby brother or sister has the greatest impact on the older child, and a 2- to 4-year difference in age appears to be most threatening.

Culture and Religion. Culture influences everything people do, produce, know, and believe in as they grow and develop as members of social groups. As children become familiar with the patterns of behavior associated with their culture, they also develop distinctive personalities, thoughts, and feelings, as suggested in Box 16-3. Religious development refers to the acceptance of specific beliefs, values, rules of conduct, and rituals.

Discipline. The term *discipline* refers to adherence to a set of rules for conduct, and it also describes actions taken to enforce the rules after noncompliance. Limit setting means establishing guidelines for behavior. Children want and need limits. These limits must be clear and enforced consistently for children to adhere to the rules.

Community. Children and their families reside in a community in which residents share and are influenced by a common environment. The community can encourage a positive outcome for children, or it can stunt it. Children living in high-risk neighborhoods have more social and behavioral problems than those in low-risk neighborhoods.

Socioeconomic Factors. Income, educational level, and single parenthood influence the growth and development of children. A child who grows up in an economically deprived home may have impairments in physical, psychosocial, and cognitive development. Inadequate educational resources can influence parenting skills, finances, and basic knowledge of a child's developmental needs. One of the most adverse influences on health is low socioeconomic status. People whose socioeconomic status is low suffer from more health problems at any one time than people in any other group. These families often have poor medical care, higher mortality rates, and higher rates of psychological and mental illnesses.

Nutritional Factors. Nutritional concerns for the child begin during pregnancy and continue after birth, when the parents decide what method of feeding to choose. Human milk is the most desirable for the first 12 months of life.

Solid foods are introduced gradually, beginning at about 4 months. Iron-fortified cereals are usually recommended by 6 months. After that, strained, pureed infant foods are gradually added, one at a time, usually one every 5 days. As each new food is added to the infant's diet, the parent should observe for signs of intolerance or allergy. The toddler's growth rate slows, decreasing slightly the need for calories, fluids, and protein. Most toddlers are eating the same food prepared for the family and using a cup. Nutrition continues to be important as the child grows and develops.

Poor nutrition may cause a child to tire easily, have a poor appetite, experience slower growth, or become ill because of an inability to resist pathogens and infections. As children grow, poor eating habits can contribute to the development of obesity. Discuss with parents the importance of providing children with nutritious, appealing foods.

PHYSIOLOGICAL FACTORS

Most children grow and develop without problems. However, a variety of physiological factors may influence a child's growth and development. One of the most difficult and most costly stems from preterm birth; these infants may experience developmental delay and chronic illness as complications. Physiological factors that affect the child's growth and development may include respiratory ailments such as recurrent colds and asthma, as well as ear infections (most commonly otitis media). Other common childhood occurrences include enuresis (recurrent involuntary urination), head lice, and animal or insect bites.

Parents should encourage their children to exercise and become involved in enjoyable and vigorous activities that promote their physical development, preferably with other children at the same developmental level. Activities should help children develop motor skills that will enable them to reach their full physical potential and should provide them with basic skills and habits that will make fitness an enjoyable, lifelong activity.

The number of hours per day spent sleeping varies with individual children and with different age-groups. The preschool-age child sleeps approximately 11 hours; this gradually decreases during the school-age years to 9 or 10 hours.

LIFESTYLE FACTORS

Attention Deficit/Hyperactivity Disorder. Attention-deficit/hyperactivity disorder (ADHD) is a neuropsychological disorder associated with disturbances in attention, impulsivity, and hyperactivity. ADHD is estimated to affect 6% to 9% of children and adolescents, and it is more prevalent in boys. Children with ADHD are at risk for developing emotional and behavioral problems, such as misconduct or antisocial behaviors, substance abuse, depression, and anxiety disorders. Frequently however, children with ADHD have intuitiveness and creativity, which helps them to be successful in other areas. Differences may also be found in the child's memory, social skills, and listening, speaking, and writing skills (DuPaul & Stoner, 2003).

Learning Disability. According to the Learning Disabilities Association of America (2005), a learning disability is a lifelong disorder that affects the manner in which people of normal or above-average intelligence select, retain, and express information. It has been estimated that approximately 20% of public school children have a learning disability (Edelman & Mandle, 2006). The deficiency usually occurs in specific areas such as reading, although related skills such as writing and mathematical concepts may also be affected. An evaluation may reveal that overall ability as measured by IQ tests is not abnormal, but standardized academic achievement tests may demonstrate areas of weakness.

Substance Abuse. When children begin to experiment with drugs, they often mistakenly think they can control their use. Children at risk for drug use are those who have poor self-concept or a strong need for acceptance and approval of their peers. Children who have school or family stresses may find relief in the use of controlled substances. Substance abuse is quite prevalent in the school-age population. Studies indicate that as children get older they have experimented with more substances. By the time they are high school seniors, 40% have tried marijuana, 9% cocaine, 12% inhalant use of glue or paint, 8% methamphetamines, 11% ecstasy, and 3% heroin. By the age of 9, 47% have had their first drink of alcohol (MMWR, 2004).

Tobacco Use. The use of tobacco, both smoking and smokeless, is also found in the middle school age-group. The most recent statistics indicate that 12% of students reported using some form of tobacco at least twice a month with cigarettes being the most prevalent form of tobacco use. The younger a child begins to smoke, the more likely he or she is to be addicted to nicotine as an adult. Nearly half of these children will die from a smoking-related disease (American Cancer Society, 2004).

Action Alert! Encourage parents to discuss the risks of tobacco, alcohol, and other drugs with their children.

Obesity. Over the last 20 years the problem of overweight and obese children has increased in the United States to become the most common health problem facing children. In the United States, 20.6% of children between the ages of 2 to 5 and 30.3% of children ages 6 to 11 are overweight. This figure has shown a steady increase since the 1960s (Fowler-Brown & Kahwati, 2004). The fact that children eat high-fat meals at both home and school compounds the problem. These foods have become the acceptable norm in our society. Children are also spending more time indoors in the front of the television or computer and not engaging in physical exercise.

ASSESSMENT

Assessment of the physical, cognitive, and psychosocial capabilities of the newborn, infant, toddler, preschool and school-age child is completed at initial and follow-up visits to the physician or advanced practice nurse. The purpose of these examinations is health promotion and disease prevention.

GENERAL ASSESSMENT

Newborns, Infants, and Toddlers. The examination for newborns, infants, and toddlers, called the well-baby examination, includes the health history and the physical examination. A comprehensive health history includes many components (Box 16-4). Typically, the health care provider obtains a complete history during the initial health care visit and updates it on subsequent visits. For an ill child, the history focuses on the current complaint. The health history closes with a review of systems. Before beginning the physical examination, make sure the child is warm and comfortable. Proceed to examine each body system thoroughly and accurately, using inspection, palpation, percussion, and auscultation.

Instruments used to assess growth include a tape measure, a height marker, and a scale. Use a tape measure to obtain height (or length) and head circumference. At age 2 years, measure the child's standing height.

Weigh an infant or small child without clothing on a hygienic paper liner, because the weight of the diaper can add 10% or more to the child's weight. By age 3 years, the child, dressed only in underpants, should be weighed on a standing scale. Scales used for weighing children may be self-adjusting, or they may need to be balanced before each use.

Measure the head circumference of the newborn and until the child is 3 years old. Place the measuring tape around the largest circumference of the head, just above the eyebrows and the posterior prominence of the occiput. The tape should remain horizontal from front to back.

Compare the child's height and weight with growth charts to detect risks from slow or accelerated growth. Initial measurements are done immediately after birth and compared with a graph of the relationship between gestational age in weeks and birth weight to determine if the newborn is average, small, or large for gestational age. During frequent health visits from the newborn through the toddler stage, the relationships between height and weight continue to be measured and recorded on charts to diagnose any disorders related to physical, emotional, environmental, or social deficiencies.

The simplest and most efficient method of assessing developmental milestones is to obtain a developmental history and observation. Ask parents to recall when developmental events occurred in their child's life. Various methods and instruments are available to ascertain developmental milestones in children, such as the Denver Developmental Screening Test II.

Preschool and School-Age Children. Optimal childhood growth and development and prevention of accidents and illness are the objectives of pediatric health supervision. The aim of the health history is to review the child's past physical and psychosocial history and to determine whether the parents or the child has any complaints or concerns. It includes a complete assessment of nutrition, exercise habits, sleep patterns, and growth and development milestones. Progress in school and the child's social interactions with family and peers should also be evaluated.

The depth and extent of a nursing health history vary with its intended purpose. The format used for history taking is usually a combination of direct and indirect techniques to elicit information about each of the functional health patterns. The school-age child should be able to cooperate fully with you, whereas the younger child may be more challenging.

Preschoolers and school-age children should have routine well-child examinations. The well-child examination involves several evaluations. The immunization history is reviewed to be sure the child is current. Measurements of

BOX 16-4 *Example of Health History Questions*

- *Reason for contact:* Why did the child come to the health care provider? Was it for a health maintenance visit, or was there a complaint of illness?
- *Present illness, chief concern:* What are the signs and associated symptoms? What makes them better or worse? Which over-the-counter drugs were taken? How long did the symptoms persist? What was done for the problem?
- *Family history:* What is the health status of siblings, parents, and grandparents? Are there significant illnesses or genetic problems in the family? Any heart, kidney, or congenital diseases? Does anyone in the family have seizures, mental retardation, or mental illness? Is there a family history of tuberculosis, diabetes, or sexually transmitted disease? Do allergies run in the family? If they do, inquire further about specific symptoms.
- *Prenatal and childbirth history:* Were there any medical, surgical, or pregnancy problems? Has the mother had any miscarriages or stillbirths? Ask the mother about the pregnancy with this child. Did she use cigarettes, alcohol, or drugs while pregnant? If so, how much? Was this pregnancy planned? What was the labor like? How long was it? Were there any complications? What type of analgesia or anesthesia was used?
- *Neonatal history:* Were there any unusual circumstances during the newborn period? When did the baby sleep through the night? Was the baby unusually fussy? At what time of the day was the baby most fretful?
- *Social history:* What is the home situation like? Who are the significant others in the child's life? In what activities is the child engaged? Does the child attend day care? How does the child like it?
- *Nutritional history:* What type of infant feeding is or was being done? What is a typical menu for 24 hours? What foods does the child like or dislike? Are there any food allergies?
- *Developmental history:* Were typical developmental milestones achieved? When did they occur? Were there any significant developmental delays?
- *Immunization history:* What immunizations were given? Do they need to be updated? Were there any untoward reactions?

the child's height, weight, and blood pressure are obtained, and vision and hearing are screened. A complete physical examination is performed.

Additional diagnostic tests may be performed, but there is some variability in the tests performed at each visit. The following are examples of such tests.

Cholesterol Screening. Parents are becoming increasingly aware that risk factors for cardiovascular disease, particularly coronary artery disease related to dietary cholesterol intake, may be present in their children. However, there is no consensus regarding the efficacy of universal cholesterol screening in children.

Action Alert! Advise parents of young children to provide diets low in cholesterol and saturated fat. Recommend an active lifestyle for children and the avoidance of smoking, including exposure to secondhand smoke.

Blood Testing for Lead Poisoning. According to the Centers for Disease Control and Prevention (CDC), 310,000 U.S. children between the ages of 1 and 5 have lead blood levels greater than the CDC recommended level of 10 micrograms of lead per deciliter. Children from all socioeconomic and ethnic groups can be affected by lead poisoning; however, children living at or below the poverty line and African American children are at greater risk. The CDC estimates 3% of African American children compared to 1.3% of white children have elevated blood lead levels. The major sources of lead exposure are deteriorated lead-based paint in older housing and dust and soil that are contaminated with lead from old paint and from past emissions of leaded gasoline. Lead poisoning can cause learning disabilities, behavioral problems, and, at very high levels, seizures, coma, and even death. The CDC recommends that at-risk children undergo a blood test for lead (CDC, 2005a).

Tuberculosis Screening. In the United States, tuberculosis (TB) occurs in less than 1% of children. However, all children should have a careful history to ascertain their risk and should be screened three times during childhood for TB: at 12 to 15 months of age, before entering kindergarten, and at 14 to 16 years of age. The multipuncture Mono-Vac is adequate for routine screening rather than the purified protein derivative (PPD) test. Children found to be at risk should be identified and screened yearly.

FOCUSED ASSESSMENT FOR DELAYED GROWTH AND DEVELOPMENT

Assessment of growth and development is a routine part of a well-child assessment from birth through school-age. It is based on knowledge of normal growth and development and the methods of eliciting information from the child and the parent. Important historical information beginning with birth records will provide the nurse critical data needed such as any preexisting conditions that may affect delay.

Defining Characteristics. The defining characteristics related to the nursing diagnosis *Delayed growth and development* are observed behaviors that indicate that the individual is experiencing an alteration in growth and development. Signs and symptoms that may indicate a delay might include the inability to perform basic self-care activities such as bathing or toileting, difficulty in performing motor skills such as ambulation, and altered physical growth.

Related Factors. Children are at risk for problems of growth and development from both internal and external factors. Physical development requires health, nutrition, and exercise. Psychosocial development requires opportunities to complete developmental tasks with a warm, caring adult to guide the way.

Children who have chronic illnesses such as congenital heart defects, inadequate nutrition or cerebral palsy, unstable family lives, teenage mothers, or multiple caregivers are at risk for *Delayed growth and development*. If you practice in a hospital, you will know that a child who is withdrawn or whose behavior is inappropriate for the age may be reacting to the hospital or may have a larger developmental problem. During the child's health maintenance visit in the clinic, you can pick up cues by listening to the parent's description of the child and by observing the child's behavior.

Related factors for *Delayed growth and development* can be divided into two categories: those of the parent and those of the child. You need to decide whether the problem of *Delayed growth and development* can best be solved by working directly with the child or with the parent. Parenting style and parenting skills are basic related factors for *Delayed growth and development.* Physiological factors should be considered if a disability or chronic disease is present. The care plan would then include modifications that take the disability into account.

If the parents lack the skills to provide a lifestyle conducive to healthy growth, or if they are just indifferent to the child's needs, development may be hampered. Consistency is important in parenting. Parents who respond sporadically to the child's needs or vacillate between positive and negative responses will not provide the child with a consistent pattern of caring that is needed to enable the child to choose healthy behaviors. Related factors in the child category include separation from family members and environmental stimulation, whereas factors in the parent or caregiver category include multiple caregivers and inadequate caretaking.

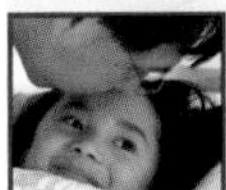

Upon assessment of Yung Hi, you see many of the related factors characteristic of a child with *Delayed growth and development.* Yung is a toddler in a private room and is on complete bed rest. She must depend totally on others. She is separated from her home and usual routine. Yung's physical disability limits her level of activity, and she cannot speak English. Her mother spends most of the day with her; however, when her father comes to visit in the evenings, he takes Yung's mother home with him. Have you determined any other related factors?

FOCUSED ASSESSMENT FOR *INEFFECTIVE HEALTH MAINTENANCE*

The nursing diagnosis *Ineffective health maintenance* refers to an alteration in health due to lack of knowledge or an unhealthy lifestyle. An alteration in health maintenance is almost never under the control of infants or toddlers; therefore you will need to assess the parent or family. As the child grows, you will begin to do health teaching with the child. Signs and symptoms of ineffective health maintenance in a child or infant may include diaper rash, poor nutrition, or exposure due to inappropriate clothing.

Defining Characteristics. The defining characteristics for *Ineffective health maintenance* include practice of an unhealthy lifestyle, lack of interest in health maintenance, and inability to take responsibility for meeting basic health needs. Other characteristics may include an inability to follow instructions, impaired cognitive functioning, and a lack of coping with environmental changes.

For the infant, toddler, and child, altered health maintenance is a reflection of family health practices. Parents who lack education, have a history of substance use or abuse, are single parents, lack support systems, have financial distress, or have a chronic illness may present problems for the child's health and wellness. You can pick up further cues when discussing child immunization schedules with the parent, such as the parent's inability to concentrate or follow instructions or a lack of interest in making the next scheduled well-baby visit that includes immunizations.

Related Factors. Related factors for *Ineffective health maintenance* involve the parents and the child and may include lack of communication skills, ineffective family coping, and the inability to identify and seek health care.

FOCUSED ASSESSMENT FOR *IMPAIRED PARENTING*

The nursing diagnosis *Impaired parenting* refers to the inability to provide a nurturing and caring environment for the infant or child. A health maintenance visit for the school-age child includes an assessment of the parent's ability to provide a constructive environment that nurtures the growth and development of the child. During the health maintenance visit, look for cues by observing the interaction between the child and the parent and by listening to their descriptions of developmental issues and concerns.

Defining Characteristics. The defining characteristics of the nursing diagnosis *Impaired parenting* are assessment of a nonnurturing environment with delays in growth and development, observed inappropriate parenting behaviors, or concern with parenting skills expressed by the parent. Evidence of child abuse is a clear defining characteristic of *Impaired parenting* and requires *immediate intervention.*

Related Factors. Difficulties in parenting can be related to a lack of knowledge or lack of exposure to positive parenting practices. Situational or personal factors may contribute to parental role conflicts and may include the lack of knowledge and resources.

DIAGNOSIS

Once the components of the assessment are completed, you will determine a nursing diagnosis, as demonstrated in Table 16-3. The choice of a nursing diagnosis involving a child's growth and development in the first 3 years after birth depends on the problems identified and the etiological factors of the diagnosis. When the history and physical examination reveal abnormal growth or development parameters resulting from environmental deprivation, physical disability, or an acute problem, *Delayed growth and development* is an appropriate choice for a nursing diagnosis.

Because parenting style and parenting skills are related factors for *Delayed growth and development,* you will need to distinguish between the diagnoses *Impaired parenting, Ineffective family coping,* and *Delayed growth and development.* If the problem involves family functioning, such as an alcoholic or abusive family, you may choose *Ineffective family coping.* The approach to treatment then becomes centered on the family.

If you are working primarily with the parent and indirectly with the children, the diagnosis is more likely to be *Impaired parenting.* The defining characteristics of *Impaired parenting* suggest that the diagnosis refers to the more serious behaviors that define a parent's inability to relate positively to the child.

The nursing diagnosis *Ineffective health maintenance* is directly related to growth and development, but it has a different focus. Positive health practices help to ensure that growth and development proceed normally. Although this diagnosis is typically used for a well child who has no obvious problems, family health practices may place the child at risk for growing up unhealthy or for contracting specific illnesses or health problems of childhood, such as measles or dental caries.

Deficient diversional activity may be the appropriate nursing diagnosis for a child experiencing a restriction in,

Table 16-3 Clustering Data to Make a Nursing Diagnosis

DATA CLUSTER	DIAGNOSIS
Growth and Development Problems	
30-month-old boy admitted to hospital for malnutrition. Height and weight below 15th percentile on growth charts. Child is lethargic and nonverbal. Mother reports withholding food when he cries.	*Delayed growth and development* related to inappropriate caregiving and possibly parental indifference
Unemployed teenage mother of 2-year-old unable to present immunization health record. Mother expresses lack of knowledge about "kids needing shots." Toddler diagnosed with mumps.	*Ineffective health maintenance* related to lack of knowledge and possibly lack of financial resources
Parents make and meet each scheduled well-child appointment for their school-age child. Child's immunizations are complete.	*Health-seeking behaviors* related to desire to obtain higher level of wellness through prevention
An 11-year-old who had above-average grades until this year. When his friends made the football team, he started hanging out with a different group. He has been arrested for shoplifting and possession of marijuana. His physician referred him to a psychiatric nurse practitioner for counseling.	*Ineffective individual coping* related to establishing peer relationships through reckless behavior

or decreased stimulation from, recreational or play activities. *Deficient diversional activity* influences developmental growth. It is associated with any prolonged hospitalization. It is also an appropriate diagnosis for a homebound child with a chronic or disabling condition. Defining characteristics include isolation with limited ability to leave the room; lack of age-appropriate toys at the bedside; physical limitations affecting participation in usual activities; and irritability, moodiness, and inactivity.

You may find that *Deficient diversional activity* is also a related factor for other nursing diagnoses.

PLANNING

Planning a comprehensive, consistent care plan for wellness will include elements of the nursing diagnoses *Delayed growth and development* and *Ineffective health maintenance*.

Expected Outcomes for *Delayed Growth and Development*. The expected outcome criteria for a child with altered growth and development are an increase in the child's weight, height, or both, and a demonstration of social, language, cognitive, or motor activities appropriate for the child's age. Additional outcome criteria for children or parents are the following:

- Child participation in daily physical activities is appropriate for his or her age.
- The child experiences no injuries (other than normal cuts and bruises) from play activities or other activities of daily living.
- Parents will bring their child to a dentist at least once a year, and the child brushes and flosses teeth (under adult supervision) at least once daily.
- Parents will bring their child for recommended screening tests at appropriate times.
- An older school-age child understands his or her growth and development patterns.

Expected Outcomes for *Ineffective Health Maintenance*. The overall expected outcome criteria for a client with altered health maintenance are that the child is present for all scheduled health maintenance visits and maintains health status. Other outcomes for this diagnosis are the following:

- Parents describe an appropriate health maintenance program.
- Parents demonstrate behaviors needed to manage the child's health alteration.
- Parents identify health resources available, such as pediatric nurse practitioner, nutritionist, and dentist.
- Child receives all scheduled immunizations.
- Parents use appropriate safety measures, such as car seats and age-appropriate toys.
- Child progresses to at least average performance levels in schoolwork and activities.

INTERVENTION

NEWBORNS, INFANTS, AND TODDLERS

Implementation of your care plan to promote healthy growth and development as well as health maintenance will involve working closely with the child's parents. Education of parents is the primary choice of intervention for both diagnoses.

Interventions to Promote Growth and Development. Nurses play an important role in promoting healthy growth and development through informing and teaching parents of newborns, infants, and toddlers. Appropriate parenting skills in relation to attachment, play, nutrition, toilet training, rest and sleep, caring for a sick child, and referrals are the realms of the interventions discussed.

Promoting Attachment. Attachment is an ongoing process that begins during pregnancy and intensifies during the months after birth. Once established, it is a constant and consistent relationship. Attachment is strengthened by intense communication between parent and child through eye-to-eye contact, touch, voice, odor, and reciprocal, synchronous activity.

Teaching Parenting Skills. These days there are fewer opportunities to teach parents basic baby-care techniques. Another opportunity for parent education occurs during each well-child visit. Take time to answer parents' questions about childcare and child-rearing issues, such as discipline, sleep disturbances, and nutritional needs. Suggest classes, support groups, literature, and other resources.

Creative Play. Each newborn, infant, and toddler is a unique individual. Encourage parents to respect and enjoy their baby's individuality. This will help parents establish the best possible foundation for their child's development, high self-esteem, and healthy relationships with others. Discuss with parents appropriate toys available to stimulate the infant's and toddler's nervous systems to achieve developmental milestones (Table 16-4).

Feeding and Elimination. Instruct parents that an infant should have six to eight wet diapers a day, sometimes more. Whether their infant is fed at the breast or by bottle will determine how many bowel movements there are in a day: breastfed babies have more frequent stools. Tell parents that they will begin to notice a regular pattern in bowel and bladder elimination at around 8 months.

Inform parents that, when their child reaches 12 to 18 months, the growth rate begins to slow, decreasing the child's need for fluids and calories. Because of this decrease in nutritional needs, most children exhibit a decrease in appetite. Toddlers begin to feel a need to be in control of their abilities. By about 18 months, most toddlers become more picky and fussy about foods. Inform parents that good eating habits are established in the first 3 years after birth. By giving their child nutritious meals and snacks, they will be helping to set the stage for future food consumption.

Inform parents that, as their infant becomes a toddler, they can begin to assess for toilet-training readiness. Not only does their toddler have to show signs of physical, mental, and psychological readiness, but the parents must also be ready. Toddlers show physical signs of readiness by having regular bowel movements, being able to remove their own clothes, and staying dry for at least 2 hours or waking up dry from a nap. Mental readiness consists of being able to recognize the urge to urinate or defecate and to communicate, either verbally or nonverbally, the need to use the toilet. Psychologically, the toddler will show curiosity about siblings' or adults' toilet habits. The toddler tends to become impatient with a soiled or wet diaper and wants to be changed immediately.

Table 16-4 Age-Appropriate Toys

AGE	APPROPRIATE TOYS
0 to 3 months	• Mobiles • Soft toys
4 to 7 months	• Toys with sounds and fingerholds • Rattle • Vinyl books
8 to 12 months	• Toys that float, squirt, or hold water • Busy boxes • Different-size containers or cup • Books
1 to 2 years	• Kitchen and tool sets with large parts • Dress-up clothes • Trucks, cars, and dolls • Books • Sandbox
2 to 3 years	• Pegboards with large pegs • Shape sorters • Nontoxic paints, crayons • Simple jigsaw puzzles • Tricycle

Besides recognizing the child's readiness for toilet training, the parents need to be willing to invest the time needed for toilet training. Parents should make this process as positive, natural, and nonthreatening as possible. Instruct parents that their toddler should be ready to begin between the ages of 18 and 24 months. Bowel training is usually accomplished before bladder training because it is more predictable and has a more regular pattern.

Rest and Sleep. Inform parents that, at first, newborns sleep about 16 hours a day in 3- to 4-hour stretches between feedings. Parents should be instructed to position newborns on their backs at all times. Research has shown this position appears to prevent sudden infant death syndrome (SIDS). As they get older and their stomachs grow, they go longer between feedings. By 2 months, they are more alert and social and will be awake more during the day. Because of the increased stomach capacity, they may skip a night feeding. By 3 months, parents will be happy to know, their child may be sleeping through the night.

At 4 months, parents should expect their infant to need only two naps a day, each lasting 1 to 3 hours. A consistent bedtime routine will help their infant to wind down at the end of the day. Such a routine may consist of a warm bath, rocking, stories, or soft music.

As the infant approaches 8 months, separation anxiety begins to increase. The child may resist going to bed and may wake up more often, looking for a parent. This is the time to introduce a transitional object (such as a blanket or teddy bear) to comfort the child when parents are not present. Stress the importance of following a consistent pattern or bedtime ritual.

As the child becomes a toddler, delaying tactics may be used. Tell parents to stick to the bedtime routine. During this age, dreams begin. Cutting teeth, a change in routine, or illness can also make an infant or toddler awaken more frequently in the night. Encourage parents to give attention to children's distress, but to let the children know they are to keep to their bedtime routine.

At 2 to 3 years, the child may take a single 1- to 2-hour nap around lunchtime. Some children may give up naps entirely. Again, inform parents that their child may begin to resist going to sleep. Part of this is from separation anxiety and part from the negativity stage of development. Giving the child choices at bedtime helps. A night-light may become necessary. Nightmares may also awaken toddlers. Parents should hold and comfort their child until they are calm enough to fall back to sleep.

Interventions to Promote Health Maintenance. Interventions related to health maintenance include assisting parents with scheduling health maintenance visits so their children can receive preventive health care. Also, teach parents about immunizations, child safety, and dental care. Again, education of the parents is the primary intervention.

Immunizations. One of your most important tasks is to inform parents of the reasons for routine immunizations. Children are susceptible to disease because they have an immature immune system. Immunization protects the child from being infected and prevents the infection of others at day care centers.

When administered properly, immunizations provide the most cost-effective contribution to the health of children worldwide. They are recommended in an established schedule for healthy infants and children (Figure 16-7). Instruct parents in the importance of completing all scheduled immunizations. Give them an immunization schedule. Inform them of the common side effects of each vaccine. Although most side effects are mild, the parents need to know what to expect. Mild discomfort is normal, with slight fever, rash, or soreness at the site of injection. Serious reactions to vaccines are rare. If the child is immunodeficient because of acquired immunodeficiency syndrome (AIDS), an organ transplant, or immunosuppressive therapy, the parents should consult their physician about vaccines.

Parents should retain a vaccination record and have it updated each time the child receives a scheduled vaccination. A vaccination and health record will help the parents when they move to a new area or have a change of health care provider or when their child attends day care, preschool, or elementary school. Work closely with parents to establish and maintain a schedule of immunizations.

Safety. Accidents are a leading cause of death of infants and toddlers. Many accidents result from a child's natural curiosity and exploration of the environment. Some common accidents are aspiration, choking, falls, burns, car accidents, and drowning. A vital part of assessing for potential accidents is to ask parents about safety hazards in the child's environment. For example, do the parents ever leave their baby or toddler unattended in the bath?

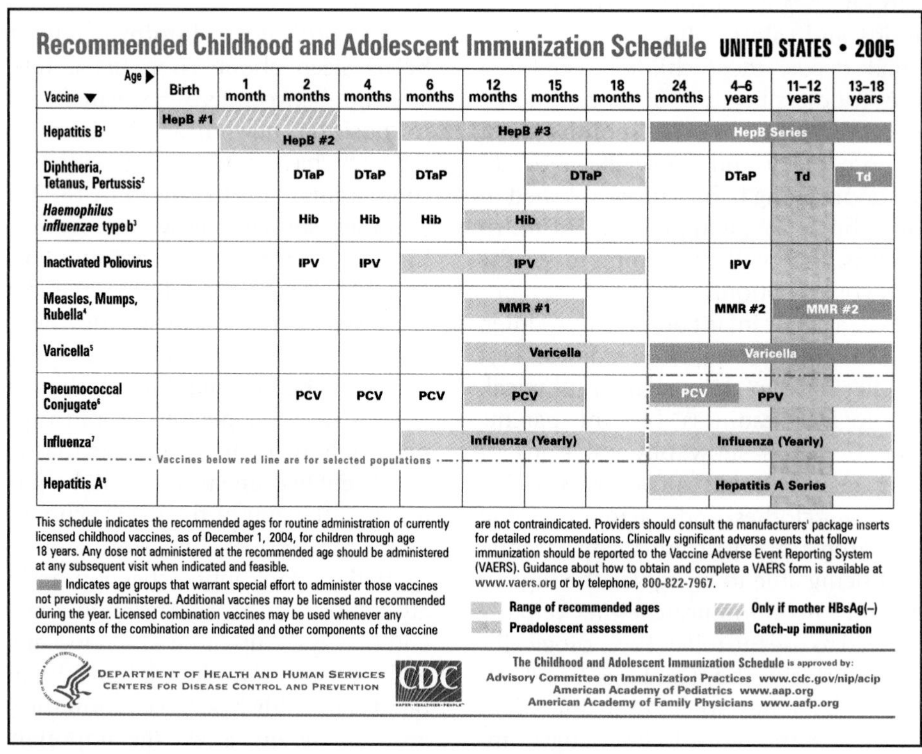

Recommended Childhood and Adolescent Immunization Schedule UNITED STATES • 2005

Vaccine ▼ / Age ▶	Birth	1 month	2 months	4 months	6 months	12 months	15 months	18 months	24 months	4–6 years	11–12 years	13–18 years
Hepatitis B[1]	HepB #1	HepB #2			HepB #3				HepB Series			
Diphtheria, Tetanus, Pertussis[2]			DTaP	DTaP	DTaP		DTaP			DTaP	Td	Td
Haemophilus influenzae type b[3]			Hib	Hib	Hib	Hib						
Inactivated Poliovirus			IPV	IPV	IPV					IPV		
Measles, Mumps, Rubella[4]						MMR #1				MMR #2	MMR #2	
Varicella[5]						Varicella			Varicella			
Pneumococcal Conjugate[6]			PCV	PCV	PCV	PCV			PCV	PPV		
Influenza[7]					Influenza (Yearly)				Influenza (Yearly)			
Vaccines below red line are for selected populations												
Hepatitis A[8]									Hepatitis A Series			

This schedule indicates the recommended ages for routine administration of currently licensed childhood vaccines, as of December 1, 2004, for children through age 18 years. Any dose not administered at the recommended age should be administered at any subsequent visit when indicated and feasible.

Indicates age groups that warrant special effort to administer those vaccines not previously administered. Additional vaccines may be licensed and recommended during the year. Licensed combination vaccines may be used whenever any components of the combination are indicated and other components of the vaccine are not contraindicated. Providers should consult the manufacturers' package inserts for detailed recommendations. Clinically significant adverse events that follow immunization should be reported to the Vaccine Adverse Event Reporting System (VAERS). Guidance about how to obtain and complete a VAERS form is available at www.vaers.org or by telephone, 800-822-7967.

Range of recommended ages
Preadolescent assessment
Only if mother HBsAg(–)
Catch-up immunization

DEPARTMENT OF HEALTH AND HUMAN SERVICES
CENTERS FOR DISEASE CONTROL AND PREVENTION
CDC

The Childhood and Adolescent Immunization Schedule is approved by:
Advisory Committee on Immunization Practices www.cdc.gov/nip/acip
American Academy of Pediatrics www.aap.org
American Academy of Family Physicians www.aafp.org

FIGURE 16-7 Recommended childhood immunization schedule, United States, 2005. (Retrieved October 20, 2005, from http://www.cdc.gov/nip/recs/child-schedule.PDF.)

To give yourself a baseline for educational interventions, determine the parents' knowledge about safety and accident prevention. Many parents are unaware of the potential dangers that can be found in a home. The potential for serious injury is ever-present. If parents are made aware of these dangers, they may be able to prevent devastating consequences.

Action Alert! Infants lying unattended on raised surfaces such as counters and beds are at risk for falling and suffering severe injury. Keep crib rails up at all times, and use barriers to block stairways to prevent injuries to toddlers.

Exploration plays an integral part in the psychological development of the infant and toddler. As soon as locomotion is established, the parents should use gates as a means to control the infant's access to various areas. Instruct parents about safety latches that can be applied to drawers and cupboards that contain dangerous materials. Give parents the telephone number of the local poison control center and emergency department, and tell them to post the number near the telephone. Also, tell parents to discard any syrup of ipecac because the American Academy of Pediatrics (2003) no longer recommends its use at home.

Playthings, although valuable in enhancing a child's development, may also cause injuries, accidents, or death. Teach parents to screen toys for age appropriateness. Children younger than age 3 should not have toys with small, removable parts on which they could choke. Instruct parents to check toys routinely for loose parts or sharp edges. All paints, crayons, molding clays, and other craft items should be nontoxic.

Accidents can occur when food is ingested too quickly or is too large to be swallowed safely. Therefore, food should also be age appropriate. As the infant progresses from liquids to solids, parents may mash, grind, or cook food until it is soft enough to swallow without chewing. When foods are prepared appropriately, toddlers can eat many of the same things their parents eat.

Action Alert! Prevent aspiration of foreign objects such as buttons, coins, and food (such as hot dogs) by not giving such small, hard objects to infants and toddlers. Choking can lead to respiratory arrest and death.

Accidental drowning is responsible for approximately 4200 deaths (including all age-groups) per year in the United States. Males are affected two to three times more than females. Older infants and toddlers are disproportionately represented in these accidents. Warn parents that an infant or toddler can drown in only a few inches of water. Bathtubs, toilets, water buckets, and swimming pools are the usual sites of drowning (Safe Kids Worldwide, 2004).

Burns are another source of injury common to infants or toddlers. Instruct parents that they should never hold an infant or toddler when smoking, holding hot liquids, or cooking. Hot liquids or food should never be left near the edge of tables or counters. Tell parents to test bath water before putting a child into it. Also tell them to set their hot water heater at 120° F or lower.

Just as safety is important in the home, it is also important when traveling. A federally approved, properly installed car seat must be used at all times. Infants should sit facing backward in the car until they can sit independently. No infant or child should sit in the front seat of a car with a passenger-side air bag. A car seat should be used throughout the toddler stage of development.

Dental Care. Dental health is important even for infants and young children. By age 3, some children already show alarming tooth decay. Neglected dental problems can lead to infection and subsequent tooth loss. Teach parents that healthy "baby teeth" influence the formation of healthy gums and permanent teeth. Ask the parents if the child has any history of dental problems or mouth pain. Ask if the infant or child is given fruit juice when put to bed. To prevent cavities, instruct parents to never let their child fall asleep with a bottle. This habit promotes decay because fluid pools around the teeth.

Action Alert! Inform parents that early childhood dental caries occur when a bottle of juice or milk is used as a pacifier at night.

Inform parents that dental hygiene is essential from the time of their child's first feeding. Even before the first teeth erupt, the child's mouth should be cleaned with a damp gauze or cloth after each feeding. On average, the first tooth erupts at 6 months. Some children show mild signs of drooling and increased finger sucking when teething. Other children become irritable and may refuse to eat. At the eruption of the first tooth, parents should begin to brush the tooth with a soft toothbrush and continue to assist their child with brushing through age 3.

Early screening for signs of caries or cavity development, starting during the first year after birth, could identify infants and toddlers who are at risk of developing early childhood caries. High-risk children include those with early signs of tooth decay, poor oral hygiene, limited exposure to fluorides, and frequent exposure to sugary snacks and drinks.

PRESCHOOL AND SCHOOL-AGE CHILDREN

Through the use of a thorough assessment process, you identify problems that affect children's growth and development. Your interventions will be based on establishing a trusting relationship with your clients and their families and incorporating their cultural beliefs in your interventions. The main interventions for *Delayed growth and development* and *Impaired parenting* are health education and counseling.

Interventions to Promote Health. Education and anticipatory guidance are the best preventive measures for parents of preschool and school-age children. Families need to understand normal growth and development and nurturing child care practices. Teaching parents how to determine when it is necessary to contact health care providers promotes good decision making about self-care. Box 16-5 lists selected reasons for parents to contact a health care provider.

- Teach parents the importance of teaching children to eat nutritious foods by using MyPyramid: milk and dairy products; lean meat, fish, and poultry; fruits and vegetables; and breads and cereals.
- Parents should encourage their children in lifetime fitness activities such as walking, running, bicycling, and swimming.

Action Alert! Encourage parents whose children are obese to participate in physical activities. Obese children tend to be less active, which reduces metabolism and increases fat accumulation.

- Parents are responsible for seeing that their children get 10 to 12 hours of sleep to function effectively during the day (Behrman et al., 2004). They must promote regular sleeping habits in their children.
- Antismoking efforts must begin before adolescence. It is important to talk with school-age children about the adverse health effects of smoking and how children can resist peer pressures. Instead of just going along with the crowd, the child needs the skills and confidence to make correct decisions.
- Children's early years are a critical time for the socializing effects of television, computer games, movie, and video game viewing habits. Encourage parents to set reasonable limits on the amount of time their children watch television, use a computer, or play video games. Encourage them to watch programs with their children.

BOX 16-5 *Reasons for Parents to Contact a Health Care Provider*

- Routine well-child examinations and immunizations
- Drastic changes in their child's behavior
- Severe pain
- Severe or worrisome injury
- Prolonged high fever (over 102°F [38.9°C])
- Persistent cough
- Foul-smelling drainage from the nose, eyes, ears, or anywhere else
- Persistent vomiting
- Unexplained persistent rash
- Prolonged diarrhea
- Blood in urine or stool

Action Alert! Advise parents that when their children spend hours in front of a television, computer, or video game, they are missing the opportunity to develop their physical and social skills by playing with siblings or friends instead of being sedentary and solitary.

Interventions to Promote Effective Parenting. The purpose of discipline is to instruct children in proper conduct or action rather than to punish children. The ultimate goal of disciplinary action is to teach children to develop a sense of inner control so that they can follow generally accepted standards of behavior and live in accord with the rules and regulations established by the group (Hockenberry et al., 2003). Disciplinary methods recommended by the American Academy of Pediatrics include showing children the natural consequences of their actions, as long as they do not place the child in danger. The Academy also recommends withholding privileges, and as a last resort, a time-out.

During the preschool years, it is important that a child have opportunities for peer interaction. A preschool child who has learned to be comfortable in groups is better able to learn in kindergarten. Explain to parents that interacting with older siblings is not the same as interacting in a group experience with peers.

The most important task for children in early school years is learning to read. Parents can serve as role models by reading books, magazines, and newspapers instead of watching television. Encourage parents to read aloud to their children at bedtime, to play word games with them, and to have them read simple directions to them. Some children may experience school phobia, the fear of attending school. Because fear is one of the most powerful negative human emotions, children may use physical symptoms such as vomiting, headache, or abdominal pain as an excuse to stay home from school. Explain to parents that they must determine the reason for their child's resistance to school before they can help the child to overcome the fear. Refer the child and family to a counselor if the phobia persists.

Interventions to Prevent Injury. No child can be considered free from risk of injury. Your awareness of some injury patterns may be helpful in counseling parents. The type of injuries to which a child is most vulnerable varies with personal circumstances and the child's age, size, and developmental ability. Parents of preschool-age children must realize that although their children's skills are becoming sophisticated, their judgment is not. Preschoolers cannot be relied on to recognize danger. In contrast, school-age children are less likely to experience unintentional injuries because they have developed more refined muscular coordination and have the cognitive abilities to avoid injuring themselves. It is often difficult for parents to maintain a balance between the level of supervision and restriction and their children's need for independence.

Promoting Home Safety. There are many safety tips you can share with parents during well-child visits to prevent future injury.

Action Alert! Teach parents about child safety as part of every well-child visit. Most accidents occur because parents overestimate or underestimate their child's abilities.

Fires present a special danger to young children, who cannot be depended on to react quickly in an emergency. When a fire occurs, children who have not been trained for a fire emergency may mistakenly try to hide in a "safe place." Smoke detectors should be placed in all hallways adjacent to bedrooms, as well as near the kitchen area and the garage. Children should be instructed to leave the house at once in the presence of smoke or fire, even if the fire is small. Calls to 911 can be made from another home. Ask the family if fire drills are held regularly so that children can plan and rehearse all possible escape routes. Children should be taught to "stop, drop, and roll" if their clothing should catch fire. House fires are not the only threat. Many children are burned when they accidentally upset a cooking pot, touch a hot grill, or play with fireworks. Portable heaters are another source of danger.

Action Alert! Teach children to avoid playing with matches, to know fire escape routes, and to practice fire escape drills at home. Teach them to avoid hot stoves and to avoid playing with flammable substances.

Ask parents about whether they own guns. If so, instruct them that guns should be locked away unloaded and separate from the ammunition.

The term *latchkey children* describes children in elementary school who spend some part of their time before or after school without adult supervision. The name arose from children who carried keys to let themselves into their homes before the parents returned from work. Inform parents of community resources available to latchkey children.

Promoting Safety at Play. Bicycling injuries begin to take their toll during the early school-age years. Children of this age are still not capable of making accurate judgments about speed and distance. To fit in with their peer group, these children may neglect to wear helmets. Children should demonstrate safe riding skills and understand traffic safety laws before being allowed to ride a bicycle on the street. Inform parents of community guidelines for bicycle safety. Pamphlets and videos can help parents teach bicycle safety to their children.

Action Alert! Remind parents that they must select the proper equipment and see that their child learns and obeys traffic laws when riding a bicycle.

If a child uses a skateboard, scooter, or in-line skates, a helmet is mandatory because these activities take place on hard surfaces such as concrete and there is great risk of head injury. Wrists, knees, and elbows also need protective gear. Children under the age of 5 should not use skateboards or in-line skates because they are not developmentally prepared to protect themselves from injury.

Action Alert! Advise parents to enforce safety guidelines such as prohibiting their children to use their in-line skates or skateboards on streets and highways.

Drowning is a leading cause of death among preschool and school-age children. Advise parents that their children should learn how to swim from an experienced and qualified swimming instructor. When children ride in a boat, they should always wear a personal flotation device. Remind parents that children learn by example, so it is important that adults also follow safety guidelines.

EVALUATION

To objectively evaluate the degree of success in achieving a goal or outcome, assess the infant, toddler, or child for the presence or absence of the desired behavior or response, and determine the level of agreement between the outcome criteria and the actual response. If the overall outcome were not met, reassessment and changes in the plan of care would be warranted. It may be that another nursing diagnosis would be a better choice. Refer to Box 16-6 to see an example of nursing process in action. A discharge note for Yung Hi might look like this:

Sample Documentation Note for Yung Hi

Discharged with parent to return home per automobile. Happy to be going home. Behavior is age appropriate. Parents will encourage physical activity and age-appropriate play within the confines of a spica cast. Has appointment with pediatrician in 1 week.

At this time you and the parents review the problems identified at the last visit and discuss whether and how they were resolved. It is not unusual for some problems to be resolved and replaced by new and different concerns. Finally, as part of the well child's annual evaluation, you should assess how the parents are adjusting to their changing role as their child grows and develops. It is important that the parents' expectations be realistic and that they promote their child's growth and development.

BOX 16-6

Nursing Care Plan

A Client at Risk for Altered Growth and Development

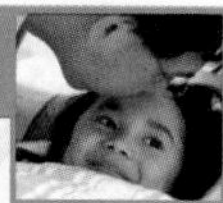

Admission Data

Yung Hi is admitted from the postanesthesia care unit to the orthopedic unit. The unit nurse receives the following report:

33-month-old Asian female child admitted to ER with greenstick fracture of the right femur. No known allergies or medical conditions. Toddler had been playing in playground of apartment complex when she fell, and her older brother tripped and fell on her outstretched leg. No reported loss of consciousness. Mother witnessed the fall and (through translation) said that the child did not hit her head. The father attempted to move the child and, when unable, called for an ambulance. Right thigh slight edema with obvious guarding due to pain. Placement of spica cast under general anesthesia in OR. Stable during procedure and while in recovery. Vitals: BP 92/48, pulse 146, respirations 38. Popliteal, posttibial, and pedal pulses present bilaterally with right pulses 12 and left 13. No other significant physical findings.

Physician's Orders

Admitting diagnosis: greenstick/incomplete fracture of right femur.
Surgical procedure: spica cast application.
Neurovascular checks to right leg every 30 minutes × 4; every 1 hour × 4, then every 4 hours.
Diet as tolerated.
Children's Tylenol with codeine 5 mL PO q3-4h prn pain.
Colace elixir 30 mg PO every day.

Nursing Assessment

Drowsy and nonverbal. Mother at bedside. Mother reports no pain expressed. Vital signs stable. Able to wiggle toes. Leg and foot pink and warm to touch, capillary refill approximately 2 seconds. Pedal and posttibial pulses strong (+2) bilaterally. Lung sounds clear bilaterally A & P. Positive bowel sounds, voiding adequate amounts clear, yellow urine in diaper.

NANDA-I Nursing Diagnosis	NOC Expected Outcomes With Indicators	NIC Interventions With Selected Activities	Evaluation Data
Risk for Delayed Growth and Development	***Play Participation***	***Activity Therapy***	***After 24 Hours of Care***
Related Factor: • Diversional activity deficit and immobility secondary to cast	• Continue to demonstrate physical, psychosocial, and cognitive skills of previous stage of growth and development.	• Ask family members to bring child's favorite toys, family pictures, and other objects from home to place at bedside.	• Parents brought in favorite stuffed bunny and blanket, pictures of each family member, and favorite book.
	• Maintain range of motion and strength.	• Consult physical therapist (PT) for strength and range-of-motion exercises.	• PT consulted. Will work with client tid. Asked parents to be present to learn exercises and to help translate to client.
	• Participate in age-appropriate play.	• Consult play therapist, and have therapist come when both parents present.	• Play therapist met with parents and child. Favorite toys, music, and activities discussed.
	• Demonstrate increased understanding of treatments.	• Provide child with opportunities for therapeutic play.	• Played nurse and doctor, with favorite stuffed rabbit as the client in spica cast.
	• Select and play with age-appropriate toys.	• Place developmentally appropriate toys conducive to immobility at the bedside.	• Crayons, paints, pegboard, books, and stuffed animals at bedside.
	• Express enjoyment in selected play activities.	• Schedule times to engage child in developmental play during day and early evening shift.	• Met with client and played at 10 AM, 1 PM, and 7 AM. Parents, PT, and play therapist also engaged client in play and physical activity.
	• Achieve developmental tasks appropriate to age.	• Monitor developmental status and progress at regular intervals.	• Age-appropriate play, talks with mother and father, sings. Says "thank you" in English and nods head at same time.

Critical Thinking Questions

1. Which developmental theory would you apply to Yung Hi to assist you in caring for her?
2. Why would you choose one theory over the other?
3. Yung Hi wanted to cast the leg of her stuffed rabbit after the therapeutic play session was over. Why do you think Yung Hi wanted to do this?
4. What role does the family play in her care during hospitalization?
5. How can you as the nurse facilitate this?

Nursing outcome and intervention labels from Johnson, M., Bulechek, G., Butcher, H., Dochterman, J. M., Maas, M., Moorhead, S., et al. (Eds.). (2006). *NANDA, NOC, and NIC linkages: Nursing diagnoses, outcomes, & interventions.* St. Louis, MO: Mosby.

▼ KEY PRINCIPLES

- Although the terms *growth* and *development* are often used synonymously, they have separate and distinct definitions. Growth refers to a physiological process, whereas development involves the maturation of body organs and the acquisition of appropriate cognitive, linguistic, and psychosocial skills.
- Developmental theories attempt to explain how the human organism matures and acquires appropriate cognitive, linguistic, and psychosocial skills.
- Nursing process guides nursing care for the well infant and well child.
- The use of nursing diagnoses guides the management of problems involving growth and development or altered health maintenance.
- Children progress through similar stages of growth and development, but the rate of progression and the behaviors observed vary with the individual.
- Understanding children's growth and development enables the nurse to individualize approaches to the child's health care needs on the basis of developmental variations in each stage.
- The nursing diagnosis *Delayed growth and development* is appropriate for the infant or child who is not achieving normal physical growth or is not accomplishing the developmental tasks of the particular age-group.
- The nursing diagnosis *Impaired parenting* is used when the family environment does not provide the basic needs for a child's physical growth and development.
- Evaluation of the well child is a systematic, ongoing process in which the nurse evaluates the child's progress toward attainment of goals. The nurse and the child's parents review the problems identified at the last visit, discuss their resolution, and make adjustments as needed.
- Substance abuse and cigarette smoking are serious health problems among children and have profound implications for their adult health.
- Primary prevention is a key issue to child health.

■ REVIEW QUESTIONS

1 By 1 month of age an infant following normal growth and development patterns should:
1. Sit erect for 5 minutes
2. Have doubled his or her birth weight
3. Grasp the handle of a spoon briefly
4. Reach for a ball

2. Which of the following instructions regarding normal growth and development patterns of the infant is accurate? The infant should:
1. Double his or her birth length by 1 year of age
2. Double his or her birth weight by 3 months of age
3. Demonstrate reflexive behavior only
4. Demonstrate whole-hand carry

3. A more thorough medical examination of a 30-month-old child is indicated when the nurse observes that the child has difficulty:
1. Kicking a ball
2. Dressing himself or herself
3. Tying his or her shoes
4. Brushing his or her teeth

4. According to Erikson, which of the following developmental crises is faced by the 7-year-old child?
1. Trust versus mistrust
2. Industry versus inferiority
3. Autonomy versus shame and doubt
4. Identity versus identity diffusion

5. To assess a 5-year-old child using Piaget's developmental theory, the nurse should focus on the child's:
1. Simple reflexes
2. Ability to draw
3. Genital fixation
4. Sense of industry

Bibliography

*Allshouse, M., Rouse, T., & Eichelberger, M. (1993). Childhood injury: A current perspective. *Pediatric Emergency Care, 9*(3), 159-164.

American Academy of Pediatrics. (2003). Handling a poison emergency. Retrieved October 28, 2006, from http://asp.org/healthtopics/safety.htm.

American Academy of Pediatric Dentistry. (2005). *Dental care for your baby.* Retrieved October 29, 2006, from www.aapd.org/publications/brochures/ babycare.asp.

American Cancer Society. (2005). *Child and teen tobacco use.* Retrieved March 30, 2006, from www.cancer.org/docroot/PED/content/PED_10_2X_Child_and_Teen_Tobacco_Use.asp?sitearea=PED.

Ball, J. W., & Bindler, R. C. (2006). *Child health nursing: Partnering with children and families.* Upper Saddle River, NJ: Prentice Hall.

Baum, C. R. (2000). Environmental emergencies. In G. R. Flisher & S. Ludwig (Eds.), *Textbook of pediatric emergencies* (4th ed., pp. 943-963). Philadelphia: Lippincott Williams & Wilkins.

Bee, H., & Boyd, D. (2002). *Lifespan development* (3rd ed.). Boston: Allyn & Bacon.

Behrman, R., E., Kliegman, R., M., & Jenson, H. B. (2004). *Nelson textbook of pediatrics.* Philadelphia: Saunders.

*Bowlby, J. (1969). *Attachment and loss.* New York: Basic Books.

Centers for Disease Control and Prevention. (2005a) *General lead information.* Retrieved October 30, 2005, from www.cdc.gov/nceh/lead/faq/about.htm.

Centers for Disease Control and Prevention. (2005b). *Preventing lead poisoning in young children.* Atlanta: Author.

Cunningham, F. G. (2001). *Williams obstetrics* (21st ed.). Norwalk, CT: McGraw-Hill.

DuPaul, G. J., & Stoner G. (2003). *ADHD in the schools: Assessment and intervention strategies.* New York: Guilford.

Edelman, C. L., & Mandle, C. L. (2006). *Health promotion throughout the lifespan.* St. Louis, MO: Mosby.

*Elkind, D. (1992). Cognitive development. In S. B. Friedman, M. Fisher, & S. K. Schoenberg (Eds.), *Comprehensive adolescent health care* (pp. 24-26). St. Louis, MO: Quality Medical.

*Asterisk indicates a classic or definitive work on this subject.

*Erikson, E. H. (1968). *Childhood and society* (2nd ed.). New York: Norton.

Fowler-Brown, A., & Kahwati, L. C. (2004). Prevention and treatment of overweight in children and adolescents. *American Family Physician, 69*(11), 2591-2598.

*Havighurst, R. J. (1972). *Developmental tasks and education.* New York: David McKay.

Hockenberry, M., Wilson, D., Winkelstein, M. L., & Kline, N. (2003). *Wong's essentials of pediatric nursing* (7th ed.). St. Louis, MO: Mosby.

Johnson, M., Bulechek, G., Butcher, H., Dochterman, J. M., Maas, M., Moorhead, S., et al. (Eds.). (2006). *NANDA, NOC, and NIC linkages: Nursing diagnoses, outcomes, & interventions.* St. Louis, MO: Mosby.

Jorde, L. B., Carey, J. C., Barnshad, M. J., & White, R. L. (2000). *Medical Genetics* (2nd ed.). St. Louis, MO: Mosby.

Kavanaugh K., Savage, T., Kilpatrick, S., Kimura, R., & Hersberger, P. (2005) Life support decisions for extremely premature infants: Report of pilot study. *Journal of Pediatric Nursing, 20*(5), 347-357.

Kenny, T. J., & Nitz, K. (2000). Mental retardation. In R. A. Hoekelman, S. B. Friedman, N. M. Nelson, M. L. Weitzman, & M. H. Wilson (Eds.), *Primary pediatric care* (4th ed., pp. 409-412). St. Louis, MO: Mosby.

*Klaus, M. H., & Kennell, J. H. (1982). *Parent-infant bonding* (2nd ed.). St. Louis: Mosby.

*Kohlberg, L. (1966). A cognitive developmental analysis of children's sex role concepts and attitudes. In A. Macroby (Ed.), *The development of sex differences.* Palo Alto, CA: Stanford University.

*Kohlberg, L. (1981). *Philosophy of moral development: Moral stages and the idea of justice.* New York: Harper & Row.

Learning Disabilities Association of America. (2005). Defining learning disabilities. Retrieved October 28, 2006, from http://www.ldaamerica.org/new_to_ld/defining.org.

*Mercer, R. (1982). Parent infant interaction. In L. Sonstegard (Ed.), *Women's health and childrearing,* vol. 2. New York: Grune & Stratton.

MMWR. (2004). Youth risk behavior surveillance—United States, 2003. *Morbidity and Mortality Weekly Report, 53*(SS2), 1-95.

NANDA International. (2005). *Nursing diagnoses: Definitions and classification, 2005-2006* (6th ed.). Philadelphia: Author.

*Piaget, J. (1950). *The psychology of intelligence.* London: Routledge & Kegan Paul.

*Piaget, J. (1980). Intellectual evolution from adolescence to adulthood. In R. E. Muuss (Ed.), *Adolescent behavior and society: A body of readings* (3rd ed.). New York: Random House.

*Piaget, J. (1997). *The moral judgement of the child.* Glencoe, IL: Free Press.

*Piaget, J., & Infelder, B. (1958). *The growth of logical thinking from childhood to adolescence.* New York: Basic Books.

*Piaget, J., & Infelder, B. (1969). *The psychology of the child.* New York: Basic Books.

Pillitteri, A. (in press). *Maternal and child health nursing: Care of the childbearing and childrearing family* (5th ed.). Philadelphia: Lippincott Williams & Wilkins.

Roberts, D. A. (2005). Childhood diabetes: Implications for the home health nurse. *Home Health Care Management and Practice, 17,* 243-245.

Robertson, J., & Shilkofski, N. (Eds.). (2005). *The Harriet Lane Handbook.* Philadelphia: Mosby.

Safe Kids Worldwide. (2004). *Facts about childhood drowning.* Retrieved April 7, 2006, from http://usa.safekids.org/tier3_cd.cfm?folder_id=540&content_item_id=1032.

*Singer, D., & Revenson, T. (1978). *A Piaget primer: How a child thinks.* New York: New American Library.

Sugarman, L. (2001). *Life-span development frameworks, accounts and strategies* (2nd ed.). New York: Psychology Press.

*Winer, G. A. (1986). Cognitive and psychosocial development during adolescence. In C. S. Shuster & S. S. Ashburn (Eds.), *The process of human development* (pp. 527-546). Boston: Little Brown.

*Asterisk indicates a classic or definitive work on this subject.

Chapter 17

THE ADOLESCENT AND YOUNG ADULT

Media Resources

- evolve Evolve Website http://evolve.elsevier.com/Harkreader/
- Companion CD

Learning Objectives

After studying this chapter, you should be able to do the following:

- Discuss the developmental tasks of adolescence and young adulthood
- Identify a variety of factors affecting adolescent and young adult development
- Describe the assessment of the adolescent and young well adult for normal function and risk factors
- Differentiate among the variety of nursing diagnoses appropriate for adolescents and young adults seeking knowledge or health care related to development or health maintenance
- Plan nursing interventions for health maintenance and reduce risk factors as appropriate to the adolescent's and adult's developmental level
- Evaluate the outcomes that describe progress toward the goals of health maintenance

Key Terms

adolescence
constitutional delay of puberty
egocentrism
formal operations
gynecomastia
menarche
nocturnal emission
young adulthood

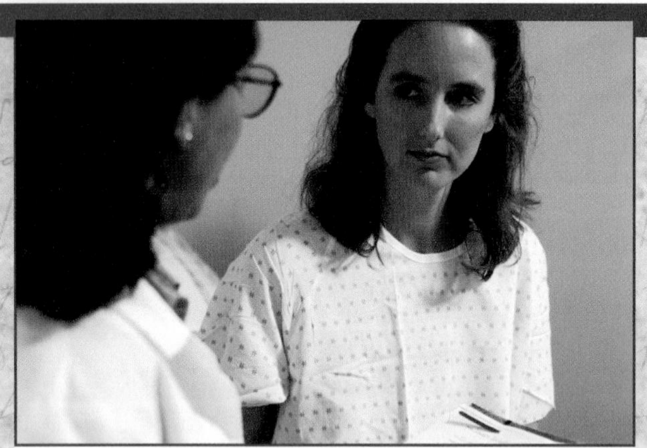

Jamie King is a 19-year-old with type 2 diabetes. Jamie has recently moved into the dorms at college away from home for the first time. The nurse at the student health center is seeing her for complaints of weakness, lethargy, and high stress levels. School started 10 weeks ago. She has been taking her blood glucose level regularly and knows it has been "high." Today it is 214. While she lived at home, her mother made all the meals, and now she visits the dorm cafeteria two to three times each day and eats quick foods between classes. Her normal physical exercise routine has been interrupted by classes and studying. See Key Nursing Diagnoses for the Adolescent and Young Adult.

KEY NURSING DIAGNOSES FOR THE ADOLESCENT AND YOUNG ADULT

Readiness for enhanced age-appropriate attainment of developmental milestones: Seeks assistance to manage age-appropriate developmental milestones

Ineffective health maintenance: Inability to identify, manage, and/or seek out help to maintain health

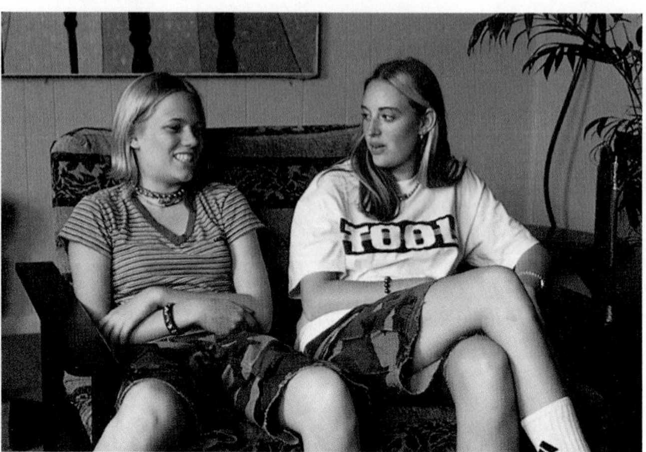

FIGURE 17-1 Peers have a strong influence on adolescents' clothes, hairstyle, and manner of speech.

CONCEPTS OF ADOLESCENCE AND YOUNG ADULT DEVELOPMENT

Nurses need to be knowledgeable about human development to understand the client's health needs in relationship to the person's life stage. Human development is the scientific study of quantitative and qualitative ways adults change and do not change over time. These changes are influenced by internal (hereditary) and external (environmental) factors (Figure 17-1). By understanding development, you can help people cope with life's transitions and help them manage their health problems in a manner appropriate to their developmental stage.

Adolescence is the period of transition between childhood and adulthood. It is a period of rapid growth and dramatic change, both physically and psychologically. For the purpose of discussion, this chapter defines adolescence as being between the ages of 12 and 21. Keep in mind, however, that children grow and develop at different rates, and any definition of adolescence should be flexible on both ends. The three stages of adolescence are the following:

- Early adolescence, from about age 12 to 14, when the adolescent has not entirely left the world of childhood
- Middle adolescence, from about age 15 to 17, when the adolescent undergoes a time of consolidation
- Late adolescence, from about age 18 to 21, when adolescents reach the threshold of adulthood and begin to establish themselves as independent persons

Young adulthood refers to the period of life from age 21 to 34. Although physical growth is complete by the early 20s, the adult continues to develop. Each adult's development is unique and complex because genetics, socioeconomic status, ethnic group, religious faith, and social expectations influence it. The 2000 U.S. Census Bureau reported that approximately 59 million people, almost 21% of the population, were between the ages of 20 and 34 (U.S. Census Bureau, 2002).

This developmental stage ranges from the end of adolescence to the beginning of middle adulthood. Young adults face a variety of developmental tasks that center around the assumption of adult roles and responsibilities (Figure 17-2). During this period, most people are in search of self. They need to establish autonomy from parents or parent surrogates, develop philosophies of life and personal lifestyles, choose and prepare for employment, enter the workforce, marry or establish other types of significant relationships, develop parenting behaviors, and become participatory citizens. There is considerable variability in how and when different people accomplish these tasks. Young adults are expected to perform many roles, including those of parent, spouse or companion, son or daughter, citizen, civic leader, friend, and employee or employer.

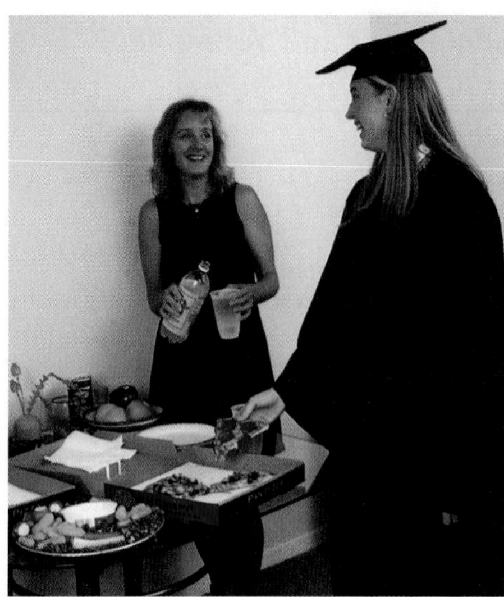

FIGURE 17-2 For many young adults, graduation from college is an important milestone that marks the end of adolescence and the beginning of adult roles and responsibilities.

DEVELOPMENTAL THEORIES OF THE ADOLESCENT AND YOUNG ADULT

During early adolescence, most youngsters acquire the stage of thinking that Piaget and Infelder (1958) call **formal operations,** which is the ability to reason abstractly. For example, the adolescent can engage in "if, then" deliberations, recognizing that if one event has occurred, another will likely follow. For example, if Mom's car will not start in the morning and she says that the battery is probably dead, then the adolescent will realize that other accessories in the car such as the radio and lights also will not function.

Similarly, adolescents develop the ability to reason and question constructs that they previously took for granted, such as the belief that parents are always correct. They begin to question others. They also develop the ability to see another person's perspective. In addition, they begin to think about *thinking* and their own thoughts.

Another hallmark of adolescents' cognitive development is **egocentrism,** which refers to their tendency to spend so much time thinking about and focusing on their own thoughts and changes in their own body that they come to believe that others are focused on them as well. As a result, young adolescents construct what Elkind (1992) has termed the "imaginary audience." This is a belief that everyone in your proximity is deeply interested in your every thought and action. This leads adolescents to believe that they must be very special because everyone else is so fascinated by them. Several types of "typical" adolescent beliefs result from this type of thinking, such as "No one has ever experienced what I'm feeling" and "Other people will die, but not me." The belief in the uniqueness of oneself is referred to as the personal fable. Although most people never completely lose their personal fables, the fables decline in influence as adolescents grow older and share experiences with others. Egocentrism similarly decreases from early through late adolescence.

Psychosocial Development. In his theory of psychosocial development, Erik Erikson (1963) identified eight stages of development from birth through death (Table 17-1). He believed that psychosocial development is a continuous process and that delays or crises in one stage can delay or diminish the achievement of other stages. They also serve as an impetus to the next stage. In Chapter 16, you learned about the stages through school-age.

The adolescent makes a transition into adulthood and does not stop developing until death. As they try to establish identities, adolescents encounter *identity versus identify diffusion,* which is Erickson's fifth stage of development, in which adolescents try to figure out who they are but are confused as to which of the many roles to adopt. Attainment of identity is established by reconsidering the goals and values set by the parents and culture, then accepting some and rejecting others.

Erikson's young adult stage focuses on intimacy versus isolation. During the stage of intimacy versus isolation, young adults are in an intense search for self; they focus on developing their capacity for reciprocal love and close personal relationships based on commitment to others. They experience conflicting values as they try to sort out what life means to them. They must resolve the conflict of balancing independence and intimacy as they form significant relationships with partners, with the aim of providing a nurturing environment for children. These tasks are relevant in a variety of lifestyles, including heterosexual marriage, homosexual and heterosexual cohabitation, and voluntary childlessness (Figure 17-3).

Levinson (1978, 1986) conceived of development as a sequence of qualitatively distinct eras or seasons (Table 17-2). Each of these eras in adult life has its own time and brings certain psychological challenges to the forefront of a person's life.

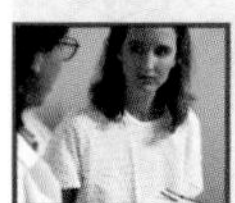

Review the opening case study and consider Jamie's stage of development. What questions might you ask to determine if her struggle with the developmental tasks of her stage of life are affecting her health?

Physical Development. The hallmark of adolescence is a physical process known as puberty, the sequence of physiological events that cause the reproductive organs to mature, making conception and childbirth possible. In girls, menarche is the hallmark event of this change. **Menarche** is the time of the first menstrual period; it occurs at an average age of 12 years and 4 months,

Table 17-1 Erikson's Stages of Development for the Adolescent and Young Adult

STAGE	AGE	DESCRIPTION
V	Adolescent	• Development of identity versus identity diffusion. • Must be able to integrate past, present, and future selves. • Teen becomes less reliant on family and more reliant on self. • Sense of group identity becomes strong.
VI	Young adult years	• Intimacy versus self-absorption, later called intimacy versus isolation. • Significant relationships are partners in friendship, sex, and competition and cooperation and ability to engage in a trusting fellowship. • The young adult seeks a permanent life partner with whom to give and receive love and support. • The primary issue is love.

Reprinted with permission from Erikson, E. H. (1963). *Childhood and society* (2nd ed.). New York: W. W. Norton & Company, Inc.; and by permission of The Random House Group Limited, London.

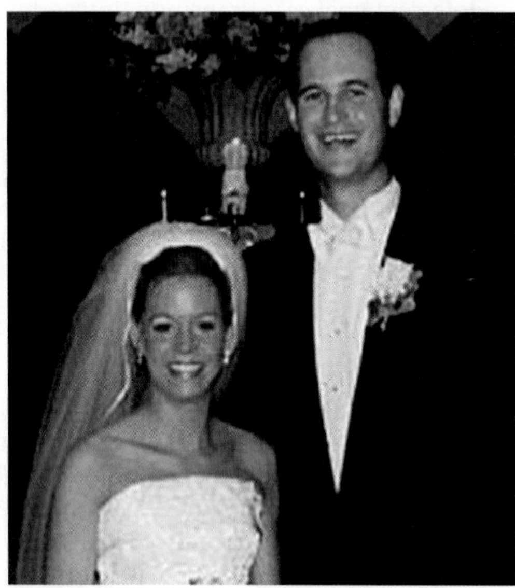

FIGURE 17-3 The stage of generativity involves seeking a permanent life partner with whom to give and receive love and support.

Table 17-2 Levinson's Development Phases for the Young Adult

APPROXIMATE AGE	TASKS
20 to 24	• Leaving the family. • Making the transition between adolescence and the adult world. • Those who go to college or military service have an intermediate experience.
25 to 29	• Getting into the adult world. • Building an initial life structure, deciding on an occupation, and working on intimacy versus isolation.
30 to 35	• A time of exploration and initial choice. • Age 30 transition. • Person either confirms earlier choices or may choose to modify or change the initial structure. • Person has vision of the future. • Person realizes extent to which he or she is dependent on and shaped by others, a disillusioning process. • A mentor can be very helpful at this stage.
36-39	• Settling down; becoming one's own person. • Moves from being mentored to being able to mentor. • Person may build a second, and more stable, early adult life structure.

Data from Levinson, D. J. (1978). *The seasons of a man's life.* New York: Knopf; and Levinson, D. J. (1996). *The seasons of a woman's life.* New York: Knopf.

although the age may range from 9 to 17 years. In boys, the first nocturnal emission marks the transition to puberty. A **nocturnal emission** is a discharge of semen during sleep; it occurs at an average age of 13 years and 4 months, but the age may range from 11 to 15 years.

During adolescence, secondary sexual characteristics appear. These changes in bodily features, such as pubic hair, axillary hair, and fully developed breasts and penis, are induced by sex hormones. Secondary sexual characteristics develop in the same sequence in all adolescents, although the timing differs from person to person. The sexual maturity scale developed by Tanner identifies five stages of pubertal development that focus on breasts in girls and scrotal and penile development in boys (Figure 17-4). Pubic hair can be assessed in both sexes but offers less important information in the overall physical assessment.

Adolescents experience a rapid growth in height called the pubertal growth spurt. It begins before menarche or the first nocturnal emission and accounts for 15% to 25% of the final adult height. Body fat is also affected. In girls, the amount of adipose tissue increases, reducing the proportion of lean body mass. In boys, the lean body mass increases during this time.

Girls begin their growth spurt at an earlier age than boys but commonly reach a shorter adult height because of a lower velocity of growth and a shorter period of growth. The cardiorespiratory system grows at a disproportionate rate to the rest of the body, making aerobic activity at this age an important part of physical fitness.

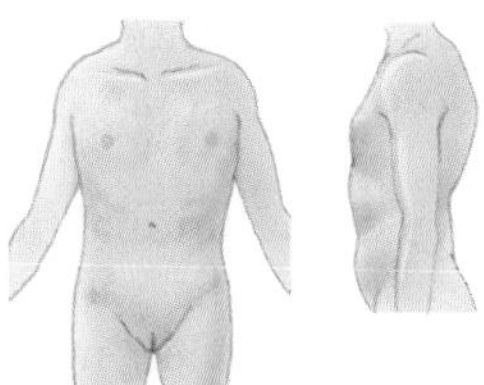

Stage I
Breasts: Preadolescent; elevation of the papilla only
Pubic hair: None

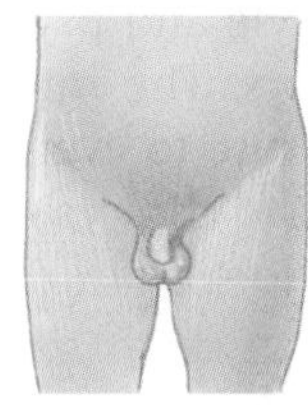

Stage I
Penis: Childhood size and proportion
Testes and scrotum: Childhood size and proportion
Pubic hair: None

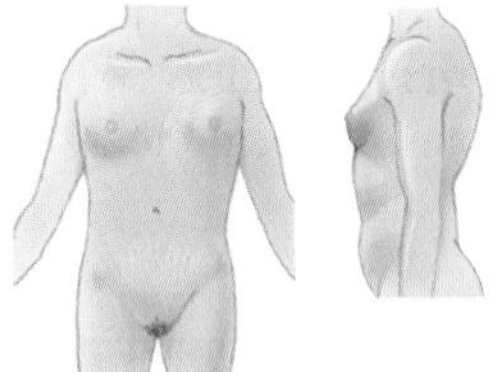

Stage II
Breasts: Breast budding (thelarche); small mound formed by elevation of the breast and papilla, with enlargement of the areolar diameter
Pubic hair: Sparse growth of long, downy pubic hair over mons veneris or labia majora; may occur with breast budding or several weeks or months later (pubarche)

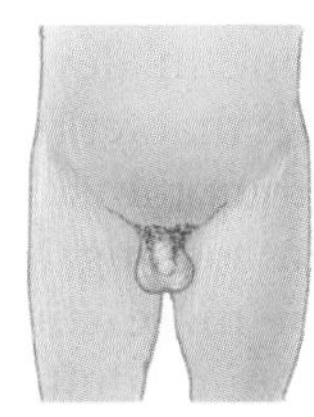

Stage II
Penis: Slight or no enlargement
Testes and scrotum: Enlargement; scrotal skin reddens, changes in texture
Pubic hair: Sparse growth of long, downy pubic hair mainly at the base of the penis

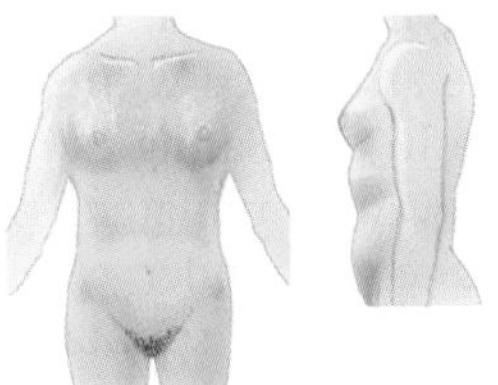

Stage III
Breasts: Further enlargement of breast tissue and areola with no separation of their contours
Pubic hair: Increased amount of hair and changes in the character of the hair (darker, coarser, and more curly), spread sparsely over junction of pubes

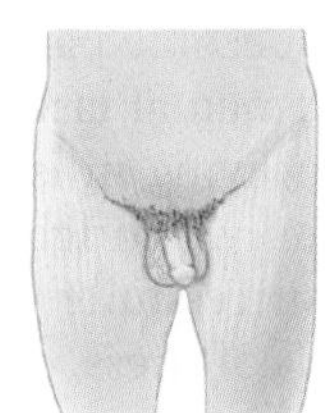

Stage III
Penis: Enlargement, particularly in length
Testes and scrotum: Further enlargement
Pubic hair: Darker, coarser, curlier hair spread sparsely over the pubic symphysis

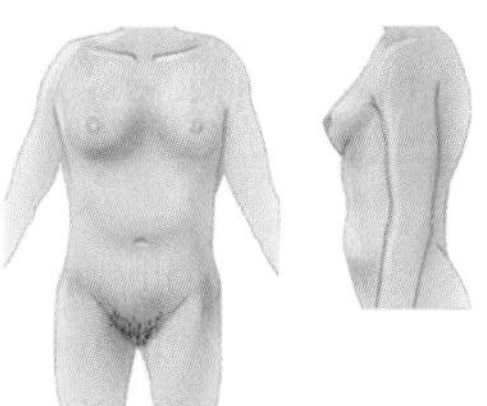

Stage IV
Breasts: Double contour form: projection of areola and papilla form a secondary mound on top of breast tissue
Pubic hair: Adult appearance but less area covered; no spread to medial aspects of thighs

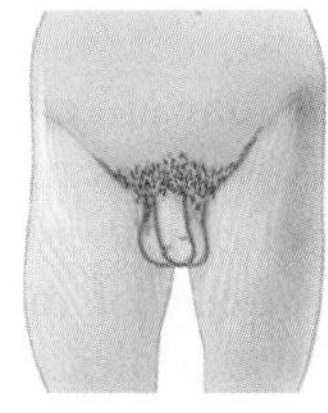

Stage IV
Penis: Further enlargement in length and breadth, with development of the glans
Testes and scrotum: Further enlargement
Pubic hair: Coarse and curly hair; greater area covered than in stage III, but still less than in an adult, with no spread to thighs

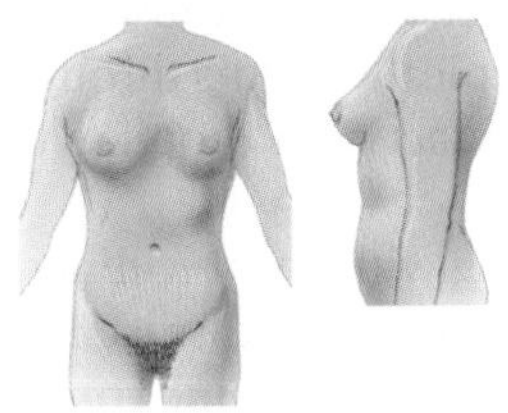

Stage V
Breasts: Larger, more mature breast with single contour form
Pubic hair: Adult distribution and quantity, with spread to medial aspect of thighs

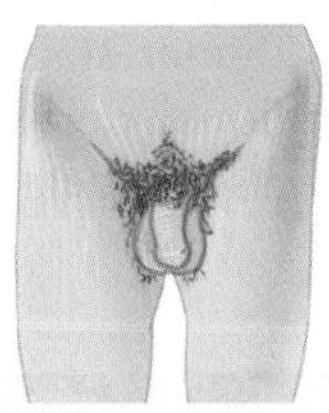

Stage V
Penis: Adult in size and shape
Testes and scrotum: Adult in size and shape
Pubic hair: Adult distribution and quantity, with spread to thighs but not to abdomen

FIGURE 17-4 Tanner stages of physical development.

Motor Development. During early puberty, many adolescents experience some awkwardness because the feet, legs, and arms begin the growth spurt before the height catches up. This gives many young teens a gangly appearance. The musculoskeletal system is also most vulnerable to injury during the period of peak height velocity, which occurs during Tanner stage III.

Moral Development. Adolescents must establish their own set of morals and values in order to gain autonomy from adults. Their decisions involving moral dilemmas are based on an internalized set of moral principles, which enables them to evaluate the situation and plan a course of action consistent with their ideals. Late adolescence involves serious questioning of existing moral values and their relevance to the individual and society.

FACTORS AFFECTING GROWTH AND DEVELOPMENT OF THE ADOLESCENT AND YOUNG ADULT

Many factors, such as environment, socioeconomic status, nutrition, and physiological status, influence growth and development. In adolescence and young adulthood, as in other stages of development, lifestyle and psychological factors influence health behaviors. The interaction of these factors greatly affects response to everyday situations. These factors also influence the choices caregivers make regarding health care behaviors.

DEVELOPMENTAL RISK FACTORS

Adolescents have a strong group identity and are frequently called upon to make choices within that group. During this time an important milestone in development for the adolescent is to make choices that represent the ability to reason and question the group think.

Young adults who have difficulty in making adult choices and accepting responsibility for those choices are at risk for developmental delays. Young adults are expected to separate from their family of origin, establish viable careers, develop an intimate adult relationship with a significant other, marry, and become parents (Figure 17-5). Failure to achieve developmental tasks of young adulthood can result in a person living in isolation and/or dependent on his or her family of origin or society. A young adult unable to cope successfully with changing roles may experience high levels of stress, demonstrate substance abuse behaviors, or express unworthiness and depression.

PHYSIOLOGICAL RISK FACTORS

Physiological and acute or chronic illness may affect the adolescent's growth and development as well. As mentioned earlier, the average age of the onset of puberty is 12 years in girls and 13 years in boys. A delay of more than 2 or 3 years from this norm may cause adolescents tremendous anxiety. **Constitutional delay of puberty** is defined as an absence of early signs of puberty (Tanner stage II breasts by age 13 for girls or Tanner stage II genitalia by age 14 for boys). Constitutional delay of puberty is the basis of more than 90% of cases of delayed puberty; it does not indicate an underlying pathological process but simply that the adolescent is a "late bloomer."

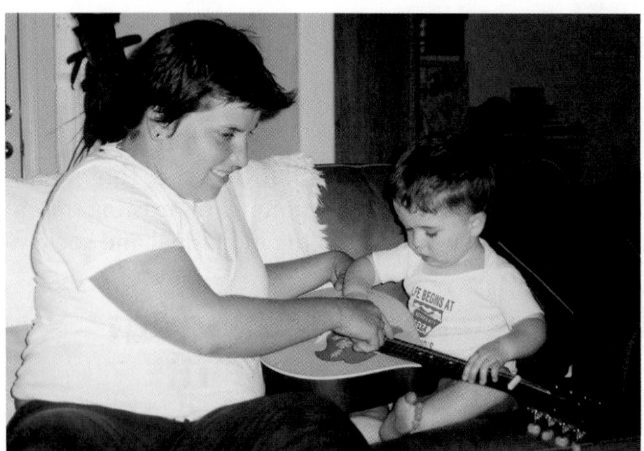

FIGURE 17-5 Young adulthood is a time for child rearing and establishing their own family traditions.

Although benign and self-limiting, constitutional delay of puberty can cause psychological problems, such as body image disturbance, self-esteem disturbance, negative emotional reactions, long-term dependency on parents, and failure to acquire appropriate social skills. It is important to reassure adolescents and their parents that this condition is self-limiting and that the adolescent is normal. Disorders that cause a pathological delay of puberty are all rare.

Action Alert! Reassure adolescents with constitutional delay of puberty that they are normal.

A concern of adolescent boys is **gynecomastia,** which is a benign increase in breast tissue associated with puberty. It results from an imbalance in circulating estrogens and androgens. Gynecomastia can be unilateral or bilateral, and the breasts are frequently tender when touched, even by clothing. Most cases resolve spontaneously within 12 to 18 months.

Action Alert! Assure boys with gynecomastia that the condition is a normal part of puberty and that it usually goes away by itself within about 12 to 18 months.

Fortunately, most acute illnesses during adolescence are short-lived and easily treated. However, mononucleosis deserves special mention because it is most prevalent during the adolescent and young adult years. The vast majority of cases of mononucleosis are caused by Epstein-Barr virus. Transmission typically occurs through saliva during direct, prolonged contact with oropharyngeal secretions.

The number of adolescents living with chronic illness has increased, not because the incidence of disease has changed but because more children with chronic conditions are surviving. The most common are asthma, diabetes mellitus, congenital heart disease, sickle cell disease, chronic renal disease, epilepsy, and hemophilia.

Leading Causes of Death. The leading causes of death for adults younger than 25 are unintentional injuries, suicide, and homicide. For adults between the ages of 25 and 44, they are unintentional injuries, cancer, and heart disease (Office of Disease Prevention and Health Promotion [ODPHP], 2002).

Action Alert! Living healthfully and avoiding behaviors that increase the risk of chronic disease will result in longer, healthier lives and lower health care costs.

Heart Disease. High blood cholesterol is an important modifiable risk factor for coronary artery disease, which is the leading cause of death for men and women in North America. Risk factors include a family history of very high cholesterol levels, premature coronary artery disease in a first-degree relative (before age 50 in men or age 60 in women), diabetes, smoking, and hypertension. Heart disease is a leading cause of morbidity and mortality in the United States. Approximately 1.3 million cases of nonfatal heart attacks are reported each year, for an annual incidence of approximately 600 per 100,000 people.

Internationally, cardiovascular diseases account for 12 million deaths annually throughout the world. Heart disease continues to be a significant problem in industrialized countries and is becoming an increasingly significant problem in developing countries. Approximately 500,000 to 700,000 deaths are caused by ischemic heart disease annually in the United States (National Center for Health Statistics, 2005).

LIFESTYLE/CULTURAL RISK FACTORS

Violence. Adolescents today are faced with higher rates of exposure and risk of injury and death from violence. Homicide, for the second decade in a row, is the second leading cause of death among white teens and young adults and the leading cause of death for African American and Hispanic populations of the same age-group (Hockenberry, Wilson, Winkelstein, & Kline, 2003). Exposure to violence both personal and witnessed may occur at home, school, and the workplace (Edelman & Mandle, 2006).

Sexual Behavior. Risky sexual behavior among adolescents is one of the major public health concerns in the United States. The prevalence of sexual activity in the United States for the age-group 15 to 17 is 42.7% (Le & Kato, 2006). Asian American teens are at the low end of the statistics at 27.9%, whereas African American males are the highest at 85%. Condom use in this age-group was reported at 63%. Sexually transmitted diseases (STDs) in the adolescent population have changed over the last decade. The cases of gonorrhea have decreased by 58%, while the cases of chlamydia have steadily risen 46%. Human immunodeficiency virus/acquired immunodeficiency syndrome (HIV/AIDS) has decreased in the 13- to 19-year-old population (Irwin, 2006).

Provide teens with the information on the risks of sexual activity in a nonjudgmental and informative manner, including discussions of both abstinence and methods of birth control.

Diet/Obesity. As children grow, poor eating habits and limited physical activity can contribute to the development of obesity. Assessment of weight in the teen is based on body mass index (BMI) as plotted on gender-specific growth charts. Current recommendations define overweight as children with a BMI at or above the 95th percentile for the gender-specific BMI growth charts. During the years 1999 to 2002, 16% of adolescents, ages 16 to 19 were estimated to be overweight. This represents a 45% increase in the overweight estimates during the years 1988 to 1994 (NHANES, 2003).

Factors contributing to obesity are complex. These include an increase in sedentary activities such as TV viewing, video and computer games, lack of social support for exercise, lack of access to physical activity facilities, and lack of access to appropriate foods. Due to the magnitude of the problem, prevention of obesity has become a major national health issue. School is often an ideal environment for offering programs to promote healthful lifestyles. Counseling should include teaching nutrition as well as promotion of exercise. Because teens are not usually buying and preparing meals, involvement of the parents is essential.

Inge et al. (2004) maintain that 50% to 77% of obese children will remain obese into adulthood, increasing risks for developing other serious and life-threatening illnesses. One example is the recent increase in type 2 diabetes among adolescents who are obese.

In 2004 the rate of obese adults in the United States had risen from 23% in 2000 to 30% for ages 20 and older (U.S. Department of Health and Human Services [USDHHS], 2004). Obesity is more frequent in certain racial groups, with half of African American and Mexican American women defined as overweight (Centers for Disease Control and Prevention [CDC], 2005). Recommended behaviors include decreasing fat intake, increasing fruits and vegetables, and incorporating physical activity into a daily routine.

Four of the ten leading causes of death in North America are linked to diet: heart disease, stroke, diabetes, and certain cancers, especially colorectal, endometrial, and ovarian cancer. The risks of developing hypertension or type 2 diabetes nearly triple for adults who are 20% or more overweight. Being overweight also increases the risk of gout, gallbladder disease, hip fractures, and osteoarthritis (USDHHS, 2004). Obese individuals may suffer from social stigmatization, discrimination, and lowered self-esteem.

Being too thin can also raise the risk of health problems. Anorexia nervosa, loss of appetite, and similar disorders are linked to menstrual irregularities and osteoporosis in women and to a greater risk of early death in both women and men.

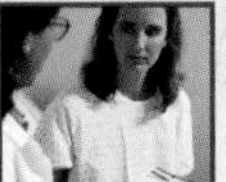

Our client, Jamie King, needs help with her diet. What do you know about the dietary needs of a young adult with type 2 diabetes? How could you find out more about Jamie's pattern of eating? How can you assist her in incorporating these lifestyle changes in her new environment?

Action Alert! Clients should eat a diet with plenty of grain products, vegetables, and fruits—a diet that is low in saturated fat and cholesterol, moderate in sugars, and moderate in sodium.

Exercise. Regular physical activity is associated with lower death rates for adults of any age. It decreases the risk of death from heart disease, it lowers the risk of developing diabetes, and is associated with a decreased risk of colon cancer. It also helps prevent high blood pressure and helps reduce blood pressure in persons with elevated levels. Physical activity is an important factor in the adult's ability to maintain health and independence. Regular exercise promotes appetite, improves mental health, and decreases stress.

Rest and Sleep. Just as activity is important to the adolescent and young adult, so too is rest. According to the National Sleep Foundation (2005), adults need 8 hours of uninterrupted, quality sleep each night for optimum health, safety, and productivity. Young adults become fatigued by stress, work, school, and other life challenges.

Poverty. Poverty is associated with limited access to heath care, poor nutrition, substandard housing, and inadequate prenatal care. If clients have no health insurance, they tend to receive substandard medical care, putting them at risk for medical problems. In 2004, more than 37 million people in the United States (about 12.7% of the population) lived below the poverty line (U.S. Census Bureau, 2004). More specifically, poverty levels for the African American population were 24.7%, Mexican American population 21.9%, and Asian Americans 9.8%. Better-educated and more-affluent clients can afford a healthier diet, better preventive health care, and more prompt medical treatment. However, these advantages do not mean that their lifestyle practices will prevent chronic diseases and premature morbidity and mortality.

Health Insurance. Adult clients in the United States may have health insurance coverage through their employer, by private pay, or by federal or state health plans.

In 2003, most of the U.S. population (64.1%) was covered by a health plan related to employment. An estimated 45 million Americans, or 15.6.% of the population, were without health insurance coverage during the entire year of 2003. The percentage of people with employment-based health insurance dropped to 61% in 2004. Because not all businesses offer health benefits, 27 million workers were uninsured. Young adults ages 18 to 24 remained the least likely of any age-group to have health insurance in 2003. Of this age-group, 30.2% did not have health insurance (National Coalition on Health Care, 2004). Among the general population between ages 18 and 64, full-time and part-time workers were more likely to be insured than nonworkers. Among the working poor, however, there was less probability of being insured than among nonworkers. The primary reason was either that the employer failed to provide health insurance or that the financial burden on employees to buy their company's plan was prohibitive. Canada is looking at similar issues resulting from the high cost of health care in relation to the gross national product. Cheaper health care insurance alternatives are being sought.

The cultural group most likely to be uninsured in the United States is Mexican Americans at 40%, followed closely by Hispanics and Native Americans at 38% and Asian Americans at 20%. Those living below poverty are three times more likely than any other group to be uninsured (National Center for Health Statistics, 2005).

Employment. In 2006, the U.S. Department of Labor's Bureau of Labor Statistics (2006) reported that 4.8% of our nation's workforce was unemployed. Furthermore, 7.2% of adult men, 4.2% adult women, 4.1% of whites, 9.3% of African Americans, and 5.5% of Mexican Americans were unemployed. Unemployment can cause great stressors not only on the individual but on the family, adding to numerous other health-related problems.

Work-Related Injuries and Deaths. The National Institute for Occupational Safety and Health (NIOSH) (2004) estimates that over 90,000 people die annually from work-related illnesses, many of which go unreported. To add to these statistics, the age-group most likely to die on the job are 25- to 34-year-olds. Men are twice as likely to sustain a fatal injury on the job as women. More then 50% of these fatal injuries are related to some form of transportation. The amount of days lost to workplace-related illnesses is even more staggering. It is reported that 1.5 million days of work are lost to due illness or injuries from the workplace. These include musculoskeletal, hearing loss, poisoning, exposure to blood-borne pathogens, respiratory distress, skin disorders and anxiety/stress. Identification and remediation of causal or exacerbating workplace factors are necessary to prevent the recurrence of these disorders (NIOSH, 2004).

Cultural Risk Factors. Culture and ethnic origin are likely to be important influences on adolescents and adults, especially when the person is a first-generation North American. The beliefs and norms of the group to which each client belongs have shaped ideas about health, diet, education, illness, pain, silence, symptom reporting, family support, death, health care providers, and older adults. Within the context of the assessment, you need to determine the strength of the client's affiliation to an ethnic group, health practices, and beliefs about health care. Unless you incorporate these belief patterns into your care plans, you may create a conflict between your nursing interventions and your clients' cultural backgrounds.

Chronic disease continues to have an increased impact on racial and ethnic minority groups. For example, the prevalence of diabetes among African Americans, Hispanics, Native Americans, and Native Alaskans is significantly higher than for white Americans (National Center for Health Statistics, 2005). The cancer survival rate among African Americans, American Indians, Native Alaskans, and Hawaiian Natives is lower than for white Americans. It is about 44%, compared with 59% for white Americans. This difference can be attributed largely to late diagnosis in minority groups (Clegg, Li, Hankey, Chu, & Edwards, 2002).

PSYCHOLOGICAL FACTORS

Suicide. It is difficult to estimate how many adolescents commit suicide because of the number that go unreported. Many single-car accidents are actually suicides or suicide attempts, for example. Adolescent girls make more suicide attempts than boys; however, boys are more successful in their attempts.

Eating Disorders. *Anorexia nervosa* is a complex disorder characterized by self-induced weight loss driven by a morbid fear of becoming fat. Of the adolescents suffering from this affliction, 90% are girls. These teenagers are preoccupied with food and weight and have a distorted body image. They have a revulsion for food that results in a weight loss of 25% or more of the normal body weight with no other apparent illness or psychiatric disorder. They may exercise compulsively to work off any food eaten. Anorexia is the third most common chronic condition among adolescent girls (after obesity and asthma). The syndrome can begin in children as young as age 9 years.

Bulimia nervosa is a disorder characterized by binge eating coupled with purging via emetics, laxatives, or self-induced vomiting. It may be a subtype of anorexia, and it has a similar etiological pattern. Although they may experience mild weight loss or gain, girls with bulimia often have a stable weight. They may suffer from gastric or esophageal rupture, parotid gland enlargement, hypokalemia, erosion of dental enamel from induced vomiting, scars on the knuckles of one hand, and amenorrhea or irregular menses.

Stress. Stress is the most common cause of illness in our society, and it is a major risk factor for the development of physical and psychological problems. It encompasses the negative cognitive and emotional states that result when clients feel that the demands placed on them exceed their ability to cope. It can be caused by external and internal influences. External stressors may stem from the following:

- The physical environment, such as loud noises, bright lights, excessive heat, and confined spaces
- The social environment, such as aggressiveness on the part of someone else
- The work environment, such as deadlines or "red tape"
- Major life events, such as the death of a relative, a lost job, a promotion, or a new baby
- Daily stressors, such as heavy traffic, misplaced keys, or a flat tire

Internal stressors commonly stem from lifestyle choices, such as drinking caffeinated beverages, getting too little sleep, or overloading the daily schedule. Stress may also stem from negative self-talk, such as pessimistic thinking and self-criticism, or from stressful personality traits, such as being a workaholic.

Only if clients cannot successfully handle situations alone do you step in to help them strengthen their weaknesses so they can overcome their restrictions and draw on a lifetime of experiences to meet current challenges. Allowing clients as much participation as possible ensures the success of this strategy.

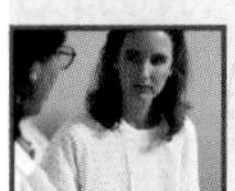

Think about Jamie again. She has just started life at college. Can you list possible stressors in her life?

Action Alert! Reduce the negative effects of stress by reducing perceived pressures, increasing coping resources, or both.

Smoking. Cigarette smoking is another serious health problem among adolescents and young adults that has profound implications for their later adult health. They may believe that the use of cigarettes is better than alcohol or marijuana, which is illegal. The prevalence of smoking remains high among all groups of adolescents.

At least one in every five deaths in North America is related to cigarette smoking–related causes, such as lung cancer; cancer of the larynx, oral cavity, esophagus, pancreas, and urinary bladder; respiratory diseases, such as emphysema; and heart disease (National Center for Health Statistics, 2005; USDHHS, 2004). Cigarette smoking is a major cause of death among Native Americans, Native Alaskans, blue-collar workers, and military personnel (USDHHS, 2004).

Action Alert! Help your clients prevent premature death by helping them to stop smoking.

Alcohol Abuse. The abuse of alcohol and other substances is a major health problem. Usually, it is difficult to detect alcohol abuse. Alcohol typically is metabolized more slowly in an older adult, resulting in a longer exposure time and a higher rate of tissue damage. Signs and symptoms of alcohol misuse may be similar to, or mistaken for, other clinical concerns. Often, however, alcoholism simply goes undetected by health care providers.

Adults who abuse alcohol increase their risk for hypertension, stroke, heart disease, certain cancers, accidents, violence, suicides, birth defects, and overall mortality. Alcohol abuse may cause cirrhosis of the liver, inflammation of the pancreas, damage to the brain and heart, and malnutrition. It may alter the effectiveness of medicines or increase the risk of toxic reactions. Some medications may increase blood alcohol levels or increase the adverse effect of alcohol on the brain.

Action Alert! Help your client avoid drinking alcohol when taking any medications, because it can interact with medications and alter the way they are metabolized.

Illicit Drug Use. Illicit drug use and its consequences threaten North Americans of every socioeconomic background, geographic region, educational level, and ethnic or racial identity. Accidents, crime, domestic violence, illness, lost opportunity, and reduced productivity are the direct consequences of substance abuse. Drug abuse and drug trafficking hurt families, businesses, and neighborhoods; impede education; and burden the criminal justice, health, and social service systems.

Chronic drug users are particularly susceptible to infectious diseases and are considered high-risk transmitters. They and their sexual partners have higher risks of contracting hepatitis, tuberculosis, gonorrhea, syphilis, and other sexually transmitted diseases. High-risk sexual behavior associated with crack cocaine and the injection of illegal drugs enhances the transmission and acquisition of HIV.

Substance abuse is a common problem among families reported for child maltreatment. Researchers have found that 25% to 50% of men who commit domestic violence also have substance abuse problems. In addition, women with substance abuse problems are more likely to become victims of domestic violence. To make matters worse, North Americans who lack access to comprehensive health care and have smaller incomes may be less able to afford treatment to overcome drug dependence.

ASSESSMENT

ASSESSMENT OF THE ADOLESCENT

Many health problems encountered by well adolescents are caused by health-risk behaviors. If possible, interview an adolescent client without the parents present, and reassure the client that your conversation will be confidential (unless the teen is suicidal or homicidal). Most adolescents would prefer not to divulge certain information in front of their parents, such as grades, drug use, sexual behavior, and suicidal thoughts. You may want to interview the parents separately to determine their concerns.

Do not be afraid to ask adolescents about illegal, unsafe, or otherwise undesirable behavior. Research has shown that they will not interpret the question as tacit approval to engage in that behavior. For example, asking adolescents whether they have ever had a sexual relationship will not encourage them to begin a sexual relationship.

Adolescents are more likely to be honest when respected and questioned honestly. They are very sensitive not only to what you actually say to them but to what they think your perceptions are of them. It is important for you to remain nonjudgmental. Teens who believe they are being criticized are unlikely to return for care.

When you assess adolescents, ask the least personal questions first to allow them to become comfortable talking with you. For example, ask about home, education, and other activities before you ask about drug use, sexuality, and suicide risk (Box 17-1). Ask teens about their perceptions of their own weight and their ideal weight, and what measures, if any, they have taken to alter their weight. Finally, question their risk for injury. Also assess adolescents' developmental level. Are they operating at an earlier cognitive level than you would expect? Are they more physically mature than the average teenager of the same age?

Make sure to assess the adolescent's physical, cognitive, and psychological functioning, beginning with a general assessment of appearance. Monitor the teen's vital signs, vision, and hearing, and obtain the results of any other diagnostic screening tests. Obtain height and weight, and assess for anorexia or bulimia if the client has a weight loss of more than 10% of previous weight or if the body weight is in the 5th percentile.

Pay particular attention to the adolescent growth spurt, which peaks in girls at about age 12 years and in boys at about age 14 years. During this period, adolescents experience many physical changes. Boys gain an average of 8 inches (20 cm) in height and more than 40 pounds (18.2 kg) in weight, whereas girls gain somewhat less height and weight. Boys' voices begin to deepen, and facial hair appears on the upper lip and then on the cheeks and lower lip. Pubic hair begins to develop, and the penis, testes, and scrotum enlarge. Some boys experience gynecomastia. Girls' breasts and pubic hair begin to develop. Menarche usually takes place during Tanner stage III or IV (see Figure 17-4).

Depending on the reason for your examination, you should pay particular attention to certain areas. For example, if the adolescent is undergoing a sports physical, you assess the heart, lungs, and abdomen for any abnormalities, and you test all the joints for range of motion, flexibility, strength, and reflexes.

Scoliosis is a structural lateral curvature of the spine. More than 60% of cases occur in girls. It often first ap-

BOX 17-1 *Sample Health History Questions for an Adolescent*

Home
- Where do you live, and who lives there with you?
- Do you get along?
- Do you have privacy in your home?

Education
- What grade are you in?
- What are you good at in school? What is hard for you?
- What kinds of grades do you get?

Activities
- What do you do after school?
- What do you do with your friends?

Alcohol
- Do you know anyone who has tried drugs, alcohol, or cigarettes?
- Have you ever tried drugs or alcohol?
- Do you drink alcohol? What do you usually drink, and how often? Alone or with friends?

Sexual Behavior
- Many young people become interested in sexual relationships at your age. Do you currently have, or have you ever had, a boyfriend or girlfriend? (Include both options for all clients.)
- Have you ever been worried that you had a sexually transmitted disease or that you were (or were responsible for someone becoming) pregnant?
- Have you used anything to prevent disease or pregnancy?
- What did you use?

Suicidal Tendencies
- Everybody feels sad or depressed sometimes. Do you think that you feel that way more often than other young people your age?
- Have you ever felt that life was not worth living?
- Have you ever wanted to kill yourself? (If yes:) Have you made a plan to kill yourself?

Weight
- Do you feel that your weight is just right, too low, or too high?
- Have you ever tried to do anything to change your weight?
- Do you think about food a lot?

Injuries
- Have you ever been the victim of violence or seen someone being assaulted?
- Do you or any of your friends drive a car? Do they ever drive after drinking?
- Have you ever gotten in a car with a driver who has been drinking?
- Do you ever drive after having had something to drink?
- Do you know students in your school who have guns or other weapons?
- Do you have a gun? Are there guns in your home?

pears during late childhood or adolescence, so all adolescents should be appropriately screened. Many states mandate scoliosis screening in the schools.

All teens should have hearing, vision, and blood pressure screenings annually and should be encouraged to have dental checkups and perform good dental care. They should be up-to-date with immunizations, including tetanus, pertussis and diphtheria, hepatitis B, measles, mumps, rubella (the second inoculation), varicella (if there is no history of chicken pox), and meningococcal vaccine. See Chapter 16 for immunization schedule. They should also be screened for tuberculosis.

Iron deficiency anemia is a relatively common problem in adolescents, especially girls. This usually results from menstrual blood loss and lack of iron in the diet. All teens should have their hemoglobin or hematocrit level measured yearly to check for this condition. Adolescents whose parents have a serum cholesterol level greater than 240 mg/100 mL and adolescents who are over 19 years of age should be screened for total blood cholesterol level at least once (Ozer, Adams, & Lustig, 2005).

Testicular cancer is a disease of adolescents and young men. It is readily treatable when detected early. Adolescent males should be screened for this disorder and taught how to examine their testicles so they can perform a self-examination regularly.

Although breast cancer is exceedingly rare in adolescents, all girls who have reached Tanner stage II (see Figure 17-4) of breast development should have a breast examination as part of their regular physical. This also enables you to monitor breast development during puberty. All adolescent girls should be taught to perform a breast self-examination and to make it a routine part of their health behaviors.

All adolescents should be asked annually about involvement in sexual behaviors that may result in unwanted pregnancy and STDs, including infection with HIV. Sexually active adolescent girls should have a cervical culture, and boys should have urine leukocyte esterase analysis to screen for gonorrhea. The frequency of screening for STDs depends on the sexual practices of the adolescent involved. All sexually active girls or any young women 18 years or older should be screened annually for cervical cancer with a Papanicolaou (Pap) test. Adolescents at risk for HIV infection should be offered confidential HIV screening (Ozer, Adams, & Lustig, 2005).

ASSESSMENT OF THE YOUNG ADULT

Assessment of the well adult is a process of holistic assessment across all functional health patterns. Well adults are assessed for many reasons and in many settings: at a physician's office, community health clinic, nursing center, college health center, or occupational health center.

Health History. Any nursing assessment normally begins with a health history. It includes the client's biographical data, past health history, chief complaint, and present health status, and it may include a family history and dynamics. You can create a balance between allowing clients to talk and gathering relevant data.

The completeness of the health history is determined by clients' health status, their ability to answer your questions, and their trust in the relationship they have with you. Start by asking them to describe their health. In their opinion, is it poor, good, or excellent? Assess for past health history that is relevant to understanding their current health status. Take a history of their lifetime health-seeking behaviors. Ask how much control they believe they have over their own health. Inquire about any illnesses within the past year that have prevented them from pursuing normal activities. Ask what they do to keep healthy. Specifically mention breast or testicular self-examinations. Ask whether they use alcohol or other drugs, and how much. Ask whether they smoke, how much, and for how long.

Physical Examination

Techniques for Age Differences. The type of physical examination you perform for a well adult depends largely on the reason for the examination and on the age of the person. For example, when you give a person a sports physical, you screen for previous and current injuries, sexually transmitted diseases, and alcohol and other substance abuse. You assess all joints for range of motion, flexibility, strength, and reflexes. You listen to the person's heart and lungs and examine the eyes, ears, and abdomen for any abnormalities.

An annual physical examination for a woman of childbearing age includes questions about possible domestic violence and increased risks for sexually transmitted diseases. You take her vital signs, including an accurate height for osteoporosis prevention. You assess her heart, lungs, thyroid gland, breasts, abdomen, and genital and rectal areas for any abnormalities. She will need a Papanicolaou test (the Pap test) if it has been 3 years since her last test—or fewer years if she has an increased risk for cervical cancer.

For all well adult clients, you should also assess general health and cognitive and emotional functioning. Begin by assessing their appearance. Observe their behaviors and apparent mental status.

General appearance. By their mid-20s, most adults are fully developed and at peak functioning (Figure 17-6). Young adults enjoy maximum muscle tone and coordination, a high energy level, and optimal mental power. From then on, they will experience a gradual decline in touch sensitivity and in respiratory, cardiovascular, and immune system functions.

Diagnostic Tests. A key to wellness for the adult is appropriate screening, especially for clients in high-risk groups. You may be directly involved in screening or in teaching clients about the importance of screening tests (Table 17-3).

Total cholesterol level in the adolescent and young adult is a significant predictor of heart disease later in life. Diet and exercise can be modified to decrease cholesterol levels. If the total cholesterol level is increased, then the client should be tested for other lipid abnormalities as well.

Hypertension is a risk factor for coronary artery disease, congestive heart failure, stroke, ruptured aortic aneurysm, retinopathy, and renal disease. All adults should be screened for hypertension at least every 2 years. If the diastolic reading is 85 mm Hg and the systolic reading is 140 mm Hg or below, screening every 2 years is sufficient. Hypertension is never diagnosed on the basis of a single reading.

The annual incidence of breast cancer increases with age. In addition to breast self-examination monthly, screening also includes a breast examination by a health practitioner during annual examinations. Screening in younger women is recommended when there is a family history of breast cancer, especially premenopausal breast cancer. All women should be taught the proper technique for monthly breast self-examination.

Screening for cervical cancer is recommended for all women with a cervix who are sexually active or have reached age 18, whichever comes first. A Pap test should be performed every 1 to 3 years for women with a cervix (Office of Disease Prevention and Health Promotion [ODPHP], 2002). Risk factors of multiple

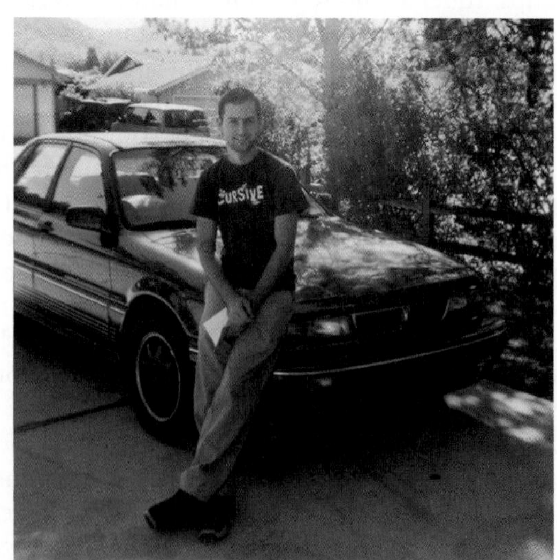

FIGURE 17-6 By the mid-20s, most young adults are fully developed and at peak functioning.

sex partners, an early onset of sexual intercourse, low socioeconomic status, and HIV infection suggest the need for more frequent screening.

All adults should be screened for problem drinking of alcohol. Heavy drinking is defined as more than five drinks per day, five times per week. Medical problems due to alcoholism include hepatitis, cirrhosis of the liver, cardiomyopathy, withdrawal syndrome, mental changes, and, in older adults, a dementia observed during the last stages of severe chronic alcoholism. Heavy drinking and alcoholism (dependency) have dire social consequences as well, including suicide, divorce, depression, domestic violence, unemployment, and poverty.

All clients should be screened for tobacco use, and those who use tobacco products should be advised to quit and encouraged to develop a plan to quit. Many methods are used to help tobacco users quit the habit, but success is directly related to the person's determination to quit rather than to the method itself. Most people try more than once before actually quitting.

All clients should be assessed for their immunization status. All clients need a diphtheria-tetanus vaccination every 10 years. Adults who have not had chickenpox should receive the varicella (chickenpox) immunization.

Young, normal-risk adults should have a comprehensive eye and vision examination every 2 to 3 years.

Table 17-3 Health Screening Guidelines for Well Young Adults

TEST	YOUNG ADULTHOOD (AGES 20 TO 35)
Body measurement	Measure height and weight periodically.
Blood pressure	At least every 2 years for normotensive adults or annually for borderline hypertension. Others should seek the advice of a physician.
Breast examination	Every 3 years. More frequent for high-risk groups.
Cholesterol level	Should seek the advice of a physician. High-risk groups may need screening.
Papanicolaou test	All women who are age 18 or older or sexually active and who have a cervix should have a Pap test every 3 years.
Prostate-specific antigen test	Recommended only if family history.
Tuberculosis	Skin testing for all persons at high risk.
Vision	Comprehensive eye and vision examination every 2 to 3 years; more often if increased risk factors present.

Based on recommendations from U.S. Department of Health and Human Services, Public Health Service, Office of Disease Prevention and Health Promotion. (1998). *Clinician's handbook of preventive services* (2nd ed.). Retrieved January 18, 1998, from http://text.nlm.nih.gov/ftrs/tocview; Report of the U.S. Preventive Services Task Force. (1996). *Guide to clinical preventive services* (2nd ed.). Baltimore: Williams & Wilkins.
NOTE: Recommendations of other groups will differ.

High-risk clients should be screened for tuberculosis. These include people who have close contact with someone known or suspected to have tuberculosis, people infected with HIV, people who inject illicit drugs, people who live or work in high-risk group settings (such as a nursing home or child care center), and people who are medically underserved. Controlling tuberculosis depends on thorough screening of high-risk populations and on providing preventive therapy.

FOCUSED ASSESSMENT FOR *READINESS FOR ENHANCED AGE-APPROPRIATE ATTAINMENT OF DEVELOPMENTAL MILESTONES*

Defining Characteristics. When a client seeks help with psychosocial development, you should consider the diagnosis of *Readiness for enhanced age-appropriate attainment of developmental milestones.* The reasons a person might seek assistance include a history of difficulty with a previous developmental stage or task or the potential for a transitional crisis, such as one associated with childbirth, parenting, midlife, or retirement.

However, this is highly individualized; therefore your assessment should include the client's perception of appropriate behavior and whether or not the behavior is causing difficulty in the person's life.

Related Factors. For the adolescent and young adult, a primary related factor in failure to attain developmental milestones is lack of knowledge. The diagnosis *Readiness for enhanced age-appropriate attainment of developmental milestones* assumes the client is seeking help; thus you can ask the client to identify the cause of this need for help. Related factors could include lack of knowledge, lack of motivation, ineffective coping skills, or inadequate role models.

However, the client could also have environmental or physical factors, such as a chronic illness, physical disability, or mental disability, that have prevented achievement of an adult task. In this case, the related factors would include prescribed dependence (such as protected living), or physical or mental disability (such as mental retardation or a mental illness), deficiencies of environment (such as homelessness), or inadequate caretaking.

FOCUSED ASSESSMENT FOR *INEFFECTIVE HEALTH MAINTENANCE*

A focused assessment for clients with *Ineffective health maintenance* includes looking at their ability to identify, manage, or seek help to maintain health (NANDA International, 2005). Ask questions that will provide cues to their ability and motivation to take responsibility for their own health. For example, "Have you engaged in a healthy lifestyle in the past? For what reasons did you seek health care in the past? Did you adopt the recommended interventions? Why or why not? Do you receive support from your family or significant other? How do family members or friends make it easy (or difficult) to maintain good health practices? To what extent do you believe that maintaining and improving health is possible? Do you need financial assistance to obtain medication?"

Review common causes of adolescent and young adult illness and injury, and discuss ways to reduce their risks. Determine clients' level of interest in improving their health and reducing their risks. This will also help you assess their level of knowledge. Assess whether the clients face barriers to taking effective health actions, such as finances or health care resources.

Keep in mind the common causes of illness and death for these age-groups. They include the following:

- Accidents, AIDS, homicide, and suicide
- Substance abuse that interferes with productivity and relationships and raises the risk of injury, especially domestic violence, and death
- Unsafe sexual practices, which raise the risk of unwanted pregnancies and sexually transmitted diseases, including HIV infection
- Family, lifestyle, or occupational risk factors for cancer or heart disease (such as obesity, a sedentary lifestyle, tobacco use, alcohol abuse, and poor nutrition)
- History of a lack of health-seeking behaviors

Defining Characteristics. Defining characteristics for *Ineffective health maintenance* include the inability or lack of ability to receive and seek necessary health care, a knowledge deficient in basic health care needs, and/or high-risk lifestyle behaviors.

Related Factors. Factors related to the onset of *Ineffective health maintenance* include ineffective coping, functional impairment, inaccessibility or lack of resources, and/or impaired judgment regarding health care or lifestyle issues.

DIAGNOSIS

Although adolescents continue to be influenced by family health practices, they are beginning to make health decisions for themselves and should be encouraged to develop healthy practices. Adolescents have an increased risk for the diagnosis *Ineffective health maintenance* because of their high-risk health behaviors, such as substance abuse, poor nutrition, and reckless driving. They often have feelings of invulnerability, coupled with peer pressure to engage in high-risk behaviors, which puts them at risk for physical illness, psychosocial problems, or death.

Keep in mind that the diagnosis *Delayed growth and development* is a broad category applicable to a client with multiple issues. Often, however, a single issue is the focus of nursing care. When this is the case, you will want to use a more specific nursing diagnosis. Group the client's diagnostic cues to help determine the best nursing diagnosis, as described in Table 17-4.

When the client needs to make dietary modifications (for example, to improve health), the diagnosis *Imbalanced nutrition: more than (less than) body requirements* is used. When the person needs knowledge to accomplish a change in lifestyle, the diagnosis *Deficient knowledge* is used. When the person is a parent who needs help with parenting skills, use the diagnosis *Impaired parenting.* When the person is overwhelmed with the stress of caring for a dependent person, the diagnosis is *Caregiver role strain.* When the person is not managing an acute or chronic illness effectively, the diagnosis is *Ineffective therapeutic regimen management.* There may be justification for more specific nursing diagnoses of problems that will require management to be able to effectively resolve *Ineffective health maintenance.* Examples include *Ineffective coping, Disabled family coping, Complicated grieving,* and *Spiritual distress.*

PLANNING

Each plan of care must be individualized to a client's needs, age, and culture. Address the client's concerns first. Then, together with the client, develop a care plan that includes achievable short- and long-term goals designed for success. For clients at risk for *Ineffective health maintenance,* the goal is for them to demonstrate the knowledge they need to improve their health behaviors and take ac-

Table 17-4 Clustering Data to Make a Nursing Diagnosis

High-Risk Lifestyle Choices	
DATA CLUSTER	**DIAGNOSIS**
A 32-year-old male client smokes two packs of cigarettes daily. He has not exercised regularly since he was in college, and he cannot remember when he last had a physical examination.	*Ineffective health maintenance* related to lifestyle/habits
A 24-year-old female client has had three consecutive blood pressure readings above 140/90 mm Hg. She says she feels fine and finds it hard to believe that anything is wrong.	*Knowledge deficit regarding causes of hypertension* related to perception
A 17-year-old male client, 5 feet 10 inches in height, weighs 237 pounds. He reports eating fast food every day for breakfast and lunch. He says that he eats fresh vegetables and fruits about three times a week.	*Imbalanced nutrition: more than body requirements* related to lifestyle management

tion to change the behavior. For example, for adolescents and young adults who are sedentary, the goal would be to engage regularly, preferably daily, in moderate physical activity for at least 30 minutes per day.

Plan primary prevention strategies with adolescents, with the goal of discouraging them from participating in high-risk behaviors. When planning care for well adolescents, focus your teaching on specific high-risk behaviors while incorporating teaching about all risk behaviors in an effort to prevent them. Because adolescence is normally a time of risk taking, chronically ill teens may have the additional problem of engaging in risk-taking behavior by failing to comply with their treatment regimen. It is essential to include the adolescent as an active partner in developing appropriate responses to the risk situation.

Some examples of expected outcomes for the well adolescent and young adult are the following:

- Outlines a realistic plan for increasing healthy behaviors (specify: exercise, diet, weight loss)
- Includes positive social interactions in daily schedule
- Establishes a target date for beginning a healthy behavior
- Seeks health-related information from valid sources
- Describes strategies to eliminate unhealthy behavior
- Performs activities of daily living consistent with energy and tolerance

Explore options with clients to help them achieve goals by changing behaviors (reducing weight, stopping tobacco use, increasing exercise, and so on). With your assistance, clients should prioritize their goals and specify time frames for achieving them.

Jamie decided that her primary goal was to start an exercise program. This along with better diet choices in the dorm cafeteria would lower her blood glucose levels to a normal level. She planned to go to bed earlier in order to awaken earlier to exercise before class at the school gym. How would you respond to Jamie? Is her plan reasonable or unrealistic? How would you help her implement and evaluate her plan?

INTERVENTION

ADOLESCENTS

Interventions to Prevent Illness. Primary prevention is clearly a key issue in adolescent health because most of the morbidities of adolescents are behavioral and therefore preventable. Client teaching is important, but research has repeatedly shown that knowledge alone does not result in behavior change. You must also be skilled in the techniques of primary prevention. These include yearly health checkup with complete blood count, vital signs, and Tanner stage, immunizations, and health education about possible teens risks of weapons, dangers of alcohol and drug use and driving while under the influence of any substance or with others under the influence (Box 17-2).

Action Alert! Consider the factors that motivate adolescents to change their high-risk behaviors as you develop your health education strategies.

Interventions to Overcome Health Care Barriers. A barrier to implementing care for adolescents is their perceived lack of access to health care providers. Some adolescents do not seek health care because they feel uncomfortable both in their pediatrician's office, where they were treated as a child, and in clinics that primarily serve adults. They may also be uncomfortable divulging personal information about a potentially embarrassing topic, such as a suspected pregnancy, to either their parents or health care providers. Some adolescents are unaware of where to obtain care. Others may not live where clinics are conveniently located. Still others have parents who may not be aware of the health needs or concerns of their adolescents.

An important goal of care for working with adolescents is to withhold judgments about teens' behaviors and to treat them with respect. Consult with them on treatment decisions instead of dealing only with their parents, because they are in the process of gaining independence from their families. They will be more likely to comply with the treatment regimen when they take part in the decision-making process.

Although an important goal is to help adolescents establish independence, you also need to consider the importance of parents in the care of adolescents and their concerns about their adolescents. Many parents are overly protective and very anxious. You can help them understand normal adolescent developmental needs so that parents can avoid impeding the teen's growth.

Interventions Through School-Based Clinics. Studies have shown that school-based clinics are an effective means of providing care to adolescents. They are often an integral part of the school where adolescents seek care, and teachers and administrators often refer students with health problems to them.

BOX 17-2 *Primary Prevention for Adolescents*

- Yearly health checkup, including complete blood count, blood pressure, height, weight, Tanner stage
- Immunizations, including tetanus and diphtheria every 10 years, hepatitis B series, measles, mumps, rubella, hepatitis A for high-risk persons (including those traveling to endemic areas), and tuberculosis
- Health education about the risks of weapons, dangers of alcohol and drug use, drunk driving

Many clinics are multidisciplinary, with on-site social workers and health educators. In most clinics, primary care health services are provided by nurse practitioners who consult with physicians. They provide reproductive health services aimed at reducing rates of teen pregnancy and sexually transmitted diseases, and they often provide primary care health services, care for chronic and episodic illnesses (such as asthma and ear infections), health education, and mental health services. Most school districts mandate health education programs. In addition to one-to-one care, the group approach used in schools is very effective for teens because they are peer oriented.

YOUNG ADULTS

Educating for Lifestyle Changes. When teaching young adults about interventions to change lifestyle choices, give specific, informational instructions to help maximize compliance. Fully explaining the regimen and its rationale, demonstrating it clearly, and writing down the instructions will enhance behavior change. Providing clients with written pictorial material for them to keep and review reinforces the teaching session and will build on their ability to retain information (visually and auditory). For example, explain the purposes and expected effects of the interventions you recommend to the clients, and tell them when to expect these effects. This is especially important if the benefits of an intervention will not be immediate (for example, the benefits of a regular exercise program may not be apparent for several months). Otherwise, clients may become discouraged and abandon the intervention.

Suggest small changes rather than large ones. Ask clients to do only slightly more than they are already doing. By achieving a small goal, clients initiate a positive change that will encourage them to continue; this helps to avoid noncompliance.

Successful persuasion involves not only increasing clients' belief in their capacities but also structuring interventions so that they are likely to be successful. Sometimes, rather than eliminating established behaviors, it is better to add new ones. For example, it might be better to suggest to overweight clients that they add exercise to their day rather than that they eat less. Also, link clients' new behaviors with old ones. For example, if clients forget to take their daily medication, you might suggest that they take their medication in the morning while brushing their teeth or with an evening meal. This is the beginning of incorporation of the new lifestyle changes with the old.

Finally, use a combination of strategies to help educate clients, such as oral and written instructions, audiovisual aids, individual and group counseling, and community resources. Multiple techniques are more likely to foster success than single strategies. Refer clients to community agencies, voluntary health organizations (such as the American Heart Association), instructional references (such as books, videotapes, or the Internet), or to support groups for clients with similar problems.

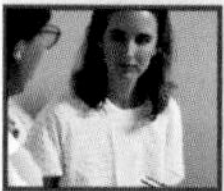

If Jaime succeeds in going to the school gym three times a week for a month but makes no other changes, she may not reach her blood glucose level goals. However, she may have achieved other benefits. Can you think of any?

Once clients fully understand the intervention, ask them for a specific commitment. Ask them to describe specifically what they plan to achieve. Doing this encourages them to begin thinking about how to integrate a new behavior into their daily schedule.

Diet. Nutritional assessments ascertain whether young adults, are able to obtain and/or prepare food and whether they consume the recommended amounts of protein, calories, minerals, and vitamins. A daily diet log has been proven in many cases to help clients make their own assessments and evaluation of all the foods they truly consume in a day. Teaching can begin after careful assessment and mutual goal setting has occurred.

Exercise. An appropriate exercise program for adolescent and young adult clients should take into consideration their current level of activity, which is determined by careful assessment.

Following the assessment, clients should engage regularly, preferably daily, in moderate physical activity for at least 30 minutes.

Rest and Sleep. Clients and their family members should keep a regular sleep schedule, which means going to bed and getting up at nearly the same time each day, even on weekends, within a 30-minute time frame. Encourage clients to make their bedroom conducive to sleep, such as cool, quiet, and dark. It is better if they read or watch television in another room. Encourage clients to engage in a relaxing, nonstimulating activity at bedtime such as reading or listening to music. A warm bath or hot tub may promote sleep. Encourage clients not to bring their problems to bed and to avoid eating and drinking before bedtime. A bedtime routine will prepare the mind and body for sleep.

Stress. Because stress is associated with increased disease susceptibility, stress management is an important component of health promotion activities. Daily stressors are associated more with health problems than are stressful life events because they result in a high level of stress being maintained over a long period.

Exercise can be successfully used not only to maintain activity but also to decrease stress. Physical activity is an important factor in the adult's ability to maintain health and independence. Regular exercise promotes appetite, mental health, and balance. Adults quickly realize the benefits of a program of activity and exercise because the change in energy level can be quick and dramatic.

Supportive relationships and friendships are critical to well-being. Developing support systems can be a beneficial effect of health promotion groups.

Action Alert! Talking only of failures in life is a sign of possible despair.

EDUCATING FOR HEALTH MANAGEMENT

Medication Management. Nursing interventions for young adults may involve education about medications. After performing an assessment, you must educate clients about any misconceptions they might have about prescribed medications. Teach them about the interactions of prescribed drugs and about the effects of taking them concurrently with over-the-counter drugs.

Health Maintenance Visits. Plan with clients for regular visits with a primary health care provider for screening and evaluation, including vision checks, physicals, and immunizations (Box 17-3). Teaching clients to arrange annual checkups and immunizations at the same time yearly helps them remember their immunizations. Consistent scheduling helps clients arrange appointments in advance.

Counseling for Lifestyle Behaviors. Research suggests that clients have only a few important beliefs about any one subject. To persuade clients to change their behavior, it is first necessary to identify their beliefs that are relevant to the high-risk behavior and to provide information based on this foundation. Counseling is used to help clients with problems related to illicit drugs and alcohol abuse, smoking, personal loss, and stress.

Changing a client's high-risk behaviors involves more than giving information. Knowledge is necessary but not sufficient to change health behaviors. One set of interventions is not effective for all clients; you will need to adapt your teaching and recommendations to each client's perceptions of health and ability to change. Use the power of your profession. Research studies have indicated that your individual attention and feedback to the client are more useful than news media or other communication media in changing the client's knowledge and behavior. Most clients respect nurses and believe that what you say is important. However, some clients lack confidence in their ability to make lifestyle changes. Be empathic and supportive while providing firm, definite recommendations for changing high-risk behaviors. For example, you can say, "I want you to quit smoking." The message is simple and specific. You also need to monitor the client's progress through follow-up contact, by appointment or telephone call within a few weeks, to evaluate progress, reinforce successes, and identify and respond to problems. You can also assist clients in monitoring their own progress through journals. Writing activities help to clarify and reward positive behaviors.

Many barriers exist to making a change in unhealthy lifestyle behaviors. The client may feel unwilling to take responsibility for accomplishing day-to-day preventive behaviors for many reasons. Such unwillingness may result from lack of motivation, lack of readiness, inadequate health care teaching, lack of support, and lack of resources.

BOX 17-3 *Teaching for Wellness*

Helping a Young Adult Maintain Health

Purpose: To maintain a healthy lifestyle.
Expected Outcome: The client will maintain his or her present level of functioning.

Client Instructions

Your client can do many things to maintain his or her health well into old age. You can help him or her by offering these suggestions:

- Maintain your social relationships. Use the telephone to call your family and friends. Attend family functions, church, activities, and senior citizen events in your community.
- Exercise every day. Walking is one of the best exercises. Wear sturdy shoes, and work up to walking three to four times a week for 20 minutes each time.
- Relax. Take deep breaths and practice relaxation exercises. Visualize a peaceful outdoor scene or a happy family event. Decrease stressors in your life, and share problems with a trusted person, such as your clergy.
- Eat sensibly. Eat from the five food groups. It may be easier—and better—to eat six small meals and one or two snacks than three meals each day. Drink plenty of fluids, especially water.
- Stop smoking. Do not be afraid to seek help, such as a smoking cessation class or a nicotine replacement plan, to help reduce the need for smoking. See your physician for help.
- Sleep well at night. To do so, try not to nap in the late afternoon or evening. Do not eat right before bed. Limit fluids in the evening hours to reduce the need to urinate during the night. If you wake up at night and do not fall back to sleep right away, get up and read or watch television until you become sleepy.
- Maintain a comfortable environment. Use your heating and cooling system for adequate warmth in winter and a cool environment in very hot, humid weather.
- Practice health maintenance. Take medication as ordered. Schedule and keep appointments with your physician. Comply with suggested standards for screening tests, immunizations, and so on. Be alert to changes in your body, and seek help from your health care provider as soon as possible.

In clinics and other health care settings, barriers to implementing a preventive health program include an emphasis on curing illness and injury rather than prevention. You or your agency may not have an adequate system for tracking, monitoring, and following up on a client's progress. Your clients may lack health insurance, or their insurance may not pay for preventive services.

Development Issues. The main interventions for *Delayed development* are counseling and health education. Counseling is entering into a therapeutic relationship to help the client achieve personal development and avoid a crisis. The goals are to help clients solve their problems and to assist them in mobilizing their resources and regaining equilibrium. Their usual coping mechanisms do not work, and counseling can help them develop new coping mechanisms, such as identifying relatives or friends they can talk with about their problem. Education can provide information to enable clients to gain a better understanding of their developmental issues. For example, having a new mother take parenting classes can give her confidence to be a parent.

EVALUATION

Evaluation is a systematic, ongoing process of evaluating the client's progress toward the attainment of goals, as suggested in Box 17-4. With many of the behavioral problems of adolescence, you will not have an objective,

BOX 17-4 *Nursing Care Plan*

An Adolescent/Young Adult With Type 2 Diabetes

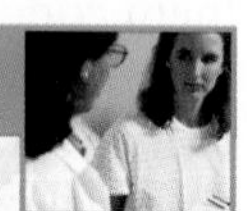

Assessment Data

After performing an assessment at the university student health center, the nurse records the following report: *Jamie King, age 19, presents with history of type 2 diabetes and complaints of fatigue, weakness, and increased stress. Regular blood glucose measurements indicate hyperglycemia. She reports a decrease in physical exercise, increase in eating "on the run," and poor food choices in the dorm cafeteria. Her blood glucose level is currently 214. Vital signs: temperature 98.4° F, pulse 67, respirations 16, blood pressure 112/58.*

Nursing Orders

Health teaching about regular exercise and stress level and food choices to regulate blood glucose level
Recommendations for nutrition journal and exercise
Follow-up appointment in 1 month
Refer to health center physician for follow-up care and routine health maintenance

NANDA-I Nursing Diagnosis	NOC Expected Outcomes With Indicators	NIC Interventions With Selected Activities	Selected Evaluation Data
Ineffective Health Maintenance **Related Factors:** • Blood glucose level 214 • 0 regular exercise • Poor diet choices	***Health-Promoting Behaviors***	***Counseling***	
	• Client will have appropriate screenings and immunizations done within the next 6 months.	• Review appropriate screening tests and immunizations for client's age-group.	• Client has scheduled an appointment for a physical examination with student health center physician.
	• Client will eliminate high-risk behaviors within 1 year.	• Counsel client on recognizing high-risk behaviors and understanding their connection to chronic illness.	• Client can describe connection between high blood glucose levels, lack of exercise, and poor diet choices to increased stress levels and other chronic diseases.
	• Client will be knowledgeable about health promotion activities within 1 month.	• Review Jamie's exercise and diet plan to promote decreased blood glucose levels and stress level.	

Critical Thinking Questions

1. How might dorm living affect Jamie's compliance with the treatment regimen?
2. What other resources might be useful for her?
3. What approach would you use to help Jamie to select better foods?
4. How is stress related to Jamie's blood glucose levels?
5. How can Jamie permanently incorporate these changes into her school lifestyle?
6. What help could her family offer her?

Nursing outcome and intervention labels from Johnson, M., Bulechek, G., Butcher, H., Dochterman, J. M., Maas, M., Moorhead, S., et al. (Eds.). (2006). *NANDA, NOC, and NIC linkages: Nursing diagnoses, outcomes, & interventions.* St. Louis, MO: Mosby.

accurate measure of the outcome. For example, to evaluate a change in drinking habits, you will need to rely on the adolescent's report. However, if the adolescent does not feel completely comfortable with you, you may receive an inaccurate report. One objective way to look for a change in a teen's weekend drinking would be to check his or her attendance record on Mondays. Likewise, an objective way to evaluate an increase in condom use would be to check for a change in how often the client seeks treatment for sexually transmitted diseases.

Before evaluating altered development in the adult, you need to have set long-term goals that are in keeping with the client's abilities and lifestyle. Also, the expected outcomes that you have chosen need to let the clients experience progress toward the long-term goals. Clients and their families, when appropriate, should be involved in the process. If the expected outcomes are not achieved within the defined time frame, reassessment is needed to examine the impediments to the progress. The ongoing assessment data you gather are used to revise nursing diagnoses, outcomes, and the plan of care, in consultation with clients and significant others. Evaluate the effectiveness of your interventions by considering your clients' responses to them as well as the attainment of the goals.

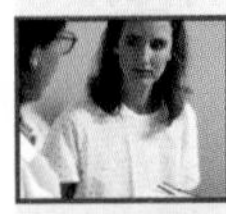

The nurse at the student health center calls Jamie 1 week after her appointment and records the following evaluation information in her chart.

SAMPLE DOCUMENTATION NOTE FOR JAMIE KING

Reports that she has visited the school gym three times during the week since her visit. She has been able to make better choices at the dorm cafeteria for five of the seven days and has kept track of her food choices in her nutrition journal. Her blood glucose level was slightly elevated to 200 on two of the days.

▼ KEY PRINCIPLES

- The developmental tasks of adolescents and young adults are influenced mainly by genetics, socioeconomic status, ethnic group, religious faith, and social expectations.
- Erikson's stages of psychosocial development of the adolescent are to achieve a sense of identity, whereas the young adult is centered around developing adult relationships, contributing to society, and developing satisfaction.
- Lifestyle risk factors for the adolescent and young adult are poor diet, lack of exercise, inadequate rest and sleep, stress, and engaging in risky behaviors.
- Each psychosocial stage of adolescence and young adulthood is associated with choices that can lead to health problems.
- Socioeconomic factors create risk for illness and injury at any developmental stage.
- The risk for illness increases with physical decline and is related to lifestyle choices.
- Assessment of the adolescent and well young adult is a process of holistic assessment of all functional health patterns.
- Problems of adolescent and young adult development are diagnosed as *Delayed growth and development* or a more specific diagnosis to address individual problems.
- Planning for the well adolescent and young adult is centered on the goals of maintaining health and preventing illness.
- Intervening with adolescents and well young adults to enable them to maintain health requires education for change in lifestyle.
- Intervening with the adolescent and young adult with health problems includes education for health management.
- Evaluation is a systematic, ongoing process.

■ REVIEW QUESTIONS

1. Accurate information regarding the growth and development patterns for adolescents would include which of the following?

1. A growth spurt occurs 2 years later in boys compared with girls.
2. Concerns over body image and peer relationships characterize adolescence.
3. Complete skeletal maturational development occurs by age 16 years.
4. Girls plateau in height around the average age of 12.

2. To assess growth and development patterns in young adults, the nurse knows they typically have:

1. Complete dental maturity
2. Decreased near-vision acuity
3. Tremendous emotional strain
4. Identity diffusion

3. When assessing a 25-year-old obese male client, the nurse recognizes that the client is at greatest risk for the development of:

1. Chronic respiratory infections
2. Osteoporosis
3. Hypertension
4. Mental deterioration

4. Lack of health care access for uninsured adults in the United States would be of most concern to the nurse because:

1. Clients do not receive well adult care
2. Clients may limit health care to emergencies only
3. Clients may wait to receive any care until they become extremely ill
4. Clients may not follow recommended health care providers' advice

5. Obesity in adolescents has proved to be:

1. A declining problem in the United States
2. Problematic due to the health risks that do not begin until adulthood
3. Overreported due to the concern of health care providers
4. Placing the child at greater risk for developing chronic diseases during childhood

Bibliography

American Psychiatric Association. (2000). *Diagnostic and statistical manual of mental disorders* (4th ed.) [text revision, DSM-IV-TR]. Washington, DC: Author.

America's Children in Brief. *Key national indictors of well-being, 2004.* Retrieved November 7, 2005, from http://childstats.gov.

Centers for Disease Control and Prevention. (2005). *Overweight and obesity: Obesity trends among U.S. adults between 1985 and 2004.* Retrieved November 11. 2005, from http://www.cdc.gov/nccdphp/dnpa/obesity/trend/index.htm.

Clegg, L. X., Li, F. P., Hankey, B. F., Chu, K., & Edwards, B. K. (2002). Cancer survival among U.S. whites and minorities. *Archives of Internal Medicine, 162,* 1985-1993.

*Cumming, E., & Henry, W. E. (1961). *Growing old: The process of disengagement.* New York: Basic Books.

Daniels, S. R. (2005). *Overweight in children and adolescents: Pathophysiology, consequences, prevention, and treatment.* AHA scientific statement available at www.cirulationaha.org.

Edelman, C. L.. & Mandle, C. L. (2006). *Health promotion throughout the lifespan.* St. Louis, MO: Mosby.

*Elkind, D. (1992). Cognitive development. In S. B. Friedman, M. Fisher, & S. K. Schoenberg (Eds.), *Comprehensive adolescent health care* (pp. 24-26). St. Louis, MO: Quality Medical.

*Erikson, E. (1959). Growth and crises of the healthy personality. *Psychological Issues, 1,* 50-100.

*Erikson, E. H. (1963). *Childhood and society* (2nd ed.). New York: Norton.

*Erikson, E. H. (1982). *The life cycle completed.* New York: Norton.

*Folstein, M. F., Folstein, S. E., & McHugh P. R. (1975). Mini-Mental State: A practical method for grading the cognitive state of patients for the clinician. *Journal of Psychiatric Research, 12,* 189-198.

Gordon, M. (2002) *Manual of nursing diagnosis* (10th ed.). St. Louis, MO: Mosby.

Hockenberry, M., Wilson, D., Winkelstein, M. L., & Kline, N. (2003). *Wong's essentials of pediatric nursing* (7th ed.). St. Louis, MO: Mosby.

Inge, T. H., Krebs, N. F., Garcia, V. F., Skelton, J. A., Guice, K. S., Strauss, R. S., et al. (2004). Bariatric surgery for severely overweight adolescents: Concerns and recommendations. *Pediatrics, 114*(1), 217-223.

Irwin, C. E. (2006). Beyond abstinence: What we need to do to decrease the risks of sexual behavior during adolescence. *Journal of Adolescent health, 38,* 165-168.

Johnson, M., Bulechek, G., Butcher, H., Dochterman, J. M., Maas, M., Moorhead, S., et al. (Eds.). (2006). *NANDA, NOC, and NIC linkages: Nursing diagnoses, outcomes, & interventions.* St. Louis, MO: Mosby.

Le, T. N., & Kato, T. (2006). The role of peer, parent, and culture in risky sexual behavior for Cambodian and Lao/Mien adolescents. *Journal of adolescent health, 38,* 288-296.

*Levinson, D. J. (1978). *The seasons of a man's life.* New York: Knopf.

*Levinson, D. J. (1986). A conception of adult development. *American Psychologist, 41,* 3-13.

*Levinson, D. J. (1996). *The seasons of a woman's life.* New York: Knopf.

*Levinson, D., Darrow, C., Klein, E., Levinson, M., & McKee, B. (1986). Periods in the adult development of men: Ages 18-45. *Counseling Psychologist, 6* (12), 21-25.

NANDA International. (2005). *Nursing diagnoses: Definitions and classification, 2005-2006.* Philadelphia: Author.

National Center for Health Statistics. (2005). *Health, United States, 2005, with chartbook on trends in the health of Americans.* Hyattsville, MD: U.S. Government Printing Office.

National Coalition on Health Care. (2004). *Facts on health insurance coverage.* Washington, DC: Author.

National Institute on Aging, U.S. Department of Health and Human Services. (2000). *Life expectancy in G-7 industrialized nations may exceed past predictions, study suggests.* Retrieved November 7, 2005, from http://www.nia.nih.gov/news/pr/2000/06%2D14.htm.

National Institute for Occupational Safety and Health. (2004). *CDC Health work chartbook.* Retrieved November 1, 2005, from http://www.2a.cdc.gov/NIOSH-chartbook/ch1-4.asp.

National Sleep Foundation. (2006). *How much sleep do we really need?* Sleep Matters. Retrieved October 10, 2006 from http://www/sleepfoundation.org/sleepmatters.

Office of Disease Prevention and Health Promotion, U.S. Department of Health and Human Services, Public Health Service. (2002). *Guide to clinical preventive services, 2000-2002* (3rd ed.). Retrieved November 1, 2005, from http://www.ahrq.gov/clinic/uspstfix.htm.

Ozer, E. M., Adams, S. H., & Lustig, J. L. (2005). Increasing the screening and counseling of adolescents for risky behaviors: Primary care intervention. *Pediatrics,115,* 960-968.

*Pfeiffer, E. (1975). A short portable mental status questionnaire for the assessment of brain deficits in elderly patients. *Journal of the American Geriatric Society, 23,* 433-441.

*Piaget, J., & Infelder, B. (1958). *The growth of logical thinking from childhood to adolescence.* New York: Basic Books.

Statistics Canada. (2002a). *Changes in unmet health care needs 2000/01.* Retrieved November 1, 2005, from http://www.statcan.ca/Daily/English/ 020313/d020313a.htm.

Statistics Canada. (2002b). *High blood pressure.* Retrieved November 11, 2005, from http://www.statcan.ca/english/freepub/82-221-XIE/ 00502/high/canada/cblood.htm.

Statistics Canada. (2002c) *Labour force characteristics by age and sex.* Retrieved November 7, 2005, from http://www.statcan.ca/english/Pgdb/People/ Labour/labor20a.htm.

U.S. Census Bureau. (2002). Population tables: U.S. Census Bureau 2000 Census. Washington, D.C.: U.S. Department of Commerce.

U.S. Census Bureau. (2004). Population tables: U.S. Census Bureau 2000 Census. Washington, DC: Department of Commerce.

U.S. Department of Health and Human Services. (2004). *The health consequences of smoking: A report of the surgeon general.* Publication No. 017-024-01685-3. Atlanta: U.S. Department of Health and Human Services, Centers for Disease Control and Prevention, National Center for Chronic Disease Prevention and Health Promotion, Office on Smoking and Health. Retrieved March 12, 2006, from http://www.cdc.gov/tobacco/sgr/sgr–2004.

U.S. Department of Health and Human Services. (n.d.) *Overweight among U.S. children and adolescents.* Data briefs: National Health and Nutrition Examination Survey. Hyattsville, MD: Centers for Disease Control and Prevention, National Center for Health Statistics.

U.S. Department of Labor, Bureau of Labor Statistics. (2006). *Employment situation summary.* Retrieved March 12, 2006, from http://www.bls.gov/news.release/empsit.nr0.htm.

*Asterisk indicates a classic or definitive work on this subject.

Chapter 18

The Middle and Older Adult

Media Resources

- evolve Evolve Website http://evolve.elsevier.com/Harkreader/
- Companion CD

Learning Objectives

After studying this chapter, you will be able to do the following:

- Discuss aging and the developmental tasks of middle and older adulthood
- Identify factors affecting the health and well-being of middle and older adults
- Describe the assessment of a well middle and older adult for normal function and risk factors
- Describe modifications of the health history and physical examination for the older adult
- Differentiate among the variety of nursing diagnoses appropriate for adults seeking knowledge or health care practices to increase the likelihood of successful aging
- Plan nursing interventions for health maintenance, and reduce risk factors as appropriate to the adult's developmental level
- Evaluate the outcomes that describe progress toward the goals of health maintenance

Key Terms

ageism
geriatric nursing
gerontology
menopause
middle adulthood
midlife crisis
older adult
retirement
sandwich generation

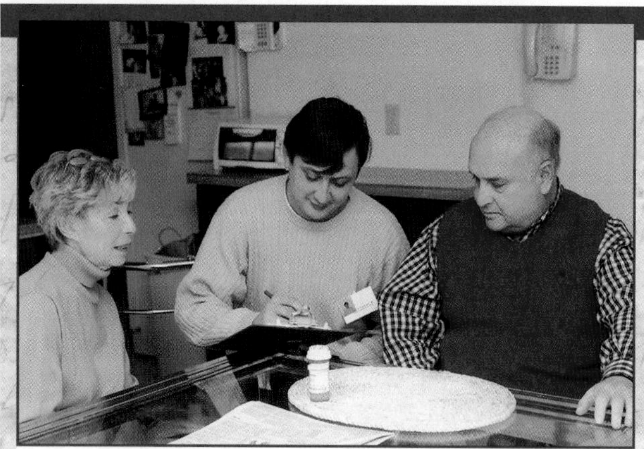

From Maurer, F. A. (2005). *Community/public health nursing practice: Health for families and populations* (3rd ed.). St. Louis, MO: Mosby.

Mr. Alessandro Cognomi, a 70-year-old obese Italian American man, is married with a son age 50 and a daughter age 45. He has three grandchildren, ages 25, 20, and 15. He recently retired from a job as a chief accountant at a large insurance company. He has a history of adult-onset diabetes and borderline hypertension. His current blood pressure is 148/96 mm Hg. He is 5 feet 10 inches tall and weighs 227 pounds.

He has not been hospitalized since he had his appendix removed as a small child. He smokes two packs of cigarettes a day and reports, "I don't eat many fruits and vegetables. I just never liked them." His diet is high in fat, and he has not exercised for "years." Mr. Cognomi says that he is surprised he has high blood pressure because he is not feeling bad. He knows he should lose a little weight, quit smoking, and get some exercise.

Possible nursing diagnoses for Mr. Cognomi's situation are listed in the nursing diagnoses box.

KEY NURSING DIAGNOSES FOR THE MIDDLE AND OLDER ADULT

***Readiness for enhanced age-appropriate attainment of developmental milestones:** Seeks assistance to manage age-appropriate developmental milestones

Ineffective health maintenance: Inability to identify, manage, and/or seek out help to maintain health

*Not currently on approved NANDA International (NANDA-I) list.

The baby boom generation is currently in middle adulthood and on the brink of older adulthood. Nurses who are grounded in knowledge of a healthy adult lifestyle and optimal geriatric care can affect prevention, diagnosis, treatment, and rehabilitation of age-related health problems for this generation. Nurses have an obligation to improve the quality of life for people as they grow older by reducing the impact of disease and disability.

Baby boomers will enter **retirement** more optimistic economically than the previous generation partly because they have been two-income families and will have two-income retirements. However, economic certainty is not guaranteed because baby boomers have faced downsizing and layoffs in their peak employment years and they have not been a generation of savers. Entering retirement as a more educated generation, especially women, baby boomers are likely to have different expectations for retirement, health care, and quality of life. They are an individualistic generation, with a tendency to reject the stereotypical expectations of aging. They may continue to work at least part-time into older adulthood and use technology to enhance their work life and their health. Aging baby boomers are expected to be a knowledgeable group of health care consumers who place high demands on the health care system for specialists, such as orthopedic surgeons, cardiovascular surgeons, and plastic surgeons with the hope of maintaining their vitality well into old age.

The specialty of geriatric nursing will come of age as baby boomers age. **Geriatric nursing** is a branch of nursing that deals with the problems and diseases of old age and aging people. **Gerontology** is the comprehensive study of aging and the problems of older adults. Because the baby boom generation is a large cohort and because the life expectancy is increasing, the group age 65 and older is expected to reach 20% of the population by the year 2040.

Healthy aging is a prerequisite for allowing people a range of personal choices and aspirations that facilitate the pleasures of family, career, friendship, spiritual growth, travel, learning, productivity, and service to the community (Figure 18-1). Increasing the span of healthy life is more important than increasing the years of life without regard to quality of life. High-quality health care, informed by best geriatric practices, as well as access to the newest and most effective medications, treatments, therapies, and medical technologies without discrimination based on age may help achieve the goal of a longer period with quality of life.

CONCEPTS OF ADULT DEVELOPMENT

Aging is a process of gradual change in the physical, mental, social, and emotional self, resulting in maturation by the mid 20s followed by a gradual decline into old age and death. Physical age is only one determinant of people's health care needs as they grow older.

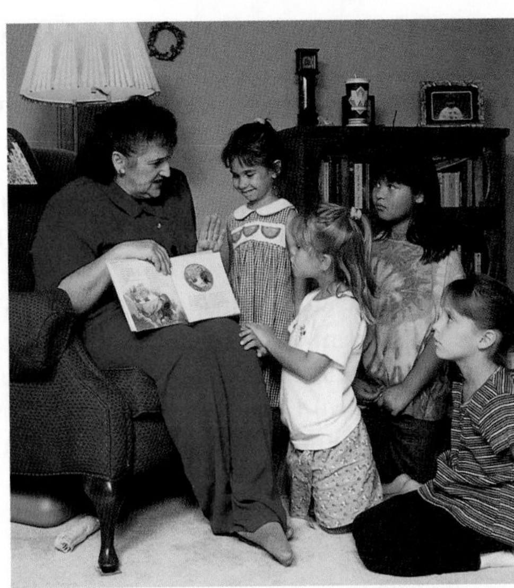

FIGURE 18-1 Healthy aging allows for personal choices of lifestyle changes such as contributing to the lives of younger generations.

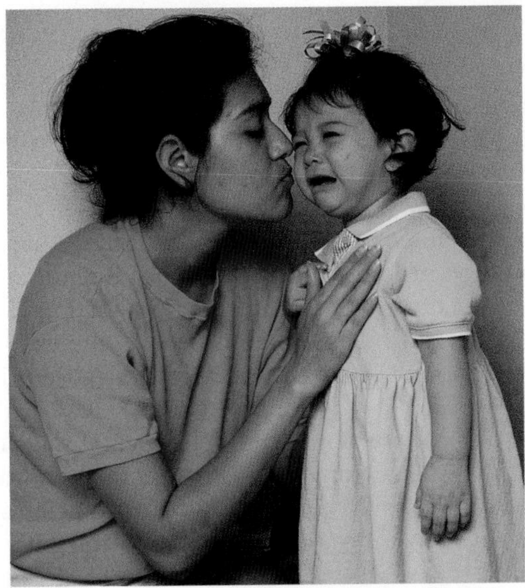

FIGURE 18-2 The stage of generativity involves the development of a capacity to care for others.

Human development is a continuous, lifelong process occurring gradually over time and involving both gains and losses. Development is plastic, that is, individuals are adaptable or resilient to a variety of biological, personal, and social influences. Middle and older adults continue to develop socially, intellectually, emotionally, and in the use of principled behavior even as they make adjustments to the physical changes that occur with age.

Knowledge about a client's stage in human development is necessary to understanding the client's perspective of his or her health needs and goals for health care. By understanding adult development, you can help people cope with life's transitions and help them manage their health problems in a manner appropriate to their developmental stage.

Because middle adulthood is more a concept that a specific age, **middle adulthood** can refer broadly to the period from age 35 to 64. Because our society expects ever-increasing longevity and requires more years of education, the tasks of young adulthood and middle adulthood are being delayed. In 2006, the United States Census Bureau (U.S. Census Bureau) reported that more than 73 million people were between the ages of 45 and 64 (U.S. Census Bureau, 2006).

Although the age of 65 is a commonly accepted benchmark for old age, the working definition for an individual is dependent on the person's health status, functional status, mental attitude, and genetics. **Older adult** describes a wide range of physical, mental, and psychosocial status. In 2006, the U.S. Census Bureau reported that approximately 42 million people were age 65 and older (U.S. Census Bureau, 2006). The fastest-growing segment of the U.S. population is the group who are over age 85. The number of centenarians could reach 550,000 by 2040.

THEORIES OF PSYCHOSOCIAL AGING

Developmental tasks of adulthood are generally described as either a process in the development of relationships with others or as based on stereotypical life events associated with the person's age. Each theory makes a contribution to understanding aging while recognizing there are multiple patterns for adult development and successful aging.

Psychosocial Theory. The best-known theory of psychosocial development in adulthood is Erik Erikson's (1963) eight-stage theory of psychosocial development, which describes stereotypical challenges that each person must successfully balance over a lifetime. Erikson suggested that successful aging lies in achieving a coherent identity in one's life by mastering certain developmental challenges. He believed that psychosocial development is a continuous process and that delays or crises in one stage can delay or diminish the achievement of other stages. However, these delays or crises may also serve as an impetus to the next stage. Although in general these stages occur in sequence from childhood through adulthood, adult development is complicated by the idea that people may reconfront these issues as they proceed through life.

Erikson describes the psychosocial development of middle adulthood as primarily one of balancing generativity and stagnation (Figure 18-2). Within generative activity the capacity for love matures as the adult's ability to look outside oneself and care for others grows (Table 18-1). The adult also focuses on other generative activities of creativity, productivity, teaching, mentoring, writing, social activism, producing music or anything that satisfies the need to be useful to society and develop a capacity to care for others. This theory describes a process in which middle-age individuals critically evaluate the meaning of the structures they use to make sense of the world and self and transform these schemes into personal relevance. Generativity begins early in adulthood, particularly with childbearing, child rearing, and establishing a career and may well continue beyond the age of 65.

The individual must balance the feeling that life is personally satisfying and socially meaningful with the feeling that life is without meaning. Stagnation is caring for no one and being self-absorbed. To the extent that stagnation occurs, the person becomes egocentric and self-absorbed.

In Erikson's psychosocial developmental stage of ego integrity versus despair, the older adult works toward accepting responsibility for his or her life and being able to reflect on it in a positive manner. Ego integrity is the ego's accumulated assurance of its capacity for order and meaning. According to Erikson, achieving ego integrity means fully accepting oneself and coming to terms with death. Ego integrity is achieved by older adults who see themselves as having lived a productive life and having few regrets. Failure to achieve ego integrity results in feelings of hopelessness, despair, and fear of death (see Table 18-1).

Seasons of Life Theory. Levinson (1978, 1986) conceived of development as a sequence of qualitatively distinct eras or seasons (Table 18-2). Each of these eras in adult life has its own time and brings certain psychological challenges to the forefront of a person's life. Levinson's model emphasizes that development of life structures is a continuous life process. Each era is an opportunity for learning and growth.

Table 18-1 Erikson's Stages of Development for the Middle and Older Adult

STAGE	AGE	DESCRIPTION
VII	Middle adult years	• Generativity versus stagnation, which is a creative giving of the self to the world in a participatory way. Generativity is helping and guiding the next generation. • Unless such concern develops, the person focuses on self, stagnates, and commonly regresses. • Middle adults share tasks and divide necessary labor. • The primary issue is care.
VIII	65 to death	• Ego integrity versus despair. • Reflects on and accepts one's life. • Feels a sense of fulfillment about life and accepts death as an unavoidable reality. • If unable to obtain a feeling of fulfillment and completeness, will despair and fear death.

Reprinted with permission from Erikson, E. H. (1963). *Childhood and society* (2nd ed.), New York: W. W. Norton & Company, Inc.; and by permission of The Random House Group Limited, London.

Table 18-2 Levinson's Development Phases

APPROXIMATE AGE	TASKS
40 to 42	• Midlife transition. • Person realizes that earlier choices cannot fulfill all of the self and that parts of the self were repressed or dormant. At some point, life must be restructured to express more of the self. • The adult reappraises, modifies, and rediscovers important neglected parts of the self and makes choices that provide for a new life structure. There may be a sense of compromise of the dream as person searches for what he or she really wants. • There is a sense of bodily decline and a need to confront one's mortality. The person recognizes that he or she is no longer young.
43 to 46	• Restabilization. • The fullest and most creative period of life. • Time represents both the possibility for further development and a threat to the self. • Person is building and living with a first provisional life structure for middle adulthood.
47 to 59	• Stable period of fulfillment.
60 to 65	• Preparing for retirement; work no longer the central focus. More time spent pursuing personal interests, such as travel, grandchildren, community services.
65 to death	• Creates new life structure that suits person's retirement and health. Must deal with no longer being young and preparing for death.

Information from Levinson, D. J. (1978). *The seasons of a man's life.* New York: Knopf; and Levinson, D. J. (1996). *The seasons of a woman's life.* New York: Knopf.

Disengagement Theory. Cumming and Henry's disengagement theory (1961) pertains to adults past the age of 65. They proposed that in the normal course of aging, older adults gradually withdraw or disengage from social roles as a natural response to lessened capabilities and diminished interest and to societal disincentives for participation. This theory argues that it is beneficial for both the aging individual and society that such disengagement take place, to minimize the social disruption caused at an aging person's eventual death.

Disengagement does appear to happen for some older adults; for example, some happy, healthy older adults disengage when they move to retirement communities, contentedly taking to a rocking chair or pursuing other solitary, passive activities while preparing for death. However, many older adults, even after retiring, remain highly involved in the life of their communities, their children and grandchildren, and friends, and the disengagement theory does not seem applicable to them.

Activity Theory. Activity theory is diametrically opposed to disengagement theory (Havighurst, 1952). It suggests that the route to successful aging is to remain actively engaged with people and life events. Activity theory would explain the tendency of retirees to find alternative sources of activity to replace those lost when children become adults and the person separates from a place of employment. The activity may be travel, volunteer work, raising grandchildren, or paid employment.

Continuity Theory. As an extension of activity theory, continuity theory also suggests that disengagement is not universally a path to successful aging. Personality traits and coping styles do not change as a person ages, rather the process of adaptation to old age has continuity with ways the person managed past experiences, decisions, and behaviors; thus the past forms the foundation for the present behaviors. Disengagement may be the preferred style for the person who enjoyed solitary activities in his or her youth (Atchley, 1989).

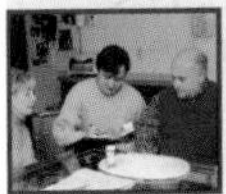

Review the opening case study, and compare Mr. Cognomi's stage of development to Levinson's developmental phases. What questions might you ask to determine if his struggle with the developmental tasks of his stage of life are affecting his health?

THEORIES OF BIOLOGICAL AGING

To the extent that successful aging means maintaining independent living, a high functional status, an active mind, and the capacity for self determination, then the physical status of the person will be an important predictor of successful aging. Both heredity and environment are necessary to explain physical changes with aging and variations in life span.

Wear-and-Tear Theory. Wear-and-tear theories have to do with the toll on the body as it reacts to internal and external stressors associated with living. The accumulation of metabolic waste products or nutrient deprivation damages deoxyribonucleic acid (DNA) synthesis, leading to molecular and eventually organ malfunction. Diet and lifestyle may be factors in the accumulation of normal injury that results in the changes of age. However, as we grow older, our body chemistry changes. The body ends up overusing and working overtime in a way it was not meant to do, accelerating the aging process. Taking vitamins and supplements to ease the overuse and overworking of your body is one way to diminish the wear and tear of aging.

As a wear-and-tear theory, the immunity theory specifically focuses on stress and the accumulated effects of illness and contaminants in our environment. As the immune system declines with age, eventually, the body loses its ability to protect itself from stress and disease, such as cancer and infections. Similarly, the rate-of-living theory assumes a fixed amount of metabolic potential for every living organism (live fast, die young).

Similarly, the neuroendocrine theory hypothesizes that reduction of neuroendocrine control of homeostasis results in age-related physiological changes. As we get older, our production of many hormones is significantly reduced. For example, growth hormone is a production of the anterior pituitary and affects everything in the body. After it is secreted, it passes from the pituitary to the liver, changing to insulin-like growth factor I (IGF-I). IGF-I goes all over the body to reverse some of the first signs and symptoms we see in aging. It affects brain cells, hair color, and even cellulite.

Free-Radical Theory. The free-radical theory of aging states that every time you consume something, you generate chemicals known as free radicals. A structure in the cell called the mitochondrion is a powerhouse to the cell. The mitochondrion generates energy and, as a by-product, gives off an oxygen ion with a negative charge that is called a free radical. These free radicals bombard the muscle cells and cause atrophy or bombard the brain cells and cause diseases like Parkinson's and Alzheimer's disease. The body fights back, refusing to just give in to the barrage of free-radical assaults. Antioxidants are one of the major weapons against free-radical aging.

Genetic Theory. Proponents of the genetic theory of aging believe that life span is determined by the genes we inherit. Aging is much more a matter of destiny; that is, our life span is in part programmed even before our birth. They believe that aging is caused by our genes or by the predictable decline in the functioning of various organ systems. The pacemaker theory of aging is based on the notion of "biological clocks," systems or processes that are set at birth to run for a specified period of time and then wind down, leading to aging and death. Genetic theories include DNA theory, error-and-fidelity theory, somatic mutation, and glycogen theory. The current evidence suggests that how we age may be 30% genetics.

FACTORS AFFECTING ADULT DEVELOPMENT

Although most scientists agree there is a maximum life span, no one really knows the limit of human life. Life expectancy in the United States has risen to 78.9 years primarily because of advances in public health, such as improved housing, sanitation, and immunizations. For those who reach the age of 65, life expectancy is longer. Today, risk factors that contribute to premature adult morbidity and mortality include high-risk lifestyle practices and other physiological, psychosocial, socioeconomic, and environmental factors.

Action Alert! Assist clients in living healthier and longer lives by avoiding behaviors that increase their risk for chronic diseases.

LIFESTYLE RISK FACTORS

Diet. In the United States, 30% of adults age 20 and older (U.S. Department of Health and Human Services [USDHHS], 2006c) are overweight. Minority populations, especially women, are affected disproportionately: nearly half of African American, Mexican American, and Native American adults are overweight.

Four of the ten leading causes of death in North America are linked to diet: heart disease, stroke, diabetes, and certain cancers, especially colorectal, endometrial, and ovarian cancer (USDHHS, 2006a). Being overweight also increases the risk of gout, gallbladder disease, hip fractures, and osteoarthritis. Obese individuals may suffer from social stigmatization, discrimination, and lowered self-esteem.

Being too thin can also raise the risk of health problems. Anorexia nervosa, loss of appetite, and similar disorders are linked to menstrual irregularities and osteoporosis in women and to a greater risk of early death in both women and men.

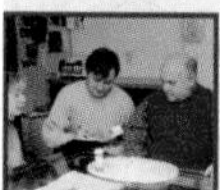
Our client, Mr. Cognomi, needs help with his diet. What do you know about the dietary patterns in the Italian culture? How could you find out more about Mr. Cognomi's pattern of eating? How can you motivate him to change?

Several factors can contribute to poor nutritional status in the older adult. They include poor oral health; use of multiple medications, which can alter the absorption of vitamins and minerals; reduced mobility; economic issues; and diminished taste and smell. Obtaining food and preparing meals can be challenging, especially for the older adult who lives alone.

Action Alert! Clients should eat a diet with plenty of grain products, vegetables, and fruits—a diet that is low in saturated fat and cholesterol, moderate in sugars, and moderate in sodium.

Exercise. Regular physical activity is associated with lower death rates for adults of any age. It decreases the risk of death from heart disease, lowers the risk of developing diabetes, and is associated with a decreased risk of colon cancer. It also helps prevent high blood pressure and helps reduce blood pressure in persons with hypertension. Physical activity is an important factor in the adult's ability to maintain health and independence. Regular exercise promotes appetite, improves mental health, and decreases stress. We probably have not fully learned the extent to which physical mobility problems with aging could be prevented by the right kind of exercise.

Rest and Sleep. Just as activity is important to the adult, it should be balanced with adequate rest. According to the National Sleep Foundation (2006), adults need 7 to 9 hours of uninterrupted, quality sleep each night for optimum health, safety, and productivity.

Age-related changes that can affect a person's ability to sleep at night include nocturia, muscle cramps, and anxiety. The length of deep restful sleep and psychologically refreshing rapid eye movement (REM) sleep may decrease with age. To improve the quality of sleep, the older person may benefit from avoiding physical exertion near bedtime, practicing effective toileting, avoiding stimulants (such as caffeine) after supper, and obtaining needed pain relief before trying to fall asleep.

Stress. Stress is the most common cause of illness in our society, and it is a major risk factor for the development of physical and psychological problems. It encompasses the negative cognitive and emotional states that result when clients feel that the demands placed on them exceed their ability to cope. It can be caused by external and internal influences. External stressors may stem from the following:

- The physical environment, such as loud noises, bright lights, excessive heat, and confined spaces
- The social environment, such as aggressiveness on the part of someone else
- The work environment, such as deadlines or "red tape"
- Major life events, such as the death of a relative, a lost job, retirement, birth of a grandchild
- Daily stressors, such as heavy traffic, an unsafe neighborhood, misplaced keys, or a flat tire

Internal stressors commonly stem from lifestyle choices, such as drinking caffeinated beverages, getting too little sleep, or overloading the daily schedule. Stress may also stem from negative self-talk, such as pessimistic thinking and self-criticism, or from stressful personality traits, such as being a workaholic.

Only if clients cannot successfully handle situations alone do you step in to help them strengthen their weaknesses so they can overcome their restrictions and draw on a lifetime of experiences to meet current challenges. Allowing clients as much participation as possible ensures the success of this strategy.

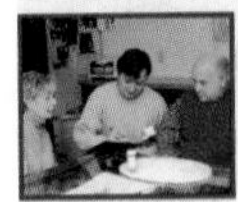

Think about Mr. Cognomi again. He has just retired from a job where he had an important position. Can you list possible stressors in his life?

Action Alert! Reduce the negative effects of stress by reducing perceived pressures, increasing coping resources, or both.

Risky Behaviors

Smoking. At least one in every five deaths in North America is related to cigarette smoking–related causes, such as lung cancer; cancer of the larynx, oral cavity, esophagus, pancreas, and urinary bladder; respiratory diseases, such as emphysema; and heart disease. Cigarette smoking is a major cause of death among Native Americans, Native Alaskans, blue-collar workers, and military personnel (CDC, 2005).

Action Alert! Help your clients prevent premature death by helping them to stop smoking.

Alcohol Abuse. The abuse of alcohol and other substances is a major health problem. Usually, it is difficult to detect alcohol abuse. Alcohol typically is metabolized more slowly in an older adult, resulting in a longer exposure time and a higher rate of tissue damage. Signs and symptoms of alcohol misuse may be similar to, or mistaken for, other clinical concerns. Often, however, alcoholism simply goes undetected by health care providers.

Adults who abuse alcohol increase their risk for hypertension, stroke, heart disease, certain cancers, accidents, violence, suicides, and overall mortality. Alcohol abuse may cause cirrhosis of the liver, inflammation of the pancreas, damage to the brain and heart, and malnutrition. It may alter the effectiveness of medicines or increase the risk of toxic reactions. Some medications may increase blood alcohol levels or increase the adverse effect of alcohol on the brain. The use and abuse of alcohol in older adults may be underrecognized. Although many people drink less alcohol as they age, others may turn to alcohol to cope with declining physical and mental function.

Action Alert! Help your client avoid drinking alcohol when taking any medications, because it can interact with medications and alter the way they are metabolized.

Illicit Drug Use. Illicit drug use and its consequences are not just a problem in teenagers and young adults. Elder drug abuse is complicated by declining physical status and interactions with both over-the-counter drugs and prescription drugs. Some reports say unrecognized drug and alcohol abuse in older adults is a hidden national epidemic.

DEVELOPMENTAL RISK FACTORS

Midlife Adults

Midlife Crisis. Some adults experience a midlife crisis, also called a midlife transition. **Midlife crisis** is a stressful life period during middle adulthood, precipitated by the review and reevaluation of one's past, including goals, priorities, and life accomplishments, during which the person experiences inner turmoil, self-doubt, and major restructuring of personality. Typically, a midlife crisis occurs in the early to middle forties, but it may not occur until the fifties.

As a group, middle-age adults are commonly called the **sandwich generation** (Figure 18-3). They are caught between the needs of adjacent generations, caring for ill or frail parents while handling the competing demands of children and employment. Their responsibilities may range from financially supporting a retired parent to taking physical care of a frail, demented, dependent parent, while at the same time caring for their own children. Depending on the family's financial situation and the type of health insurance the older adult family member has, home health care services can ease some of the middle-age adult's caregiving tasks. Individual counseling and participation in support groups can help to relieve some of the family's stress and provide encouragement in difficult times.

All generations feel the effects of this sandwiching. For example, some older adult parents may feel that they have become a burden or inconvenience to their families, but they try to help their families any way they can. The children may feel neglected by their parents and resentful or jealous of their grandparents. The middle-age adult is caught in the middle, trying to please everyone, but feels unsupported and unappreciated.

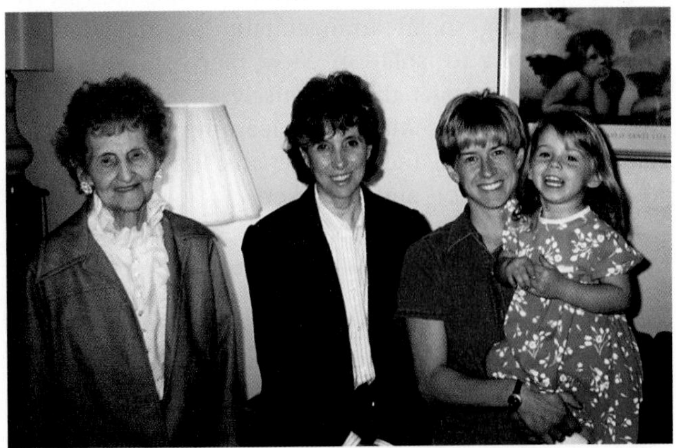

FIGURE 18-3 Middle-age adults are often "sandwiched" between the competing needs of adjacent generations.

Onset of Chronic Illness. Chronic illnesses, such as arthritis, hypertension, heart disease, and diabetes, can be major concerns for adults. An adult's level of hope, life satisfaction, and self-concept can be influenced by the adjustment to such a disease process. The goals for adults who have chronic illness are to maintain self-care, prevent complications, delay decline, and achieve the highest possible quality of life.

Older Adults

Ageism. Self-concept in the older adult is dependent on self-concept throughout life. However, it is also affected by society's image of aging. **Ageism** is a stereotype, prejudice, or discrimination against people, especially older adults, based on their age and on a very narrow definition of how a certain age-group is or lives. That definition is then used to view all members of this group as having the same characteristics, behaviors, or both.

Ageism is deeply embedded in Western culture. In a society that values youth and beauty to an obsessive degree, being old can be seen as a negative. Older adults, as they have aged, have been participants in their culture. As is true for victims of other prejudices, the effects of discriminatory thinking about being old can damage self-esteem. It is not uncommon to have ageist thinking present in older adults who are successfully adjusting to developmental changes but who see themselves as disconnected from their age cohort.

Personal Loss. For the older adult, the role of the spouse changes from earlier configurations. Although long marriage may result in a strong relationship, age-related health changes can bring new challenges for a couple. The death of a spouse is a common consequence of a long life; it is one of the most stressful passages for the older adult, causing profound loss and sense of change.

Living alone because of the death affects more women than men, both because women have a longer life span and because most men remarry. Men and women adjust to the loss of a spouse in different ways. The wife may have been in charge of monitoring her husband's care and of making social arrangements, so the widower might be prone to isolation. Most men remarry (often with women younger than themselves). For a woman, the loss of a spouse may mean learning to manage finances, less income, and home repairs. It also means the loss of a companion and caretaker.

> ***Action Alert!*** Assess the ability to cope with loss. A bereaved widow or widower who feels unable to live without the deceased spouse may be suffering from dysfunctional grieving.

Depression. About 1 in 4 women and 1 in 10 men suffer from depression at some point in life. Only about a third of these seek medical help (American Psychiatric Association, 2000; Thobaben & Buxton-Blake, 2005). Depression is a potential killer: as many as 15% of those who develop it commit suicide each year. The Centers for Disease Control and Prevention (CDC) listed suicide among the leading causes of death in the United States (USDHHS, 2005). Most researchers, however, think this number is too small.

Depression, although not a normal part of aging, is the most common problem in older adults. Older Americans are disproportionately likely to die by suicide. Constituting only 13% of the U.S. population, individuals age 65 and older accounted for 18% of all suicide deaths in 2000 (Office of Statistics and Programming, 2005). Because depression commonly coexists with medical conditions and, in particular, dementias, it can be misdiagnosed or overlooked. Also, depressive disorders may cause or contribute to medical illnesses. Rates of depression for older persons hospitalized with medical conditions such as hip fracture or heart disease is 12%, and for those living in nursing homes it ranges from 15% to 25% (USDHHS, 2005). Increasingly, findings indicate that severe depression heightens the risk of dying after a heart attack or stroke and reduces the quality of life for clients who have cancer and might reduce their survival time.

Another possible source of depression is drug therapy. The type of drug an adult may be taking, or a number of drugs taken to treat multiple problems, can contribute to depression. Several drugs taken for high blood pressure, heart disease, and insomnia are known to cause depression in some people. When assessing for depression and its causes, make sure you take a thorough drug history.

Clients who are depressed experience a great deal of functional impairment, resulting in lost work time, decreased job performance, and decreased family and social functioning. The stigmatization and misunderstanding associated with mental illness prevents many people from seeking help. Encourage clients to seek treatment for depression; effective treatment is available.

SOCIOECONOMIC RISK FACTORS

Poverty. Poverty is associated with limited access to heath care, poor nutrition, substandard housing, and inadequate prenatal care. The poverty rate in 2004 was 12.7% for whites, 24.7% for African Americans, and 21.9% for Hispanics (U.S. Census Bureau, 2004). Better-educated and more-affluent clients can afford a healthier diet, better preventive health care, and more prompt medical treatment. However, these advantages do not mean that their lifestyle practices will prevent chronic diseases and premature morbidity and mortality.

Health Insurance. Adult clients in the United States may have health insurance coverage through their employer, by private pay, or by federal or state health plans.

In 2004, 68% of the U.S. population was covered by a private health plan, which was most often related to employment. Also, more than 45.8 million people in the United States (about 15.7% of the population) were without health insurance, and 12.9% of the population was covered by Medicaid, which includes people at 125% of the poverty level (U.S. Census Bureau, 2004). Despite Medicaid coverage, the poor are less likely to be covered by health insurance. Hispanics, Native Americans, and Native Alaskans were the least likely of all racial groups to have health insurance. Among the general population between ages 18 and 64, full-time and part-time workers were more likely to be insured than nonworkers. Among the working poor, however, there was less probability of being insured than among nonworkers. The primary reason was either that the employer failed to provide health insurance or that the financial burden on employees to buy their company's plan was prohibitive.

Medicare covered 99.3% of people age 65 and over (USCB, 2004). In spite of this, health care for older adults is becoming increasingly expensive and complex. The levels of health care deductibles are increasing, making it more difficult for even employed older adults to pay them. For those not working, paying the deductibles takes a larger percentage of their income. For both groups, the rising cost and use of medications is unpredictable. Older adults who now live in poverty will have a more difficult time meeting their basic survival needs, as well as their health care needs. Increasingly, working older adults are discovering that more of their after-tax dollars are spent on health care.

Housing Safety. People who are more affluent can afford better housing than those with lower incomes. In addition, if the neighborhood around the home declines as the house and the adult age, the person's safety may suffer. Without any hope of an increase in income, however, the person may be forced to remain in that area. Older adults may be forced to stay indoors more if they fear moving about in the neighborhood. Some have begun to share housing to address the problems of aging on fixed or decreasing incomes. This can be accomplished by home sharing—renting portions of the home to other older adults who have similar needs and interests. Some older adults sell their houses and move in with family members. If the husband dies first, the wife may be forced to sell the home and move to another, cheaper location or apartment.

As adults age, they may spend more time at home because of retirement or altered health and mobility. Age-related changes and the increased amount of time spent at home make it increasingly important to ensure the safety of an older adult's environment. Often, safety can be enhanced simply by encouraging the use of health aids already in place. Your goal is to mitigate the effects of age-related changes while helping the older client maintain as much independence as possible. For example, regular battery replacement in smoke and carbon monoxide detectors will improve warning systems to support safety. Encourage the older client to wear a hearing aid and glasses, if needed, to increase sensory awareness. Ensure that the home environment is free of hazards, such as throw rugs, that contribute to falls.

Employment. In 2004, the U.S. Department of Labor's Bureau of Labor Statistics (2006) reported that 82.3% of U.S. families had at least one employed member. Both parents were employed in 61.3% of married-couple families with children under 18; the father, but not the mother, was employed in 30.9% of these families. The proportion of "traditional" families—that is, families in which the father, but not the mother, is employed—was much larger among couples with preschool children (under 6 years of age) than among families whose youngest child was 6 to 17 years old.

The U.S. Department of Labor's Bureau of Labor Statistics (2006) reported that the unemployment rate was 4.6% as of September. Among the families with unemployment, white and Hispanic families were more likely than African American families to have at least one employed member.

Work-Related Injuries and Deaths. According to the Survey of Occupational Injuries and Illnesses by the Bureau of Labor Statistics (BLS), U.S. Department of Labor, nonfatal workplace injuries and illnesses for full-time workers among private industry employers in 2005 was 4.2 million. The Census of Fatal Occupational Injuries, part of the BLS occupational safety and health statistics program, compiles a count of all fatal work injuries occurring in the United States and in 2005, 5702 fatal work injuries were recorded. Many others remain unreported. Those that often go unrecognized include musculoskeletal disorders of the upper extremity, irritant or allergic dermatitis, asthma, chronic obstructive lung disease, reproductive abnormalities, hearing loss, and cancers of the lung, skin, and bladder.

PHYSIOLOGICAL RISK FACTORS

Leading Causes of Death. The leading causes of death for adults are heart disease, cancer, cerebrovascular diseases, chronic respiratory diseases, accidents, diabetes, Alzheimer's disease, and influenza and pneumonia (USDHHS, 2006b).

> ***Action Alert!*** Living healthfully and avoiding behaviors that increase the risk of chronic disease will result in longer, healthier lives and lower health care costs.

Major Health Problems. Older adults must adapt to a number of physiological changes associated with aging

(Figure 18-4). These changes include chronic illnesses, sensory deficits, cognitive and intellectual changes, and changes in mobility. Chronic diseases account for 70% of all deaths in the United States, more than 60% of total medical care expenditures, and decreased quality of life for millions of Americans (National Center for Chronic Disease Prevention and Health Promotion, 2004).

For people in their 70s, chronic disease becomes more probable. If they have not yet had cataract surgery or a need for hearing aids, this decade carries a high likelihood that these aids will be needed. However, because cataract surgery has become relatively simple and hearing aids more effective, their lifestyle is not necessarily hampered.

Major surgery is common at this time, with such procedures as total hip and knee replacement, coronary artery bypass, and endarterectomy being used to help extend the period of active living. A change in motor coordination is noticeable, and the incidence of Alzheimer's disease and related dementias increases. For many, the 80s are associated with the giving up of driving a car, a major loss of freedom and independent living.

As people grow older, activities and the contribution to the family's general welfare, at least in terms of physical labor, gradually become more limited. Maintaining mobility and activity becomes more difficult. Major surgery is performed successfully on people in their 90s, but a decision to manage a health problem conservatively is more likely. Maintaining independent healthy living in the 90s requires the use of alternative strategies for managing the tasks of daily living, such as housekeeping, grocery shopping, cooking, and obtaining medical care.

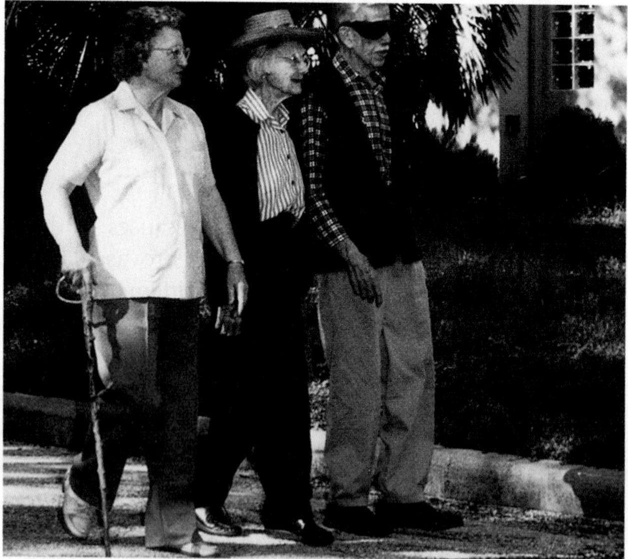

FIGURE 18-4 These older adults demonstrate some common adaptations to the physiological changes of older adulthood.

Heart Disease. High blood cholesterol is an important modifiable risk factor for coronary artery disease, which is the leading cause of death for men and women in North America. Risk factors include a family history of very high cholesterol levels, premature coronary artery disease in a first-degree relative (before age 50 in men or age 60 in women), diabetes, smoking, and hypertension. In addition, obesity and sedentary lifestyle add to the risk factor.

Hypertension. An estimated one in three Americans have high blood pressure. They are at increased risk for coronary artery disease, peripheral vascular disease, stroke, renal disease, or retinopathy. Treatment of hypertension is generally effective, although it must commonly be tailored to meet individual needs and responses.

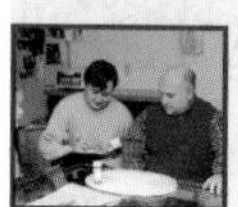

Mr. Cognomi is advised to lower his blood pressure with diet and exercise. How often would you suggest that he have his blood pressure checked?

Sensory Deficits. Visual changes with aging include a decrease in visual acuity and accommodation (the ability to focus at various distances). This loss of accommodation is called presbyopia, and it results from a loss of flexibility in the lens. Commonly, it begins to appear in 40-year-olds, when reading glasses become necessary. A variety of techniques can help you interact most effectively with an adult who has a visual or other sensory deficit (Box 18-1).

Other visual changes may occur as well. For example, older people's pupils may become less responsive to light, reducing their ability to see well in dimly lit areas or at night. They may need more light for reading and fine work. Difficulty in seeing at night can change or decrease the older adult's level of independence. If night driving becomes too challenging, for example, the person may need to make plans, or alter them, to avoid driving at night.

Action Alert! Teach your clients to position a 300-watt bulb so that it shines forward from behind their shoulder if they have difficulty reading.

Cataracts, or clouding of the lens, are a common age-related change. They can cause blurring and decreased light and color perception. Correction of this condition, the surgical removal of the clouded lens, commonly can be performed as same-day surgery. Afterward, the person may receive a lens implant or wear corrective lenses.

Glaucoma, also common in the older adult, is a degenerative disease of increasing intraocular pressure that arises when the aqueous humor is unable to drain properly from the anterior chamber of the eye. Glaucoma can lead to optic nerve damage if untreated. Yearly checks of intraocular pressure should be encouraged for all people age 40 and older, but especially for African Americans, who have a high risk for this condition. Medication commonly controls the disease process, but careful monitoring is essential for the rest of the person's life.

Loss of hearing is not a normal part of aging. However, it is not uncommon to gradually lose the ability to hear high-frequency sounds. Because of the gradual nature of this change, many older adults adapt to it without much difficulty. However, reduced hearing in older adults can also result from secretion of a drier type of cerumen than was produced when they were younger. These secretions can be more difficult to remove and, if they accumulate, can cause difficulty in hearing. Many individuals at this time have been exposed to unacceptable noise levels during their working years and are presently experiencing hearing deficits because they failed to use appropriate safety apparel.

Action Alert! Face the hearing-impaired person, and use short, direct phrases while you assess hearing acuity. The failure of an older adult to answer your questions appropriately may indicate hearing loss.

Cognitive and Intellectual Development. It has been documented that healthy older adults do not demonstrate a decline in such intellectual abilities as wisdom, judgment, and common sense. They may have a slight, gradual decline in short-term memory, calculation ability, word fluency, and abstraction, beginning at about age 60. Older adults can learn new skills, but it may be at a slower pace. Sensory deficits and lack of relevance to their daily life must be factored into the teaching plan when working with older adult clients. Cognitive performance remains difficult to predict because of the many factors that can affect cognition in the older adult.

When tests are judiciously chosen and test-taking conditions are conducive to the older adult, the results typically show that intelligence does not decrease with age. Two of the more reliable and validated tools for assessing cognitive function in the older adult are the Mini-Mental State Examination developed by Folstein, Folstein, and McHugh (1975), and the Short Portable Mental Status Questionnaire developed by Pfeiffer (1975).

Mobility Concerns. Normal aging does not necessarily limit mobility. The extent to which age-related changes affect movement is often determined by movement patterns established before entering old age. Thus remaining active throughout life is a way to maintain healthy movement in old age (Figure 18-5).

As a person ages, gait changes can result from changes in muscles and joints. Muscle strength, flexibility, stability, and cognition are factors that contribute to mobility. When illness affects any of these factors, mobility may decline and the risk of falls may rise. Hip fracture is the most common fall-related injury leading to hospitalization in older adults. Roughly

BOX 18-1 *Tips for Interacting Effectively With Adults Who Have Sensory Deficits*

The Visually Impaired Adult

- Identify yourself each time you enter the client's space.
- Tell the client when you are leaving.
- Maximize available lighting.
- Use color-contrasted toiletries and kitchen utensils as visual cues.
- Do not move objects in the client's space without permission.
- Verbally cue the client before you hand him or her an object.
- Describe objects, such as food on a plate, as if they were on a clock face, to enhance communication.
- Make sure the client's glasses are clean and positioned properly.

The Hearing-Impaired Adult

- When talking with the client, face him or her at his or her level. Make sure the area is well lit, and keep your hands away from your face.
- Eliminate as much competing noise as possible.
- Speak at a moderate speed, articulate clearly, and use short sentences.
- Pause between sentences.
- Make sure that only one person speaks at a time.
- Use creative facial and hand gestures.
- Assess the use and function of hearing aids.
- Do not shout.

Modified from Ebersole, P., Hess, P., & Schmidt, A. (2003). *Toward healthy aging: Human needs and nursing response*, St. Louis, MO: Mosby.

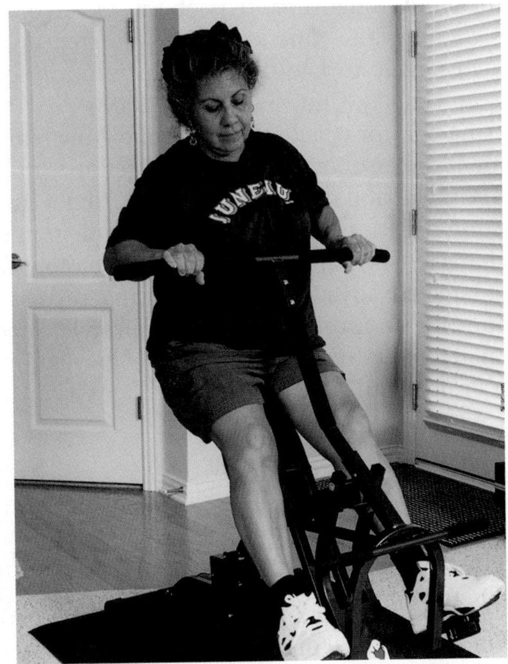

FIGURE 18-5 Remaining active throughout life is a way to maintain healthy movement in old age.

half of all persons sustaining hip fractures never regain full function; many must then walk with assistance or assistive devices. Falls are the second leading cause of injury death for adults between 65 and 84 years and the leading cause of injury death for those 85 years and older. Therefore, prevention of falls has a great influence on keeping older persons healthy. Through public health or community agencies, many communities have a falls-prevention program in place, which helps to support older adults living at home.

CULTURAL RISK FACTORS

Culture and ethnic origin are likely to be important influences on adults, especially when the person is a first-generation North American. The beliefs and norms of the group to which each client belongs have shaped ideas about health, diet, education, illness, pain, silence, symptom reporting, family support, death, health care providers, and older adults and aging. Within the context of the assessment, you need to determine the strength of the client's affiliation to an ethnic group, health practices, and beliefs about health care. Unless you incorporate these belief patterns into your care plans, you may create a conflict between your nursing interventions and your clients' cultural backgrounds.

Chronic disease has an increased impact on racial and ethnic minority groups. For example, the prevalence of diabetes among African Americans, Hispanics, Native Americans, and Native Alaskans is significantly higher than for white Americans (National Center for Chronic Disease Prevention and Health Promotion, 2004). The cancer survival rate among African Americans, American Indians, Native Alaskans, and Hawaiian Natives is lower than for white Americans. It is about 44%, compared with 59% for white Americans. This difference can be attributed largely to late diagnosis in minority groups (Clegg, Li, Hankey, Chu, & Edwards, 2002).

No single factor negatively affects the growth and development of people in racial and ethnic minority groups. Growth and development result from a complex interaction of factors, such as socioeconomic status, cultural characteristics, acculturation, stress, biological elements, targeted advertising, and varying capacities of communities to promote healthy lifestyle practices (National Center for Chronic Disease Prevention and Health Promotion, 2000).

ASSESSMENT

GENERAL ASSESSMENT OF THE WELL ADULT

Assessment of the well adult is a process of holistic assessment across all functional health patterns. Well adults are assessed for many reasons and in many settings: at a physician's office, community health clinic, nursing center, or occupational health center.

Annual or periodic assessment of the asymptomatic adult is designed to identify and reduce risk factors or to detect disease in the earliest, most treatable stage. The nature of the screening diagnostic tests depends on the risk factors present in the person. By assessing a well adult, you can help to prevent acute illness or manage chronic diseases.

Gerontologists have been concerned about the assessment of older adults because of some important differences between responses of younger and older adults. Older adults need a quiet, well-lit, and temperate environment, with no distractions. The testing environment should also be emotionally nonthreatening to reduce the client's anxiety. Before testing, it may be beneficial to both you and the older adult to have some relaxed time together to get to know one another. Under these conditions, the older adult client will be comfortable and more likely to trust you. If the client uses eyeglasses or a hearing aid, be sure these are functional before beginning.

A printed assessment form will help you be organized, and it will conserve the client's energy. Being efficient and client centered helps build trust between you and your client (Figure 18-6). The purpose of the assessment is to identify strengths and limitations so you can plan nursing interventions to optimize function and independence. For older adults, focus your assessment on function, not on the changes of aging. Structure your questions to elicit functional data. Make sure that older clients understand the purpose of the assessment; their understanding is vital to the success of your assessment. At the end of the assessment, allow time for them to ask questions and clarify any confusing aspects of your conversation.

One limitation may be long-held beliefs about health that are not longer true. Approach misconceptions with care and respect for the dignity of the individual.

Health History. The health history for the older adult should allow extra time for the client to respond. The examiner should consider that older adults may under-

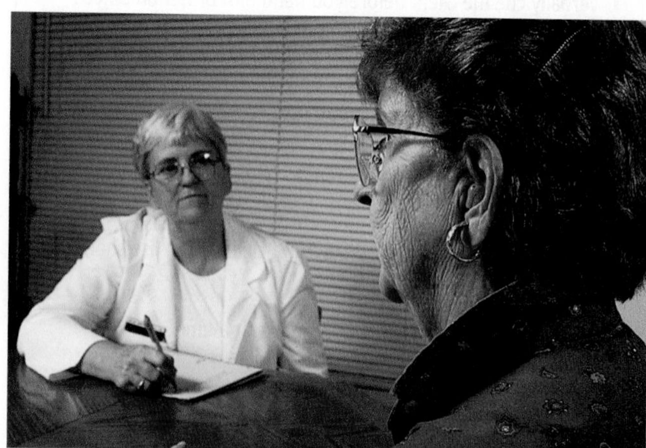

FIGURE 18-6 Establishing a trusting relationship with the client is an important component of assessing the older adult. This nurse takes the time to develop a relationship with the client before beginning the assessment.

report symptoms, thinking that their symptoms are a normal part of aging coupled with a desire to mask the physical and mental changes with age. For older adults, structure questions to gather information in a focused manner, and help them concentrate on events that might influence their current health. You can create a balance between allowing clients to talk and gathering relevant data.

The completeness of the health history is determined by clients' health status, their ability to answer your questions, and their trust in the relationship they have with you. Start by asking them to describe their health. In their opinion, is it poor, good, or excellent? Assess for past health history that is relevant to understanding their current health status. Take a history of their lifetime health-seeking behaviors. Ask how much control they believe they have over their own health. Inquire about any illnesses within the past year that have prevented them from pursuing normal activities. Ask what they do to keep healthy. Specifically mention breast or testicular self-examinations. Ask whether they use alcohol or other drugs, and how much. Ask whether they smoke, how much, and for how long. Be aware that the health history may include illnesses that are no longer prevalent, such as poliomyelitis, and treatments that are not longer done.

Medication History. Review the client's current medications, times taken, purpose, and side effects to determine the client's level of knowledge about the medication and safety in using the medications. It is best to have the client bring in the prescription bottles, so you should look at the medications in their labeled containers to confirm drug name, dosage, and times per day. Encourage clients to talk with you about their prescriptions and any over-the-counter medications they take. Also you should determine their level of understanding and beliefs about the drugs they take. Be alert to prescriptions from multiple physicians; sometimes the same medication is ordered by more than one physician or medications that are incompatible are ordered.

FUNCTIONAL ASSESSMENT

With older and disabled adults, you will need to do a functional assessment to identify their strengths and weakness in the activities of daily living (ADLs). Changes in functional status may lead you to discover cardiovascular or respiratory problems manifested as activity intolerance or dyspnea on exertion. Functional activities are those involved with eating, grooming, dressing, toileting, mobility, social interaction, and problem solving. An older adult person may stop attending social functions rather than admit to not being able to drive. Have the client describe a typical day to gain information about how physical status affects quality of life, thought processes, and physical activity. Also assess the person's ability to shop for food and prepare meals. You can use Gordon's functional health patterns as a framework to obtain the client's specific health history (see Chapter 6).

Illness may be detected by verbal and nonverbal cues. How the client says something rather than what the client says may provide a cue to depression or pain; loose-fitting clothes may be a sign of poor appetite, digestive problems, and weight loss.

Physical Examination

Techniques for Different Ages. The type of physical examination you perform for a well adult depends largely on the reason for the examination and on the age of the person. For all well adult clients, you should also assess general health and cognitive and emotional functioning. Begin by assessing their appearance. Observe their behaviors and apparent mental status. Measuring cognitive function in older adults should be done carefully because some potential problems are caused by physical needs. For example, if the older adult tires easily, it may be advantageous to perform the testing in several sittings at different times.

> **Action Alert!** Do not assume confusion is a normal part of aging. For example, confusion in an older adult can signify the presence of an infection even before body temperature changes.

Age-Related Changes. Disease is not a normal part of aging. However, as a person ages, there are gradual declines in all body systems. These changes make the person more vulnerable to disease, disability, and complications of illness, surgery, and medical treatments.

General Appearance. Skin changes, especially lines and sagging, become more pronounced in the 40s and 50s. Age spots begin in the 50s and 60s. Many of the changes in the skin are due to chronic sun exposure earlier in life. The skin becomes thin and is vulnerable to skin tears from minor assaults. Hair begins to gray and thin in the early 40s, a process that continues throughout adulthood. An adult's height begins to decline in the 30s and 40s; because of compression of disks in the spinal column, height may drop an inch during the 50s and 60s.

Vision and Hearing. During the 30s and 40s, vision and hearing begin to change. The accommodative ability of the ocular lens declines; by the 50s and 60s, it may no longer exist. Color discrimination declines as well, and most people have an increased sensitivity to glare during their 40s and 50s. Hearing begins to decline in the 30s and 40s, initially involving mostly high frequencies. By the 50s and 60s, hearing loss may include all frequencies, although it is still most pronounced at high frequencies.

Taste and Smell. The total number of taste buds declines and the sense of smell diminishes. The older adult is vulnerable to not recognizing the warnings normally received through taste and smell. Nutrition deficits may be secondary to the loss of taste and smell.

Cardiovascular Function. Age-related changes that occur in the cardiovascular system include thickening and stiffening of the heart valves, changes in the conduction system, atherosclerosis of the coronary vessels, and reduction in the force of the cardiac contraction. From a functional point of view, the cardiovascular system has a reduced ability to increase output in response to increased demand. More time is needed for the maximum heart rate to return to its resting rate. Any illness can add stress or demand that compromises cardiac function.

Respiratory Function. Age-related changes in the older adult include increased airway resistance, a decreased exchange of oxygen and carbon dioxide (caused by diminished pulmonary circulation), and decreased strength in the respiratory accessory muscles, which causes rigidity in breathing. These changes can lead to other changes:

- A decrease in vital capacity, which is the maximum amount of air that can be expired after maximal inspiration
- A decrease in residual volume, which is the volume of gas left after maximal expiration
- A decrease in functional capacity, which is the amount of air left in the lungs after normal expiration

Musculoskeletal Function. Age-related changes in bones include a loss of bone mass and density, increased bone reabsorption, and decreased calcium absorption. Height can actually diminish. As they age, muscles become smaller and have decreased numbers of muscle fibers, which presents as less muscle mass and decreased strength. Cell membrane deterioration results in a loss of fluid and potassium from cells. Slower body movements may be from diminished muscle mass and changes in the joints, as well as balance problems. To some extent, declining musculoskeletal function may be prevented or slowed through continued activity and exercise..

Gastrointestinal Function. Gastrointestinal function is strongly related to the client's nutritional status. Examination of the oral cavity may reveal changes, such as retraction of the gingivae, exposing the roots of teeth. These preventable changes can lead to degeneration of tissues around the teeth, leading to loss of teeth. Although tooth loss is not a normal part of aging, a high percentage of elders have lost their teeth or have dental problems. Determine the client's ability to swallow without choking.

Age-related gastrointestinal changes may include some atrophy and slowing of the gastrointestinal tract. The older adult is more at risk for inflammation of the gastric membrane from food or medication, which can lead to gastritis. Although highly seasoned foods may provide the taste to improve enjoyment of food, these same foods can cause indigestion and aggravate gastroesophageal reflux disease (GERD).

Bowel Function. Assessment of the abdomen may reveal loss of abdominal muscle tone, and decreased muscle tone in the colon may result in hypoactive bowel sounds. Loss of muscle tone increases the risk for constipation. Weakness of the internal anal sphincter and the presence of hemorrhoids may be a factor in controlling intestinal elimination. Assess for an abdominal mass in the left lower quadrant suggesting constipation. Diverticular disease is present in about 80% of older adults, but it often is benign. An age-related contributing factor can be a decrease in the colon's muscular strength.

Urinary Function. Keep in mind that urinary incontinence (involuntary urination) is not a normal age-related change in the older adult. There are several types of urinary incontinence. They can be identified through a good health assessment and history, including a drug history. When taking the health history, check the client's daily pattern of urinating, including amount, times, frequency, and whether incontinence occurs. If it does occur, assess precipitating factors, time of day, and presence of blood in urine. If the older adult takes a medication with diuretic effects, that could contribute to the risk of incontinence; consult with the physician who prescribed the medication.

Sexual Function. Include an assessment of the adult's sexual activity and function. Sexuality and interest in sexual intercourse do not necessarily decrease as a person ages; however, physical problems that limit sexual activity do increase. Having a relationship that meets the adult's sexual needs is important to a wellness lifestyle. Older adults may be as interested in sexual activity as they were throughout their life.

Sexual activity begins to decline in the 30s and 40s. Men experience a decrease in the quality of semen and sperm after age 40. The inability to obtain an erection can occur at any age, but it becomes more common in midlife. As basal metabolism declines in the 40s and 50s, weight increases, and muscle and bone mass decline. This process accelerates in women after menopause. **Menopause** is the stage in the female climacteric during which hormone production is reduced, the ovaries stop producing eggs, and menstruation ceases. The woman's reproductive ability has now ended. Menopause usually occurs between ages 50 and 55, although the range is from 40 to 59. After menopause, the rate of osteoporosis increases.

Diagnostic Tests. A key to wellness for the adult is appropriate screening, especially for clients in high-risk groups. You may be directly involved in screening or in teaching clients about the importance of screening tests (Table 18-3).

Coronary artery disease is the leading cause of death in the United States and Canada. Consequently, clients should be screened regularly, at least every 5 years for men between the ages of 35 and 65 and for women between 45 and 65, for elevated cholesterol level, a major modifiable risk factor for heart disease (ODPHP, 2002). If the total cholesterol level is increased, then the client should be tested for other lipid abnormalities as well.

Table 18-3 Health-Screening Guidelines for Well Adults

TEST	MIDDLE AND OLDER ADULTHOOD	COMMENTS
Body measurement	Measure height and weight periodically.	Obesity is a major public health problem.
Blood pressure	At least every 2 years for normotensive adults or annually for borderline hypertension. Others should seek the advice of a physician.	About 50 million Americans have hypertension that warrants monitoring or drug therapy.
Breast examination	Mammography and clinical breast examination every 1 to 2 years (ages 50 to 75). Breast self-examination alone is useful but not reliable.	Breast cancer is the most common type of cancer in women and the second leading cause of death.
Cholesterol level	Periodic screening for men ages 35 to 75 and women ages 45 to 75. High-risk groups should seek the advice of a physician.	High blood cholesterol is a modifiable risk factor for heart disease.
Papanicolaou test	All women who are age 18 or older or sexually active and who have a cervix should have a Pap test every 3 years.	The major risk factor for cervical cancer is sexually transmitted infection with human papillomavirus.
Prostate-specific antigen test	Annual test together with rectal examination beginning at age 50; earlier for men at high risk.	Prostate cancer is the second leading cause of cancer death in men.
Sigmoidoscopy	Every 3 to 5 years beginning at age 50 (age 40 for those with a family history of colorectal cancer, along with fecal occult blood tests, sigmoidoscopy, colonoscopy, or barium enema).	Colorectal cancer is the third leading cause of cancer death in the United States, most often among people older than age 40.
Tuberculosis	Skin testing for all persons at high risk.	Control depends on screening high-risk populations and providing preventive therapy.
Vision	Comprehensive eye and vision examination every 2 years; more often if increased risk factors present.	Control depends on screening high-risk populations and providing preventive therapy.

Based on recommendations from U.S. Department of Health and Human Services, Public Health Service, Office of Disease Prevention and Health Promotion. (1998). *Clinician's handbook of preventive services* (2nd ed.). Retrieved Jan. 18, 1998, from http://text.nlm.nih.gov/ftrs/tocview; Report of the U.S. Preventive Services Task Force. (1996). *Guide to clinical preventive services* (2nd ed.). Baltimore: Williams & Wilkins.
NOTE: Recommendations of other groups will differ. Measure height and weight periodically.

Hypertension is a risk factor for coronary artery disease, congestive heart failure, stroke, ruptured aortic aneurysm, retinopathy, and renal disease. All adults should be screened for hypertension at least every 2 years. If the diastolic reading is 85 mm Hg and the systolic reading is 140 mm Hg or below, screening every 2 years is sufficient. Hypertension is never diagnosed on the basis of a single reading.

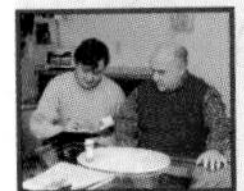

Mr. Cognomi, from our case study, was being monitored by the nurse in his primary care clinic after he was diagnosed with borderline hypertension. He is self-monitoring his blood pressure and has obtained readings of 140/90, 160/88, and 150/92 mm Hg in a single day. He says, "See, it isn't too bad for a man my age." How would you respond?

The annual incidence of breast cancer increases with age. Screening for breast cancer is recommended every 1 to 2 years for women over the age of 50. Screening includes a breast examination by a health practitioner and a mammogram. Screening in younger women is recommended when there is a family history of breast cancer, especially premenopausal breast cancer. All women should be encouraged to do breast self-examination every month.

All people older than age 50 should annually have a fecal occult blood test done for colorectal cancer, and a sigmoidoscopy every 3 to 5 years beginning at age 50 (or 40 if they have a family history of colorectal cancer). When the finding is positive, a colonoscopy may be performed. Other screening methods include a digital rectal examination and a barium enema. For people who have first-degree relatives with colorectal cancer, a more thorough screening may be recommended.

Screening for cervical cancer is recommended for all women with a cervix who are sexually active or have reached age 18, whichever comes first. A Papanicolaou test should be performed every 1 to 3 years for women with a cervix. Risk factors of multiple sex partners, an early onset of sexual intercourse, low socioeconomic status, and human immunodeficiency virus (HIV) infection suggest the need for more frequent screening.

All men should have an annual prostate-specific antigen test and an annual rectal examination beginning at age 50, or earlier if at high risk.

All adults should be screened for problem drinking of alcohol. Heavy drinking is defined as more than five drinks per day, five times per week. Medical problems due to alcoholism include hepatitis, cirrhosis of the liver, cardiomyopathy, withdrawal syndrome, mental changes, and, in older adults, a dementia observed during the last stages of severe chronic alcoholism. Heavy drinking and alcoholism (dependency) have dire social consequences as well, including suicide, divorce, depression, domestic violence, unemployment, and poverty.

All clients should be screened for tobacco use, and those who use tobacco products should be advised to quit and encouraged to develop a plan to quit. Many methods are used to help tobacco users quit the habit, but success is directly related to the person's determination to quit rather than to the method itself. Most people try more than once before actually quitting.

All clients should be assessed for their immunization status. All clients need a diphtheria-tetanus vaccination every 10 years. Adults who have not had chickenpox should receive the varicella (chickenpox) immunization. Adults 65 and older should have a pneumococcal immunization once in their lifetime and an influenza vaccination annually. Seniors should be screened for tuberculosis because of its increasing incidence and their more vulnerable status.

Vision loss is common in adults, and the prevalence increases with advancing age. Young, normal-risk adults should have a comprehensive eye and vision examination every 2 to 3 years. Middle-age and older, normal-risk adults should have such an examination every 2 years.

High-risk clients should be screened for tuberculosis. These include people who have close contact with someone known or suspected to have tuberculosis, people infected with HIV, people who inject illicit drugs, people who live or work in high-risk group settings (such as a nursing home or child care center), and people who are medically underserved. Controlling tuberculosis depends on thorough screening of high-risk populations and on providing preventive therapy.

FOCUSED ASSESSMENT FOR *READINESS FOR ENHANCED AGE-APPROPRIATE ATTAINMENT OF DEVELOPMENTAL MILESTONES*

Defining Characteristics. *Readiness for enhanced age-appropriate attainment of developmental milestones* is a wellness diagnosis for the client who expresses concerns about managing life changes such as menopause, retirement, assuming the caregiving role for a parent, physical changes with aging, children leaving the home, or making a transition to supportive living arrangements for elder care. The client may need advice about diet, exercise, sleep, or family relationships. Your assessment should include the client's perception of appropriate behavior and whether or not the behavior is causing difficulty in the person's life.

Related Factors. The diagnosis *Readiness for enhanced age-appropriate attainment of developmental milestones* assumes the client is seeking help; thus you can ask the client to identify the cause of this need for help. Related factors could include lack of knowledge, lack of motivation, ineffective coping skills, or inadequate role models.

However, the client could also have environmental or physical factors, such as a chronic illness, physical disability, or mental disability, that have prevented achievement of an adult task. In this case, the related factors would include prescribed dependence (such as protected living), or physical or mental disability (such as mental retardation or a mental illness), deficiencies of environment (such as homelessness), or inadequate caretaking.

FOCUSED ASSESSMENT FOR *INEFFECTIVE HEALTH MAINTENANCE*

A focused assessment for clients with *Ineffective health maintenance* includes looking at their ability to identify, manage, or seek help to maintain health (NANDA International, 2007). This diagnosis may be more appropriate for a person living with a chronic illness or an older adult who is no longer able to meet his or her own needs independently. Ask questions that will provide cues to the client's ability and motivation to take responsibility for his or her own health. For example, Have you engaged in a healthy lifestyle in the past? For what reasons did you seek health care in the past? Did you adopt the recommended interventions? Why or why not? Do you receive support from your family or significant other? How do family members or friends make it easy (or difficult) to maintain good health practices? To what extent do you believe that maintaining and improving health is possible? Do you need financial assistance to obtain medication?

Determine clients' needs for assistance and the level of functional independence in meeting self-care needs. Assess their level of knowledge. Assess whether clients face barriers to taking effective health actions, such as finances or health care resources.

Defining Characteristics. Evidence for *Ineffective health maintenance* in the older adult may include the following:

- Evidence of not taking medications as prescribed or a new medication regimen
- Unkempt appearance or poor personal hygiene
- Evidence of malnutrition
- Not reporting for scheduled health care visits
- Concerns reported by family members
- Reported or observed inability to take responsibility for meeting basic health practices in any or all functional pattern areas
- Demonstrated lack of adaptive behaviors to internal or external environmental changes
- Self-report of inability to maintain self-care

Related Factors. Factors related to the onset of *Ineffective health maintenance* include the following:

- Ineffective individual or family coping
- Perceptual or cognitive impairment
- Impaired gross or fine motor skills
- Lack of or significant alteration in communication skills
- Unachieved developmental tasks, such as ineffective coping with the loss of a spouse
- Lack of material resources
- Dysfunctional grieving or disabling spiritual distress
- Lack of ability to make deliberate and thoughtful judgments

DIAGNOSIS

Group the client's diagnostic cues to help determine the best nursing diagnosis, as described in Table 18-4. *Ineffective health maintenance* may be used when there are multiple problems; when there is a single problem, a more specific diagnosis is used. When the client needs to make dietary modifications, the diagnosis *Imbalanced nutrition: more than (less than) body requirements* is used. When the person needs knowledge to accomplish a change in lifestyle, the diagnosis *Deficient knowledge* is used. When the person is overwhelmed with the stress of caring for a dependent person, the diagnosis is *Caregiver role strain.* When the person is not managing an acute or chronic illness effectively, the diagnosis is *Ineffective therapeutic regimen management.* Other examples include *Ineffective coping, Disabled family coping, Complicated grieving,* and *Spiritual distress.*

PLANNING

Each plan of care must be individualized to a client's needs, age, and culture. Address the client's concerns first. Then, together with the client, develop a care plan that includes achievable short- and long-term goals designed for success. For clients at risk for *Ineffective health maintenance,* the goal is for them to demonstrate the knowledge they need to improve their health behaviors and take action to change the behavior. For example, for middle-age adults who are sedentary, the goal would be to engage regularly, preferably daily, in moderate physical activity for at least 30 minutes per day.

Some examples of expected outcomes for the well adult are the following:

- Outlines a realistic plan for increasing healthy behaviors (specify: exercise, diet, weight loss)
- Includes positive social interactions in daily schedule
- Establishes a target date for beginning a healthy behavior
- Seeks health-related information from valid sources
- Describes strategies to eliminate unhealthy behavior
- Performs activities of daily living consistent with energy and tolerance
- Makes a plan for long-term care in anticipation of declining health and self-care ability
- Demonstrates evidence of accepting the need for long-term care

Explore options with clients to help them achieve goals by changing behaviors (reducing weight, stopping tobacco use, increasing exercise, preventing unwanted pregnancy, and so on). With your assistance, clients should prioritize their goals and specify time frames for achieving them.

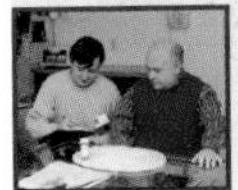

Mr. Cognomi decided that his primary goal was to start an exercise program. He thought he would feel better about himself by taking brisk walks 3 days per week after dinner. He felt he would then be able to try to stop smoking because he would have more confidence in his ability to quit. How would you respond to Mr. Cognomi? Is his plan reasonable or unrealistic?

INTERVENTION

Client interventions are based on trusting relationships. Your client relationships must be based on honesty, acceptance, respect, empathy, and cultural sensitivity. First, assess your own cultural beliefs, and become aware of regional, ethnic, and religious beliefs as well as of practices

Table 18-4 Clustering Data to Make a Nursing Diagnosis

High-Risk Lifestyle Choices

DATA CLUSTER	DIAGNOSIS
A 52-year-old male client smokes two packs of cigarettes daily. He has not exercised regularly since he was in college, and he cannot remember when he last had a physical examination.	*Ineffective health maintenance* related to lifestyle/habits
A 64-year-old female client has had three consecutive blood pressure readings above 140/90 mm Hg. She says she feels fine and finds it hard to believe that anything is wrong.	*Deficient knowledge regarding causes of hypertension* related to perception
A 36-year-old male client, 5 feet 10 inches in height, weighs 237 pounds. He reports eating fast food every day for breakfast and lunch. He says that he eats fresh vegetables and fruits about three times a week.	*Imbalanced nutrition: more than body requirements* related to lifestyle management

of groups in the area where you work. This aids you in the development of culturally specific interventions. Your interventions are to help clients improve their quality of life, maintain function, and delay or prevent age-related conditions.

The selection of interventions will depend on clients' cognitive and perceptual abilities, as well as on the level of gross and fine motor skills needed to engage in health maintenance behaviors. If they are forgetful, they may need strategies to remind them about medications, meals, or exercise. Their communication skills (written, verbal, or gestural) are important in selecting health maintenance strategies.

EDUCATING FOR LIFESTYLE CHANGES

To maximize compliance when teaching to change lifestyle choices, give specific, informational instructions. Fully explaining the regimen and its rationale, demonstrating it clearly, and writing down the instructions will enhance behavior change. Providing clients with written pictorial material for them to keep and review reinforces the teaching session and will build on their ability to retain information (visually and auditory). For example, explain the purposes and expected effects of the interventions you recommend to the clients, and tell them when to expect these effects. This is especially important if the benefits of an intervention will not be immediate (e.g., the benefits of a regular exercise program may not be apparent for some clients for several months). Otherwise, clients may become discouraged and abandon the intervention.

Suggest small changes rather than large ones. Ask clients to do only slightly more than they are already doing. By achieving a small goal, clients initiate a positive change that will encourage them to continue; this helps to avoid noncompliance.

Successful persuasion involves not only increasing clients' belief in their capacities but also structuring interventions so that they are likely to be successful. Sometimes, rather than eliminating established behaviors, it is better to add new ones. For example, it might be better to suggest to overweight clients that they add exercise to their day rather than that they eat less. Also, link clients' new behaviors with old ones. For example, if clients forget to take their daily medication, you might suggest that they take their medication in the morning while brushing their teeth.

Finally, use a combination of strategies to help educate clients, such as oral and written instructions, audiovisual aids, individual and group counseling, and community resources. Multiple techniques are more likely to foster success than single strategies. Refer clients to community agencies, voluntary health organizations (such as the American Heart Association), instructional references (such as books, videotapes, or the Internet), or to support groups for clients with similar problems. Nursing interventions that can help homebound adults include connecting them with community services that can provide transportation to shopping areas, or with agencies that deliver prepared meals, such as Meals on Wheels.

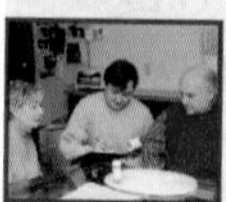

If Mr. Cognomi succeeds in taking brisk walks three times a week for a month but makes no other changes, he is not likely to lose much weight. However, he may have achieved other benefits. Can you think of any?

Once clients fully understand the intervention, ask them for a specific commitment. Ask them to describe specifically what they plan to achieve. Doing this encourages them to begin thinking about how to integrate a new behavior into their daily schedule.

Also, ask clients if they are willing to carry out the commitment. Clients with a high degree of certainty are more likely to follow through. If your clients express uncertainty, you can explore the problems that they might be encountering in carrying out the regimen.

Diet. Nutritional assessments ascertain whether adults, particularly older adults, are able to obtain and prepare food and whether they consume adequate protein, calories, minerals, and vitamins. For adults, cultural influence on diet usually does not change with aging. Older adults who have followed dietary laws throughout their lives will continue to choose foods according to that diet. Decrease in taste and smell can reduce appetite. In addition, decreased income, difficulty getting to the market, and decreased mobility can affect an adult's eating habits. Once the clients' concerns and an understanding of their issues are apparent, you can appropriately focus your teaching.

Exercise. An appropriate exercise program for adult clients should take into consideration their current level of mobility, which is determined by careful assessment. Even chair-bound older adults can do range-of-motion exercises. Adults who are more mobile can benefit from more advanced exercise programs that have been adapted to their needs. They should engage regularly, preferably daily, in moderate physical activity for at least 30 minutes. Tai chi is an effective exercise for cardiovascular fitness.

Rest and Sleep. Clients and their family members should keep a regular sleep schedule, which means going to bed and getting up at the same time each day, even on weekends. Encourage clients to make their bedroom conducive to sleep, such as cool, quiet, and dark. It is better if they read or watch television in another room. Encourage clients to engage in a relaxing, nonstimulating activity at bedtime such as reading or listening to music. A warm bath or hot tub may promote sleep. Encourage clients not to bring their problems to bed and to avoid eating and drinking before bedtime (National Sleep Foundation, 2006).

Stress. Because stress is associated with increased disease susceptibility, stress management is an important component of health promotion activities. Daily stressors are associated more with health problems than are stressful life events because they result in a high level of stress being maintained over a long period.

Estate planning can be a source of stress for an older person who has spent a lifetime accumulating wealth or possessions and feels that it is important to leave something of value to others. It is important to be remembered, and, if the amount of money or property is small, it is important that it not have to go to pay for lawyers and court costs. Planning and making advance arrangements for burial or cremation, and so on, is another important topic.

The threat of an illness that results in hospitalization is a source of stress. Hospitalization is disruptive and frightening, and it has the potential to significantly reduce any savings that may have been accumulated. Even though private health insurance, Medicare, and supplemental health insurance pay a significant portion of medical expenses, hospitalization is expensive. Perhaps the greatest source of stress associated with hospitalization is the vulnerability to death or the loss of independence. Hospitalization for a fractured hip is particularly frightening, because most older adults know someone who sustained a fracture and had to enter a nursing home. The concept of loss of independence is a threat, and nursing homes are associated with death in their thoughts.

Exercise can be successfully used not only to maintain activity but also to decrease stress. Physical activity is an important factor in the adult's ability to maintain health and independence. Regular exercise promotes appetite, mental health, and balance. Many adults soon realize the benefits of a program of activity and exercise because of their change in energy level.

For older adults who live alone or even with another person, loneliness can be a problem. Supportive relationships and friendships are critical to well-being. Developing support systems can be a beneficial effect of health promotion groups.

Action Alert! Talking only of failures in life is a sign of possible despair.

Home Safety. Collaboratively, you, the client, and the client's family can increase home safety, often without much cost, through environment assessment. Teaching adults to use their spaces wisely is often all it takes for them to focus on current needs and age-related changes. Controlling clutter, using available lights, and repositioning electrical cords may be a change from how they are used to thinking about moving through their space, and it can be the start of placing a higher value on safety. The client might need teaching about the use of nonslip shoes and slippers, as well as the importance of protecting the feet by wearing shoes.

EDUCATING FOR HEALTH MANAGEMENT

Medication Management. Many of the nursing interventions for adults involve education about medications. At home, adults need to be assessed by the home health care nurse regarding their understanding about their drug regimen and compliance with it. After performing an assessment, you must educate clients about any misconceptions they might have about prescribed medications. Teach them about the interactions of prescribed drugs and about the effects of taking them concurrently with over-the-counter drugs. Teach clients how to avoid medication errors and interactions, as outlined in Box 18-2.

Teach clients to drink plenty of fluids when taking medications. Explain that with aging, there is decreased absorption, and it takes longer for drugs to take effect. In addition, kidney function decreases, so drugs take longer to leave the body. In addition, because albumin (protein) levels are decreased, there is less protein for drugs to bind to, so there may be more of the drug floating in the blood, which may lead to drug toxicity.

Instruct adults to carry a complete list of all the medications they are taking (both prescription and over-the-counter), so that all health care providers stay informed about the medication regimen. Work with them to monitor their medications and, when possible, help them to use the least amount for the greatest effect. This takes effective communication between you, the client, the client's family, and the client's physician.

Make sure clients are aware of their allergies and that they communicate this information to all health care providers. When you care for a client in a short- or long-term facility, you will work together with pharmacists, physicians, and the other members of the multidisciplinary team to identify interactions, adverse reactions, and duplication of drug effects. If there is a possibility that clients will experience side effects from an intervention, such as those of medication for depression, tell the clients what to expect and under what circumstances they should stop the intervention and consult a health care provider.

The presence and use of support systems is directly related to the success of health maintenance activities. For the well older adult, belonging to a group of senior citizens who are experiencing similar problems in maintaining health can be a major source of support.

Health Maintenance Visits. Plan with clients for regular visits with a primary health care provider for screening and evaluation, including vision checks, physicals, immunizations, and foot care. Teaching clients to arrange annual checkups and immunizations at the same time yearly helps them remember their immunizations. Consistent scheduling helps clients arrange appointments in advance, making it possible for

BOX 18-2 *Teaching for Wellness*

Helping an Adult Maintain Health

Purpose: To maintain a healthy lifestyle.
Expected Outcome: The client will maintain his or her present level of functioning.

Client Instructions

Your client can do many things to maintain his or her health well into old age. You can help him or her by offering these suggestions:

- Maintain your social relationships. Use the telephone to call your family and friends. Attend family functions, church, activities, and senior citizen events in your community.
- Exercise every day. Walking is one of the best exercises. Wear sturdy shoes, and work up to walking three to four times a week for 20 minutes each time.
- Relax. Take deep breaths, and practice relaxation exercises. Visualize a peaceful outdoor scene or a happy family event. Decrease stressors in your life, and share problems with a trusted person, such as your clergy.
- Eat sensibly. Eat from the five food groups. It may be easier—and better—to eat six small meals and one or two snacks than three meals each day. Drink plenty of fluids, especially water.
- Stop smoking. Do not be afraid to seek help, such as a smoking cessation class or a nicotine replacement plan, to help reduce the need for smoking. See your physician for help.
- Sleep well at night. To do so, try not to nap in the late afternoon or evening. Do not eat right before bed. Limit fluids in the evening hours to reduce the need to urinate during the night. If you wake up at night and do not fall back to sleep right away, get up and read or watch television until you become sleepy.
- Avoid constipation. Eat fruits and vegetables, drink fluids, and maintain a walking program, if possible. A stool softener, if suggested by your physician, can help with gentle elimination of stool.
- Maintain a comfortable environment. Use your heating and cooling system for adequate warmth in winter and a cool environment in very hot, humid weather.
- Practice health maintenance. Take medication as ordered. Schedule and keep appointments with your physician. Comply with suggested standards for screening tests, flu shots, and so on. Be alert to changes in your body, and seek help from your health care provider as soon as possible.

them to take advantage of support services provided by the community; this in turn improves client compliance in keeping appointments.

Counseling for Risky Behaviors. Research suggests that clients have only a few important beliefs about any one subject. To persuade clients to change their behavior, it is first necessary to identify their beliefs that are relevant to the high-risk behavior and to provide information based on this foundation. Counseling is used to help clients with problems related to illicit drugs and alcohol abuse, smoking, personal loss, and stress.

Changing a client's high-risk behaviors involves more than giving information. Knowledge is necessary but not sufficient to change health behaviors. One set of interventions is not effective for all clients; you will need to adapt your teaching and recommendations to each client's perceptions of health and ability to change. The best way to improve clients' health status and health behavior is by enhancing their self-efficacy (that is, their conviction that they can carry out a recommended action).

Use the power of your profession. Research studies have indicated that your individual attention and feedback to the client are more useful than news media or other communication media in changing the client's knowledge and behavior. Most clients respect nurses and believe that what you say is important. However, some clients lack confidence in their ability to make lifestyle changes. Be empathic and supportive while providing firm, definite recommendations for changing high-risk behaviors. For example, you can say, "I want you to quit smoking." The message is simple and specific. You also need to monitor the client's progress through follow-up contact, either by appointment or telephone call, within a few weeks to evaluate progress, reinforce successes, and identify and respond to problems.

Many barriers exist to making a change in unhealthy lifestyle behaviors. The client may feel unwilling to take responsibility for accomplishing day-to-day preventive behaviors for many reasons. Such unwillingness may result from lack of motivation, lack of readiness, inadequate health care teaching, lack of support, and lack of financial resources.

In clinics and other health care settings, barriers to implementing a preventive health program include an emphasis on curing illness and injury rather than prevention. You or your agency may not have an adequate system for tracking, monitoring, and following up on a client's progress. Your clients may lack health insurance, or their insurance may not pay for preventive services.

Other barriers may be related to you and other health care providers. You may lack training in preventive health services, or you may be confused over conflicting recommendations for adult health screening tests, personal beliefs, values, and assumptions. You may not have confidence that prevention interventions work. In addition, you may lack time in the face of competing demands to do follow-up care with essentially well adults.

LONG-TERM CARE

Long-term care is a broad spectrum of nursing, medical, and other services for clients with functional limitations resulting from a chronic illness or condition that is expected to be ongoing. It is designed for the client who is not capable of independent living.

If clients have periods of confusion, totally independent living may not be possible. The lack of ability to make deliberate and thoughtful judgments is a determining factor for independent living. Clients may need to be referred for long-term care services. The types of services available in most communities include assisted living, adult day care, respite care, home care, subacute care/rehabilitation, and nursing home care.

CARE AND LIVING ARRANGEMENTS

Independent Living. Most older adults prefer independent living in their own home or relocating to a retirement community or assisted living apartment where they can maintain independence for an extended period. Retirement communities and assisted living apartments may have contracted services available that provide support to extend the period of independent living. Assisted living apartments generally provide one to three meals a day, activities, and transportation for medical appointments and may have onsite health care services. Other elders maintain residence in their own homes with support provided by families.

Continuing Care Retirement Communities. These housing communities have different levels of care based on residents' needs. Where a person lives depends on the level of care needed. In the same community, there may be individual homes or apartments for residents who still live on their own, an assisted living facility for people who need some help with daily care, and a nursing home for those who require higher levels of care. Residents move from one level of care to another based on their needs but still stay in the continuing care retirement community.

Community Care. In addition to family support, older adults may turn to community support services to maintain living in their own home or in the home of a family member who is employed. In some cases these services are provided by volunteers, but they may be provided on a sliding scale fee for service. Such services include Meals on Wheels, transportation services, personal care, chore services, adult day care, telephone reassurance, and a variety of activities in senior centers. The local Area Agency on Aging often coordinates such services.

Home Care. Home care is provided by home care agencies. Help is available for a fee for medication administration, medical treatments, physical therapy, and occupational therapy and with activities such as laundry, bathing, dressing, cooking, and cleaning. Some home care can only be given by licensed health care workers, such as skilled nursing care and certain other health care services that are provided in the home for the treatment of an illness or injury. Insurance or Medicare may pay for some services for a limited time when the elder is recovering from an illness. Home care could also include medical equipment, hospice, respite care, and even home repair and modification.

Home Modifications to Support Caregiving. The National Resource Center on Supportive Housing and Home Modification received a grant award from the Administration on Aging, U.S. Department of Health and Human Services, as part of the National Family Caregiver Support Program. This grant makes funds available to modify a home to assist in caregiving. Modifications may include such items as a ramp for wheel chair access, roll-in showers, and widened doorways. An in-law apartment is a separate housing arrangement within a single-family home or on the lot. It may also be referred to as a second unit, accessory apartment, or accessory dwelling unit. An in-law apartment is a complete living space and includes a private kitchen and bath.

Housing for Aging and Disabled Individuals. The federal government and most states have programs that help pay for housing for older adults with low or moderate incomes. Some of these housing programs also offer help with meals and other activities such as housekeeping, shopping, and doing the laundry. Residents usually live in their own apartments in the complex.

Board and Care Homes. A board and care home or group home is a group living arrangement that provides help with activities of daily living such as eating, bathing, and using the bathroom for people who cannot live on their own but do not need nursing home services. Insurance or Medicaid may provide some services in these homes.

Nursing Homes. Nursing homes are the traditional long-term care for older adults. Originally nursing homes were operated more like a hospital than a residence for older adults. They usually have semiprivate rooms, often equipped with a hospital bed, a nightstand, and a small closet. Nursing homes provide a wide range of personal care and health services. For most people, this care generally is to assist people with support services such as dressing, bathing, and using the bathroom, for people who cannot take care of themselves due to physical, emotional, or mental problems. Care in a nursing home may be skilled care provided by Medicare or private insurance for recovery from an acute illness or custodial care that is either private pay or Medicaid supported.

Subacute Care/Rehabilitation. Subacute care is inpatient care designed for adults who have an acute illness, injury, or exacerbation of a disease process. The client is well enough not to need the intensive monitoring and medical care of a hospital setting (the acute crisis has been resolved) but has ongoing medical and nursing needs for an unstable condition, such as regulation of blood pressure medications, improving nutritional status, or monitoring of oxygen therapy. Physical and occupational therapy are begun in a subacute care setting. Rehabilitation provides occupational and physical therapy for people who are physically able to participate in an intensive therapy program with a reasonable chance of improving their functional status.

EVALUATION

Evaluation is a systematic, ongoing process of evaluating the client's progress toward the attainment of goals, as suggested in the nursing care plan (Box 18-3). Before evaluating altered development in the adult, you need to have set long-term goals that are in keeping with the client's abilities and lifestyle. Also, the expected outcomes that you have chosen need to let the client experience progress toward the long-term goals. Clients and their families, when appropriate, should be involved in the process. The older adult client who needs support and assistance requires some special considerations. The need for safety must be balanced with meeting the need for independence, self-determination, and the personal wishes of the client. You should consider the following factors in the care of older adults:

- The client maintains the maximum level of independence that is possible with the presenting physical and mental limitations.

BOX 18-3

Nursing Care Plan

An Older Adult With Hypertension

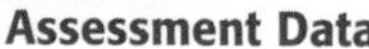

Assessment Data

After performing an assessment, the nurse records the following report: *"Mr. Cognomi is a 70-year-old obese Italian American man who is married with two adult children and three grandchildren. He recently retired from a job as a chief accountant at a large insurance company. He has a history of adult-onset diabetes and mild hypertension. He smokes two packs of cigarettes per day, eats a diet high in fat, and has not exercised for 'years.' 'I don't many eat fruits and vegetables. I just never liked them.' Mr. Cognomi states he does not understand why he has high blood pressure and that he is not feeling bad. He knows he should lose a little weight and get some exercise. He knows that smoking is not good for him, but he has been unable to quit in the past. BP is 148/96. Height is 5 feet 10 inches, and weight is 227 pounds."*

Nursing Orders

Health teaching about hypertension, low-salt diet, and weight reduction
Recommendations for smoking cessation and exercise
Follow-up appointment in 1 month
Refer to private physician for follow-up care

NANDA-I Nursing Diagnosis	NOC Expected Outcomes With Indicators	NIC Interventions With Selected Activities	Selected Evaluation Data
Ineffective Health Maintenance	***Health Promoting Behaviors***	***Counseling***	
Related Factors: • Wt 227 lb • Ht 5 ft 10 in. • BP 148/96 • Smokes 2 packs cigarettes/day • 0 fruits/vegetables	• Client will have appropriate screenings and immunizations done within the next 6 months.	• Review appropriate screening tests and immunizations for client's age-group.	• Client has scheduled an appointment for a physical examination with his private physician.
	• Client will eliminate high-risk behaviors within 1 year.	• Counsel client on recognizing high-risk behaviors and understanding their connection to chronic illness.	• Client can describe connection between smoking, high-fat diet, lack of exercise, and hypertension, heart disease, cancers, and other chronic diseases.
	• Client will be knowledgeable about health promotion activities within 1 month and begin an exercise program.	• Review Mr. Cognomi's eating habits, including who cooks and how the food is prepared.	• Has scheduled an appointment at a gym for an evaluation.

Critical Thinking Questions

1. How might the family affect Mr. Cognomi's compliance with the treatment regimen?
2. What other resources might be useful for him?
3. What approach would you use to help Mr. Cognomi stop smoking?
4. How is smoking related to Mr. Cognomi's hypertension?

Nursing outcome and intervention labels from Johnson, M., Bulechek, G., Butcher, H., Dochterman, J. M., Maas, M., Moorhead, S., et al. (Eds.). (2006). *NANDA, NOC, and NIC linkages: Nursing diagnoses, outcomes, & interventions.* St. Louis, MO: Mosby.

- The client controls the decision-making process.
- The client feels respected and understood.
- Care is provided with respect to cultural and personal values.
- The client is safe within the environment of care.

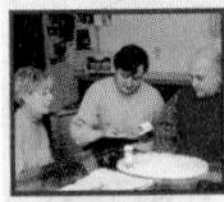

The nurse in Mr. Cognomi's primary care clinic calls him 1 week after his appointment and records the following evaluation information in his chart.

SAMPLE DOCUMENTATION NOTE FOR MR. COGNOMI

Reports that he has reduced his smoking to one pack a day for the week since his visit. Walked three times this week. His wife wants him to go with her to a nutrition class, but he is not sure about that.

▼ KEY PRINCIPLES

- The developmental tasks of adults are partially related to age but are influenced by genetics, socioeconomic status, ethnic group, religious faith, and social expectations.
- Biological development in the adult includes periods of stability and decline.
- Erikson's stages of psychosocial development of the adult are centered around developing adult relationships, contributing to society, and developing satisfaction.
- Lifestyle risk factors for the adult are poor diet, lack of exercise, inadequate rest and sleep, stress, and engaging in risky behaviors.
- Each psychosocial stage of adulthood is associated with choices that can lead to health problems.
- Socioeconomic factors create risk for illness and injury at any developmental stage.
- The risk for illness increases with physical decline and is related to lifestyle choices.
- Assessment of the well adult is a process of holistic assessment of all functional health patterns.
- Cognitive function should be assessed carefully, in an environment that supports maximum function, using tools that are specifically designed for accuracy with older adults.
- Medication history is a part of health assessment.
- Problems of adult development are diagnosed as *Delayed growth and development* or a more specific diagnosis to address individual problems.
- Planning for the well adult is centered on the goals of maintaining health and preventing illness.
- Intervening with well adults to enable them to maintain health requires education for change in lifestyle and education for health management.

■ REVIEW QUESTIONS

1. Which of the following data would be representative of a theory of aging based on developmental tasks? (Select all that apply.)

1. A 67-year-old woman volunteers for assisting school-age children with reading.
2. A 70-year-old man talks to his son about his satisfaction in his career in advertising.
3. An 80-year-old woman talks to a nurse about her regret for not having children.
4. A 65-year-old man is experiencing severe depression as the day of retirement approaches.

2. Which of the following should be part of routine screening in older adults based on common risk factors in this age-group? Select all that apply.

1. Depression secondary to being in the sandwich generation
2. Cancer
3. Heart disease
4. Acquired immunodeficiency syndrome (AIDS)

3. Which of the following would be most likely to be effective in teaching an older adult about managing a new diet?

1. Give the person a book to read, and allow privacy for reading.
2. Give small amounts of information at a time, and teach over multiple sessions.
3. Teach the content at a sixth-grade level.
4. Find a family member, and present the information to the family.

4. A 90-year-old woman is not able to shop for groceries and cook her own meals. She is fully ambulatory, enjoys socializing with friends, can take her own medicines if the pills are in boxes labeled by the days of the week, and enjoys solitary activities of reading and watching television, but she feels unsafe getting into the bathtub by herself. Which type of housing would you recommend for her?

1. Assisted living with medication and bathing support
2. Home health care weekly for physical therapy and medication monitoring
3. Nursing home care
4. Community-based day care

5. A 75-year-old fell in her home and fractured her hip. She is ready for discharge from the hospital but can only take a few steps with a walker. She is mentally alert, has no other medical problems, and expects to return to her own home with the support of her daughter. Which of the following would be most appropriate for her discharge plan?

1. A subacute care unit in the hospital
2. An inpatient rehabilitation unit
3. A nursing home
4. Her own home

Bibliography

*American Psychiatric Association. (2000). *Diagnostic and statistical manual of mental disorders* (DSM-IV-TR). (4th ed), Text Revision. Washington, D.C.: Author.

*Atchley, R. C. (1989). A continuity theory of normal aging. *The Gerontologist, 29*(2): 183-190.

Averill, J. B. (2005). Multicultural aging. Studies of rural elderly individuals: Merging critical ethnography with community-based action research. *Journal of Gerontological Nursing, 31*(12), 11-88.

Bauer, J. (Ed.). (2005). Clinical highlights. Few elderly patients have their BP under control. *RN, 68*(11), 24.

Bauer, J. (Ed.). (2005). Clinical highlights. For the elderly, flu vaccine isn't all it's cracked up to be. *RN, 68*(12), 24, 26.

Butcher, H. K., & McGonigal-Kenney, M. (2005). Depression & dispiritedness in later life: a 'gray drizzle of horror' isn't inevitable. *American Journal of Nursing, 105*(12), 52-62.

Centers for Disease Control and Prevention, National Center for Chronic Disease Prevention and Health Promotion. (2004). *Tobacco-related mortality fact sheet.* Retrieved October 28, 2006, from http://www.cdc.gov/tobacco/factsheets/Tobacco_Related_Mortality_factsheet.htm.

*Clegg, L. X., Li, F. P., Hankey, B. F., Chu, K., & Edwards, B. K. (2002). Cancer survival among US whites and minorities. *Archives of Internal Medicine, 162*:1985-1993.

Cresci, M. K. (2005). Home health care: Older adults living in the community: Issues in home safety. *Geriatric Nursing, 26*(5), 282-286.

Cumming, E., & Henry, W. E. (1961). *Growing old: The process of disengagement.* New York: Basic Books.

Danilova, V. (2005). Serving nutrition education through Meals on Wheels Program. *Nursingmatters, 16*(10), 18-19.

Dolansky, M. A., Moore, S. M., & Visovsky, C. (2006). Older adults' views of cardiac rehabilitation programs: Is it time to reinvent? *Journal of Gerontological Nursing, 32*(2), 37-44.

Dulak, S. B. (2005). Consult stat: Screen older drivers to evaluate their risk for an accident. *RN, 68*(11), 65.

*Erikson, E. (1963). *Childhood and society* (2nd ed.). Revised and enlarged. New York: W. W. Norton & Co.

*Erikson, E. H. (1982). *The life cycle completed.* New York: Norton.

Fakouri, C., & Lyon, B. (2005). Perceived health and life satisfaction among older adults: The effects of worry and personal variables. *Journal of Gerontological Nursing, 31*(10), 17-24.

Flowers, L. (2006). Are your elderly patients safe to go home? *OR Manager, 22*(1), 21, 23, 25.

*Folstein, M. F., & Folstein, S. E. (1975). Mini-Mental State: A practical method for grading the cognitive state of patients for the clinician, *Journal of Psychiatric Research, 12*:189-198.

Furman, E. F. (2006). Undernutrition in older adults across the continuum of care: Nutritional assessments, barriers, and interventions. *Journal of Gerontological Nursing, 32*(1), 22-27.

Johnson, M., Bulechek, G., Butcher, H., Dochterman, J. M., Maas, M., Moorhead, S., et al. (Eds.). (2006). *NANDA, NOC, and NIC linkages: Nursing diagnoses, outcomes, & interventions.* St. Louis, MO: Mosby.

*Levinson, D. J. (1978). *The seasons of a man's life.* New York: Knopf.

*Levinson, D. J. (1996). *The seasons of a woman's life.* New York: Knopf.

Litwack, K. Healthier aging: caring for older adults. Adjusting postsurgical care for older patients. *Nursing, 36*(1), 66-67.

NANDA International. (2007). *Nursing diagnoses: Definitions and Classification,* 2006-2007. Philadelphia: Author.

National Center for Chronic Disease Prevention and Health Promotion (U.S. Department of Health and Human Services, Public Health Services, Centers for Disease Control and Prevention). (2004). *The burden of chronic diseases and their risk factors.* Available from http://www.cdc.gov/nccdphp/burdenbook2004/pdf/burden_book2004.pdf.

National Sleep Foundation. (2006). *Sleep myths—fact or fiction.* Available from http://www.sleepfoundation.org/quiz/quiz.php?id=6.

Office of Statistics and Programming, National Center for Injury Prevention and Control, Centers for Disease Control and Prevention. (2005). Web-based Injury Statistics Query and Reporting System (WISQARS): http://www.cdc.gov/ncipc/wisqars/default.htm.

Pfeiffer, E. (1975). A short portable mental status questionnaire for the assessment of brain deficits in elderly patients. *Journal of the American Geriatric Society, 23,* 433-441.

Thobaben, M., & Buxton-Blake, P. (2005). *Honor society of Sigma Theta Tau international nursing's online case studies for nursing: Ms. Florence Luke's road to recovery from a major depressive episode—Case Study LB0003.* Available from http://www.nursingsociety.org/education/case_studies/cases/LB0003.html#issues.

Troxel, D. (2005). The last great frontier in long-term care: Let's get our elders outside. *Alzheimer's Care Quarterly, 6*(4), 332-334.

U.S. Census Bureau (U.S. Department of Commerce). (2004). *Health insurance coverage: 2004.* Available from http://www.census.gov/prod/2005pubs/p60-229.pdf.

U.S. Census Bureau, Population Division. (2006). *Table 2: Annual Estimates of the Population by Selected Age Groups and Sex for the United States: April 1, 2000 to July 1, 2005* (NC-EST2005-02). Retrieved October 28, 2006, from http://www.census.gov/popest/national/asrh/NC-EST2005/NC-ET2005-02.xls.

U.S. Department of Health and Human Services. (2005). *Healthy People 2010: Understanding and improving health* (2nd ed.). Washington, DC: U.S. Government Printing Office.

U.S. Department of Health and Human Services (Public Health Services, Centers for Disease Control and Prevention). (2005). *Suicide.* Available from http://www.cdc.gov/nchs/fastats/suicide.htm.

U.S. Department of Health and Human Services (Centers for Disease Control and Prevention: National Center for Health Statistics). (2006a). *Deaths: Preliminary data for 2004.* Retrieved October 26, 2006, from http://www.cdc.gov/nchs/products/pubs/pubd/hestats/prelimdeaths04/preliminarydeaths04.htm.

U.S. Department of Health and Human Services (Centers for Disease Control and Prevention: National Center for Health Statistics). (2006b). *Deaths/mortality.* Retrieved October 27, 2006, from http://www.cdc.gov/nchs/fastats/deaths.htm.

U.S. Department of Health and Human Services (Centers for Disease Control and Prevention). (2006c). Overweight and Obesity: Frequently Asked Questions (FAQs). Retrieved October 22, 2006, from http://www.cdc.gov/nccdphp/dnpa/obesity/faq.htm.

U.S. Department of Labor, Bureau of Labor Statistics. (2006a). *Employment characteristics of families summary.* Available from http://stats.bls.gov/news.release/famee.nr0.htm

U.S. Department of Labor (U.S. Bureau of Labor Statistics, Division of Labor Force Statistics). (2006a). *Labor force statistics from the current population survey.* Retrieved October 26, 2006, from http://www.bls.gov/cps/.

U.S. Department of Labor (U.S. Bureau of Labor Statistics, Divison of Labor Force Statistics). (2006c). *National census of fatal occupational injuries in 2005.* Retrieved October 27, 2006, from http://www.bls.gov/news.release/osh.nr0.htm.

U.S. Department of Labor (U.S. Bureau of Labor Statistics, Division of Labor Force Statistics). (2006d). *Workplace injury and illness summary.* Retrieved October 27, 2006, from http://www.bls.gov/news.release/osh.nr0.htm.

Yu, F., & Richmond, T. (2005). Factors affecting outpatient rehabilitation outcomes in elders. *Journal of Nursing Scholarship, 37*(3), 229-236.

---

*Asterisk indicates a classic or definitive work on this subject.

Chapter 19

HEALTH PERCEPTION

Media Resources

- evolve Evolve Website http://evolve.elsevier.com/Harkreader/
- Companion CD

Learning Objectives

After studying this chapter, you will be able to do the following:

- Describe the perception of health for individuals, families, and communities
- Identify factors that affect health for individuals, families, and communities
- Understand the focus of assessment of health in the individual, family, and community
- Identify health goals and expected outcomes when planning for individuals, families, and communities
- Discuss the use of the nursing diagnosis *Health-seeking behaviors*
- Identify methodologies of intervention for improving the health of individuals, families, and communities
- Evaluate health outcomes in individuals, families, and communities

Key Terms

disease
etiology
health goals
health-illness continuum
health perception
health promotion
health within illness
illness
population health
preventive health care
primary health care
primary prevention
secondary prevention
tertiary prevention
well-being
wellness

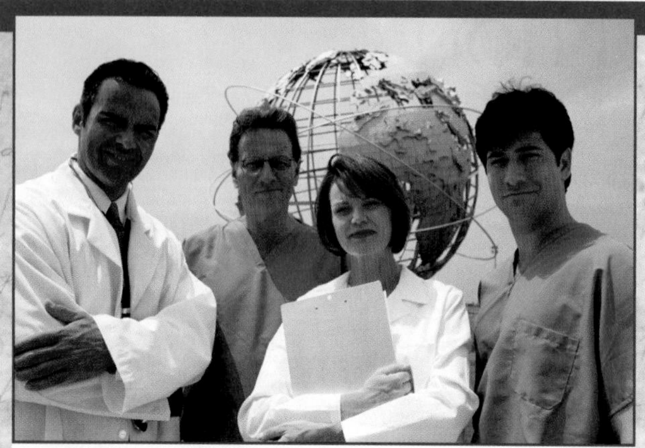

A medium size city in the southeastern United States has had an influx of older adults in the last 10 years. Because this population had begun to tax the community's health services, the city authorized a new senior citizens center with the goal of maintaining optimal health of the aging population. The board members of the senior center requested the local health education center's assistance with completing a survey of the health perception and needs of senior citizens. The survey asked specifically, "What is health?" "What does health mean to you?" and "What are your current health needs?"

The survey results identified the priority needs of increasing preventive health care and wellness activities available to senior citizens. The Morgantown Task Force on Preventive and Wellness Services for Senior Citizens was formed consisting of interested volunteers, including two senior citizens, a health department nurse, the community hospital outreach director, the community outreach program coordinator, two parish nurses, and two religious leaders. The task force was scheduled to meet biannually to develop a program and evaluate the success of the program in meeting health needs of the community. The nurses on the task force considered the nursing diagnoses in the accompanying nursing diagnosis box.

KEY NURSING DIAGNOSES FOR HEALTH PERCEPTION

Health-seeking behaviors (specify): Active seeking (by an individual, family, or community in stable health) of ways to alter personal health habits and/or the environment to move toward a higher level of health

Readiness for enhanced community coping: Pattern of community activities for adaptation and problem solving that is satisfactory for meeting the demand or needs of a community but can be improved for management or improvement of current and/or future problems or stressors

CONCEPTS OF HEALTH

Health is important to individuals, families, and communities. It is important to individuals to feel good, to be able to perform needed work, and to enjoy life. It is important to families to meet the needs of their members by providing love, belonging, food, shelter, and safety and by helping family members achieve their highest potential. Health is important to the community, from the standpoints of both quality of life and the economic well-being of its citizens. In addition, health has been described as the bedrock on which social progress is built. Healthy people can do things that make life worthwhile, and as the level of health increases, so does the potential for happiness. **Health perception** is the knowledge and experience of one's state of wellness and well-being.

Nurses are involved in health care planning and decision making for individuals, families, and communities. To fulfill this nursing role, you will need to understand the meaning of health to the individual, the family, and the community. As you begin to study this chapter on the perception of health, consider your own perception of health. Ask yourself important questions about health, such as these: What does it mean when I say I am healthy? How could I be healthier? What are the benefits and risks of seeking better health? Are there factors in my environment that would hinder me from becoming a healthier person?

Also think about your family and community. What factors would you use to describe a healthy family or community? What would need to change in your community to increase the health of the people with whom you live and work? To answer these questions, you need to consider the influences of biology, behavior, physical environment, social environment, and public policies and interventions (Figure 19-1).

Our ideas about health and illness have changed over the past century. At the beginning of the twentieth century, society thought in terms of a dichotomy of health or illness. Health care was focused on conquering the most prevalent diseases. Around the middle of the century, the death rate from acute disease declined below that of chronic illness. Thus it became more important to identify the risk factors of chronic illnesses and to change lifestyle factors to prevent them. In the 1980s, the emphasis in health care shifted to changing behaviors and health habits as a way to prevent illness and prolong life. Today, the importance of a comprehensive program of health promotion is recognized as a means of managing the factors that determine whether or not we are healthy and live in a healthy community. Three areas of health care are important to this change in philosophy: health promotion, prevention, and primary health care.

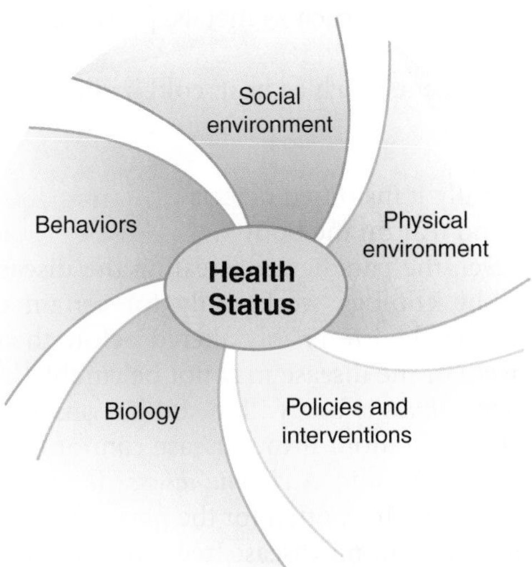

FIGURE 19-1 Determinants of health. (Data from U.S. Department of Health and Human Services. [2000]. *Healthy People 2010* [2nd ed]. Washington, DC: U.S. Government Printing Office.)

Health promotion is the advancement of health through the encouragement of activities that enhance the wellness of individuals, families, and communities. Health in the context of health promotion is a dynamic rather than a static state, in which individuals and communities strive to maintain or regain a positive state of physical and psychological being. It is a basic force in daily life, influenced by circumstances, beliefs, culture, and the social, economic, and physical environment. Health promotion enables people to be responsible for improving their health in keeping with its personal meaning.

Preventive health care is the recognition of the risk for disease and the actions taken to reduce that risk. Preventive health care has the potential to reduce the incidence of disease.

Primary health care means all care necessary to people's lives and health, including health education, nutrition, sanitation, maternal and child health care, immunizations, prevention, and control of endemic disease (World Health Organization, 1978). Primary health care is a comprehensive array of services designed to improve the health of a society.

HEALTH AS A NATIONAL AND AN INTERNATIONAL GOAL

As citizens of the world, we can no longer view health only from an individual or a local community perspective. A global economy and growing international mobility suggest that all countries must share the health concerns of any one country. The industrialized nations of the world look to each other for ideas about how to improve the health of their citizens and those in less-developed countries. They also must monitor the threat of pathogen transmission across international boundaries.

BOX 19-1 Healthy People 2010: *What Are Its Goals?*

Healthy People 2010 is designed to achieve two overarching goals:

GOAL 1. INCREASE QUALITY AND YEARS OF HEALTHY LIFE: To help individuals of all ages increase life expectancy and improve their quality of life.

GOAL 2. ELIMINATE HEALTH DISPARITIES: To eliminate health disparities between different segments of the population.

The World Health Organization (WHO) has defined health as a "state of complete physical, mental, and social well-being, and not merely as the absence of illness." This holistic definition recognizes that being healthy involves more than physiological functioning. The need for comprehensive health goals to address these determinants of health has been well recognized. **Health goals** broadly outline what needs to be done to achieve health for individuals, families, and communities.

WHO also declared that health is a fundamental human right and initiated a movement toward a social goal to attain the highest possible level of health by all people by the year 2000 (WHO, 1978). This goal was subsequently adopted by many nations, including the United States, and has been renewed for the year 2010 (Box 19-1). WHO further promoted primary health care as the key to attaining the target of health for all. In 2000, the U.S. Public Health Service released updated target health objectives for the United States in a document entitled *Healthy People 2010: National Health Promotion and Disease Prevention Objectives.* This document outlined 28 priority areas and established scores of specific health objectives for the country (Box 19-2).

Box 19-3 lists some facts that form the basis for the targets of *Healthy People 2010.* The first year of *Healthy People 2010* was a time of listening, and it began a broad consultation process for a decade-long agenda. The overarching goal of *Healthy People 2010* is "increasing the quality and years of healthy life," but the agenda also strengthened the *Healthy People 2000* goal of "reducing health disparities" to read "elimination of health disparities" among the different groups in society.

DEFINITIONS OF HEALTH

Whether a client is an individual, a family, or a community, your understanding of different perspectives of health will help you to manage health and health care from the client's perspective. The client's goals for health are derived from a personal definition of health.

Health as the Absence of Disease. Health and illness can be viewed as a dichotomy, with health being defined as the absence of disease. A **disease** is a specific disorder characterized by a recognizable set of signs and symptoms and attributable to heredity, infection, diet, or environment. A disease is an interruption in the continuous process of health. A disease may disrupt the person's ability to function, and it may even shorten life.

Using this definition of health, health care is the diagnosis and treatment of disease based on identification of a specific disorder and its etiology. **Etiology** is the cause of the disease. If the cause of the disease can be removed, the person will often be cured of the disease. For example, using antibiotics to remove the cause of a disease will cure an infection caused by bacteria. Etiologies of diseases include the following:

- Biological agents, such as viruses, bacteria, fungi, rickettsia, protozoa, and helminths
- Chemical agents, such as metals, poisons, and strong irritants
- Physical agents, such as heat, cold, radiation, and electricity
- Stress
- Genetically transmitted defects
- Wear and tear on the body

However, the paradigm of treating the disease by removing the etiology works only for certain diseases. Function may be irreversibly altered before the etiology is removed, or the disease may not be curable.

An *acute illness* is one with a sudden onset and, usually, a short duration. If the disease cannot be cured, it may become chronic. A *chronic disease* is one that lasts for an extended time, often for the person's lifetime. The definition of a chronic disease frequently specifies that it lasts 6 months or longer. Chronic diseases can have periods of *remission* in which symptoms disappear or are

BOX 19-2 *Focus Areas for* Healthy People 2010

Access to quality health services
Arthritis, osteoporosis, and chronic back pain
Cancer
Chronic kidney disease
Diabetes
Disability and secondary conditions
Educational and community-based programs
Environmental health
Family planning
Food safety
Health communication
Heart disease and stroke
Human immunodeficiency virus (HIV)
Immunization and infectious diseases
Injury and violence prevention
Maternal, infant, and child health
Medical product safety
Mental health and mental disorders
Nutrition and overweight
Occupational safety and health
Oral health
Physical activity and fitness
Public health infrastructure
Respiratory diseases
Sexually transmitted diseases
Substance abuse
Tobacco use
Vision and hearing

BOX 19-3 *Health Indicators*

- Regular physical activity throughout life is important for maintaining a healthy body, enhancing psychological well-being, and preventing premature death.
- Cigarette smoking is the single most preventable cause of disease and death in the United States. Smoking results in more deaths each year in the United States than AIDS, alcohol, cocaine, heroin, homicide, suicide, motor vehicle crashes, and fires—all combined.
- Alcohol and illicit drug use are associated with many of this country's most serious problems, including violence, injury, and HIV infection.
- Unintended pregnancies and sexually transmitted diseases (STDs), including infection with HIV, which causes AIDS, can result from unprotected sexual behaviors. Abstinence is the only method of complete protection. Condoms, if used correctly and consistently, can help prevent both unintended pregnancy and STDs.
- Nearly 700,000 cases of AIDS have been reported in the United States since the HIV/AIDS epidemic began in the 1980s. The latest estimates indicate that 800,000 to 900,000 people in the United States are currently infected with HIV. The lifetime cost of health care associated with HIV infection, in light of recent advances in HIV diagnostics and therapies, is $155,000 or more per person.
- Depression is associated with other medical conditions, such as heart disease, cancer, and diabetes, as well as with anxiety and eating disorders. Depression has also been associated with alcohol and illicit drug abuse.
- More than 400 Americans die each day from injuries due primarily to motor vehicle crashes, firearms, poisonings, suffocation, falls, fires, and drowning. The risk of injury is so great that most persons sustain a significant injury at some time during their lives. Motor vehicle crashes are the most common cause of serious injury.
- An estimated 25% of preventable illnesses worldwide can be attributed to poor environmental quality.
- In 1998, influenza immunization rates were 64% in adults aged 65 years and older—almost double the 1989 immunization rate of 33%. In 1998, only 46% of persons aged 65 years and older had ever received a pneumococcal vaccine.

From U.S. Department of Health and Human Services. (2000). With understanding and improving health and objectives for improving health. In *Healthy People 2010* (2nd ed.). Washington, DC: U.S. Government Printing Office. Retrieved from http://www.health.gov/healthypeople/Document/html/uih/uih_bw/uih_4.htm.
AIDS, Acquired immunodeficiency syndrome; HIV, human immunodeficiency virus.

minimal and periods of *exacerbation* in which symptoms reappear or become worse.

Chronic illness makes us less comfortable with a definition of health as an absence of disease. People with chronic illnesses may define themselves across a continuum of health from very poor health to even excellent health. The definition of health becomes less a matter of "Do I have a disease?" and more a matter of "How well can I function?" People with arthritis, muscular dystrophy, psoriasis, and even heart disease may believe themselves to be healthy and may describe themselves as ill only during an exacerbation of the disease. That is why **illness** refers to the personal experience of feeling unhealthy, caused by changes in a person's state of well-being and social function.

Health as a Continuum. If health is not merely the absence of disease, then perhaps we should think of it as a continuum. A **health-illness continuum** ranges from high-level wellness—an optimal state of mental and physical well-being—to premature death (Figure 19-2). Every person exists at some point on the continuum and may move back and forth between the two extremes. A person at any point on the continuum can be focused in the direction of wellness.

Thinking of health as existing on a continuum has several advantages. For one, the health-illness continuum recognizes that few people are in an optimal state of health, thus providing the philosophy of optimal health as a goal and health care as a way of helping people move toward this goal. For another, the continuum discounts the notion that disease and health are dichotomous terms.

The health-illness continuum recognizes that more than one factor is necessary to determine a person's state of health. A person with arthritis who walks 3 miles a day, eats a well-balanced diet, and has a positive outlook on life may be closer to optimal health on the continuum than a person with no identifiable illness but with a sedentary lifestyle, a junk-food diet, a lack of energy, and a fear of the world.

The health-illness continuum makes room for health within illness. **Health within illness** is a state that can expand human potential by providing an opportunity for personal growth and well-being despite having an illness. The outcome of an illness is that the person becomes stronger as a human being, even though the disease may not be cured. Many people who suffer from chronic illness or life-threatening acute illness can develop a heightened sense of self and of personal potential, can feel greater spiritual inner peace, and can discover new meaning and purpose in life.

Health as High-Level Wellness. Health as high-level wellness includes both positive physiological function and a sense of well-being. **Well-being** is a subjective perception of a good and satisfactory existence in which the individual has a positive experience of personal abilities, harmony, and vitality. Like illness, well-being is a relative, changing state experienced in the course of everyday living.

Wellness is a state of optimal health or optimal physical and social functioning. Wellness includes optimal physical function, successful and satisfying relationships with others, emotional stability, managing feelings comfortably, intellectual growth, and a spiritual element that gives meaning and purpose to life (Figure 19-3). In addition, several assumptions underlie the concept of wellness to give it meaning as a framework for health care (Travis & Ryan, 2004).

Individuals possess their own optimal level of functioning, which represents the best state of well-being that is possible for them. Each person sets individual goals that are compatible with body build, age, and physical state. Not everyone can jog 5 miles a day, nor would everyone enjoy the benefits associated with long-distance jogging.

Wellness is a choice that cannot be passively achieved. To achieve optimal health, a person must choose to engage in positive health actions and behaviors to achieve wellness. A person purposefully engages in actions to attain and maintain health. These actions can be in response to internal drives, stressors, or bodily functions, or they can be in response to environmental risk factors that threaten health and well-being.

Wellness is a process; thus the achievement of wellness is ongoing. Wellness is not a finite state to be achieved, with the present being a time of constant struggle to attain this utopian state. Rather, the process itself is wellness when the person recognizes and experiences the possibility for health and happiness in each moment.

Wellness is an efficient channeling of energy received from the environment, transformed within you, and

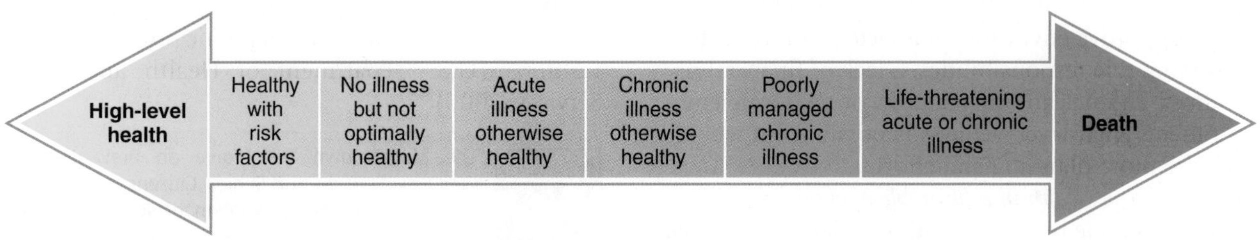

FIGURE 19-2 Health as a continuum.

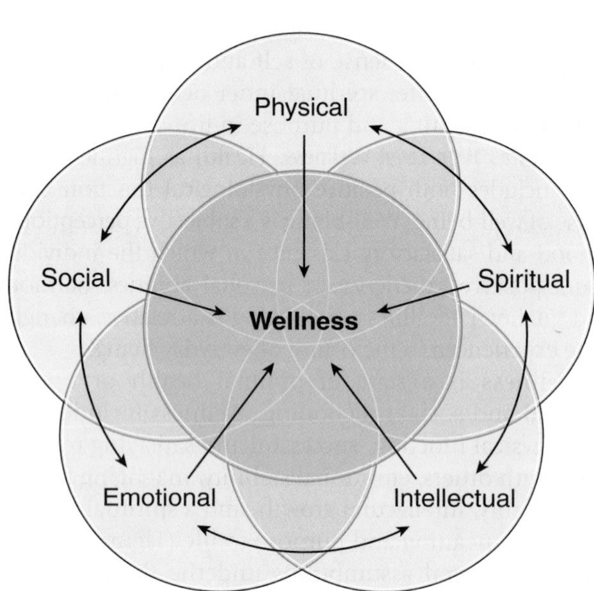

FIGURE 19-3 Dimensions of wellness.

Very favorable environment

Protected poor health (in favorable environment, i.e., through social and cultural institutions)

High-level wellness (in favorable environment)

Environmental Axis

Death — Health Axis — Peak wellness

Poor health (in unfavorable environment)

Emergent high-level wellness (in unfavorable environment)

Very unfavorable environment

FIGURE 19-4 Dunn's concept of well-being. (Redrawn from Dunn, H. L. [1959]. High-level wellness for man and society. *American Journal of Public Health, 49*[6], 786-792.)

sent on to affect the world outside. Wellness is the integration of body, mind, and spirit, the appreciation that everything you do, think, feel, and believe has an impact on your state of health. Accepting yourself as a worthwhile person and recognizing the value in your personal attributes is necessary for high-level wellness. High-level wellness is associated with a good feeling about yourself in relationship to other people.

Knowledge of the environment in which wellness is achieved is necessary to understanding wellness. Dunn (1959) uses a grid to depict a concept of wellness (Figure 19-4). The horizontal axis is the continuum from peak wellness to death. The vertical axis is the environment, from very favorable to very unfavorable. The four quadrants in the grid represent the interactions of the state of wellness with the environment.

- *High-level wellness in a favorable environment.* This quadrant represents a person who is in an optimal state of health. The environment supports the person's efforts to achieve high-level wellness.
- *Emergent high-level wellness in an unfavorable environment.* This person has the knowledge, motivation, and physical stamina to achieve high-level wellness. Nonsupportive environmental factors could be demanding role responsibilities, a lack of financial resources, an unclean water supply, or an unsafe environment. High-level wellness is possible but would require more planning and effort.
- *Protected poor health in a favorable environment.* This person has one or more health problems but is able to manage them because the environment is supportive. The person has access to high-quality medical care, nursing services, and social services. Financial resources allow the person to engage home maintenance services as needed.
- *Poor health in an unfavorable environment.* This person has one or more health problems—such as old age, diabetes, and obesity—and an environment unfavorable to wellness. For example, the person might live in a rural farming community without medical services, might lack health insurance to pay for medicine, and the diabetes may frequently be uncontrolled, making complications likely.

Health in Populations. Health in a community is defined by the parameters of population health (Box 19-4). **Population health** considers health problems encountered as a result of being a part of a group and focuses intervention on the population rather than on the individual. A population can be a subgroup within a community, such as teenage mothers in the local high school, or a larger group, such as men at risk for heart disease. Population health addresses the five determinants of health: biology, behaviors, physical environment, social environment, and public policies and interventions (U.S. Department of Health and Human Services, 2000).

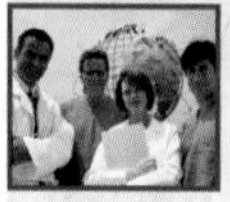

The Morgantown Task Force on Preventive and Wellness Services for Senior Citizens is concerned with health of the population of senior citizens in Morgantown.

BOX 19-4 *The Population Health Approach*

A population health approach has two major differences from an individual health approach.

RANGE OF HEALTH DETERMINANTS: Health problems cannot be totally explained by individual characteristics and behaviors. Individual health is also determined by factors that affect populations as a whole. Population health strategies address the entire range of factors that determine health.

POPULATIONS AS TARGET: Individual health care solves health problems or improves health one person at a time. Population health strategies are designed to affect the entire population.

FACTORS AFFECTING HEALTH

Our understanding of the five determinants and how they relate to one another, coupled with our understanding of how individual and community health affects the health of the national community, is perhaps the most important key to achieving our *Healthy People 2010* goals of increasing the quality and years of life and of eliminating the nation's health disparities.

BIOLOGY

Biology refers to the individual's genetic makeup (those factors with which one is born), family history (which may suggest risk for disease), and the physical and mental health problems acquired during life.

Heredity, or genetic makeup (in this case, predisposition to specific illnesses), raises known health risks. Family histories of diabetes mellitus, cancer, and coronary artery disease are examples of known genetic risk factors. The methods of managing genetically transmitted disease include case-finding and treating the manifestations of the illness. However, genetics as a cause of disease is not clear-cut. The onset of many genetically transmitted diseases requires an interplay of environmental and lifestyle factors with heredity.

BEHAVIORS

Behaviors are individual responses or reactions to internal stimuli and external conditions. Behaviors can have a reciprocal relationship to biology; in other words, each can react to the other. Personal choices and the social and physical environments surrounding individuals can shape behaviors. The social and physical environments include all factors that affect the life of individuals, positively or negatively, and many may not be under their immediate or direct control.

In recent years, lifestyle factors have received major attention for their influence on health. Lifestyle includes diet, exercise, stress level, health practices, coping skills, education, work, interpersonal relationships, and cultural practices. They are the sum of a person's life experiences.

Family health practices play an important role in the health of individuals and communities. Families can promote a positive perception of health by providing a supportive environment, by promoting positive health practices, by appropriate use of health services, and by seeking safety and security for family members.

Cultural factors influence individual beliefs and values. Cultural folkways and customs influence entry into the health care system, personal health practices, social environment, and physical environment, which may exacerbate any biological differences among persons of various cultures. The serious health disparities that exist in the United States between the minority and majority cultures must be addressed from all five determinants of health.

In addition, economic factors such as income, layoffs, the cost of housing, the cost of health services, community design, education and training, social services, and public policy can all affect health status. In fact, these economic factors affect individual, family, and community health status in many ways. Thus economic factors must be addressed if citizens are to achieve improved health.

SOCIAL ENVIRONMENT

Social environment includes interactions with family, friends, co-workers, and others in the community. It also encompasses social institutions, such as law enforcement, the workplace, places of worship, and schools. Housing, public transportation, and the presence or absence of violence in the community are other components of the social environment.

Individual, family, and community health is affected by a variety of intellectual factors. In individuals, cognitive abilities, educational level, and past experience all play a role in shaping a person's attitude toward health care. A family's knowledge about health and illness influences its members' ability to understand disease patterns, factors involved in health and illness, and the importance of personal health practices. Likewise, the community's health status is influenced by the knowledge of its citizens. As citizens become more informed through modern communication and technology, more communities are calling for improved health standards and practices.

Social networks have a profound influence on the health status of individuals, families, and communities. The organization of the community and health care system can determine how clients can access and obtain health care. Recreational facilities, churches, and social organizations are part of the community social network that affects health and health status. You, along with other individuals, families, and communities, need to work toward shared values and collective actions that will ensure equitable health practices and treatment for all citizens.

PHYSICAL ENVIRONMENT

Physical environmental factors contribute to the health status of individuals, families, and communities. The quality of one's work life, safety and security factors, and environmental ecosystem issues are examples of the many possible environmental factors that can influence health. It is important for you to assess the client's physical environment, recognize possible risk factors, and work with other health disciplines and team members to address the health risks identified.

Physical environment can be thought of as that which can be seen, touched, heard, smelled, and tasted. However, the physical environment also contains less tangible elements, such as radiation and ozone. The physical environment can harm individual and community health, especially when individuals and communities are exposed to toxic substances, irritants, infectious agents, and physical hazards in homes, schools, and worksites. The physical environment can also promote good health—for example, by providing clean and safe places for people to work, exercise, and play.

PUBLIC POLICY AND INTERVENTION

Public policies and interventions can have a powerful and positive effect on the health of individuals and the community. Examples include health promotion campaigns to prevent smoking; policies mandating child restraints and safety belt use in automobiles; disease prevention services, such as immunization of children, adolescents, and adults; and clinical services, such as enhanced mental health care. Policies and interventions that promote individual and community health may be implemented by a variety of agencies, such as transportation, education, energy, housing, labor, justice, and other venues, or through places of worship, community-based organizations, civic groups, and businesses.

The health of individuals and communities also depends greatly on access to quality health care. Expanding access to quality health care is important to eliminating health disparities and to increasing the quality and years of healthy life for all people living in the United States. Health care in the broadest sense includes not only services received through health care providers but also health information and services received through other venues in the community.

Good health depends on equitable access to all necessary and appropriate health services. These consist of prevention and health promotion services, services to reduce pain and suffering and restore health, and services to enhance quality of life for those with chronic diseases and limitations. For example, adequate perinatal care can result in healthier babies.

ASSESSMENT

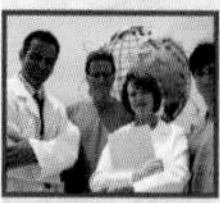

The Morgantown Task Force on Preventive and Wellness Services for Senior Citizens reviewed other community senior health programs to determine which programs might best meet their needs. A review of the survey identified that many seniors walk at the local mall for exercise and many attend religious services. The task group determined that the development of a parish nurse program and a nurse available at the local mall could be an effective method of affecting health. The Morgantown Task Force on Preventive and Wellness Services for Senior Citizens identified the nursing diagnosis of *Readiness for enhanced community coping.*

A community planning group is concerned with health primarily from the broad perspective of the needs of the community. A health assessment of an individual, family, or community shares a common definition of health but requires different data. Notice the differences in data used for assessment for the dimensions of health for individuals, families, and communities.

INDIVIDUAL HEALTH

Assessment of individual health includes physical, social, emotional, intellectual, and spiritual dimensions. Specific individual health assessment is addressed throughout this book and may include characteristics of individual health such as these:

- Presence of disease and symptomatology
- Coping skills
- Capacity for making healthy lifestyle decisions
- Physical, mental, social, and emotional limitations
- Education and training
- Quality of work life
- Positive and supportive interpersonal relationships and social networks

FAMILY HEALTH

Assessment of family health includes physical, social, emotional, intellectual, and spiritual dimensions. Family strengths and problems are identified to provide a basis and direction for further assessment of individual family members (Figure 19-5).

Your nursing care plan for family health may address many factors that relate to family health. Those factors may belong to broad characteristics such as these:

- Positive and supportive interpersonal family relationships
- Consequences of family employment opportunities
- Consequences of family level of poverty
- Consequences of lower-status occupations
- Impact of job loss
- Safety and security issues
- Access to and appropriate use of health care services

The many other factors that relate to family health and function are addressed in other areas of this text.

COMMUNITY HEALTH

Assessment of community health includes physical, social, emotional, intellectual, and spiritual dimensions.

Community health assessment commonly uses statistics on populations and uses data to compare community needs with available services. Some examples include mortality and morbidity studies, annual health reports from multiple agencies, and health inventories and resource reports. Traditional methods of measuring the health of a community have centered on mortality (death rate), longevity (life expectancy), and morbidity (illness).

When assessing community health, your plan may address broad social issues of community health, such as the following:

- A safe environment
- Affordable housing
- Community design
- Social services and public policy
- Cost-effective health services
- Preventive health practices
- Joint action for minority and cultural health issues

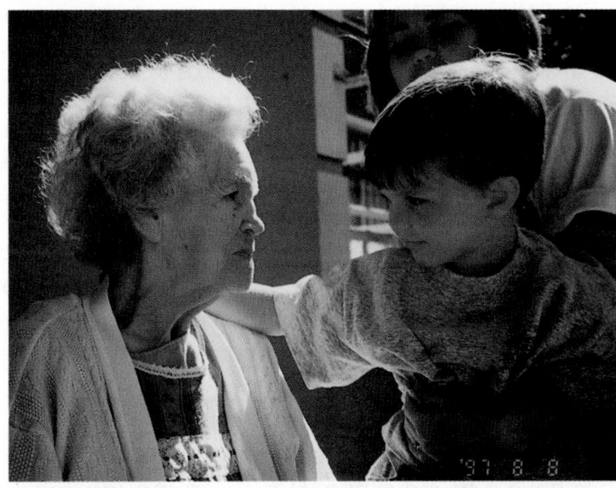

FIGURE 19-5 Family strength is seen in the contribution of a great-grandmother to the emotional development of a child. (Courtesy David A. Zerr.)

Community health is complex and specific to the community involved. No one pattern of community health can be understood without knowing the multitude of relevant environmental, social, and economic factors that affect it.

FOCUSED ASSESSMENT FOR *HEALTH-SEEKING BEHAVIORS*

The nursing diagnosis *Health-seeking behaviors* is observed in individuals, families, and communities. The key element of *Health-seeking behaviors* is choice. The individual, family, or community expresses the desire to seek a higher level of wellness, or you may observe behaviors that indicate a motivation to attain a higher level of wellness. Additional defining characteristics include the following:

- Expression of concern about the effects of current environmental conditions on health
- Stated or observed unfamiliarity with community wellness resources
- Demonstrated or observed lack of knowledge about health promotion behaviors

You will need to look for specific indicators of health-seeking behaviors in individuals, families, and communities to recognize opportunities to support health promotion activities and provide teaching (Box 19-5).

BOX 19-5 *Examples of Health-Seeking Behaviors*

INDIVIDUALS

- Having periodic physical examinations
- Seeking counseling for weight loss
- Requesting a health evaluation before starting an exercise program
- Using a seat belt
- Using a bicycle helmet
- Using sunscreen
- Using condoms
- Joining a support group to help break an addictive behavior pattern, such as the use of nicotine, alcohol, or illicit drugs
- Participating in recreational, social, and cultural community activities

FAMILIES

- Obtaining a family membership at a fitness center
- Seeking family therapy to manage addictive behavior in a teenager
- Making a commitment to reduce the incidence of colds and flu in the family
- Asking for assistance in managing the care of an older adult family member
- Expressing a need for information about caring for a new infant
- Expressing a need for information about making the home safe for all family members, especially children and older adults
- Seeking opportunities to enhance an employment situation

COMMUNITIES

- Petitioning of the city council by a neighborhood association for a new park in the area
- Organizing a group of concerned citizens to form a health clinic in a neighborhood with poor access to health care
- Seeking volunteers for a community action group to reduce violence in the public schools
- Initiating a public outcry over an incidence of hepatitis in the community and organizing a petition for better testing of community water supplies
- Attending a public hearing to discuss the provision of health services by schools
- Forming a committee in a community action group to study the need for affordable housing for disadvantaged groups
- Meeting to explore the possibilities of providing an education program to young parents about the importance of prenatal care and parenting skills
- Working with the community to address problems of low-income families, single-parent families, and gender-gap inequities in the labor force

DIAGNOSIS

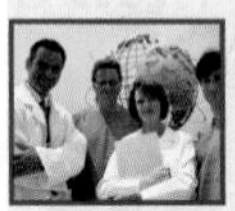

The Morgantown Task Force on Preventive and Wellness Services for Senior Citizens identified the nursing diagnosis of *Readiness for enhanced community coping.*

NANDA International (NANDA-I) recognizes the need for both wellness nursing diagnoses and risk nursing diagnoses for individuals, families, and communities. Wellness nursing diagnoses describe human responses to the state or quality of being healthy in an individual, family, or community, especially as a result of deliberate effort (NANDA-I, 2007). Risk nursing diagnoses describe human responses that may develop in a vulnerable individual, family, or community resulting from exposure to factors that increase the chance of injury or loss (NANDA-I, 2007).

Nursing diagnoses can occur along the entire health-illness continuum. The individual, family, or community can be described as having a deficiency, dysfunction, or decrease in health behaviors that creates risk for diminished health. In addition, the individual, family, or community at any point on the continuum can be recognized as having a potential for enhancing a state of wellness. The client—whether individual, family, or community—starts from a state of wellness and has the desire to increase that level of wellness.

PLANNING

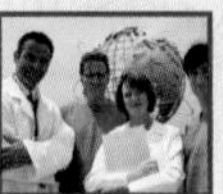

The Morgantown Task Force on Preventive and Wellness Services for Senior Citizens decided to focus on two outcomes: (1) screening for cholesterol and diabetes will be available to all seniors in the community at locations consistent with daily activities of senior citizens, and (2) the availability of wellness activities will increase by 20% over a 2-year period. This group has chosen to focus on preventive health behaviors.

A statement of health goals flows from the perception of health and an understanding of related factors (the determinants of health, see Figure 19-1) that contribute to health. The expected outcomes provide specific guidelines for implementation. Thus planning includes designing interventions that can realistically be expected to achieve the goals.

Health promotion is expected to result in an improved quality of life. Quality living is in part being able to do what you want to do, do it well, and derive a sense of satisfaction from the effort. It is described in terms of effective functioning in areas of life that are important to each person. Through improved health, people can have the opportunity to maintain vigor and stamina throughout their life span. In addition, better health will contribute to an increase in both individual and social productivity.

The outcomes for health promotion are described in practical, situation-specific results. For an occupational health effort, the expected outcomes include increased worker satisfaction, increased productivity, and a lower cost of employee health care. In a school setting, the expected outcomes are decreased absence from school, improved learning, increased motivation, and increased self-esteem.

INTERVENTION

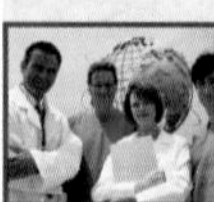

The Morgantown Task Force on Preventive and Wellness Services for Senior Citizens contacted the local hospital, which agreed to provide a nurse to perform mini health assessments in the mall for 2 hours on Monday, Wednesday, and Friday (1 hour in the morning and 1 hour in the afternoon), including free blood pressure checks, with quarterly glucose and cholesterol checks available for a small fee. An assessment and survey was to be completed with each visit to continue to assess the health and wellness of the individual. Nurses who were recruited for the parish nurse program were trained to perform the same assessment and screening at sites in local churches.

Designing interventions to improve health requires both health promotion and preventive health care. Although (from a philosophical perspective) these two concepts are different, they are not mutually exclusive.

INTERVENTIONS TO PROMOTE HEALTH

From a community perspective, health promotion activities have a broad scope. Health promotion can include educational, political, organizational, regulatory, and environmental supports for actions and conditions of living conducive to the health of individuals, families, and communities. Health promotion includes modifying the individual and collective lifestyle, modifying environments to support health, strengthening community action, reordering health services, and using public policy to enhance health. The activities that can be labeled as health promotion recognize the interrelationship of the person and the environmental, biological, social, and political determinants of health. *When the expected outcome is a higher level of wellness, the activity is health promotion.*

From an individual perspective an activity can be labeled *health promotion* if it provides people with tools or knowledge to take control of their own health. This paradigm for health promotion recognizes the potential impact of the self-care movement that has been occurring since the 1970s. The paradigm for wellness includes self-reliance, person-centered activities, and client participation. Thus the paradigm for health promotion, by its very nature, must include decisions about who is responsible for decision making in health care. The philosophy of health promotion places the responsibility for health on the individual and family rather than on the professional.

However, if individuals are solely responsible for their own health, there is a danger that the biological, social, political, and environmental determinants of health may be ignored. Considering broad determinants of health, society as a whole bears some responsibility for the health of its members. The question is, then, whether health promotion is a responsibility of the public or private sector. If it is society's responsibility, and the public sector assumes some or all of the responsibility, should the decision making and program support lie with the local, state, or national government? To the extent that health is a national resource serving a common national interest, perhaps the responsibility is best placed in the federal government. To the extent that health needs reflect local conditions and interests, the responsibility may be best held at the local and state level.

Health promotion is expected to provide the means to revolutionize public health as a means to manage chronic illness in the same way infection control practices revolutionized public health in the first half of the twentieth century.

INTERVENTIONS TO PREVENT ILLNESS OR DISABILITY

Prevention is a concept across the continuum of health care from wellness to illness. This comprehensive approach to prevention can be best understood by describing health care activities as primary, secondary, and tertiary levels of prevention.

Levels of Preventive Care. **Primary prevention** consists of actions that are considered true prevention because they precede disease or dysfunction and are applied to clients considered physically and emotionally healthy to protect them from health problems. Activities are aimed at decreasing the probability of specific illnesses or dysfunction. They may include health education programs, immunizations, and physical and nutritional fitness activities. Primary prevention can be applied to an individual or to a general population, or it can focus on individuals at risk for developing specific diseases. An example is a public health nurse providing health education programs in high schools to inform teenagers about sexually transmitted diseases.

Secondary prevention consists of actions that focus on the early diagnosis and prompt treatment of people with health problems or illnesses who are at risk for developing complications or worsening conditions. Activities are directed at diagnosis and prompt intervention to reduce the severity of the disease and to enable the client to return to normal function as quickly as possible. Secondary prevention includes nursing care delivered at home, at a hospital, or at a nursing center for screening techniques and treatment of early stages of disease. An example is a public health nurse who carries out screening tests for postpartum depression on mothers attending well-baby clinics or the nurse who recognizes complications in a hospitalized client and takes action before the complications become worse.

Tertiary prevention involves minimizing the effects of a permanent, irreversible disease or disability through interventions directed at preventing complication and deterioration. Activities are directed at rehabilitation rather than diagnosis and treatment. Care at this level is aimed at helping the client achieve as high a level of functioning as possible, despite the limitations caused by illness or impairment. The term *preventive* is applied to this level of care because it involves prevention of further disability or reduced functioning or making maximum use of the remaining functions. An example is a nurse working in a geriatric care center who refers a diabetic client with diabetic neuropathy to a foot-care education program.

Methods of Prevention. The concept of disease prevention is based on identifying risk factors and using those factors to identify persons at risk for a specific disease. The value of prevention is a reduction in morbidity or mortality rates for the specific disease. However, not all diseases can be prevented. Hence prevention is often aimed at early detection of the disease to prolong life and reduce suffering.

The decision to implement widespread prevention strategies requires that multiple factors be considered: the prevalence of the disease, whether the disease can be prevented, the degree of devastation resulting from the effects of the disease, and the availability of treatment options that can eradicate the disease or prolong the client's life.

Another consideration is the availability and accuracy of methods to screen for risk factors and for the disease. If prevention demands major lifestyle changes or requires costly, risky, toxic, or unpleasant preventive measures, the benefits of prevention may not outweigh the risks. In addition, screening tests need to have an acceptable margin of error. That is, the tests should produce a low number of false-positive or false-negative results. False-positive results can cause unnecessary worry and, sometimes, unnecessary procedures. False-negative results give a false sense of security that the disease is not present and may delay treatment.

Preventive measures can be difficult to administer. If clear cost savings cannot be shown, reimbursement for prevention may not be available. In addition, a well-coordinated system of health care delivery is needed to ensure optimum use of money available for prevention.

Disease prevention is derived only in part from the hard sciences. Clinical interventions should address personal health practices and engage the client in joint decision making. Chapter 20 discusses the methods of promoting lifestyle changes. Although a one-to-one relationship with a clinician gives the client and clinician the opportunity to selectively make choices about screening tests, some problems may be more effectively prevented through prevention strategies at the community level. Examples include sexually transmitted diseases, acquired immunodeficiency syndrome (AIDS), teenage pregnancies, and child abuse.

PRIMARY HEALTH CARE

With the present social concern for financing health care that is affordable and accessible for all, the question arises about what is meant by a package of essential health care. This package of health care is what a society defines as primary health care.

Primary health care focuses on comprehensive care with a much broader perspective than just medical and nursing care; it includes prevention and health promotion. Primary health care includes the care provided at the point at which a client first enters the health care system. Thus the common use of the term *primary care* refers to the use of a primary care physician. Primary medical care is the first contact for the provision of coordinated care for a wide range of health concerns within a sustained relationship with a health care provider. If the range of concerns truly encompasses a comprehensive view of health care, it can be labeled primary health care.

In the definition of primary health care created by WHO (Box 19-6), there are six principles:

- There are essential services that should be available to all members of a society.
- There should be equitable access to health services for all members of a society.
- Individual and community involvement in the planning and operation of health services will result in socially acceptable methods and technology.
- The health of a society will improve with emphasis that includes prevention and promotion services rather than only curative services.
- Technology should be used appropriately.
- Health development should be integrated with social and economic development.

The essence of the WHO definition combines a focus on individuals and families with a focus on the health of a defined population within a community. Primary health care is delivered by a variety of health professionals and providers working collaboratively with clients to maintain health, support wellness, and treat illness. Full participation of clients and accountability to clients and the community for high-quality comprehensive services are essential features of primary health care.

Primary health care is an important shift from a "medical" focus to a "health" focus in health care. The WHO definition identifies the multidisciplinary nature of the primary health contact, the collaborative nature of relationships between consumers and health care workers, and the accountability of consumer and community to strive for a high level of health.

The need for changes to primary health care is fundamental to a reform of the health care system in both the United States. Nursing as a profession has the expertise to play a vital role in this change. Emerging roles and expanded nursing functions are part of this reform.

BOX 19-6 *World Health Organization Definition of Primary Health Care*

Primary health care is "essential health care based on practical, scientifically sound and socially acceptable methods and technology made universally accessible to individuals and families in the community through their full participation and at a cost that community and country can afford to maintain at every stage of their development in the spirit of self-reliance and self-determination. It forms an integral part both of the country's health system, of which it is the central function and main focus, and of the overall social and economic development of the community. It is the first level of contact of the individual, the family, and the community with the national health system bringing health care as close as possible to where the people live and work, and constitutes the first element of a continuing health care process."

From World Health Organization. (1978). *Primary health care: Report on the international conference on primary health care,* p. 21, Alma Ata, USSR, 6-12 September 1978. Geneva: Author.

EVALUATION

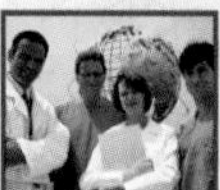

The Morgantown Task Force on Preventive and Wellness Services for Senior Citizens arrived at six health priority/action statements: (1) promote a perception of health for individuals, families, and community; (2) pursue a process to gather and analyze health data; (3) promote collaborative planning and coordination of health promotion decisions and strategies; (4) promote education on health issues and community involvement with the issues identified; (5) make an effort to break down established stereotypes that hinder health promotion, such as multicultural issues and youth issues; and (6) promote efforts to provide adequate resources for preventive health initiatives.

The last step for the workshop participants is to work toward measurable outcomes for the health priorities identified. The hour is late, and participants have exhausted their energies with the identification of health priority/action statements. They agree to draft action plans for each of the six statements. Plans are made for the next meeting, when future steps in the quest to develop health goals for the citizens of Morgantown will be addressed.

The case situation that appears throughout this chapter provides the community context that illustrates the significance of health promotion. The importance of a perception of health for establishing goals and actions for individuals, families, and communities emerged as the top health priority in the workshop scenario.

To evaluate health goals fully, those goals must be explicit, and they must provide specific implementation guidelines and evaluation criteria. For example, consider the goal of improving nutrition by reducing saturated fat intake. During the planning process for a community, you might establish as an expected outcome that community members would reduce their fat intake by reading food labels properly. As one step of the evaluation process for this outcome, you could demonstrate by survey that foods available in the community's grocery stores have fat content listed on their labels. If the survey finds that foods are not clearly labeled with fat content, then your expected outcomes will need revision.

The concept of health perception relates to all health disciplines and to the many factors and determinants of health. For this reason, a plan of action specific to nursing may not be appropriate. The plans developed may need to be broad and multidisciplinary in scope. As a result, the plan will help to develop a perception of health for the individual, family, and community.

▼ KEY PRINCIPLES

- Because we are all citizens of the world, health cannot be viewed from only an individual or a local perspective.
- Health is more than the absence of disease.
- Health exists on a continuum.
- Wellness includes positive physiological function and a sense of well-being.
- Population health considers health problems encountered by being a part of a group and focuses intervention on the population rather than on the individual.
- An individual's health is affected by many personal, family, and community factors.
- Families are the primary unit of health.
- Community health studies have revealed that health is also affected by changing conditions in communities.
- Influences from internal and genetic factors and from external sources affect health.
- Assessment of individual health includes physical, social, emotional, intellectual, and spiritual dimensions.
- Family health assessment requires gathering health data on each member of the family and on the function of the family as a whole.
- Community assessment uses statistics on population data, statistics on the use of services, and data that compare community needs with available services.
- The nursing diagnosis *Health-seeking behaviors* addresses the desire or need for positive health action by individuals.
- Primary health care consists of all care necessary to people's lives and health, including health education, nutrition, sanitation, maternal and child health care, immunizations, prevention, and control of endemic disease.
- Nurses carry out preventive health care and health promotion in a multitude of ways each day of nursing practice.

■ REVIEW QUESTIONS

1. Which of the following distinguishes high-level wellness from good health?

1. A 60-year-old woman who has no major health problems
2. A 50-year-old man who actively pursues good health through diet and exercise
3. A 20-year-old who has no health problems and feels well despite a sedentary job
4. A 3-year-old who spends 6 hours a day watching television and eats healthy snacks

2. Which of the following describes health promotion rather than disease prevention?

1. Immunizing a sexually active population for genital herpes
2. Ensuring clean air and water quality in a city
3. Giving a beta blocker to all people who have had a heart attack
4. Screening a high-risk population for tuberculosis

3. Select the health service that represents tertiary prevention:

1. Physical therapy to reduce the residual paralysis from a cerebrovascular accident
2. A public health campaign to increase the use of pap smears as a screening tool for early detection of cervical cancer
3. Teaching high school students about the effects of marijuana
4. Administering a vaccine after an outbreak of bird flu

4. A 60-year-old man says he is healthy. However, he has been having chest pain for the last year. When it happens, he stops and rests until the pain goes away. One day the pain does not go away, and he drives himself to the emergency department, where he finds out the pain is from coronary artery disease. Now he believes his health is poor. What do you think this man believes is the definition of health?

1. The absence of disease
2. Being able to do what you need and want to do
3. A subjective perception of a good and satisfactory existence
4. A state of optimal physical and social functioning

5. A 50-year-old woman realizes she no longer feels optimally well and wants to plan a program to improve her physical fitness and sense of well-being. Because of her financial circumstances, she lives in an area of the city with a high crime rate, prostitutes on several major street corners, and no city park or swimming pool in the area. She rides the city bus to work every day. Her husband of 30 years smokes two packs of cigarettes a day. He talks about how fat his wife is but also laughs at her for wanting to improve her health. Which best describes her state of well-being?

1. Protected poor health in a favorable environment
2. Poor health in an unfavorable environment
3. High-level wellness in a favorable environment
4. Emergent high-level wellness in an unfavorable environment

Bibliography

Allison, K. G., Duran, M., & Pena-Purcell, N. (2005). Cervical cancer screening practices among Hispanic women: Theories for culturally appropriate interventions. *Hispanic Health Care International, 3*(2), 61-67.

Bennett, J. A., Perrin, N. A., Hanson, G., Bennett, D., Gaynor, W., Flaherty-Robb, M., et al. (2005). Healthy Aging Demonstration Project: Nurse coaching for behavior change in older adults. *Research in Nursing & Health, 28*(3), 187-197.

Carter, M., Gaskins, S., & Shaw, L. (2005). Employee wellness program in a small rural industry: Employee evaluation. *AAOHN Journal, 53*(6), 244-248.

Chwedyk, P. (2005, Fall). Vital signs. Administration on Aging awards grants to tribal elders. *Minority Nurse, 15*,1.

Clemen-Stone, S., McGuire, S., & Eigsti, D. (2002). *Comprehensive community health nursing: Family aggregate and community practice* (6th ed.). St. Louis, MO: Mosby .

Davila, Y. R. (2005). The social construction and conceptualization of sexual health among Mexican American women. *Research and Theory for Nursing Practice, 19*(4), 357-368.

Dunn, H. L. (1959). High-level wellness for man and society. *American Journal of Public Health, 49*(6), 786-792.

Farrell, A., & Geist-Martin, P. (2005). Communicating social health perceptions of wellness at work. *Management Communication Quarterly, 18*(4), 543-592.

Ferrari, A., & Rideout, B. (2005). The collaboration of public health nursing and primary care nursing in the development of a nurse managed health center. *Nursing Clinics of North America, 40*(4), 771-778.

Goins, R., Williams, K., Carter, M., Spencer, S., & Solovieva, T. (2005). Perceived barriers to health care access among rural older adults: A qualitative study. *Journal of Rural Health, 21*(3) 206-213.

Gordon, E., Golanty, E., & McCormak Brown, K. (2004). *Essentials for health and wellness* (8th ed.). Sudbury, MA: Jones & Bartlett.

Gordon, M. (2006). *Manual of nursing diagnosis* (11th ed.). St. Louis, MO: Mosby.

Grindel C. (2005). From AMSN. Influencing health care policy with our children in mind. *Medsurg Nursing, 14*(5), 277-278.

Hendricks, D. L., & Hendricks, C. S. (2005). The relationship of hope and self-efficacy to health promoting behaviors among student-athletes attending historically black colleges and universities. *Journal of Multicultural Nursing & Health, 11*(3), 23-34.

Keller, L. O., Strohschein, S., Lia-Hoagberg, B., & Schaffer M. A. (2004). Population-based public health interventions: practice-based and evidence-supported. Part I. *Public Health Nursing, 21*(5), 453-468.

Leifer, G., & Hartston, H. (2004). *Growth and development across the lifespan: A health promotion focus*. Philadelphia: Saunders.

NANDA International. (2005). *Nursing diagnoses: Definitions and classification, 2005-2006* (6th ed.). Philadelphia: Author.

Nyamathi, A., Sands, H., Pattatucci-Aragon, A., Berg, J., Leake, B., Hahn, J., & Morisky, D. (2004). Perception of health status by homeless U.S. veterans. *Family and Community Health, 27*(1), 65-74.

Oliver, M. (2005). Clinicians' forum. Reaching positive outcomes by assessing and teaching patients self-efficacy. *Home Healthcare Nurse, 23*(9), 559-562.

O'Rourke, T. W. (2005). Promoting school health: An expanded paradigm. *Journal of School Health, 75*(3), 112-114.

Smeltzer, S. C., & Zimmerman, V. L. (2005). Health promotion interests of women with disabilities. *Journal of Neuroscience Nursing, 37*(2), 80-86.

Strunk, C. (2005). Innovative workplace influenza program: Boosting employee immunization rates. *AAOHN Journal, 53*(10), 432-437.

Travis, J. W., & Ryan, R. S. (2004). *Wellness workbook* (2nd ed.). Berkeley, CA: Celestial Arts.

*U.S. Department of Health and Human Services. (2000). With understanding and improving health and objectives for improving health. In *Healthy People 2010* (2nd ed.). Washington, DC: U.S. Government Printing Office. Retrieved from http://www.health.gov/healthypeople/Document/html/uih/uih_bw/uih_2.htm#determinants.

*World Health Organization. (1978). *Primary health care: Report on the international conference on primary health care.* Alma Ata, USSR, 6-12 September, 1978. Geneva: Author.

Yousey, Y., & Carr, M. (2005). A health care program for homeless children using Healthy People 2010 objectives. *Nursing Clinics of North America, 40*(4), 791-801.

*Asterisk indicates a classic or definitive work on this subject.

Chapter 20

Health Maintenance: Lifestyle Management

Media Resources

- Evolve Website http://evolve.elsevier.com/Harkreader/
- Companion CD

Learning Objectives

After studying this chapter, you should be able to do the following:

- Describe world views of health and health care and models of behavioral change that underlie decision making about lifestyle changes to manage a therapeutic regimen
- Describe factors affecting behavioral change
- Assess the client who is experiencing problems in maintaining health when a therapeutic regimen requires alterations in lifestyle
- Write diagnoses for clients who need to manage a therapeutic regimen to maintain health
- Plan nursing interventions that assist the client in effectively managing lifestyle changes needed to implement a therapeutic regimen
- Evaluate the behavioral outcomes of lifestyle changes made to maintain health through a therapeutic regimen

Key Terms

action stage
contemplation stage
counseling
emic dimension
etic dimension
lifestyle
maintenance stage
perceived barriers
perceived benefits
perceived severity
perceived susceptibility
precontemplation stage
preparation stage
referral
self-efficacy
social support
termination stage

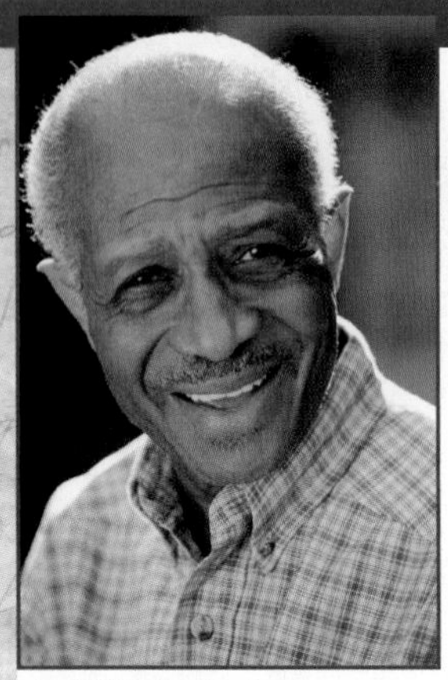
© 2007, JupiterImages Corporation.

Mr. Oscar Kitchen is a 69-year-old African American widower who keeps house for himself. His only living relatives are distant cousins living in another state. He receives a monthly Social Security check and a small retirement check from his former employment as a janitor in a public school.

Six weeks ago, Mr. Kitchen became short of breath and reluctantly went to a primary health care clinic. The nurse assessed that he had an irregular pulse and pitting edema of the lower extremities. The doctor prescribed digoxin (Lanoxin) for his heart and furosemide (Lasix), a diuretic. After the first week of medication, Mr. Kitchen felt better and decided to stop the medication. He missed his follow-up clinic appointment.

Two weeks ago, Mr. Kitchen once again became short of breath. He awakened soon after going to bed and was unable to breathe when lying supine. He slept very little during the night. Mr. Kitchen returned to the clinic the next morning.

The nurse discovered that Mr. Kitchen had discontinued medications on several occasions and that he continues to smoke. The nurse makes the diagnosis *Ineffective therapeutic regimen management* related to (1) knowledge deficit regarding current diagnosis, medications, and consequences of failure to comply with treatment, and (2) unwillingness to modify or change an unhealthy lifestyle. Other possible nursing diagnoses relating to lifestyle management are listed in the nursing diagnoses box.

KEY NURSING DIAGNOSES FOR HEALTH BEHAVIORS

Ineffective therapeutic regimen management (individuals, family, or community) A pattern in which the individual experiences or is at risk for experiencing difficulty integrating into daily living a program for treatment of illness and the sequelae of illness that meets specific health goals

Noncompliance (specify): The state in which an individual or group desires to comply, but factors are present that deter adherence to health-related advice given by health professionals

Effective therapeutic regimen management: A pattern in which the individual integrates into daily living a program for treatment of illness and its sequelae that is satisfactory for meeting health goals

Decisional conflict (specify): The state in which an individual or group experiences uncertainty about a course of action when the choice of options involves risk, loss, or challenge to values and beliefs

CONCEPTS OF BEHAVIORAL CHANGE

A person's **lifestyle** is a behavior or group of behaviors chosen by the person that may have a positive or a negative influence on health. A healthy lifestyle is evident when one avoids poor health habits, such as smoking and overeating, engages in good habits, such as achieving adequate nutrition and rest, and effectively manages a therapeutic regimen prescribed by a physician (Figure 20-1).

Lifestyle choices are connected to the incidence of heart disease, diabetes, and other chronic illnesses. Pender, Murdaugh, and Parsons (2006) believe that healthy lifestyle choices are the foundation for preventing chronic diseases. Health promotion, disease prevention, and monitoring of chronic illnesses are all part of improving life expectancy and maintaining health into old age.

The experience of an acute or chronic disease may demand changes in a person's lifestyle and behavioral patterns as part of management of the disease. For an acute illness, these changes are only temporary. For a chronic illness, permanent lifestyle changes are the only avenue to successful living with the illness.

However, helping a client change well-established health and lifestyle habits is challenging. The development of health habits begins in early childhood, and once developed, they become patterns of behavior that are difficult to change. To understand some of the complexities involved in changing lifestyle behaviors, you will need to reconsider the definitions of health in conjunction with theories about behavioral changes.

In Chapter 19, you learned that health may be defined from the multiple perspectives of the individual, the family, and the community. Furthermore, a person's definition of health stems in part from a personal worldview. This is true for the health care provider's definition as well. When client and provider have different worldviews, the result may be misunderstandings and differences in the selection of expected outcomes for health promotion and prevention (Spector, 2004).

Tripp-Reimer (1984) conceptualized health as two-dimensional, having an etic dimension and an emic dimension. **Etic dimension** refers to the objective interpretation of health by a scientifically trained practitioner. **Emic dimension** refers to an individual's or a social group's subjective perception and experiences related to health. Understanding health from the perspective of the client is critical to the development of health services (Jones, Zhang, Jaceldo-Siegl, & Meleis, 2002).

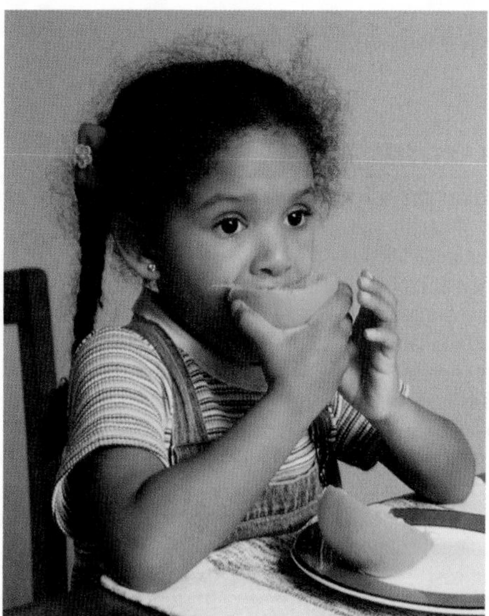

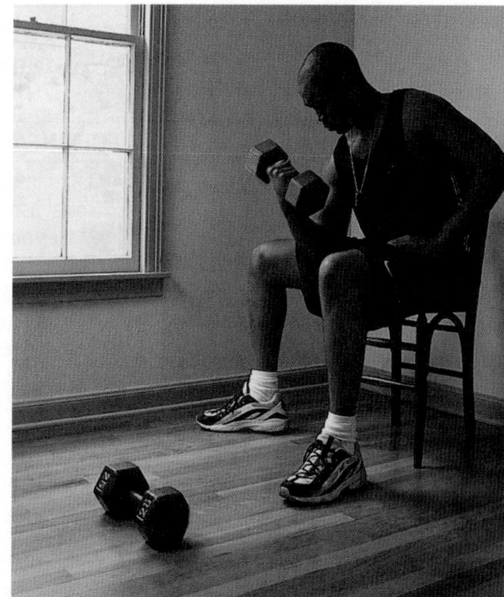

FIGURE 20-1 Lifestyle patterns associated with health include good nutrition and exercise.

To effectively help others, health care professionals must first understand the health and quality-of-life perspective of the client. A person's identity, role assignment, health, and opportunities in life are greatly influenced by such factors as sex, skin color, age, income, and culture. In addition, health-related quality of life is defined not only by the signs and symptoms of disease or its effects on survival but also by functional status, opportunity, and one's perception of relative well-being.

WORLDVIEWS OF HEALTH AND HEALTH CARE

Culture refers to the learned, shared, and transmitted values, beliefs, norms, and lifeways of a particular group that guides their thinking, decisions, and actions in patterned ways (Leininger, 2006). These ways of living, or lifestyles, reflect a person's understanding of health and health practices, as well as the person's view of illness. The experience of illness is determined in part by how illness is defined by one's culture, as well as by the individual or sick person (Spector, 2004).

All cultures have concepts of health and illness. They also have theories of disease causation, which may differ widely from group to group. These concepts and theories define the nature of illness, its treatment, and the type of relationships that should occur between client and health care provider. In addition, ethnic groups with different cultural histories have different approaches to reality, socialization, and health practices. Ideas and beliefs related to health and illness are integral parts of a culture's worldview (Table 20-1).

Table 20-1 Comparison of Nonwestern and Western Worldviews

NONWESTERN	WESTERN
Emphasizes group cooperation	Emphasizes individual competition
Values achievement as it reflects group	Values achievement for the individual
Values harmony with nature	Values mastery and control of nature
Sees time as relative	Adheres to rigid time schedule
Accepts affective expression	Limits affective expression
Embraces extended family	Prefers nuclear family
Thinks holistically	Thinks dualistically
Religion permeates culture	Holds religion distinct from other parts of culture
Accepts worldviews of other cultures	Feels own worldview is superior
Emphasizes social orientation	Emphasizes task orientation

Modified from Anderson, A. (1988). Cognitive styles and multicultural populations. *Journal of Teacher Education, 39*(1), 2-9.

A client's worldview is important because ideas related to health and illness originate from everyday experiences, family, social network, and the community. Most people seek advice from family, friends, or lay sources before seeking professional advice. Clark (2003) suggests that there are two domains of health care: the folk or generic form and the scientific or professional form (Table 20-2). In current American society, a blending of traditional and nontraditional medicine is becoming increasingly popular and is referred to as complementary and alternative therapies.

Table 20-2 Similarities and Differences Between Folk (Alternative) and Scientific Health Care Systems

	Differences	
SIMILARITIES	**FOLK HEALTH SYSTEM**	**SCIENTIFIC HEALTH SYSTEM**
• Employ similar diagnostic techniques, including observation and listening	• Takes into account the religious and social aspects of health	• Focuses primarily on the personal implications of disease
• Use verbal and nonverbal communication	• Makes no definite distinction between mental and physical illness	• Makes a definite distinction between mental and physical illness
• Engage in naming of illnesses and creation of positive expectations	• Oriented to the community	• Oriented to the individual
• Employ suggestion, interpretation, emotional support, and manipulation of the environment as therapeutic modalities	• Takes place in familiar surroundings	• Takes place in unfamiliar surroundings
	• Emphasizes humanistic care	• Emphasizes impersonal care
	• Emphasizes familiar, practical, and concrete behavior	• Emphasizes abstract concepts
• Use medicinal substances and employ some form of laying on of hands in the care of the sick	• Provides holistic care	• Provides fragmented care
• Based on asymmetric relationships between experts and laypersons	• Emphasizes caring	• Emphasizes curing
	• Stresses prevention	• Stresses diagnosis and treatment
• Provide an explanation of disease, a rationale for treatment, and a rationale for social and moral norms	• Emphasizes cultural support	• Does not emphasize cultural support
	• Is of moderate cost	• Is of high cost

From Clark, M. J. (2003). *Community health nursing: Caring for populations* (4th ed.). Upper Saddle River, NJ: Prentice Hall.

The folk medicine system classifies illnesses into two parts, natural and unnatural, and is common among some groups from Central America and in the United States among Mexican Americans, African Americans, and some southern white Americans (Giger & Davidhizar, 2004). Illnesses treated by folk medicine tend to be described as chronic, nonincapacitating maladies and those believed to be caused by supernatural agents (Clark, 2003). Natural illnesses in the folk medicine system relate to events that have to do with the world as God made it or as God intended it (Giger & Davidhizar, 2004). Unnatural illnesses relate to events that cause disharmony with nature. Therefore unnatural illnesses may be viewed as forces of evil or as events that interrupt the plan intended by God (Giger & Davidhizar, 2004).

Western medicine focuses a biopsychosocial, cultural, and spiritual approach to explain illness, with an emphasis on cure. Folk medicine focuses on personal data and experiences rather than on scientific persuasion (Giger & Davidhizar, 2004). Health care is provided in dyads (nurse-client or physician-client relationships), whereas in the folk medicine system, people tend to seek health care from multiperson health care networks, including relatives and nonrelatives (Giger & Davidhizar, 2004).

Clark (2003) suggests that many similarities exist between folk (alternative) and scientific health care systems. One such similarity is the way people initially approach a health problem. According to Kavanagh and Kennedy (1992), "Virtually no one runs for professional help at the first hint of a symptom. Traditional and folk remedies . . . might be used and a homemade diagnosis and etiology tentatively constructed. The next resort may be to popular or over-the-counter resources, which may or may not be associated with allopathic medicine. Finally, if relief is not in sight, professional consult is likely to be undertaken" (pp. 19-20).

A person's culturally acquired worldview of health and illness can be modified by social and economic conditions, with the economically disadvantaged forced to adopt lifeways that may be more a product of poverty than of culture.

MODELS OF BEHAVIORAL CHANGE

In addition to using culturally specific lifestyle knowledge to promote health, you need to understand theories of behavioral change to explain and predict health-related behaviors. However, these models were not developed as culturally specific models, so no one model is likely to explain the behaviors and belief systems of all specific cultural groups.

Theory of Reasoned Action. The theory of reasoned action is a human behavior framework designed to explain a person's intention to perform a behavior. The theory is based on the assumption that people are reasonable and, in deciding which actions to take, systematically process and use the information available to them (Poss, 2001). The theory further assumes that behavior is totally under voluntary control and that barriers to performance of the intended behavior do not exist (Pender et al., 2006).

The theory of reasoned action does not rely solely on facts and logic. It also considers the relations between beliefs, attitudes, and intention in determining behavior. To change or reinforce a given intention, the person must change or strengthen the attitude toward performing that behavior.

The theory further holds that a behavioral intention is determined both by attitudes toward the specific behavior and by subjective norms (what others think) regarding the behavior. Thus people intend to perform a behavior when they evaluate that behavior positively and when they believe significant others think they should perform it. Compelling as it is, the theory of reasoned action is, by itself, not sufficient to explain health behaviors.

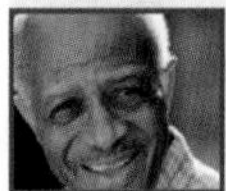

Remember Mr. Kitchen? A reasonable person might be expected to associate shortness of breath with smoking, to see that the medication caused a decrease in leg swelling, and to take the actions necessary to improve health. Why do you think Mr. Kitchen stopped taking his medication and continued to smoke?

Transtheoretical Model for Behavioral Change. The transtheoretical model for behavioral change provides stages of change in behavior. People must change their behavior to make major reductions in risks for chronic disease. Prochaska et al. (1994) describe six stages of behavioral change: precontemplation, contemplation, preparation, action, maintenance, and termination. People move through these stages as they consider, and then act on, reducing risky behaviors. Assessing a client's stage of behavioral change can help you determine appropriate interventions to assist the person in reducing risky behavior.

In the **precontemplation stage,** the person does not intend to change a high-risk behavior in the foreseeable future (the next 6 months), primarily because he or she is unaware of the long-term consequences of the behavior. Furthermore, the person may feel demoralized about his or her inability to change and defensive because of social pressures to change (Prochaska et al., 1994). Although unconvinced of the need for change, the person may agree to make changes under pressure from family and friends. These changes are usually minimal and last only as long as pressure continues to be applied.

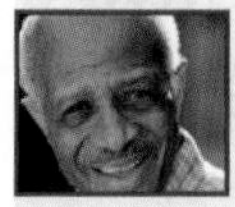

Do you think that Mr. Kitchen was in the precontemplation stage at the time of his first visit to the clinic? Why or why not?

In the **contemplation stage,** the person intends to change within the next 6 months. However, despite this good intention, the person usually stays in this stage for at least 2 years. He tells himself that he is going to change, but he keeps putting it off. The person is ambivalent about changing and usually substitutes thinking for acting (Prochaska et al., 1994).

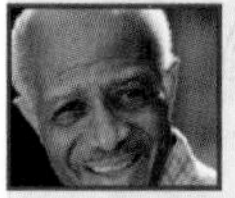

Because Mr. Kitchen's health problem had a sudden onset and required immediate behavior change, it is not likely that this stage initially applied to him. Under what circumstances might this stage apply to him in the future?

In the **preparation stage,** the person intends to take action in the very near future, usually within the next month. This stage has both intention and action. The person usually develops a plan of action and may take small steps toward behavioral change. Furthermore, the person evaluates the advantages and the disadvantages of the risky behavior and decides that the disadvantages outweigh the advantages (Prochaska et al., 1994).

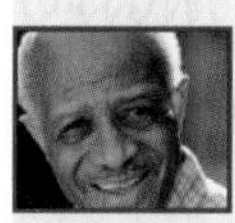

Could this stage apply to Mr. Kitchen and, if so, how?

In the **action stage,** the person changes risky behaviors and the context of the behavior (environment, experience) and makes significant efforts to reach goals. This is the busiest but most risky stage because of the chance for relapse. The person is considered to be in the action stage if the behavior is changed for 1 day to 6 months. This stage offers the most external recognition because others become aware of the effort that the person is making toward the change.

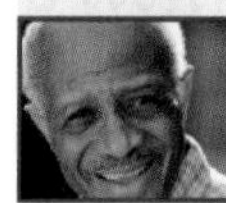

When was Mr. Kitchen in this stage? What factors in his life will influence whether he remains in this stage after the second clinic visit or returns to an earlier stage?

The **maintenance stage** takes place during the 6 months after the person changes the high-risk behavior. This stage is characterized by a period of continuing change, with fewer mechanisms needed to prevent relapse. However, the time frame for continuous maintenance is 5 years. Prochaska et al. (1994) discovered that people must continuously abstain from the high-risk behavior for 5 years to prevent the fear of relapse. For example, they found that, even after 12 months of continuous abstinence from smoking, 37% of people will return to regular smoking. After 5 years of continuous abstinence, only 7% will return to regular smoking.

In the **termination stage,** the person is no longer tempted to engage in old behavior. He has confidence in no longer being tempted by previous situations.

Most people go through some or all of these stages several times before conquering an addiction, despite professional help. Movement through the stages occurs in a spiral pattern as the person moves backward into previous stages and forward through later stages. The upward and forward spiral movement toward elimination of the behavior occurs as the person learns from previous experience. The greater the number of successes the person has over time in this spiral movement, the greater the possibility of sustained change.

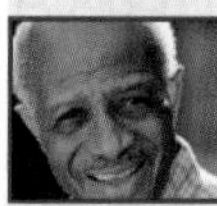

When the nurse expresses her concern to Mr. Kitchen, he pats her on the hand and says, "Don't you worry none, the good Lord will take care of me." Which of these stages describe Mr. Kitchen's frame of mind concerning his health behaviors? Are any of these stages relevant?

Health Belief Model. The health belief model is a health protection model that provides a framework to explain why some people take specific actions to avoid or treat illness, whereas others fail to protect themselves (Stanhope & Lancaster, 2004; Pender et al., 2006). The model has been used to predict and explain health behavior on the basis of value-expectancy theory and Kurt Lewin's cognitive theory.

Lewin is a cognitive theorist who conceptualized that certain aspects of a person's life space have negative, positive, or neutral values. He believed that disease has a negative value and, as a result, exerts a force to move the person toward health behaviors. He also believed that behavior is a function of the subjective value of an outcome and of the subjective expectation that a particular action will achieve that outcome (Rosenstock, 1974).

The health belief model states that the probability that a person will take appropriate health care actions depends on the person's value of health, perceptions about disease, and perceived threat of disease. In addition, action is motivated by perception about the medical team and therapy plans, past experience, contact with risk factors, level of participation in regular health care, life aspirations, and factors in the environment.

Four components of the health belief model have been identified: perceived susceptibility, perceived severity, perceived benefits, and perceived barriers (Rosenstock, 1974). People will take action to ward off, to screen for, or to control ill health if they regard themselves as susceptible to the condition, if they believe it to have potentially serious consequences, or if they believe that actions available to them would reduce either their susceptibility to or the severity of the condition. Action is more likely if they also believe that the anticipated barriers to (or costs of) taking the action are outweighed by its benefits.

Perceived susceptibility refers to a person's subjective perception of the risk of contracting a health condition. For example, with cigarette smoking, the person might not perceive the risk of getting lung cancer. **Perceived severity** refers to the perceived seriousness of contracting an illness or leaving it untreated. In cigarette smoking, the person might not perceive that serious personal harm will occur as a result of smoking. **Perceived benefits** refers to the person's perceptions and beliefs about the effectiveness of the recommended actions in preventing the health threat. **Perceived barriers** refers to perceived negative aspects of a health action or the perceived impediments to undertaking the recommended behaviors (Rosenstock, 1974). Key components of the health belief model can be found in Box 20-1.

Self-efficacy is a central concept in the health belief model. **Self-efficacy** is defined as the conviction that one can successfully execute the behavior required to produce the outcomes (Rosenstock, 1974, p. 40). Bandura (1977) believes that efficacy expectancies differ from outcome expectancies in that efficacy expectancies refer to one's capacity to perform the behavior, whereas outcome expectancies refer to beliefs about what will happen as a result of engaging in the behavior. For example, for a person to quit smoking, the person must believe that cessation will benefit his or her health (outcome expectation) and also that he or she is capable of quitting (efficacy expectation). According to Bandura, self-efficacy judgments are based on four major sources of information: the individual's own performance accomplishments, vicarious observation of the performance of others, the influence of external persuasion and social influence, and states of emotional arousal. A person's success with coping in a variety of high-risk situations increases his or her sense of self-efficacy and decreases the probability of relapse.

Health Promotion Model. The health promotion model, developed by Pender et al. (2006), describes the multidimensional nature of a person's interactions with the environment in the pursuit of health. This model combines nursing and behavioral science perspectives with factors that impact health behaviors. Unlike the health belief model, the health promotion model does not rely on "personal threats." The model uses constructs from the value-expectancy theory and the social cognitive theory.

The value-expectancy theory suggests that behavior is rational and economical. This means that people will not waste their time and resources on behavior changes that have little value to them (Pender et al., 2006). Furthermore, people will not invest in a goal that they believe is impossible to achieve. The motivational significance of successfully changing behavior is based on the person having some past experiences with success. In other words, the person must have some confidence in the achievement of the goal. This is why, for some peo-

BOX 20-1 *Key Components of the Health Belief Model*

THREAT
- Perceived susceptibility to an illness (or acceptance of a diagnosis)
- Perceived seriousness of the condition

OUTCOME EXPECTATIONS
- Perceived benefits of specified action
- Perceived barriers to taking that action

EFFICACY EXPECTATIONS
- Conviction about one's ability to carry out a recommended action (self-efficacy)
- Sociodemographic factors (such as education, age, sex, race, ethnicity, and income) are believed to influence behavior indirectly by affecting perceived threat, outcome expectations, and efficacy expectations.

From Rosenstock, J. (1974). Historical origins of the health belief model. *Health Education Monograph, 2*(4), 328-335.

ple, achieving small steps is more successful than attempting major change (e.g., cutting down on the number of cigarettes rather than quitting).

Social cognitive theory focuses on the person's beliefs interacting with environmental influences (Pender et al., 2006). Behavior is not solely driven by inner forces or automatically shaped by external stimuli. Rather, there is an interaction between cognitive factors, personal factors, and environmental events.

Beliefs about oneself formed through self-observation and self-reflective thought have the greatest potential for influencing behavior. These beliefs, according to Pender et al., include self-attribution, self-evaluation, and self-efficacy. Perceived self-efficacy "is a judgment of one's ability to carry out a particular course of action. The greater the perceived self-efficacy, the more persistent individuals will be in achieving the behavior outcome" (Pender et al., 2006).

FACTORS AFFECTING BEHAVIORAL CHANGE

In helping a client make behavioral changes to manage health, you need to understand possible areas that can influence the relationship with the client. Some areas are open to the influence of the nurse and the client, whereas others are not.

COMMUNICATION

Impaired verbal skills or language differences prevent a client from expressing health needs or communicating effectively with health care professionals. Comprehension and meaning vary among cultures. Words and their meanings carry different nuances and significances, depending on a person's culture, values, and beliefs. Language barriers, whether from foreign languages or varying dialects of the same language, can result in anxiety, fear, and frustration for people who need to communicate, especially when health care is required. Because communication involves body language along with verbal language, the meaning of body position and expression can further facilitate or impede communication. A person's values regarding what personal thoughts and feelings are appropriate to share with others also affect communication.

A client's inability to provide a health care provider with accurate information may result in erroneous or ineffective treatment of illness or disease. Likewise, a client's ability to communicate with health care providers can improve the treatment of illness—and the client's satisfaction with treatment. For example, a client who is confused is likely to be a poor historian about the onset of an acute urinary tract infection or may be completely unable to provide a history of symptoms. This could delay diagnosis of the infection and initiation of antimicrobial therapy.

COGNITION AND PERCEPTION

Cognition is the systematic way in which a person thinks, reasons, and uses language. Perception of information includes sensing and interpreting stimuli from the external and internal environments. The person's cognitive-perceptual functioning refers to the ability to understand and follow directions, retain information, make decisions, solve problems, and use language appropriately. Cognitive-perceptual impairments include limitations of the senses (such as blindness or deafness) or brain dysfunction (such as memory loss or confusion). These impairments may reduce the level of knowledge a person acquires about a health condition or prescribed treatment.

Inability to make deliberate and thoughtful judgments can create a delay in seeking professional assistance. Signs and symptoms may not be understood by the client as being relevant to the disease. Health education or discharge instructions may be misinterpreted instead of being assimilated and remembered, leading to a failure to implement them and ultimately to inadequate health maintenance or exacerbation of disease.

AGE AND DEVELOPMENTAL LEVEL

The age and developmental level of the client influence health beliefs and practices. A person's health status can be significantly altered by unachieved developmental tasks. Inadequate education or resources regarding nutrition, safety, fitness, or health protection practices during childhood or adolescence can adversely affect adult health.

Age may also significantly affect a person's ability to manage and maintain health. The very young and the very old are at greatest risk for inadequate health maintenance. For example, infants and very young children rely on parents and guardians for the management of health, whereas school-age children can be taught to manage some health-related self-care activities. Older adults may experience changes that may negatively affect health maintenance. For example, loss of teeth may impede proper nutrition, arthritis may limit the ability to exercise, and slowed cognitive processes may affect safety practices, cognitive and perceptual abilities, and the ability to solve problems and conceptualize. In addition, a decline in visual acuity, hearing, touch, and taste occurs with increasing age.

Advancing age increases susceptibility to certain health risks. For example, the risk of cardiovascular disease increases with age for both sexes. The risks of birth defects and complications of pregnancy increase among pregnant women over age 35. Age-related risk factors increase in association with other risk factors, such as family history and personal habits. For example, a man at age 60 who has smoked for 40 or more years is at greater risk of developing lung cancer than a man at age 30 who has smoked for 10 years.

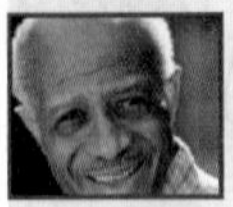

What health risks would you anticipate for Mr. Kitchen, who is 69 years old?

LIFESTYLE AND HABITS

Lifestyle and health are closely related. Changes in one usually create changes in the other. The family plays a critical role in the development of health-promoting and health-protective behaviors.

Health-related decisions regarding diet and leisure activities affect all family members, with health practices of children and adolescents influenced by actions of adults. Those behaviors that are most satisfying are retained and reinforced and largely determine their pattern for health maintenance. Inappropriate health habits, such as overeating, lack of exercise, use of alcohol and tobacco, and ineffective coping patterns may also be established in early childhood and adolescence and carried through adulthood.

Health practices and behaviors can have positive or negative effects on health. Practices with potential negative effects are labeled risk factors. Overeating or poor nutrition, insufficient rest and sleep, poor personal hygiene, smoking, alcohol or drug abuse, and activities involving a threat of injury, such as skydiving, mountain climbing, or bungee jumping, are all examples of risk factors. Some habits are risk factors for specific diseases—for example, skin tanning increases the risk of skin cancer, and being overweight increases the risk of cardiovascular disease.

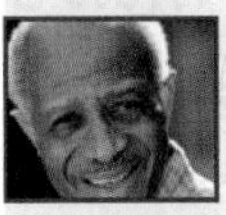

Does Mr. Kitchen have any risks to health that arise from his lifestyle and habits?

ECONOMIC RESOURCES

Economic factors can affect a client's level of health by influencing how or at what point the client enters the health care system, or the ability to comply with a prescribed treatment plan. People who have fewer economic resources are more likely to have barriers to health care, with the result of being underserved. Government-sponsored health insurance programs such as Medicare try to provide a baseline level of insurance for those over age 65, and state-sponsored programs such as Medicaid assist those who meet income guidelines. Nonetheless, a segment of the population continues to be uninsured or underinsured, making economic resources (or their lack) a key factor that has an impact on health care.

People who have health insurance have easier access to health care with less financial burden than those who do not, increasing the likelihood of seeking early treatment for symptoms. People who have no health insurance may need to fulfill basic needs, such as food, rather than obtaining health care, or may seek treatment at later stages of a health problem. Access to health care facilities generally requires transportation, which may be unaffordable or unavailable. Some people may not be able to afford the loss of wages if they leave work for health care appointments with health care providers.

A person's compliance with a treatment plan designed to maintain or improve health is also affected by economic status. A person who has a high utility bill, a large family, and a low income must give higher priority to the greater good of food and shelter for everyone rather than to costly drugs, treatments, or special diets for one family member.

Crowded living conditions contribute to an increased incidence of illness and disease because of the close proximity of people, the sharing of utensils and belongings, and poor sanitation. Isolation, language or communication difficulties, seasonal work occupations, and migration patterns could also adversely affect a person's health status.

Compared with the poor population, middle-class people work in more protected jobs, are better educated, and are more able to seek treatment for minor illnesses. Members of the upper-income group are able to obtain assistance more easily in promoting and maintaining health.

CULTURAL VALUES AND BELIEFS

Cultural background influences individual beliefs, values, and customs, including entry into the health care system and personal health practices (Box 20-2). The range of health definitions, practices, and beliefs about prevention manifested by various ethnic groups is infinite. There are variations in health definitions, beliefs, and practices even within a given ethnic group.

Action Alert! Treat the basic needs of all human beings, regardless of cultural background, the same. How people seek to meet these needs is influenced by their culture and their personal beliefs. Each person is the best source of how he or she would like to be treated.

Spiritual values and beliefs are integrated into all other dimensions of human beings—physical, mental, psychological, and social. The spiritual dimension helps a person find meaning in all aspect of life, including suffering, pain, illness, and death. Religious beliefs can influence lifestyle choices, attitudes, and feelings about illness, and these may conflict with interventions to promote, maintain, or restore health. These conflicts are often revealed when clients describe the course of an illness, refuse recommended medical intervention, or refuse to comply with treatment modalities for spiritual reasons.

BOX 20-2 *Cross-Cultural Care*

Caring for an African American Client

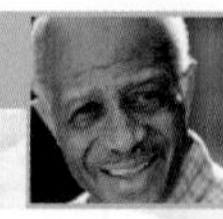

Oscar Kitchen is an African American man who ascribes to the traditional definition of health held by many African Americans. Like people of many other cultures, African Americans have a unique way of classifying illness that aids in diagnosis and treatment. Likewise, many beliefs and values held by African Americans can influence health behaviors and lifestyle. Some of these beliefs include the following:

- Health as harmony with nature, feeling good (no pain), ability to engage in activities of daily living and go to work
- Illness as feeling bad, inability to work or engage in activities of daily living, and disharmony of mind, body, and spirit
- Prayer and a well-balanced diet as helpful in avoiding illness and recovering from illness
- Group orientation
- Spirituality as an influence on perception of health and illness
- Close personal space
- Strong family and kinship ties
- Family resources as a source of support rather than outside assistance
- Health values and beliefs that vary with age, socioeconomic status, and location (rural/urban)
- Dietary pattern that reflects many cultures
- Home remedies accepted for their effectiveness, decreased cost, and lack of segregation and racism that can be found in formal health care
- Distrust of "the system"

During a focused assessment, Ms. Emanuel, the nurse, engaged Mr. Kitchen in a conversation about his health during the past few weeks. He informed Ms. Emanuel he had been fine, "just a little short of breath," which had begun the day before. He revealed that he had stopped taking his medications because he was "feeling fine and no longer needed it."

ROLES AND RELATIONSHIPS

Social relationships within the family, social group, work setting, and community are significant to one's well-being. The inability to engage in satisfying relationships or to feel comfortable in social interactions may lead to social isolation. Social isolation may prevent the seeking of preventive health services. Conflicting role expectations within the family, social group, and work setting produce stress. Communication patterns, decision-making skills, feelings of self-worth and autonomy, and perceived support will influence patterns of health maintenance.

COPING AND STRESS TOLERANCE

Stress can affect health and well-being in any of the adaptive modes: physiological, psychological, spiritual, developmental, and social. In the physical dimension, stress can have a negative affect on homeostasis. In the emotional dimension, stress can threaten the way a person normally perceives information and solves problems. In the social dimension, stress can threaten interpersonal relationships, the support received from others, and a sense of belonging. In the spiritual dimension, stress can threaten a person's view of life and attitude toward a supreme being. In essence, stress can affect a person in all areas of basic human needs.

WORKPLACE AND ENVIRONMENTAL CONDITIONS

The environment has many influences on health and illness. The physical environment in which a person works or lives can increase the likelihood that certain illnesses will occur. Industrial workers exposed to certain chemicals are more likely to develop some kinds of cancer and other diseases. In some environments, high noise levels, increased emotional stress, environmental pollution, violence, or overcrowding are risk factors.

ASSESSMENT

A thorough assessment of health, attitudes, cultural beliefs, and health practices is critical to developing an effective health promotion plan for your clients (Pender et al., 2006). Collect information about nutrition, elimination, rest and sleep, activity and exercise, and hygiene. Patterns of psychological health can be determined by assessing coping, interactions, and self-concept. Sociocultural health can be assessed through cultural practices, recreation, and significant relationships. Religious beliefs and values are determinants of spiritual health.

GENERAL ASSESSMENT OF HEALTH PROMOTION

The health history may be the most important part of the database. Cues from the nursing history can alert you to traits that increase the client's vulnerability to a certain condition or disease. In addition to the health history, you can identify the client's risk factors by using health risk appraisal tools.

Health Practices. Pender et al. (2006) describe several components of health assessment that focus on wellness, including physical fitness evaluation, health risk appraisal, social support systems, and lifestyle assessment.

Physical fitness evaluation is divided into skill-related physical fitness and health-related physical fitness. Skill-related fitness relates to agility, speed, power, and reaction time, the qualities that contribute to successful athletic performance. Health-related fitness relates to cardiorespiratory endurance, muscular strength and endurance, body composition, and flexibility, the qualities found to contribute to general health (Pender et al., 2006). Health-related fitness also includes qualities that contribute to a person's general well-being.

Health risk appraisal includes assessment data that provide clients with essential information about health threats from hereditary factors, lifestyle, and family history (Pender et al., 2006). Risk factors include genetics, age, biological characteristics, personal health habits, lifestyle, and environment.

The health risk appraisal provides an average indication of risk. Clients can provide information regarding their own health experience and what improvements they could make in their mortality profile if they adopted more positive behaviors (Pender et al., 2006).

Social support systems are important in enhancing successful coping and promoting comfortable and effective living. These factors reduce stress and improve health and well-being. **Social support** can be defined as the subjective feeling of belonging, or being accepted, loved, esteemed, valued, and needed for oneself, not for what one can do for others (Pender et al., 2006). All people need some type of social support, but the amount and type vary on the basis of the person's age, situation, and personal desires. Types of social support that have been clearly documented in the literature include emotional support, informational support, family support, and instrumental support, which includes assistance with specific tasks (Pender et al., 2006).

When obtaining assessment data related to cultural beliefs and attitudes, follow these four basic principles (Clark, 2003):

- View all cultures in the context in which they developed.
- Examine underlying premises for culturally determined beliefs and behaviors.
- Interpret the meaning and purpose of behavior in the context of the specific culture.
- Recognize the potential for intercultural variation.

Lifestyle assessment is closely related to assessment of cultural beliefs and attitudes. Assess life events, dietary patterns, and health habits. "The desired outcomes of health assessment are to (1) identify health assets, (2) identify health-related lifestyle strengths, (3) determine key health-related beliefs, (4) identify health beliefs and health behaviors that put the client at risk, and (5) determine how the client wants to change to improve the quality of life" (Pender et al., 2006).

> ***Action Alert!*** Base risk appraisal on current referent group (personal risk age) and the predicted improvement in mortality profile if they were to adopt more positive health-promoting behaviors. A total risk for developing any disease increases on the basis of the number of risk factors present and the intensity of each risk factor.

Illness Practices. A person experiencing a health problem may be told to make adjustments in many aspects of day-to-day living. These changes may be for treatments to restore optimal health, prevention of additional health problems, or early detection of other health concerns. Your assessment should include identifying factors and cues that would indicate ineffective management.

Factors to be considered in a therapeutic regimen include the following:

- The client's knowledge of the disease, including severity and prognosis
- Disease history and previous treatment patterns (including the number of previous admissions for acute care)
- Previous history of accessing health care resources
- Treatment and preventive measures
- Pattern of adhering to prescribed therapeutic regimen
- Factors that prevent full implementation of or adherence to recommended therapeutic regimen
- Missing knowledge or information that prevents comprehension of the recommended treatment program and its subsequent implementation
- The extent to which adherence to the treatment program has altered the person's life and relationships

In addition, attention should focus on financial resources, health care resources, presence of sensory deficit, and expressed feelings regarding illnesses or disease process.

Knowledge of Disease. Knowledge of the disease process includes the client's understanding of the onset of symptoms, causes and consequences of the current condition, and level of overall health knowledge. Solicit the following information: the effects of this illness on present health, personal ideas about the cause of the symptoms, factors that aggravate or alleviate the symptoms, how the present illness affects the performance of role expectations and activities of daily living, and the health promotion and illness prevention activities engaged in since onset.

Disease History. The length of time of the disease process and the frequency of exacerbation of symptoms are cues to the extent to which the client has been able to manage the therapeutic regimen. Soliciting and recording this information in the client's own words will give vital clues when clustered with data collected during the assessment of cognitive-perceptual abilities.

History of Accessing Health Care Resources. A person's perception of health and illness, culture and spiritual beliefs, roles, relationships, and support systems are among the many factors that influence the person's use of health care resources. Each person has a personal definition of health. It may be defined as "good" even though the person has hypertension or symptoms of a respiratory infection. The extent to which a condition has a negative impact will influence the decision to seek health care or engage in health maintenance practices.

The attitudes and behaviors of significant others in the family, social groups, place of employment, or community have an impact on the person's beliefs and actions. When significant others express apathy or distrust in a particular treatment regimen or health promotion practices, the client may have difficulty adhering to the regimen. The family's sociocultural beliefs influence not only how a client perceives illness but also from whom assistance is sought and what types of treatment will be considered most advantageous.

FOCUSED ASSESSMENT FOR *INEFFECTIVE THERAPEUTIC REGIMEN MANAGEMENT*

Defining Characteristics. Several subjective factors may emerge from the health history that suggest that the client is having difficulty managing a therapeutic regimen. The initial defining characteristic is the person's or family member's verbal expression of a desire to adhere to the therapeutic program. Subsequently, the client may report difficulty in carrying out proposed activities or in making choices to incorporate the activities of the regimen into daily living, or the client may report making no attempt to incorporate these activities into patterns of daily living. The difficulty may reflect the person's lifestyle, work patterns, or roles and relationships.

An exacerbation of symptoms is an objective characteristic in making this diagnosis. Failure to seek out health care and related support, to make needed appointments, or to keep appointments would be additional defining characteristics.

Related Factors. Related factors contributing to the diagnosis of *Ineffective therapeutic regimen management* include those related to aspects of the treatment regimen, to the health care system, and to personal factors. Factors related to treatment include the complexity of the therapeutic regimen, negative side effects, the financial cost, and the complexity of maneuvering through the health care delivery system. Therapeutic regimens may be complex technological advancements that, although they are useful devices for managing health problems, can create confusion for the clients who must use them. Many electronic devices are used in the home to assist the client in monitoring blood sugar level, blood pressure, urinalysis, and so on. The client's cognitive-perceptual level must be assessed to detect cognitive or sensory deficits that may contribute to the inability to incorporate a complex therapeutic regimen.

Access to care is a factor in the health care system. Some clients enter the system easily through physician's offices, clinics, or hospital emergency departments. Other clients experience difficulties in entering the system because of confusion or unfamiliarity with the various agencies or because of low income status. Some geographical locations lack adequate health care resources.

Fragmentation of services is a second factor within the system. Specialization and technological advancement throughout the health care system have led to fragmentation in the provision of care. During the course of an illness, a person may be seen by several health care providers that treat, prescribe, and initiate separate health maintenance programs, each of which requires a follow-up visit. This process may overwhelm the client and family and lead to failure to initiate any or all health maintenance activities.

Personal factors also affect a client's adherence to a therapeutic regimen. Individual decisional conflict, family conflict, or excessive demands on the client or family can lead to failure to incorporate the planned program into activities of daily living. A client's unrealistic expectations of care by family members can produce conflict or role strain, which can lead to a breakdown in communication as well as anger.

You must give attention to the premise that a person's health beliefs, locus of control, and self-efficacy influence motivation, learning, and the capacity for behavioral changes needed to manage a therapeutic regimen and maintain health. By assessing the client's health beliefs, you can determine the extent to which the client's ineffective management of a therapeutic regimen relates to mistrust of the regimen, a feeling that the health problem is not serious, or a belief that he or she is not susceptible to disease. Assess the client's level of self-efficacy by investigating the level of personal confidence the client has about initiating proposed activities and reaching desired outcomes. Remember that the perceived value of the proposed therapeutic program will influence the client's willingness to follow it. If the client believes an activity will be very effective in preventing the development of a health problem, compliance is more likely. In addition, the perceived benefits of the activities, when weighed against the adverse reactions and the cost, should be assessed as a causative factor.

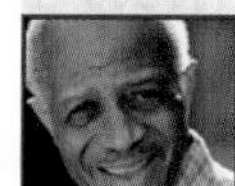

What questions would you ask Mr. Kitchen to determine his problems with adhering to his therapeutic regimen? Do you think knowledge is a factor? Cost? The need to change his usual pattern of living? His beliefs about health?

DIAGNOSIS

When the objective of care is primarily that the client learns behaviors to improve health maintenance, cluster data (Table 20-3) to help select a diagnosis from the list of related health maintenance diagnoses. The list includes *Health-seeking behaviors, Ineffective health maintenance, Noncompliance, Deficient knowledge, Decisional conflict,* and *Ineffective therapeutic regimen management.* Related or contributing factors that influence the health status change are listed in Box 20-3.

The diagnosis *Health-seeking behaviors* is appropriate when a person is in a state of wellness but is seeking ways to achieve a higher level of wellness. A person of normal weight, for example, may wish to improve his or her physical fitness and stamina and may verbalize his or her unfamiliarity with community resources or a lack of knowledge about how to achieve this goal. The defining characteristics in making this diagnosis include an expressed or observed desire to seek information for health promotion (Carpenito, 2005).

Ineffective health maintenance is appropriate for a person who expresses a desire to change an unhealthy lifestyle.

Examples of an unhealthy lifestyle are excessive dissatisfaction with occupation; lack of exercise; failure to be refreshed after rest; diet high in fat, salt, simple carbohydrates; tobacco use; obesity; excessive alcohol use; and insufficient social support. Because individuals are responsible for their own health, *Ineffective health maintenance* represents a diagnosis that the individual is motivated to treat. This nursing diagnosis is applicable to both well and ill populations. The assessment for *Ineffective health maintenance* includes both subjective and objective data defining general health status and data on related factors, including familial and environmental risk factors and preventive health activities (Carpenito, 2005). This diagnosis can also be used for a client who must alter health maintenance activities to manage an illness.

The diagnosis *Noncompliance* is used for a state in which an individual or group desires to comply but factors are present that deter adherence to health-related advice given by health professionals. Compliance depends on a variety of factors, including the person's motivation, perception of vulnerability, and beliefs about controlling or preventing illness; environmental variables; quality of health instruction; and the ability to access resources. Because each individual has the freedom to make choices, do not use *Noncompliance* to describe a person who has made an informed autonomous decision not to comply. In this situation, assess for and validate that all required elements for an informed consent are present (Carpenito, 2005).

Table 20-3 Clustering Data to Make a Nursing Diagnosis

Health Behaviors

DATA CLUSTER	DIAGNOSIS
An 83-year-old diabetic man lives by himself and prepares his own food when he is feeling well. He feels that family members have abandoned him because they are busy with their own families and jobs. He self-administers insulin when he thinks about it or is feeling "bad."	*Ineffective therapeutic regimen management* related to feelings of abandonment and isolation
A 20-year-old woman has a history of obesity since childhood. She desperately wants to be thin to please her boyfriend. She smokes two packs of cigarettes per day to decrease appetite. She eats a lot of fried and spicy foods and goes on "crash" diets to lose weight quickly. She frequently states, "I can't ever seem to lose weight."	*Ineffective health maintenance* related to poor self-esteem interfering with health care regimen
A 42-year-old woman has four children and works part-time outside the home. She feels no need for exercise because she is always chasing the kids around. She loves to bake desserts for her family. She would like to regain her prepregnancy figure but states that she "isn't ready to diet or exercise."	*Ineffective therapeutic regimen management* related to altered self-concept and resistance to adopting healthy behaviors at this time
A 50-year-old man is head of a household that includes his spouse, two children, and his aging mother. He has just been informed that he will be let go from his job because the company must show a profit. He immediately made plans to change the family's lifestyle and health care standards because there will be no health insurance. He feels particularly bad because his mother and children will suffer from the lack of money to purchase food and medicines.	*Ineffective health maintenance* related to unexpected change in financial status

BOX 20-3 ***Contributing or Related Factors for Nursing Diagnoses***

INEFFECTIVE HEALTH MAINTENANCE
- Information misinterpretation
- Lack of motivation
- Lack of education
- Lack of access to adequate health care services
- Inadequate health teaching

HEALTH-SEEKING BEHAVIORS
- Anticipated role changes, such as marriage, parenthood, retirement
- Lack of knowledge

DEFICIENT KNOWLEDGE
- Lack of exposure
- Lack of recall
- Cognitive limitation
- Misinterpretation

NONCOMPLIANCE
- Impaired ability to perform, for example, because of poor memory or motor or sensory deficits
- Side effect of therapy
- Financial issues
- Nonsupportive family
- Lack of access to health care

DECISIONAL CONFLICT
- Risk versus benefits of therapeutic regimen
- Lack of relevant information, or information is confusing
- Conflict with personal values or beliefs

INEFFECTIVE THERAPEUTIC REGIMEN MANAGEMENT
- Complexity of the therapeutic regimen
- Financial cost of regimen
- Complexity of health care system
- Side effect of therapy
- Insufficient knowledge
- Cognitive deficit
- Mistrust of health care system or therapeutic regimen

Deficient knowledge is best used when the client lacks knowledge about the relationship between an unhealthy behavior or habit and the use of community resources to assist in changing it. Use this diagnosis when the knowledge deficiency is the direct cause or a potential cause of a problem. Defining characteristics that may be exhibited by the client include verbalizing a deficiency of knowledge or skill (e.g., a request for information), expressing inaccurate perception of health status, or failure to correctly perform a desired or prescribed health behavior (Carpenito, 2005).

Decisional conflict is the state in which an individual or group experiences uncertainty about a course of action when the choice of options involves risk, loss, or challenge to personal life values. Many situations can contribute to decisional conflict, particularly those that involve complex medical interventions of great risk. Defining characteristics for making this diagnosis include verbalized uncertainty about choices, verbalization of undesired consequences of alternative actions being considered, vacillation between alternative choices, and delayed decision making (Carpenito, 2005).

The diagnosis *Ineffective therapeutic regimen management* describes individuals or families who are experiencing difficulty in achieving positive outcomes. Individuals or families experiencing a variety of health problems, acute or chronic, are usually faced with a treatment program that require changes in previous functioning or lifestyles. When an individual is faced with a complex regimen to follow or has compromised functioning that impedes successful management, the diagnosis *Risk for ineffective therapeutic regimen management* is appropriate (Carpenito, 2005).

Use care to differentiate between *Ineffective therapeutic regimen management, Noncompliance,* and *Ineffective health maintenance* (Figure 20-2).

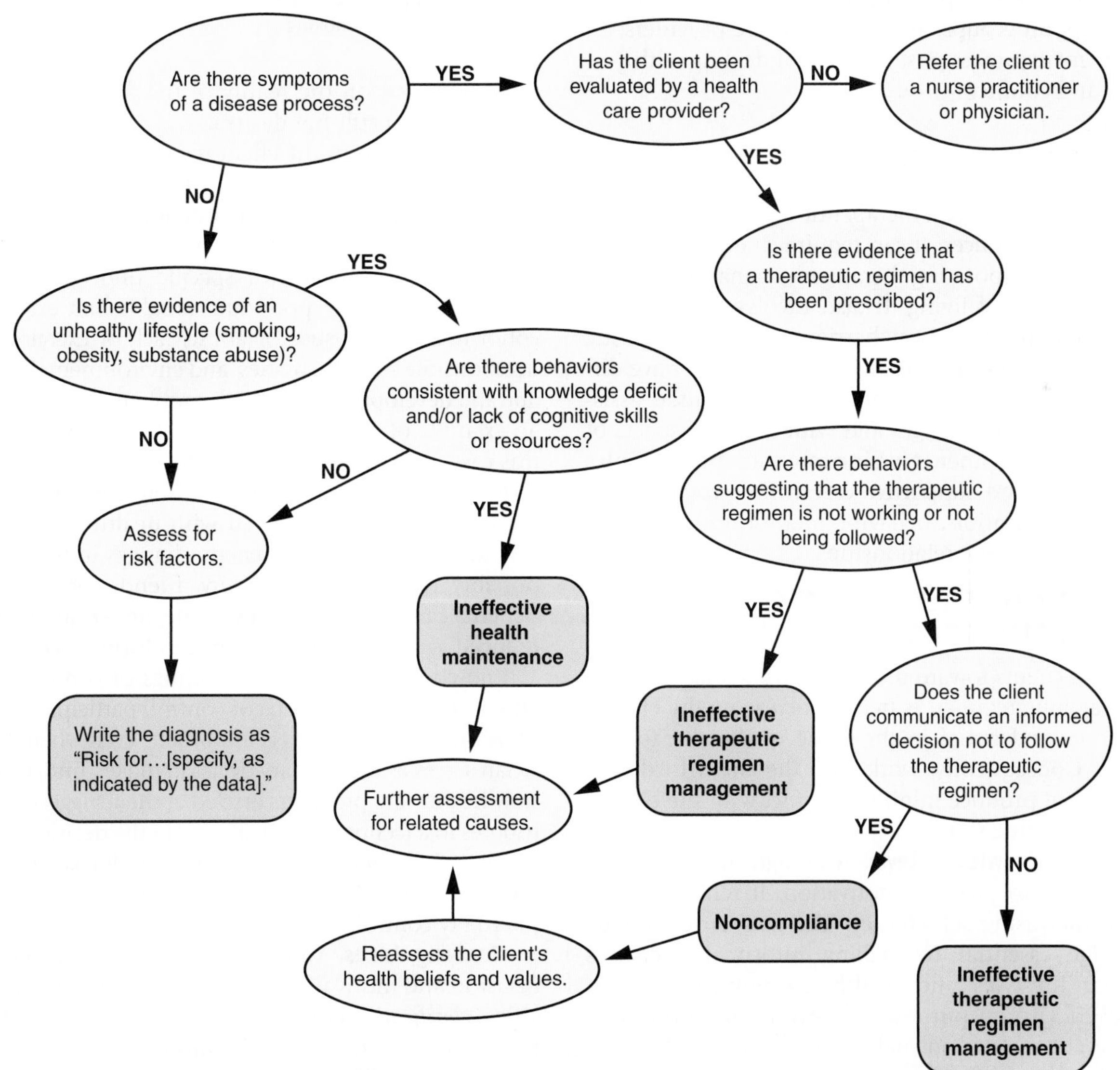

FIGURE 20-2 Decision tree for health maintenance/lifestyle management nursing diagnoses. Diagnoses are shown in rectangles. Within these rectangles, diagnoses shown in **bold** type are NANDA-International (NANDA-I)–approved nursing diagnoses; diagnoses shown in regular type are not NANDA-I–approved nursing diagnoses.

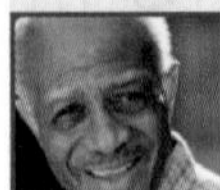

Which of the diagnoses just described would you use for Mr. Kitchen? Consider whether he lacks knowledge, is unsuccessful in his efforts, or has chosen not to comply with the therapeutic regimen. Do you believe Mr. Kitchen has made an informed decision not to follow the therapeutic regimen?

PLANNING

The overall expected outcome for intervention to help the client manage a therapeutic regimen is that the client achieve the desired goals of the treatment plan. Outcomes related to successful movement toward achievement of treatment goals are the following:

- The client makes effective choices in integrating the treatment plan into activities of daily living and actively participates in the regimen as prescribed.
- The client seeks help as needed from family members, support groups, and/or health care providers.
- The client expresses positive ways of dealing with stress and conflict.

INTERVENTION

A person must manage a therapeutic regimen in the context of lifestyle choices. It can require changing patterns of living or incorporating therapeutic management into present patterns of living. It also involves overcoming physical and psychological barriers to the therapeutic regimen. Nursing interventions for clients who have difficulty managing a therapeutic regimen include assistance with lifestyle changes and with specific aspects of the therapeutic regimen. Nursing care uses the principles of motivation and supportive care while providing the client with education, behavior modification, motivation, and therapeutic relationships.

INTERVENTIONS TO MOTIVATE HEALTH BEHAVIORS

Motivating clients toward more effective management of the therapeutic regimen is tied to increasing the client's self-efficacy and belief in the value of the therapeutic regimen. Consequently, work with the client to design activities that produce minimal conflict with the client's lifestyle and value system.

Increasing Knowledge Level. Although knowledge is not sufficient to produce motivation, it remains a key issue in increasing self-efficacy. The goal is to provide knowledge essential to making informed decisions regarding lifestyles and health promotion practices (Figure 20-3). The purpose of health education is to facilitate client decision making about personal health behaviors, use of health resources, and general health issues. Teaching a client to plan meals is one example of educating the client. However, appropriate education

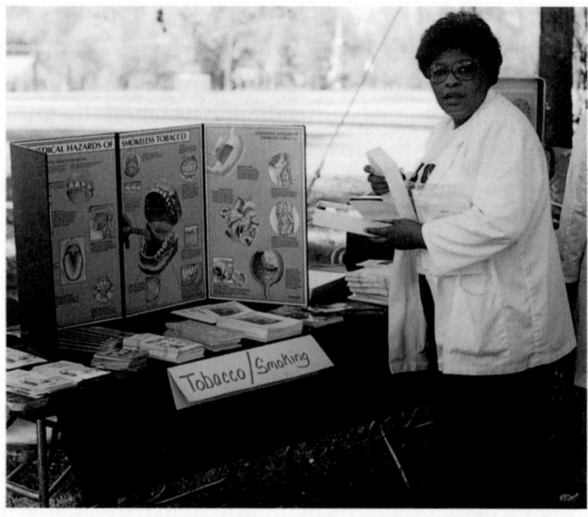

FIGURE 20-3 Health education is the primary intervention for promoting and maintaining health in individuals, families, groups, and communities. This nurse is participating in a community health fair to educate participants about the far-reaching physical changes caused by cigarette smoking.

must be based on the reality of the foods a client may obtain and on cultural desires.

Knowledge helps the client recognize susceptibility to an illness, or the consequences of an illness along with their potential severity. An individualized educational plan must focus on increasing awareness of the relationships between the client's specific unhealthy lifestyles (such as tobacco use, poor nutritional habits, excessive alcohol use, drug misuse or abuse, lack of exercise, stress, irresponsible sexual activities, and environmental hazards) and the development of health problems. Box 20-4 offers an example of a way to increase a client's knowledge—in this case about how to lose weight.

Knowledge helps the client weigh benefits against risks. Possible risks involved with health care regimens are side effects, inconveniences, changes in lifestyle, and possibly criticism from family, friends, or co-workers. Benefits can include prolonged life, better quality of life, reduced symptoms, and a return to former activities.

Knowledge contributes to feelings of control. For clients with an internal locus of control, participation in the decision-making process is important. Even when the physician serves as the primary decision maker, understanding how health care providers arrived at their suggestions contributes to a feeling of participating in the decision-making process. For clients with an external locus of control, knowledge may help them recognize factors that can be internally controlled, thus increasing self-efficacy.

Clarifying Values. Values and beliefs play a role in the decision and motivation to follow a health care regimen. *Values clarification* is a self-discovery process that allows a person to find answers to situations or to arrive at freely chosen values. This process allows the person to determine what choices to make when faced with alternatives. Your primary goal is to help the client sort out feelings

BOX 20-4 *Teaching for Wellness*

Helping a Client Lose Weight

Purpose: To support the client's motivation to lose weight through recognition of risk factors and a simple regimen. Teaching supports the client's maintenance of a healthy diet and exercise program.

Expected Outcome: The client will develop a plan to lose weight.

Client Instructions

- In planning for weight loss, make nutritional adequacy your top priority. Most people cannot maintain nutritional adequacy on less than 1200 calories a day, so plan to consume no less than that. To maintain weight, most adults need 2200 to 2500 calories per day, although older adults need less.
- Keep in mind that you will experience a healthier, more successful weight loss with a small energy deficit that provides an adequate intake than with a large energy deficit that creates feelings of starvation and deprivation. These feelings can lead to an irresistible urge to binge. Note the following suggestions:
  - Keep meals small, and avoid long periods without food.
  - Choose a diet with plenty of vegetables, fruits, and grain products.
  - Drink plenty of fluids between meals.
  - Avoid foods that are greasy, fried, or highly spiced.
- Weight loss alone can lower your cholesterol level, decrease your blood pressure, increase your energy level, and lessen joint pain. However, a regular exercise program will enhance these benefits, as well as promote self-esteem, reduce the risk of heart disease, and encourage the loss of extra pounds. Note the following suggestions:
  - If you are over 35, have heart trouble, or are taking medicine for high blood pressure, see a doctor before you start a physical exercise program.
  - Initiate your exercise program slowly, and build up your activity level gradually.
  - Exercise at least for 20 minutes, four times a week.
  - Listen to your body. Pay attention to warning signals, such as sudden dizziness, cold sweats, fainting, or pressure in the chest.

and clarify meanings by listening to the client's comments and appreciating the reason for them.

Lifestyle management involves helping the client develop self-awareness related to attitudes and beliefs regarding smoking, overeating, or other unhealthy lifestyle habits. Help the client identify and examine all available alternatives when faced with choices regarding an unhealthy lifestyle. Guide the client in examining consequences associated with each choice to help promote informed decision making. The goal is to get the client to recognize and assume primary responsibility for making healthy lifestyle choices.

Action Alert! Accept the client's choice or point of view, even if it appears to be self-destructive, such as a decision to continue smoking. Confrontation is not beneficial and may actually be detrimental to further cooperation and goal achievement.

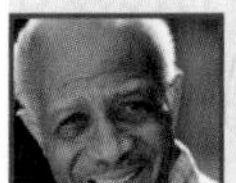

Recall that Mr. Kitchen continues to smoke despite his problems with edema and shortness of breath. Although Mr. Kitchen would benefit from a smoking cessation class, the nurse should also recognize that he may be depressed and lonely. Because his wife managed his health care, he may also lack the knowledge to follow through on his care. If he is depressed, he may lack the ability to act. It may be difficult for him to relate to the clinic staff, and he may believe it is acceptable to stop medications if he feels better.

The clinic staff might try a follow-up telephone call a week before Mr. Kitchen's scheduled appointment to determine how the therapeutic regimen is progressing. Can you think of other ways to help Mr. Kitchen?

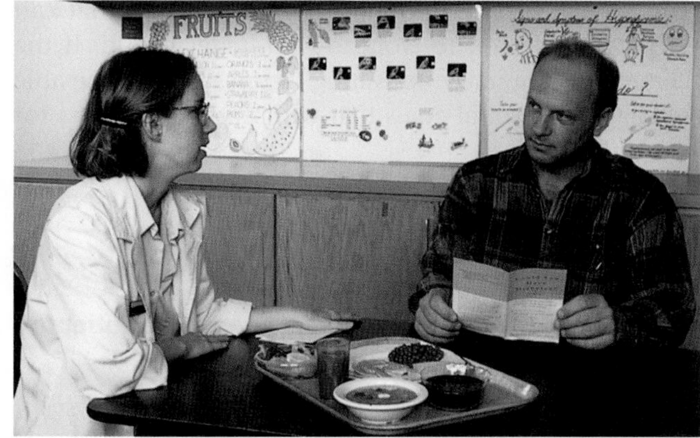

FIGURE 20-4 Counseling is a method of communication that helps clients recognize personal risk factors and manage necessary behavioral changes.

Engaging Participation. Active participation in learning typically increases learning and motivation. **Counseling** is a method of communication that actively involves the client in recognizing personal risk factors and managing necessary behavioral changes (Figure 20-4). Counseling is different from education in that it guides the client through decision making rather than merely ensuring that he has the knowledge to make a decision.

During counseling, the client plays the major role in identifying and clarifying the problem to be solved. Engage the client in a dialogue to identify the problem and examine factors that contribute to it and those that may enhance or block its resolution. Do not tell the client what to do to solve the problem but instead assist and guide the problem-solving or decision-making process.

Because many people lack the knowledge or skills to approach a problem systematically, teaching and counseling can be combined to help the client solve the dilemma successfully. If the health history reveals that the client is at risk for a sexually transmitted disease, health education involves providing didactic information to help the person avoid infection. Counseling involves greater interaction and entails helping the person identify risky behaviors and developing a plan to reduce the risk. Counseling is tailored to the individual risk factors, needs, and abilities of each client.

Anticipating Problems. Anticipate problems the client may have in managing the therapeutic regimen. If the client is illiterate, has poor eyesight, has decreased mobility, or has decreased manual dexterity, you can help plan for alternative methods of managing the therapeutic regimen. Also, anticipate side effects of medication and help plan ways to manage them.

Providing Reinforcing Factors. Help the client find motivation from life goals or desirable activities. Playing with grandchildren, traveling to Europe, attending a child's graduation from college, or caring for an older adult parent are among the important activities of life that can motivate a person to work toward better health. If the client does not have motivating factors, you may be able to suggest personal goals that will serve as a reward for effective management of the therapeutic regimen. Rewards can be achieving a major long-term goal or engaging in small daily or weekly pleasures.

INTERVENTIONS TO PROVIDE SUPPORTIVE CARE

Changing lifestyle behaviors to manage a therapeutic regimen can be a complex problem. Although the client may initially have strong motivation and expect to be able to make the changes, continued support from family and health care providers is often necessary to sustain the changes.

Establishing a Therapeutic Relationship. The most influential factor in increasing the client's participation in effective management of a therapeutic regimen is the relationship with the health care provider. Give the client individual attention by providing information in a face-to-face, two-way communication process.

Probe for the client's level of understanding of and perspective on the problem. A common and sometimes mistaken practice is to wait for the client to ask questions. The assumption is that the client may not want to know everything and will ask the questions that are of the most concern. However, the client may not know what to ask and may not have enough information even to form the questions. Only after you have learned how the client perceives the problem can you offer information that deals with the client's often unspoken concerns (Box 20-5).

BOX 20-5 *A Patient's Perspective*

"Nurses Need To Be Aware That Patients Depend on Them to Come in Closer Than Most Doctors Will"

Eight years ago I was dying, hospitalized with *Pneumocystis jiroveci* pneumonia. I was 36 years old and alone with my secret: HIV/AIDS. I had lived with that secret for 2 years, fearing discovery by my family, my company, the government. Disclosing my diagnosis would also mean disclosing that I am gay to my co-workers. Feeling that it was a death sentence anyway, I didn't seek treatment until I got really sick.

Today, I am healthy, perhaps not the way some people would define it, but I am living, not dying. New drugs and new connections to the community have made all the difference. All my fears of disclosure proved to be unfounded. My family, my friends, my co-workers have all been totally supportive, even though some of them had never known a gay or HIV-positive man before. And though I live alone, every area of my life is filled with support.

Living with AIDS gives new meaning to "continuing education." Survival means continuing to learn about your disease and about treatment options. The AIDS community has taught me to be a fully informed participant in treatment decisions, a partner with my doctor and with my nurse practitioner. You need to have health professionals you get along with and feel close to.

Nurses have been some of my greatest supporters, not just when I was hospitalized but afterward. Maybe I'm just lucky, but I've never encountered homophobia among nurses. When I went home after pneumocystosis, I needed nightly infusions for 2 weeks. My Korean nurse had never met a gay man before, but she couldn't have been more supportive and understanding. She would bring me home-cooked Korean food and spend time with me. We exchanged cards and letters for a long time afterward.

My nurse practitioner is the one I'm closest to–I look forward to seeing her every month. Nurses need to be aware that clients depend on them to come in closer than most doctors will and that this helps not only physically but emotionally as well. One of the most important things nurses do is teach–providing practical information about HIV-friendly doctors and about resources in the community. Just a list of phone numbers can make a huge difference, especially when you're alone and afraid.

HIV, Human immunodeficiency virus; *AIDS,* acquired immunodeficiency disease syndrome.

Guiding the Client Through the Health System. A major focus of nursing care is to promote and assist the client in receiving the health care necessary to achieve and maintain health. Lifestyle behavioral changes may require the client to seek services from several health care agencies. Getting to and through these systems can prove difficult for many clients.

Helping the client identify services to assist in achieving desired goals should be the initial step. Determine the client's eligibility, as well as the fees involved and methods of payment, to ensure that services are available and affordable. Identify constraints, such as lack of transportation, cultural beliefs, and the ability to communicate. Preparing the client for what will be encountered will help to make the best use of the services available.

The initial step is to help the client recognize the need for these services. A client who is in denial will not see the need for or benefit of services. After the client has acknowledged the problem, discuss the services that are available.

Planning for Discharge. As defined in Chapter 10, *Discharge planning* is the preparation for moving a client from one level of care to another within or outside the current health care agency. It is a systematic process of preparing clients and family members to manage therapeutic regimens and to engage in health maintenance activities once they leave the hospital or other health care delivery system. The objectives of discharge planning are to do the following:

- Make sure that there will be no interruption in the implementation of the therapeutic regimen.
- Provide adequate teaching and instruction or additional demonstrations of procedures to manage the therapeutic regimen.
- Identify or familiarize the client and family with appropriate resources to ensure continuity of care.
- The client and the family should be actively involved in the planning process, goal setting, and all decision making.

Although discharge planning should begin at the time of admission to allow for adequate teaching and preparation, an assessment of the needs of the client and family is ongoing, and final plans are made immediately before discharge. Because most clients stay fewer days in the hospital than they once did, the scope and complexity of the discharge planning has increased. Different clients have different complexities of need, as well. For example, a client being discharged from a substance abuse treatment center would require a more complex discharge plan than a middle-age client being discharged from an emergency department with a fractured wrist. The substance abuser will require additional community resources, such as substance abuse counselors, a support group, and family members, to assist in managing the treatment plan and the related lifestyle changes needed to remain free of drugs.

During your predischarge assessment, pay attention to any statements that could indicate a potential for ineffective management of health or the health plan, such as an unwillingness or inability to modify personal habits and integrate necessary treatments into the lifestyle. Failure to adhere to a treatment plan while hospitalized (such as refusal to take medication, walk, or follow dietary modification) would suggest a potential for the diagnosis *Ineffective therapeutic regimen management* after discharge.

Referring to Health Services. Referral is a process designed to provide the client with access to health care and supportive services that are not available from the sending institution. The referral process begins after assessment data reveal a need for additional services. A client with chronic obstructive pulmonary disorder who continues to smoke, for example, may be referred to a smoking cessation class. When altered nutritional intake appears to be a family problem, the family may be referred to a nutritionist. An adolescent who shows evidence of anorexia nervosa may be referred to a clinical psychologist or physician. If the assessment data indicate that the client has not completed immunizations for the age-group, the client should be referred to the local health department.

As in discharge planning, the client and family should be involved in the decision for referral. This is important to facilitate the client's follow-through. If the referral is recognized by the client as being insignificant, the client probably will not follow through.

Several factors must be taken into consideration when planning for referral. The referred source must be acceptable to the client, and it must be specific to the needs of the client. Some clients will not use services that are perceived as "charity" or "demoralizing." For example, a client who is overweight may perceive different implications if referred to Overeaters Anonymous instead of Weight Watchers. Also, the client must be eligible for the services. Services that are designed for Medicare or Medicaid clients will not provide services to people who do not meet the appropriate criteria.

To be effective in making referrals, you will need to know about resources in the client's community, including the location of services, name and telephone number of a contact person, types of services provided, eligibility criteria, operating hours, and a general overview of fees required. When making a referral, give the client all the necessary information. If the client agrees, call ahead to make the appointment.

Promoting Social Support. An assessment of social support involves an analysis of the client's social network to ascertain actual and potential sources of support, the client's perception of need for social support, and the specific helping behaviors that would be of assistance to the client. Help the client make this assessment and develop the social support structure to facilitate the expected lifestyle behavioral changes or to incorporate the therapeutic regimen into daily life. Help the client clarify expectations of support persons and the type of support needed. Encourage open communication of needs among family members, goal setting, and identification of strategies to be implemented to achieve goals.

> **Action Alert!** Assess current actions of significant others and how they are received by the client. When significant others try to be helpful, does the client perceive them as being helpful? Also assess whether significant others are withdrawn or overly protective.

In addition to family and friends, a support group may be helpful with smoking cessation, adjusting dietary habits, or participating in an exercise program. Social support can be provided through groups that provide an opportunity for clients to share the experiences of others in changing behaviors.

EVALUATION

Evaluation involves reassessing the client to determine whether all outcomes were achieved. The outcomes will have been achieved if the client reports participation in activities to increase knowledge of health promotion. Participation in these activities could entail attending classes at the local health center or health department; seeking health information through the media, such as newspaper or television; and building knowledge of preventable diseases and related risk factors.

In addition, the client may express a desire to achieve better health by participating in health screening clinics (Figure 20-5) or learning to perform self-examinations. Reducing the number of risk factors or being successful in integrating the treatment plan into daily life indicates that the client has achieved the outcomes for effective management of the therapeutic regimen. The client should be reassessed for the establishment of new goals.

If no noticeable change occurs in unhealthy behaviors within a reasonable period, or if the client returns with an exacerbation of symptoms, reassess the client to determine what prevented the progress. For example, a client who has successfully followed a reduced-calorie nutritional program may not show a weight loss during the first week because of medications that have fluid-retention properties or other physiological alterations. Mr. Kitchen is an example. Box 20-6 illustrates how the clinic nurse worked with him to improve his management of the therapeutic regimen. Before he left the clinic the nurse wrote the note below.

SAMPLE DOCUMENTATION NOTE FOR MR. KITCHEN

Demonstrates concern for his health and intention to comply with medication schedule. However, he relies on a neighbor for cooking and feels he has no means to control his diet. Instructed to avoid highly salty foods like bacon and not to add salt at the table. Given a written schedule of his medications. Will do telephone follow-up to reinforce need for compliance.

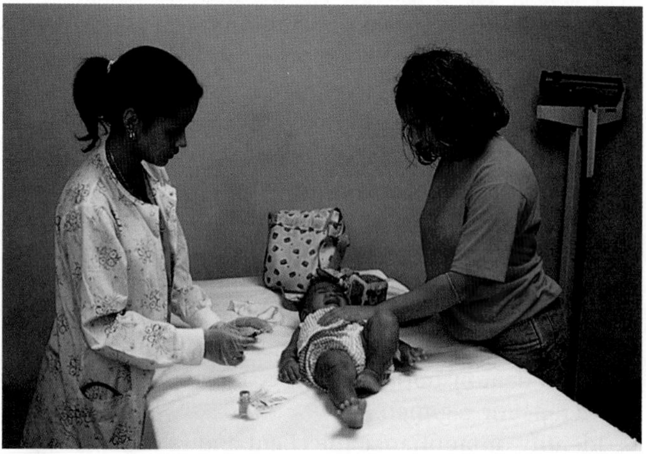

FIGURE 20-5 Health screening is a primary strategy used to promote health. The young mother *(at right)* understands the importance of health screening in achieving optimal health for her child. During a routine screening visit, the nurse has identified the need to update the child's immunizations.

BOX 20-6 *Nursing Care Plan*

A Client With Heart Failure

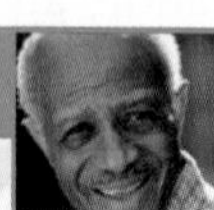

Admission Data

Mr. Oscar Kitchen is a 69-year-old African American man who is being seen in a primary health care center. This is the second time he has come in with shortness of breath and edema of the lower limbs. The doctor has told him to stay on the same medication for his heart and on diuretics. With proper instructions, he believes Mr. Kitchen can manage the therapeutic regimen at home.

Physician's Orders

Admitting diagnosis: Chronic heart failure
Lasix 20 mg PO daily every morning
Digoxin 0.125 mg PO daily every morning
Low-sodium diet
Hygroton 25 mg PO daily every morning
Return to clinic in 2 weeks

Nursing Assessment

BP 160/98, pulse 98, respiration 32 and labored. Height 5 feet 11½ inches, weight 220 pounds, 3+ pitting edema of lower extremities. Widower of 3 months. Wife previously assisted in management of health care regimen. No close relative living near. Very little interaction with neighbors. Smokes two packs of cigarettes each day. He has smoked for 55 years.

BOX 20-6 *Nursing Care Plan—cont'd*

A Client With Heart Failure

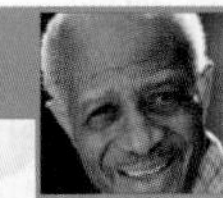

NANDA-I Nursing Diagnosis	NOC Expected Outcomes With Indicators	NIC Interventions With Selected Activities	Evaluation Data
Ineffective Therapeutic Regimen Management	***Compliance Behavior***	***Medication Management***	***At 1-Month Follow-up Visit***
Related Factors: • Shortness of breath • 3+ pitting edema • Pulse 98 and irregular • BP 160/98	• Takes medications daily as prescribed.	• Assists in making a schedule to take medications at planned times that work best for him.	• States medication is taken daily as prescribed. • Pitting edema decreased to less than +1 or eliminated. • Pulse regular and within normal range for client.
Deficient Knowledge Related to Treatment Regimen	***Knowledge***	***Teaching***	
• Made a decision to stop taking medications after the first week because he "feels better."	• Treatment regimen.	• Prescribed medication.	• Voices no misconception about illness or purpose for medications.
	• Asks questions to clarify understanding of treatment regimen.	• Determine client's understanding of illness and medications.	
	• Statements reflect an understanding of the implication of not following the prescribed treatment.	• Explain the disease process of chronic congestive heart failure in very simple terms.	• Answers questions correctly about the disease process.
	• Statements reflect an understanding of the effect of sodium on his conditions.	• Explain purpose of medications and consequences if medications are not taken.	• Reports he takes his medication every day.
		• Explain low-sodium diet and assist in developing a list of low-sodium foods that he likes.	• Gives a 3-day recall of food eaten, and foods are determined (by the nurse) to be appropriate for a low-sodium diet.

Critical Thinking Questions

1. Which is the priority nursing intervention? What is the rationale for your choice?
2. Can you think of other ways the nurse could have incorporated Mr. Kitchen's culture into his care? How would you change your approach if the client was of Hispanic or Vietnamese origin?
3. How could the client be motivated to change behavior and accept responsibility for a healthier lifestyle?

Nursing outcome and intervention labels from Johnson, M., Bulechek, G., Butcher, H., Dochterman, J. M., Maas, M., Moorhead, S., et al. (Eds.). (2006). *NANDA, NOC, and NIC linkages: Nursing diagnoses, outcomes, & interventions.* St. Louis, MO: Mosby.

▼ KEY PRINCIPLES

- Understanding health from the perspectives of the client and the provider is critical to the development of health services and nursing interventions.
- Concepts that differ across cultures include an explanatory model of illness that defines the nature of illness, its treatment, and the type of relationships that should occur between client and health care provider.
- There are two domains of health care: the folk, or generic, form and the scientific form.
- The theory of reasoned action is based on the assumption that people are reasonable and, in deciding what action to take, systematically process and use the information available to them.
- The transtheoretical model of behavioral change is useful across all theories to plan interventions that are appropriate to the stage of change: precontemplation, contemplation, preparation, action, maintenance, and termination.
- In the health belief model, behavior is a function of the subjective value of an outcome and of the subjective expectation that a particular action will achieve that outcome.

Continued

- The health promotion model uses concepts from the health belief model but decreases the focus on threats as an avenue to behavioral change.
- Factors affecting behavioral change affect the relationship with the health care provider. They include communication, cognition and perception, age and developmental level, lifestyle and habits, economic resources, cultural values and beliefs, roles and relationships, coping and stress tolerance, and workplace and environmental conditions.
- Lack of education about nutrition, safety, fitness, or health-protecting practices during early childhood or adolescence can have a significant impact on adult health.
- Wellness assessment focuses on physical fitness evaluation, health risk appraisal, social support systems, and lifestyle assessment.
- Assessment for behavioral change requires assessing the client's level of knowledge.
- Assessment for *Ineffective therapeutic regimen management* often relies on indirect cues suggesting that the client needs to improve the management of the therapeutic regimen.
- The health care system can be a related factor for *Ineffective therapeutic regimen management.*
- Educational interventions aimed at improving behavior can reduce at-risk behaviors.
- Motivation, locus of control, health perception, and a sense of self-efficacy affect participation in activities to promote or maintain health.
- Nursing interventions for *Ineffective health maintenance* include activities to help the client promote and maintain health through education, health screening, and counseling.
- Nursing interventions for *Ineffective therapeutic regimen management* include teaching the client about the current illness and treatment regimen, supporting the client's well-being through stress management skills, and promoting health management choices through values clarification.
- Although knowledge is not sufficient to produce motivation, it remains a key issue in increasing self-efficacy.
- Knowledge helps the client recognize susceptibility to an illness or the consequences of an illness, along with the potential severity of the consequences.
- Values clarification is a self-discovery process that allows the person to make choices when faced with alternatives.
- Active participation in learning is expected to increase learning and motivation.
- Anticipation of problems is an effective teaching tool for complex health care regimens.
- The most influential factor in increasing the client's participation in effective management of a therapeutic regimen is the relationship with the health care provider.
- The objectives of discharge planning are to ensure that there will be no interruption in implementation, to provide adequate teaching, and to familiarize the client with appropriate resources.
- Social support is a key element in health promotion activities.

■ REVIEW QUESTIONS

1. The nurse is counseling a client who has high blood pressure about the need to stop smoking cigarettes. The client indicates that family and friends are also urging him to stop. He states he does not want to quit but may try because of the "pressure" he is getting from family and health care providers. The nurse would characterize this client as being in which of the following stages of change?

1. Precontemplation
2. Contemplation
3. Planning
4. Action

2. A client who is overweight has received dietary teaching about nutrition that will help with weight loss and may also reduce risk of developing type 2 diabetes, which is a familial risk factor. The client says to the nurse, "It's going to be really hard for me to change my eating habits after all these years." The nurse realizes that, using the health belief model, the client is focusing on which of the following?

1. Perceived susceptibility
2. Perceived severity
3. Perceived benefits
4. Perceived barriers

3. A client who has been trying unsuccessfully to maintain a steady exercise program at a local gym says to the nurse, "It makes no sense for me to make these big plans that I can never stick to. I work too many hours, and I am too tired both in the morning and at night. I am going to start walking for 20 to 30 minutes a day after work instead, so I at least do something." The nurse interprets that this client is exemplifying which of the following that relates to health promotion?

1. Social cognitive theory
2. Value-expectancy theory
3. Health belief model
4. Termination stage of change

4. A healthy young man in his early 20s tells the occupational health nurse during routine health screening that he has obtained membership in a gym and is thinking about requesting a personal trainer to help him get the most benefit from his workouts. The nurse concludes that which nursing diagnosis applies to this client?

1. Ineffective therapeutic regimen management
2. Deficient knowledge
3. Health-seeking behaviors
4. Risk for injury

5. The nurse assesses that an older adult client newly diagnosed with diabetes who lives alone might benefit from increased social support to adhere to the treatment plan. Which of the following suggestions by the nurse may be most effective?

1. Keep a daily log of all activities to share with the nurse at each visit to the clinic.
2. Join a support group for people with diabetes that meets in the client's neighborhood.
3. Telephone a daughter who lives out of state at least once per month.
4. Telephone the nurse twice weekly to report blood glucose levels and weight loss.

Bibliography

*Bandura, A. (1977). Self-efficacy: Toward a unifying theory of behavioral change. *Psychological Review, 84,* 191-215.

Bendelius, J. (2005). Pediatric weight issues: What are health-care providers and parents to do? *School Nurse News, 22*(4), 16-17.

Carpenito, L. J. (2005). Nursing diagnosis: *Application to clinical practice* (11th ed.). Philadelphia: Lippincott.

Centers for Disease Control (Division of Health Education). (1984). *CDC health risk appraisal user manual* (Publication No. 746-011/15233). Washington, DC: U.S. Government Printing Office.

Clark, M. J. (2003). *Community health nursing: Caring for populations* (4th ed.). Upper Saddle River, NJ: Prentice Hall.

Colella, C., & Laver, J. (2005). Setting the stage for changing health behavior. *Nurse Practitioner, 30*(10), 68-70.

Davis, T. K. (2005). Beyond the physical examination: The nurse practitioner's role in adolescent risk reduction and resiliency building in a school-based health center. *Nursing Clinics of North America, 40*(4), 649-660, viii.

Giger, J. N., & Davidhizar, R. E. (2004). *Transcultural nursing: Assessment and intervention* (4th ed.). St. Louis, MO: Mosby.

Gleason, A. M. (2006). Racial disparities in testicular cancer: Impact on health promotion. *Journal of Transcultural Nursing, 17*(1), 58-64.

*Henderson, J. W. (2002). *Health Economics and policy* (2nd ed.). Cincinnati, OH: South-Western/Thomson Learning.

* Johnson, M., Bulechek, G., Butcher, H., Dochterman, J. M., Maas, M., Moorhead, S., et al. (Eds.). (2006). *NANDA, NOC, and NIC linkages: Nursing diagnoses, outcomes, & interventions.* St. Louis, MO: Mosby.

*Jones, P. S., Zhang, X. E., Jaceldo-Siegl, K., & Meleis, A. I. (2002). Caregiving between two cultures: An integrative experience. *Journal of Transcultural Nursing, 13*(3), 202-209.

*Kavanagh, K. H., & Kennedy, P. H. (1992). *Promoting cultural diversity: Strategies for health care professionals.* Newbury Park, CA: Sage.

*Leininger, M. M. (1970). *Nursing and anthropology: Two worlds to blend.* New York: John Wiley.

*Leininger, M. M. (1991). *Culture care diversity & universality: A theory of nursing.* New York: National League for Nursing Press.

Leininger, M. M. (2006). *Culture care diversity & universality: A worldwide nursing theory* (2nd ed.). Boston: Jones & Bartlett.

Masters, J. A. (2005). Moderate drinking and cardiovascular disease. *Annual Review of Nursing Research,* 23, 65-97.

McCabe, B. W., Hertzog, M., Grasser, C. M., & Walker, S. N. (2005). Practice of health-promoting behaviors by nursing home residents. *Western Journal of Nursing Research, 27*(8), 1000-1016.

NANDA International. (2007). *Nursing diagnoses: Definitions and classification, 2006-2007* (7th ed.). Philadelphia: Author.

Ott, C. H., Plach, S. K., Hewitt, J. B., Cashin, S. E., Kelber, S., Cisler, R. A., et al. (2005). Smoking-related health behaviors of employees and readiness to quit: Basis for health promotion interventions. *American Association of Occupational Health Nurses Journal, 53*(6), 249-256.

Pender, N. J., Murdaugh, C. L., & Parsons, M. A. (2006). *Health promotion in nursing practice.* (5th ed.). Upper Saddle River, NJ: Prentice Hall.

*Poss, J. E. (2001). Developing a new model for cross-cultural research: Synthesizing the health belief model and the theory of reasoned action [Review]. *Advances in Nursing Science, 23*(4), 1-15.

*Prochaska, J. O., Velicer, W. F., Rossi, J. S., Goldstein, M. G., Marcus, B. H., Rakowski, W., et al. (1994). Stages of change and decisional balance for 12 problem behaviors. *Health Psychology, 13*(1), 39-46.

*Rosenstock, J. (1974). Historical origins of the health belief model. *Health Education Monograph, 2*(4), 328-335.

Spector, R. (2004). *Cultural diversity in health and illness* (6th ed.). Upper Saddle River, NJ: Prentice Hall.

Stanhope, M., & Lancaster, J. (2004). *Community and public health nursing* (6th ed.). St. Louis, MO: Mosby.

*Swanson, E. A., Tripp-Reimer, T., & Buckwalter, K. (2001). *Health promotion and disease prevention in the older adult: Interventions and recommendations.* New York: Springer.

*Thomas, S. (1992). The health of the black community in the twenty-first century: A futuristic perspective. In R. L. Braithwaite & S. E. Taylor (Eds.), *Health issues in the black community.* San Francisco: Jossey-Bass.

*Tripp-Reimer, T. (1984). Reconceptualizing the concept of health: Integrating emic and etic perspectives. *Research, Nursing & Health,* 7, 101-109.

Underwood, S. M., Buseh, A. G., Canales, M. K., Powe, B., Dockery, B., Kather, T., et al. (2005). Nursing contributions to the elimination of health disparities among African-Americans: Review and critique of a decade of research. *Journal of National Black Nurses Association, 16*(1), 31-47.

*Walker, S. N., Sechrist, K. R., & Pender, N. J. (1987). The health-promoting lifestyle profile: Development and psychometric characteristics. *Nursing Research, 36*(2), 76-81.

*Asterisk indicates a classic or definitive work on this subject.

Chapter 21

Health Maintenance: Medication Management

Media Resources

- Nursing Skills Online
- evolve Evolve Website http://evolve.elsevier.com/Harkreader/
- 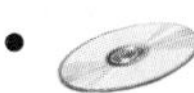 Companion CD
- 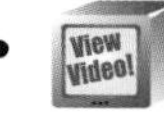 Skills Video Clips

Learning Objectives

After studying this chapter, you should be able to do the following:

- Identify important concepts related to safe and effective medication management
- Describe a variety of factors that influence drug actions in individual clients
- Explain how to assess a client who is receiving medication therapy
- Formulate appropriate nursing diagnostic statements for a client receiving medications
- Plan appropriate expected outcomes for a client taking medications
- Incorporate safe and effective nursing interventions in the care of a client receiving medications
- Evaluate the effectiveness of medication therapy in helping to achieve health-related expected outcomes

Key Terms

adverse effect
anaphylaxis
antagonistic effect
bioavailability
biotransformation
chemical name
controlled substance
generic name
hypersensitivity reaction
idiosyncratic response
intradermal (ID) route
intramuscular (IM) route
intravenous (IV) route
loading dose
official name
parenteral route
pharmacokinetics
prescription
side effect
subcutaneous (subcut) route
synergistic effect
target organ
teratogenic potential
therapeutic effect
topical route
toxic effect

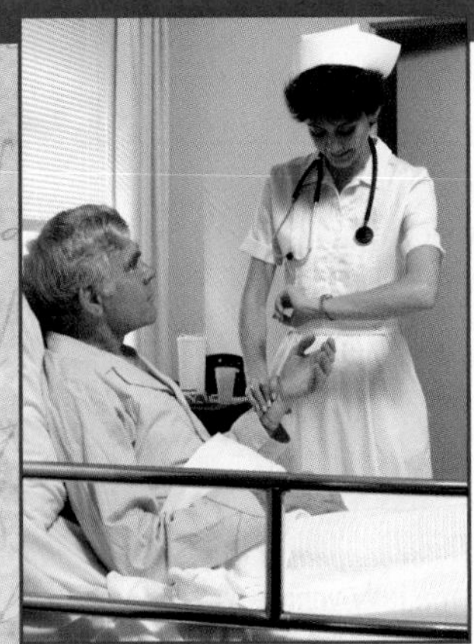
© 2007, JupiterImages Corporation.

Daniel Connell is a married 62-year-old Irish American. He came to the emergency department (ED) after experiencing chest pain while carrying an air conditioner up two flights of stairs. Upon arrival at the ED, vital signs were pulse 96, blood pressure 166/96, respirations 22, and oral temperature 98.8° F. Mr. Connell described the chest pain as a "pressure," and rated it as 6 on a 0-10 pain scale. The pain did not worsen with inspiration and was relieved with rest and nitroglycerin.

Results of serum laboratory studies and electrocardiogram showed that Mr. Connell did not have a myocardial infarction (heart attack). By taking a more thorough history, the ED nurse learns that Mr. Connell has hypertension but has not been taking prescribed medications. His diet is high in sodium, and he does not exercise regularly. Knowing that Mr. Connell is not taking action to control his health problems, the nurse considers the diagnosis of *Ineffective health maintenance.* The nurse also considers other nursing diagnoses that may apply, such as *Ineffective therapeutic regimen management* and *Noncompliance,* as shown in the Nursing Diagnoses box.

CONCEPTS OF MEDICATION MANAGEMENT

Medication administration is a critically important part of the nurse's role. Many clients take medication as part of a therapeutic regimen for health problems. This chapter examines concepts, clinical judgments, and practices needed for safe, effective medication therapy.

DRUG NAMES AND FORMS

The terms *drug* and *medication* are often used interchangeably, although technically they differ. A *drug* is a chemical substance that alters an organism's function and may or may not have a therapeutic effect. A *medication* is a drug used for an intended therapeutic effect. Most drugs or medications can be called by several different names. The **chemical name,** often long and complex, is of interest to pharmacists and precisely describes the chemical and molecular structure of a medication. For example, the chemical name for acetaminophen (Tylenol) is *N*-acetyl-*para*-aminophenol.

KEY NURSING DIAGNOSES FOR MEDICATION ADMINISTRATION

Ineffective health maintenance: Inability to identify, manage, and/or seek out help to maintain health

Ineffective therapeutic regimen management: A pattern of regulating and integrating into daily living a program for treatment of illness and the sequelae of illness that is unsatisfactory for meeting specific health goals

The **generic name,** or *nonproprietary name,* is the name assigned to a drug by the United States Adopted Names Council when it is first manufactured. Subsequent manufacturers of the drug then use the same generic name. The **official name** is the name assigned by the Food and Drug Administration (FDA) after approval of a drug and is often the same as the generic name. The official name of a drug is how it is listed in the *United States Pharmacopeia* (USP) and *National Formulary* (NF), two publications officially approved by the FDA.

The **trade name,** also known as the brand name or *proprietary name,* is a copyrighted name for a medication given by a specific manufacturer. Because a medication may be produced by several manufacturers, it may have several trade names. For example, acetylsalicylic acid is the generic name for Bayer Aspirin, which has other trade names, including Ecotrin and Empirin. Alarmingly for international nurses, one trade name might indicate two entirely different generic drugs depending on the country one is in.

Although it is important to be familiar with both the generic and trade names of medications, this may be difficult because of the sheer number of trade names on the market and because generic names are often complex or foreign. First try to learn the generic name of a drug and its classification, and then try to learn trade names as you are able.

Prescription and Nonprescription Medications. Medications are commonly grouped into two categories, prescription and nonprescription (also called over-the-counter, or OTC). A **prescription** is an order for a medication that contains the client's name, medication name, dose, route, frequency, amount of medication to be dispensed, number of refills allowed (if any), and the physician's signature. The physician must sign the prescription and indicate whether a generic interchange may be substituted. Prescription drugs should be used under the supervision of a health care provider. Taking a prescription drug without supervision could lead to harm or result in abuse.

In some states, revised nurse practice acts allow selected groups of advanced practice nurses to write

Table 21-1 Common Forms for Drug Preparations

PREPARATION	GENERAL DESCRIPTION
Caplet	Tablet coated with gelatin that dissolves in the stomach
Capsule	Powder or gel form of drug encased in a hard or soft outer casing that dissolves in the stomach
Elixir	Drug dissolved in a clear liquid containing water, varying amounts of alcohol, and a sweetening agent or flavor
Emulsion	Drug in which one liquid is spread by means of small droplets through another liquid
Enteric-coated tablet	Tablet coated with a substance that blocks drug absorption until the tablet reaches the small intestine
Extract	Highly concentrated form of drug made when the active portion is removed from the other drug components
Liniment	Drug combined with alcohol, soap, or oil that is applied to the skin
Lotion	Drug that is dissolved in liquid and applied to the skin
Lozenge or troche	Drug in a flavored or sweet base that is released as the base dissolves in the mouth
Ointment	Semisolid form of a drug that is applied to and absorbed by the skin
Oil based paste	Semisolid form of a drug that is applied to and absorbed by the skin, solids dispersed in a fatty vehicle
Patch (transdermal)	Drug encased in a manufactured material that allows continuous drug absorption through the skin at a steady rate
Pill	Drug in powder form mixed in a cohesive material
Powder or granules	Finely ground form of a drug
Solution	Drug that has been dissolved in a liquid, commonly water
Suppository	Drug mixed in a firm base that melts easily when inserted into the rectum, vagina, or urethra
Suspension	Undissolved particles or powder placed in a liquid that must be shaken vigorously before use
Syrup	Drug dissolved in a solution containing water and sugar
Tablet	Solid drug that is compressed or molded into a particular shape and may be swallowed whole, chewed, or placed in the cheek or under the tongue, depending on its purpose
Tincture	Type of solution in which a drug is dissolved in alcohol or a water-alcohol base

prescriptions. Prescriptive privileges are limited to certified nurse practitioners, nurse anesthetists, nurse midwives, and clinical nurse specialists who work in collaboration with a physician.

Action Alert! Know which groups of health care providers have legal authority to write prescriptions in the state in which you are practicing nursing.

A *nonprescription* or *OTC medication* can be purchased without a prescription and can be used to enhance personal health (e.g., vitamins) or treat common health problems (e.g., constipation or diarrhea). Nurses and pharmacists have an important role in teaching clients about possible interactive effects between medications.

Classification. Medications with similar characteristics may be classified together according to therapeutic effect (bronchodilators), symptoms relieved (antianxiety agents), or clinical actions and composition (opioid analgesics). Classifications have characteristics in common that can help you understand medications. Some medications have more than one classification, so it is important in your clinical practice to understand its purpose for each client.

Drug Forms. Medications are manufactured in a variety of forms to make them more useful or easy to administer. Some examples of drug forms include tablets, suspensions, suppositories, and ointments (Table 21-1). The form of a drug guides its route of administration. Do not interchange one form with another without a specific physician order because the rate of absorption or **bioavailability** (amount available for use by target tissues) may differ among forms or even among brand names (McKenry, Tessier, & Hogan, 2006).

LEGISLATION AND STANDARDS

Because medications have a great impact on the health and well-being of clients, their manufacture and use is highly regulated. This protects clients from harm and provides a common set of guidelines for those in the pharmaceutical and health care industries. All drugs produced in the United States and Canada must meet legal standards for quality control. Health care personnel rely on these standards to provide safe, effective medication therapy.

Pure Food and Drug Act of 1906. In the United States, the Pure Food and Drug Act of 1906 set the first standards for drug quality and purity. This act empowered the FDA to monitor drug standards, such as chemical composition, quality, purity, strength, and form. The standards further required that drugs be adequately packaged and labeled. The U.S. standards have been updated over time with various pieces of legislation. Current standards have been broadened to include drug safety and effectiveness. State laws may be even stricter than federal standards. Refer to a pharmacology textbook for detailed information about key drug legislation.

Food and Drug Administration. The FDA is the official government agency responsible for determining that drug manufacturers maintain standards set by law. Its scope of authority spans several areas, including drug testing, approval of drugs for use, and control of drug sale and distribution. It also specifies whether a medication is classified as prescription or nonprescription.

Table 21-2 Controlled Substance Schedule

SCHEDULE	EXPLANATION	EXAMPLES
I	Not accepted for medical use because of their high potential for abuse	• Heroin • LSD • Marijuana
II	Have acceptable medical uses but also have a high potential for abuse or physical or psychological dependency	• Amphetamines • Codeine • Meperidine (Demerol) • Methadone • Morphine • Oxycodone
III	Have acceptable medical uses and a potential for abuse or dependence that is less than Schedule II drugs	• Propoxyphene • Some codeine preparations
IV	Have acceptable medical uses with limited risk of abuse or dependence	• Benzodiazepines • Nonnarcotic analgesics • Phenobarbital
V	Have medically acceptable uses with minimal risk for abuse or dependence	• Opioid-containing antidiarrheals • Opioid-containing cough remedies

If a pharmaceutical company wishes to produce a new drug, it submits a written proposal to the FDA. Controlled studies, called clinical trials, are then undertaken in four phases to test the drug. If it meets required standards, it may be approved for use. This rigorous process explains why drugs that are available in some countries may not be authorized for use in the United States.

Controlled Substances. Control of opioid analgesics and other select drugs is an important element of drug legislation. **Controlled substances** are drugs that affect the mind or behavior, may be habit forming, and have a high potential for abuse. They include opioids (also called narcotics), barbiturates, and illegal drugs. Controlled drugs are assigned to a specific category ranging from Schedule I to Schedule V. Their distribution and use is either highly regulated or prohibited (Table 21-2).

The Drug Enforcement Agency (DEA) is empowered to enforce narcotics laws. Violations may result in fines, imprisonment, or loss of a nurse's license. Health care facilities have detailed policies and procedures for storage, distribution, and record keeping of controlled substances. Sample guidelines for controlled substance administration by nurses are outlined in Box 21-1. Adhere to these guidelines to ensure that your behavior is within the law.

Institutional Policies. Hospitals, extended-care facilities, home health care agencies, and other health care facilities have policies and procedures for medication administration that are unique to that facility. You have an obligation to be aware of and comply with them.

Institutional policies must be congruent with the nurse practice act for the state in which the facility is located. The nurse practice act includes specific regulations about the nurse's role in medication administration. It is your legal and professional responsibility to understand the legal foundations of your nursing practice.

BOX 21-1 *Controlled Substance Administration and Control Guidelines*

- Place all controlled substances in the facility-approved, double-locked storage area.
- Count controlled substances according to facility policy at the beginning and end of each work shift. Have an off-going and an on-coming nurse sign that the count is correct.
- Follow facility protocols for reporting discrepancies in the count.
- Obtain a key from the designated RN or LPN to gain entry to the storage cabinet, or use your assigned code if you have a computerized storage system.
- Make an entry in the controlled substance inventory when removing a medication, unless your computerized system does so automatically. This ensures an ongoing record of the number of drugs used and remaining.
- When you sign out a controlled substance, record the client's name, the date, the time of administration, the drug name, and the dose needed. Make sure to sign the record. If you have a computerized system, your entry code will serve as your signature.
- Have a second nurse witness the disposal of a partial dose of a controlled substance. Both of you should sign the record or use your entry codes as your signatures.

SOURCES OF INFORMATION

Printed Materials. General information about many medications and their classifications is found in pharmacology texts and other printed references. Several textbooks have been written with nurses as the primary audience; also published are several drug reference handbooks for easy use.

Detailed information about medications can be found in sources such as the *American Hospital Formulary Service Drug Information* (AHFS DI), *Physician's Desk Reference* (PDR), and the *United States Pharmacopeia: Drug Information for the Health Care Professional* (USP DI).

Most health care institutions use one of these as the facility's official drug reference book.

People. Certain key people are good sources of drug information. Other experienced nurses and advanced practice nurses are knowledgeable and available to answer questions during everyday nursing practice. The health care provider who prescribes a medication can explain its expected action or benefit and why it was ordered for a particular client.

Pharmacists are a primary source of medication information. Larger institutions, such as hospitals, commonly employ pharmacists who are readily available on site. Smaller facilities, such as extended-care facilities, usually have a contract with a specific pharmacy; these pharmacists are generally available by telephone. Pharmacists employed in local pharmacies are yet another source of information and are the resource most often used by consumers.

Pharmaceutical sales representatives often have detailed information about medications produced by a specific company. Keep in mind that their primary objective is sales, not education. Thus they may readily identify the positive aspects of a medication while being less vocal about negative ones. They are best used for information about a medication's benefits and how to use it for maximum effect.

Computer-Based Resources. Computer-based resources are increasingly available for drug reference. Use caution when selecting Internet sites, however, because accuracy of information posted on a website is not guaranteed. Some facilities have computer-based resources for medication information available within the facility, such as *Micromedex,* which provides information about drugs, their dosing, drug interactions, and aftercare instructions that can be printed and given to clients.

DRUG ACTIONS

Mechanism of Action. The mechanism of action is the physiological change caused by a medication that results in the body's response to that medication. This change alters either the chemistry of the cell environment or the cell itself to either increase or decrease the function of the cell.

Many medications exert a therapeutic effect by interacting with cell receptor sites that have a similar chemical shape. When a medication is linked to the receptor site, similar to a lock and key, a chain of physiological events occurs that ends with the intended therapeutic effect. Because the "shape" of some cell receptor sites may be unique to a certain type of tissue, some medications exert an effect only on that tissue. Others have more systemic or widespread effects. When a medication has a specific effect on one type of body tissue, the tissue is said to be the **target organ** for that medication. An example is a diuretic, which targets the kidneys. The route of administration aids in determining whether a medication exerts a local or systemic effect. For example, a topical medication is more likely to exert a local effect on skin, whereas an intravenous (IV) medication rapidly exerts a systemic effect.

Therapeutic Effect. The **therapeutic effect** is the medication's intended effect. It is accomplished when a drug interacts with cell mechanisms, producing a change in cellular function. Effective drug therapy helps to cure or control disease (antibiotics), relieve pain or other aggravating symptoms (analgesics or decongestants), prevent disease (immunizations), or promote health (vitamin or mineral supplements). Every medication has at least one therapeutic effect, and some have several. For example, acetaminophen is an analgesic, but it also is an antipyretic (reduces fever).

Side Effects. **Side effects** of a medication are those that are not intended or planned but may occur as a result of use. Side effects can range from mildly unpleasant to harmful. Although all side effects cannot be avoided, teaching a client how to reduce common side effects may help the client tolerate the medication (Box 20-2).

Adverse Effects. An **adverse effect** is a more serious medication side effect that is potentially harmful to a client. Adverse effects can occur even when taking normal drug doses.

Toxic effects are serious adverse effects of medications that may even threaten life. Some examples are a low heart rate with a cardiac glycoside or wheezing or rash with an antibiotic. Be sure to inform clients about important adverse effects and which ones should prompt a call to the primary care provider or emergency services.

A toxic effect occasionally results from a single ingestion of a large amount of a drug (an overdose). When this occurs, the drug must be inactivated or removed from the body to prevent organ damage or death. This is done using activated charcoal in the gastrointestinal (GI) tract (to bind the incompletely absorbed drug) or hemodialysis (for drugs that are already absorbed or cannot be cleared via the GI tract). Another drug known as an *antidote* may be used to reverse the toxic effect of a drug.

Action Alert! If a client is exhibiting toxic effects of a medication, do not administer the next scheduled dose. Immediately report signs and symptoms of toxicity to the physician.

Allergic Responses. An allergic response is an antigen-antibody response to a medication. Although this can occur with the first administration, the body requires previous exposure to the antigen to develop antibodies. The allergic response could be triggered by the drug itself, a preservative, or a metabolite.

A **hypersensitivity reaction** is a mild allergic reaction to a drug. Symptoms vary according to the drug and the client, but they typically include skin manifestations,

BOX 21-2 *Teaching for Wellness*

Avoiding Common Side Effects of Medication Therapy

Purpose: To help the client remain free of the most common side effects of a variety of medications by encouraging health-promoting behaviors.

Expected Outcome: The client will remain free of common medication side effects or will have less severe side effects if they occur.

Client Instructions

Constipation. Many groups of medications, such as opioid analgesics, antispasmodics, and iron supplements, slow the action of the gastrointestinal tract. The following are helpful hints about actions you can take to decrease the risk of getting constipated while taking these medications:

- Drink increased fluids unless contraindicated by another health problem. Because foods also contain fluid, you will probably obtain a sufficient fluid intake by drinking 6 to 8 glasses of water each day in addition to the normal diet, to total 2 to 3 quarts of fluid per day.
- Walk or do some other activity that moves and stretches the abdominal muscles each day. This movement "massages" the intestines and increases peristaltic activity.
- Increase the amount of fiber in your diet. Eat plenty of fruits and vegetables, and include whole grains whenever possible instead of refined carbohydrates.

Sedation. Many medications, such as decongestants, some cough preparations, narcotics, and antianxiety agents, cause drowsiness. Although you may not be able to prevent this side effect, you can modify your activities to reduce the risk of injury while taking these medications.

Some suggestions include the following:

- Do not drive or do any other activity that requires concentration for approximately 2 to 3 hours after taking the medication. Resume these activities only after the drowsiness has worn off.
- Make sure travel paths, such as the hallway leading to the bathroom, are sufficiently lighted at night to prevent falls caused by sedation or reduced vision. Remove scatter rugs or other objects that increase the risk of falls.
- If you take the medication once a day, do so at bedtime if possible, to minimize the risks associated with sedation.
- Do not drink alcohol or take any other over-the-counter (OTC) drugs with a sedative effect while taking this medication. Consult with your physician about specific questions to obtain individualized advice.

Dizziness. Because of their effects on blood vessels, many medications taken for cardiovascular problems cause dizziness (vertigo) when you sit up or stand up. The most common ones are antihypertensives and diuretics. If you are taking one of these medications, try to do the following (especially within the first few hours after taking a dose):

- Sit or stand up slowly when rising from the bed or chair.
- Avoid extremely warm environments or hot baths because they can aggravate the problem by dilating the blood vessels.
- Do not drink alcohol while taking the medication because alcohol dilates blood vessels and causes excessive lowering of blood pressure.
- If you take an antihypertensive medication once a day, do so at night to reduce your dizziness or light-headedness. If you are taking a diuretic, however, continue to take it in the morning. Taking it at night would interfere with sleep by making you have to get up to urinate.

such as rash, urticaria, and pruritus. Headache, rhinitis, or nausea and vomiting may also occur.

Anaphylaxis is a life-threatening allergic reaction that requires immediate intervention to prevent possible death. It is a medical emergency. Symptoms are typically cardiorespiratory in nature and include dyspnea, wheezing, stridor, tachycardia, and hypotension. They are caused by bronchoconstriction, laryngeal edema, and widespread vasodilation. Treatment includes supportive care and administration of epinephrine, bronchodilators, antihistamines, and corticosteroids to reduce the allergic response.

Action Alert! **If a client begins to exhibit signs of anaphylaxis after receiving a medication, maintain the client's airway and call for help immediately.**

Because allergic responses can be serious, carefully question clients about a history of drug allergy. For drugs commonly known to be antigenic, such as penicillin, also inquire about a family history of drug allergy. Inquire not only about the drug but also about specific symptoms of the allergic response. This information helps determine whether the client could safely receive the drug if given with another drug (such as an antihistamine) or whether it must not be used at all. All clients with a history of drug allergy should wear or carry identification noting the drug allergy. They should also be taught to inform all future caregivers about the allergy.

Idiosyncratic Responses. An **idiosyncratic response** is an unexplained and unpredictable response to a medication. It may be a suboptimal response, an exaggerated response, or an abnormal type of response. For example, some medications that normally produce drowsiness may cause excitability in children. Idiosyncratic responses may be listed in the drug literature as rare types of adverse effects. Because these are so unpredictable, skilled and conscientious nursing assessment is warranted.

Drug Tolerance. Drug tolerance refers to a diminishing therapeutic drug effect at the same dosage over time, a trend that requires increasing the dosage to achieve the same therapeutic effect. Tolerance occurs as the body becomes accustomed to a drug from prolonged use. A classic example involves pain medication. Over time, a client taking an opioid analgesic for chronic pain may require larger doses to control the pain, even if there is no drug addiction. Carefully monitor the degree of symptom relief from a specific dose of a medication, especially if it will be used on a long-term basis.

Drug Interactions. Drug interactions can be either synergistic or antagonistic. A **synergistic effect** occurs when one drug enhances or increases the effect of another drug. This may be either accidental or planned purposefully by the prescriber. An **antagonistic effect** occurs when one drug reduces or negates the effect of another. Antagonistic effects can also be accidental or purposeful. A client who takes multiple medications (called polypharmacy) is more likely to experience accidental drug interactions; thus the medication regimen must be reviewed carefully.

Other substances, such as alcohol or sodium, can also enhance or interfere with drug action. Teach clients about the effects of these substances on prescribed medications. The resurgence of interest in "natural" or "herbal" remedies provides yet another area for assessment. Interactions between medications and these alternative remedies are increasingly of concern and are active areas of research.

Pharmacokinetics. The term **pharmacokinetics** refers to a drug's activity from the time it enters the body until it leaves. This process has four parts: absorption, distribution, biotransformation (metabolism), and excretion. All health care professionals responsible for managing client medications should understand these processes.

Absorption. Absorption refers to the transference of drug molecules from the point of entry in the body into the bloodstream. Most medications are absorbed systemically to exert their effects. Drug absorption is influenced by many factors, including route of administration, drug dosage and form, and conditions at the absorption site.

The route of administration directly affects the extent and speed of medication absorption and is related to the physical structure of the tissues. The IV route is fastest because the medication is injected directly into the bloodstream, but it also carries risks to client safety (Nicholas & Agius, 2005). Medications are also absorbed rapidly through mucous membranes of the mouth, nose, and respiratory tract because these tissues are highly vascular. Injected medications are absorbed fairly rapidly, but their action also depends on conditions at the injection site. Absorption from the oral route can be affected by dose form and conditions in the GI tract. The topical route has the slowest absorption rate because the skin is a natural barrier.

The dosage and form of a medication commonly affect its absorption. Higher-than-average doses may be purposefully ordered when giving a **loading dose,** which is an initial medication dose that exceeds the maintenance or therapeutic dose. A loading dose may be ordered when the client has not recently received the medication and must rapidly achieve a therapeutic serum level. Examples of drugs commonly initiated with loading doses are digitalis and aminophylline. The loading dose is followed by therapeutic doses, and drug levels in the serum may be periodically monitored.

The form of the medication and conditions in the GI tract greatly affect absorption. Liquid forms, such as solutions or suspensions, are absorbed more quickly than solid forms, such as capsules or tablets. Extended-release products gradually release medication for absorption over a period of time. They can usually be recognized by letters at the end of the medication name, such as ER (extended release), SR (sustained release), SA (sustained action), or XL (extended length). Enteric-coated drugs are coated to prevent them from dissolving until they reach the alkaline environment of the small intestine; usually a drug is enteric coated if it would otherwise irritate the stomach lining. Most drugs are absorbed in the small intestine because of the numerous villi there.

Medications are often administered in relationship to meals. Most are better absorbed when taken between meals. Selected medications are given with food to decrease the irritating effect on the stomach. Be sure to read drug reference material to determine whether a medication should be given with food or between meals (1 hour before or 2 hours after a meal).

Medications not given via the GI tract are greatly affected by conditions at the site of absorption, especially the blood supply to the area. Muscles have a rich supply of blood, making the intramuscular (IM) route the second choice after the IV route when rapid absorption is desired. The subcutaneous (subcut) route is slower than the IM route and is a better choice when slower absorption is needed. Local site conditions that interfere with parenteral drug absorption include bruising, scarring, and edema. Local circulatory impairment may also impede absorption.

Distribution. The process of drug distribution begins with absorption of a drug into the circulation and ends with its arrival at the site of action. The health and makeup of the client, as well as the chemical and physical properties of the medication, affect the degree and speed of distribution.

Various circulatory dynamics affect medication distribution. The more blood vessels supplying a tissue, the better the distribution, and vice versa. Blood vessel tone also affects distribution. Vasoconstriction reduces drug distribution, whereas vasodilation enhances it. Thus distribution of a drug to target tissues may be poorer in clients with impaired circulatory status or with edema.

The body also has physiological barriers to certain medications. The blood-brain barrier permits transport of lipid-bound medications while preventing transport of many water-soluble ones. This has important implications when prescribing medications meant to affect the brain. The placental barrier also inhibits transport of some drugs, but it is less selective than the blood-brain barrier. Prescribers ordering drug therapy for a pregnant client carefully consider this variable when selecting a medication. This decision is crucial because many medications have a high **teratogenic potential,** which is the possibility that a medication will harm a developing fetus (McCarter-Spaulding, 2005). The FDA, therefore, classifies medications according to a pregnancy category to reflect teratogenicity (Table 21-3).

Most medications are partially bound to proteins such as albumin in the bloodstream, making that portion inactive and unable to be used by body tissues. The active, unbound, or "free" portion exerts the therapeutic effect. Clients with low albumin levels have greater circulation of the "active" drug and require decreased dosages. Low albumin levels are typically found in infants, older adults, and those with poor nutrition or liver disease.

Biotransformation. Drug **biotransformation,** or metabolism, is the process of inactivating and breaking down a medication. Enzymes chemically alter a drug's structure, converting it to a less potent substance.

Most drug biotransformation occurs in the liver by microsomes that trigger the enzymatic breakdown of drugs. The liver can oxidize and transform many substances before they reach the body tissues, called a *first-pass effect.* However, liver function can decrease with age or disease, allowing active drug to accumulate in the body. For this reason, infants, older adults, and those with cirrhosis or other liver diseases experience the same effect even with reduced medication doses. Standard doses would place them at risk for drug toxicity.

Less frequent sites of drug biotransformation are the kidneys, lungs, blood, and intestines. Pathologic conditions in these areas also requires reduced drug doses to prevent toxicity. Know the sites of biotransformation for the medications being given, and monitor the client for intended and adverse drug effects.

Excretion. Excretion is the movement of a drug from the site of biotransformation back into the circulation and its transport to the site of exit from the body. The route of excretion is determined by the drug's chemical properties. The kidneys are responsible for excreting most drugs. Other organs of excretion are the lungs, exocrine glands, and GI tract.

The nephrons of the kidneys secrete unwanted substances into the urine when there is an adequate glomerular filtration rate. Most medications undergo biotransformation before excretion; some are eliminated in their original form. It is important to know how a drug is excreted to anticipate its effectiveness. For example, when a client has a urinary tract infection, the drug of choice is one that is excreted relatively unchanged in the urine. Otherwise, the drug will not effectively treat the infection.

Adequate fluid intake (6 to 8 glasses per day) is generally beneficial to aid excretion, except when the client retains fluid, such as with renal or heart failure. A medication dose may be reduced if the client has renal disease that impairs drug excretion.

The lungs, sweat glands, mammary glands, and GI tract excrete drugs to a lesser degree. The lungs excrete volatile gases such as alcohol, nitrous oxide, and ether. The sweat glands help excrete lipid-soluble drugs. Because the mammary glands excrete drugs, women who breastfeed infants should use medications only when advised by a primary care provider, who carefully weighs the benefits to the mother and risks to the infant. The GI tract eliminates medications in bile. The rate of medication excretion by this route can be slowed or accelerated by the same conditions that cause constipation or diarrhea, respectively.

Impaired clearance through any route of excretion could result in drug toxicity. Review the results of

Table 21-3 FDA Pregnancy Categories Used to Assess Fetal Risk

RISK CATEGORY	RISK LEVEL	INTERPRETATION
A	No risk	Study results have not shown evidence of fetal harm from use of this medication.
B	Little or no risk	Results of animal studies show no risk, but no well-controlled studies have been performed with pregnant women.
C	Uncertain risk	Results of animal studies indicate that there is risk to the fetus, but no well-controlled studies have been performed with pregnant women. The risks and benefits of using the drug must be assessed.
D	Proven risk	The risks and benefits of using the drug must be assessed and should be considered in the event of life-threatening situations.
X	Proven risk	This drug should be avoided during pregnancy because the risks outweigh any benefits.

FDA, Food and Drug Administration.

periodically drawn laboratory studies, such as liver enzymes or blood urea nitrogen and creatinine (which monitor kidney function), for elevations.

Blood Level. To be effective, the active component of a medication must be present in the blood within a therapeutic range—that is, the blood level that effectively treats a health problem without creating toxic effects. When a medication is within its therapeutic range, various doses are in different phases of being absorbed, distributed, metabolized, and excreted.

The blood (or serum) level of a medication is the amount circulating in the bloodstream at a given time. The *peak serum level* of a drug is its highest concentration in the blood, which usually occurs just as the last bit of the most recently administered dose is being absorbed. After this, absorption stops and only distribution, biotransformation, and excretion continue. The serum level then falls progressively until the next dose begins to be absorbed. The *trough level* is the term for the lowest circulating level of a drug.

The route of drug administration also influences the blood level. For example, the level of an oral drug typically peaks about 2 hours after ingestion and then tapers steadily (Figure 21-1). Medications given by the IV route reach their peak almost immediately and then taper steadily. In general, therapeutic drug levels are easier to maintain with IV administration, especially when using a continuous pump or drip, because this route avoids the pronounced peaks and valleys of oral administration.

> ***Action Alert!*** Monitor the results of peak and trough serum drug levels, and report values outside the therapeutic range immediately. Assess the client for signs and symptoms of toxicity if results are high, and for symptoms of the original disorder if results are low.

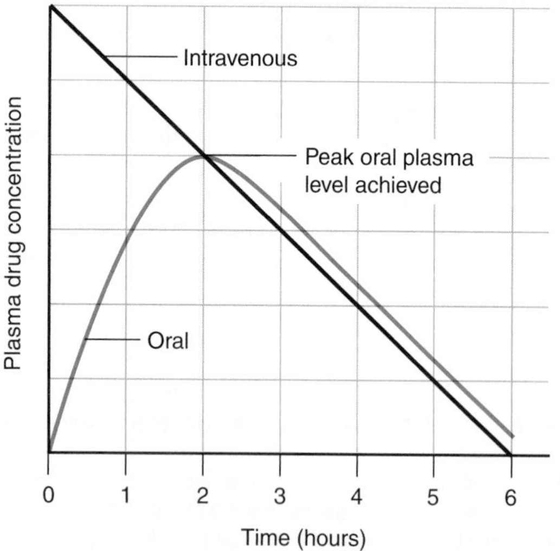

FIGURE 21-1 The blood level of an oral drug typically peaks about 2 hours after ingestion and then tapers steadily, whereas a drug given by the IV route reaches its peak almost immediately and tapers steadily.

Half-Life. Every drug has a half-life, which is the amount of time the body needs to lower by half the drug's serum concentration by biotransformation and excretion. A drug's half-life helps determine how frequently it should be given. Drugs with a long half-life are given less frequently, whereas drugs with a short half-life require more frequent administration.

Onset, Peak, and Duration. *Onset, peak,* and *duration* are terms frequently used to describe the times of the anticipated effects of a drug. The onset is the amount of time needed after drug administration to produce the desired effect. The peak is the amount of time needed for a drug to reach the highest concentration for effectiveness. The duration is the span of time during which the serum drug concentration is high enough to produce the intended effect.

Plateau. The term *plateau* refers to the serum concentration or level of a drug that has been reached and sustained with a series of fixed doses. When the plateau is achieved and maintained, the client should receive the optimal therapeutic benefit.

SYSTEMS OF DELIVERY

Nurse-Administered Medications. When a client is admitted to a hospital or extended-care facility, the responsibility for medication administration usually shifts from the client to the nurse. Expect to obtain a medication history on admission (including use of OTC drugs and herbal remedies), review current medication orders, and consult with the health care provider about any discrepancies. Anticipate that new medications may be ordered to treat the current health problem. Realize also that medications routinely taken at home are sometimes not reordered in the hospital. This may be intentional, as in the case of digitalis toxicity, because the blood level of the drug needs to decrease. Because nurses share the responsibility for ensuring that the client receives medication for ongoing health problems as well as medications ordered for the current problem, consult with the health care provider whenever discrepancies are noted. Be aware also that certain drugs, such as steroids or antihypertensives, cannot be stopped abruptly.

Once admitted to a health care facility, most clients receive medications only when the nurse provides them. In other words, you assume responsibility for obtaining the correct medication, dispensing the correct dose and form at the correct time, and recording administration in the client record. Use extreme caution to avoid errors, which can be harmful to the client, distressing to you, and costly to the institution (Beyea, 2005).

Both institutional factors and nurse-related factors can contribute to the medication error rate in any institution. For this reason, institutions are moving away from a culture of individual nurse blame to a culture of system solutions to reduce medication error rates (Lewis, 2005). Computerized medication systems and bar coding of medications are system safeguards that have been demonstrated to be effective in reducing medication error rates (Doyle, 2004; Patterson, Rogers, & Render, 2004; Southard, 2005). Standard protocols for medication administration may reduce nurse-related errors, and signage placed in medication preparation areas may reduce interruptions by others that interfere with the nurse's focus when preparing medications for administration (Pape, 2003; Pape et al., 2005). Adequate math skills may also reduce dosage calculation errors (Polifroni, Allchin, & McNulty, 2005). A heightened focus on medication safety practices in nursing school curricula may reduce medication errors made by student nurses, which most frequently related to performance deficits in the form of omitted dose or incorrect dose (Wolf, Hicks, & Serembus, 2006).

In your practice, prepare medications for administration in an environment that is conducive to safety and accuracy. Plan to work alone to avoid errors that could result from interruptions and distractions. Make sure there is adequate lighting in the work area to promote accuracy. Ask another nurse to double-check doses for injection, such as digoxin and insulin.

Maintain the security of medications being dispensed. Do not leave medications unattended after beginning their preparation. If you must leave the area briefly, place medications in a locked drawer, cart, or cabinet until you return. The medication cart or storage area should always be locked when unattended.

Action Alert! Lock the medication cart after use. Do not leave medications unattended on top of a cart during or after preparation.

Client-Administered Medications. Sometimes a client self-administers medications after admission to a health care facility, with a corresponding order from the health care provider. This decision is made after considering the client's reliability, the nature and purpose of the medication, and whether client independence should be promoted. Examples of clients who can benefit from self-administration are alert postpartum women who require analgesics, clients with diabetes who regularly take insulin and know how to administer it, older adult clients who take inhalation medications at home, and clients who take oral contraceptives.

General guidelines should be followed when allowing a client to self-administer medications. First, the client should be alert and reliable. The client should also be able to state when he or she has self-administered a medication (so you can document it) or reliably record self-medication on a special form placed at the bedside. This form becomes part of the medical record upon discharge. The client should not keep any medications at the bedside other than those permitted for self-administration.

COMPONENTS AND PROCESSING OF MEDICATION ORDERS

Medication orders must be legally entered into the medical record. When a physician or advanced practice nurse enters a medication order, it must include the date and time of the order; medication name, dose, route, and frequency; and the signature of the prescriber (Table 21-4). A complete order not only fulfills the legal standard but also gives sufficient direction to the pharmacist, nurse, and client.

Once a drug order has been written, it must be communicated to others. Ideally the pharmacist has direct access to the physician's order without transcription, such as with computerized order entry. In a system using manually written orders, agency policy and procedure will dictate how the order is transcribed and communicated to the pharmacy. Your legal responsibility includes accurately interpreting the order and administering the medicine. Note any special conditions or parameters for administration, such as withholding an

Table 21-4 Components of a Drug Order

COMPONENT	EXPLANATION
Date and time of order	Includes month, day, and year. Also includes time of day on orders for inpatients (written on order sheet instead of prescription pad). Time of day indicates AM or PM if military time is not used. Time of order is especially important for drugs with automatic stop times.
Name of medication	Should be clearly and precisely written. Most facilities use generic names, but sometimes both generic and trade names are identified. Prescription orders state the trade name if no interchange is permitted.
Dose of medication	Lists exact amount of the drug ordered.
Route of administration	Lists exact route by which to give the drug. This is very important because many medications can be given by more than one route.
Frequency of administration	May specify the number of times per day (such as qid for four times a day) or may state the number of hours between doses (such as q6h for every 6 hours) depending on the drug and its purpose.
Signature of prescriber	Required by law. An unsigned prescription will not be filled in a pharmacy, and you should not implement an unsigned drug order. For a narcotic prescription, the prescriber's DEA number must be provided in addition to the signature.

DEA, Drug Enforcement Agency.

Table 21-5 Abbreviations Commonly Used in Medication Orders

ABBREVIATION	MEANING
ac	Before meals
ad lib	As desired
ASAP	As soon as possible
bid	Twice daily
$\bar{c}$	With
cap	Capsule
elix	Elixir
gtt	Drop(s)
ID	Intradermal
IM	Intramuscular
IV	Intravenous
IVP	IV push
IVPB	IV piggyback
KVO	Keep vein open
pc	After meals
PO	By mouth, oral
PR	Per rectum
prn	When needed, as necessary
q	Every
qh	Every hour
q3h	Every 3 hours
qid	Four times a day
qs	Quantity sufficient
Rx	Take
$\bar{s}$	Without
subcut	Subcutaneous
SL	Sublingual
stat	Immediately
supp	Suppository
susp	Suspension
tid	Three times a day
tab	Tablet

antihypertensive medication for a systolic blood pressure less than 100 mm Hg. If handwritten orders are illegible or an abbreviation is unclear, clarify the order, because nurses can be held accountable for drug administration errors based on faulty interpretation. Table 21-5 lists commonly used abbreviations in medication orders, and Table 21-6 lists several of the more common abbreviations that are no longer recommended or approved for use by the Institute for Safe Medication Practices (ISMP) or The Joint Commission (TJC) because of risk for error in interpretation.

Verbal or telephone orders may be given in emergency or unusual situations. Facility policy usually dictates whether and under what conditions these types of orders may be taken. (Nursing students generally cannot take verbal or telephone orders.) When verbal or telephone orders are allowed, record the date and time of the order, and the drug name, dose, route, and frequency. Write "T.O." or "V.O." to indicate a telephone or verbal order, respectively, and write the name of the ordering physician after the medication order. Record your own signature, followed by title (RN, LPN). Verbal and telephone orders must be cosigned by the prescriber within a specified time, usually 24 hours or less. To prevent communication errors, always repeat back the order to the prescriber after taking a verbal or telephone order, including the client's name and room number. These types of orders pose the greatest liability for nurses and prescribers. At no time should a medication be administered without an order.

It is an ethical and legal responsibility to clarify any questions you have about a medication order. You could place yourself in legal jeopardy if an error *should* have been noted on the basis of your education and experience. If the prescriber does not respond appropriately to an inquiry, report the problem following the facility's chain of command to prevent the medication error. If you believe the client could be harmed by the medication as ordered, withhold the medication, document this on the medication administration record, and document the rationale carefully on the nursing progress notes.

TYPES OF ORDERS

Several types of medication orders exist; it is critically important to understand what type of order is being carried out. The type of order used depends on the goal of the medication therapy.

Standing Orders. A standing order indicates that a medication should be given on a routine basis. It may be written for a specified number of days, or it may carry no time limit. If there is no limit, follow the order until another order is specifically written to discontinue it. Facility policy sometimes dictates when standing orders are no longer in effect. For example, opioid analgesics often have a "stop date" that is 3 to 7 days after the original order date. In many institutions, any previously written medication orders are canceled when a client goes to surgery, is transferred to another facility, or is discharged. In these circumstances, new orders must be written because the client's status may have changed and the old orders may no longer be appropriate. Facility policy may also dictate how frequently standing orders must be reviewed.

A special type of standing order may be found in specialty nursing units such as cardiac care or maternity units. In these areas, one or more standardized written medication orders are activated or followed when special circumstances occur (such as cardiac dysrhythmias). These orders are medically safe, time saving for the nurse, and potentially lifesaving for the client. Once activated, these medications are charted just as any other medication would be.

Prn Orders. A prn order is an order for a medication that is given as needed. The label derives from the Latin *pro re nata,* meaning "as necessary." It lists the minimum amount of time that must elapse between doses, and it may also specify the symptoms it is used to treat. This

Table 21-6 Common Abbreviations No Longer Approved in Medication Orders

DANGEROUS ABBREVIATION	MEANING AND MISINTERPRETATION	CORRECTION
μg	Microgram; mistaken for mg	mcg
AD, AS, AU	Right ear, left ear, each ear; mistaken for eye	right ear, left ear, each ear
OD, OS, OU	Right eye, left eye, each eye; mistaken for ear	right eye, left eye, each eye
cc	Cubic centimeters; mistaken as "u" (units)	mL
D/C	Discontinue or discharge; mistaken for each other	discontinue or discharge
IN	Intranasal; mistaken for IM or IV	intranasal or NAS
HS or hs	Half-strength and bedtime or hour of sleep; mistaken for each other	half-strength or bedtime
IU	International unit; mistaken for IV or 10	units
o.d. or OD	Once daily; mistaken as right eye	daily
OJ	Orange juice; mistaken for right or left eye	orange juice
Per os	By mouth, orally; os mistaken for left eye	PO, by mouth, or orally
q.d., QD, or q1d	Every day; mistaken for q.i.d	daily
qhs or qn	Nightly or at bedtime; mistaken for every hour	nightly or at bedtime
q.o.d. or QOD	Every other day; mistaken for daily or q.i.d.	every other day
SC, SQ, sub q	Subcutaneous; mistaken for SL, 5 every, and subcutaneously every, respectively	Subcut or subcutaneously
ss	Sliding scale (insulin) or ½ (apothecary measure); mistaken for 55	Sliding scale, one-half, or ½
U or u	Unit; mistaken for 0 or 4 and sometimes cc	Unit
×3d	For three days; mistaken for 3 doses	For three days
> and <	Greater than and less than; mistaken for each other	Greater than and less than

Selected from Institute for Safe Medication Practices. (2003). *List of error-prone abbreviations, symbols, and dose designations.* Retrieved June 12, 2006, from http://www.ismp.org/Tools/abbreviationslist.pdf.
In addition, drug names should be written out and not abbreviated.
See http://www.ismp.org for the full list.

type of drug order allows you to use discretion in administering a medication. It also requires that you have good assessment skills, noting both the situation and clinical condition of the client. An example of a prn order is *droperidol (Inapsine) 2.5 mg IV q6h prn for nausea or vomiting.* This tells you that it may be given for nausea or vomiting, provided the client has not received a dose for at least 6 hours.

Single Orders. A single order is a medication order carried out one time only. It identifies the drug, dose, route, and time for administration. Preoperative and preprocedure orders are commonly written as one-time orders. An example is *nafcillin (Nafcil) 1 g IVPB on call to OR.* This order states to infuse a specific antibiotic attached to a mainline IV when the client is called to the operating room. (IVPB will be described later.)

Stat Orders. A stat order (from the Latin *stat*) is one that is implemented immediately. These orders are frequently given during an emergency or near-emergency situation, such as an impending cardiac or respiratory arrest. Stat orders are more likely to be given as verbal or telephone orders. Most institutions have policies and guidelines stating the time period within which a stat order must be completed.

MEDICATION DISTRIBUTION SYSTEMS

Medication distribution systems are designed to promote safety and accuracy, conserve time and money, and promote client self-care. Within a facility, a single system is used and all personnel and support structures work together to provide streamlined delivery.

Unit-Dose System. The most commonly used system today is the unit-dose system. A unit dose is a single dose of a medication that is prepackaged and labeled by the manufacturer or pharmacist. A new supply of unit doses for each client is delivered to the nursing unit every 24 hours. You then take a single dose of each medication to the bedside at the appropriate time.

Computer-Controlled Dispensing Systems. The most recently developed unit-dose system is the computer-controlled dispensing system. The system is menu driven, and access is limited to users having personal identification codes. The unit contains medications stored in specific containers that are labeled and coded in the machine. The computer is programmed with the number of unit doses stocked for each medication. After drug removal, the computer records the transaction and the user, and charges the drug to the client. This system is time saving for you and is cost-effective because of better inventory control. It is used most frequently for controlled substances and prn medications, but some facilities use it for all medication dispensing.

ROUTES OF ADMINISTRATION

Oral Routes. Oral or PO (from the Latin *per oris*) means given by mouth. There are three oral routes for medication administration: the oral, sublingual, and buccal routes.

Oral. A medication given by the oral route is placed in the mouth and swallowed. A client with a nasogastric (NG) tube connected to suction cannot receive oral medications. Confused clients or those who are unwilling to swallow should be carefully assessed to determine if this route is appropriate. Clients with an impaired or absent swallow reflex cannot use this route but may have a feeding tube in place. If so, medications may be given by NG, gastrostomy, or jejunostomy tube and are called enteral medications. A client who is on NPO (nothing by mouth) status may not receive oral medications unless the order specifically states *NPO with/except meds.*

Sublingual. A medication given by the sublingual (SL) route is placed under the tongue and allowed to dissolve. The medication is quickly absorbed through the mucous membranes into the systemic circulation. Tell the client not to swallow a tablet ordered for SL use because it will not be effective. The client should avoid eating, swallowing liquids, or smoking while the tablet is dissolving. An example is nitroglycerin, which is used to treat chest pain of cardiac origin.

Buccal. A tablet or lozenge given by the buccal route is placed against the mucous membranes of the mouth, between the cheek and the gums, near the molars. The drug dissolves and acts either locally on mucosa or systemically after being absorbed from saliva swallowed into the stomach. Teach clients using this route to avoid swallowing liquids while the medication is dissolving and to alternate cheeks with succeeding doses to minimize mucosal irritation.

Parenteral Routes. A **parenteral route** is one that is outside the GI tract. Parenteral medications are given by injection into a body tissue using sterile technique. The four routinely used parenteral routes are intradermal, subcutaneous, intramuscular, and intravenous. These routes provide for faster drug action but are associated with risks of discomfort, infection, and even bleeding in some clients. Other, less frequently used parenteral routes are the epidural and intrathecal routes. These routes are initiated by physicians or advanced practice nurses.

Intradermal. The **intradermal (ID) route** involves injection into the dermal layer of the skin. It is commonly used to test for allergic reactions to a substance planted in the dermis. Examples of ID injections are purified protein derivative for tuberculosis and skin testing for mumps and *Candida.*

Subcutaneous. The **subcutaneous (subcut) route** involves injection into subcutaneous tissue just under the dermis. It is commonly used by nurses and by clients self-administering insulin or small amounts of other medications that do not need to be rapidly absorbed. The former abbreviations for this route, SC SQ, and sub q are no longer recommended because these abbreviations contribute to medication errors (ISMP, 2003).

Intramuscular. The **intramuscular (IM) route** involves injection into muscle tissue, specifically the body of a muscle. Medications are absorbed quickly, making this a popular route when faster absorption is needed. It is frequently used to administer opioid analgesics, antiemetics, and some antibiotics.

Intravenous. The **intravenous (IV) route** involves injection of a medication into a vein. This route provides the most rapid effect, with distribution throughout the body in a few minutes. For this reason, smaller drug doses are needed. A disadvantage is that the route is potentially dangerous because drugs given incorrectly cannot be retrieved; this is true for all parenteral medications, but here there is less time to intervene. Antibiotics, histamine-receptor antagonists, and selected pain medications are examples of medications commonly given by the IV route. This route is also used for patient-controlled analgesia (see Chapter 37).

Topical Route. The **topical route** is used to deliver a medication directly to a body site, such as the skin, eyes, ears, nose, throat, vagina, or rectum. A skin preparation may be applied by manually spreading it over an area, applying a patch, placing the drug in a medicated dressing, soaking the area in solution, or using a medicated bath.

Topical drugs often have a local effect, although some are absorbed systemically as well. The length of exposure to a topical application directly correlates to the amount absorbed. Remove a previous dose before applying the next dose, and wash the area to prevent further absorption.

Suppositories are the drug form often used for insertion into the rectum or vagina. Drops may be instilled into the eyes, nose, or ears. Irrigations may be ordered for the eye, ear, bladder, rectum, or vagina. Medications can also be sprayed into the nose or throat, or throat gargles may be used.

Inhalation Route. Inhalation is used to bring medications into the respiratory tract via the nose or throat. Most medications given by this route exert local effects on the bronchial mucosa. They are administered via metered-dose inhaler, nebulizer (see Chapter 34), or the newer turbo-inhaler.

Clients may also receive inhaled medications via an endotracheal tube or a tracheostomy, such as anesthetic gases and some emergency resuscitative drugs. This route allows for rapid systemic absorption because the lungs have a very large and highly vascular surface area.

A nasal inhaler may be used to administer certain medications. The most common example is the use of a decongestant nasal spray to constrict nasal blood vessels and relieve cold symptoms. Another type of nasal medication uses a nasal canister with a thin tube attached. The tube is inserted into the nares and is either squeezed or blown in to deliver a dose of medication.

An example is desmopressin (DDAVP), which is used to treat diabetes insipidus.

FACTORS AFFECTING DRUG ACTIONS

A number of client-related factors can influence the action of a medication. These include risk factors that are present across the life span, physiological factors, and cultural/lifestyle factors.

RISK FACTORS ACROSS THE LIFE SPAN

Age. A client's age significantly influences medication actions. Infants have immature function of the renal, hepatic, and GI systems. They also lack certain metabolic enzymes needed for proper drug biotransformation. Finally, they have relatively more body water and less body mass. These factors cause the infant's system to be highly responsive to medications.

Older adults can also have an altered response to medications because of changes that occur with the aging process (Ebersole et al., 2004). Absorption, biotransformation, and excretion are reduced by slowed or decreased organ function. Drug distribution is altered by decreased size, protein-binding sites, body water, and lean muscle mass. Each of these factors increases the risk for drug toxicity. Older adults also have a higher risk of adverse effects from polypharmacy or from taking medications incorrectly. Nurses play an important role in preventing these occurrences (Frazier, 2005).

Psychological Factors. Psychological factors can influence whether a client chooses to take a medication and whether the drug is ultimately effective. These factors include the client's acceptance of medication use, prior experience with medications, fear, motivation, secondary gain, and the behavior of the nurse administering the medication. Chapter 20 discusses factors affecting compliance with a health care regimen.

PHYSIOLOGICAL FACTORS

Genetic Differences. Genetic factors can influence the manner in which the body uses, metabolizes, or reacts to a drug (Lea, 2005). Deficiencies in natural body enzymes used to biotransform drugs may be responsible for these events. Genetics helps to explain why allergies to penicillin, for example, can run in families and why people of one ethnic origin may not obtain the same benefits from a medication dose as those of another origin.

Gender Differences. Men and women have different amounts of body fat, body water, and muscle mass. They also have different circulating levels of male and female hormones. These factors influence drug actions by affecting one or more pharmacokinetic processes. Much clinical drug research is done with male subjects, so drug effects on women may sometimes be unexpected.

Height and Weight. Height and weight are important factors affecting drug actions. Standard drug doses are published for average-sized adults, who range in age from 18 to 65 and weigh about 150 pounds. Overweight adults may require an increased dose to achieve therapeutic results. Drug doses for infants and children are calculated according to body weight or body surface area. Record height and weight at the time of hospital admission (or during the intake process in an ambulatory care setting) to provide a ready reference for the prescriber to determine drug dosages.

Diseases. Diseases that adversely affect any one of the pharmacokinetic processes ultimately affect drug action. For example, impaired GI function may reduce absorption. Heart failure or other edema-causing conditions may impair drug distribution. Liver or renal disease limits drug biotransformation and excretion, putting the client at risk for toxic effects.

Reactions to Environment. Physical agents in the environment can directly affect a client's response to a medication. Heat and cold produce vasodilation and vasoconstriction, which in turn alter drug distribution or even its effects (e.g., antihypertensives). Advise clients to dress appropriately for the weather and to avoid temperature extremes. Ionizing radiation, such as sunlight, can affect enzyme activity in the body, altering drug actions. Many medications have photosensitivity as a side effect, so warn clients to avoid prolonged exposure or to use a strong sunscreen when outdoors.

CULTURAL AND LIFESTYLE FACTORS

Dietary Factors. Dietary factors and overall nutritional state can either positively or negatively affect medication actions in the body. Recall that cells manufacture proteins and enzymes. Because most drugs bind with proteins, sufficient protein intake is needed for proper drug distribution. Both proteins and enzymes are also needed for drug biotransformation.

Specific foods can trigger drug-food interactions that either increase or decrease a drug's effectiveness. The diet may have to be changed somewhat to manage these nutrients. For example, liver or green leafy vegetables rich in vitamin K should be limited or maintained at a steady level when taking warfarin (Coumadin) because they antagonize the drug's action. Clients who take potassium-wasting diuretics should increase intake of high-potassium foods.

Fluid balance also influences drug effects. Sufficient body fluid is necessary to carry drugs to their site of action and to excrete them after use. Thus dehydration can limit the transport of drugs and their metabolites, reducing the effectiveness of drug therapy.

Cultural and Religious Beliefs. Cultural and religious beliefs can influence a client's thoughts about medication effectiveness and whether to comply with therapy.

If the client has a cultural heritage in which medication is commonly used to treat health problems, the medication is more likely to be accepted because it is a form of traditional medicine for that client. If the client's cultural heritage does not typically use medication freely, this form of treatment is likely to be viewed instead as an alternative therapy (Spector, 2004) and may not be well accepted. Non-Western healing practices, such as herbal therapy, talismans, and use of spiritual advisors or healers, may complement or interfere with the intended effects of prescribed medications, depending on specific circumstances. Assess the client in a culturally sensitive fashion to build a sufficient database for evaluating drug effectiveness. Become familiar with the basic beliefs and health practices of clients of other cultures to help you to communicate medication information more effectively (Box 21-3).

Socioeconomic Factors. Socioeconomic factors play an indirect role in influencing drug therapy. Financially disadvantaged clients may not seek care for a health problem as quickly as those with adequate finances or health insurance. When a disadvantaged client does seek treatment, the medication regimen may be more complex because the health problem was not identified at an early stage. The client may be unable to afford continued medication therapy after the initial episode resolves and may not refill prescriptions or may take partial doses to help the medication last longer.

The Institute for Safe Medication Practices (ISMP) (2001) indicates that more than 40% of clients with a chronic illness are functionally illiterate, that almost one quarter of American adults read at or below the fifth-grade level, and that most medical information leaflets are written at or above the tenth-grade level. An inability to understand medication instructions will have consequences for the client at some point in the health-illness trajectory.

BOX 21-3 *Communicating Effectively With Clients of Other Cultures About Medication Therapy*

- Become informed about the health practices and beliefs of cultural groups in your community. Be aware that diversity may exist within subgroups of a larger cultural group.
- Encourage clients of other cultures to communicate their concerns and ask questions related to medication therapy.
- Provide printed or audiovisual medication information in the client's language if possible.
- Question the client directly about the use of remedies prescribed by a healer within the culture.
  These remedies may have an interactive effect with prescribed medication therapy.
- Watch for atypical drug responses or unexpected side effects in clients in certain cultural groups. Cultural influences such as diet, complementary therapies, or even genetic factors can precipitate unusual responses to medication therapy.

ASSESSMENT

A client receiving medication therapy deserves a thorough and multifaceted assessment to determine both the need for medication and the likelihood of response. The assessment process is twofold and includes general assessment and focused assessment.

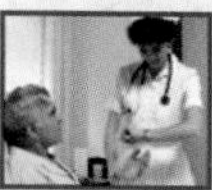

Mr. Connell was diagnosed with hypertension (high blood pressure) 5 years ago. At that time, atenolol (Tenormin, a beta-adrenergic blocking agent) was prescribed. Within a few months, furosemide (Lasix, a diuretic) was also prescribed because his blood pressure was not effectively reduced. This regimen was effective, and he continued with therapy for a little over a year. At that time, he felt quite well and decided that he did not need the medication any longer. He has not seen a physician in more than 3 years. Box 21-4 provides information useful to the nurse working with Mr. Connell and adds to the assessment database gathered thus far.

GENERAL ASSESSMENT FOR MEDICATION ADMINISTRATION

Health History. A client's health history provides information about existing health problems being managed with medications and illnesses or organ dysfunction that may increase the risk of toxicity or other adverse drug

BOX 21-4 *Cross-Cultural Care*

Caring for an Irish American Client

Daniel Connell, the client whose story we've been following through this chapter, is of Irish American descent. His family came to Boston, Massachusetts, in the late 1800s. Although there are always individual differences among clients, Irish Americans as a group tend to have the following characteristics (Wilson, 1998):

- Believe and expect that life is a difficult process.
- Understate their symptoms when ill and delay seeking health care until symptoms are severe or cannot be ignored.
- Are stoic and resist expressing emotions associated with illness or pain.
- Use facial expressions to communicate nonverbally rather than more expressive gestures, such as hand and arm movements.
- Use traditional home remedies to treat minor illnesses but seek out a traditional health care provider if these fail or if a larger health problem emerges.

effects. Inquire about any significant surgical procedures performed in the past. If a hormone-secreting organ has been removed, such as ovaries or thyroid, the client may take hormone replacement therapy. These medications should be continued during inpatient care.

History of Allergies. It is critically important to assess for drug allergies, especially when a client is being treated for the first time. Even if the client has an existing medical record from previous admissions or visits, verify allergies at each encounter. Assess the following factors whenever possible: drug, dose and route, number of times taken before allergy symptoms occurred, and onset and nature of the reaction. Assess for both drug and food allergies because some foods contain ingredients that are also found in medications. For example, clients who are allergic to shellfish cannot receive injectable radiocontrast dye during diagnostic studies because both contain iodine. Some vaccines are made from substances in chick embryos and should not be given to a client allergic to eggs.

Record allergies in large print on the cover of the client's medical record. If handwritten physician order forms are used, place an allergy sticker on each new blank order page as it is inserted into the chart. You may also find allergy notations in nursing admission notes, physician history-and-physical notes, medication administration records, and possibly on or over the bed. On admission, put a bracelet listing all pertinent allergies on the client's wrist, and leave it in place until discharge.

> **Action Alert!** Always check for an allergy bracelet before giving medication to a client. If a bracelet falls off or becomes illegible, replace it at once.

Medication History. On admission, document the name of each drug the client routinely takes, the dose, the route (usually oral), and time of the last dose. Document whether any medications have been brought to the hospital and their disposition (e.g., sent home or stored on the nursing unit). In addition to questioning the client about prescription and OTC drug use, ask about the use of herbal or nutritional supplements (Fontaine, 2005). Many clients will not mention OTC or herbal drugs unless specifically asked. Assess the dose, frequency, and reason for use.

Medication reconciliation is a process that requires health care providers to create an accurate list of a client's medication on admission (Barnsteiner, 2005). The list must include the drug name, dose, frequency, route, and time of last dose and is compared to current medication orders at the time of admission, transfer to another unit or facility, and at discharge. The purpose is to eliminate oversights, duplication, or other discrepancies in the medication record that could lead to errors or adverse drug events (Manno & Hayes, 2006). Medication reconciliation became one of the 2006 National Patient Safety Goals set by TJC.

Diet History. Because most medications are administered orally, assess the client's usual dietary intake, food preferences, and meal patterns. Several medications are better absorbed when taken either with or without food. Adjust the medication schedule accordingly. This may be more difficult than it seems because most facilities have policies and procedures governing routine medication administration times for standard drug therapy.

Client's Knowledge of Drug Therapy. Increased knowledge of drug therapy should positively influence compliance. Assess the client's knowledge of the following:

- What the drug is being taken for
- How and when it should be taken
- If any doses have been skipped and why
- Any side effects experienced
- Other specific information unique to the drug

Inadequate knowledge in any of these areas should guide you to develop an individualized teaching plan. If the client cannot learn the necessary information, obtain assistance from others (family or friends), who then become the focus of teaching. Older adults, in particular, are at risk for medication-related problems after discharge, which may be influenced by client teaching (Curry, Walker, Hogstel, & Burns, 2005; Foust, Naylor, Boling, & Cappuzzo, 2005).

Physical Examination

Current Condition. Use knowledge of the client's ongoing condition or health status to assess whether current orders for drug therapy are sufficient and appropriate. Depending on changes in physical assessment data, new medications may be ordered and existing medications may be placed on hold, undergo a change in route, or be discontinued. Assess each client carefully, and report changes in condition to the prescriber.

Be aware of any specific parameters to assess before giving a medication. For example, you might withhold a dose of digoxin if the client's pulse rate is less than 60 beats per minute. In contrast, you may implement a medication order on the basis of client assessment. For example, you may administer a prn medication for nausea, pain, or high blood pressure if the client's condition warrants.

Perception and Coordination. Assess whether the client has any difficulty with perception or coordination. Sensory perceptual deficits usually relate to vision or hearing. Problems with coordination could result from arthritis, muscle weakness or paralysis, or reduced sensation in the hands or fingertips. These clients could have difficulty reaching a medication cabinet, opening medication packages or bottles, splitting scored tablets, or self-administering injections.

Problems with perception or coordination may not seem as important while the nurse is administering drugs, but they become significant as the client prepares for self-management at discharge. An example is a client newly started on insulin therapy who has poor vision and cannot see syringe markings. Another is a client with myasthenia gravis who cannot coordinate or control muscle movements. In such cases, assess whether family members, friends, or close neighbors can assist. If not, the client may require the services of a home health care agency.

FOCUSED ASSESSMENT FOR *INEFFECTIVE HEALTH MAINTENANCE*

Defining Characteristics. Assess the client's knowledge about the need for the medication, the instructions for self-administration, and the need for a temporary or permanent change in lifestyle. Although seemingly simple, for some clients this is complex. For example, an antibiotic prescribed to treat an infection must generally be taken for 5 to 10 days, depending on the antibiotic. Although taking an antibiotic is a temporary change in lifestyle, the client needs to understand that the medication must be taken exactly as prescribed for the full amount of time ordered, even if symptoms disappear. Otherwise, the infection could reoccur and the client's condition could become worse than when originally diagnosed.

Note the client's reported or observed ability to take responsibility for managing medication therapy. Also assess the client's interest in following medication instructions, which may be evidenced by the client's reviewing instructions and asking questions.

Assess whether the client has an adequate support system—that is, one or more other persons to turn to if problems arise in taking or obtaining medications. Clients with no support system are more likely to have difficulty with medication therapy. Remember that this could also involve assistance for follow-up laboratory work needed with some medications (e.g., the international normalized ratio, or INR, for anticoagulant therapy). Home health care assistance may be required.

Assess the client for inadequate financial and other resources, which can also influence adherence to medication therapy (Curry et al., 2005). Assess whether the client can physically obtain the medication and has insurance or other financial resources to pay for it. Some medications are expensive, and the client may stop taking them because of cost. Some clients have no transportation to a pharmacy. Determine whether the client could benefit from referral to a social worker for financial matters or whether resources are available to deliver medication refills to the client.

Related Factors. In general, related factors are those things that increase the likelihood that a nursing diagnosis will apply, although there may not be a cause-and-effect relationship. Examples of assessing and responding to related factors for *Ineffective health maintenance* include the following:

- *Misinterpretation of medication-related information.* A client who inadequately understood previous instructions has *Ineffective health maintenance,* despite prior teaching. Assess the current level of understanding to plan remedial teaching.
- *Inability to take responsibility for medications.* Sometimes clients cannot take their own medications. Two examples are a young child and a client who is not ready to learn because of anxiety. In such situations, assess whether other people in the client's support system could be taught about medication therapy.
- *Cognitive impairment.* Assess the client's ability to take in and retain information. A client who has a disorder that impairs cognitive function, such as stroke, closed head injury, or dementia, may not be able to respond adequately to medication teaching. For example, a cognitively impaired client may be unable to remember to take a medication at specified times. This client may benefit from a 7-day medication dispenser, which can be prefilled by a family member or home health care nurse. If needed, the teaching plan is again directed to others.
- *Physical impairment.* Some clients are physically unable to administer their own medications, open a pill bottle, or manipulate a syringe. They may be paralyzed or have some other limitation that prevents mobility in the environment. Assess whether environmental changes are likely to enable the client to take medications. Determine whether special adaptive devices such as syringe holders or pillboxes could help the client become independent. Some clients with physical impairments must have their medications administered by others.
- *Inadequate communication skills.* A client who cannot comprehend directions will have difficulty taking in and retaining medication information. Examples include clients with a language barrier or receptive aphasia (inability to understand the spoken word). When working with such clients, obtain an interpreter or give the instructions to someone who will be assisting the client after discharge.

If medication therapy is to be effective, the client must be able to obtain the medication, store it properly, take it as directed, watch for expected drug effects, and notice and report important side effects. Difficulty in any of these areas leads you to consider *Ineffective health maintenance* as a nursing diagnosis.

FOCUSED ASSESSMENT FOR *INEFFECTIVE THERAPEUTIC REGIMEN MANAGEMENT*

Defining Characteristics. Clients' beliefs about their ability to regain health or their desire to do so may influence their willingness to take medication. Assess their desire to utilize medication therapy as part of an overall treatment plan. Assess for difficulty in integrating medication therapy into the daily routine. Also, note evidence of compliance with other aspects of the health care regimen and the acceptance of responsibility for self-care as supportive data in determining motivation to comply with medication therapy.

Assess clients' ability to understand and follow the drug regimen. Sometimes clients who are labeled as noncompliant actually have barriers to effective self-administration. These barriers can stem from lack of comprehension, family conflicts, mistrust of the health care team, or the complexity of the medication regimen.

Each of these factors requires a different approach on your part. For example, older adults and those with multiple health problems are most likely to have complex medication schedules. Develop calendars, charts, or other visual reminders for use as needed. Some clients benefit from using prefilled weekly or monthly medication boxes to prevent them from taking the wrong medication or dose. At times, you may enlist the help of family, friends, or a home health care agency to ensure that the client receives correct medications.

Related Factors. The related factors for *Ineffective therapeutic regimen management* overlap to some degree with those listed under *Ineffective health maintenance* in relation to perceived barriers, social supports, and economic difficulties. Additional factors include the following:

- *Deficient knowledge.* Assess the client's current level of knowledge and understanding.
- *Perceived susceptibility, seriousness, and benefits.* Clients who believe that they are not susceptible to a worsening of the condition, that the condition is not serious, or that there are no benefits to medication therapy may not adhere to the medication schedule. They may display no interest in managing medication therapy and may not pay attention to instructions or follow them even if properly understood. Try to assess why the client is not interested so you can include information in the teaching plan that may help change these client beliefs.

DIAGNOSIS

A useful approach for selecting nursing diagnoses is to think about the goal of care for a particular client. For example, consider an otherwise healthy 68-year-old woman who has been hospitalized with a myocardial infarction. She is concurrently diagnosed with hypertension and shows early signs of heart failure. She is started on daily oral doses of furosemide (a diuretic) and metoprolol (an antihypertensive, antianginal). Nitroglycerin sublingual tablets (antianginal) are prescribed for prn use. The client is scheduled for discharge within 24 hours and says that she does not understand how these medications will help her. The most logical nursing diagnosis with the information given is *Ineffective health maintenance.* These medications are newly ordered for this client, who was healthy before admission. A sample nursing diagnostic statement could be *Ineffective health maintenance related to insufficient knowledge of newly prescribed medications.* The goal of care is to return the client to independent living, and the client requires the usual information about medication therapy before discharge.

If this client had mild dementia and could not retain information, you might select *Ineffective therapeutic regimen management.* A sample nursing diagnostic statement might be *Ineffective therapeutic regimen management related to cognitive impairment.* The goal of care in this case would be to put safeguards in place to ensure that the client receives both of her daily medications and the prn nitroglycerin as well.

If an oriented client experienced orthostatic intolerance from the vasodilating effect of metoprolol and fluid loss from furosemide, you might select the nursing diagnostic statement *Risk for injury related to orthostatic hypotension secondary to medication effect.* The goal of care in this instance would be to keep the client from self-injury or experiencing a fall during periods of dizziness and hypotension. The focus of care would be teaching the client to change position slowly, avoid concurrent use of alcohol, and use other standard measures outlined in pharmacology references.

Even if medication use is not the driving force in formulating a nursing diagnosis, administration of medications may be included in the nursing interventions listed for other nursing diagnoses. A client with emphysema may have a nursing diagnosis of *Activity intolerance.* Teaching proper use of bronchodilators may be part of the plan of care for that nursing diagnosis.

The issues and problems that could arise during medication therapy are so broad that several other nursing diagnoses could be relevant. The following is a list of other nursing diagnoses that may apply to individual clients.

- *Constipation* or *Diarrhea related to GI effects of medication therapy.* Opioid analgesics frequently cause constipation, whereas antibiotics may cause diarrhea. Determine any changes in the client's usual pattern of bowel elimination, and analyze these changes in relation to the onset and timing of medications. The focus of nursing care is reducing or eliminating the disturbance.
- *Ineffective sexuality patterns related to altered libido secondary to medication therapy.* Common medications that decrease libido are antidepressants, antihistamines, antihypertensives, sedatives, and tranquilizers (chronic use). Medications that increase libido include testosterone, sedatives (low-dose), and tranquilizers. The focus of nursing care is teaching clients about these side effects and about coping mechanisms.

- *Insomnia related to medication effects.* Some medications, such as benzodiazepines or skeletal muscle relaxants, cause drowsiness, whereas others, such as stimulants, cause nervous system excitation. The focus of nursing care is to analyze whether the scheduling of medications could be changed to allow more normal sleep, and to implement these changes whenever possible. Otherwise, reduce interfering stimuli, such as noise, temperature, a full bladder, pain, fear, or stress.
- *Risk for injury related to adverse medication side effects on mobility or sensorium.* Clients with reduced mobility may be at risk for falls from a decreased ability to move purposefully in the environment. Clients with altered sensorium may harm themselves either by falling or by climbing out of bed. Drugs that could cause these effects include sedatives, vasodilators, diuretics, antidiabetics, antihypertensives, and psychotropics. Assess the risk of injury, and put precautionary measures in place, such as a call bell, ambulation aids, a night-light, and a clutter-free environment. In general, clients also need to know to avoid drinking alcohol or taking OTC drugs with sedative effects concurrently with many types of medications to avoid adverse interactive effects.
- *Risk for infection related to possible superinfection as a consequence of antibiotic therapy.* Superinfection is an overgrowth of pathogens normally kept in balance by the organisms killed by the antibiotic. Assess for signs of superinfection, such as oral lesions (thrush), diarrhea *(Clostridium difficile)*, or vaginal itching (yeast infection). Report these manifestations to the prescriber so that the new infection(s) may be treated.
- *Risk for infection related to medication-induced immune system depression.* Clients with cancer who receive chemotherapy or radiation therapy and clients taking immunosuppressant drugs after organ transplant are at greatest risk for this diagnosis. Monitor vigilantly these clients' vital signs (especially temperature), white blood cell counts, and other signs and symptoms of infection. Remember that infection may be occurring in immunosuppressed clients when the white blood cell count is too low, not only when it is elevated. Report signs and symptoms of infection immediately.
- *Disturbed sensory perception related to adverse effects of medication therapy (sedatives and tranquilizers).* These medications reduce or change the perception of incoming stimuli. Assess clients for such indicators as disorientation, restlessness, blurred vision, and sometimes auditory or visual hallucinations. Refer back to the nursing diagnosis *Risk for injury.* This diagnosis may also apply when there are toxic drug effects (such as hearing loss from ototoxicity with aminoglycosides). Check the drug literature for adverse neurological effects, and report them if noted. Reorient affected clients as needed, and take measures to maintain client safety.
- *Imbalanced nutrition: less than body requirements related to medication-induced anorexia, GI discomfort, or diarrhea.* Teach clients about the proper timing of medications in relation to meals to reduce the incidence of this problem. Report abdominal discomfort that the client cannot tolerate (such as severe abdominal pain caused by erythromycin). The prescriber may order a change to a different drug with fewer GI side effects.
- *Impaired swallowing related to cranial nerve impairment.* This diagnosis often applies after cerebrovascular accident (CVA or stroke) or other central nervous system problems. Use this nursing diagnosis if the client has an impaired gag reflex, if food remains in the mouth after swallowing, or if the client coughs when swallowing medications, liquids, or food (see Chapter 25). The focus of care is to give medication in a form that the client can manage (crushed medications, getting an order for a liquid form rather than solid). At times, the physician may need to change the route from oral to enteral (by tube). A client who cannot swallow medications is at risk for aspiration, which could lead to pneumonia.

In summary, clinical diagnostic reasoning is a complex process that becomes easier with time and practice. Assess each client carefully, and cluster the data to form possible alternative nursing diagnoses (Table 21-7).

Table 21-7 Clustering Data to Make a Nursing Diagnosis

Medication Therapy	
DATA CLUSTER	**DIAGNOSIS**
A client with a newly prescribed medication does not know what effects to expect or how to use the medication properly but has expressed an interest in learning about it.	*Ineffective health maintenance* related to insufficient knowledge of medication use and effects
An older adult client with arthritis in her hands and fingers has been changed from an oral hypoglycemic drug to insulin therapy. Although she expresses interest in managing her insulin therapy, she is unable to draw up the insulin or manipulate the syringe.	*Ineffective therapeutic regimen management* related to poor manual dexterity secondary to inflammation of joints
An older adult client has not refilled a needed prescription because of inability to afford the medication and lack of transportation to a local pharmacy	*Noncompliance* related to medication therapy secondary to financial and physical barriers

Select the ones that have the best "fit" with the goal or intended outcome of care. *Ineffective health maintenance* is often appropriate to use with a client receiving medication therapy.

PLANNING

During the planning phase of the nursing process, establish the expected outcomes or goals for the selected nursing diagnosis. Next, write the specific nursing interventions that will help the client achieve the identified outcomes.

EXPECTED OUTCOMES FOR *INEFFECTIVE HEALTH MAINTENANCE*

Sample expected outcomes for the client receiving medication therapy with a nursing diagnosis of *Ineffective health maintenance* are the following:

- Identifies the need to take medication for treatment of health problem
- Verbalizes an understanding of medication purposes, actions, adverse effects, and comfort and safety measures
- Demonstrates initiative in beginning to manage medication therapy
- Utilizes support systems as needed to adhere to medication therapy, such as getting prescriptions from pharmacy or keeping follow-up appointments with health care provider

EXPECTED OUTCOMES FOR *INEFFECTIVE THERAPEUTIC REGIMEN MANAGEMENT*

Sample expected outcomes for the client receiving medication therapy with a nursing diagnosis of *Ineffective therapeutic regimen management* are the following:

- Verbalizes an understanding of medication purposes, actions, adverse effects, and comfort and safety measures
- Verbalizes an intention to take medications as prescribed to promote health and limit disease progression
- Correctly self-administers medications
- States proper information about drug procurement, storage, and handling
- States an appropriate plan for medical follow-up for monitoring of medications

These expected outcomes could apply to the client being discharged from nursing care in any setting, including a hospital, an extended-care facility, or a home health care agency. The expected outcomes may be modified or made more specific depending on individual client need. For example, a client who is learning to self-inject insulin may need additional intermediate goals to assist in meeting these expected outcomes. The goals developed for a specific client drive the selection of nursing interventions, which are then implemented to provide quality nursing care.

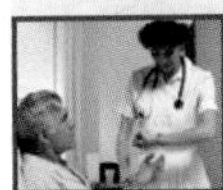

Mr. Connell will be discharged to home from the ED. His wife has been quietly waiting with him during his evaluation. The diagnosis of myocardial infarction has been ruled out, but he has been diagnosed with hypertension and stable angina. He is being restarted on atenolol and furosemide and is being given a prescription for nitroglycerin for prn use to relieve chest pain. As the nurse preparing Mr. Connell for discharge, what is your nursing diagnosis? What are your goals? What would you teach him about his medications, and how would your teaching be different knowing he has taken two medications before? What factors should you assess about his home environment and lifestyle? How would you modify your teaching because Mrs. Connell is present?

INTERVENTION

INTERVENTIONS TO ADDRESS *INEFFECTIVE HEALTH MAINTENANCE*

The interventions that help a client meet the expected outcomes for *Ineffective health maintenance* are driven by the goals established for the client. They often include the following:

- Explain the medication's purpose, action, dose, and timing in clear and simple terms. Determine the client's prior knowledge, and reinforce or reeducate. Provide instruction in an unhurried manner to allow the client time to process information and ask questions.
- Describe key side effects, and stress the ones the client should report immediately.
- Determine the client's ability to obtain the medication after discharge and how the client plans to take it correctly and safely. Make referrals as needed to ensure that the client has the assistance required.
- Instruct selected clients to carry an identification card or wear a bracelet identifying the medications being used.
- Give written materials, and encourage questions, both at the time of teaching and later.

INTERVENTIONS TO ADDRESS *INEFFECTIVE THERAPEUTIC REGIMEN MANAGEMENT*

The interventions that help a client meet the expected outcomes for *Ineffective therapeutic regimen management* include those listed in the preceding section and also include interventions that assist the client in understanding how medication therapy can help to prevent exacerbations of illness or prevent complications from developing. Box 21-5 summarizes important instructions that will enable a client to manage the medication regimen effectively.

INTERVENTIONS TO PROVIDE SAFE AND EFFECTIVE MEDICATION THERAPY

Measuring the Dose. To correctly administer medications, you must be able to accurately calculate and measure the drug dose. Computation errors, such as incorrect

BOX 21-5

Teaching for Wellness

Self-Administering Medications Effectively

Purpose: To obtain optimal effects from medication therapy because of knowledge of proper use and enhanced compliance, which in turn should promote and maintain health and decrease overall health care costs by minimizing the number and severity of exacerbations.

Expected Outcome: The client will demonstrate proper use and handling of medications and will adhere to the medication regimen.

Client Instructions

- Take all medications according to the directions on the package.
- Finish all prescriptions given for short-term use (such as antibiotics). Do not stop taking prescription medication unless you are told to do so by the prescriber. Discard unused portions properly.
- Follow any guidelines given about follow-up blood work, measuring vital signs or weight, or visits to the physician. Some medications must be monitored periodically to make sure you have the correct level in your bloodstream. In other cases, the physician may need to examine you to determine whether the medication is effective.
- Follow any guidelines given about foods, alcohol, or over-the-counter drugs to be used or avoided while taking the medication. This will help the medication to work most effectively and will reduce the risk of food or drug interactions.
- Obtain all medications from the same pharmacy so that the pharmacist will be familiar with your total medication regimen. This will enable the pharmacist to give you the most complete and thorough advice about taking your medications.
- Call the prescriber if you feel that the medication is causing adverse effects.
- Store medications properly to maintain their potency. Keep them in a cool, dry place, out of direct sunlight and out of the reach of children.
- If needed, use some form of reminder system to help you to remember to take medications as directed. Use a calendar, pill box, or paper clock if these would be helpful. Ask your nurse or physician to help you decide what method would be best for you.
- Do not change brand names of a medication without checking first with the prescriber. Sometimes different brand names have different added ingredients, and the real strength of the medication (bioavailability) may vary slightly from brand to brand.
- Keep all medications in their original containers. Check the expiration dates regularly, and obtain a new supply before the expiration date arrives so that medications exert their full intended effects.
- Do not take medications that have been prescribed for another person, and do not give another person a medication that was prescribed for you.

placement of a decimal or addition of an extra zero, can be harmful or possibly lethal to the client. Inability to draw up a medication to the correct calibration unit on a syringe could have equally disastrous consequences. To ensure accuracy in drug calculation and measurement, become comfortable working with the three systems of weight and volume measurement currently in use. These systems are the metric, apothecary, and household systems. In the United States and Canada, the metric system is the primary system used. Because the United States has not formally adopted the metric system as the official standard of measurement, some drugs are ordered using the apothecary system. When a client is given a prescription for home use, the order might be written using household measures for convenience.

Metric System. The metric system is a logical, easy-to-understand measurement system based on units of 10. Move from one metric unit to another by multiplying or dividing by 10. The decimal point moves to the right when multiplying, and to the left when dividing.

There are three basic units of measurement in the metric system. These are the meter (measuring length), the liter (measuring volume), and the gram (measuring weight). Volume and weight measurements are the ones most commonly computed as part of medication therapy (Figure 21-2).

Apothecary System. The apothecary system is familiar to most people in the United States and Canada, even if it is not the most widely used system for drug measurement. It originated in colonial England and is based on the weight of a single grain of wheat. The basic unit for weight, then, is called the grain. In this system, Roman numerals are used to denote numbers that are equal to or larger than 1 (grains X = 10 grains). Progressions or increases in weight are labeled dram, ounce, and pound.

The basic unit of measure for volume in the apothecary system is the minim, which is the approximate amount of water that weighs a grain. Progressions or increases in volume are labeled fluid dram, fluid ounce, pint, quart, and gallon. Abbreviations were often made using special symbols, which were confusing and could lead to error because they resemble other abbreviations. The ISMP (2003) has placed the symbols for dram and minim on the *ISMP List of Error Prone Abbreviations, Symbols, and Dose Designations*.

Household Measurements. The household system of measurement is familiar to most people. The basic units of measure for weight are the ounce and the pound. The basic units of measure for volume are the teaspoon (tsp), tablespoon (tbsp), ounce (oz), pint (pt), quart (qt), and gallon (gal). There is some overlap between the apothecary and household measurement systems.

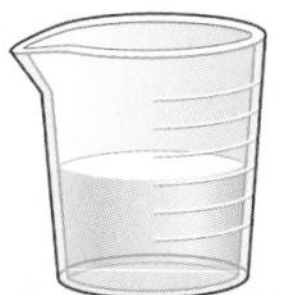

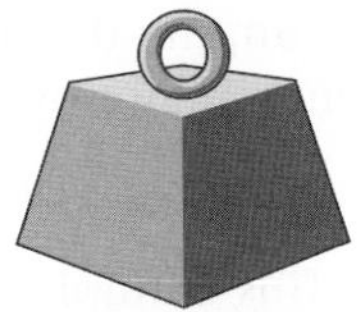

Units	Measures of volume	Measures of weight
Thousands		Kilograms (kg)
Hundreds		
Tens		
Ones	Liters (L)	Grams (g)
Tenths		
Hundredths		
Thousandths	Milliliters (mL)	Milligrams (mg)
Ten thousandths		
Hundred thousandths		
MIllionths	Microliters (μL)	Micrograms (μg)

FIGURE 21-2 Measures of volume and weight in the metric system.

Table 21-8 Approximate Equivalents Among Metric, Apothecary, and Household Measurement Systems

METRIC	APOTHECARY	HOUSEHOLD
	VOLUME	
5 mL	1 fluid dram	1 teaspoon
10 mL	2 fluid drams	2 teaspoons
15 mL	4 fluid drams	1 tablespoon
30 mL	1 fluid ounce	1 ounce
60 mL	2 fluid ounces	1 wine glass
120 mL	4 fluid ounces	1 teacup
240 mL	8 fluid ounces	1 tumbler
500 mL	1 pint	1 pint
1000 mL	1 quart	1 quart
4000 mL	1 gallon	1 gallon
	WEIGHT	
1 mg	1/60 grain	
4 mg	1/15 grain	
10 mg	1/6 grain	
15 mg	1/4 grain	
30 mg	1/2 grain	
60 mg	1 grain	
1 g	15 grains	
4 g	1 dram	
30 g	1 ounce	1 ounce
500 g	1.1 pound	1 pound
1000 g (1 kg)	2.2 pounds	2.2 pounds

The household system is the least precise because household utensils used to measure liquids, such as cups and teaspoons, vary in size. Household scales (if used) may not be well calibrated. The use of utensils to measure liquid prescription medication can be hazardous, especially for children who require precise doses because of smaller body size. Teach clients to use the measuring device supplied with a medication whenever one is available. Table 21-8 compares approximate equivalent measurements using each of the three systems.

Solutions. Solutions contain a specific amount of either a liquid or a solid substance dissolved in a known amount of liquid. You will use solutions frequently in clinical practice for procedures such as injections, infusions, and irrigations. Carefully check the concentration of any solution before using it. The concentration is best described as the amount of solute per unit of solvent (such as mg/mL or g/mL) and is sometimes expressed as a percentage. Common examples include IV solutions containing 5% dextrose in water or an irrigating solution of 0.9% sodium chloride. Occasionally, solutions are expressed as a proportion, such as 1:1000 solution, which has 1 g of a solid dissolved in 1000 mL of a liquid.

Converting Measurement Units. Nurses occasionally convert drug doses from one form of measurement to another. For example, if an opioid analgesic is ordered in grains and the drug is supplied in milligrams, you must correctly convert between the apothecary and metric systems to administer the correct dose. Other examples of more common conversions include recording ounces of fluid intake as milliliters, and body weight as kilograms instead of pounds.

Conversion within a system. Making conversions within a system is relatively easy. Within the metric system, either multiply or divide by 10 or one of its multiples. To convert grams to kilograms, divide the number of grams by 1000 by moving the decimal point three places to the left (for example, 480 g = 0.480 kg). To convert grams to milligrams, multiply the number of milligrams by 1000 by moving the decimal point three places to the right (for example, 0.75 g = 750 mg). To reduce the risk of error if decimal points are not seen, always place a leading zero before the decimal point when the number is less than one, such as 0.75, and do *not* use a trailing zero (such as 1.0; use 1 instead) (Institute for Safe Medication Practices, 2003).

Within the apothecary system, use or memorize a conversion table. This enables you to know, for example, that there are 32 ounces in a quart and 64 ounces in a half gallon. Because this system is used so frequently in the United States, you will often make these conversions by memory.

Conversion between systems. In clinical practice, you may occasionally need to convert between the metric and apothecary systems to calculate drug doses. Begin the conversion process by comparing the ordered measurement with what is available. Identify the equivalent needed to make the conversion. For example, an older surgeon has ordered *morphine sulfate gr. 1/6 IM q4h prn for pain.* The unit dose of morphine is labeled 10 mg/mL. To calculate the dose, you must convert the grains to milligrams. Recall that there are 60 mg in a grain. Set up the conversion as follows:

$$60 \text{ mg/grain} \times \tfrac{1}{6} \text{ grain} = 10 \text{ mg}$$

When you have calculated correctly, you know that one unit dose of the opioid analgesic must be used for the injection. Review a pharmacological math text for ready access to multiple examples and sample problems for converting from one unit of measure to another.

Dosage Calculations. Standard mathematical formulas or calculations are used to compute medication dosages. They may involve dimensional analysis (a variation of ratio and proportion) or other traditional formulas.

Traditional formulas. Formulas commonly used to solve medication dosage problems are the following:

$$\frac{\text{Dose ordered}}{\text{Dose on hand}} \times \text{Amount on hand} = \text{Amount to administer}$$

or

$$\frac{\text{Desired}}{\text{Have}} \times \text{Quantity} = \text{Dose}$$

The dose that is "ordered" or "desired" is the amount of drug prescribed that the client should receive. The dose that is on hand (the "have") is the drug measurement (weight or volume) available from the pharmacy. The dose on hand can be determined by reading the label, which states the amount of drug present in each tablet or capsule or in a certain volume of liquid. The "amount on hand" or "quantity" is the actual unit that contains the dose on hand. This could be "1 tablet" if the medication is a solid, or it could be "5 mL" if the medication is a liquid. For the most part, the "amount on hand" (quantity) is the most confusing part of the equation for nursing students. Some students repeatedly try to put the value of "1" into the equation for "amount on hand" instead of carefully reading the label and inserting the true unit. The following sample problem using a solid medication form illustrates how to calculate a drug dose using this method:

Example: The order states to give *diltiazem (Cardizem) 30 mg PO.* The tablets are labeled 60 mg/tablet. After comparing the order to the medication, reason that 30 mg is the dose "desired," whereas 60 mg is the dose available, or the "have." Set up the calculation as shown:

$$\frac{30 \text{ mg}}{60 \text{ mg}} \times 1 \text{ tablet} = \text{No. of tablets to administer}$$

Simplify the fraction by dividing the numerator and denominator by 30 to get

$$\tfrac{1}{2} \times 1 \text{ tablet} = \tfrac{1}{2} \text{ or } 0.5 \text{ tablet to administer}$$

This example illustrates that a portion of a solid drug may be given. However, this can be done only if the tablet or pill is scored (has an indented line) to allow it to be broken easily into two equal halves. A tablet that is not scored may not be broken into a partial dose because it is highly likely that the dose of the broken pill will be inaccurate. The client could then receive either a high or a low dose of the medication. Both situations are equally dangerous.

Dimensional analysis. The use of dimensional analysis by nurses as a method for calculating medication dosages is growing. This method is already popular in the physical sciences as a problem-solving method (Olsen, Giangrasso, & Shrimpton, 2004). It involves setting up the problem so that all of the units for the entries in the calculation (called factors) cancel each other out except the one being solved for. Use the following steps to solve a problem using dimensional analysis:

- Identify the unit of measure or drug form being calculated (such as mL or tab/cap) to the left of the equation, followed by an equal sign.
- Locate the factor in the problem that contains the unit of measure (such as 500 mg/mL or 325 mg per tab)
- Set up the remainder of the problem so that all units cancel from the numerator and denominator except the one being solved for (again, the mL or tab/cap). Multiply one side of the equation by a conversion factor as needed to help cancel out extra units (this will not change the value of the equation).

The following sample problem illustrates how to calculate a drug dose using this method. Beyond this, consult a pharmacological math text for additional practice.

Example: The order states to give *Potassium chloride elixir 20 mEq PO.* The label on the bottle states a drug concentration of 40 mEq/15 mL. After comparing the order with the drug label, reason that the mL is the unit of measure that needs to be calculated. Set up the problem so that the mL is on the left side of the equation and all other conversion factors are on the right side, until all unnecessary units cancel each other out:

Perform the calculation by multiplying 20 by 15 to get 300, then divide by 40 to obtain the dose of 7.5 mL to administer. Note that the mEq units cancel each other out, leaving only the mL.

$$\text{mL} = 20 \text{ mEq} \times \frac{15 \text{ mL}}{40 \text{ mEq}}$$

When performing drug calculations, make it a habit to perform a "commonsense check" at the end of the problem. Compare the answer obtained in relationship to the dose required and the amount of drug available. If the answer seems oddly high or low, recheck the answer, then have another nurse check the dose as needed before giving the dose to the client. It is rare for a dose to be higher than three pills or tablets, and an injectable dose should not be higher than the maximum volume recommended for that route.

Pediatric Dosages. It is particularly important to calculate dosages correctly for pediatric clients because of their smaller body size and weight and possible differences in biotransformation. Physicians usually calculate the safe dose when ordering the medication. Most drug references include the safe dose range for pediatric clients as well. Your additional responsibility when giving medications to pediatric clients is to recheck the client's dosage to ensure that it is in the safe dose range.

One method for calculating a dose is based on the child's weight. For example, a drug may be ordered in mg/kg of body weight. Determine the client's weight in kilograms and multiply it by the number of mg/kg ordered. Your answer is the child's dose in milligrams.

Regardless of the method used to calculate a pediatric dose, remember that these methods only provide the best *estimate* of the required dose. It is imperative to evaluate the pediatric client's response to medication as the final check of the appropriateness of a drug dosage. Note and report any adverse effects immediately so that dosage adjustments can be made if needed.

Administering the Dose. Safety and accuracy in medication administration are of paramount importance. During the course of a normal work shift, you may administer multiple medications to several clients. There is a risk of error each time a medication is administered. Do not become lulled by habit when preparing medications. Each drug administration requires alertness and purposeful action. Use a systematic method of checking medications during preparation to prevent possible errors. The new gold standard system of checking used by nurses is called the "six rights" (the original five rights plus a sixth, documentation). The following paragraphs briefly describe each of them.

Right Drug. Make sure that you have selected the right drug by comparing the drug name on the container with the medication administration record (Figure 21-3) or computer-generated list. In fact, you should check the medication label against the administration record three times while preparing the medication:

- When first taking the medication out of the container or unit-dose package
- Just before opening the medication package or pouring the dose
- Just before replacing the container in the storage area or giving a unit dose to the client

Never administer a medication prepared by someone else, because the person administering it is responsible for its effects. Take seriously any client concerns about the drug. If a client questions a drug or expresses any other form of concern, stop and verify the order before administering it. Often, you will find that the prescriber has changed the order, but this last check *can* prevent an error. If the order is correct, it provides an opportunity for client teaching. If the client refuses a drug, discard it if it was taken from a bulk container. Unopened unit doses may be returned for storage. Finally, remove medications only from packages or bottles with clearly marked labels.

Right Dose. The widely used unit-dose drug distribution system minimizes the chance of errors in drug dose. Occasionally the unit dose supplied by the pharmacy does not match the total dose ordered by the prescriber. In this instance, you must calculate the needed amount. For example, the client may have an order for digoxin (Lanoxin) 0.25 mg. The available supply is 0.125 mg. To give the correct dose, you must calculate that two tablets must be given.

At other times, a drug is ordered using one measurement system but has a label from another. Make the correct conversion to administer the correct dose. For example, the client may have an order for codeine grain ½. The medication supply area has codeine 30-mg tablets available. Calculate or recall that 60 mg = 1 grain. Therefore 30 mg equals ½ grain. You would then administer 1 tablet.

To ensure that a correct dose is given, carefully handle a medication that will be crushed or broken. If tablets are to be split, cut them evenly with a sharp implement into two pieces; if they are uneven, discard them and begin again with a new tablet. This limits the chance of underdose or overdose. Completely remove crushed medications from the crushing device and carefully clean it before the next use. Giving the correct dose may require using a syringe for accuracy—for example, when giving drugs such as digoxin (Lanoxin, a cardiac glycoside) or phenytoin (Dilantin, an anticonvulsant) in liquid form.

Finally, there are instances when it is prudent to check the dose of an ordered medication with another nurse, such as when the calculated dose seems unusual. Some nurses routinely check all insulin and heparin doses with another nurse. Many drugs have powerful effects on the body; this added check decreases the risk of dosage error.

Right Client. Check the client's identity using two unique identifiers before giving medication to make sure that the correct client receives the dose (JCAHO, 2006). In most facilities, clients wear identification (ID) bracelets. Carefully check the name and medical record number on the bracelet against the medication administration record or name on the computer sheet before administering medications. This practice should be strictly followed even if you recognize the client (e.g., in extended-care facilities). Any ID bracelet that is smudged or cannot be easily read should be replaced immediately. In hospitals using bar-code technology, scan both the client ID bracelet and the medication label to ensure accuracy.

Medication Administration Record

The Medical Center

MEDICATIONS	0100	0200	0300	0400	0500	0600	0700	0800	0900	1000	1100	1200	1300	1400	1500	1600	1700	1800	1900	2000	2100	2200	2300	2400
Ceftriaxone 1 g Rocephin 30 min Q12H Start : 09/06 Stop : 09/13 IVPB 06, 18						X 06 CW												X 18 AL						
Famotidine 20 mg ORAL Pepcid 20 mg BID Start : 09/06 Stop : 08, 20								X 08 BM												X 20 AL				
Furosemide 40 mg ORAL Lasix 40 mg Daily Start : 09/06 Stop : 08								X 08 BM																
Potassium chloride ORAL 20 mEq Daily Start : 09/06 Stop : 08								X 08 BM																
Zolpidem ORAL Ambien 10 mg At bedtime Start : 09/06 Stop : 22																						X 22 AL		

SIGNATURE	INITIALS
Carl Washington	CW
Betty Marsh RN	BM
Ann Lake RN	AL

DIAGNOSIS : Pneumonia

ALLERGIES : ADR : NKA

COMMENTS :

PAGE : 1

ABBREVIATIONS

A - LUOQ	G - L. deltoid
B - RUOQ	H - R. deltoid
C - L. ventrogluteal	I - Abdomen
D - R. ventrogluteal	NN - Other - SEE NURSES' NOTES
E - L. thigh	
F - R. thigh	

ACCT # : 0650312 2303–B AGE : 72Y
ADMITTED : 09/06/2006 SEX : F
PHYSICIAN : James, Margaret

FIGURE 21-3 Sample medication administration record.

Another widely accepted method of client identification is to ask the client to state his or her name and date of birth. This method is frequently used in the home or in extended-care facilities that do not use ID bracelets. Avoid using a question that could be answered with a nod of the head, such as, "Are you Mr. Cook?" Clients who are confused or not fluent in the language used by the nurse could misunderstand and nod inappropriately.

In the home, teach clients not to share their medications with others. Because the medication and dose are specifically ordered for one client, others cannot be expected to have the same response to the drug. In fact, it could be hazardous to another person taking it. Include this point as part of your teaching about general medication safety.

Right Route. Check the medication order carefully to see that the route is specified. Clarify if the route is illegible or missing. If you know that a medication is not usually given by the specified route, question the order.

Because pharmaceutical companies manufacture drugs to be given by different routes, take care to have the correct preparation on hand. For example, oral solutions may not be injected, and parenteral medications are not administered orally. Medications manufactured for parenteral use usually state "for injection only" or something similar. Incorrectly used preparations can cause harm.

Right Time. A scheduled medication is given at specified frequencies or times. Be sure to give it at the correct time, which is generally within 30 minutes before or after the ordered time.

Medications given once daily should be given at the same time each day to maintain a therapeutic blood level. Medications that are quickly metabolized are spaced evenly around the clock for the same reason. Most health care agencies have policies indicating standard times for medication administration. For example, one institution may schedule bid (Latin *bis in die,* or twice a day) medications for 8 AM and 8 PM (0800 and 2000 using military time), whereas another may choose 10 AM and 10 PM (1000 and 2200). The use of standardized times helps to decrease the number of omitted or doubled doses. It also helps to organize the nurses' work so that most of the shift is not spent administering medications to a group of clients.

Know the nature and purpose of a medication so you can ensure optimal timing. The prescriber indicates the frequency for drug administration as part of the order; however, you must use critical thinking skills in scheduling the medication. For example, a medication that is ordered qid (*quater in die,* or four times daily) and one that is ordered every 6 hours are both given four times a day. The qid medication, however, may be given before or after meals and at bedtime, whereas the medication ordered every 6 hours must be timed so doses are spaced evenly around the clock. Question an order if the timing does not seem optimal based on principles of pharmacokinetics and maintaining consistent serum drug levels.

The timing of prn medications is of special concern. If a medication is ordered *q4h prn,* you may not administer it more frequently than every 4 hours without obtaining a new order from the prescriber. Before administering a prn medication, check the time the last dose was given. If more time has elapsed since the last dose than the interval specified by the order, the medication may be safely given. Analgesics are commonly ordered on a prn basis.

In the home setting, you may assist the client in planning the medication schedule within the parameters of the prescription order. Consider both drug variables and client variables, such as personal preference and the ability to remember to take the dose.

Right Documentation. After administering a medication to a client, chart it immediately on the medication administration record (MAR) or computerized medical record. Chart the site of a parenteral medication also. When an MAR is used, initial the medication in the appropriate area on the form. Write your full signature once, and put your initials in the signature box. When a computerized record is used, your computer access code serves as your signature. Your name is printed at the bottom of the sheet along with the computer signature when a copy is printed for the medical record.

If a client refuses a medication, or if a dose was omitted, document that the dose was not taken. It is common to circle the scheduled time on the MAR to indicate a refused or missed dose. Write a follow-up note in the medical record indicating the reasons for the omission. When a computerized record is used, you may use a mouse to select "given" or "not given." When "not given" is selected, indicate on a follow-up screen why it was omitted. Provide follow-up charting in the medical record as required by agency policy.

There are various reasons for not giving a scheduled medication. The client may not think the dose is necessary (e.g., a client who has diarrhea refuses a stool softener). A client who routinely took the medication before admission may have a medication time schedule that does not match institutional policy. (Client preferences should be respected if appropriate and possible.) At times, clients do not understand the importance of the medication and client teaching can resolve the problem.

Occasionally, a medication dose must be omitted because the client was not available at the scheduled time, such as when the client leaves the unit for a procedure or diagnostic testing. Use critical thinking when administering delayed doses of medications such as insulin, considering the timing of the dose in relation to a meal. Use agency policy and medication knowledge as guides when rescheduling doses.

Developmental Considerations. Both younger and older clients may have special needs with regard to medications. Assess their unique needs to facilitate safe and effective medication administration. Children under age 5 may have trouble swallowing pills, tablets, and capsules and thus require a liquid form. If a special measuring device accompanies a liquid form, use it in dosage preparation and clean it after use. If no liquid form is available, crush the solid form and add it to a soft food such as applesauce or pudding (Box 21-6).

When giving parenteral medications to children, use proper injection sites for the client's age. For example, avoid the gluteus maximus muscle when giving an infant an intramuscular injection because it is in close proximity to major nerves and blood vessels. Use knowledge of the child's developmental level to plan an effective approach. For instance, give a fearful toddler or preschool child a toy or blanket to hold for security. Some may cry, and you should allow them to do so. Comfort the client during and after the injection, and use rewards as appropriate.

Parents are often responsible for giving medications to children once they leave the hospital or physician's office. Teach the parents how to give the medication correctly and how to store it after use. Often antibiotics, commonly given to children, require refrigeration. Medications are now routinely packaged in containers with child-resistant caps. Teach parents to replace the cap securely for the child's safety and to keep all medications in the original containers.

Older adults commonly require smaller doses because of age-related changes, and they may need other special considerations as well. Utilize the following suggestions when giving medications to older clients:

- Allow sufficient time to administer medications to older clients. They may require additional explanations of the medications being given and may have slower reflexes and body movements.
- Offer a small amount of liquid before giving medications to ease swallowing. Administer only one or two medications at a time for the same reason.
- Encourage the client to drink an additional 5 or 6 ounces of fluid after taking all medications to ensure that they have reached the stomach and to enhance medication absorption.
- Obtain a liquid form of the medication if possible for those who have trouble swallowing. If not possible, crush non–enteric-coated tablets or empty the contents of capsules into soft foods or liquids. Gently massaging the laryngeal prominence or the area just under the chin stimulates swallowing.
- Teach clients to identify medications by name, not by the color of the tablet. Generic drugs could vary in color according to manufacturer, and visual changes associated with aging could make it difficult for the client to use color as a guide.
- Assess all older adults for special needs, especially in the home setting. Help diabetic clients with motor or visual problems to draw up and inject insulin. Provide prefilled medication boxes to those with memory deficits so medications are taken at correct times.

Avoiding Errors. According to the National Coordinating Council for Medication Error Reporting and Prevention (NCCMERP), a medication error is any preventable event that could lead to inappropriate medication use or harm while that medication is in the control of the health professional, client, or consumer (NCCMERP, 2006). There are four global categories of errors:

- No error, although circumstances or events could have led to an error
- Medication errors without harm
- Medication errors causing harm
- Medication error resulting in death

Multiple checks and balances should be used to prevent medication errors. The prescriber must write legible and complete orders. You must check the order during transcription and question any area of concern. The

BOX 21-6 *Helpful Hints for Administering Medications to Children*

- Hold a very young child or infant in an upright or semi-upright position with his or her back against your chest or abdomen. Using a dropper, place the medication between the gum and cheek to promote swallowing and prevent the medication from being aspirated or spit out.
- Crush pills or tablets (unless they are enteric coated) and mix them with a small amount of soft food, such as cereal or applesauce, to make them easier to swallow. Avoid using a favorite food or an essential dietary item (such as formula), so that the child will not refuse the food in the future. Avoid using large volumes to ensure that the child takes the full dose.
- Use a calibrated device supplied with the medication to accurately measure liquid doses less than 10 mL. If a measuring device is not provided, use a disposable syringe without the needle attached. Do not use a teaspoon to measure the dose or to give the medication.
- Be honest when administering medications to children who are old enough to communicate. Tell them if the medication has an unpleasant taste or that an injection may hurt briefly. Failure to do so can damage the child's trust in you.
- Give injections quickly. Distract the child using toys or conversations as appropriate. Be prepared to briefly restrain the child if necessary. Encourage the child to look away from the site during an injection. Also encourage the child to pretend to "blow away" the pain.
- Praise the child for taking the medication, and offer rewards if available and appropriate, such as stickers or lollipops.
- Monitor the child carefully for side effects after medication administration. Young children, especially, may be unable to report reactions to medications.

pharmacy technician or pharmacist must check the order while dispensing the medication. You must check the order again when preparing the medication for administration. Consistent use of the six rights of medication administration substantially reduces the likelihood of a medication error.

If a medication error does occur, it is your professional responsibility to report it. Follow facility policies and procedures for reporting and documenting the incident. Report the error to the physician and appropriate nursing management personnel. The physician will order any follow-up procedures or tests that are indicated or may prescribe an antidote.

Your highest priority after a medication error is the client's physiological status and safety. Carefully assess the drug's effects, and quickly carry out new orders given to counteract them.

Document the error carefully. Write factual information about the error in an accurate, thorough, and objective manner on the medical record. Avoid the use of judgmental words such as "error" in the documentation. Instead, chart the medication administered, the actual dose given (not the ordered dose), and any observable client effects. Also document that the physician was notified, any follow-up actions or orders that were implemented, and the client's condition after both the medication error and any corrective actions.

Most facilities require additional documentation when a medication error occurs, usually with a form called an *incident report* or *unusual occurrence report*. Follow facility policies and procedures for completing an incident report. Document factual information about the error and corrective actions taken. Complete any additional sections of the form, which may help during investigation of the incident. This report is used by the institution's risk management department. Do not document on the medical record that an incident report was filled out, and do not keep a copy of incident reports. Incident reports are not placed in the medical record.

INTERVENTIONS SPECIFIC TO DRUG ROUTE

Managing Oral Medications. The oral route is most commonly used for medication administration. Orally administered medications have a slower onset of action and a more prolonged, less potent effect. They are less expensive to manufacture, easy to administer, and do not interrupt the skin and mucous membrane barriers.

Oral medications are most frequently given in solid forms, such as tablets, capsules, and pills. Liquid forms are helpful for clients who have trouble swallowing tablets, and they can be poured using a variety of aids. When pouring a dose into a calibrated measuring cup, hold it at eye level and measure the dose at the base of the meniscus (Figure 21-4).

Remember the following safety points when preparing oral medications for administration:

- If a medication must be removed from a bottle, make sure the label is intact and legible. Return an unlabeled bottle or one that is difficult to read to the pharmacy.
- Pour medications carefully to prevent unnecessary loss. If too much medication is poured, discard the excess. Never return unused medication to a container.
- If pouring a dose from a stock supply, do not return a solid medication to the container if it has been taken out of the cap.
- Do not move medications from one bottle to another, because bottles can be identified by a code number or lot number assigned by the manufacturer. This number may be needed to track medications with quality control problems.

A key concern when giving an oral medication is preventing aspiration. Place clients in an upright position, either on the back or turned to one side. This reduces the risk of medication accumulating at the back of the throat. Provide fluid to drink, and give only one pill or tablet at a time. Allow clients enough time to swallow each medication before giving the next one. If they begin to cough, wait until they have recovered before giving additional medications. Remain with them until all medications have been taken. Do not leave medications at the bedside for clients to take after you leave the room. Make sure that they drink at least 50 or 60 mL of fluid with the last tablet to ensure that the medication reaches the stomach and does not stick in the esophagus. If the client's intake and output are being measured, record all fluid taken with medications on this record. Specific guidelines for administering medications by the oral route are given in Procedure 21-1.

Managing Parenteral Medications. Parenteral routes are differentiated by the angle of injection and depth of penetration. To give these medications safely, you must be familiar with the equipment, follow accepted proce-

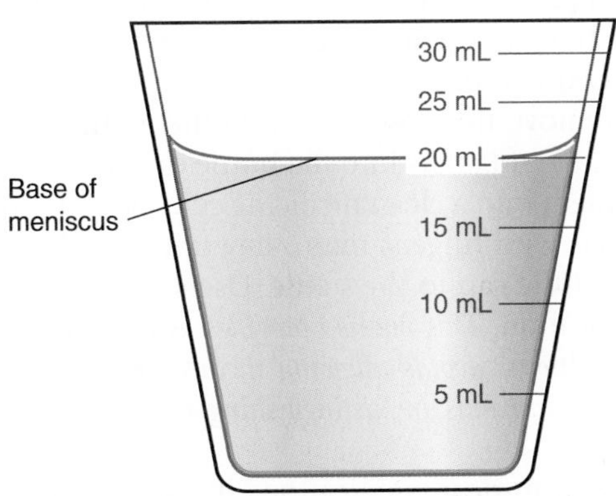

FIGURE 21-4 When using a calibrated measuring cup, measure the dose at the base of the meniscus.

TIME TO ALLOW: NOVICE: 10 min. EXPERT: 5 min.

PROCEDURE 21-1 ADMINISTERING ORAL MEDICATIONS

Nursing Skills Online: Safe Medication Administration, Lesson 5

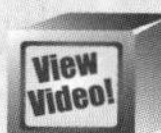

Oral medications are administered to provide a pharmacological benefit or effect for a client. They are given carefully, using strict guidelines to prevent error.

DELEGATION GUIDELINES

At no time is it appropriate to delegate medication administration to a nursing assistant. Your knowledge of pharmacological agents, their administration, and ongoing client assessment necessitate that you perform this procedure.

EQUIPMENT NEEDED

- Medication order sheet, computer-generated medication administration record, medication Kardex or cards
- Medication cart or tray
- Disposable medication cups (calibrated plastic or souffle)
- Glass of water, juice, or other preferred fluid
- Drinking straw
- Pill-crushing device (as needed)
- Medications or medication cart (unit-dose system)

1 Follow preliminary actions (see inside front cover).

2 Assess the client to verify that the oral route is appropriate. Notify the physician if you find contraindications for giving medications by this route.

3 Confirm the medication order sheet against the original physician orders.

a. Clarify inconsistencies if found.
b. Check the client's record for allergies.
c. Determine any assessments needed (e.g., blood pressure or pulse) before the dose can be given.

4 Dispense medications one at a time, for one client at a time.

a. Unlock the drawer of the medication cart or storage area.
b. Select the correct medication, and compare its label with the order sheet.
c. Calculate the dose needed.
d. Recheck the dose to be sure it is correct.
e. Place a solid medication into a disposable souffle cup.
f. For a partial dose, use a gloved hand or a cutting device to split a scored medication in half. Discard the unused half of a divided tablet.
g. To remove the dose from a bottle, pour the correct number of tablets into the bottle cap and then transfer them into a clean medicine cup. Do not touch the tablets with fingers; return any untouched extra tablets in the cap to the bottle. Use a new cup for each medication. *This method provides aseptic preparation of medications, avoids allowing medications to touch your hands, and aids in distinguishing one medication from another.*
h. Leave unit-dose medications in their original packaging, and place them together in one cup. Do not open the wrappers until you get to the client's bedside. Keep medications that require special assessments in a separate cup. *This approach makes it easier to return refused medications to the pharmacy or to withhold medications as needed on the basis of client assessment.*
i. To give a liquid medication, pour it into a calibrated, disposable medication cup.
   (1) Mix the medication thoroughly, and discard it if it has changed color or become cloudy.
   (2) Remove the lid from the bottle or container, and place it upside down. *This position prevents contamination of the container lid.*
   (3) Hold the bottle so that the label is facing up, under the palm of your hand. *This position ensures that the medication label does not become soiled or faded by spilled liquid.*
   (4) Hold the medication cup at eye level, and use your thumbnail to mark the level of the correct dose. Pour medication into the cup until the bottom of the meniscus reaches the level of your thumbnail. Do not return any excess medication to the bottle; instead, discard it.
   (5) Wipe the lip of the container with a clean paper towel before recapping.
   (6) Bring a unit dose of a liquid to the bedside without opening it, unless the client needs a partial dose.

5 For medications of all types, recheck the medication and the dose after it is poured but before it is given to the client.

6 Lock the medication cart or storage area, and bring the medications to the client.

7 Identify the client.

a. Read the name on client's identification bracelet.

b. Ask the client to tell you his or her name. *This step requires that client be alert and able to cooperate.*

c. Verify the client's identity with another staff member who knows the client. *Perform this step only if the client does not have an identification bracelet and is confused or unable to communicate.*

8 Perform final assessments (parameters for administration, such as hold Toprol if pulse is less than 55), and explain the purpose of the medications to client.

9 Give the medications to the client.

a. Allow the client to choose whether to take one or more than one medication at a time and whether to take them in a certain order. *Clients' needs and preferences should be respected if they do not threaten health or safety.*

b. Recheck the accuracy of any medication that the client questions. *Doing so may help to prevent a medication error.*

c. Remove unit-dose medications from their wrappers, and give them to the client in a cup or in the hand according to the client's preference. *This method allows the client to see the medication, become familiar with it, and notice any discrepancies from the usual dose.*

d. Offer a full glass of fluid. Have client moisten the mouth with fluid, bow the head slightly to aid swallowing, and follow the medications with an additional 60 to 100 mL. *You may need to use less fluid if the client is on fluid restriction.*

e. Give liquids, chewable medications, lozenges, and sublingual or buccal medications separately from oral tablets, pills, or capsules.

f. Make sure the client has swallowed all medications by questioning the client or checking the mouth. Stay with the client until all medications have been taken.

10 Document the medication administration on the client's medication administration record or computerized medication record.

11 Recheck the client when the medication has had time to take effect to assess the client's response to the medication.

PEDIATRIC CONSIDERATIONS

Children under the age of 5 may need liquid forms of medication because of difficulty in swallowing tablets or capsules. Whenever possible, a child should be allowed to take medication with a beverage of choice. Explanations about medication therapy should be given at an age-appropriate level.

GERIATRIC CONSIDERATIONS

Older adults may need more time than younger individuals to take oral medications. They may also require additional liquid to ensure that all medications are swallowed.

A variation of the oral route used for some clients is an enteral tube, such as a nasogastric (NG) tube, gastrostomy tube (G-tube), or jejunostomy tube (J-tube). Important guidelines to follow when administering medications by the enteral route are given in Box 21-7.

BOX 21-7 *Guidelines for Administering a Medication Through an Enteral Tube*

- Whenever possible, obtain medications in liquid form to lessen the risk of obstructing the tube.
- Crush medications carefully; do not administer large particles or whole medications. Dissolve in warm water first.
- Do not crush enteric-coated, extended-action, sublingual, or buccal medications.
- Administer medications at room temperature rather than chilled. Also, warm the fluids used to flush the tube.
- Put on disposable gloves. Access the tube using standard procedure. Check tube placement before administering a medication. Sit the client upright or semi-upright to reduce risk of aspiration.
- Place a waterproof pad on the bed linens under the area of the tube. Flush the tube with 15 to 60 mL of warm water before and after giving the medication, or as directed by facility policy.
- Administer medications by gravity, pouring them into an irrigation syringe with the plunger removed. Hold the syringe approximately 18 inches high to ensure a slow, steady flow rate. Monitor how the client tolerates the procedure.
- Do not administer a medication through the air vent of a feeding tube.
- After the final flush, clamp the tube that was attached to suction for 20 to 30 minutes. If the client was receiving continuous tube feedings, clamp the tube for a few moments before resuming, if directed by facility policy.
- Help the client to a right-side-lying position with the head elevated for at least 30 minutes after administering the medication.
- Clean up the work area, remove gloves, and perform hand hygiene.
- Document the medication and fluid intake on appropriate charting forms.

dures, and have manual dexterity. When preparing medications to be given by this route, keep the equipment and medication sterile.

Medications given by a parenteral route are absorbed more rapidly than those given orally. They cannot be removed or retrieved once given, making safety and accuracy key concerns.

Equipment. Needles and syringes are used to give parenteral medications. They are available in many sizes and are selected according to the medication dose and site to be injected. All needles have a bevel (an angled end), a shaft, and a hub. All syringes have a tip, a barrel, and a plunger (Figure 21-5).

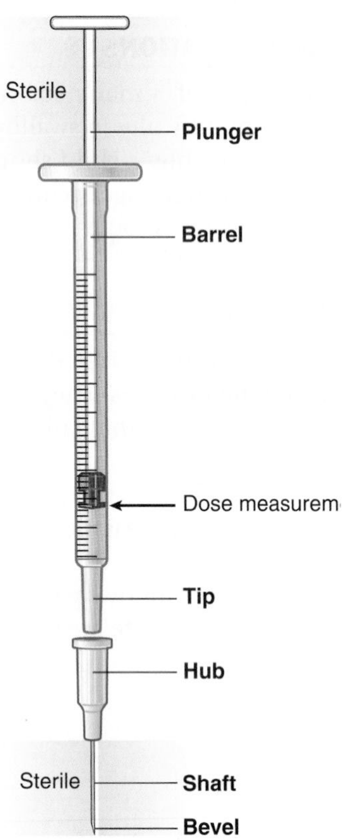

FIGURE 21-5 The needle and the syringe each have three parts.

Syringes. Syringes must be kept sterile with the exception of the outside barrel and the top edge of the plunger. This means that the syringe tip, barrel interior, and most of the plunger cannot be touched. The plunger moves up and down in the barrel of the syringe so that medication can be withdrawn and injected. The barrel holds the medication, and the barrel tip connects to a needle. Barrel tips may be either straight-end or Luer-Lok.

Most syringes used today are disposable and made of plastic. They are individually packaged to ensure sterility. They are clearly labeled with size (1 mL, 2 mL, 3 mL, 5 mL, 10 mL, 20 mL) and may be identified by their use (tuberculin, insulin). Many syringes are prepackaged with a specific-size needle attached, which is also clearly labeled.

The barrel of a syringe is calibrated by volume (Figure 21-6). For example, a tuberculin syringe can hold up to 1 mL of volume and is calibrated in units of 0.01 mL. An insulin syringe is calibrated in units of insulin. Most insulin manufactured in the United States and Canada contains 100 units per milliliter and is therefore called U100 insulin. An insulin syringe may hold up to either 1 mL (most common) or 0.5 mL. Most subcutaneous and IM injections do not exceed 2 or 3 mL. A 3-mL syringe is calibrated in units of 0.1 mL. Larger syringes, such as 5 mL, 10 mL, and 20 mL, are calibrated in increments of 0.2 mL. Larger syringes may be used occasionally to draw up IV medications.

Needles. Most needles used today are disposable and made of stainless steel. In selected areas, such as operating rooms, needles may be reused, but they must be resterilized after each use and inspected frequently for wear and tear.

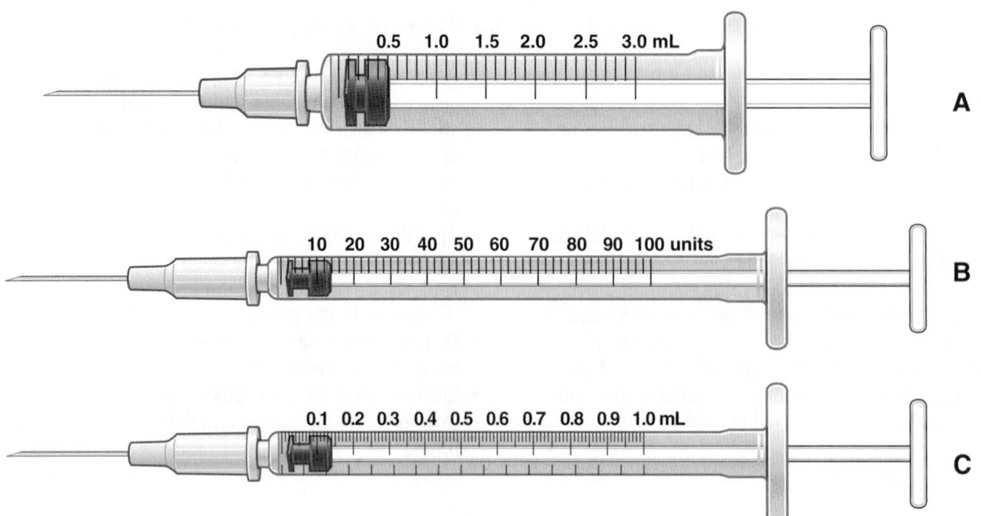

FIGURE 21-6 Three types of syringes. **A,** 3 mL. **B,** Insulin. **C,** Tuberculin.

Needles are measured by length and diameter. Lengths range from 1/4 to 5 inches (with 5/8 to 1 1/2 inches most common). A shorter needle is used when the client is smaller in size or when more superficial tissues are being injected (such as insulin and intradermal injections). Longer needles are used to inject deeper tissues (such as IM injections).

The angle at which the needle is inserted also affects the tissue depth reached. In general, IM injections require the use of 1- to 1 1/2-inch needles, whereas subcutaneous injections require use of 3/8- to 5/8-inch needles. Longer needles also have longer bevels, which helps to decrease discomfort at the injection site. Insulin syringes are specially manufactured with a small needle attached to the syringe to meet the needs of clients who must inject themselves regularly.

The diameter of a needle is referred to as its gauge. The diameter size is inversely related to the gauge number. Gauges range from 28 (small) to 14 (large). Smaller-gauge needles are used with smaller drug volumes and produce less tissue trauma. Larger-gauge needles are used when larger volumes are injected, when the medication is viscous, or when the medication must penetrate to deeper tissues.

Prefilled syringes. Some parenteral medications are manufactured in prefilled, single-dose, disposable syringes (Figure 21-7). These medication systems are available with a preattached needle or in a Luer format (without needle). You simply bring the prefilled syringe to the bedside, remove the needle shield, inject the medication, and dispose of the syringe. However, do not confuse this system with a unit-dose system. You may need to discard excess medication if the ordered dose is smaller than that supplied in the syringe. The purpose of prefilled syringes is to simplify and ease the injection process while decreasing the risk of needlestick injury during medication preparation. Some prefilled syringes may require you to assemble a prefilled cartridge into a holder device and then disassemble the system after use.

Safe use of needles and sharps. Preventing needlestick injuries is a vital concern in the health care industry. The Occupational Safety and Health Administration (OSHA) mandates the use of standard precautions, which include proper handling and disposal of sharp instruments including needles. After administering an injection, discard the syringe and needle, without recapping the needle, in a rigid container that has been specifically labeled and provided for that purpose (Figure 21-8). The container should be leakproof and punctureproof. Rigid containers are kept on medication carts in all client care settings and are wall-mounted in client rooms and treatment areas in many acute care institutions. To prevent the risk of needlestick injury, do not try to place a used syringe into an overfilled container.

If you must recap a needle, do so using the one-handed (or scoop) method. Slide the needle into the needle cover as it lies on a flat surface. Lift the syringe, and twist the cover into place near the base of the needle. Never push the cap onto the needle using a finger on the end of the needle cover.

Action Alert! Avoid recapping needles whenever possible. If you must recap, use the one-handed (or scoop) method.

If you cannot discard a syringe immediately, encase it in a protective sheath temporarily. An increasing number of facilities are using safety syringes that cover or encase

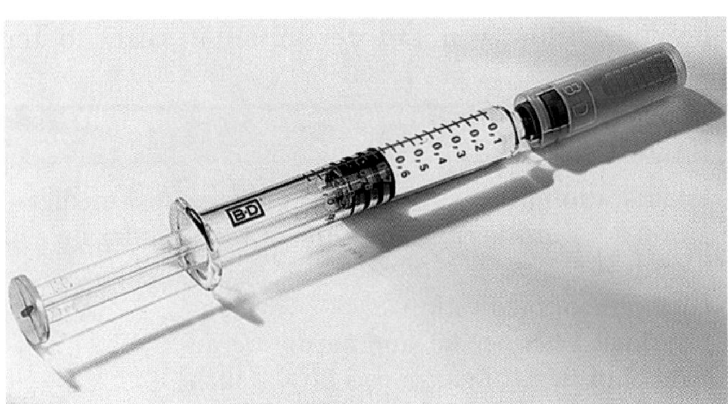

FIGURE 21-7 The Hypak injection system is an example of a prefilled, single-dose, disposable syringe. It consists of a cartridge holder and a prefilled medication cartridge with a needle. (Courtesy Becton Dickinson Pharmaceutical Systems, Franklin Lakes, NJ.)

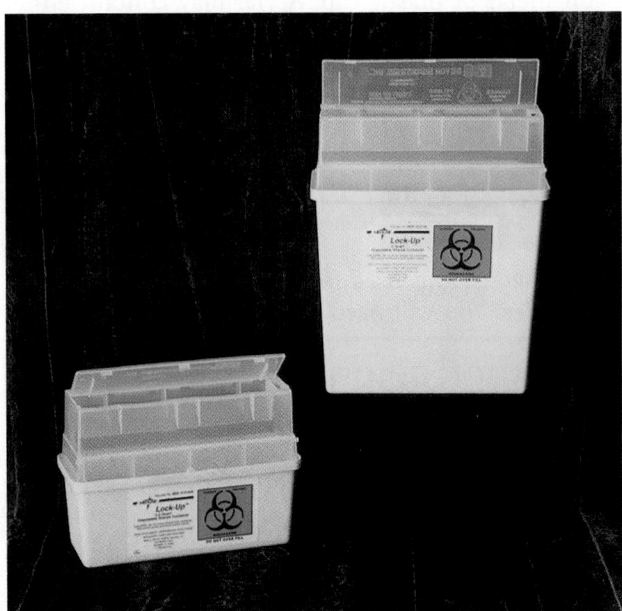

FIGURE 21-8 Proper use of rigid disposal containers ("sharps" containers) for used needles helps prevent accidental needlesticks. (Courtesy Medline Industries, Mundelein, IL.)

the needle after use. Follow manufacturer's guidelines and facility procedures if using these devices.

Do not leave needles and syringes (even temporarily) in a pocket, on a client's meal tray, at the bedside, or in the client's bed. Do not discard them in wastebaskets or in a rigid container that is full. Doing so increases the risk of needlestick injury, with possible infection from a number of pathogens, including hepatitis B and human immunodeficiency virus (HIV).

When clients need to give themselves injections at home, teach them safe methods of syringe and needle disposal. The United States Environmental Protection Agency (2004) recommends that used syringes generated at home be disposed of through use of at-home needle destruction devices, sharps mail-back programs, community drop-off programs, or household hazardous waste facilities. Do not teach clients to dispose of used needles and syringes in the household trash.

Preparing an Injection From an Ampule. An ampule is a glass container that holds a single drug dose and ranges in size from 1 mL to 10 mL or larger. The neck of the ampule is narrow and may have a colored ring indicating where it is prescored for opening. Because bits of glass sometimes found in ampules can be drawn into the syringe, it is prudent to use a filter needle to withdraw the medication (Heiss-Harris & Verklan, 2005). The used filter needle is discarded before administering the medication to the client. The steps for withdrawing medication from an ampule are given in Procedure 21-2.

Preparing an Injection From a Vial. A vial is a glass or plastic container with a rubber seal at the top. The seal is sterile before being opened and is protected by a soft metal or plastic cap. A vial may contain either liquid or powder medication. If a powder is used, product literature indicates the type and amount of diluent (such as sterile normal saline solution or sterile water) to use for reconstitution. Read the label carefully to determine the end concentration of the medication to avoid drawing up the wrong dose. Inject the solvent into the vial using the same technique that you would use to inject air. A powdered medication may dissolve easily, or you may have to gently roll or agitate the vial. If needed, the syringe may be removed from the vial before doing this.

Vials are labeled for a single dose or for multiple doses. A single-dose vial must be discarded after one use. A multiple-dose vial may be reused but must be labeled with the date and time opened and your initials. A used vial must be discarded 30 days after being opened, or less according to manufacturer's directions, even if it is not empty. Reconstituted medications in multiple-dose vials often require refrigeration after initial use. The steps for withdrawing medications from a vial are given in Procedure 21-3.

Mixing Medications. Two medications may be mixed in one syringe if they are compatible with each other and if their total volume does not exceed the amount that may be given in one parenteral site. Most nursing units and pharmacology texts have charts identifying compatible medications. Consult a pharmacist if the medication is not identified or if you have any questions about compatibility.

Mixing medications from an ampule and a vial. When a medication from an ampule must be mixed with one from a vial, first withdraw from the vial and then from the ampule. This prevents the vial from being contaminated with medication from the ampule. It also is easier because

TIME TO ALLOW: NOVICE: 5 min. EXPERT: 1 TO 2 min.

PROCEDURE 21-2 WITHDRAWING MEDICATION FROM AN AMPULE

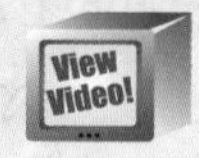

Nursing Skills Online: Injections, Lesson 2

Liquid medications used for injection may be supplied in ampules. You will need to withdraw the medication properly before you can administer it safely to the client.

DELEGATION GUIDELINES

The withdrawal and preparation of medication is yours alone. You may not delegate this task or any of the component parts of medication preparation to a nursing assistant.

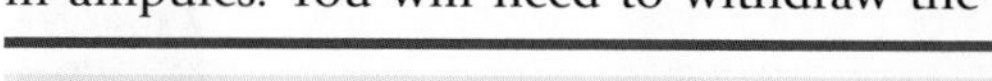

EQUIPMENT NEEDED

- Medication order sheet, computer-generated medication administration record, medication Kardex or cards
- Ampule of medication
- Syringe, filter needle, and needle
- Alcohol swab or gauze pad (2 × 2 inch)
- Container for disposing of sharps and ampule

1 Follow preliminary actions (see inside front cover).

2 Open the ampule.

a. Tap the upper chamber of the ampule quickly but lightly until all the fluid drops into the lower chamber. *This action ensures that all medication is available for use.*

b. Wrap the alcohol swab or gauze pad around the neck of the ampule. *Doing so will protect your fingers from small glass fragments as you open the ampule.*

c. Snap the neck of the ampule so that it opens away from your body (see illustration). *This directs any fragments of glass away from you rather than toward you.*

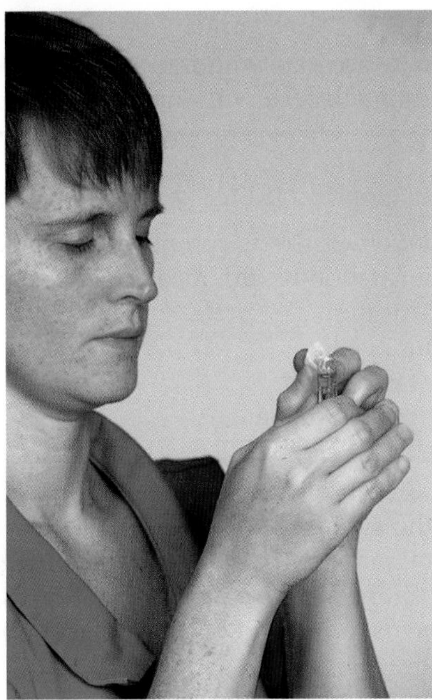

Step 2c. Snapping the neck of the ampule away from your body.

3 Place the ampule upright on a flat surface, and withdraw medication into a syringe (see illustration).

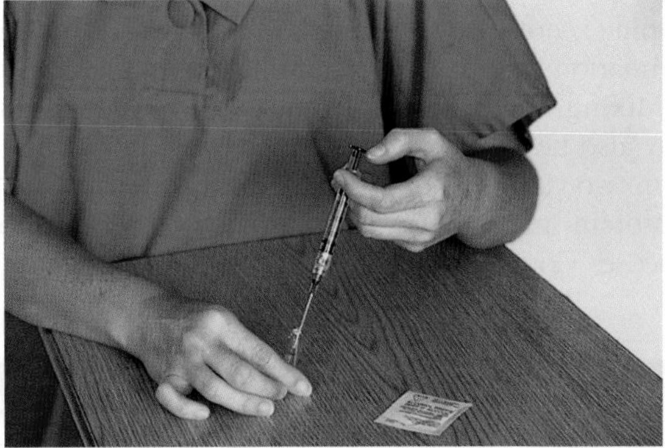

Step 3 Withdrawing medication into the syringe with the ampule upright.

a. Attach the filter needle (if used) to the syringe. Hold the ampule while inserting the filter needle into the center of the opening on the ampule. Do not allow the tip or shaft to touch the rim of the ampule. *This prevents contamination of the needle or filter needle, because the rim is considered contaminated.*

b. Gently pull back on the plunger to aspirate medication into the syringe.

c. Tilt the ampule as needed to keep the needle tip below the level of medication. *This step keeps you from withdrawing air into the syringe.*

d. If air enters the syringe, do not inject it into the ampule. Instead, remove the needle from the ampule, hold the syringe with the needle pointing upward, and eject the air (not the fluid). Then reinsert the needle into the center of the ampule and withdraw fluid again. *These steps provide sufficient room in the syringe to withdraw the full dose needed, prevent loss of medication from excess air pressure, and ensure withdrawal of the complete dose.*

4 Eject excess air or fluid as needed.

5 Replace the needle or filter needle with a new needle, and secure it tightly. Discard the used filter needle properly. Replacing the needle prevents needle contamination and irritation of the client's tissues caused by tracking of medication through dermal and subcutaneous layers.

6 Compare the volume of fluid in the syringe with the ordered dose.

the syringe partially filled with medication from the ampule is not used to inject air into the vial. (This recommendation assumes use of a multidose vial.)

Mixing medications from two vials. Medications may also be mixed in one syringe by withdrawing them from two vials. Insulin is a good example. Insulin is both a protein and a hormone needed by the body to use glucose. Clients with diabetes mellitus produce either insufficient amounts of insulin or no insulin at all, and many require daily insulin injections. Insulin manufactured in the United States and Canada contains 100 units per milliliter of solution, and a 1-mL U100 syringe holds up to 100 units of insulin.

Several types of insulin are available that have variable onset and duration of action. Insulin is identified as long-acting, intermediate-acting, or short-acting (also

PROCEDURE 21-3 WITHDRAWING MEDICATION FROM A VIAL

TIME TO ALLOW: NOVICE: 5 min. EXPERT: 1 TO 2 min.

Nursing Skills Online: Injections, Lesson 2

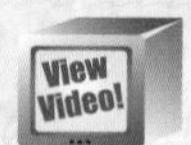

Liquid medications used for injection may be supplied in sealed, airtight vials. You will need to add air to the vial to facilitate accurate withdrawal; otherwise you will create a vacuum effect by withdrawing the medication.

DELEGATION GUIDELINES

As in the previous procedures in this chapter, medication preparation is the sole responsibility of you, the RN. You may never delegate this procedure to a nursing assistant.

EQUIPMENT NEEDED

- Medication order sheet, computer-generated medication administration record, medication Kardex or cards
- Vial of medication
- Syringe and needle
- Alcohol swab
- Glass disposal container

1 Follow preliminary actions (see inside front cover).

2 Prepare the vial.

a. Remove the plastic or metal top of a new vial to expose the rubber seal.

b. Cleanse the rubber seal with an alcohol swab.

c. Check the expiration date of a previously opened vial. Do not use the medication if the vial has been opened longer than manufacturer's directions. Check the medication for appropriate color and clarity.

3 Prepare the syringe.

a. Check for a tight connection between the needle hub and syringe barrel. *This action ensures a tight seal and a closed system.*

b. Remove the needle cover.

c. Draw back on the plunger to fill the syringe with a volume of air equal to the dose of medication you will be giving.

4 Withdraw the medication.

a. Insert the needle into the center of the vial's rubber seal using gentle but firm pressure. The center of the seal is thinner and designed for penetration.

b. Inject air from the syringe into the vial. This step creates positive pressure inside the vial to ease medication withdrawal and prevent creation of a vacuum after removing the medication.

c. Invert the vial while holding it with the first two fingers of your nondominant hand. Use your thumb and last two fingers to brace the barrel of the syringe. Use the thumb of your dominant hand to hold the end of the syringe barrel steady. Use the fingers of your dominant hand to withdraw the plunger. Proper hand position allows easier medication withdrawal and prevents movement of the plunger or bending of the needle.

d. Withdraw the medication slowly and steadily while holding the vial at eye level. Keep the tip of the needle in the solution at all times. Touch only the syringe barrel and plunger tip. This method prevents air bubbles from entering the syringe and prevents contamination of the syringe.

e. Remove excess air in the syringe by tapping the side of the syringe with a finger and pushing air back into the vial. Remove additional fluid as needed to ensure the full dose.

f. Return the vial to an upright position, and remove the needle by pulling back on the syringe barrel, not the plunger. Remove any excess air if present. This ensures that the correct amount of medication remains in the syringe.

5 Replace the needle with a new one. Secure the new needle tightly, and discard the used needle properly. *Replacing needle prevents needle contamination and irritation of client tissues from medication tracking through dermal and subcutaneous tissue layers.*

6 Compare the volume of fluid in the syringe with the ordered dose.

known as rapid-acting). A client may require more than one type of insulin. The most common example is a client who needs NPH insulin (intermediate-acting) mixed with regular insulin (short-acting) to achieve stable blood glucose levels over the course of a day (Procedure 21-4). Regular insulin is clear in color and may be given by either subcutaneous or IV route. NPH insulin is cloudy because protein has been added to slow its absorption; it is given only by the subcutaneous route.

A key concept to remember when mixing regular and NPH insulin is to withdraw them "clear to cloudy." This means that the clear (regular, unmodified) insulin is withdrawn from the vial first, and the cloudy (NPH, modified) insulin is withdrawn second (Figure 21-9). This technique prevents the NPH insulin from inadvertently being mixed into the regular insulin vial. Be aware that glargine (Lantus) insulin and lispro insulin are also clear but cannot be mixed with other forms of insulin. In addition, lispro and Lantus insulin, although clear, are not recommended for use by the IV route. See a pharmacology text for further information.

Warm insulin that was refrigerated before use by rolling it between the palms of your hands. Insulin can be safely stored for 1 month at room temperature but should be refrigerated if it will be kept for longer periods. In general, insulin should be stored in a cool location. A plan to rotate the site of injection should be developed and followed.

Administering Injections. The name of the injection route identifies the tissue into which the medication is injected. The characteristics of these tissues affect the depth of injection and the rate of absorption. Before administering an injection, become familiar with the site's landmarks, the nature and viscosity of the medication, and the maximum volume that can be safely given at that site.

Incorrect administration can have serious negative effects for the client. Excess volume causes pain or discomfort and can irritate tissues. Some medications

PROCEDURE 21-4

TIME TO ALLOW: **NOVICE:** 10 min. **EXPERT:** 5 min.

MIXING INSULINS IN A SINGLE SYRINGE

Some clients require doses of short-acting (unmodified, regular) and intermediate-acting (modified, NPH) insulins at the same time. Mixing them in one syringe allows a single injection.

DELEGATION GUIDELINES

You may not delegate the preparation of insulin to a nursing assistant. The preparation of any medication, including insulin, is your duty alone.

EQUIPMENT NEEDED

- Medication order, medication administration record or computerized medication order sheet
- Insulin vials
- Insulin syringe with attached needle
- Alcohol swabs

1 Follow preliminary actions (see inside front cover).

2 If the insulin is in suspension, rotate the vial between the palms of your hands. *This step mixes the solution without forming tiny air bubbles that could interfere with accurate measurement of the dose.*

3 Prepare the vials.

a. Remove the metal covers if you are using new vials.

b. Wipe the rubber seals with alcohol swabs.

c. Check the expiration date.

4 Add air to both vials.

a. Remove the needle cover.

b. Draw up a volume of air equal to the dose of modified (NPH) insulin and inject it into the NPH vial without letting the needle touch the solution (see illustration). Remove the needle from the vial. *Insertion of air prevents creation of a vacuum when you withdraw the fluid.*

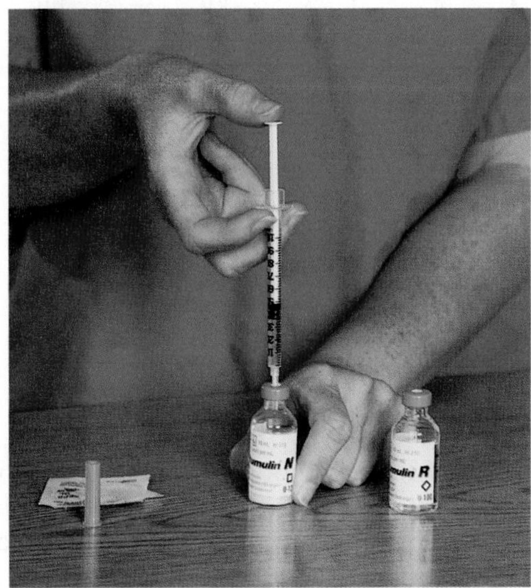

Step 4b. Injecting air into the NPH vial.

Continued

c. Draw up a volume of air equal to the dose of unmodified (Regular) insulin, and inject into regular insulin vial. Do not remove the needle from this vial.

5 Remove insulin from the two vials.

a. Invert the vial of regular insulin, and withdraw the correct dose. Make sure you draw no air bubbles into the syringe. Turn the vial upright, and remove the needle from the vial. *Turning the vial upright prevents solution from leaking out of the vial.*

b. Cleanse the rubber seal of the NPH insulin vial again, and insert the needle into the vial. Invert the vial, and carefully withdraw the correct dose. Turn the vial upright again, and remove the needle.

c. Recap the needle using the scoop technique, being careful not to contaminate the needle. *The needle is preattached to the syringe and must be brought to the bedside; in this case, recapping helps prevent needlestick injury.*

6 Double-check the dose. You may also ask another licensed nurse to check your dose. Then return the vials to their storage areas. Administer the mixed insulin dose to the client within 5 minutes of preparing it. *Double-checking verifies the correct dose. Returning the vials to storage maintains the potency of the insulin. Administering the medication within 5 minutes reduces the risk that the mixture will separate.*

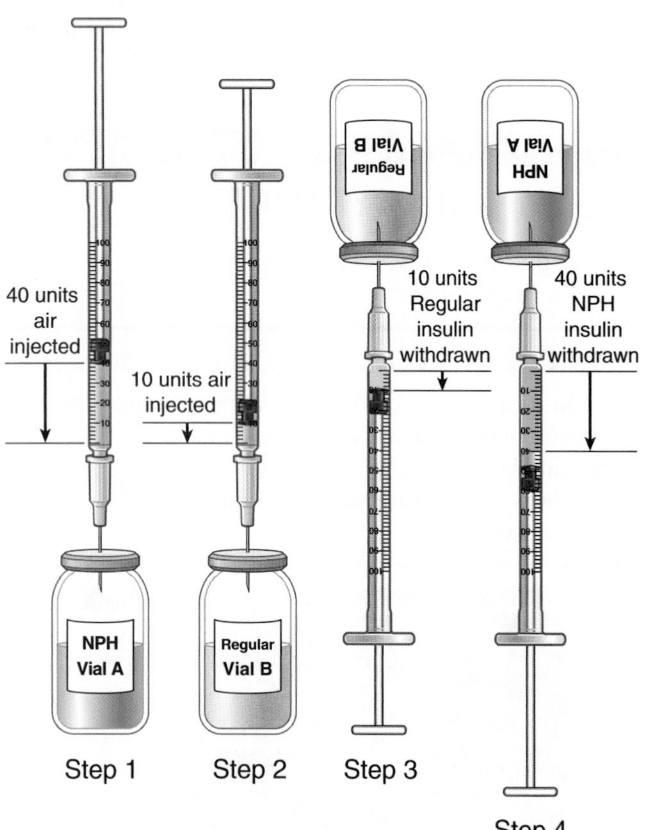

FIGURE 21-9 Mixing two medications in one syringe.

stain tissues if they are not given deeply enough or if incorrect technique is used. Failure to aspirate before injecting could result in a medication being inadvertently injected into a blood vessel. Incorrect site selection can cause damage to bones or nerves (McGrath, 2004). You are liable for medications that are given incorrectly.

BOX 21-8 *Minimizing the Discomfort of Injections*

- Use a needle with the smallest appropriate length and gauge.
- Make sure that the needle has a sharp bevel.
- Use anatomical landmarks to select a correct injection site and avoid unintended tissues.
- If necessary, change the position of the limb to be injected to relax the muscles at the site.
- Distract the client with conversation to relieve anxiety, but tell the client just before you insert the needle.
- If the client is very anxious, numb the site briefly with ice before administering the injection.
- Put on gloves; use smooth but quick hand movements when inserting the needle to minimize discomfort from tissue trauma.
- Hold the syringe steady while injecting the medication; do not rotate the syringe and needle while it is in the tissue.
- Apply gentle pressure to the injection site for about 10 seconds after withdrawing the needle unless doing so is contraindicated.

Receiving an injection is not a pleasant experience; however, you can reduce a client's fear and discomfort (Box 21-8). Strategies to reduce the discomfort of injections may be particularly useful with children or clients who need multiple injections over time.

Intradermal injections. The ID route has the slowest absorption of all parenteral routes. An advantage of this route for diagnostic testing is that the site is superficial, making it easy to determine positive reactions. Commonly used sites include the inner aspect of the forearm, the upper chest, and the upper back (Figure 21-10). Use a site that is free of bruises or other lesions and is relatively hairless to allow accurate follow-up assessment. Note the date, time, and location of the injection on the medical record as well as when the test should be "read" for a reaction (usually 48 to 72 hours later). If multiple injections are given, sites should be rotated and clearly marked. If there is a reaction (a positive test result), record and report it quickly.

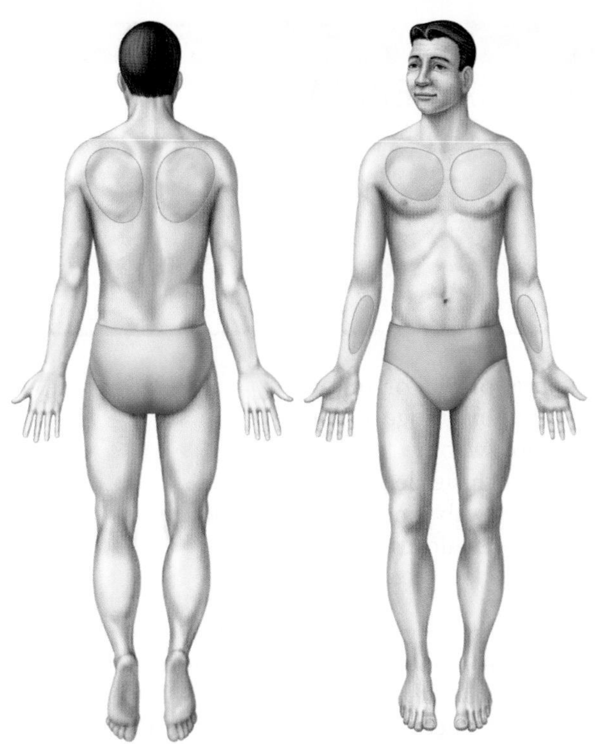

FIGURE 21-10 Frequently used sites for intradermal injection.

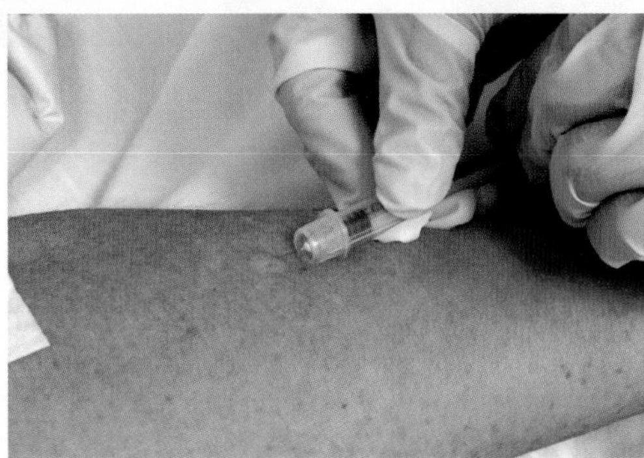

FIGURE 21-11 Intradermal injection. Insert the needle bevel up, with the syringe almost parallel to the skin at a 10- to 15-degree angle. As the medication is injected, a small wheal should form under the skin.

ID injections are administered using a tuberculin syringe, which holds up to 1 mL of medication and is calibrated in 0.1 mL and 0.01 mL. Use a small needle (25 to 27 gauge) with a short bevel that is 1/4- to 1/2-inch long. The usual medication dose is small (0.1 to 0.01 mL). Angle the needle at 10 to 15 degrees from the skin to deposit the medication below the epidermis (Figure 21-11). A wheal forms under the skin with proper administration. The procedure for administering ID injections is given in Procedure 21-5.

Subcutaneous injections. Subcutaneous tissue is not as vascular as muscle tissue, so medication is absorbed more slowly with subcutaneous injection than with IM injection. The slower absorption rate allows for a more prolonged drug effect.

The body is well supplied with subcutaneous tissue. Common injection sites include the anterolateral upper arms, anterior thighs, and lower abdominal wall between the costal margins and the iliac crests (Figure 21-12). Other acceptable sites are the scapular area of the back and the upper ventral or dorsal gluteal areas. Drugs commonly given by this route include heparin, insulin, and selected immunizations and analgesics.

As with any other injection, the site should be anatomically correct and free of infection, lesions, scars, or bruises. When giving injections frequently, rotate the sites to prevent local complications, such as sterile abscesses (painful lumps), lipohypertrophy (thickening of the skin), and lipodystrophy (atrophy or dimpling of the skin). This is especially important for diabetic clients who self-inject insulin daily. Identify the site rotation plan on the client's care plan, and note the sites of previously administered injections on the medication administration record. Use an injection diagram to help the client remember the site rotation pattern. It is currently common practice to systematically rotate injections within an anatomical site before moving to another site. Individual sites should be separated from each other by 1 inch. Give heparin in the abdomen (unless contraindicated by the client's condition).

Action Alert! Do not aspirate heparin or insulin injection sites. Do not massage heparin or insulin sites, which could lead to bleeding after heparin injection or increased speed of absorption after insulin injection.

The equipment used for subcutaneous injection depends on the medication to be given and the client's body size and weight. The amount of medication injected into one site is commonly 0.5 to 1.0 mL but should not exceed 1.5 mL. Insulin syringes are used to administer insulin, whereas tuberculin syringes are commonly used to administer heparin. For other medications, up to a 3-mL syringe may be used. The needle should be 25 to 29 gauge with a 3/8- to 5/8-inch needle. Within this range, use shorter needles for smaller clients and longer needles for larger clients. In most cases, you may adjust the angle of insertion according to needle length. Shorter needles (1/2 inch and smaller) are usually inserted at a 90-degree angle, whereas 5/8-inch needles may be inserted at a 45-degree angle or a 90-degree angle, depending on whether the client has a smaller or a larger body mass, respectively (Figure 21-13). Further adjustments may be made for very small or pediatric clients according to need and facility policy. Administration techniques for subcutaneous injections are described in Procedure 21-6.

Intramuscular injections. The IM route may be chosen when rapid absorption is desired or when the medi-

Time to Allow: **Novice:** 10 min. **Expert:** 5 min.

PROCEDURE 21-5 ADMINISTERING AN INTRADERMAL INJECTION

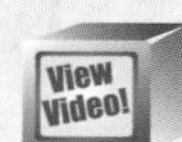

Nursing Skills Online: Injections, Lesson 4

Intradermal injections are done most often to test for allergies or for diagnostic purposes. The site is evaluated within a specific time period after the injection is given.

DELEGATION GUIDELINES

You may not delegate the administration of an intradermal injection to a nursing assistant.

EQUIPMENT NEEDED

- Medication order, medication administration record, computerized medication order sheet, or medication Kardex or cards
- Medication vial or ampule
- Tuberculin syringe and needle
- Alcohol swab
- 2 × 2 inch sterile gauze pad
- Acetone swab if needed for oily skin
- Disposable gloves

1 Follow preliminary actions (see inside front cover).

2 Check the medication order, and note any client allergies.

3 Withdraw medication from the vial as described in Procedure 21-3. Take the syringe and other supplies to the client's room, and place them on a clean, flat surface.

4 Prepare the client for the intradermal injection.

a. Identify the client using an identification bracelet or other agency-accepted means.

b. Explain the procedure to the client in a calm and confident manner.

c. Put on disposable gloves, and open the swab(s) and gauze package using aseptic technique.

d. Provide privacy, and position the client comfortably. Select and expose the injection site. *These steps reduce client tension and provide a view of the area to be used.*

5 Prepare the injection site and the syringe.

a. Make sure area is free of bruises, redness, or lesions.

b. Clean the site with an alcohol swab, wiping skin gently from top to bottom. Allow the alcohol to air dry. Use an acetone swab as well if the client's skin is oily. *Avoids circular motion that could stimulate capillary blood flow. Alcohol reduces the number of pathogens on the skin that could be pushed into the tissues by the needle. Allowing the alcohol to dry prevents tissue irritation.*

c. Remove the needle guard or cap with your nondominant hand by pulling it straight off. *This action helps prevent a needlestick injury.*

d. Check the syringe to make sure that the volume of medication is correct and that it contains no air bubbles.

6 Inject the medication.

a. Hold the syringe in your dominant hand, and spread the skin taut with your nondominant hand. *The dominant hand has better fine motor control. It is easier to inject into taut skin.*

b. Insert the needle bevel-up at a 10- to 15-degree angle into skin for 1/8 inch or until the bevel disappears from view. The needle should be visible below the skin surface, and you should feel resistance. *This step places the needle under the epidermal layer of skin but not into subcutaneous tissue.*

c. Inject the medication slowly while watching for formation of a small bleb, wheal, or blister (see Figure 21-11). If none is visible, withdraw the needle slightly and continue injecting. *This procedure deposits medication into the dermis.*

d. Withdraw the needle at the same angle used for insertion. *Doing so will reduce tissue trauma and client discomfort.*

e. Pat the area dry using the gauze pad. Do not massage the area. *Avoiding massage prevents the medication from spreading beyond the intended injection site.*

7 Dispose of used equipment properly, and clean the area.

a. Discard the needle and syringe in a rigid container without recapping the needle. Dispose of the alcohol swab, gauze, wrappers, and other used materials in a trash receptacle.

b. Position the client comfortably.

c. Remove gloves, and discard them in a proper receptacle. Perform hand hygiene.

8 Document the procedure carefully.

a. Observe the site and the client for any immediate allergic reaction. *Anaphylaxis could occur suddenly if the client has a severe allergy to the substance you injected.*

b. Use a skin pencil or a ball point pen (according to facility policy) to circle area of the wheal. *Doing so will provide an easy way to identify the site when performing follow-up readings.*

c. Document the date, time, substance, and site of the injection on the client's medication administration record. Document the date and time of follow-up observations, and inform the client and caregivers about their roles. *This will provide clear direction for caregivers responsible for interpreting test results.*

PEDIATRIC CONSIDERATIONS

Provide explanations about medication therapy at an age-appropriate level.

GERIATRIC CONSIDERATIONS

Older adults may display anergy and need a second round of testing to mount a detectable immunological response when allergens such as for tuberculosis are administered by the intradermal route.

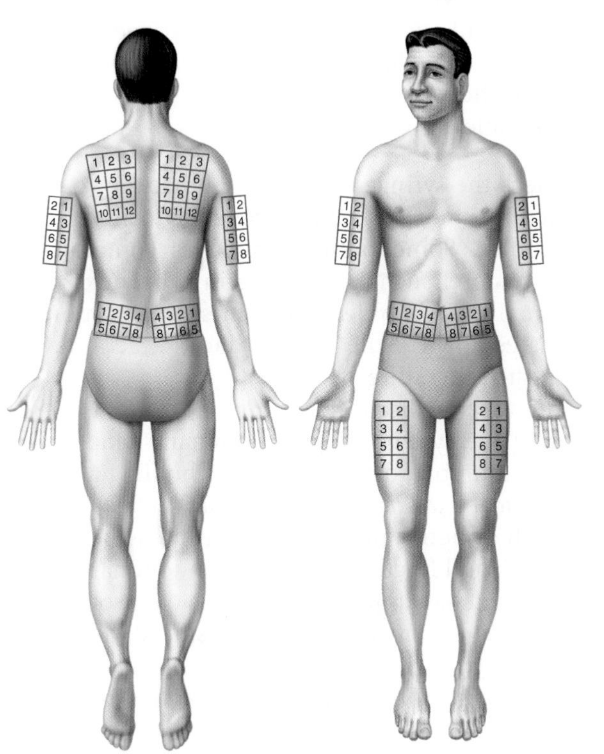

FIGURE 21-12 Common subcutaneous injection sites.

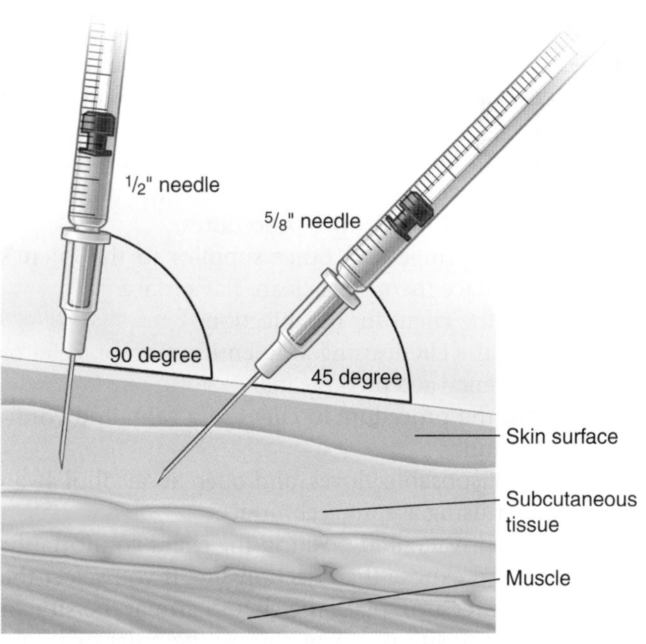

FIGURE 21-13 Technique for subcutaneous injection.

cation is irritating to subcutaneous tissue (Procedure 21-7). There are fewer nerve endings in muscle tissue, making this area more comfortable when irritating substances are injected. Nonetheless, clients can experience discomfort with IM injections. For this reason, do not inject into muscles that are tender to the client or that are contracted, hard, or tense. Complications of inappropriate site selection or improper technique include abscess formation, skin sloughing and necrosis, continued site pain, nerve injury, and periostitis (inflammation of the membrane over bone).

The volume that can be safely given by the IM route varies with the client's age and the site selected. An adult can receive a maximum of 4 mL in a large muscle, such as the gluteus. Children and older adults should not receive more than 1 or 2 mL because their muscles are less developed. The deltoid should be limited to 0.5 or 1 mL, depending on client size.

The appropriate needle size greatly depends on client size and drug viscosity. The average needle used for IM injection is 21 to 23 gauge and 1 to $1^1/_2$ inches long. A 2-inch needle may be used for very large clients so the medication reaches the muscle. Give all IM injections at a 90-degree angle.

There are four common sites for giving IM injections: ventrogluteal, dorsogluteal, vastus lateralis, and deltoid. These sites are safe because they do not lie near blood vessels, nerves, or bones. The gluteus muscles are particularly large and accept medication easily (Figure 21-14). As with subcutaneous injections, rotate sites if giving

TIME TO ALLOW: NOVICE: 10 min. EXPERT: 5 min.

PROCEDURE 21-6 ADMINISTERING A SUBCUTANEOUS INJECTION

View Video!

Nursing Skills Online: Injections, Lesson 3

Subcutaneous injections are given to administer medication into subcutaneous tissue with a written health care provider's order. This route provides faster medication action than the oral route.

DELEGATION GUIDELINES

You may not delegate the performance or administration of subcutaneous injections to a nursing assistant.

EQUIPMENT NEEDED

- Medication order, medication administration record, computerized medication order sheet, or medication Kardex or cards
- Medication vial or ampule
- Sterile, 3-mL insulin or tuberculin syringe and needle (5/8 inch or smaller)
- Two alcohol swabs
- Disposable gloves

1 Follow preliminary actions (see inside front cover).

2 Check the medication order, and note any client allergies.

3 Check the medication for appropriate color and clarity, and withdraw the medication from the ampule or vial as described in previous procedures.

4 Take the syringe and other supplies to the client's room, and place them on a clean, flat surface.

5 Prepare the client for the injection.

a. Identify the client using an identification bracelet or other agency-accepted means.

b. Explain the procedure to client in a calm and confident manner.

c. Put on disposable gloves, and open an alcohol swab wrapper using aseptic technique.

d. Provide privacy, and position the client comfortably. Select and expose the injection site. If you select the upper outer arm, place the client's arm at the side in a relaxed position. If you choose the anterior thigh, have the client sit or lie down with the leg muscle relaxed. If you choose the abdomen, have the client lie in a recumbent or semirecumbent position. If you choose the scapula, have the client sit or lie prone or on his or her side. *These positions give you a clear view of the area to be used.*

6 Prepare the injection site and syringe.

a. Make sure the area is free of bruises, redness, or lesions.

b. Identify the exact site of the injection. Clean the site with an alcohol swab using a circular motion, moving outward from injection site. Allow the alcohol to air dry. Leave the swab in a clean area so you can reuse it when withdrawing the needle.

c. Remove the needle guard or cap with your nondominant hand by pulling it straight off.

d. Check the syringe to make sure that the volume of medication is correct and generally contains no air bubbles. Some prefilled syringes containing the exact dose, such as enoxaparin (Lovenox) require that the air bubble be left in so medication does not escape via the needle track. Read individual product literature.

7 Inject the medication.

a. Hold the syringe in your dominant hand between your thumb and forefinger, as if holding a dart. *The dominant hand has better fine motor control.*

b. Pinch or bunch up subcutaneous tissue between the thumb and forefinger of your nondominant hand. If the client has ample subcutaneous tissue or if you are injecting an anticoagulant drug, spread the skin taut. *Bunching the tissue aids needle insertion into tissue. Use needle length, the amount of tissue, and tissue turgor as a guide.*

c. Quickly insert the needle up to the hub at a 45- to 90-degree angle, depending on the length of the needle. *This action positions the needle in subcutaneous tissue.*

d. Release the bunched tissue, and grasp the distal end of the syringe with your nondominant hand. *Holding the syringe with your nondominant hand steadies it in the tissue, reducing movement and client discomfort.*

e. Unless injecting insulin or heparin, aspirate for a blood return by pulling back gently on the tip of plunger with the thumb and forefinger of your dominant hand. *A blood return indicates that the needle has entered a blood vessel. Avoid aspiration with insulin or heparin because aspiration could cause local trauma.*

f. If a blood return is noted, pull the needle from the injection site, discard the syringe and needle, and begin the procedure again. *This prevents administering the medication intravenously and prevents hematoma formation from blood being introduced into the tissue.*

g. If no blood return is noted, inject the medication slowly and steadily. *Slow, steady injection disperses the medication evenly in the tissues to enhance absorption.*
h. Withdraw the needle quickly at the same angle used for insertion. Massage the area gently with the alcohol swab. Do not massage after injecting insulin or heparin. *Massage reduces tissue trauma and client discomfort, but it could increase the rate of insulin absorption or cause bleeding from heparin.*

8 Dispose of used equipment properly.

a. Discard the needle and syringe in a rigid container without recapping the needle. Dispose of the alcohol swab, wrapper, and other used materials in a trash receptacle.
b. Position the client comfortably.
c. Remove your gloves, and discard them in the proper receptacle. Perform hand hygiene.

9 Document the procedure carefully.

a. Record the date, time, substance, and site of injection on the client's medication administration record.
b. Check on the client within 30 minutes to assess the effects of the medication.

PEDIATRIC CONSIDERATIONS

Children are often fearful of injections. Use strategies outlined in Box 21-6.

GERIATRIC CONSIDERATIONS

Older adults may have reduced amounts of subcutaneous tissue. Select equipment and injection sites carefully.

HOME HEALTH CARE CONSIDERATIONS

Subcutaneous injections commonly administered in the home include insulin, heparin, and allergy injections. Subcutaneous injections are easier for the client or family to administer than are intramuscular injections. Teach about the medication, injection technique, site rotation, and management of adverse effects.

repeated injections. Identify the site rotation plan on the care plan, and chart sites used on the medication administration record.

Ventrogluteal site. The ventrogluteal site uses the gluteus medius and minimus muscles in the area of the hip. This is a preferred site for adults and for children and infants over 7 months old. It is particularly useful because it does not lie near major bones, blood vessels, or nerves; is relatively free of microorganisms from fecal contamination; and allows the client to lie on the back, side, or abdomen during injection.

Locate the site by placing the palm of your hand over the greater trochanter with your fingers pointed in the direction of the client's head (Figure 21-15). Use your left hand to identify landmarks when the client is receiving the injection in the right hip, and vice versa. Place your index finger on the anterior superior iliac spine at the midaxillary line, and extend your middle finger dorsally to the iliac crest. Give the injection in the center of the triangle created by these fingers.

Dorsogluteal site. The dorsogluteal site uses the gluteus maximus muscles in the buttocks and is another commonly used site for IM injection. This site is recommended for adults and children over age 3 because these muscles are developed by walking. It is not recommended for infants and children under age 3 because the gluteal muscles are small and underdeveloped. This site is not the preferred site for administering IM injections—there is a potential for injury because of the proximity of the sciatic nerve, major blood vessels, and bone.

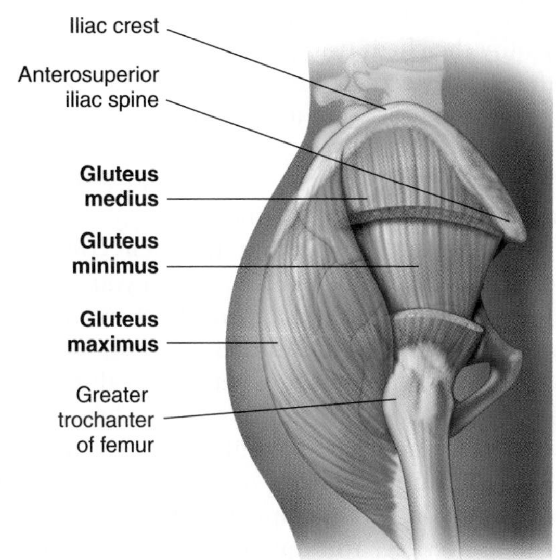

FIGURE 21-14 The three gluteus muscles are particularly large and accept intramuscular medication easily.

To expose the site, the client may lie on the side with the top leg flexed and in front of the lower leg. The client may also lie prone with the toes pointed inward. These positions reduce muscle tension and promote relaxation.

TIME TO ALLOW: NOVICE: 10 min. EXPERT: 5 min.

PROCEDURE 21-7 ADMINISTERING AN INTRAMUSCULAR INJECTION

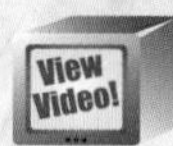

Nursing Skills Online: Injections, Lesson 5

Intramuscular injections are used to administer medication into muscle tissue with a written physician's order. This route provides faster action than the oral or subcutaneous route.

DELEGATION GUIDELINES

You may not delegate the administration of an intramuscular injection to a nursing assistant.

EQUIPMENT NEEDED

- Medication order, medication administration record, computerized medication order sheet, or medication Kardex or cards
- Medication vial or ampule
- Sterile, 3-mL syringe and needle (1 to 2 inches, 20 to 22 gauge, long bevel)
- Two alcohol swabs
- Disposable gloves

1 Follow preliminary actions (see inside front cover).

2 Check the medication order, and note any client allergies.

3 Check the medication for color and clarity, and withdraw the medication from the ampule or vial as described in previous procedures. Take the syringe and other supplies to the client's room, and place them on a clean, flat surface.

4 Prepare the client for the injection.

a. Identify the client using an identification bracelet or other agency-accepted means.

b. Explain the procedure to client in a calm and confident manner.

c. Put on disposable gloves, and open the alcohol swab wrapper using aseptic technique.

d. Provide privacy, and position the client comfortably. Select and expose the injection site. If you choose the upper arm (deltoid), place the client in a sitting or lying position with the arm relaxed at the side of the body. If you choose the anterolateral thigh (vastus lateralis), place the client in a sitting or lying position with the leg muscle relaxed. If you choose the dorsogluteal location (gluteus maximus), select a side-lying position with the upper leg flexed and in front of the lower leg. You can also use a prone position with the client's toes pointed inward. If you choose the ventrogluteal location (gluteus medius), place the client in a supine position with legs relaxed or a side-lying position with hip and knee flexed. *These positions reduce muscle tension and allow you to clearly see the area to be used.*

5 Prepare the injection site and the syringe.

a. Make sure the area is free of bruises, redness, or lesions.

b. Identify the exact site of the injection. Clean the site with an alcohol swab using a circular motion, moving outward from injection site. Allow the alcohol to air dry. Leave the swab in a clean area so you can reuse it when withdrawing the needle.

c. Remove needle guard or cap with your nondominant hand by pulling it straight off.

d. Check the syringe to make sure that the volume of medication is correct.

6 Inject the medication.

a. Hold the syringe in your dominant hand between your thumb and forefinger as if holding a dart (see illustration).

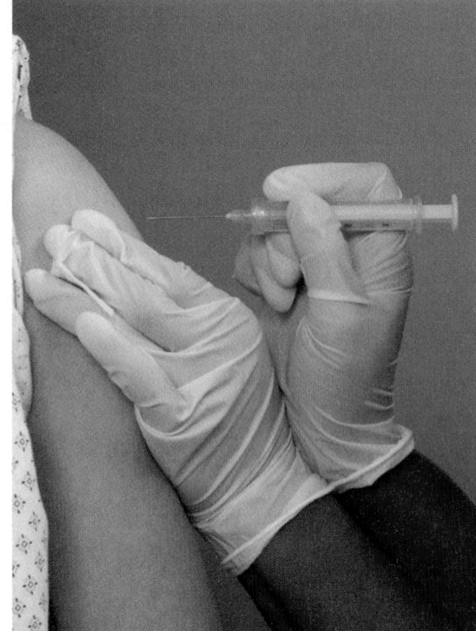

Step 6a. Holding the syringe like a dart and spreading the skin taut (here, over the deltoid).

b. Spread the skin taut between the thumb and forefinger of your nondominant hand, or displace the skin using a Z-track technique (see Figure 21-20). *Making the skin taut aids insertion of the needle into the muscle tissue.*
c. Insert the needle quickly at a 90-degree angle up to the hub. *This action positions the needle in the muscle tissue.*
d. Release the skin, and grasp the distal end of the syringe with your nondominant hand. *Grasping the syringe steadies it in the tissue, thus reducing movement and client discomfort.*
e. Aspirate for a blood return by pulling back gently on tip of the plunger with the thumb and forefinger of your dominant hand. *Blood return indicates that the needle has entered a blood vessel.*
f. If blood return is noted, remove the needle, discard the syringe, and begin the procedure again. *Beginning again prevents the medication from being injected intravenously and prevents the reinjection of aspirated blood.*
g. If no blood return is noted, inject the medication slowly and steadily, taking about 10 seconds to inject each 1 mL. *Slow, steady injection disperses the medication evenly in the tissue to enhance absorption.*
h. Wait a few seconds, then withdraw the needle quickly at the same angle used to insert it. Apply gentle pressure to the site with an alcohol swab or 2 × 2 inch gauze. *These steps allow the medication to diffuse into the muscle while reducing tissue trauma and discomfort.*

7 Dispose of the used equipment.

a. Discard the needle and syringe in a rigid container without recapping the needle. Dispose of the alcohol swab, wrapper, and other used materials in an appropriate trash receptacle.
b. Position the client comfortably. If medication was injected into a leg muscle, encourage the client to flex and extend leg muscles. *These actions promote client comfort and enhance absorption of medication from sites in the leg.*
c. Remove gloves, and discard them in the proper receptacle. Perform hand hygiene.

8 Document the procedure carefully.

a. Record the date, time, substance, and site of injection on the client's medication administration record.
b. Check on the client at an appropriate time after giving the injection (2 to 4 hours for many medications) to assess the client's response to the medication.

PEDIATRIC CONSIDERATIONS

Children are often fearful of injections. Use strategies outlined in Box 21-6.

GERIATRIC CONSIDERATIONS

Older adults may have reduced subcutaneous tissue and muscle mass, allowing the use of a shorter needle. Select equipment and injection sites carefully.

HOME HEALTH CARE CONSIDERATIONS

The need for intramuscular injections in a homebound client is justification for a home health care nurse. Intramuscular injections given in the home include iron, vitamins, antibiotics, and ketorolac tromethamine (Toradol) and other pain medications. The home health care nurse must plan for the management of side effects and adverse effects. If a family caregiver is taught to administer intramuscular injections, client teaching should include recognizing and managing emergency reactions such as anaphylaxis. Consider whether the client needs to have injectable epinephrine (Adrenalin) at home for possible emergency use. Teach about the medication, injection technique, site rotation, and the management of adverse effects.

Do not allow the client to stand when injection is done in the dorsogluteal site. Make sure you can see the area well. Have the client lower the undergarment, or move aside the hospital gown. Locate the site by drawing an imaginary line between the anatomical landmarks of the posterior superior iliac spine and the greater trochanter. Administer the injection lateral and slightly superior to the midpoint of this line (Figure 21-16).

Vastus lateralis site. The vastus lateralis muscle is a thick, well-developed muscle located on the anterolateral aspect of the thigh. In the adult, it extends from a handbreadth above the knee to a handbreadth below the greater trochanter. It measures in width from the midline of the top of the thigh to the midline of the lateral thigh. It is easiest to use this site by injecting the outer middle third of the thigh (Figure 21-17). This is a preferred injection site for adults, children, and infants. It is especially useful in children whose gluteal muscles are poorly developed. There are no large nerves or blood vessels in the area, and the muscle does not lie over a joint. The client may lie supine or be in a sitting position during injection as long as the leg muscles are relaxed.

The rectus femoris muscle is located on the midanterior thigh and is another well-developed muscle that lies away from blood vessels and nerves (Figure 21-18). It can safely be used in adults, children, and infants. This site is not as popular, however, because it can cause discomfort. In general, it is only used if other sites are contraindicated.

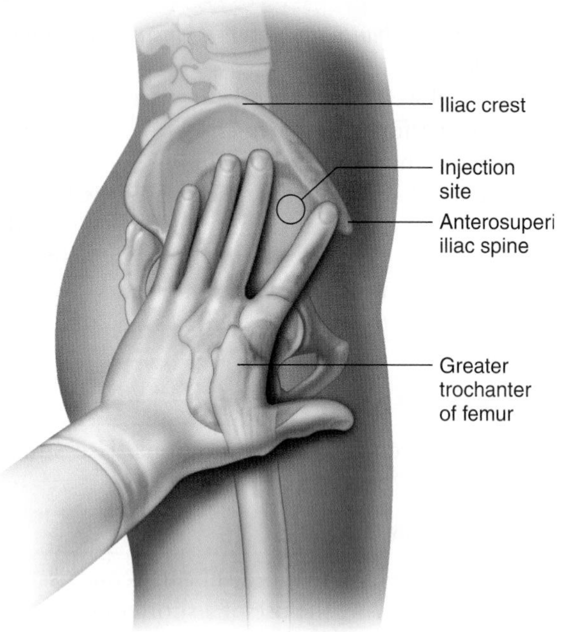

FIGURE 21-15 Ventrogluteal intramuscular injection site. Place the palm of your hand over the greater trochanter, with your middle finger pointed toward the iliac crest and your index finger toward the anterosuperior iliac spine. Administer the injection in the center of the triangle formed by your fingers.

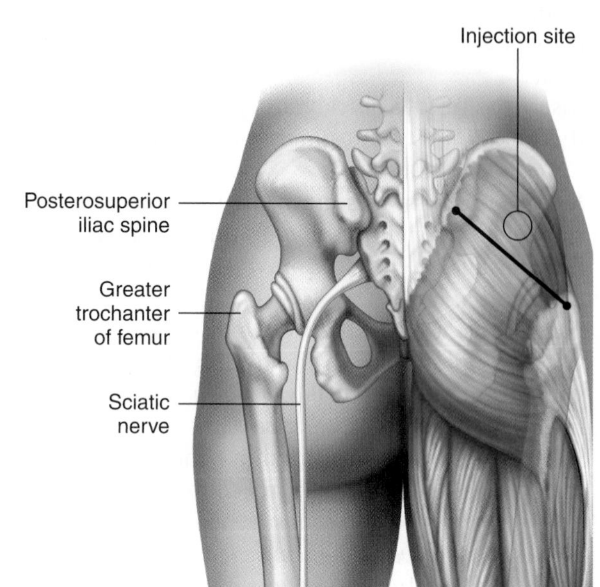

FIGURE 21-16 Dorsogluteal intramuscular injection site. Identify an imaginary line between the greater trochanter and the posterosuperior iliac spine. Give the injection superior and lateral to that line.

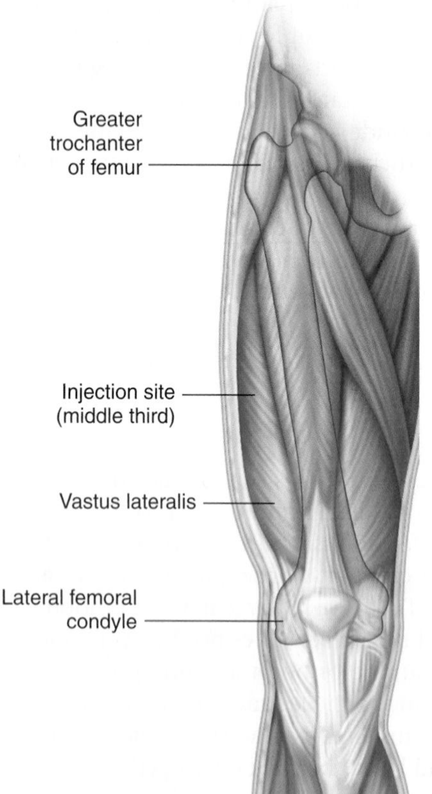

FIGURE 21-17 Vastus lateralis intramuscular injection site on the right thigh. Divide the thigh into thirds; give the injection in the middle third.

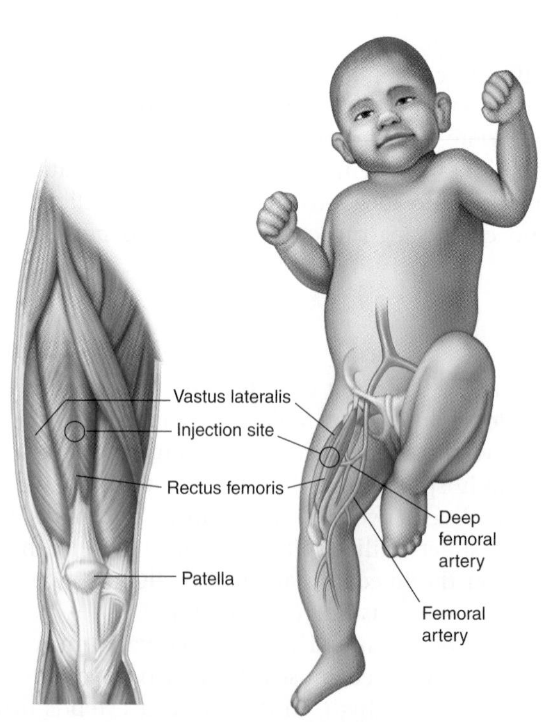

FIGURE 21-18 Rectus femoris intramuscular injection site on the anterior part of the thigh (used in adults only if other sites are contraindicated). In children, the site is located one-third the distance from the patella to the greater trochanter in the center of the anterior thigh.

Deltoid site. The deltoid muscle is found on the lateral aspect of the upper arm. It is not used as often as other sites because it is a small muscle, incapable of absorbing large medication volumes. The deltoid muscle should not be used in infants and children because of its size. In adults, injected volumes should not exceed 1 mL. The client may sit or lie down during injection as long as the arm is relaxed against the body to minimize muscle tension and resistance.

Locate the site by palpating the lower edge of the acromion process. Inject the area that lies 2 to 3 fingerbreadths below the acromion process in adults. An alternative method is to locate the triangular muscle area that extends from 2.5 to 5 fingerbreadths below the acromion process (Figure 21-19). In a child, locate the site 1 fingerbreadth below the acromion process.

Air-lock technique. Some clinicians use an air lock when giving IM injections. A 0.2-mL air bubble may be drawn into a syringe and injected to prevent tracking of irritating medication through subcutaneous tissue when the needle is withdrawn. Determine and follow agency policies and procedures about use of air locks. When giving a Z-track medication, use an air lock according to agency policy (see next paragraphs).

Z-track method. The Z-track method for giving IM injections seals the medication within muscle tissue. It minimizes tissue irritation by preventing tracking of medication through subcutaneous tissue with needle removal after injection. Although previously used only when giving irritating or tissue-staining medications such as iron dextran (Imferon), Z-track is now being used more frequently to minimize pain and discomfort at any IM injection site.

Use the Z-track technique when giving injections in the ventrogluteal or dorsogluteal areas (Figure 21-20). After drawing up the medication and adding a 0.2-mL air lock, change the needle to ensure that medication is not tracked into subcutaneous tissue during needle insertion. The needle should be at least $1\frac{1}{2}$ inches long. Pull the skin and subcutaneous tissue about 1 to $1\frac{1}{2}$ inches (2.5 to 3.5 cm) to one side using your nondominant hand. Inject the medication as usual, count to 10 to allow for distribution of medication, withdraw the needle, and release the tissue. The tissue glides back into normal position, eliminating the needle track. Apply gentle pressure over the area, but do not massage (to avoid forcing medication back into the needle track).

Intravenous Medications. The IV route is chosen when medication effect is needed within 1 to 2 minutes or when the medication is irritating to subcutaneous or muscle tissue. Use extreme caution, and follow the six rights of medication administration when using the IV route. If there is an antidote to an IV medication, it should be readily available for emergency use.

Generally, there are three possible methods for giving an IV medication: added to an IV solution, IV piggyback, and IV push. When medication is added directly to a bag or bottle of IV solution, it infuses slowly but continuously into the client. When available, special transfer devices simplify the transfer of medication to an IV solution. See Procedure 21-8 for the correct method for adding medication to an IV solution.

A second method of IV medication administration is the intermittent IV piggyback (IVPB) setup (most common) or an IV tandem setup (Figure 21-21). The

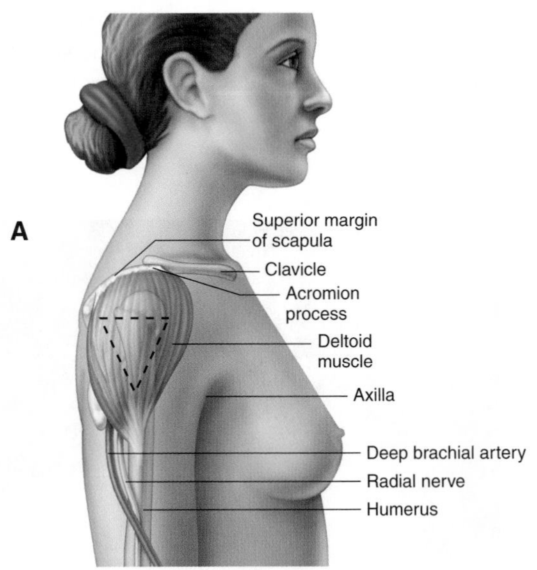

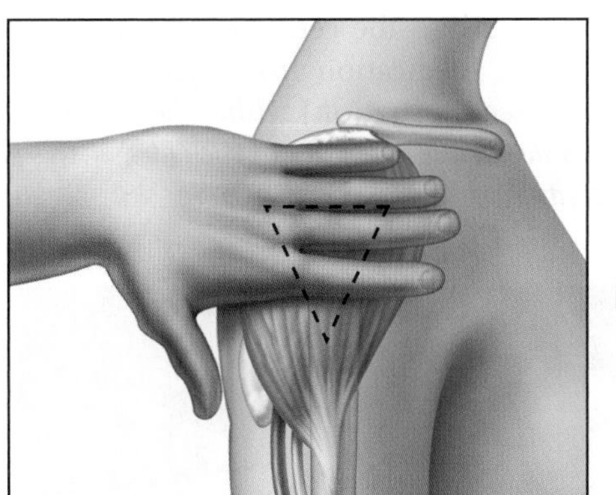

FIGURE 21-19 A, Deltoid muscle injection site in the upper arm. **B,** Locate the site in the triangular area 2.5 to 5 fingerbreadths below the acromion process.

IVPB method uses gravity to determine flow rate. A roller clamp is used to adjust the flow rate of these infusions as well. The secondary solution (Table 21-9) is plugged into an intermittent IV infusion device using long tubing, or it is added to a primary IV line using either a needle or a needleless system. Preparation and administration of an intermittent IV medication are described in Procedure 21-9.

Use an infusion control pump to control the infusion rate of an intermittent IV medication. Make sure the alarm is always turned on to alert you if the line infiltrates or other problems arise. Remember that these de-

TIME TO ALLOW: **NOVICE:** 8 min. **EXPERT:** 3 min.

PROCEDURE 21-8 ADDING MEDICATION TO AN IV BAG

Nursing Skills Online: Intravenous Medication Administration, Lesson 4

Some medications are given to clients as part of an intravenous (IV) infusion. The pharmacy may add the medication to the IV infusion bag, or you may need to do it.

DELEGATION GUIDELINES

You may not delegate the addition of medication to an IV bag to a nursing assistant.

EQUIPMENT NEEDED

- Medication order, medication administration record, computerized medication order sheet, or medication Kardex or cards
- Medication vial or ampule
- IV solution
- Medication label
- Sterile syringe and needle of appropriate size (3 to 20 mL and 1 to 1½ inch, 19 to 21 gauge)
- Needle filter, if appropriate
- Two alcohol swabs
- Disposable gloves

1 Follow preliminary actions (see inside front cover).

2 Check the medication order.

3 Withdraw the medication from the ampule or vial as described in Procedures 21-2 and 21-3.

4 Inject the medication into the bag of IV solution.

a. Close the roller clamp on the tubing attached to the IV solution. *This step prevents fluid loss from the IV bag.*

b. Wipe the medication port of the bag containing the IV solution. *Doing so prevents contamination of the needle by microorganisms on the outside of the port.*

c. Insert the needle into the center of the medication port, and inject medication from syringe into the solution bag (see illustration). *Using the center of the port prevents accidental puncture of the sides of the port or the IV container.*

d. Withdraw the needle, and discard the needle and syringe, without recapping the needle, in an approved receptacle.

e. Rotate the solution bag gently but thoroughly (see illustration). Rotation distributes the medication evenly throughout the IV solution.

f. Write the name and dose of the medication, the date, the time, and your initials on a medication label. Affix the label to the IV bag without obstructing the name of the solution or the IV time tape. The label clearly identifies what you added to the IV solution without hampering your ability to identify the solution or determine whether the IV is infusing on time.

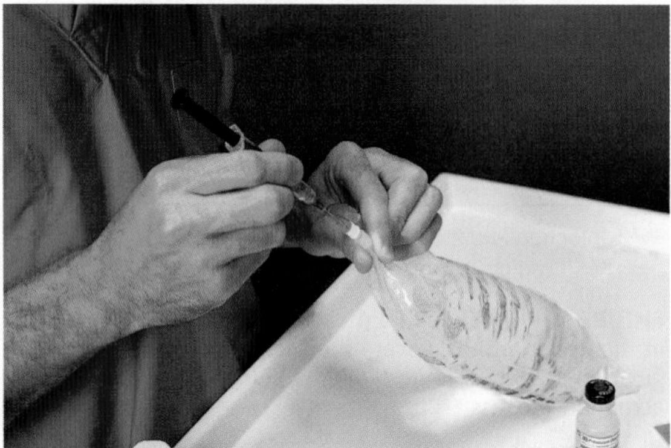

Step 4c. Inserting the needle into the center of the medication port.

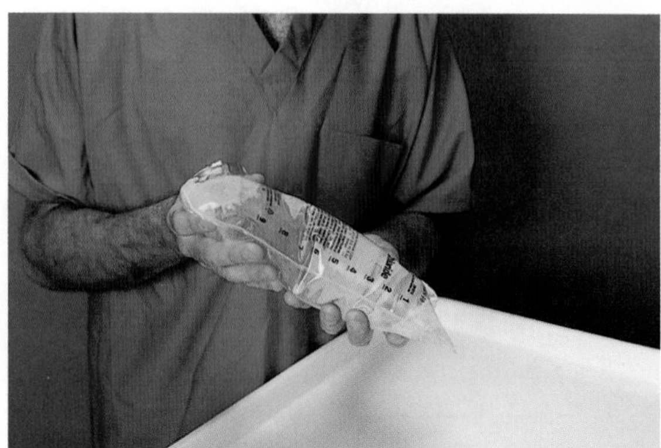

Step 4e. Rotating the solution bag.

Continued

g. Dispose of the medication container, alcohol swab, wrapper, and any other used materials in an appropriate receptacle.

5 Prime the tubing, bring the container to the client's room, and hang the solution bag according to standard procedure. Set the drip rate carefully. Follow all procedures needed to monitor IV therapy properly. *This step prevents medication error and possible fluid overload.*

6 Document the date, time, IV solution used, and additive used on the client's medication administration record or other IV charting form.

HOME HEALTH CARE CONSIDERATIONS

The administration of IV medications is a growing trend in home health care. Clients include people with acquired immunodeficiency syndrome (AIDS), cancer, and other serious illnesses. In home health care settings today, you may administer chemotherapy, acyclovir, total parenteral nutrition, blood, and medications that were at one time administered only in a hospital setting. You will need to assess for the effects and side effects of medications, recognize serious or life-threatening reactions, and know how to respond. Clients receiving IV medications at home may have prefilled epinephrine (Adrenalin) syringes in the event of an anaphylactic reaction.

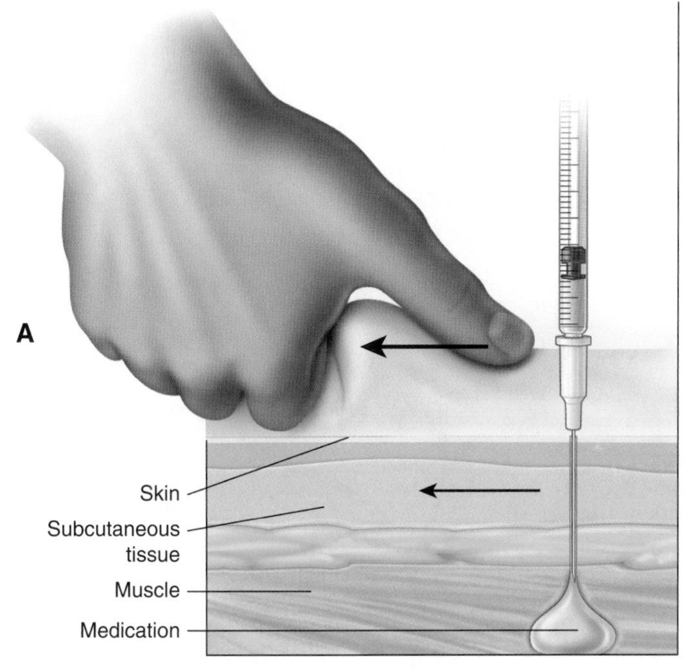

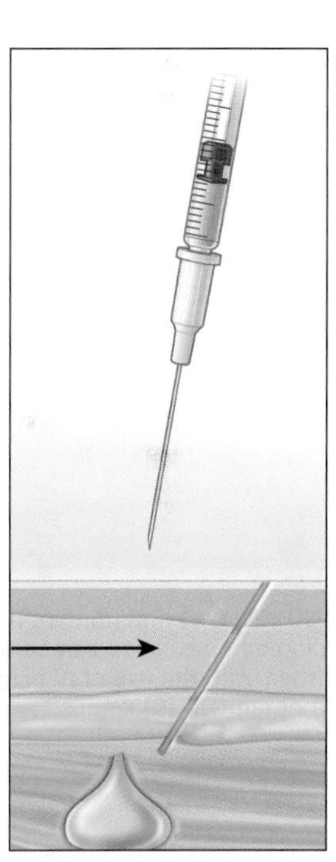

FIGURE 21-20 Intramuscular injection using the Z-track technique. **A,** Pull the skin and subcutaneous tissue 1 to 1½ inches (2.5 to 3.5 cm) to the side with the thumb or the side of the hand, and inject the medication. **B,** Withdraw the needle, and release the tissue to seal the medication in the muscle.

vices are adjuncts to nursing care, not substitutes for careful nursing assessment.

The third method for administering an IV medication is IV push. As with an intermittent IV infusion, you may give IV push medications through a mainline IV or an intermittent infusion device. Medications are usually injected over 1 minute or longer, according to drug literature. If an intermittent infusion device is used, flush the line with normal saline (or, occasionally, heparin) according to facility policy to verify that the line is patent. Procedure 21-10 describes how to administer an IV push medication. When administering IV push medications or flushes via a central venous catheter, be sure to use a 10-mL syringe, even if the volume to be used is smaller. The larger syringe size reduces the pounds per square inch pressure of the injection on the blood vessels and thereby reduces risk to the client.

Regardless of the specific method used, universal principles apply to the preparation and administration of IV medications. Be especially careful to select the correct medication and to draw up the correct dose. Use proper technique when withdrawing medication from a vial or ampule, and wipe the IV port with an alcohol swab before adding the medication or entering the IV line. Label the syringe or bag according to facility policy with the medication name, dose, date, time, and your name or initials. Do not apply a label until you have actually added a medication.

Before giving an IV medication, assess the IV line for patency and the site for signs of phlebitis (local tenderness, redness, and warmth) or infiltration (local coolness, firmness, pain, and swelling). Refer to Chapter 26 for further discussion of IV site assessment. If signs of phlebitis or infiltration are found, do not use the line; start a new IV line before proceeding. Severe tissue damage could result if irritating medications are injected into an infiltrated IV line. A vein with signs of phlebitis could be damaged further by injection of an IV medication, or the line may be resistant to flushing. Periodically assess the status of the client and the line during the infusion to detect early signs of complications or untoward reactions.

Clients who have veins of poor quality or who require IV medication therapy for prolonged periods may undergo percutaneous insertion of a central venous catheter. Such a catheter may have multiple lumens or a single lumen. Other central venous lines are implanted surgically and are accessed using specific techniques. Such lines may be implanted in clients who need chemotherapy. Adhere to facility policies and procedures when giving IV medications through these catheters. Use strict surgical aseptic technique when accessing these lines, because organisms introduced into a central line could lead rapidly to sepsis.

Managing Topical Medications. Topical medications are often used to produce an anesthetic effect, create a systemic effect, or relieve local irritation or infection. Most are given two to three times a day.

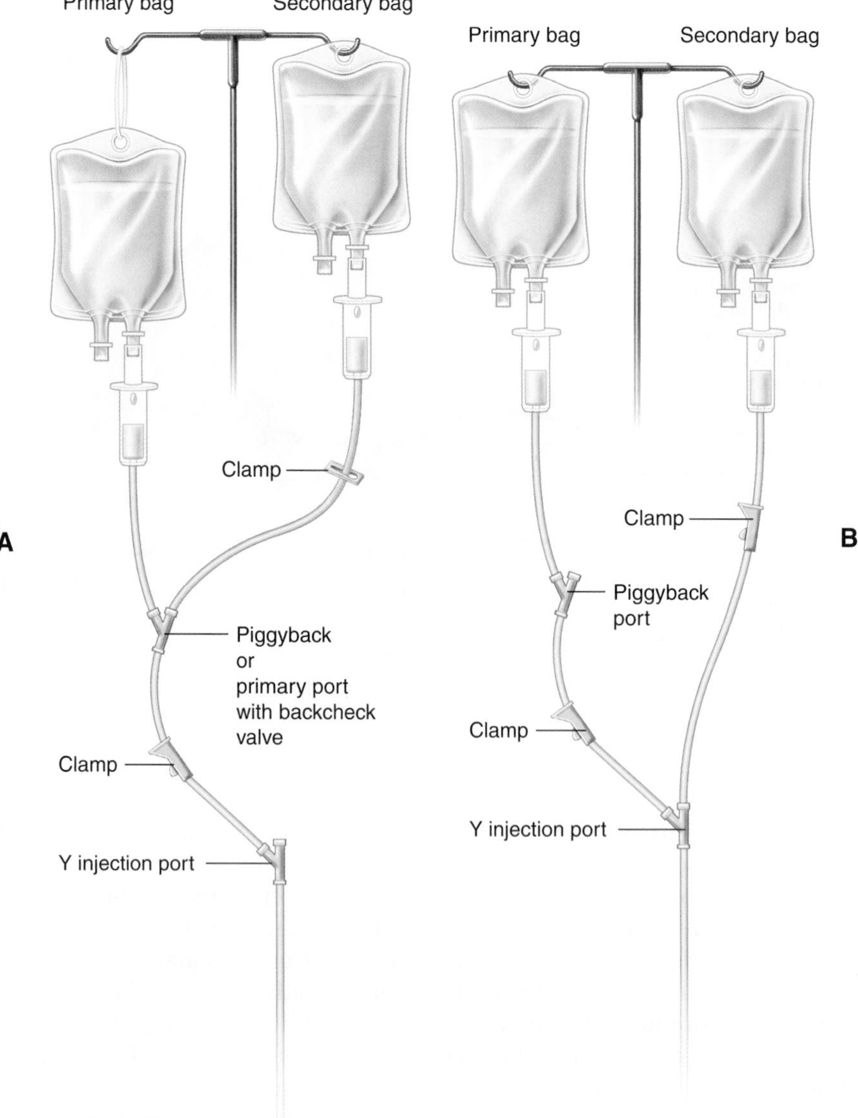

FIGURE 21-21 Intermittent IV medication administration can be accomplished with the use of IV piggyback **(A)** or tandem **(B)** setups.

Skin Applications. A medication applied to the skin is manufactured in the form of a cream, lotion, ointment, powder, paste, or patch (also called a disk). Before giving a topical medication, assess the client's skin for breakdown, lesions, rashes, or erythema. The medication may be ordered to treat one of these conditions, or the condition may indicate that the medication should not be applied to that surface, depending on the medication and client circumstances. Use standard precautions when administering a topical drug to

Table 21-9 Systems for Administering a Drug by IV Piggyback

SYSTEM	PROCEDURE	SYSTEM	PROCEDURE
Ready-to-use Premix 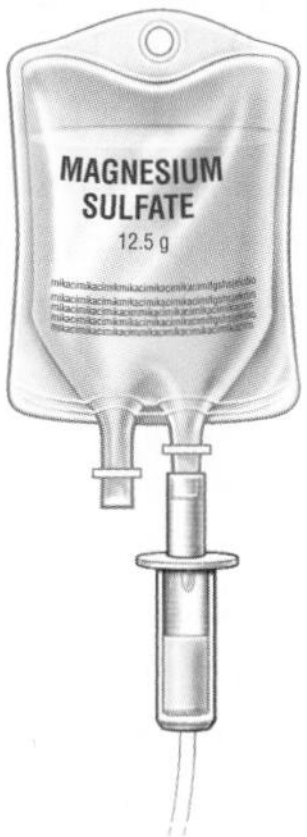	A plastic bag contains both medication and diluent. Unstable drugs may be frozen to preserve them and are thawed before use.	Drug manufacturer's piggyback 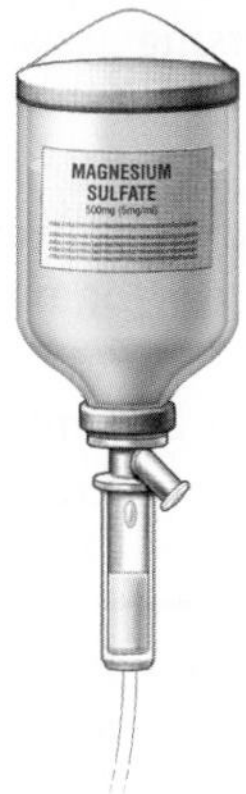	A medication dose is prefilled in a container that must be diluted before use.
Add Vantage 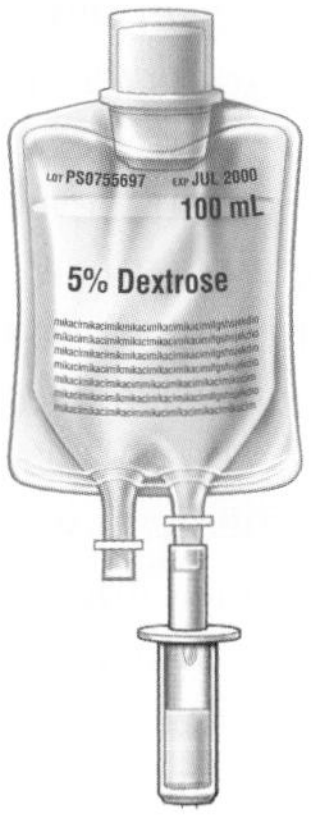	A drug is reconstituted and then added to diluent in a small plastic bag.	Minisyringe pump 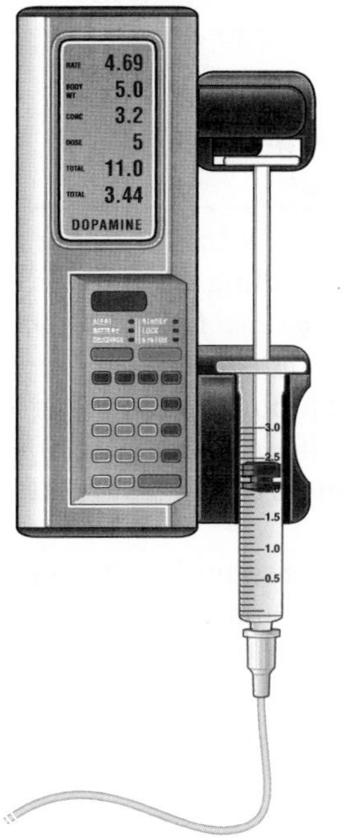	The medication is injected using a pressurized syringe plunger.
Minibag 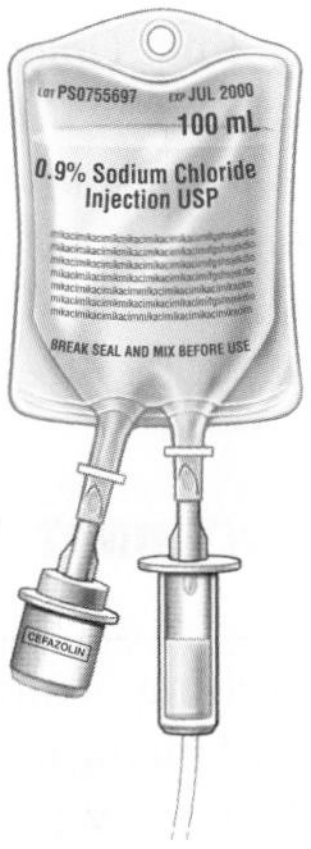	A medication vial is attached to an IV bag. You break an internal seal and mix the drug and diluent just before administration.		

TIME TO ALLOW: **NOVICE:** 10 min. **EXPERT:** 5 min.

PROCEDURE 21-9 ADMINISTERING AN IV MEDICATION BY INTERMITTENT INFUSION

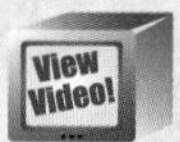

An intermittent intravenous (IV) infusion is administered when a medication to be given by the IV route requires a longer infusion time (typically 30 to 90 minutes) than IV push provides. It is connected into a primary IV line by intravenous piggyback (IVPB) or tandem setup or connected to an intermittent infusion device (saline lock).

DELEGATION GUIDELINES

You may not delegate the administration of IV medication by intermittent infusion to a nursing assistant.

EQUIPMENT NEEDED

- Medication order, medication administration record, computerized medication order sheet, or medication Kardex or cards
- Medication premixed in a 50-mL to 250-mL infusion bag (usually 50 to 150 mL), clearly labeled
- Macrodrip or microdrip tubing of appropriate length (primary tubing if attaching to a heparin lock, secondary tubing if attaching to a primary IV line)
- Needleless IV connector or 21- to 23-gauge needle
- Metal or plastic hook (if adding to a primary IV line) or a vial of sterile normal saline and two 3-mL syringes with attached needles (if giving medication through a heparin lock)
- Alcohol swab
- Disposable gloves
- Tape (optional)

1 Follow preliminary actions (see inside front cover).

2 Check the medication order, and assess the client's allergies.

3 Prepare the medication at the medication cart or another designated area. Label the IV medication bag/bottle if the pharmacy has not done so already.

4 Administer the medication.

ADMINISTRATION THROUGH AN EXISTING IV LINE (IVPB OR TANDEM SETUP)

a. Attach secondary tubing to the IV bag or bottle that contains the medication according to standard IV therapy protocol. *Tubing may be used for 48 to 96 hours from the time of initial use in most facilities.*

b. Make sure to use nonvented tubing for an IV bag and vented tubing for an IV bottle. Also make sure that the roller clamp on the tubing is closed before attaching the tubing.

c. Prime the tubing, and label the secondary IV bag and the tubing with the date, time, and your initials.

d. Bring the medication administration record, IV bag with medication, needle or needleless device, alcohol swab, metal hook, gloves, and tape to client's room.

e. Identify the client using an identification bracelet or other acceptable means.

f. Assess the IV site, and put on gloves if the facility requires it.

g. Remove the cap from the distal end of the IV tubing, and attach the needle or needleless device.

h. Wipe the IV additive port on the primary line with an alcohol swab, and attach the needle or needleless device. Make sure to attach the medication above the flow regulator clamp on the primary line. Although needleless systems are typically manufactured to secure tightly to the IV port, tape the connection if needed for stability. *Cleaning with alcohol prevents the IV line from contamination with microorganisms from the exterior IV port. Attaching above the regulator clamp allows you to regulate the flow rate.*

i. Lower the primary IV solution below the level of the IV medication bag using the metal or plastic hook provided with the secondary tubing set. *The IV medication flows and the primary bag stops flowing because of the effects of gravity.*

j. Regulate the drip rate of the IV medications as ordered, or set the infusion pump rate and volume. Check to be sure that it is running, and monitor to determine that the client is tolerating the medication. *If you use a regulator clamp below the site where the IVPB is connected, the primary bag will start flowing when the IVPB is empty.*

k. Come back when the medication has infused, and reset the drip rate on the primary line. *Unless readjusted, the primary line will continue to infuse at the rate set for the secondary infusion. If you use an infusion pump, the primary rate should resume once secondary medication is infused.*

l. Reassess the IV site and the client's tolerance of the medication.

ADMINISTRATION THROUGH AN INTERMITTENT INFUSION DEVICE (SALINE LOCK)

a. Close the roller clamp, and attach tubing of adequate length (70 inches or longer) to the IV medication bag or bottle according to standard IV therapy protocol.

Use nonvented tubing for an IV bag and vented tubing for an IV bottle. Prime the tubing. *Closing the clamp prevents loss of the medication through the tubing. Choosing correctly vented tubing ensures that solution will flow through the tubing. Priming the tubing removes air from the system.*

b. Using standard procedure, draw 3 mL of sterile normal saline solution into a 3-mL syringe (or another solution or amount according to facility policy). *An intermittent infusion device is flushed both before and after use to ensure patency.*
c. Bring the medication administration record, IV medication bag, needle or needleless device, syringe with flush, alcohol swab, gloves, and tape to client's room.
d. Identify client using an identification bracelet or other acceptable means.
e. Assess the IV site, and put on gloves if required by your facility.
f. Remove the cap from the distal end of the IV tubing. Attach the needle or needleless device and prime the tubing. *Priming removes air from the system.*
g. Wipe the port of the intermittent infusion device with an alcohol swab.
h. Assess the site, and flush the infusion device port with sterile saline solution or other ordered solution.
i. Attach the IV medication bag to the infusion device port using the needle or needleless device (see illustration). Tape the connection if needed.

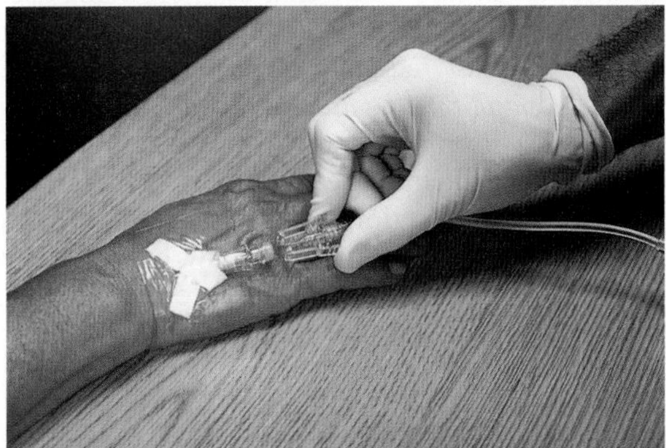

Step 4i. **Intermittent device.** Using a needleless device, attach the IV medication bag to the infusion device port.

j. Regulate the drip rate of the IV medication as ordered. Monitor the client to ensure the client is tolerating the medication.
k. Once the medication has infused, close the roller clamp, and remove the tubing from the port. Recap or attach a clean needle or needleless device to the tubing according to facility policy. *Most facilities allow IV tubing to be reused for 48 to 96 hours after the initial use, if sterility has been maintained.*
l. Reassess the IV site, and flush the infusion port with a second syringe filled with the ordered flush solution (often normal saline). Evaluate client response to the medication.

5 Document the date, time, and IV medication given on the client's medication administration record or computerized medication record.

PEDIATRIC CONSIDERATIONS

Children are often fearful of injections, even into an intravenous line. Reassure children they will not feel pain with insertion of the syringe into an existing IV line.

GERIATRIC CONSIDERATIONS

Older adults may have fragile veins, so use extra caution when administering medications via the IV route.

PROCEDURE 21-10 ADMINISTERING AN IV PUSH MEDICATION

TIME TO ALLOW: NOVICE: 10 min. EXPERT: 5 min.

Push means the medication is mixed in a small amount of fluid (usually 1 to 10 mL) and administered directly into the vein (not mixed with intravenous [IV] fluid) over a short time (usually 1 to 5 minutes). The bolus of medication is given by the IV push method when the client needs an immediate effect or the medication cannot be mixed with the fluid. Product literature indicates whether a specific medication can be given using this method.

DELEGATION GUIDELINES

You may not delegate the administration of IV push medication to a nursing assistant.

EQUIPMENT NEEDED

- Medication order, medication administration record, computerized medication order sheet, or medication Kardex or cards
- Medication vial or ampule
- Syringe of appropriate size for the medication dose ordered, with a 21- to 23-gauge needle attached
- Vial of sterile normal saline and two 3-mL syringes with attached needles (if using an intermittent infusion device)
- If a needleless system is used, one needleless device if injecting through a mainline IV and three devices if injecting via an intermittent infusion device
- Alcohol swabs
- Disposable gloves

1 Follow preliminary actions (see inside front cover).

2 Check the medication order, and assess the client's allergies. Also check the compatibility of the medication with the current IV fluid, if one is infusing.

3 Prepare the medication at the medication cart or other designated area. *Preparing the medication before going to the bedside helps to reduce the client's anxiety.*

4 Administer the medication.

ADMINISTRATION THROUGH AN EXISTING IV LINE

a. Draw up the medication from an ampule or a vial as described in previous procedures. Be certain it reads "for IV use." Recap the needle using one-handed technique. Label the syringe with the medication and dose.

b. Remove the capped needle, and attach a needleless device if a needleless system is in use.

c. Bring the medication administration record, IV medication, alcohol swab, and gloves to the client's room.

d. Identify the client using an identification bracelet or other acceptable means.

e. Assess the IV site, and put on gloves if the facility requires it.

f. Wipe the IV additive port of the primary line with an alcohol swab. Make sure that the port being used is the port nearest to the client. *Using the closest port ensures the least resistance to flow of medication and helps to control the rate at which the medication reaches client's bloodstream.*

g. Insert the needle into the port, and pinch off the tubing above the injection port (see illustrations). As a final check for compatibility, draw back slightly to pull a small amount of IV fluid into the syringe and watch for precipitation if incompatible. *Pinching ensures that the medication flows into the client's vein and*

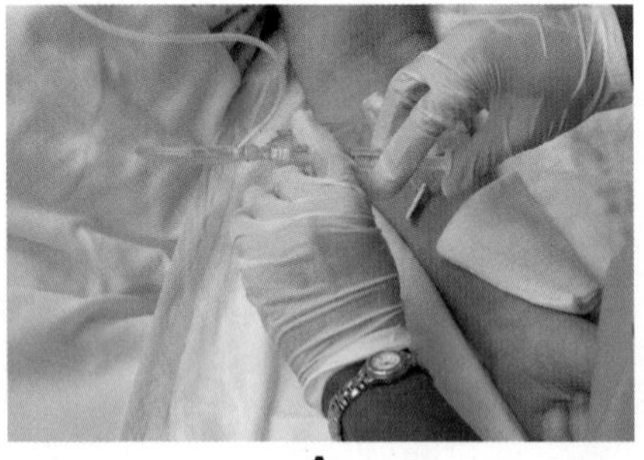
A

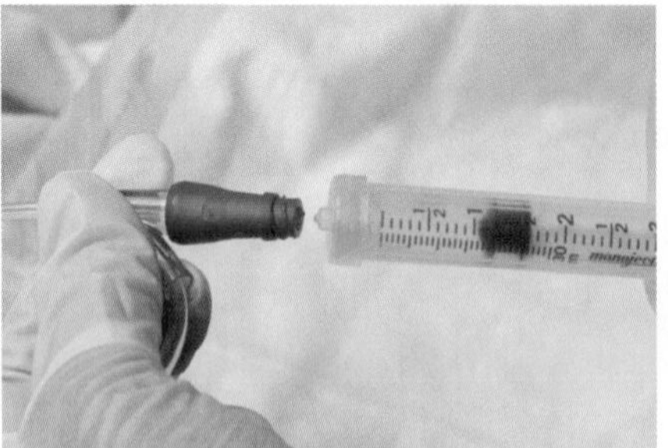
B

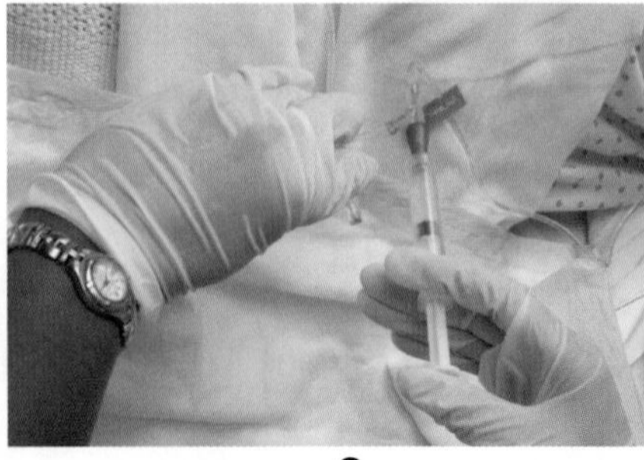
C

Step 4g. A, Blunt-tip plastic access device inserted into needleless port. **B,** Using a syringe to access a needleless access container. **C,** Clamping the tubing to ensure forward injection of medication.

not upward into the IV tubing. If the medication is not compatible with the IV fluid, the precipitation occurs in the syringe rather than the IV catheter or client's vein. If incompatible, remove the IV tubing from the infusion device port; flush the port with a compatible solution, give the medication, then flush the port again, and reconnect the IV tubing.

h. Inject the medication slowly and steadily at the rate recommended by the manufacturer. Use a watch to ensure accurate timing. Assess the IV site during injection. *Overly rapid injection could be harmful to the client or cause IV infiltration. Injection that is too slow is not useful and could produce anxiety.*
i. Release the tubing, remove the syringe, and assess the client's tolerance of the medication.

ADMINISTRATION THROUGH AN INTERMITTENT INFUSION DEVICE (HEPARIN LOCK)

a. Draw up sterile normal saline (or another ordered flush solution) into two syringes of 3 mL each (or another ordered volume) according to facility policy using Procedure 21-3 for drawing medication out of a vial. Label the syringes. *An intermittent infusion device is flushed with normal saline both before and after use to ensure patency.*
b. Draw up the ordered medication into a syringe from an ampule or a vial (see Procedure 21-2 or 21-3). Recap the needle using one-handed technique. Label the syringe.
c. Bring the IV medication, needle or needleless devices, syringes with flush solution, alcohol swabs, and gloves to the client's room.
d. Identify the client using an identification bracelet or other acceptable means.
e. Assess the IV site, and put on gloves if the facility requires it.
f. Wipe the port of the intermittent infusion device with an alcohol swab.
g. Insert one syringe filled with flush solution, and inject it slowly into the client. Remove the syringe. *If the line does not flush, evaluate it for patency and placement.*
h. Wipe the port again with an alcohol swab.
i. Insert the syringe containing the medication, and inject it slowly and steadily at the rate recommended by the manufacturer. Use a watch with a second hand to ensure accurate timing. Assess the IV site during the injection. Remove the syringe. *Overly rapid injection could be harmful to the client or cause IV infiltration. Injection that is too slow is not useful and could produce anxiety.*
j. Wipe the port again with another alcohol swab.
k. Insert the second syringe containing flush solution, and inject it slowly into the client. Remove syringe, and continue to assess the client's tolerance of the medication.
l. Dispose of supplies properly, and discard syringe in rigid needle disposal container.

5 Document the date, the time, and the IV medication given on the medication administration record or computerized medication record.

PEDIATRIC CONSIDERATIONS

Children are often fearful of injections, even into an intravenous line. Reassure children they will not feel pain with insertion of the syringe into an existing IV line.

GERIATRIC CONSIDERATIONS

Older adults may have fragile veins, so use extra caution when administering medications via the IV route.

protect yourself from contact with the medication and the client's secretions. These precautions also protect the client from microorganisms on your hands.

Before giving a topical medication, cleanse the area with soap and water unless contraindicated. Use sterile procedure as indicated for cleansing an open wound. Medication does not absorb as readily if the skin has accumulated oils, dead cells, or encrustations from lesions. Body oil also reduces the adhesive properties of patches, disks, or tape. Unless there is an open wound or lesion, apply topical medications to dry skin.

Use principles of asepsis when handling topical medications. Use a tongue depressor or swab to remove creams, pastes, or ointments from the original container, such as a jar. Use a new swab or depressor to remove additional medication from the container. If the medication comes in a tube, squeeze the medication onto an applicator before use. Do not squeeze it directly onto the skin. Apply medication evenly using long, smooth strokes, moving in the direction of hair growth to prevent the medication from accumulating in hair follicles. Assess the skin within 2 to 4 hours of the application to assess the medication's effects and possible allergic reaction.

Depending on the type of application, special techniques may be used to enhance medication effectiveness or to protect the client or nurse. Powders are usually applied to prevent friction on the skin and to promote drying. When using powder, apply it lightly and evenly, being careful not to inhale the particles.

Ointments remain in contact with skin for a long time and tend to soften the skin. Massage ointments into skin that is intact. Creams or oils are often used to treat dry or cracked skin. When applying these products to large areas, warm them in your hands before use to keep the client from becoming chilled. Lotions protect and soothe irritated skin. Shake lotions well before use, and apply them with gauze or cotton balls if appropriate.

Pastes (such as nitroglycerin) may be applied for the purpose of systemic absorption. Remove the old dose before applying a new one, and rotate sites to avoid skin irritation. Measure these doses carefully using paper supplied by the manufacturer to avoid underdosing or overdosing.

The newest form of topical administration is the transdermal patch or disk, which allows for time-release medication absorption through the skin. This limits the number of applications needed to maintain the therapeutic effect and reduces fluctuations in circulating drug levels. A transdermal patch may be applied daily or may be left in place as long as 7 days. Examples of drugs administered by this route include nitroglycerin, estrogen, fentanyl, and scopolamine. Box 21-9 outlines important guidelines for using a transdermal patch.

Eye Applications and Irrigations. Ophthalmic (eye) medications are available as drops, ointments, and disks. They are commonly used for diagnostic reasons or to treat problems such as glaucoma or eye infection. Although the eye is not a sterile area, conjunctival secretions protect the eye against many pathogens, and eye medications are administered as a sterile procedure. Eyedrops have a water base and are easily instilled. Ointments have an oily base and stay in place longer. Because of their composition, eye ointments can cause blurred vision for a period of time after application. If both an eyedrop and an eye ointment are scheduled to be given at the same time, give the eyedrop first.

Disks, which may resemble a contact lens, are the newest form of ocular medication. Disks have prolonged action and can stay in place for up to a week. They are best inserted at bedtime because they may cause temporary blurred vision after insertion.

Because the cornea is sensitive and easily damaged, eye medications are placed in the lower conjunctival sac, not directly on the eyeball. Methods for instilling eyedrops, ointments, and disks are described in Procedure 21-11.

Cross-contamination is a major concern with the use of ocular medications. Follow these guidelines, and teach them to clients as appropriate to decrease the risk of infection:

- Do not use eyedrops prescribed for one client on another client. Teach the client not to share them with family or friends.
- Apply ointments from the inner canthus to the outer canthus.
- Apply drops into the lower conjunctival sac.
- Apply medication only to the affected eye.
- Avoid touching the eye with the dropper or tube. Discard and replace contaminated items.
- Discard unused solution that remains in the dropper after instillation.
- Once opened, try to keep the drug at the bedside rather than replacing it on medication cart.

At times, an eye irrigation is needed to remove secretions from an eye before giving an ophthalmic medication. Irrigation can also be done in an emergency if the eye sustains chemical injury by caustic chemicals. In most emergency situations, the eye should be irrigated for at least 15 minutes with sterile eyewash, if available, or with copious amounts of tap water. The client should obtain professional follow-up after an emergency irrigation. Never irrigate an eye if there is a penetrating eye injury. Procedure 21-12 describes how to perform a routine eye irrigation.

BOX 21-9 *Teaching for Wellness*

Using Transdermal Patches

Purpose: To maintain optimal medication effect by using a transdermal patch correctly.

Expected Outcome: The client verbalizes and demonstrates correct application and removal of a transdermal patch.

Client Instructions

- Clean the skin before application. Apply the patch to a hairless site on your body. Avoid sites at the ends of your arms and legs. Also avoid areas with cuts or calluses that could interfere with absorption of the medication.
- Use firm pressure when applying the patch, especially around the edges, to ensure good contact with the skin.
- If the patch loosens or falls off, apply a new one. The medication is time-released through the special backing on the patch, so you cannot overdose by replacing a loose patch.
- Do not cut or trim the patch, because doing so would interfere with the time-release absorption of the medication through the special backing.
- Because transdermal patches are waterproof, you may shower or bathe as usual.
- Do not change brands of a transdermal patch without checking first with your physician. The dosage may or may not be equivalent.
- Apply and remove the patch as directed. Some patches remain in place for 12 to 14 hours and then are removed for 10 to 12 hours to prevent tolerance from developing (such as with nitroglycerin). Others can be left in place for 3 days (scopolamine) to 7 days (clonidine). Ask your physician, nurse, or pharmacist if you have questions about how to use your patch.

TIME TO ALLOW: NOVICE: 10 min. EXPERT: 5 min.

PROCEDURE 21-11

ADMINISTERING AN EYE MEDICATION

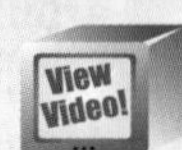

Nursing Skills Online: Nonparenteral Medication Administration, Lesson 3

A client with glaucoma, an eye infection, or a number of other ocular disorders will need ophthalmic (eye) medications instilled directly into the eye. Following this procedure will allow you to administer the medication without injuring sensitive eye tissue.

DELEGATION GUIDELINES

The administration of eye medications may not be delegated to a nursing assistant.

EQUIPMENT NEEDED

- Medication order, medication administration record, computerized medication order sheet, or medication Kardex or cards
- Medication bottle, tube, or disk
- Tissue or cotton ball
- Warm water and facecloth, as needed
- Disposable gloves

1 Follow preliminary actions (see inside front cover).

2 Check the medication order, noting especially the eye to be treated. Note any client allergies.

3 Prepare the client for instillation of the medication.

a. Identify the client using an identification bracelet or other agency-accepted means.

b. Explain the procedure to the client in a calm and confident manner. Help the client to sit or lie down with the head slightly hyperextended. Put on gloves. *This head position assists in correct medication placement and minimizes drainage through the tear duct.*

c. Assess the condition of the client's eye. Wash away any exudate using the facecloth and warm water, wiping from the inner canthus to the outer canthus. *This observation provides baseline assessment data to evaluate the medication's effect. Removing exudate also removes microorganisms and provides a clean surface to apply the medication.*

4 Administer the medication.

EYEDROPS

a. Remove the cap from the bottle, and place it on its side. Fill the medication dropper (if used) to the prescribed amount. *This position prevents contamination of the cap.*

b. Place your nondominant hand on the client's cheekbone just under the eyelid, and pull downward against the bony orbit to expose the lower conjunctival sac. Hold tissue or a cotton ball under the eyelid, and apply slight pressure to the inner canthus. *This action exposes the lower conjunctival sac while preventing pressure and trauma to the eye. Pressing on the inner canthus blocks the tear duct temporarily and prevents the medication from leaving the eye through the duct and possibly causing systemic effects.*

c. Rest your dominant hand against the client's forehead for stability, and hold the medication bottle or dropper ½ to ¾ inch above the conjunctival sac. *Resting on the client's forehead stabilizes your hand and reduces the risk of contact between eye structures and the medication bottle, preventing trauma, infection, or both.*

d. Ask the client to look up at the ceiling, and then instill the prescribed number of drops into the lower conjunctival sac (see illustration). If the client closes the eye or blinks, or if a drop lands on the eyelid, repeat the missed drop. *Looking up reduces stimulation of the blink reflex and thus promotes accurate delivery of the dose into the conjunctival sac.*

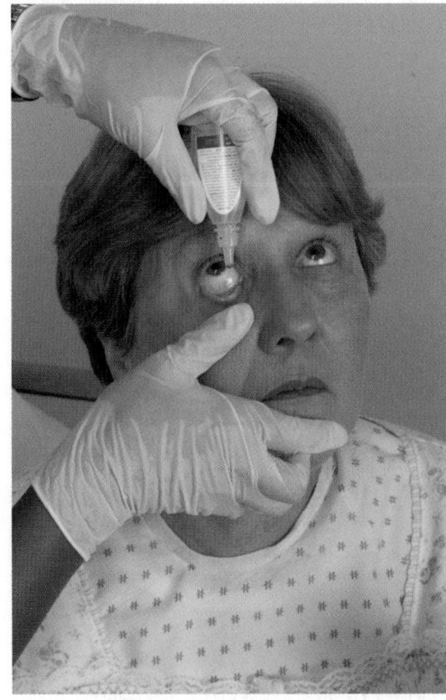

Step 4d. Eyedrops. Administering the prescribed number of drops into the lower conjunctival sac.

Continued

e. Ask the client to gently close the eye and move it around. Apply gentle pressure over the lacrimal duct for 1 minute, or ask the client to do so if possible. *Moving the eye behind the closed lid helps to distribute the medication over the conjunctiva and eyeball. Gently closing it (not squinting or squeezing) prevents loss of medication from conjunctival sac. Pressing the lacrimal duct helps to prevent systemic absorption of the medication.*

EYE OINTMENT

a. Remove the cap from the tube, and place it on its side. Squeeze and discard a small bead of medication. Placing the cap on its side helps to prevent contamination. The first bead of an ointment is considered contaminated.
b. For instillation in the lower lid, separate client's eyelids with the thumb and forefinger of your nondominant hand, pulling lower lid downward over the bony prominence of the cheek. (For instillation in the upper lid, draw upper lid up and away from eyeball.)
c. Ask the client to look up for instillation in the lower lid or down for instillation in the upper lid. Looking up or down reduces stimulation of the blink reflex and rotates the sensitive cornea away from the medication.
d. Apply a thin line of ointment along the inside edge of the lower or upper lid as ordered (see illustration), moving from the inner canthus to the outer canthus. This method ensures aseptic and even distribution of medication as well as the proper dosage.

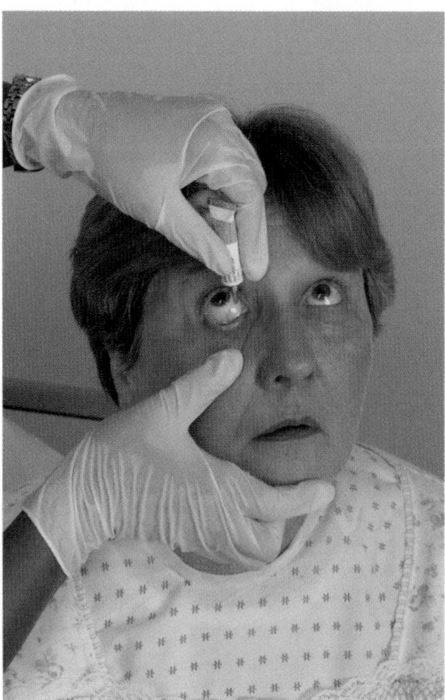

Step 4d. **Eye ointment.** Applying a thin line of ointment along the inside edge of the eyelid.

e. Ask the client to gently close the eye and move it around. Moving the eye behind closed lids helps to distribute medication over the conjunctiva and eyeball. Gently closing it (not squinting or squeezing) prevents loss of medication from conjunctival sac.

MEDICATED EYE DISK

a. Open the package, and press the tip of the index finger of your dominant hand against the convex part of disk. Doing so helps the disk adhere to your fingertip.
b. Pull the client's lower eyelid away from the eye with your nondominant hand, and ask the client to look up. *This exposes the conjunctival sac and reduces the blink reflex.*
c. Place the disk horizontally in the conjunctival sac between the iris and the lower eyelid.
d. Pull the lower eyelid out, up, and over the disk. Ask the client to blink a few times. If the disk is visible, repeat this step. Otherwise, have the client press his or her fingers against the closed lids, without rubbing the eyes or moving the disk. *This action ensures proper disk position.*
e. If the disk falls out, rinse it with cool water and reinsert it. *Rinsing the disk reduces the risk of infection.*
f. To remove a disk, pull or invert the client's lower eyelid so you can see the disk, then use the thumb and index finger of your dominant hand to pinch the disk and lift it from the conjunctival sac. If it is in the upper eye, stroke the client's closed eyelid with your fingertip, gently and in long circular motions. Ask the client to open the eye, and look for the disk in the corner of the eye. Slide the disk to the lower lid and remove it as noted earlier. *This minimizes risk of trauma or infection while aiding removal of the disk.*

5 Remove gloves, and perform hand hygiene.

6 Document the medication administration on the medication administration record or computerized medication record.

PEDIATRIC CONSIDERATIONS

Provide explanations about medication therapy at an age-appropriate level.

GERIATRIC CONSIDERATIONS

Allow sufficient time for medication administration, and encourage client to self-administer eye medication if able and appropriate.

PROCEDURE 21-12

TIME TO ALLOW: NOVICE: 15 min. EXPERT: 8 min.

IRRIGATING AN EYE

Eye irrigation is used to remove infection or other foreign matter from the eye. It should not be done when the client has a penetrating eye injury because it could cause further injury. It can be done on a short-term intermittent basis or as a one-time order based on client need.

DELEGATION GUIDELINES

The performance of this procedure requires your expertise and skill and may not be delegated to a nursing assistant.

EQUIPMENT NEEDED

- Sterile irrigating solution warmed to body temperature
- Sterile irrigation set with irrigating or bulb syringe and a sterile container
- Emesis or curved irrigation basin
- Waterproof pad if not supplied with irrigation set
- Towel
- Cotton balls
- Disposable gloves

1 Follow preliminary actions (see inside front cover).

2 Prepare the client for the irrigation.

a. Identify the client using an identification bracelet or other agency-accepted means.

b. Explain the procedure to the client in a calm and confident manner.

c. Help the client to sit or lie with the head tilted toward the eye that will be irrigated. Place the waterproof pad under the affected side. Put on gloves. *This head position enlists the aid of gravity so solution flows from inner canthus to the outer canthus without flowing through the unaffected eye.*

d. Pour irrigant into the container, and draw it into the syringe using aseptic technique.

e. Clean the client's eyelids and eyelashes with a cotton ball moistened with irrigant or normal saline solution. Wipe from the inner canthus to the outer canthus using a new cotton ball with each pass. *This step removes material on the lids and lashes that could be washed into the eye with irrigation.*

f. Place the curved basin under the affected cheek to catch the irrigating solution as it flows from the client's eye. Ask the client to hold the basin if possible.

3 Irrigate the eye.

a. Use your nondominant hand to hold the client's upper lid open, and expose the lower conjunctival sac. Using the conjunctival sac reduces stimulation of the blink reflex and prevents irrigant from injuring the cornea.

b. Hold the irrigation syringe about 1 inch above the eye. Do not touch the eye with the syringe. Push fluid gently into the conjunctival sac, directing the flow from the inner canthus to the outer canthus. If agency policy allows, you may use approved intravenous (IV) solution (normal saline) with IV tubing, allowing the fluid to gently flow from the medial to the lateral side. This process uses the least amount of pressure necessary to cleanse the eye while reducing the risk of injury to the eye or contamination of the eye.

c. Repeat the irrigation until the secretions are gone or the irrigant is used up. Allow the client to close the eyes intermittently during procedure as needed. Closed eye movements help to move secretions from the upper to the lower conjunctival area.

d. Dry the area with cotton balls, and offer the client a towel to dry the face and neck.

4 Remove gloves, and perform hand hygiene.

5 Document the irrigation in the client's medical record. Also record the appearance of the eye, characteristics of drainage, and the client's response to treatment.

PEDIATRIC CONSIDERATIONS

Provide explanations about the procedure at an age-appropriate level.

GERIATRIC CONSIDERATIONS

Allow sufficient time for the procedure, and encourage client to assist with positioning and use of disposable tissues following as appropriate.

Ear Instillations and Irrigations. The external ear is not sterile and consists of the external auditory canal and the pinna. The middle and inner ear lie behind the tympanic membrane and are sterile areas. Because a rupture of the tympanic membrane would create an opening between these areas, sterile solutions should be used prophylactically for instillation or irrigation of the ear.

Ear instillations require special care. Warm the solution to body temperature before use if possible, but at least give it at room temperature to prevent vertigo and nausea. Avoid using excessive force when instilling medication or irrigating an ear, to avoid rupturing the tympanic membrane. Do not occlude the auditory meatus during these procedures for the same reason. Assess ear drainage carefully to detect possible infection (see Chapter 38).

Otic (ear) medications exert a local effect and are commonly used to soften earwax, fight infection, relieve pain, or destroy an insect trapped in the canal. Different approaches are used when administering otic medications to adults and to children because of differences in the shape of the ear canal. Pull the pinna of an adult's ear up and back to straighten the canal before administering eardrops or ear irrigation. In contrast, pull the pinna of an infant or young child down and back. The recommended methods for administering an ear medication are given in Procedure 21-13.

Nasal Instillations. Medications are given by the nasal route to relieve the symptoms of sinus colds and congestion, shrink swollen mucous membranes, loosen nasal secretions, and treat nasal or sinus infection. Occasionally, medications are used for a systemic effect (such as vasopressin). Nasal medications are generally available in the form of sprays (decongestants, vasopressin) or drops (antiinfectives).

Clients have ready access to a number of OTC nasal medications, so teach their use carefully. Decongestants, in particular, cause rebound nasal congestion when used to excess. Teach clients how to properly administer them for maximum effect. Warn clients about other active ingredients in these products. For example, many nasal decongestants contain sympathomimetics (adrenergic agonists) that exert a systemic effect and are not suitable for use with children or others who could be adversely affected. In these instances, suggest saline drops.

Use clean technique to administer a nasal medication unless the client has undergone nasal or sinus surgery; then use sterile technique. Properly position the client by tilting or hyperextending the head. Procedure 21-14 describes how to give an intranasal medication.

Vaginal Instillations. Vaginal medications are commonly used for contraception or to treat itching, pain, or discomfort from inflammation or infection. They are supplied as gels, creams, foams, or suppositories. Keep suppositories refrigerated to prevent them from melting. Depending on the product, you will administer the medication using a gloved hand and possibly an applicator. Allow the client to self-administer the medication if appropriate.

Before administering the medication, offer the client an opportunity to void. Administer it using standard precautions and aseptic technique as outlined in Procedure 21-15. Once the medication is in the body, it will melt and may produce drainage. For this reason, administer it at bedtime if possible. Offer the client a perineal pad to help absorb drainage. Especially when treating infection, provide meticulous perineal hygiene and carefully assess the characteristics of any drainage.

Rectal Instillations. Rectal instillations are usually used to produce a local effect, such as stimulation of a bowel movement. Less often, they are used for systemic effects, such as relief of fever or nausea when the client cannot tolerate oral medication. Rectal medications typically come as suppositories, but they are often thinner and longer than vaginal suppositories for easier insertion. Many rectal suppositories are kept refrigerated until use.

Use standard precautions when administering a rectal suppository, and place it properly for adequate results. Do not place the suppository into a fecal mass because it will not be effective. Administer a small cleansing enema beforehand if needed. The proper method for administering a rectal suppository is described in Procedure 21-16.

Administering Inhalation Medications. Medications administered by inhalation are absorbed into the bloodstream via the alveolar epithelium in the lower respiratory tract. To be effective, a medication must be dispersed in very small droplets, such as a mist, and must be inhaled deeply. Common types of medications administered by inhalation are bronchodilators and mucolytics.

Inhalation agents are delivered either by nebulizer (or atomizer) or by metered-dose inhaler (MDI). A nebulizer uses a forceful flow of oxygen or compressed air to break up liquid medication into tiny particles that can be inhaled. Teach the client to form a tight seal around the mouthpiece and to breathe through the device until the medication has been completely inhaled (often 15 to 20 minutes). Clean the mouthpiece, or teach the client to wash it after each use.

An MDI delivers a preset dose of medication when the client discharges the canister. Teach the client the proper method for positioning the mouthpiece. Make sure that the client has manual dexterity and enough strength to push with 5 to 10 pounds of pressure, the amount of pressure needed to depress the medication

PROCEDURE 21-13

Time to Allow: Novice: 8 min. Expert: 3 min.

ADMINISTERING AN EAR MEDICATION

Nursing Skills Online: Nonparenteral Medication, Lesson 4

Ear infections are relatively common among children and are one of the most common reasons for administering a medication into the ear canal.

DELEGATION GUIDELINES

As with all medication administration procedures, you may not delegate the administration of ear medications to a nursing assistant.

EQUIPMENT NEEDED

- Medication administration record, computerized medication order sheet, or medication Kardex or cards
- Medication (eardrops)
- Tissue or cotton ball
- Cotton-tipped applicator
- Disposable gloves

1 Follow preliminary actions (see inside front cover).

2 Check the medication order, and note any client allergies.

3 Prepare the client for instillation of the medication.

a. Identify the client using an identification bracelet or other agency-accepted means.

b. Explain the procedure to the client in a calm and confident manner. Help the client to a side-lying position with the affected ear upward. Put on gloves. *This position assists in correct placement of medication and minimizes its drainage from the ear canal.*

c. Assess the condition of the ear. Gently wash away any cerumen or exudate using cotton-tipped applicators. Do not force wax or drainage into the ear canal. *This step provides baseline assessment data and cleans the area before application of the medication.*

4 Administer the medication.

a. Remove the cap from the bottle, and place it on its side. Fill the medication dropper (if applicable) to prescribed amount. *Placing cap on its side prevents its contamination.*

b. Pull the pinna up and back in an adult client or down and back in a child (see illustration). *This step straightens the ear canal.*

c. Hold the dropper or bottle 1/2 inch above the ear canal, and instill as many eardrops as ordered. *Holding the bottle above the ear canal avoids excess pressure in the canal.*

d. Ask the client to maintain the side-lying position for 2 to 3 minutes. Apply gentle pressure with your finger to the tragus of the ear or ask the client to do so. *Staying in the side-lying position helps to distribute the medication. Because ear infections are painful, the client may prefer to apply the pressure.*

e. Place a cotton ball into the outermost portion of the ear canal. *This helps to prevent medication loss when the client changes position.*

f. Remove your gloves, and perform hand hygiene.

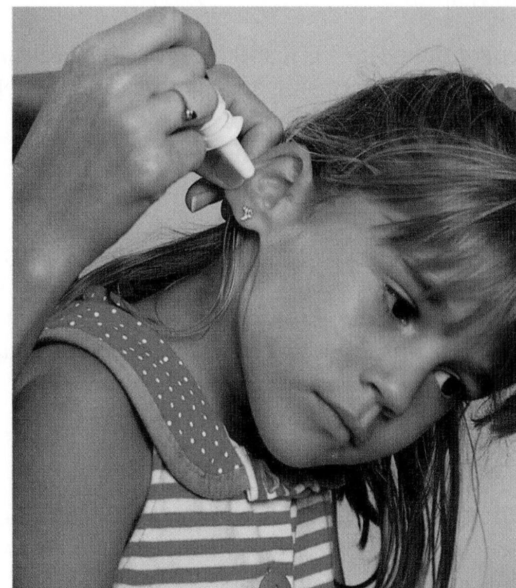

Step 4b. Pulling the pinna down and back in a child.

5 Document the medication administration in the medication administration record or computerized medication record.

6 Check on the client in 15 minutes to remove the cotton ball from the ear, assess the client's condition, and help him or her to a comfortable position.

PEDIATRIC CONSIDERATIONS

Provide explanations about the procedure at an age-appropriate level.

GERIATRIC CONSIDERATIONS

Allow sufficient time for medication administration, and encourage client to assist with positioning as appropriate.

PROCEDURE 21-14

Time to Allow: Novice: 8 min. Expert: 3 min.

ADMINISTERING AN INTRANASAL MEDICATION

Intranasal medications may be ordered to produce local vasoconstriction of blood vessels or for administration of medications for rapid absorption through nasal mucous membranes.

DELEGATION GUIDELINES

You may not delegate the administration of intranasal medication to a nursing assistant.

EQUIPMENT NEEDED

- Medication order, medication administration record, computerized medication order sheet, or medication Kardex or cards
- Nasal spray or drops
- Facial tissue
- Disposable gloves

1 Follow preliminary actions (see inside front cover).

2 Check the medication order, and note any client allergies.

3 Prepare the client for instillation of the medication.

a. Identify the client using an identification bracelet or other agency-accepted means.

b. Explain the procedure to the client. Mention that the solution may cause choking, stinging, or burning as it drips into the throat. Put on gloves.

c. Ask the client to the blow the nose unless contraindicated because of risk of nosebleed or increased intracranial pressure. Assess the resulting discharge. *Blowing the nose removes secretions that could interfere with the effectiveness of the medication.*

4 Administer the medication.

ADMINISTRATION OF A NASAL SPRAY

a. Remove the cap from the bottle, and place it on its side. *This position prevents contamination of the medication's cap.*

b. Ask an adult client to tilt the head backward, and support the head with your nondominant hand. Keep a child's head in an upright position. *This position allows the medication to reach nasal passages without causing the client to swallow it. Supporting the client's head reduces neck strain.*

c. Hold the medication container just inside the tip of the nostril without touching nasal tissue (see illustration). Ask the client to occlude the opposite nostril and inhale while you administer the spray. *Avoiding contact between the container and the nasal tissue prevents contamination of container. Occluding the opposite nostril while inhaling through the target nostril provides maximum effectiveness of the medication.*

d. Assist the client to a comfortable position.

ADMINISTRATION OF NASAL DROPS

a. Remove cap from bottle, and place on its side.

b. Position the client to accommodate the intended site of action, and support the head with your nondominant hand. For the posterior pharynx, tilt the client's head backward. For the ethmoid or sphenoid sinus, either tilt the client's head back and place a pillow under one shoulder or tilt the head back over the edge of the mattress while supporting the back of the head with your nondominant hand. For the frontal or maxillary sinus, assume the position just described and turn the client's head toward the affected side.

c. Hold the tip of the dropper just above the intended nostril and pointed toward the midline of the ethmoid bone (see illustration). Do not touch the client's nasal tissue with the dropper. Ask client to

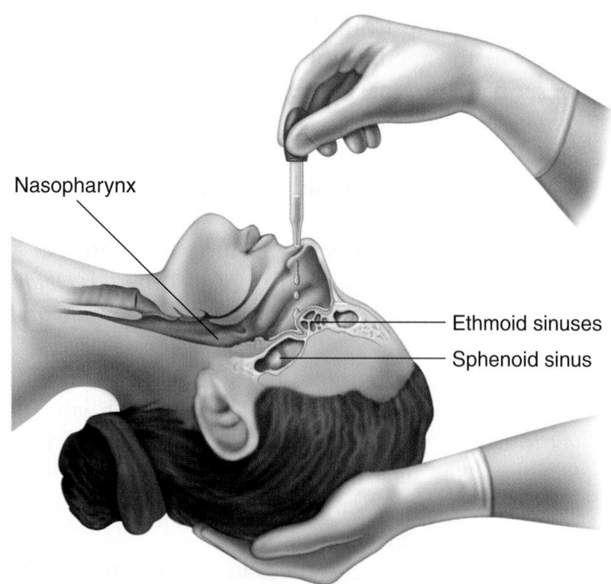

Step 4c. **Nasal drops.** Proper position for instillation of nasal medication.

mouth-breathe, and instill the ordered number of drops. *This process provides the greatest medication effectiveness and prevents contamination of the container.*

d. Ask the client to maintain this position for 5 minutes, and then assist to a comfortable position. *Maintaining position prevents leakage of medication from the nose and promotes medication absorption.*

5 Remove gloves, and perform hand hygiene.

6 Document the medication administration on the medication administration record or computerized medication record.

7 Wash nasal spray devices daily in lukewarm water. If used for infection, the remainder should be discarded when no longer needed.

PEDIATRIC CONSIDERATIONS

Provide explanations about the procedure at an age-appropriate level.

GERIATRIC CONSIDERATIONS

Allow sufficient time for medication administration, and encourage the client to self-administer if able and appropriate.

canister into the device to release a dose. This is an important consideration when working with older or debilitated clients. A turbo-inhaler is a variation of an MDI that must be assembled for use. A spacer may be ordered when a client has difficulty in coordinating the acts of depressing the canister and inhaling at the same time; it attaches to the mouthpiece of the inhaler and holds the medication dose until the client inhales. Important teaching points for using an MDI are found in Chapter 34.

PROCEDURE 21-15

TIME TO ALLOW: **NOVICE:** 15 min. **EXPERT:** 7 min.

ADMINISTERING A VAGINAL MEDICATION

Nursing Skills Online: Nonparenteral Medication Administration, Lesson 6

Vaginal instillations are usually performed to treat infection. They may also be used by the client as part of a contraceptive method.

DELEGATION GUIDELINES

You may not delegate the administration of vaginal medication to a nursing assistant.

EQUIPMENT NEEDED

- Medication administration record, computerized medication order sheet, or medication Kardex or cards
- Vaginal medication and applicator, if needed
- Water-soluble lubricant
- Perineal pad, if needed
- Cotton balls or facecloth and towel for cleansing, if needed
- Disposable tissue
- Disposable gloves

1 Follow preliminary actions (see inside front cover).

2 Check the medication order.

3 Prepare the client for instillation of the medication.

a. Identify client using an identification bracelet or another agency-accepted means.

b. Explain the procedure to the client. Offer her an opportunity to void. Close the curtain or door, and help her to a supine position with the abdomen and legs draped. *Maintaining privacy is an important step in this type of medication administration.*

c. Put on gloves.

d. Inspect the client's external genitalia, and provide perineal hygiene as needed.

4 Administer the medication using clean technique.

Continued

ADMINISTRATION OF A SUPPOSITORY

a. Remove the suppository from its wrapper, and insert into the applicator, if used. *Use of either a gloved finger or an applicator is acceptable.*
b. Lubricate the rounded end of the suppository with water-soluble lubricant. If you will not be using an applicator, also lubricate the index finger of your gloved, dominant hand. *Lubrication allows easier insertion by reducing friction.*
c. Separate the client's labia with your nondominant hand, and insert the rounded end of the suppository along the posterior vaginal wall for an entire finger-length (see illustration). *This distance ensures complete insertion of the medication and distribution through the entire vagina.*
d. Withdraw your finger or the applicator, and wipe away excess lubricant from the genitals.

ADMINISTRATION OF A FOAM, JELLY, OR CREAM

a. Fill applicator with medication according to the package directions.
b. Separate the client's labia with your nondominant hand, point the applicator toward her sacrum, and use your dominant hand to insert it 2 or 3 inches into the vagina.
c. Depress the plunger on the applicator to push the medication out of the applicator.
d. Withdraw the applicator, and place it on a tissue or paper towel. Wipe away excess medication from the genitals. *The applicator may contain microorganisms from the client's vagina.*

5 Help the client to a comfortable position, and ask her to remain supine for 5 to 10 minutes or for time frame recommended by medication directions. If needed, offer her a perineal pad. *Lying supine prevents loss of the medication from melting and gravity. The perineal pad absorbs excess drainage.*

6 Wash the applicator with soap and water, and store for future use.

7 Remove your gloves, and perform hand hygiene.

8 Document the medication administration on the medication administration record or computerized medication record.

GERIATRIC CONSIDERATIONS

Assist with client positioning, and recognize that this position and procedure may not be comfortable for client.

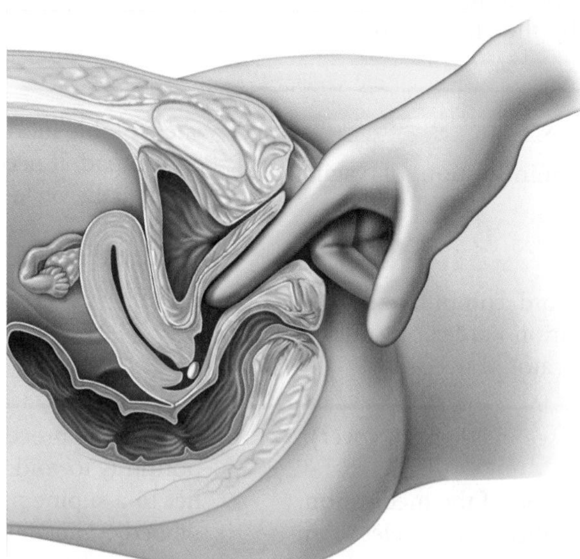

Step 4c. Inserting the vaginal suppository.

TIME TO ALLOW: NOVICE: 15 min. EXPERT: 7 min.

PROCEDURE 21-16

ADMINISTERING A RECTAL MEDICATION

Nursing Skills Online: Nonparenteral Medication Administration, Lesson 6

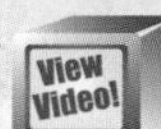

Rectal medications can be used to stimulate a bowel movement or to administer medications when the client cannot take them orally.

DELEGATION GUIDELINES

You may not delegate the administration of rectal medication to a nursing assistant.

EQUIPMENT NEEDED

- Medication administration record, computerized medication order sheet, or medication Kardex or cards
- Rectal medication
- Water-soluble lubricant
- Facecloth and towel for cleansing, if needed
- Disposable tissue
- Disposable gloves

1 Follow preliminary actions (see inside front cover).

2 Check the medication order.

3 Prepare the client for instillation of the medication.

a. Identify the client using an identification bracelet or another agency-accepted means.

b. Explain the procedure to client. Offer an opportunity to void. Close the curtain or door.

c. Put on gloves. Help the client to a left lateral (Sims') position with the upper leg flexed. Drape the client to expose only the anal area. *This position helps to retain the suppository and promotes relaxation of the external anal sphincter.*

d. Inspect the anal area, and provide perineal hygiene as needed.

4 Administer the medication using clean aseptic technique.

a. Remove the suppository from the packaging, and lubricate the rounded end. Also lubricate the index finger of your gloved dominant hand. *Lubrication eases insertion by reducing friction.*

b. Instruct the client to breathe slowly and deeply through the mouth. *This promotes relaxation of the client's rectal area and anal sphincter to prevent pain.*

c. Separate the buttocks with your gloved nondominant hand. Use your dominant hand to insert the rounded end of the suppository about 4 inches (10 cm) into the rectal canal along the rectal wall (see illustration). Insert the suppository 2 inches (5 cm) for a child. *This distance ensures insertion of the suppository past the external and internal anal sphincters.*

d. Withdraw finger, and wipe away fecal material or excess lubricant at the client's anus.

e. Ask the client to remain side-lying for 5 minutes (up to 30 minutes for a laxative). Give an immobile client the call bell, and ask the client to call you when he or she feels the need for a bowel movement. *Remaining in position prevents the medication from being expelled.*

5 Remove gloves, and perform hand hygiene.

6 Return after 5 minutes to see if the suppository has been expelled. *If so, reinsert it.*

7 Document the medication administration on the medication administration record or computerized medication record.

8 Return 30 minutes after administration to assess effectiveness. Assist the client as needed.

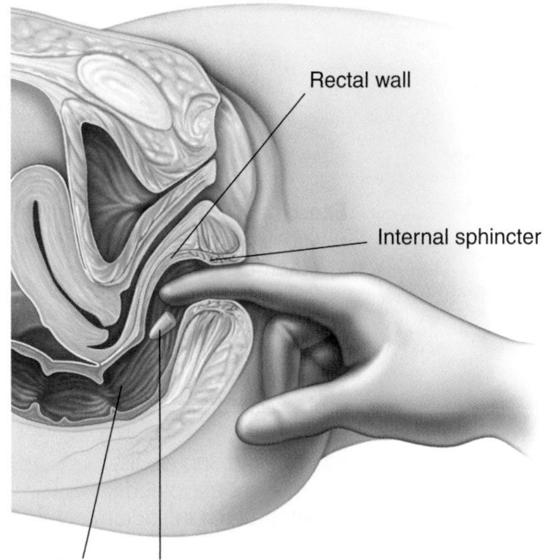

Step 4c. Inserting the rectal suppository.

PEDIATRIC CONSIDERATIONS

Provide age-appropriate explanation. Assist with client positioning, and recognize that this position and procedure may not be comfortable for client.

GERIATRIC CONSIDERATIONS

Assist with client positioning, and recognize that this position and procedure may not be comfortable for client.

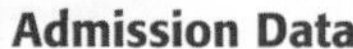

BOX 21-10

Nursing Care Plan

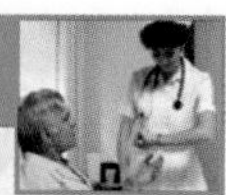

A Client Beginning Medication Therapy

Admission Data

Mr. Connell was admitted to the emergency department following an episode of chest pain. His condition has stabilized and he will be discharged within an hour.

Physician's Orders

Atenolol 50 mg PO daily
Furosemide 20 mg PO daily
Nitroglycerin 1/150 grain SL prn for chest pain, may repeat twice

Nursing Assessment

Before Mr. Connell goes home, he should receive initial instructions to address learning needs he has demonstrated in a variety of areas. He requires information about each of the medications ordered. He would benefit from information about exercise to slow progression of his cardiovascular disease. He could also benefit from initial information on stress management. His understanding and his wife's understanding of sodium restriction should be evaluated and reinforced. He has a definite identified need to understand the importance of continued medical supervision.

NANDA-I Nursing Diagnosis	NOC Expected Outcomes With Indicators	NIC Interventions With Selected Activities	Evaluation Data
Ineffective Health Maintenance **Related Factor:** • Insufficient knowledge of treatment regimen	***Knowledge: Treatment Regimen*** **Medications** • Verbalizes purpose, actions, and directions for use of all ordered medications.	***Teaching: Procedure/Treatment*** • Provide information about atenolol, furosemide, and nitroglycerin. Describe purpose and actions using clear and simple terms. • Review directions for use of each medication (atenolol at night, furosemide in the morning, nitroglycerin at the first sign of chest pain). • Describe handling and storage, especially for nitroglycerin (out of light and away from heat). • Outline common side effects of each medication. • Give instructions about when to call physician.	• States he knows "all about atenolol and furosemide" but has never taken nitroglycerin. Reviews the printed material and asks several questions.
	Exercise • Verbalizes the benefits of aerobic exercise to diminish the risk of cardiovascular disease and states intention to begin exercise with physician approval.	• Discuss the benefits of aerobic exercise on the heart, and develop a tentative plan for exercise subject to physician approval.	• States he and his wife will start walking after the evening meal.
	Diet • Client and spouse list foods to be avoided that are high in sodium.	• Review foods to avoid (those that are naturally high in sodium). Discuss that foods from animal sources (meats, dairy products) are naturally high in sodium because of physiological saline.	• Is able to list foods high in sodium but expects compliance to be difficult.
	Knowledge: Health Behavior **Stress Management** • Verbalizes the importance of stress management as an adjunct to blood pressure control.	***Teaching: Individual*** • Begin initial teaching about the effects of stress on blood pressure. Develop an initial plan to manage stress effectively to aid in blood pressure reduction. • Stress the importance of continued medical supervision, and develop a specific plan for medical follow-up.	• Has his own business and cannot reduce working hours. • Will visit doctor in 1 week.

BOX 21-10 *Nursing Care Plan—cont'd*

A Client Beginning Medication Therapy

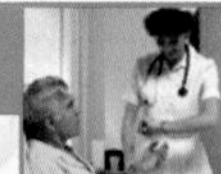

Critical Thinking Questions

1. How would you proceed as a follow-up to Mr. Connell's statement that he knows "all about atenolol and furosemide"?
2. Do you have suggestions to help with planning for diet and exercise?

Nursing outcome and intervention labels from Johnson, M., Bulechek, G., Butcher, H., Dochterman, J. M., Maas, M., Moorhead, S., et al. (Eds.). (2006). *NANDA, NOC, and NIC linkages: Nursing diagnoses, outcomes, & interventions.* St. Louis, MO: Mosby.

EVALUATION

Evaluation of a client's response to medication therapy is just as important as other aspects of administration. Reassess the client to determine whether the original symptoms have been relieved, and gather objective data to further evaluate the effects of medication. For example, evaluate urine output, breath sounds, and peripheral edema to determine the effectiveness of diuretic therapy. Document and report medication effects as appropriate.

Use data from laboratory studies as an adjunct in evaluating medication effectiveness. For example, serum drug levels provide useful information about the client's status. Report abnormal values at once so that further adjustments can be made to the medication regimen. Finally, assess for adverse medication effects and report them promptly so corrective action may be taken.

Box 21-10 suggests an initial plan of care that would help meet this Mr. Connell's need for information. Below is a sample documentation note pertaining to his medication management at the time of his discharge. When Mr. Connell is discharged, the part of the discharge note that pertains to medication management reads as shown below:

Sample Documentation Note for Mr. Connell

Instructions given to client and wife about atenolol, furosemide, and nitroglycerin; they are able to repeat back indications, key actions, adverse effects of medications, and when to call for emergency cardiac care. Client states an intention to follow up with primary care physician. First appointment made by telephone for client before discharge.

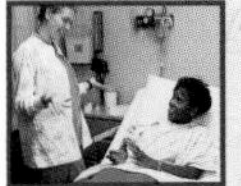

Mr. Connell was ultimately discharged to home with his wife. One month later, he still takes his medications regularly and has started to exercise. His job is still stressful, but he verbalizes satisfaction with his lifestyle and his health. As the nurse working in the physician's office where he is receiving follow-up care, consider the following questions:

- What measures will you use to determine the continued effectiveness of therapy?
- What suggestions can you make to further reduce his risk factors for heart disease?
- What should you teach Mr. Connell, specifically considering his Irish American cultural beliefs and practices, concerning health?

▼ KEY PRINCIPLES

- Drugs have a variety of names, including the official name, chemical name, generic name, and trade name or names. Become familiar with the generic and trade names of medications.
- A client's knowledge base for successful self-administration of medication should include information about therapeutic effect, dose, side effects, adverse effects, directions for use, drug interactions, and storage and expiration.
- Drug manufacture and use is highly regulated in the United States and Canada. There are stringent controls over the distribution and use of highly addictive substances, such as opioids.
- The nurse functions within legal guidelines when administering medications. The nurse practice act in each state specifies the responsibility a nurse has in administering medications.
- Pharmacokinetics refers to the processes of absorption, distribution, biotransformation, and excretion. A variety of client-related factors influence a drug's effectiveness.
- Drugs can elicit a variety of responses. Each drug may have a therapeutic effect, adverse effects, and toxic effects. Drugs can also elicit an allergic response or an idiosyncratic response in some clients. Be aware of potential responses to adequately assess the client.
- Some drugs can cause physiological or psychological dependence in the client. These drugs are labeled as controlled substances and require special precautions.
- Each drug has a specific onset, peak, and duration of action. Each drug also has a specific half-life, which determines how often it must be given to maintain a therapeutic blood level.
- There are various types of drug orders. A standing order is given routinely at prescribed times. A prn order is given as needed but cannot be given more often than specified. A single or one-time order is carried out once only. A stat order is completed immediately.

- Numerous client-related factors affect drug actions, including life span considerations and various physiological, cultural, and lifestyle factors.
- Medication may be given by the oral, parenteral, topical, or inhalation route. The route has a significant effect on the timing and duration of action. Specific procedures are followed when each of these routes is used.
- All five steps of the nursing process are used when administering medications to clients.
- Many client factors should be considered to safely administer medications: health history, allergies, medication and diet histories, current condition, problems with perception and coordination, knowledge about drug therapy, and individual learning needs.
- *Ineffective health maintenance* is a useful nursing diagnosis for clients receiving medication therapy. Other nursing diagnoses, such as *Ineffective therapeutic regimen management,* may also apply. Assess each client individually to determine whether defining characteristics of one or more nursing diagnoses are exhibited.
- Drug doses are measured using one of three systems: metric, apothecary, and household. Familiarity with all three systems is needed to administer drugs safely.
- It is imperative to give medications correctly to protect the client's safety. Adhere to the "six rights" when giving medications: right client, right drug, right dose, right route, right time, and right documentation.
- The nurse is responsible for safely and accurately administering all medications and documenting administration using established policies and procedures.
- If a medication error does occur, it is your legal and ethical responsibility to report it promptly. Health care facilities have specific policies and procedures to follow if an error occurs. Client safety is the paramount concern.
- Special populations, such as children and older adults, have unique needs with regard to drug therapy. Incorporate your knowledge of these needs when giving medications to these groups.
- Standard precautions are used when administering medications. Use extreme caution when handling needles and other sharps, which can transmit pathogens (such as HIV or hepatitis) from an infected client if a needlestick injury occurs.

■ REVIEW QUESTIONS

1. A client has a new diagnosis of renal failure. The nurse concludes that medication dosages will likely need to be reduced for several medications because of impairment of which pharmacokinetic phase?

1. Absorption
2. Distribution
3. Biotransformation
4. Excretion

2. The nurse cannot read a newly written medication order on the physician order sheet. Which of the following actions by the nurse would be most appropriate?

1. Consult a unit secretary who has seen this writing many times before.
2. Fax the order to the pharmacist for interpretation.
3. Write an incident report.
4. Contact the physician to clarify the order.

3. During a history taken at the time of hospital admission, the client reports using herbal supplements to maintain health. Which action is most important for the nurse to take next?

1. Report this information to the physician.
2. Advise the client that this practice could counteract the effectiveness of prescribed medications.
3. Obtain information about the herbs used, amounts and type of preparation, and frequency of use.
4. Tell the client that they will not be used during the hospital admission.

4. A client has an order for dexamethasone (Decadron) 6 mg orally this morning, followed by a 4-mg dose in the afternoon. Available are tablets containing 2 mg of dexamethasone. How many tablets should the nurse administer for the morning dose?

1. ½
2. 1
3. 2
4. 3

5. An adult client who is 5 feet 2 inches tall and weighs 250 pounds has an order for an intramuscular injection. The nurse should select which of the following needle sizes to attach to the syringe?

1. ⅜ inch
2. ½ inch
3. 1 inch
4. 1½ inches

Bibliography

American Hospital Formulary Service. *AHFS drug information 2006 (annual).* Bethesda, MD: American Society of Hospital Pharmacists.

Barnsteiner, J. H. (2005). Medication reconciliation: Transfer of medication information across settings—keeping it free from error. *American Journal of Nursing, 106*(Suppl. 3), 31-36, 48-51.

Beyea, S. (2005). Patient safety first. Best practices for safe medication administration. *AORN Journal 81*(4), 895, 897-898.

Curry, L., Walker, C., Hogstel, M., & Burns, P. (2005). Teaching older adults to self-manage medications: Preventing adverse drug reactions. *Journal of Gerontological Nursing, 31*(4), 32-42.

Disposal of medical sharps. (2004). *Waste Industry News.* Retrieved October 30, 2006, from http://www.epa.gov/epaoswer/other/medical/sharps.htm.

Doyle, M. (2004). Generating knowledge to decrease medication administration errors. 37th Annual Communicating Nursing Research Conference. *Communicating Nursing Research, 37,* 336.

Ebersole, P., Hess, P., Touhy, N., & Jett, K. (2005). *Gerontological nursing & healthy aging* (2nd ed.). St. Louis, MO: Elsevier Mosby.

Environmental Protection Agency. (2004). *Disposal of medical sharps.* Retrieved June 16, 2006, from http://www.epa.gov/epaoswer/other/medical/sharps.htm.

Fontaine, K. L. (2005). *Complementary and alternative therapies for nursing practice* (2nd ed.). Upper Saddle River, NJ: Pearson Prentice Hall.

Foust, J., Naylor, M., Boling, P., & Cappuzzo, K. (2005). Opportunities for improving post-hospital home medication management among older adults. *Home Health Care Services Quarterly, 24*(1-2), 101-122.

Frazier, S. (2005). Health outcomes and polypharmacy in elderly individuals: an integrated literature review. *Journal of Gerontological Nursing, 31*(9), 4-11.

Heiss-Harris, G., & Verklan, M. (2005). Maximizing patient safety: Using filter needles with glass ampules. *Journal of Perinatal and Neonatal Nursing, 19*(1), 74-81.

*Institute for Safe Medication Practices. (2001). *To promote understanding, assume every patient has a health literacy problem.* Retrieved June 12, 2006, from http://www.ismp.org/msaarticles/promote.html.

Institute for Safe Medication Practices. (2003). *List of error-prone abbreviations, symbols, and dose designations.* Retrieved June 12, 2006, from http://www.ismp.org/Tools/abbreviationslist.pdf.

* Johnson, M., Bulechek, G., Butcher, H., Dochterman, J. M., Maas, M., & Moorhead, S., et al. (Eds.). (2006). *NANDA, NOC, and NIC linkages: Nursing diagnoses, outcomes, & interventions.* St. Louis, MO: Mosby.

*Johnson, M., Maas, M., & Moorehead, S. (2000). *Nursing outcomes classification (NOC)* (2nd ed.). St. Louis, MO: Mosby.

Joint Commission on Accreditation of Healthcare Organizations (2006). Joint Commission announces 2007 patient safety goals for hospitals and critical access hospitals. Retrieved June 16, 2006, at http://www.jointcommission.org/NewsRoom/NewsReleases/nr_npsg_hap.htm.

Lea, D. (2005). Tailoring drug therapy with pharmacogenetics. *Nursing, 35*(4), 22-23.

Lehne, R. (2007). *Pharmacology for nursing care* (6th ed.). Philadelphia: Saunders.

Lewis L. (2006). Technology and safe medication administration. *American Journal of Nursing. 106*(Suppl. 3), 37, 48-51.

Manno, M., & Hayes, D. (2006). Best practice interventions: How medication reconciliation saves lives. *Nursing, 36*(3), 63-64.

McCarter-Spaulding, D. (2005). Medications in pregnancy and lactation. *MCN American Journal of Maternal Child Nursing, 30*(1), 10-17.

*McCloskey, J., & Bulechek, G. (2000). *Nursing interventions classification* (3rd ed.). St. Louis, MO: Mosby.

McGrath, J. (2004). Sciatic nerve damage from intramuscular injections: The preventable injury. *Journal of Legal Nurse Consulting, 15*(4): 3-5.

McKenry, L., Tessier, E., & Hogan, M. (2006). *Mosby's pharmacology in nursing* (22nd ed.). St. Louis, MO: Mosby.

Micromedex. (2006). *2006 USP DI Volume 1: Drug information for the health care professional.* Greenwood Village, CO: Thomson Micromedex.

NANDA International. (2007). *Nursing diagnoses: Definitions and classification, 2006-2007* (7th ed.). Philadelphia: Author.

National Coordinating Council for Medication Error Reporting and Prevention. *About medication errors.* Retrieved June1, 2006, from http://www.nccmerp.org.

Nicholas, P. K., Agius, C. R. (2005). Toward safer IV medication administration: The narrow safety margins of many IV medications make this route particularly dangerous. *American Journal of Nursing, 106*(Suppl. 3), 25-30, 48-51.

Olsen, J., Giangrasso, A., & Shrimpton, D. (2004). *Medication dosage calculations* (8th ed.). Upper Saddle River, NJ: Prentice Hall.

Pape, T. (2003). Applying airline safety practices to medication administration. *Medsurg Nursing, 12*(2), 77-94.

Pape, T., Guerra, D., Muzquiz, M., Bryant, J., Ingram, M., Schranner, B., Alcala, A., et al. (2005). Innovative approaches to reducing nurses' distractions during medication administration. *Journal of Continuing Education in Nursing, 36*(3), 108-116, 141-142.

Patterson, E. S., Rogers, M., & Render, M. L. (2004). Fifteen best practice recommendations for bar-code medication administration in the Veterans Health Administration. *Joint Commission Journal on Quality and Safety, 30*(7), 355-365.

Polifroni, E. C., Allchin, L., & McNulty, J. (2005). Limited math skills: A prescription for change. *Journal for Nurses in Staff Development, 21*(2), 79-81.

Southard, K. (2005). Bar coding medication administration: Preparing the culture for change. *Nurse Leader, 3*(3), 53-55.

Spector, R. (2005). *Cultural diversity in health & illness* (6th ed.). Upper Saddle River, NJ: Prentice Hall.

State of the Science on Safe Medication Administration. (2005). *American Journal of Nursing, 106*(Suppl. 3), 2-51.

Wilson, S. (1998). Irish Americans. In L. Purnell & B. Paulanka (Eds.), *Transcultural health care: A culturally competent approach,* pp. 353-370. Philadelphia: Davis.

Wolf, Z., Hicks, R., & Serembus, J. (2006). Characteristics of medication errors made by students during the administration phase: A descriptive study. *Journal of Professional Nursing, 22*(1), 39-51.

*Asterisk indicates a classic or definitive work on this subject.

Chapter 22

HEALTH PROTECTION: RISK FOR INFECTION

Media Resources

- Nursing Skills Online
- evolve Evolve Website http://evolve.elsevier.com/Harkreader/
- Companion CD
- 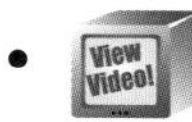 Skills Video Clips

Learning Objectives

After studying this chapter, you should be able to do the following:

- Discuss the course of an infection, physiological defenses against infection, and chain of infection in relationship to infection control
- Describe the assessment of a client who is at risk for infection, an actual infection, and responses to infection
- Identify appropriate nursing diagnoses for a client with either an active infection or an increased risk for infection
- Plan for goal-directed interventions to prevent infection or control the spread of infection
- Identify specific interventions needed to prevent transmission of infection, manage a client with a compromised immune system, and reduce the personal risk for infection
- Evaluate the outcomes that describe progress toward the goals of health protection nursing care
- Identify work restriction guidelines for client and care provider protection
- Identify cultural beliefs that may influence care

Key Terms

antibacterial
antibiotic
antibody
antimicrobial
bacterium
differential cell count
Gram stain
iatrogenic infection
immunization
immunocompromised
immunosuppressant
infection
infection control
inflammatory response
isolation
medical asepsis
nosocomial infection
pathogen
quarantine
septicemia
standard precautions
surgical asepsis
virulence
virus

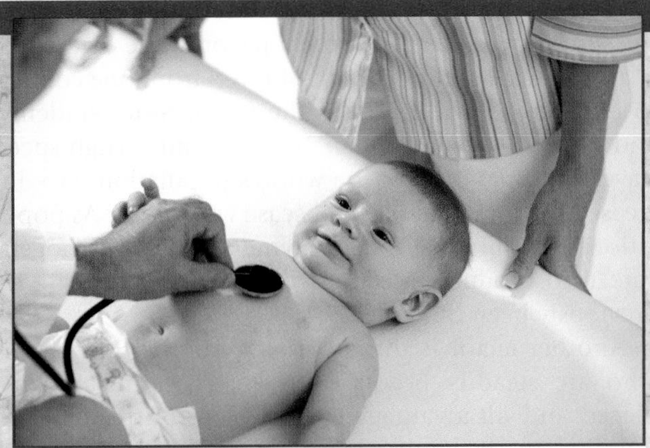

Eight-month-old Colleen Brown lives with her parents and two siblings: Sarah, 5 years old, and James, 3 years old. The Brown family was relocated to the Washington, D.C., area from New Orleans, Louisiana, after living in an evacuation center for 2 weeks following a devastating hurricane.

Colleen and her siblings have been complaining of stomach cramps, fever, and diarrhea, which began 2 days after the family left the shelter in Louisiana. When Colleen's mother took her axillary temperature, the thermometer registered 102° F. Mr. and Mrs. Brown took the children to the local emergency department. Each child was evaluated and, based on the recent travel history, stool samples were obtained. Colleen was admitted to the children's unit with a diagnosis of dehydration secondary to possible infection. In addition to being frightened and under extreme stress due their current life situation, Colleen's parents appeared to be fearful of the hospital setting and were confused about the admission process. The parents did not understand why one child was being admitted and not the others. There was also concern over the cost and payment for the hospital stay. Mr. Brown had insurance coverage from his job but was no longer employed after the hurricane. The nurse therefore makes a referral to a client representative to facilitate the management of Colleen's illness, recovery, postdischarge follow-up, and financial assistance. Because of Colleen's age, health status, and the risk for hospital-acquired infection, the nurse considers the nursing diagnoses *Risk for infection* and *Ineffective protection* (see nursing diagnoses box). Colleen will continue to have *Risk for infection* on discharge because she lives with two older siblings and has altered immunity related to her infancy.

KEY NURSING DIAGNOSES FOR INFECTION

Risk for infection: At increased risk for being invaded by pathogenic organisms

***Risk for infection transmission:** A state in which a person is at risk for transferring a pathogenic or opportunistic infection to others

Ineffective protection: Decreased ability to guard self from internal or external threats such as illness or injury

*Not currently on approved NANDA International (NANDA-I) list

CONCEPTS OF INFECTION CONTROL

Nurses have played a major role in preventing infectious diseases since Florence Nightingale demonstrated the effectiveness of nursing care in reducing the infection rate in military hospitals during the Crimean War. Nursing management of infectious and communicable diseases encompasses three levels of prevention. In primary prevention, nurses teach health promotion strategies to stay well. Primary prevention includes practices in the home and in health care institutions that prevent the spread of infection. In secondary prevention, nurses monitor clients both as individuals and in groups to detect infection early, obtain prompt treatment for infection, and prevent the spread to other members of a group. In tertiary prevention, a nurse helps the client manage the medical interventions of bacterial illnesses (commonly with an **antibiotic,** a medication that kills bacteria) to ensure complete recovery from the infection.

An **infection** is a disease state caused by the invasion and multiplication of a **pathogen,** a disease-producing microorganism, in body tissues. Pathogens may be bacteria, viruses, fungi, or parasites. Bacterial pathogens cause local cellular injury through their metabolism, toxin production, intracellular replication, or antigen-antibody response. The body responds to the invasion of causative organisms by forming antibodies and by a series of physiological changes known as inflammation.

Infections can be either localized or systemic. A localized infection is restricted to a well-defined or limited area of tissue. A systemic infection is one that affects the body, including organ systems, as a whole.

COURSE OF INFECTION

To control the spread of infection, it is important to understand the clinical course of infection, especially the period when it can be transmitted to others. The clinical course of an infection varies with the causative organism, dose and virulence of the causative organism, mode of entry of the organism, the site of infection, and the overall host resistance (health status) of the infected person. In general, however, the course of an infection can be described in four phases that are important to **infection control** in many cases.

Phases of an Infection. The *incubation period* extends from the time of a client's exposure to the organism to the appearance of the first symptoms. Depending on the disease, an exposed client might transmit the disease to others during this time. The incubation period varies in length with each disease. Knowing the incubation period may be helpful in knowing when to initiate postexposure prophylaxis, isolate the client, or expect symptoms to occur.

The *prodromal phase* is a period of vague, nonspecific symptoms that may precede the full manifestation of some infections. Depending on the infection, symptoms may include general malaise, low-grade fever, nausea, weakness, and general aches. A different example of the prodromal phase is the tingling sensation that occurs before a herpes lesion is noted.

The period of *clinical illness* is the time when the symptoms are fully manifested and most clearly recognized as representing a specific infection. The diagnosis is made from an assessment of signs and symptoms and confirmed after obtaining cultures to identify the specific organism.

The period of *convalescence* is the time following the acute symptoms to the time the person experiences a return to normal health. It is common for a person recovering from an infection to complain of decreased energy or feeling tired before full recovery from an illness.

An infectious disease is the term used to describe illness caused by a pathogen. Not all infections are communicable. A communicable disease is one that can be transmitted from one person to another under certain circumstances during one or more phases of the infection. For example; a client who has a urinary tract infection has an infectious process but will not transmit it to the nurse caring for the client, because it is not a communicable disease. A client diagnosed with human immunodeficiency infection (HIV) infection, however, has a communicable disease that could be transmitted to the nurse if the nurse sustains a needlestick injury or blood or body fluid splatter to the eye, mucous membranes, or nonintact skin.

Other communicable diseases may be spread by direct contact or via airborne route or respiratory droplets. It is important to note that exposure does not mean infection has immediately occurred; rather, it means that one was exposed and may be at risk for developing the disease if not treated prophylactically following the exposure.

Socioeconomic Factors Affecting Infection. With the development of antibiotics, antiviral agents, and immunization or vaccinations, health care practitioners had hoped that infectious diseases would become a problem of historic interest. However, several communicable diseases remain an ongoing health concern, even in developed countries such as the United States and Canada. Since the 1970s, there has also been emergence of new or more virulent infectious diseases with the threat of increased incidence in the near future. Acquired immunodeficiency syndrome (AIDS) and severe acute respiratory syndrome (SARS) are two examples of newer diseases. An example of a more virulent disease is multidrug-resistant tuberculosis.

Factors within the social structure can contribute to the spread of disease. A primary factor in the emergence of new disease is the amount of travel from one country to another, as evidenced by the recent SARS epidemic and concerns for an Avian flu pandemic. High-speed travel and migration of the world's population have increased the transmission of disease worldwide. As populations intermingle, both evolving and new pathogens spread to produce infectious diseases where they have previously been unknown.

Another factor is the increasing number of persons who are steadily becoming more economically displaced and disadvantaged. The recent hurricanes and flooding in the Gulf Coast is a current example reflected in this chapter's case study. Natural disasters can lead to overcrowded living conditions and destroy sanitation and clean water facilities, which in turn can result in outbreaks of diarrhea and increase transmission of hepatitis, tuberculosis, and influenza. The growth of large inner-city ghettos, where public and private services are inadequate or lacking and overcrowding is common, also creates conditions for the spread of infection. Although it is easy to assume that the risk for infection could be contained in areas where risk is the greatest, a highly mobile population means that the risk can spread rapidly.

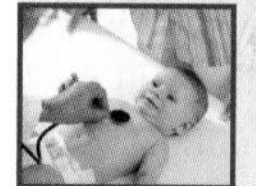

Colleen's family is large and shares a relatively small living area in an apartment with the extended family after being housed in an overcrowded shelter. What impact would these living conditions have on her risk for infection?

Another factor is the potential for disease to spread through the food supply, which is perhaps greater than it was in the recent past. The overuse of antibiotics in animal feed may increase the risk of drug allergies. The high demand for fresh fruits and vegetables year-round has resulted in an increase in the importation of these food items, often requiring transportation over great distances and handling at multiple points in the distribution system. With current concerns about bioterrorism, the government is increasing efforts to reduce the opportunity for contamination of the food system. The Department of Homeland Security (DHS) will work in conjunction with the Department of Agriculture toward this goal.

Because health policy in the United States is trying to become more prevention oriented, increased resources are now being funneled to address concerns related to bioterrorism and the effects of natural disasters. This reallocation of funds has actually led to cuts in funding for typical public health services, which now have greater demands but fewer financial resources.

Infection and Health Care Institutions. The health care system itself is yet another factor in infectious disease transmission. How antibiotics are prescribed has been identified as a major factor in the development of resistant strains of organisms. The overuse and misuse of antibacterial products has also led to the development of resistant organisms. Medical facilities now have pharmacy formularies that guide the use of antibiotics by physicians. The continuous development of equipment for invasive procedures has in turn created new problems in cleaning and sterilizing equipment. The rise in organ and tissue transplants has further increased the risk of transmission of disease because of the need for **immunosuppressant** therapy (drugs to suppress the body's immune system). These agents prevent the transplanted organ from being rejected by the body as foreign, but they also limit the body's ability to fight infection. Immunosuppression is also an adverse effect of several drugs used to treat cancer.

The public has a right to expect that the risk for acquiring an infection during hospitalization be minimal; however, controlling hospital-acquired infection rates is a major problem. Such infections not only adversely affect clients but also increase health care costs and lengths of hospital stay. Because of this concern, medical facilities are now required to report their infection rates, which could influence choice of site and provider of care for those with sufficient financial resources. In July of 2005, the state of Pennsylvania became the first state to begin reporting health care infection rates and the costs associated with their treatment.

A **nosocomial infection,** or hospital-acquired infection is any infection that was not present or incubating at the time of admission. An **iatrogenic infection** is the direct result of treatments such as invasive procedures. In 1970, the Centers for Disease Control (CDC) began the National Nosocomial Infections Surveillance (NNIS) system to monitor trends in rates, pathogens, and antibiotic susceptibility in the United States. It has been estimated that 5% to 10% of clients experience health care–acquired infections and, of these, multiple resistant organisms infect 25%. Depending on the site of infection and causative organism, hospital stays may be lengthened by 1 to 30 days, costing the health care system over $5 billion annually. As many as 90,000 persons die each year from health care–acquired infections. Up to 70% of these infections may be preventable if staff members adhere to basic infection prevention and control procedures such as hand washing.

DEFENSES AGAINST INFECTION

Primary Defenses. The human body has a number of refined defenses against infection. Primary defenses include the skin and mucous membranes, respiratory tract, gastrointestinal (GI) tract, genitourinary (GU) tract, and circulatory system.

Skin and Mucous Membranes. The skin and mucous membranes are the primary physical barrier to prevent organisms from entering the body through the intact dermis and epidermis. Although the skin harbors many different kinds of microorganisms (normal flora), we rarely become infected from these organisms if the skin remains intact. The surface of the skin also has **antimicrobial** properties, which enhances the protective barrier and limits the spread of microorganisms. Dryness of the skin promotes desiccation of microorganisms, and the ongoing desquamation of skin cells rids the skin surface of remaining organisms. The skin surface has additional protection from a low pH, which results from fatty acids that occur as a byproduct of lipid conversion by normal skin flora. The mucous membranes of the urinary system, vagina, and the respiratory and GI tracts produce mucus that traps and removes organisms. Mucous membranes also destroy bacteria through the action of macrophages and lysozymes.

Respiratory System. The respiratory tract filters and warms the air that we breathe. Hairlike structures called cilia that line the respiratory tract continuously sweep debris up and out of the respiratory tract. Cells lining the respiratory tract secrete lysozymes that can destroy certain bacteria. Macrophages engulf and destroy bacteria found in the alveoli. All of these mechanisms serve as the first line of protection from respiratory droplets and airborne transmissible diseases such as tuberculosis.

Gastrointestinal System. The GI tract is a hostile environment for many microorganisms because of the pH extremes of the highly acid stomach and the highly alkaline small intestine. Nonetheless, bacterial colonies found normally in the colon aid digestion and provide needed vitamins. They can also provide resistance to colonization by pathogenic organisms by competing for nutrients and by producing inhibitors in the form of proteins that limit the growth of other, possibly pathogenic, bacteria. Goblet cells lining the GI tract produce secretions that form barriers, preventing penetration by bacteria. These cells also produce enzymes that lyse, or break apart, bacterial cell walls.

Circulatory System. The circulatory system is essential to the inflammatory and immune response. Blood carries the components of cellular and humoral immunity and removes waste products of tissue destruction from sites of injury.

Secondary Defenses. The immune and inflammatory responses constitute the second line of defense against infection. The **inflammatory response** is a localized reaction to injury and is activated when tissue damage occurs. The immune response is activated in the presence of foreign substances or pathogens. It has various specific and nonspecific mechanisms to respond to invasion by microorganisms. The very complexity of the immune response gives it enormous flexibility and effectiveness.

Inflammatory Response. The inflammatory response should not be confused with infection. The inflammatory response is the local reaction to an infectious agent. It serves to localize, destroy, dilute, neutralize, or remove a pathogen or damaged cells to prepare for the healing process. There is a direct relationship between the degree of inflammation and the time needed for repair to take place. Inflammation is identified by the use of the suffix *-itis.* When this reaction is fast and severe, it is described as being acute. Any type of traumatic injury, including surgery, initiates the inflammatory response, for which redness, heat, swelling, and pain are classic signs.

The inflammatory response involves blood vessels, fluid and cellular components of the blood, the lymphatic system, and surrounding tissues. Local tissue injury releases substances from the damaged cells that cause arterioles, vesicles, and capillaries to dilate. Fluid then leaks from the capillaries into the interstitial space, along with proteins and enzymes that inactive viruses and destroy bacteria.

Other cells present in this fluid-filled space include red blood cells (RBCs) and white blood cells (WBCs). White blood cells are of various types and have specific roles in fighting infections. Those involved in the nonspecific or innate system include polymorphonuclear leukocytes, macrophages, granulocytes, and null cells. This represents the first stage in the development of immunity.

Immune Response. Although inflammation is a general protective response, the immune response is specific to an antigen or foreign substance that has invaded the body. The activation of this response, then, requires that the body has had previous contact with the organism or antigen. Immunity (see Box 22-1 for terminology) is a measure of a person's ability to fight disease by forming immunoglobulins (antibody cells that destroy antigens), developing immunologically competent cells, or, in the case of viral infections, producing interferon. The immune response consists of two closely interrelated components: the humoral and cell-mediated immune response.

Cell-mediated immunity is the cellular response that is the result of the activity of *T lymphocytes* or *B lymphocytes* in action. When a pathogenic organism or toxin is recognized by the body's immune system, these cells can be found at the site of infection. There are three types of T lymphocytes; some may attack a specific antigen whereas others may secrete substances that attract other leukocytes to destroy the invading pathogen. Cellular immunity provided by sensitized T lymphocytes remains indefinitely in the host. Because these cells help the B cell recognize an antigen, they are called helper T cells. Suppressor T cells also exist that prevent the reaction to the antigen from becoming an overreaction or hypersensitivity. A third type of T cell, natural killer (NK), is able to kill tumor cells and virus-infected cells. The B and T cells work together to fight infections that they recognize and, thus, require previous contact with the invading organism.

Humoral immunity is the antigen-antibody immune response that takes place in body fluids. An **antibody** (immunoglobulin) is a circulating protein that recognizes and destroys foreign invaders (antigens). When B cells contact an antigen, they divide into immunoglobulins (antibody cells that destroy antigens) and memory cells that can recognize a repeated invasion by the antigen. There are five types of immunoglobulins: IgM, IgG, IgA, IgD, and IgE.

IgM is the first to form and is the initial response to a current infection.
IgG is slower to respond but will remain present for years.
IgA represents a secretory antibody that is found in blood, saliva, and tears.
IgD is found in serum, but its role is not fully identified.
IgE releases histamine.

The immune response and its components provide the basis for medications to provide protection against a specific disease or disease agent. An **immunization** or vaccination is a medication administered to activate an immune response before exposure to the disease agent. Immunizations are available to protect most of the world's population from many communicable diseases. In the United States, all families have access to childhood immunizations to protect against vaccine-preventable diseases through routine well-child visits to health care providers or through free clinics.

BOX 22-1 *Terminology of Immunity*

- **Active immunity:** A form of long-term acquired immunity that protects the body against a new infection as a result of antibodies that develop naturally after an initial infection or artificially after a vaccination.
- **Passive immunity:** A form of acquired immunity resulting from antibodies that are transmitted naturally through the placenta to a fetus, through the colostrum to an infant, or artificially by injection of antiserum for treatment or prophylaxis. Passive immunity is not permanent and does not last as long as active immunity.
- **Natural immunity:** The immunity achieved when an animal or human is infected with an organism; the antigenic response occurs naturally within the body.
- **Artificial immunity:** Immunity induced by man-made vaccines or immunoglobulins.
- **Acquired immunity:** A form of immunity that is not innate but is obtained during life. It may be natural or artificial, and actively or passively induced.

CHAIN OF INFECTION

The process of infection can best be illustrated as a chain. Understanding the components of the chain assists in understanding the risk for infection in a specific situation and identifying measures to prevent infection (Figure 22-1). The elements are the characteristics of the organism (pathogen), portal of entry, reservoir, portal of exit, mode of transmission, and characteristics of the host (the client).

Characteristics of the Organism (Pathogen). The causative organism is an entity that is capable of causing infection. Biological agents include bacteria, viruses, fungi, para-

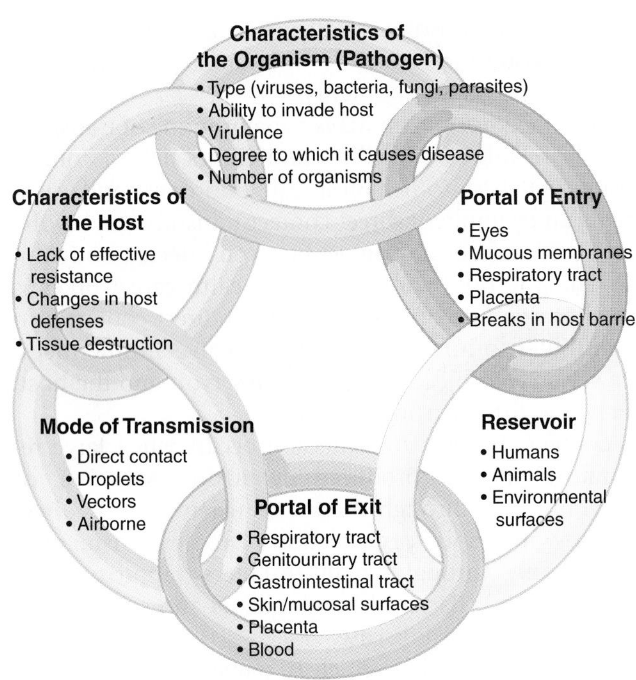

FIGURE 22-1 Chain of infection.

sites, and protozoa. The ability of an organism to cause disease is affected by the type of organism and its level of **virulence**—the power of an organism to cause disease or its ability to survive outside the body.

The number of organisms present is a key factor. There are a certain number of organisms that must be present in order for infection to occur; this number varies with each disease. Host resistance (the client's health status) also plays a role in risk for disease transmission. Table 22-1 lists common pathogens responsible for health care–acquired infections and the usual mode of transmission for each.

Types. Agents that commonly cause infection are viruses, bacteria, fungi, and parasites. Each is briefly discussed here.

Viruses. A **virus** is a tiny microorganism, much smaller than a bacterium, that can only replicate inside the cell of a host, such as a human. A virus is a packet of genetic material covered with protein coats. A virus functions by taking over the metabolism of the cell to make more copies of itself. The invaded cell can then no longer function normally. The new viral particles are released slowly through the cell membrane and continue to infect other cells without necessarily killing them. Some viruses do kill cells and release large numbers of viral particles with cell lysis. Other viruses have the characteristic of latency, which allows the cell to continue with some or all of its normal functions, while the virus has integrated itself into the genetic material of the cell.

Because viruses use the host cell to reproduce, any medications used to kill them must be specific for the viruses and not the host's metabolism. Examples of antiviral medications are those used to reduce symptoms of herpes infections and HIV. Immunizations, such as those against chicken pox and hepatitis, are important in preventing viral infection.

Table 22-1 Common Pathogens in Health Care–Acquired Infections and Usual Mode of Transmission

PATHOGEN	MODE OF TRANSMISSION
Staphylococcus	Contact usually but depends on strain
Antibiotic-resistant *Staphylococcus aureus*	Contact
Pseudomonas	Contact usually but depends on strain
Escherichia coli	Contact usually but depends on strain
Shigella	Contact

Bacteria. A **bacterium** is a small, single-celled organism that can grow independently outside of cells. Bacteria can survive and multiply outside the human cell in the presence of the right temperature and nutrients. An example would be salmonella in chicken salad or in eggs. Many bacteria are actually beneficial to humans, such as normal flora in the GI tract; however, some are pathogenic (capable of causing disease). Bacteria cause disease by invading and multiplying in the tissues of the host and forming toxins. The body's defense system for specific and nonspecific immune reactions is important in fighting these infections. Many antibiotics have been developed to kill specific types or strains of bacteria.

Fungi. Fungi are eukaryotic organisms with cell walls, which can contain chitin, cellulose, or both. Like bacteria, they can replicate very rapidly given the right growing conditions. Fungi require nutrients from organic materials. Therefore most fungal infections are acquired from contact with decaying organic matter or from airborne spores in the environment. These are divided into two groups—molds and yeasts. Yeasts are unicellular organisms that produce budding and/or circular mucoid colonies on culture. They can also cause disease by overgrowing and damaging tissues as they grow. Unlike bacteria, their cell walls contain the substance chitin, which makes them very resistant to destruction by the body's resistant mechanisms.

Parasites. A parasite is an organism living in or on another living creature and taking advantage of that creature while the host is disadvantaged. Parasites feed off cells and tissues, depriving them of nutrition and causing tissue destruction. This can be life threatening, depending on where the parasite is lodged and which tissues are destroyed. Common examples include scabies and pathogenic worms.

Virulence. Virulence is a measure of the organism's ability to invade and create disease in a host. Virulence also refers to the ability of the organism to survive in the environment. Virulence of microorganisms is a growing concern with the development of antibiotic-resistant organisms such as vancomycin-resistant enterococci (VRE) and methicillin-resistant *Staphylococcus aureus* (MRSA).

The first element of virulence is invasiveness, which has three parts. The first is the ability of the organism to survive in the environment while transferring between hosts. The second is the method of transfer to another host, and the third is the ability to grow once attached to the new site.

The second element of virulence is toxigenicity, the ability to produce toxic substances that can damage the host. Much of an organism's disease-causing capability and its ability to cause tissue damage results from the production of enzymes and toxins. Toxins are proteins or complexes of proteins, polysaccharides, and lipids that microorganisms release to cause tissue damage or destruction. Enzymes may assist in the rapid spread of an organism through tissues.

Portal of Entry. Organisms can enter a host through the eyes, mucous membranes (including those of the GI and GU tracts), respiratory tract, placenta, and any breaks in the host's mechanical barriers, such as nonintact skin, or chemical barriers. Controlling the *portal of entry* involves maintaining the integrity of the protective tissues in the host.

Reservoir. A *reservoir* is a place where the infectious agent can survive and, possibly, multiply until it can invade a susceptible host. Three common reservoirs include humans, animals, and environmental surfaces. Reservoirs inside the hospital include clients, health care personnel, equipment, the hospital environment, and sometimes visitors. When an individual develops a hospital- or health care–acquired infection, it is acquired from a reservoir in that environment.

To grow and multiply, organisms need a food supply and optimal conditions for growth. Many organisms grow best in a warm, moist, dark environment at some optimal pH. Some are aerobic (requiring oxygen), whereas others are anaerobic (not requiring oxygen). Common reservoirs in the home are improperly stored food, improperly cleaned counter surfaces where food has been prepared, and surfaces in bathrooms. In hospitals, hands of health care workers and improperly cleaned client care equipment are common reservoirs for infection. In addition, the materials used to contain wound drainage and collect urine create additional reservoirs, requiring the use of standard precautions.

Portal of Exit. Organisms can exit a host through the respiratory tract, GU tract, GI tract, skin or mucosal surfaces, placenta (mother to infant), and blood. Controlling the portal of exit involves management of body fluids and wastes.

Mode of Transmission. Modes of transmission are the mechanisms by which pathogens are transferred from an agent to the host. The three main modes are direct contact, droplet, and airborne spread. Other possible modes are by vector (mosquitoes, flies, rats, and other vermin) and by common vehicle (contaminated food, water, medications, and equipment).

Direct Contact. Contact is a major mode of transmission in health care facilities and clinics. Direct contact results in person-to-person spread. Improper hand washing is an example of direct contact transmission involving MRSA infection. Contact between infected body fluids and the nonintact skin of a health care worker is another example of direct contact. Indirect contact also contributes to infection and may involve an intermediate surface or object between the reservoir and the host, such as a dirty instrument.

Droplet. Droplet transmission occurs when large respiratory droplets produced by talking, sneezing, or coughing pass through the air or when there is direct contact with respiratory secretions. Droplet transmission occurs only through small distances (approximately 3 feet or less). Bacterial meningitis is an example of a droplet-transmitted disease.

Vector. A vector is a vehicle to transmit infection from a reservoir to a host. One example of a common vector is food. Organisms, such as *Salmonella,* can multiply in food before infecting the host. Other organisms do not multiply in the food but are carried on the food, such as the hepatitis A virus.

An important mode of transmission is via a living vector, such as an insect or arthropod. Organisms can be transmitted externally on the vector, such as on the legs of flies. Some vectors carry the organism internally, such as the malarial parasites or yellow fever virus in a mosquito. West Nile virus is a current example of a vector-borne disease.

Airborne. Airborne diseases such as varicella (chickenpox) are spread by airborne droplet nuclei that can remain suspended in air for extended periods of time. The infection is acquired by breathing in air contaminated with the microorganisms.

Characteristics of the Host. Once an organism has exited a reservoir, infection can occur in a susceptible host—a nonimmune person who is capable of developing the infectious disease. Any changes in the natural defenses of the host increase the likelihood of infection by a pathogenic agent. Tissue destruction, either accidental or through medical or surgical intervention, increases the possibility of infection. Factors that have been identified as affecting host resistance include age, smoking, the presence of chronic disease (such as diabetes or cancer), and nutritional status.

ASSESSMENT

GENERAL ASSESSMENT

Prevention of infection in clients is a primary nursing concern. All clients entering a health care agency should be assessed for *Risk for infection.*

Health History. The health history is the primary tool for detecting *Risk for infection*. It should include questions about immunization, possible exposure to communicable disease, current and past illness, travel history, and the general health status of the client. The client's history will give you clues about behaviors that may be associated with the incidence of infections and health teaching that should be done. Include assessment of the client's knowledge level and factors in the environment that increase the risk for infection. Allergy status is also an important factor to note on assessment. In this time of emerging diseases, travel history is a newer tool to be added to a client's health history. This proved to be very important during the SARS epidemic and will be important in assessing and monitoring other infections, such as the Avian influenza.

Physical Examination. Follow up on findings obtained from the health history in your physical examination, which can help tie information from the health history to the physical status of the client. For example, if the client is on immunosuppressants such as cortisone, you will look for the physical effects of the long-term use of cortisone.

Diagnostic Tests

Blood Cell Count. Because blood cells are important components of the immune system, a blood sample can help determine whether your client has an infection or is at increased risk for infection. The hemoglobin and hematocrit are red blood cell measurements that reflect cell nutrition and repair; white blood cell count reflects the ability to fight actual infections.

Hemoglobin and Hematocrit. RBCs are called erythrocytes, and their main function is transporting oxygen. The oxygen attaches to hemoglobin, the iron-containing component of the cell. The hematocrit identifies the percentage of RBCs present in whole blood. A decreased number or size of RBCs indicates anemia or blood loss. As a reflection of nutritional status and thus overall health, anemia helps define the risk for infection. Certain genetic diseases or infections can alter the numbers or form of RBCs, increasing risk for infection.

White Blood Cell Count. The total WBC count reflects the body's response to infection. An increased number of WBCs may indicate infection. A decreased number indicates a reduction in infection-fighting ability. An individual's risk for infection increases as the WBC count decreases. The cause of the decrease is sometimes an active infection. Some viral infections, such as HIV, and some cancers, such as leukemia, cause decreases in the WBC count.

When evaluating a WBC count, look at what is called the "differential." The **differential cell count** shows the numbers of the different types of WBCs. These include neutrophils, eosinophils, basophils, lymphocytes, and monocytes (Table 22-2). The largest group is the neutrophils. Immature or nonfilamented neutrophils are called bands. A left shift, which is an increased number of immature neutrophils, is a possible indication of infection.

Other diagnostic tests can measure the function of the immune system. Immunoglobulin levels can be used to evaluate the integrity of the humoral immune system or B-cell function. Delayed hypersensitivity tests (skin tests) are used to test T-cell function.

Culture and Sensitivity. Determining the actual organism causing an infection enables the treatment plan to be specific to the infecting organism. For this reason, a culture is an important diagnostic test and can be performed on sputum, spinal fluid, skin, blood, and urine. A culture of microorganisms can be grown from samples taken from a site of obvious infection, such as pus draining from a wound or from a site that does not have yet obvious signs of infection, such as lung secretions of an intubated client. Because urinary tract infections are common in hospitalized clients who have an indwelling catheter, a urine sample may be cultured once an infection is suspected.

Culturing of bacteria requires growing the bacteria on a medium that supports their growth. Usually within 3 to 5 days there will be enough organisms to identify the specific species of bacteria that is causing the infection. The growing bacteria can then be exposed to different antibiotics to determine which one will be most effective in fighting the infection. This is called a *sensitivity test*, and it is needed to determine the organism's resistance to a medication. Resistance is the ability of a microorganism to make genetic changes in response to environmental pressures, such as medications. The sensitivity test, then, is a very important tool for identifying which antibiotics will kill the microorganism cultured.

Polymerase chain reaction (PCR) or blanched-chain deoxyribonucleic acid (DNA) assay are new tests that can detect genetic material present in infections such as

Table 22-2 Interpreting a Differential White Blood Cell (WBC) Count

CELL TYPE	NORMAL PERCENTAGE OF 100 WBCs	USUAL REASON FOR INCREASE
Neutrophil	32 to 62	Acute infections, especially localized infections, such as tonsillitis or otitis media
Lymphocyte	31	Certain acute viral infections with early increase; chronic infections
Basophil	0.6	Infrequently increased; when elevated, most often associated with myeloproliferative disorders
Eosinophil	2.2	Allergic reactions and drug reactions
Monocyte	0 to 4	Certain bacteria, such as brucellosis; tuberculosis; protozoa; rickettsiae

HIV or tuberculosis (TB). These tests have replaced viral culture testing for some diseases and assist in a more rapid diagnosis.

Various terms are used to describe drug treatment for microorganisms. The term *antimicrobial* is a broad term and generally refers to the ability to limit the spread of microorganisms. This term, then, can also apply to soaps and other chemicals, as well as medications. The term **antibacterial** refers to the killing of all bacteria. The term *antibiotic* typically refers to a drug that is able to kill a bacterial pathogen. Antiviral drugs are used to treat viral infections. Antifungal agents are used to treat fungal infections.

Gram Stain. The **Gram stain** is a specific microscopic test used to obtain rapid results on a sample sent to the laboratory. Although the Gram stain specifically tests the nature of the bacterial cell walls, it can also indicate the presence of cell types, such as epithelial cells or polymorphonuclear leukocytes. The Gram stain divides bacteria into two basic groups depending on whether the cell walls take up the stain (gram-positive) or does not (gram-negative). The shape and arrangement of the bacteria are also indicated by this test. Shapes can be round (cocci), rodlike (bacilli), or spiral (spirochetes). Furthermore, the arrangement can be single, in pairs (diplococci), in chains *(Streptococcus)*, clusters *(Staphylococcus)*, or tetrads *(Sarcina)*. This test can quickly give direction for preliminary treatment with antibiotics until culture results are available to indicate the most effective antibiotic agent. A Gram stain is the test of choice in the initial diagnosis of meningitis. It can distinguish viral from bacterial illness in 10 minuets instead of waiting 2 to 3 days for a culture report. Thus, treatment can be started more quickly and assist in a positive outcome for the client.

Viral cultures are more difficult because viruses must be grown inside cells, not just on culture media. Many times, if a virus is suspected to be the cause of an infection, the culture is sent for antibody testing and not for culturing. The presence of the viral antibody can be determined relatively rapidly, so that therapy can be started.

The presence of fungi can often be determined from the Gram stain if the laboratory is specifically looking for it; however, fungi grow under much different conditions in the laboratory than on the host. If a fungal infection is suspected, the sample for culture should be collected and placed in a special growth medium at the time of specimen collection.

FOCUSED ASSESSMENT FOR *RISK FOR INFECTION, RISK FOR INFECTION TRANSMISSION,* AND *INEFFECTIVE PROTECTION*

As mentioned earlier, several risk factors make a client more susceptible to infection. These include invasive procedures, trauma, some medications, malnutrition, inadequate primary or secondary defenses, drug treatment, smoking, and certain chronic diseases. Assess your clients carefully for these and other factors to better anticipate if they have an increased *Risk for infection.* Assess the environment as well; it too can raise a client's risk.

Characteristics of the Host

Primary Defenses. Assess the condition of the skin, respiratory tract, and GI and GU systems as the primary defenses against infection. Assess also for tissue damage and circulatory status. Assess the skin for lesions or breaks in the skin and trauma.

Any breaks in the protective barriers of the skin or membranes surrounding tissues will impair an individual's protection against infection. Trauma can break the skin barrier and nearby blood vessels and tear other tissues in the area. This has several immediate results. Any infective organisms that were on the surface of the skin or membranes are now closer to the exposed tissue. The ability of the circulation to provide oxygen and remove debris is disrupted. Any immune response is also altered as a result of interrupted circulation. Finally, tissue functioning may be hampered or destroyed.

The rupture of the amniotic membranes of a pregnant woman often signals the beginning of an end of pregnancy; however, the fetus now loses this defense against invasion of microorganisms in the immediate environment, including the nonsterile environment of the vagina. Thus a prolonged break of these membranes before the birth of the child can put the infant at increased risk for infection.

Assess the amount of trauma caused by invasive procedures. The amount of ineffective protection depends on the amount and location of the trauma. The risk for infection from a hangnail is considerably less than from a gunshot wound to the abdomen. Invasive medical procedures performed by a health care worker can also alter protection. Intravenous (IV) lines, especially central venous lines, allow exposure of the circulatory system and tissues surrounding the placement site to infection. Similarly, providing pulmonary support by endotracheal intubation alters a client's risk for infection. The procedure itself can cause trauma to the airway, but there is also ineffective protection from presence of the tube, which blocks the natural mechanisms that clear the airway. Artificial suctioning further increases risk for infection by providing a vehicle for introducing pathogens into the airway. Other procedures that alter protection against infection include insertion of nasogastric tubes, other GI tubes, and urinary catheters; spinal taps; and invasive radiographic examinations. Any surgical procedure alters an individual's protection against infection.

Review the client's history for problems in the GI, respiratory, circulatory, and GU systems that can contribute to infection. Some examples are given in Box 22-2.

Assess the person's nutritional status. Malnutrition resulting from malabsorption of nutrients or inadequate intake reduces the body's ability to protect against infection as well as to repair itself after infection.

BOX 22-2 *How Selected Diseases Affect Infection Risk*

CROHN'S DISEASE

Crohn's disease is a genetic disease that causes chronic inflammation of the gastrointestinal (GI) tract, putting those with the disease at increased risk for infections of the GI tract. They may require hospitalization and antibiotic treatment for food poisoning, although someone with a normally functioning GI tract who ate the same food would not become ill. Other examples of chronic illnesses that increase the risk for GI infections are human immunodeficiency virus (HIV) infection and cystic fibrosis.

CARDIOVASCULAR DISEASE

People with cardiovascular disease may have reduced circulation and thus a poor inflammatory response in the extremities. An ingrown toenail can become severely infected, possibly leading to amputation. Diabetes, sickle cell disease, and multiple sclerosis are other chronic diseases that can result in reduced circulation and thus increase the risk for infection.

ASTHMA

Clients with asthma can have chronic inflammation of their bronchial passages. Because of this alteration in the airways, what would ordinarily be a minor cold and inconvenience can lead to severe pulmonary pneumonia, requiring hospitalization. Other chronic conditions that can alter the airway and increase the risk for infection include cystic fibrosis, emphysema, smoking, and residual lung disease in premature infants.

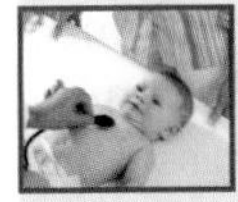

Colleen and her family were without adequate food and water for several days before being rescued from floodwaters and taken to the shelter. What was the impact on her overall risk for infection?

Altered Immunity. Review the client's history for problems that are known to alter immunity. Any alteration in the immune response can increase the risk for infection. Immunosuppression can result from any disease process that removes the secondary defenses against infection. *Leukemia* is a term for a group of infections that alter the populations of the infection-fighting WBCs. *Lymphoma* is a cancer that can affect the lymph system, an important component of the immune response. Chronic diseases that alter the numbers of WBCs put these people at increased risk for infection. HIV infection reduces the number of T4 (CD4) cells that can function normally. Diabetes mellitus, especially type 1, has also been associated with decreased functioning of the immune system. Cirrhosis of the liver or removal of the spleen can also result in reduced functioning of the immune system.

Take a medication history because pharmaceutical agents can alter the immune system. A common example is corticosteroid administration, which affects the functioning of WBCs in the immune response and reduces the inflammatory response. This can be a positive effect. For example, these medications can be lifesaving by reducing swelling from trauma or from allergic reactions in the airway. At the same time, however, they also have some negative consequences. For example, persons on corticosteroid therapy for chronic diseases such as arthritis, asthma, inflammatory bowel disease, or multiple sclerosis may experience alleviation of disease symptoms but also do not have an inflammatory response to infection. Corticosteroids also decrease the delayed hypersensitivity response of the immune system that involves T-cell activity. Furthermore, any antibiotics used to fight infection can themselves increase the risk for infection through their effects on WBCs and the bone marrow.

Many chemotherapeutic drugs used to treat some forms of cancer can attack WBCs or inhibit bone marrow activity, the site of production for many of the cells needed for an immune system response. As a result, the client receiving chemotherapy will have reduced protective mechanisms and increased risk for infection because of a decrease in the number of WBCs available to respond to infection.

An immunosuppressed client is not only at increased risk for infection but, because of immunosuppression, may not display typical manifestations of infection. Increased vigilance is needed to reduce the risk for infection and to observe for signs of infection in these clients.

Finally, review the client's recent history of medical therapies. Radiation therapy, another treatment for cancer, can alter primary defense systems against infection, causing immunosuppression.

Health Practices. Assess a client's health practices for factors that contribute to the risk for infection. Contributing factors for clients with the diagnosis *Risk for infection* include contacts with infectious organisms, the environment, and personal health practices. Health practices that increase risk for infection include personal hygienic practices. Young children may not take the time or know the importance of performing hand hygiene. Persons with impaired mental capabilities or physical limitations may not have optimal personal hygiene because of their knowledge base or because of a physical inability to bathe, wash hands, and maintain a clean environment that does not promote growth of microorganisms.

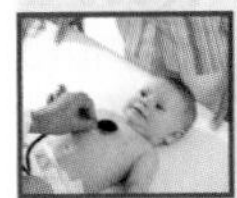

What are the implications of being in contaminated floodwaters on Colleen's risk for infection? What is the risk her diarrhea could be contagious to others?

Age. The client's age should be considered a factor in assessing the client as a susceptible host. An individual's level of immunity is related to age. A newborn infant has no antibodies of its own at the time of birth. Maternal antibodies that have crossed the placenta are the only defenses against infection at the time of birth. The infant, if breastfeeding, continues to receive antibodies from its mother in breast milk. The protective antibodies received from the mother before birth drop rapidly in the newborn period and are almost gone by 4 to 6 months of age. The infant begins to make its own antibodies but does not begin to approach adult levels until about age 2. These levels continue to rise gradually over the first 10 years of life.

The unborn fetus has multiple means to guard against infection. Although the immune response is not well developed until after birth, the mother's immunoglobulins cross the placenta and provide protection for the fetus. The placenta and the amniotic sac that contains the fetus are physical barriers that prevent the passage of infective organisms to the fetus. It is normal for the amniotic membrane to rupture at the time of delivery; however, once rupture occurs, the fetus is at increased risk for infection. If the amniotic membranes rupture more the 24 hours before delivery, there is ineffective protection and the fetus is at risk for infection.

After age 65, clients lose some of their infection-fighting abilities. Normal age-related changes can alter the protection of those over 65 years of age. The skin becomes more friable, losing some connective tissue layers, and there are changes in the protective oils and layers of outer skin cells. Some older adults also have reduced mobility that can make minor infections more severe. For example, an upper respiratory infection can rapidly lead to pneumonia. Older persons are at higher risk for falls. Failing eyesight can also be a contributing factor. Mental changes can further contribute to ineffective protection. The ability to provide for personal hygiene and maintain a clean environment can become impaired, altering their protection and leading to an increased risk for infection.

Heredity. Heredity can play a role in *Ineffective protection.* Hereditary diseases should be part of the medical history; it is pertinent to ask about family history. Infants who lack proper immune response, such as severe combined immunodeficiency disease (SCID), are unable to destroy invading organisms and are great risk of infection.

Immunizations/Vaccinations. Ask clients about immunizations that are appropriate to their situation. Much of modern success in preventing infections has resulted from the development of immunizations that protect against a specific agent or toxin. According to the American Academy of Pediatrics, immunizations should begin in the newborn period, with a second round occurring at 2 months of age. See the 2006 Recommended Childhood and Adolescent Immunization Schedule (Centers for Disease Control and Prevention) in Chapter 16. Some adolescents will be offered boosters to some previous vaccines, and adults should receive periodic tetanus boosters. Other adult vaccinations are often based on need, such as when planning travel abroad.

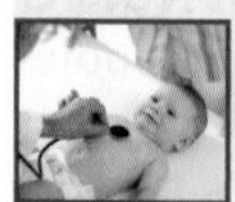

If Colleen has not begun her immunizations, she will be at risk compared with infants her age who have started their immunizations.

Immune Status. Clients who are **immunocompromised** are more likely to experience opportunistic infections, which result from overgrowth of organisms that do not normally cause disease. An example is *Pneumocystis carinii* pneumonia in a person infected with HIV. A reduced immune response can alter the client's protective system so that these normally nonpathogenic organisms can reproduce and cause disease. Another common cause of immunosuppression is cancer or its related therapies. Persons with myeloma have defects in humoral immunity, resulting in deficiencies of antibodies. Other malignancies have an impact on cell-mediated immunity. Hodgkin's disease is an example of a malignancy that alters the ability to fight intracellular infections. Chemotherapy and radiation therapy can also impair immunity.

Presence of Congenitally Acquired Conditions. Review the history for congenitally acquired conditions. Any disease that alters the nutritional status increases the risk for infection. Physical defects present at birth can alter many of the defenses against infection. Lung disease in premature infants puts them at risk for pneumonia. Infants with cardiac defects have circulatory changes that impair their ability to deliver oxygen to tissues and remove debris and waste products, altering the tissue's ability to prevent infection. Anomalies such as spinal defects that expose internal tissues alter the protection of these tissues from possible infection.

Presence of Acquired Conditions. Acquired infections can alter the immune system's response to infection. These infections alter the cell-mediated immune response. Viral infections associated with decreased cell-mediated immunity include measles, mumps, varicella, influenza, Epstein-Barr virus, and rubella. Bacterial and fungal infections include tuberculosis, leprosy, syphilis, coccidioidomycosis, histoplasmosis, and blastomycosis. HIV destroys the immune system cells that are active against infection and that would normally destroy mutated cells that could lead to cancer.

Presence of Mental Illness. People with mental health problems may have increased risk for infection if they lack the ability or judgment to protect themselves from infection. Decreased ability to recognize or respond to illness alters their protection. Persons with dementia may be unable to protect themselves from infection. Their inability to maintain nutrition, personal hygiene (bathing, dental hygiene, and hand hygiene) or a safe environment puts them at increased risk.

Characteristics of the Environment Characteristics of the environment can raise the risk for infection as well and deserve careful assessment.

Community. For clients in the community, assess the home and community environment for risk factors. Some clients are at increased risk because of contacts with infectious organisms. Visitors to foreign countries come into contact with microorganisms to which they have no immunity. Persons living in milder climates of the United States are more at risk for mosquito vector–borne diseases. Lifestyles can put people at increased risk for some infections. IV drug abusers are at increased risk for the blood-borne infections of HIV and hepatitis B and C. People with multiple sexual contacts are at risk for sexually transmitted diseases, as well as blood-borne pathogens. Homeless persons are at increased risks for airborne infections such as tuberculosis because of crowded conditions in shelters.

Environmental factors that contribute to increased risk for infection can include overcrowded living conditions, which can lead to increased contact with individuals who may have an infection. Environments that harbor pests, such as rats or roaches, raise the risk for infection because the pests harbor infectious agents. Lack of screens in mild weather can lead to increased infections caused by mosquitoes or flies. Lack of insect repellent and insufficient coverage of skin by clothing can increase risk of tick bites that can lead to Lyme disease.

Health Care Institutions. Assess the health care institution's environment for risk factors. Hospital environments require more stringent rules of cleanliness and sanitation because the clients as a group are at high risk for infection. They may have weakened defenses to infection because of illness and may be in close proximity to others who harbor infectious agents. In addition to multiple individual risk factors, hospitalized clients come into contact with antibiotic-resistant organisms not present in other places, and they may undergo multiple invasive procedures.

Assessing the hospital environment includes being aware of the infections that are currently present in the hospital. When a hospital has an unexpected increase in the number of health care–acquired infections (compared to either own past performance or current performance of other hospitals), especially those caused by resistant organisms, efforts at infection control should be reviewed and refined to eliminate the spread of these organisms. An example would be an outbreak of *Clostridium difficile* on a nursing unit. The infection control department may be consulted to review individual client cases and make recommendations for control on that specific nursing unit.

It is also important to be aware of the legal and regulatory requirements for the protection of clients and health care workers. Various standards have been set by the Centers for Disease Control and Prevention (CDC), the Occupational Safety and Health Administration (OSHA), and The Joint Commission (TJC).

FOCUSED ASSESSMENT FOR INFECTION

Localized Infection. The clinical appearance of a localized or contained infection has basic components: fever (may be low-grade), *redness* (erythema), *swelling* (edema), *pain,* and *heat.* Often a fifth component, *loss of function,* also is present. This response occurs whether or not the body has experienced this type of infection previously. After an initial decrease of circulation to an infected area, increased permeability of blood vessel (vascular) walls allows fluid and cells to flow into the affected tissue to aid in fighting the infection. The presence of fluid and RBCs causes the redness, edema, and increased temperature common at the site of infection. The WBCs result in the formation of pus, a familiar sign of infection found on skin surfaces.

Note pain of any kind: head, chest, abdominal, or in the extremities. Frequently, infants with acute otitis media pull or rub the affected ear. Increased nasal secretions or abnormal breath sounds indicate the possibility of respiratory infection.

Systemic Infection. Systemic infections, those that progress to involve more than one organ system, are more difficult to treat and generally result in poorer outcomes. These infections might result from lack of treatment of a localized infection. Clients who are at increased risk for infection because of decreased primary defenses or inadequate secondary defenses may experience a systemic infection.

Systemic infections are manifested by signs and symptoms that affect the entire body. These signs and symptoms define a clinical syndrome that determines the diagnosis of infection. Clients with these infections frequently present with a general malaise, fever, myalgia, arthralgia, and nonspecific GI symptoms, such as nauseas, vomiting, cramping, or diarrhea. However, GI symptoms can indicate a localized GI infection as well. Fever, although common with infections, may not always be present with systemic infection. If unrecognized, systemic infections can lead to dehydration, acidosis, septic shock, and possibly death within a short period.

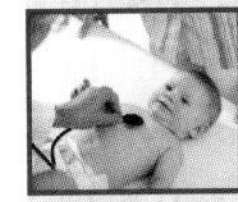

What symptoms did Colleen exhibit that might indicate the presence of systemic infection? What factors put her more at risk for localized GI infection instead of systemic infection?

Septicemia, or infection in the bloodstream, may result more often from surgery or contaminated central venous catheters. It may be accompanied by nonspecific client complaints, such as tiredness and fever, but can also include chills, sweats, myalgia, and arthralgia. Central nervous system infections can present with general malaise and fever but can also include headache and stiff neck. Urinary frequency, urgency, and dysuria can be presenting symptoms of a urinary tract infection (common in clients with indwelling urinary catheters), but these signs may be absent, especially in older adults. Fever is not usually a symptom in such an infection and, if present, along with flank pain, chills, and sweats, probably indicates that pyelonephritis has developed.

Vaginal or other genital organ infections frequently cause symptoms and can result in severe infections involving the uterus and ovaries. Abnormal discharge (changes in color, consistency, and odor), itching, and pain with intercourse can be signs of vaginal infection. These infections sometimes lead to pelvic inflammatory disease (PID), which can result in problems with fertility and childbearing.

Symptoms in Immunocompromised Clients. An immunocompromised client may present with a modified clinical picture of infection. The pace of the illness may be more rapid, which may lead to more serious infection as well as a spread of infection from the initial site to other sites.

Assess all clients for *Risk for infection*, and include three major areas in your assessment. First, obtain a history and physical examination, including questions about the characteristics of the host (client) that contribute to the person's vulnerability to infection. Remember that smoking is a factor in decreased immune response. Second, obtain information about exposure to infection, the type of organisms to which the individual is exposed, or the characteristics of the agent of infection. This could involve ascertaining the signs of infection in other family members. Finally, examine the environment for factors that contribute to the spread of infection. This might involve questions related to the type of housing client and or family has.

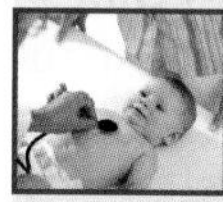

To assess Colleen's risk for infection before the present illness, what questions would you ask her parents?

DIAGNOSIS

When a client presents with either an infection, increased risk for infection, or ineffective protection against infection, evaluate the client based on the health history and physical examination, including any sign of inflammatory response. If the risk factors are present without signs of infection, write the diagnosis as *"Risk for infection related to . . ."* If the client has ineffective protection due to physical causes of tissue damage or to altered immune response, write the diagnosis as *"Ineffective protection against infection related to . . ."* An active infection puts the client at increased risk for further infection. Some infections that alter the immune system of the client, such as HIV, actually result in ineffective protection. As another example, infants in a day-care center are at increased risk for infection because of the frequent exposure to many children. If those infants have not been immunized as recommended by the American Academy of Pediatrics, they have ineffective protection compared with the infants with proper immunization history. Consider *"Risk for infection transmission related to . . ."* when a client has been exposed or colonized with an infectious agent, has a contaminated wound or treatment devices with contaminated drainage, or has environmental factors that increase risk (including but not limited to natural disasters, unsanitary living conditions, and areas at high risk for vector-borne infections). Table 22-3 gives examples of client data with appropriate nursing diagnoses.

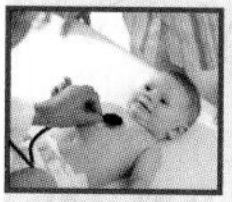

How would you determine the appropriate nursing diagnosis or nursing diagnoses for Colleen? To what extent, if at all, does her family share her risk?

Write nursing diagnoses appropriate to the stage of the client's illness and the focus of care. Persons in whom HIV infection is initially diagnosed may need counseling about how to effectively communicate with their partners, and they may not need interventions based on ineffective health protection at this time. The focus of care for persons with HIV admitted to the hospital for *Pneumocystis carinii* pneumonia would initially be improved oxygenation. With recovery, though, the focus of care could shift to that of *Ineffective protection*. Be aware, however, that although the focus of care differs, some of the specific interventions may be similar.

Table 22-3 Clustering Data to Make a Nursing Diagnosis

Injuries	
DATA CLUSTER	**DIAGNOSIS**
Client presents with pain, redness, swelling on leg injured during previous week. He is 86 years old and has diabetes.	*Risk for infection* secondary to poor wound healing
A 60-year-old client, living by himself, is readmitted for antibiotic treatment for infected surgical incision. He lacks knowledge of wound care.	*Ineffective health maintenance* related to need to manage wound care
A 2-year-old admitted for dehydration is refusing PO foods, fluids on day 2 of hospitalization. Parents not visiting.	*Ineffective health maintenance* related to fear and lack of social support
Infant at first well-baby visit 6 weeks after delivery. Has normal axillary temperature, respirations 40, and heart rate 100. Appears fussy in mother's arms. Mother expresses concern about the infant receiving immunization.	*Risk for infection* related to age and mother's lack of knowledge regarding immunizations
A 40-year-old woman receiving chemotherapy for cancer of the uterus. White blood cell count 500. Complaining of vaginal dryness and itching.	*Risk for infection* related to decreased WBC count and altered vaginal mucous membranes
A 25-year-old man with AIDS. Critically low T-cell count. Rents a room with no cooking facilities. Weight loss 30 pounds.	*Ineffective protection* related to decreased immunity and inadequate nutrition

AIDS, Acquired immunodeficiency syndrome; *PO*, by mouth; *WBC*, white blood cell.

Individuals can and often do respond differently to the same medical diagnosis. The type of response can determine the outcomes for the client in terms of both a willingness to undergo treatment and the actual response to that treatment. It is important to assess the client's and family's responses to the diagnosis. Their responses will form the basis for formulating nursing diagnoses and planning appropriate interventions. A client's culture can significantly influence the response to diagnosis and treatment as well, as suggested in Box 22-3.

Ineffective Health Maintenance. Determine whether a client's health practices are helpful in preventing a recurrence of a previous illness. Previous experience helps shape one's attitude toward health maintenance. If a previous illness did little to interfere with life or caused minimal discomfort, the client may be unwilling to undertake health maintenance practices to prevent a recurrence. If, however, the previous illness was perceived to cause extreme distress or was life threatening, the client might take major steps to maintain health and prevent a recurrence.

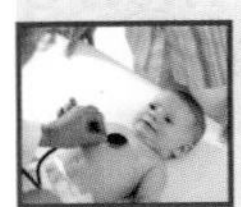

Colleen's siblings also have diarrhea, but they gave a history of diarrhea illness in the past. How might this family history have had an impact on the parents' response to Colleen's current symptoms?

Anxiety. Assess for concerns about the risk for infection that may produce anxiety. Concerns about emerging infections and hospital-acquired infection have been publicized and may result in alarm. Concern over loss of home and possessions and family income will increase anxiety as well. Clients whose immunity is suppressed from illness or medical therapy need information about common ways to protect themselves. The increased state of anxiety itself can reduce one's protection against infection.

Fear. Fear of a diagnosis can be reality based but also can be greater than is warranted in a particular situation. Evaluate client fears, and provide a climate in which the client feels comfortable in verbalizing them. Knowledge of a particular diagnosis and usual outcomes may help allay fear of the unknown. At times, you must simply acknowledge your client's fears as being true and feel comfortable in assisting them and their families with accessing coping mechanisms to assist them through the illness. Your ability to assess the level of fear and help the client cope can help determine the client's outcome. Again, the mind-body connection can be very significant in the healing process.

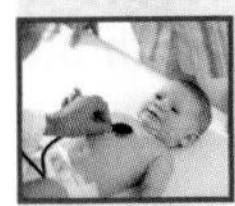

What factors might put the Brown family at risk for fear?

Impaired Social Interaction. Many times nursing diagnoses pertaining to infection require a support system in order for clients to carry out activities of daily living. Without support of friends or family, an infection may develop needlessly into a life-threatening situation. In the past, homeless persons diagnosed with active tuberculosis who were unable or unwilling to seek therapy not only endangered their own health but also that of those with whom they came in contact. Now, with the provision of Direct Observed Therapy (DOT), public health nurses visit these clients on a daily basis and offer care and support while administering drug therapy. Clients living alone who are unable to seek medical attention and have no one to call for help lack a system of support not only for seeking care but also for treatment.

BOX 22-3 *Cross-Cultural Care*

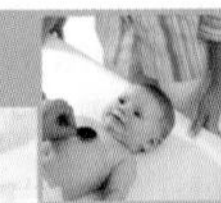

Caring for a Cajun Client

Colleen's father is Cajun. He was employed in a local restaurant in New Orleans, and his entire family continues to live with his brother and his family. In Mr. Brown's culture, it is not unusual for extended families to continue to live together, and this arrangement is not based on financial need.

The family's confusion with the admission process was the result of (1) a lack of understanding about the infant's medical diagnosis and (2) the different health practices of many traditional Cajuns. Cajuns believe in faith healing. They have strong cultural ties, and healing may begin with practices of incantation, plant cures, and prayer. Colleen's extreme dehydration at the time of admission was probably the result of delay in getting medical care in the wake of a national disaster, and possibly related to Cajun traditions, which have shown that they are less likely to take prevention measures.

Colleen's mother stays throughout her hospitalization. Other family members care for their other children. Her mother is devoted to her care and follows the agreed-upon plan. The father blames the government for the status of his children's health.

Colleen improves dramatically with intravenous (IV) hydration and antibiotic therapy. Because of the Browns' sense of not having control over their environment, adherence to an immunization schedule begun during this hospitalization will require family- and community-based support. Although every client is unique, Cajuns, like those in Colleen's family, tend to have the following characteristics (Waldmeier, 2002):

- They are tactile, communicating with touch and preferring a close personal space during interview.
- They believe in faith healing and the "joy of life."
- They use the family as the major support system and view the family as more important than the individual.
- They are less likely to take prevention measures.
- They exhibit strong cultural ties.
- They are honest and dignified.
- They are focused on relationships rather than tasks.
- They have a belief in fatalism.

Situational Low Self-Esteem. Self-esteem is another component of a client's mental health that plays a role in determining individual outcomes. Low self-esteem can be influenced by society's response to a particular illness. A diagnosis of HIV infection can carry stigma in society, despite public campaigns designed to eliminate these prejudices. The client, as a part of society, requires support from you to maintain a positive sense of self-worth. The infection may not even be one that is sexually transmitted (e.g., HIV can also be acquired by other means). An adult may contract chickenpox and be ridiculed by others for having a childhood disease. Even though these examples differ in many respects, the client can have situational low self-esteem in both cases. Because this could hinder the healing process and interfere with client outcomes, it is important to assess for low self-esteem and work with the client to alleviate or eliminate it.

PLANNING

EXPECTED OUTCOMES FOR THE CLIENT WITH *RISK FOR INFECTION*

The goal of care for the client at risk for infection is to prevent that client from getting an infection. To achieve this goal you must work to reduce risk factors. The expected outcomes are based on primary and secondary prevention strategies (i.e., elimination of those risk factors and early recognition and treatment). Sample client outcomes for the nursing diagnosis *Risk for infection* include the following. The client will do the following:

- Have intact skin and mucous membranes
- Have containment of any infection after the initial diagnosis
- Verbalize knowledge of measures to avoid infection
- Remain free of exposure to organisms causing infection
- Verbalize early signs of infection and seek appropriate treatment
- Demonstrate no signs or symptoms of infection secondary to medical or nursing procedures

EXPECTED OUTCOMES FOR THE CLIENT WITH *INEFFECTIVE PROTECTION*

The goal of care for the client with the nursing diagnosis *Ineffective protection* is that the client will have increased ability to safeguard from internal or external threats such as illness or injury. The expected outcomes depend on the specific threat, but the things the client will do may include the following:

- Verbalize knowledge of how to self-protect from infection (if immunocompromised)
- Verbalize knowledge of how to self-protect from damage to tissue (if anticoagulated)
- Remain free of infection or injury
- Verbalize knowledge of wound management (open wounds due to trauma or surgery)
- Show evidence of wound healing without experiencing an infection
- Reduce the risk factors to minimize the risk for health care–acquired infection
- Be able to identify an infection in its early stages when it can be treated minimally before the infection may become life threatening

Other goals may be formulated, knowing that it is more desirable to treat an infection with oral antibiotics (when able) than with IV antibiotics and to treat clients at home rather than in the hospital. At times, however, clients with infections cannot be treated in the home setting. A plan of care is then developed to meet the client's needs during hospitalization.

INTERVENTION

INTERVENTIONS TO PREVENT TRANSMISSION OF INFECTION

Interventions to prevent the transmission of infection are discussed in two categories: hospital infection control and infection control in the home. Infection control measures used in the hospital include medical asepsis, standard precautions, isolation precautions, antibiotic treatment review, proper nutrition, and proper hydration. Reducing the number of pathogenic organisms in the environment provides a more sanitary environment. Proper hand hygiene is the single most effective way to stop the spread of microorganisms between individuals. To prevent the spread of airborne organisms, an isolation room and the use of personal protective equipment are required.

Implementing Medical Asepsis. **Medical asepsis** consists of practices designed to reduce the numbers of pathogenic microorganisms in the client's environment. The desired result is to prevent or reduce the transmission of microorganisms from one person to another. **Surgical asepsis** is the protection of the client against infection before, during, and after surgery using sterile technique. The term *sterile* means free of all microorganisms, whereas the term *medical asepsis* implies freedom from pathogenic organisms.

Hand Hygiene. The first line of defense in medical asepsis is good *hand hygiene,* which refers to any method approved by the CDC for decontaminating the hands. Alcohol-based hand rubs are approved for use when hands are not visibly soiled. Hand washing still refers to the mechanical action of hand antisepsis using soap and water to clean the hands. Friction or rubbing increases the amount of soil and microorganisms removed. When performing hand hygiene, wash from areas of clean to less clean. Procedure 22-1 describes the correct method for hand hygiene using principles of medical asepsis.

TIME TO ALLOW: NOVICE: 30 seconds EXPERT: 30 seconds

PROCEDURE 22-1 HAND WASHING

Nursing Skills Online: Infection Control, Lesson 2

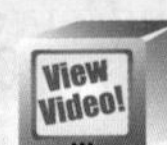

Performing hand hygiene is one of the most important ways to prevent transmission of infectious organisms. Make sure you perform hand hygiene properly before and after contact with each client, following glove removal, after using the restroom, before eating, and between dirty and clean tasks. Perform hand washing when you first come on duty and when hands are visibly soiled.

DELEGATION GUIDELINES

All staff members are expected to comply with proper hand hygiene technique and adherence to standard precautions. Nursing assistants or medical assistants should follow this hand hygiene procedure.

EQUIPMENT NEEDED

- Sink with running water
- Antimicrobial soap
- Paper towels
- Alcohol-based hand rubs

1 Perform preliminary actions (see inside front cover).

2 Turn on the faucet so that warm water is running. *Warm water leaves more protective skin oils in place than hot water and is less chafing to the skin over time, when frequent hand hygiene is done.*

3 Wet your hands, and lower arms under running water while holding your hands lower than your elbows (see illustration). *This position helps microbes run off your hands rather than up your arms.*

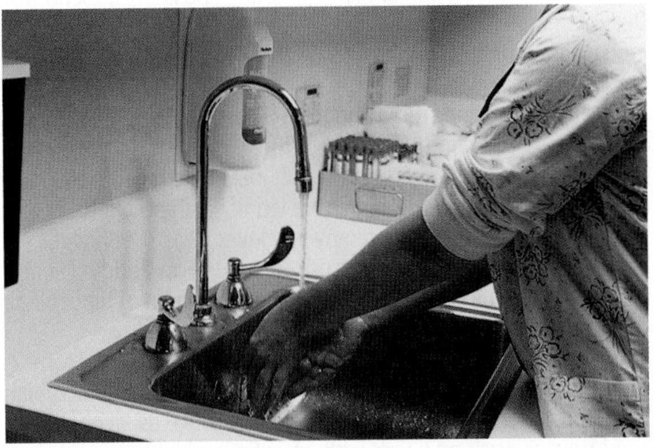

Step 3. Wetting the hands while holding them lower than the elbows. Amount of jewelry worn should be limited.

4 Using soap, thoroughly rub all surfaces of your hands, including your palms, backs of your hands, and wrists (see illustration). Work the soap into a foamy lather while rubbing both hands together using circular movements. *Because bar soap can provide an environment for bacterial growth if left to sit in a continually we environment, liquid soap from a dispenser is recommended. Friction aids in mechanical removal of microorganisms.*

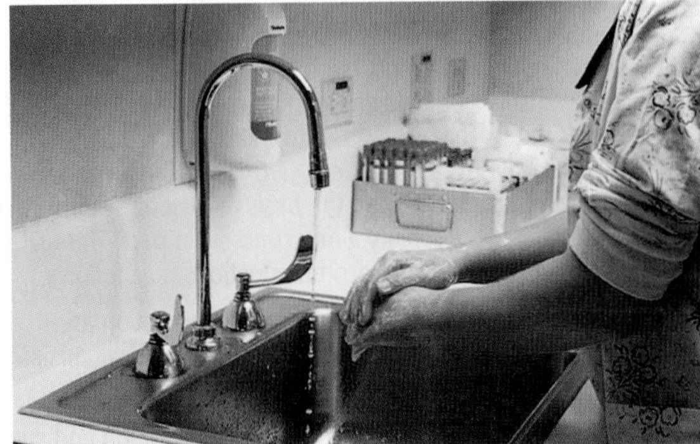

Step 4. Thoroughly rubbing all surfaces of the hand with soap.

5 Pay special attention to cleansing the following areas that can concentrate microorganisms: between the fingers, at creases and breaks in the skin, at the nail beds, and under the nails (see illustration). Spend 15 to 30 seconds performing hand hygiene. *A cuticle or orangewood stick can be used to assist in properly cleansing under the nails.*

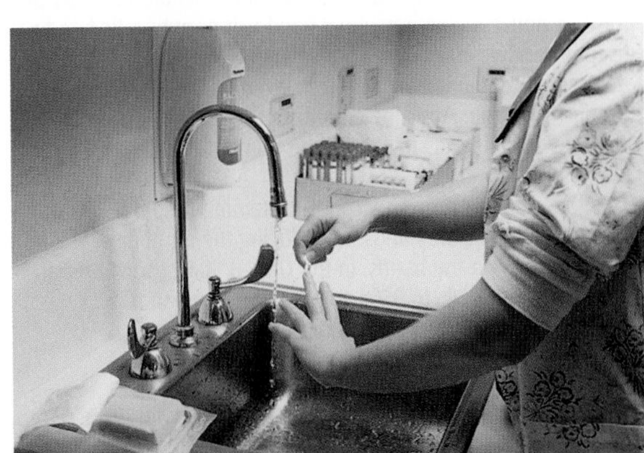

Step 5. Cleaning under the fingernails and under rings.

Continued

6 Rinse your hands with warm running water under the faucet, allowing the water to wash down your hands and over your fingertips.
7 Dry hands thoroughly with a *paper towel.*
8 If sink is not foot-operated, turn off the faucet with the used towel, and then discard the towel in the appropriate designated receptacle. *The towel acts as a barrier between your clean hand and the faucet.*

HOME HEALTH CARE CONSIDERATIONS

If you work in home health care, bring antimicrobial soap or alcohol-based hand rubs and paper towels with you to the client's home. Unless hands are visibly soiled, use alcohol-based hand rubs. These now contain cosmetic emollients and will not dry the skin.

BOX 22-4 *Hand Hygiene Guidelines From the Centers for Disease Control and Prevention*

CATEGORIES

These recommendations are designed to improve the hand-hygiene practices of health care workers and to reduce transmission of pathogenic microorganisms to clients and personnel in health care settings. As in previous Centers for Disease Control/Healthcare Infection Control Practices Advisory Committee (CDC/HICPAC) guidelines, each recommendation is categorized on the basis of existing scientific data, theoretical rationale, applicability, and economic impact. The CDC/HICPAC system for categorizing recommendations is as follows:

Category IA. Strongly recommended for implementation and strongly supported by well-designed experimental, clinical, or epidemiological studies.

Category IB. Strongly recommended for implementation and supported by certain experimental, clinical, or epidemiological studies and a strong theoretical rationale.

Category IC. Required for implementation, as mandated by federal or state regulation or standard.

Category II. Suggested for implementation and supported by suggestive clinical or epidemiological studies or a theoretical rationale.

No Recommendation. Unresolved issue. Practices for which insufficient evidence or no consensus regarding efficacy exist.

DEFINITION OF TERMS

Handwashing: Washing hands with plain (i.e., non-antimicrobial) soap and water or an antimicrobial soap and water when hands are visible dirty or contaminated with proteinaceous material

Decontaminate hands: To reduce bacterial counts on hands by performing antiseptic/antimicrobial hand rub or antiseptic handwash.

Antiseptic handwash: Washing hands with water and soap or other detergents containing an antiseptic agent.

Antiseptic hand rub: Applying an antiseptic hand-rub product to all surfaces of the hands to reduce the number of microorganisms present.

Alcohol-based hand rub: An alcohol-containing preparation designed for application to the hands for reducing the number of viable microorganisms on the hands. In the United States, such preparations usually contain 60% to 95% ethanol or isopropanol.

RECOMMENDATIONS

1. Indications for Handwashing and Hand Antisepsis

A. When hands are visibly dirty or contaminated with proteinaceous material or are visibly soiled with blood or other body fluids, wash hands with either a non-antimicrobial soap and water or an antimicrobial soap and water (IA).
B. If hands are not visibly soiled, use an alcohol-based hand rub for routinely decontaminating hands in all other clinical situations described in items 1C-1J (IA). Alternatively, perform hand hygiene with an antimicrobial soap and water in all clinical situations described in items 1C-1J (IB).
C. Decontaminate hands before having direct contact with clients (IB).
D. Decontaminate hands before donning sterile gloves when inserting a central intravascular catheter (IB).
E. Decontaminate hands before inserting indwelling urinary catheters, peripheral vascular catheters, or other invasive devices that do not require a surgical procedure (IB).
F. Decontaminate hands after contact with a client's intact skin (e.g., when taking a pulse or blood pressure, and lifting a client) (IB).
G. Decontaminate hands after contact with body fluids or excretions, mucous membranes, nonintact skin, and wound dressings if hands are not visibly soiled (IA).
H. Decontaminate hands if moving from a contaminated body site to a clean body site during client care (II).
I. Decontaminate hands after contact with inanimate objects (including medical equipment) in the immediate vicinity of the client (II).
J. Decontaminate hands after removing gloves (IB).
K. Before eating and after using a restroom, perform hand hygiene with a non-antimicrobial soap and water or with an antimicrobial soap and water (IB).
L. Antimicrobial-impregnated wipes (i.e., towelettes) may be considered as an alternative to washing hands with nonantimicrobial soap and water. Because they are not as effective as alcohol-based hand rubs or washing hands with an antimicrobial soap and water for reducing bacterial counts on the hands of health care workers, they are not a substitute for using an alcohol-based hand rub or antimicrobial soap (IB).
M. Wash hands with non-antimicrobial soap and water or with antimicrobial soap and water if exposure to *Bacillus anthracis* is suspected or proven. The physical action of washing and rinsing hands under such circumstances is recommended because alcohols, chlorhexidine, iodophors, and other antiseptic agents have poor activity against spores (II).
N. No recommendation can be made regarding the routine use of non-alcohol–based hand rubs for hand hygiene in health care settings. Unresolved issue.

BOX 22-4 *Hand Hygiene Guidelines From the Centers for Disease Control and Prevention—cont'd*

2. Hand-Hygiene Technique

A. When decontaminating hands with an waterless alcohol-based hand rub, apply product to palm of one hand and rub hands together, covering all surfaces of hands and fingers, until hands are dry (IB). It should take 15 to 25 seconds for hands to dry. Follow the manufacturer's recommendations regarding the volume of product to use.

B. When washing hands with soap and water, wet hands first with warm water, apply the amount of product recommended by the manufacturer to hands, and rub hands together vigorously for at least 15 seconds, covering all surfaces of the hands and fingers. Rinse hands with water and dry thoroughly with a disposable towel. Use towel to turn off the faucet (IB). Avoid using hot water, because repeated exposure to hot water may increase the risk of dermatitis (IB).

C. Liquid, bar, leaflet, or powdered forms of plain soap are acceptable when washing hands with a non-antimicrobial soap and water. When bar soap is used, soap racks that facilitate drainage and small bars of soap should be used (II).

D. Multiple-use cloth towels of the hanging or roll type are not recommended for use in health care settings (II).

OTHER ASPECTS OF HAND HYGIENE

A. Use hand lotions to minimize the occurrence of contact dermatitis associated with hand antisepsis or hand washing.

B. Do not wear artificial fingernails or extenders when providing patient care (IA).

C. Keep natural nail tips less than ¼-inch long (II).

D. Wear gloves when contact with blood or other potentially infectious materials, mucous membranes, and non-intact skin could occur (IC).

E. Remove gloves after caring for a client. Do not wear the same pair of gloves for the care of more than one client, and do not wash gloves between uses with different clients (IB).

F. Change gloves during client care if moving from a contaminated body site to a clean body site (II).

G. No recommendation can be made regarding wearing rings in health care settings. Unresolved issue.

Modified from Guidelines for hand hygiene in health-care settings: Recommendations of the Healthcare Infection Control Practices Advisory Committee and the HICPA/SHEA/APIC/IDSA Hand Hygiene Task Force, Centers for Disease Control and Prevention. (2002). *MMWR Morbidity and Mortality Weekly Report, 51*(RR-16). Retrieved October 29, 2006, from http://www.cdc.gov/handhygiene.

Box 22-4 provides guidelines from the CDC for frequency of performing hand hygiene.

Action Alert! Perform hand hygiene before and after every contact with a client and after glove removal. Performance of hand hygiene by care providers is the first line of defense to prevent infection.

Environmental Controls. Minimizing the spread of infection requires the use of appropriate environmental precautions. Routine cleaning of the environment should be done daily. Any spills, especially those involving infectious materials, should be cleaned immediately to avoid spreading the infectious organisms. The use of clean materials and Environmental Protection Agency (EPA)–registered hospital disinfectants for daily cleaning and cleaning between clients is important to reduce the spread of infection.

The housekeeping or environmental services department is responsible for cleaning client rooms, bathrooms, halls, waiting rooms, utility rooms, and the nurses' station. Daily cleaning of the client's room includes removing trash, wiping sinks and countertop with disinfectants, using disinfectants in the bathroom, and sweeping or vacuuming the floor. Disinfectants remove most microorganisms from surfaces, which are then considered clean. They do not prevent microorganisms from returning to these surfaces. Due to the increased incident rate for MRSA in hospitals, environmental cleaning is extended to doorknobs and other frequently touched areas to reduce the risk of spread through contact with contaminated surfaces.

Nursing personnel help the client keep the room clean. The sink and bathroom are generally considered to be dirty areas. When using the sink, consider that it has been used for washing dirty hands and disposing of dirty bathwater. Clean objects that come in contact with the client should not touch dirty surfaces. It is inappropriate to place urinals, bedpans, and even potted plants on a surface that will be used for eating or storing eyeglasses, hearing aids, and dentures.

For even more stringent control of microorganisms, various disinfection methods can be used. Disinfection removes microorganisms sensitive to the disinfectant used. It does not limit reintroduction of microorganisms to the surface that was cleaned. Sterilization is a process that removes all microorganisms from a piece of equipment. The sterilized object, however, can be easily contaminated by contact with an unsterile surface, equipment, or air currents. Table 22-4 outlines the use and limitations of various methods used to control or eliminate the growth of microbes.

Sharps Disposal. Needles and other sharps used in delivering care are considered to be infectious wastes and must be disposed of according to the individual state regulations. Sharps containers should be located in every hospital room and in all medication preparation

Table 22-4 Disinfection and Sterilization Methods

METHOD	USE	LIMITATIONS
Steam	Kills microorganisms sensitive to heat and moisture	• Some bacterial spores seem resistant to this treatment. • Some equipment cannot withstand the high temperatures and moisture.
Gas (ethylene oxide)	Kills microorganisms on products that cannot be steam-sterilized	• Articles must be allowed to release gas by aeration before use. • Cannot use to sterilize liquids, which would absorb gas. • Is expensive and time consuming (2 to 5 hours).
Radiation	Kills microorganisms	• Many spores are resistant, although equipment is not damaged
Ultraviolet light	Sensitizes microorganisms to other treatments	• May have to be used with other methods to kill additional microorganisms but does not damage equipment.

areas. Home health care nurses should carry a sharps container to collect all sharps used in client care. For family members who are administering medications or testing blood glucose, sharps must be handled in accordance with state law. For example, they may be placed into leakproof, rigid, puncture-resistant, and shatterproof containers and brought to a local approved treatment and disposal facility.

Disposing of Bodily Wastes. Feces and urine are of course flushed through the bathroom toilet into the sewage system. If the client uses a bedpan, urinal, or bedside commode, use care to prevent spills, and clean the container after disposing of urine or feces. Change any soiled linen as necessary. Rinsing with a bleach/water solution of 1:100 (1 tablespoon bleach to 1 gallon of water) or rinsing with vinegar will also assist in the reduction of bacteria.

Promoting Air Quality. Designated hospital personnel monitor the institution's ventilation system to ensure that the quality of air is healthy. Maintenance of the system prevents the growth of molds and bacteria that could be circulated throughout the hospital, causing disease. Negative pressure rooms also need to be monitored for proper functioning.

Implementing Standard Precautions. The concept of standard precautions was developed a number of years ago with the developing awareness that any client has the potential for carrying an unknown infection in his or her blood or secretions. Standard precautions include the use of hand hygiene and barrier precautions to prevent the caregiver from exposure to pathogens. Any bodily substance has the potential for harboring infectious organisms, which can be transmitted from client to caretaker and then possibly to another client.

Standard precautions are a set of CDC-mandated actions, including hand hygiene and the use of barrier precautions, designed to reduce transmission of infectious organisms; they are applied to every client regardless of whether an infection has been identified. Standard precautions are also known as CDC Tier 1 precautions and include the use of gloves (preferably nonlatex), water-impermeable gowns, masks or respirators, and eye protection if splashes are possible. Standard precautions are specific to the task. They should be implemented whenever contact with a client's blood, excretions, secretions, or nonintact skin is anticipated. These precautions are used to protect the caregiver from exposure to pathogens, but they also reduce the risk of transmitting infection to other clients.

BOX 22-5 *Common Infections Managed With Standard Precautions*

- Abscess with minor or limited drainage contained by a sterile dressing
- Acquired immunodeficiency syndrome (AIDS)
- Most pneumonias, including those caused by gram-negative bacteria
- Acute bacterial conjunctivitis, including gonococcal and chlamydial
- Salmonella (use contact precautions if client diapered, incontinent, <6 years of age)
- Hepatitis A, B, C, E (for hepatitis A, use contact precautions if client diapered or incontinent)
- Herpes zoster (localized lesions in immunocompetent client)

Action Alert! *Always* use standard precautions, not just with clients whose infections are known.

The CDC guidelines are enforced by OSHA. JCAHO also monitors compliance during inspections. Box 22-5 lists common infections that are managed using standard precautions. Not all protective equipment needs to be used in all care situations, but Box 22-6 provides information about each of these components.

Employing Barriers. Another component of medical asepsis and standard precautions is the use of barriers that can reduce the transmission of organisms. Gloves can be used to avoid direct contact with infectious material. Gloves should never be used as a substitute for good hand hygiene. Gloves should not contain latex. Nonlatex gloves can be used for all but surgical procedures and protect the caregiver from developing latex allergy or sensitivity. Always ask clients if they may have latex allergy, and note it on the medical record. A clean gown or

BOX 22-6 *Components of Standard Precautions*

HAND HYGIENE
Perform hand hygiene before having any contact with clients and before preparing any items that will be used in client care. Perform hand hygiene again after any contact with a client, especially after touching any blood, body fluids, secretions, excretions, and contaminated items. Even if you wore gloves, you must still perform hand hygiene. When needed, perform hand hygiene during the care of a client to prevent cross-contamination of body sites.

GLOVES
Wear gloves to handle blood, body fluids, secretions, excretions, and contaminated items. Although blood-borne pathogens are the basis for wearing gloves, the blood does not have to be visible in the body fluids for gloves to be required. Remove the gloves immediately, and perform hand hygiene before proceeding with the next task or touching noncontaminated items, even on the same client. Change your gloves between tasks on the same client if different body sites are involved.

MASK, EYE PROTECTION, FACE SHIELD, GOWN
Use as needed if you could be exposed to splashes or sprays of blood, body fluids, secretions, and excretions. The risk for splashes or sprays is higher in emergency departments and operating rooms; however, the risk exists with some clients in general care areas as well.

CLIENT-CARE EQUIPMENT
Handle equipment in a manner that prevents personal skin and mucous membrane exposure and cross contamination to other clients. Ensure that reusable equipment is cleaned and reprocessed before using it in the care of another client.

ENVIRONMENT
Review hospital procedures for routine care, cleaning, and disinfection of environmental surfaces. Spills of blood and body fluid may need to be handled with special procedures. The facility's exposure control plan will state who is responsible for this task.

LINEN
Linen should be handled in a way that keeps it from contaminating skin, mucous membranes, and clothing. Fold soiled linen with the contamination to the inside. Hold it away from your body, place it directly in a plastic bag, tie the bag, and take it directly to the soiled-linen area.

SHARP OBJECTS
Take all possible precautions to prevent needlesticks or cuts with sharp objects (called *sharps* for short). Needles are the primary concern on a general client unit; however, scalpels, lancets, and other sharps are sometimes used. After using a sharp, immediately discard it in a punctureproof container.

apron can be used to protect clothing from contamination in situations where uniforms may come in direct contact with client wound drainage or bodily discharge. Another technique used as part of medical asepsis is cohorting, a process in which clients with similar diagnoses are placed together to minimize the spread of their infections to clients not infected by that organism. In nursing units and other departments that have more than one bed unit per room, the beds for these clients may be grouped together in the case of an outbreak of infection.

Implementing Transmission-Based Precautions. Historically, health care agencies have instituted procedures for **isolation,** the separation of clients who have a specific communicable disease from those who do not, and have restricted client movements to stop the spread of that infection. The CDC has replaced the term *isolation* with the term *transmission-based precautions,* and these are collectively called CDC Tier 2 precautions. The three main categories are *airborne, droplet,* and *contact precautions.* If a large-scale communicable disease were to strike, such as after a natural disaster, public health officials would need to determine whether to **quarantine** (isolate) large groups of people affected.

Airborne Precautions. Airborne precautions are used to prevent infection when the infectious organism is capable of remaining in the air for prolonged periods of time and of being transported in the air for distances greater than 3 feet. The most recognized organism in this group is the tuberculosis bacterium, although the chickenpox and SARS viruses are also included in this category. Besides standard precautions, clients with these infections should be placed singly in an airborne infectious isolation room (AIIR) with negative pressure, if possible. The room should vent directly to the outside and have a designated minimum number of air exchanges (6 to 12) per hour. Anyone entering the room must wear a special particulate filter mask (N95 or greater). The use of these respirators requires individual fit testing for all personnel. The CDC also recommends limiting visitors and, in the cases of chickenpox, limiting caretakers to those already immune. The door to the room should remain closed unless entering or exiting.

Droplet Precautions. Droplet precautions refer to precautions used for organisms that can be spread by respiratory droplets but are unable to remain in the air farther than 3 feet. Thus a standard surgical mask (without a special filter) must be worn when entering the client's room, in addition to standard precautions. Many respiratory viral infections, including influenza, require droplet precautions.

Figure 22-2 compares three different types of masks. The first is the individually fitted particulate filter respirator mask required as part of airborne precautions. The second is a standard surgical mask that also contains a face shield to guard against exposure to splashes (it is often used in operating rooms). The third is a standard surgical mask that is routinely used as part of droplet precautions.

Contact Precautions. Contact precautions include standard precautions and the use of barrier precautions such as gloves and impermeable gowns. They are used when working with clients who have infections that are spread by direct or indirect contact. Examples are diarrhea, draining wounds not contained by the sterile dressing, or acquired antibiotic-resistant infections, such as

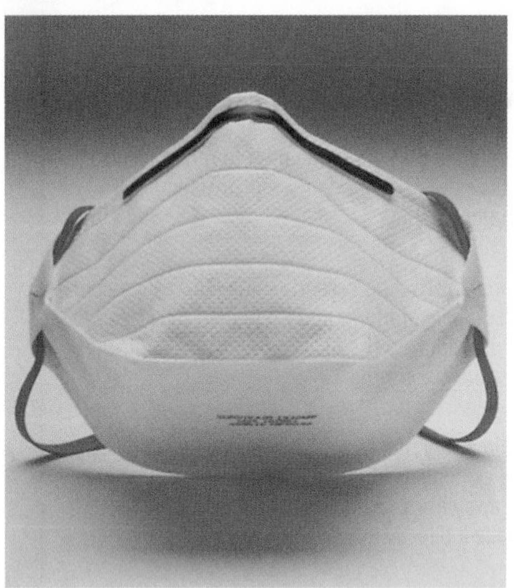

A

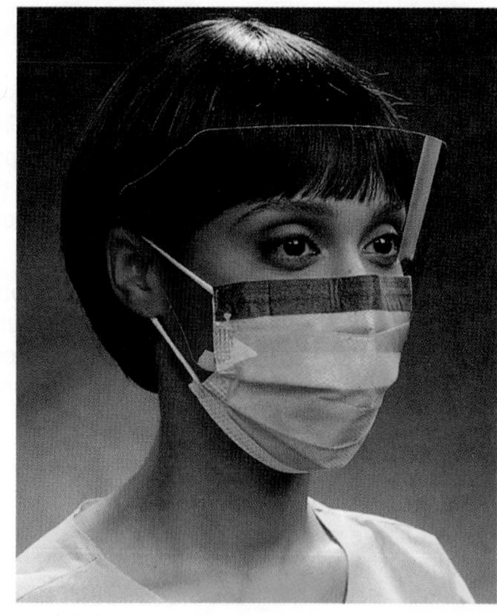

B

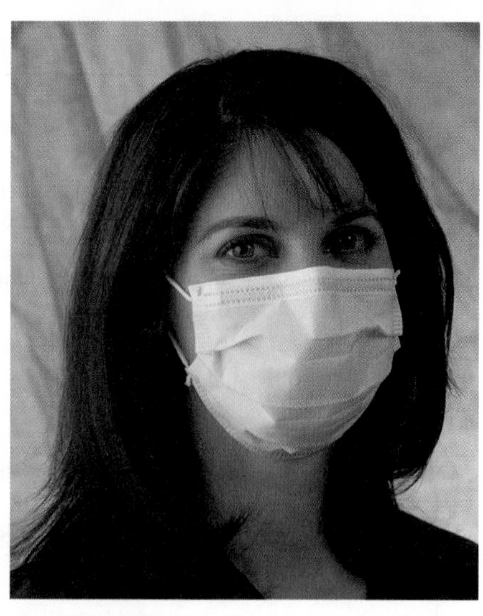

C

FIGURE 22-2 Masks/respirators used as barrier methods of infection control. **A,** Individually fitted N95 respirator. **B,** Surgical mask with face shield. **C,** Surgical mask. (**A** courtesy Uvex Safety, Smithfield, RI; **B** courtesy Kimberly-Clark, Roswell, GA; **C** courtesy Medline Industries, Mundelein, IL.)

Table 22-5 Precautions for Specific Clinical Syndromes or Conditions

CLINICAL SYNDROME OR CONDITION	POTENTIAL PATHOGENS	PRECAUTIONS
DIARRHEA		
Acute diarrhea with a likely infectious cause in an incontinent or diapered client	Enteric pathogens	Contact
Diarrhea in an adult with a history of recent antibiotic use	*Clostridium difficile*	Contact
RESPIRATORY INFECTIONS		
Cough, fever, upper-lobe pulmonary infiltrate in an HIV-negative client or a client at low risk for HIV infection	*Mycobacterium tuberculosis*	Airborne
Cough, fever, pulmonary infiltrate in any lung location in an HIV-infected client or a client at high risk for HIV infection	Atypical tuberculosis	Airborne
Respiratory infections, particularly bronchiolitis and croup, in infants and young children	Respiratory syncytial or parainfluenza virus	Contact
RISK OF MULTIDRUG-RESISTANT MICROORGANISMS		
History of infection or colonization with multidrug-resistant organisms	Resistant bacteria	Contact
Skin, wound, or urinary tract infection in a client with a recent hospital or nursing home stay in a facility where multidrug-resistant organisms are prevalent	Resistant bacteria	Contact

HIV, Human immunodeficiency virus.

MRSA. The goal of these precautions is to eliminate disease transmission resulting from either direct contact with the client or indirect contact through an intermediary infected object or surface that has been in contact with the client, such as instruments, linen, dressing materials, or any horizontal surface.

Table 22-5 outlines common clinical conditions that require some form of isolation and identifies the potential pathogens for these disorders and the precautions that are warranted. Procedure 22-2 describes how to appropriately don and remove gown, gloves, and face protection when working with a client in isolation.

AIIR rooms should be used to isolate clients with airborne infections. Private rooms can be used to isolate because of hygiene or to provide a protective environment. When available, rooms with negative pressure are useful for airborne infections such as tuberculosis or chickenpox. Negative-pressure rooms vent

TIME TO ALLOW: NOVICE: Variable EXPERT: Variable

PROCEDURE 22-2 CARING FOR A CLIENT ON ISOLATION PRECAUTIONS

Appropriate protective equipment should be used whenever you face a risk for exposure to infectious substances or nonintact client skin or mucous membranes. Likewise, in the case of protective isolation, appropriate protective equipment should be worn to protect the client from exposure to possibly infectious substances.

DELEGATION GUIDELINES

You may delegate aspects of your client's care to a nursing assistant or medical assistant who has received training in the performance of isolation procedures, consistent with your institution's policies and procedures.

EQUIPMENT NEEDED

- Gown; if fluid penetration is likely, use impenetrable gown
- Mask/respirator
- Goggles or face shield (if risk of splash is present)
- Gloves, well fitting
- Trash receptacle
- Laundry receptacle (if gown is nondisposable)

APPLICATION OF BARRIERS

1 Perform preliminary actions (see inside front cover).

2 Put on gown.

a. Pick up the gown by its collar, and allow it to unfold without touching the floor.

b. Put your arms through the sleeves, and pull the gown up over your shoulders (see illustration).

c. Fasten the neck ties (see illustration).

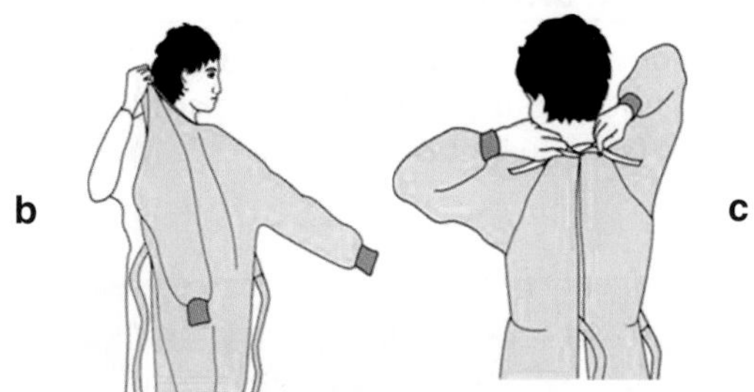

Step 2b & c. Lapping the gown over itself and fastening the waist ties. (From Department of Health and Human Services, Centers for Disease Control and Prevention. *Personal protective equipment (PPE) in healthcare settings.* Retrieved December 26, 2006, from http://www.cdc.gov/ncidod/dhqp/ppe.html.)

d. Make sure the gown laps over itself at the back, and fasten the waist ties. *Overlapping the back reduces the chance of contaminating the back of your clothing underneath the gown, especially when you are removing the gown.* Use second gown if necessary to cover back.

3 Put on the mask or respirator. Respirator masks should be well fitted.

a. Position the mask over your nose and mouth (see illustration).

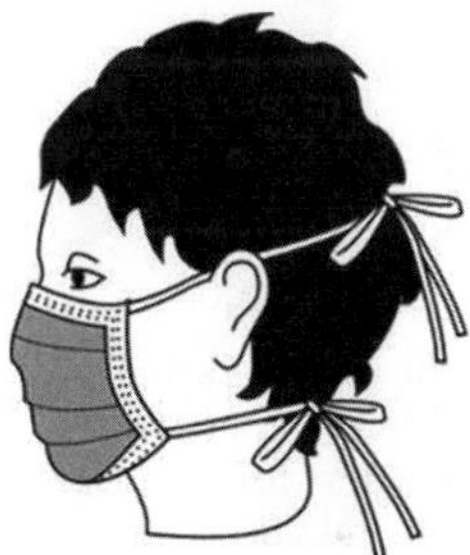

Step 3a. Surgical mask positioned over the nose and mouth. (From Department of Health and Human Services, Centers for Disease Control and Prevention. *Personal protective equipment (PPE) in healthcare settings.* Retrieved December 26, 2006, from http://www.cdc.gov/ncidod/dhqp/ppe.html.)

b. Bend the nose bar over the bridge of your nose for a snug fit. Eliminates air entering around the mask rather than through the mask.

c. Fasten the elastic bands, or tie the mask securely in place if it has strings. A mask reduces potential exposure to respiratory droplets. Plan to change your mask every 30 minutes because its effectiveness dramatically drops after that time period.

4 Put on eyewear, if indicated, after your mask or respirator is in place (see illustration). Protective eyewear is indicated in situations where splattering of blood or secretions is possible. If you wear prescriptions eyeglasses, protective face shield may be applied instead of goggles.

Continued

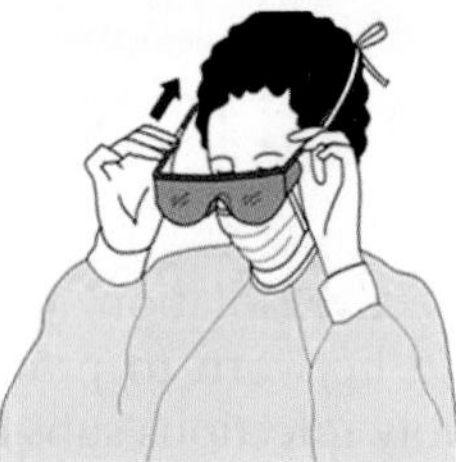

Step 4. Putting on eyewear. (From Department of Health and Human Services, Centers for Disease Control and Prevention. *Personal protective equipment (PPE) in health-care settings.* Retrieved December 26, 2006, from http://www.cdc.gov/ncidod/dhqp/ppe.html.)

5 Put on disposable gloves.

a. Pull the cuff of each glove over the edge of the gown sleeve (see illustration). *Prevents transmission of microorganisms between you and the client.*

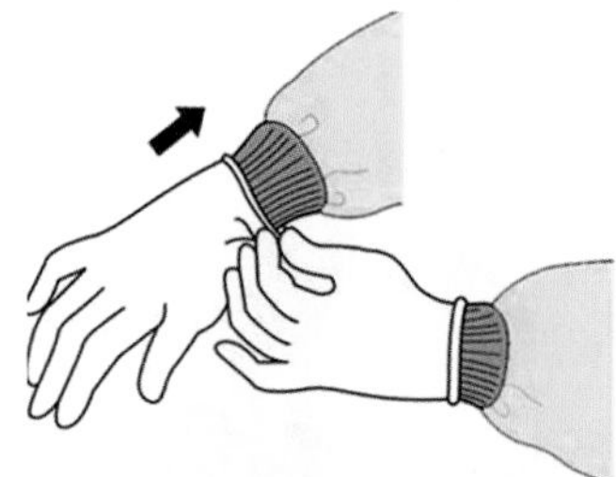

Step 5a. Pulling the cuff of each glove over the edge of the gown sleeve. (From Department of Health and Human Services, Centers for Disease Control and Prevention. *Personal protective equipment (PPE) in health-care settings.* Retrieved December 26, 2006, from http://www.cdc.gov/ncidod/dhqp/ppe.html.)

b. Interlace your fingers, if needed, to adjust the fit of the gloves.

6 Administer care to client. After disposing of soiled items used in client care, tie the bag securely (see illustration). If special disposal methods are used, and the bag is not prelabeled, mark the bag appropriately. Each state has a medical waste law that outlines what is considered medical waste and needs to be placed into a red or orange bag.

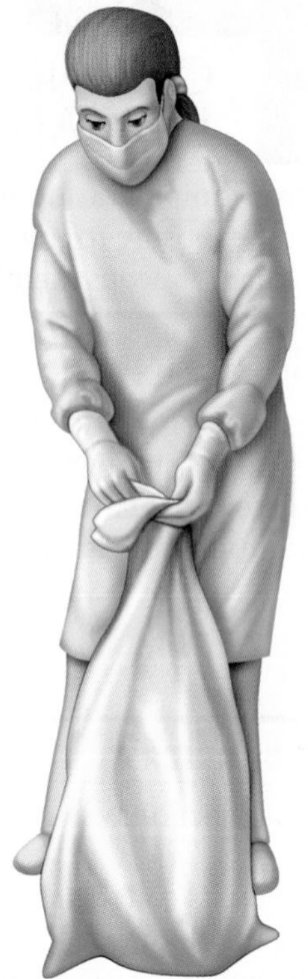

Step 6. Tying the bag securely.

REMOVAL OF BARRIERS

1 At the door to the client's room and next to a trash container, untie your gown at the waist but do not remove it yet (see illustration).

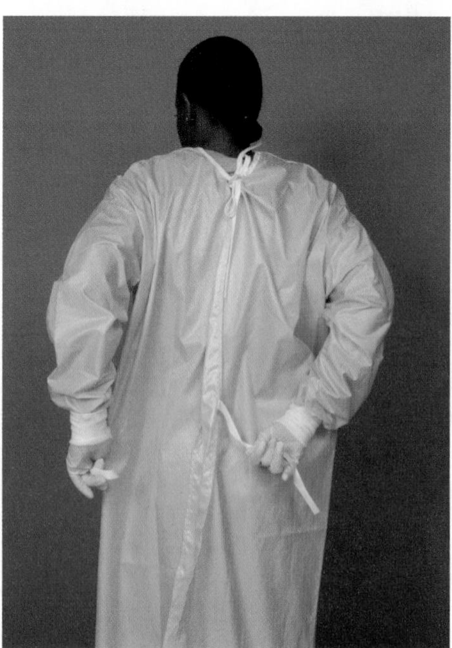

Step 1. Untying the gown at the waist.

2 Remove your gloves.

a. Grasp the outside of the cuff of one glove, and pull the glove inside out over your hand (see illustrations). Hold the removed glove in the second hand.

b. Tuck an ungloved finger inside the cuff of the remaining glove.

c. Pull the second glove off inside out (see illustration), and discard both gloves. *This method prevents contamination of your hands by microorganisms.*

1

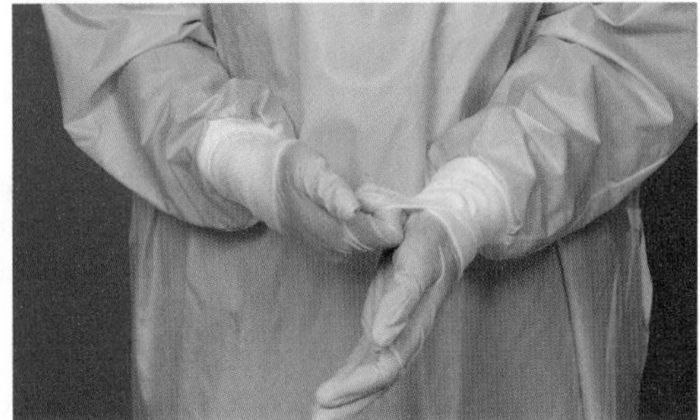

2

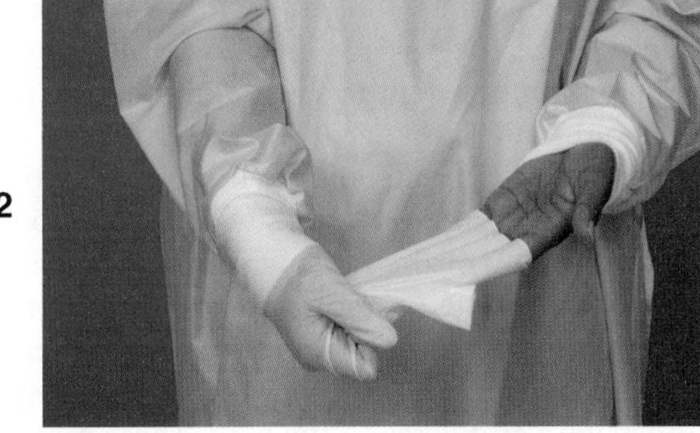

Step 2a. (1) Grasping the cuff. (2) Pulling the first glove inside out.

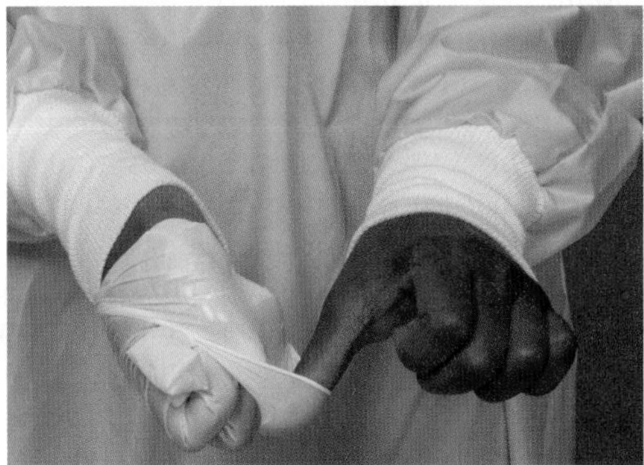

Step 2c. Pulling the second glove inside out.

3 Remove your gown.

a. Untie your gown at the neck, and allow it to fall forward from your shoulders (see illustration).

b. Slide your hands through the sleeves, and remove them without touching the outside of the gown.

c. Hold the gown at the inside shoulder seams and away from your body, allowing it to turn inside out.

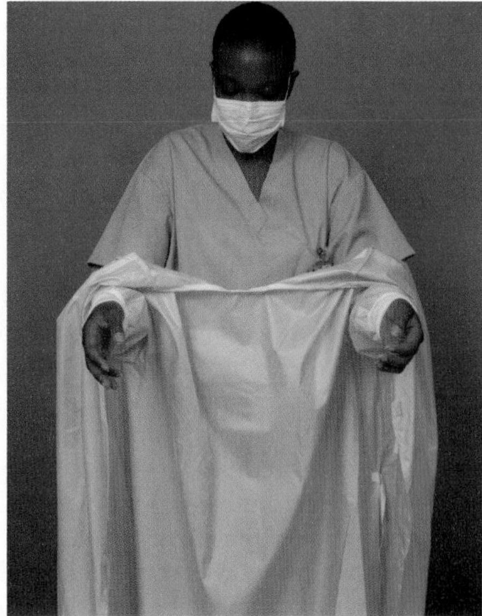

Step 3a. Allowing the gown to fall forward from the shoulders.

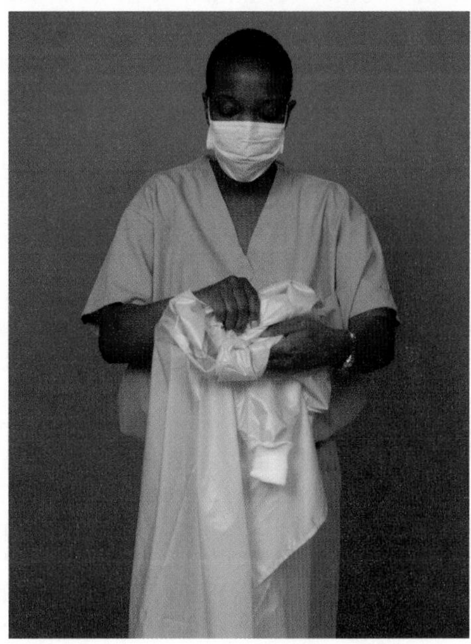

Step 3c. Folding the contaminated side of the gown to the inside.

Fold the contaminated side of the gown to the inside (see illustration).

d. Discard the gown in an appropriate receptacle.

4 Remove your mask or respirator and goggles (if used).

a. Pull the elastic or untie the strings from the back of the head without touching the mask's outer surface. Touch only the strings or elastic.

b. Place the mask or respirator in an appropriate receptacle. *These steps prevent cross-contamination. Unless covered in blood, masks or respirators are not considered to be medical waste.*

5 Perform hand hygiene.

directly to the outside and must have air exchanges with outside air, not with air circulated from the rest of the ventilation system unless it is filtered before recirculation. Positive-pressure rooms are those rooms that prevent the air from the rest of the agency from entering the room, thereby minimizing the possibility of introducing infectious agents to the client. To be effective, doors to both negative- and positive-pressure rooms should be kept closed.

Many health care facilities use a special cart placed outside the client's room to conveniently store personal protective equipment (PPE) needed when caring for clients on transmission-based precautions. PPE includes gloves (preferably nonlatex), impermeable gowns, masks, and protective eyewear. Whenever droplet, airborne, or protective precautions are implemented, PPE must be available to all of the client's visitors as well.

Because standard precautions require that all bodily fluids except sweat be treated as potentially infectious, laboratory specimens are now treated as if they are infectious. This usually requires placing the specimen container in another container, such as a bag that is clean on the outside and has not come into contact with the laboratory specimen. The bag is labeled with a biohazard alert symbol to indicate that the specimen may be potentially infectious (Figure 22-3). Health care personnel should wear gloves when handling the actual specimen containers. Laboratory personnel should use gloves and barrier precautions when actually handling the material.

The CDC discusses a fourth type of isolation, known as protective isolation. This is used for immunocompromised clients, who would have a nursing diagnosis of *Ineffective protection.* This type of isolation is discussed further when we look at interventions for clients with this nursing diagnosis. Here, it is especially important that the nurse follow work restriction guidelines and not present for client care if ill. If a nurse works when ill, this poses an increased risk for infection for the client and an increased risk for the nurse. OSHA is enforcing the CDC work restriction guidelines as a means to protect both client and care provider.

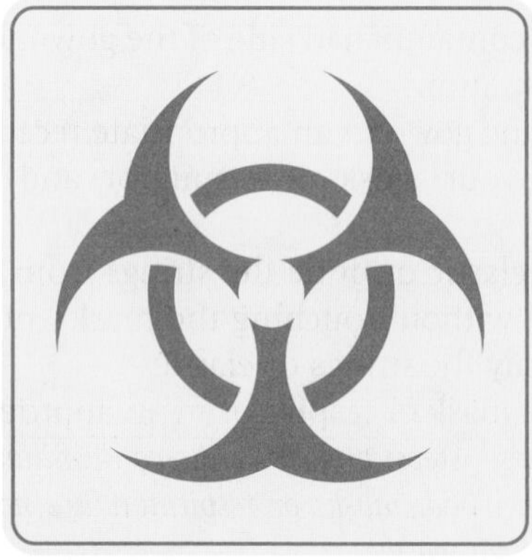

FIGURE 22-3 Biohazard alert symbol.

Action Alert! Use protective isolation for clients with compromised immune systems.

The infection control methods used when transporting clients on isolation depend on the isolation category. For clients requiring just standard precautions, there are no special precautions. Those with additional precautions should have limited movement and be transported as infrequently as possible out of their room. If it becomes necessary to transport these clients from their room, it is essential to maintain precautions to minimize the risk of transmitting the infecting organism to other clients or to the environment. Clients with droplet precautions or airborne precautions should wear a common surgical mask when outside their room. Never place a respirator mask on a client. Respirator masks filter the air that comes in through a mask. A surgical mask filters the air that goes out through the mask.

Controlling Infection in the Home. Whenever a nurse delivers care in the home, interventions must include the input of the client and any other residents into the plan of care. Because the nurse has less control over interventions to minimize the risk for infection, it is critical to have participation of both the client and others living in the household to develop needed interventions to reach the agreed-upon client outcomes. Without the participation of the entire group, outcomes will certainly be less than optimal. Many of the nursing interventions in the home revolve around education and the understanding of the residents. Because the nurse is usually there for only a prescribed period of time, the main caregivers must understand and agree to the plan. These caregivers may consist of family members or family plus home health care workers, depending on the client's situation and ability to provide self-care.

Managing Risk For Infection. The basic element of infection control to prevent the spread of infection in the home is the same as in the hospital: good hand hygiene. It is also important for the home health caregiver to know how the infection is transmitted to reduce the potential for infecting others. Basic hygiene, proper food preparation, and pest control might also be issues that may require attention. Principles of good nutrition and signs and symptoms of infection are other educational issues for the nurse working in home health care (Box 22-7).

Action Alert! Teach the home health care client about the importance of hand hygiene as a basic infection control measure.

The client who is discharged to home after a surgical procedure is often responsible for daily self-monitoring of wound status and self-care for the wound until a follow-up appointment has been scheduled with the surgeon.

However, as part of the campaign to monitor health care–acquired infection rates, many medical facilities are telephoning clients post discharge and asking questions to determine possible postoperative infection. Because an incision is a break in the skin, a first line of defense, surgical clients are at increased risk for infection by virtue of the surgery. Box 22-8 provides information for clients on how to manage a wound to prevent postoperative infection. The principles of medical asepsis also apply.

Managing Ineffective Protection. Good hand hygiene is an educational issue that can never be addressed too many times and should be reviewed periodically when caring for immunocompromised clients in the home setting. A clear understanding of why their protection for infection is ineffective is essential to minimizing their risk. Assess for situations or practices that should be changed because of the ineffective protection, and address these issues with the client and caregivers. Box 22-9 provides instructions for methods to minimize the risk of an immunocompromised client's acquiring an infection in the home.

A health care worker in the home must use the same precautions to prevent the spread of infection from the client to others. Good hand hygiene is still required, but unfortunately some homes may not have running water and soap as readily available resources. In these instances, you must use alcohol-based hand rubs. Use barrier precautions as you would in the health care setting if contact with potentially infectious material is possible. The barrier precautions used in the home are the same: gloves, water-impermeable gown, mask or respirator, and eye protection (appropriate to the task being performed.). If occupants of the home, other than the client, need to use selected barriers, ensure that the necessary items are available to them and give instructions on their correct use.

BOX 22-7 *Teaching Tips for Preventing Infection in the Home*

Food Handling

- Good hand hygiene is the best defense against infection.
- Perform hand hygiene after using the bathroom and before preparing or eating food.
- When cleaning and cutting chicken, perform hand hygiene before preparing other foods.
- Clean work area after cleaning or cutting chicken, or use separate areas for preparing chicken versus other foods.
- Wash all fresh fruits and vegetables before eating them.
- Store leftover food in the refrigerator. Use airtight containers.
- Do not refreeze uncooked meat that has been thawed.
- Cook ground meat, chicken, and pork thoroughly. Wash chicken before preparing.

Respiratory Etiquette/Hygiene

- Keep tissues handy to catch sneezes and coughs.
- Keep a wastebasket/paper bag close to the sick person.
- Perform hand hygiene often to help reduce the chance of spreading a cold or the flu.

Caring for Minor Scrapes and Cuts

- Clean the wound with mild soap and water, and pat it dry.
- Cover it with a bandage if it is bleeding or likely to become contaminated.

BOX 22-8 *Teaching for Self-Care*

Wound Care

Purpose: To keep a wound from getting infected.
Expected Outcome: The client will clean the wound and experience complete healing without incurring an infection.

Client Instructions

- Assemble the supplies you'll need, such as fresh sterile gauze, saline, antibiotic cream (if appropriate), tape, and a trash can.
- Perform hand hygiene.
- Remove your old dressing, and place it in the trash.
- Look to see if the wound has any new redness, tenderness, or drainage. If it does, tell your doctor or nurse about it.
- Using some sterile gauze moistened with saline, wipe your incision from the center out to an edge one time. Then throw the gauze in the trash.
- Using a new piece of moistened sterile gauze, wipe your wound one more time from the center to the edge. Go in a different direction this time.
- Repeat the preceding step until you have cleaned the entire wound.
- Allow the wound to air dry.
- Apply antibiotic cream if your doctor told you to.
- Cover the incision with sterile gauze, and tape it in place.

BOX 22-9 *Teaching for Self-Care*

Preventing Infection in Immunosuppressed Clients

Purpose: To prevent the client from acquiring an infection at home.
Expected Outcome: The client will continue to function at home without acquiring an infection.

Client Instructions

- Gather as many of your friends and family as possible to learn about keeping you free from infection.
- Perform hand hygiene often with soap and water. This is the best means to prevent infection.
- If you have pets, consult your physician. The presence of pets has been documented to assist clients in health improvement.
- Have any dusting or vacuuming done when you are not in the room.
- If you have living plants in the house, have someone else water them.
- You may need to alter what you eat. For example, all meats should be cooked thoroughly until well done. Also, eat no thin-skinned fresh fruits or vegetables unless they are canned. This includes grapes, peaches, and apples. (Ask clients for their own examples to ensure understanding of this point.)
- Ask your friends to visit you at another time if they feel ill.

Implementing Sterile Technique. Sterile technique refers to those practices used to prevent the introduction of microorganisms that could cause infection. This is sometimes called *surgical aseptic technique.* Sterile technique is used when there is a break in the first line of defense (i.e., the skin and mucous membranes) and may be indicated for selected procedures performed by the nurse or other health care personnel at the bedside or during surgical procedures. Sterile technique as used during surgery requires extensive procedures for preventing microorganisms from entering surgical wounds. There are three areas of application of this technique: the skin, physical barriers (sterile field), and the environment.

Skin. The client's skin is thoroughly cleansed before any invasive procedure. This may involve washing first with soap to remove soil. The area is then thoroughly painted with an antimicrobial agent that is left on the skin as an antimicrobial barrier. Hair is sometimes removed with hair clippers or depilatory preparations; if so, it should be done before cleansing.

Aside from surgery, sterile technique is used whenever host defenses are interrupted, such as during catheter insertion (e.g., IV and urinary), dressing changes for many surgical wounds, or endotracheal suctioning. It should also be used during IV fluid or medication administration. Box 22-10 outlines the principles of sterile technique.

Sterile Field. Using sterile technique for limited procedures outside the operating room involves setting up a small sterile field with a few pieces of equipment and using sterile gloves to handle sterile equipment. Procedure 22-3 describes how to apply and remove sterile gloves.

When setting up a sterile field, you may open a tray that already contains sterile materials wrapped in a drape. At other times, you may be required to use a drape to set up the sterile field and then place sterile supplies onto that sterile drape. Procedures 22-4 and 22-5 review how to prepare a sterile field using a tray wrapped in a sterile drape and how to set up a sterile field using a sterile drape.

BOX 22-10 *Principles of Sterile Technique*

- Sterile means the absence of all microorganisms.
- The skin cannot be sterilized, but thorough cleaning can significantly reduce the number of microorganisms present.
- Sterile objects that come in contact with unsterile objects are no longer sterile.
- When a sterile field is wet, capillary action will draw microorganisms from the surface underneath a permeable drape. This is called *strike-through.* A wet drape is not a sterile drape.
- Consider anything below the waist to be unsterile.
- Consider any part of the sterile field that falls or hangs below the top of the table to be unsterile. Waist level is the limit of a good visual field.
- Consider the edge of a sterile field and 2 inches inward as unsterile, but do not touch it.
- Do not cough, sneeze, or talk excessively over a sterile field.
- Do not reach across a sterile field.
- Always face a sterile field. If you turn your back on it, you cannot guarantee its sterility.
- Use a sterile package immediately once it has been opened. Otherwise, it cannot be considered sterile.
- Consider a bottle of sterile liquid no longer sterile once it has been opened. If you save it to repeat a procedure, you may be performing a clean procedure, but you will not be performing a sterile procedure.
- Sterile packages have expiration dates determined by the manufacturer or the method of sterilization. Do not use packages that have passed their expiration date.
- Sterile packages are labeled as sterile. If a package is not so labeled, consider it unsterile.
- If there is any doubt about the sterility of an object, consider it unsterile.
- If a sterile package is wet or damaged, or if there is evidence that moisture has dried on it, consider it unsterile.

TIME TO ALLOW: NOVICE: 2 min. EXPERT: 15 seconds

PROCEDURE 22-3 DONNING AND REMOVING STERILE GLOVES

Nursing Skills Online: Infection Control, Lesson 4

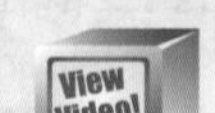

Sterile gloves should be used when performing procedures requiring surgical asepsis. This will eliminate the risk of introducing microorganisms from the caregiver to a sterile object or to the client.

DELEGATION GUIDELINES

Some of the tasks that you will delegate to your nursing assistant or medical assistant may require the use of sterile gloves. Nursing assistants or medical assistants should receive appropriate training in this skill before the delegation of such tasks.

EQUIPMENT NEEDED

- One package sterile gloves of appropriate hand size
- Flat work surface
- Other supplies as needed according to procedure being performed

DONNING STERILE GLOVES

1 Perform preliminary actions (see inside front cover). Remove rings with stones or irregular surfaces. Reduces microorganisms and the risk of puncturing the gloves with the rings.

2 Grasp the package at the tabs above the upper sealed edge. Peel down to open the outer wrapper to display the gloves. Discard the outer wrapper.

3 Place the inner package on a flat surface. Open the inner package at the first fold, touching the outside of the folded edge and pulling outward. Then open the next fold, pulling that edge outward without touching the inside of the package. The package is usually labeled "up" and "down," or "left" and "right." Opening in this manner creates a sterile field. The outside of the wrapper is now contaminated. Gloves are now laid out with the left glove on the left and the right glove on the right.

4 Put on the first glove.

a. Grasp the folded edge of the cuff of one glove (see illustration). Usually, the dominant hand is gloved first.

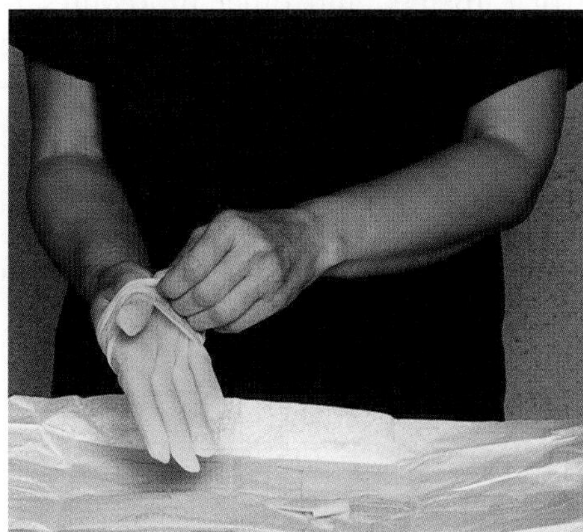

Step 4a. Grasping the folded edge of the cuff of one glove.

b. Lift the glove above the wrapper and away from your body. Lift the glove straight up (perpendicular to the wrapper) to avoid dragging the gloves over the contaminated edge of the wrapper. Step back if necessary to give yourself room to glove without touching a contaminated surface.

c. Do not adjust the cuff or fingers now or let your ungloved hand touch the outside of the glove. *This technique maintains sterility by preventing contact of the gloves with unsterile objects, such as the hand, uniform, or other surfaces.*

d. Place your thumb inside the top cuff edge. Stretch the glove over your fingertips.

5 Put on the second glove.

a. Pick up the second glove by sliding your sterile gloved fingers under the edge of the cuff (see illustration). Avoid the tendency to let your gloved thumb touch the (to become) unsterile surface of the cuff of the second glove. *Prevents the gloved thumb from coming in contact with a surface that will also be touching the ungloved hand.*

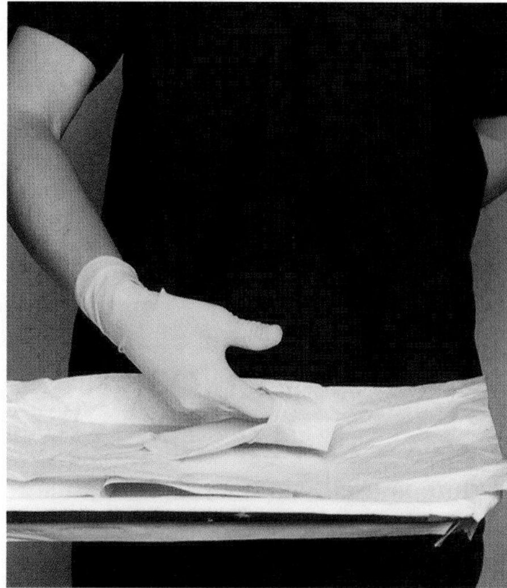

Step 5a. Picking up the second glove.

b. Keep your fingers straight. Slide the fingers of your opposite hand into the glove (see illustration). Let go of the edge when your hand is in the glove. As you slide your hand into the glove, the hand that is holding the glove should stretch the edge of the glove out to avoid touching the unsterile wrist.

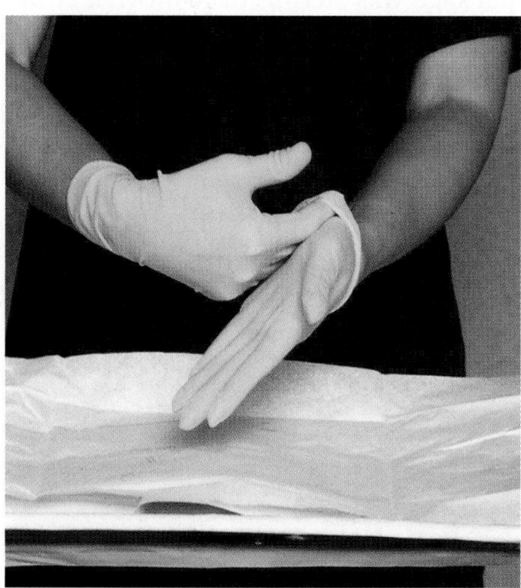

Step 5b. Sliding the fingers of the opposite hand into the glove.

Continued

c. Adjust the gloves for comfort and fit. Your fingers are touching the outside of the glove that will remain sterile. Keep sterile surface to sterile surface. The edges of the glove touching your wrist are not sterile.

REMOVING STERILE GLOVES

1 Grasp the first glove just below the wrist. Prevents the used and contaminated glove from coming in contact with the skin of your wrist.

2 Fold it over and peel it back, turning it inside out. Once it is almost off hold it in the palm of the gloved hand.

3 Slide your ungloved thumb or fingers inside the second glove, and remove it by pulling it inside out also. If you held the first glove in your hand, they are now wrapped together.

4 Discard into appropriate receptacle.

5 Perform hand hygiene.

PROCEDURE 22-4 PREPARING A STERILE FIELD BY OPENING A TRAY WRAPPED IN A STERILE DRAPE

TIME TO ALLOW: **NOVICE:** 1 min. **EXPERT:** 15 seconds

This procedure is used when a microorganism-free surface is needed to hold materials for dressing changes, insertion of catheters, and other procedures requiring that sterility of objects on the field be maintained.

DELEGATION GUIDELINES

You may delegate the preparation of a sterile field to a nursing assistant or medical assistant who has been appropriately trained in the performance of this task. You would generally not delegate the actual performance of a sterile procedure to a nursing assistant.

EQUIPMENT NEEDED

- Wrapped sterile package
- Flat work surface
- Sterile gloves and other items required to perform the intended procedure on an actual client

1 Perform preliminary actions (see inside front cover).

2 Check the integrity of the package. If using nondisposable items, note whether the indicator tape shows that the package was sterilized. Remove a commercially packaged kit from the outer wrapper. Dispose of wrapper in general trash.

3 Position the inner package in the center of the work surface so that the outer flap of the wrapper is facing away from you.

4 Reach around (but not over) the package to open the flap away from yourself (see illustration). Touch the outside of the flap only. *Maintains sterility of the package.*

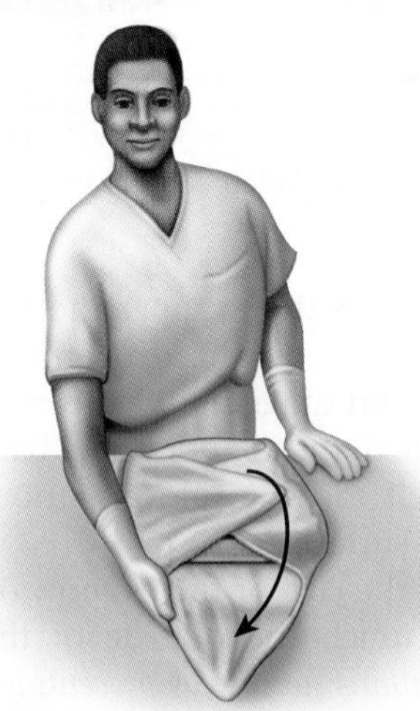

Step 4. Opening the first flap away from yourself.

5 Open the side flaps one at a time, in the same manner as the first, with the uppermost side flap being opened first (see illustration). Remember not to let your hands cross over the sterile field.

6 Open the innermost flap that faces you last (see illustration). Be sure to stand back sufficiently so that the flap does not touch you during opening.

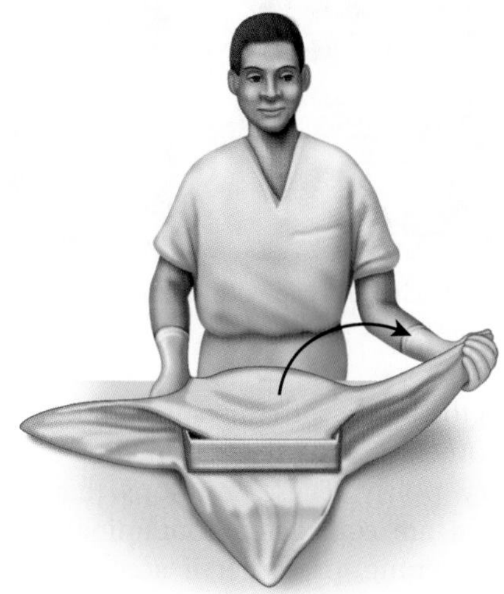

Step 5. Opening the side flaps.

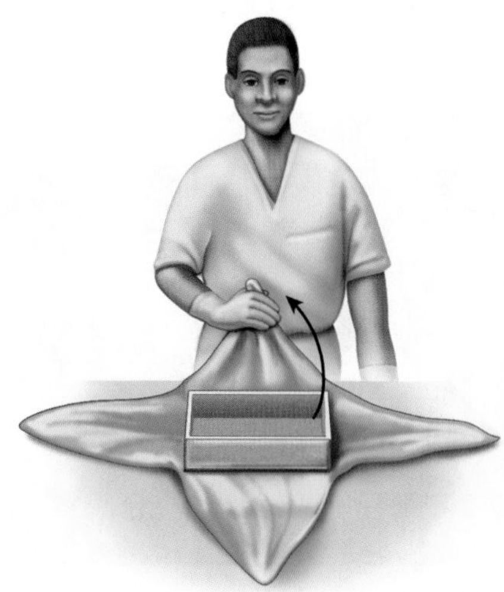

Step 6. Opening the last flap toward yourself.

PROCEDURE 22-5

PREPARING A STERILE FIELD

TIME TO ALLOW: NOVICE: 6 min. EXPERT: 3 min.

This procedure is used when a microorganism-free surface is needed to hold materials for dressing changes, insertion of catheters, and other procedures requiring the sterility of the objects on the field.

DELEGATION GUIDELINES

You may delegate the preparation of a sterile field to a nursing assistant or medical assistant who has been appropriately trained in the performance of this task. You would generally not delegate the actual performance of a sterile procedure to a nursing assistant.

EQUIPMENT NEEDED

- Sterile drape
- Sterile gloves
- Sterile supplies and/or solutions as needed for the planned procedure
- Protective barrier equipment as needed according to the planned procedure

1 Perform preliminary actions (see inside front cover).

2 Arrange your work area. Use a clean, dry, flat, uncluttered surface at waist level. The sterile field should be close to the client. *You should position the field in a manner that allows you to work with the client and keep the field within your line of vision.*

3 Ensure that supplies are sterile by checking the expiration date and for the integrity of the package. *If the package is damaged in any way or shows signs of moisture, it cannot be used. This protects the client from being touched by contaminated supplies.*

4 Set up a drape as a sterile field.

a. Prepare a sterile field or surface that is at least 2 inches larger on all sides than the area you need to work with the supplies.
   (1) Open the outer wrapping of a sterile cloth drape, keeping the drape itself sterile.
   (2) Pick up the drape by the loose corner edge, and lift the drape into the air and away from your body.
   (3) With your other hand, grasp another corner edge and spread the drape in the air.

Continued

(4) Decide which surface is to remain sterile, and spread the drape on the table, with the side that will remain sterile facing up (see illustration). *Alternatively, if you are setting up this field without access to sterile gloves, touch only corner flap that is folded inward and lay the drape on the table.*

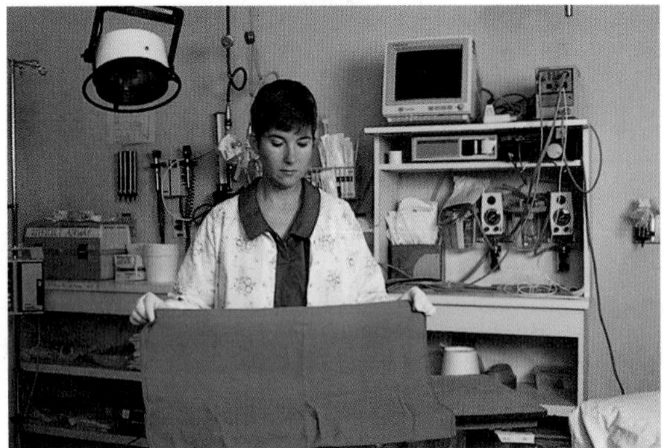

Step 4a(4). Spreading the drape on the table, with the side that will remain sterile facing up

5 Add sterile supplies.

a. **Peel-Apart Packages**

(1) Use both hands and grasp the edges designed to be peeled open.

(2) Open the package over the sterile field so materials can fall freely from the package onto the field without touching your hands (see illustration).

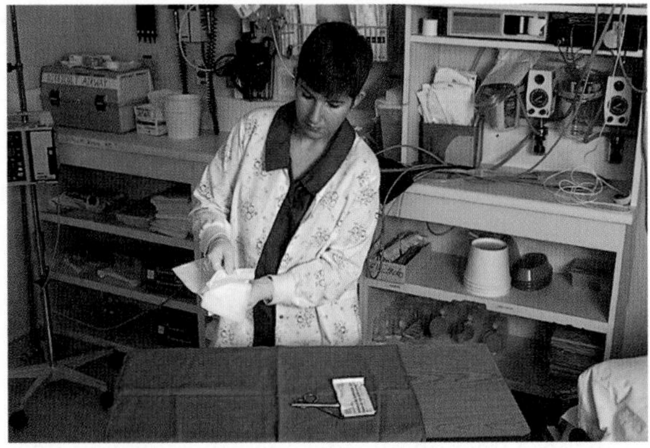

Step 5a(2). Opening the package over the sterile field.

b. **Sterile Liquids**

(1) Remove or loosen the cap from the bottle of liquid. Do not touch the inside of the cap or the rim of the liquid. Place the cap so the inside is face-up on a flat, unsterile surface to prevent its contamination (see illustration).

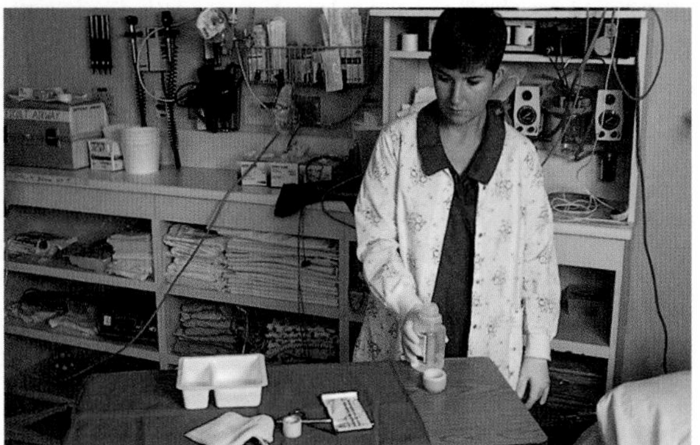

Step 5b(1). Placing the cap with the inside face up on the unsterile surface.

(2) Label the bottle with the date and time. Solutions are sometime reused after opening according to agency policy. These solutions that have been opened are considered contaminated 24 hours after opening, or earlier if according to agency policy. When this policy is followed, the procedure is a clean procedure, not a sterile procedure.

(3) If the container that will hold the liquid needs to be adjusted, put on one sterile glove.

(4) Use the other ungloved hand to pick up the bottle of liquid so that the label is in the palm of your hand. This prevents the solution from damaging the label if fluid drips or runs down the side of the bottle. This is only important when the solution is used within 24 hours for a clean procedure.

(5) Hold the bottle of solution about 10 cm (4 inches) above the container that will receive the liquid. Pour carefully to avoid spills or splashes (see illustration). Do not touch the field with the lid of the bottle. *If you get the surface of a permeable sterile field wet, it is no longer sterile. The bottle cannot touch the sterile field for the same reason.*

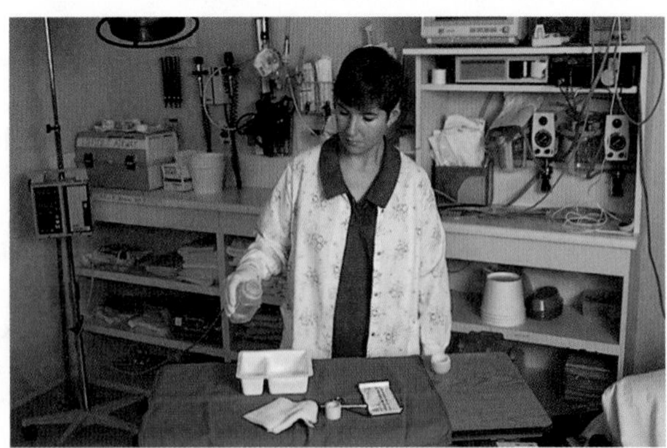

Step 5b(5). Pouring the sterile liquid.

(6) Replace the lid on the bottle tightly. Eliminates the risk of spilling the bottle during the procedure.
(7) Put on the second (or both) sterile glove(s).

c. **Wrapped Packages**
(1) Hold the object in one hand by the bottom or underside of the wrapping.
(2) Unwrap the first corner away from you, then each side, then the last corner toward you.
(3) Stabilize the corners against your wrist. This prevents the corners from touching the sterile object.
(4) Turn the object toward the sterile surface and drop it onto the field without touching the field itself.

A member of the surgical team who will work within a sterile field scrubs the hands and arms before entering the operating room to put on sterile attire. The hands and arms are first washed with soap and water to remove gross soil. Hands and arms are then washed with an antimicrobial soap using a sponge to remove as many microorganisms as possible. The use of scrubbing has been eliminated. Studies have shown that this process raises unwanted organisms to the surface. The soap leaves an antimicrobial residual that continues to prevent the presence of microorganisms after the washing. Note, however, that the friction from using a sponge is the most effective component of reducing the organisms on the skin. The objective is to remove microorganisms without destroying tissue. Procedure 22-6 describes how to perform surgical hand asepsis.

To maintain the area free of microorganisms, sterile gloves, gowns, and drapes are used to create a barrier between the environment (including the members of the team) and the client. To achieve an outer surface that is sterile, a gown and gloves are put on to cover the body. The technique for putting on a gown and gloves requires not touching the outer surface of the attire. After the procedure, careful removal of the gown and gloves is important to prevent contamination of the clothing under the gown. Procedure 22-7 describes how to don a sterile gown and use closed gloving technique. The basics of setting up a sterile field in the operating room include covering the client with sterile drapes, covering work surfaces with sterile drapes, and laying out sterile instruments on the sterile field.

PROCEDURE 22-6

TIME TO ALLOW: NOVICE: Determined by agency policy; usually 10 minutes **EXPERT:** Determined by agency policy; usually 10 minutes

PERFORMING A SURGICAL HAND SCRUB

This procedure removes as many microorganisms from your hands as possible before entering a surgical field.

DELEGATION GUIDELINES

The scope of nursing assistant duties in a surgical arena does not generally require the completion of a surgical hand scrub. Nursing assistants or medical assistants may be responsible for the assembly of scrub supplies and should be familiar with this procedure for this purpose alone.

EQUIPMENT NEEDED

- Agency-approved antimicrobial agent
- Deep sink with knee or foot controls for water and soap—operating room area

1 Perform preliminary actions (see inside front cover).

2 Apply surgical attire, including shoe covers, cap or hood, face mask, and protective eyewear (possibly a mask with a face shield).

3 Turn on the water using the control lever, and adjust it to a comfortably warm temperature.

4 Wet your hands and arms, keeping your elbows flexed so that your hands remain higher than your elbows. Water will flow off your arms at the elbows. *Keeps the hands as the cleanest part of the extremities.*

Continued

5 Clean under your nails on both hands (see illustration). *Removes materials under the fingernails that could harbor a variety of microorganisms.*

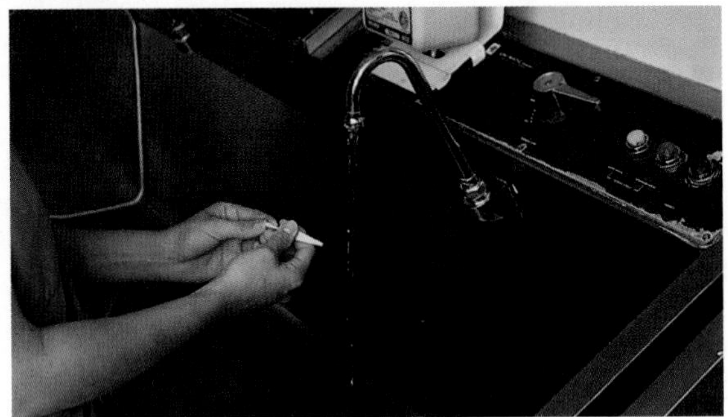

Step 5. Using a plastic nail stick to clean under the fingernails.

6 Apply antimicrobial liquid or alcohol-based foam or gel or according to agency policy.

7 When using antimicrobial soap, wash hands and forearms for the amount of time recommended by the manufacturer. Usually 2 to 6 minutes is appropriate. *Longer times are not necessary and may result in the development of dermatitis*

8 When using an alcohol-based product, prewash hands with soap and water. Dry completely. Use alcohol-based product according to the manufacturer's instruction. Allow hands to dry before applying gloves.

9 Turn backward to open door into the operating room with your hands elevated in front of you and away from your body. *Allows you to keep cleansed hands above waist level and in your line of vision. Reduces the possibility that your hands will become contaminated.*

10 If using an antimicrobial soap, go to the sterile set-up area. Pick up a sterile towel without dripping water onto the sterile field. Using one end of the towel, dry one hand completely using a rotating motion and moving from fingers to elbow. *Dries from cleanest area (fingers) to less clean (elbows).*

11 Using other end of the towel, repeat with other hand and drop the towel into the designated receptacle or an assistant's hand.

Time to Allow: **Novice:** Variable **Expert:** 7-10 min.

PROCEDURE 22-7 DONNING A STERILE GOWN AND CLOSED GLOVING

This procedure is done before entering a surgical (sterile) field.

DELEGATION GUIDELINES

The scope of nursing assistant duties in a surgical arena does not generally require the donning of a sterile gown and closed gloving. A nursing assistant may be responsible for the assembly of these supplies and should be familiar with this procedure for this purpose alone.

EQUIPMENT NEEDED

- Surgical shoe covers, cap, mask, and protective eyewear
- One package sterile gloves of appropriate size
- One sterile pack containing sterile gown
- Clean, flat, dry surface for opening gown and gloves (such as a Mayo stand)

1 Follow preliminary actions (see inside front cover).

2 Don surgical attire, and scrub your arms and hands as described in Procedure 22-6.

3 Have the circulating nurse or other designated person open the sterile gown and gloves.

4 Don the gown.

a. Hold your arms out straight in front of you, and the scrub nurse will slip the gown over your hands and arms. If no scrub nurse is available,
   (1) Identify the inner surface of the gown, and pick up the gown beneath the neckband without touching the sterile field or the outer surface of the gown.
   (2) Make sure you have control of all the folded layers to avoid dangling the gown against unsterile surfaces.

(3) Move away from the table, holding the gown away from your body at arm's length, and allow it to unfold from the top down (see illustration). Do not let the gown touch the floor. *Maintains sterility of the gown.*

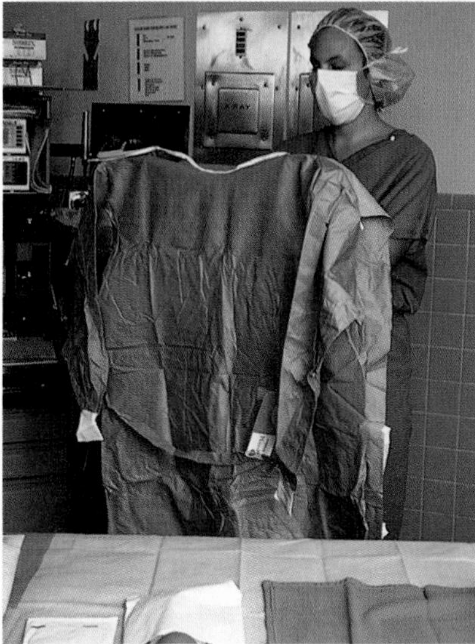

Step 4a(3). Holding the gown at arm's length and allowing it to unfold.

(4) Hold the gown just below the neckband near the shoulders, and slide both hands into the sleeves until the fingers are at the end of the cuffs but not through the cuffs (see illustration). The fingers remain covered to prepare for closed gloving.

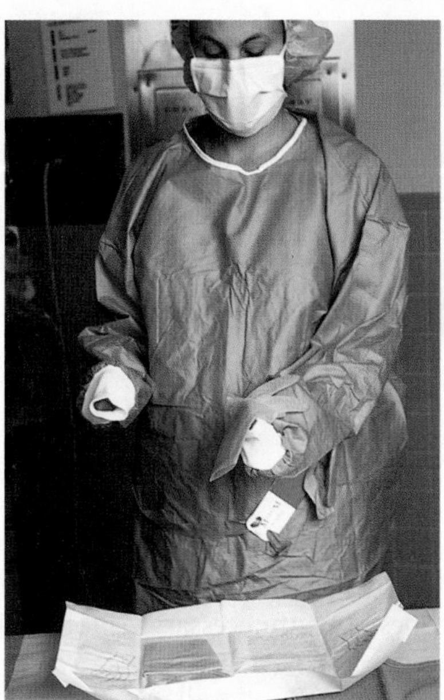

Step 4a(4). Sliding the hands into the sleeves.

(5) Have someone tie the gown. *The gown should be lapped over itself in the back. The person tying the gown should take care to touch only the ties and not the front or sides of the gown. The front of the gown is sterile.*

5 Put on the gloves.

a. Apply the first glove.

(1) With your hands covered by the sterile gown cuffs, open the inner sterile glove package and pick up the first glove by the cuff (see illustration). The first glove goes on the dominant hand.

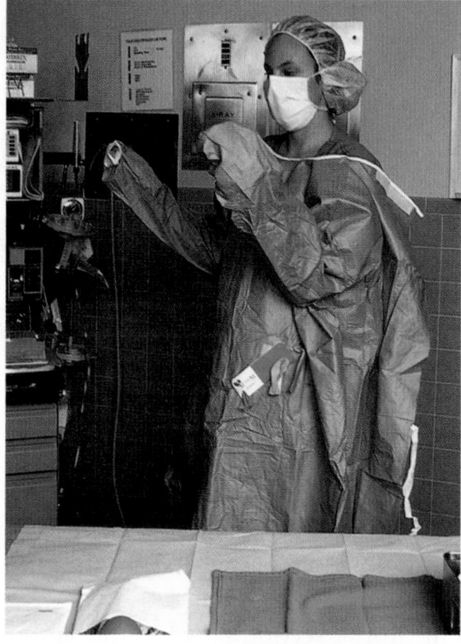

Step 5a(1). Picking up the first glove by the cuff.

(2) Position the glove on the forearm so the cuff faces the hand and the fingers face the elbow.

(3) Begin to put the opposite hand into the glove. Hold the cuff edge of the glove with the sleeve cover of the hand to be gloved. Grasp the back of the glove cuff with the sleeve-covered second hand and turn the cuff over the sleeve. *The fingertips of the hand you are gloving remain inside the sterile sleeve until the sleeve is covered by the sterile glove.*

Continued

(4) Push your fingers into the glove (see illustration).

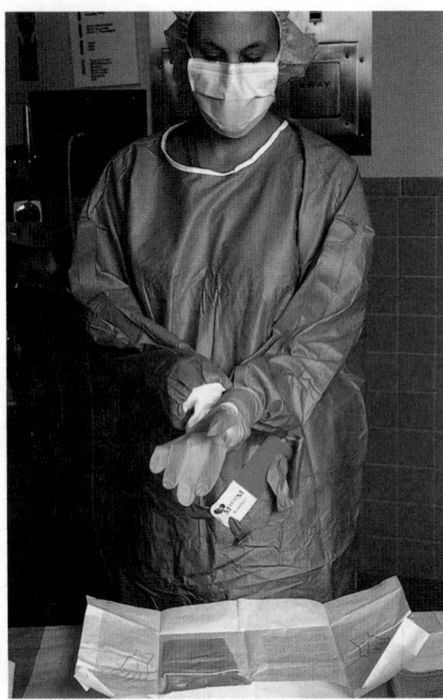

Step 5a(4). Pushing the fingers into the first glove.

b. Apply the second glove.
   (1) Use your sterile hand to pick up the second glove (see illustration). Put the second glove in the same position as the first on the opposite forearm.
   (2) Put on the second glove in the same manner as the first (see illustration).
c. Adjust the gloves for fit and comfort.

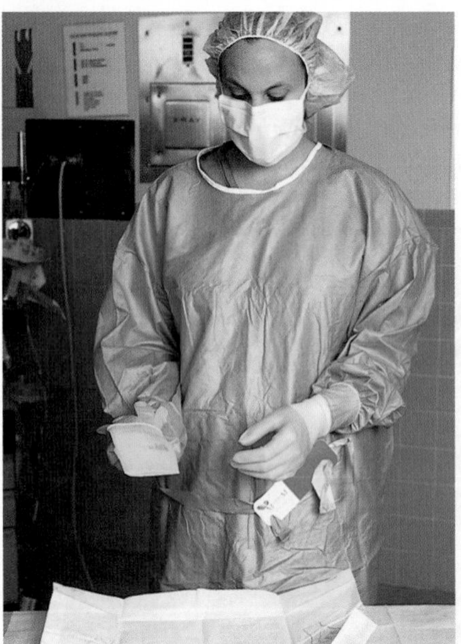

Step 5b(1). Positioning the second glove with the cuff facing the hand and the fingers facing the elbow.

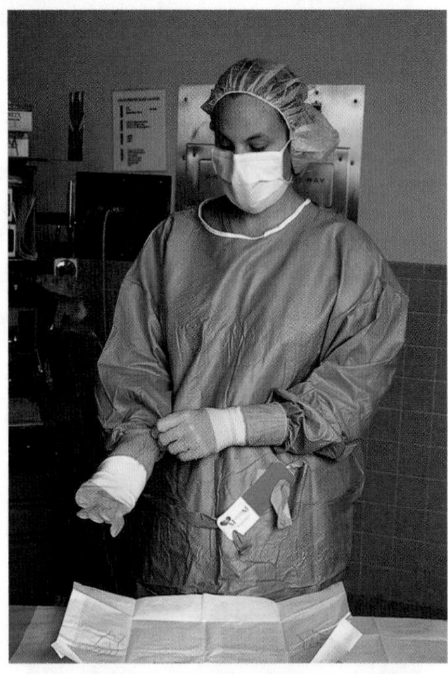

Step 5b(2). Putting on the second glove.

Environment. Environmental controls contribute to reducing the presence of microbes. Special areas may be set aside for special use, such as operating or procedure rooms. These rooms, when not in use, are cleaned using germicidal detergents. The area may have positive-pressure airflow to minimize the introduction of microorganisms into the air, and the ventilation system may have more frequent air exchanges to remove any introduced microbes. Any unnecessary visitors and personnel are excluded.

If a special room is not available, the designated area for a procedure can be cleaned ahead of time using a germicidal detergent. Then traffic or other activity in the area can be curtailed during the procedure to minimize the number of microbes deposited on the procedural area by air currents. Screens can be used to designate the area and remind personnel to avoid the area. After a sterile procedure is completed, the area is cleaned using CDC guidelines.

Cleaning of nondisposable equipment used in sterile procedures involves removing any visible soil and then disinfecting with a germicidal cleaner. Any materials used in invasive procedures that are not disposable must be sterilized after cleaning. Items are generally sterilized in autoclaves that utilize steam at high heat and pressure over a period of time. Items that could be destroyed by moisture or high heat and pressures can be sterilized by gas. Many disposable items are bought presterilized. The sterility of these items is guaranteed over a specified time period, assuming no breakage in the packaging has occurred. As a nurse, you are responsible for ensuring that sterilized equipment is properly stored to maintain sterility for use in future procedures and checking the integrity of sterile packages before use.

Action Alert! You are responsible for storing sterilized equipment in a manner that maintains its sterility for future use.

INTERVENTIONS TO PROTECT CLIENTS WITH DEFICIENT IMMUNITY

Using Environmental Safeguards. Because clients with a compromised immune system have ineffective protection, their entire environment must be altered to minimize their risk for infection. This begins with the type of food that they are able to eat. Fresh fruits and vegetables have been shown to carry organisms that could pose an additional risk to the immunocompromised client. The neutropenic diet, also known as the "cooked-food diet" or the low-bacterial diet, has been recommend for these clients.

The physical environment should be maintained in as clean a state as possible. Not only should these clients avoid dusting and other chores related to cleaning, they should try as much as possible to avoid being in the room when these chores are done. Household pets can be perilous and are not recommended for some clients. This needs to be evaluated on a case-by-case basis. Living plants are also not recommended, but if there are living plants in the home, they should not be watered by immunocompromised clients.

Preventing Feelings of Isolation. While in the hospital, immunocompromised clients are usually placed in isolation rooms with the door closed. If available, a room with positive-pressure ventilation to minimize airflow into the room from the rest of the hospital is recommended. Many institutions have special requirements for visitors of these clients. Visitors may be required to perform hand hygiene before entering the room and to wear gloves, gown, and possibly a mask when inside the room to minimize the spread of normally harmless microbes to the client with ineffective protection. After discharge, because of the extreme risk for infection to those with an altered immune system, these clients should avoid public places, especially those with crowds. Visitors should not be allowed if they think they might have an infection.

Children or adults who have up-to-date immunizations and no signs of infection may be allowed to visit in the home. An exception is if they have recently been vaccinated with polio vaccine, measles, mumps, and rubella (MMR), smallpox, varicella (chickenpox), or FluMist inoculations (live virus flu vaccine); in this case they should not be allowed to visit. These vaccines are live viral preparations, and although they do not put persons with normal immune systems at risk, those with ineffective protection against infection can become seriously ill from shed viral particles.

To prevent a sense of isolation, encourage clients to have visitors who have no signs of infection. Assess the support systems available to these clients once they go home. Although the number of visitors may be limited at any one time, visiting by friends and relatives is beneficial to the client. Encourage activities that can be done in the home while maintaining relationships with friends and family through telephone conversations and intermittent visits.

Providing Client and Family Teaching. As a starting point for client education, recall that teaching should include any family or friends who will be involved in the client's care. Teach the client about the disease process and its underlying basis. This must include information about the change in ability to fight infections of any kind. Teach the client the basics of infection control and about the importance of keeping the environment as clean as possible, even though all germs cannot be eliminated.

Other important topics for client teaching can then follow. Explain that infections that might be considered a nuisance to some will be life threatening for the client. Teach about the signs and symptoms of infection to watch for, and remind the client that these may be subtle. Tell the client to report any physical changes in general health to the primary health caregiver immediately, so that the client can be evaluated as soon as possible. Subtle signs might include a change in ability to tolerate activity and quite possibly will not include fever or pain. Any rashes or skin breakdown should be reported as well. Changes in bowel habits should be noted, as well as any increase in respiratory secretions. Any earache or continuing headache could also be an underlying symptom of infection. The timeliness of reporting these subtle signs is important to reduce the risk for severe infection in the immunocompromised client.

INTERVENTIONS TO REDUCE YOUR OWN RISK OF INFECTION

To reduce the risk for infection for the health care worker, strict adherence to guidelines provided by the CDC is necessary. By using hand hygiene and barrier precautions when necessary, health care workers can minimize the risk for infection. Health care workers should use the same precautions to protect themselves that they use for their clients. Use clean technique when in contact with the client to prevent the spread of infection to health care personnel. Perform thorough hand hygiene after client contact to reduce the risk of spreading the infection. Hospital-purchased lotions may be used during the work shift, but any lotion brought from home should be used only at the end of the work day. If you do have a possible exposure, comply with recommended health service follow-up to minimize the potential risk. Table 22-6 provides an overview of the follow-up treatment recommended after exposure to blood-borne pathogens.

EVALUATION

Evaluation of goal achievement in limiting or preventing infection involves reassessing the client to determine whether the criteria for evaluation have been met.

If the outcomes do not progress as anticipated, a reassessment could provide information as to why. If a client who has received antibiotics for 7 days continues to show signs of inflammation and general malaise, the culture and sensitivity should be reassessed. This may involve reculturing the primary site of infection and looking for additional or new sites of infection.

Evaluation allows continual review of the nursing care. By connecting outcomes to the interventions, nurses can evaluate the effectiveness of those interventions, as suggested in Box 22-11. In most instances, this requires the active participation of the clients and their families. If a client has been instructed to clean a wound twice a day and to re-dress it applying antibiotic ointment and then arrives 2 days later in the emergency department with odorous, green drainage from the wound, the nurse may question the client's understanding or willingness to participate in the procedure.

A discharge note for Colleen after her treatment for her dehydration secondary to effects of *Shigella* infection might look like the note below.

SAMPLE DOCUMENTATION NOTE FOR COLLEEN BROWN

Infant with diarrhea, stomach cramps. Tympanic temperature 98.6° F without receiving acetaminophen during the past 12 hours. Infant appears alert but lethargic. Intake has been PO without IV fluids for the last 12 hours. Skin turgor elastic. Infant appears free of pain without any noticeable distress when parents are present. Mr. and Mrs. Brown accurately verbalized the instructions to continue the antibiotic until all of the medication is complete. In addition, they have stated that they will follow up with the pediatrician at the local clinic within 1 week. At this appointment they will ask for information on Colleen's immunizations, request that they be updated, and request a record of all their children's immunizations.

Table 22-6 Follow-up for Health Care Workers Exposed to Blood-Borne Pathogens

PATHOGEN	FOLLOW-UP
Unknown	• Contact should be tested for known blood-borne diseases utilizing the rapid HIV screening test (result in less than 1 hour), HBV antigen, HCV antibody, possible syphilis if source client is HIV or HCV positive. Each state has laws governing the right to test a source for HIV. Consult the facility exposure control plan for information on testing. • If contact tests positive for HIV, immediate prophylaxis with anti-HIV medications may be considered based on client's viral load and the type of exposure. • CDC recommendations should be reviewed and followed. • If contact does not test positive and health care worker has never undergone hepatitis B vaccine series, hepatitis B gamma globulin should be administered and immunizations should be offered and started per agency protocol. • After the source client tests are reviewed, health care worker should be screened and/or counseled. Tests ordered will depend on the source client test results.
HIV	• If the client was positive for HIV, the health care worker should also be screened and be possibly started on HIV prophylaxis, which could include up to three antiviral drugs. This is only after extensive counseling about side effects and after baseline blood work. • The health care worker exposed to a positive HIV client with high viral load should be tested at 6 weeks, 3 months, and 6 months after the exposure. • If the source is negative for HBV, no treatment for health care worker is indicated.
Hepatitis B	• If the health care worker is nonimmune, hepatitis B immune globulin will be offered and the vaccination series begun.
Hepatitis C	• If the source is HCV positive, the health care worker should have a baseline HCV antibody test and a hepatitis C-RNA test in 4-6 weeks.

CDC, Centers for Disease Control and Prevention; *HBV*, hepatitis B virus; *HCV*, hepatitis C virus; *HIV*, human immunodeficiency virus.

BOX 22-11

Nursing Care Plan

An Infant With Sepsis

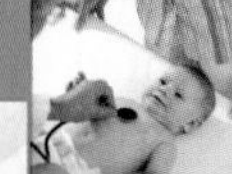

Admission Data

Colleen is admitted through the emergency department to a general pediatric floor. The emergency department nurse telephones the following report. *"Colleen is an 8-month-old Cajun infant presenting with dehydration. IV fluids have been started. Blood cultures have been drawn, as well as a CBC. Infant is lethargic. Her parents are at the bedside. She appears to have a GI infection. A stool culture has been done. She is reported to have had a seizure in the emergency department.*

Physician's Orders

Admitting diagnosis: Dehydration, diarrhea with possible sepsis
R/O Shigellosis
IV fluids $D_{10}W$ to infuse at 25 mL/hr
Ampicillin IV q 12 hr
Tylenol PO 50 mg prn q 3-4 hr for temp greater than 100.4° F
Contact precautions

Nursing Assessment

Color pale, skin dry, with "tenting" noted, lethargic. Heart rate regular with no murmur audible, rate = 90/min. Peripheral pulses weak but palpable, equal bilaterally. Bowel sounds active. Diaper dry (no urine output since admission). Tympanic temperature 103° F. Mother and father at bedside, quiet, appear frightened.

Colleen recovers with prescribed medical and nursing intervention. When Colleen is ready for discharge the nurse would like to give the parents information about prevention, makes the diagnosis of *Risk for infection,* and implements the following care plan.

NANDA-I Nursing Diagnosis	NOC Expected Outcomes With Indicators	NIC Interventions With Selected Activities	Evaluation Data
Risk for Infection	***Immunization Behavior***	***Infection Protection*** • Teach parents about the recommended childhood immunization schedule; direct them how to contact local health department.	• Mr. Brown says they do not have a family physician and do not have health insurance. States will contact health department.
Risk Factor: • Immune status associated with age and presence of siblings in home	***Knowledge: Infection Control***	***Teach Parents:*** • Mode of transmission of disease among siblings and practices to prevent transmission. • Monitor playmates for signs of infectious disease. • Monitor child's general health. • Signs and symptoms of infection. • Diet, rest, and exercise to increase resistance. • Maintain fluid intake during illness. • Follow physician's recommendation about reporting signs of illness.	• Mrs. Brown expresses gratitude for the information. She asks questions about how much fluid a child should have when she is ill and what temperature she should report to the physician. She says she does not have a thermometer at home. The nurse provides a thermometer to take home and shows her how to use it. Reports diarrhea has cleared in siblings. • Read instructions about fluid needs for all three children and parameters for calling the physician. • Reports understanding of written instructions.

Critical Thinking Questions

1. What other interventions can you think of to make the care delivered more culturally specific?
2. What should the nurse be thinking about in order to incorporate cultural considerations in discharge planning?
3. What specific teaching would you provide to Colleen's mother to ensure that another episode such as this does not occur?

Nursing outcome and intervention labels from Johnson, M., Bulechek, G., Butcher, H., Dochterman, J. M., Maas, M., Moorhead, S., et al. (Eds.). (2006). *NANDA, NOC, and NIC linkages: Nursing diagnoses, outcomes, & interventions.* St. Louis, MO: Mosby.

With the sample documentation, the nurse has documented the data that demonstrate the resolution of the initial diagnosis of *Ineffective protection.* In addition, the nurse, through a translator, has established new goals for the parents to attain. The nurse can assist the parents in establishing new goals with statements such as "With Colleen more like herself, we need to focus on keeping her healthy and at home with her family."

▼ KEY PRINCIPLES

- We are all at risk for infection. There is no environment without organisms' having the potential for causing disease.
- We have important physical and physiological mechanisms to protect ourselves from disease-causing organisms.
- Primary defenses against infections include the skin and the membrane barriers of the respiratory, GI, and GU tracts.
- Additional defenses against infection include molecules secreted by skin and membrane cells that provide additional barriers and may break down disease-causing organisms.
- Secondary defenses in the immune system have both nonspecific disease-fighting components and very specific components in the immunoglobulin system.
- Clients with breaks in the primary defenses have the nursing diagnosis *Risk for infection;* those with inadequate secondary defenses have *Ineffective protection.*
- Using the initial assessment of the client, the nurse develops plans of care to provide for the health protection of the client. The assessment includes physical findings and an evaluation of the client's mental status and social support system.
- Interventions may include education, modification of the client's physical environment, administration of antibiotics to eliminate or prevent the spread of infection, and psychosocial support.
- The outcome goals for any client are to minimize the risk for infection and to protect against further spread of infection for both the client and those caring for or associating with the client.
- Cultural influences play a major role in client education and follow-up of care.

■ REVIEW QUESTIONS

1. A client has a respiratory infection that can be transmitted during coughing and sneezing via respiratory secretions. The nurse would consider that this client should be placed on which of the following types of isolation precautions?

1. Contact
2. Airborne
3. Droplet
4. Protective

2. If all of the following pieces of protective equipment are needed, which of them would the nurse put on first when preparing to enter the room of a client on isolation precautions?

1. Gown
2. Gloves
3. Mask
4. Goggles

3. Which nursing diagnosis related to infection would the nurse formulate for a client admitted to the nursing unit who is taking corticosteroid medications and has diabetes mellitus?

1. Risk for infection
2. Risk for infection transmission
3. Ineffective health maintenance
4. Ineffective protection

4. The nurse would become concerned that a client with an infected leg ulcer was developing a systemic infection if which of the following client symptoms were assessed?

1. Redness
2. Swelling
3. Malaise
4. Heat

5. When opening a sterile tray wrapped in a drape, which piece of the drape would the nurse open last?

1. The flap that is away from the nurse.
2. The left flap
3. The right flap
4. The flap that is toward the nurse

Bibliography

Centers for Disease Control and Prevention. (2002). Guideline for hand hygiene in healthcare settings: Recommendations of the Healthcare Infection Control Practices Advisory Committee. *MMWR, 51*(RR-16), 1-45.

Centers for Disease Control and Prevention. Updated U.S. Public Health guidelines for management of occupational exposures to HIV: Recommendations for postexposure prophylaxis. *MMWR*. Retrieved October 29, 2006, from http://www.cdc.gov/mmwr/preview/mmwrhtml/rr5409a1.htm.

Centers for Disease Control and Prevention. (2005). *Shigellosis in the evacuation center environment.* Atlanta, GA: Author.

Centers for Disease Control and Prevention. (2005). Foodborne illness. Retrieved October 29, 2006 from http://www.cdc.gov/ncidod/dbmd/diseaseinfo/foodborneinfections_g.htm.

Centers for Disease Control and Prevention. (2006). TB facts for health care workers 2006. Retrieved October 29, 2006 from http://www.cdc.gov/nchstp/tb/pubs/TBfacts_HealthWorkers/default.htm.

Creedon, S. A. (2005). Healthcare workers' hand decontamination practices: Compliance with recommended guidelines. *J Adv Nurs 51*(3):208-216.

Fast facts about hospital-acquired infections. (2005). Retrieved October 29, 2006, from www.consumersunion.org/campaigns/learn_more/001544indiv.html.

Garner, J. S. (2005). Guideline for isolation precautions in hospitals. Retrieved October 29, 2006 from http://www.cdc.gov/ncidod/dhqp/gl_isolation_ptI.html.

Gerding, D. N. (2005). Pseudomembranous colitis *(Clostridium difficile)*. In *APIC Text of Infection Control & Epidemiology* (pp. 75-1-75-6). Washington, D. C.: Association for Professionals in Infection Control and Epidemiology.

Girouard, S., Levine, G., Goodrich, K., Jones, S., Keyserling, H., Rathore, M., et al. (2001). Infection control programs at children's hospitals: A description of structures and processes. *American Journal of Infection Control, 29*(3), 145-151.

Johnson, M., Bulechek, G., Butcher, H., Dochterman, J. M., Maas, M., Moorhead, S., et al. (Eds.). (2006). *NANDA, NOC, and NIC linkages: Nursing diagnoses, outcomes, & interventions.* St. Louis, MO: Mosby.

Kyne, L., Hamel, M. B., Polavaram, R., & Kelly, C. P. (2002). Health care costs and mortality associated with nosocomial diarrhea due to *Clostridium difficile. Clinical Infectious Diseases, 34*(3), 346-353.

Larson, E. (2004). A tool to assess barriers to adherence to hand hygiene guideline. *American Journal of Infection Control, 32,* 48-51.

Mandram, A. J. (1999). Hospital Infection Control Practices Advisory Committee (HICPAC) and Centers for Disease Control and Prevention (CDC). 1999 Guidelines for prevention of surgical site infection. *Infection Control & Hospital Epidemiology, 24*(4), 247-278.

Millman, S. (2002). The emerging threat of antibiotic resistance: A hidden cost of factory farming. *The Humane Society of the United States, 4*(1), 1-2.

NANDA International. (2007). *Nursing diagnoses: Definitions & classification, 2006-2007,* Philadelphia: NANDA-I.

Needlestick Safety & Prevention Act. (2000). Pub. L. No. 106-430, U.S. Congress, Washington, DC.

Neutropenic diet. (2002). Baltimore, MD: Johns Hopkins Bayview Medical Centre.

Preliminary FoodNet data on the incidence of infection with pathogens transmitted commonly through food—10 sites, United States, 2004. *MMWR, 54*(14), 352-356.

Snow, M., White, G. L., Alder, S. C., & Stanford, J. B. (2006). Mentor's hand hygiene practices influence student's hand hygiene rates. *Am J Infect Control 34*(1):18-24.

Stelfox, H. T. (2003). Safety of patients isolated for infection control, *JAMA, 290,* 1899-1950.

Underwood, M. A. (2005). Hand hygiene. In *APIC text of infection control and epidemiology* (pp. 19-1-19-7). Washington, D. C.: Association for Professionals in Infection Control and Epidemiology.

Waldmeier,V. (2002). Laissez les bon temps rouler (let the good times roll): Can embedded Cajun cultural health beliefs be changed through traditional health education? *Journal of Cultural Diversity, 9*(4):113-117.

---

*Asterisk indicates a classic or definitive work on this subject.

Chapter 23

Health Protection: Risk for Injury

Media Resources

- Nursing Skills Online
- evolve Evolve Website http://evolve.elsevier.com/Harkreader/
- Companion CD
- 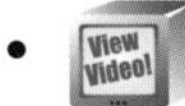 Skills Video Clips

Learning Objectives

After studying this chapter, you should be able to do the following:

- Discuss the epidemiology of common injuries from falls, asphyxiation, and poisoning
- Discuss the epidemiology of trauma from burns, electricity, motor vehicle accidents, and radiation
- Identify the behavioral, environmental, socioeconomic, developmental, cognitive, and physiological factors that affect safety
- Assess the client's risk for injury
- Distinguish between related nursing diagnoses for the client at risk for injury
- Plan interventions to prevent injury and promote safety in the acute care setting, the client's home, and the community
- Evaluate client outcomes and nursing interventions used to help the client reduce the risk for injury

Key Terms

asphyxiation
aspiration
burn
choking
injury
poisoning
restraint
strangulation
trauma

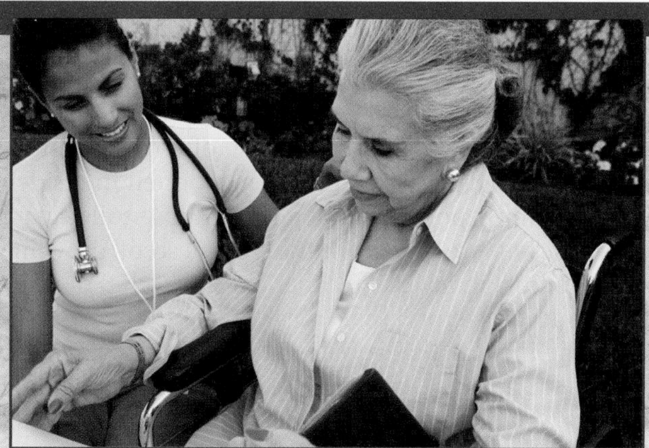

Juanita Soto is a 75-year-old widow who lives alone in a two-story house. Her sons and daughters live in distant cities and visit her whenever they can. She relies primarily on her neighbors and friends for help. Juanita has been relatively healthy most of her life and has been able to keep up her home despite the fact that 5 years ago she was diagnosed with osteoarthritis. During the last 4 months, however, her condition has worsened. She now uses her wheelchair to get around the house, although she sometimes uses a cane to navigate the flight of stairs that leads downstairs to the washer and dryer. She complains of pain and weakness in her hands and legs. At her last physician visit, she was referred to a local home health care agency for evaluation of her condition and her needs.

During the initial assessment visit, the home health care nurse notes that, in addition to having limited hand and leg movement, Juanita is partially blind in one eye. The nurse also notes that Juanita's home needs some repairs—especially the stairs, which are old and have no railing for support. Because of the many physical and environmental factors identified, the nurse considers the diagnosis of *Risk for injury.* The nurse also considers related nursing diagnoses for clients with safety needs (see nursing diagnoses box).

KEY NURSING DIAGNOSES FOR HEALTH AND SAFETY

Risk for injury: At risk for injury as a result of environmental conditions interacting with the individual's adaptive and defensive resources

Risk for trauma: Accentuated risk for accidental tissue injury (e.g., wound, burn, fracture)

Risk for poisoning: Accentuated risk for accidental exposure to, or ingestion of, drugs or dangerous products in doses sufficient to cause poisoning

Risk for suffocation: Accentuated risk for accidental suffocation (inadequate air available for inhalation)

Risk for aspiration: At risk for entry of gastrointestinal secretions, oropharyngeal secretions, solids, or fluids into tracheobronchial passages

Risk for falls: Increased susceptibility to falling that may cause physical harm

CONCEPTS OF SAFETY

Every person has an inherent need to be and feel safe. Feeling safe allows us to think and act with confidence. Although at birth we depend on someone else for our safety, as we mature we become responsible for our own safety, and eventually we may become responsible for the safety of others. Injuries from behavioral, environmental, or physiological hazards affect people of all ages, developmental stages, and socioeconomic groups. No matter the cause, injuries can have devastating effects from pain, emotional distress, financial hardship, permanent disability, and even death. Thus safety is a need that remains with us throughout our lifetime.

Client safety is a priority issue in all health care settings. Prevention of injury can reduce the need for hospitalizations, the risk for complications from medical treatment, the hardship of long-term care, and even the loss of life. Together with your clients, you can develop a plan of action to ensure the safest possible environment.

EPIDEMIOLOGY OF INJURY

An **injury** is damage to some part of the body resulting from physical, mechanical, biological, or chemical agents. According to the National Center for Health Statistics, unintentional injuries are among the leading causes of death in the United States for individuals age 1 to 34 years and in the top 10 for all other age-groups. Suffocation is the leading cause of unintentional injury death in infants. Motor vehicle accidents lead the list up to age 65, and then falls are the most common cause of unintentional injury deaths (Centers for Disease Control and Prevention [CDC], 2005b; data from 2001).

Falls. Older people form the group affected most often by falls, both at home and in institutional settings. Falls are the leading cause of injury-related deaths among people age 65 years and older, accounting for 11% of the deaths from unintentional injury in older adults (CDC, 2005a). When a fall occurs, a fracture can result in prolonged hospitalization and lead to immobility, early nursing home placement, or death. When older clients fall, the biggest concern is the threat of a hip fracture. Hip fractures result in approximately 300,000 hospital admissions each year. In most cases, the affected person is age 65 or older and is more likely to be female (CDC, 2005a). Because falls occur frequently and have serious consequences, the risk for falls is one of the most serious problems that acute and long-term care facilities must manage.

Falls occurring in the home account for most reported home accidents in people age 75 and older. Because older adults are more likely to have muscle weakness, joint stiffness, slowed reflexes, altered gait, decreased mobility, incontinence, or confusion, older adults are at risk for falling. Falls tend to occur in the home when the person is in a hurry, stressed, or faced with obstacles. Stairways, lighting, and bathrooms are common sources of hazards.

Action Alert! Assess older clients and their environment to identify the risk for falling.

Falls in the hospitalized client account for up to 10% of fatal falls (Fuller, 2000). Hospital falls occur most commonly in the client's room when the client is alone and trying to get to the bathroom unassisted. The use of bed side rails and restraints do not necessarily prevent falls, because clients who fall had either removed the restraints or exited the bed safely, only to fall while walking without assistance. Polypharmacy (use of multiple medications) is often a factor in clients who fall.

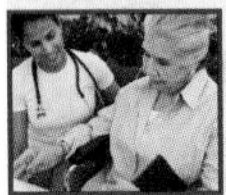

One day when the home health care nurse comes to visit with Mrs. Soto, her daughter is there. The daughter is telling Mrs. Soto that she should sell her home and come to stay with the daughter's family. Can you list the possible concerns that prompted Mrs. Soto's daughter to make this suggestion?

Asphyxiation. **Asphyxiation** is an interruption in breathing from a severe lack of oxygen (asphyxia) because there is either no source of air, an inadequate supply of oxygen in the air, or inadequate inhalation. Causes of asphyxia include aspiration, choking, or strangulation. **Aspiration** is the inspiration of foreign material into the airway. **Choking** is an internal obstruction of the airway by food or a foreign body. Choking can result from aspiration. **Strangulation** is constriction of the airway from an external cause.

Choking on food or objects and aspirating them into the airway, as well as asphyxiation caused by materials that block the external airway, are of special concern in young children and older adults. The death rate from choking is especially high during the first few years of life. Asphyxiation can result when a child is caught in an airtight compartment from which the oxygen is gradually depleted by the child's breathing; when airtight material, such as plastic, covers the nose and mouth; or when the chest is compressed so that breathing is impossible, as in some crushing injuries. Causes of strangulation include hanging from highchair straps or drapery cords and wedging of the head between crib slats, in accordion-style safety gates, between a bed and wall, and in electrically operated car windows.

In the older adult or neurologically impaired client, choking and aspiration can result from the loss or absence of protective airway reflexes. Choking and aspiration also can occur in clients who are unconscious from drugs, alcohol, a cerebrovascular accident (stroke), or cardiac arrest. Tube feedings, ill-fitting dentures, and overzealous feeding contribute to the risk for aspiration.

Accidental drowning is a significant cause of injury and death for toddlers and teenagers. For children under 1 year old, drowning occurs most often in bathtubs. Children ages 1 to 4 years drown most often in residential swimming pools, although bathtubs, toilets, and water buckets are also common. Adolescent drowning usually occurs in lakes and other natural bodies of water. Contributing factors that may increase the risk for drowning include inadequate supervision, lack of safety devices, hazardous swimming conditions, careless boating and water sports, and the use of alcohol and drugs (Figure 23-1).

Poisoning. **Poisoning** is clinically defined as an adverse condition or physical state resulting from the administration or ingestion of a toxic substance. Toxic substances enter the body through ingestion, inhalation,

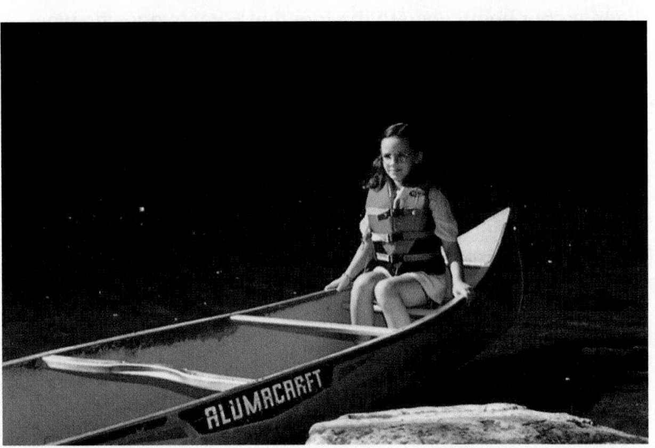

FIGURE 23-1 The use of a life jacket can promote water safety.

BOX 23-1 *Causative Agents in Deaths From Poisoning*

The following list presents suspected causative agents in 705 deaths reported to poison control centers in the United States in 1992:

- Antidepressants, such as amitriptyline, desipramine, doxepin, imipramine, and nortriptyline
- Analgesics, such as acetaminophen, aspirin, codeine, morphine, and propoxyphene
- Cardiovascular medications, such as digoxin and verapamil
- Street drugs, such as cocaine, heroin, and methamphetamine
- Sedatives and hypnotics, such as phenobarbital
- Antiasthmatic medications, such as theophylline
- Fumes, gases, and vapors, such as carbon monoxide and hydrogen sulfide
- Chemicals, such as cyanide and strychnine
- Insecticides, such as diazinon
- Household cleaners, such as sodium hypochlorite (bleach)
- Hydrocarbons, such as butane
- Alcohol, especially the ethanol form
- Automotive products, such as ethylene glycol and methanol

From Loomis, T. A., & Hayes, A. W. (1996). *Loomis' essentials of toxicology* (4th ed., p. 14). San Diego, CA: Academic Press.

injection, application, or absorption of the noxious material and produce injury or death through chemical action. For example, poisoning can result from accidental medication overdose, gases produced when household cleaners are mixed, leaking carbon monoxide, and use of tainted street drugs. Box 23-1 provides examples of potentially harmful chemicals that have been adequately documented as having caused serious health problems in humans (Loomis & Hayes, 1996).

The reasons for and types of poisonings vary with age. The people most at risk for poisoning include toddlers, young children, and adults with sensory impairment and communication barriers. Lack of adequate supervision and improper storage of toxic household substances are major factors in poisonings in children. Among adolescents and adults, poisoning most often results from snakebites, recreational drugs, or suicide attempts. Poisonings among older adults may result from medication overdose associated with mental impairment, polypharmacy, poor eyesight, illiteracy, or a language barrier (Figure 23-2).

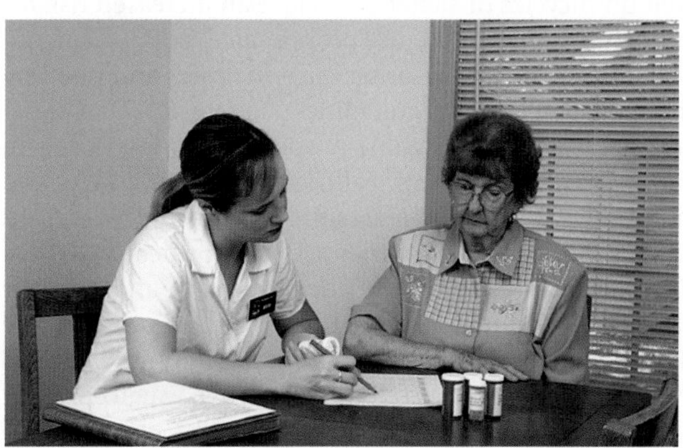

FIGURE 23-2 Teach a homebound client that the proper labeling and storage of medications can help prevent accidental poisoning.

Proper storage, labeling, and use of chemicals and other toxic agents can prevent poisoning, especially in children (Table 23-1).

Action Alert! Teach prevention of accidental poisoning through proper storage and labeling of containers. For hospitalized clients, triple-check all medications before administering them.

EPIDEMIOLOGY OF TRAUMA

Clinically, **trauma** is a physical injury or wound caused by a forceful, disruptive, or violent action. Trauma is the leading cause of potential years of life lost and the fourth leading cause of death in the United States. Traumatic injury causes morbidity, disability, lost productivity, and medical costs. It has been estimated that each year 57 million Americans (1 in 4) are injured seriously enough to require medical treatment.

Fires and Burns. Institutionalized clients are especially at risk for injury in the event of a fire because they may be debilitated and unable to escape without assistance. Also, the health care environment contains flammable gases, materials, and equipment that may increase the risk of fire. Oxygen is not flammable but will increase the rate of combustion of flammable materials; therefore oxygen increases the risk for fire in the presence of anesthetics and electrical equipment, such as monitors, heating and cooling units, and respiratory equipment. Equipment that is malfunctioning or used improperly may cause sparks that could easily ignite linens, especially in an oxygen-rich environment.

House-fire death rates are highest for children younger than 5 years and for adults older than 65. Older adults are at increased risk for fire death because sensory impairment (e.g., blindness or hearing loss) may prevent them from noticing a fire or hearing a

Table 23-1 Preventing Childhood Poisoning

COMMON SOURCES OF POISONING	CLIENT INSTRUCTIONS TO PREVENT POISONING
Medications	• Keep all medications out of the reach of children, preferably in locked cabinets. • Make sure that medication containers have childproof caps. • Store and label medications properly in their original containers. • Read medication labels carefully before administering a medication. • Do not share medications. • Use appropriate measuring devices when administering medications to ensure proper dosing. • Destroy expired medications promptly and appropriately. • Keep emergency numbers–including the local poison control center–near the phone and in plain view. • Never tell a child that a medication is candy. • Keep emergency medications (such as syrup of ipecac) in the home.
Chemicals, cleaning solutions, and other toxic substances	• Keep chemicals, cleaning solutions, and other toxic substances in locked cabinets. • Keep all such substances in their original containers with proper labels. • Maintain adequate ventilation when using chemicals and cleaning solutions. • Do not mix cleaning products, chemicals, and other such substances together.
Houseplants	• Keep out of reach of children. • Provide adequate supervision for young children and infants.

smoke alarm, and mobility impairment may keep them from escaping a fire (CDC, 2000a). Most house-fire deaths result from the poisoning effects of smoke inhalation rather than from burn injuries. The most common cause of house-fire deaths is cigarette smoking. The most common causes of house fires are cooking and heating equipment fires (CDC, 2000a). In house fires where deaths occur, smoking and alcohol use are often contributing factors.

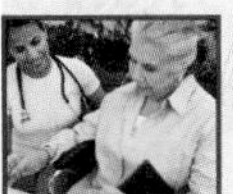

Think again about Mrs. Soto. Is she at risk for injury from a fire? What would you assess about her home to determine the level of risk?

Action Alert! Urge clients to keep a portable heater at least 36 inches away from anything that might be flammable. Also, recommend that clients install a smoke detector with working batteries on each level of the home. Instruct clients to test the batteries monthly, to change batteries every 6 months, and to keep a multipurpose fire extinguisher on hand in case of fire (Figure 23-3).

A **burn** is clinically defined as any injury caused by excessive exposure to electricity, chemicals, gases, radioactivity, or thermal agents. Besides fire, some of the most common causes of burns in the home or health care institution include exposure to hot bath water, overly hot moist dressings, heat lamps, and other forms of equipment.

People at highest risk for burns include children age 14 and younger, the handicapped, and older adults with sensory impairments. Children are at risk for burns from misuse of matches and exposure to hot liquids or vapors, and the risk is increased by inadequate parental supervision. Handicapped persons or older adults with sensory impairments risk being burned from the unsafe use of space heaters, water heaters, stoves, and irons.

Electrical Shock. Injury from electrical shock can range from trivial burns to charring and destruction of the skin and underlying tissues. Hazards occurring from electrical shock are of concern in both the home and the health care environment.

The most common type of electrical injuries involve electrical equipment, household appliances, or tools. Electrical shock results when current travels to the ground via the body instead of traveling through the electrical wiring. Fatalities from electrical hazards are relatively uncommon.

Motor Vehicle Accidents. Motor vehicle accidents are the leading cause of accidental death in the United States (CDC, 2000b). Unsafe driving practices and the use of alcohol and drugs contribute to the occurrences. Depending on the circumstances of the accident, persons at risk for sustaining injuries may include the driver, passengers, pedestrians, bicyclists, and skateboarders. Children on bicycles or skateboards face an increased risk for injury when they fail to use proper safety equipment and precautions, such as wearing safety helmets and padding and following safety guidelines (Figure 23-4). Guidelines include using signals properly and not riding in traffic or near driveways. Failure to use safety belts and infant car seats also increases the risk for injury.

Back Injuries. Back injuries account for nearly 20% of all injuries and illnesses in the workplace and cost the nation an estimated 20 to 50 billion dollars per year. The National Institute for Occupational Safety and Health (NIOSH) believes that the most effective way to prevent back injury is to implement an ergonomics program that focuses on redesigning the work environment and work

FIGURE 23-3 All smoke and fire detectors in the home should be installed properly and maintained with fresh batteries.

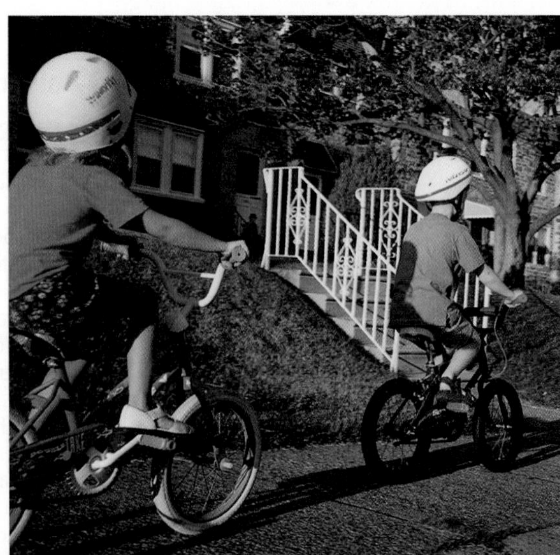

FIGURE 23-4 Recommend appropriate safety equipment to help prevent head injuries in school-age children.

tasks to reduce the hazards of lifting. OSHA recommends minimizing manual lifting of clients in all cases and eliminating lifting when possible (NIOSH, 2006).

Back injury can often be prevented by following guidelines such as those in Box 23-2. Occupational back injury accounts for a significant number of workers' compensation claims. Back injuries are the main reason for prolonged absence from work; the lost productivity creates substantial costs.

Back pain and injuries can be caused by disk degeneration, obesity, postural problems, structural problems, and overstretching of the spinal supports. The consequences of injury may include prolonged pain and suffering, decreased quality of life, and a reduced potential for future earnings or job opportunities.

Certain job tasks and personal characteristics increase the probability of back injury. Job tasks include heavy lifting, repetitive lifts (especially while bending or twisting), prolonged sitting, working in a stooped or awkward position, and operating vibrating machinery. Personal characteristics may include lack of job experience, obesity, smoking, alcohol consumption, job dissatisfaction, recent back injury, and lack of strength and overall physical fitness. Most back injuries probably result not from a single, stressful lifting event but rather develop gradually over time. Improper lifting techniques lead to a significant number of back injuries.

Radiation. Exposure to radiation in the form of energy, rays, or waves can lead to a variety of injuries, including radiation burns and radiation dermatitis. Radiation burns result from exposure to radiant energy in the form of sunlight, x-rays, or nuclear emissions or explosion. Exposure to ionizing radiation, as from cancer radiation therapy, can lead to an acute or chronic inflammation of skin known as radiation dermatitis. The signs of redness, blistering, and sloughing of the skin usually appear 3 weeks after exposure.

Exposure to radiation can occur in the community or the health care environment. Community risk increases near nuclear power plants and manufacturing industries that produce radioactive wastes.

In the health care setting, you and other clinicians may be at risk when assisting with diagnostic procedures that use radioactive materials or when caring for clients who have radioactive implants. Injury can occur if you fail to use lead shielding or fail to follow the necessary safety procedures involving exposure time and distance from the radioactive source. Radiation can injure the skin, reproductive organs, bone marrow, gastrointestinal tract, and other parts of the body. The international

BOX 23-2 *Teaching for Wellness*

Protect Yourself From Job-Related Back Injuries

Purpose: To prevent back injuries when lifting and moving clients in the acute care setting.

Expected Outcome: The worker will not experience work-related back injuries.

Instructions

- Maintain your health. Eat a well-balanced diet, get a good night's sleep, and reduce stress in your life.
- Maintain your level of physical fitness. Get regular exercise. Exercise for cardiovascular fitness through aerobic exercise and for muscle strength through weight-bearing exercises. Exercise 20 minutes a day to strengthen your back, leg, and abdominal muscles. Include stretching exercises before and after your exercise session.
- Before you lift or move a client, assess the client's ability to help. Can the client move in bed, bear weight when standing, and cooperate with your instructions? How much does the client weigh? Is the range of motion sufficient to accomplish the move?
- Assess your ability to bear the load. How much weight can you lift? Ask for assistance if necessary.
- Arrange the environment to facilitate the move. For example, put the chair close to the bed when you are transferring a client to a chair. Move the furniture to allow you to get close to the client without twisting your back.
- Use assistive devices to lessen your workload. A mechanical lift is suggested when the client is immobile and exceeds the weight you can lift. A gait belt is used to increase leverage and provide a firm grasp. A walker assists the client to balance and bear part of the body's weight.
- Use principles of body mechanics when lifting and moving objects or clients:
  1. Lift using the longest and strongest muscle group; hold your back in the neutral position, and use your arm and leg muscles rather than your back muscles.
  2. Face the object or person to be lifted or moved; avoid twisting as you move. It is easier to pull, push, or roll an object than it is to lift it.
  3. Movements should be smooth and coordinated rather than jerky.
  4. Keep the work as close as possible to your body. It puts less of a strain on your back, legs, and arms.
  5. Rock backward or forward on your feet to use your body weight as a pushing or pulling force.
  4. Avoid working against gravity. Keep the work at a comfortable height to avoid excessive bending at the waist.
  5. In general pushing is safer than pulling. Pulling is more likely to involve twisting. Use your body weight to help push an object. It is easier to pull, push, or roll an object than it is to lift it.
  6. Less energy or force is required to keep an object moving than to start and stop it.
  7. Stability and balance is greater with a wide base of support and the center of gravity over the base of support. Widen your stance, and keep objects close to your body.
  8. Avoid standing in one position for prolonged periods of time. Take regular breaks to stretch and restore the neutral position of your back.

radiation symbol notifies you and other health care workers of the danger of radiation injury (Figure 23-5). The principle of protection from radiation exposure involves three elements: time, distance, and shielding. Reducing the time of exposure, increasing the distance from the source, and using appropriate shielding will reduce the dose of radiation.

FACTORS AFFECTING SAFETY

LIFESTYLE FACTORS

A person's lifestyle can raise the risk for injury. Pertinent factors include not taking appropriate safety precautions, choosing a sedentary lifestyle, abusing chemical substances, and being unable or unwilling to provide self-care.

Lack of Safety Precautions. Careless behaviors are associated with highly stressful situations or a general disregard for safety. Speeding while driving, smoking in bed, entering high-crime areas at night, riding a bicycle without a helmet, and other risky behaviors invite accidents and injuries. Lack of safety precautions can affect people of all ages and walks of life.

Activity and Exercise. A lack of activity and exercise will negatively affect each body system and predispose the person to physiological as well as emotional hazards. Limited mobility and reaction time increases the risk for falls and decreases the ability to flee from dangerous situations, including fires and other external hazards. Despite the fact that activity and exercise are known to be beneficial, many people choose to live relatively inactive lives.

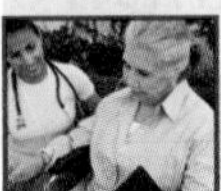

Mrs. Soto has gradually become less active. You will need to suggest that she gets her arthritis evaluated by a physician before planning a program to increase her activity. How would you approach this situation with her daughter?

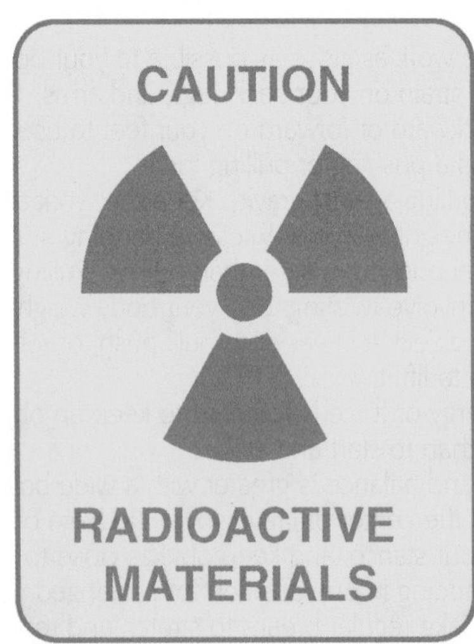

FIGURE 23-5 The international radiation symbol is commonly used in health care facilities.

Substance Abuse. The use of drugs and alcohol can affect safety in every aspect of a person's life. Substance abuse can reduce judgment and coordination and the ability to complete typical tasks. Operating heavy equipment, driving a car, climbing a ladder, and using a chain saw while under the influence of alcohol are associated with a high risk for injury.

ENVIRONMENTAL FACTORS

Our surroundings, no matter where we live, work, or play, are never completely hazard free. Even when we take all the necessary precautions, there is no guarantee of our safety because we cannot be in total control of our home, community, and workplace environments.

Home. The home environment contains hazards or potential hazards both inside and outside. Potential hazards may involve inadequate lighting, steps or handrails that are missing or in poor repair, clutter, throw rugs, electrical cords, or slippery surfaces. Features that suggest a safe home environment include grab bars in the tub or shower, nonskid rugs, covered electrical plugs, and locked storage cabinets.

Work. The work environment may contain a variety of overt or covert occupational safety hazards. Potential occupational hazards may result from noise, dust, or air pollution; working at heights; working with dangerous machinery; and being exposed to toxic substances. Occupations that raise the risk for injury include those that involve exposure to radiation or high-voltage electricity or the use of heavy equipment. Farm workers, electrical line workers, construction workers, and workers in power plants are a few examples of people at increased risk for injury. Both employers and employees should be aware of potential hazards and the need for precautions, such as wearing appropriate protective apparel.

Community. Hazards that can affect the community environment include crime, landfills, busy intersections, unsafe roads or bridges, dilapidated houses, cliffs, unprotected creeks and swimming pools, toxic waste dumps, air pollution, water pollution, noise from nearby construction, railroad crossings, and airports. Other environmental concerns include a clean water supply, an adequate sewage system, and insect and rodent control. Lack of sanitation in impoverished or less-developed areas increases the risk for disease and infection.

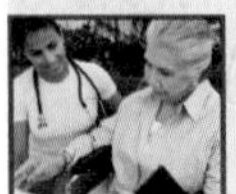

We know that Mrs. Soto's house needs repairs, but we do not know anything about the community in which she lives. How would you assess the community to determine Mrs. Soto's level of safety in her home?

Institution. Potential dangers to health care workers and clients within health care institutions are addressed by safety committees, infection control committees, and hazardous waste committees. For example, each institution is required to have up-to-date written policies to address such problems as chemical spills, infectious outbreaks, exposure to infectious blood and body fluids, and disposal of hazardous wastes. You must be familiar with your institution's policies and procedures to ensure your own safety and that of your clients.

SOCIOECONOMIC FACTORS

A frequently cited reason for ignoring safety is a lack of financial resources. Buying car seats for children and making repairs to protect the home from a faulty furnace can be expensive. A family may not have the financial means to obtain smoke detectors, fire extinguishers, or carbon monoxide detectors for their home.

However, the cost of *not* preventing accidents can be devastating. When someone is injured or involved in an accident, the costs can be astonishing. They involve lost wages and productivity, medical expenses, administrative expenses, employer costs, vehicle damage, and property losses.

DEVELOPMENTAL FACTORS

Each stage of human development has its own unique risks (Table 23-2). Preventing injury and promoting safety are major concerns and the responsibility of the nurse, client, family, and caregiver. Promoting awareness of potentially hazardous situations is a lifelong process that should begin early (Figure 23-6). Infants and toddlers are particularly vulnerable to accidents and injuries because of their limited awareness of potential dangers, oral activity, mobility, and inherent curiosity. School-age children face potential dangers as their environment expands from the home to the school. Box 23-3 is an example of teaching preventive measures. In adolescents, the need for independence, peer pressure, and the high-risk behaviors common in this age-group greatly increase the risk for accidents and injury. In adults, the risk for injury tends to result from lifestyle. The physiological changes of aging increase the risk for older adults.

COGNITIVE FACTORS

A person's cognitive and perceptual abilities are crucial to promoting safety. The ability to acquire and interpret in-

Table 23-2 Risk for Injury by Age-Group

AGE-GROUP	RISKS	POSSIBLE CAUSES
Developing fetus	• Maternal exposure to smoke • Maternal use of alcohol or other drugs • X-rays received during first trimester • Exposure to certain pesticides	• Mother cannot or will not assume responsibility for the safety of fetus, or she lacks the knowledge to do so. • Radiograph ordered by physician without inquiry about possible pregnancy. • Mother lives in proximity of fields of crops where the use of pesticides may be common.
Newborn	• Falling • Suffocating in crib • Choking or aspiration of formula • Burns, especially with bath water • Injuries in automobile accidents • Injuries in crib or playpen	• Failure to use approved car seats, cribs, and playpens correctly. • Inappropriate supervision. • Propping bottles while feeding. • Using a microwave oven to warm formula.
Infant or toddler	• Physical trauma from falling • Banging into objects • Falling down stairs • Being cut by sharp objects • Injuries in automobile accidents • Burns • Posioning • Drowning • Electric shock from household outlets	• Environment not childproofed. • No gate at the top of stairs. • Obstructed passageways. • Unsafe window protection. • Improper use of car seats. • Highly flammable toys or clothing. • Pot handles facing front of stove. • Unsupervised bathing. • Unsupervised backyard swimming pool. • Unused electric outlets not blocked.
Preschool and school-age	• Injuries in automobile accidents • Injuries on playground equipment • Choking • Suffocation • Obstruction of airways or ears by foreign objects • Poisoning • Drowning • Electrical shock	• History of hyperactivity; attention deficit disorder. • Experimenting with chemicals or gasoline. • Playing with matches, cigarettes, candles, or fireworks. • Improper storage of knives, guns, and ammunition. • Improper use of car seats or seat belts. • Unsupervised activities around the pool, electrical outlets, etc.

Continued

Table 23-2 Risk for Injury by Age-Group—cont'd

AGE-GROUP	RISKS	POSSIBLE CAUSES
Adolescents	• Sports injuries • Automobile accidents • Drug or alcohol use	• Lack of proper athletic training. • Lack of experience driving. • Failure to use or misuse of seat belts.
Older adults	• Falls • Burns • Pedestrian and automobile accidents	• *Physical:* Weakness, poor vision, disturbed balance, reduced sensations, poor coordination, impaired eye-hand coordination. • *Environmental:* Slippery floors, snow or ice on walkways, unanchored rugs, no handgrips or rails in shower or bathtub, unsteady ladders or chairs, poor lighting, electrical cords in walkways, clutter or spills, unsteady or absent stair rails, inadequate method to call for assistance, cognitive or emotional disturbance.
All ages	• Fires	• Gas leaks. • Delayed lighting of gas burners. • Unscreened fires or heaters. • Flowing clothes around open flame. • Inappropriately stored combustibles or corrosives. • Faulty wiring or frayed cords. • Smoking in bed.

A

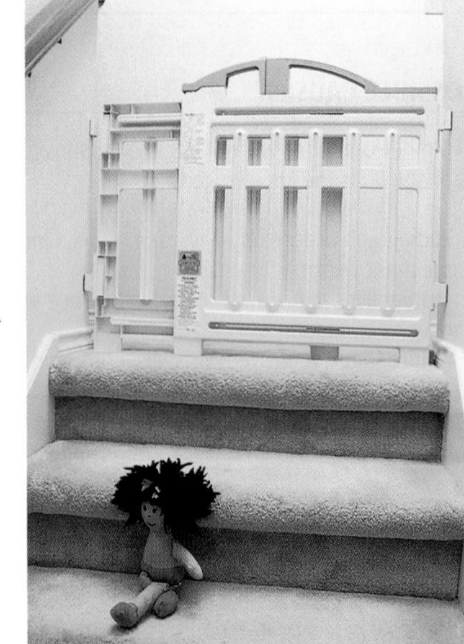

B

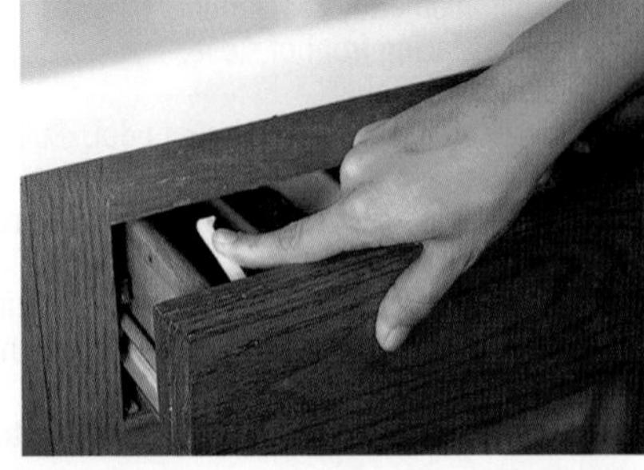

C

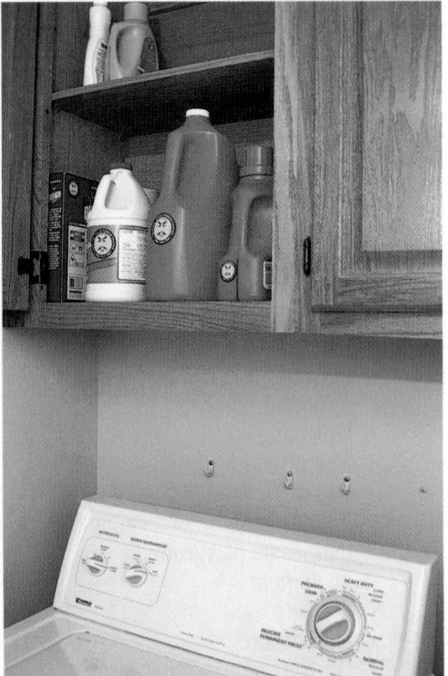

FIGURE 23-6 Childproofing a home. **A,** Toddler gates on stairs and doors. **B,** Childproof locks for cabinets. **C,** Chemicals labeled with "Mr. Yuk" stickers and placed out of reach.

BOX 23-3 *Teaching for Wellness*

Preventing Lead Poisoning

Although there has been significant progress in the reduction of exposure to lead, there are approximately 38 million homes in the United States that contain lead-based paint, representing about 25% of all U.S. housing. Other sources of lead include, but are not limited to, jewelry, soil, and playground equipment.

Purpose: To educate families about strategies for the prevention of lead poisoning in very young children.

Expected Outcomes: Families will initiate action to detect the presence of and prevent ingestion of lead.

Client Instructions

Sources of Lead

- Although houses built before 1950 contain the greatest threat, over 80% of houses built before 1978 contain lead-based paint.
- Although all children are at risk, those who live in dilapidated housing face the greatest danger, especially children under age 2.
- Houses in coastal towns may have been painted with paint intended for boats, which has a high lead content.
- Soil near mines, industries that use lead, and smelters can have high lead levels.
- Solder on older plumbing and brass fixtures can contain lead.
- Food grown in soil with a high lead content can contain lead.
- Ceramic tableware and toys from some countries contain lead.
- Ethnic folk remedies, such as the Hispanic remedies *azarcon* and *greta* and the Southeast Asian remedy *pay loo lah,* may contain lead.
- Hobbies that involve working with leaded glass, artist paints, bullets, and jewelry are sources of lead.

Actions

- If you suspect a high level of lead in your home or environment, have your children tested even if they seem healthy.
- Keep your house clean; dust and dirt may contain lead.
- Do not attempt to remove lead-based paint yourself. Improper removal can increase the amount of lead in the environment.
- If you have older plumbing, have your water tested.

Data from National Lead Information Center, U.S. Environmental Protection Agency. (2005). Retrieved from http://www.nsc.org; and Centers for Disease Control and Prevention, National Center for Environmental Health, Childhood Lead Poisoning Prevention. (2005). *Screening young children for lead poisoning: Guidance for state and local public health officials.* Retrieved from http://www.cdc.gov/nceh.

formation is a prerequisite for judgment, orientation, and socially appropriate behaviors. Promoting safety requires a person to think clearly, recall past problems and solutions, and create solutions to current problems. To remain safe, the person must also be able to perceive impending danger. Often the ability to perceive danger is based on knowledge or learning from past experiences.

PHYSIOLOGICAL FACTORS

Impaired neurological function is a major component of risk for injury. To be safe, a person must have the judgment to recognize the presence of danger and the ability to move away. Many physiological factors can raise a person's risk for injury, including poor nutrition, clotting problems, a compromised immune system, a long history of alcohol and drug abuse, a debilitating disease, difficulty swallowing, and a need for tube feedings.

ASSESSMENT

General assessment of a client's safety requires gathering subjective data by interviewing the client and family about their safety needs. Gather objective data through physical examination, risk assessment tools, and environmental appraisals.

A home hazard appraisal tool allows you to elicit information objectively about the client's safety (Box 23-4). Variables used to categorize the client's risk include unsteady gait, dizziness or imbalance, impaired memory or judgment, weakness, and a history of falls. Many health care agencies also use tools that specifically identify a client's risk for falls (Box 23-5).

HEALTH HISTORY

Begin the safety assessment by identifying the client's lifestyle and health status factors that affect safety. Take a complete health history, emphasizing areas most likely to reveal issues of safety. They include lifestyle, medications, cardiovascular and respiratory systems, neurological function, and mobility.

Lifestyle. Assess the client's lifestyle for safety risk factors based on the developmental risk factors in Table 23-2. To elicit a subjective response, ask questions pertaining to the client's awareness of safety practices or plans for management of hazards. Also, ask about the client's occupation, home environment, and habits that may entail a risk for injury.

Medications. Include in your assessment questions about medications the client is currently taking and any side effects that may have been experienced.

BOX 23-4 *Home Assessment*

To help prevent injuries in the home, assess the client's home and immediate surroundings thoroughly. Make sure your assessment includes the following areas:

- General layout of the home
- Type of access into the home
- Availability of adequate lighting, including night-lights
- Availability of adequate ventilation
- Presence of uneven walkways, stairs, or pathways
- Presence of loose steps on stairways
- Presence or absence of railing on stairways
- Repairs needed to make walkways, stairs, and pathways safe
- Sturdiness and security of all stairs, stepstools, ladders, and handrails
- Potential dangers from cluttered or obstructed hallways, stairways, and walkways
- Presence of unanchored carpet, mats, or throw rugs
- Types of furniture, including sharp or jutting corners, heights in relationship to client, and support provided
- Types of floors, including those in bathrooms, showers, and bathtubs
- Presence or absence of grab bars around tubs, showers, and toilets
- Use of or need for a raised toilet seat or bath chair in tub or shower
- Condition of electrical appliances
- Loose or frayed electrical cords, overloaded outlets or extension cords, and proximity of electrical cords to water
- Presence and condition of smoke alarms and carbon monoxide detectors
- Presence and condition of fire extinguishers and plans for an escape route to be used in case of fire
- Appropriate disposal of expired foods and medications
- Proper storage and labeling of medications, cleaning solutions, combustibles (such as paint thinner and gasoline) or corrosives (such as rust remover [phosphoric acid]), and other toxic substances
- Presence of a fence around the pool
- Presence of a reliable heating system
- Accessibility of emergency telephone numbers, such as for the fire department, police department, ambulance, poison control center, and hospital

BOX 23-5 *Determining an Adult Client's Risk for Falls*

A person may have an increased risk for falling if he or she has one or more of the following risk factors:

- Age 65 or over
- A history of falling
- Decreased mobility or difficulty walking
- Need for assistance when getting out of bed or transferring to and from a chair
- A history of dizziness or seizures
- Impaired vision, hearing, or speech
- Need for assistive devices, such as a cane, walker, wheelchair, crutches, or braces, for mobility
- Weakness or fatigue caused by a disease process or prescribed therapy
- Confusion, disorientation, impaired memory or judgment, or impaired cognitive function
- Use of certain medications, such as diuretics, laxatives, or those that can alter the client's level of consciousness, including sedatives, hypnotics, tranquilizers, and analgesics

Cardiovascular medications, sedatives, antidepressants, and other medications that affect the central nervous system are particularly pertinent.

Cardiovascular and Respiratory Systems. Assessment of the cardiovascular and respiratory systems provides information about the client's activity tolerance. Assess changes in the client's blood pressure, pulse, and respirations with activity. Orthostatic hypotension and dizziness are factors in client safety.

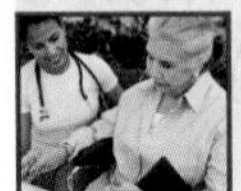

Mrs. Soto's arthritis has kept her from remaining active, but she is determined to keep trying. How would you assess her cardiovascular status to determine her ability to tolerate an exercise program?

Neurological Function. Assessment of the neurological system can provide information about the client's mental status, sensory function, reflexes, and coordination. Level of consciousness; orientation to time, person, and place; attention span; and decision-making abilities are also included in the neurological assessment. Testing of the senses (vision, hearing, taste, and smell) should be conducted to detect any deficits or alterations. This is important to determine the client's risk for injury with medication administration and while climbing stairs, reading warning labels, and listening for cars, smoke alarms, or other warning sounds.

Mobility. Assessment of the client's mobility is the key element of a safety assessment. Clients who experience impaired mobility because of paralysis, muscle weakness, poor balance, or poor coordination are at increased risk for injury.

PHYSICAL EXAMINATION

The collection of objective data allows you to assess the client's safety function and to assess for injuries and risk factors. You are also looking for evidence of past injuries. Examples of objective data include the client's muscle strength, joint range of motion, gait characteristics, pulse rate, skin color, skin turgor, and posture. The physical assessment should focus on the neurological system, skin integrity, and mobility. Ask the client about any history of accidental injuries while you inspect the skin. Inspect all areas of the client's skin for bruises, cuts, scratches, and scars. If lesions are present, describe the lesion and the client's explanation of their cause.

FOCUSED ASSESSMENT FOR *RISK FOR INJURY*

To assess the general category of *Risk for injury,* you need to observe the client's physical and psychological status and elements of the environment that are unsafe. Often, a combination of factors from the internal and external environments defines the client's risk.

Defining Characteristics. Internal risk factors for injury are classified as biochemical, physical, and psychological (NANDA International [NANDA-I], 2007). Biochemical factors of the neurological system include sensory, integrative, and motor dysfunction. In addition, hypoxia affects the ability to form reasoned judgments. Immune/autoimmune dysfunction, malnutrition, and an abnormal blood profile can make even minor injuries serious. Physical factors include altered mobility and the client's developmental status, with the very young and very old being the most vulnerable. Depression and anxiety are psychological factors that affect a person's ability to reason or to be alert to environmental hazards.

External risk factors are characterized as biological, chemical, physical, and people/provider. These may be found in the person's home, workplace, or community (NANDA-I, 2007).

FOCUSED ASSESSMENT FOR *RISK FOR TRAUMA*

Defining Characteristics. *Risk for trauma* is the nursing diagnosis that indicates the presence of any factor that increases the client's risk for accidental traumatic injury, such as a wound, burn, or fracture. Internal risk factors involve the individual. They include weakness, balancing difficulties, reduced coordination of large or small muscles, lack of safety education or precautions, cognitive or emotional difficulties, poor vision, reduced temperature or tactile sensation, reduced hand-eye coordination, insufficient finances to purchase safety equipment or make repairs, and a history of previous trauma (NANDA-I, 2007).

External risk factors involve hazards in the client's environment that can result in fires, burns, electrical shock, or accidents, particularly from falls. (NANDA-I, 2007).

Related Factors. For the client who is at risk for injury or trauma, nursing care may be aimed at reducing the risk or at helping the client compensate for the risk factors. In addition, care may be aimed at one or more of the following related factors.

Lack of Knowledge. Knowledge is an important factor to help prevent accidents. The knowledge of parents, caregivers, and other family members should be assessed.

Lack of Self-Care Ability. The client must have the physical and mental ability to appraise hazardous situations and make the necessary changes to prevent injury. People with physical limitations may be unable to recognize a high-risk situation or take corrective actions. Assess the client's ability to remove risk factors independently. Is there a potential to improve health or make the client more independent by introducing behaviors that reduce risk? For example, could teaching the client how to use a walker prevent falls?

Lack of Adequate Support Systems. If your client is cognitively, emotionally, or physically impaired, assess the support systems available. The client may be receiving support from a variety of sources, such as family, friends, volunteer agencies, and professional services. Determine any gaps in service that may leave the client vulnerable to injury.

FOCUSED ASSESSMENT FOR *RISK FOR POISONING*

Both internal and external factors are required to produce the *Risk for poisoning.* Internal factors may make clients unable or unwilling to prevent poisoning in the presence of external factors that place them at risk. Assess clients for these factors.

Defining Characteristics. Internal characteristics that increase the *Risk for poisoning* include the use of multiple medications, disability, and reduced vision. Also, assess the client's knowledge of poisonous substances and storage of household chemicals. For young children, the cognitively impaired, and persons with emotional difficulties, assessment should include the level of supervision and precautions taken to prevent accidents related to harmful substances (NANDA-I, 2007).

The environment should be assessed for external factors associated with the *Risk for poisoning* (NANDA-I, 2007).

Related Factors. Factors related to an increased *Risk for poisoning* are the same as those just listed. Nursing interventions are aimed at reducing the risk that these factors create.

FOCUSED ASSESSMENT FOR *RISK FOR SUFFOCATION*

Defining Characteristics. Assess for internal and external risk factors for *Risk for suffocation,* which include reduced olfactory sensation, reduced motor abilities, lack of safety education and precautions, cognitive or emotional difficulties, altered consciousness, and the presence of disease or injury. Assess the environment for external risk factors, especially the level of supervision of children and dependent adults (NANDA-I, 2007).

Related Factors. Factors related to an increased *Risk for suffocation* are the same as those just listed. Nursing interventions are aimed at reducing the risk that these factors create.

Lack of adequate supervision is a significant factor in preventing asphyxiation in infants and young children. To prevent asphyxiation in young children, hazards must be removed, and the child must be supervised. No environment can be made completely hazard free.

Supervision is also an important factor in preventing asphyxiation in neurologically, cognitively, or physically impaired people. Assess the client's ability to move in bed and maintain a body position that ensures a patent airway.

FOCUSED ASSESSMENT FOR *RISK FOR ASPIRATION*

Defining Characteristics. Aspiration is the inhalation of a foreign body or substance into the lungs. Physiologically, it occurs because the epiglottis fails to close completely. A person who does not have a gag reflex, who cannot produce a strong cough, or who is comatose has a high risk for aspiration. A nasogastric tube interferes with the gag reflex and with the lower esophageal sphincter. Any condition in which the lower esophageal sphincter is incompetent can raise the risk of regurgitation of stomach contents into the esophagus.

Related Factors. Aspiration is often associated with feedings through a nasogastric tube. It is not uncommon for these clients to have impaired swallowing. A distended stomach from any cause increases the chance of vomiting and aspiration. Lying flat in bed with a full stomach adds to the risk. Other conditions that can impair swallowing are wired jaws or oral surgery.

The outcome of aspiration can be fatal and usually depends on the amount of aspirant, the depth to which it is aspirated, and the person's ability to cough. Massive aspiration usually causes death. A small, localized aspiration from regurgitation may result in pneumonia or respiratory distress. Small aspirations that go unobserved (silent aspiration) are probably the most common type.

Every precaution needs to be taken to ensure the client's safety and prevent or reduce the *Risk for aspiration.* For example, food should be appropriate for the age, developmental stage, and condition of the client. The type of feeding (e.g., tube feeding or oral feeding) will determine the proper client positioning, the need for assistance or supervision, and the type of teaching that will be included in the client's plan of care.

> ***Action Alert!*** Aspiration is a medical emergency. Tachycardia, dyspnea, inability to speak, cyanosis, and hypertension may signal inhalation of gastric contents. Place the client in the best position for respiration (most often with head elevated), suction the trachea, and provide supplemental oxygen.

DIAGNOSIS

The main nursing diagnosis used to describe alterations in safety is *Risk for injury.* This diagnosis can be used for clients in the home setting, in long-term care facilities, and in the hospital or acute care setting. Depending on the safety issue involved, a diagnosis can be written to address the specific risk for an individual client. Examples include *Risk for trauma, Risk for poisoning, Risk for asphyxiation,* and *Risk for aspiration.*

Risk for trauma and *Risk for injury* are closely related concepts. *Risk for injury* is useful in an institutional setting, where you can protect clients from a broad array of risk. *Risk for trauma* is used more often in the community setting, where you would be helping to prevent accidents in individuals or groups of clients. Use the major risk factors identified so far and Table 23-3 to help you select the most appropriate nursing diagnosis for a client with a safety need.

Other diagnoses may be useful in the client who is at risk for injury. These include the following:

- Disturbed thought processes: The nursing diagnosis *Disturbed thought processes* suggests a high risk for injury.

Table 23-3 Clustering Data to Make a Nursing Diagnosis

INJURIES	
DATA CLUSTER	**DIAGNOSIS**
Maria Martinez is 85 years old and lives alone. She takes blood pressure medications and has osteoarthritis. Her physician recommended a total hip replacement, but she does not want to have surgery.	*Risk for injury* related to limited mobility, lack of assistance in the home, and possible orthostatic hypotension from blood pressure medications
Patrick, 6 months old, lives with his mother in a one-room apartment. He sleeps in the bed with his mother. She pads the bed with pillows to keep him from rolling off. He sleeps face down most of the time.	*Risk for asphyxiation* related to lack of resources for safe bedding and lack of knowledge about infant asphyxiation
Andrea, 5 years old, lives with her great-grandmother, who takes several medications and keeps them handy on the kitchen sink. The pills include a bright red tablet and a bright green one. Andrea thinks they look like Christmas.	*Risk for poisoning* related to unsafe storage of medications
Millie Kendall is 72 years old and in the wandering stage of Alzheimer's disease. She walks constantly in the nursing home and cannot identify her room. If not monitored, she leaves the building. She was once found a half-mile from the nursing home.	*Risk for injury* related to inability to make judgments about the environment
Richard King is 92 years old, lives alone, and manages his own care. A corner grocery store delivers supplies to his door. After being admitted to the hospital, he wakes from naps or during the night and thinks he is at home. He has been found in the hall looking for the bathroom.	*Risk for injury* related to unfamiliar environment, disorientation

Assess the client for impaired memory, confusion, judgment, and unusual patterns of thinking. Altered patterns of thinking can result from sleep deprivation or the use of medications that affect thinking. Therefore assessment should include all factors that have the potential to cause *Disturbed thought processes.*

- *Impaired home maintenance*: Impaired home maintenance can cause safety hazards. If the client is unable to keep the home in good repair, accidents can involve faulty furnaces, broken stairs, and other environmental hazards. Assess the client's home environment for safety hazards.
- *Deficient knowledge:* Lack of knowledge about health and safety practices may be the primary diagnosis, particularly with parents of young children. Assess the parents' knowledge of childhood safety, growth and development parameters, and measures for preventing accidents. Use this nursing diagnosis—*Deficient knowledge*—when the client has the skills and resources needed but does not have the knowledge of health and safety practices.
- *Impaired physical mobility:* Impaired mobility always causes an increase in the risk for injury. The degree of impairment and the client's knowledge of and use of safety measures should be assessed.

PLANNING

Planning involves identifying appropriate nursing interventions for clients who have actual or potential safety risks. Nursing interventions are individualized for each client and take into consideration the severity of the risk and the client's developmental stage, level of health, and lifestyle. The goal for the diagnoses of *Risk for injury* and *Risk for trauma* is that the client will remain free from injury. The care plan for *Risk for injury* focuses on prevention. You can prevent injuries by identifying potential hazards and measures to address them.

EXPECTED OUTCOMES FOR *RISK FOR INJURY*

The client will be able to do the following:

- Identify safety measures to prevent falls, such as removing safety hazards in the home, using assistive devices correctly, installing ramps or safety bars as needed in the home
- Use medical equipment correctly, employing recommended safety precautions
- Use protective measures to prevent falling while performing usual activities of daily living
- Be protected from injury by medical or other hospital equipment, therapeutic interventions, or other hazards in the environment during hospitalization
- Understand and utilize methods of calling for assistance in the hospital
- Recognize internal risk factors that increase vulnerability to injury
- Be protected from risk for fire, electrical hazards, and other environmental hazards in a health care facility

EXPECTED OUTCOMES FOR *RISK FOR TRAUMA*

The client will be able to do the following:

- Identify high-risk practices, such as speeding, alcohol or drug use, and smoking in bed
- Verbalize knowledge of the rationale for the use of seat belts, infant and toddler car seats, and bicycle and motorcycle helmets
- Commit to consistent use of seat belts, infant and toddler car seats, and bicycle and motorcycle helmets
- Identify safety measures and practices needed to decrease the risk for fires, electrical hazards, and burns from hot water bottles or heating pads
- Avoid high-risk practices such as diving in unknown places, speeding, and driving while intoxicated
- Describe the safe use of machinery or tools

EXPECTED OUTCOMES FOR *RISK FOR POISONING*

The client will be able to do the following:

- Recognize potential poisons in the home
- Properly label and store poisonous substances, including medications
- Develop a system for ensuring correct self-administration of medications
- Consult with a physician before combining over-the-counter medications or herbal supplements with prescription medications

EXPECTED OUTCOMES FOR *RISK FOR SUFFOCATION*

The client will be able to do the following:

- Identify risk factors for suffocation
- List preventive measures for suffocation
- Commit to implementation of prevention of suffocation
- Demonstrate correct use of oxygen and other respiratory equipment in the home
- Be protected from hazards associated with oxygen therapy equipment in the health care agency

EXPECTED OUTCOMES FOR *RISK FOR ASPIRATION*

The client will be able to do the following:

- Sit upright for eating
- Eat small bites of foods of the appropriate consistency
- Select foods that can be easily and safely swallowed
- Be evaluated for factors contributing to aspiration, such as nausea and competency of swallowing mechanisms

INTERVENTION

When a client is at risk for injury, nurses intervene to reduce hazards and prevent injury, trauma, suffocation, poisoning, and aspiration. Nursing interventions should be individualized and holistic, taking into consideration age, developmental level, health care needs, abilities, support systems, strengths, and weaknesses. Preventing hazards, trauma, and illness can be done by providing a safe environment, preventing falls, enhancing safety efforts, identifying risk factors, and increasing environmental awareness, knowledge, and a sense of physical and psychological safety and well-being.

INTERVENTIONS TO PROMOTE A SAFE ENVIRONMENT

Nursing interventions promote a safe environment at home and in the health care institution. Promoting safety at home can be accomplished by creating a safe home environment, especially for infants, children, and older adults. Creating a safe institutional environment, orienting clients to the environment, and monitoring clients can ensure safety in the hospital.

Promoting Safety at Home. When a client requires care in the home, the environment may need modifications to maintain ongoing safety. The environment may have been safe when the client was well and able to freely move about to manage the activities of daily living and necessary maintenance and repairs. However, when a client becomes physically or mentally compromised, even on a short-term basis, home safety becomes an issue.

Creating a Safe Home Environment. The home should be free of hazards that could result in falls. Measures to promote home safety include using nonskid rugs or tacking down throw rugs to prevent slips and falls, installing and using grab bars in the tub or shower, installing ramps to allow easier access, and keeping rooms, halls, and stairs free of clutter.

Safety practices to prevent burns or electrical shocks should be in place. Potential electrical hazards in the home environment include frayed cords, overloaded outlets and extension cords, use of electrical appliances near water, and lack of supervision of children near uncovered electrical outlets or electrical appliances. Covering electrical outlets when not in use, positioning pans with handles toward the back of the stove while cooking, and avoiding open-flame heaters are examples of prevention strategies.

Proper storage and labeling of bottles containing poisonous substances is essential. Have emergency telephone numbers, including the number for poison control, readily available (Figure 23-7). Instruct the client and family about medication administration, including information about the type of medication, dosage, reason for taking, expected effects, and possible side effects.

Encourage the client to call the poison control hotline for immediate access to information about appropriate first aid in a possible poisoning. Emetic agents should be given only after contacting the poison control center and ascertaining the guidelines for the specific poison. Although several emetic agents are available, syrup of ipecac is the most effective one to use in the home setting; administration within 30 minutes is best, but it can be effective for up to 1 hour after ingestion of poison. Syrup of ipecac is contraindicated after ingestion of gasoline, fuel oil, paint thinner, cleaning fluid, or strychnine. Also, children under 6 months old, people with severe heart disease, and pregnant or lactating women should not use syrup of ipecac.

Teaching may also involve instructing the client and family in the use of safe techniques for mobility of the physically impaired client. Provide instructions in the proper use of assistive devices, such as walkers, wheelchairs, or crutches. Teach the client and family ways to prevent back injury, including proper lifting techniques, back exercises to prevent back injury, and proper use of body mechanics.

Teaching may need to address the client's lifestyle as well. For example, the client may need to stop drinking and smoking. The family may need instruction in how to recognize signs and symptoms of choking and carbon monoxide poisoning and how to perform the Heimlich maneuver and cardiopulmonary resuscitation.

Safety precautions are essential for preventing injuries in older adults and in mentally ill or disabled clients. Ways to prevent injury include proper labeling of medications, assessing the home environment for potential hazards, and teaching appropriate safety measures. Establishing an open line of communication

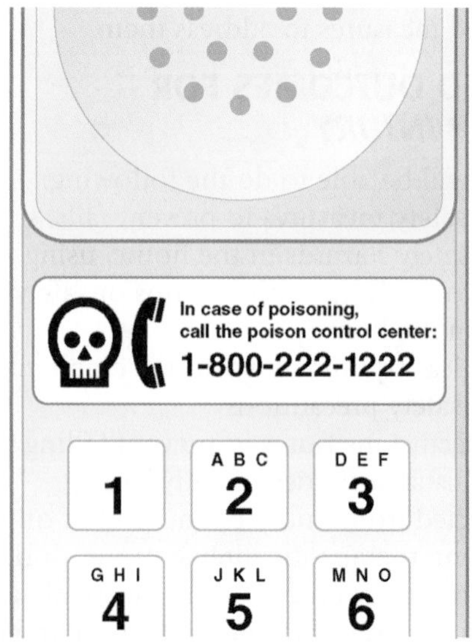

FIGURE 23-7 An example of a poison label on a telephone.

with the client or primary caregiver is of utmost importance in enhancing and promoting the safety of all those involved.

At times you may need to refer a dependent older adult to a home health care agency so that a home safety assessment can be performed before the client is discharged from the hospital. If a referral is necessary, it should be done 3 days before discharge to allow appropriate planning and implementation of safety measures. Make every attempt to accommodate the client's cultural needs, as outlined in Box 23-6.

Promoting Safety for Infants and Children. Involvement of clients and their families increases the likelihood of positive outcomes and the long-term lifestyle changes required. Referral to community resources may be helpful. Child safety is taught as part of parenting classes. Nurses may organize parenting classes for populations at risk or as part of a wellness program in a health care facility.

To promote a safe environment for infants and children, teach the family ways to childproof a home. Families can employ a number of important safety measures to prevent accidents. For example, plastic bags should be stored in a cabinet out of the child's reach. Covering an infant's or a child's mattress or pillow with plastic should be avoided. Crib design should follow federal safety regulations, and the mattress should be the appropriate size for the crib frame. Discourage parents from sleeping with their infant or putting the infant down to sleep with a bib, bonnet, or other snug-fitting garment tied around the neck. They should be taught never to tie a pacifier around the infant's neck. To avoid choking accidents, parents should inspect toys for removable parts and avoid feeding the infant such foods as grapes, nuts, and popcorn. When giving medication to a child, parents should avoid trying to entice the child by calling it candy.

Other safety measures that can be taken to ensure a child's safety include keeping doors of large appliances, especially unused refrigerators or freezers, closed at all times. Areas around a swimming pool should be fenced, and children should be supervised and wear protective gear when swimming. Instruct parents to avoid leaving pails of water or cleaning solutions accessible to children. Tell parents to use seat belts or car seats appropriate for the child's age and weight. Sharp objects, such as knives and other kitchen utensils, matches, and toxic substances should be kept out of children's reach.

Most accidents are preventable. By educating yourself, your clients, and their families, you can help reduce the risk in the home.

Providing Safety in Institutions

Creating a Safe Institutional Environment. In a health care institution, the client, especially one who is incapacitated by illness or disability, depends on the staff to provide a safe environment. This requires a team effort by nursing services, housekeeping, maintenance—indeed, every employee of the institution. Safety issues are similar to those in the home, but a hospital has more equipment, hazardous chemicals, and a large number of people using the facility. Every employee should be trained in electrical safety and fire safety as well as in safe interactions with clients.

Stay aware of the risk for electrical injury, especially in situations that combine moisture with electrical equipment. These situations may involve spills on the floor, a leaking or disconnected intravenous line, or a client with moist skin caused by diaphoresis.

BOX 23-6 *Cross-Cultural Care*

Caring for an Older Mexican American Client

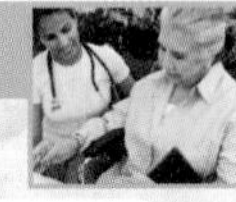

Mrs. Soto, the client described in this chapter's case study, lives in a city on the border of Texas and Mexico. She was born in Mexico and maintains close ties with family in Mexico. The following are some key facts to keep in mind when caring for Mexican American clients:

- Mexican Americans are the most successful of all ethnic groups at retaining their culture and language.
- In southwestern cities, Mexican Americans often live in *barrios* (Hispanic ethnic neighborhoods), where their primary interactions are with members of their own ethnic group.
- More than half (51%) of older Mexican Americans were born in Mexico.
- Older adults constitute less than 4% of the population of Mexican Americans.
- Mexican Americans tend not to retire; they tend to work as long as they are able.
- Mexican American culture values respectful behavior toward older persons and absolute obedience to their commands.
- Mexican American women tend to become more outgoing and domineering as they get older.
- Older Mexican Americans tend to function in the role of teacher, delineating proper conduct, relating historic events, and explaining the origin of things.
- Mexican American grandparents are unlikely to live alone.
- Older Mexican Americans are rarely placed in nursing homes by their families.

Data from Holmes, E. R., & Holmes L. D. (1995). *Other cultures, elder years.* Thousand Oaks, CA: Sage.

You can help prevent electrical injuries by making sure that electrical equipment stays in good working order and by using devices equipped with three-pronged grounded plugs (Figure 23-8). The third prong of the plug is called the *ground* because it is specifically designed to carry any stray electrical current into the earth. The two regular prongs carry power to the equipment being used. However, simply having a three-pronged plug does not ensure that the plug is grounded. The maintenance department should check the grounding periodically. Box 23-7 includes additional ideas to reduce the risk for electrical injury. Identifying and correcting potential sources of danger can prevent electrical shock.

Action Alert! Prevent electrical shocks by using grounded equipment. Teach others to avoid the use of faulty equipment and to never overload electrical outlets or extension cords.

Although fires are uncommon in modern buildings when safety precautions are followed, fire safety programs increase the readiness to respond correctly to a fire. Any fire that arises in a health care setting requires quick actions in response. A common response plan incorporates the acronym RACE to help prioritize those actions. It stands for *rescue, alarm, confine,* and *extinguish.*

The first priority in case of fire is to rescue or remove all clients from immediate danger. The second priority is to call for help. Be familiar with the protocol for activation of the fire alarm in your hospital or health agency.

The third priority is to confine the fire. Close nearby doors and windows, and turn off oxygen and electrical equipment. Close fire doors to confine the fire to an area of the building. Do not use elevators during a fire. The fourth priority is to extinguish the fire. Be sure to use the proper type of extinguisher for the type of fire involved (Box 23-8).

Also take steps to prevent back injuries—both your back and the client's. Back injuries can lead to lifelong pain, suffering, and disability. Taking care of your back is of vital importance to ensuring a healthy, productive life. Many general rules and principles can be applied to home and work environments to reduce the risk for back injuries. Make sure to follow safety guidelines to prevent back injuries from occurring, such as using proper lifting techniques and body mechanics and engaging in appropriate exercise and activity to promote strong bones and muscles.

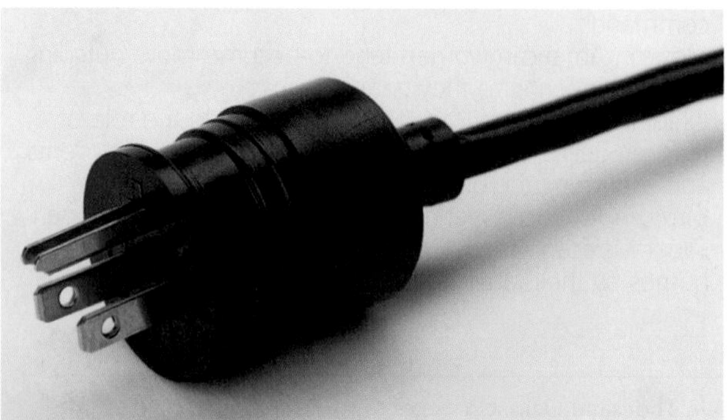

FIGURE 23-8 A three-pronged grounded plug, used to prevent electrical injuries. (Courtesy Lion Electric, South Norwalk, CT.)

Action Alert! Prevent back injuries from occurring. Use proper body mechanics and proper lifting and pushing techniques, and always ask for help when needed.

Orienting the Client to the Environment. A client newly admitted to a hospital or nursing home needs to be oriented to the new environment. The client and family should know how to operate the bed and any other equipment that the client will be using. One of the most important features of the safety orientation is teaching the client how to call for help using the call light at the bedside and the emergency call light in the bathroom. If the client needs the side rails raised for safety, make a point of saying so; give instructions for calling for help to get out of bed.

Some older clients, very ill clients, and clients under the influence of sedative medications may need ongoing orientation. A client with mild dementia may function

BOX 23-7 *Teaching for Self-Care*

Preventing Electrical Shocks

Purpose: To provide information about electrical safety.
Expected Outcome: The client will demonstrate electrical safety practices.

Client Instructions

Equipment

- Make sure that equipment is grounded; the use of a three-prong outlet does not ensure that the outlet is grounded.
- Do not use electrical cords that are frayed or that have visible damage.
- Repair or replace all malfunctioning equipment. If you drop a piece of electrical equipment, have it tested before reusing it.
- Experiencing shocks while using equipment means that it is not safe; have it tested before continuing to use it.
- Learn about all electrical equipment that you intend to use before attempting to use it.

Electrical Outlets

- Do not overload.
- Cover outlets not currently in use, especially if small children are present.
- Install outlets with ground fault circuit interrupters near sources of water, such as bathroom and kitchen sinks.
- Never pull a plug from the socket by the cord. Grip the plug firmly, and pull it straight out of the socket.

Extension Cords

- Avoid using extension cords when possible.
- Anchor extension cords to the floor using specially designed covers to prevent tripping over the cord.

well at home but become confused in a strange environment. To maintain a client's orientation, provide information about time, person, place, and environment at regular intervals. Use clocks, calendars, even family pictures to help keep the client oriented, especially if there is an impaired awareness of time, place, or person.

Preventing Ingestion of Toxic Substances. To prevent the accidental ingestion of toxic substances in the health care environment, take precautions to not leave medications or toxic solutions in the client's room. Using disposable cups and containers that can be immediately discarded can prevent accidental poisonings.

Monitoring the Client. While clients are in your care, take every precaution necessary to ensure their safety. By assessing their risk for injury, you can make sound judgments about the type and frequency of monitoring needed to maintain their safety. Clients who need frequent monitoring include those with the following conditions:

- At risk for compromised airway from muscle weakness or sedation
- Impaired mobility, especially when trying to get out of bed
- Unstable (fluctuating) vital signs
- A tendency to be restless in bed, especially if medical therapy includes intravenous lines or nasogastric tubes
- Cognitive impairment, especially if it reduces cooperation with the treatment plan
- Sensory impairments

Monitor totally dependent clients at least once an hour. If they have a high risk for injury, either have someone stay with them or place them in a room close to the nurses' station where you can monitor them frequently. A family member or private sitter can be used to provide constant surveillance.

If a client has a high risk for falls, consider using an identification system (colored tape on an arm band, a note in the chart and on the head of bed) to alert other staff members of the client's status. A warning system such as an Ambularm can be attached to the client's leg to alarm when the client tries to get out of bed (Figure 23-9). The device is sensitive to position changes and is activated when the client's leg goes over the side of the bed. The problem with an electronic monitoring system is that multiple false alarms desensitize staff members to the sound, resulting in a slow response.

Frequent monitoring increases the likelihood of detecting risk factors if you form the habit of looking for potential hazards each time you enter the client's room. Assess the client's environment to make sure the bed stays in the low position, side rails are up, bed wheels are locked, and items such as tissues, water, urinal, bedpan, glasses, and call light are within the client's reach. Note the client's level of consciousness, especially if an analgesic, a hypnotic, a sedative, or a tranquilizer has been administered.

The frequent presence of a nurse in the client's room contributes to a sense of security that may prevent the client from trying to get out of bed independently. Inform the client that you are nearby and will respond quickly to a call for help. It may be helpful to inform the client that you will return in a given period of time. However, make sure that you are indeed available when you say you will be.

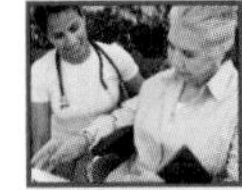

Think again of Mrs. Soto. Imagine that she is admitted to the hospital. We know she uses a wheelchair and walks with extreme difficulty. She is partially blind. How would you help her be safe in the hospital?

BOX 23-8 *Fire Extinguishers and Indications for Their Use*

A–Use on wood, cloth, paper, and rubbish fires. Do not use on electrical fires or burning liquids.
B–Use on oil, paint, propane, and flammable liquid fires.
C–Use on electrical equipment fires. Nonconductive.

WATER PUMP EXTINGUISHER

Use for type A fires, which involve paper, wood, or cloth.

CARBON DIOXIDE (CO_2) EXTINGUISHER/ DRY CHEMICAL EXTINGUISHER

Use for type B fires, which involve such flammable liquids as fuel oil, cooking oil, grease, paint, solvents, and anesthetic gases, and for type C fires, which involve electrical sources.

FOAM EXTINGUISHER

Use for type B fires.

MULTIPURPOSE EXTINGUISHER

Use for type A, B, and C fires.

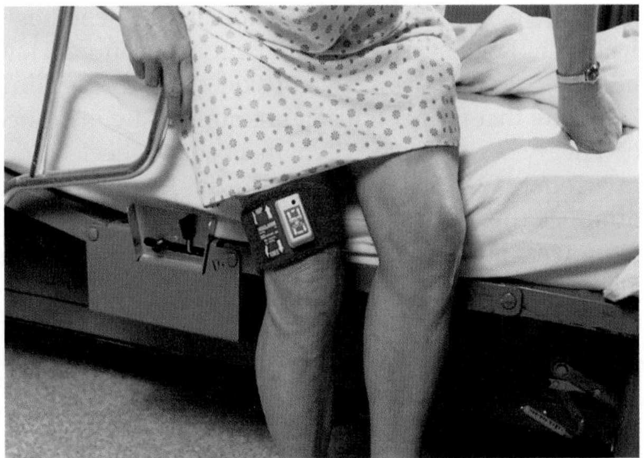

FIGURE 23-9 An Ambularm is a position-sensitive electronic device that is placed on the client's leg. Because it sounds a warning when the client attempts to get out of bed, it may provide a useful alternative to restraints. (Courtesy Alert Care, Mill Valley, CA.)

Infants and Children in the Hospital. In the hospital setting, all necessary precautions must be taken to keep children safe. Examples of common safety practices include the following:

- Never leave an infant unattended.
- Keep a bulb syringe readily available in case an infant's oropharynx needs to be suctioned.
- Make sure that periodic safety checks have been performed on emergency response equipment such as suctioning devices.
- Check the infant's or child's arm band before giving medications; remember that young children may answer to any name.
- Keep small objects out of reach to help prevent infants and small children from putting them into their mouth, nose, or ears.
- Keep the side rails of the crib up, and inspect all attachments on the crib or bassinet to make sure that they are fastened securely.
- Check the temperature of bath water to prevent scalding or chilling.
- Maintain bodily contact at all times when bathing an infant or toddler; never leave a child unattended during a bath.
- Always check the temperature of food or formula before feeding an infant.
- Never microwave an infant's formula to warm it.

INTERVENTIONS TO PREVENT FALLS

Interventions to prevent falls, especially in older adults, are of major concern. The environment should be free of potential hazards and equipped with safety devices. Certain basic safety measures should be incorporated into any prevention plan. The use of restraints can be included but only as a last resort and only under a physician's order.

Modifying the Environment. Health care environments are often crowded with equipment and people. Modifying this environment can reduce the risk for falls. For example, make sure that the ambulatory client has a clear path. Remove excess equipment or furniture. Have the client wear shoes with nonskid soles for walking. Make sure that proper transfer precautions are instituted for a heavy or debilitated client in a bed or wheelchair or on a toilet. Teaching safeguards to the family can also minimize the client's risk for falls in the health care environment. Box 23-9 describes measures for preventing falls in the hospital setting.

Using Equipment Safely. Equipment used in the hospital should be in proper working order. Proper training in the use of equipment commonly used in the home or hospital (suctioning machines, monitors, and so on) should be conducted on a regular basis. To ensure proper use of newly acquired equipment, qualified personnel should present training sessions.

BOX 23-9 *Preventing Falls in the Hospital Setting*

On admission, assess each client's risk for falls, and assign one of the following risk levels:

Low Risk: Assign this risk level if the client is alert, ambulates with a steady gait, can perform self-care activities without assistance, has no history of falls, and is cognitively intact and cooperative.

Medium Risk: Assign this risk level if the client may need some assistance or supervision when performing certain daily activities. The person may be alert and cooperative but may have a chronic physical ailment or a barrier (e.g., language) that could prevent calling for help.

High Risk: Assign this risk level if the client experiences periods of confusion or denies obvious problems of ambulation or mobility. This client may refuse to call for assistance and may attempt to perform activities independently. The client may have a history of falls and noncompliance with safety measures.

General Interventions for All Clients

No matter what your client's risk level, always take the following precautions to help avoid falls:

- When your clients arrive in their room, orient them to their new surroundings.
- Keep the two side rails in the raised position (per agency policy), regardless of age. Clients at low risk for falls may choose to have the side rails down during the day.
- Keep the call light, bedside table, water, glasses, and so on within the client's easy reach.
- Use a night-light.
- Make sure the client has and wears footwear with nonskid soles when out of bed.
- Use restraints and bed monitors as ordered by the physician.
- Keep the client's bed in the low position at all times except during procedures.
- Teach fall prevention techniques, such as sitting up for a moment before rising from the bed.

Specific Interventions for At-Risk Clients

- If your clients have a medium risk for falling, allow them to ambulate only with assistance. Make sure their family and other visitors understand this restriction. Anticipate and meet the clients' needs as much as possible. Offer assistance frequently.
- If your clients have a high risk for falling, try to locate them in a room close to the nurses' station. Answer these clients' call lights as quickly as possible. Assess them more frequently than usual. Maintain their scheduled toileting routine, and provide assistance with all activities of daily living. Encourage family members or other visitors to stay with them.

Equipment such as wheelchairs, beds, commode chairs, and shower chairs should have brakes that are working properly. Bed wheels should be locked, and the bed should be kept in the low position. The use of side rails varies by health care agency policy, although many hospitals use two side rails for most clients. Other measures include installing grab bars in the bathroom, applying safety strips in the tub or shower, and not leaving the client unattended while in the bathtub or shower (Figure 23-10).

Using Restraints. Restraints are used as a protective measure when clients are in danger of harming them-

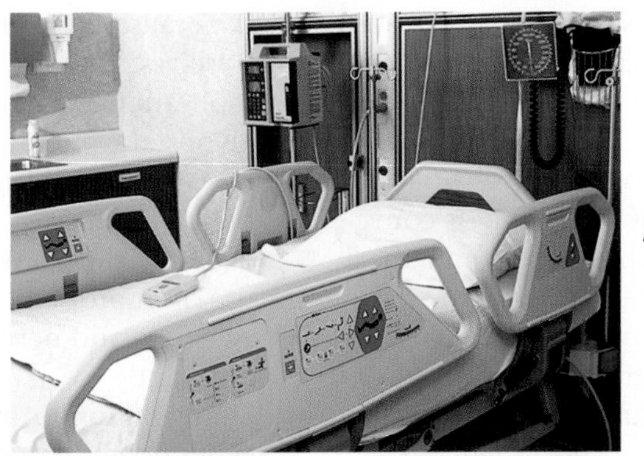
A

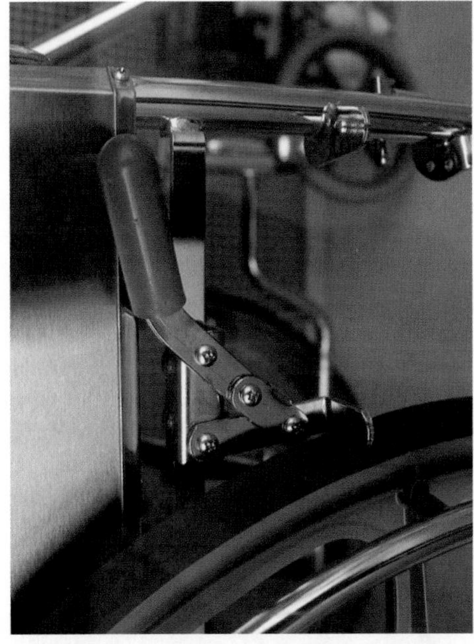
B

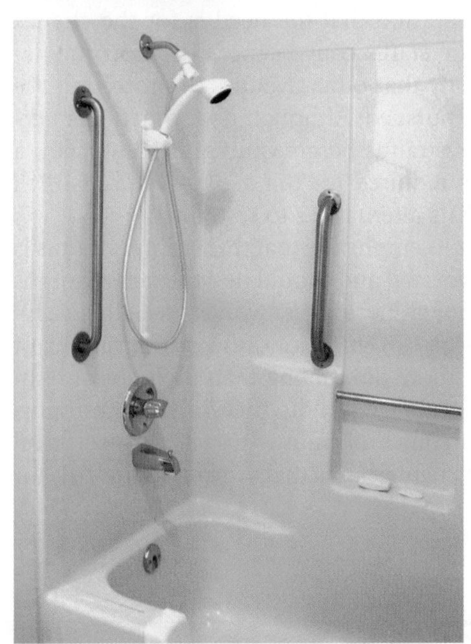
C

FIGURE 23-10 Safety devices help prevent falls in health care institutions and in the client's home. **A,** Side rails on beds. **B,** Locking devices on wheeled equipment. **C,** Grab bars in showers.

selves or others. The U.S. Food and Drug Administration, which regulates medical devices, defines a **restraint** as a device (usually a wristlet, anklet, or other type of strap) intended for medical purposes that limits movement to the extent necessary for treatment, examination, or protection of the client. Restraints also can be chemical (medications to calm the person's behavior) or environmental (side rails on beds, locked psychiatric units, or quiet rooms).

In the hospital or nursing home setting, the primary use of restraints is to prevent a client from falling and sustaining an injury. The client must be at high risk for falling or injury, be unable to understand that risk, and have no other avenues of prevention available.

The second major reason for restraints is to prevent the client from interrupting therapy, especially when the therapy is life sustaining. When a client is confused or sedated and therefore unable to understand the presence of an intravenous line, nasogastric tube, wound dressing, or other medical device, it is a natural human instinct to attempt to remove the irritant. Then the client's hands may need to be restrained.

The third major reason for restraints is to prevent the client from self-harm or from harming others. Although violent or self-destructive behavior is more often associated with psychiatric units, it occasionally occurs in general medical or surgical units. Usually, combative behavior results from the confusion and fear that arises in a situation the client cannot understand or control. It sometimes occurs after withdrawal from certain drugs (Procedure 23-1).

The appropriate use of restraints is controversial in the health care setting. Physical restraints are used in health care institutions, especially with confused clients who interfere with medical treatments or devices, demonstrate disruptive behaviors, or face an increased risk for falls. Psychiatric facilities have adopted policies of treating the client in the least restrictive manner possible. In 1987, the Omnibus Reconciliation Act extended this philosophy to nursing home residents, using the following language: "The client has the right to be free from any physical restraints imposed or psychoactive drug administered for purposes of discipline or convenience, and not required to treat the resident's medical condition."

All health care facilities have well-defined written policies regarding the use of restraints. Unnecessarily restraining a person may be construed as assault or false imprisonment. You must be able to document a clear need for a restraint and that the need is for the client's safety, not for the staff's convenience. The documentation should specify that other avenues of protecting the client have been pursued. Although it is sometimes necessary to apply restraints before calling the physician, a medical order is required for the use of restraints. Box 23-10 (p. 559) lists alternatives to restraints.

It is important to emphasize that the use of restraints is generally not advocated and should be considered only as a last resort. Although health care workers usually use restraints with the best of intentions, the complications of restraints can be more devastating than their absence. In spite of the belief that restraints prevent falls, restraints themselves are a source of injury. In fact, the use of restraints in older clients can actually increase the risk for falls because the clients may struggle desperately to free themselves from the perceived bondage. Other potential complications include the following:

- Hypostatic pneumonia from failure to turn and move in bed or from the inability to take a deep breath because of a constricting device
- Skin abrasions, edema, or pressure injuries from the use of improperly padded restraints
- Ischemia and nerve damage if the restraint is applied too tightly
- Strangulation from a vest restraint when the client slides down in bed and is unable to move or call for help
- Contractures from immobility
- Shoulder dislocation from struggling against a restraint
- Aspiration pneumonia

Side rails provide the simplest and least restrictive method of restraint used in the health care environment. If the client needs traditional restraints, several types are available, such as jacket and vest restraints, belt restraints, mitt or hand restraints, and wrist and ankle restraints. Some commonly used restraints must be tied to another object, such as a stable heavy chair, wheelchair, or bed. They must be tied securely enough to prevent the client from releasing them but in a manner that allows quick release in case of an emergency.

Text continued on p. 559

Time to Allow: **Novice:** 10 min. **Expert:** 5 min.

PROCEDURE 23-1 USING PROTECTIVE RESTRAINTS

Nursing Skills Online: Safety, Lesson 2

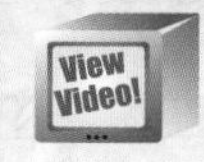

Restraints are any physical or chemical method used to restrict or control behavior for the purpose of protecting the client from harm or from causing injury to others. A person can be restrained by confinement to a room, a chair, or a bed or restrained by the use of drugs that decrease angry or aggressive behavior.

DELEGATION GUIDELINES

The decision to restrain a client may not be delegated to a nursing assistant. Physical restraint requires a physician's order. As a registered nurse, you will be able to determine whether to restrain a client when the client is deemed to be in immediate danger of causing harm to self or others and no other more appropriate means of managing the behavior exist. However, you must inform the physician and receive an order to continue the restraints. You may delegate observation of the restrained client to a nursing assistant. You may delegate assistance with eating or toileting and repositioning including reapplication of restraints. However, you must provide specific criteria for observation and supervision of the client.

POSSIBLE COMPLICATIONS MAY RESULT FROM:

Improper application: skin damage, ischemia/nerve damage, strangulation; and **enforced immobility:** hypostatic pneumonia or contractures; or **secondary to struggling to be free:** fall secondary to climbing over side rails.

EQUIPMENT NEEDED

- Restraints: jacket, vest, waist, wrist, or ankle restraint
- Padding as needed

1 Follow preliminary actions (see inside front cover).

2 Assess the need for restraints. *The client's behavior could cause self-harm (risk for fall, risk for suicide, risk for wandering into unsafe areas) or injury to others. Alternatively, it could interrupt medical therapy, thus increasing the risk for complications, delaying the healing process, or causing an early death.*

3 Consider alternatives to restraints. *Discuss with the physician and with the client's family.*

4 Choose the least restrictive type of restraint.

a. A *jacket restraint* allows the client to turn from side to side in the bed but prevents getting out of bed or a chair. It secures both the shoulders and the waist (see illustration).

b. A *belt restraint* secures the person at the waist only. Less restrictive than a jacket, it is also not as protective. It also allows the client to turn from side to side in bed (see illustration).

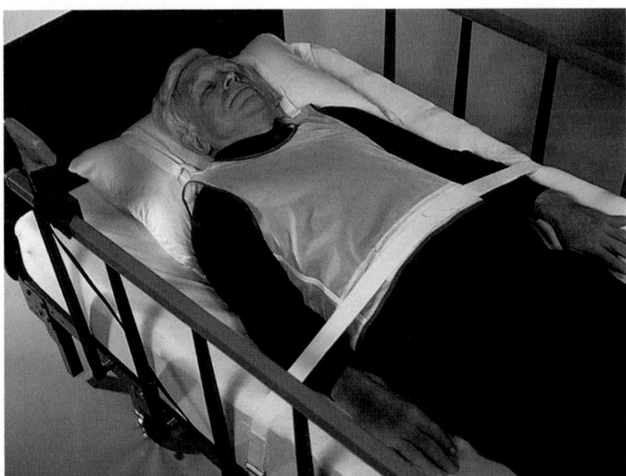

Step 4a. Jacket restraint. (Courtesy Medline Industries, Mundelein, IL.)

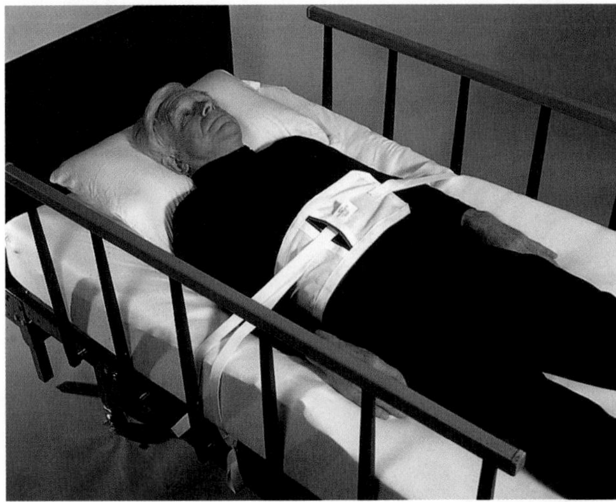

Step 4b. Belt restraint. (Courtesy Medline Industries, Mundelein, IL.)

c. A *wrist restraint* secures one or both of the client's hands. By positioning the client's hand or hands away from tubes and dressings, the wrist restraint prevents the client from removing an intravenous line, a nasogastric tube, an indwelling urinary catheter, or a wound dressing. It also can prevent infiltration of an intravenous drug by immobilizing the client's arm. Finally, it can prevent the client from striking people standing nearby (see illustration).

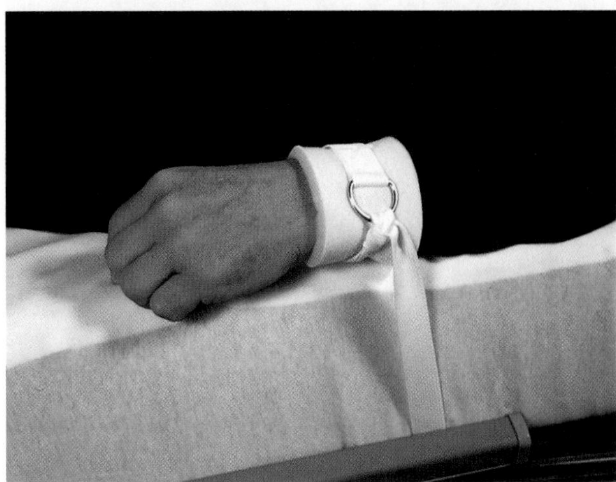

Step 4c. Wrist restraint. (Courtesy Medline Industries, Mundelein, IL.)

d. An *ankle restraint* secures one or both ankles and prevents injury caused by thrashing about in bed. It also prevents the client from dislodging a femoral arterial line (see illustration).

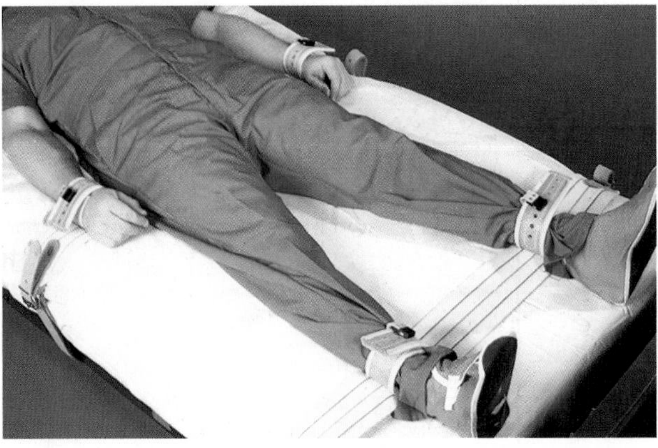

Step 4d. Ankle restraints. (Courtesy Humane Restraint Company, Waunakee, WI.)

Continued

e. A *mitten restraint* prevents use of the hands while allowing free arm movements. It is useful for a client who is disturbed by wrist restraints but needs to be prevented from dislodging an intravenous line, an indwelling urinary catheter, a nasogastric tube, or a wound dressing (see illustration).

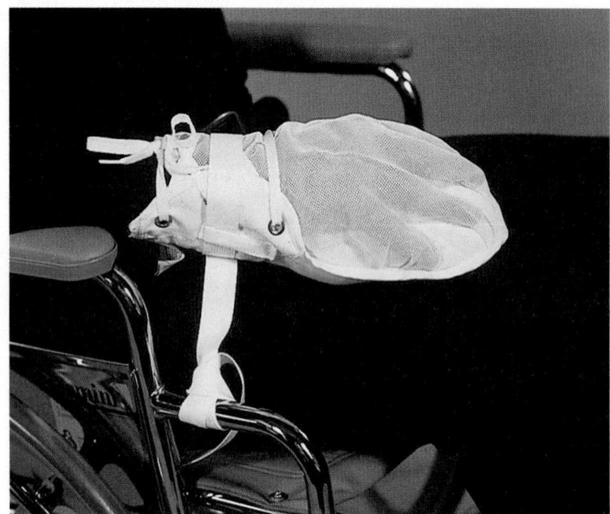

Step 4e. Mitten restraint. (Courtesy Medline Industries, Mundelein, IL.)

5 Apply the restraint.

a. Approach the client in a calm, reassuring manner. Avoid sudden or threatening movements.
b. If the client can understand, explain the need for restraint.
c. If the client cannot understand the need for restraint, proceed by applying it in a gentle but firm manner.
d. Pad the skin under the restraint, especially over bony prominences.
e. Allow room for two fingers to be inserted between the restraint and the client's limb. *Doing so will prevent circulatory constriction.*
f. Avoid constricting the client's breathing.
g. Allow the client freedom to turn in bed, if possible.
h. Tie the restraint to the bed frame rather than a side rail (see illustration). *The side rail can be moved, which may make the restraint too tight (and harmful to the client) or too loose (ineffective).*
i. Tie the restraint in a location where the client cannot reach it but where an attendant can quickly and easily release it in an emergency.
j. Use a slipknot for quick release. Never tape a restraint knot.

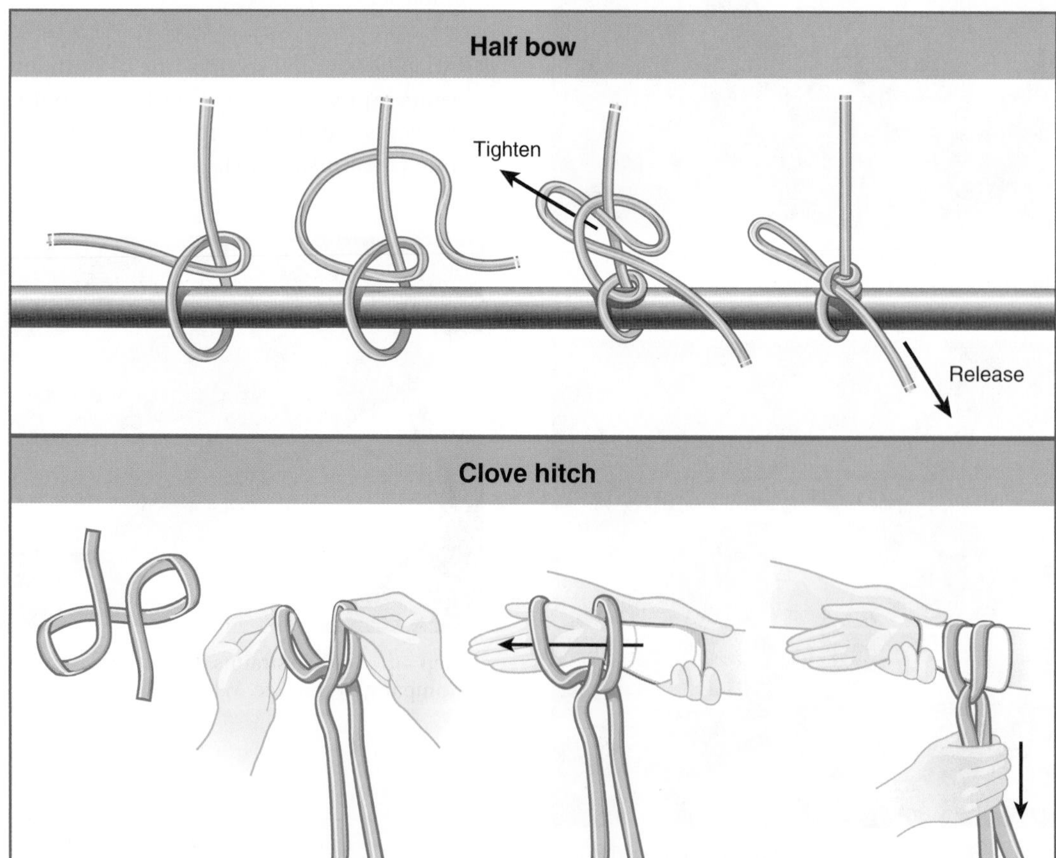

Step 5h. Tie the restraint to the bed frame.

6 Monitor the client, and intervene to prevent complications.

a. Observe the client every 30 minutes.
b. Check the client's skin and circulation every 30 minutes.
c. Provide a regular schedule of toileting.
d. Turn the client at least every 2 hours; position for comfort.
e. Orient the client to the environment every time you check.
f. Assess the client's respirations, cough, and deep breathing every 2 hours.
g. Reassess the need for restraints every 2 hours.
h. Help the client with food and fluid intake as needed.

7 Document the following properly:

a. Rationale or behavior that led to restraint
b. Type of restraint and time it was applied
c. Ongoing assessment and interventions to prevent complications
d. Time restraints are discontinued and client's response

PEDIATRIC CONSIDERATIONS

Restraints for children depend on the age of the child. Provide the least restrictive environment possible, but maintain safety. For some procedures the infant may be held in the mother's arms. For the infant or toddler, a mummy or papoose style of restraint is used for short procedures when it is important that the child be still (e.g., when passing a nasogastric tube, inserting an intravenous catheter, or suturing a laceration).

GERIATRIC CONSIDERATIONS

The older client should receive care in the least restrictive environment possible. Seek alternatives to maintain dignity and respect. Also exercise caution to avoid injury to delicate skin.

HOME HEALTH CARE CONSIDERATIONS

When the client's behavior in the home requires protection to prevent falls or other self-harm, you should work with the family to provide the protection in the least restrictive manner. If the client needs frequent personal care, a hospital bed may be helpful to family caregivers because of the ease of raising the bed to a working height and of lowering the bed to transfer the client to a chair. If the side rails are sufficient restraint, a hospital bed is a good solution. Otherwise, placing the mattress on the floor may give freedom from restraints and afford protection from falling when trying to get out of bed. Also talk to the family about supervision, and help them work out a schedule to ensure that the client is attended closely.

BOX 23-10 *Finding Alternatives to Restraints*

Increase Monitoring Frequency

- Assign the client a room near or within view of the nurses' station.
- Perform hourly safety checks.
- Use an electronic monitoring device, such as an Ambularm, which sounds an alarm when the client's leg reaches a 45-degree angle. An ankle alarm can be used to reveal when an ambulatory client wanders off the nursing unit.
- Have family members or a sitter remain with the client.

Provide a Familiar Environment

- Familiarize the client with the immediate surroundings.
- Provide continuous orientation to person, place, time, and environment. Remind the client to use the call light.
- Use colors as environmental cues.
- Allow the client to use personal belongings, such as a pillow or clothing, when possible.
- Assign familiar personnel, if possible, to help the client feel secure and provide a more accurate needs assessment.
- Encourage the family's participation in the client's care.

Prevent the Need to Get Out of Bed Unassisted

- Promote a restful environment by minimizing noise, maintaining appropriate lighting, playing relaxing music, and so on.
- Provide comfort measures, such as pain relief and proper positioning.
- Assist with toileting on a regular schedule.

Institute Safety Measures

- Use stabilizing devices, slanted seats, or positioning devices (such as pillows, rolled blankets, and wedge cushions) on wheelchairs to keep the client positioned safely.
- Use bed, chair, or position-sensitive alarms.
- Keep the client's bed in the low position; use half rails or keep the side rails down.
- Increase lighting in the room; use night-lights.

Change The Treatment Plan

- Consult with the physician to review the need for intravenous catheters, urinary catheters, or nasogastric tubes.

EVALUATION

The effectiveness of nursing interventions used to promote safety and prevent injury is evaluated by comparing the expected outcomes to the goals devised during the planning phase. Nursing interventions are considered effective if the client remains free from injury and the client's personal freedom and dignity are optimally maintained.

You should continuously reevaluate the client's situation and determine whether new threats to safety have developed or previous ones remain. Continuous reevaluation will help you make judgments about discontinuing

BOX 23-11

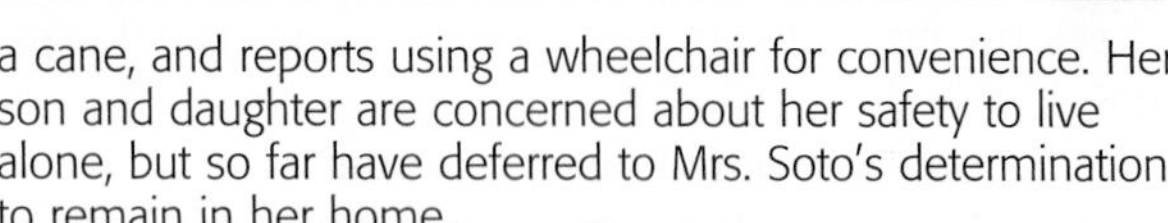

Nursing Care Plan

An Older Adult Client With a History of a Fall

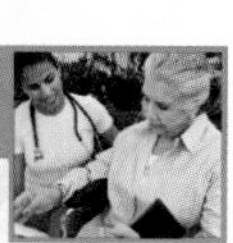

Hospital Admission Note

Mrs. Soto is a 75-year-old Hispanic woman admitted through the emergency department to 4N after sustaining a head contusion when she fell in her bathroom at home and hit her head on the wastebasket. She also has a bruised knee and wrist. Apparently she put out her hand in an attempt to stop the fall. Mrs. Soto informed the nurse, "I never have hurt myself this much before. Usually I catch myself before I fall all the way. Since my husband died, I have lived by myself, but I manage okay. I just hurried too fast this morning." Mrs. Soto lives alone in a two-story wood frame house.

Discharge Nursing Report to Home Health Care Agency

Mrs. Soto was admitted to be evaluated for a head injury following a fall at home in the bathroom. The findings for a head injury were negative, but she did sustain several bruises. Her son was with her in the hospital and will stay with her a few days at home. She reports a history of falling without serious injury. She is fully oriented, ambulatory with a cane, and reports using a wheelchair for convenience. Her son and daughter are concerned about her safety to live alone, but so far have deferred to Mrs. Soto's determination to remain in her home.

Physician's Referral Request

Evaluate ability to perform activities of daily living and instrumental activities of daily living. Monitor BP for orthostatic hypotension, and monitor compliance with medications. Arrange for home health care aide and Meals on Wheels if needed. Physical therapy to teach isometric exercises and use of cane. Home paraffin therapy daily before exercise.

Home Health Care Nursing Initial Visit Assessment

Minimally safe in home environment. No apparent cognitive deficits. Cooking would be difficult because of mobility and vision deficit. An older two-story house with no safety equipment in the bathroom, some throw rugs, inadequate lighting at night, cluttered hallways, and broken stairs to basement with no handrails. Moves slowly but can safely ambulate in house with cane. No orthostatic hypotension.

NANDA-I Nursing Diagnosis	NOC Expected Outcome With Indicators	NIC Interventions With Selected Activities	Evaluation Data

Risk for Injury: Fall
Related factors:
• Limited mobility from arthritis
• Blind in one eye
• History of multiple falls
• Lives alone
• Alternates between using a cane and a wheelchair
• Age 75
• Determined to remain in her own home
• Home has stairs that need repairs, handrails and grab bars needed in bathroom
	Safety Status: Fall Occurrence
	• Record number of falls:
	  • While standing
	  • While walking
	  • While sitting
	  • While transferring
	  • Climbing stairs
	  • Descending stairs
	• Client will institute measure to improve safety of home environment.
		Fall Prevention: Surveillance: Safety
		• Identify cognitive or physical deficits that may increase risk for falls at home.
		• Assess gait, balance, and fatigue level with ambulation.
		• Provide a walker, and teach her to use it.
		• Remove hazards from home: throw rugs and clutter.
		• Arrange for installation of grab bars for tub and nonslip floor.
		• Increase lighting in home.
		• Home health care aide twice a week for assistance with bathing.
			Second Home Visit
			• Clutter and throw rugs have been removed.
			• Son will return on weekend to repair stairs to basement.
			• Daughter plans to come weekly to do laundry.
			• Meals on Wheels has started delivery of a daily meal consistent with Hispanic food preferences.
			• Mrs. Soto expresses gratitude that she will be able to stay at home.
			• Physical therapist reports that she can be expected to increase mobility with strengthening exercises, balance exercises, and learning to use a walker.
			• A referral has been made to obtain home modifications.
			• Mrs. Soto maintains order in her home and is familiar with environment.
			• She has neighbors who are willing to visit frequently and perform small tasks.
			• She has limited range of motion in lower extremities but demonstrates proper use of walker.
			• She has shoes with nonskid soles.
			• Her home is about 50 years old; it has four bedrooms and two baths. The bathroom floor has tile, and she usually has throw rugs on the floor because it tends to be cold. She expressed concern over the cost of grab bars.

BOX 23-11

Nursing Care Plan—cont'd

An Older Adult Client With a History of a Fall

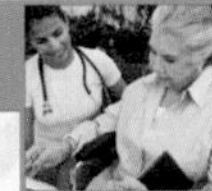

Critical Thinking Questions

1. How would you handle the subject of using a copper bracelet rather than the medication the physician has ordered?
2. How would you approach the subject of having a caretaker live with Mrs. Soto?
3. Would adult day care be helpful in this situation?

Nursing outcome and intervention labels from Johnson, M., Bulechek, G., Butcher, H., Dochterman, J. M., Maas, M., Moorhead, S., et al. (Eds.). (2006). *NANDA, NOC, and NIC linkages: Nursing diagnoses, outcomes, & interventions.* St. Louis, MO: Mosby.

unnecessary restrictions, especially the use of restraints. The evaluation phase requires frequent assessment of the client's situation to identify specific needs for support services, such as home health care, nursing home placement, or physical and occupational therapy. A care plan for Mrs. Soto can be found in Box 23-11.

It is important to be aware of all the different categories of accidents and hazards that create the potential for risks. Also of importance is an awareness of the people most at risk, such as children and older adults, the handicapped, and the debilitated. You can make a significant difference in the lives of many individuals, especially when safety issues are concerned. Nurses are in a unique position to teach preventive measures, promote safety guidelines, and alleviate alterations in safety.

SAMPLE DOCUMENTATION NOTE FOR MRS. SOTO

Discharge per wheelchair to son's automobile. Alert and oriented, able to walk the length of the hall without dizziness. Son has acquired a walker for his mother's use. Referred to Spring Valley Home Health for evaluation of home setting for safety needs, ability to perform activities of daily living, correct use of walker, need for Meals on Wheels, and physical therapy services. Will see primary physician on Friday for follow-up.

▼ KEY PRINCIPLES

- To feel safe and to be safe in the home setting or health care facility is a basic human need.
- Nurses are in a prime position to help prevent accidents, promote safety, and alleviate alterations in safety.
- Falls, asphyxiation, choking, and poisoning are preventable.
- Traumatic injuries can result from fires, electrical shock, motor vehicle accidents, and exposure to radiation.
- Falls are the second leading cause of death in people over the age of 74 years.
- The risk for falls is significantly higher in hospitalized older adults.
- Asphyxiation, or suffocation, is a leading cause of mortality during childhood.
- People most at risk for poisoning include toddlers, young children, and adults with sensory impairment.
- Cigarette smoking and the use of alcohol are common factors that can increase the risk for fire injuries.
- Factors that determine the type and extent of an electrical injury include voltage, type of current, area and duration of contact, skin resistance, and path of current flow.
- Motor vehicle accidents are the leading cause of accidental death in the United States.
- Measures to prevent back injuries include using proper lifting techniques and proper body mechanics and performing proper exercises and activities to promote strong bones and muscles.
- Prevent exposure to radiation by using lead shielding and by observing the increased distance/decreased time rule when caring for a client with radioactive implants.
- Factors affecting a person's risk for injury can be identified in the person's home, work, and community.
- The nurse's role in home safety includes education appropriate for age and developmental status; it also includes making referrals to help the family attain and maintain safe housing.
- The nurse's role in institutional safety involves the safe use of equipment, appropriate client education, and collaboration with the housekeeping and maintenance departments to ensure a safe environment.
- Clients should be restrained only in the absence of viable alternatives and when there is clear evidence that failure to restrain could lead to client harm.

■ REVIEW QUESTIONS

1. Falls most often occur in the hospital when the client is alone in the room. Your nursing unit has a policy that the beds should be left in a low position and have two side rails up for clients who should not get out of bed unassisted. Which of the following is the best rationale for this policy?

1. It satisfies the hospital legal department that precautions are taken to prevent falls.
2. It guarantees that the client will not get out of bed unassisted.
3. It reminds the client to call for assistance when getting out of bed.
4. It reduces the frequency of needing to monitor the client's behavior.

2. You are on the night shift at the hospital. Which of the following clients is at greatest risk for falling in the hospital?

1. A 90-year-old with mild memory deficit who goes to the bathroom several times a night
2. A 45-year-old with a fractured femur and a full leg cast who ambulates with crutches
3. An active 10-year-old who continues to have a problem with bed wetting
4. A 70-year-old who had major abdominal surgery 2 days ago

Continued

3. You enter a client's room and find her using a hair dryer from home. It has a frayed cord. Which of the following is the safest initial action?

1. Take the hair dryer, and tell her you will have the maintenance department check it for safety.
2. Inform the client that the hairdryer does not appear to be safe to use, but leave it in the room.
3. Obtain some electrical tape, and wrap it around the frayed cord.
4. Make sure that the cord is not touching any metal parts of the bed.

4. You smell smoke, and enter a client's hospital room. The client is fully ambulatory. The room is full of smoke, and there is a fire in wastebasket. Your first action should be:

1. Activate the hospital fire alarm.
2. Get a fire extinguisher, and put out the fire.
3. Escort the client out of the room.
4. Close the door to all the rooms on the unit.

5. Your client is 1 day post surgery for a bladder tumor. She has a Foley catheter that is bothering her. She becomes confused and is trying to pull the catheter out. You believe she should be restrained. Select the best initial action.

1. Call the physician for an order to restrain her.
2. Call her husband to come and stay with her.
3. Apply wrist restrains to prevent her from dislodging the catheter.
4. Attempt to orient her to the environment and the need for the catheter.

Bibliography

Birks, Y. (2003). A multifactorial intervention after a fall did not prevent falls in elderly patients with cognitive impairment and dementia. *Evidence-Based Nursing, 6*(4), 114-115.

Bright, L. (2005). Strategies to improve the patient safety outcome indicator preventing or reducing falls. *Home Healthcare Nurse, 23*(1), 29-38.

Bush, T. (2003). More than gravity: Falls in the elderly mentally ill patient with dementia—increasing nurses' awareness of the risk factors. *Nurse 2 Nurse, 3*(9), 36-38.

Capezuti, E. (2004). Minimizing the use of restrictive devices in dementia patients at risk for falling. *Nursing Clinics of North America, 39*(3), 625-647.

Centers for Disease Control and Prevention. (2000a). Fire related injuries. *Fact book for the year 2000.* Retrieved from http://www.cdc.gov/ncipc/factsheets/fire.htm.

Centers for Disease Control and Prevention. (2000b). Motor-vehicle-related injuries. *Fact book for the year 2000.* Retrieved from http://www.cdc.gov/ncipc/pub-res/FactBook/fkmve.htm.

Centers for Disease Control and Prevention. (2004). *A tool kit to prevent senior falls: The costs of fall injuries among older adults.* Retrieved January 31, 2005, from http://www.cdc.gov/ncipc/factsheets/fallcost.htm.

Centers for Disease Control and Prevention. (2005a). Falls and hip fractures among older adults. *Fact book for the year 2005.* Retrieved from http://www.cdc.gov/ncipc/pub-res/Factsheets/falls.htm.

Centers for Disease Control and Prevention. (2005b). Web-based Injury Statistics Query and Reporting System (WISQARS) [Online]. National Center for Injury Prevention and Control, Centers for Disease Control and Prevention (producer). Retrieved August 7, 2005, from http://www.cdc.gov/ncipc/wisqars.

Centers for Disease Control and Prevention, National Center for Environmental Health, Childhood Lead Poisoning Prevention. (2005). *CDC Childhood Lead Prevention Program.* Retrieved August 7, 2005, from http://www.cdc.gov/nceh.

Clark, M. A. (2005). Involuntary admission and the medical inpatient: Judicious use of physical restraint. *Medsurg Nursing, 14*(4), 213-219.

Farrell, M. K. (2004). Using functional assessment and screening tools with frail older adults. *Topics in Geriatric Rehabilitation, 20*(1), 14-20.

Folkes, K. Is restraint a form of abuse? *Paediatric Nursing, 17*(6), 41-44.

Hildreth, R. (2002). Review: Hip protectors reduce hip fractures after falls in elderly people living in institutions or supported home environments. *Evidence-Based Nursing, 5*(1), 23.

Hoffman, S. B., Powell-Cope, G., MacClellan, L., & Bero, K. (2003). BedSAFE: A bed safety project for frail older adults. *Journal of Gerontological Nursing, 29*(11), 34-42, 54-55.

*Holmes, E. R., & Holmes L. D. (1995). *Other cultures, elder years.* Thousand Oaks, CA: Sage.

Insomnia, not medications, are related to falls in elderly. (2005). *Senior Care Management, 8*(4), 47.

Johnson, M., Bulechek, G., Butcher, H., Dochterman, J. M., Maas, M., Moorhead, S., et al. (Eds.). (2006). *NANDA, NOC, and NIC linkages: Nursing diagnoses, outcomes, & interventions.* St. Louis, MO: Mosby.

Letizia, M., Babler, C., & Cockrell, A. (2004). Repeating the call for restraint reduction. *Medsurg Nursing, 13*(1), 9-13.

*Loomis, T. A., & Hayes, A. W. (1996). *Loomis' essentials of toxicology* (4th ed.) San Diego, CA: Academic Press.

McCarter-Bayer, A., Bayer, F., & Hall, K. (2005). Preventing falls in acute care: An innovative approach. *Journal of Gerontological Nursing, 31*(3), 25-33.

NANDA International. (2007). *Nursing diagnoses: Definitions and classification, 2006-2007* (7th ed.). Philadelphia: Author.

National Lead Information Center, U.S. Environmental Protection Agency. (2004). *Health Effects on Children.* Retrieved from http://www.nsc.org.

*National Institute for Occupational Safety and Health, U.S. Department of Labor. (2006). *Ergonomics: Guidelines for nursing homes.* Retrieved August 7, 2005, from http://www.osha.gov/.
ergonomics/guidelines/nursinghome/index.html.

Nurmi, I. S., Luthje, P. M. J., & Kataja, J. M. (2004). Long-term survival after falls among the elderly in institutional care. *Archives of Gerontology and Geriatrics, 38*(1), 1-10.

Reyes-Ortiz, C. A., Al Snih, S., & Markides, K. S. (2005). Falls among elderly persons in Latin America and the Caribbean and among elderly Mexican-Americans. *Pan American Journal of Public Health, 17*(5/6), 362-369.

Saufl, N. M. (2004). Restraints use and falls prevention. *Journal of PeriAnesthesia Nursing, 19*(6), 433-436.

Sweeney-Calciano, J., Solimene, A. J., & Forrester, D. A. (2003). Finding a way to avoid restraints: Learn how simple interventions can help keep a wandering or agitated patient safe. *Nursing, 33*(5): Hospital Nursing, 32hn1-2, 32hn4.

Tomlinson, D. (2004). Physical restraint during procedures: Issues and implications for practice. *Journal of Pediatric Oncology Nursing, 21*(5), 258-263.

*Asterisk indicates a classic or definitive work on this subject.

Chapter 24

PROMOTING HEALTHY NUTRITION

Media Resources

- Evolve Website http://evolve.elsevier.com/Harkreader/
- 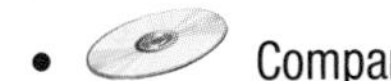 Companion CD

Learning Objectives

After studying this chapter, you should be able to do the following:

- Describe the elements of a nutritious diet and how the body uses nutrients
- Distinguish among various guidelines for normal nutrition
- Discuss the factors that affect nutritional status, such as lifestyle, culture, life span, pregnancy and lactation, and psychological and physiological states
- Describe the assessment of a client's nutritional status
- Identify nursing diagnoses applicable to the client with a normal nutritional balance
- Plan for goal-directed interventions to promote optimal nutrition and reduce nutritional risk factors
- Describe specific interventions and strategies to promote optimal nutrition and reduce nutritional risk factors throughout the life span
- Evaluate the outcomes of nutritional interventions

Key Terms

amino acids
anthropometric measurements
calorie
carbohydrate
disaccharide
fiber
glycogen
metabolism
minerals
monosaccharide
nutrient
nutrition
nutritional status
polysaccharide
protein
recommended dietary allowance (RDA)
starch
triglycerides
vitamin

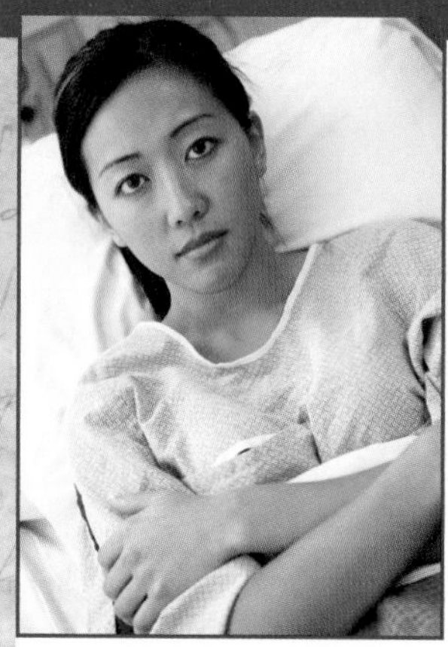
© 2007, JupiterImages Corporation.

Joan, a 20-year-old woman, arrives in the nurse practitioner's office for a wellness examination, stating that she feels good and has "no problems." She is of "normal weight" at 115 pounds for her 60-inch (5-foot) frame. Joan says that she has never been hospitalized and has had no serious illnesses. She is an office secretary and participates in many church activities but engages in very little physical activity. Previous medical records reveal that her cholesterol was elevated at an examination 1 year ago.

Joan never eats breakfast but begins a continuous eating pattern beginning about 11:00 AM. She says that she does not really eat a meal at lunch but snacks continually until dinner on cookies, candy, rolls, cheese, potato chips, and other snack foods. For dinner she eats fried foods, potatoes, bread, and dessert, and she admits disliking fruits and vegetables.

The clinical evaluation reveals no abnormalities or specific alterations. The triceps skinfold measure is within normal limits. Joan's total cholesterol is still elevated, and she wants to know how she can reduce it. In analyzing Joan's status, the nurse considers *Risk for imbalanced nutrition: more than body requirements* from the list of nursing diagnoses that relate to nutrition (see nursing diagnoses box).

KEY NURSING DIAGNOSES FOR NUTRITION

Imbalanced nutrition: more than body requirements: An intake of nutrients that exceeds metabolic needs
Imbalanced nutrition: less than body requirements: An intake of nutrients insufficient to meet metabolic needs
Risk for imbalanced nutrition: more than body requirements: Being at risk for experiencing an intake of nutrients that exceeds metabolic needs
Risk for imbalanced nutrition: less than body requirements: Being at risk for experiencing an intake of nutrients insufficient to meet metabolic needs

CONCEPTS OF NUTRITION

The human body constantly builds, maintains, and heals itself with molecules it derives from food. For this reason, there is no single factor that influences a person's health more than decisions about the types and amount of food to eat. It is important for optimal health that the daily diet be balanced and high in quality. Health professionals, such as nurses, physicians, and dietitians, are key sources of information about the role of nutrition in promoting health.

NUTRITION AND NUTRIENTS

Nutrition is the science of food and nutrients and of the processes by which an organism ingests them and uses them for energy to grow, maintain function, and renew itself. To the layperson, the term *nutrition* is synonymous with food or diet. The building block of the diet is a **nutrient**, a biochemical substance used by the body for growth, maintenance, and repair. For optimal health, the diet must be sufficient in a variety of nutrients.

Nutritional status is the condition of the body resulting from use of available essential nutrients. A client's nutritional status may be good, fair, or poor, depending on the intake of dietary essentials, the relative need for them, and the body's ability to use them. Good nutritional status is essential for normal organ development and function; for normal reproduction, growth, and maintenance; for optimal activity and working efficiency; for resistance to infection; and for the ability to repair bodily damage or injury. Poor nutritional status exists when the body is deprived of adequate amounts of essential nutrients over an extended period.

Nutritional status is relative because the body's stores of some nutrients last longer than others. In addition, at certain times, demands for particular nutrients may rise. If intake remains constant, stores of these nutrients may be depleted. This may happen, for instance, if a pregnant woman fails to increase her intake of iron, calcium, and certain vitamins.

THE GASTROINTESTINAL SYSTEM

The gastrointestinal (GI) or digestive system converts food into elemental materials that build, maintain, and repair the body's cells. These materials are then absorbed through the intestinal membranes into the bloodstream for use by the body.

Structure. The organs of the GI system include the mouth, pharynx, esophagus, stomach, small intestine, and large intestine (Table 24-1). Ancillary organs that play a role in digestion include the liver, gallbladder, and pancreas. Food enters through the mouth, passes into the pharynx and is swallowed, and then passes through the esophagus into the stomach.

The stomach is much wider than the rest of the GI tract and has a J-shaped curve at the bottom. It holds food until the food is digested to the right consistency

Table 24-1 Digestive Functions of Gastrointestinal Structures

STRUCTURE	FUNCTION
Mouth	Chews food and mixes it with saliva
Salivary glands	Produce enzymes to begin the breakdown of carbohydrates
Epiglottis	Closes when food is swallowed to prevent aspiration
Esophagus	Transports food bolus from mouth to stomach
Lower esophageal sphincter	Protects the esophagus from regurgitation of hydrochloric acid
Stomach	Mixes food with hydrochloric acid, pepsin, and lipase to form chyme
Pyloric sphincter	Prevents backflow of alkaline intestinal contents into stomach
Liver	Secretes bile for the emulsification of fat
Gallbladder	Stores and releases bile when fat is present in food
Bile duct	Transports bile to duodenum
Pancreas	Produces trypsin, chymotrypsin, amylase, and lipase for digestion of carbohydrates, fats, and proteins
Pancreatic duct	Collects pancreatic enzymes and transports them to duodenum
Duodenum	Mixes chyme with digestive enzymes and begins nutrient absorption across numerous villi
Jejunum	Provides the main area for digestion and absorption across a great number of villi
Ileum	Finishes digestion of chyme and absorption across a smaller number of villi, especially at distal end
Ileocecal sphincter	Slows absorption time and prevents bacteria from entering small intestine
Appendix	Function unknown
Colon	Reabsorbs water and electrolytes and prepares waste for excretion
Rectum	Stores wastes until peristalsis produces urge to defecate
Anus	Controls bowel elimination by means of internal and external sphincters

before allowing it to flow into the small intestine. The C-shaped duodenum is the first and shortest portion of the small intestine, followed by the jejunum (the longest portion), and the narrow ileum. The ileocecal valve joins the small intestine to the large intestine, which continues to the rectum and anus.

Function. The four main functions of the GI system are digestion, absorption, metabolism, and excretion. This chapter focuses on the first three. Concepts related to excretion are discussed in Chapter 29.

Digestion is a mechanical and chemical process by which the body changes food into elemental nutrients for absorption. The process begins in the mouth, where food is chewed and mixed with saliva. Ptyalin, the enzyme in saliva, begins the breakdown of starches into simpler sugars. The powerful peristaltic action of the stomach churns, liquefies, and mixes food with gastric juices. Pepsin and hydrochloric acid in the stomach break down proteins into proteases, peptones, and polypeptides. Gastric lipase, which is most active in infants for milk digestion, is a weak, fat-splitting enzyme secreted in the stomach.

Food exits the stomach at the pyloric sphincter and enters the small intestine, where most enzymatic digestion and virtually all absorption occur. The pancreatic enzymes—amylase, trypsin, and lipase—are secreted into the small intestine to break down carbohydrates, proteins, and fats into sugars, amino acids, and fatty acids, respectively. Bile from the liver, which is concentrated and stored by the gallbladder, emulsifies fats for the action of the fat-splitting enzymes. Once digested material reaches the large intestine, it contains very few nutrients. Here, water and electrolytes are absorbed from this mass, resulting in semisolid feces.

Absorption is the passage of the end products of carbohydrate, protein, and fat digestion, as well as many vitamin and mineral molecules, through the intestinal wall into the bloodstream for distribution throughout the body. Absorption takes place through diffusion or active transport. The intestinal lining is designed for absorption because it has multiple folds and villi that yield a large surface area.

Metabolism is the process by which energy from nutrients is used by the cells or stored for later use. Individual cells convert chemical energy from molecular bonds into energy for growth, maintenance, and repair as well as for muscle contraction and nerve function. Metabolism can be either anabolic or catabolic. Anabolic processes build up substances and body tissues, whereas catabolic processes break them down. Body reserves are used when a person does not eat sufficient amounts of nutrients or when the body has an increased need for them.

MAJOR COMPONENTS OF FOOD

The body's main nutrients are carbohydrates, proteins, fats, vitamins, and minerals. An adult's metabolism requires 9 amino acids, 1 fatty acid, 13 vitamins, and 12 minerals. All major energy-yielding nutrients are composed of smaller units. Carbohydrates, proteins, and fats must be hydrolyzed into their smaller characteristic units before absorption. Water is another important component of all foods and is also necessary for life. The body's need for water is discussed in Chapter 26.

Energy and Calories. Carbohydrates, proteins, and fats are collectively called the energy nutrients because they contribute the energy value (calories) from food. Their primary physiological function is the production of energy for health and activity. *Energy* is power that can be translated into motion, can overcome resistance, or can effect physical change. Energy production in the body is a chemical process that indirectly involves the use of vitamins, minerals, and water.

The human body may be likened to a machine or engine that must constantly be refueled to enable it to perform work. The fuel needed by the body for both external and internal work is, of course, food. The chemical energy available from food is converted in the body to electrical energy for impulse transmission in the brain and nervous system, to thermal energy for regulation of body temperature, and to other forms of chemical energy for synthesis of body compounds. Chemical energy from food is also converted into mechanical energy, which allows muscles to contract and work to be accomplished in the external environment.

Foods are frequently discussed in terms of the calories they contain. **Calorie** is the common term used to refer to the more accurate *kilocalorie* (kcal), a measure of the potential energy of the carbohydrate, protein, and fat content of food. The calorie used in nutrition is defined as the amount of heat needed to raise the temperature of 1 kg of water 1° C. This unit (the kilocalorie) is 1000 times larger than the calorie used in either biology or chemistry.

Three major factors determine a human's daily energy requirement: the *basal metabolic rate* (BMR), the degree of *physical activity*, and the *specific dynamic action* of food. The BMR is the amount of energy needed to maintain essential body functions expressed as calories per hour per square meter of body surface. Essential body functions include respiration, circulation, peristalsis, muscle tone, body temperature, glandular activity, and the other vegetative functions of the body. For infants, children, and pregnant women, growth is an additional factor. Energy requirements are stated in calories.

Carbohydrates. A **carbohydrate** is a simple or complex compound composed of carbon, oxygen, and hydrogen. A **monosaccharide** is a six-carbon sugar (a subunit of carbohydrates). Glucose, fructose, and galactose are examples of monosaccharides. A **disaccharide** is a molecule that forms when two monosaccharides join together to form a double sugar. These include sucrose (glucose and fructose), maltose (two units of glucose), and lactose or milk sugar (glucose and galactose). Notice that glucose is a component of all disaccharides. A **polysaccharide** is a group of monosaccharides joined together in a chain. They can be converted back to monosaccharides through a process called acid hydrolysis.

Carbohydrates are stored differently in plants and animals. **Glycogen** is the form in which carbohydrates are stored in the muscle tissue of humans and animals. When the body needs quick energy, it uses glycogen stores, which can be broken down into glucose by enzymes. **Starch** is the form in which plants store glucose. They use this energy for growth. When a person eats a plant, the plant starch is hydrolyzed by enzymes into glucose, which can then be used for energy or rearranged to form glycogen for storage. Carbohydrate as an energy source provides 4 kcal/g. The body needs a sufficient daily intake of carbohydrates for energy production to avoid breakdown of proteins and fats. The recommended percentage of dietary carbohydrates is approximately 50% to 60% of total caloric intake.

Fiber. **Fiber** is the structure of which plants are composed, which includes cellulose, hemicellulose, pectins, gums, and mucilages. A diet high in fiber contains foods such as cereals (especially bran), whole wheat bread, and raw fruits and vegetables. Although most fibers begin as polysaccharides, human enzymes cannot further digest or break down the bonds between monosaccharide units of fiber, leading to reduced absorption. Because fiber retains water and increases the rate at which residue moves through the large intestine, people who consume sufficient fiber have fewer problems with constipation.

Other advantages of a high-fiber diet include delayed absorption of glucose and lower blood cholesterol levels. A high-fiber diet also may prevent diverticulosis from developing later in life and may decrease the risk of colon cancer. People who increase fiber in their diet should do so gradually to prevent diarrhea caused by the added bulk and water. They should also drink plenty of fluids to prevent stool impaction.

Protein. **Protein** is a compound containing polymers of *amino acids*, linked together in a chain to form polypeptide bonds. There are over 20 **amino acids,** which are composed of carbon, hydrogen, oxygen, and an amino group. Amino acids can be classified as essential or nonessential depending on whether or not the body can manufacture them from other sources. Essential amino acids cannot be adequately synthesized by the body to meet metabolic needs and therefore must be supplied by the diet. The body needs a sufficient daily dietary intake of essential amino acids to meet bodily maintenance and growth needs. Similarly, proteins can be classified as complete or incomplete, depending on whether or not they contain all nine essential amino acids. Some diets, such as a strict vegetarian diet, have a high proportion of incomplete proteins, but incomplete proteins can be successfully combined to form complete proteins (for example, a peanut butter sandwich contains a grain and a legume). See a nutrition text for a more detailed discussion of complete and incomplete proteins in the diet.

Proteins form the structure of the body and regulate bodily processes. Skin, hair, and eyes are made of protein, as are the enzymes needed for digestion and absorption. The antibodies that defend against disease, hormones that regulate body functions, and red and white blood cells are all made of protein. Even lipoproteins, molecules that carry fat and cholesterol in the blood, have a protein core. Proteins also help to maintain fluid, electrolyte, and acid-base balance.

Enzymes break down dietary proteins or *polypeptides* into individual amino acids or *peptides*. In this form, they can be absorbed through the intestinal wall. Some dipeptides (two amino acid chains) and tripeptides (three amino acid chains) are also transported this way. Protein as an energy source provides 4 kcal/g. When the body is storing protein (anabolism), the person is said to have a positive nitrogen balance. In contrast, when the body is breaking down protein (catabolism), it is said to be in negative nitrogen balance. Nitrogen that is released during protein catabolism can be measured in the bloodstream as *blood urea nitrogen (BUN)* and is excreted through the kidneys.

Lipids. Lipids, or fats, are a family of compounds that includes *triglycerides* (fats and oils), phospholipids, and steroids. Like carbohydrates and protein, fat is composed of carbon, oxygen, and hydrogen. A key difference, however, is that there are more carbon and hydrogen atoms in proportion to oxygen atoms, so lipid molecules yield more energy: 9 kcal/g. Lipids are a source of fuel for the body, add flavor to food, and assist with satiety.

Triglycerides, each composed of three fatty acids and a glycol unit, are the chief form of fat in the diet and the main form of fat transport in the blood. Ninety-nine percent of body fat is stored as triglycerides. Enzymes and bile salts are needed to break down triglycerides into smaller units (fatty acids, monoglycerides, and glycerol) for use by the body. Small units of digested fat can be absorbed through cells of the small intestine and into the bloodstream. Larger units are released into the lymph system to enter the bloodstream at the thoracic duct. The body can manufacture many fatty acids, but two essential fatty acids (linolenic acid and linoleic acid) must be obtained from the diet.

Vitamins. A **vitamin** is an organic substance found in food that serves as a coenzyme in enzymatic reactions. Vitamins are essential nutrients required in small amounts for physiological and metabolic functioning (Table 24-2). Vitamins cannot be synthesized by the body and must be obtained from foods. No single food contains all vitamins.

Unlike carbohydrates, proteins, and fats, vitamins are not linked together in long chains. They are individual units that release energy from food but do not add energy themselves. Vitamins are measured in very small units, such as milligrams and micrograms.

There are 13 different vitamins, and they are classified as either water soluble or fat soluble. Water-soluble vitamins are the B vitamins and vitamin C; these need to be replenished daily in the diet because they are easily excreted via the kidneys. Fat-soluble vitamins include vitamins A, D, E, and K. Because the body can store these, it is important to avoid excessive intake, which could lead to toxic levels.

Minerals. Minerals are inorganic elements present in small amounts in virtually all body fluids and tissues (Table 24-3). There are 16 minerals essential to human

Table 24-2 Overview of Important Vitamins

VITAMIN AND ITS ADULT RDA*	SOURCES	FUNCTIONS
Vitamin A (retinol, retinal, retinoic acid) *RDA:* 800 to 1000 retinol equivalents	Dark-green and yellow vegetables, broccoli, carrots, winter squash, sweet potatoes, liver, egg yolks, breakfast cereals, dairy products, margarine, fortified milk, peaches, apricots, cantaloupe.	• Better vision in dim light. • Formation and maintenance of skin and mucous membranes. • Normal growth and development of bones and teeth.
Vitamin B_1 (thiamine) *RDA:* 1.0 to 1.4 mg	Pork, organ meats, liver, enriched and whole grains, eggs, nuts, dried peas, dried beans.	• Energy metabolism, especially of carbohydrates. • Normal nervous system functioning.
Vitamin B_2 (riboflavin) *RDA:* 1.2 to 1.7 mg	Dairy products, milk, eggs, organ meats, enriched grains, green leafy vegetables.	• Carbohydrate, protein, and fat metabolism. • Other metabolic functions.
Niacin (nicotinic acid) *RDA:* 13 to 19 mg	Lean meat, kidney, poultry, liver, fish, enriched and whole grains, nuts, yeast, peanut butter, and dried peas and beans.	• Carbohydrate, protein, and fat metabolism.
Vitamin B_4 *RDA:* 2.0 to 2.2 mg	Organ meats, pork, egg yolks, potatoes, whole grain cereals, wheat germ, yeast.	• Amino acid metabolism. • Blood formation. • Maintenance of nervous tissue. • Conversion of tryptophan to niacin.
Folic acid *RDA:* 400 mcg	Organ meats, milk, eggs, green leafy vegetables, broccoli, asparagus, wheat germ, yeast.	• RNA and DNA synthesis. • Formation and maturation of red blood cells. • Amino acid metabolism.

DNA, Deoxyribonucleic acid; *RDA,* recommended dietary allowance; *RNA,* ribonucleic acid.
*Others include vitamin B_{12} (cobalamin), 3.0 mcg; pantothenic acid, 4 to 7 mg; and biotin, 100 to 200 mcg.

Continued

Table 24-2 Overview of Important Vitamins—cont'd

VITAMIN AND ITS ADULT RDA*	SOURCES	FUNCTIONS
Vitamin C (ascorbic acid) *RDA:* 60 mg	Citrus fruits and juices, brussels sprouts, broccoli, green peppers, strawberries, tomatoes, cabbage, greens, guava.	• Collagen formation. • Protection of other nutrients from oxidation. • Enhancement of iron absorption. • Conversion of folic acid to its active form. • Metabolism of certain amino acids.
Vitamin D (cholecalciferol ergosterol) *RDA:* 5 to 10 mcg	Sunlight, liver, egg yolks, fish-liver oils, breakfast cereals, margarine, butter, fortified milk.	• Metabolism of calcium and phosphorus. • Stimulation of calcium absorption. • Mobilization of calcium and phosphorus from bone. • Stimulation of reabsorption of calcium and phosphorus by kidney.
Vitamin E (tocopherol) *RDA:* 8 to 10 mg	Vegetable oils, wheat germ, whole-grain products.	• Protection of vitamin A and polyunsaturated fatty acids from oxidation. • Maintenance of cell membrane integrity. • Heme synthesis.
Vitamin K *RDA:* 70 to 140 mcg	Dark-green leafy vegetables, vegetables of the cabbage family. Also produced by gut bacteria in the intestines.	• Synthesis of certain proteins needed for blood clotting.

DNA, Deoxyribonucleic acid; *RDA,* recommended dietary allowance; *RNA,* ribonucleic acid.
*Others include vitamin B_{12} (cobalamin), 3.0 mcg; pantothenic acid, 4 to 7 mg; and biotin, 100 to 200 mcg.

Table 24-3 Overview of Important Minerals

MINERAL AND ITS ADULT RDA*	SOURCES	FUNCTIONS
MACROMINERALS		
Calcium *RDA:* 800 mg	Milk and dairy products, canned fish with bones, green leafy vegetables.	• Bone and tooth formation. • Blood clotting. • Nerve transmission. • Muscle contraction. • Cell membrane permeability. • Activation of certain enzymes.
Phosphorus *RDA:* 800 mg	Milk and milk products, meat, poultry, fish, eggs, dried peas, dried beans, nuts, soft drinks, processed foods.	• Bone and tooth formation. • Acid-base balance. • Energy and metabolism. • Cell membrane structure. • Component of nucleic acids. • Regulation of hormones and coenzymes. • Fat absorption and transport. • Glucose absorption.
Magnesium *RDA:* 350 mg	Green leafy vegetables, nuts, dried peas, dried beans, grains, seafood, cocoa, chocolate.	• Bone and tooth formation. • Smooth muscle relaxation. • Carbohydrate metabolism. • Protein synthesis. • Hormonal activity. • Cell reproduction and growth.
Sodium *RDA:* 1100 to 3300 mg	Salt, sodium-containing preservatives and additives, processed foods, canned meats and vegetables, condiments, pickled foods, ham, soft water, foods prepared in brine solutions, milk, meat, carrots, celery, beets, spinach.	• Fluid balance. • Acid-base balance. • Muscular irritability. • Cell permeability. • Nerve impulse transmission.
Potassium *RDA:* 1875 to 5625 mg	Whole grains, legumes, fruits, leafy vegetables, broccoli, sweet potatoes, potatoes, meat, tomatoes.	• Fluid balance. • Acid-base balance. • Nerve impulse transmission. • Striated skeletal and cardiac muscle activity. • Carbohydrate metabolism. • Protein synthesis. • Catalyst for many metabolic reactions.

Table 24-3 Overview of Important Minerals—cont'd

MINERAL AND ITS ADULT RDA*	SOURCES	FUNCTIONS
MICROMINERALS		
Iron *RDA:* 10 to 18 mg	Liver, lean meats, enriched and whole-grain breads and cereals.	• Oxygen transport via hemoglobin and myoglobin. • Constituent of enzyme systems.
Iodine *RDA:* 150 mg	Iodized salt, seafood, food additives, dough conditioners, dairy disinfectants.	• Component of thyroid hormones.
Zinc *RDA:* 15 mg	Oysters, liver, meats, poultry, dried peas, dried beans, nuts.	• Tissue growth, development, and healing. • Sexual maturation and reproduction. • Enzyme formation. • Immune response.

RDA, Recommended dietary allowance.
*Others include copper, 2 to 3 mg; manganese, 2 to 5 mg; fluoride, 1.5 to 4 mg; chromium, 0.05 to 0.2 mg, selenium, 0.05 to 0.2 mg; molybdenum, 0.15 to 0.5 mg.

nutrition. Minerals do not yield energy, and they are not metabolized. The major minerals regulate fluid, electrolyte, and acid-base balance and help form the structure of bone. They are also important in the function of muscle and nerve cells.

The major minerals include sodium, chloride, potassium, calcium, phosphorus, magnesium, and sulfur. In addition to major minerals, the body needs trace minerals in smaller amounts. They include iron, zinc, iodine, selenium, copper, manganese, fluoride, chromium, and molybdenum.

A balanced diet composed of a wide variety of foods is the best source of all nutrients needed for good health. Dietary vitamin and mineral supplements, if used, should only supplement nutrients obtained from a balanced diet.

FACTORS AFFECTING NUTRITIONAL STATUS

Despite increasing public awareness, good nutrition typically ranks low in priority when most people are making food choices. Consequently, you must fully appreciate the meanings and values associated with food because they commonly are more important than the nutrient content and health impact of food in the minds of clients.

A person's dietary pattern is usually slow to change because food habits are deeply rooted in the past. Even among those who want to change, social pressures may make it difficult. Food choices have always been influenced by nonnutritional factors, including religious taboos, ethnicity, gender roles, and social status. Meal preparation, for example, can reflect relatedness, obligation, self-fulfillment, creativity, or love. Mealtimes have historically been viewed as social occasions, bringing together family and friends. Nonetheless, if national nutrition statistics accurately indicate emerging trends, we are experiencing a dietary revolution unprecedented in the history of nutritional science.

RISK FACTORS ACROSS THE LIFE SPAN

Infants and Children. Sufficient calorie and protein intake is important in meeting a child's nutritional needs. Growth is especially rapid during infancy, and it is slower but steady during toddlerhood and childhood. Toddlers may also experience physiological anorexia and food jags, in which one or a few foods are preferred to the exclusion of others. Because growth patterns vary at different stages of infancy and childhood, the need for carbohydrates, fats, and other minerals and vitamins is constantly changing. As a health professional, you can support the growth process by supervising the diet and providing dietary teaching to parents.

Adolescents. Adolescents vary in their growth patterns; however, their rapid physical growth requires increased calories to meet their metabolic demands. Specific nutrients also assume added importance, such as calcium (for the support of long-bone calcification) and iron (for maintaining increased red blood cell mass).

Vitamins A and C are necessary at this stage as well, and intake of both vitamins may be inadequate if food intake is erratic. Typically during adolescence, peer group pressure leads to increased snacking, which can then reduce intake of a balanced diet.

Menstrual blood loss in pubescent girls further increases iron needs and puts girls at risk for iron deficiency anemia. Young boys may suffer from the same condition if they are growing rapidly.

Middle Adults. Maintaining health for the middle adult includes eating a well-balanced diet. Appropriate calorie intake depends on each person's body type and physical activity. An adequate nutritional program should include balanced nutrients, vitamins, adequate fiber, and sufficient water.

Older Adults. Many nutrition-related changes occur with aging, including decreases in salivation, chewing efficiency, number of taste buds, GI secretions, calcium absorption, renal function, glucose tolerance, and hemopoiesis. The risk of constipation tends to increase. The rate at which these changes occur varies; however, they are common enough to influence general dietary recommendations for older adults.

Many older adults have dietary deficiencies in protein, iron, calcium, and zinc. Individual differences may vary and depend on mobility, financial status, and socialization. Other factors that affect nutrient needs and nutritional status include chronic or acute diseases, medication use, and mental health problems.

Drug-nutrient interactions are important in older adults because medications may alter nutrient needs. For example, a client taking a potassium-sparing diuretic should limit or avoid food sources that are high in potassium, because this could lead to excessively high potassium levels. Clients taking warfarin (Coumadin) should avoid ingesting foods high in vitamin K because this vitamin reduces the drug's effect. The timing of food ingestion in relationship to medication administration is another important consideration, particularly among clients who take several drugs. Many older adults take 3 or more medications daily, while institutionalized clients may take up to 10 or more.

Pregnant and Lactating Women. Pregnancy and lactation increase a woman's need for calories and fluid. Furthermore, physiological changes that occur during pregnancy can alter body status. For example, increased intravascular volume can cause a pseudoanemia from hemodilution. The overall increase in blood volume and total body fluid can also cause fluid retention and edema, which may be treated in part with diet.

It is especially important during pregnancy that the diet be well balanced, include high-nutrient foods, and exclude low-nutrient foods. This helps promote optimal fetal growth and development while minimizing excess maternal weight gain. It is also important to take a daily prenatal multivitamin supplement that contains the added vitamins needed during pregnancy. An adequate intake of folic acid, for example, is very important in preventing fetal neural tube defects.

PSYCHOLOGICAL FACTORS

People eat for many reasons, only one of which is hunger. Emotional states—such as boredom, anger, depression, or loneliness—can influence the quality and quantity of a person's intake. Emotions can overpower subtle physiological cues that regulate hunger and can lead some people to undereat or overeat. Emotions can also influence poor eating habits.

Food is often used unintentionally as reward or punishment. We can offer food to express love and approval or withhold it to express disapproval. In the United States, it is acceptable to give children candy, cookies, or ice cream when they are good. Adults may continue this symbolism established in childhood by rewarding themselves with a special food or by going out to dinner if they have worked hard or achieved an important goal.

Good eating behavior continues when it is positively reinforced. Reinforcement may be physiological, as when hunger is eliminated. Eating behavior may also be situational, such as eating at the same time each day or when guests come to visit.

Children sometimes rebel against their parents through food. A daughter who develops anorexia nervosa or a son who feels unloved and tends to overeat at mealtime is communicating with his or her parents.

> ***Action Alert!*** Recognize anorexia nervosa or overeating as a possible attempt to cope with frustration, anger, aggression, depression, or unmet needs for affection. Become aware of the behavior exhibited and try to understand the meaning of that behavior in relation to food.

Nutritional Problems in Well Populations. The typical American diet is often abundant in quantity but poorer in quality, containing excess fat and animal proteins and inadequate fresh or unprocessed foods. Even with use of fresh, unprocessed foods, there are concerns about the health consequences of pesticide residues left on many of those foods. A high-calorie and high-fat diet can lead to obesity over time, especially if coupled with a sedentary lifestyle. It can also lead to high serum cholesterol levels, which increase an individual's risk for atherosclerotic heart disease, stroke, or peripheral vascular disease. A diet high in sodium can lead to hypertension, which increases risk of heart disease, stroke, and renal disease. It can also exacerbate existing heart failure by increasing fluid retention.

An important factor when considering diet is the concept of *nutrient density.* Nutrient-dense foods have a high ratio of important nutrients in relation to calories. An increase in these types of foods overall is still needed in the American diet, despite educational initiatives such as *Healthy People 2000* and *Healthy People 2010.*

PHYSIOLOGICAL FACTORS

Healthy body functioning promotes optimal digestion and absorption of food. Healthy teeth and gums or well-fitting dentures are important for chewing, which is needed to break down food for digestion. The GI system must function well for optimal use of ingested nutrients. Normal production of insulin and digestive enzymes is also important for food use.

Physical factors can affect a person's ability to buy, transport, cook, and eat food. Physical mobility and energy are needed for shopping, cooking, and eating.

When a person physically cannot complete such tasks, assistance may be needed to ensure adequate nutrition.

CULTURAL, ECONOMIC, AND LIFESTYLE FACTORS

Cultural Factors. Cultural agents of society (those that promote adaptation to a culture and assimilation of its values), such as family, religion, and schools, are all very complex and interrelated. It is difficult to determine the extent to which one agent is more influential than another in determining food habits. Family, particularly parents, usually plays the most significant role in determining foods that are served and eaten.

Certain generalizations can be made about cultural influences on eating habits. The first is that most cultures design meals using a complex mixture of foods along with a staple, such as potatoes, rice, or pasta, which forms the basis of the meal. Second, spices or herbs are used to augment the flavor of foods, and herbs can have medicinal effects as well as dietary value. Third, every cultural group tends to have its unique preparation of foods, such as the beef bourguignon of the French or the beef Wellington of the English. The continual use of certain foods and their combinations through cultural, technological, and geographical changes shows their value to that cultural group.

Characteristic eating habits and patterns of cultures are observed among different nationalities and religious groups. A Jewish client might become ill after eating pork unintentionally, or a Seventh Day Adventist might become upset after drinking punch that has been made with alcohol. To be able to provide or suggest meals that are acceptable as well as promoting good nutrition, it is important to understand the food preferences and taboos of various cultural and religious groups.

Economic Factors. Cost is another influence on food selection, with economics playing a major role in determining food habits. People living in poverty have an increased risk of malnutrition, not because they lack the knowledge to eat nutritious foods (such as fresh fish, organic fruits and vegetables, and fiber-rich breads) but because these products are more costly.

An increasing number of people are making changes in what they purchase in supermarkets to save money. They may buy in larger quantities or use generic products rather than brand names. They are also more likely to look at unit pricing and information on food labels regarding calories and nutrients, which is a favorable change that over time may result in better nutritional status.

Lifestyle Factors. Lifestyle factors are closely related to food habits. The term *food habits* refers to what people eat and the way they eat. Food habits are derived from total life experience and are very resistant to change. Strong rejections of or desires for foods are learned through either role modeling or compliance (a strong desire to please the caretaker or food distributor, usually the mother). Thus food habits are more closely linked to associations with others and attitudes toward food than to food nutrient value.

A fast-paced lifestyle is consistent with increased consumption of snack foods and fast foods, which are low-nutrient-density foods. The increased dietary fat, decreased complex carbohydrate, and increased simple-sugar components of fast foods are clearly contradictory to nutritional goals. In addition, the typical fast-food meal is high in calories, ranging from 900 to 1300 kcal per meal, which represents a large percent of a typical person's daily calories. The risk for adverse long-term health effects from excess ingestion of these foods is of growing concern to health professionals.

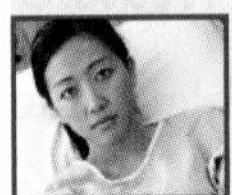

Remember Joan, who was introduced at the beginning of this chapter? What aspects of her nutritional lifestyle could put her at risk for health problems later in life, even if she is healthy at the present time?

ASSESSMENT

Most people could benefit from an assessment of their nutritional status and dietary patterns. The three purposes of a screening nutritional assessment are to identify clients who need in-depth nutritional assessment, to establish baseline values for evaluating the efficacy of nutritional regimens, and to provide a system for early recognition of increased health risk caused by nutritional factors.

GENERAL ASSESSMENT OF NUTRITIONAL STATUS

Because a client's nutritional status has an effect on well-being, growth, performance, and resistance to disease, a thorough and accurate nutritional assessment is important. This assessment involves measuring how well the physiological need for nutrients is being met and also the balance between nutrient intake and nutrient expenditure. The components of a nutritional assessment include the health history (including diet history), evaluation of food intake, and physical examination and diagnostic tests.

Health History. Refer a client with a severe problem or an unusual eating pattern to a registered dietitian who is trained to evaluate nutritional states and to provide recommendations and sample meal plans. The registered dietitian can be an excellent consultant for you and a resource for your clients, especially if you work in home health care. Following referral, your role is to reinforce the information provided by the dietitian.

To take a diet history, collect and analyze data about the type and amount of food the client eats. It can be difficult and frustrating to accurately record and evaluate dietary intake for several reasons. First, it is difficult to record clients' food intake without influencing it. When people are watched, questioned about what they eat, or asked to write down what they eat, eating patterns tend to change. The extent of change depends on how well clients understand the dietary history and to what extent they are influenced by what they think you want to see or hear.

Second, many people simply cannot remember the types or amounts of food eaten. Third, it can be difficult to accurately evaluate the nutrient composition of food unless the specific ingredients are known. Carefully reading food labels on manufactured foods can be helpful. Food labels are required by law to list, among other things, the calories and specific nutrients in each product. Be aware that methods of cooking can greatly affect nutrient values. Even the area in which a fruit or vegetable is grown can affect its nutrient content.

24-Hour Recall. The most popular and easiest method for obtaining data about a dietary intake is the *24-hour recall.* The client completes a questionnaire or is interviewed by you, a dietitian, or a nutritionist experienced in dietary interviewing. The client is asked to recall everything eaten the previous day or within the last 24 hours. When performing this assessment, keep in mind that it has three significant sources of error:

- The client may not be able to recall accurately the amounts of food eaten.
- The previous day's intake may not represent the usual intake.
- The client may not tell the truth for a variety of reasons, including possible embarrassment.

Clients have a tendency to underestimate intake as the portion size increases and overestimate intake as the portion size decreases. Foods that are least likely to be accurately reported are sauces, gravies, fruits, and snack items.

When conducting an interview for a 24-hour recall, compare an actual day (the previous day is best) with a typical day. Be objective, and use open-ended questions, such as *When did you get up? What was the first thing that you ate? What did you drink? What time did you eat next?* This type of questioning may elicit information on snacks and unusual patterns of eating. It is less likely to encourage incorrect information because it avoids giving clients clues about what answers are considered appropriate. To foster accurate reporting, do not react negatively to any response from the client.

Food Frequency Questionnaire. To help overcome inherent weaknesses in the 24-hour recall method, a *food frequency questionnaire* may also be completed. Using this tool, you can collect information about how many times per day, week, or month a client eats particular foods. This information can help validate the accuracy of the 24-hour recall data and clarify the client's real food consumption pattern. The food frequency questionnaire may be general, containing questions concerning all foods, or selective, containing questions about suspected deficient or excessive foods in the diet.

Food Diary. A *food diary* is a written record of food intake maintained for a specified period of time, usually 3 to 7 days. The time frame depends on the purpose, the nutrients being assessed, and the interest level of the client. This assessment may also be used to determine food allergies. Consider carefully the days chosen to observe intake. Food consumption on weekends and holidays may differ from that on weekdays. A combination of weekday and weekend recordings often reflects a more accurate picture. In the hospital or extended-care setting, you may be required to keep track of food intake on a calorie count sheet kept at the bedside or on the chart.

For best results, client teaching must be clear. For each day the food diary is kept, ask the client to record the names of foods eaten, the way the food was prepared, and (if indicated) the time and place the food was eaten. A legitimate concern with the food diary is that the client may change eating patterns on the days of the recording. Encourage clients to eat the foods and amounts that are normal for them on these days. Again, a nonjudgmental manner helps.

When a very accurate record of food consumption is required, the *weighed intake record* is best. Teach the client to weigh all food consumed during the recording and to correct for food waste (food served but not eaten). Disadvantages are that this method is tedious, the client must be well motivated to achieve accurate results, the client may use shortcuts in preparation to make the weighing less time-consuming, and the client's eating patterns may change. The weighed intake method is used in controlled laboratory studies and hospital settings.

Household Food Consumption. This method involves visiting a household periodically and recording the amounts and types of food purchased for that household and the disappearance of that food. It assumes that the family has eaten any food that is unaccounted for. Household food consumption is most commonly used in large population surveys. It is not a good evaluation of individual intake because it does not record food waste or food consumed by each household member. It is helpful, however, in trying to gain insight into the nutritional status of a community.

Food in the household can vary with household income, foods available in the marketplace, and other factors. For example, foods available in the market may be limited for some inner-city dwellers, such as frail older adults, who may have to shop at a corner market that does not carry items such as soy milk, salt-free crackers, or fresh fruits and vegetables.

Evaluation of Food Intake. There are two methods by which food intake information is evaluated for adequacy: the food group method and the nutrient composition method. When a client is hospitalized, a calorie count may be done, which evaluates both of these.

Food Group Method. The simplest and fastest way to evaluate food intake data is to determine how many servings from each food group were consumed during the recorded day. The number of servings per group is then compared with the number of servings suggested in MyPyramid (Figure 24-1). It becomes more difficult to use this method if the diet has many food mixtures or unusual cultural foods that do not fit into one of the food groups. For many people, however, gross deficiencies of protein and of a number of vitamins can be detected using this method.

Vitamin deficiencies can often be linked to deficiencies in specific food groups. Intake of folic acid and vitamins A and C is most variable because they are not widely present in foods, except for particular fruits and vegetables. Intake of these nutrients is frequently seasonal, with

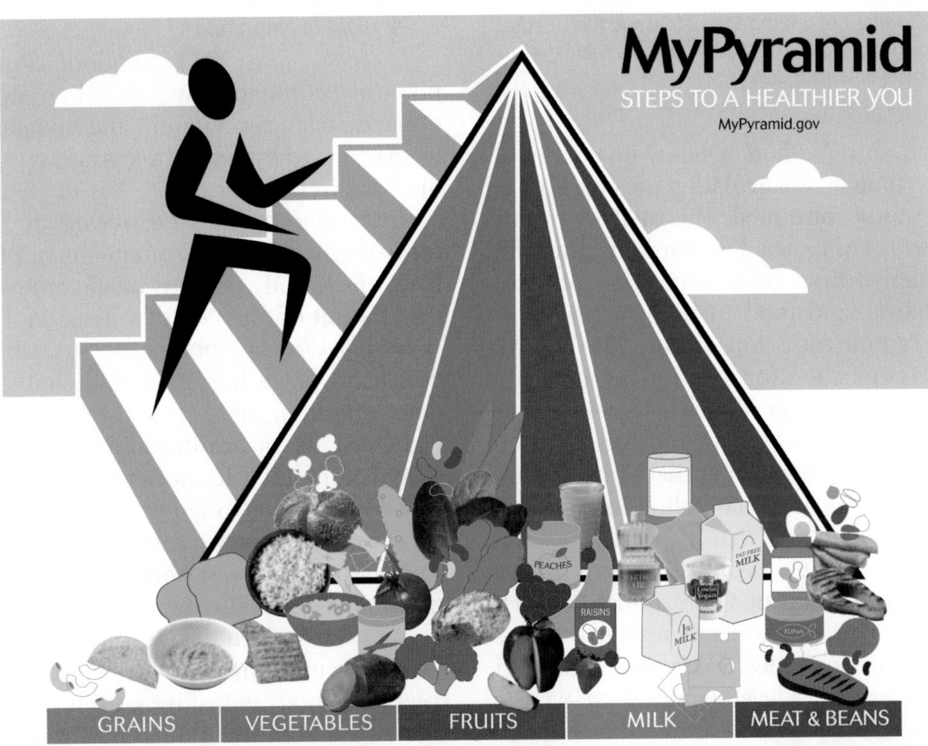

GRAINS Make half your grains whole	VEGETABLES Vary your veggies	FRUITS Focus on fruits	MILK Get your calcium-rich foods	MEAT & BEANS Go lean with protein
Eat at least 3 oz. of whole-grain cereals, breads, crackers, rice, or pasta every day 1 oz. is about 1 slice of bread, about 1 cup of breakfast cereal, or ½ cup of cooked rice, cereal, or pasta	Eat more dark-green veggies like broccoli, spinach, and other dark leafy greens Eat more orange vegetables like carrots and sweetpotatoes Eat more dry beans and peas like pinto beans, kidney beans, and lentils	Eat a variety of fruit Choose fresh, frozen, canned, or dried fruit Go easy on fruit juices	Go low-fat or fat-free when you choose milk, yogurt, and other milk products If you don't or can't consume milk, choose lactose-free products or other calcium sources such as fortified foods and beverages	Choose low-fat or lean meats and poultry Bake it, broil it, or grill it Vary your protein routine — choose more fish, beans, peas, nuts, and seeds
For a 2,000-calorie diet, you need the amounts below from each food group. To find the amounts that are right for you, go to MyPyramid.gov.				
Eat 6 oz. every day	Eat 2½ cups every day	Eat 2 cups every day	Get 3 cups every day; for kids aged 2 to 8, it's 2	Eat 5½ oz. every day

Find your balance between food and physical activity

- Be sure to stay within your daily calorie needs.
- Be physically active for at least 30 minutes most days of the week.
- About 60 minutes a day of physical activity may be needed to prevent weight gain.
- For sustaining weight loss, at least 60 to 90 minutes a day of physical activity may be required.
- Children and teenagers should be physically active for 60 minutes every day, or most days.

Know the limits on fats, sugars, and salt (sodium)

- Make most of your fat sources from fish, nuts, and vegetable oils.
- Limit solid fats like butter, stick margarine, shortening, and lard, as well as foods that contain these.
- Check the Nutrition Facts label to keep saturated fats, *trans* fats, and sodium low.
- Choose food and beverages low in added sugars. Added sugars contribute calories with few, if any, nutrients.

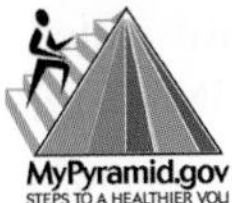

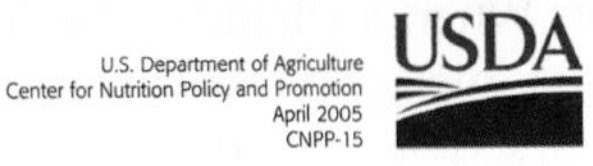

USDA

USDA is an equal opportunity provider and employer.

FIGURE 24-1 MyPyramid. (U.S. Department of Agriculture. Retrieved July 30, 2006, from http://www.mypyramid.gov/downloads/MiniPoster.pdf.)

higher intake in the summer and fall when fresh fruits and vegetables are abundant and less expensive.

Riboflavin, calcium, and vitamin D intake largely depends on the intake of milk and milk products. Daily intake of protein, thiamine, niacin, phosphorus, iron, and vitamins E, B_6, and B_{12} is more consistent because these nutrients are present in a wide variety of foods.

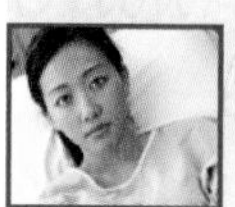

Use the food group method to determine the degree to which Joan, our case study client, is taking in a nutritionally balanced diet.

Nutrient Composition Method. Dietary intake can be evaluated more accurately by calculating the amounts of a nutrient in each food consumed. This analysis can be done manually or by computer. The nutrient values for foods can be obtained from several nutrition publications, nutrition labels, and food manufacturers' information on a food's nutrient composition. After recording the nutrient composition for individual foods, you can determine the composition of the total diet.

Once the nutrient composition of the diet is determined, the amount of an individual nutrient can be compared with the **recommended dietary allowance (RDA).** The RDA is the level of a nutrient that is adequate to meet the needs of almost all healthy people as determined by the Food and Nutrition Board of the National Research Council. Although the RDA is frequently used to evaluate the components of a person's diet, this is theoretically an improper use. RDAs are set at a level slightly above average requirements so they can include everyone in the population who might have an increased need for a particular vitamin or mineral. Because the RDAs include this "safety factor," they are probably higher than a typical person needs. Nutrition textbooks typically contain published tables of RDAs for fat- and water-soluble vitamins and minerals according to age-group, height, and weight.

Energy and protein intake should be evaluated on the basis of body weight or, in the case of an underweight or overweight person, on the basis of height. This increases the usefulness of the RDA in individual assessment, especially with children, who at any particular age may differ greatly in size.

RDAs are not meant to be applied to people who are ill, whose requirements may be very different from those who are healthy. At present, however, there are no established nutrient requirements for various disease states. With these limitations in mind, you can use nutrient RDAs as a general evaluation of the dietary intake of clients who are ill.

Calorie Count. When a client who is hospitalized is nutritionally at risk, dietary intake can be monitored using a calorie count. For each dietary tray, record the amount of food consumed on a form or on the menu for that meal. Record the client's intake in measurable amounts (such as ounces, teaspoons, tablespoons, or cubic centimeters) or the percentage (%) of the food or beverage portion ingested. Record also any additional foods or fluids consumed during the 24-hour period. Return the forms to the dietitian for analysis, which usually consists of calorie and protein intake. A calorie count is often ordered for a 3-day period. Accurate results depend on your careful assessment of intake and accurate completion of the forms.

Physical Examination

Clinical Signs of Nutritional Status. A thorough physical examination will reveal physical signs of nutritional deficiencies. Vitamin and mineral deficiencies can be manifested by clinical signs and symptoms, which are included in Chapter 25.

Anthropometric Measurements. **Anthropometric measurements** are measurements of physical characteristics of the body (such as height and weight), as well as the amount of muscle or fat tissue in the body.

Height-Weight Tables. Various tables are available that list average heights and desirable weights for infants, children, men, and women. All suggest approximate weights for healthy adults. Charts listing desirable weights for adults according to frame size are also available. These charts, often produced by insurance companies, list the weight for each inch of height that is associated with the lowest morbidity and mortality. These charts are commonly found in nutrition textbooks.

Another frequently used height-weight figure is the "usual weight." In an older adult, the "usual weight" might be more indicative of nutritional health than a figure based on the optimal height-weight tables.

Remember that these tables are guides and should be used for screening purposes. To obtain a quick estimate useful for basic screening, use the following:

- A man of 5 feet 0 inches should weigh about 106 pounds. Add 6 pounds for each additional inch.
- A woman of 5 feet 0 inches should weigh about 100 pounds. Add 5 pounds for each additional inch.

Being either underweight or overweight may be associated with increased risk of morbidity and mortality. In particular, increased mortality rates have been associated with underweight status or more extreme levels of obesity (Flegal, Graubard, Williamson, & Gail, 2005).

A disadvantage of height-weight tables is that they group all adults together without considering age. Because they are based on mortality rates, they also may not reflect weights at which people are healthiest, look their best, or have peak performance.

Body Mass Index. Because of the disadvantages of height-weight methods, many health professionals prefer to use a mathematical standard called body mass index (BMI). Determine a person's BMI using this formula:

$$\text{BMI} = \text{weight (kg)} \div \text{height}^2 \text{ (meters)}$$

To do this calculation, recall that 1 kilogram equals 2.2 pounds and 1 meter equals 39.37 inches. The desired

BMI for healthy adults is 18.5 to 24.9. A BMI of less than 18.5 indicates underweight status and is associated with a health risk such as respiratory or digestive diseases. A result of 25.0 to 29.9 indicates overweight status, and a BMI of 30 or greater indicates obesity. Obesity is a growing and significant concern in the United States. Between 1960 and 2000, there was an 8% increase in adults age 20 years and over who are overweight and a 17.6% increase in those who are obese (Ogden, Flegal, Carroll, & Johnson, 2002). This trend has continued, with an additional growing concern about obesity in children and adolescents, as well as adults (Ogden, Carroll, Curtain, McDowell, Tabak, & Flegal, 2006). Obesity leads to increased risk of high blood pressure, type 2 diabetes mellitus, coronary heart disease, gastroesophageal reflux disease, degenerative joint disease, sleep apnea, and colon, breast, and prostate cancers (O'Brien & Dixon, 2002).

Body Composition. Various body compartments (fat stores or lean tissue) can be affected by overnutrition or undernutrition. To estimate the degree to which these compartments are affected, use fat-fold measurements and midarm muscle circumference.

Because about half the body's fat is located directly beneath the skin, skinfold measurements reflect total body fat. The fat-fold measure is useful when performed by a trained person following a standard procedure and using reliable calipers to reduce errors in measurement. The most easily accessible area is the triceps fat fold, making it the most practical in clinical settings (Figure 24-2, *A*).

The midarm muscle circumference is an indicator of lean tissue stores (Figure 24-2, *B*). It can be derived by measuring the midarm circumference and the triceps fat fold, and then using the following equation:

$$\text{Midarm muscle circumference} = \text{Midarm circumference (cm)} - [0.314 - \text{triceps fat fold (mm)}],$$

where 0.314 is a conversion factor. The 50th percentile value for midarm muscle circumference is 281 for middle-age men and 222 for middle-age women.

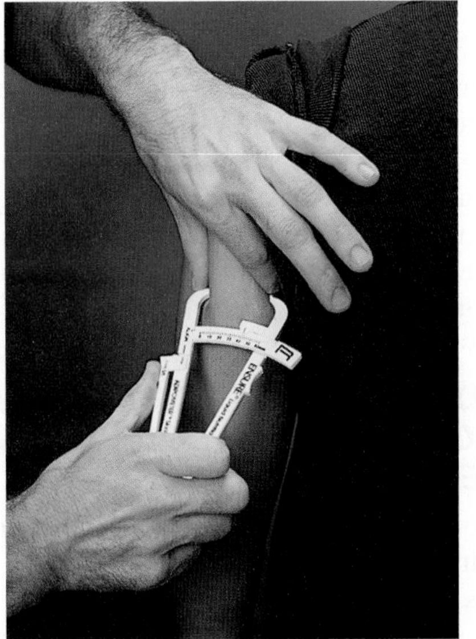

A

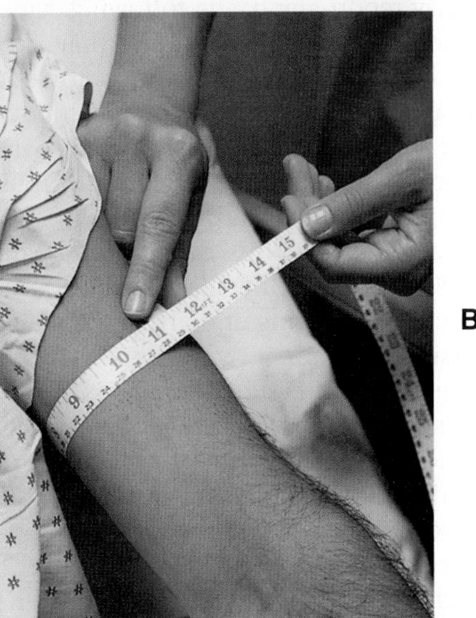

B

FIGURE 24-2 Anthropometric measurements. **A,** Using calipers to measure triceps fat fold. **B,** Measuring midarm muscle circumference.

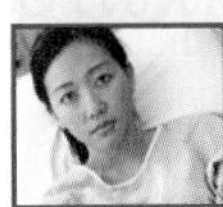

Joan's triceps fat-fold measure is within normal limits. Remember also that her clinical evaluation revealed no specific abnormalities. What does this tell you about the impact of her eating habits to this point?

Diagnostic Tests. The most common laboratory indexes of nutritional status are serum prealbumin, albumin, transferrin, lymphocyte count, hemoglobin, hematocrit, and urine specific gravity.

Albumin and *prealbumin* indicate visceral protein status. Albumin is most useful when monitoring long-term nutritional status because normal levels (3.5 to 5.0 g/dL) may be found even in those who are malnourished. Prealbumin (normally 20 to 50 mg/dL) is useful in measuring short-term changes in protein status because of its short half-life of 2 days. The *lymphocyte count* (normally > 1500 cells/mm^3) is a measure of immune function used in conjunction with other assessments to determine overall nutritional status.

Transferrin and *hematocrit* are measures of iron status. Transferrin is a trace protein needed for iron absorption and transport and is calculated as a percentage (normally 30% to 40%) using both serum iron level and iron-binding capacity. The *hematocrit* is the percentage of whole blood that is composed of red blood cells (RBCs), and values differ for adult men (37% to 49%) and women (36% to 46%). An increase or decrease in either RBC count or plasma volume affects the hematocrit. Conditions that increase RBC production increase the hematocrit, whereas anemia can lower both hemoglobin and hematocrit. Extracellular fluid volume deficit (e.g., dehydration) may increase the hematocrit (called hemoconcentration), whereas fluid volume excess decreases it (hemodilution).

With normal fluid intake, *urine specific gravity* is usually 1.010 to 1.020. Concentrated urine has a higher specific gravity, and dilute urine has a lower one. These findings correlate with hypovolemia and hypervolemia, respectively.

FOCUSED ASSESSMENT FOR *IMBALANCED NUTRITION: LESS THAN BODY REQUIREMENTS*

Some populations at risk for nutritional deficiencies are older adults, adolescents, children, pregnant women, and infants.

Defining Characteristics. Clients with nutritional deficiencies may report any of the following: satiety immediately after eating, food intake less than the RDA for nutrients, lack of interest or aversion to food, altered taste sensations, or inadequate or inaccurate information about diet. Physical signs may include pale conjunctival or mucous membranes; weakness of muscles used for chewing or swallowing; soreness or inflammation of the oral cavity; weight loss despite food intake; body weight 20% or more below ideal for height, frame, and age; abdominal cramping or diarrhea; capillary fragility; and excessive hair loss.

Because this nursing diagnosis from NANDA International (NANDA-I) refers globally to insufficient nutrients to meet metabolic demands, it is often used when the overall diet is inadequate. It might also be useful, however, whenever specific deficiencies arise, such as deficiencies of vitamins, minerals, or proteins. The defining characteristics do not clearly address the healthy client with a poor diet that could be improved.

Related Factors. Related factors for this nursing diagnosis include inability to ingest food, digest food, or absorb nutrients. This inability can result from biological, psychological, or economic factors.

In the well client, nutritional deficiencies may not be severe enough to produce actual signs and symptoms of deficiency; however, general signs may result from a diet that is deficient in one or more nutrients.

Action Alert! Be alert to the presence of fatigue, irritability, frequent colds and flu, and stress-related symptoms as cues to the possibility of mild nutritional deficiency.

Assess the client's lifestyle and dietary pattern for other risk factors, such as overuse of snack foods or processed foods, using fast foods as a main dietary source, and using cooking methods that destroy nutrients. The nutritional deficiency may be related to lack of knowledge, money, motivation, or time to prepare food.

FOCUSED ASSESSMENT FOR *IMBALANCED NUTRITION: MORE THAN BODY REQUIREMENTS*

Defining Characteristics. The client may report a sedentary activity level, greatest food intake at the end of the day, eating in response to external cues (time of day, social situation), internal cues other than hunger (anxiety), or a dysfunctional eating pattern that pairs food with another activity (such as watching television). Anthropometric measurements show a weight that is 10% or more above ideal for height and frame, and a triceps skinfold of more than 25 mm for women or 15 mm for men.

Assess the client's intake of nutrients, and cluster the data to recognize obesity, high fat intake, and high sodium intake, all of which are linked to negative health consequences, as discussed earlier.

Related Factors. Related factors are any situations in which there is excessive intake in relationship to metabolic need. Lifestyle, knowledge, and motivation could also be related factors for this nursing diagnosis.

Factors that increase the risk of obesity are those that apply to *Risk for imbalanced nutrition: more than body requirements.* They include the following:

- Reported use of solid food as a major food source before 5 months of age
- Concentrated food intake at the end of the day
- Reported or observed obesity in one or both parents
- Reported or observed higher baseline weight at the beginning of each pregnancy
- Rapid transition across growth percentiles in infants or children
- Pairing food with other activities
- Observed use of food as a reward or comfort measure
- Eating in response to internal cues other than hunger, such as anxiety
- Eating in response to external cues, such as time of day or social situation
- Dysfunctional eating patterns

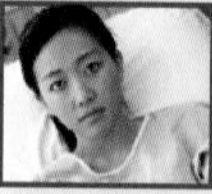

Although Joan is not overweight, why might the nursing diagnosis *Risk for imbalanced nutrition: more than body requirements* be appropriate? Joan has indicated an interest in reducing her elevated cholesterol level, which should help to motivate her to make healthy changes in her nutritional habits.

DIAGNOSIS

Several options exist in the NANDA-I nursing diagnosis system for addressing nutritional problems. Diagnostic labels are needed for the well client who seeks a higher level of wellness, the client who has risk factors for nutritional problems, and the client who has an actual deficit or excess in one or more nutrients.

The diagnosis *Health-seeking behaviors: nutrition* can be used for a client who is well but seeks an optimal state of physical and mental well-being. The goals of *Health-seeking behaviors* suggest the need for health promotion activities, one of which is proper nutrition.

The diagnosis *Imbalanced nutrition: less than body requirements* indicates that the client has one or more nutritional deficiencies. The diagnosis *Imbalanced nutrition: more than body requirements* indicates obesity or a diet high in nutrients such as fat, carbohydrates, or sodium.

Clients who have related factors for a nursing diagnosis, but not the actual defining characteristics, are stated to be at risk for a specific nursing diagnosis. The client may be at risk for imbalanced nutrition that is either more than or less than body requirements.

PLANNING

Planning for clients with a specific nutritional imbalance involves using assessment data to identify nutritional needs. Goals for nutritional status can then be chosen within the parameters of the specific nursing diagnosis. Guidance, supervision, and education may be incorporated into the plan to help improve the client's nutritional knowledge. Direct nursing care may also be part of the plan.

EXPECTED OUTCOMES FOR *IMBALANCED NUTRITION: LESS THAN BODY REQUIREMENTS*

Sample expected outcomes for the client with *Imbalanced nutrition: less than body requirements* are the following:

- Explains the importance of adequate nutrient intake in the daily diet
- Ingests sufficient nutrients to meet daily needs, considering activity level and metabolic needs
- Implements shopping and cooking methods for economical food preparation, such as using beans and legumes as a protein source, using powdered milk for cooking, and making soups or stews with leftover food

EXPECTED OUTCOMES FOR *IMBALANCED NUTRITION: MORE THAN BODY REQUIREMENTS*

Sample expected outcomes for the client with *Imbalanced nutrition: more than body requirements* are the following:

- Identifies elements of the daily diet that do not meet nutritional standards
- Plans meals using the MyPyramid guide
- Eats the bulk of calories early in the day
- Eats only when seated at the dining table
- Increases activity level by using stairs instead of elevators, parking the car in more remote parking spots, and taking a daily walk

INTERVENTION

To succeed in national efforts to promote wellness, prevent disease, and improve quality of life, all nurses must work cooperatively with educators, researchers, industrial and political leaders, and informed consumers to continue to develop positive strategies to improve nutrition. It is also important to be aware of the ever-expanding body of nutritional knowledge generated by research.

INTERVENTIONS TO PROMOTE A HEALTHY DIET

Knowledge of the nutritional value of foods and their relationship to wellness is essential but is clearly not enough to induce clients to eat appropriate foods. Otherwise, health professionals themselves would be by far the slimmest, best-exercised, optimally nourished group in the nation! What can be done, then, to get clients to change their nutritional patterns?

One key is providing nutritional education throughout the life span. Health professionals too often encounter adolescents and adults who have well-established eating patterns that are far from ideal. As a nurse working with clients at varying points in the life span, you are in a unique position to assess cultural, economic, and environmental factors influencing their food choices. This information is crucial to successful dietary intervention. Although not yet evidence based, interventions to prevent obesity from childhood include not only nutritional education, but also dietary counseling, parent training and modeling, promoting physical activity, and behavioral counseling (American Dietetic Association, 2006).

For adults, most nutritional counseling takes place in acute or long-term care facilities and community-based clinics. Most nutrition education begins with assessment of dietary intake. A broad knowledge of food, nutrition, pathophysiology, and biochemistry is important in analyzing food habits and making recommendations for improved or modified eating behaviors. As in all types of teaching and counseling, you must identify instructional objectives, devise or select evaluation tools, assess the learner's knowledge, screen for and organize information needs, select education materials, implement the teaching, and critique and revise your instruction. It is also essential to keep the learner's needs in the forefront and work to maintain rapport with the client.

To successfully educate clients, include information about the types and amounts of foods to eat. To maintain an appropriate body weight and prevent obesity, food intake and physical activity must be balanced. The need for calories can be calculated from the resting energy expenditure (REE), which is calculated as 15.3 times body weight (kg) plus 679 (for men age 18 to

30), and 11.6 times body weight (kg) plus 879 (for men age 30 to 60).

For women age 18 to 30, the formula is 14.7 times body weight (kg) plus 496. For women age 30 to 60, it is 8.7 times body weight (kg) plus 829. Very light physical activity requires 1.5 times the REE, light physical activity uses 2.5 REE, moderate physical activity burns 5.0 REE, and heavy physical activity requires 7.0 REE.

Using Recommended Dietary Allowances. An RDA is the level of intake of an essential nutrient that, based on available scientific knowledge, is adequate to meet the known nutritional needs of practically all healthy persons. Nutrient requirements during illness may be higher than the RDA. Requirements are also higher when one is under stress or recovering from trauma, infection, or surgery.

To optimize nutrition for relatively healthy clients, teach them to read nutrition labels that appear on manufactured foods, in accordance with the Nutrition Labeling and Education Act of 1990. These labels, titled "nutrition facts," contain information about the percentage of "daily value" that a specific product has for fat, cholesterol, sodium, carbohydrate, protein, vitamins, and minerals. The reference daily intakes (RDIs) are based on the RDA. Another type of labeling is the reference daily value (RDV), which is identified for important nutrients for which an RDA has not yet been established.

Developing Healthy Dietary Patterns. A healthy diet can be obtained by following MyPyramid, the Food Guidance System developed by the U.S. Department of Agriculture (2005). MyPyramid helps to implement the *2005 Dietary Guidelines for Americans* (Box 24-1) and is also based on the Dietary Reference Intakes from the National Academy of Sciences. MyPyramid alters the typical American diet in three ways:

- Intake of vitamins, minerals, fiber, and other essential nutrients is increased.
- Intake of saturated fats, *trans* fats, and cholesterol is decreased, whereas intake of fruits, vegetables, and whole grains is increased.
- Calorie intake is balanced with energy needs to prevent weight gain and/or achieve a healthy weight (USDA, 2005).

MyPyramid also provides Internet-based print materials for consumers and has an interactive page that uses an individual's age, sex, and physical activity level to calculate the amounts of foods from the various food groups needed by a particular person. A key difference between MyPyramid and the former Food Guide Pyramid is that there are no universal guidelines for intake from various food groups. Instead, portions are individualized based on the factors just described.

The five food groups included in MyPyramid are grains, vegetables, fruits, milk, and meat and beans. At

BOX 24-1 *Evidence-Based Practice*

Promoting Nutrition

Problem: Many factors can affect a client's nutritional status. Emotions such as boredom, anger, depression, and loneliness (emotional/psychological factors) can negatively affect food intake. Some view food as a reward or punishment. Other physiological factors include the client's ability to digest and absorb nutrients. Physical, cultural, and economic factors can affect one's ability to procure, shop for, and cook food. A client's lifestyle can affect what the client eats. "Poor diet and a sedentary lifestyle contribute to about 400,000 of the 2 million or so annual deaths in the United States. Specific diseases and conditions linked to poor diet include cardiovascular disease (CVD), hypertension, dyslipidemia, type 2 diabetes, overweight and obesity, osteoporosis, constipation, diverticular disease, iron deficiency anemia, oral disease, and malnutrition" (HHS, 1996; U.S. Preventive Services Task Force, 1996).

Evidence

The *Dietary Guidelines for Americans 2005* is intended to be a resource for policymakers, nutrition educators, and health care providers and is based on the latest scientific evidence. The analysis of new scientific information is performed every 5 years by the Dietary Guidelines Advisory Committee appointed by the Secretaries of the U.S. Department of Health and Human Services and the U.S. Department of Agriculture. A summary of the methodology and sources can be found at http://www.health.gov/dietaryguidelines/dga2005/report/.

Application to Practice

As health care providers, we must be able to assess our clients' nutritional status and provide scientific and evidence-based information about the role of nutrition in promoting health across the life span and reducing the risks for major chronic diseases. In the guidelines, the dietary chapter is summarized with these key recommendations:

- "Consume a variety of nutrient-dense foods and beverages within and among the basic food groups.
- Limit intake of saturated and *trans* fats, cholesterol, added sugars, salt, and alcohol.
- Meet recommended intakes within energy needs by adopting a balanced eating pattern such as the USDA Food Guide or the DASH Eating Plan."

There are other key recommendations for specific population groups such as people over age 50, women of childbearing age, and older adults.

These guidelines can be found at http://www.healthierus.gov/dietaryguidelines/.

References

U.S. Department of Health and Human Services and the U.S. Department of Agriculture. *Dietary Guidelines for Americans 2005.* (n.d.). Retrieved May 16, 2006, from http://www.healthierus.gov/dietaryguidelines/index.html.

U. S. Preventive Services Task Force, Sax, H. S., Chairman (1996). *Guide to clinical preventive services,* Report of the U. S. Preventive Services Task Force. Baltimore, MD: Williams & Wilkins.

least half of the grains should be whole grains, which supply more nutrients and fiber than refined grains. Vegetables should be varied, and include dark green vegetables, orange vegetables, dry beans and peas, starchy vegetables, and other vegetables. Any fruit or fruit juice is included in the fruit food group. The milk food group includes milk, cheese, yogurt, and milk-based desserts. The meat and beans food group consists of meats, poultry, eggs, fish, nuts and seeds, and dry beans and peas (these also belong to the vegetable group). Meats should be lean and low fat, whenever possible. MyPyramid also recommends the amount of oils and number of discretionary calories based on individual data.

Using General Nutrition Recommendations to Reduce Risk of Disease. Various government agencies and programs in the United States and Canada provide nutritional guidelines for consumers. These include recommendations for nutrient intake, food guides, menu plans, and sample diets. Teaching these recommendations can help clients establish their own goals for improved nutrition; however, knowledge of the recommendations is not usually sufficient to change a dietary pattern.

The importance of dietary habits in preventing disease and maintaining health is becoming more apparent. A diet high in fat and calories has been associated with heart disease, stroke, and cancer, the three major causes of death in the United States. Fortunately, the incidence of heart disease and stroke has declined in recent years, possibly in part because of improved dietary habits. Increasing intake of fruits, vegetables, and whole grains as part of a healthy diet may offer some protection against development of cancer (Holmes, 2006). As increased evidence emerges about the relationships between diet and chronic diseases, several organizations are promoting healthier diets, including the American Heart Association, the American Cancer Society, and American Dietetic Association, in addition to the U.S. Department of Agriculture. Nutritional guidelines published in Canada are similar in concept to guidelines used in the United States.

Fat intake should be 30% or less of caloric intake. Saturated fat intake should be less than 10% of calories, and the intake of cholesterol should be less than 300 mg daily. Polyunsaturated fats (fats that are liquid at room temperature) have a cholesterol-lowering effect, and vegetable oils containing polyunsaturated fats are the best source of vitamin E. Hydrogenated vegetable oil has a cholesterol-elevating effect. Overall, clients should modify fat intake to keep the cholesterol level below 200 mg/dL, with low-density lipoprotein level (LDL, or "bad" cholesterol) below 130 mg/dL and high-density lipoprotein (HDL, or "good" cholesterol) greater than 60 mg/dL.

Although not all persons are sensitive to salt, limiting salt intake may help prevent high blood pressure. In addition, eating large quantities of foods pickled or preserved in salt is associated with cancer of the stomach.

Action Alert! Advise clients to limit salt intake to 6 g/day or less. Salt-sensitive clients should restrict salt intake to 4.5 g/day or less. Most Americans consume more than 6 g of salt daily.

Calcium-containing foods (such as dairy products and dark leafy vegetables) promote bone growth just before the onset of puberty and during adolescence. They also protect against osteoporosis later in life. The RDA for calcium is 800 mg for adult men and nonpregnant adult women. The best sources of calcium are milk and milk products. Calcium in dietary supplements is often present in the poorly soluble forms of phosphate or carbonate, which are not well absorbed.

Alcohol consumption should be avoided. Some studies have shown that small amounts of daily alcohol may reduce the risk of coronary disease; however, there are other ways to reduce this risk. If a client must drink, keep the amount to less than 1 ounce of pure alcohol each day. The "proof" identified on the bottle represents twice the percentage of alcohol it contains; in other words, 80 proof means 40% alcohol.

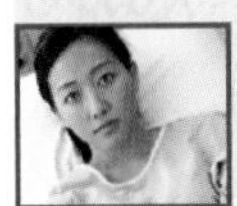

How would you use MyPyramid in teaching Joan how to improve her diet?

Using Dietary Supplements Safely. Fluoride intake is recommended to prevent tooth decay, particularly when consumed before permanent teeth erupt. This benefit persists throughout life as long as fluoride intake continues. Some communities fluoridate the water supply, making supplements unnecessary.

Controversy exists about the advantages and risks of dietary supplements. Food continues to be the best source of nutrients. Dietary supplements should be unnecessary if a client eats a balanced diet that contains the recommended servings in each food group. Although a single multivitamin with 100% of the RDA is not known to be harmful, it has also not been proven to be decidedly beneficial for the vast majority of people. It may be most useful for those whose diet does not supply the recommended intake of vitamins.

When people take vitamins in megadoses, they are using them as drugs, not as nutrients. Research to date has failed to support the original claims for using megavitamins, for example, curing the common cold, lowering cholesterol levels, and decreasing risk of cancer.

Because fat-soluble vitamins, especially vitamin A, are stored largely in the liver, toxicity from megadoses could possibly lead to liver and brain damage. Most people believe large doses of water-soluble vitamins are not harmful because they are readily excreted, but this is not always true. Prolonged vitamin B_6 therapy at 5 g/day to treat premenstrual syndrome has been shown to cause lack of muscle coordination and occasionally nerve damage, and ascorbic acid (vitamin C) in doses above 2 g/day can cause

GI pain, increase the risk of kidney stone formation, and reduce effectiveness of white blood cells against bacteria.

Principles of Nutrient Supplementation. The following principles may be used to guide personal decisions about the use of nutrient supplements:

- Read the labels on dietary supplements as manufacturers of these products supply them, consistent with the Nutrition Labeling and Education Act of 1990.
- Any nutrient can be harmful if taken in excessive amounts; large doses are best used in cases of severe deficiency or problems with absorption or utilization.
- Choose supplements according to personal dietary needs and health care provider recommendations.
- Be aware that excessive intake of one vitamin may lead to deficiency symptoms if that supplement is suddenly discontinued.

Phytochemicals. Phytochemicals are plant chemicals that under close scrutiny in current nutritional research. Foods containing combinations of phytochemicals are sometimes called healing foods, superfoods, or power foods. Generally, they refer to fruits, vegetables, legumes, grains, nuts, and seeds. Expect to read more about the possible benefits of these chemicals as research results become available:

- *Antioxidants* include selenium; vitamins A, C, and E; carotenoids; and flavonoids. They are found in yellow to red and green leafy vegetables, yellow or orange fruits, citrus fruits, nuts, unrefined grains, and seafood. Potential benefits include preventing cancer.
- *Carotenoids* are plant pigments found in cruciferous vegetables, red and yellow fruits and vegetables, green leafy vegetables, and sea vegetables (kelp). Potential benefits are as antioxidants, precursors to vitamin A, eye protection from excessive light, and reducing risk of prostate cancer.
- *Flavonoids* are plant chemicals that give fruits and vegetables their color. They may help reduce the risk of cancer, act as antioxidants, or have antiallergenic and antiinflammatory properties.
- *Phytoestrogens* are hormonelike substances found in whole grains, legumes, and soy. They may reduce the risk of hormone-related cancers, enhance immunity, inhibit platelet aggregation (blood clotting), and mimic some estrogen effects.
- *Polyphenols* are plant compounds found in red wine, tea, apples, grapes, strawberries, onions, and yams. They may reduce the risk of heart disease and cancer.

INTERVENTIONS FOR SPECIAL POPULATIONS

Promoting Nutrition During Pregnancy and Lactation. The recommendations for dietary management during pregnancy emphasize an increase in total calories, protein, vitamins, and minerals. Poor nutrition is a factor in excessive maternal weight gain, preeclampsia, postpartum infections, and an increased incidence of premature babies, low-birth-weight babies, anomalies, developmental disabilities, and stillbirths.

Although the mother's preconception nutrition also affects the outcome of pregnancy, most nutritional care begins during the first trimester of pregnancy. Three well-planned meals, plus one or more snacks, provide the RDA for all nutrients with the possible exceptions of iron and folic acid. Daily supplementation of 30 to 60 mg of ferrous iron and 400 mg of folic acid are recommended. Depending on preferences and tolerance, adequate calcium and zinc may be difficult to achieve in the diet and may require supplementation as well. Prenatal vitamin-plus-mineral supplements are commonly prescribed for pregnant women to minimize the risk of micronutrient (vitamin and mineral) deficiency.

Adequate calories and weight gain are necessary throughout pregnancy. For women entering pregnancy at or near their ideal body weight, a total weight gain of 25 to 35 pounds over the course of the pregnancy is recommended, at a rate of 2 to 4 pounds in the first trimester and 3/4 to 1 pound per week thereafter (roughly an increase of 300 kcal/day). Underweight women should gain the amount they are underweight plus a normal pregnancy gain of 25 pounds. Women whose weight is 120% to 130% of their ideal body weight are encouraged to gain about 20 pounds, whereas those whose weight is more than 135% of the ideal body weight are urged to gain 15 to 16 or 18 to 20 pounds, depending on the source. Most authorities discourage dieting for weight loss during pregnancy. Instead, the emphasis is on high-quality food choices to meet nutrient needs.

> ***Action Alert!*** Teach pregnant women the importance of appropriate weight gain during pregnancy. Advise them that pregnancy is not the time for dieting to lose weight.

All pregnant women should be counseled to avoid potentially harmful substances, including smoking, alcohol, and caffeine during pregnancy. They should also avoid nonprescription drugs, saccharin and other artificial sweeteners, all fad-diet products or regimens, pica (nonnutrient items such as clay or ice), and all recreational drugs.

During lactation, the need for a well-balanced diet continues. Caloric needs are increased by 500 kcal/day from the woman's baseline needs. At least six to eight glasses of water are needed to provide a sufficient volume of milk. Vitamin and mineral supplementation may continue. Harmful substances should still be avoided to prevent transmission to the infant via breast milk.

Promoting Nutrition in Infants. Breast milk or iron-fortified formula is the only source of nourishment needed for the first 4 to 6 months after birth. The infant who is ready to start solid food has doubled the birth weight, can control head movements, and sits up with support.

Vitamin and mineral recommendations are based on the contents of human milk. Daily water requirements are usually met with breast milk or infant formula, except when the weather is hot or the infant has diarrhea or vomiting. Supplemental water is needed at these times to prevent dehydration.

Action Alert! Watch for signs of dehydration (such as decreased urine output, decreased skin turgor, weight loss) in infants with diarrhea or vomiting. With persistent diarrhea or vomiting, severe dehydration can develop quickly in infants.

Promoting Nutrition in Children. Children need adequate calories, protein, water, vitamins, and minerals. Meals should be selected using foods from MyPyramid. Children 1 to 2 years old require smaller servings, more frequent snacks, and 3 cups of whole milk each day (Table 24-4). A good rule of thumb is 1 to 2 tablespoons of a food group with each meal or snack. When planning a child's meals, have the caretaker select from a variety of foods from each food group. Serving sizes increase with age.

A child grows 2 to 3 inches and gains about 5 pounds each year. A standard weight gain–growth chart reflects the child's nutritional health. Weight gain out of proportion to height may reflect overeating or inactivity. If the child's weight-to-height ratio drops below the normal curve, it may indicate malnutrition. By periodically comparing weight to height, you can plot the child's progress on the standard growth curve over time.

Promoting Nutrition in Adolescents. Growth rate increases with the onset of adolescence. In girls, the growth spurt begins at about age 10 and peaks at age 12. Boys begin their growth spurt at about age 12, and it peaks at age 14. Body composition in girls includes a higher percentage of fat tissue. The boys' growth spurt results in a higher proportion of lean body mass, such as muscle and bone.

Two minerals of special concern include iron in girls from the time they begin menstruation and calcium in both boys and girls for bone growth and optimal bone mass. Adequate calcium remains one of the best protectors against age-related bone loss and fractures.

Promoting Nutrition in Older Adults. Older adults require fewer calories because of reduced activity levels and because the basal metabolic rate slows as one ages. Caloric intakes for adults over 51 years are 1900 kcal for women and 2300 for men. The RDAs for individual nutrients remain the same after age 51, except that increased vitamin D is needed because of reduced bodily synthesis. Proper vitamin and mineral intake is needed to reduce the risk of osteoporosis caused by deficiencies in vitamin D and calcium and to reduce the risk of anemia due to inadequate iron intake. Older adults benefit from a low-fat, plant-based diet including fruits, vegetables, whole grains, eight glasses of water per day, and a vitamin and mineral supplement (Topp, Fahlman, & Boardley, 2004).

Specific dietary recommendations may be made for individual clients who have disease processes requiring dietary management. These commonly include reduced sodium for hypertension, reduced fat intake for those at risk for atherosclerosis, reduced caloric intake to achieve weight reduction for those with type 2 diabetes mellitus, and other limitations according to the specific health problem.

Nutrition education for older adults requires careful planning because common techniques may not be appropriate. Group discussion, as opposed to lecture, is often more beneficial in teaching normal nutrition. Counseling on strict diet modifications may be less successful because of resistance to changing lifelong eating habits. To simplify instruction, teach an older adult with

Table 24-4 Child's Daily Food Plan

		Average Size of Serving		
FOOD GROUP	**SERVINGS PER DAY**	**AGE 1 TO 3**	**AGE 4 TO 6**	**AGE 7 TO 10**
Bread and cereals (whole-grain or enriched)[a]	6 or more	1 slice	1 slice	1 slice
Vegetables[b]	3 or more	2 to 4 tablespoons or ½ cup juice	¼ to ½ cup or ½ cup juice	½ to 1 cup
Fruits[b]	2 or more	2 to 4 tablespoons or ½ cup juice	¼ to ½ cup or ½ cup of juice	½ to 1 cup
Meat and meat alternatives[c]	2 or more	½ ounce	1 to 2 ounces	2 to 3 ounces
Milk and milk products[d]	3 to 4	¼ to ½ cup	¾ cup	¾ to 1 cup

Modified from Queen, P. M., & Henry, R. R. (1987). Growth and nutrient requirements of children. In R. J. Grand, L. Sutphen, & W. H. Dietz, Jr. (Eds.), *Pediatric nutrition: Theory and practice* (p. 347). Boston: Butterworth.
[a]1 slice bread = ¼ cup dry cereal, ½ cup cooked cereal, or ½ cup potato, rice, or noodles.
[b]Sources of vitamin C (weekly) include citrus fruits, berries, tomatoes, broccoli, cabbage, and cantaloupe. Sources of vitamin A (3 to 4 times weekly) include spinach, carrots, squash, and cantaloupe.
[c]1 ounce of meat, fish, or poultry = 1 egg, 1 frankfurter, 2 tablespoons peanut butter, or ½ cup cooked legumes.
[d]½ cup milk = ½ cup cottage cheese, pudding, or yogurt; ¼ ounce cheese; or 2 tablespoons dried milk.

diabetes that the diet is a normal, healthy diet that restricts concentrated sweets and simple sugars.

Action Alert! Teach older adults with diabetes to eat a normal diet while restricting simple sugars, to establish regular meal times, and to distribute foods consistently among meals.

Improved nutrition at home may also reduce hospitalization rates for older adults and decrease the number hospitalized who have signs of malnutrition. A dietitian can provide you with valuable information about feeding programs for older adults, low-cost nutritious foods, foods that have a longer shelf life and minimal preparation, and programs that provide shopping assistance.

EVALUATION

Nutritional education is not complete until learning has been evaluated. Formal and informal tools may be used to measure learning against established nutritional teaching objectives. In general, the client should be able to state the components of the healthy diet and any necessary restrictions needed because of disease processes. In addition, the client must have the ability or resources to procure food, store it, cook it properly, and eat it. Difficulty in any of these areas indicates the need for some type of home health care or social service support.

A sample note documenting the outcomes of dietary teaching for Joan, the case study client in this chapter, could be as follows:

Sample Documentation Note for Joan

Client verbalizes understanding of the food groups in MyPyramid and the proper number and sizes of food portions for each group. States she is motivated to change her food intake habits to adopt a healthier lifestyle. Indicates an intention to reduce dietary fat and to return for periodic follow-up monitoring of cholesterol level.

KEY PRINCIPLES

- Good nutritional status is essential for normal organ development and function, for optimal activity and working efficiency, for resistance to infection, and for the ability to repair bodily damage or injury.
- The four functions of the GI system are digestion, absorption, metabolism, and excretion.
- Carbohydrates, proteins, fat, vitamins, minerals, and water are essential nutrients.
- Factors that affect nutrition include life-span considerations, culture and lifestyle, and physiological state.
- General assessment of nutritional status includes a complete health history, diet history, evaluation of food intake, and physical examination.
- The nursing diagnosis *Health-seeking behaviors: nutrition* may be used to promote optimal nutrition for the well client.
- The nursing diagnoses *Imbalanced nutrition: less than body requirements* and *Imbalanced nutrition: more than body requirements* may be used when the diet contains deficient or excess nutrients, respectively.
- Planning for expected outcomes should focus on individual client needs and sound dietary principles.
- The nurse's role in nutritional intervention includes teaching and counseling about appropriate dietary modifications.
- Reading nutrition labels can help relatively healthy clients optimize their nutritional status, and it can improve the nutritional status of those with poor nutrition.
- A healthy diet is based on MyPyramid, which includes individualized recommendations based on age, sex, and physical activity regarding intake of grains, vegetables, fruits, milk, and meat and beans.
- Proper diet habits can reduce the risk of heart disease, stroke, and cancer, three leading causes of death in the United States.
- There may be special dietary needs depending on age, pregnancy status, or disease state.
- Evaluation is necessary to review and improve or change dietary or nutritional plans.

REVIEW QUESTIONS

1. The nurse who is counseling a client about proper intake of vitamins would stress that it is important to avoid excess intake of which of the following vitamins as a diet supplement?

1. Niacin
2. Folic acid
3. Vitamin A
4. Vitamin C

2. The nurse working in a health clinic is concerned about the nutritional status of a client who is underweight and has poor condition of the hair and nails. Which method could be used by the nurse as a quick and easy measure to assess dietary intake?

1. 24-hour recall
2. Food diary
3. Calorie count
4. Household food consumption

3. The nurse is participating in a nutritional screen at a local health fair. The nurse recommends that the attendee who has which body mass index should see a health care provider for further follow-up?

1. 18.7
2. 21.6
3. 24.8
4. 27.5

4. The nurse is working with a 17-year-old girl who says she wants to follow a healthy diet and remember to take a multivitamin, but she often forgets because of a busy school and work schedule. The nurse would stress that it is especially important to take in sufficient amounts of which of the following minerals for unique needs at this age?

1. Copper and zinc
2. Selenium and calcium
3. Iron and calcium
4. Zinc and iron

5. The nurse is evaluating health teaching done with a client about selecting foods from the MyPyramid food guidance system. The nurse concludes that the client has a working knowledge of the groups after selecting an egg as a food choice for which good group?

1. Grains
2. Vegetables
3. Milk
4. Meat and beans

Bibliography

Albert, N. (2005). We are what we eat: Women and diet for cardiovascular health. *Journal of Cardiovascular Nursing, 20*(6), 451-460.

American Dietetic Association. (2006). Position statement of the American Dietetic Association: Individual-, family-, school-, and community-based interventions for pediatric overweight. *Journal of the American Dietetic Association, 106* (6), 925-945.

Cole, K., Waldrop, J., D'Auria, J., & Garner, H. (2006). An integrative research review: Effective school-based childhood overweight interventions. *Journal for Specialists in Pediatric Nursing, 11*(3), 166-177.

Dudek, S. G. (2006). *Nutrition essentials for nursing practice* (5th ed. Revised reprint). Philadelphia: Lippincott Williams & Wilkins.

Flegal, K., Graubard, B., Williamson, D., & Gail, M. (2005). Excess deaths associated with underweight, overweight and obesity. *Journal of the American Medical Association, 293*(15), 1861-1867.

Fontaine, K. (2005). *Complementary and alternative therapies* (2nd ed., pp. 121-142). Upper Saddle River, NJ: Pearson Prentice Hall.

*Food and Nutrition Board, Subcommittee on the Tenth Edition of the RDAs. (1989). *Recommended dietary allowances* (10th ed.). Washington, DC: National Academy Press.

Ford, F. (2004). A guide to nutrition during pregnancy. *The Practising Midwife, 7*(11), 24, 26.

Grodner, M., Anderson, S. L., & DeYoung, S. (2004). *Foundations and clinical applications of nutrition: A nursing approach* (3rd ed.). St Louis, MO: Mosby.

Holmes, S. (2006). Nutrition and the prevention of cancer. *Journal of Family Health Care, 16*(2), 43-46.

Lutz, C., & Przytulski, K. (2006). *Nutrition and diet therapy: Evidence-based applications* (4th ed.). Philadelphia: F. A. Davis.

Miller, E. (2006). Embracing the problems of obesity. *Rehabilitation Nursing, 31*(4), 134-135.

Morin, K. (2005). Water-soluble vitamins. *MCN: The American Journal of Maternal Child Nursing, 30*(4), 271.

Nix, S. (2005). *Williams' basic nutrition and diet therapy* (12th ed.). St Louis, MO: Mosby.

O'Brien, P. E. & Dixon, J. B. (2002). The extent of the problem of obesity. *American Journal of Surgery, 184*(6B), 4S-8S.

Ogden, C., Carroll, M., Curtin, L., McDowell, M., Tabak, C., & Flegal, K. (2006). Prevalence of obesity and overweight in the United States, 1999-2004. *Journal of the American Medical Association, 295*(13), 1549-1555.

*Ogden, C., Flegal, K., Carroll, M., & Johnson, C. (2002). Prevalence and trends in overweight among U.S. children and adolescents, 1999-2000. *Journal of the American Medical Association, 288*(14), 1772-1773.

Sitzman, K. (2005). Vitamin D: an essential nutrient. *American Association of Occupational Health Nurses, 53* (6), 280.

Topp, R., Fahlman, M., & Boardley, D. (2004). Healthy aging: Health promotion and disease prevention. *Nursing Clinics of North America, 39*(2), 411-422.

*U.S. Department of Health and Human Services. (2000). *Healthy People 2010* (2nd ed.). Washington, DC: U.S. Government Printing Office. Available at http://web.health.gov/healthypeople.

Watts, S., & Anselmo, J. (2006). Nutrition for diabetes: All in a day's work. *Nursing, 36*(6), 46-48.

Yen, P. K. (2005). Depression: The diet connection. *Geriatric Nursing, 26*(3), 143-144.

*Asterisk indicates a classic or definitive work on this subject.

Chapter 25

Restoring Nutrition

Media Resources

- Nursing Skills Online
- evolve Evolve Website http://evolve.elsevier.com/Harkreader/
- 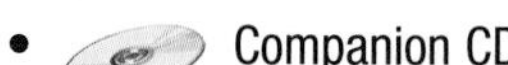 Companion CD

Learning Objectives

After studying this chapter, you should be able to do the following:

- Describe the physiology of malnutrition and starvation
- Discuss factors affecting nutritional deficits
- Assess clients who are experiencing severe nutritional deficits
- Formulate nursing diagnoses for nutritional deficits
- Plan goal-directed interventions for clients with nutritional deficits
- Employ a variety of interventions to facilitate optimal nutrition for clients
- Evaluate the achievement of measurable outcomes for clients with nutritional deficits

Key Terms

anorexia
catabolism
deglutition
dysphagia
enteral nutrition
malnutrition
parenteral nutrition

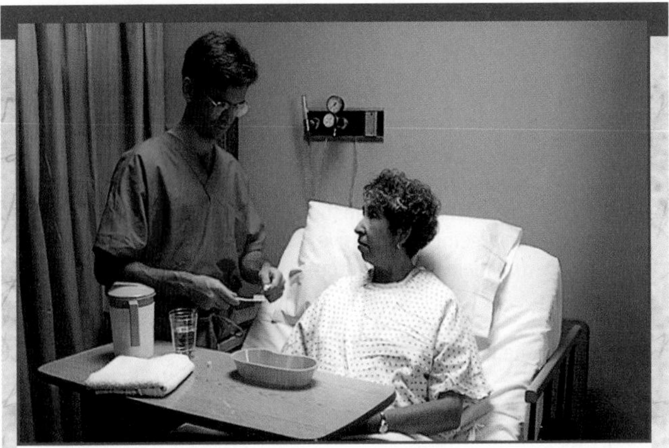

Mrs. Rosalie Goldman is a 54-year-old lawyer whose parents came to the United States from Russia in the early 1900s. She has had surgery for cancer of the breast and now is receiving outpatient chemotherapy. Because of her treatments, she experiences early satiety and anorexia and says that food does not have much taste. Mrs. Goldman is 5 feet 4 inches tall, and her usual weight is 140 pounds. Currently she weighs 115 pounds. Her serum albumin level is 2.7 g/100 mL.

The clinic nurse is concerned with Mrs. Goldman's weight loss and considers her at risk for malnutrition. She makes the diagnosis of *Imbalanced nutrition: less than body requirements* from the list of nursing diagnoses related to nutrition (see the key nursing diagnoses box).

KEY NURSING DIAGNOSES FOR IMBALANCED NUTRITION

Imbalanced nutrition: less than body requirements: An intake of nutrients insufficient to meet metabolic needs
Impaired swallowing: Abnormal functioning of the swallowing mechanism associated with deficits in oral, pharyngeal, or esophageal structure or function
Risk for aspiration: Being at risk for entry of GI secretions, oropharyngeal secretions, solids, or fluids into the tracheobronchial passages

CONCEPTS OF NUTRITIONAL PROBLEMS

As a nurse, you will observe nutritional problems in clients across care settings: homes, rehabilitation or long-term care settings, clinics, and hospitals. Collectively, nutritional problems create a condition known as **malnutrition,** which is any nutritional disorder caused by imbalanced, insufficient, or excessive diet or by impaired absorption or metabolism of nutrients. To care for clients with malnutrition, you will need a sound understanding of inadequate and excessive nutrition and the many factors that affect nutritional status.

Nutritional deprivation results from inadequate intake, which may be caused by nausea and vomiting, difficulty swallowing, or inability to obtain food. It can also result from problems that raise energy needs, such as infection, trauma, stress, or surgery.

Extreme malnutrition can lead to death through starvation, the physiological response to chronic food deprivation. During starvation, the body attempts to reduce its energy use first by lowering voluntary activity and the basal metabolic rate (BMR). When nutrient intake fails to meet the body's energy expenditure, the body first converts glycogen stores in the liver to glucose (glycogenolysis), but these stores last for only a few hours. Next, the body breaks down muscle and lean body mass. This phenomenon, called **catabolism,** yields glucose from protein in a process called gluconeogenesis. Protein can supply about 2 weeks of calories; however, this protein breakdown negatively affects the body by decreasing lean body mass. After 10 to 14 days of starvation, the body breaks down fat for energy through lipolysis. The liver makes ketone bodies from fatty acids for use as fuel by most tissues, including the brain. Fatty acids may also be used directly by many tissues for fuel. Ketosis occurs as ketone bodies accumulate in the body as end products of fat metabolism. Figure 25-1 summarizes the

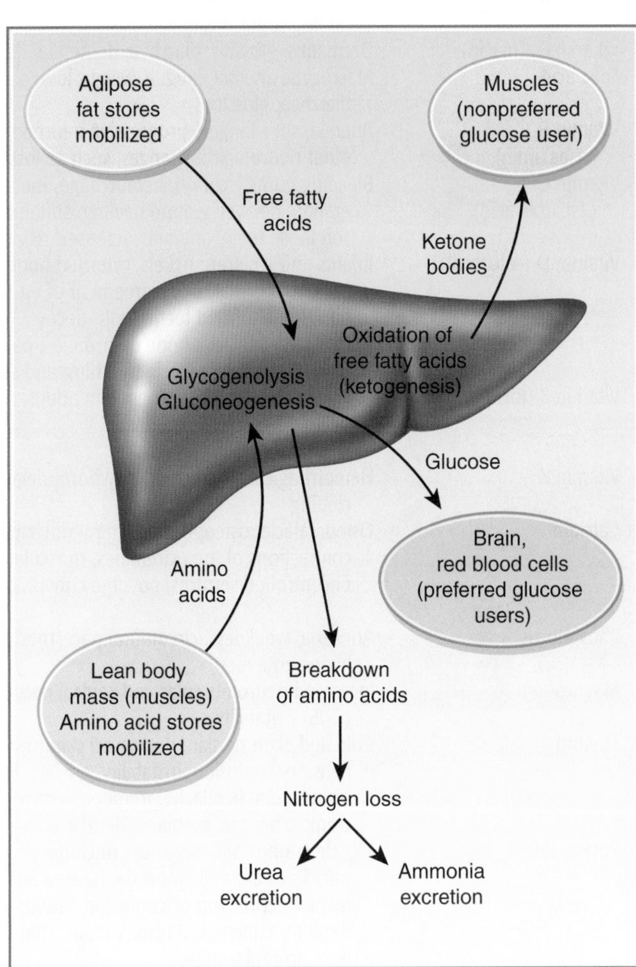

FIGURE 25-1 Metabolic changes that occur when the body uses endogenous fuels to meet energy needs. (Modified from Lemoyne, M., & Jeejeebhoy, K. N. [1985]. Total parenteral nutrition in the critically ill patient. *Chest, 89*[4], 568.)

Table 25-1 Manifestations of Nutritional Imbalances

NUTRIENT	EVIDENCE OF DEFICIENCY	EVIDENCE OF EXCESS
Vitamin A	Night blindness, dry rough skin, dry eyes (xerosis), dry mucous membranes, decreased saliva secretion leading to difficulty chewing and swallowing, impaired digestion and absorption, diarrhea, increased susceptibility to respiratory, urinary, and vaginal infections, impaired development of bones and teeth	Anorexia, nausea, vomiting, abdominal pain, diarrhea, weight loss, irritability, fatigue, portal hypertension, loss of hair, dry skin, bone pain and fragility, spleen enlargement, extensive liver damage, hydrocephalus (in infants and children)
Vitamin B_1 (thiamine)	Anorexia, edema, enlarged heart, heart failure, mental confusion, peripheral paralysis, fatigue, beriberi, painful calf muscles	None known
Vitamin B_2 (riboflavin)	Reddening of the cornea, dermatitis, cheilosis, glossitis, photophobia, ariboflavinosis	None known
Vitamin B_3 (niacin)	Dermatitis, glossitis, diarrhea, dementia, death	None known
Folic acid	Macrocytic anemia, fatigue, weight loss, pallor, diarrhea, glossitis	None known
Vitamin B_{12} (cobalamin)	Anemia, sore tongue, progressive neuropathy and other neurological changes, such as loss of memory	None known
Vitamin C (ascorbic acid)	Bleeding gums (scurvy), hemorrhage, muscle degeneration, delayed wound healing, softening of bones, soft loose teeth, anemia, increased risk of infection	Kidney stones, scurvy upon withdrawal, nausea, abdominal cramps, diarrhea, false-positive test for urinary glucose
Vitamin D (calciferol)	Infants and children: rickets, retarded bone growth, bone malformation, enlargement of ends of long bones, malformed teeth, tooth decay Adults: osteomalacia, bone deformities, pain, easy fracture, involuntary muscle twitching and spasms	Excessive calcification of bones, kidney stones, nausea, vomiting, headache, weakness, weight loss, constipation, polyuria, polydipsia, mental and physical growth retardation (children), failure to thrive (children), drowsiness, and coma (in severe cases)
Vitamin E (tocopherol)	Possible mild hemolytic anemia in adults, macrocytic anemia in premature infants	With large doses, possible depression, fatigue, diarrhea, cramps, blurred vision, headaches, interference with normal blood clotting and vitamin A metabolism
Vitamin K	Hemorrhagic disease of the newborn, delayed blood clotting	Hemolytic anemia and liver damage with synthetic vitamin K
Calcium	Osteomalacia, osteoporosis, tetany (intermittent, tonic contractions of the extremities, muscular cramps, uncontrolled seizures, possible convulsions)	Nausea, abdominal pain, vomiting, constipation, anorexia, polydipsia, polyuria, calcium kidney stones, excessive calcification of bones and soft tissues, possible coma and death
Phosphorus	Anorexia, weakness, circumoral paresthesia, hyperventilation	Symptoms of hypocalcemic tetany
Magnesium	Increased neuromuscular and central nervous system (CNS) irritability	CNS depression, hypotension, coma
Sodium	Cold and clammy skin, decreased skin turgor, apprehension, confusion, irritability, anxiety, hypotension, tachycardia, headache, tremors, seizures, abdominal cramps, nausea, vomiting, diarrhea	Edema, weight gain, hot flushed dry skin, dry red tongue, intense thirst, restless agitation, oliguria or anuria
Potassium	Muscle cramps and weakness (including cardiac muscle weakness), anorexia, nausea and vomiting, mental depression or confusion, lethargy, abdominal distention, increased urine output, shallow respirations, irregular pulse	Irritability, anxiety, listlessness, mental confusion, nausea, diarrhea, poor respirations, gastrointestinal (GI) hyperactivity, muscle weakness, numbness of the extremities, hypotension, cardiac arrhythmias, heart block, cardiac arrest
Iron	Microcytic anemia, pallor, decreased work capacity, fatigue, weakness, intolerance to cold, pica, spoon-shaped fingernails	Acute iron poisoning from accidental overdose, which leads to GI cramping, nausea, vomiting, possible shock, seizures, coma
Iodine	Goiter	Acne-like skin lesions, "iodine goiter"
Zinc	Impairments of growth, sexual maturation, and immune system functioning; skin lesions; decreased sense of taste and smell	Anorexia, nausea, vomiting, diarrhea, muscle pain, lethargy, drowsiness, bleeding gastric ulcers, decreased serum levels of high-density lipoproteins

metabolic changes that occur when the body uses endogenous fuels to meet energy needs. In nonobese adults, fat (the body's main stored fuel) is depleted in about 1 to 2 months.

Catabolism results in a negative nitrogen balance. Although protein intake is low, the blood urea nitrogen (BUN) and serum creatinine, which represent end products of protein breakdown, will rise. Later in starvation, these levels begin to decline as fats are utilized to a greater extent for energy needs. Ketosis can be detected by testing the urine by dipstick.

Protein-calorie malnutrition in hospitalized clients may be present at time of admission or may develop during hospitalization because of the hypercatabolic state caused by stress, infection, or impaired organ function (Winaver & Williams, 2001). Unless this is recognized and treated, these clients are likely to remain nutritionally depleted during their hospital stay and are at risk for complications and longer lengths of stay (Pichard et al., 2004).

Marasmus is a chronic condition of starvation with severe fat and muscle loss that results from deficient caloric intake over months or years. Clients appear starved and weigh less than 80% of their ideal body weight (IBW) but have a normal serum albumin level. Fortunately, they respond fairly well to therapy as long as they are not refed too quickly.

Kwashiorkor is a condition of starvation, usually in young children after weaning, caused by decreased protein intake; symptoms can develop in a few weeks. A client with kwashiorkor may appear well nourished but is at tremendous risk. The serum albumin level falls below 2.8 g/100 mL, leading to significant edema. Wounds heal more slowly, and the client risks infection from decreased immunity. The mortality rate is high because of weakened immune status and poorer response to refeeding than with marasmus.

Vitamin and mineral deficiencies can also result from decreased intake or increased loss (as with diarrhea or vomiting). Table 25-1 summarizes manifestations of the major imbalances. Vitamin and mineral imbalances commonly affect the skin, peripheral nervous system, hematopoietic system, immunity, calcification of bones, and vision.

FACTORS AFFECTING NUTRITIONAL STATUS

RISK FACTORS ACROSS THE LIFE SPAN

Throughout the life cycle, a complex balance exists between the anabolism of growth and the catabolism of aging. Energy expenditure and nutrient requirements are higher early in life, are stable during the middle years, and decline with aging. Specifically, metabolism peaks during the first 5 years and then rises again during puberty. After age 20, the BMR declines steadily. During pregnancy, the BMR increases by about 13%. Uncomplicated stressors (changes in food intake or activity level) or more severe stressors (such as trauma or disease) can increase a client's energy needs significantly.

Infants and Children. Low-birth-weight infants are at risk for undernutrition and need close monitoring (Anderson, 2004). These newborns weigh less than 2500 g ($5^1/_2$ pounds) and are classified as small for gestational age (restricted intrauterine growth rate) or premature (shortened length of gestation). These infants have fewer nutritional reserves because fetal nutrient stores are deposited in the last 3 months of pregnancy. Premature infants may be given enteral feedings by tube in carefully controlled amounts (Gregory, 2005) because the suck-swallow reflex does not develop until 32 to 34 weeks of gestation.

Infants or children may need extra nourishment if they experience hypermetabolism or decreased growth. Trauma, burns, and failure to thrive are examples of conditions that require special nutritional support. Children who have a low weight for age are also have higher mortality rates when physiological stressors, such as with diarrhea or measles, are added (Caulfield, deOnis, Blossner, & Black, 2004).

Malnutrition in children incorporates overnutrition (excess energy intake) as well as undernutrition. Children who are overweight may still ingest inadequate amounts of vitamins, minerals, and protein, while taking in higher than recommended levels of fat, sugar, and overall calories. Contributing factors are increased visits to fast-food restaurants, increased portion sizes, food choices made at school (cafeteria meals, a la carte, and vending machines), inactivity, and eating during sedentary leisure activities, such as watching television or computer usage (Lucas, 2004).

Adolescents. Eating disorders tend to occur during adolescence (often with onset at 13 and 20 years), a time of emotional and physical turmoil. Adolescents gain 20% of adult height and 50% of adult weight during this time. They are also developing a sense of self and may feel uncomfortable about their changing bodies. In a society that favors slimness, these factors all promote development of eating disorders. Females are affected more than males at a ratio that ranges from 6:1 to 10:1. Eating disorders in the United States occur with relatively equal incidence in white and Hispanic females, occur more frequently among Native Americans, and occur less frequently among African Americans and Asians. Eating disorders consist of anorexia nervosa, bulimia nervosa, and eating disorders not otherwise specified (American Psychiatric Association, 2000). Girls and boys who compete in sports requiring low body fat, such as track, dance, rowing, gymnastics, or wrestling, are more at risk for eating disorders in the unspecified category.

Obesity and overweight status in adolescents follows the pattern found in children. It is significant because it adds to the risk of diabetes, heart disease, stroke, and peripheral vascular disease in later life.

Older Adults. In general, aging causes an increased proportion of connective tissue and a loss of functioning cells. Although the etiology is uncertain, one theory is that free radicals attack the cells and impair energy production in mitochondria. Antioxidant nutrients (such as vitamin C, vitamin E, and selenium) may reduce free-radical damage to tissues.

Some nutritional deficits may be linked to aging. For example, deficiencies of calcium, iron, zinc, thiamine, vitamin B_{12}, and folate are common in the older adult and may be secondary to problems with chewing, swallowing, and digesting foods. Reduced secretion of gastric hydrochloric acid limits absorption of calcium, iron, and vitamin B_{12}. About half of clients age 65 and older wear dentures, which can create problems with chewing and limit intake if they do not fit well. Finally, many older adults take multiple prescription and over-the-counter drugs, increasing the risk of potentially dangerous drug-nutrient interactions (Brownie, 2006).

PHYSIOLOGICAL FACTORS

Illness can impair the body's ability to maintain normal nutrition by affecting ingestion, digestion, absorption, or metabolism.

Ingestion. Factors that affect food ingestion are those that influence appetite and disorders of the mouth and esophagus that affect swallowing. **Anorexia** is a reduced desire for food, leading to decreased intake and possibly malnutrition if prolonged. It is a hallmark of the disorder anorexia nervosa that most frequently affects girls and young women. Anorexia is also caused by liver disease, medications, depression, acquired immunodeficiency syndrome (AIDS), or gastrointestinal (GI) problems. AIDS further inhibits ingestion when lesions occur in the mouth and throat (stomatitis). Nausea with vomiting impairs intake and causes loss of certain minerals. This condition may be self-limiting but, if prolonged, may require hydration with intravenous (IV) fluids and possible parenteral nutritional support. Even minor disorders such as upper respiratory infection can cause anorexia by reducing the sense of taste and smell.

Swallowing, or **deglutition,** is the reflex passage of food and fluids from the mouth to the stomach (Figure 25-2). Swallowing is initiated by voluntary action and is controlled by the central nervous system. The term **dysphagia** refers to difficulty in swallowing.

Involuntary control of swallowing is coordinated from the swallowing center in the reticular formation of the medulla and lower pons in the brain. The process uses cranial nerves V, IX, X, and XII. After food is propelled to the back of the throat by the tongue and palate muscles, an involuntary wave of pharyngeal muscle contraction pushes food into the esophagus. Meanwhile, the glottis and epiglottis move to close off the trachea and suspend breathing. When this mechanism malfunctions (such as with a cerebrovascular accident [CVA] or stroke), food is aspirated into the lungs.

Muscle tension at the upper esophageal (hypopharyngeal) sphincter and the lower esophageal sphincter (LES) normally keeps these sphincters tightly closed except during swallowing, when they relax to allow food passage into the stomach by peristalsis. Increased pressure at the LES can cause dysphagia. Decreased pressure can cause reflux of acidic stomach contents back into the esophagus. Pressure at the LES is increased by parasympathetic drugs and gastrin. It is decreased by anticholinergics, cigarettes, fatty foods, alcohol, and certain digestive substances, such as cholecystokinin and secretin.

Several factors may hinder swallowing. Damage to the cranial nerves that innervate the tongue and pharynx may interfere with initiation of the swallowing reflex, effective chewing, and pushing food back into the pharynx and esophagus. The discomfort of an inflamed throat, obstruction, and decreased muscular contraction of the esophagus also can impede swallowing.

Clients who have neurological disease or a CVA (stroke) often have problems swallowing because of decreased level of consciousness (LOC) or partial paralysis of the tongue, mouth, or throat. Examples of difficulties include drooling, inability to form a seal around a cup or straw, uncoordinated tongue movements, and pocketing of food in the mouth. All of these problems raise the risk of aspiration.

Aspiration occurs when the client cannot protect the airway. This may result from difficulty swallowing, decreased LOC, seizures, impaired gag or cough reflexes, or a compromised immune system. Weakness of muscles in the soft palate, pharynx, and upper esophagus hinder the cough reflex.

Digestion and Absorption. Certain diseases alter the digestive process and impair food absorption, a condition called malabsorption. Some examples include inflammatory bowel disease (Crohn's disease or ulcerative colitis), diarrhea caused by infection, and cystic fibrosis. *Lactose intolerance* is a condition in which the intestinal villi do not produce lactase, the enzyme that breaks down lactose, a carbohydrate found in milk. The lactose remains in the GI tract and draws water into the intestine by osmosis, leading to diarrhea. These disorders require specific management to promote optimal nutrition.

Metabolism. Liver diseases also affect food metabolism. Vitamins normally stored (A, B, C, K) or activated (D) in the liver may be deficient. Liver disease impairs protein metabolism because the liver cannot transform ammonia to urea.

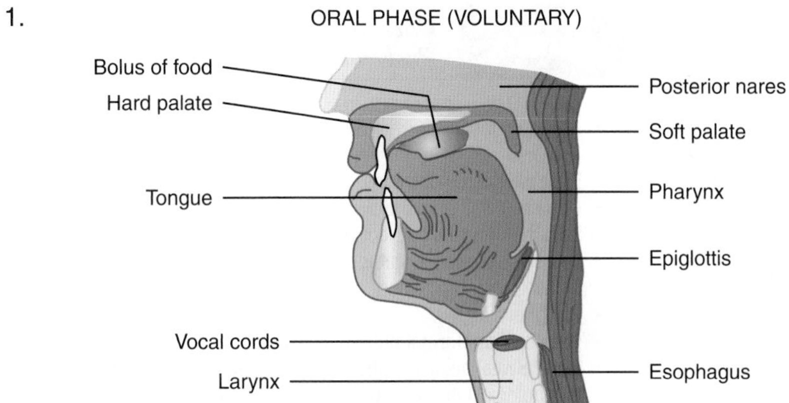

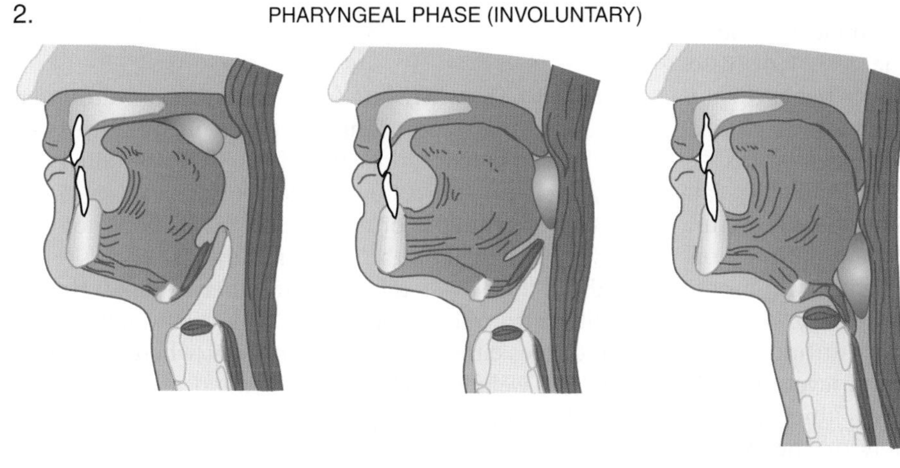

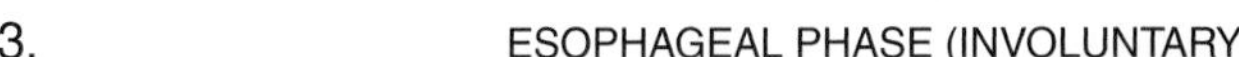

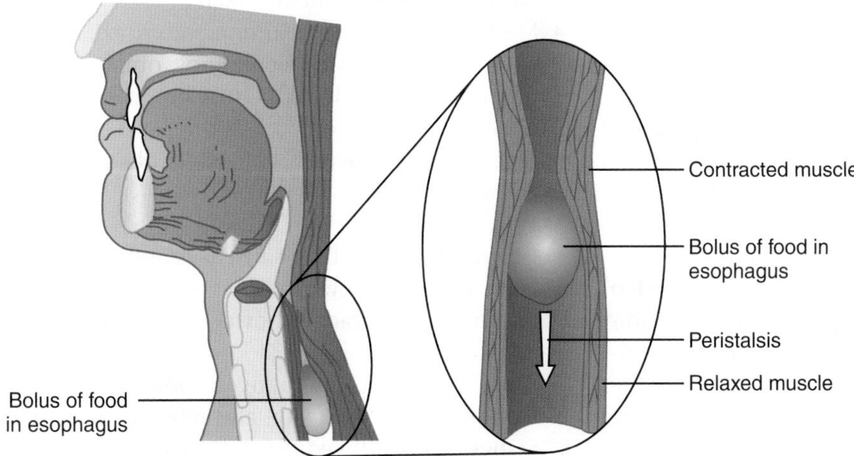

FIGURE 25-2 Mechanics of swallowing. Swallowing occurs in three phases: (1) *Voluntary* or *oral* phase. The tongue presses food against the hard palate, forcing it toward the pharynx. (2) *Involuntary, pharyngeal* phase. *Early:* A wave of peristalsis forces the bolus between the tonsillar pillars. *Middle:* The soft palate draws upward to close posterior nares, and respirations cease momentarily. *Late:* The vocal cords approximate and the larynx pulls upward, covering the airway and stretching the esophagus open. (3) *Involuntary, esophageal* phase. Relaxation of the upper esophageal (hypopharyngeal) sphincter allows a peristaltic wave to move the bolus of food down the esophagus. (From Black, J. M., Hawks, J., & Keene, A. [2001]. *Medical-surgical nursing: Clinical management for positive outcomes* [6th ed.]. Philadelphia: Saunders.)

Infection and trauma cause hypermetabolism and catabolism, requiring added calories, protein, vitamins, and minerals. Infection may also cause anorexia and electrolyte imbalances. Anemia may be associated with chronic infection, but the mechanism of this association is not fully understood.

When calculating energy needs from predictive equations for clients who have infections, be sure to consider body temperature. Fever increases metabolic needs by 7% for each degree Fahrenheit (13% for each degree centigrade). Clients with massive trauma or burns have very high calorie needs.

CULTURAL AND LIFESTYLE FACTORS

Intake of an imbalanced diet, low income that limits access to affordable nutritious food, and physical difficulty with obtaining or preparing food place clients at risk for malnutrition. It is important to conduct nutritional assessments to detect any of these factors. Inadequate nutrition over time can impair health, delay recovery from illness or surgery, and decrease overall well-being.

ASSESSMENT

GENERAL ASSESSMENT FOR NUTRITIONAL PROBLEMS

Nutritional assessment and screening can identify cues to nutritional problems (Box 25-1). Chapter 24 discusses general assessment of nutritional status. When a client is identified as having a nutritional problem, further assessment focuses on etiology, severity, and related factors.

Laboratory test results can provide valuable data about a client's nutritional status (Table 25-2). Serum studies will likely be ordered if the client unintentionally loses 10% of his or her body weight in a 6-month period or has signs of a nutritional deficiency. However, no single laboratory test will diagnose nutritional problems. For example, creatinine and BUN levels are reliable as long as clients do not have kidney disease. When a client has kidney disease, rely on the ratio of BUN to serum creatinine. Serum albumin levels may be measured, but albumin has a 20- to 24-day half-life, so it does not provide data about the short-term effectiveness of diet therapy. Instead, look to increases in prealbumin (for improved protein status) or transferrin (improvement in anemia).

Laboratory tests are rarely done to measure vitamin deficiencies. Instead, use the nutritional history, physical examination, and anthropometric measurements. Electrolyte levels are commonly measured, and they can provide general information about nutrition as well.

Swallowing and aspiration may be evaluated using videofluoroscopy, a procedure also known as a video swallow esophagography, cine-esophagography, modified barium swallow, or swallow study. The client swallows barium, which is observed passing through the oropharynx during swallowing. This study is done in the radiology department and exposes the client to a minimal amount of radiation.

FOCUSED ASSESSMENT FOR *IMBALANCED NUTRITION: LESS THAN BODY REQUIREMENTS*

Although weight loss is the most commonly identified cue to nutritional deficiency, more subtle cues need to be considered. Cluster various cues to make this diagnosis.

BOX 25-1 *Cues to Possible Nutritional Problems*

- Anorexia
- Artificial airway
- Diarrhea
- Increased metabolic need
- Compromised immune system
- Less-than-normal nutrient consumption
- Low socioeconomic status
- Malabsorptive condition
- Polypharmacy
- Greater-than-normal nutrient consumption
- Muscle weaknesses in pharynx, soft palate, or esophagus
- Psychological disturbance (low self-esteem, depression)
- Reduced level of consciousness
- Nausea and vomiting

Defining Characteristics. Clients who have nutritional problems may report weight changes, inability to swallow or eat, fatigue, and skin lesions. Take a detailed history, including the following elements:

- Body weight 20% or more below ideal; assess for weight changes in the last 6 months; ask clients about their *usual weight* and whether current weight differs from the usual weight; abnormal weight gain indicates either fluid gain or obesity, whereas involuntary weight loss indicates disease or malnutrition and can be a grave sign
- Changes in appetite: anorexia, early satiety, lack of interest in food, aversion to food, loss of taste
- Motor symptoms, such as an inability to eat independently
- Nutritional supplements taken
- Medications taken, including prescribed, over-the-counter, and herbal preparations; obtain a history of other health problems to correlate with the medication list
- Difficulty swallowing or chewing; obstructed esophagus or pharynx
- Pale conjunctiva
- GI symptoms, such as nausea, vomiting, constipation, abdominal cramping or pain with or without pathology, hyperactive bowel sounds, diarrhea or steatorrhea
- A perceived inability to ingest food
- Condition of skin, teeth, and mucous membranes: rashes, scaling, bleeding, poor wound healing, capillary fragility, pale or ulcerated mucous membranes, depapillation of the tongue, bleeding, gum disease, cracks in the mouth, and dental caries; a sore or inflamed mouth or altered taste sensation
- Hair condition, such as brittleness and how easily it can be plucked
- Fingernail condition, including ridges, clubbing, and brittleness

Table 25-2 Implications of Laboratory Tests for Nutritional Status

LABORATORY TEST	NORMAL RANGE OF VALUES	POSSIBLE NUTRITIONAL IMPLICATIONS OF ABNORMAL VALUES
Blood urea nitrogen	8-23 mg/100 mL	Decreased: Low protein intake Increased: Possibly either excessive protein intake or catabolism
Hematocrit	Female: 34%-44% Male: 39%-49%	Decreased: Anemia (deficiency of iron, pyridoxine, folate, vitamin B_{12}, protein) Increased: Possible dehydration (hemoconcentration)
Hemoglobin	Female: 12-15 g/100 mL Male: 14-17 g/100 mL	Decreased: Anemia (deficiency of iron, pyridoxine, folate, vitamin B_{12}, protein)
Ratio of blood urea nitrogen to serum creatinine	12 or above	If 8 or below, poor protein intake
Serum albumin	3.5-5.5 g/100 mL	Decreased: Compromised protein status (levels under 2.8 are associated with edema and possible kwashiorkor); half-life is 20 to 24 days
Prealbumin (PA) antibody assay or transthyretin (TTR)	17-40 mg/100 mL	Decreased: Malnutrition, zinc deficiency, protein-wasting diseases; half-life is short (2 to 4 days), so rising values toward normal indicate effective nutritional therapy
Serum creatinine	0.6-1.6 mg/100 mL	If decreased: Muscle wasting
Total lymphocyte count	1500/mm^3 or above	If decreased: Not specific for any particular nutritional deficiency, but correlates best with protein deficit

- Neck characteristics, including enlarged lymph nodes, enlarged thyroid
- Musculoskeletal conditions, such as bone deformities and muscle wasting, muscle weakness, decreased muscle tone
- Central nervous system dysfunction, including difficulty walking and peripheral neuritis
- Other medical conditions: liver, heart, or kidney disease; diabetes; cancer; or AIDS

Related Factors. Other related factors may include the following:

- Economic factors in obtaining food
- Misconceptions, lack of information, or misinformation
- Inadequate caregivers or support systems

FOCUSED ASSESSMENT FOR *IMPAIRED SWALLOWING*

Defining Characteristics. Defining characteristics for *Impaired swallowing* may pertain to any of the three phases of swallowing and include the following:

- Oral phase: lack of tongue action to form a bolus; weak sucking in an infant; incomplete lip closure; food pushed out or falls out of mouth; slow bolus formation; premature entry of bolus; nasal reflux; inability to clear the mouth; coughing, choking, or gagging before swallowing; abnormal results of swallow study; lack of chewing; pooling, drooling, or excessive saliva formation
- Pharyngeal phase: altered head positions, inadequate laryngeal elevation, refusal of food, unexplained fevers, delayed swallowing, recurrent pulmonary infections, a gurgly voice, nasal reflux, choking, coughing, gagging, multiple swallows, abnormal swallow study results
- Esophageal phase: heartburn or epigastric pain, acidic-smelling breath, unexplained irritability at mealtime, vomitus on pillow, repetitive swallowing or ruminating, wet burps, bruxism (teeth grinding), nighttime coughing or awakening, observed difficulty swallowing, hyperextension of head during or after meals, abnormal swallow study, painful swallowing, limiting or refusing food, complaints of "something stuck," vomiting (including blood)

Related Factors. Factors related to *Impaired swallowing* may include the following:

- Weakness or tiredness
- Lack of or decreased motivation
- Severe anxiety
- Neuromuscular or musculoskeletal impairment
- Perceptual or cognitive impairment
- Pain or discomfort
- Environmental barriers

FOCUSED ASSESSMENT FOR *RISK FOR ASPIRATION*

Defining Characteristics. Because this is a risk nursing diagnosis, there are no defining characteristics. Instead, assess the client for related factors.

Related Factors. Factors related to *Risk for aspiration* include the following:

- Conditions that result in decreased GI motility, delayed gastric emptying, increased gastric residual (contents remaining from previous meal or feeding), or increased intragastric pressure
- Presence of an enteral feeding tube or other GI tubes

- Presence of an artificial airway, such as a tracheostomy or endotracheal tube
- Reduced level of consciousness or depressed cough or gag reflexes
- Insufficient elevation of upper body or impaired swallowing
- Trauma or surgery to the face, mouth, or neck
- Medication administration

DIAGNOSIS

It is relatively easy to identify *Imbalanced nutrition: less than body requirements,* but it may be more difficult to distinguish between *Impaired swallowing* and *Risk for aspiration.* If the client has a swallowing disorder but also has reduced intake, use the *Imbalanced nutrition* diagnosis until the nutritional state has stabilized. This allows you to focus your care on improving the client's nutritional state.

Remember that impaired swallowing increases the risk of aspiration. Focus your efforts first on preventing aspiration, since it can be life threatening. Review data from the history and physical examination to find cues to an increased risk for aspiration. If you cannot make a definitive diagnosis of *Risk for aspiration,* then focus on impaired swallowing. Remember that interventions to improve swallowing also help prevent aspiration.

Make the diagnosis that focuses on priority nursing care. For example, if a client with anorexia nervosa is acutely ill in the emergency department, use *Imbalanced nutrition: less than body requirements* until the acute episode resolves. If there are life-threatening fluid and electrolyte imbalances, use *Deficient fluid volume.* As treatment continues and the client gets psychological help, focus on *Chronic low self-esteem* or *Disturbed body image.* Table 25-3 shows how to select nursing diagnoses according to clustered data.

RELATED NURSING DIAGNOSES

Noncompliance may be diagnosed if clients do not follow nutritional advice because of identifiable barriers; it is not appropriate to use if the client freely chooses not to adhere to the dietary plan. Obese clients may have trouble following the prescribed dietary regimen. Clients with eating disorders see themselves in a distorted way and have difficulty thinking about food and weight in a customary way. A related nursing diagnosis to consider would be *Ineffective therapeutic regimen management.*

Clients who are not receiving sufficient fluid may be at risk for dehydration. Consider the diagnosis *Deficient fluid volume,* especially for older adults or those with swallowing difficulty, anorexia, or eating disorders.

Use the diagnosis *Impaired skin integrity* for a client with skin breakdown associated with nutritional problems, such as low serum albumin and decreased protein. Because dehydration causes dry skin and mucous membranes, another related nursing diagnosis to consider is *Impaired oral mucous membrane.*

Use the diagnosis *Diarrhea* for a client with nutritional problems caused by diarrhea, which leads to a loss of fluids and decreased absorption of nutrients. Diarrhea is a common complication of enteral feedings.

The diagnosis *Fatigue* may be appropriate when a client receives insufficient nutrients for metabolism and energy production and, as a consequence, feels tired. Fatigue can also be a risk factor for both impaired swallowing and aspiration.

Table 25-3 Clustering Data to Make a Nursing Diagnosis

Nutritional Problems	
DATA CLUSTER	**DIAGNOSIS**
A 27-year-old client presents with a weight 120% of normal; has been overweight since age 10; preoperative for gallbladder surgery and referred for weight loss.	*Imbalanced nutrition: more than requirements* related to unknown etiology
A 45-year-old client is 120% above his ideal body weight; has been coming to the weight-control clinic for 6 months and continues to gain weight. Refuses to exercise and to keep a food diary.	*Noncompliance* with weight control program related to lack of motivation
A 14-year-old bulimic client comes to the emergency department with a weight of 55 pounds, height of 5 feet 2 inches, blood pressure of 70/20, pulse of 124, respiratory rate of 30, decreased skin turgor, weakness, and thirst.	*Deficient fluid volume* related to frequent vomiting without sufficient fluid replacement
A 76-year-old man has had a stroke and is comatose. He is receiving nasogastric feedings and has developed pneumonia.	*Risk for aspiration related to esophageal reflux and pharyngeal muscle weakness*
A 52-year-old woman receiving chemotherapy for cancer has developed stomatitis, early satiety, anorexia, and decreased taste. Her serum albumin is 2.7 g/100 mL and she has recent unintentional weight loss.	*Imbalanced nutrition: less than body requirements* related to stomatitis, early satiety, anorexia, and decreased taste
An 81-year-old client with Parkinson's disease is drooling and pocketing food. Recently he has lost 5 pounds unintentionally. His lungs are clear, and he is ambulatory and alert.	*Impaired swallowing* related to muscle rigidity

PLANNING

Devise a plan for the client to use during the hospital or clinic stay, but also begin discharge planning for the client upon admission. Set general goals with the client, as well as specific outcome criteria that are objective and measurable. For example, "weight gain of 3 pounds" is objective and easy to measure, whereas "client appears better" is subjective and difficult to measure.

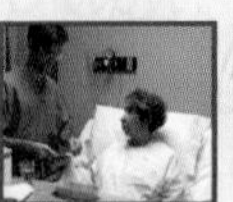

The clinic nurse sets goals with Mrs. Goldman and her daughter to prevent further nutritional deterioration and to gain 2 pounds per month. The nurse assesses Mrs. Goldman's food preferences and notes that she maintains a kosher diet. What foods would you recommend including in Mrs. Goldman's diet? How would you encourage her to monitor her progress toward her nutritional goals?

EXPECTED OUTCOMES FOR THE CLIENT WITH *IMBALANCED NUTRITION: LESS THAN BODY REQUIREMENTS*

Goals for *Imbalanced nutrition: less than body requirements* focus on an improved nutritional state; weight gain is a typical outcome criterion. Generally, if a client gains 2 to 4 pounds a month, the plan is considered successful; however, this rate is individualized to each client. For some clients, such as those with eating disorders, the initial plan may be simply to avoid further weight loss. A maximum of 1.5 kg per week weight gain can be expected from intensive parenteral nutrition. Rapid weight gain is an indicator of fluid retention rather than an increase in lean body mass.

Action Alert! Check daily weights, and report a weight gain of more than 1 pound per day.

Laboratory test results may also be used to determine the plan's success. Prealbumin or transferrin levels are good short-term indicators. Albumin levels take about 3 weeks to reflect results of refeeding.

If pretreatment physical assessment findings are consistent with nutritional deficiency, then cite improvement in these as outcome criteria. For example, outcome criteria could include that a wound begins to heal, edema resolves, or petechiae disappear.

EXPECTED OUTCOMES FOR THE CLIENT WITH *IMPAIRED SWALLOWING*

The client should maintain a stable weight, show no signs of dehydration, and report no difficulty swallowing. Outcome criteria indicating normal hydration are the following:

- Good skin turgor (no tenting)
- Normal vital signs (no hypotension, tachycardia, or fever)
- Skin and mucous membranes moist, not dry
- Denies thirst
- Normal hematocrit (not elevated)

EXPECTED OUTCOMES FOR THE CLIENT WITH *RISK FOR ASPIRATION*

The client should not experience actual aspiration. The client should also be able to identify and avoid risk factors for aspiration. Examples include positioning self upright before eating and drinking, selecting foods according to swallowing ability, and thickening liquids to appropriate consistency.

INTERVENTION

Interventions for nutritional problems in any setting require a team approach. Hospital standards require performance-based interdisciplinary delivery of nutritional support, so you can expect to obtain assistance from nutritional support teams in these institutions. Nurses working in home health care agencies may initiate referrals to a dietitian as appropriate. See Figure 25-3 for general guidelines for selecting nutritional interventions.

INTERVENTIONS TO INCREASE NUTRIENT INTAKE

Make sure that the client is comfortable during meals. Clients who are fatigued, immobilized, or paralyzed will need assistance. Until they can eat independently, feed them and teach the family or caregiver about feeding (Figure 25-4). Tell a client who is blind the location of food on a plate in relation to a clock face (e.g., mashed potatoes at 6 o'clock). Consider food preferences, and serve food in an attractive manner to improve intake. Young children generally like their food less spicy, whereas older adults (with diminished taste) prefer food that is seasoned. Fresh herbs are a good choice. Assess an older client's ability to chew, and grind or puree the food as needed if the teeth are in poor condition.

Often, an evaluation team will recommend treatment for complex feeding problems. The team works to improve the client's hand-to-mouth coordination, vision, or ability to suck, chew, swallow, or grasp. Special feeding equipment may be used, including weighted utensils, two-handed cups, and unbreakable dishes with suction cups. Battery-powered machines are also available.

Enriching the Insufficient Diet. The diet should be the primary source of good nutrition, but sometimes it is insufficient. Pregnant women need extra folic acid, calcium, and iron. Clients with osteoporosis need extra calcium and magnesium, and many chronically ill clients require multiple vitamin or mineral supplements (Mahan & Escott-Stump, 2004).

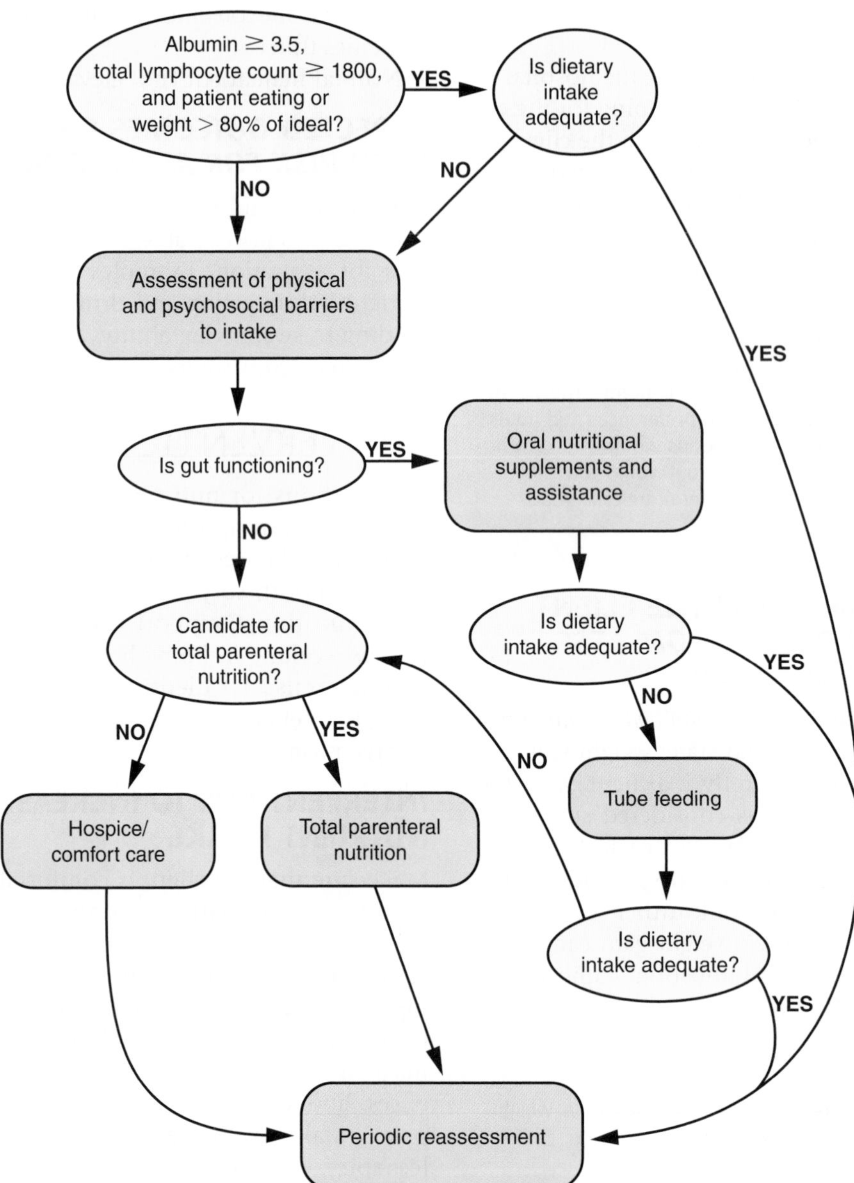

FIGURE 25-3 Decision tree for nutritional assessment and support.

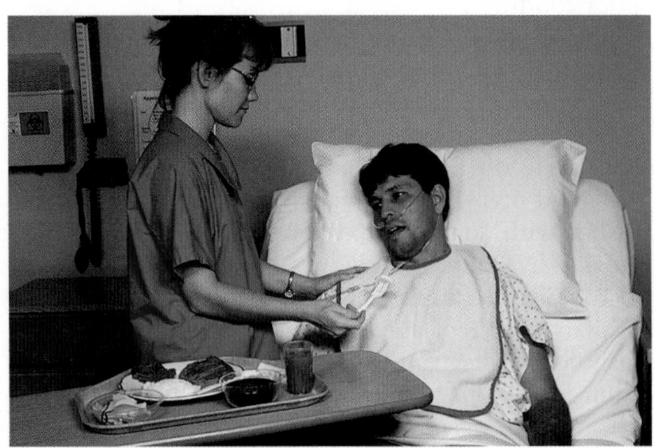

FIGURE 25-4 Until clients can eat independently, feed them, and teach the family or caregiver about feeding.

Some clients cannot eat enough at mealtime and begin to lose weight. To remedy this, give supplemental feedings to increase calories and nutrients. The extra food should be nutritious and something the client enjoys. Generally, six small meals are preferable to three larger ones.

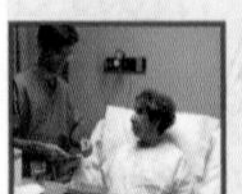

Encourage Mrs. Goldman to eat small, supplemental meals. Which types of food would you consider offering her?

Liquid foods are less filling and easier for debilitated people to handle. Milkshakes, puddings, and instant breakfast drinks are nutritious. Adding powdered milk, yogurt, or tofu to foods provides extra protein. Adding sugar or corn syrup provides calories, but be aware that sweet additives increase the solution's osmolality and thus increase the risk of GI distress. Commercial supplements can add protein, fat, carbohydrate, and calories.

Managing Therapeutic Diets. In the hospital setting, the physician prescribes the diet. The diet may meet therapeutic needs or be based on the client's ability to tolerate food.

Hospitalized clients may be on *NPO* (*nil per os*, meaning nothing by mouth) status to prevent complications from diagnostic tests, surgery, trauma, or acute illness. Intravenous fluids are prescribed, often with 5% dextrose, to prevent dehydration but do not provide nutrition because 1000 mL (1 L) of a 5% dextrose solution yields only *170 kcal*. This amount is thought to prevent catabolism. Most healthy people can tolerate a few days of NPO status but should receive enteral nutrition if the need persists longer than 5 days; infants and children should receive it even sooner.

When a diet order is resumed, clients are often started on a *clear liquid diet*, which is a temporary diet that generally consists of any fluid that you can see through. These liquids are thin and have no pulp. Check hospital policy because there may be different guidelines as to what constitutes a clear liquid. This diet provides about 400 to 500 kcal, 5 to 10 g of protein, 100 to 120 g of carbohydrate, no fat, and very few vitamins and minerals. Do not give red clear liquids to a client soon after surgery in the head or neck area, such as tonsillectomy, to avoid confusing residual liquid with bloody drainage from the surgical site.

The client may then progress to a *full liquid diet*, which contains as much as 1500 calories and has more nutrients than a clear liquid diet. Although mainly used briefly as a transitional diet, with careful planning and the addition of fiber, it could be used indefinitely.

A *soft diet* is sometimes used as a transition to a general diet or for clients who have difficulty eating. This diet is low in fiber and is devoid of bran, grains, strong vegetables (such as cabbage), and raw fruits or vegetables. However, institutions sometimes differ in their definition of a soft diet, and the trend is to define it more liberally, allowing more whole-grain products, cereals, and vegetables. See Box 25-2 for an overview of commonly ordered therapeutic diets.

Anorexia. A client with anorexia benefits from smaller, more frequent meals that include nutritious foods that the client enjoys. Keep the environment clean and odor-free to enhance intake. A client with anorexia nervosa needs psychological treatment and medical nutrition therapy using the services of a dietitian with experience in treating this disorder.

Nausea and Vomiting. When nausea and vomiting occur secondary to infection (such as flu), withhold food until nausea and vomiting subside. Encourage sips of fluids (totaling 2 to 4 ounces per hour) to prevent dehydration. When nausea occurs as a drug side effect, encourage the client to drink liquids between meals or to drink only small amounts with meals. Cold, carbonated, and clear liquids are easier to tolerate than others.

Lactose Intolerance. Dietary interventions for lactose intolerance consist of eliminating lactose-containing foods, such as dairy products or prepared foods that have lactose.

Action Alert! Teach lactose-intolerant clients to read food labels for hidden sources of lactose.

Because the degree of lactose intolerance varies from person to person, small amounts (up to 5 to 8 g, or 1 to 2 cups of milk per day) might be gradually added back to the diet. Lactose is better tolerated when consumed with other foods or beverages, rather than alone. Dietary

BOX 25-2 *Medical Nutrition Therapy: Typical Therapeutic Diets*

Clear Liquid
Includes apple juice or other clear juices, ginger ale or other carbonated beverages, gelatin, frozen ice pops, broth, bouillon, coffee or tea (without added milk or cream)

Full Liquid
Includes all clear liquids plus milk and milk shakes, all fruit and vegetable juices, refined cooked cereals or gruels, ice cream, custards, puddings, and eggnog

Regular
Consists of a typical balanced diet

Low Cholesterol
Reduces total cholesterol intake to less than 300 mg/day; uses fish, poultry that has skin removed, and lean meats; uses reduced-fat dairy products; limits eggs, fats and oils; and increases intake of fruits, vegetables, and dietary fiber

Low Sodium
Varies in degree from 4 g (no added salt) to 2 g, 1 g, or 500 mg daily; uses fresh fruits and vegetables freely, while reducing intake of foods with physiological saline (meats and dairy products) and packaged or processed foods that contain sodium as the restriction becomes more severe

High Fiber
Includes fresh or steamed vegetables, fresh fruits, bran, whole grains, oat bran or oatmeal, nuts and seeds, and dried beans or legumes

Low Residue
Includes low-fiber foods such as pastas and other refined carbohydrates, canned fruits and vegetables, and casseroles; prohibits or limits foods found in a high-fiber diet

Mechanical Soft
Includes meats that are finely cut or diced and foods that are already soft or easy to chew, such as cooked or canned vegetables or fruits, soft cheeses, rice, breads, and soups

Pureed
Includes full liquids plus mashed potatoes, scrambled eggs, sauces and gravies, and blenderized meats, vegetables, or fruits

supplements such as Lactaid, Lactrase, or Dairy Ease may be taken before eating or added to milk 24 hours before use. Restriction of lactose-containing foods may place clients at risk for calcium, vitamin D, and riboflavin deficiency, so mineral and vitamin supplementation is needed unless lactase-treated milk products are used.

Malabsorption. Dietary interventions for malabsorption syndromes depend on the specific disorder. In celiac disease (gluten-sensitive enteropathy), damage to the intestine is caused by *gliadin,* a protein fraction of gluten. Thus foods that contain gluten, such as wheat, oats, rye, and barley, must be restricted, whereas rice and corn are allowed. Dietary interventions for ulcerative colitis (an inflammatory bowel disease, or IBD) include reducing dietary fiber, such as seeds, nuts, and dried beans (low-residue diet). Dietary interventions for Crohn's disease, another IBD, vary according to its severity and may include reducing fiber intake, limiting fat and lactose-containing foods, increasing protein intake, giving vitamin and mineral supplements, and providing bowel rest using enteral feeding with elemental formulas or total parenteral nutrition (see sections that follow).

Diabetes Mellitus. Clients with diabetes should eat a well-balanced, carbohydrate- and calorie-controlled diet, and avoid concentrated sweets. A dietitian develops the dietary prescription based on a physician's order. With the development of newer rapid-acting insulins, medication therapy can be planned to accommodate the client's dietary needs, rather than the reverse. The newest recommendations by the American Diabetes Association (2004) focus on planning for a consistent carbohydrate intake for each meal (e.g., all breakfasts) but it does not need to be identical across meals in a single day (e.g., breakfast, lunch, and supper). This approach broadens the dietary focus beyond just restricting calories and sugars. It is still important for the client to avoid skipping meals or planned snacks.

Action Alert! Urge clients with diabetes, especially type 1, to immediately report any illness that prevents them from eating.

AIDS and Cancer. Clients with AIDS or cancer may have cachexia (a syndrome of anorexia, anemia, fatigue, and muscle wasting). They also may have a decreased sense of taste (which may respond to zinc supplements). These clients tend to eat better in the morning and tolerate smaller, more frequent feedings during the day. Serve foods cool or at room temperature, and avoid serving foods with strong odors.

Encourage foods that contain protein, especially milk shakes, poultry, and eggs, but remember that clients may have an aversion to red meats. Immunosuppression may lead to a sore mouth and throat, as well as to xerostomia—mouth dryness caused by insufficient saliva. Encourage fluids, limit spicy or acidic foods, and emphasize good oral hygiene.

Heart Disease. Clients with heart disease require a diet low in saturated fat, cholesterol, and salt. Foods to be avoided include butter, whole milk, eggs, red meat, and cheese. Skim milk, poultry, fish, and fresh fruits and vegetables are encouraged, along with foods high in soluble fiber, such as apples, citrus fruits, oats, and barley. This diet also promotes weight loss and may help reduce obesity and overweight status in many adult clients.

A 2-g sodium diet (moderate restriction) is common for clients with hypertension. Teach clients on this diet not to add salt while cooking or at the table and to avoid foods high in sodium, such as canned, prepared, and processed foods. Encourage hypertensive clients to increase the amount of calcium and potassium in their diet.

Kidney Disease. Therapeutic dietary management of kidney disease depends on the type and stage of disease. Protein is generally restricted as the disease advances. Fluid, sodium, potassium, and phosphorus are restricted because the kidneys cannot maintain adequate fluid and electrolyte balance. Vitamin D and calcium levels may be low, causing fractures and bone softening. Administer vitamin D and calcium supplements as ordered. With less erythropoietin to stimulate production of red blood cells, iron supplements and possibly the drug epoetin (Epogen) are needed to treat anemia.

Liver Disease. Protein intake in liver disease should be normal to maintain nitrogen balance; however, with impending liver failure, protein is restricted. When the liver fails, ammonia (a by-product of protein metabolism) is not converted to urea, and serum ammonia levels rise to toxic levels, causing encephalopathy. The diet should provide adequate kilocalories and carbohydrates, as well as vitamins normally stored in the liver (especially vitamins K and B_{12}, thiamine, pyridoxine, folate, and niacin). Sodium and fluid may be restricted because the liver no longer breaks down aldosterone.

Providing Enteral Feedings. When a client cannot eat sufficient nutrients to sustain life and health, enteral feedings may be initiated. Although **enteral nutrition** can refer to any form of nutrition delivered to the GI tract (orally or by tube), it is generally used to mean tube feedings. Feeding a client through a tube inserted into the GI tract can help to keep it functioning normally. Table 25-4 identifies clinical situations in which such artificial nutrition may be necessary. See Box 25-3 for current evidence-based practice guidelines for both enteral and parenteral nutrition.

Feeding Tubes and Routes of Access. A feeding tube may be inserted through the nose and placed into the stomach, duodenum, or jejunum. These are known as nasogastric, nasoduodenal, or nasojejunal tubes, respectively. The tube can also be inserted surgically into the esophagus, stomach, or jejunum. These are known as esophagostomy, gastrostomy, and jejunostomy tubes, respectively (Figure 25-5, *A*). When endoscopy is used to insert the tube, it is referred to as a percutaneous endoscopic gastrostomy (PEG) or percutaneous endoscopic jejunostomy (PEJ) tube (Figure 25-5, *B*). PEG and PEJ often use low-profile tubes because they are comfortable underneath clothing. Figure 25-6 provides some examples of low-profile gastrostomy tubes.

The choice of enteral nutrition support depends on the client's status, anticipated length of use, the cost, and availability of a person experienced in placing the feeding tube, as diagrammed in Figure 25-7. The gastric site is preferred to the jejunal site because the stomach has a larger reservoir. However, the jejunal site may be used if the client has significant esophageal reflux, a history or risk of aspiration, or a dysfunctional stomach from gastric surgery or gastritis. Also, function returns to the small intestine faster than to the stomach after stress or trauma.

Endoscopic feeding tube placement is less invasive and less expensive than surgical placement. Surgical placement is done under general or local anesthesia using a laparoscopy or open laparotomy.

Tube feedings are usually initiated with a nasogastric tube. A pliable, small-bore tube is used because it causes less discomfort and less interference with the lower esophageal sphincter than a large-bore tube. To place a feeding tube, follow the relevant procedure in Chapter 26, with the modifications shown in Box 25-4.

The definitive way to make sure a tube has reached the stomach is by radiography. To date, the most reliable nurse-initiated indicator of tube placement is checking the pH of fluid withdrawn through the tube. If the pH is less than 5.0, the tube is most likely in the stomach, unless the client is taking acid-inhibiting medications (pH often 4.0 to 6.0). With duodenal tube placement, you should note a change of drainage color from green to golden and the pH is generally greater than 6.0 (Metheny et al., 2005). To measure pH, flush the tube with 30 mL of air to clear enteral feedings, medications, or other flushes. A sample of 5 to 10 mL is usually sufficient. Flush the tube afterward with 30 mL water to prevent clogging (Edwards and

Table 25-4 Clinical Situations in Which Artificial Nutrition May Be Necessary

SITUATION	POSSIBLE CAUSE
Inability to ingest food	• Cancer of the mouth, tongue, esophagus • Facial trauma • Unconsciousness • Severe stomatitis • Impaired swallowing • Muscle weakness in mouth or esophagus
Inability to digest or absorb food	• Pancreatitis • Cancer of the stomach • Crohn's disease or ulcerative colitis • Biliary disease
Inability to meet nutritional needs	• Increased resting energy expenditure from major trauma or surgery, burns, or severe infection • Anorexia nervosa or bulimia nervosa

BOX 25-3 Evidence-Based Practice

Restoring Nutrition: Guidelines for Enteral or Parenteral Nutrition

Problem: Some clients are unable to eat sufficient nutrients to sustain life due to events such as infection or trauma, complications of age-related changes, gastrointestinal inflammation or obstructions, psychological disturbances, anorexia, nausea and vomiting, cultural barriers, inability to eat by mouth due to disease processes, or impaired swallowing.

Evidence

Guidelines were developed for clients for whom enteral or parenteral specialized nutrition support is indicated. A search of electronic databases was the method used to collect and select the evidence. A weighting according to a rating scheme was the method used to assess the quality and strength of the evidence. This was a modified version of the method used by the Agency for Healthcare Research and Quality (AHRQ), U.S. Department of Health and Human Services. Expert consensus was the method used to formulate the recommendations. Both internal and external peer review was the method used for guideline validation.

Application to Practice

These guidelines:

- Serve as tools to help guide policy makers, health care organizations, and insurers
- Assist clinical practitioners who provide specialized nutritional support to clients in all care settings
- Provide recommendations and specific strategies that have been shown to reflect current, evidenced-based, best approach practice of nutritional support
- Considered the safety and efficacy of specialized nutrition support
- Considered the rates of complications
- Considered cost-effectiveness

These were written to revise the 1993 American Society for Parenteral and Enteral Nutrition Clinical Guidelines.

The guidelines can be found at http://www.guideline.gov/summary/summary.aspx?ss=15&doc_id=3630&nbr=2856

Reference

Access for administration of nutrition support. (2002). *JPEN Journal of Parenteral and Enteral Nutrition 26*(1 Suppl.), 33SA-41SA [125 references].

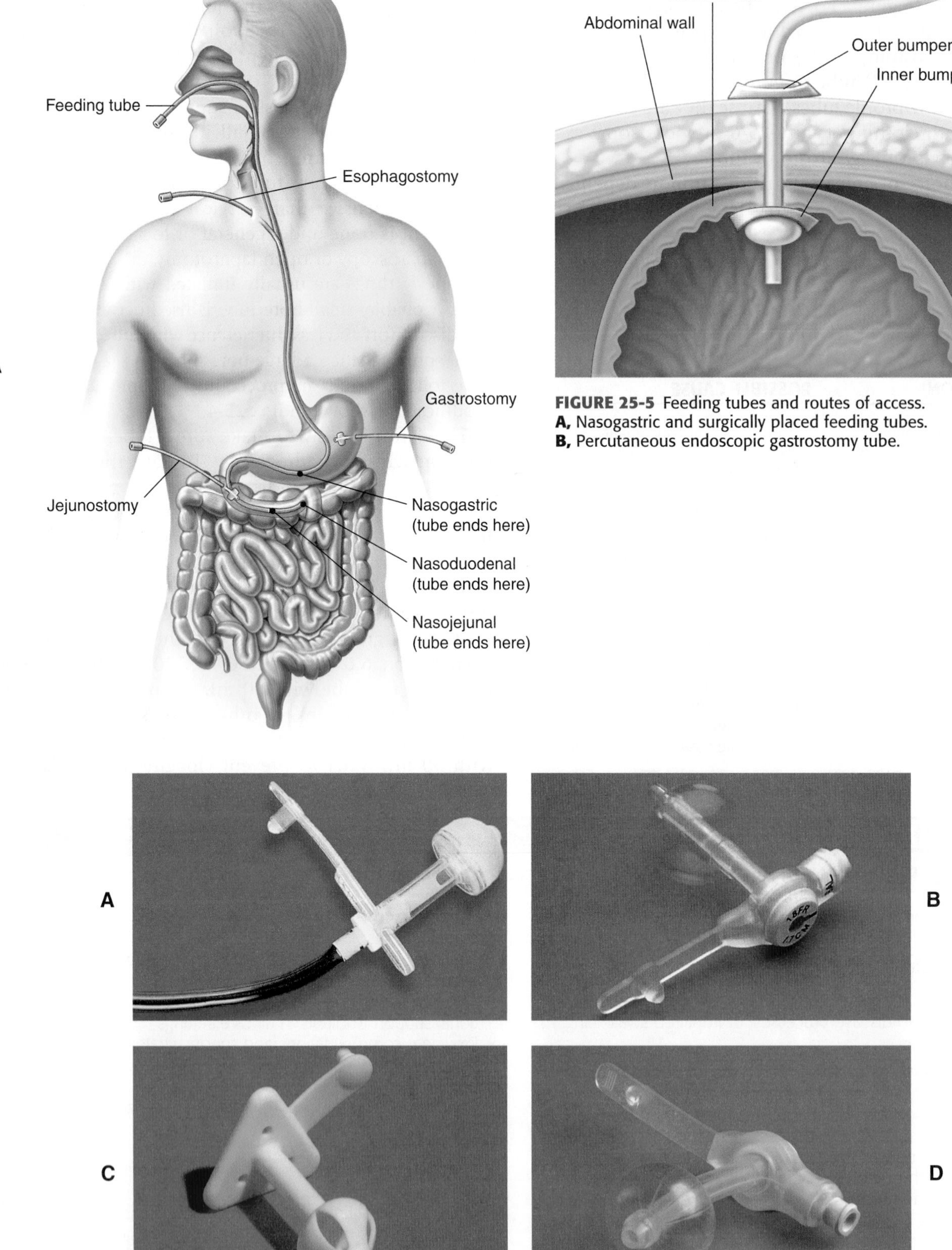

FIGURE 25-5 Feeding tubes and routes of access. **A,** Nasogastric and surgically placed feeding tubes. **B,** Percutaneous endoscopic gastrostomy tube.

FIGURE 25-6 Examples of low-profile gastrostomy tubes. **A,** Bard Button. **B,** Ballard Mic-Key. **C,** Ross Stomate. **D,** Ross Hide-a-Port. (**A** courtesy C. R. Bard, Inc., Billerica, MA; **B** courtesy Ballard Medical Products, Draper, UT; **C** and **D** used with permission of Ross Products Division, Abbott Laboratories, Columbus, OH.)

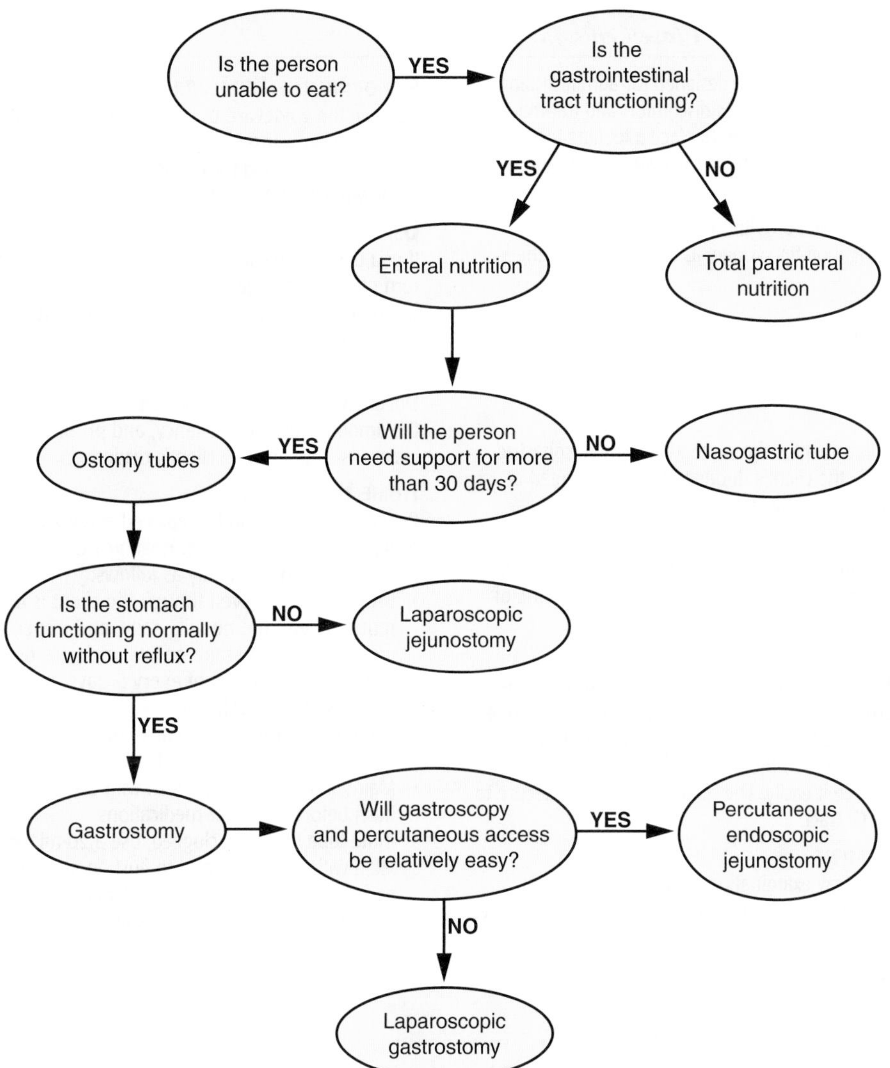

FIGURE 25-7 Decision tree for route of enteral nutrition support. (Modified from Duh, Q. Y. [1996]. Decision tree for route of enteral nutrition support: Placement techniques. *Current issues in enteral nutrition support: Report of the first Ross Conference on Enteral Devices* (pp. 9-16). Columbus, OH: Ross Products Division, Abbott Laboratories. Used with permission of Ross Products Division, Abbott Laboratories, Columbus, OH. Copyright 1996, Ross Products Division, Abbott Laboratories.)

Metheny, 2000). In the hospital setting, one barrier to using pH to check tube placement might be agency policy. Because pH testing is considered a point-of-care laboratory test, requiring validation in the skill and annual competency update (similar to blood glucose monitoring), it is more expensive and resource intensive to allow this practice at the bedside.

Although not 100% reliable, a persistent common method for checking tube placement is to insert 10 to 30 mL of air into the tube while listening with a stethoscope over the left upper quadrant for a popping or "swooshing" sound (Box 25-5). Because this sound may be heard when the tube is inadvertently placed in the lungs, it is unreliable as the sole method of determining placement. In summary, radiography is the definitive method of determining tube placement, and nursing research is ongoing in this area.

Action Alert! When placing a feeding tube, be sure that a radiograph is ordered, because it is the definitive method of confirming gastric placement. Determining placement by pH measurement and auscultation does not eliminate the need for an abdominal radiograph.

Types of Enteral Formulas. Enteral formulas are labeled as polymeric, modular, elemental, or specialty. Polymeric formulas can be commercial formulations or can be made by blenderizing regular foods in a milk base. Blenderized formulas should be refrigerated and the bag hung only long enough to be infused. Baby foods could also be used for clients who will receive tube feedings indefinitely. Commercial polymeric feedings are milk based or lactose free and are similar to oral supplements (1 to 2 kcal/mL). They contain whole protein, long-chain fatty acids, and complex carbohydrates

BOX 25-4 *Modifications for Placement of a Feeding Tube*

A feeding tube can be a small-bore tube designed for administration of enteral feedings. This type of tube reduces discomfort and trauma and can thus be safely used for a longer time. To place a feeding tube, follow Procedure 26-1 (next chapter), with the following modifications.

EQUIPMENT

- No. 6-10 Fr feeding tube with or without guidewire
- 60-mL Luer-Lok or irrigation-tip syringe, as indicated, to fit the specific tube
- Cup of tap water
- Water-soluble lubricant
- pH strips
- Clean gloves

MEASURING

Measuring for gastric placement is the same as for any nasogastric tube. To place the tube in the client's duodenum, you will need at least 75 cm of tube to reach the ligament of Treitz.

LUBRICATION

Use water-soluble lubricant, or moisten the surface with water. For some tubes, follow the manufacturer's directions to insert 10 mL of water into tube with a syringe to activate the lubricant.

USING A GUIDEWIRE

A guidewire is provided with small-bore feeding tubes to make the tube rigid during insertion. After you become experienced with tube placement, you may be able to place a tube without a guidewire. If you use a guidewire, insert it into the tube, make sure it fits, and make sure you can remove it easily. The guidewire must be secure to prevent damage to the GI tract.

CHECKING FOR PLACEMENT

Check for placement by x-ray examination with the guidewire in place. Thereafter, check for placement by determining pH of aspirate, bilirubin content, and using air instillation.

REMOVING THE GUIDEWIRE

Remove the guidewire only after the placement of the tube is confirmed. Never reinsert a guidewire after removing it unless the tube is specifically designed for reinsertion of the guidewire. Reinserting a guidewire could puncture the tube and injure the client.

USING A TOPICAL ANESTHETIC

If you used a topical anesthetic on the client's throat, test for the return of the client's gag reflex with a tongue blade when finished. The use of a topical anesthetic may be contraindicated when a client has dysphagia.

DOCUMENTATION

Document the time you inserted the tube; the type of tube inserted; the amount, color, consistency, and pH of secretions; the amount of water instilled; and the client's response.

HOME HEALTH CARE

Pediatric tubes should be replaced every 2 to 6 weeks and adult tubes every 6 weeks to 3 months. Health care agencies establish differing protocols. Teach the family as follows:

- Brush the teeth even though the client is taking nothing by mouth. Clean the nostrils daily, and inspect for irritation or incrustations. The tape or fixator device on the nose should be changed a minimum of every 5 days. Inspect for any allergic response to the adhesive.
- Some clients can take small amounts of soft foods and swallow around the tube. The tube feeding supplements the diet.
- Maintain tube patency. Flush with water at regular intervals. Always flush before and after medications.
- If the tube becomes clogged, use a 20-mL or larger syringe half filled with water. Attempt to flush in and out. Flushing with a clear carbonated beverage instead of water may help unclog the tube. Use caution because it is possible to exert enough pressure to puncture the tube.

and require an intact intestine for digestion. Modular formulas (3.8 to 4 kcal/mL) are single macronutrient preparations containing protein, glucose, lipids, or polymers that are added to other foods as supplements; these formulations are nutritionally incomplete by themselves. Elemental or hydrolyzed formulas (1 to 3 kcal/mL) contain short-chain peptides or amino acids for easy digestion, as well as short-chain fatty acids and simple carbohydrates. These formulas are partially digested and are used for clients with abnormal bowel function. Specialty formulas (1 to 2 kcal/mL), such as Pulmocare or Hepatic-Aid, are designed for use in clients with specific diseases.

Their components can vary, but enteral formulas usually provide recommended amounts of vitamins and minerals. Many formulas now have fiber added to maintain normal GI function. The osmolarity of the formula also varies. Hyperosmolar (e.g., hydrolyzed) formulas pull water into the GI tract and can cause diarrhea. Standard formulas provide only 80% to 85% of the client's water needs, so tube-fed clients who do not have another source of fluid require additional water to meet their physiological needs.

Administration of Enteral Feedings. Initiate tube feedings slowly, especially if the client has not eaten for a period of time. Monitor for decline in serum phosphorus level as an indicator of refeeding syndrome after the metabolism begins to rise. The administration of feedings through various types of tubes at different time intervals is described in Procedure 25-1. Continuous feedings are given over 24 hours. Intermittent feedings deliver no more than 250 mL of feeding over 30 minutes periodically during the day. Bolus feedings of up to 400 mL of formula are given by the nurse or client over approximately 10 to 15 minutes. Because the small intestine tolerates bolus feedings poorly, tube placement in the duodenum or jejunum necessitates continuous feedings.

Disadvantages of bolus or intermittent feedings include diarrhea and increased resting energy expenditure. The diarrhea results from an osmotic effect and is more common in older adults. The resting energy expenditure increases by 5% to 10% daily because of the fluctuation in fuel reserves with periodic feeding; it does not occur with continuous feedings. Disadvantages of continuous feedings include tube clogging and a lower serum protein synthesis. Clogging generally re-

BOX 25-5 *Checking Placement of Feeding Tubes*

1. Always check placement before instilling anything into a nasogastric tube (NGT). The purpose of confirming the placement of the NGT after inserting is to prevent the high-risk complications that can occur from inadvertent entry into the lungs or from perforation of the esophagus. Airway cannulation may occur in as much as 25% to 30% of clients.
2. Use more than one method of checking placement. No nonradiological method is 100% reliable.
3. Problems exist with all methods of checking placement:

   Air injection and auscultation: Inability to distinguish sound coming from the lungs, esophagus, or intestine; may only be accurate 30% to 40% of the time. Very-small-bore tubes are easily regurgitated into the esophagus and may be coiled there or enter the lungs. Assess the oropharynx for the presence of coiled tubing.

   Aspiration of gastric fluid and testing pH: The most reliable method. Normal pH is from 1 to 4, it is higher if in the small intestine and even higher if in the lungs. However, pH can be altered by last intake of fluids, feeding. formulas (feeding would need to be stopped for 1 hour to insure accuracy), H_2 receptor blockers, other antacids, and illnesses such as human immunodeficiency virus (HIV), pernicious anemia, and gastroesophageal reflux disease (GERD). Quality control must be maintained on the procedure for measuring pH. Different guidelines are necessary for neonates.

   Observing for choking, coughing, dysphagia, and the ability to speak: If a gastric tube enters the lungs, the client will generally cough and cannot speak. However, this does not help if the client is unconscious.

   Aspiration and visual assessment of the aspirate: Normal gastric aspirate color is clear to slightly yellow. If client has gastrointestinal (GI) bleeding or obstruction, there will naturally be different colors.

TIPS

1. When placing a tube, document the length of the tube inserted or note the external length of tube. Check for migration or displacement of the tube before putting anything down a tube.
2. A pH of 5 or less suggests that the tip of the tube is in a gastric location.
3. The pH of aspirate should be checked just before medication or feeding administration to maximize the predictive power.
4. Gastric juices are clear, grassy green, light yellow to tan, or brown if blood is present. Respiratory secretions may look the same. Intestinal juices are bile colored, dark yellow or amber, or greenish-brown in color.
5. Check external markings and external tube length to determine if the tube seems to have moved since initial placement if previously documented to be in proper position by pH and/or radiograph.
6. For intestinal feeding tubes, injection of 10 mL of air should be well tolerated and difficult to aspirate back out. If able to aspirate more than 2 mL of air, the tip may be in the stomach.
7. If a child is receiving continuous feedings and tolerating them well and other cues (above) suggest proper placement, the tip is likely in correct position, and feedings can continue.
8. If pH results and/or additional cues do not suggest proper position, tubes whose placement has not been confirmed by radiography should be replaced (unless contraindicated). Repeat verification process.
9. If uncertain of proper placement, consult physician about getting radiographic confirmation before using the tube.
10. For an intestinal tube, a sudden drop in pH to 5 or less or increase in vomiting when feedings have been previously well tolerated may indicate the tube has likely migrated into the stomach even if the external length is unchanged.
11. Children and adults who are comatose or semicomatose, have swallowing dysfunction, or have vomiting are at higher risk for placement error or migration of the tube.
12. Residual volume from a jejunal tube should be less than 10 mL. A sudden increase in residual volume to 50 mL or more may mean the tube has moved up to the stomach.
13. To facilitate aspiration through a small-bore tube, inject 30 mL of air into the tube via a 60-mL syringe immediately before aspirating.
14. To prevent clogging of the tube after checking for residual volume, flush the tube with 30 mL of water (or normal saline, if indicated for clients with hyponatremia).

sults from a slow feeding rate through a small-bore tube. Decreased protein synthesis occurs because continuous feedings increase insulin and glycogen levels, favoring the use of protein for fuel rather than tissue storage. Bolus and intermittent feeding methods are more natural and allow greater client mobility. Seriously ill clients are often fed continuously, with a goal of intermittent or bolus feedings.

Regardless of the method used, always ensure correct tube placement and the presence of bowel sounds before giving a feeding. Raise the head of the bed as much as the client can tolerate, and keep it elevated for 30 minutes after a bolus or intermittent feeding.

When administering enteral feedings using a feeding bag, perform good hand hygiene to prevent bacterial contamination. Change the bag and tubing as indicated by agency policy, usually every 24 hours. Identify on the bag the date and time it was hung.

Complications of Enteral Feedings. Monitor any client receiving tube feedings to prevent or minimize complications (Box 25-6). As discussed previously, the most serious complication is aspiration. To minimize it, follow the procedures described for confirming tube placement. Check gastric residual volume (GRV) before giving a feeding, or every 4 hours with continuous feedings. There is no consensus in the literature about when to withhold feedings (Zaloga, 2005), but this should be done if the GRV is greater than 400 mL. Assess this client also for sensations of fullness or nausea and vomiting, abdominal distention, and reduction or absence of bowel sounds. Volumes between 200 mL and 400 mL indicate the need for bedside assessment and analysis of trends. Obtain specific parameters from the physician, and follow agency policy. In general, volumes less than 400 mL should be returned to the client to prevent fluid and electrolyte imbalance, but this may also vary. Assess

TIME TO ALLOW: NOVICE: 15-25 min. EXPERT: 10-15 min.

PROCEDURE 25-1

ADMINISTERING AN ENTERAL FEEDING

Nursing Skills Online: Enteral Nutrition, Lesson 4

Enteral feedings can be administered into the stomach, duodenum, or jejunum through a tube inserted in the client's nose or inserted via the abdominal wall (gastrostomy or jejunostomy tubes). These feedings are administered on a time schedule specified in the physician's order to provide nutrition to a client who cannot eat or swallow. Complications include aspiration, tube blockage, nausea and vomiting, diarrhea, hyperglycemia, and tube dislodgment.

DELEGATION GUIDELINES

Client assessment and the administration of enteral nutrition via gastric, duodenal, or jejunal tube require the expertise of a licensed nurse. You may delegate to a nursing assistant with special training the gathering and assembly of necessary equipment and preparation of the tube feeding formula. You are then responsible for initiating the enteral infusion and evaluating the client's response. Institutions vary in their approach to the nursing assistant's role in delivering enteral nutrition; some allow nursing assistants to deliver tube feeding via the bolus method only. Be sure to follow your institution's policies and procedures regarding delegation of this task.

EQUIPMENT NEEDED

- 60-mL syringe
- Cup of water
- Stethoscope
- Clean gloves
- Feeding pump and IV pole if feeding will be continuous
- pH tape
- Prescribed formula
- Adapter for gastrostomy or jejunostomy tube, if needed
- 4 × 4 inch gauze pads (possibly precut), nonallergenic tape, and soap to clean and dress a gastrostomy or jejunostomy tube site

1 Perform preliminary actions (see inside front cover).

2 Make sure the client is comfortable and has privacy. Raise the head of bed to 30 to 45 degrees. *These steps help the procedure go smoothly and reduce the risk of aspiration.*

3 Assess the client.

a. Listen to bowel sounds.

b. Observe for abdominal distention or distress. *Distention and absence of bowel sounds may indicate paralytic ileus.*

c. Inquire about diarrhea, or check with other assigned caregivers if client is nonverbal. *Diarrhea is not always a reaction to the tube feeding; always assess for the cause. If you detect any of these problems, report them and confirm that you should still give the feeding.*

4 Prepare for the feeding.

a. Make sure the formula is at room temperature and within its expiration date. Also check manufacturer's information because some formulas are stable for only a limited time after opening (such as 4 to 8 hours). *Cold formula can cause cramping. Formula left open too long may promote growth of microbes.*

b. Confirm placement, and check for residual volume. With the tube clamped, insert a syringe into the end of the tube, unclamp the tube, and aspirate residual fluid from the client's stomach. For a small-bore tube, use a 10-mL syringe. For a large-bore tube, use a 60-mL syringe. Return the gastric aspirate to the stomach. *If the residual exceeds an amount identified by the physician, withhold the feeding for a prescribed time as ordered. Remember that a jejunostomy tube typically has the smallest residual volume.*

c. Test the pH of the gastric fluid.

5 Flush with water. Remove the plunger from the irrigating syringe, and insert the barrel into the end of the tube. The barrel is then used as a funnel to pour the water through. For small-bore tubes, the water is injected slowly with a syringe. *Flushing with water helps keep the tube patent and prevents stomach acid from clumping the formula.*

6 To give a bolus feeding with a syringe, follow these steps:

a. Using the barrel of the syringe as a funnel, add formula until it nearly fills the syringe. *Feedings flow by gravity and may take up to 15 minutes.*

b. When the syringe is almost empty, refill it with formula until the total amount has been instilled. By refilling the syringe before it empties, you avoid instilling air into the tube. Do not force feedings by using the plunger, because the client will be at increased risk for aspiration, diarrhea, and bloating.

c. Instill 50 mL water after the feeding is complete (or other amount as ordered by physician). *Instilling water helps to avoid clogging in the tube.*

d. Clamp the tube.

e. Remove the syringe, wash it with tap water, and store it for future use.

f. Cover the end of the tube with clean gauze.

7 To give an intermittent feeding with a bag and tubing, follow these steps:

a. After instilling water into the tube in Step 5, clamp the tube and attach the feeding tube.
b. Fill the feeding bag with the prescribed amount of formula, and prime the tubing.
c. Hang the feeding bag on an IV stand.
d. Unclamp the feeding tube.
e. Regulate the flow so the formula is instilled over 20 minutes.
f. When formula has finished flowing, clamp the tube and remove the feeding bag. Instill 50 mL water into the feeding tube.
g. Wash out the feeding bag with tap water, and store it for future use. Hints: Change the bag and tubing every 24 hours, or according to agency policy, to avoid bacterial contamination. Fresh formula should be hung after 4 to 8 hours. Consult agency policy.
h. When hanging a new feeding bag, label it with the time, the date, and your initials.

8 To give a continuous feeding, follow steps 1 through 7 but use an infusion pump (see illustration) to regulate the flow of formula. *The infusion pump ensures a regular rate.*

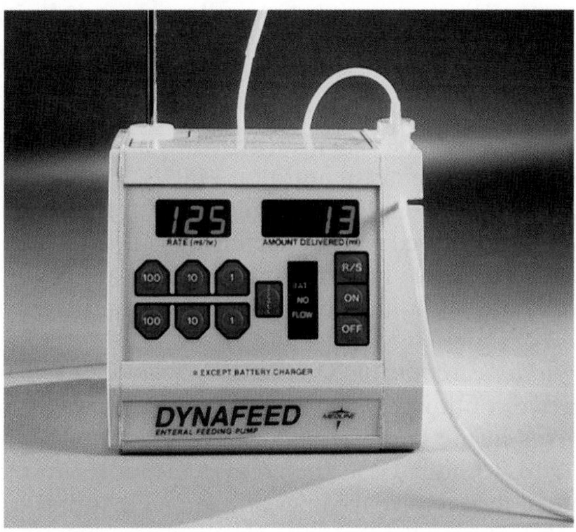

Step 8. Feeding infusion pump. (Courtesy Medline Industries, Mundelein, IL.)

a. Thread the tubing from the feeding bag through the infusion pump. *Read manufacturer's pump instructions because they vary.*
b. Set the infusion pump at the prescribed rate.

9 Before giving a medication through a nasogastric tube, make sure it is available in liquid form or can be finely crushed. *Medication that is not crushed finely enough could clog the tube.*

10 If necessary, clean and dress the entrance site of a gastrostomy or jejunostomy tube. Most clients do not require a dressing over the site. If leaking gastric acid is a problem, a hydrocolloid dressing will protect the skin.

a. Use clean technique to clean the entrance site unless the client is in the immediate postoperative period. Use soap and water to remove all leakage of gastric contents and crusty drainage. Dry the area well. *Using careful cleaning technique and teaching the client thoroughly about cleaning these long-term feeding tubes can help avoid problems and the need for surgical replacement.*
b. Observe for and report any unusual drainage (thick, green, yellow, or foul-smelling), redness, puffiness, or pain at the site.
c. To dress the site, use a precut 4 × 4 inch gauze pad, or make a cut to the middle of a pad. Place the pad around the tube so the tube protrudes from the middle of the pad, and use nonallergenic tape to affix the pad in place.

11 Monitor the client.

a. Make sure the tube is taped securely to the client's nose and pinned safely to the gown when you finish with the feeding.
b. Assess the client for gastric distress, distention, cramping, and diarrhea.

12 Tidy the client's environment, and discard any used materials. Discard your gloves, and perform hand hygiene.

13 Document the amount and type of feeding delivered on an intake and output sheet, the time of the feeding, your assessment findings, residual gastric contents and its pH, and the client's daily weight.

PEDIATRIC CONSIDERATIONS

Provide age-appropriate explanations to the client. Carefully monitor the effectiveness of feedings to promote normal growth and development.

GERIATRIC CONSIDERATIONS

Recognize that mealtimes may provide opportunities for socialization, so do not ignore the psychosocial needs of an older adult who is receiving enteral feedings.

HOME HEALTH CARE CONSIDERATIONS

Teach family caregivers to administer feedings. Include feeding technique, cleaning and storing equipment, preventing and managing complications, skin care, and monitoring nutritional status.

BOX 25-6 ***Monitoring Clients Receiving Tube Feedings***

- Measure residual gastric contents every 4 hours. If the amount is greater than half the feeding given in the last 4 hours, stop the feeding, assess the abdomen, and consult the physician.
- Weigh the client daily to detect fluid retention; weekly to detect actual weight gain.
- Assess for signs of edema daily.
- Assess for signs of dehydration daily.
- Obtain fingerstick glucose readings daily.
- Assess intake and output daily.
- Record stool output daily.
- Assess calorie, protein, fat, mineral, and vitamin intake twice weekly.
- Check levels of serum electrolytes, serum phosphorus, blood urea nitrogen, and creatinine and complete blood count two or three times weekly (by physician's order).
- Obtain a chemistry profile weekly (by physician's order).
- Check nitrogen balance weekly (optional).

respiratory status at least every shift, and note any changes. If a blue dye is added to the feedings and respiratory secretions become blue, stop the feeding immediately because aspiration has occurred.

To prevent clogging of a feeding tube, flush it with water before and after giving all feedings and medications. Flush also when adding new formula or at least every 4 hours (even when not in use) to avoid obstruction. Record the volume of the flush on the intake and output record. If the client is on a fluid restriction, consult with the nutrition support team about methods to keep the tube patent. Request an order for liquid formulations of medications to be given by tube, whenever possible. If they are not available in liquid form, dissolve finely crushed pills in warm water, but be aware that even finely crushed medications can clog small-bore nasoenteric tubes. Do not give enteric-coated or extended-release tablets through enteral tubes because crushing them destroys the coating.

If the tube does occlude, various methods can be used to reopen it. Flushing with very warm water is a common method. Pancreatic enzyme or sodium bicarbonate crushed in 5 mL of water may be helpful. Some sources suggest the use of meat tenderizer, cola, or cranberry juice, but others discourage their use, so follow agency policy. The best treatment is prevention with adequate flushing.

Diarrhea can result from hyperosmolar feedings, medications, or bacterial contamination of the feeding. Assess the cause of diarrhea carefully rather than simply stopping the feeding, decreasing the rate, or diluting the formula. Send a stool specimen as ordered, and evaluate all medications, especially laxatives and those containing sorbitol or magnesium.

If the feeding itself is causing the diarrhea, the rate can be lowered, although doing so also lowers calorie intake. Once the problem is resolved, the rate should be gradually increased as tolerated. The formula may also be changed to one that is more elemental or has a lower osmolality. Antidiarrheal medication can be given for symptom management while the cause is treated.

Other complications of enteral nutrition include infection at the ostomy site, nausea and vomiting, hyperglycemia, and tube dislodgment. Continually assess the skin around a gastrostomy or jejunostomy site for infection. If the client is nauseated, stop the feeding and report the finding. Nausea and vomiting can stem from contaminated formula or feeding bag or from completely unrelated factors. Contamination can be reduced by use of closed systems and minimal handling of systems (Williams & Leslie, 2004). Perform fingerstick glucose readings daily to detect hyperglycemia. If the tube becomes dislodged or clogged beyond repair, it must be replaced.

Home Enteral Nutrition. Shortened lengths of hospital stay have increased the provision of enteral nutrition at home. Adequate home health care, professional and family supports, and teaching are needed for this to be effective (Box 25-7). General training for caregivers should include stoma assessment and monitoring of devices.

Parenteral Nutrition. **Parenteral nutrition** provides total nutrition through a central or peripheral intravenous catheter. When a central vein (such as the subclavian) is used, this procedure is known as total parenteral nutrition (TPN), hyperalimentation, or central venous nutrition. Sometimes, parenteral nutrition is given in a smaller peripheral vein in an extremity and is then called peripheral parenteral nutrition (PPN). The peripheral approach is being used more widely for hospitalized clients who need parenteral nutrition for less than 14 days. Parenteral nutrition is indicated for any client who does not have a functional GI tract for an extended period of time.

Administration of Parenteral Nutrition. Most clients receive continuous parenteral nutrition; however, some clients in the home setting receive cyclic feedings on a 12- to 18-hour cycle to increase their quality of life. Often, they receive feedings at night so that they can be mobile during the day.

Initiate parenteral nutrition slowly to avoid the refeeding syndrome, triggered by a drop in serum phosphate levels as phosphorus moves into cells (Hearing, 2004). A suggested regimen is to start the feedings at 42 mL/hr or 1000 mL/day, and then increase slowly over a 2- to 3-day period. Watch for changes in serum glucose, potassium, magnesium, and calcium levels caused by increased cellular metabolism of these nutrients. Assess for both cellular dehydration and signs of heart failure, because the hyperosmolar serum attracts water from cells. Box 25-8 has recommendations for monitoring a client receiving parenteral nutrition.

BOX 25-7 Teaching for Wellness

Home Enteral Nutrition

Purpose: To teach a client or family member to deliver feedings through a gastrostomy tube and to care for the tube properly.

Expected Outcome: The client or a family member will be able to successfully feed the client through a gastrostomy tube and will prevent infection at the entrance site.

Client Instructions

Giving a Feeding

1. If your feeding formula is refrigerated, allow it to come to room temperature before using it, because cold feeding formula can cause cramping.
2. Perform hand hygiene, and put on clean gloves.
3. If your doctor wants you to, check for residual gastric contents before delivering a feeding. To do so, insert a syringe into the tube, unclamp the tube, and use the plunger to remove and measure the volume of gastric secretions. If the amount of residual contents is too great, you may have to withhold the feeding for a while.
4. Measure the prescribed amount of feeding formula.
5. After removing the plunger from a 60-mL syringe, insert the syringe into the end of the tube.
6. Unclamp the tube. If you unclamp the tube before inserting the syringe, gastric contents may leak out.
7. Pour enough of the formula into the syringe to nearly fill the syringe.
8. When the syringe is still about a quarter full, refill it with formula. Refilling before the syringe is empty will prevent air from entering the tube.
9. After instilling all of the formula, flush the syringe and tube with about 60 mL of water.
10. Before removing the syringe from the tube, clamp the tube. Clamping the tube keeps gastric contents from leaking out.
11. Expect this entire process to take about 15 minutes.
12. Wash the syringe after each feeding, and change syringes daily.
13. Store the formula according to the package directions.

Caring for the Gastrostomy Site

1. To clean the area where the tube enters your skin, use a washcloth or a 4 × 4 inch gauze pad. Wet it with warm, soapy water, and clean around the site. Rinse with clear water, and dry thoroughly with a soft towel.
2. Usually, a gastrostomy tube needs no dressing. If your doctor tells you to use one, use a precut 2 × 2 inch gauze pad or use scissors to cut to the middle of the pad. Slide the slit in the pad over the tube so that the tube protrudes from the middle of the pad. Affix the pad in place with nonallergenic tape.
3. Tell your doctor right away if you notice redness, swelling, abnormal drainage (thick, foul smelling, yellow or green), or pain at the tube's entrance site. Also report any abdominal pain, bloating, cramping, or diarrhea.

Procedure 25-2 describes administering parenteral nutrition through a central line. Ongoing site care is especially important because the client is at risk for infection at the site and in the bloodstream (sepsis). Sepsis is a life-threatening complication with a high mortality rate.

Change the client's central catheter dressing at least every 72 hours—more often if facility policy dictates or if the dressing is wet or no longer occlusive. There is controversy about the correct technique for this dressing change, but generally it includes the use of sterile technique (including sterile gloves and masks) in the hospital setting to avoid hospital-acquired infection. In the home, clients can use clean technique when changing their own dressing. Most hospitals use transparent polyurethane dressings. The catheter site is scrubbed with an antiseptic, such as povidone-iodine. Some clinicians use an antiseptic ointment at the site as well, but current recommendations from the Centers for Disease Control and Prevention are not to use such an ointment. If used with a transparent dressing, the amount should be small because the dressings are designed to adhere to the skin and promote visualization of the site.

BOX 25-8 Monitoring a Client Receiving Parenteral Nutrition

To monitor the nutritional status of a client receiving parenteral nutrition, make sure to complete the following steps. You may need to measure some values more frequently than shown here until the client stabilizes.

Growth Variables

- Weigh the client daily.
- Measure an infant's head circumference weekly.
- Measure an infant's length weekly.

Metabolic Variables

- Assess for signs of edema or dehydration daily.
- Obtain fingerstick glucose levels daily or as ordered.
- Assess intake and output daily.
- Assess calorie, fat, protein, carbohydrate, vitamin, and mineral intake twice weekly.
- Check serum sodium, potassium, chloride, CO_2, phosphorus, blood urea nitrogen, creatinine, and triglyceride levels twice weekly.
- Assess complete blood count, prothrombin time, albumin, calcium, magnesium, copper, zinc, and liver function tests weekly.
- Obtain a urinalysis weekly.
- Check nitrogen balance weekly (optional).

TIME TO ALLOW: NOVICE: 20 min. EXPERT: 10 min.

PROCEDURE 25-2 ADMINISTERING PARENTERAL NUTRITION THROUGH A CENTRAL LINE

Parenteral nutrition is administered to provide fluids and balanced nutrition to a client who cannot eat and who cannot receive such nutrition via the GI tract. Total parenteral nutrition is infused into either a central or a peripheral vein according to a physician's order. Major complications are hyperglycemia, infection, and refeeding syndrome. Hypoglycemia can occur if the solution is terminated abruptly. This procedure describes using a central line.

DELEGATION GUIDELINES

The assembly of the necessary equipment to perform this procedure may be delegated to a licensed practical or vocational nurse or nursing assistant. The verification of the solution with the physician's order, preparation of the tubing and catheter, and initiation of the infusion are your responsibility and may not be delegated.

EQUIPMENT NEEDED

- Prescribed infusion
- IV tubing with extension tubing
- 0.22-μm filter (if solution contains lipids or albumin)
- Alcohol sponges
- Infusion pump
- Sterile dressing package
- Labels
- Clean gloves
- Sterile gloves

1 Perform preliminary actions (see inside front cover).

2 Confirm the physician's order, and check it against the listed ingredients. *Parenteral nutrition usually requires special physician orders that are written daily, specifying all ingredients and the rate of infusion.*

3 Check the solution.

a. Remove the solution from the refrigerator at least 1 hour before using it.

b. Observe the solution for cloudiness, turbidity, particles, or cracks in the container.

c. If the solution has a brown layer, return it to the pharmacy, because the lipid emulsion has separated from the solution.

4 Assess the client.

a. Know client's potassium, phosphorus, and glucose values. Glucose and electrolyte values can change dramatically on parenteral nutrition.

b. Look for any signs of inflammation or swelling at the infusion site.

c. Assess the client's frame of mind and, to ease any fears, reassure that the procedure is not painful. *Clients associate eating with positive feelings and may be upset by not being able to eat.*

5 Prepare the tubing in the infusion pump.

a. Connect tubing, extension tubing, and filter. *Place the filter close to the client.*

b. If the tubing does not have Luer-Lok connections, tape all connections. *Accidental separation of IV tubing could cause air embolism or infection.*

c. Prime the tubing, and clamp it.

d. Thread the tubing through the infusion pump.

e. Time and date the IV tubing. *The tubing should be changed every 24 hours or according to your facility's policy.*

6 repare the central line catheter.

a. Flush the catheter, according to your facility's policy, with saline.

b. Put on sterile gloves. *Asepsis at the site* (see illustration) *prevents infection.*

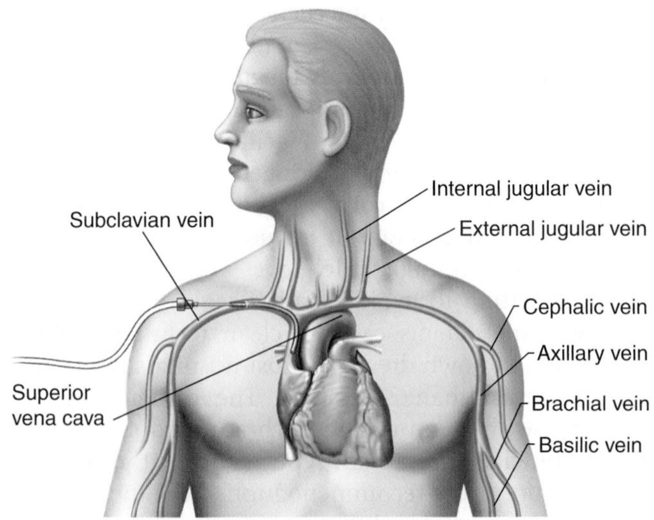

Step 6b. Subclavian infusion site for parenteral nutrition through a central line.

c. Clean the catheter cap with alcohol.
d. Using aseptic technique, insert the needle into the injection cap.
e. Unclamp the tubing.

7 Set the infusion pump at the prescribed rate. Start the flow slowly, and monitor the rate carefully.

8 Do not use a single-lumen central line to infuse blood or draw blood. Also, if possible, avoid giving any IV medication during parenteral nutrition. Before adding a piggyback medication to parenteral nutrition, check with the pharmacist to make sure it is compatible. Never add a medication to a parenteral nutrition solution.

9 Monitor and document the client's vital signs, laboratory values (including electrolytes), vital signs, glucose levels, daily weight, urine output, and catheter site. Use sterile technique for dressing changes. *Continued assessment is essential because extravasation of the solution can cause tissue necrosis.*

10 Document the type of solution used, the time and date the bag was hung, the client's response, and the amount of solution added on the intake and output sheet.

HINT

If for any reason you must remove the gummed rubber cap from the central line, *be absolutely sure* the catheter is clamped or the client is performing the Valsalva maneuver. Otherwise, the negative intrathoracic pressure can draw air into the vein, leading to air embolism in a pulmonary artery.

PEDIATRIC CONSIDERATIONS

Provide age-appropriate explanations to the client. Carefully monitor for fluid and electrolyte imbalance and the effectiveness of therapy in promoting normal growth and development.

GERIATRIC CONSIDERATIONS

Be aware that older adults are at greater risk for fluid imbalance than younger adults. Monitor intake and output carefully as well as monitoring for electrolyte imbalances.

Composition of Parenteral Nutrition. Various combinations of protein, fat emulsions, and carbohydrates are used to meet clients' energy needs. The dextrose concentration of parenteral nutrition given through a central vein can vary from 5% to 70%, but it is usually 25%. The dextrose concentration of PPN is usually limited to 10% to avoid irritation of vessel walls.

Protein is given in ranges from 3% to 15%. Fat emulsions of 10% or 20% are given to avoid fatty acid deficiency. An all-in-one mixture includes lipids, protein, and carbohydrate and helps to reduce solution osmolarity. Nutrition given through a central vein may consist of a carbohydrate and protein solution in one bag and fat emulsion in another. Vitamin and mineral contents are slightly lower than the recommended daily amount because they do not undergo digestive processes. The client's fluid needs are calculated and factored into the solution requirements.

Complications of Parenteral Nutrition. Refeeding syndrome is an important complication of parenteral nutrition. Assess for a drop in serum phosphorus level, which can cause a weakened diaphragm and respiratory failure. Hyperosmolar fluids can cause extracellular fluid overload and pulmonary edema or heart failure. Auscultate the lungs for crackles, and watch the urine output carefully. If the urine output increases significantly, the flow rate may be too fast or erratic. Use an infusion pump to deliver the TPN, and do not try to "catch up" if the infusion has fallen behind.

Obtain fingerstick glucose levels at least daily because hyperglycemia can result from high glucose loads (Box 25-9 for an overview of blood glucose monitoring). Insulin may be added to the solution or given subcutaneously on a sliding scale as needed. TPN should be discontinued slowly to avoid rebound hypoglycemia.

Infection is a major complication of parenteral nutrition. An early sign of sepsis is glucose intolerance. Others include fever or hypothermia, shaking chills, hypotension, and tachycardia. A significant advantage of PPN is that infection, if it occurs, is local rather than systemic. The signs include pain, redness, edema, and warmth at the site.

Some clients react to lipid emulsions. Adverse reactions include fever, chills, vomiting, and pain in the chest or back. A milder symptom is an itchy skin rash. Alert the nutrition support team if these reactions occur. Lipid overload is accompanied by increased triglyceride levels, an enlarged liver, and altered liver function test results. Lipid emulsions are usually discontinued if these reactions occur.

Home Parenteral Nutrition. Information about home health care for clients receiving parenteral nutrition is found in Box 25-10. This therapy is often quite successful with proper professional support to monitor for potential complications and provide information to clients and caregivers.

BOX 25-9 *Teaching for Self-Care*

Blood Glucose Monitoring

Purpose: Blood glucose monitoring is useful whenever a client is at risk for hyperglycemia or hypoglycemia or to monitor the effects of insulin therapy.

Expected Outcome: The client will demonstrate correctly the ability to measure capillary blood glucose and read and record the results accurately.

Client Instructions

- Assess the skin of the area to be used for puncture (most frequently fingers). Avoid areas with ecchymosis (bruising) or that are broken (open).
- Gather all necessary equipment: glucose meter, reagent strip, sterile lancet or Autolet device, alcohol or povidone-iodine swab, and cotton ball. Although health care providers wear clean disposable gloves, it is unnecessary for a client to wear them for self-testing.
- Wash hands with soap and warm water. Assume a comfortable position, such as sitting in a chair.
- Remove the reagent strip from the container, being sure to handle it according to the manufacturer's directions. Place it on a clean, dry surface.
- Select the finger to be punctured, and massage it gently while holding it in a dependent (downward) position to increase circulation to the area.
- Wipe the site with alcohol or povidone iodine swab, and allow it to dry completely.
- Remove the cover of the lancet or Autolet device; hold the lancet perpendicular to the side of the finger and pierce the skin quickly; if an Autolet is used, push the release button to trigger the puncture.
- Use the cotton ball to wipe away the first drop of blood; gently squeeze or massage the skin toward the puncture site to obtain a large drop of blood.
- According to manufacturer's directions, either allow the blood to drop onto the reagent pad or touch the drop of blood onto the pad; in either case, the blood should cover the pad completely. Be sure not to smear the blood.
- If indicated by manufacturer, begin the timer on the meter and wipe the blood from the test strip after the specified amount of time; note that all meters do not require this.
- According to manufacturer's directions, place the reagent strip into the glucose testing meter. Read the results after waiting the specified period of time.
- Remove the reagent strip from the meter, turn off the meter, and dispose of used equipment.
- Record the results per primary care provider directions, and store the meter for future use.

BOX 25-10 *Home Health Care for Clients Receiving Parenteral Nutrition*

ASSESS

- Confirm the physician's order. (Will the parenteral nutrition be given only at night or also during the day? For what length of time will the client need it?)
- Does the client have a support system, such as family?
- What motivation level do the client and family have?
- Can client and family understand the complexities of parenteral nutrition?
- Do the client and family have adequate financial resources to maintain safe, accurate therapy? (Consult a social worker about solving financial problems.)
- Is the client mobile? (If so, consider suggesting that the client wear a lightweight vest with large pockets to hold parenteral nutrition supplies if feedings will occur during the day.)
- What safety problems are present in the client's home?
- Does the client have access to nursing services or a hospital?

TEACH

- Find a quiet space where the client and family can concentrate.
- Include family in all teaching sessions.
- Because the material is complex and important, begin with simple content and use drawings or models as needed. For example, use a teddy bear with a central line site to show procedures.
- Make sure to fully teach the following concepts:
  1. Strict hand-hygiene techniques
  2. How to hang the solution
  3. Setting the feeding rate (operating an infusion pump)
  4. Cleaning the site and changing the dressing
  5. Flushing the catheter
  6. Taking fingerstick glucose readings, if needed
  7. Which problems to report, such as redness, swelling, drainage, or pain at the site; fever; inability to flush the catheter; shortness of breath; increased urinary output; hyperglycemia; chest pain
- When teaching procedures, avoid placing time limits on the client or family members, because manual dexterity can vary from client to client.
- Provide written handouts with specific directions, important adverse responses, and actions to take.
- Provide client with list of phone numbers for reporting problems.

EVALUATE

- Ask the client (and family) to give you a return demonstration of cleaning the site, changing the dressing, and hanging the solution.
- Have the client or a family member keep a record of the amount of parenteral nutrition taken in a 24-hour period and any abnormal responses or symptoms that develop.

INTERVENTIONS TO MANAGE *IMPAIRED SWALLOWING*

Positioning the Client. The position that best facilitates swallowing is 90-degree flexion at the hips and 45-degree flexion at the neck. Have the client sit as upright as possible and remain there for at least 30 minutes after eating.

If the client has partial paralysis (as from a stroke), rotate the chin toward the weaker side to improve swallowing. Encourage neck flexion to enhance the pharyngeal phase of swallowing and facilitate closure of the glottis. Place food in the unaffected side of the mouth.

You can also enhance the swallowing reflex by using an ice collar or by brushing the client's neck with a small brush, such as a small paint brush, just before he eats. Place food behind the client's front teeth and instruct the client to tilt his or her head before swallowing.

Encouraging Appropriate Foods. Certain foods are easier to swallow than others (Box 25-11). Thin liquids are most difficult for clients with dysphagia because they require greater oral coordination and finer motor movements of the swallowing muscles. Dysphagic clients should never "wash food down" with thin liquids. Fluid requirements for clients with dysphagia must be met with fluids that are thickened with potato flakes, corn starch, fruit, or commercial products.

Flavorful foods that are either warm or cold stimulate the swallowing reflex better than bland, lukewarm foods. Flavoring also stimulates the flow of saliva. Sauces and gravies are good choices because they are flavorful and they lubricate food. Fragmented foods, such as corn kernels, peas, rice, and ground meat, are easily aspirated and should be moistened. Moist pastas, casseroles, and egg dishes are good choices.

Clients with dysphagia sometimes report increased mucus production or phlegm after ingesting milk, but this may result from impaired swallowing rather than a change in mucus production (Remig & Romero, 2004). The client should follow milk intake with thickened liquids to flush the throat, rather than decrease milk intake.

Pureed foods are not tolerated as well as textured foods because they fail to stimulate swallowing. Sticky foods (such as peanut butter) or bulky foods (such as raw fruits and vegetables) are also more difficult to swallow and should be avoided. Foods with a combination of textures should also be avoided because they are difficult to control. These include chunky soups, although blenderized soups are good.

INTERVENTIONS TO REDUCE *RISK FOR ASPIRATION*

Many interventions for *Risk for aspiration* have already been discussed, because two major risks for aspiration are impaired swallowing and enteral feedings. Carefully monitor clients because silent aspiration may produce only subtle cues, such as change in respiratory rate, temperature, breath sounds, or oxygen saturation levels. Also assess the client's bowel sounds, and check for abdominal distention that could indicate increased gastric residual volume. Keep the client's head positioned to at least a 30-degree angle. If the head cannot be elevated, place the client in a right lateral position to facilitate gastric emptying. Suction oral secretions to keep the oropharynx patent. Treat nausea to prevent vomiting. The physician may order H_2 receptor antagonists to reduce gastric acidity and prokinetic agents as needed.

BOX 25-11 *Comparing Easy-to-Swallow and Hard-to-Swallow Foods*

EASY TO SWALLOW	HARD TO SWALLOW
Warm or cold foods	Lukewarm foods
Flavorful foods (salted or mildly sweetened)	Bland foods
Thickened liquids	Thin liquids and milk
Sauces and gravies	Foods that fall apart (such as peas or rice)
Moist pastas, casseroles, egg dishes	Pureed foods, which do not stimulate swallowing
Blenderized soups	Slippery foods, sticky or bulky foods

EVALUATION

During evaluation, determine if the plan and interventions were successful in achieving the established outcomes, such as those in Box 25-12. If goals are not met, revise the plan, implement it, and reevaluate. Document the extent to which expected outcomes are met.

A partial documentation note for Mrs. Goldman at a 1-month follow-up visit might be as follows.

SAMPLE DOCUMENTATION NOTE FOR MRS. GOLDMAN

Weight 116 pounds, increased from 115 pounds 1 month ago. Serum albumin 2.8 mg/100 mL, up from 2.7 mg/100 mL 1 month ago. Goals of 117 pounds for weight and 3.0 mg/100 mL serum albumin level not yet met, although progress has been made.

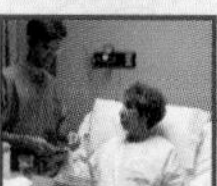

How might you revise the interventions? What intervening variables might have interfered with Mrs. Goldman's reaching her goals? What would you add to the documentation note to reflect the changes you would make in the plan of care?

BOX 25-12 *Nursing Care Plan*

A Client With Inadequate Nutritional Intake During Chemotherapy

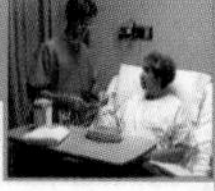

Outpatient Clinic Data

Mrs. Goldman is halfway through her 6 months of chemotherapy. She uses prochlorperazine (Compazine) for nausea for 3 days after her treatments, has experienced a 25-pound weight loss, and has signs of depression.

Physician's Orders

Assist with diet planning to maintain ideal body weight.

Nursing Assessment

Client is 54 years old, is 5 feet 4 inches tall, and weighs 115 pounds. Adheres to a kosher diet. Reports weighing 140 pounds before chemotherapy; weight/IBW = 95%; energy needs from Harris-Benedict equation plus 10% for activity = 2000 calories; serum albumin 2.7 g/100 mL; hemoglobin 11.5 g/100 mL and hematocrit 32%; client describes feeling fatigued and has decreased interest in eating. Client is concerned about recent weight loss.

Continued

BOX 25-12

Nursing Care Plan—cont'd

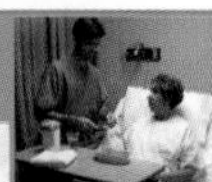

A Client With Inadequate Nutritional Intake During Chemotherapy

NANDA-I Nursing Diagnosis	NOC Expected Outcomes With Indicators	NIC Interventions With Selected Activities	Evaluation Data
Imbalanced Nutrition: Less Than Body Requirements	***Weight Control***	***Weight Gain Assistance***	***After 1 Month of Care***
Related factors:			
• A 25-pound weight loss	• Weight gain of at least 2 pounds in 1 month.	• Offer choices of good-tasting protein supplements to be taken between meals.	• Weight has increased by 1 pound. Reports that supplement is nauseating.
• Nausea	• Eats at least 2000 calories daily.	• Have client keep a calorie diary; consider suggesting zinc for increasing taste.	• Client reports that she has been eating better and has kept a record of her food intake. Eating 1500 calories.
	Nutritional Status	***Nutritional Monitoring***	
	• Increase in hemoglobin and hematocrit by 1 month.	• Include a source of iron in diet. Select culturally agreeable foods.	• Hemoglobin and hematocrit show moderate increase after 1 month.
	• Increase in albumin by 3 weeks.	• Select high-protein foods that are culturally agreeable.	• Albumin has begun to slowly increase by 3 weeks.
	• Decreased fatigue in 1 month.	• Establish a contract with client to engage in one pleasurable activity a day. Limit rest periods to one or two per day.	• Has increased number of ple asurable activities. Takes an afternoon nap. Otherwise engages in light activities. Reports that fatigue has improved.

Critical Thinking Questions

1. How frequently does Mrs. Goldman need follow-up once her nutritional status stabilizes?
2. Who is the most desirable member of the health care team to provide this follow-up?
3. What further dietary teaching might be needed if current interventions are not successful?

Nursing outcome and intervention labels from Johnson, M., Bulechek, G., Butcher, H., Dochterman, J. M., Maas, M., Moorhead, S., et al. (Eds.). (2006). *NANDA, NOC, and NIC linkages: Nursing diagnoses, outcomes, & interventions.* St. Louis, MO: Mosby.

▼ KEY PRINCIPLES

- Nutrition inadequate to meet the body's needs results from energy needs that exceed the amount taken in and may have many physical and psychological causes.
- Impaired swallowing typically results from neuromuscular problems or a decreased level of consciousness.
- The risk for aspiration is high in clients who receive tube feedings, are intubated, or have decreased consciousness or impaired swallowing.
- There is no single marker for nutritional problems. To detect them, you must review the collected assessment data. Unintentional loss of 10% of body weight within a 6-month period is a red flag for *Imbalanced nutrition: less than body requirements.*
- *Impaired swallowing* can be definitively diagnosed with evidence of aspiration.
- Refeeding of malnourished clients must be done carefully to prevent serious metabolic complications.
- Enteral feeding is a major risk factor for aspiration.
- When making a differential diagnosis for nutritional problems, choose the diagnosis that will best focus care on the client's most immediate needs.
- Interventions for nutritional problems require a team approach, whether carried out in the client's home or in the clinic, hospital, or other health care setting.
- Parenteral and enteral nutritional support includes specialized nursing procedures important for clients with *Imbalanced nutrition: less than body requirements.*
- Interventions for *Impaired swallowing* focus on providing foods and techniques that will encourage the swallow reflex, and on preventing aspiration.
- When evaluating outcome criteria for *Imbalanced nutrition: less than body requirements,* expect a weight gain of at least 2 pounds/month; a weight gain of 1 pound/day or more indicates fluid gain.

REVIEW QUESTIONS

1. The school nurse would anticipate that which of the following adolescents is most at risk for developing an eating disorder?
1. A 13-year-old girl who plays softball
2. A 14-year-old boy who plays football
3. A 15-year-old girl who does gymnastics
4. A 16-year-old boy who enjoys hiking

2. A client with anorexia nervosa would most likely have which of the following nursing diagnoses?
1. Noncompliance
2. Impaired swallowing
3. Risk for aspiration
4. Imbalanced nutrition: less than body requirements

3. The nurse would most likely remove the salt packet on the meal tray for the client with which of the following health problems?
1. Asthma
2. High blood pressure
3. Lactose intolerance
4. Diabetes mellitus

4. The nurse would raise the head of the bed for a client receiving enteral feedings to a minimum of how many degrees?
1. 10
2. 30
3. 60
4. 90

5. The nurse would assess which of the following most closely to detect a serious complication of total parenteral nutrition (TPN)?
1. Temperature
2. Pulse
3. Oxygen saturation
4. Blood pressure

Bibliography

American Diabetes Association. (2004). Diabetes nutrition recommendations for health care institutions. *Diabetes Care, 27*:S55. Retrieved from http://care.diabetesjournals.org/cgi/content/full/diacare;27/suppl_1/s55.

American Psychiatric Association. (2000). *Diagnostic and statistical manual of mental disorders* (4th ed. text revision). Washington, DC: Author.

Anderson, D. (2004). Nutrition for low-birth-weight infants. In K. McMahon & S. Escott-Stump, *Krause's food, nutrition, & diet therapy* (11th ed., pp. 234-258), St. Louis, MO: Elsevier Science.

*ASPEN Board of Directors & The Clinical Guidelines Taskforce. (2002). Guidelines for the use of parenteral and enteral nutrition in adult and pediatric patients. *Journal of Parenteral and Enteral Nutrition, 26*(1), Supplement.

Braga, J., Hunt, A., Pope, J., & Molaison, E. (2006). Implementation of dietitian-recommendations for enteral nutrition results in improved outcomes. *Journal of American Dietetic Association, 106*(2), 281-284.

Brownie, S. (2006). Why are elderly individuals at risk of nutritional deficiency? *International Journal of Nursing Practice, 12*(2), 110-118.

Caulfield, L., deOnis, M., Blossner, M., & Black, R. (2004). Undernutrition as an underlying cause of child deaths associated with diarrhea, pneumonia, malaria, and measles. *American Journal of Clinical Nutrition, 80*(1), 193-198.

*Duh, Q. Y. (1996). Decision tree for route of enteral nutrition support: Placement techniques. *Current issues in enteral nutrition support: Report of the first Ross conference on enteral devices* (pp. 9-16). Columbus, OH: Ross Products Division, Abbott Laboratories.

*Edwards, S., & Metheny, N. (2000). Measurement of gastric residual volume: State of the science. *MedSurg Nursing, 9*(3), 125.

Gregory, K. (2005). Update on nutrition for preterm and full-term infants. *Journal of Obstetric, Gynecological, and Neonatal Nursing, 34*(1), 98-108.

Hearing, S. (2004). Refeeding syndrome. *British Medical Journal, 328(*7445), 908-909.

*Johnson, M., Bulechek, G., Butcher, H., Dochterman, J. M., Maas, M., Moorhead, S., et al. (Eds.). (2006). *NANDA, NOC, and NIC linkages: Nursing diagnoses, outcomes, & interventions.* St. Louis, MO: Mosby.

*Kohn-Keeth, C. (2000). How to keep feeding tubes flowing freely. *Nursing, 30*(3), 58-59.

*Lemoyne, M., & Jeejeebhoy, K. N. (1985). Total parenteral nutrition in the critically ill patient. *Chest,* 89(4), 563-569.

*Livingston, A., Seamons, C., & Dalton, T. (2000). If the gut works use it. *Nursing Management, 31*(5, part 1), 39-42.

Lucas, B. (2004). Nutrition in childhood. In K. McMahon & S. Escott-Stump, *Krause's food, nutrition, & diet therapy* (11th ed., pp. 259-283). St. Louis, MO: Elsevier Science.

Mahan, K., & Escott-Stump, S. (2004). *Krause's food, nutrition, & diet therapy* (11th ed.). Philadelphia: Saunders.

Metheny, N., Schnelker, R., McGinnis, J., Zimmerman, G., Merritt, B., Banotai, M., et al. (2005). Indicators of tube site during feedings. *Journal of Neuroscience Nursing, 37*(6), 320-325.

Pichard, C., Kyle, U., Morabia, A., Perrier, A., Vermeulen, B., & Unger, P. (2004). Nutritional assessment: Lean body mass depletion at hospital admission is associated with an increased length of stay. *American Journal of Clinical Nutrition, 79*(4), 613-618.

Remig, V., & Romero, C. (2004). Medical nutrition therapy for neurologic disorders. In K. McMahon & S. Escott-Stump, *Krause's food, nutrition, & diet therapy* (11th ed., pp. 1081-1120). St. Louis, MO: Elsevier Science.

*Welch, S. (1996). Certification of staff nurses to insert enteral feeding tubes using a research-based procedure. *Nutrition in Clinical Practice, 11*(1), 21-27.

Williams, T., & Leslie, G. (2004). A review of the nursing care of enteral feeding tubes in critically ill adults: Part I. *Intensive Critical Care Nursing, 20*(6), 330-343.

Williams, T., & Leslie, G. (2005). A review of the nursing care of enteral feeding tubes in critically ill adults: Part II. *Intensive Critical Care Nursing, 21*(1), 5-15.

Winaver, N., & Williams, M. (2001). Nutritional support. In *Making health care safer: A critical analysis of patient safety practices* (Agency for Healthcare Research and Quality Evidence Report/Technology Assessment No. 43). Retrieved October 31, 2006, from http://www.ahrq.gov/clinic/ptsafety/pdf/ptsafety.pdf.

Zaloga, G. (2005). The myth of the gastric residual volume. *Critical Care Medicine, 33*(2), 449-450.

*Asterisk indicates a classic or definitive work on this subject.

Chapter 26

MAINTAINING FLUID AND ELECTROLYTE BALANCE

Media Resources

- Nursing Skills Online
- evolve Evolve Website http://evolve.elsevier.com/Harkreader/
- 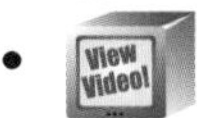 Companion CD
- Skills Video Clips

Learning Objectives

After studying this chapter, you should be able to do the following:

- Describe the normal physiology of fluid balance, including fluid compartments, functions of body fluids, and types of electrolytes
- Identify mechanisms that contribute to the regulation of fluid, electrolyte, and acid-base balance
- Discuss five common problems related to fluid balance
- Identify the factors affecting fluid balance, including physiological problems and associated therapeutic interventions
- Describe the general assessment of a client's fluid, electrolyte, and acid-base balance
- Describe the focused assessment of clients at risk for fluid, electrolyte, or acid-base problems, manifestations of actual problems, and client responses
- Diagnose the problems of clients with fluid, electrolyte, or acid-base imbalances that are within the domain of nursing
- Plan and carry out goal-directed interventions to prevent or correct fluid, electrolyte, or acid-base imbalances
- Evaluate outcomes regarding progress or lack of progress toward the goals of fluid, electrolyte, or acid-base balance with revision of the care plan as appropriate

Key Terms

active transport
anion
cation
colloid
colloid osmotic pressure
diffusion
electrolyte
filtration
hydrostatic pressure
hypertonic
hypotonic
isotonic
metabolic acidosis
metabolic alkalosis
milliequivalent
milliosmole
nonelectrolyte
osmolality
osmolarity
osmosis
respiratory acidosis
respiratory alkalosis
third spacing

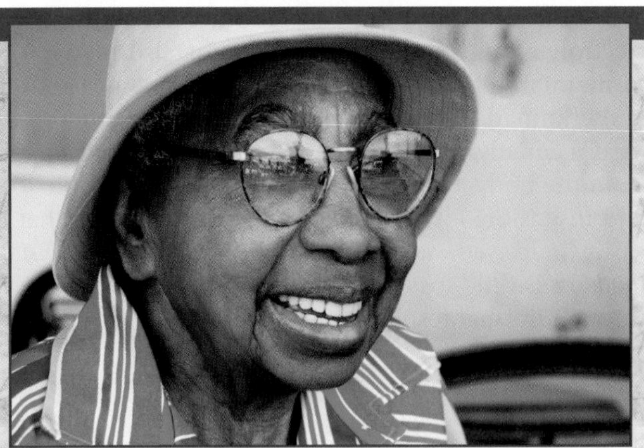

Elli Thompson, an 81-year-old African American woman, has lived independently in her own home since her husband died 4 years ago. She has one daughter, who lives 500 miles away, and two sons, one within 10 miles and one within 100 miles. She lately has developed arthritic joint changes and visual changes that interfere with her activities as well as with her ability to drive, cook, and maintain her usual standard of hygiene.

Her physician prescribed a nonsteroidal antiinflammatory drug (NSAID), a BP medication, and an ophthalmic medication. Mrs. Thompson has found these medications helpful, but she still has problems meeting her everyday needs. She still tries to make three meals for herself, even though cooking has become difficult. The inconvenience has led her to choose foods other than the foods she so dearly loves. In addition, she becomes so full with smaller amounts of food that she has stopped drinking in order to make room for the food. Her fatigue has also resulted in fewer trips to the kitchen for more fluids.

Mrs. Thompson's son Gerald stopped by for a visit and noticed that his mother looked thin and listless. Mrs. Thompson's physician, Dr. Kline, found her to be severely dehydrated. He believed that her lack of energy and change in self-care and social activity were related to the dehydration. Mrs. Thompson also said that the medication "makes me tired."

Dr. Kline recommended a change in her prescription and a home visit from a nurse. The visiting nurse's evaluation supported the diagnosis of *Deficient fluid volume.*

Mrs. Thompson progressed well. To increase Mrs. Thompson's ability to detect problems in the early stages, the nurse reviewed with her a written list of signs and symptoms that should be reported to Dr. Kline.

Mrs. Thompson was on her own again, with support from her family and friends. But she was so concerned about not getting in "this shape" again that she forced herself to drink fluids almost continuously. A week later, Gerald stopped by to check on his mother. This time, she looked puffy and was having trouble breathing. He became alarmed and immediately called Dr. Kline, who admitted Mrs. Thompson to the hospital with a diagnosis of acute congestive heart failure. In analyzing Mrs. Thompson, the nurse considers *Excess fluid volume* from the list of possible nursing diagnoses that relate to fluid imbalance (see key nursing diagnoses box).

KEY NURSING DIAGNOSES FOR FLUID IMBALANCE

Risk for imbalanced fluid volume: A risk of a decrease, an increase, or a rapid shift from one to another fluid state—intravascular, interstitial, and/or intracellular

Risk for deficient fluid volume: The state in which an individual is at risk for experiencing vascular, cellular, or intracellular dehydration

Deficient fluid volume: The state in which an individual experiences decreased intravascular, interstitial, and/or intracellular fluid; refers to dehydration, water loss alone without change in sodium

Excess fluid volume: The state in which an individual experiences increased isotonic fluid retention

Although older adults such as Mrs. Thompson represent the age-group most often endangered by fluid imbalance, this risk exists at any age and is associated with many conditions. Consider the child who becomes dehydrated from vomiting or diarrhea, the pregnant woman who develops abnormal swelling in her legs and feet, or the middle-age man with alcoholism who has an increasingly large abdomen from liver disease.

Fluid and electrolytes are critical to maintain a state of homeostasis. The body maintains this state by responding to continuous changes imposed by both internal physiological processes and the external environment. As a person takes in fluid and nutrients, the body's chemical equilibrium is disrupted by the processes of digestion, absorption, and metabolism of nutrients and the excretion of wastes. In addition, environmental conditions such as temperature and humidity cause changes in physiological functions to maintain a constant body temperature.

Through continuous internal change and adaptation, the body maintains precise control over fluids and electrolytes. When faced with conditions such as a hot day, high humidity, or a temporary delay of a meal, the healthy body responds through chemical reactions and hemodynamic changes to maintain normal physiological processes. Both acute and chronic illness can upset this delicate balance. The client may be too ill to respond to the need for fluid or electrolytes by increasing intake or excreting excess fluid, or there may be abnormal losses that exceed the body's ability to compensate.

The body functions by keeping the total input of water and electrolytes relatively equal to the amount lost. Therefore fluid and electrolyte balance means that total body water and electrolytes are normal, as is their distribution within body compartments.

Fluid and electrolytes are interdependent, meaning that an abnormality in one causes an abnormality in the other. In these situations, supportive medical therapy and nursing care is provided to help the body attain and maintain fluid and electrolyte balance.

The nurse's role is to monitor the client for fluid and electrolyte balance, administer prescribed medical therapy, and teach the client health practices to prevent recurrence of the problem. Monitoring is multifaceted because the regulation of fluid and electrolytes is a complex physiological process involving multiple organs and systems.

CONCEPTS OF FLUID BALANCE

Water is not found in its pure state in the body; rather, it is the medium in which all chemical products of nutrition, metabolism, and excretion are found. The term *fluid* is used to mean water and the components it contains. Chemical compounds are the principal components of most body fluids. An **electrolyte** is any compound that, when dissolved in water, separates into electrically charged particles, which are called *ions.* Positively charged ions are called **cations;** negatively charged ions are called **anions.**

The most common compound that becomes an electrolyte in solution is table salt, or sodium chloride (NaCl). Important cations in body metabolism are sodium (Na^+), potassium (K^+), calcium (Ca^{2+}), magnesium (Mg^{2+}), and hydrogen (H^+). Important anions are chloride (Cl^-), bicarbonate (HCO_3^-), sulfate (SO_4^{-2}), proteinate, and phosphate (PO_4^-). **Nonelectrolytes** are substances that do not ionize and thus do not carry an electrical charge. Glucose is an example of a nonelectrolyte compound in body fluids.

Fluid balance depends on the chemical and physical properties of electrolytes and plasma proteins. Thus, from a practical perspective, fluid deficit or fluid overload cannot be addressed in isolation from electrolytes and proteins because they are so interrelated. In other words, when a client has a fluid imbalance, you will also need to assess the client's electrolyte and protein status. Therefore this chapter presents an overview of major electrolytes as they relate to the person's risk or actual state of fluid imbalance.

You need to understand many fundamental physiological concepts to anticipate a fluid imbalance or understand the nature of fluid deficit or fluid excess. These include the functions of body fluids, the storage of fluids in different compartments, the role of electrolytes, the shifting of fluid between compartments, the regulation of fluid balance, and common problems of fluid balance.

FUNCTIONS OF BODY FLUIDS

The body needs at least 1200 to 1500 mL of water every day in addition to water that comes from foods we eat (about 800 mL) and the oxidation of food (about 300 mL). Why does the body need so much fluid?

The answer is partly because fluid makes up over half of the normal adult's weight. Fluids transport nutrients and wastes to and from cells and act as a solvent for electrolytes and nonelectrolytes. Fluids also play a role in maintaining body temperature, facilitating digestion and elimination, and lubricating joints and other body tissues. Finally, fluids need to be restored as they are lost from the body. Fluid output includes both sensible loss and insensible loss. *Sensible fluid loss* is fluid loss that is easily perceived, such as through urination. *Insensible fluid loss* is fluid loss that is not easily perceived, such as through normal respiration.

FLUID COMPARTMENTS

Fluids exist in several compartments in the body. Although fluid is in a continual state of exchange between compartments, the amount of fluid and the relative components in each compartment remain relatively constant.

Body fluid is in a state of balance when the following occurs:

- The water and electrolyte components are present in the proper proportions.
- Fluids are distributed normally between compartments.
- Lost body water and electrolytes are replaced.
- Excess water and electrolytes are eliminated.

For body cells to function normally, the composition of body fluids must remain constant and the distribution among compartments must remain normal. In the average adult, 50% to 60% of body weight is from fluid, 70% of which is intracellular and 30% extracellular. Homeostasis depends on the relationship of the components within the intracellular and extracellular fluid compartments (Figure 26-1).

Intracellular Fluid Compartment. Intracellular fluids provide cells with the internal aqueous medium necessary for their chemical functions. Therefore anything that affects fluid loss at the cellular level has significant implications for the entire body.

Extracellular Fluid Compartment. Extracellular fluids are found outside body cells and serve as the body's transportation system. They carry water, electrolytes, nutrients, and oxygen to the cells and remove waste products of cellular metabolism. The extracellular compartments are further divided as follows: intravascular (6% of the total), interstitial (22%), and transcellular (2%).

Intravascular Fluids. The term *intravascular* refers to the spaces within the arteries, veins, and capillaries, whose major function is to carry blood. Blood consists of the fluid known as *plasma* and cells (white and red blood cells and platelets) carried in that plasma. Plasma contains **colloids** (macromolecules that are too large to pass though a cell membrane and that do not readily dissolve into a solution, such as proteins) and byproducts of cellular function and metabolism.

Having too little blood (fluid) in the intravascular space affects the nutrient and oxygen supply to all tissues. Tissues that have a high demand for oxygen and

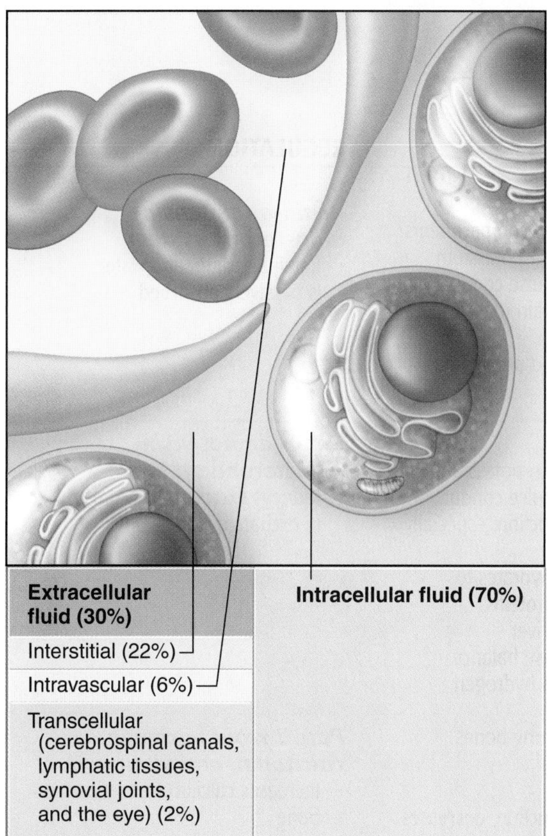

FIGURE 26-1 Distribution of fluid by compartments in the average adult.

nutrients, such as the brain, heart, and kidneys, are compromised first. A familiar example is the loss of intravascular fluid that occurs with a hemorrhage and results in a drop in blood pressure. Changes in fluid volume in the vascular space trigger a series of compensatory neuroendocrine responses (discussed later in the chapter).

Interstitial Fluids. Fluid is everywhere in the body, even between the cells and vascular compartments, in spaces known as the *interstitial spaces.* Interstitial fluid transports nutrients and waste products between the cells and the blood vessels. Too much or too little fluid in this space affects bodily functions.

A sprained ankle is a familiar example of an increase in interstitial fluid. The swelling of the tissue around the ankle bones results from damage to the vessel walls and the release of byproducts of tissue injury. These alter the permeability of the vessel walls, allowing excess fluid to seep into the interstitial spaces. Excess fluid in the interstitial spaces is called *edema.*

Transcellular Fluids. Transcellular fluids are found in spaces in the cerebrospinal canals in the brain, and in the lymph tissues, synovial joints, and eyes. Although these fluids contribute only about 2% of the total body fluid volume, even small changes in fluid volume in these compartments can have a major impact on the health of these organs.

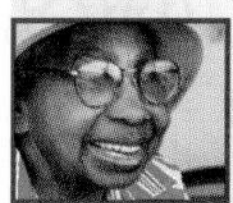

If Mrs. Thompson, from our case study, was eating three meals a day, why didn't the food sustain her? Is drinking water and other fluids really that important?

ELECTROLYTES

As noted earlier, electrolytes are ionized substances that perform their functions within a fluid environment. Extracellular and intracellular fluids contain the same electrolytes but in different amounts. For example, about 98% of the body's potassium is found in the intracellular compartment, compared with 2% in the extracellular compartment. In contrast, 99% of the sodium is found in the extracellular compartment, and the remaining 1% is in the intracellular compartment.

The electrolytes that are most plentiful inside the cells are potassium, magnesium, phosphate, and protein. Sodium, calcium, chloride, hydrogen, and bicarbonate are the most plentiful electrolytes in the extracellular fluid. Electrolytes exert a major influence on the movement of water between compartments, on enzyme reactions, on neuromuscular activity, and on acid-base regulation. The specific functions of protein, hydrogen, bicarbonate, and other electrolytes as they affect acid-base balance will be discussed later.

It is through complex regulatory systems that the body maintains electrical neutrality. This means that the number of negative ions (anions) equals the number of positive ions (cations) in the body. Table 26-1 lists the functions and regulators of ions important in the body.

An example of fluid and electrolyte relationships occurs daily when a person eats. Water, proteins, fats, and carbohydrates are ingested, and minerals, including sodium, potassium, calcium, magnesium, chloride, and phosphate, are consumed. When these minerals are consumed, they ionize and become electrolytes. For example, table salt (NaCl) separates into Na^+ and Cl^- when it dissolves in body fluid.

Sodium. The osmotic role of sodium is essential to maintaining the proper amount of water in and between compartments. Vascular volume, which affects blood pressure, is a direct response to the level of sodium ions (where sodium goes, water follows). Sodium is also critical to nerve impulse conduction because of its effect on the electrical potential of cells. The sodium-potassium pump is an active transport mechanism that promotes the opening of sodium and potassium channels during different phases of impulse propagation. In **active transport,** molecules move from an area of lower concentration to an area of higher concentration with an expenditure of energy. These changes in sodium and potassium concentrations are critical to nerve conduction; and without them, cells would die.

Potassium. Potassium plays a key role in maintaining the sodium-potassium pump and thus the transmission of nerve impulses. Potassium balance is critical to the

Table 26-1 Electrolyte Functions and Regulators

ELECTROLYTE	NORMAL SERUM LEVELS (mEq/L)	FUNCTIONS	REGULATION
Sodium (Na^+)	135-145	• Maintains blood volume • Controls water shifting between compartments • Major cation involved in sodium-potassium pump necessary for nerve impulse conduction • Interacts with calcium to maintain muscle contraction • Major cation in bicarbonate and phosphate acid-base buffer system	***Renin-angiotensin-aldosterone system*** • Retains sodium and water is passively absorbed
Potassium (K^+)	3.5-5.0	• Affects osmolality • Major cation involved in sodium-potassium pump necessary for nerve impulse conduction • Promotes nerve impulse conduction, especially in heart and skeletal muscles • Assists in conversion of carbohydrates to energy and amino acids into proteins • Promotes glycogen storage in liver • Assists maintenance of acid-base balance through cellular exchange with hydrogen	***Renin-angiotensin-aldosterone system*** • Kidneys excrete potassium in exchange for sodium
Calcium (Ca^{2+})	4.5-5.5 (or 9-11 mg/mL)	• Nonionized form promotes strong bones and teeth • Promotes blood coagulation • Promotes nerve impulse conduction, decreases neuromuscular irritability • Strengthens and thickens cell membrane • Assists in absorption and utilization of vitamin B_{12} • Activates enzymes for many chemical reactions • Inhibits cell membrane permeability to sodium • Activates actin-myosin muscle contraction	***Parathyroid hormone, calcitonin, and vitamin D*** • Increases calcium resorption from bone • Increases calcium reabsorption by inhibiting phosphate reabsorption from kidney tubules • Increases calcium absorption from gastrointestinal tract
Magnesium (Mg^{2+})	1.5-2.5	• Promotes metabolism of carbohydrates, fats, and proteins • Activates many enzymes (B_{12} metabolism) • Promotes regulation of Ca, PO_4, K • Promotes nerve impulse conduction, muscle contraction, and heart function • Powers sodium-potassium pump • Promotes conversion of adenosine triphosphate (ATP) to adenosine diphosphate (ADP) for energy release	***Kidneys*** • Increases or decreases magnesium reabsorption in kidney tubules according to need
Chloride (Cl^-)	98-106	• Inhibits smooth muscle contraction • Regulates extracellular fluid volume • Promotes acid-base balance through exchange with bicarbonate in red blood cells (chloride shift) • Promotes protein digestion through hydrochloric (HCl) acid; acid pH required for activation of protease	***Renin-angiotensin-aldosterone system*** • Kidneys excrete chloride if body fluids are acidic and reabsorb it if body fluids are alkalotic
Phosphate (HPO_4^-)	1.2-3.0 (or 2.5-4.5 mg/mL)	• Nonionized form promotes bone and teeth rigidity • Promotes acid-base balance through phosphate buffer system • Necessary for ATP production	***Parathyroid hormone, calcitonin, and vitamin D*** • Increases phosphate resorption from bone • Inhibits phosphate reabsorption in kidney tubules • Increases phosphate absorption in gastrointestinal tract as needed

See http://www.ismp.org for the full list.

normal function of all cells but especially that of cardiac and skeletal muscles.

Calcium. Calcium plays a primary role in the formation of healthy bones and teeth. It promotes normal blood coagulation and is critical to nerve conduction. The slow calcium channels open after the more rapid sodium and potassium channels to maintain the electrical potential necessary for the transmission of nerve impulses across the cell membrane.

Magnesium. Although magnesium is present in low concentration, it also is critical to the function of many body systems through its effect on over 300 enzyme systems. It promotes the release of a phosphate bond (conversion of adenosine triphosphate [ATP] to adenosine diphosphate [ADP]), which provides the energy source for the sodium-potassium pump.

A change in any of these four cations (sodium, potassium, calcium, magnesium) can make the cell more or less responsive to stimuli. The degree and acuteness of the imbalances, as well as the client's adaptive mechanisms, determine the client's responses.

Chloride. Because chloride is the major anion associated with sodium, its role in osmolality and nerve conduction is also critical. Chloride also plays a key role in the process of digestion because it is the anionic part of hydrochloric acid.

Phosphate. Phosphate works with calcium to promote the integrity of bones and teeth. It is an integral part of ATP and ADP, which maintain our energy sources for all cell functions.

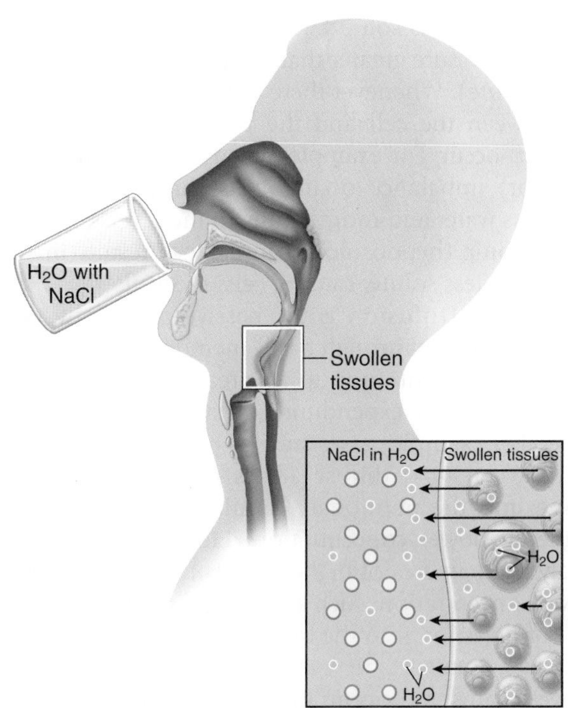

FIGURE 26-2 Osmosis. When a client uses a saline solution as a gargle for swollen tonsils, the gargle provides a feeling of comfort. This is because of the process of osmosis. The excess water in the swollen tonsils moves from the area of lesser concentration of particles (in the swollen cells) to the extracellular spaces that now have a higher concentration because of the added sodium.

MOVEMENT OF FLUIDS AND ELECTROLYTES

To maintain homeostasis, fluid shifts constantly between compartments, exchanging nutrients and waste products. For example, nutrients from ingested food are transported from the bloodstream to cells for use in cell maintenance, repair, and growth. Waste products from cellular metabolism of these nutrients are then transported to the bloodstream for removal from the body. Water is the medium that allows the transport of essential particles to the cells and waste products from the cells.

The factors that regulate the movement of water between compartments are discussed next. Understanding the normal mechanisms of fluid transport will enhance your ability to identify potential or actual fluid and electrolyte problems. Remember that fluid movement depends on the *relationships* between these factors, not on one factor alone.

Osmosis. The cell wall is a semipermeable membrane that selectively allows water and smaller particles to pass through it. Larger particles, such as proteins and glucose, are transported by more complex processes. The movement of fluid between compartments is influenced by osmosis and various pressure forces. **Osmosis** is the movement of water through a semipermeable membrane from an area containing a lesser concentration of particles to an area of greater concentration of particles.

Osmolality and osmolarity are expressions of the osmotic force of a solution. Osmotic force can be illustrated by considering ordinary table salt, sodium chloride (NaCl), as a gargle for a sore throat. The salt particles in the water create an osmotic force that draws fluid from the tissues and reduces swelling (Figure 26-2). The force from the dissolved particles (such as salt) in a solvent (such as water) can be represented as **milliosmoles,** the number of dissolved particles needed to produce one unit of force. **Osmolality** is the number of milliosmoles per kilogram of water. The term **osmolarity** is similar but is the measurement of milliosmoles per liter of solution. The term *osmolality* is used to describe body fluids, whereas the term *osmolarity* is used more often in reference to solutions measured by volume, such as an intravenous (IV) fluid.

To illustrate osmolality even further, consider two clients, one receiving a hypotonic IV solution and the other receiving an isotonic solution, with both solutions given at a fairly rapid rate. An **isotonic** solution has an osmotic pressure equal to that of plasma (solute is evenly distributed within the water). A **hypotonic** solution has an osmotic pressure less than that of plasma (more water, less solute). A **hypertonic** solution has an osmotic pressure greater than that of plasma (less water, more solute). Whenever there is a difference in osmolality between the cell and the plasma, fluid shifting is likely to occur. For example, when a hypertonic (hyperosmolar) imbalance occurs, cells shrink because they have less water and more solute. In the reverse situation, a hypotonic (hypoosmolar) imbalance results in more water and less solute, causing cells to swell.

Diffusion. **Diffusion** is the passive process by which molecules move through a cell membrane from an area of higher concentration to an area of lower concentration without an expenditure of energy (passive transport). For example, gases such as carbon dioxide (CO_2) and oxygen (O_2) diffuse across the respiratory membrane into the pulmonary capillaries from an area of higher to lower concentration. Electrolytes move passively from an area of higher concentration to an area of lower concentration, such as from the small bowel at the end of digestion into the bloodstream.

Active Transport. In contrast, when an electrolyte moves against a concentration gradient, from an area of lower concentration to an area of higher concentration (active transport), energy is required. This process is used by the sodium-potassium pump, which is critical to the maintenance of electrical impulses, such as in the heart. It is the active movement of sodium from inside the cell to the outside of the cell by this pump that results in a negativity on the inside of the cell.

This electrical difference between the outside and the inside of the membrane results in a resting potential, so that the cell can respond to an impulse. When it does so, the response is called an action potential because the cell is no longer in a state of rest but is in a state of action.

Filtration. **Filtration** pressure is the sum of (1) the forces tending to move water and dissolved substances out of the blood vessels and (2) the opposing forces. The balance of fluids within the capillaries depends on both hydrostatic pressure and colloid osmotic pressure. **Hydrostatic pressure** is the pressure exerted by the weight of fluid within a compartment or closed system. Tissue hydrostatic pressure pushes fluid into the capillary. Capillary hydrostatic pressure pushes fluid out of the capillary. **Colloid osmotic pressure** is the osmotic pressure exerted by large molecules, such as proteins. Tissue colloidal osmotic pressure pulls fluid into the interstitial spaces. Capillary colloidal osmotic pressure pulls fluid back into the capillary.

Hydrostatic Pressure. Arterial hydrostatic pressure is greater than colloid osmotic pressure. On the arterial end of the capillary, the hydrostatic pressure (approximately 32 mm Hg) is greater than the colloid osmotic pressure (approximately 22 mm Hg). This +10 difference is known as filtration pressure and results in the movement of fluid from the arterial end of the capillary into the interstitial compartment in the process known as filtration (Figure 26-3).

In the venous end of the capillary, the pulling force of the colloids draws fluids into the capillaries. The hydrostatic pressure (approximately 12 mm Hg) is less than the colloid osmotic pressure, approximately a −10 difference in filtration pressure. This pulling pressure results in reabsorption of the fluid back into the venous end of the capillary. In other words, a positive filtration pressure at the arterial end leads to fluid being "pushed" into the interstitial compartment, whereas a negative filtration pressure at the venous end leads to fluid being "pulled" back into the capillary, called *reabsorption*.

Factors that affect arterial or venous blood pressure or blood flow through the capillary network can affect hydrostatic pressure. These include blood volume, size of the vessel lumen, and the opposing forces from all osmotic molecules. Refer to Figure 26-3 again for the approximate pressures in a healthy adult.

Colloid Osmotic Pressure. Colloid osmotic pressure is the osmotic force created by colloids, which are large molecules such as proteins. This pressure draws fluid into the capillary or interstitial space. Colloid osmotic pressure is the major force opposing hydrostatic pressure in the capillary. It maintains a relatively constant value of 22 mm Hg. It is this opposition that affects how much fluid filters from the arterial end of the capillary to the interstitial spaces and the cell itself.

Proteins are the only dissolved substances that do not readily diffuse through the capillary membrane. Thus they exert a greater osmotic force than smaller molecules. The term *oncotic pressure* is used interchangeably with the

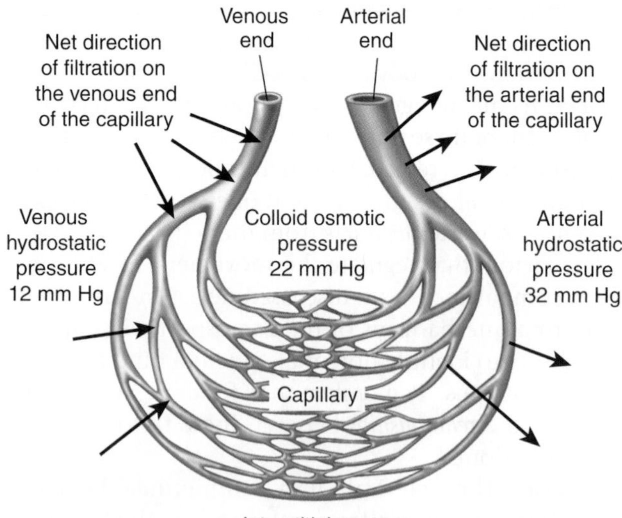

FIGURE 26-3 Filtration. Complex factors affect the movement of water and nutrients between the plasma, interstitium, and cellular spaces. Two critical factors are hydrostatic pressure and colloid osmotic pressure. Filtration on the arterial end, and reabsorption on the venous end, result in fluid shifting. The lymphatic tissues transport any remaining fluid or proteins to the right atrium.

term *colloid pressure,* and they both refer specifically to the osmotic force of protein and its superior ability to pull in water.

Proteins found in the plasma include albumin, globulin, and fibrinogen. Albumin has the greatest influence on the "pulling" pressure in the capillary. It constitutes 50% of the plasma proteins but is responsible for 80% of the colloid osmotic pressure in plasma. Although proteins play a vital role in fluid shifting, they cannot manage fluid homeostasis by themselves. When a person has a deficiency in protein, more fluid stays in the interstitial spaces. This abnormality, called edema, will be discussed later in the chapter.

In a healthy person, the interstitial compartment contains electrolytes and some proteins that have leaked through the capillary membrane; thus it has its own colloid osmotic pressure. However, the concentration of proteins is always greater in the plasma compartment than in the interstitial compartment, which helps maintain fluid volume in the intravascular compartment.

REGULATION OF FLUID BALANCE

Thirst. Why do you drink fluids? Is it because of habit or socialization, or are you thirsty? All of these factors probably affect your fluid intake. Western culture emphasizes the provision of beverages at social activities and in the home. Health publications remind us continually to drink plenty of fluids each day. But although habit and culture certainly influence our fluid consumption, our internal thirst mechanism is also a powerful stimulant that encourages us to drink.

The thirst center is located in the hypothalamus. The stimulation or inhibition of the thirst response depends on changes in local serum osmolality. For example, when the osmolality of the blood flowing around the lateral preoptic cells of the hypothalamus increases, the cells sense the change and trigger the thirst response. Situations that promote increased osmolality include a decrease in fluid intake, excessive fluid loss, or an excessive sodium intake either orally or intravenously. On the other hand, a high intake of fluids, fluid retention, a low sodium intake, and excessive IV infusion of hypotonic solutions inhibit the thirst mechanism.

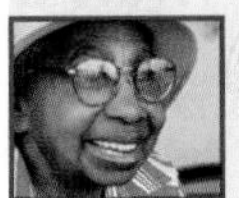

To return to our case study, why didn't Mrs. Thompson's thirst mechanism stimulate her to drink more? Recall that Mrs. Thompson is 81 years old. Like all older adults, she has a decrease in thirst as a normal consequence of aging. This will be addressed later in the chapter.

Lymphatic System. The lymphatic system performs the essential role of "sponging up" excess fluid that is not reabsorbed into the capillaries. The lymphatic ducts return fluid and some protein to the subclavian veins, which in turn empty into the right atrium of the heart. When the lymphatic system is not functioning properly, fluid excess occurs in the interstitial compartments. Severe lymphatic dysfunction can lead to localized tissue ischemia and cell death. It can also lead to systemic sepsis caused by metabolites from necrotic tissue.

Neuroendocrine System. Another very powerful regulator of fluid intake is the neuroendocrine system. It regulates body fluid volume by producing and secreting hormones that stimulate or inhibit osmotic receptors in the carotid arteries and aortic arch (Figure 26-4). These receptors are very sensitive to blood volume. The neuroendocrine system also uses specialized nerve endings (chemoreceptors) in the walls of the large blood vessels and atria to respond to changes in intravascular fluid volume.

Hormones. One of the most influential hormones affecting fluid balance is antidiuretic hormone (ADH). This hormone opposes (i.e., it is "anti") fluid loss (or "diuresis"). ADH is produced by the hypothalamus and stored in the vesicles in the posterior pituitary gland. The osmolality of extracellular fluid as it passes through the hypothalamus is the major stimulant or inhibitor of the secretion of ADH.

The osmolality of Mrs. Thompson's plasma was increased when she was in a state of fluid deficit. It makes sense, then, that her body, in an attempt to compensate, promoted a decrease in water loss. Increased secretion of ADH caused the pores in the distal and collecting tubules of her kidney nephrons to become larger. This resulted in increased reabsorption of the water back into the capillaries and a decrease in urinary output (oliguria). Conversely, under conditions that would decrease the plasma osmolality (fluid overload), ADH secretion would be inhibited and urine output would increase.

Aldosterone is another hormone that has a major effect on fluid balance. Although low sodium levels, high potassium levels, and the release of adrenocorticotropic hormone (ACTH) affect the release of aldosterone, the major stimulant for its release is the hormone angiotensin II (the renin-angiotensin-aldosterone [RAA] system). Unlike ADH, aldosterone has only an indirect effect on water. When it is released, aldosterone promotes reabsorption of sodium and excretion of potassium in the distal tubules and collecting ducts of the kidney. Sodium reabsorption results in the passive reabsorption of water.

When fluid excess is present, the opposite occurs: aldosterone secretion is decreased, resulting in sodium and water excretion and potassium retention. Note that when one cation (sodium) is retained, another (potassium) is excreted. This is one way in which the delicate balance of electrical neutrality is maintained. Also recall that changes in cations affect the movement of anions. Usually, the chloride ion passively accompanies its leader, the sodium ion, to its destination.

Thyroid hormones (thyroxine [T_4] and triiodothyronine [T_3]) affect fluid volume by influencing cardiac output. An increase in thyroid hormones causes an

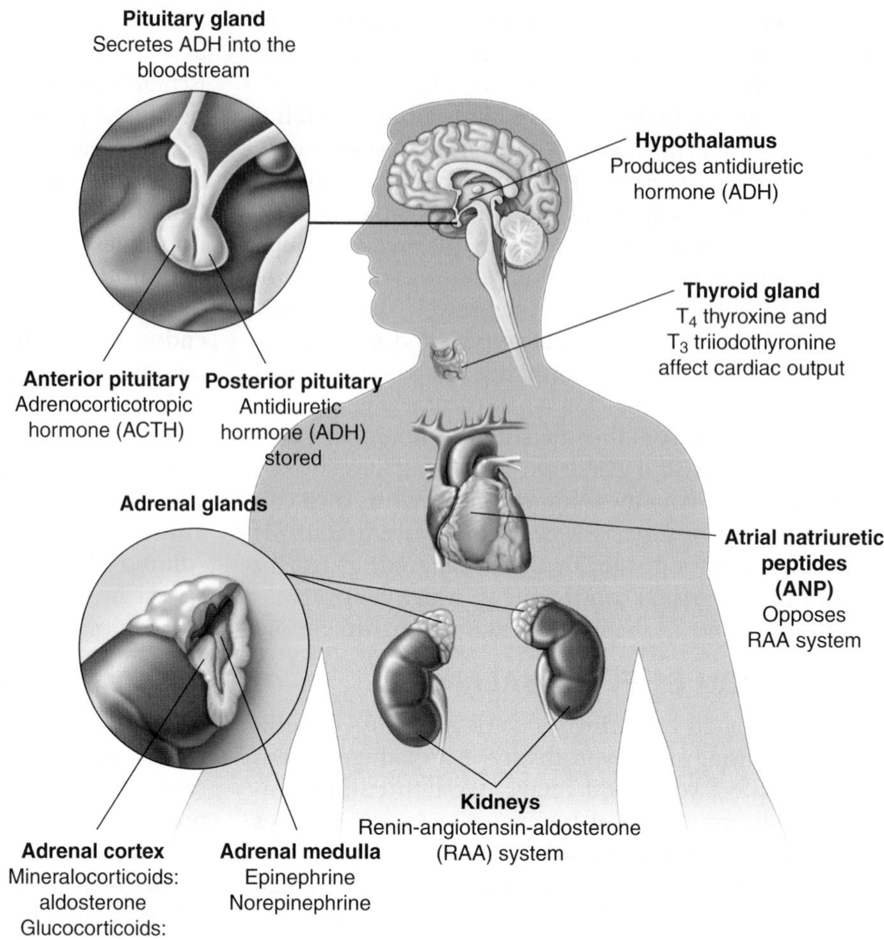

FIGURE 26-4 Effect of hormones on fluid balance.

increase in cardiac output, which in turn increases glomerular filtrate and thus urinary output. A decrease in these hormones has the opposite effect.

The cardiovascular system also plays a role in fluid balance through the release of atrial natriuretic peptides (ANPs) whenever the atrial cells are overloaded with fluid. Any condition that causes fluid overload, vasoconstriction, or direct cardiac damage stimulates an increase in the release of ANPs. Their release has an effect opposite to that of the renin-angiotensin-aldosterone system, causing dilation of the arterioles and venules, sodium excretion (natriuresis), and diuresis. In contrast, any situation that cause fluid deficit leads to inhibition of ANP.

Baroreceptors. Have you ever felt your heart pounding after a stressful event? If someone took your blood pressure at that time, it would be much higher than normal. However, this rise does not cause a problem in a healthy person because of the "minute-to-minute" control of the blood pressure by baroreceptors. These receptors are specialized nerve endings in the walls of the large veins and arteries and in the atria of the heart. They respond to the slightest changes in pressure inside the blood vessels and relay this information to the vasomotor centers in the medulla. Anything that affects the relationship of the size of the blood vessels or the volume inside the blood vessels affects these receptors.

Gastrointestinal System. Besides the fluid absorbed from dietary intake, the gastrointestinal (GI) tract produces about 7 to 9 L of glandular and tissue secretions per day. All but about 100 mL of this fluid is reabsorbed. About every 90 minutes, a volume of blood equivalent to the total body plasma level (about 3000 mL in a person who weighs 70 kg) passes through the intestinal mucosa. The GI fluid contains many nutrients, including electrolytes. Understanding the relationship between fluid balance and normal GI function is essential to anticipating fluid and electrolyte imbalances in a state of altered GI function.

Renal System. The renal system works interdependently with the neuroendocrine system to regulate extracellular fluid volume. Recall that the kidney is the target organ for ADH and aldosterone. ADH (through the regulation of water) and aldosterone (through the regulation of water, sodium, and potassium) play a major role in fluid and electrolyte homeostasis.

The renin-angiotensin-aldosterone (RAA) system functions to maintain homeostasis between sodium and water as well as regulate the blood pressure. Juxtaglomerular cells secrete renin, an enzyme that converts angiotensinogen to angiotensin I in the liver. Angiotensin I then travels to the lungs, where it is converted to angiotensin II (a potent vasoconstrictor). Angiotensin II has two effects: (1) it raises blood pressure by vasoconstriction, and (2) it stimulates the production of aldosterone from adrenal glands, which also raises the blood pressure by increasing blood volume. The amount of renin secreted depends on the volume of blood and the sodium level in the bloodstream. In response to a decreased sodium level or a decrease in plasma volume, the RAA system is triggered.

The kidneys also affect many other electrolytes, including calcium, magnesium, phosphate, hydrogen, chloride, and bicarbonate. The renal nephrons regulate electrolyte balance by secreting excess ions into the tubules, where they are later excreted as urine. When a deficit occurs, electrolytes are reabsorbed from the renal tubules back into the capillary network surrounding the tubules of the nephron.

PROBLEMS WITH FLUID BALANCE

The regulators of fluid balance are important to consider when a client is at risk for or has an actual fluid volume deficit or excess. Compare the following definitions to get a clearer picture of basic concepts related to fluid imbalance.

Deficient Fluid Volume. *Deficient fluid volume* refers to a state of hypovolemia (low blood volume), or dehydration, in either the extracellular fluid (intravascular or interstitial) compartment or the intracellular fluid compartment. The defining characteristics are a direct or an indirect result of a rapid change in fluid output or a lack of intake without compensation by fluid shifts or other homeostatic mechanisms.

Excess Fluid Volume. *Excess fluid volume* refers to a state of hypervolemia, or water intoxication, in the vascular compartment, the presence of edema in the interstitial compartment, or excess fluid in the intracellular spaces. The defining characteristics are a direct or indirect result of an increase in fluid intake or decrease in excretion without compensation by intercompartmental fluid shifts or other regulatory mechanisms.

Electrolyte Imbalance. *Electrolyte imbalance* means that a person has either a deficit or an excess of one or more electrolytes. Table 26-2 lists the risk factors and manifestations of common imbalances of sodium, potassium, calcium, magnesium, and phosphorus. Note the similarity of some manifestations, as well as the manifestations that are unique to each ion. A client often has more than one electrolyte imbalance, as well as an accompanying fluid imbalance.

Acid-Base Balance. Normal cellular function depends on the maintenance of hydrogen ion concentration within very narrow limits. The normal range of pH (a negative logarithm used to express the H^+ ion concentration) is 7.35 to 7.45. Cellular function is seriously affected when pH drops to 7.20 or lower or rises to 7.50 or higher. Ranges outside of 6.80 and 7.80 are usually incompatible with life.

In a healthy state, four systems interactively maintain the body within this narrow margin: cellular buffers, chemical buffers, the lungs, and the kidneys. The cellular buffers work as follows. Most dissolved CO_2 from tissue cell metabolism diffuses into the red blood cells, combines with water to form carbonic acid, and dissociates into hydrogen and bicarbonate. The bicarbonate shifts across the plasma membrane in exchange for chloride, and the hydrogen combines with hemoglobin and thus is buffered. Any pathological condition that leads to a deficit of sodium, phosphate, or protein impairs the base component of the chemical buffer systems, resulting in excess hydrogen. A decrease in hemoglobin or chloride can also increase the risk for acid-base imbalances by altering the buffering process.

Chemical buffer systems, chiefly the bicarbonate buffer system, neutralize excess acids and bases within the body by attaching or releasing hydrogen ions, respectively. Excess hydrogen ions combine with bicarbonate to form carbonic acid, which can then dissociate into water and CO_2 (called the hydrolysis reaction).

The lungs and kidneys are called physiological buffers because they can actually eliminate chemicals from the body. The lungs increase elimination of CO_2 (an acid) when the body has excess acid and decrease its elimination when there is base excess. The kidneys can eliminate either acids or bases depending on the body's need, which is therefore a powerful homeostatic mechanism.

Cellular and chemical buffer systems act within seconds to restore acid-base balance, the lungs act within minutes to hours, and the kidneys respond within hours to a few days. Figure 26-5 illustrates acid-base balance.

Respiratory acidosis results from retention of CO_2, an acid, and a subsequent decrease in pH (Table 26-3). Any pulmonary insufficiency resulting in hypoventilation (which causes the CO_2 level to build up) will result in respiratory acidosis. Conditions that depress the respiratory center (lung diseases, airway obstruction, and situations in which the chest wall and respiratory muscles are hindered) also cause respiratory acidosis. Manifestations include weakness, tremors, confusion, depression of the central nervous system, and even coma. Potassium and bicarbonate are retained, and hydrogen and chloride are lost in order to compensate.

Respiratory alkalosis is a result of rapid or excess elimination of CO_2, resulting in an increase in pH with a decrease in the partial pressure of CO_2 ($PaCO_2$). Any

Table 26-2 Common Electrolyte Imbalances: Risk Factors and Manifestations

IMBALANCE	RISK FACTORS	MANIFESTATIONS
HYPONATREMIA • Sodium <135 mEq/L • Chloride <98 mEq/L • Serum osmolality <285 mOsm/kg	• Low-salt diet, especially when taking diuretics at same time • Excess sweating • Athletic events • Vomiting and diarrhea in excess • Dilutional from taking in too much water	*General:* fatigue, weight loss *Musculoskeletal:* weakness *Cardiac:* orthostatic hypotension; rapid, thready, weak pulse; peripheral vein filling takes more than 5 seconds *Respiratory:* tachypnea *Gastrointestinal:* nausea, vomiting, diarrhea *Renal:* oliguria, anuria *Neurological:* hypothermia, decreased thirst, confusion, stupor, seizures
HYPERNATREMIA • Sodium >145 mEq/L	• Increased intake, especially the presence of renal disease • Excessive IV saline solutions • Increased retention from cardiac disease, renal disease, liver disease, Cushing's disease, hyperaldosteronism • Conditions in which water loss exceeds sodium loss, such as diabetes mellitus, diabetes insipidus, hyperventilation, hypertonic feedings, diaphoresis, decreased water intake	*General:* fatigue, pitting edema, puffy eyelids, ascites, weight gain *Musculoskeletal:* weakness *Cardiac:* rapid, bounding pulse; third heart sound; hypertension; peripheral vein emptying takes more than 5 seconds; neck vein distention *Respiratory:* dyspnea, crackles, pulmonary edema, pleural effusion *Gastrointestinal:* anorexia, nausea, vomiting *Renal:* oliguria, anuria *Neurological:* fever, restlessness, confusion
HYPOKALEMIA • Potassium <3.5 mEq/L	• Certain medications, such as diuretics and laxatives • Excess vomiting, diarrhea • GI suctioning • Diet low in potassium • Diuretic phase of renal failure	*General:* malaise, fatigue, alkalosis *Musculoskeletal:* weakness *Cardiac:* hypotension; arrhythmias; cardiac arrest; peaked P waves, depressed S-T segments, and flattened T and U waves on ECG *Respiratory:* shallow breathing, apnea, respiratory arrest *Gastrointestinal:* anorexia, nausea, vomiting, distention, paralytic ileus *Neurological:* dysphasia, lethargy, disorientation, irritability, hyporeflexia, paresthesias, tetany, seizures
HYPERKALEMIA • Potassium >5.0 mEq/L	• Increased oral or IV intake, especially in renal disease; stored blood • Decreased output, as from taking angiotensin-converting enzyme inhibitor with potassium-rich salt substitutes or potassium-sparing diuretics, renal failure, postoperative oliguria, Addison's disease • Excessive cellular loss, as from metabolic or respiratory acidosis (except diabetic acidosis) or during first 3 days after a severe burn or cellular trauma	*General:* restlessness, acidosis *Musculoskeletal:* severe weakness *Cardiac:* hypotension, arrhythmias; cardiac arrest; depressed P waves, wide QRS complexes, depressed S-T segments, and tall, tented T waves on ECG *Respiratory:* dyspnea *Gastrointestinal:* nausea, colic, diarrhea *Renal:* oliguria, anuria *Neurological:* restlessness, paresthesias, dysphasia, seizures
HYPOCALCEMIA • Calcium <4.5 mEq/L	• Certain medications, such as diuretics and laxatives • Hypoparathyroidism • Renal failure	*General:* bleeding *Musculoskeletal:* muscle cramps, pathological fractures *Cardiac:* hypotension; palpitations; arrhythmias; prolonged QT intervals on ECG *Respiratory:* laryngospasm, stridor *Neurological:* paresthesias, positive Trousseau's and Chvostek's signs, diplopia, tetany, seizures

Table 26-2 Common Electrolyte Imbalances: Risk Factors and Manifestations—cont'd

IMBALANCE	RISK FACTORS	MANIFESTATIONS
HYPERCALCEMIA • Calcium >5.5 mEq/L • Phosphorus decreased	• Rarely, from excessive intake of milk, calcium-based medications, or vitamin D • Increased loss from bone due to immobilization, cancer (bone, lung, breast, leukemia), multiple fractures, hyperparathyroidism • Decreased opposition, from Addison's disease, hypophosphatemia • Any condition producing acidosis • Decreased loss, from thiazide diuretics	*General:* dehydration, polydipsia *Musculoskeletal:* weak, relaxed muscles; osteoporosis; osteomalacia; bone pain; pathological fractures *Cardiac:* dysrhythmia, cardiac arrest, short QT intervals on ECG *Gastrointestinal:* nausea, vomiting, constipation *Renal:* polyuria, calculi, renal colic, flank pain *Neurological:* confusion, lethargy
HYPOMAGNESEMIA • Magnesium <1. 5 mEq/L	• Certain medications, such as diuretics • Alcoholism • Malnutrition • Hyperparathyroidism	*General:* refractory hypokalemia, hypocalcemia, or both *Musculoskeletal:* weakness *Cardiac:* tachycardia, arrhythmias *Neurological:* nystagmus, diplopia, disorientation, tremors, hyperactive reflexes, tetany, seizures
HYPERMAGNESEMIA • Magnesium >2.5 mEq/L	• Certain medications, such as magnesium antacids • Kidney disease	*General:* flushing *Musculoskeletal:* weakness, dysarthria *Cardiac:* hypotension, arrhythmias, cardiac arrest *Respiratory:* bradypnea, apnea, respiratory arrest *Gastrointestinal:* nausea, vomiting *Neurological:* thirst, hyporeflexia, lethargy, coma
HYPOPHOSPHATEMIA • Phosphate <1.2mEq/L	• Certain medications, such as aluminum antacids and diuretics • Hyperparathyroidism • Malnutrition	*General:* fatigue *Musculoskeletal:* weakness, bone pain, pathological fractures *Cardiac:* decreased cardiac function *Neurological:* confusion, seizures
HYPERPHOSPHATEMIA • Phosphate >3.0 mEq/L • Calcium decreased	• Certain medications, such as phosphate antacids and sodium phosphate enemas • Massive trauma, strokes • Renal failure	*Cardiac:* tachycardia *Gastrointestinal:* anorexia, nausea, vomiting *Neurological:* hyperreflexia, tetany

ECG, Electrocardiogram; *GI,* gastrointestinal; *IV,* intravenous.

pulmonary insufficiency or state resulting in hyperventilation will cause CO_2 to be blown off, leaving an alkalotic state. Manifestations include cardiac dysrhythmias, dizziness, light-headedness, tingling of fingers and toes, tetany, and possibly seizures. Hydrogen and chloride are retained, and potassium and bicarbonate are lost in order to compensate.

Metabolic abnormalities are secondary to imbalances in nonvolatile acids (those that cannot be eliminated by exhaling additional carbon dioxide) or in the amount of alkali and are often more difficult to diagnose. Bicarbonate shifts in the same direction as the pH (hence the memory hint: metabolic equal). Table 26-3 identifies the shifts in pH and HCO_3 in metabolic abnormalities.

Metabolic acidosis is a pathological condition caused by an increase in noncarbonic acids or a decrease in bicarbonate in the extracellular fluid, or both. Any pathological process that results in ineffective tissue perfusion and the accumulation of lactic acid leads to lactic acidosis, a type of metabolic acidosis. Because the kidneys are primarily responsible for excreting acids and reabsorbing bicarbonate, any state of severe renal insufficiency leads to metabolic acidosis.

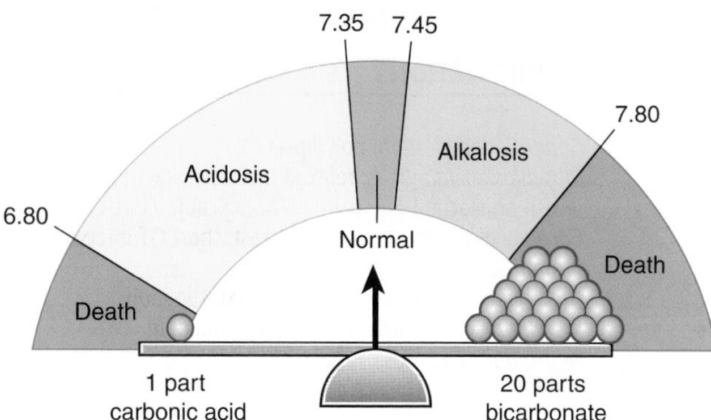

FIGURE 26-5 Acid-base balance. In the healthy state, a ratio of 1 part carbonic acid to 20 parts bicarbonate provides a normal serum pH between 7.35 and 7.45. Any deviation to the left of 7.35 results in an acidotic state. Any deviation to the right of 7.45 results in an alkalotic state.

Table 26-3 Acid-Base Imbalances

IMBALANCE	COMPENSATORY STATE	pH	CO_2	HCO_3^-
Respiratory acidosis	U	↓	↑	N
	PC	↓	↑	↑
	C	N	↑	↑
Respiratory alkalosis	U	↑	↓	N
	PC	↑	↓	↓
	C	N	↓	↓
Metabolic acidosis	U	↓	N	↓
	PC	↓	↓	↓
	C	N	↓	↓
Metabolic alkalosis	U	↑	N	↑
	PC	↑	↑	↑
	C	N	↑	↑

C, Compensated; *N*, normal value; *PC*, partially compensated; *U*, uncompensated.

An increase in potassium ions also increases the risk of metabolic acidosis. Whenever serum potassium rises, the protective cellular buffer attempts to decrease the risk of hyperkalemia by exchanging potassium for hydrogen across the cell membrane. Thus potassium enters the cell in exchange for hydrogen, which enters the plasma.

The most common manifestations of metabolic acidosis are neurological (headache, lethargy), GI (anorexia, nausea, vomiting, diarrhea), cardiovascular (dysrhythmias), and respiratory. The client may develop deep, rapid (Kussmaul's) respirations as the body attempts to blow off carbonic acid. Severe acidosis can lead to coma and death.

In contrast, metabolic alkalosis occurs when the pH rises above 7.45. This is a pathological condition caused by an increase in bicarbonate or a decrease in acid in the extracellular fluid, or both. Conditions such as excessive vomiting (with loss of hydrochloric acid) increase the risk for metabolic alkalosis. Potassium deficiency, regardless of the cause, promotes the shifting of hydrogen into cells and potassium into plasma—thus metabolic alkalosis. An overingestion of bicarbonate (as in antacids), especially in the presence of renal insufficiency, can result in metabolic alkalosis.

Common manifestations of metabolic alkalosis include generalized weakness, muscle cramps, neurological problems (hyperactive reflexes, tetany, confusion, seizures), cardiac dysrhythmias, and respiratory changes. As in metabolic acidosis, the respiratory system attempts to compensate. In this state, however, the respirations become slow and shallow in an attempt to conserve carbonic acid.

FACTORS AFFECTING FLUID BALANCE

Many variables influence a client's risk of fluid, electrolyte, and acid-base imbalance, including lifestyle, developmental stage, physiological state, and clinical factors. Table 26-4 lists the many etiologies of fluid deficit and fluid excess and the contributing factors for each variable. A client at risk for fluid deficit does not present with the actual signs and symptoms of an imbalance. However, recognizable risk factors can indicate that the person has a high probability of developing a fluid deficit if preventive actions are not taken.

LIFESTYLE FACTORS

Nutrition. An alteration in fluid intake increases risk. Although most fluid intake comes from water or other liquids, do not underestimate the importance of the water obtained from foods (Figure 26-6). The water byproduct of food oxidation in the cell also contributes to fluid balance, but to a lesser degree. The amounts listed in Figure 26-6 are for a healthy, relatively inactive person exposed to a temperate climate. People require at least 1500 mL of fluid daily to maintain essential cellular functions. The usual recommendation for fluid intake is six to eight glasses of water daily and other fluids to total about 2000 to 2400 mL.

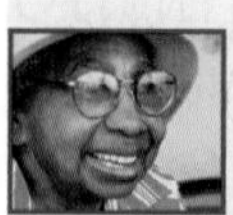

Now it makes sense that Mrs. Thompson became ill when she stopped drinking an adequate amount of fluid.

In a healthy person, the body compensates for excess fluid, sodium, or both by increasing excretion. However, if the person has cardiac, renal, or liver disease, excess intake only prompts more fluid retention. Excess fluid compromises the exchange of nutrients and wastes across the membrane between the cell and the plasma.

Table 26-4 Risk Factors for Fluid Volume Imbalance

RISK FACTOR	CONTRIBUTING FACTORS
DEFICIENT FLUID VOLUME	
Life Span	
Children	• Decreased ability to concentrate urine (immature kidneys). • Higher metabolic rate. • Greater body surface area relative to weight. • Hormonal and growth demands. • Compensatory responses less stable. • Fevers higher and last longer.
Pregnancy	• Increased need for fluid (fetal and supportive tissue changes).
Older adults	• Decreased thirst mechanism, even in healthy older adults. • Decreased ability to concentrate urine.
Weight Extremes	• Fatty tissue contains less fluid. • Excess fluid may be in compartments outside the blood vessels, making it unavailable. • Thirst may be an indicator of plasma deficit. • Women have larger proportion of fat tissue.
Altered Intake	
Decreased thirst	• Older adult population. • Hypoosmolality of the plasma inhibits thirst. • Decreased level of consciousness impairs perception of thirst.
Pain	• Alters desire or perception of thirst.
Dysphagia	• Increases time required for fluid intake. • Makes swallowing more difficult. • Requires thickened fluids.
Decreased access	• Lack of transportation, limited finances, ill health.
Increased Gastrointestinal (GI) Loss	
Diarrhea, vomiting, GI suctioning, ileostomy, fistula	• Rapid movement of fluid through GI tract decreases absorption of water, nutrients, and electrolytes. • Massive amounts of fluid can be lost via these sources regardless of etiology.
Hypertonic feedings (osmolarity >300 mOsm/kg)	• Increased osmolarity of feeding pulls water into bowel, which can cause diarrhea and dehydration.
Lactose-based feedings	• Lactose intolerance is common and may cause diarrhea.
Medications	• Many medications cause GI side effects, including anorexia, nausea, vomiting, and diarrhea. • Many elixirs are made with sorbitol, which can cause osmotic diarrhea.
Environmental	• Intolerance to toxins causing vomiting, diarrhea, or both. • Exposure to high temperature or humidity.
Increased Urinary Loss	
Decreased antidiuretic hormone	• May result from hypoosmolality of extracellular fluid, increased blood volume, exposure to cold, acute alcohol ingestion, carbon monoxide poisoning.
Hyperglycemia	• Causes osmotic diuresis.
Diuretic phase of renal failure	• Excess fluid lost through urine.
Medications	• Diuretics are a common cause.
Increased Integumentary Loss	
Environmental	• Temperature above 30° C (86° F) and humidity above 50%.
Fever	• Insensible water loss, can be large amounts.
Wounds/burns	• Loss of fluid, protein, electrolytes. • Damage to capillary membrane with direct fluid loss and secondary fluid loss due to loss of protein.
Increased Respiratory Loss	
Hyperventilation	• Increased loss of water through expired air.
Other Losses	
Hemorrhage or trauma	• Increased loss of fluid, nutrients, electrolytes.
Addison's disease	• Decreased sodium retention, thus decreased water reabsorption.
Third spacing	• Abnormal amounts of fluid accumulation in compartments that normally have minimal fluid decreases availability of fluids needed to maintain blood volume and cellular function.

Continued

Table 26-4 Risk Factors for Fluid Volume Imbalance—cont'd

RISK FACTOR	CONTRIBUTING FACTORS
EXCESS FLUID VOLUME	
Excessive Intake	
Excess fluid	• Increased oral or intravenous volume. • Electrolyte-free infusion, such as dextrose 5% in water.
Excess sodium	• Increased sodium promotes water reabsorption.
Decreased Excretion	
Renal disease	• Kidney cannot excrete excess fluid.
Increased antidiuretic hormone	• More chronic disease in older adults. • Increase in osmolality of extracellular fluid (water loss, sodium gain), reduced blood volume, pain, stress (emotional and physiological), medications (such as morphine, barbiturates, general anesthetics). • Excessive stress activates hypothalamic center, causing release of both antidiuretic hormone and adrenocorticotropic hormone.
Increased Capillary Permeability	
Sepsis, inflammatory processes, major trauma and burns, acid-base imbalance	• Increased capillary permeability allows more fluid to leak into the interstitial spaces, causing fluid excess or edema.
Hypoproteinemia	
Decreased intake or increased loss	• Any state of decreased protein, regardless of etiology, results in a decrease in capillary colloid osmotic pressure that impairs reabsorption. Excess fluid is left in the interstitial spaces, causing edema.

Fluid intake

Ingested water	1200-1500 mL
Ingested food	800-1100 mL
Metabolic oxidation	300 mL
TOTAL	2300-2900 mL

Fluid output

Kidneys	1500 mL
Insensible loss through skin	600-800 mL
Insensible loss through lungs	400-600 mL
Gastrointestinal tract	100 mL
TOTAL	2600-3000 mL

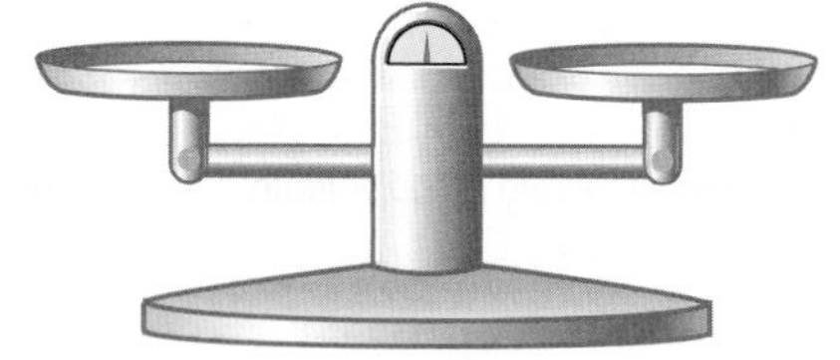

FIGURE 26-6 Sources of fluid intake and fluid output.

Hypoproteinemia, or decreased protein in the plasma, either from decreased intake or increased loss, results in decreased intravascular oncotic pressure. This ultimately leads to hypotension because of reduced fluid reabsorption at the venous end of the capillary.

Exercise. Exercise, especially in a hot, humid environment, is a risk factor for fluid deficit. In fact, a water loss of only 1.2% has been found to impair thermoregulation. A fluid loss of only 2% can cause increased heart rate, increased body temperature, and decreased plasma volume. It is not just one factor but the relationship of the temperature and humidity that determines a person's response. In an athlete, a low temperature with a high humidity or a high temperature with a low humidity can cause fatal heat strokes (see Chapter 28).

Stress. Regardless of whether a stressor stems from a physiological, psychological, environmental, or other cause, the body's response will vary with the client's perception of the seriousness of the stressor, degree of physical damage, and ability to adapt to the insult. Any significant stressor activates the general adaptation system, which trigger hypothalamic releasing factors that stimulate the anterior pituitary to release ACTH. ACTH, in turn, stimulates the adrenal cortex to release cortisol and aldosterone. Cortisol heals damaged capillary membranes to decrease capillary leaking and increases sodium and thereby water retention. Aldosterone has an even stronger influence on sodium retention. Both promote the loss of potassium. If the stressor results in marked hypokalemia, metabolic alkalosis may also result. This occurs because when potassium moves from cells into the plasma, hydrogen ions move from the plasma into cells, increasing the risk for metabolic alkalosis.

DEVELOPMENTAL FACTORS

Everyone is at risk for fluid and electrolyte imbalance, but older adults and the very young are at greatest risk because of their varying water distribution (Table 26-5).

Infants and Children. The younger the child, the greater the risk for fluid deficit. This is partly because after fetal development, the highest growth rate, and thereby the

Table 26-5 Proportion of Body Water by Age

AGE	PERCENT OF BODY WEIGHT
Neonate	77
6 months	72
2-16 years	60
20-39 years	59 (women) to 60 (men)
40-59 years	47 (women) to 55 (men)
65 years and older	45 to 50

greatest metabolic activity, is during infancy. Infants and children also have immature kidneys with a decreased ability to concentrate urine. In addition, an increased body surface area compared with weight leads to increased fluid loss through the skin. Compensatory mechanisms are also less efficient.

Adolescents and Middle-Age Adults. Adolescents have an increased risk for fluid deficit because of an increase in hormonal activity and increased loss with exercise-related activities. Teenagers who become pregnant further compromise their health because of the increased demands of the fetus during a time when their own bodies have an increased need.

Middle-age adults are the age-group least at risk for fluid imbalance. Developmentally, however, the demands of work-related activities and family rearing can increase the risk for self-care deficit. Pregnancy does increase the need for fluid because of fetal demands and tissue changes.

Older Adults. The older adult is more at risk for fluid imbalances because of the increased incidence of chronic diseases. Fluid deficit, or dehydration, is the most common fluid and electrolyte problem in the older adult population. Even healthy older adults have a decreased thirst mechanism. The older adult kidney also has a decreased ability to concentrate urine. Lack of access to food purchasing because of financial, health, or transportation barriers also lead to decreased intake. Older adults usually take more medications, over-the-counter (OTC) or prescribed, than any other age-group. The most common side effects of most of these medications are nausea, vomiting, and diarrhea.

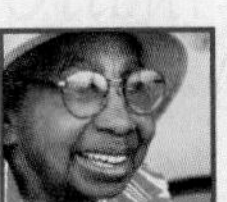

Referring to the case study, Mrs. Thompson was drinking less. She should be assessed for losing fluid by four routes. Increased perspiration, diarrhea, vomiting, and, to a lesser extent, rapid respiration each contributed to the dehydration she experienced. Remember that in the early phases of Mrs. Thompson's fluid deficit, her body compensated. Recall that thirst was not a compensatory mechanism for her because of advancing age. Possible manifestations of oliguria, constipation, and dry skin are expected responses to her body's need to conserve fluid. As her regulatory systems could no longer compensate, she became very ill.

PHYSIOLOGICAL FACTORS

The most common physiological factors that increase the risk for fluid, electrolyte, and acid-base problems are pathological processes, stressors, or treatments that affect the cardiovascular, respiratory, GI, renal, and integumentary systems. Trauma can affect any one or a combination of these systems.

Uncommon, but just as serious, is the risk for fluid deficit caused by alterations in adrenal gland function. Hypoaldosteronism can lead to severe sodium deficit and thus fluid loss. Hyperaldosteronism and Cushing's syndrome both increase the risk for fluid retention secondary to sodium retention. Certain cancers (some lymphomas and bronchogenic, pancreatic, and prostatic cancers) also increase the risk for fluid overload secondary to the increased secretion of ADH (also called vasopressin) from the tumor cells.

Cardiovascular Problems. Cardiovascular diseases can lead to a state of weakness or inability to access fluids and food products so that a deficit results. More common, however, is fluid overload caused by heart disease. When the left ventricle cannot contract efficiently, the buildup of fluid pressure has a retrograde effect, causing an increase in left atrial pressure followed by increased pulmonary pressure, which leads to pulmonary congestion.

The most critical consequence of left ventricular failure is pulmonary edema. This can lead to a subsequent increase in right ventricular pressure, followed by systemic fluid overload. Excess fluid or sodium intake in a person who has cardiac or renal dysfunction will only further exacerbate the fluid overload.

Respiratory Problems. Any situation or pathological condition that increases the respiratory rate also increases the amount of fluid and CO_2 lost in expired air.

Gastrointestinal Problems. Many GI problems, including vomiting, diarrhea, ileostomies, and fistulas, lead to fluid loss. Prescribed therapies such as gastric or bowel suction also increase fluid loss. Decreased fluid intake, as in dysphagia, is a common factor in dehydration. The most common GI pathological process that causes fluid overload is liver disease.

Renal Problems. End-stage renal disease is usually characterized by polyuric, oliguric, and anuric phases. During the polyuric phase, a client is at risk for *Deficient fluid volume.* In the oliguric and anuric phases, *Excess fluid volume* predominates because of excessive retention of fluid.

Integumentary Problems. Loss of the protective skin barrier results in increased fluid loss. Blisters that accompany partial-thickness burns are filled with fluid that is no longer available to the body. This process by which fluid moves into an area that makes it physiologically unavailable is known as **third spacing.** Other examples of third spacing include the movement of fluid into the peritoneal space (ascites), the pericardial space (pericardial effusion), and the pleural space (pleural effusion).

Protein loss from burn wounds into the interstitial spaces results in decreased plasma colloid osmotic pressure. The etiology of the resulting edema is twofold: impaired reabsorption of water into the capillaries and increased interstitial oncotic pressure. Hypoproteinemia is a common example of how an extracellular fluid deficit (in the plasma) can exist at the same time as an extracellular fluid excess (in the interstitium).

Trauma. As with burns, tissue damage from any type of trauma can lead to fluid loss. Metabolites released at the time of cell damage trigger the inflammatory process, which in turn stimulates release of byproducts that increase capillary permeability. Increasing permeability allows more fluid to shift from plasma into the interstitial space. This extra interstitial fluid is not available to aid in maintaining body functions, and it alters gas and nutrient exchange in the involved tissues.

Protein loss from traumatized tissues is also a consequence of increased capillary permeability and has the same manifestations as burn trauma. Sepsis, a possible complication of trauma, promotes increased capillary permeability and more fluid, electrolyte, and protein loss.

A client with head trauma may develop either fluid deficit or fluid excess. Head trauma can result in diabetes insipidus or a syndrome of inappropriate antidiuretic hormone (SIADH). Diabetes insipidus manifests with polyuria (2 to 15 L of urine daily), which can lead to severe fluid deficits. SIADH results in an obligatory increase in ADH, a secondary decrease in urinary output, and thus a risk for fluid overload.

CLINICAL FACTORS

Many interventions can increase a client's risk for fluid imbalance. They include surgery, chemotherapy, medications, suctioning, and long-term use of IV therapy.

Surgery. Clients are at risk both before and after surgery. The longer the client has had nothing by mouth or has had a decreased intake or increased loss before surgery, the greater the risk of intraoperative and postoperative complications. For example, preoperative preparations such as cathartics or enemas, as well as excessive blood loss during or after surgery, can cause a fluid volume deficit. Infection is still one of the most common postoperative complications. The fever, diaphoresis, and tachypnea that accompany infection increase fluid loss.

Chemotherapy. Many chemotherapeutic drugs cause GI cell damage, leading to frequent complications of stomatitis, anorexia, taste changes, nausea, and vomiting. These effects promote fluid deficit through a decreased intake or an increased loss. Fluid volume excess is also a risk with chemotherapeutic drugs that increase the release of ADH, such as vincristine (Oncovin), cyclophosphamide (Cytoxan), vinblastine (Velban), cisplatin (Platinol-AQ), and oxytocin (Pitocin).

Medications. Medications that cause fluid loss (such as diuretics) and adverse effects that result in fluid loss (such as vomiting and diarrhea) are common causes of fluid deficit. For example, elixirs that contain sorbitol, which may be used to promote bowel elimination, can cause diarrhea in some people.

Medications such as insulin and oral antidiabetics are commonly used to control the hyperglycemia of diabetes mellitus. Hyperglycemia, regardless of the cause, increases fluid loss secondary to the osmotic effect of the glucose molecule in the renal tubules.

General anesthetics, barbiturates, and some opioids (such as morphine) increase the secretion of ADH, which increases the risk for fluid excess. Glucocorticoids and mineralocorticoids increase sodium retention and, consequently, water retention. Taken in excess, any medication that contains sodium, such as an OTC antacid, increases the risk of water retention. Some medications increase the secretion of ADH and thus increase fluid retention. They include carbamazepine (Tegretol), many opioids (including morphine), and several barbiturates.

Gastrointestinal Intubation. GI intubation is performed for one of two reasons: to empty the stomach contents or to provide an alternative route for nutrients (Procedure 26-1). When a nasogastric (NG) tube is placed for purposes of gastric emptying (decompression), it increases the client's risk for fluid deficit. After insertion, you will need to monitor the client for fluid and electrolyte deficit and metabolic alkalosis. Once therapy is successful, the tube can be removed (Procedure 26-2).

The second most common use for an NG tube is to provide a route for foods or fluids for a client who cannot take them by mouth (see Chapter 25). Diarrhea resulting in fluid deficit is a common complication of tube feedings. The two most common sources of diarrhea secondary to tube feedings are the use of hypertonic feedings and a rapid delivery rate. The increased osmolality of hypertonic feedings promotes fluid shifting into the small bowel, which can result in diarrhea and dehydration. Likewise, the client may not tolerate a rapid delivery of a feeding and may develop diarrhea. Giving water boluses with hypertonic feedings and either giving feedings slowly or diluting them will decrease these risks.

Intravenous Therapy. Many clients receive IV therapy as part of their treatment. If the client's IV fluid intake is not adequate to meet maintenance and replacement needs, a risk for fluid deficit exists. For example, a client who is receiving IV therapy over several days with no other source of intake is at risk for fluid deficit as well as electrolyte deficit. Fluids, sodium, and potassium are required on a daily basis to maintain homeostasis. When a client has been 3 or more days without food through the oral or enteral route, an IV approach is chosen to provide these nutrients.

When an IV route is used to provide carbohydrates, proteins, fats, and other electrolytes, it is known as total parenteral nutrition (see Chapter 25). You must monitor the client for hyperglycemia and secondary polyuria because of the risk for osmotic diuresis from the high glucose levels in the solution. Frequent monitoring of capillary glucose readings and administration of regular insulin on a sliding scale will prevent this syndrome.

TIME TO ALLOW: **NOVICE:** 20 min. **EXPERT:** 5 min.

PROCEDURE 26-1 INSERTING AND MAINTAINING A NASOGASTRIC TUBE

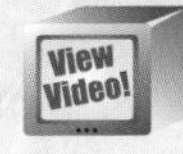

Decompression relieves pressure by removing gas and fluids from the stomach. It can be used to prevent nausea, vomiting, and gastric distention when GI tract motility is slow or absent, when the client has a bowel obstruction, or when the client has a fresh abdominal suture line that must be protected.

DELEGATION GUIDELINES

The complex assessment and potential risks associated with inserting and maintaining nasogastric (NG) tubes dictate that this procedure may not be delegated to a nursing assistant. However, you may delegate the gathering and assembly of the necessary equipment, along with the measurement, recording, and testing of nasogastric drainage. The temporary discontinuation of suction for purposes of toileting or ambulation may be appropriate for delegation under RN supervision. Reconnection of the NG tube to the suction device necessitates RN verification of the suction pressure settings.

EQUIPMENT NEEDED

- Single-lumen or double-lumen nasogastric tube
- Water-soluble lubricant or water to be used as lubricant
- Portable suction machine or wall suction outlet
- Collection device, short tubing to attach collection device to suction, and long tubing to attach suction to distal end of nasogastric tube
- Five-in-one connector to connect nasogastric tube to suction tubing
- Clean gloves
- Tongue blade and penlight
- Glass of water with a straw
- Towel or drape to place across the client's chest
- Emesis basin
- 50- or 60-mL cone-tipped syringe
- Specified dressing for securing tube to nose (tape, Y-shaped dressing, or clear, 2 × 2 inch dressing)
- Safety pin and rubber band
- pH test strip

1 Perform preliminary actions (see inside front cover).

2 Prepare the equipment.

a. Arrange all equipment on a small table or bedside stand.

b. Prepare the dressing needed to secure the tube to the client's nose. If using tape, tear a 3-inch strip of 1-inch tape and make a 1½-inch horizontal tear up the center of this strip. If using a clear occlusive dressing, open the package.

c. Check the suction apparatus. Attach the collection device to the suction apparatus and the tubing. Make sure the lid is on the canister tightly and turn on the suction to confirm a pressure of 80 to 100 mm Hg.

3 Prepare the client.

a. Place the client in a position that enhances the client's ability to assist you by swallowing. Usually, high Fowler's position (head of the bed elevated 60 to 90 degrees) is the best position to allow the client to bring his or her head forward to swallow. If this position is contraindicated or the client is unconscious, it may be necessary to keep him in a recumbent position.

b. Determine which of the client's nostrils is most open. Occlude one of the client's nostrils and listen while he or she breathes through the other nostril. Repeat the process on the opposite side to compare openness. Also inspect the nose for septal deviation, ask the client about any history of a broken nose or problems with past intubations, if applicable.

Continued

4 Pass the tube.

a. Find the proper length for the nasogastric tube by measuring from the client's nose to the earlobe and then to the xiphoid process (see illustration).

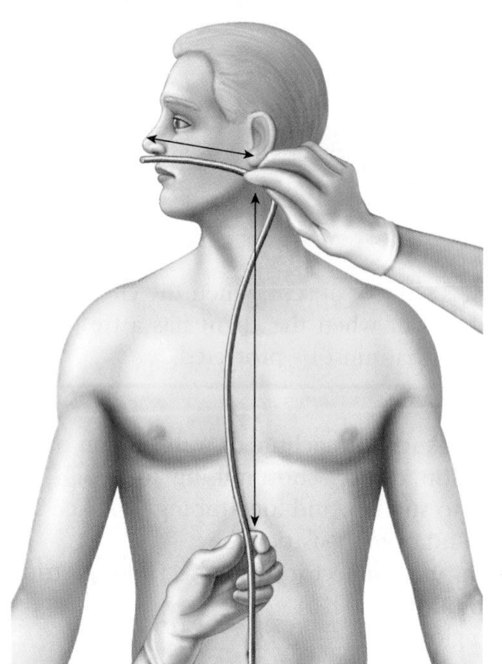

Step 4a. Measuring the insertion length of the nasogastric tube.

b. Mark the length of tube to be passed with a small piece of tape partially around the tube, and then lubricate the final 3 inches at the tip of the tube.
c. With the client's head in a neutral position, insert the tube through the client's most patent nostril and pass it through to the nasopharynx. Have the client tilt the head slightly forward while holding the water glass in one hand. Grasp the lubricated tube with your dominant hand about 6 inches from the end. Place your forefinger on the top and your thumb on the bottom. When you reach the posterior part of the nostril, press your thumb and forefinger together to bend the tube, thus facilitating advancement past the sharp curvature of the nasopharynx.
d. Once you clear the client's epiglottis, have the client bend the head forward (touching chin to chest), advance the tube until you reach the tape marker, indicating that the tube has reached the stomach. *The client's epiglottis must be closed as the tube passes to prevent the tube from entering the trachea. Ask the client to sip water through the straw and, each time the client swallows, advance the tube. If the client cannot swallow, have the client hold his or her breath to close the epiglottis. If the client is unconscious, watch his or her respirations. If the client begins coughing or becomes cyanotic at any time, remove the tube immediately. If the client gags or vomits, stop advancing the tube but leave it in place if possible. Give the client an emesis basin, if appropriate, and allow the client to rest for a moment.*

5 Connect the tube to suction, and ensure client safety.

a. Tape the tube to the nose using only one side of the split tape to maintain the position while verifying placement (see illustration).

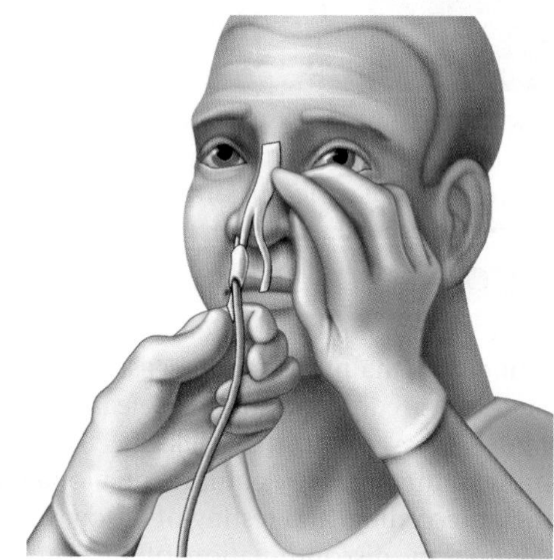

Step 5a. Taping the nasogastric tube to decrease trauma to the nares.

b. Verify tube placement in the stomach. Attach the cone-shaped syringe to the tubing, and aspirate for gastric secretions. If no gastric secretions appear, advance the tube 2 inches more and repeat the test. *Gastric secretions are usually greenish to off-white unless a bleeding problem exists, which may be presented as bright red or brownish secretions.*
c. Check for gastric pH by aspirating stomach contents and dipping the pH test strip into the contents. *Contents from the stomach usually have a pH of less than 5. Although usually a good indicator, medications as well as blood can alter the pH.*
d. Use the five-in-one connector to attach the distal end of the tube to the tubing marked "to patient" on the lid of the suction collection device.
e. Finish taping the tube to the client's nose using the method specified by your facility.
f. Attach the tubing to the gown with a rubber band and safety pin. *By leaving some slack in the tube when you affix it to the gown, you can prevent accidental pulling on the tube when the client turns his or her head.*
g. Set the suction control at the prescribed level. *Usually, you will use low intermittent suction (80 to 120 mm Hg) for an adult. Only with a double-lumen tube can you safely use high suction (>120 mm Hg). This is because the sec-*

ond lumen allows constant air exchange and thus prevents gastric tissue trauma from the high suction pressure. The second lumen must be kept clear of secretions to decrease this risk. If you notice secretions in the second lumen, instill about 10 to 20 mL of air into it to displace the secretions.

6 Finish the procedure.

a. Document the reason for the NG tube, your collaboration with the physician, the actual procedure, and the client's response. *Documentation is essential to validate care and provide data for future comparison and follow-up.*

b. Provide comfort care for the client's nose and mouth at least every 8 hours and as needed. Use a clean cotton-tipped swab and water-soluble lubricant to clean the client's nostril. Assess the amount and characteristics of the nasogastric drainage as you provide care. Avoid alcohol-based mouth care agents for oral care because they tend to promote dryness.

7 Monitor the client.

a. Inspect the client's abdomen, and auscultate bowel sounds at least every 8 hours. To decrease the possibility of mistaking suction sounds for bowel sounds, pinch the suction tubing as you auscultate the client's abdomen.

b. Monitor and document the amount and characteristics of the client's NG output, manifestations of deficient fluid volume, low electrolyte levels (especially sodium, potassium, calcium, chloride, and magnesium), or plasma levels that suggest deficient fluid volume (elevated sodium, blood urea nitrogen, and hematocrit).

c. Notify the physician if the client's NG output exceeds 100 mL/hr, if total output exceeds total intake, or if there are new or worsening signs of deficient fluid volume. *Signs of deficient fluid volume include hypotension, a pulse of more than 20 beats per minute above the client's baseline when resting, urine production of less than 30 mL/hr for 2 consecutive hours or more, seizures, confusion, sudden behavioral changes, and abnormal electrolyte levels.*

d. If the client's NG tube stops draining well, first assess the equipment for function errors. If this is not the problem, consult a physician for an irrigation order. Irrigate the tube using a 50- or 60-mL cone-shaped syringe with 30 to 60 mL of normal saline. Repeat as necessary. *Normal saline is the only acceptable irrigating solution because its isotonicity will not further compromise the client's fluid and electrolyte balance. Make sure to compute the difference in the amount of irrigant instilled and the amount removed; subtract or add that figure to the client's 8-hour nasogastric drainage total.*

PEDIATRIC CONSIDERATIONS

Measurement of the tube in an infant or young child is from the nose to the tip of the earlobe and then to the point midway between the umbilicus and the xiphoid process. It is often easier for the child to have the tube placed quickly rather than taking pauses. Another nurse or caregiver (even restraints) may be needed to help hold the hands of a child during placement to keep the child from pulling the tube out. The neck of an infant should remain neutral during placement. Taping the tube to the cheek rather than the gown usually works better in a pediatric client.

GERIATRIC CONSIDERATIONS

A geriatric client may need to rest after the tube has been inserted to the posterior part of the nostril (between steps 4c and 4d) before advancing further into the stomach, especially if the procedure is extremely difficult. In very debilitated older adults, another individual may need to hold the head of the client in a forward position while placement is attempted. An older adult taking antacids or gastric reflux medicines may have a higher pH because of the medications.

PROCEDURE 26-2 REMOVING A NASOGASTRIC TUBE

TIME TO ALLOW: NOVICE: 10 min. EXPERT: 5 min.

This procedure is used to discontinue gastric decompression therapy.

DELEGATION GUIDELINES

The necessity for assessment before discontinuation of a nasogastric (NG) tube, the risk of aspiration associated with tube removal, and the short nature of this procedure suggest that this procedure not be delegated to a nursing assistant.

EQUIPMENT NEEDED

- Clean gloves
- Towel
- Emesis basin
- Plastic bag
- 50- or 60-mL syringe
- Tissue
- Stethoscope

Continued

1 Perform preliminary actions (see inside front cover).

2 Prepare the client.

a. Before removing the tube, assess for the presence of bowel sounds. *Do not remove the tube if bowel sounds are absent.*

b. Place the emesis basin and opened plastic bag on a nearby table, put on clean gloves, and place the towel across the client's upper chest.

c. Turn off the suction machine, and disconnect the NG tube from the suction tubing.

d. Unpin the NG tube from the client's gown, or untape from the cheek.

e. Prevent stomach contents from leaking from the tube as it passes the glottis. Instill 20 mL of air into the NG tube to displace secretions back into the client's stomach, or pinch the tube as you remove it. *Doing so decreases the client's risk of aspiration.* Don't flush with air or saline if there is doubt about placement.

f. Loosen the tape on the client's nose while holding the distal end of the NG tube.

3 Remove the tube. Instruct the client to hold his or her breath, and then pull the tube out in one quick, steady motion. Note the intactness of the tip of the tube.

4 Finish the procedure.

a. Assist with or provide skin and mouth care.

b. Document the presence of bowel sounds, the tube removal procedure, and the client's response.

c. Continue to monitor the client's bowel status.

ASSESSMENT

GENERAL ASSESSMENT OF FLUID BALANCE

Perform a general health history to gather baseline data that will help you screen for specific risk factors. Also, focus your physical assessment on systems that are related to the fluid imbalance.

Health History. Because fluid and electrolyte imbalances affect so many systems, a complete history and a physical examination are necessary. Begin the health history by gathering more data about the client's chief complaint. When the problem is related to fluid and electrolyte deficit, the client's chief complaint is usually related to one of the following: nausea, vomiting, diarrhea, anorexia, increasing fatigue and weakness, weight loss, fever, blood loss, excess urine output, or a change in mental status. Or the client's chief complaint may be a condition or a traumatic injury, such as a burn, in which manifestations of a fluid and electrolyte imbalance might be hidden by the more obvious problem of the injury itself.

When the problem is related to fluid and electrolyte excess, the client's chief complaint is usually related to one of the following: weight gain, cough, dyspnea, cardiac palpitations, pitting edema, decreased urinary output, or mental status changes.

Whatever the chief complaint, determine the characteristics of the client's symptoms, including the onset, location and radiation if applicable, frequency, severity, associated signs and symptoms, and aggravating or alleviating factors, and the client's previous history or treatment of this problem.

Also, assess the client's past history of illnesses, hospitalizations, surgeries, trauma, allergies, current or recent medication, and currency of immunizations. Obtain an obstetrical history if applicable. Collect data related to family history and psychosocial history, and then complete the review of systems. If the client's condition is acute, collect data pertinent to the immediate problem, and intervene quickly. When possible, obtain additional history from family members or old records and complete the history when the client's condition stabilizes.

Physical Examination. A full head-to-toe physical examination may be necessary for an accurate diagnosis. Again, if the client's condition is critical, collect only the data needed for safe and immediate intervention. In addition to the initial physical examination, an accurate diagnosis of fluid and electrolyte imbalances often requires monitoring the client's intake and output, weight trends, edema levels, diagnostic tests, and ongoing physical assessments.

Standard Clinical Measurements. A basic understanding of standard measurements related to fluid balance is essential to assessing and evaluating a client's fluid status. Volume is commonly measured in liters (L) and milliliters (mL). Weight is commonly measured in grams (g) and milligrams (mg). See Chapter 21 for additional information on volume and weight measurements. Protein is reported on a laboratory result in g/100 mL of fluid. The normal serum protein range is 6 to 8 g/100 mL.

The **milliequivalent** (mEq), one thousandth of a chemical equivalent, is the measurement used to express the chemical activity or chemical combining power of an ion. Although electrolytes have variable milligram weights, the weight has no relationship to its chemical combining power. One mEq of any electrolyte is chemically equal to 1 mEq of any other electrolyte. Chemical neutrality, an equal number of milliequivalents of cations and anions, must be present for normal neuromuscular excitability to occur.

Weighing the Client. When the accuracy of intake and output measurements is uncertain, or when the client has generalized body edema, a client's weight is a better and more critical indicator of fluid loss or gain. One kilogram (kg) or 2.2 pounds is equal to 1 liter (1000 mL) of fluid loss or gain.

Because interventions are based on the data obtained from weight assessments, standardization is very important. Standardization includes weighing the client at the same time of day (preferably early morning after voiding but before food or fluid intake), with the same amount of clothing, and on the same scale. When any of these standards are unavoidably changed, the documentation should reflect this change.

Measuring Intake and Output. Measure intake and output (I&O) whenever a fluid imbalance exists or the client is at risk. This can initiated by nurses and does not require an order by a health care provider. The decision requires knowledge of who is at risk for fluid imbalance and who has an actual imbalance, as well as appropriate assessment skills. Measurement of I&O will be used most often in acute care settings, where clients have higher acuity levels and are at greater risk for complications, but should be done whenever there is a need for careful monitoring of fluid balance.

Most clients in a chronic care setting are older adults. Because dehydration is the most common fluid imbalance in this group, prevention is the key. Give fluids frequently throughout the day and early evening to help prevent this problem. Monitor I&O for any client at risk for or experiencing an actual fluid volume deficit or excess.

When the problem is fluid overload, assessing the specific systems should be made in addition to measuring I&O. For example, if the client's primary problem is pulmonary congestion, an increase in lung crackles would indicate a worsening condition. In contrast, a decrease in crackles is a positive response to interventions.

Remember to measure I&O from all sources. Intake includes fluids taken orally, by tube, or by IV. Fluid output includes urine, diarrhea, vomitus, suction, wound drainage, diaphoresis, hyperventilation, and other drainage. Insensible fluid loss (through normal breathing and the skin) and sensible fluid loss (through hyperventilation or diaphoresis) should also be considered in analyzing data about fluid balance.

In situations where I&O is critical and normal urinary output cannot be measured, it may be necessary to compare the weight of the clean or dry product that is used (e.g., linens, pads, diapers) with the weight of the soiled or wet product. The difference in grams is equal to the output in milliliters.

To perform an I&O measurement accurately, use the appropriate measurement device for the quantity being measured (e.g., a medicine cup for amounts less than 30 mL, or a graduated cylinder to measure 100 to 1000 mL). Other tools include appropriate documentation forms, such as an I&O form (Figure 26-7). Add the intake recorded at various times during the shift in each column (oral, IV, tube feedings, other) to determine the total shift intake of the item in that column. Add the shift totals for all intake columns to determine total shift intake. Use the same process to record and measure output. Add together the shift totals for intake and then for output to determine the 24-hour intake and output totals for a specific client.

Action Alert! Note 24-hour fluid intake and output trends over days of time to determine whether the client is maintaining or regaining fluid balance.

It is essential to document and communicate the amount of IV fluid that is left hanging for the next shift to count. This is known as the "credit" or "claim." For example, if a client receives 1000 mL IV every 8 hours and had 600 mL from the current bag and 350 mL from the previous IV bag, the client received 950 mL. The credit for the next shift, from the current 1000 mL bag, is 400 mL (difference of 1000 − 600). If you use a pump form of delivery, you may just clear the 8-hour intake of feeding or IV fluid and leave the next shift with a starting base of 0 instead of a credit.

Other essential tools include appropriate elimination collection devices (fracture pan or regular bedpan, specimen collection devices for toilet or commode, or urinal) and clean disposable gloves. Some fluid collection devices have graduations marked on the container. It is acceptable to use these if the measurement can be made accurately.

Adaptation to the home setting includes teaching the client and family how to keep a diary of fluid intake and output. Suggest a simple notebook with a column for the client's sources of intake, a column for measured output, a column for date and time (if appropriate), and a column for other essential data (such as a description of drainage). Graduated measuring cups normally used for cooking purposes will facilitate accuracy. Other supplies—such as a graduated cylinder, specimen pan, bedpan, or urinal—may need to be purchased at a local pharmacy or medical supply outlet.

Your assessment should include the client's and family's willingness and readiness to learn and their level of understanding of the importance of I&O monitoring. It also includes assessing functional abilities, financial resources and barriers, and developmental, cultural, and religious variables. Collaborate closely with the social worker to maximize care, such as purchasing a bedside commode or other equipment that is constrained by financial barriers.

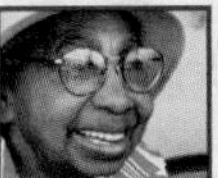

Referring to the case study, Mrs. Thompson was very willing to learn but was not capable of cooking or shopping because of extreme fatigue and weakness. Developmentally, her decreased thirst mechanism interfered with her perception of fluid need. Culturally, she did not like the prepared food items available at the local grocery store. However, because she raised her children with the strong African American value of family bonding, she had them as a resource. Daily, one of the children assisted her with I&O monitoring and grocery shopping and provided many of her favorite food dishes.

Elkins Park Medical Center

Intake and Output Record

Patient Label
Patient name ____________
ID# ____________
Physician ____________

	Date:	0700 – 1900		1700 – 0900	
Intake	Oral				
	Tube feeding				
	Intravenous	Intake	Credit	Intake	Credit
	Primary				
	Secondary				
	Blood products				
	TPN				
	Other				
Output	Urine				
	Gastric				
	Emesis				
	Suction				
	Stool				
	Other				
Total 24° Intake =			**Total 24° Output =**		

FIGURE 26-7 I&O form. A standard I&O form should include all of the common sources of intake and output to provide cues to the caregiver. Compare the total intake and output over several days with weight changes to identify trends in fluid excess or deficits.

Assessing Edema. Edema scales vary among different institutions. If your facility has an edema scale, all personnel should use that scale to promote continuity in assessment. If no scale is available, measure the level of pitting edema by assessing the residual indentation left by pressing your finger into the area for 5 seconds (+1 edema is mild and +4 is severe; see Figure 26-8). Document the site, the depth of the tissue indentation in millimeters (mm), and the time needed for the tissue to spring back.

Assessment for pitting edema works well with small, localized edematous areas, such as the sacrum, feet, ankles, or tibia. In situations where the edema is more pronounced, however, such as when it involves the entire leg, thigh, or abdomen, you will need a more objective assessment. Because consistency is important, mark the site you are measuring with a marker. Use a centimeter tape to measure the circumference of the leg, thigh, or abdomen. Document the measurement and compare against earlier data for changes. When a client has generalized body edema, called anasarca, weighing is more accurate.

Diagnostic Tests. The serum levels most commonly used to indicate dehydration or fluid volume deficit are serum sodium, serum and urine osmolality, hematocrit, and blood urea nitrogen (BUN). The sodium ion is used as a direct measure of osmolality because it is the major ion in extracellular fluid. Serum sodium, osmolality, hematocrit, and BUN levels are elevated in fluid volume deficit because there is less fluid in relation to the same amount of solutes (called hemoconcentration). BUN levels may also be elevated in individuals with a high-protein diet. Urine osmolality is also increased secondary to the release of ADH and aldosterone. The kidney still excretes an obligatory amount of urine to rid the body of waste products of metabolism; this is about 30 mL of urine per hour.

Urine osmolality is measured and reported by the laboratory. Less commonly, you may be asked to test specific gravity (SG) using a test tube and a floating urinometer. If you test urine SG, obtain enough urine to half fill the test tube, spin the urinometer inside the test tube, and read the level of the calibrated mark on the urinometer as it is spinning. Normal specific gravity is 1.005 to 1.026. A specific gravity less than 1.005 indicates excess fluid intake, and greater than 1.026 indicates decreased fluid intake.

Osmolality measurement is often ordered when the concentrating ability of the kidney is being evaluated. This function is significant because, if the kidney cannot

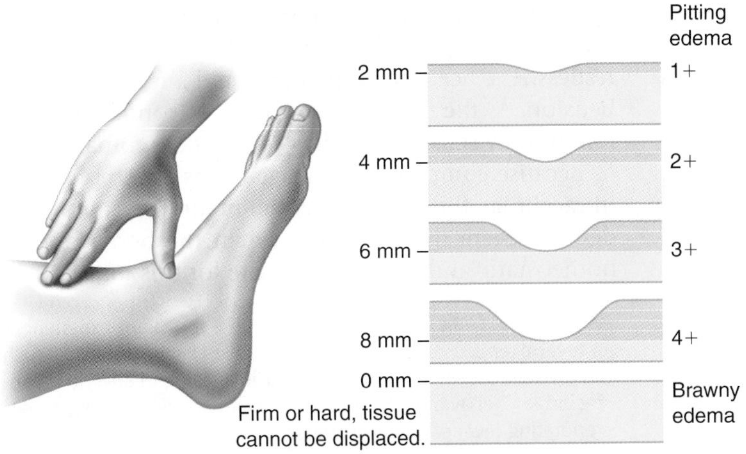

Pitting edema
2 mm 1+
4 mm 2+
6 mm 3+
8 mm 4+
0 mm Brawny edema
Firm or hard, tissue cannot be displaced.

FIGURE 26-8 Assessment of pitting edema using a four-point scale. Press on the area being assessed and note the depth in indentation. Record depth as 1+ to 4+ as shown.

concentrate urine, the client loses more fluid and develops a fluid volume deficit. Remember that, in the body, it is the *relationship* of the solute (such as sodium, protein, glucose, or urea) to the solvent (water) that determines the body's response, not the level itself.

Decreased BUN, hematocrit, sodium, and serum osmolality are classic laboratory findings with excess fluid volume. Because these levels represent the relationship of the plasma solvent to the solute, they appear to be decreased when actually they are just diluted in greater amounts of fluid (called hemodilution).

When plasma levels tend toward the unexpected or the client presents with manifestations that suggest a specific pathological process for a fluid volume deficit or excess, the physician will order other serum studies or diagnostic tests. For example, creatinine levels can help evaluate renal dysfunction, liver function studies can reveal liver pathological condition, and glucose studies can show glucose intolerance.

Serum levels are accurate indicators of potassium, sodium, and chloride levels. However, because potassium is primarily an intracellular ion, small deficits in the serum level are very reflective of a decrease in total body potassium. Indeed, a level of 3.4 mEq/L, a deficit of only 0.1 mEq/L, requires potassium replacement. On the other hand, the serum level of sodium, which is predominantly extracellular, gives a much more accurate presentation of total body sodium levels. A client rarely needs replacement if sodium levels exceed 125 mEq/L.

The serum calcium level helps identify imbalances but can become a false indicator if the client has abnormal albumin levels, an acid-base imbalance, or hypoparathyroidism. Because 99% of the calcium in plasma is bound to albumin and only 0.5% is free (ionized), the amount of albumin has an inverse relationship to the level of functional ionized calcium. For example, when a client has a protein deficit, less calcium is bound, resulting in an increase in free calcium. The serum level (the bound version) may appear normal when in reality the ionized calcium is higher. The reverse is true when a client has an excess protein intake. The client presents with signs of hypocalcemia because of the excess binding of the calcium to the protein, which leaves less free, ionized calcium.

Alkalosis and acidosis also affect the calcium binding and result in similar manifestations. For example, in alkalosis, more calcium is bound and thus less is ionized, so the client presents with signs of hypocalcemia. In acidosis, less calcium is bound, leaving more free ionized calcium. The client presents with signs of hypercalcemia. In any client with critical calcium regulation, a serum ionized calcium test should be performed to discover the true functional level of calcium.

Magnesium serum levels are not commonly ordered because they have not proved accurate as indicators of cellular levels. Assessment of tendon reflexes has been suggested as a more accurate indicator of magnesium imbalance than serum level.

Because the cardiac conduction system is so sensitive to electrolyte imbalance, an electrocardiogram (ECG) is a helpful diagnostic test. The more serious and acute the imbalance, the more grave the changes are on the ECG.

Arterial blood gases (ABGs) are essential to properly diagnose acid-base imbalances. If only oxygenation data are necessary, an oxygenation saturation level can easily be obtained using pulse oximetry.

FOCUSED ASSESSMENT FOR *DEFICIENT FLUID VOLUME*

Fluid deficit is a common problem. Many pathological processes and situations increase the risk for or result in fluid deficit. Recognizing and intervening in high-risk situations or in early phases of fluid deficit are very important to the client's outcome.

Defining Characteristics. The official definition for *Deficient fluid volume* does not differentiate between vascular, interstitial, and intracellular dehydration. Although all compartments are interactive, the cellular compartment is the last to be affected by a fluid deficit. This is because the body's homeostatic mechanisms attempt to

BOX 26-1 *Characteristics of Extracellular Fluid Deficit*

GENERALIZED
- Flattened neck veins in supine position
- Sudden weight loss, unless masked by third spacing
- Peripheral vein filling takes more than 5 seconds
- Decreased skin turgor (not accurate in older adults)
- Dry mucous membranes and furrowed tongue
- Speech changes
- Muscle weakness, especially in upper body
- Subnormal temperature if severe loss, fever if moderate loss
- Depressed fontanels in an infant
- Soft and sunken eyeballs

CARDIAC
- Orthostatic hypotension (systolic blood pressure [BP] falls more than 25 mm Hg and diastolic BP falls more than 20 mm Hg) with compensatory tachycardia (up to 120 beats per minute)
- Weak, thready pulse
- Narrow pulse pressure

GASTROINTESTINAL
- Constipation or decrease in number and moisture of stools

RENAL
- Urinary output greatly exceeding intake if this is the etiology of the deficit
- Urinary output decreased if compensatory response

correct the deficit. Therefore early recognition and intervention targeted at reversing extracellular fluid deficit will help prevent intracellular dehydration.

Extracellular. Box 26-1 provides a list of defining characteristics and age-related manifestations common in a client with extracellular fluid deficit. Muscle weakness results primarily from the altered relationship of fluid to sodium. The decreased plasma volume is responsible for the compensatory increase in pulse rate, orthostatic hypotension, prolonged peripheral vein filling, decreased central venous pressure, flattened neck veins, and compensatory conservation of fluid by the bowel and kidneys.

No single manifestation increases morbidity or mortality as long as compensatory mechanisms or planned interventions reverse the deficit. However, cerebral manifestations indicate cerebral cell involvement that could result in irreversible cerebral tissue damage.

Action Alert! Notify the physician if a client experiences a rapid, unexpected weight loss (more than 3 pounds/day); vomiting or diarrhea that lasts more than 24 hours in a child, pregnant woman, older adult, or a person with chronic disease; or unexplained tachycardia or other atypical cardiac irregularities.

Intracellular. Intracellular dehydration is much more serious than extracellular dehydration because of the potential dysfunction of mitochondrial formation of ATP; ATP is critical to all cell function and transport. Defining characteristics include fever, thirst, and central nervous system changes. Shrinkage of cerebral cells stimulates osmoreceptors in the hypothalamus, which triggers the thirst mechanism. The fluid imbalance also disrupts cortical functioning. Early cerebral manifestations include restlessness, headache, irritability, and a feeling of apprehension. As the fluid deficit progresses, confusion occurs, followed by seizures and, in severe deficit, coma.

Because compensatory mechanisms are so protective, intracellular fluid volume is maintained except in sudden or severe fluid losses or when the body loses the homeostatic ability to compensate for this loss.

Action Alert! Notify the physician if the client experiences a fever over 38.3° C (101° F) or a change in mental status, such as a headache (new, unrelenting, or increasing in severity), confusion, or behavioral changes such as irritability, seizures, or deteriorating level of consciousness.

Related Factors. Many underlying pathological and situational factors can cause fluid volume deficit. Excessive output from the urinary system, GI tract, skin, or respiratory system can result in extracellular deficit followed by intracellular deficit if not corrected. Decreased intake, whether from lack of access to fluids, financial constraints, pathological conditions impairing intake, fatigue, weakness, or the decreased thirst mechanism found in older adults, is the other major contributory factor to fluid deficit. If excess output and insufficient intake coexist, the client is at an even higher risk for more serious consequences. Four major variables determine how critical these manifestations are:
- The acuteness of the loss
- The severity of the loss
- The client's age and state of health
- The degree to which the client's compensatory mechanisms or therapeutic interventions combat the deficit

FOCUSED ASSESSMENT FOR *EXCESS FLUID VOLUME*

Defining Characteristics. Again, the official definition of *Excess fluid volume* does not differentiate between extracellular and intracellular excess. Because the cell is the last compartment to undergo shifting (unless the excess is very acute or massive), it is important to be able to differentiate between extracellular and intracellular changes.

Extracellular. Box 26-2 lists common defining characteristics with extracellular fluid excess. The excess fluid can be localized to a small area of the body and have little or no effect on overall body function. It can be localized to a specific compartment and cause alterations to specific tissues. Or it can be generalized throughout the body and cause major system dysfunction. An example of extracellular fluid excess at the local level is an ankle sprain. As the fluid accumulates around the joint, joint function is compromised.

If generalized manifestations of extracellular excess are present, they are secondary to fluid accumulation either throughout the body or in large body spaces, such

BOX 26-2 *Characteristics of Extracellular Fluid Excess*

GENERALIZED
- Weakness and fatigue
- Body edema (anasarca)
- Pitting or nonpitting edema in dependent areas such as legs, sacrum, and scrotum
- Ascites
- Sudden weight gain of more than 2 pounds/week (1 L of fluid = 2.2 pounds or 1 kg)
- Peripheral venous distention
- Peripheral vein emptying taking more than 5 seconds
- Jugular venous distention (distended neck veins with client sitting at 45 degrees or higher)
- Bulging fontanels in an infant

PULMONARY
- Progressive worsening of dyspnea, from dyspnea on exertion to orthopnea, and finally to dyspnea at rest
- Increased respiratory rate
- Respiratory rhythm may become irregular or apneic
- Crackles present from fluid congestion in alveoli
- Possible pulmonary edema from severe fluid congestion in alveoli secondary to left ventricular failure
- Possible pleural effusion with audible pleural rub from fluid congestion in pleural spaces

CARDIAC
- Tachycardia
- Bounding pulse
- Hypertension (systolic blood pressure >140 mm Hg or diastolic > 90 mm Hg)
- Possible pericardial effusion with audible pericardial rub from fluid congestion in pericardium
- Third heart sound (sometimes called an S_3 gallop) from left ventricular fluid overload

GASTROINTESTINAL
- Anorexia, nausea, and vomiting

RENAL
- Increased output if kidney can compensate
- Decreased output if kidney damage is part of etiology

as in the peritoneum. This is called ascites. As excess fluid accumulates, it interferes with the exchange of nutrients and waste products between the cells and plasma spaces. A buildup of waste products leads to feelings of generalized weakness and fatigue, as well as to manifestations of tissue dysfunction.

An example of localized tissue edema that can have systemic effects is pulmonary fluid overload, or pulmonary edema. In pulmonary overload, manifestations are related to fluid in the alveoli of the lungs, which reduces exchange of O_2 and CO_2. The fluid pressure in the lungs may also lead to shifting of fluid into the pleural spaces, a condition called pleural effusion. This condition decreases the affected lung's ability to expand during inhalation and thus can compromise the body's O_2 status even further.

As with any altered health state, the body attempts to compensate. The cardiac signs of bounding pulse, increased blood pressure, and gallop rhythm are all related to the increased volume of fluid in the heart and blood vessels. The bounding pulse and tachycardia represent the cardiovascular system's attempt to increase cardiac output by increasing the volume of blood ejected with each heart beat (stroke volume) and by increasing the rate. The same phenomenon of effusion in the lungs can occur in the pericardial spaces when the heart suffers from increased fluid overload. As with pleural effusion, pericardial effusion not only compromises cardiac function further but also affects tissue perfusion to the other body systems.

The renal response to fluid overload varies. The decreased osmolality will result in a decrease in ADH secretion. If the kidneys are healthy, this will lead to an increase in urinary output. However, if the kidneys are part of the etiology of the fluid overload, polyuria followed by oliguria and then anuria will occur as the renal function diminishes.

Action Alert! Notify the physician if the client has a rapid weight gain (more than 2 to 3 pounds/day); a new onset of severe pulmonary difficulty (respiratory rate greater than 30; irregular or apneic rhythm, marked increase in crackles or bronchial breath sounds, pleural friction rub); new onset or increased severity of cardiac manifestations (pericardial friction rub, arrhythmia, more than 5 premature beats per minute, a rate less than 50 or greater than 120 beats per minute, an S_3 gallop); or a change in urinary output (marked diuresis without taking a diuretic, output less than 30 mL/hr for 2 or more consecutive hours).

Intracellular. Recall that, in a healthy person, protective mechanisms provide a very delicate balance between intracellular and extracellular fluid compartments. However, many conditions can overpower these protective mechanisms, resulting in abnormal fluid shifting into the intracellular spaces. Because brain cells are very sensitive to minimal changes in fluid balance, the early manifestations of intracellular shifting are cerebral.

Action Alert! Notify the physician if the client shows a change in mental status or cerebral perfusion, such as a new, unrelenting, or worsening headache, confusion, lethargy, irritability, restlessness, or seizures.

The key variable that indicates the need to collaborate with the physician is *change.* This reinforces the importance of thorough and accurate communication and documentation between caregivers. Without this critical communication, client outcomes may be compromised.

Related Factors. Several variables are related to the risk for fluid volume excess. Any increase in fluid intake, sodium intake, or both, especially in the presence of altered excretion, places a person at risk for fluid volume excess. Pathological processes that result in increased capillary permeability or protein loss also increase this risk. The same four variables that determine how critical manifestations are to a person's response to fluid volume deficit also determine how critical fluid volume excess will become.

FOCUSED ASSESSMENT FOR ASSOCIATED PROBLEMS

Electrolyte Imbalances. Because fluid imbalance rarely exists without electrolyte imbalance, you will need a basic knowledge of electrolyte homeostasis to identify risk factors and intervene early. Abnormalities in one or more of the normal control mechanisms commonly cause fluid and electrolyte imbalances. Excess losses through urine, vomiting, suction, diarrhea, tachypnea, and wounds require early intervention, especially in young, older, and compromised clients. Anticipate the risk for imbalance in clients who have pathological conditions or receive medications or treatments that affect the thirst mechanism, thyroid hormones, ADH, aldosterone, baroreceptor responses, and renal or GI regulation of fluids and electrolytes.

The same major variables that affect a client's response to fluid imbalance affect the response to electrolyte imbalance. The more severe and sudden the onset of fluid or electrolyte loss or gain, the less the regulatory systems can compensate for the change. Older adults and the very young are even more at risk when sudden or severe imbalances occur because of the greater inefficiency of their regulatory systems.

Preexisting health abnormalities, especially those that affect regulatory systems—such as the brain, kidney, heart, or bowel—will only increase the client's risk for fluid and electrolyte imbalance. Anticipation of these risks through careful assessment is the key to early intervention and prevention of serious outcomes.

Metabolic Acidosis. Assess for the manifestations of metabolic acidosis in clients who are at high risk, such as those with end-stage renal disease or bicarbonate loss from severe diarrhea, and anyone with hypoxia or hyperglycemia. Neurological assessments identify early signs of metabolic acidosis, such as headaches and a decreased level of consciousness. Apical pulse assessment detects early cardiac dysrhythmias that occur secondary to hypoxia and acidosis. Monitoring for elevated serum glucose levels, urinary ketones, fruity-smelling breath, and hyperpnea in clients at risk for improper fat metabolism (such as a client with diabetes mellitus or malnutrition) will provide early indicators of metabolic acidosis. Nausea, vomiting, and diarrhea are early indicators of GI involvement. The diarrhea is secondary to increasing potassium levels. As metabolic acidosis progresses, life-threatening cardiac dysrhythmias, extreme muscle weakness, and coma ensue.

Arterial blood gas levels will show a pH below 7.35, a decreased bicarbonate level, and variable O_2 and CO_2 levels. If the client has a healthy respiratory system, a compensatory increase in respiratory rate and depth will lower the CO_2 level in an attempt to reduce the acidotic state. If the acidosis is secondary to hypoxia, the partial pressure of O_2 will be decreased. Serum potassium levels are higher because of movement of hydrogen into the cell in exchange for potassium. This is a cellular compensatory mechanism to reduce the acidosis. An exception to hyperkalemia occurs in diabetic ketoacidosis as a result of the loss of potassium that accompanies the osmotic diuresis from hyperglycemia.

Metabolic Alkalosis. Anticipate metabolic alkalosis in clients who have consumed excessive bicarbonate products, lost excessive potassium and hydrochloric acid from vomiting or gastric suction, or lost excessive hydrogen, chloride, and potassium from diuretics or other medications.

Alkalosis has a stimulating effect on the neurological system. Early manifestations include irritability, disorientation, muscle twitching, and paresthesia. Apical pulse assessment will reveal arrhythmias as evidence of early cardiac involvement. Bowel assessment will indicate a hypotonic peristalsis as the potassium level decreases. If the alkalotic state progresses, tetany, convulsions, paralytic ileus, and life-threatening arrhythmias occur.

The diagnostic findings are the opposite of those found in metabolic acidosis: a pH above 7.45, an increase in serum bicarbonate, and a decrease in serum potassium. In addition, a healthy respiratory system attempts to compensate through slow, shallow respirations. The increased retention of carbonic acid is associated with an increase in the partial pressure of CO_2.

> ***Action Alert!*** Notify the physician if the client has an electrolyte or acid-base imbalance (especially if preoperative), a high risk for imbalance, low or borderline serum levels, a urine output that decreases to less than 30 mL/hr when the client receives IV potassium, a marked change in bowel sounds in a high-risk client, a new onset of atypical cardiac irregularities or palpitations, or a new onset of confusion or other alteration in behavior.

As noted earlier, many manifestations are common to more than one imbalance. Table 26-6 lists many of these commonalities.

Respiratory Acidosis and Alkalosis. The respiratory system compensates for pH changes that occur because of metabolic conditions leading to metabolic acidosis or alkalosis. Respiratory alkalosis will occur to compensate for metabolic acidosis and respiratory acidosis will occur to compensate for metabolic alkalosis. These compensatory mechanisms will help to bring the pH back inside the normal range, although they will not correct the primary disorder. See Chapter 34 for detailed discussion of the primary respiratory conditions that cause these acid-base imbalances.

When respiratory acidosis occurs to compensate for metabolic alkalosis, the client's respiratory rate and depth will decrease to help retain CO_2, an acid, to offset the alkalosis. Although the CO_2 level will be high, the

Table 26-6 Diagnostic Clues to Fluid and Electrolyte Imbalances

DIAGNOSTIC CLUE	POSSIBLE IMBALANCE
Thirst	• Decreased blood volume resulting in hypertonic extracellular fluid • Dehydration
Weakness, fatigue	• Fluid volume deficit or excess • Potassium deficit • Protein deficit
Nausea	• Fluid volume deficit or excess • Hyponatremia • Hypokalemia or hyperkalemia • Hypercalcemia • Hypermagnesemia • Hyperphosphatemia • Alkalosis
Hypotension	• Fluid volume deficit • Hyponatremia • Hypokalemia or hyperkalemia • Hypermagnesemia • Hypoproteinemia
Hypertension	• Fluid volume excess • Hypernatremia • Hypomagnesemia
Hyperthermia Hypothermia	• Intracellular fluid deficit • Extracellular fluid excess or deficit
Bounding pulse	• Fluid volume excess • Hypernatremia
Thready, weak pulse	• Fluid volume deficit • Hyponatremia
Tachycardia	• Fluid volume deficit • Hypomagnesemia or hypermagnesemia • Hyperphosphatemia • Alkalosis or acidosis
Bradycardia	• Hyperkalemia • Hypercalcemia • Hypermagnesemia
Dysrhythmias	• Hypokalemia or hyperkalemia • Hypocalcemia or hypercalcemia • Hypomagnesemia or hypermagnesemia • Alkalosis or acidosis
Kussmaul's (deep, rapid) respirations	• Respiratory alkalosis • Compensatory response to metabolic acidosis
Shallow, slow respirations	• Respiratory acidosis • Compensatory response to metabolic alkalosis • Severe hypokalemia or hyperkalemia from respiratory muscle weakness
• Central nervous system stimulation	• Fluid volume deficit or excess • Hyponatremia or hypernatremia • Hypokalemia or hyperkalemia • Hypocalcemia • Hypomagnesemia • Hypophosphatemia or hyperphosphatemia • Alkalosis
• Central nervous system depression	• Fluid volume deficit or excess • Hyponatremia • Hypercalcemia • Hypermagnesemia • Acidosis
• Paresthesias (tingling or numbness) in fingers or extremities	• Fluid volume excess • Hypokalemia or hyperkalemia • Hypocalcemia • Hypomagnesemia • Alkalosis
• Muscle cramps	• Hypocalcemia
• Bone pain	• Hypocalcemia or hypercalcemia • Hypophosphatemia
• Swelling	• Fluid volume excess • Hypernatremia • Hypoproteinemia
• Weight changes • Acute weight loss • Chronic weight loss	• Fluid volume deficit • Hyponatremia • Hypoproteinemia
• Weight gain • Changes in urinary pattern • Oliguria	• Fluid volume excess • Hypernatremia • Fluid volume deficit
• Polyuria • Changes in bowel pattern • Constipation • Diarrhea	• Fluid volume excess • Fluid volume deficit • Hypokalemia • Hypercalcemia • Hyponatremia • Hyperkalemia

pH is either elevated (instead of low as with primary respiratory acidosis) or back down into the normal range nearer to the alkalotic end. When respiratory alkalosis occurs to compensate for metabolic acidosis, the respiratory rate and depth increase, to "blow off" excess CO_2 and thereby eliminate a different form of acid from the body. Although the CO_2 level will be low, the pH is either low (instead of high as with primary respiratory alkalosis) or back up into the normal range nearer to the acidotic end. To review other signs of primary respiratory acidosis and alkalosis, refer back to the discussion near the beginning of the chapter.

DIAGNOSIS

When a client presents with a fluid, electrolyte, or acid-base problem—or a risk for one—use the health history, physical assessment, and findings from the diagnostic tests to determine whether there is an imbalance or risk for imbalance (Figure 26-9). When the data support the presence of dehydration, the diagnosis is written as *Deficient fluid volume.* When the data support a risk for fluid loss, as in a client with gastric suction, the diagnosis could be written as *Risk for deficient fluid volume related to gastric suction.*

If the data support a state of fluid overload, the diagnosis of *Excess fluid volume* is appropriate. When fluid excess is not present but the data support a risk for it, use the *Risk for* construction. For example, in a client with a recent myocardial infarction, the diagnosis could be written as *Risk for excess fluid volume related to decreased myocardial contractility secondary to myocardial infarction.* Prevention and early detection of these imbalances improve the overall health of the client. This is especially important in clients with reduced adaptive mechanisms, such as older adults, the young, and those with chronic diseases. Note that in each of the preceding examples, it is the *related to* or etiology component of the diagnostic statement that individualizes the problem. The etiology is derived from the data and explains the pathophysiology behind the problem.

RELATED NURSING DIAGNOSES

Clients may have one or many different responses to fluid imbalances. The most common related nursing diagnoses follow. To help make appropriate nursing diagnoses, cluster these and other responses into a data set specific for your client (Table 26-7).

- *Fatigue* related to altered cellular metabolism secondary to deficient (or excess) fluid
- *Anxiety* related to altered stability of the neuroendocrine transmission secondary to deficient (or excess) fluid
- *Ineffective health maintenance* related to inability to care for basic needs secondary to fatigue
- *Imbalanced nutrition: less than body requirements* related to lack of appetite and fatigue

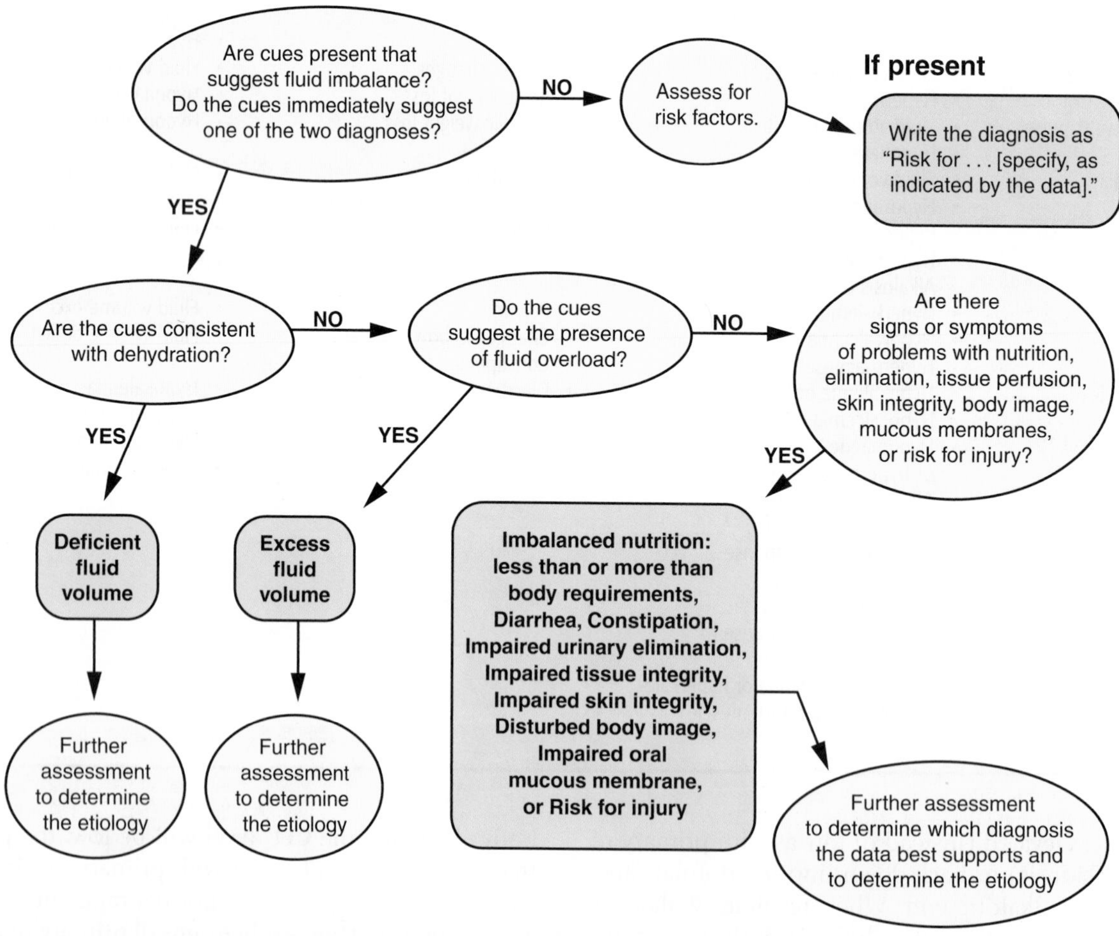

FIGURE 26-9 Decision tree for fluid balance nursing diagnoses. Diagnoses are shown in rectangles. Within these rectangles, diagnoses shown in **bold** type are NANDA-I–approved nursing diagnoses; diagnoses shown in regular type are not NANDA-I–approved nursing diagnoses.

- *Impaired skin integrity* related to lack of transport of nutrients to and waste products from the cells secondary to deficient (or excess) fluid
- *Ineffective tissue perfusion* related to impaired cellular function secondary to deficient (or excess) fluid
- *Impaired gas exchange* related to decreased volume of blood available to transport respiratory gases secondary to deficient fluid volume
- *Impaired gas exchange* related to interference with the diffusion of oxygen and carbon dioxide between the capillaries and cells secondary to excess fluid volume
- *Constipation* related to inadequate amount of fluid to provide volume for stool formation
- *Impaired oral mucous membrane* related to cellular dehydration in the mouth secondary to deficient fluid volume
- *Impaired oral mucous membrane* related to swollen tissues resulting in a breakdown of cells secondary to excess fluid volume
- *Insomnia* related to anxiety secondary to deficient fluid volume
- *Insomnia* related to inability to find a comfortable position to sleep secondary to excess fluid volume

Action Alert! Notify the physician whenever one or more of these occurs: the client's fatigue and anxiety interfere with activities of daily living and role functions, illness persists more than 48 hours, cerebral or cardiac manifestations are present, an unplanned lack of food intake leads to an unwarranted weight loss greater than 5 pounds, a wound does not heal with basic cleansing and time, a wound infection develops, or decreased tissue perfusion becomes progressively worse. In the feet, for example, you might notice that edema continues to increase, the feet are growing cooler, and pulses are barely palpable. Cerebral effects might include atypical confusion. Also notify the physician if the client develops a new productive cough accompanied by increasing dyspnea, especially at rest, constipation that lasts more than 3 days and does not respond to typical remedies, mouth sores that do not heal normally, or sleep pattern disturbances or disturbed thought processes that persist after a few weeks of treatment.

PLANNING

Planning is an essential part of nursing care. The expected outcomes must be specific to the etiology of the nursing diagnosis. The goal for a client with a fluid imbalance is to improve the existing deficit or excess. If it is not an actual problem but a risk, the goal is to reduce any risk factors that can be controlled. An example of a goal statement is *Client will improve deficient fluid volume as evidenced by . . .* or *Client will improve risk for deficient fluid volume as evidenced by . . . .* A listing of expected outcomes that are specific to the etiology follows the goal statement.

EXPECTED OUTCOMES FOR THE CLIENT WITH *DEFICIENT FLUID VOLUME*

Each expected outcome for *Deficient fluid volume* focuses on measurable data that indicate an improvement in the client's fluid deficit. Some examples include the following:

- Increase in fluid intake to at least 1500 mL/24 hr (unless contraindicated)
- Moist mucous membranes
- Absence of tongue furrows
- Absence of tenting when skin turgor assessed
- Neck veins full in a supine position
- Absence of orthostatic hypotension
- Presence of full-volume peripheral pulsations (+2 on a scale of 1-3 or +3 on a scale of 1-4)
- Serum osmolality, hematocrit, sodium, and urine specific gravity values within normal limits
- Client relates the need for, amount of, and type of increased fluid intake during periods of excess loss

Again, the expected outcomes are specific to the etiology. If knowledge deficit is part of the etiology, then *relates the need for . . .* is an example of how to write an outcome criterion focusing on lack of knowledge.

The acuteness and severity of the deficit also influence the focus of the expected outcomes. In very acute states, the expected outcomes address the return to a

Table 26-7 Clustering Data to Make a Nursing Diagnosis

Problems of Fluid Balance

DATA CLUSTER	DIAGNOSIS
A 9-month-old child has been vomiting for 24 hours. Even a sip of water does not stay down. The mother has noticed a decrease in the number of times his diaper is changed. He has a gastrointestinal virus.	*Deficient fluid volume* related to gastrointestinal effects of pathogenic organisms
A 25-year-old man has had violent emesis and diarrhea for 2 days after his chemotherapy treatment. He is weak and has dry mucous membranes. He states he is thirsty.	*Deficient fluid volume* related to side effects of medications
An 80-year-old woman arrived in the emergency department struggling for breath with audible gurgling sounds. She has crackles and rhonchi throughout the lung fields. She is in high Fowler's position, appears ashen, and has distended jugular veins. Her blood pressure is 220/110 mm Hg. Her family states that she did not refill her prescriptions last week. She is diagnosed with congestive heart failure (CHF).	*Excess fluid volume* related to inability of the heart to pump efficiently secondary to CHF and client's stopping her medication regimen
A 50-year-old man is admitted with 3+ pitting edema and decreased urinary output. He was prescribed a short-term treatment of corticosteroids for an episode of bronchitis. He has a history of congestive heart failure.	*Excess fluid volume* related to ineffective pumping action of the heart secondary to CHF and side effect of corticosteroids

hemodynamic state in the most critical tissues of the brain, heart, and kidney. Examples of expected outcomes in this situation include the following:
- Absence of confusion, lethargy, hallucinations, seizures
- Absence of cardiac dysrhythmias
- Increase in blood pressure to within normal range
- Increase in pulse volume (+2 on a scale of 1-3 or +3 on a scale of 1-4)
- Increase in urinary output with decrease in urine osmolality to within normal limits

EXPECTED OUTCOMES FOR THE CLIENT WITH *EXCESS FLUID VOLUME*

Expected outcomes for *Excess fluid volume* also focus on measurable data that indicate an improvement in the state of fluid overload. Some examples include the following:
- Decrease in peripheral edema, as from +3/5 to +2/5
- Weight loss in an amount appropriate to the aggressiveness of the treatment
- Decreasing fatigue and weakness
- Decreasing dyspnea
- Absence of jugular venous distention at a 45-degree elevation
- Serum osmolality, hematocrit, sodium level, and urine specific gravity within normal limits
- Client reports knowledge of foods and fluids limited on low-sodium diet
- Client reports correct technique and importance of self-weighing

The etiology again directs the choice of outcome criteria. The last two examples are appropriate for a client who had deficient knowledge of behaviors specific to diet and weighing.

Examples of outcome criteria that are more specific to acute fluid overload again relate to the following manifestations of involvement of the brain, heart, and kidney:
- Absence of confusion, lethargy, hallucinations, seizures
- Absence of cardiac dysrhythmias
- Absence of bounding blood pressure and pulse
- Decrease in pulmonary crackles
- Improvement in blood pressure, pulse, respiratory response to activity
- Increase in urine osmolality to within normal limits

EXPECTED OUTCOMES FOR THE CLIENT WITH ASSOCIATED PROBLEMS

Because the planning process for electrolyte and acid-base problems involves collaboration with other disciplines, the goal statement is written differently. The expected outcomes are preceded by the phrase: *The nurse will monitor the client for . . .* instead of *Client will improve . . . .* Goals and expected outcomes related to electrolyte and acid-base deficits also require focusing on the specific data obtained from the client assessment. With a diagnosis of metabolic alkalosis, the nurse will monitor the client for the following:
- Serum pH between 7.35 and 7.45
- Serum bicarbonate between 23 and 26 mEq/L
- Improved level of consciousness without seizures
- Respirations deep and regular at 16 to 20 per minute
- Less than 5 premature cardiac beats per minute
- Potassium level greater than 3.5 mEq/L

With a diagnosis of metabolic acidosis, the nurse will monitor the client for the following:
- Serum pH between 7.35 and 7.45
- Serum bicarbonate between 23 and 26 mEq/L
- Improved level of consciousness, absence of coma, improved signs of orientation
- Respirations deep and regular at 16 to 20 per minute
- Less than 5 premature cardiac beats per minute
- Potassium level less than 5.0 mEq/L

INTERVENTION

INTERVENTIONS TO REDUCE THE RISK OF DEFICIENT FLUID VOLUME

There are three main categories of interventions to consider in reducing a client's risk for deficient fluid volume: teaching the client about fluid needs, preventing excessive fluid deficits, and restoring lost fluids.

Teaching the Client About Fluid Needs. Health teaching is a primary nursing intervention to support fluid needs in well clients. This includes information to support fluid needs when the body is in a resting state as well as in a state of activity. Remind clients to increase their fluid intake during hot weather, when working or exercising in the heat, during periods of heightened stress, and during pregnancy.

For normal cellular function, a healthy adult needs approximately 2.0 to 2.5 L of water daily, school-age children need 100 to 110 mL/kg/day, toddlers need 120 to 135 mL/kg/day, and infants need 70 to 100 mL/kg/day. This amount will change when illness or other factors alter normal body functions.

Changing the fluid intake must be within the client's capabilities. Clients confined to bed, those extremely weakened or fatigued, and those confined by treatments may need assistance. Collaborate with the dietitian, the physician, the client, and the family to achieve a level of intake that maximizes the client's state of health. The accompanying self-care instructions (Box 26-3) can help your clients reduce their risk of deficient fluid volume.

Preventing Excessive Fluid Deficits. The second major intervention is to prevent excessive fluid deficits related to increased activity levels, medication use, or hypertonic feedings. Fluid needs during exercise can be met in most circumstances by following the recommendations in Box 26-4. Even clients who take medications to pro-

BOX 26-3 *Teaching for Self-Care*

Reducing the Risk for Deficient Fluid Volume

Purpose: To prevent deficient fluid volume.
Expected Outcome: The client will maintain or regain hydration.

Client Instructions

- While awake, drink 30 to 100 mL of fluid hourly when a fever or other illness causes fluid loss. Increase to 240 mL hourly if the fever rises above 37.8° C (100° F).
- Drink adequate fluids before and after exercise. Consult your physician for specific precautions if you have a chronic illness, such as cardiac disease, diabetes mellitus, renal disease, or liver disease.
- Replace fluids lost from all body sources (vomiting, diarrhea, wounds) with the approximate amount lost. Drink fluids that contain nutrients, such as juices, sport drinks, or decaffeinated cola.
- If a hypertonic food supplement or feeding has been prescribed, consume 1 mL of water for every calorie of the feeding.
- Monitor and record your weight at least weekly. Notify your physician about rapid changes, as indicated.

mote water loss need to have the recommended daily amount of water unless the physician has prescribed otherwise.

When a hypertonic feeding reaches the small bowel, it increases the risk of fluid shifting into the bowel from the other compartments in an attempt to offset the state of hypertonicity. These shifts can result in fluid deficit in those compartments, as well as in diarrhea, which further compromises the state of fluid deficit.

Fluid loss with hypertonic feedings can be avoided by providing fluid equal to 1 mL/kcal. Calculate the difference between the kilocalories in the feeding and the volume of liquid, and give the difference in water boluses divided over 24 hours. For example, for a client receiving 2160 kcal in 1440 mL of feeding over 24 hours, the difference of 720 can be divided by 6 (one bolus every 4 hours). Giving an additional 120 mL of water every 4 hours will not only keep the tube from plugging but also provide the additional water needed to prevent the dehydration that can result from hypertonic feedings.

Restoring Lost Fluids. The third major intervention is to restore fluid lost during mild illnesses to prevent an actual fluid deficit. Taking 30 to 100 mL of fluid every hour during illness can prevent a fluid deficit from occurring. Choose fluids that are enjoyed by the client, contain electrolytes, and are nonacidic. Cool fluids may be better tolerated than warm. Place fluids within the client's reach and in nonspilling cups or with covers and straws to improve access for the more debilitated client. Thickened liquids are safer for the client with dysphagia.

BOX 26-4 *Teaching for Wellness*

Preventing Exercise-Related Deficient Fluid Volume

Purpose: To maintain hydration during exercise.
Expected Outcome: The client will understand and respond to the relationship between fluids and exercise.

Client Instructions

- Avoid replacing fluid too rapidly because it only overflows to the gastrointestinal (GI) tract and kidneys.
- Drink 8 ounces of cold water 15 minutes before exercise. Cold water lowers the GI temperature faster.
- Drink 8 to 12 ounces of fluid (5 ounces for a child) for each 20 to 30 minutes of exercise. Another rule of thumb is to drink a pint of water for each pound of weight lost during exercise.
- Cold water is the preferred fluid replacement for exercise-related loss. Sports drinks do not improve intestinal absorption and have no advantage over water in maintaining plasma volume or electrolyte concentrations. However, their carbohydrate content may enhance performance.
- Take breaks during strenuous exercise, especially in hot or humid conditions.
- Avoid diuretics. If your physician has prescribed one for you, ask about its safety during exercise.
- Avoid wearing excess clothing during exercise because it reduces evaporation. If possible, wear one layer of absorbent clothing, expose as much skin as possible, and replace wet garments with dry ones.
- Follow your physician's conditioning recommendations. For example, start an exercise program with a few minutes daily. Over time, increase to 30 minutes of aerobic exercise or more at least three times weekly.
- Use extra caution if you are obese, because obesity impairs the sweating mechanism.
- Use extra caution with children because they have a less efficient thermoregulation response, decreased sweat output, and a slower rate of acclimatization.
- Use extra caution if taking medications that impair thermoregulation, such as thyroid hormones, amphetamines, haloperidol, antihistamines, anticholinergics, phenothiazines, and benztropine.

INTERVENTIONS TO INCREASE FLUID VOLUME

There are four major categories of interventions to increase fluid volume: restoring fluid balance, preventing further loss, instituting rehabilitative care, and administering IV therapy.

Restoring Fluid Balance. The normal maintenance fluid is not enough when a person is experiencing an actual moderate to severe fluid loss. The physician's directive to "encourage fluids" usually means to provide twice the amount of recommended daily intake, or 3000 mL. You will then need to calculate the client's fluid intake per shift. Usually, the goal for a 12-hour day shift is to give three fourths of the total fluid prescription; the night shift gives the remaining one fourth. For example, if the prescription is for 3000 mL/24 h, the day shift attempts to achieve an intake of about 2300 mL, and the night shift, 700 mL. The client at home may find it useful to plan the intake around three meals and three periods between meals. The client needing 3000 mL would thus drink two 8-ounce glasses of fluid with each meal and two more glasses between meals. Alternatively, for a period of 16 waking hours, the client could choose to drink 12 ounces every 2 hours. Careful measurement and documentation of I&O and daily weights are critical to evaluating the client's progress toward the goal of improved fluid balance.

If the fluid loss is related to exercise, follow these guidelines:

- Gradually rehydrate an alert adolescent or adult (cold water, 1 to 2 L over 2 to 4 hours).
- Rehydrate an unconscious client with IV fluids (5% dextrose in normal saline) up to 800 mL/hr depending on preexisting contraindications.
- If the client is hyperthermic, lower body temperature by moving the client to a shady area and applying cold packs to the neck, axilla, and groin. Establish evaporative surfaces through sponge baths with towel drying of skin and changing washcloths frequently. Use a fan to promote heat loss through convection. Administer niacin, if prescribed, to promote a cutaneous flush. Monitor I&O, vital signs, and fluid status hourly.

Remember that thirst is not a reliable indicator of the need for fluid replacement. Up to 3% of body weight can be lost before thirst is stimulated. Administering or consuming fluids only until thirst is relieved can result generally in only one half to two thirds of the lost fluid being replaced.

Preventing Further Loss. The second major intervention is to provide supportive care to prevent further fluid loss. In addition to fluid replacement, interventions should be individualized to the etiology of the fluid loss. For example, when diarrhea or vomiting is present, antidiarrheal or antiemetic medications are appropriate. When loss is secondary to diaphoresis, choose appropriate interventions such as controlling fevers with medications that fight the etiology of the fever, giving prescribed antipyretics, and removing excess bed linens.

Instituting Rehabilitative Care. The third intervention is to provide and recommend rehabilitative care to maximize client and family potential. Teach the client and family the importance of replacing lost fluids, maintaining nutrition, monitoring weight changes, and reporting significant concerns to the physician. Box 26-5 helps clients and families decide when to call a physician. Also, emphasize safety precautions if weakness or orthostatic hypotension is a problem. Safety precautions include changing positions slowly, using assistive devices as appropriate, and removing scatter rugs or other objects that increase the risk of falls.

Administering IV Therapy. Many routes are available for fluid intake: oral, tube (NG, gastric, duodenal, or jejunal tubes), or parenteral (subcutaneous or IV). The oral route is the most preferred, common, and cost efficient. Recall from our earlier discussion that maintenance of body fluid balance depends on the total amount of fluid intake from pure water as well as from other fluids and food products. When fluid homeostasis cannot be maintained through the oral route, alternative methods must be initiated to ensure cellular function. For more information on fluid given via an artificial tube, see Chapter 25.

When a client's homeostatic fluid needs cannot be met through an oral route or tube, or replacement is needed more quickly than either of these two routes can offer, IV therapy is the method of choice. Examples of clients requiring IV therapy include those who receive nothing by mouth, those unable to ingest oral fluids (possibly because of nausea, vomiting, or mental status changes), and those unable to absorb nutrients because of a dysfunctional bowel. The IV route is also used to deliver medications that would be destroyed by gastric enzymes, when rapid medication response is necessary, or when higher plasma levels are necessary. Clients with life-threatening losses of plasma volume (such as hemorrhage, shock, and severe burns) also require IV therapy.

As with any medication, you are responsible for the "six rights" (the right client, drug, dose, time, route, and documentation) of IV therapy administration. Table 26-8 lists common IV fluids, their purpose, and specific nursing implications.

Accurate IV administration requires many skills. These include the skills required for the preparatory phase of starting an IV line, the actual starting of an IV infusion, regulating the flow rate, administering IV medications, and discontinuing the IV infusion (Procedures 26-3 and 26-4).

Text continued on p. 651

BOX 26-5 *Teaching for Self-Care*

When to Call the Physician for Problems of Fluid Balance

Purpose: To recognize changes in fluid balance that would necessitate a call to the physician.
Expected Outcome: The client will seek a physician's advice when a change is recognized in fluid status.

Client Instructions

Call the physician if the following occur:

- Fluid loss (as from vomiting or diarrhea) lasting more than 24 hours, especially if it involves a child, a pregnant woman, an older adult, or a person with chronic disease
- Rapid weight loss (>3 pounds in a day if not an expected outcome of therapy)
- Rapid weight gain (>3 pounds in a week or less)
- Increased difficulty breathing or a cough of new onset
- Atypical cardiac irregularity or palpitations
- Confusion or behavioral changes

Table 26-8 Understanding Intravenous Solutions

IV FLUID	PURPOSE	NURSING IMPLICATIONS
DEXTROSE SOLUTIONS		
Hypotonic (<240 mOsm/L), such as dextrose 5% in water (D_5W)	• Provides free water • Dextrose is quickly metabolized, promotes renal excretion of solutes • Without saline in the solution, water may be drawn out of vascular space and cause edema • Adds enough calories to prevent ketosis (170 cal/L)	• Risk for hyponatremia and hypokalemia if excess free water given • Not sufficient for nutrition; need other nutrient source if used for long-term therapy • Monitor for hyponatremia (disorientation, headache, lethargy, nausea, weakness) • Never used with blood administration (increases coagulation) • Not used in head trauma because could worsen cerebral edema and increase intracranial pressure
Hypertonic (>350 mOsm/L), such as dextrose 10% (505 mOsm/L) to 50% (2525 mOsm/L) in water	• Osmotic diuretic • Treats hypoglycemia • Used in total parenteral nutrition • Hypertonic solutions may irritate vein	• Risk for phlebitis and hyperglycemia • Monitor infusion site and glucose levels • Client may need regular insulin administered on a sliding scale (based on blood glucose)
SALINE SOLUTIONS		
Hypotonic, 0.2% or 0.45% normal saline (with or without 5% dextrose)	• Water replacement without increase of osmotic pressure or serum sodium levels • Replaces loss of Na^+ through normal daily excretion • Adds 170 cal/L if dextrose included	• Risk for hyponatremia and fluid volume excess • Do not give to clients with hypotension or may decrease blood pressure further
Isotonic (310 mEq/L), 0.9% normal saline (with or without 5% dextrose)	• Replaces sodium and chloride lost through vomiting • May increase serum sodium level depending on rate of administration and sodium excretion rate • Expands extracellular fluid without changing osmolality (can expand blood volume following blood loss until blood available) • Primes an IV catheter before use and flushes it afterward, as indicated • Is a backup solution to administer blood	• Risk for fluid volume excess (sodium causes the kidneys to retain water)
Hypertonic, such as 3% to 5% normal saline	• Rarely used • Reverses severe sodium deficit	• Risk for hypernatremia, vascular volume overload, pulmonary edema, phlebitis • Give slowly to prevent cellular dehydration
POTASSIUM ADDITIVE		
Usual dose range: 20-40 mEq/L to 3L/day to meet an average daily intake of 50-150 mEq/day	• Potassium maintenance or potassium replacement; if on a diet, this amount would replace losses	• Risk for hyperkalemia, especially if client has oliguria • Phlebitis is more likely in a small vein • Mix well to prevent potassium bolus (cause of cardiac arrest); may need cardiac monitoring • Rarely administer a concentration >80 mEq/L • Never give IV push or undiluted
RINGER'S SOLUTIONS		
Ringer's (isotonic)	• Mimics electrolyte concentration of blood • Replaces fluids, sodium, potassium, calcium, and chloride • Can be used as volume expander with lower gastrointestinal tract loss or in hemorrhage until blood is available	• Risk for fluid volume excess
Lactated Ringer's	• Ringer's plus lactate-precursor bicarbonate; used for metabolic acidosis (except lactic acidosis)	• Risk for fluid volume excess
Total parenteral nutrition–hypertonic	• Provides carbohydrates, amino acids, lipids, vitamins, electrolytes • Provides energy and nutrients for cellular function and repair	• Give via a central IV line • Can give via a peripheral line if tonicity is decreased • Monitor client's glucose levels

IV, Intravenous.

Continued

Table 26-8 Understanding Intravenous Solutions—cont'd

IV FLUID	PURPOSE	NURSING IMPLICATIONS
BLOOD PRODUCTS		
• Packed red blood cells • Whole blood • Plasma	Used for symptomatic anemia; hemorrhage • Red blood cells provide cells without volume expansion of plasma • Whole blood provides cells and plasma for volume expansion; can cause volume overload • Plasma provides volume expansion	• Follow procedural guidelines exactly for validating product, assessing client, and administering product • Use of acetaminophen as a premedication may mask a fever response, which may be the only early warning of anaphylaxis
Platelets or fresh frozen plasma	• Given to client with idiopathic or therapy-induced thrombocytopenia • Provides volume expansion; reverses protein malnutrition	• As above

IV, Intravenous.

PROCEDURE 26-3

TIME TO ALLOW: NOVICE: 20 min. EXPERT: 10 min.

INITIATING PERIPHERAL INTRAVENOUS THERAPY

Nursing Skills Online: Intravenous Fluid Administration, Lesson 2

Peripheral IV therapy is the administration of fluid and possibly electrolytes through a needle or cannula inserted into a vein in the arm, which is then connected to tubing through which the fluid is administered. The term *peripheral* distinguishes this form of IV therapy from central venous therapy, which is administered via a catheter in the subclavian or jugular vein, vena cava, or right atrium.

DELEGATION GUIDELINES

Initiating IV therapy may not be delegated to a nursing assistant.

EQUIPMENT NEEDED

- Tourniquet
- Warm moist pack with warm moist towel, plastic bag, and tape (optional)
- IV catheter or needle
- IV extension tubing, if appropriate
- IV pole for gravity infusion or infusion pump, if needed
- IV lock, if needed, prefilled with saline solution
- 3-mL syringe with Luer-Lok end, prefilled with saline; needle or needleless adapter
- IV bag with appropriate tubing attached, preprimed
- Alcohol, povidone-iodine (Betadine), or chlorhexidine (Hibiclens) antiseptic
- IV dressing
- Tape or transparent dressing
- Clean gloves

1 Perform preliminary actions (see inside front cover).

2 Prepare for IV therapy.

a. Verify the six rights, investigate any client allergies, check for incompatibility between solutions or IV medications, and read the facility procedure manual for specific instructions. *The six rights, or Rs, include the right client, right medication, right rate, right time, right route, and right documentation. If solutions or medications may be incompatible, you may need to start an IV line at a second site unless an existing IV access device has more than one port.*

b. Obtain an IV strip, and mark it. Place the strip on the IV bag (see illustration).

c. Using the appropriate tubing, close the roller regulator clamp. Then remove the protective covers on the IV injection port and on the IV spike, keeping both sites sterile. Now spike the IV port. Prime the IV chamber and tubing (see illustration).

d. Prime the chamber one-third to one-half full by pressing it between your thumb and index finger. Prime the tubing on a gravity system by opening the roller clamp and allowing the IV fluid to completely

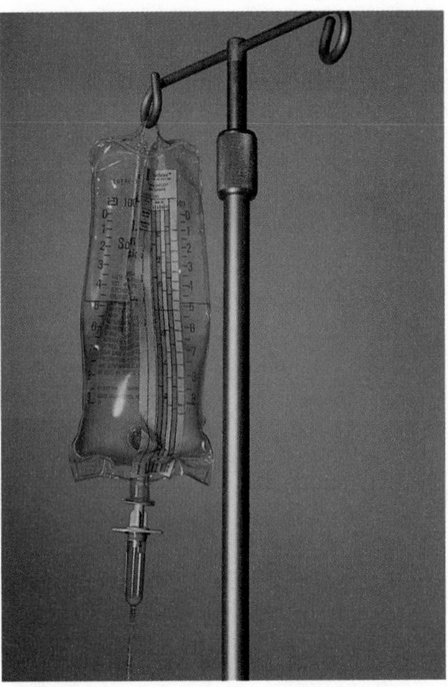

Step 2b. An IV strip on an IV bag.

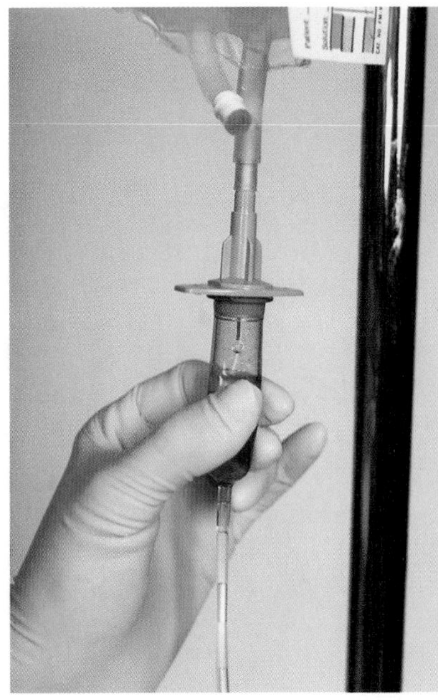

Step 2d. Priming the IV chamber and tubing.

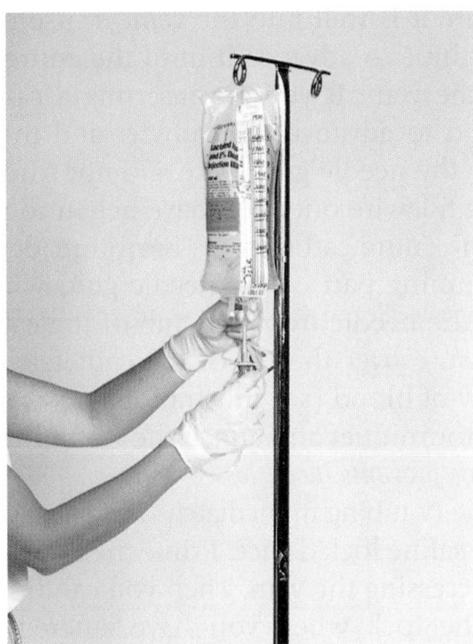

Step 2c. Spiking the IV port.

displace the air in the tubing. Then close the roller clamp. If using a pump, follow the manufacturer's guidelines to prime the IV tubing (see illustration). ***Never purge the air from the tubing while it is connected to a client's vein.*** *Doing so could cause an air embolus and tissue necrosis.*

3 Start an IV line.

a. If the client has no IV line or an existing line is not appropriate for current needs, start a new line. For example, although a 22-gauge or occasionally a 25-gauge catheter is adequate for most solutions, you will need to use a 20-gauge catheter and a 19-gauge needle or larger if preparing a client for surgery or administering blood products.
b. Put on clean gloves, and assess the client for an appropriate site to start a new IV line. Always use the most distal vein possible. Also, avoid using an arm that has had previous lymphatic problems or has been affected by surgery (such as mastectomy) or a fistula.
c. To find a suitable vein, lower the client's arm to below heart level and apply a tourniquet at least 6 inches above the projected site. Use the arm of the client's nondominant hand whenever possible. Look for a vein that is generally straight, and does not have a hardened (sclerotic) feel or a twisted (tortuous) appearance. Choose the most distal site that is not painful and where the catheter will not be inserted over, lying on, or ending near a joint such as the wrist or elbow (point of flexion) (see illustration). *Aids in successful cannulation on the first attempt and reduces risk of early infiltration because of catheter compression or dislodgment.*

Continued

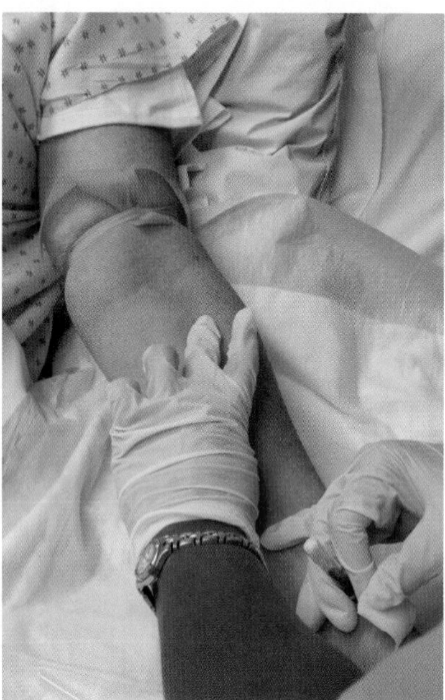

Step 3c. Finding the vein.

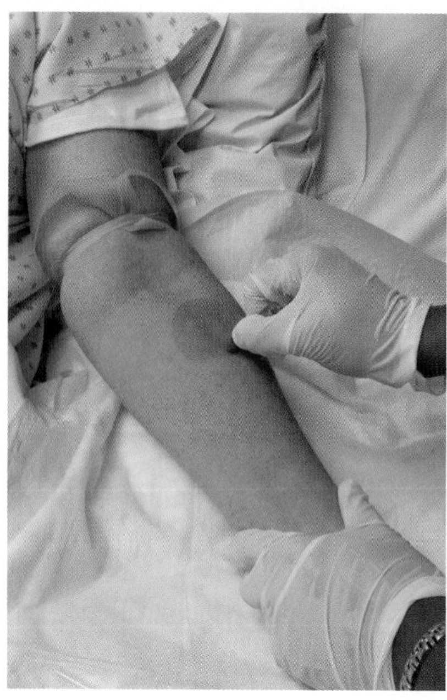

Step 3e. Preparing the site.

d. Implement as needed strategies to dilate the vein and ease IV catheter insertion. Apply a warm, moist pack over the site for 5 to 10 minutes and reassess. Lower the arm to a dependent position. Ask the client to open and close the fist several times. Stroke the arm from the elbow to the wrist (distal to proximal). Do not tap or slap the vein repeatedly. *These techniques are especially useful if the veins are difficult to see or the client is an older adult. They aid in venous dilation without causing injury to the vein.*

e. Cleanse the site as directed by your facility's procedure manual. Using alcohol, povidone-iodine (Betadine), or chlorhexidine (Hibiclens), start at the point of needle insertion and wipe in an outward spiral until you have cleaned a 3-inch circle around the site. Or, if your facility specifies, use two pledgets. Prepare the site for 30 seconds with the first one by applying friction and multidirectional cleansing around the hair follicles. Then use the second sterile pledget in the same circular method (see illustration).

f. Remove the needle or catheter from its protective cover and, with your dominant hand, hold it bevel up at a 30-degree angle to the skin, either directly over or parallel to the vein. *The direct approach usually works better for a larger vein, whereas the parallel approach often works better for a smaller one. To prevent the vein from wandering, stabilize the vein with your nondominant hand from above or below the targeted entry site.*

g. Pierce through the skin with one quick motion. As you do, decrease the angle of the needle or catheter to 15 degrees. Continue advancing toward the vein until you see blood return in the catheter or tubing. Then advance the catheter about another ¼ inch to make sure it is well into the vein. If inserting a needle, continue to advance it until the entire needle is within the vein. If you are inserting a catheter, use one hand to advance the catheter and the other to stabilize the needle guidewire. Do not readvance the needle guidewire once you have begun to remove it. When the entire catheter has been threaded, remove the remaining part of the needle guidewire. As you remove the needle from the hub of the catheter, apply pressure over the tip of the catheter to prevent backflow of blood (see illustrations).

h. Release tourniquet and attach the IV tubing immediately. *This prevents blood loss.*

i. Attach the IV tubing immediately. *This prevents blood loss.*

j. Attach a saline lock device. Prime the lock with saline before accessing the vein. Then you can immediately attach the lock when you have entered the vein. Access the IV port with the prefilled syringe. Aspirate to validate blood return, and inject the saline into the vein. If no swelling occurs, proceed to dress the site. If swelling occurs, remove the needle or catheter. *Keep in mind that some types of needleless systems require the use of the needleless device to access. Others require you to attach the prefilled syringe to the distal end of the tubing until flushing has validated correct placement. Then you place the needleless cap. Follow the manufacturer's recommendations* (see illustration).

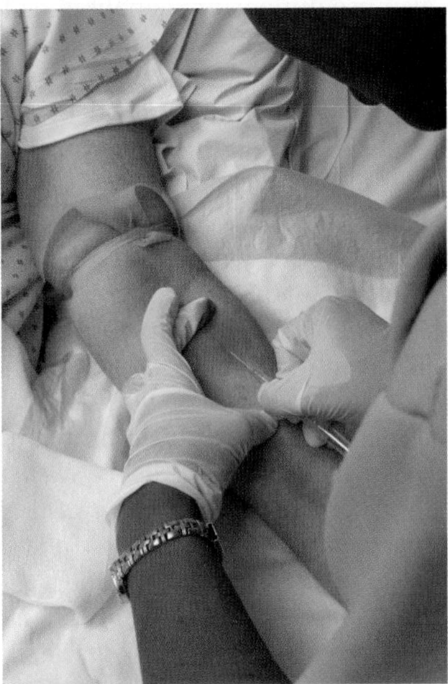

Step 3g(1). Inserting the catheter bevel up.

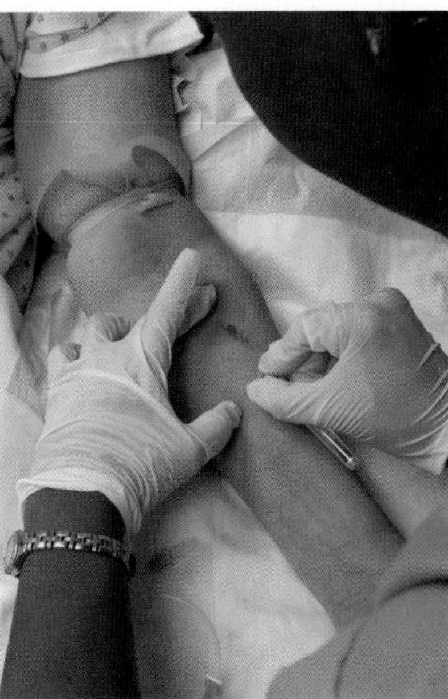

Step 3g(3). Putting pressure on the tip of the cannula to prevent blood flow.

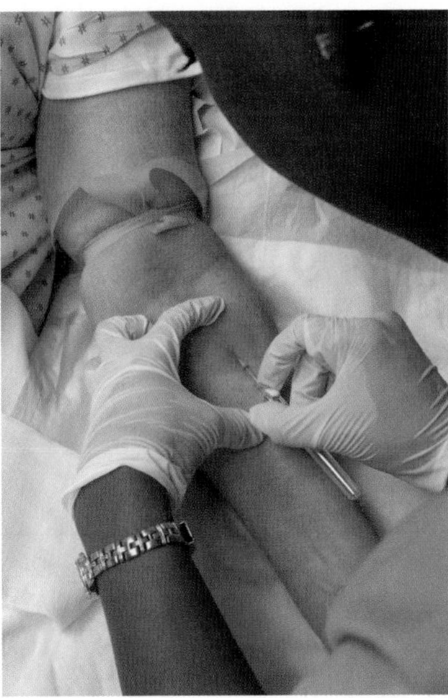

Step 3g(2). Retracting the needle (push white button) after the cannula is threaded into the vein.

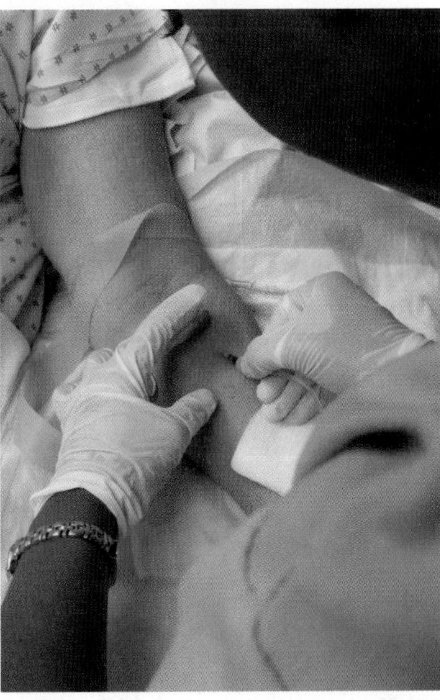

Step 3i. Attaching a primed saline lock to the cannula.

Continued

4 Dress the IV site following your facility's procedural guidelines.

a. Transparent dressing (see illustration).
b. Butterfly tape and 2 ×2 inch gauze.

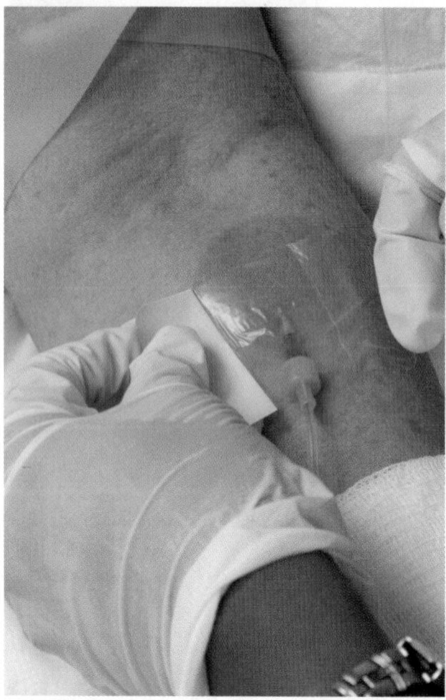

Step 4a. Applying transparent dressing.

c. Other dressing per agency policy.

5 Stabilize the tubing with an additional strip of tape if necessary. *Use an armboard to stabilize the IV site only as a last resort to prevent the risk of ineffective tissue perfusion.*

6 Label the IV site with the catheter size and date. Some institutions may require the nurse's signature.

7 Label the IV tubing and IV bag if these were attached with the date and nurse's initials.

8 Regulate the flow of the infusion as ordered. Use the following formula to help calculate the flow rate:

$$\text{Amount of solution} \times \text{gtt/mL (tubing factor)} \div \text{time in minutes}$$

For example, imagine that the physician ordered 1000 mL D_5W/0.45% sodium chloride to be given over 8 hours. The tubing drop (gtt) factor is 15 gtt/mL. The resulting formula is as follows:

$$1000\text{ mL} \times 15\text{ gtt/mL}/8 \times 60\text{ min} = 15{,}000\text{ gtt}/480\text{ min} = 31.25\text{ gtt/min (31 gtt/min)}$$

You can also use dimensional analysis, as follows:

$$(1\text{ hr}/60\text{ min}) \times (1000\text{ mL}/8\text{ hr}) \times (15\text{ gtt}/1\text{ mL}) = (15{,}000\text{ gtt}/480\text{ min}) = 31.25\text{ gtt/min (or about 31 gtt/min)}.$$

In other words, when the physician orders 1000 mL of IV fluid in 8 hours, you will be giving 125 mL/hr. Using IV tubing with a drop factor of 15 gtt/mL means that, to give 125 mL/hr, you will need about 31 drops per minute in the IV chamber. This is about 8 drops every 15 seconds. *Use the second hand on your watch to achieve precise measurement of drops per minute. Remember that movement of the client's arm or a change in arm position can alter gravity drip rates, as will changing the height of the bag. Most often a pump is ordered, the formula is in units of mL/hr. For the same problem, 1000 mL/8 hr = 125 mL/hr. You would set the pump or a flow regulator at 125 mL/hr. Be sure to use an infusion pump when an IV infusion contains additives caustic to interstitial tissues, when a change in delivery rate increases the risk of dangerous adverse effects, and when the client has an increased risk of air embolus (as with a central line).*

9 Monitor and maintain the ongoing drip rate. *You can provide ongoing monitoring by counting the drip rate each hour and by placing a time strip on the side of the IV bag. To manage precise delivery or delivery at a keep-vein-open rate, use an infusion pump.*

PEDIATRIC CONSIDERATIONS

Try to start the IV in a room other than the assigned hospital room. Secure help (not from the parents) to hold the arm of a pediatric client. The use of an armboard to stabilize the site is sometimes helpful with pediatric clients. Use of a 24-gauge needle in a scalp vein is often indicated for infants. Let parents comfort the child.

GERIATRIC CONSIDERATIONS

Secure help to hold the arm of a confused or disoriented client. A tourniquet may not be necessary in an older adult client because the veins are often superficial and can burst when the needle enters, and constricting blood flow may hinder finding the site. A more suitable vein may be palpable but not visible in a geriatric client or someone who has had multiple needlesticks as a result of frequent or long-term IV therapy. Use of an armboard is not suggested unless the client is combative.

HOME HEALTH CARE CONSIDERATIONS

IV therapy in the home is usually intermittent therapy performed by the nurse. If the medication or fluid therapy is ongoing over days, weeks, or months, it is usually administered through a central venous access route. However, peripheral IV sites are also used. The nurse may go to the home, perform a venipuncture, and administer the fluids or medications before leaving. However, the nurse may initiate the therapy and teach the family to monitor and maintain the therapy until it is complete. Nurses may also need to teach the family to maintain the venous access site and prevent infection. Teaching may include the following:

- Signs and symptoms of infiltration
- Troubleshooting an IV pump
- Discontinuing the infusion and removing the IV cannula
- Observing for side effects
- Cleaning and dressing the site
- When to call the nurse
- When to call the doctor

TIME TO ALLOW: NOVICE: 6 min. EXPERT: 3 min.

PROCEDURE 26-4 DISCONTINUING PERIPHERAL INTRAVENOUS THERAPY

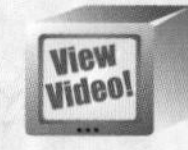

Nursing Skills Online: Intravenous Fluid Administration, Lesson 2

To discontinue peripheral IV therapy, the nurse removes the needle or cannula from the vein and takes precautions to prevent hematoma or infection.

DELEGATION GUIDELINES

Peripheral IV catheter discontinuation may be delegated to a nursing assistant who has received training in this skill.

EQUIPMENT NEEDED

- 2 × 2 gauze or cotton ball
- Band-Aid
- Clean gloves
- Tourniquet, if required by your facility

1 Perform preliminary actions (see inside front cover).

2 Prepare to discontinue IV therapy, and don clean gloves.

3 Remove the tape and dressing covering the insertion site. *Remove tape from the skin, not necessarily from the catheter.*

4 Remove the catheter.

a. Stabilize the catheter. *Stabilization prevents unnecessary trauma from an accidental removal.*

b. Hold the alcohol swab or cotton ball over the IV insertion site but do not apply pressure. *Premature pressure can cause discomfort and injure the vein. Cotton tends to work better for clients who have extra bleeding tendencies or who have been receiving anticoagulants (such as geriatric clients).*

c. Slide the catheter out of the vein and promptly apply pressure to the site. Apply pressure for 1 to 2 minutes or until the vein no longer leaks blood. *Removing pressure prematurely will result in continued bleeding and a bruise.*

d. Apply a bandage (Band-Aid) to the site.

Equipment. Proper equipment selection is essential for safe administration of IV therapy (Figure 26-10). All solutions and connecting tubing must remain sterile to decrease the risk of infection. To begin, compare the solution to the physician's order to ensure accuracy. Choose the type of tubing appropriate to the site, the type of solution, and the type of delivery. For example, basic solutions including 5% dextrose or saline solutions can be given by gravity flow in a peripheral vein; therefore gravity tubing is sufficient. The size of the drip factor in gravity tubing varies between microdrip (60 drops/mL) and macrodrip (such as 10 or 15 drops/mL). (Sometimes the measurement unit gtt is used, from the Latin *guttae,* drops.)

Microdrip tubing has less risk of flowing in too rapidly if the IV needle or catheter changes positions in the client's vein. Also, amounts less than 30 mL/hr have to be given by microdrip or on a pump. Use macrodrip tubing when a solution needs to infuse rapidly. Most institutions today routinely utilize IV pumps for delivering IV therapy. This is especially critical when administering any solution that needs precise delivery or

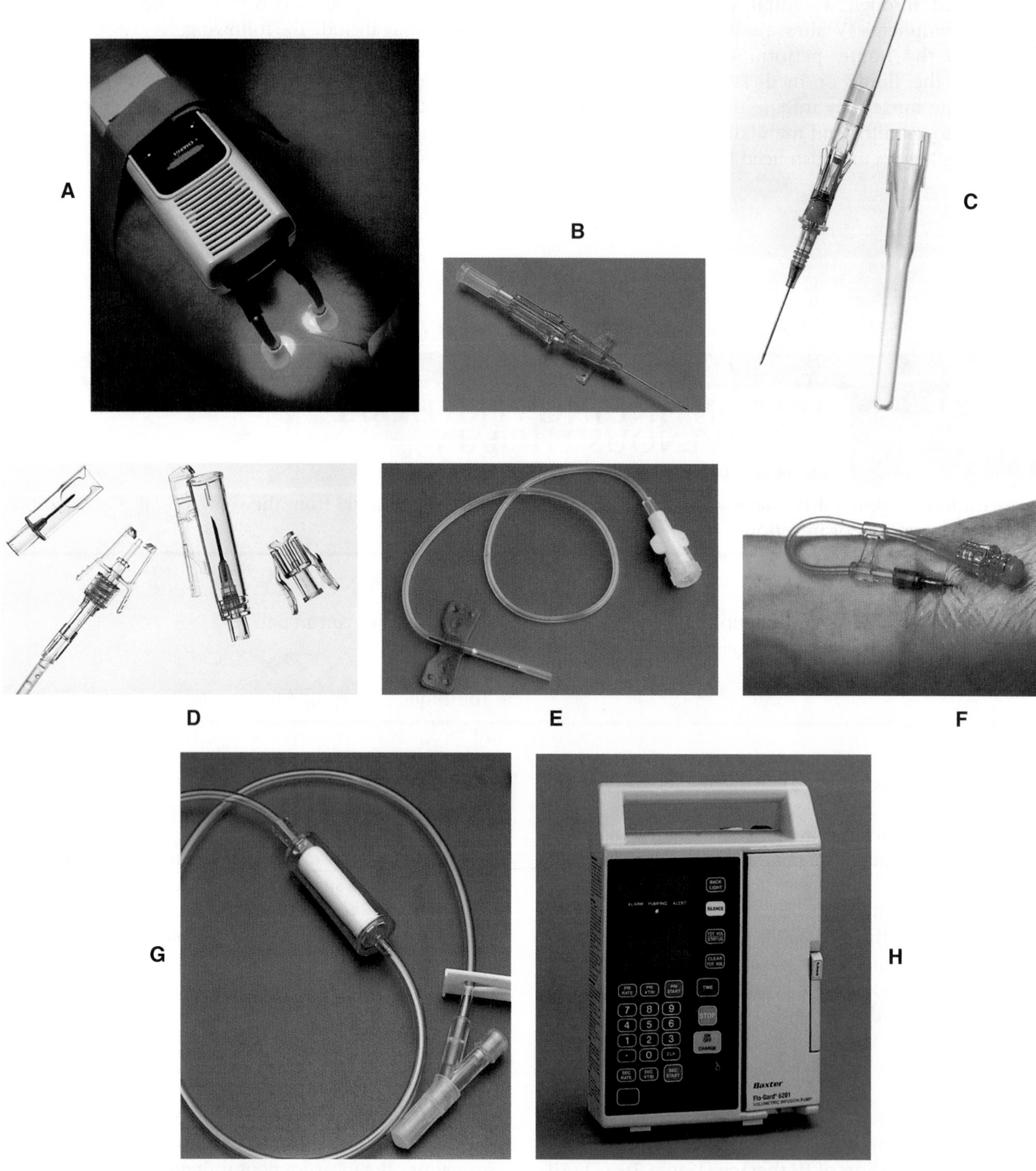

FIGURE 26-10 Examples of equipment used in IV therapy. **A,** Vein finder (Venoscope). **B,** Over-the-needle IV catheter. **C,** Insyte Autoguard IV cannula. **D,** Two types of protected needles with locking covers and two types of needleless lever locks. **E,** Butterfly infusion set. **F,** Saline lock with transparent dressing. **G,** In-line IV filter (Millipore IV Express). **H,** IV pump (Flo-Gard Volumetric). (**A** courtesy Applied Biotech Products, Lafayette, LA; **B** courtesy Becton Dickinson, Sandy, UT; **E** courtesy Medline Industries, Mundelein, IL; **G** courtesy Millipore Corporation, Bedford, MA; **H** courtesy Baxter Healthcare Corporation, Deerfield, IL).

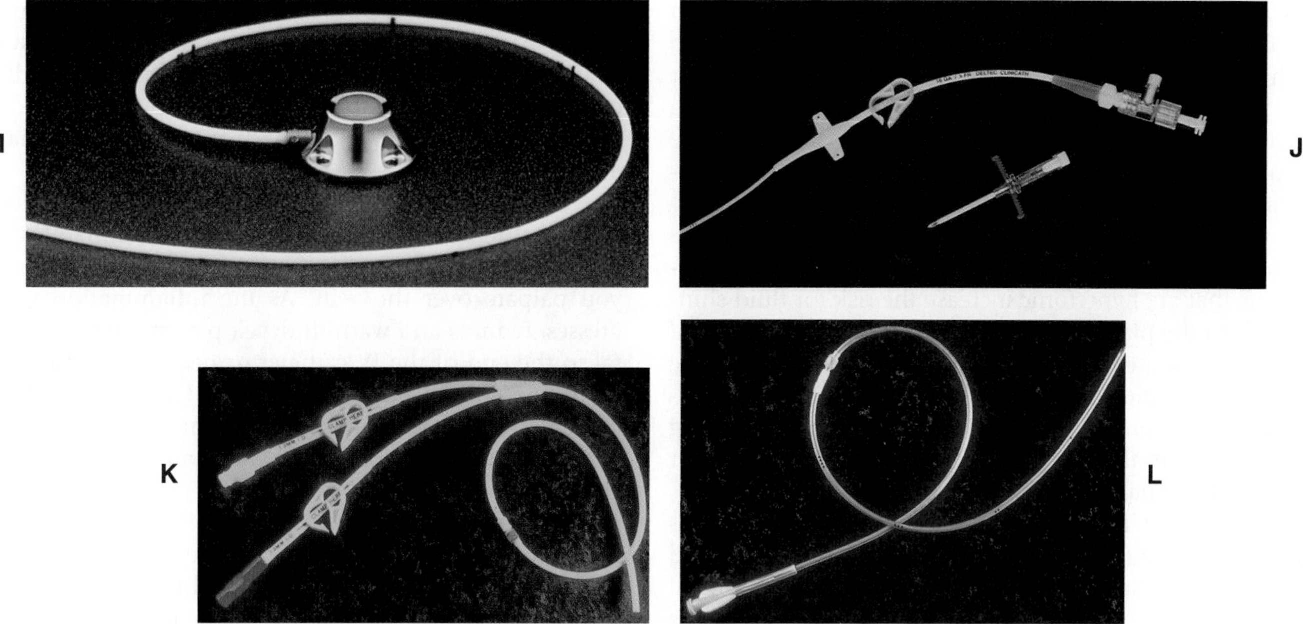

FIGURE 26-10, cont'd Examples of equipment used in IV therapy. **I,** Implantable vascular access device (Port-a-Cath). **J,** Peripherally inserted central catheter, or PICC (CliniCath). **K,** Hickman catheter. **L,** Groshong catheter. (**I** and **J** courtesy SIMS Deltec, St. Paul, MN; **K** and **L** courtesy Bard Access Systems, Salt Lake City, UT.)

contains potassium chloride or any other high-risk medication. Solutions given through a central vein (subclavian or jugular) also require an infusion pump to decrease the risk of air embolus. Many IV pumps have specialized tubing. Other solutions, such as total parenteral nutrition and some blood products, require an IV pump and filter tubing.

The type of pump also varies. Most pumps are volume specific. The most commonly used pumps deliver 1 mL or more per hour, but there are also micropumps that deliver less than 1 mL/hr. Newer volume pumps can be set for tenths. As an example, if 31.3 gtt/min is needed, the pump can be set at 31.3 and there is no need to round to 31. If precise measurement is required, but a pump is not feasible, an in-line flow regulator can be attached to the main IV line. This device adjusts the rate by mL/hr, but it is usually a one-time charge versus a daily charge for a pump.

Specialized tubing is required for some medications, such as nitroglycerin, that can be adsorbed by tubing. Tubing with volume control chambers called buretrols may be used with children and critically ill clients to precisely deliver small amounts of fluid or medication. Extension tubing is also available to increase mobility and facilitate position changes.

Often, you will need to "piggyback" a prescribed medication into the client's main IV line. Types of piggyback tubing are specific to the manufacturer. Several manufacturers have created needleless IV equipment to decrease the risk of needlesticks.

In addition to the right solution, tubing, and probably pump, you will need more equipment if you are starting an IV line. After assessing the client's veins, choose the correct needle or catheter, and a tourniquet, gloves, dressing, and site preparation agents (alcohol, povidone-iodine [Betadine], or chlorhexidine [Hibiclens]) as required by agency policy. The size of the needle or catheter is specific to the type of IV therapy. A 23- to 25-gauge needle and a 20- to 22-gauge catheter are sufficient for most IV therapy. Larger sizes, such as a 16- to 20-gauge catheter, are required if the client will receive blood products or hyperosmotic solutions, or is being prepared for surgery.

Solutions. Many types of IV solutions are available. Solutions are categorized by the *osmolarity,* or number of milliosmoles per liter of solution, or, more importantly, by their *osmolality*—how they affect the other fluids they are being compared with. Solutions come in three levels of osmolality: isotonic, hypertonic, and hypotonic. To review, an *isotonic* solution is one that has an osmotic pressure very similar to that of the solution or fluid with which it is being compared and thus does not affect fluid shifting. The amount of solute equals the amount of solution. A *hypertonic* solution is one that has a higher osmotic pressure than the one with which it is being compared. An easy way to remember this is that the *hyper* refers to the solute. This type of solution has a high solute concentration with less fluid, thus causing cells to shrink. A *hypotonic* solution is one that has a lower osmotic pressure than the one with which it is being compared. Again, the *hypo* refers to a low solute concentration, and the solution has a low solute concentration and more fluid, thus causing cells to swell.

Both the *hypertonic* and *hypotonic* solutions increase the risk of fluid shifting between compartments. IV solutions that are hypertonic increase the risk for fluid shifting into the plasma and thus for fluid excess because of the increased osmotic pull. *Hypotonic* IV fluids increase the risk of fluid shifting from the plasma to the interstitial compartments and cells because of the decreasing osmolality in the plasma. This concept is discussed later under Potential Complications.

Sites. Sites for IV therapy are categorized as peripheral or central (Figure 26-11). Any IV line that is inserted into the subclavian or jugular vein, or into a peripheral vein and threaded past the axillary line (a peripherally inserted central catheter or PICC line), is considered a central line. The subclavian veins are accessed more often than the jugular veins, especially for long-term therapy, because of the increased risk of phlebitis, catheter displacement, disconnection, and client discomfort associated with jugular IV placement. All other IV sites are considered peripheral IV sites. The most common site for peripheral IV therapy is the arm. The purpose and duration of the IV therapy, the type of solution, and the age and physical condition of the client are factors that determine the most appropriate IV site.

Avoid starting an IV over a joint to decrease the need for joint immobilization. Avoid the small, thin-walled veins in the hand if possible. This site is more painful and at greater risk for infiltration and limits the client's hand mobility. Also avoid the veins in the legs because their decreased flow rate increases the risk for thrombus or embolus formation. The most recommended site is the most distal site in the forearm above the wrist area. This allows for later venipunctures in more proximal veins. Avoid sites that are compromised by venous or lymphatic flow changes. These include veins on the same arm a mastectomy or lymphatic resection has been performed, on arms with fistulas or shunts, or on arms with varicosities or history of phlebitis or thrombosis.

Baseline Assessment. To accurately evaluate a client's response to IV therapy, complete a baseline head-to-toe assessment before initiating IV therapy. Repeat the assessment every 8 hours, and compare data. Clients with risk factors for overload may need to be assessed more frequently.

A baseline assessment includes vital signs, level of consciousness (LOC), mucous membranes for color and moisture, jugular venous distention, heart sounds, lung sounds, abdominal assessment, peripheral pulses, and urinary output. If the client experiences any changes in status, such as changes in LOC, marked changes in vital signs, shortness of breath, chest pain, or feeling that "something is wrong," initiate a thorough assessment immediately. Consult the physician about your findings.

Potential Complications. *Phlebitis* is an inflammation of the intimal layer of the vein. The earliest manifestation of phlebitis is the client's report of tenderness when you palpate over the vein. As the inflammation progresses, redness and warmth develop along the vein distal to the end of the IV catheter or needle. The catheter or needle should be removed when tenderness is first present to decrease the risk of clot formation in the vein. If the client still requires IV therapy, an alternative site will need to be selected.

The term *infiltration* means that the IV fluid has leaked through the venous wall into the interstitial tissue surrounding that vein. The area may feel hard or cold and probably will be painful. It is possible to still get blood return when you aspirate via the tubing with a syringe, even though the site is infiltrated. If there is swelling distal to the IV site that was not there when the IV infusion was initiated, you must remove the catheter or needle even if you can get blood return. The longer the infiltration continues, the more the fluid will accumulate and put pressure on the surrounding nerve endings, causing discomfort.

Infiltrated fluid is not functionally useful when it is in the interstitial tissues. Also, if the IV infusion contains medication that is caustic to tissues, it is even more critical that the infusion be discontinued immediately when infiltration is first noted. If this occurs, notify the physician of the infiltration. Depending on the medication, the physician will prescribe an antidote to be given subcutaneously in the infiltrated tissue. Use the agency procedure manual for further guidance. Table 26-9 lists the common data and nursing interventions for infiltration and other IV complications, including circulatory overload, infection, air embolism, and allergic reactions. The most common risk factors for circulatory overload include the administration of hypertonic solutions, rapid IV administration, and the presence of renal insufficiency.

Site Care

Peripheral. Review your facility's procedure manual for specific guidelines for peripheral IV site care. Studies of peripheral IV infection rates have prompted most facilities to require changing of the peripheral IV site every 72 to 96 hours. The type of IV dressing dictates whether the dressing requires changing more frequently. For example, if an occlusive, transparent dressing was applied following catheter insertion and the dressing remains intact and dry, it does not usually require changing, because it will be removed when the IV catheter site is changed. However, if the dressing is not occlusive (gauze, for example), it will

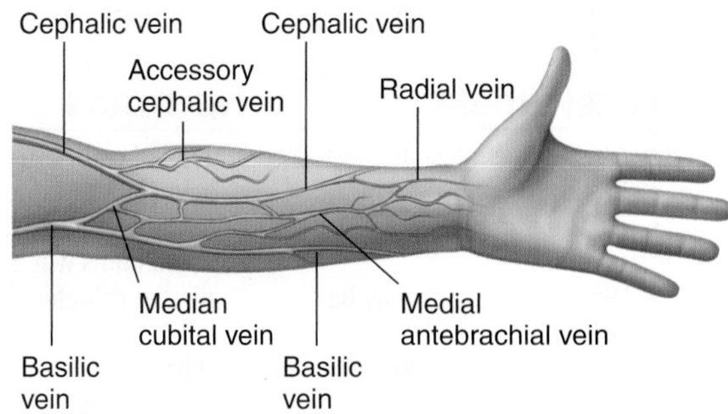

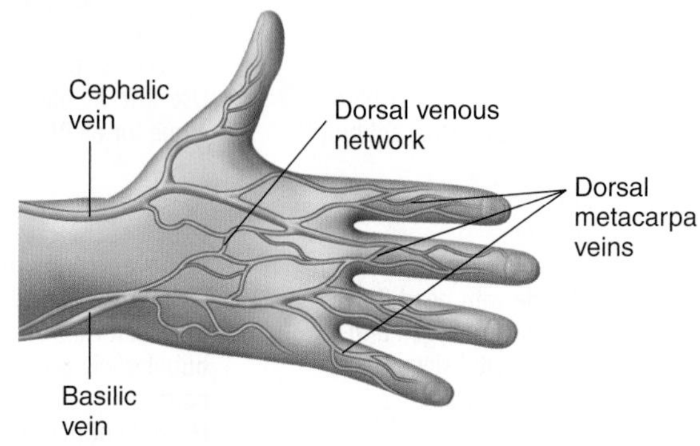

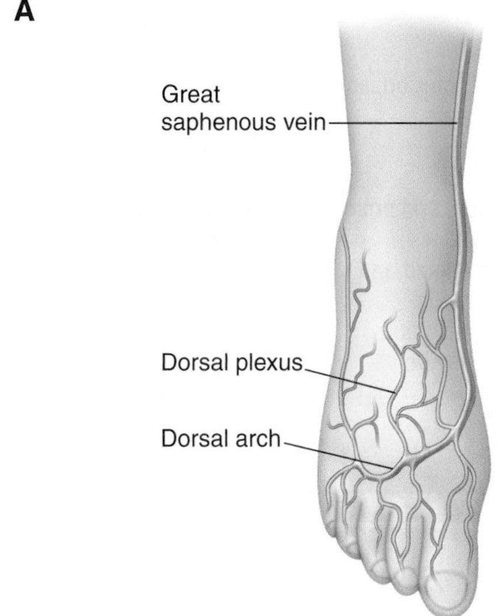

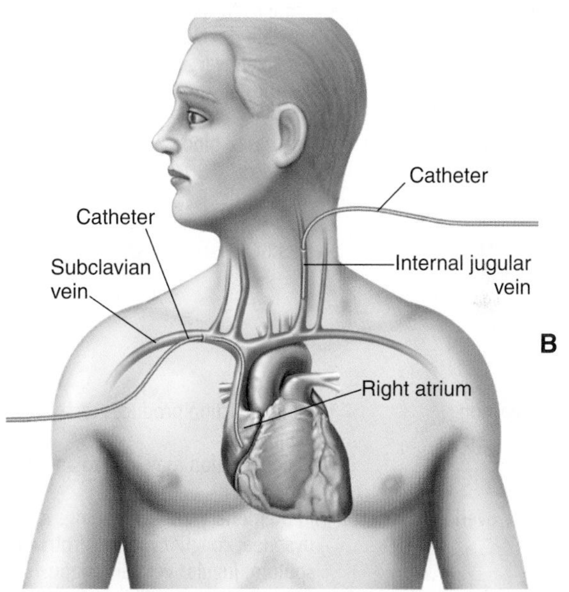

FIGURE 26-11 IV sites. **A,** Peripheral sites. Sites on the inner arm are preferred. Sites on the dorsum of the hand are often used, but the use of these sites increases the risk of vascular trauma and pain. Sites on the dorsum of the foot should be used only as a last resort because they are associated with an increased risk of thrombi. **B,** Central sites: subclavian vein and internal jugular vein.

need to be changed every 24 hours for site assessment. Many facilities require that a gauze dressing be used if a client is neutropenic, because a neutrophil count below 1000/mm^3 increases the risk for bacterial infection and gauze dressings decrease moisture retention.

When changing a dressing or starting an IV line, cleanse the site with an antimicrobial substance. Povidone iodine (1% to 2%), 70% alcohol, or chlorhexidine (Hibiclens) are the solutions recommended for IV site preparation. Agency policy dictates the type and order of cleansing. All cleansing is done in a circular motion starting at the IV insertion site and moving outward in a 2- to 3-inch circular motion. Let the antimicrobial agent dry before inserting the IV needle or catheter. Place the date and your initials on the IV dressing.

Central. Many variables influence the physician's choice for the type of IV access device. Among these are cost, ease of surgical placement, infection rates, length of therapy, client choice (when possible), quality of vascular tissue, and urgency of placement. Commonly used types include the Swan-Ganz (or introducer) catheter, triple-lumen catheter, tunneled catheter (such as Groshong or Hickman), implanted port (such as a Mediport, Infusaport, or Port-a-Cath), and a PICC line.

Table 26-9 Managing Complications of Intravenous Therapy

COMPLICATIONS	ASSESSMENT FINDINGS	INTERVENTIONS	PREVENTION
Infiltration	• Site is edematous, blanched, painful, cold. • Fluid will not flow by gravity despite confirmed patency of line (blood backflow when bag lowered below site).	• Discontinue infusion. • Restart in opposite arm. • Elevate arm if edema is severe. • Warm, moist pack may be comforting.	• Tape IV catheter securely in place and protect it from being pulled. • Avoid joints when placing catheter.
Phlebitis	• Heat, pain, redness, and edema develop around the site, or a streak running along the course of the vein may occur.	• Discontinue infusion. • Avoid massage because it might dislodge clots. • Warm, moist pack may be comforting.	• Dilute irritating medications. • Use smallest-gauge catheter appropriate. • Change site every 3 days or as specified.
Infection	• Same as for phlebitis. • Possible discharge at site. • Possible fever and sepsis. • Warmth at site.	• Physician will order blood cultures and start antibiotic therapy. • Discontinue infusion at this site	• Use strict sterile technique for all IV care.
Air embolism	• Decreased blood pressure. • Cyanosis. • Tachycardia. • Jugular vein distention. • Loss of consciousness.	• Immediately turn client on left side with head down. • Administer oxygen and monitor vital signs. • Notify physician.	• Remove air from tubing before connecting to catheter (small air bubbles will not be harmful) • Have client perform Valsalva maneuver or place head below heart level while changing tubing on central line.
Allergic reaction	• Minor reaction produces rash, redness, itching. • Major reaction may lead to anaphylactic shock	• Discontinue infusion, and notify physician.	• Assess client for history of allergies. • Monitor closely.
Circulatory overload	• In pulmonary edema, findings include dyspnea; cough; cyanosis; frothy, pink sputum; jugular vein distention. • Other findings include ascites, weight gain, edema.	• Slow infusion, and notify physician. • Verify correct fluid and rate of administration. • Diuretics and sodium restriction may be indicated.	• Take precautions to ensure correct fluid and rate of administration. • Use an IV infusion pump. • Monitor client's intake and output. • Monitor lung sounds • Monitor for edema.

IV, Intravenous.

Figure 26-12 illustrates a tunneled and an implanted central catheter.

Regardless of the type of central line used, you are responsible for following the manufacturer's and the facility's procedural guidelines for care and flushing protocols. For example, a normal saline flush maintains patency in a Groshong (close-ended) catheter and in some implanted ports, whereas heparin is recommended for a PICC line and many other types of central lines. The amount of flushing solution varies with the length and diameter of the catheter and the procedure. For instance, you may need as little as 1 to 3 mL of flush to keep a line open but as much as 10 to 20 mL of saline solution to cleanse the line after blood is drawn. If heparin is recommended, it is always the last solution in the flushing sequence because its only purpose is to prevent coagulation in the catheter system.

Follow the agency procedure manual for changing a dressing on a central line (Procedure 26-5). The frequency of dressing changes for central lines is similar to that for peripheral dressings. When a client is neutropenic, daily dressing changes with varying types of gauze may be mandated. When a transparent dressing is used without gauze, change the dressing every 72 hours or up to every 7 days, depending on agency policy. Sterile technique is required with all IV dressing changes, and a mask is also recommended when changing central line dressings. Sterile technique may be adapted to clean technique in the home setting if the client is not neutropenic.

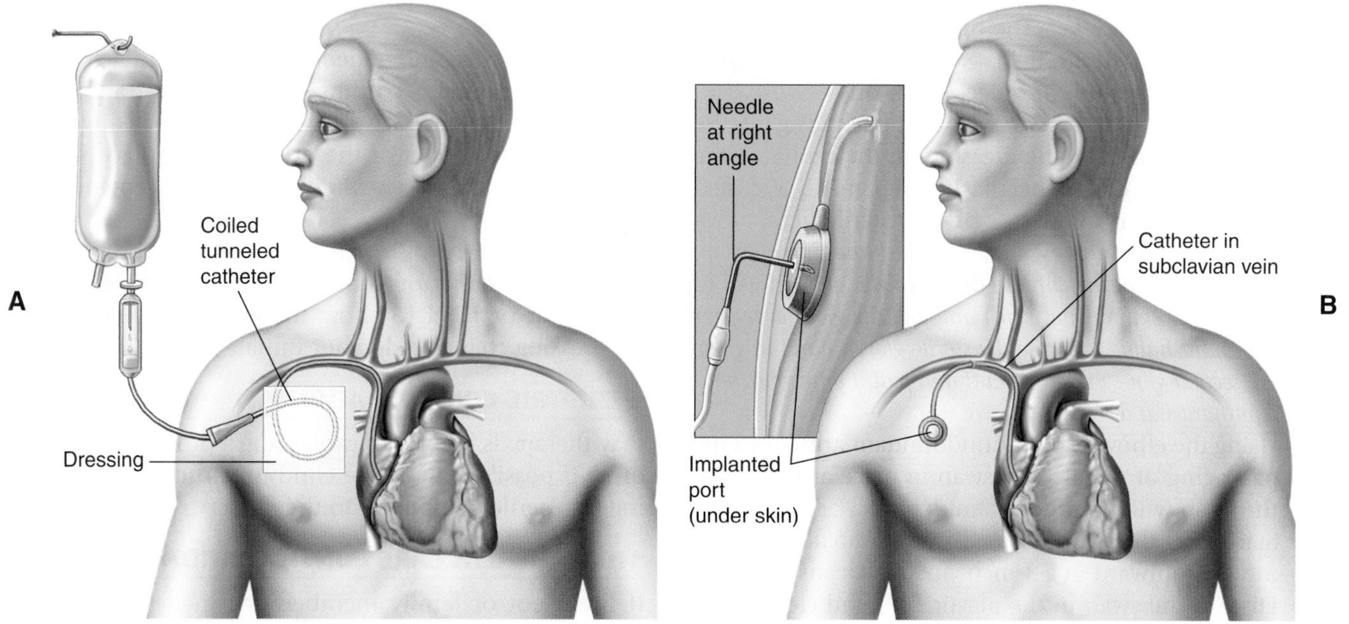

FIGURE 26-12 **A,** Placement of a tunneled central venous catheter. **B,** An implanted central port. The distal ends of both the tunneled central catheter and the implanted port are in the subclavian vein.

PROCEDURE 26-5

TIME TO ALLOW: NOVICE: 20 min. EXPERT: 10 min.

CHANGING THE DRESSING ON A CENTRAL LINE

Nursing Skills Online: Vascular Access, Lesson 3

A central venous access line is cleaned and dressed with meticulous care to prevent infection from entering the line. The old dressing is removed, the site cleaned, and the new dressing applied using sterile technique. Infection in the bloodstream (septicemia) is a life-threatening complication.

DELEGATION GUIDELINES

The indications for RN assessment and the potential risks associated with improper care of a central line suggest that this procedure not be delegated to a nursing assistant.

EQUIPMENT NEEDED

- Face mask
- Clean gloves
- Sterile gloves
- Three swabs or sticks of povidone-iodine (Betadine)
- Three swabs or sticks of alcohol
- Sterile, occlusive transparent dressing
- Cap for saline or heparin lock
- Plastic bag
- Black pen or marker
- Bedside table or flat surface for setting up a sterile field

1 Perform preliminary actions (see inside front cover).

2 Remove the soiled dressing. Remember that a client with a port that is not accessed does not require a dressing.

a. Put on the face mask, wash your hands, and put on clean gloves.

b. Remove the old dressing with your dominant hand while stabilizing the central line device with two fingers of the nondominant hand. Remove the dressing in the direction toward the catheter insertion site to prevent the risk of dislodging the catheter. *Be careful not to touch the catheter entry site.*

c. Holding the old dressing in your dominant hand, use your nondominant hand to pull the glove on your dominant hand off over the old dressing. Remove the other glove, and discard them both in the plastic bag.

d. Perform hand hygiene.

3 Clean the site.

a. Set up a sterile field. If a kit is available, open kit to create a sterile field. Put on sterile gloves, and then tear open the Betadine and alcohol swabs. Check the dressing but do not remove its backing yet. If no kit is available, open the package of sterile gloves but do

Continued

not put them on yet. The inside of the package will become your sterile field. Now, tear open Betadine and alcohol swabs and place them on the corner of the sterile field. Open the outer packaging of the dressing, and drop the dressing on the center of the sterile field. Open the plastic bag, make a cuffed edge, and set it to the side of your sterile field. Now, don the sterile gloves. *To do so, grasp the first glove on the top inside of the cuff (so the place you grasped will be against the skin of your arm) and pull the glove over your dominant hand. Now use the sterile gloved hand to grasp the second glove under the cuff and pull it onto your nondominant hand.*

b. Using the elbow of your nondominant arm, hold the packaging of the alcohol swab in place as you grasp the swab with your dominant hand.

c. Starting at the site of IV access, use a circular motion moving outward in a 3-inch circle to cleanse the site. Discard the swab in the plastic bag, and cleanse the site in the same manner with the other two alcohol swabs.

d. After the alcohol has evaporated (about 15 seconds), repeat the cleansing motion with the three Betadine swabs. *Allowing the alcohol and Betadine to mix when the alcohol is still wet can cause skin irritation and alter the bacteriostatic properties.*

4 Dress the site.

a. If gauze is recommended, apply it over the cleansed site and tape it according to policy. If a transparent dressing is being used, remove the backing and, holding the edges of the dressing taut, place it over the site so the IV access device is in the center of the dressing.

b. Use the fingers of one hand to smooth the dressing from the center outward to make a tight seal. Use a marker or label to show the date and time of the dressing change. Add your initials as well.

PEDIATRIC CONSIDERATIONS

Play therapy is helpful in explaining a procedure to children. If possible, allow the child to participate in handing nonsterile equipment to the nurse.

HOME HEALTH CARE CONSIDERATIONS

If the client or family members will perform dressing changes at home, teach them how to use clean technique unless the client is neutropenic. In that case, sterile technique is required. If the site has no dressing, teach the client or family member to cleanse the site with soap and water and to place a Band-Aid over the entry site using tape to support the tunneled catheter.

INTERVENTIONS TO DECREASE FLUID VOLUME

There are three primary interventions related to decreasing fluid volume: restoring fluid balance, preventing complications, and instituting rehabilitative care.

Restoring Fluid Balance. Limit the client's fluid and sodium intake. Instruct the client and family about the rationale for fluid and dietary restrictions to ensure compliance.

Administer prescribed medications. Diuretics are often ordered to help rid the body of excess fluid. Another focus of drug therapy is to correct the etiology of the fluid excess. If the overload is from an ineffective myocardial pump, the physician may prescribe an inotropic drug to enhance myocardial contractility, or a medication to decrease myocardial workload, such as a calcium channel blocker or angiotensin-converting enzyme (ACE) inhibitor.

If capillary permeability is the etiology, in addition to treating the underlying sepsis, acid-base imbalance, or other factors, the physician will prescribe corticosteroids to promote healing of the membrane. Carefully monitor fluid volume if corticosteroids are ordered for a client with congestive heart failure (CHF) because of added risk of fluid retention. If protein deficit is present, the source of this deficit is investigated and corrected if possible, and additional protein is given if appropriate. The etiologies of fluid volume excess are quite numerous.

Preventing Complications. To prevent complications, provide appropriate supportive care. Monitor and record I&O, and weigh the client daily. Compare your findings with previous documentation. Maintain the client's nutritional needs, consulting with a dietitian if necessary. To decrease the client's feeling of mucosal dryness that accompanies fluid restriction, you can encourage the family to bring hard candies or lozenges, provide ice chips, and give or assist with oral care frequently (up to hourly if necessary).

Perform a thorough head-to-toe assessment to determine how a client is responding to the interventions; this is essential to secondary prevention. The frequency of the assessments varies with the severity of the fluid overload. Assessments may be needed as often as hourly in a critical care setting, every 8 hours when the condition has stabilized, or weekly or monthly in a chronic-care or home setting.

Fluid retention impairs tissue perfusion. The interventions for impaired tissue perfusion are specific to the organ or system that is involved. Although the goal is to promote optimal perfusion of all body tissues, fluid overload in the heart, lungs, liver, kidneys, and brain must be treated immediately to avoid life-threatening complications.

One system that is often affected by fluid retention is the skin. One of the most common interventions to decrease the risk for impaired skin integrity is pressure relief. Repositioning the client every 2 hours or more as necessary may be enough to decrease the pressure on these tissues. However, if this is not enough, consult the physician about ordering a pressure-reducing mattress or bed. If the edema is localized to an extremity, elevate the limb to promote venous return and thus decrease swelling. Passive or active range-of-motion exercises five or more times for each joint twice a day will also promote venous return and maintain joint function.

If fluid retention has involved the pulmonary system, elevate the head of bed for client comfort and optimal diaphragmatic excursion. The more pulmonary fluid the client has, the greater the need for head of bed elevation. A client with severe pulmonary fluid overload often needs a 90-degree headrest with arms supported on pillows on a bedside table. Elevating the client's head will also decrease venous return to the right side of the heart and thus decrease cardiac workload. The greater the amount of fluid overload, the more aggressive the interventions need to be. Minimal fluid overload can often be managed with deep breathing, incentive pyrometer, repositioning, mild diuretics, inotropic medications, and calcium channel blockers or ACE inhibitors.

Fluid retention is always a risk with a postoperative client who has received general anesthesia. Administer fluids cautiously in early postoperative or posttraumatic stress periods. Increased ADH secretion during this period can cause fluid overload. The presence of or increase in crackles is an early sign of pulmonary fluid and should alert you that fluids are being given faster than the body can tolerate them. An increase in urinary output is an early sign of the end of this phase.

Instituting Rehabilitative Care. Self-care is a major component of rehabilitation from fluid volume excess. Promote self-care by teaching the client and family about restricting fluid and table salt, reading food labels, avoiding products high in sodium, keeping a diary of weights, balancing activity and rest, and calling the physician whenever significant health changes occur.

Additional interventions for fluid balance maintenance include the following:

- Control delivery of fluid by using IV and feeding pumps when appropriate.
- Monitor laboratory results specific to fluid and electrolyte homeostasis, such as BUN, creatinine, hemoglobin, hematocrit, urine or serum osmolality, and serum electrolytes.
- Monitor for expected and unexpected responses to prescribed medications.
- Provide referrals to assist with lifestyle changes and financial constraints as appropriate, such as social services, dietitian counseling, home health care nursing services, and home health care aide.
- Evaluate fluid balance in relationship to output and compare data with the client's other presenting data.
- Provide client and family teaching.

INTERVENTIONS TO BALANCE ELECTROLYTE LEVELS

When caring for a client who has an electrolyte imbalance, your goal is to decrease the risk for serious consequences. With electrolyte deficits, the goals of the intervention include replacing the lost electrolyte, decreasing the rate of further loss, or both. With electrolyte excess, the goals of intervention focus on limiting intake, increasing loss, or both.

General Interventions. Nutrition is a key intervention in most electrolyte imbalances. Consult with a dietitian for information on specific foods to include or exclude in therapeutic diets specific to each imbalance. Give your client a written handout listing these food items. Keep in mind that dietary changes are among the most difficult for clients to make. Provide resources such as the names of local dietitians or nutrition support groups to help the client with this behavioral change.

Providing practical examples of how to "eat healthier" can also be helpful. For example, you can suggest that the client use fresh lemon on foods and salads instead of prepared sauces. Or, when dining out, the client could request that food be prepared without salt and cooked by grilling, baking, or broiling. The client may also wish to carry along a seasoning that fits the prescribed diet. Also teach the client or food buyer the importance of reading the entire nutritional label for levels of sodium, potassium, and other nutrients. Bold print is often misleading.

When teaching about dietary restrictions, it is very important that the "cook" and other family members be involved. The more support the client has, the more successful the behavioral change will be. Finally, be very clear about whether the dietary restriction is a temporary change or a lifelong change.

In a client at high risk for malnutrition, especially a client unable to consume nutrients orally, the physician may prescribe a nutritional supplement that contains all of the previously mentioned electrolytes as well as some trace minerals. This may be delivered by gastric or intestinal tube for a person with long-term nutritional needs or by the IV route in the form of total parenteral nutrition for someone with short-term needs.

Whether the client is experiencing a deficit or an excess, the promptness of the intervention will depend on two key factors: the severity of the imbalance and the presenting manifestations. The following nursing interventions are appropriate to all electrolyte imbalances.

- Monitor the client's liver, kidney, and bowel functions. Normal medication processing and excretion depend on the interactive functioning of these systems. Dysfunction in any of these systems can lead to toxicity, which often includes fluid and electrolyte imbalances.

- Monitor the client's level of serum electrolytes, especially when giving medications that either affect or are affected by electrolyte levels.
- Assess the client's vital signs. Frequency varies with the severity of the alteration. You may need to assess vital signs as often as every 15 minutes when the electrolyte level is critical, or once a week or month in a more chronic situation.
- Assess an apical pulse for a full minute whenever the peripheral pulse is irregular. Remember that many electrolytes (including sodium, potassium, magnesium, and calcium) affect the rate and rhythm of the cardiac cells.
- Cardiac monitoring may be necessary with an irregular pulse. If the client is on a cardiac monitor, watch for dysrhythmias and other changes.
- Monitor I&O every hour in an acutely ill client. Teach the client and family to monitor and compare weight trends at least weekly for a stable "at home" client.
- Assess peripheral vein filling and emptying time. Normally, veins take less than 5 seconds to empty or fill.
- Because weakness is a common manifestation of many electrolyte imbalances, remember to initiate fall precautions when appropriate, such as removing obstacles from the environment and providing mobility support.
- Teach clients and families the importance of consuming foods within the prescribed diet. Encourage intake of a well-balanced diet when possible. Encourage intake of foods that replace nutrients that are lost secondary to an illness or other condition. For a state of electrolyte excess, avoid foods high in that electrolyte.
- Teach clients to follow pharmaceutical recommendations for electrolyte replacement and to avoid taking more than the recommended daily vitamin-mineral supplement without consulting with a physician. Tell the client to avoid other OTC medications unless approved by a physician, because many of these drugs can alter fluid and electrolyte balance. Implement and teach the client that antacids should be separated from other medications by 1 to 2 hours, because they can alter electrolyte balance or affect the absorption of other medications.
- Irrigate NG tubes with normal saline only; if ice chips are ordered, use sparingly.
- When "enemas till clear" are prescribed, give no more than three in a row. Hypotonic solutions can alter fluid and electrolyte status. Consult the physician before proceeding.

Interventions for Sodium Imbalance. Hyponatremia is one of the more common electrolyte imbalances. The client's response to hyponatremia varies with the cause, rate of loss, and type of associated fluid imbalance. A client can present with a sodium level of 120 mEq/L and be asymptomatic if the imbalance developed slowly. The same level, if it results from an acute loss, can cause life-threatening manifestations.

The client's amount of body water also affects response. Sodium deficit can occur in the presence of decreased, normal, or increased body water. However, one of the most common types of hyponatremia is caused by fluid overload. When this is the etiology, fluid restriction is the intervention of choice. Fluid restriction is very difficult for any client to abide by. You can help the client understand the importance of this intervention and provide suggestions that will increase compliance. Ice chips, lozenges, frequent mouth care, and small, frequent sips of fluids will provide comfort.

If hyponatremia is truly due to a sodium deficit, then the physician will prescribe additional sodium either orally, by tube, or in IV form. If the level is 125 mEq/L or greater, diet supplementation and interventions to decrease the loss are the usual treatment. Other common interventions include prescriptions to improve the function of the organs that are causing the problem, such as digitalis and diuretics for cardiac overload.

Hypernatremia is not as commonly encountered as hyponatremia. Interventions include withholding sodium in the diet and IV fluids and increasing intake of free water.

Interventions for Potassium Imbalance. Potassium imbalance can be very dangerous. Because potassium is predominantly an intracellular ion, the serum level is only an indirect reflection of the cellular level. Minor serum imbalances can indicate serious risk for cellular imbalance. Although many systems are affected by a potassium imbalance, the cardiovascular system is most critically affected. A low serum potassium level increases the risk of cardiac dysrhythmias. The risk of digitalis toxicity is also increased.

> ***Action Alert!*** Consult the physician before giving digitalis derivatives when potassium is low, when the serum digitalis level is high, or when the client has bradycardia (pulse less than 60 beats per minute).

Physicians usually prefer to be notified of the bradycardia and often will prescribe the continuance of digitalis as long as the apical pulse is above 50 beats per minute. This is because the client is at a greater risk from the complications of an ineffective myocardial pump without the digitalis. In other instances the dosage may be reduced.

If dietary replacement is insufficient, oral potassium supplements are usually prescribed. If the level is critical, then the more rapid IV replacement route is chosen.

Give oral potassium with food because it is a GI irritant. Intravenous potassium can be given *only* in diluted form; direct IV potassium has been known to cause cardiac arrest. The maintenance dose is 40 to 80 mEq/day. If the potassium level is critically low or if the client has serious cardiac dysrhythmias, up to 10 mEq/hr can be given in as little as 125 mL of solution, but the client must be on a cardiac monitor during this infusion. Use an IV pump to ensure a safer delivery of IV potassium. Potassium is a venous irritant; if the client experiences pain at the IV site, the infusion rate may need to be slowed or the potassium diluted further. Potassium is very toxic to interstitial tissues; if infiltration occurs, stop the IV infusion immediately and notify the physician. Because potassium is excreted primarily via the kidneys, it is essential to monitor urinary output. If the output is borderline (about 30 mL/hr), monitor output hourly. If the urine output drops to less than 30 mL/hr for 2 consecutive hours, notify the physician.

Hyperkalemia can be a medical emergency. If the potassium level has caused significant cardiac conduction changes, the physician may order IV glucose and insulin to promote immediate, but temporary, shifting of the potassium from the plasma into the cells. To ensure excretion of potassium from the body, a cation exchange resin such as sodium polystyrene sulfate (Kayexalate) may be ordered in oral or rectal form, or, if time is critical, peritoneal dialysis or hemodialysis may be done to remove excess potassium from the body.

Interventions for Calcium Imbalance. Calcium imbalance is less common than sodium and potassium imbalances. Therefore, as a cost-conscious effort, the physician tests this level only when a client is at high risk for imbalance or has manifestations that suggest an imbalance. You play an active role in helping the physician identify such clients.

Calcium must be taken with vitamin D to promote absorption. High-phosphate products (such as milk and carbonated beverages) promote calcium loss. Therefore it is important to teach clients to avoid these products if the hypocalcemia is caused by hypoparathyroidism. When a client has normal parathyroid functioning, parathormone is able to manage the high phosphate levels in milk products, and the client is then able to receive the full calcium benefit from the calcium in the milk product.

The bone softening that accompanies calcium deficit or excess can result in a fracture with minimal strain. Teach clients the importance of weight-bearing activities to decrease calcium bone loss. Calcium deficit also increases the client's risk for bleeding; teach clients to report signs of bleeding. If hypercalcemia is present, strain all urine and teach the client to strain urine to identify the presence of renal calculi. Teach the client that forcing fluids will decrease this risk. Also help the client understand the role of prescription medications for hypercalcemia. These include saline IV infusions, diuretics (nonthiazides), etidronate disodium (Didronel), phosphates, and corticosteroids.

Interventions for Magnesium Imbalance. When a magnesium deficit exists, increasing dietary intake is seldom sufficient. Usually an oral replacement is given unless the situation requires a more aggressive IV approach. The oral magnesium is often given in the form of a magnesium-containing antacid. The parenteral form is usually magnesium sulfate. IV magnesium must be diluted in a nonsaline solution. Monitor blood pressure for improvement and ECG for decreased dysrhythmias as top priorities. Provide safety and seizure precautions for any client who is confused or at risk for seizures; these are critically important measures. Assess the return of the deep tendon reflexes as an indication that magnesium balance has been restored.

Interventions for Phosphate Imbalance. Phosphate imbalances are rare. A deficit is treated by oral or IV replacement. A phosphate excess is treated with calcium or aluminum supplements.

INTERVENTIONS TO RESTORE ACID-BASE BALANCE

Nursing interventions for acid-base imbalances are typically driven by written orders from health care providers and aim to return the client to a state of acid-base balance. Other than monitoring for signs of specific acid-base imbalances, nursing interventions usually include supportive fluid and electrolyte replacement, support of respiratory function with primary respiratory imbalances, and administering prescribed medications, such as sodium bicarbonate to treat acidosis or insulin in diabetic ketoacidosis.

EVALUATION

The time frame for evaluating fluid or electrolyte imbalance varies with the urgency of the imbalance. For example, if the client is experiencing a life-threatening dysrhythmia, cardiac monitoring with narrow alarm parameters will be continuous. Neurological manifestations that indicate a worsening condition also require continuous evaluation. As the client stabilizes, however, the frequency of evaluation decreases, from hourly assessments to every 4 hours and every 8 hours. In extended-care facilities and in the home, clients may require evaluation of risk or actual imbalances on only a weekly or a monthly basis.

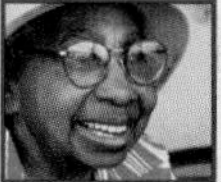

Let us return to Mrs. Thompson. After recovering from her episode of congestive heart failure, she was discharged with home health care visits weekly. A nursing progress note for this client might look like the documentation note on p. 662.

Sample Documentation Note for Mrs. Thompson

Monitoring her fluid intake and the number of voidings every 24 hours. Intake is comparable to output. Compliant with monitoring her weight daily and noting values in her diary. Weight gain of 1/2 pound in 1 week is noted. Denies edema or shortness of breath. States she feels better and less fatigued since starting current medication regime. Skin recoils rapidly, capillary refill is less than 3 seconds in nail beds, lungs are clear bilaterally. Encouraged to continue monitoring intake and output as well as weight. Reviewed food intake, and she is compliant with low-sodium diet.

If the client is not improving, collect data to help determine the reason that outcomes are not being achieved. There are many possible variables, including barriers such as nausea or lack of access to food or fluids, another etiology or underlying pathologic process that is not responding to the current treatment, or perhaps a lack of compliance with the prescribed treatments for other reasons.

If a client has an actual fluid and electrolyte imbalance, compare the current manifestations with those present on the last assessment. The desired outcome is an improvement in any of the signs or symptoms discussed in this chapter. Clearly, improvement of manifestations involving life-sustaining tissues is the highest priority. However, even a fluid imbalance at a local level, such as severe edema in an extremity, could pose a threat to the life of that tissue. Naturally, life-threatening signs and symptoms require aggressive intervention. Revise the care plan if there is no longer a risk or an actual problem, if improvement is evident, if improvement does not occur quickly enough, or if the condition worsens. See Box 26-6 for more information.

BOX 26-6

Nursing Care Plan

A Client With Fluid Volume Deficit

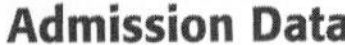

Admission Data

Mrs. Thompson was examined by her physician's nurse in the outpatient clinic. The nurse reported the following data to Dr. Kline.

Nursing Assessment

Color pale, skin dry, oral mucous membranes dry with tongue furrows, weight 110 pounds (decrease of 10 pounds in 2 weeks), blood pressure 116/50, pulse 110 and weak, respirations 24 (usually 142/70, 80, 16). Appears restless and is unable to remember when she last ate. Reports extreme fatigue and weakness over the last several weeks; states stools have been hard and infrequent.

Dr. Kline examined Mrs. Thompson and wrote the following on her chart.

Physician's Progress Note

Diagnosis: Dehydration secondary to decreased intake, extreme weakness, and fatigue. Early signs of ECF deficit with minimal signs of intracellular affect (confusion). In no acute distress at this time. Believe she can be managed at home because supportive family will assist in monitoring and care delivery. Visiting nurse three times a week for 2 weeks. Hospitalization for IV therapy only if signs worsen.

Office Care

The office nurse completed teaching with Mrs. Thompson and her son Gerald. While consulting with Mrs. Thompson, especially about her ethnic preferences, a grocery list was compiled. The nurse also reinforced the importance of Gerald's daily visits until his mother becomes stable. She also gave them a list of signs and symptoms about which Dr. Kline's office must be notified. Later, the office nurse contracted the visiting nursing agency and gave Judy Carson, RN, Mrs. Thompson's nurse, a full report with the following orders:

Initial visit today to include the following:
- Home baseline assessment.
- Instruct Mrs. Thompson and her family about schedule for oral fluid replacement.
- Plan to include increasing fluid intake to 1500 mL per day; stopping 3 hours before bedtime.
- Plan to include increasing food intake to six small meals per day.
- Validate understanding of teaching.

Additional orders:
- Contact Meals on Wheels about meal supplementation.
- Evaluate progress every 2 days for 2 weeks.

NANDA-I Nursing Diagnosis	NOC Expected Outcomes With Indicators	NIC Interventions With Selected Activities	Evaluation Data
Deficient Fluid Volume **Related Factors:** • Dry skin • Dry mucous membranes • Furrowed tongue	***Hydration*** **Fluid balance:** • Maintain moist oral mucous membranes in 48 hours. • No tongue furrows within a week. • Oriented to person, time, and place in 48 hours.	***Fluid Management*** • Assess oral mucous membranes and tongue.	***Home Visit, 48 Hours Later*** • Tongue furrows absent, but oral mucous membranes remain dry.
• Weight 110 (decrease of 10 pounds in 2 weeks)	**Weight:** • Increased by 1 pound within a week.	• Weigh with approximate amount of clothing had on at initial visit, and at same time of day.	• Weight gain of 1 pound.

BOX 26-6

Nursing Care Plan—cont'd

A Client With Fluid Volume Deficit

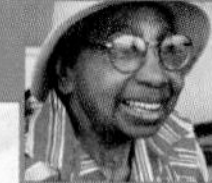

NANDA-I Nursing Diagnosis	NOC Expected Outcomes With Indicators	NIC Interventions With Selected Activities	Evaluation Data
Deficient Fluid Volume	***Hydration***	***Fluid Management***	***Home Visit, 48 Hours Later***
	Vital signs monitoring:		
• BP 116/50 (usually 142/70)	• Improvement seen in BP, systolic <120.	• Assess orientation to person, place, and time.	• Able to state name, home address, and month.
• Pulse 110, R 24 • Restless	• Pulse <100	• Assess vital signs.	• BP 118/70, P 96, R 20.
• Slightly confused	• Respirations < 20 within 48 hours		
	Constipation management:		
• Stools hard and infrequent	• Reports softer stools at least once since doctor's visit.	• Assess stool characteristics since office visit.	• Stated one stool, moderate amount, still somewhat hard.
	Fluid management:		
• Fatigue and weakness	• Reports taking 60 mL fluids per hour, six small meals per day for 1 month.	• Assess fluid and diet history since office visit.	• Diary of fluid/food intake: • Day 1: 1000 mL, four meals.
	• Reports more strength.		• Day 2: 1200 mL, four meals but one bigger; daughter-in-law, Sue, made favorite ethnic dish.
	• Improvement in self-care activities.	• Evaluate her ADLs since office visit, as well as level of fatigue and weakness.	• Able to serve self breakfast, heat up meals from Meals on Wheels; too tired to cook at supper; Gerald fixed supper; Sue helped with bath each night. Required morning and afternoon nap.

Critical Thinking Questions

1. Mrs. Thompson has made progress toward the expected outcomes but has not achieved them. When the family expresses concern about this and asks you if you think she should come to live with them or be placed in a residential home, how would you answer and why?
2. Referring to the original case study, review the changes that are seen 1 week later. What signs and symptoms is Mrs. Thompson having now? Why? What other signs and symptoms indicate fluid volume excess? Which ones are the most serious, and why?

ADLs, Activities of daily living; *BP,* blood pressure; *ECF,* extracellular fluid; *R,* respiration.
Nursing outcome and intervention labels from Johnson, M., Bulechek, G., Butcher, H., Dochterman, J. M., Maas, M., Moorhead, S., et al. (Eds.). (2006). *NANDA, NOC, and NIC linkages: Nursing diagnoses, outcomes, & interventions.* St. Louis, MO: Mosby.

▼ KEY PRINCIPLES

- Fluid and electrolyte imbalances are fairly common and often overlooked.
- Fluid and electrolyte imbalances rarely occur in isolation. It is the relationship of the solute to the solvent that determines the client's response, not the level of the deficit by itself.
- The most common fluid imbalance is dehydration, which occurs most often in the very young and in older adults.
- Fluid overload is common in clients with cardiovascular problems.
- Seventy percent of the body fluid is in the intracellular spaces. Therefore acute or severe loss can have serious consequences for cellular functioning.
- Fluid shifting occurs between the extracellular compartments first, unless the loss or excess is acute or severe. Regardless, cellular fluid shifting occurs last after the extracellular compensatory mechanisms have been exhausted.
- The most common electrolyte imbalance is hyponatremia. It is more common in the older adult population, especially in those on low-salt diets who are taking diuretics.

Continued

- Nurses must anticipate imbalances in high-risk clients: the very young; older adults; those experiencing pregnancy, especially teenage pregnancy; and those with acute or chronic illnesses.
- Thorough history and physical assessments including diagnostics are necessary for making an accurate differential diagnosis.
- The outcomes of the imbalance depend on the acuteness and severity of the condition, the age and health state of the client, and the degree to which the client's compensatory mechanisms or therapeutic interventions combat the imbalance.
- The nurse has many roles, including teaching the clients and their families positive health behaviors, promoting nutritional maintenance and replacement, collaborating with the physician for early detection of imbalances and poor responses to treatment, and collaboration with the dietitian in the promotion of positive nutritional outcomes.
- Through individualization of interventions and mutual goal setting with the clients and their families, nurses can facilitate optimal health outcomes.
- Nurses are in a key position to influence cost-effectiveness and cost efficiency through utilization of appropriate resources, delegation of appropriate interventions, promotion of primary and secondary prevention, and ongoing care plan evaluation and revision.

■ REVIEW QUESTIONS

1. The nurse is checking the serum electrolyte levels of a client with a cardiac dysrhythmia. Which of the following laboratory values is consistent with the client's cardiac status?

1. Sodium 145 mEq/L
2. Potassium 3.2 mEq/L
3. Calcium 5.0 mEq/L
4. Chloride 102 mEq/L

2. The nurse would look to which of the following assessment data as the best indicator of fluid status in a client with renal disease?

1. Neck vein distention
2. Skin turgor
3. Intake and output totals
4. Daily weight

3. The client has the following arterial blood gas results: pH, 7.32; $PaCO_2$, 49 mm Hg; HCO_3^-, 24 mEq/L; PaO_2, 86 mm Hg. The nurse should assess the client for manifestations of which of the following acid-base imbalances?

1. Respiratory alkalosis
2. Respiratory acidosis
3. Metabolic alkalosis
4. Metabolic acidosis

4. The nurse has an order to insert a nasogastric tube in a client who keeps vomiting. Which of the following steps should the nurse take first?

1. Measure the length of the tube for insertion
2. Provide the client with a cup of water and a straw
3. Explain the procedure to the client
4. Cut small lengths of tape for securing the tube after insertion

5. The nurse should take which action when caring for the client with an intravenous catheter who is receiving parenteral fluid therapy?

1. Change the intravenous tubing every 48 hours
2. Check the flow rate once per hour
3. Change the catheter site every other day
4. Use a gauze dressing on the insertion site

Bibliography

Astle, S. M. (2005). Restoring electrolyte balance. *RN, 68*(5), 34-40.

Cook, L. S. (2003). IV fluid resuscitation. *Journal of Infusion Nursing, 26*(5), 296-303, 327-330.

Davidhizar, R., Dunn, C. L., & Hart, A. N. (2004). A review of the literature on how important water is to the world's elderly population. *International Nursing Review, 51*(3), 159-166.

Diehl-Oplinger, L,. & Kaminski, M. F. (2004). Choosing the right fluid to counter hypovolemic shock. *Nursing, 34*(3), 52-54.

Elgart, H. N. (2004). Assessment of fluids and electrolytes. *AACN Clinical Issues: Advanced Practice in Acute and Critical Care, 15*(4), 607-621.

Ellet, M. L. (2004). What is known about methods of correctly placing gastric tubes in adults and children? *Gastroenterology Nursing, 27*(6), 253-259.

Infusion Nurses Society. (2003). *Core curriculum for infusion nursing* (3rd ed.). Philadelphia: Lippincott Williams, & Wilkins.

Infusion Nurses Society. (2006). *Infusion nursing standards of practice. Journal of Infusion Nursing*. Philadelphia: Lippincott Williams & Wilkins.

Johnson, M., Bulechek, G., Butcher, H., Dochterman, J. M., Maas, M., Moorhead, S., et al. (Eds.). (2006). *NANDA, NOC, and NIC linkages: Nursing diagnoses, outcomes, & interventions.* St. Louis, MO: Mosby.

Karch, A. M. (2004). Practice errors. On the rebound: Maintaining normal fluid intake is critical while on diuretics. *American Journal of Nursing, 104*(10), 73.

Khair, J. (2005). Guidelines for testing the placing of nasogastric tubes. *Nursing Times, 101*(20), 26-27.

Larson, K. (2003). Home health care. Fluid balance in the elderly: Assessment and intervention—important role in community health and home care nursing. *Geriatric Nursing, 24*(5), 306-309.

*Maughan, R. J. (1992). Fluid balance and exercise. *International Journal of Sports Medicine, 13,* S132-S135.

Mitchell D. (2004). Consult stat. Here's an easy way to make sense of IV fluid therapy. *RN, 67*(10), 65-67.

Puthoff, T. D. (2004). Fluids and electrolytes management. *Newborn and Infant Nursing Reviews,* 4(2), 98-105.

*Reherer, N. J. (1994). The maintenance of fluid balance during exercise. *International Journal of Sports Medicine, 15*(3), 122-125.

Understanding fluids and electrolytes. (2004). *Nursing, 34,*(4), 81-84.

*Asterisk indicates a classic or definitive work on this subject.

Chapter 27

Promoting Wound Healing

Media Resources

- Nursing Skills Online
- evolve Evolve Website http://evolve.elsevier.com/Harkreader/
- 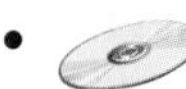 Companion CD
- 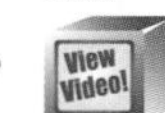 Skills Video Clips

Learning Objectives

After studying this chapter, you should be able to do the following:

- Describe skin disruptions, wound healing, and problems of wound healing
- Discuss the staging of pressure ulcers
- Explain the effects of lifestyle, age, and illness on skin integrity and wound healing
- Assess the client who is at risk for or has an actual impairment of skin integrity
- Distinguish among nursing diagnoses for clients with alterations in skin integrity
- Plan for goal-directed interventions to promote wound healing
- Evaluate the outcomes of interventions for *Impaired skin integrity*

Key Terms

abrasion
débridement
dehiscence
epithelialization
eschar
evisceration
exudate
fistula
granulation tissue
hematoma
hemorrhage
maceration
pressure ulcer
primary lesion
secondary lesion
slough
wound

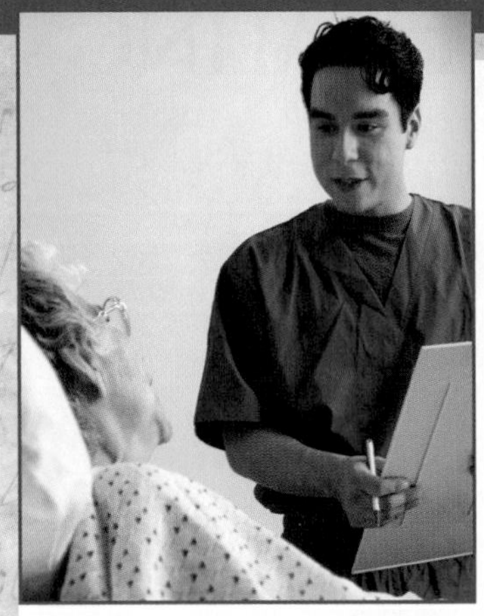

Violetta Jacan is a 72-year-old woman who has been living alone in an apartment since her husband died 3 years ago. Her daughter lives nearby. One morning while getting out of the shower, Mrs. Jacan fell onto the bathroom floor and fractured her right hip. Unable to get to the phone to call for help, she lay on the floor until her daughter checked in on her late the next day. On admission to the emergency department, Mrs. Jacan is diagnosed with a hip fracture. She also has reddened areas on her sacrum and heels.

Once Mrs. Jacan arrives on the surgical unit, the nurse prepares her for hip surgery and begins to plan for her postoperative skin care needs. He notes that Mrs. Jacan is over 70 and shows the beginning of pressure ulcer formation. He also considers that the client will have a hip incision and limited mobility during the postoperative period. As part of Mrs. Jacan's nursing care plan, the nurse considers the diagnoses in the key nursing diagnoses box.

CONCEPTS OF SKIN INTEGRITY AND WOUND HEALING

In all practice settings, nurses are concerned with skin care needs and prevention of disruptions in skin integrity. Disruptions range from minor, superficial damage, such as an abrasion or a tape blister to major disruptions, such as a deep pressure ulcer or a wound from major abdominal surgery. Throughout this range, skin care is an integral part of the overall nursing care plan.

SKIN DISRUPTIONS

The skin is the first line of defense to protect the body from mechanical, thermal, chemical, and radiant trauma. The epidermis is a tough mechanical layer that prevents microorganisms, foreign material, and chemicals from penetrating the body. The dermis (1) gives structure and flexibility to the skin, (2) supplies nutrients and removes wastes, and (3) senses pain, touch, pressure, and temperature. A break in the skin barrier creates a route for the loss of body fluids and the risk for infection.

Skin Lesions. A lesion is any pathological or traumatic discontinuity of normal tissue or loss of function of a part including wounds, sores, ulcers, tumors, cataracts, and any other tissue damage. It is a visible local abnormality in the skin caused by injuries, pathological changes, allergies, or bites. To determine the etiology of common skin lesions, you should be able to distinguish between primary and secondary lesions. A **primary lesion** is the first lesion to appear on the skin in response to a causative agent and usually has a recognizable structure. Changes can occur in a primary lesion and result in a **secondary lesion.** These changes occur in the epidermal layer and are caused by several factors including scratching, rubbing, medications, treatments, and the client's medical condition or disease process. Figure 27-1 illustrates some common skin lesions.

KEY NURSING DIAGNOSES FOR SKIN INTEGRITY

Risk for impaired skin integrity: A state in which the individual's skin is at risk of being adversely altered
Impaired skin integrity: A state in which an individual has altered epidermis and/or dermis
Impaired tissue integrity: Damage to mucous membrane, corneal, integumentary, or subcutaneous tissue

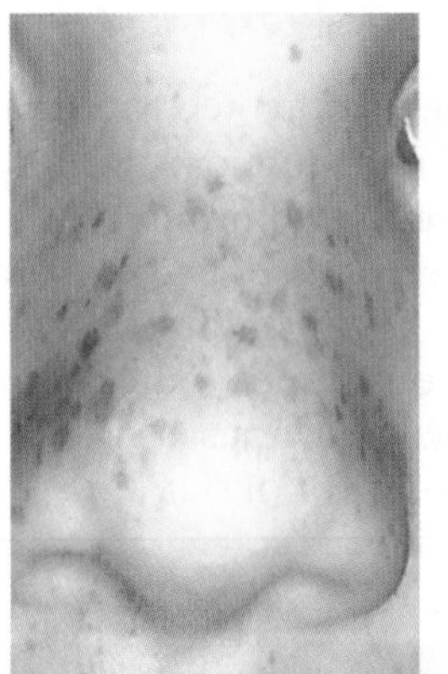

A

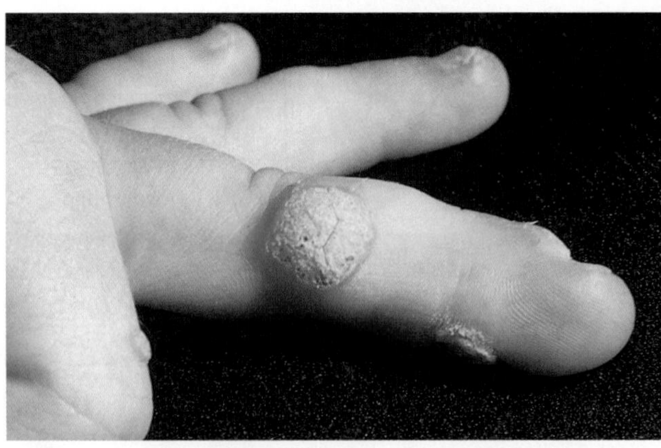

B

FIGURE 27-1 Examples of skin lesions. **A,** Macules (freckles). **B,** Papule (common wart). (**A** from Hurwitz, S. [1993]. *Clinical pediatric dermatology: A textbook of skin disorders of childhood and adolescence* [2nd ed.]. Philadelphia: Saunders; **B** from Lookingbill, D. P., & Marks, J. G., Jr. [1993]. *Principles of dermatology* [2nd ed.]. Philadelphia: Saunders)

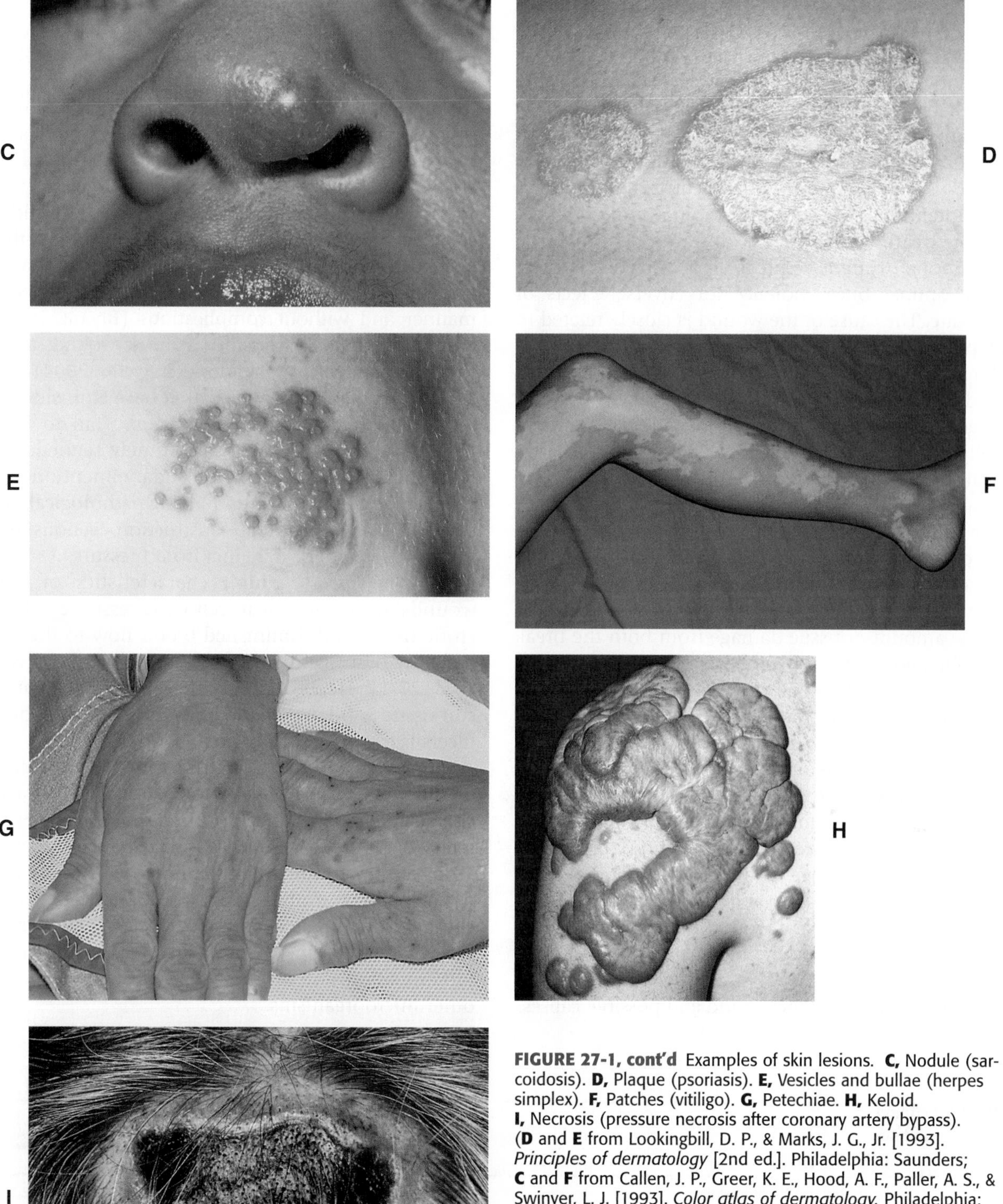

FIGURE 27-1, cont'd Examples of skin lesions. **C,** Nodule (sarcoidosis). **D,** Plaque (psoriasis). **E,** Vesicles and bullae (herpes simplex). **F,** Patches (vitiligo). **G,** Petechiae. **H,** Keloid. **I,** Necrosis (pressure necrosis after coronary artery bypass). (**D** and **E** from Lookingbill, D. P., & Marks, J. G., Jr. [1993]. *Principles of dermatology* [2nd ed.]. Philadelphia: Saunders; **C** and **F** from Callen, J. P., Greer, K. E., Hood, A. F., Paller, A. S., & Swinyer, L. J. [1993]. *Color atlas of dermatology.* Philadelphia: Saunders. **G** courtesy Dr. Beverly A. Johnson, Washington, DC; **H** from Ignatavicius, D. D., Workman, M. L., & Mishler, M. A. [1999]. *Medical-surgical nursing across the health care continuum* [3rd ed.]. Philadelphia: Saunders; **I** from Callen, J. P., Greer, K. E., Hood, A. F., Paller, A. S., & Swinyer, L. J. [1993]. *Color atlas of dermatology.* Philadelphia: Saunders.)

Wounds. A **wound** is a disruption of normal anatomical structure and function that results from bodily injury or from a pathological process that may be internal or external to the involved organ or organs. Wounds can be classified by cause and descriptors of the wound. It is important to be able to identify the cause of the wound and to describe it accurately to the health care team.

The cause of a wound may be intentional or unintentional. Intentional wounds result from a surgical procedure or treatment (such as intravenous therapy). Unintentional wounds result from accidental injury or trauma, animal bites, violence, or adverse effects of health care. The cause of the wound is closely related to the type and amount of tissue damage that results.

Wounds are classified as open or closed. In an open wound, the skin is broken and a range of soft tissue damage can be present. A surgical wound can be intentionally left open, or it may be open as a complication of healing. A closed wound involves no skin disruption.

Wounds are classified on the basis of the severity and nature of the injury. Superficial wounds involve surface layers of the skin or the body. *Deep* may refer to the deep layers of the skin or mean deep within a body cavity, penetrating internal body organs. Severity also has to do with the amount of tissue damage from both the break in the skin and trauma to surrounding tissue. It may also reflect damage to the blood supply to the site of injury.

Wounds are classified on the basis of the risk for infection. A surgical incision is created under sterile conditions, tissue damage is minimized, and healthy wound edges are approximated so that new tissue can grow and connect the tissue with minimal scarring. Wounds resulting from trauma are created under "dirty" or "clean" conditions, tissue damage is variable, wound edges may not be easily approximated, and scarring is more likely. Healing an open traumatic wound may be impeded by damage to soft tissue surrounding the open wound. Table 27-1 summarizes terms used to classify wounds on the basis of a description of the wound and possible causes.

Wounds are classified based on thickness. Partial-thickness wounds extend through the first layer of skin (epidermis) and into, but not through, the second layer of skin (dermis). Full-thickness wounds extend through both the epidermis and the dermis and may involve subcutaneous tissue, muscle, and possibly bone (Hess, 2005). These terms are often used to describe burn injuries.

An acute wound most often begins with a sudden insult that triggers a predictable cascade of events that includes growth factors and cellular stimulants that allow the wound to heal quickly in an organized, predicable manner and without complications (Bryant, in press). Surgical wounds are classified as acute wounds and heal by primary intention (Baranoski & Ayello, 2004).

Chronic wounds are those that have an insidious onset, a prolonged healing process, and fail to progress through a normal, orderly, and timely sequence of repair. These wounds heal by secondary intention and are often associated with an underlying pathological process such as diabetes, arterial obstruction, venous insufficiency, infection, or ischemia from pressure.

Pressure ulcers exhibit characteristics of chronic wounds: open, risk for infection, excessive exudate, necrotic tissue, and diminished blood flow to the wound bed. The best treatment of pressure ulcers is prevention (Box 27-1). Healing occurs through the formation of scar tissue to fill the wound bed. The etiology of pressure ulcers is discussed in Chapter 33.

Chronic wounds are often classified by a description of the wound, including color of the wound bed and characteristics of drainage. Wound drainage, or **exudate,** refers to fluid and blood cells that have escaped from blood vessels during the inflammatory response and remain in the surrounding tissues. Wound exudate also contains microorganisms and necrotic tissue; therefore it varies with the type of tissue involved, the amount of inflammation, and the presence or absence of bacteria or other microorganisms.

Table 27-1 Types of Wounds

TYPE	DESCRIPTION	POSSIBLE CAUSE
Open	Disruption or break in skin	Penetration by sharp object or instrument (such as knife, scalpel, bullet)
Closed	No disruption or break in skin	Trauma caused by blow with blunt object
Clean	Wound free of infectious organisms	Surgical incision not entering or affected by secretions from respiratory, gastrointestinal, or genitourinary tracts
Contaminated	Wound with microorganisms	Penetration of skin by dirt, bacteria
Penetrating	Wound with break through epidermis, dermis, and underlying tissues; may enter organs	Penetration by object or instrument (usually accidental)
Abrasion	Superficial injury caused by rubbing or scraping of skin against another surface	Friction injury resulting from fall or rubbing against bed linens
Laceration	Open wound with jagged edges	Penetration of skin by sharp object
Contusion	Closed wound; may be swollen, discolored, and painful	Blunt trauma, such as being hit by object

Types of wound exudate include serous, sanguineous, serosanguineous, and purulent. Serous drainage is clear and watery plasma. Sanguineous drainage (from the Latin word for blood) is red. Serosanguineous drainage, a mixture of serous and sanguineous drainage, consists of plasma and red blood cells and is pink and watery. Drainage from a surgical wound is initially sanguineous. Over several days, it changes to serosanguineous and then serous. Purulent drainage is pus, a protein-rich liquid product of the liquefaction of necrotic tissue. It is made up of cells and cellular debris and is usually caused by an infection. It is thick and yellow, green, tan, or brown.

WOUND HEALING

The human body is able to heal itself and uses complex physiological processes to aid skin and wound healing and promote restoration of function and structure. The phases of wound healing are overlapping.

Phases of Wound Healing. When an injury occurs, the body protects itself by attempting to close the wound. Hemostasis, the control of bleeding, is the process by which injured blood vessels constrict and platelets accumulate. The platelets secrete vasoconstrictive substances to aid in hemostasis, but their primary role is to form a clot to seal the damaged vessels. Hemostasis occurs within minutes of the initial injury unless there are underlying clotting disorders. The blood clot forms a fibrin matrix as a structure for further cellular repair.

The inflammatory phase begins at the time of tissue injury and lasts 3 to 4 days. The cardinal signs of inflammation are heat, erythema, edema, and pain at the wound site. Histamine is secreted by mast cells and damaged tissues, leading to capillary dilation, which increases the supply of blood and nutrients to the wound and allows migration of cells, complement, and antibodies. Polymorphonuclear leukocytes (neutrophils) migrate into the wound and begin to ingest bacteria. Then monocytes migrate, change into macrophages and, through phagocytosis, clean the wound bed of bacteria and cellular debris to prepare the wound bed for healing. Lymphocytes migrate last and are thought to stimulate *angiogenesis* (the development of new blood vessels).

Macrophages stimulate biological regulators (cytokines) and the formation of fibroblasts (connective tissue–producing cells). A fibrin network forms to provide a structure to aid the formation of fibrous bridges as well as epithelial cells that move inward from the wound edges to create an epithelial layer.

The proliferative, or reconstruction, phase of healing lasts 4 to 21 days. During this phase, collagen fills the wound bed, new blood vessels develop, and **granulation tissue** is formed by fibroblasts, giving the wound a bright red granular appearance. Also, the wound closes by **epithelialization,** a process in which epithelial cells grow to cover the wound bed. By day 5, the wound has filled with highly vascular fibroblastic connective tissue. By day 7, the surface epithelium has a normal thickness and the subepithelial layers are bridged. Progressive collagen accumulation during the second week results in

BOX 27-1 Evidence-Based Practice

Preventing Pressure Ulcers

Problem: A pressure ulcer is an injury caused by unrelieved pressure that damages the skin and underlying tissue, usually when healthy tissue is compressed between a bony prominence and an external surface. Characteristics of these chronic wounds include slow healing, resistance to healing, risk for infection, excessive exudate, and tissue necrosis.

Evidence

Guidelines were developed for the assessment of risk and strategies for prevention of pressure ulcers were developed for clients who have been identified as "at risk" for pressure ulcers. The evidence in this protocol is based upon research studies that included older adult populations. The guideline was adapted from the Agency for Health Care Policy and Research (AHCPR, now known as the Agency for Healthcare Research and Quality [AHRQ]) Clinical Guidelines. *Pressure Ulcers in Adults: Prediction and Prevention* (1992). Additional MEDLINE and CINAHL searches were conducted. The Internet was also used to access professional organizations that are involved in pressure ulcer care (e.g., National Pressure Ulcer Advisory Panel; Wound, Ostomy and Continence Nurses Society). Research articles and texts (38 references) that support these guidelines can be found at: http://www.guideline.gov/summary/select_ref.aspx?doc_id=3458.

Application to Practice

These guidelines were developed to provide evidence-based recommendations for advanced practice nurses, dietitians, health care providers, hospitals, nurses, physical therapists, physician assistants, and physicians to accomplish the following:

- Determine those clients at greatest risk for development of pressure ulcers
- Describe prevention activities which will reduce clients' risk for pressure ulcers

The guidelines can be found at http://www.guideline.gov/summary/summary.aspx?ss=15&doc_id=3458&nbr=2684#s24.

Reference

Folkedahl, B. A., & Frantz, R. (2002). *Prevention of pressure ulcers.* Iowa City: University of Iowa Gerontological Nursing Interventions Research Center, Research Dissemination Core. [38 references].

the basic structure of the scar, which is initially bright red but later fades.

The final stage of wound healing is the maturation, or remodeling, phase. Although much maturation occurs by 3 to 4 weeks, the scar may not achieve maximum strength for up to 2 years. This phase is characterized by reorganization of the collagen fibers, wound remodeling, and maturation of the tissues to approximate the skin's original strength. Although the wound is considered fully healed, the tissue will always be at risk for breakdown because the wound's tensile strength never exceeds 80% of its preinjury strength.

Types of Wound Healing. Most acute wounds and surgical wounds close by primary intention (Figure 27-2). The clinician approximates (aligns) the wound edges or margins and secures them using sutures, staples, or Steri-Strips. The wound bed that is free of **hematoma** (an accumulation of bloody fluid), debris, or exudate, then fills in with minimal granulation tissue, and the scar is usually thin and flat. Primary intention healing occurs in the first 14 days after injury. Wounds that heal by primary intention have a lower risk of infection, little tissue loss, and minimal scarring. Healing by primary intention takes a predictable course through the stages of hemostasis, inflammation, proliferation, and maturation.

In contrast, healing by secondary intention is prolonged (Figure 27-3). When the skin or wound edges cannot be approximated, as in a pressure ulcer or a wound that is large or infected, all dead (necrotic) and infectious tissue must be removed and the wound must fill with granulation tissue; some tissue regeneration (epithelialization) proceeds from the margins. Wound contraction plays a greater role in healing by secondary intention, reducing the size of the final surface scar. Secondary intention healing generally involves greater tissue loss, higher risk for infection, prolonged healing, and a large scar.

Tertiary intention, or delayed primary closure, occurs in wounds that may be contaminated, infected, or draining exudate (Figure 27-4). These wounds may be left open intentionally for 3 to 5 days to let healing begin by allowing the contaminated or infected matter or exudate to drain out. Once the infection clears, and granulation has begun, the wound is closed with sutures, staples, or Steri-Strips.

PRESSURE ULCERS

A **pressure ulcer** is any lesion caused by ischemia from unrelieved pressure that leads to necrosis of underlying tissues. Pressure ulcers develop when soft tissue is compressed between a bony prominence (such as the hip) and an external surface (such as a mattress). With prolonged pressure, the blood supply to the tissue's capillary network is disrupted, causing impeded blood flow to the surrounding tissues leading to local tissue ischemia, edema, inflammation, and cell death. The economic impact of pressure ulcers is significant for hospitals, home health care agencies, and long-term care facilities.

The National Pressure Ulcer Advisory Panel (NPUAP) (2005) identifies four stages of pressure ulcers (Figure 27-5).

- *Stage I:* An observable, pressure-related alteration of intact skin whose indicators, as compared with the

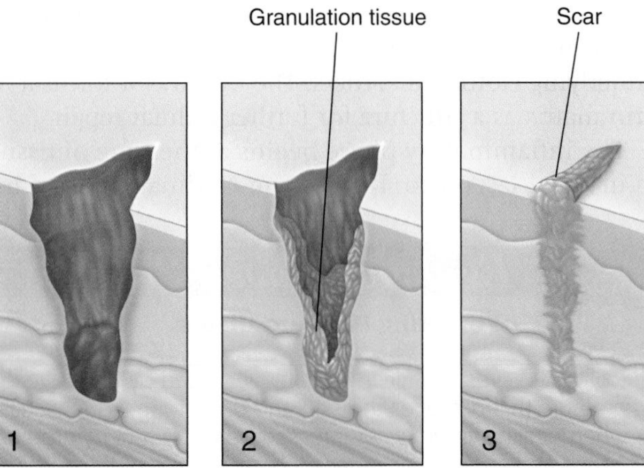

FIGURE 27-3 Wound healing by secondary intention.

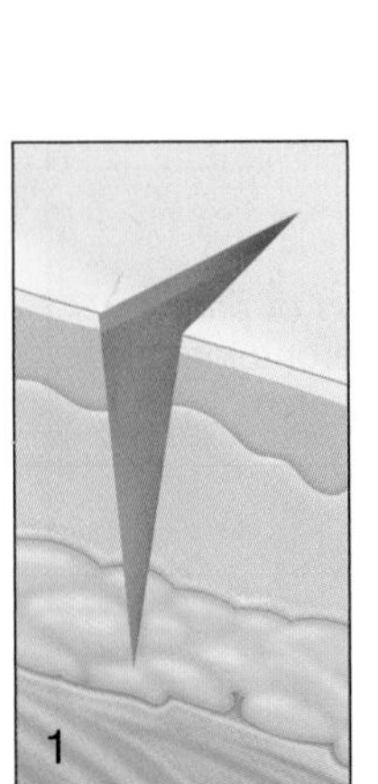

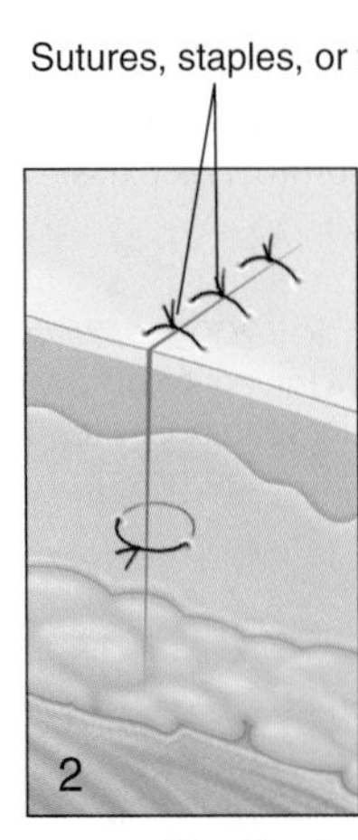

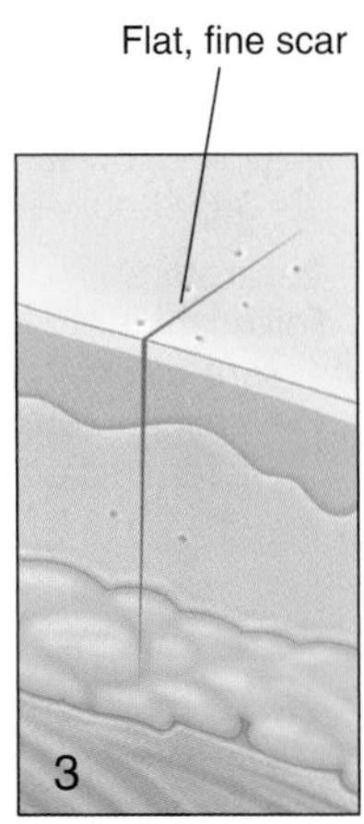

FIGURE 27-2 Wound healing by primary intention.

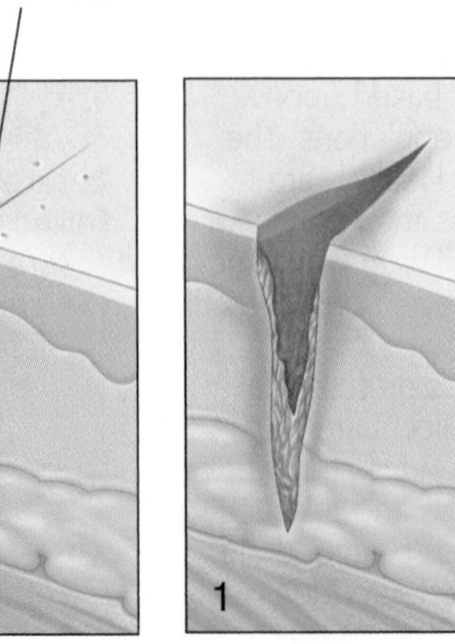

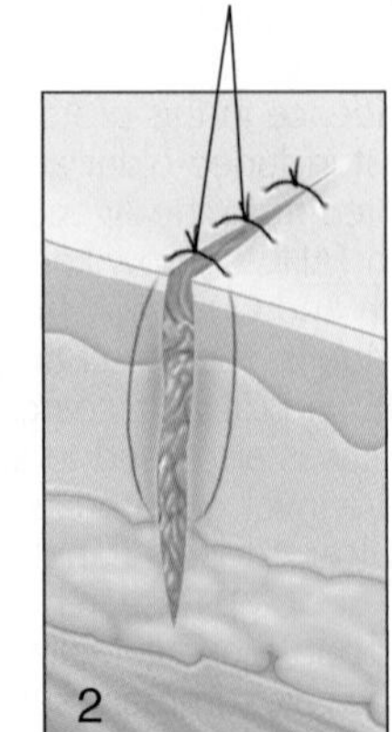

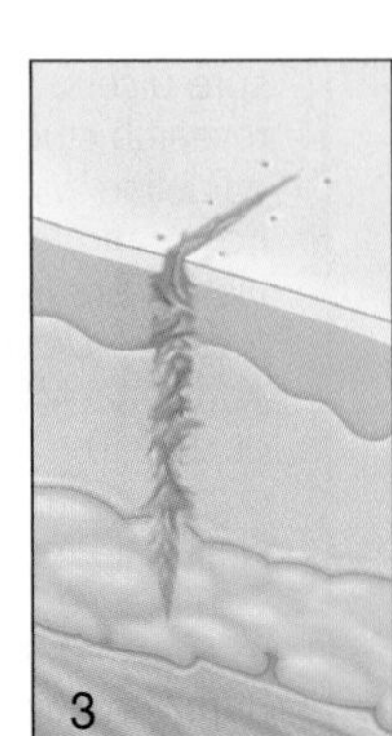

FIGURE 27-4 Wound healing by tertiary intention.

adjacent or opposite area on the body, may include changes in one or more of the following: skin temperature (warmth or coolness), tissue consistency (firm or boggy), and sensation (pain, itching). The ulcer appears as a defined area of persistent redness in lightly pigmented skin, or persistent red, blue, or purple hues in those with darker skin tones.

- *Stage II:* Partial-thickness skin loss involving the epidermis, dermis, or both. The ulcer is superficial and presents clinically as an **abrasion,** blister, or shallow crater.
- *Stage III:* Full-thickness skin loss involving damage to or necrosis of subcutaneous tissue that may extend to, but not through, the underlying fascia. The ulcer presents clinically as a deep crater with or without undermining of adjacent tissues.
- *Stage IV:* Full-thickness skin loss with extensive destruction, tissue necrosis, or damage to muscle, bone, or supporting structures (such as tendon, joint capsule).

NOTE: If the wound involves necrotic tissue, débridement is necessary before staging because staging cannot be confirmed until the wound bed is viable.

According to the NPUAP, pressure ulcer staging is appropriate only for defining the maximum depth of tissue involvement. Reverse staging (also called downstaging) does not accurately describe a healing pressure ulcer. For example, if a client has a stage IV pressure ulcer that has healed and now looks like a stage II ulcer, identify it as a healing stage IV ulcer instead of as a stage II ulcer (NPUAP, 2005).

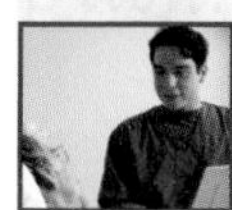

What stage pressure ulcer do you think Mrs. Jacan has on her heels and sacrum?

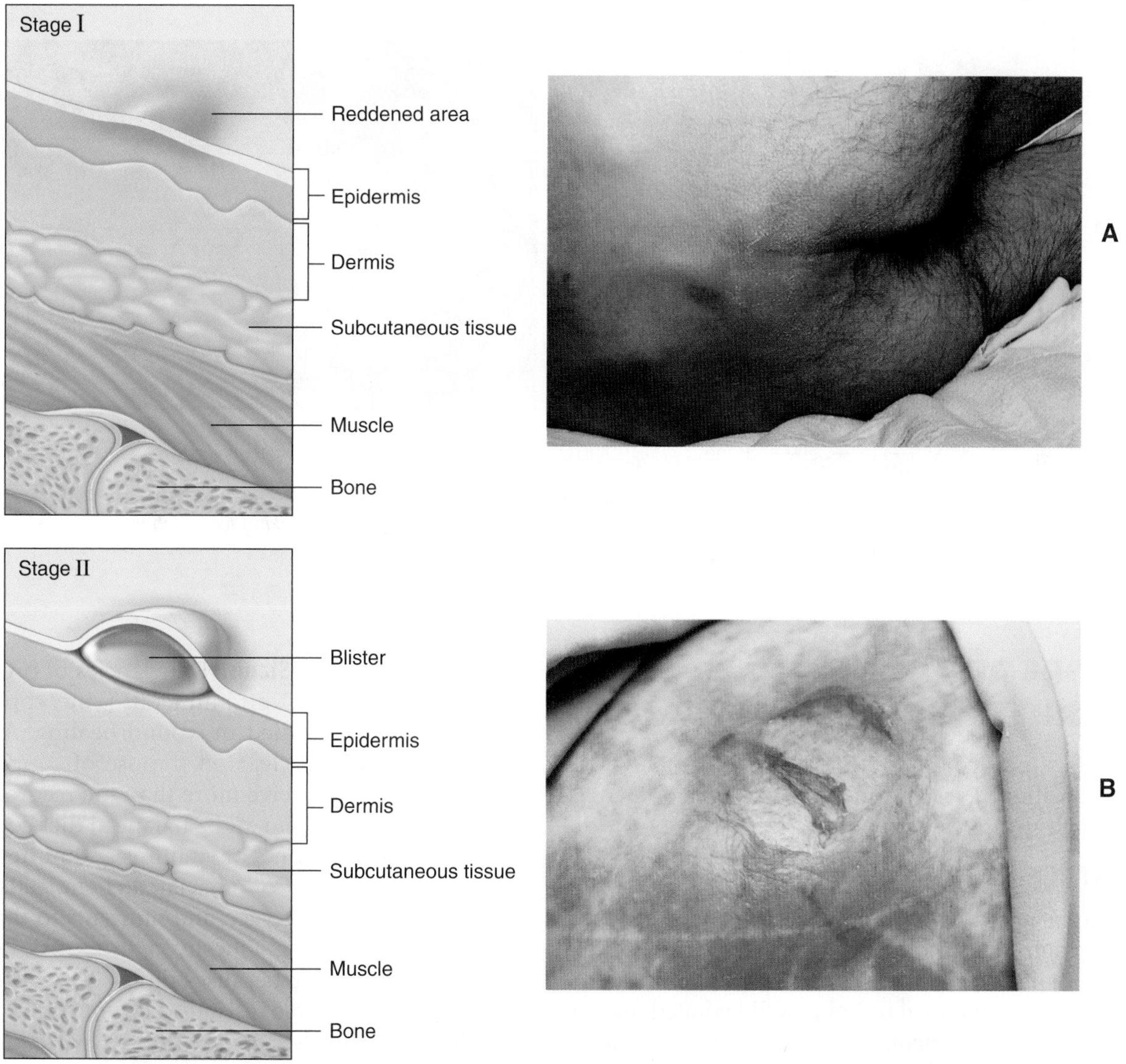

FIGURE 27-5 Stages of development of pressure ulcers. **A,** Stage I. **B,** Stage II. (From Ignatavicius, D., & Workman, M. L. [2006]. *Medical-surgical nursing: Critical thinking for collaborative care* [5th ed.]. Philadelphia: Saunders.)

Continued

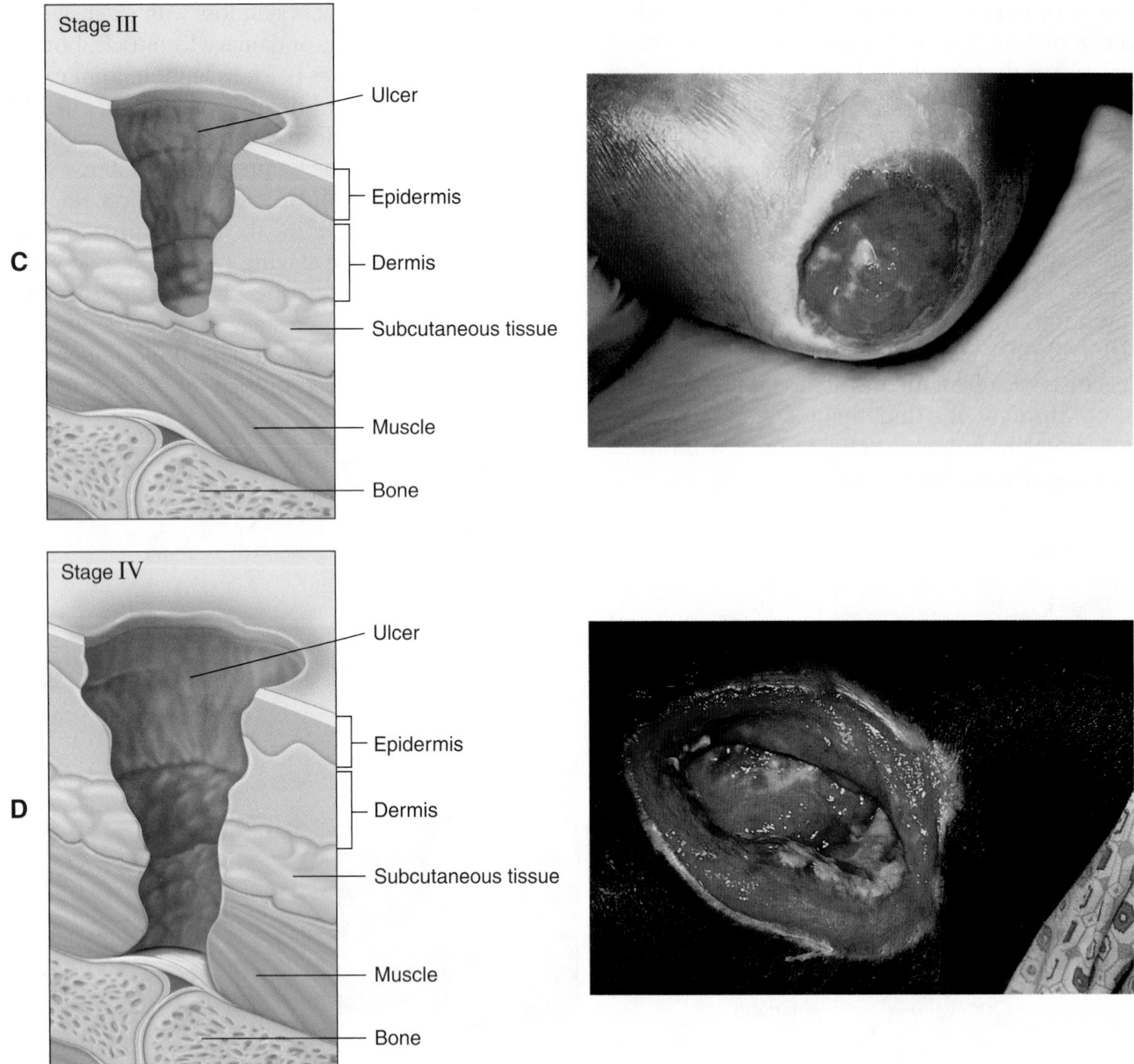

FIGURE 27-5, cont'd Stages of development of pressure ulcers. **C,** Stage III. **D,** Stage IV. (From Ignatavicius, D., & Workman, M. L. [2006]. *Medical-surgical nursing: Critical thinking for collaborative care* [5th ed.]. Philadelphia: Saunders.)

FACTORS AFFECTING SKIN INTEGRITY AND WOUND HEALING

Several factors affect skin integrity and the potential for wound healing. They include lifestyle, developmental, physiological, and environmental factors.

LIFESTYLE FACTORS

Lifestyle factors that affect skin integrity include personal hygiene, nutrition and fluid status, activity and exercise level, smoking, and substance abuse. Optimal condition of the skin is maintained by being well hydrated, having good circulation, nutrients, and being free of irritants.

Personal Hygiene. People with poor hygiene may have increased risk for a wound infection or skin disorder. Routine skin cleansing removes bacteria, sweat, and other substances that may cause skin problems.

Nutrition and Fluid Status. Deficiencies of protein, vitamins A, B, E, and C, and minerals (zinc, copper, and iron) have been studied in wound healing. Although the evidence is not clear on the use of supplements, the client should receive more than the recommended 0.8 g/kg/day of protein and a balanced diet containing recommended amounts of vitamins and minerals. In a severely underweight or emaciated client, cells cannot transport sufficient oxygen and nutrients to the tissues to aid wound healing. Obesity is also a risk factor for poor wound healing, because adipose tissue has a poor blood supply and less resistance to infection.

Activity and Exercise. Active people who get adequate exercise tend to experience fewer skin problems. On the other hand, immobilization (such as from advanced age or spinal cord injury) increases the risk for skin breakdown and other skin problems. Clients who cannot change position independently for any reason have a greater risk for pressure ulcer formation.

Smoking. Smoking constricts blood vessels and reduces the blood's oxygen-carrying capacity, resulting in decreased tissue oxygenation. Smoking also increases platelet aggregation, which in turn may cause hypercoagulability with decreased perfusion to the skin or wound.

Substance Abuse. People who abuse substances, such as alcohol or illicit drugs, often have poor nutrition, which can lead to poor wound healing and skin condition.

DEVELOPMENTAL FACTORS

Skin problems can occur at any time of life, from infancy to advanced age. However, infants and children heal faster than older adults, who may be less mobile and have more fragile, slowly healing skin than younger adults. Age plays an important role in wound healing. As a person ages, the wound healing phase can be prolonged because of decreased initial inflammatory responses. Changes in the vascular, immune, and respiratory systems can also impair wound healing.

PHYSIOLOGICAL FACTORS

Many factors affect wound healing (Box 27-2). Local factors can affect the wound site itself, whereas a systemic condition may affect overall healing. Factors such as immunosuppression, incontinence, hypoxemia, diabetes, infections, neurological impairments, medical-surgical procedures, and medications can affect wound healing. The characteristics of the wound also affect healing. Complications—such as infection, hemorrhage, fistulas, dehiscence, and evisceration—can occur during wound healing.

Immunosuppression. Immunosuppressed persons may have a slowed inflammatory response, slowed reepithelialization, and a decrease in leukocyte activity.

Incontinence. Bowel and bladder incontinence can affect and delay wound healing because contact with stool or urine can contaminate a wound, prolonging healing and providing a medium for bacterial growth and subsequent infection.

Hypoxemia. Poor or impaired blood flow to a wound and surrounding tissues impairs wound healing. Decreased tissue oxygenation impairs collagen synthesis and epithelialization.

Diabetes. Diabetic clients may have microvascular disease, which can impair tissue oxygenation and tissue perfusion. Hyperglycemia inhibits leukocyte activity, can delay formation of granulation tissue, and provides an ideal environment for the growth of yeast and fungi.

Neurological Impairment. Clients with neurological impairments, such as spinal cord injury, dementia, or diabetic neuropathy, are at greater risk for *Impaired skin integrity.* These people may be unable to care for themselves and, because they may lack sensation, cannot feel pressure or irritation to the skin. Clients with a change in level of consciousness (such as comatose or sedated clients in intensive care) also cannot protect themselves from factors that can lead to skin breakdown.

Procedures. Medical and surgical procedures, such as operative incisions, intravenous therapy, venipuncture, and radiation therapy, can raise the risk of *Impaired skin integrity.* Orthopedic clients who undergo traction or cast application to treat fractures are at increased risk for skin breakdown. Friction and pressure from medical devices, such as cervical collars, oxygen tubing around the nose and ears, and nasogastric tubes can also cause skin breakdown.

Medications. Drugs—such as steroids, antiinflammatory medications, and chemotherapy—can alter protein synthesis and cellular growth and slow the inflammatory phase of wound healing.

Infection. Wound infection causes a prolonged inflammatory response and delayed wound healing. An infected wound must be cleansed of the infecting organism and cellular debris for healing to proceed. Wound infections are more likely in the presence of obesity, debilitating conditions, advanced age, a long and complicated operative procedure, other medical conditions, long-term corticosteroid therapy, radiation therapy, and wound disruptions.

Acute wound infections most commonly occur during surgery and within 36 to 48 hours after surgery, with the manifestations of infection becoming apparent 5 to 7 days after surgery. Postoperative monitoring must include assessing for signs and symptoms of infection, such as fever, wound drainage, swelling, and heat and tenderness. Increased drainage, purulent drainage, erythema at the wound perimeter, an elevated white blood cell count, and general malaise may indicate wound infection.

When managing chronic wounds it is important to distinguish between contaminated wounds and infected wounds. Most chronic wounds have bacteria present or colonizing in the wound bed and are considered to be contaminated with bacteria. Chronic wounds that are contaminated or colonized are not necessarily infected nor is wound healing impaired by the presence of these nonreplicating surface bacteria. An infection, on the other hand, means the bacteria have invaded the tissue, are multiplying and causing a host reaction, and have a

BOX 27-2 *Factors Affecting Wound Healing*

Local Factors	Systemic Factors
• Dry environment	• Age
• Edema	• Body build
• Eschar	• Chronic disease
• Infection	• Poor nutritional status
• Pressure	• Prolonged steroid use
• Sloughing	• Smoking
• Trauma	• Vascular problems
• Wound stress	

high potential of damaging or destroying the tissue, impairing wound healing.

Many factors can affect the inflammatory response, thus making it difficult to determine the presence of an infection in a chronic wound. These factors include age, antiinflammatory medications, immune status, and underlying disease such as diabetes, impaired tissue perfusion, and autoimmune disorders. The number of bacteria, drainage, and amount of necrotic tissue—the bioburden—of a wound prolongs healing and contributes to the difficulty in assessing and diagnosing infection in chronic wounds (Baranoski & Ayello, 2004).

Hemorrhage. **Hemorrhage,** or bleeding from the wound bed or site, can occur in the immediate postoperative or initial postinjury period. Normally, hemostasis occurs quickly and clotting begins. However, significant blood loss may occur if a blood vessel continues to bleed or the client has poor clotting function. Causes include a surgical drain, a loose surgical suture, and infection.

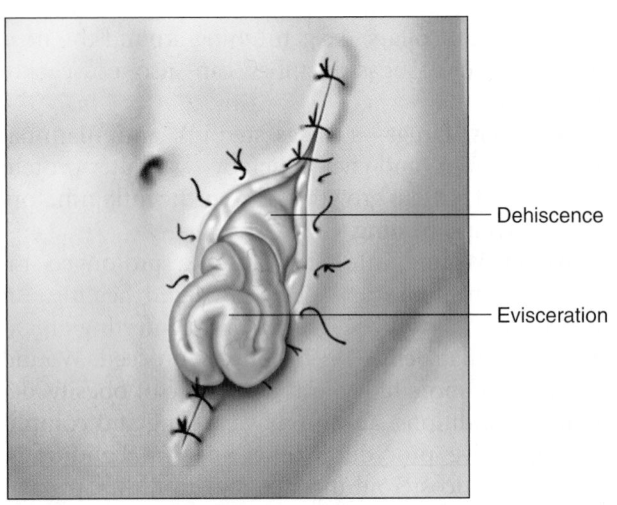

FIGURE 27-6 Wound dehiscence is the opening of the edges of a surgical wound. Evisceration is the protrusion of internal organs through the incision.

Internal hemorrhage can occur with no external evidence of bleeding. To assess for internal hemorrhage, check for distention or swelling of the affected area, a change in the amount or type of drainage from a drain, and signs and symptoms of hypovolemic shock (decreased urine output, elevated heart rate, decreased blood pressure, restlessness, thirst, and confusion).

External hemorrhage is easily detected as bloody drainage on the surgical dressing, especially if the dressing becomes saturated rapidly. However, be sure to assess not just the dressing but also the area around the dressing and posterior to the wound site. For instance, if a client has an incision and dressing on the anterior part of the neck, check the posterior neck region for drainage. A hematoma also may form during the early postoperative period. To detect a hematoma, assess for hard painful swelling around the incision site. Assess all surgical wounds closely during the first 24 to 48 hours postoperatively.

Fistula. A **fistula** is an abnormal passage between two internal organs or between an organ and the external skin surface. A fistula forms because healing tissue layers do not close. A fistula may result from an abscess or infection, traumatic injury, inflammatory process (radiation), or a disease process such as cancer.

Dehiscence and Evisceration. **Dehiscence** refers to separation of wound edges (Figure 27-6).

Evisceration is the protrusion of an internal organ (such as a bowel loop) through the incision. Wound eviscerations are medical emergencies. If one of these complications occurs, contact the physician immediately. Box 27-3 describes your role in caring for a client with wound evisceration.

ENVIRONMENTAL FACTORS

The client's environment should support a clean, dry, and intact skin condition. Skin integrity is affected by skin dryness, friction from bed linens, and moisture from incontinence, perspiration, emesis, and wound drainage. Skin may become macerated if exposed to

BOX 27-3 *Responding to Wound Evisceration*

If a client's wound eviscerates, you will need to respond swiftly and accurately, as outlined here.

1. Stay calm. Projecting a calm and confident manner will help keep the client and family calm as well.
2. Ask a colleague to obtain supplies and to notify a physician while you stay with the client.
3. Help the client into semi-Fowler's position with the knees slightly flexed after gatching the foot of the bed. This position will ease pressure on the wound, prevent further tearing of the wound edges, and reduce the risk of further evisceration.
4. Cover the protruding intestine with a sterile dressing moistened with sterile normal saline solution to help prevent wound contamination and keep the abdominal contents moist. If no sterile dressing is available, use clean towels or dressings.
5. Monitor the client closely, and assess vital signs and pulse oximetry readings. Frequent monitoring will help detect impending shock.
6. Establish intravenous access to provide fluids and prepare the client for surgery as ordered. The client will most likely need surgery to repair the wound and will not be permitted oral intake.
7. Continue to provide emotional support to client and family. Wound evisceration can be extremely frightening. A calm, supportive approach can help the client through this emergency.

moisture for a prolonged period. Friction and shear from moving across bed linens can lead to damage unless appropriate preventive strategies are implemented.

Nursing care that is consistent with a client's culture is part of the environment and can affect a client's response to care, thus affecting healing (Box 27-4).

ASSESSMENT

Assessment of the client with *Risk for impaired skin integrity* or *Impaired skin integrity* is holistic. It includes the factors affecting wound healing, as well as specific attention to the characteristics of the wound.

GENERAL ASSESSMENT OF SKIN INTEGRITY

Health History. Every hospitalized or long-term care client should be assessed for impaired skin integrity and risk for impaired skin integrity. The health history should identify factors that make the client at risk for injury, for delayed wound healing, or for pressure ulcers. The health history should prompt you to ask about previous treatment, such as radiation or surgery that may increase the risk of skin damage.

Physical Examination. A thorough skin assessment is an important part of the physical examination. See Chapter 8 for information on describing lesions. If the client cannot easily move in bed, assessment for pressure ulcers is imperative; you may need assistance to turn the client to assess all the bony prominences. Document a clear description of any lesions on the skin and any factors associated with the lesion. If your client has a wound, assess it carefully.

Assess a chronic wound for the manifestations of infection: pain, erythema, swelling, warmth, heat, and purulent drainage. In addition, assess for delayed healing, discoloration of granulation tissue, friable granulation tissue, foul odor, and serous drainage accompanied by inflammation (Baranoski & Ayello, 2004).

Diagnostic Tests. Diagnostic studies can help identify skin or wound infection, poor oxygenation, and general nutrition status—factors that can affect skin integrity and wound healing. Use these laboratory values to assess the client's hydration status, identify possible infections, and help you formulate nursing diagnoses and develop a plan of nursing care.

White Blood Cell Count. The white blood cell count is not elevated because most wound infections are local infections. An elevated white blood cell count may suggest a systemic infection.

Prealbumin and Albumin Levels. Abnormally low prealbumin and albumin levels indicate poor nutritional status, which slows wound healing. Albumin is the best indicator of long-term nutritional status.

Radiological Studies. If a client has a suspected infection in a wound over a bony prominence (such as the sacrum or heel), the physician may order radiological studies to rule out *osteomyelitis* (infection of the bone). Standard radiographs or a bone scan can be used to detect infection.

FOCUSED ASSESSMENT FOR *IMPAIRED SKIN INTEGRITY*

Defining Characteristics. Defining characteristics for *Impaired skin integrity* include invasion of body structures, disruption of the epidermis, and destruction of the

BOX 27-4 *Cross-Cultural Care*

Caring for a Filipino Client

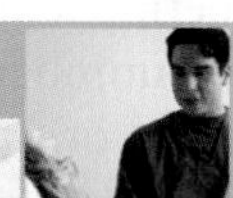

Mrs. Jacan is of Filipino descent. She came to America at age 18 after World War II with her parents and settled in the Washington, D.C., area. Mrs. Jacan lives in close proximity to her daughter, who checks in on her frequently. Postoperatively, Mrs. Jacan was quiet and cooperative but not progressing well in physical therapy. She tried to maintain a harmonious relationship with the nursing and physical therapy staff but felt that she had little privacy in a semiprivate room and little quiet time for herself. The nurse considers the possibility of assigning her to a private room. Although every client is unique, Leininger (2001) identified a number of values that Filipino Americans, like Mrs. Jacan, tend to embrace:

- Showing respect for others and deferring to authority
- Maintaining smooth and harmonious relationships with others, especially family
- Maintaining a deep sense of loyalty, mutual respect, and obligation to each other
- Preserving social relationships and maintaining a sense of self-esteem
- Believing a professional's time is valuable and not mentioning less serious problems
- Giving to others when they need assistance
- Eating fish, rice, vegetables
- Hot-cold beliefs
- Involving extended family in nursing care activities
- Privacy and quiet periods of time as essential to recovery
- Believing pain is the will of God

Data from Leininger, M. M. (2001). *Cultural care and diversity and universality: A theory of nursing.* Boston, MA: Jones & Bartlett Publishing; D'Avanzo, C., & Geissler, E. M. (2003). *Pocket guide to cultural assessment* (3rd ed.). St. Louis, MO: Elsevier.

dermis. When assessing a client's wound, you must document many characteristics of the wound and the surrounding area, including those described here.

Location. Document the exact anatomical location of a wound. For example, write "client has 4-cm abdominal incision in the right lower quadrant" or "pressure ulcer on left lateral malleolus." Alternatively you may mark the location on a figure of the human body.

Size. When measuring the wound, determine its length, width, and depth, in centimeters (cm) unless directed otherwise. Accurate wound measurement is important to evaluate wound healing.

To properly define a pressure ulcer, measure the length, width, and depth of the affected area. Use the concept of the face of a clock to help define landmarks and areas of the wound or impaired skin area. Measure wound length from head to toe (with 12 o'clock representing the client's head and 6 o'clock representing the feet). Measure the width of the wound from side to side (3 o'clock to 9 o'clock). Also assess wound depth by measuring how far the wound extends below the skin surface. Be sure to check for tunneling (a sinus tract or tunnel) or undermining of the wound or pressure ulcer.

Various measuring instruments are available to assess a wound. One of the easiest methods involves using a cotton-tipped applicator and a centimeter ruler (Figure 27-7). Another common method employs a tape measure or ruler. In the client's chart, record the wound length and width in centimeters, the measurement method used, and the client's position at the time of measurement.

Another way to measure a wound is to trace it. Hold a disposable acetate sheet, a measuring guide, or a plastic bag over the wound and trace the edges with a fine-tip permanent marker. Also write the date, the client's name or number, your name, and location markers (such as head or toes) on the tracing. Calculate the wound area, and document the area, the method of obtaining and calculating the measurement, and the client's position at the time of the measurement. Also place the tracing itself in the client's chart.

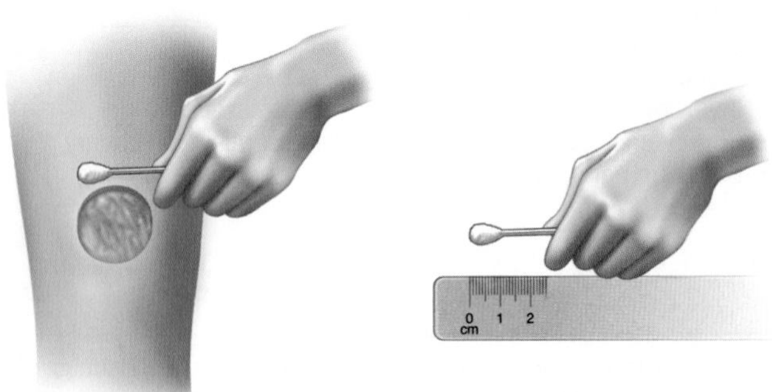

FIGURE 27-7 An easy method for measuring a wound using a cotton-tipped applicator and a centimeter rule.

The advantages of this method, especially for a large wound, are that it is easy, quick, and reliably reproduced by the same person and by other people. Wound tracings can be a valuable addition to the client's medical record, and they allow easy monitoring of changes in the wound. The expense incurred by this method depends on the materials you use. Disadvantages of this method are that it may be difficult to see the margins of the wound while tracing it, and the accuracy of the tracing declines in smaller wounds. If the transparency does not contain a grid, you will need to copy the tracing to grid paper to calculate the size of the wound.

Color. Document the color of the wound bed (Bryant, in press). For chronic wounds the color of the wound is a helpful classification system to describe the wound on a continuum of wound healing. The red-yellow-black (RYB) classification system describes the wound in a manner that helps direct treatment. Generally, red wounds are healing wounds with clean, healthy granulation tissue. Granulation tissue is any soft pink fleshy projections that form during the healing process in a wound that does not heal by primary intention. It consists of capillaries surrounded by fibrous collagen.

A yellow wound bed contains fibrinous slough. **Slough** is necrotic tissue that is moist, stringy and yellow in color. The slough must be cleansed and removed to allow the wound to heal (Baranoski & Ayello, 2004). A black wound bed indicates the presence of an **eschar** of necrotic tissue (a thick, leathery, devitalized tissue) (Hess, 2005). The red-yellow-black wound classification system can be used in conjunction with other wound classification systems.

Surrounding Skin. Note the condition of the wound edges or margins. Assess the skin around the wound for redness or induration, temperature, moisture, color, and odor. Erythema around the wound edges may indicate underlying infection. Wound edges that have been exposed to excessive moisture become soft, appear white and waterlogged, and are described as macerated. Macerated tissue is caused by inadequate management of wound drainage or an increase in drainage (Baranoski & Ayello, 2004); macerated tissue cannot heal.

Drainage. Assess any wound drainage for color, amount, consistency, and odor. Describe the drainage as serous, sanguineous, or serosanguineous. Be aware that the wound location, depth, and extent determine the amount of drainage. Noting drainage color can help identify the type of organism that may be infecting the wound. A foul, fecal, musty, or strong odor from a wound may indicate infection. Purulent drainage is a creamy, viscous fluid exudate that is the result of fluid remains of liquefactive necrosis of tissues and white blood cells usually from bacterial infection.

Action Alert! Be careful when documenting drainage and infection. Yellow drainage from a wound does not always indicate wound infection. Slough from the wound bed can be yellow and consist of wound debris, old white blood cells, and macrophages.

Temperature. To assess temperature, palpate the wound and surrounding tissues. Increased warmth of the wound bed or surrounding tissues may indicate pressure ulcer formation or an infection.

Pain. Always assess for pain at the wound site. Absence of pain may indicate nerve impairment or involvement. Although pain at the wound site indicates intact nerves, severe pain may indicate infection and underlying tissue involvement.

Wound Closures. Surgical wounds and incisions are usually closed using sutures or stainless steel staples. Suture material may be silk, nylon, cotton, linen, wire, or Dacron (polyester). When suturing, the physician sews the inner tissue layers together, usually with a suture material that is absorbed by the body during healing. Usually, skin sutures are left in place for 7 to 10 days. If sutures are removed in 3 to 4 days, Steri-Strips are used to reinforce the wound.

Several different suturing methods can be used (Figure 27-8). They include intermittent suturing (in which each stitch is knotted) and continuous suturing (in which one thread is used to create several stitches and is tied only at the beginning and the end). Retention sutures (large sutures covered by rubber tubing to prevent further skin disruption) are used for large abdominal incisions in which additional support is needed (such as in obese clients), if swelling is substantial, or when the sutures must be left in place for a prolonged period.

Stainless steel staples are commonly used to approximate incision edges (Figure 27-9). Staples have advantages over sutures because they are stronger and less irritating to the skin, and the final scar is more cosmetically acceptable. Steri-Strips (small, thin strips of tape) can be used for smaller incisions (Figure 27-10). These strips may minimize incisional irritation, swelling, and scar formation. Topical skin adhesives (glues) may be used for wound closure in the place of sutures and staples and form a fast, strong, flexible bond between the wound edges. There are no stitches to remove because the adhesive "sheds" from the skin naturally as the wound heals.

Postoperative assessment of a surgical wound should include inspecting the skin around the incision for redness, irritation, or excessive swelling. These signs may indicate a wound infection or an overly tight wound closure, which ultimately can lead to wound edge separation.

Related Factors. Factors related to the diagnosis *Impaired skin integrity* may be either internal or external. External factors include the following:

- Extreme heat or cold
- Chemical substances
- Mechanical factors, such as shear, pressure, or restraints

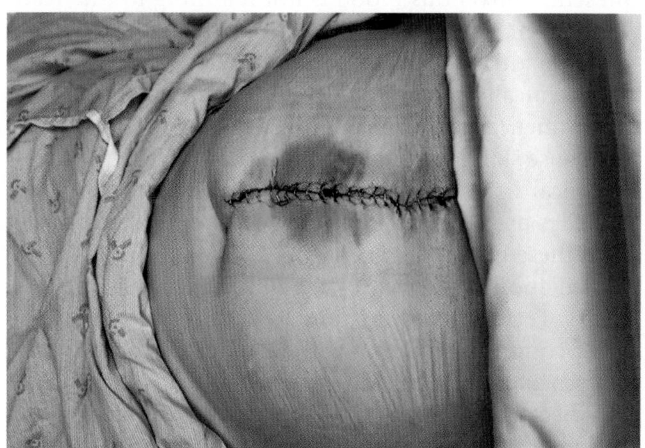

FIGURE 27-9 Staples in an incision line.

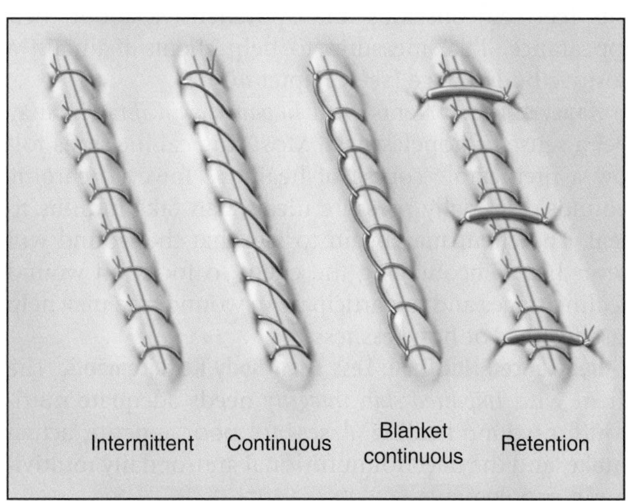

FIGURE 27-8 Types of sutures.

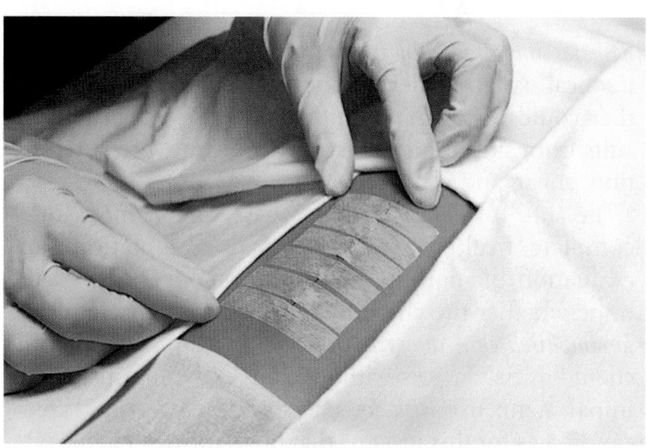

FIGURE 27-10 Steri-Strips.

- Physical immobilization
- Moisture and humidity
- Medications
- Radiation
- Diminished circulation

Internal factors include the following:

- Altered metabolism
- Skeletal prominence
- Immunological deficit
- Altered sensation, circulation, turgor, pigmentation, or nutritional state (such as obesity or emaciation)

Keep in mind that proper wound healing requires adequate perfusion. Altered circulation may lead to poor tissue oxygenation and subsequent ulceration. Decreased arterial circulation causes ulcers because the tissues fail to receive enough oxygenated blood. These ulcers most commonly appear on the bony prominences of the ankle and toes. Chronic diminished circulation produces atrophic changes, including hair loss and thin, shiny skin. Also, pulses may be absent or weak. Venous stasis ulcers, caused by poor venous return, are associated with varicose veins and thrombophlebitis. Arterial pulses are present, but venous blood is not returning to the heart. The chronic skin changes of dark pigmentation and stasis dermatitis are usually present.

Chemical irritation can result from urinary or fecal incontinence, gastric secretions, and harsh products that can cause skin irritation and breakdown. To help prevent chemical irritation, make sure the client's plan of care includes measures to protect the epidermis from contact with these irritants.

Radiation is the least common mechanism of skin injury. Excluding occupational radiation accidents, the most common type of radiation injury results from radiation therapy. The skin is vulnerable to radiation injury because the cells of the basal layer are continually and rapidly dividing. Signs of injury develop 2 to 3 days after radiation exposure and peak in 2 to 3 weeks. When the skin is severely affected, ulceration may develop.

DIAGNOSIS

Risk for impaired skin integrity applies to a client with a medical, surgical, developmental, or mobility problem that could affect skin health. *Impaired skin integrity* results from skin injury caused by moisture, pressure, friction, shear, and other factors.

Be sure to take a thorough assessment, including a complete health history, physical examination, and evaluation of mobility and nutritional status to determine whether the client has a nursing diagnosis of *Risk for impaired skin integrity* or *Impaired skin integrity*. If the client has risk factors without signs or symptoms of skin impairment, use *Risk for impaired skin integrity*. Typical candidates for this nursing diagnosis include clients who are bed-bound with poor nutrition and those with an altered level of consciousness. In contrast, a client who is being treated for pressure ulcers has a nursing diagnosis of *Impaired skin integrity*. Figure 27-11 illustrates how to choose among these nursing diagnoses.

Assigning an appropriate nursing diagnosis depends on the assessment data you collect. In some cases, another nursing diagnosis may be more suitable. For example, for a client recovering from a total hip replacement, you might choose *Impaired physical mobility* because it addresses skin integrity as well as mobility problems. *Risk for infection* may be appropriate for the postoperative client with an abdominal incision after an appendectomy. Table 27-2 provides examples of ways to formulate appropriate nursing diagnoses.

RELATED NURSING DIAGNOSES

Other client conditions and factors may affect selection of a nursing diagnosis, such as the following.

Risk for Infection. Assess the client with a pressure ulcer or postoperative surgical incision for infection. The skin opening creates an entrance site for microorganisms to enter the wound.

Impaired Tissue Integrity. Assess the tissues surrounding the client's wound for further skin breakdown or interruption. A client may have *Impaired tissue integrity* even without skin breakdown on the surface. Palpate the area around the incision or pressure ulcer to assess for bogginess or hardened tissue.

Impaired Physical Mobility. Assess for other conditions, such as visual or neurological impairment. These clients may also be at risk for *Impaired skin integrity*. For example, clients with spinal cord injury or multiple sclerosis may be unable to feel pressure and other skin sensations or to reposition themselves to decrease the risk of pressure ulcer formation.

Disturbed Body Image. Clients suffering from *Impaired skin integrity* may have a disturbance in body image. Large surgical wounds or pressure ulcers can make clients feel self-conscious and apprehensive about their appearance. Take measures to help clients maintain a positive body image (see Chapter 40).

Hopelessness. Clients with *Impaired skin integrity* may feel a sense of hopelessness. Most surgical incisions follow a predictable course of healing. However, chronic wounds, especially pressure ulcers, can take months to heal. The client may begin to feel that the wound will never heal. Encouraging the client to focus on wound healing stages and to participate in wound care may help ease feelings of hopelessness.

Imbalanced Nutrition: Less Than Body Requirements. The client with *Impaired skin integrity* needs adequate nutrition for wound healing. Assess for poor appetite, actual intake, and the need for nutritional and/or daily multivitamin supplements.

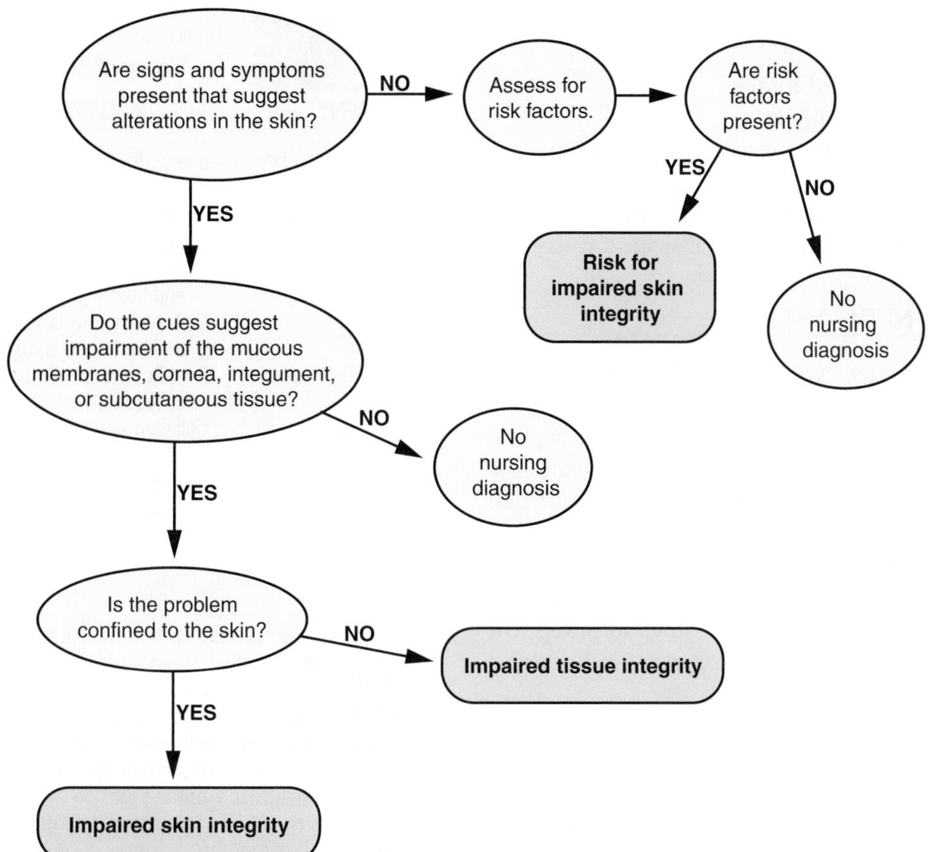

FIGURE 27-11 Decision tree for skin integrity nursing diagnoses. Diagnoses are shown in rectangles. Within these rectangles, diagnoses shown in **bold** type are NANDA-I–approved nursing diagnoses; diagnoses shown in regular type are not NANDA-I–approved nursing diagnoses.

Table 27-2 Clustering Data to Make a Nursing Diagnosis

Skin Problems	
DATA CLUSTER	**DIAGNOSIS**
A single, 44-year-old woman on the third postoperative day is very concerned about the large abdominal incision created during her hysterectomy and worries about her future cosmetic appearance.	*Disturbed body image* related to large abdominal incision secondary to hysterectomy
An 18-year-old man injured while bodysurfing at the beach sustained a C4 fracture and now is quadriplegic.	*Risk for impaired skin integrity* related to impaired physical mobility
A 72-year-old woman in a motor vehicle accident needs balanced suspended traction for a fracture of her right femur. Has a stage II pressure ulcer measuring 2 × 3 cm on left buttock.	*Impaired skin integrity* related to bed rest and traction

PLANNING

After choosing appropriate nursing diagnoses, you must develop a plan of care on the basis of the diagnoses. When planning care, assign priorities to the nursing diagnoses, select appropriate nursing interventions to achieve expected outcomes (client-centered goals), and document the nursing diagnoses, outcomes, interventions, and evaluations on the plan of care. For a client who is bed-bound after a motor vehicle accident, the goal is to prevent skin breakdown and pressure ulcer formation. For a client with a pressure ulcer, the goal is to achieve timely healing of the pressure ulcer.

EXPECTED OUTCOMES FOR THE CLIENT WITH *IMPAIRED SKIN INTEGRITY*

The expected outcome for a client with the nursing diagnosis of *Impaired skin integrity* is to achieve wound healing without complications. General outcomes for the client may include the following:

- Maintains a normal temperature or baseline vital signs

- Maintains nutritional intake to support wound healing
- Maintains adequate fluid intake
- Performs activities of daily living
- Performs wound care and dressing changes as instructed
- States the signs and symptoms of infection
- Verbalizes discharge instructions for wound care

INTERVENTION

Interventions for a client with *Impaired skin integrity* are developed by the multidisciplinary team, including the nurse, physician, physical and occupational therapists, and dietitian, as well as the client and family. A valuable resource to the medical and nursing staff is the certified wound, ostomy, and continence nurse (CWOCN). This nurse is specially trained and certified in the care and management of wound, ostomy, and incontinence issues and can assist in selecting dressings and support surfaces, planning and implementing care, and evaluating the plan of care.

INTERVENTIONS TO PROMOTE WOUND HEALING

Skin care and wound care have changed dramatically over the past 30 years. Extensive research has led to new wound care treatment protocols and products. However, wound healing cannot be approached solely from a procedural perspective. Instead, the treatment plan must take the client's entire condition into consideration. Physical condition, nutritional status, and treatment methods all affect the healing process (Hess, 2005).

Providing Adequate Nutrition. Adequate nutrition is essential for the client with *Impaired skin integrity* (Hess, 2005). Malnutrition inhibits wound healing and may increase the risk for wound infection (Table 27-3). Commonly, a client with *Impaired skin integrity* needs assistance in meeting daily nutritional requirements. Wound healing depends on the availability of adequate protein, vitamins, and minerals. Postoperative clients and older, debilitated clients with pressure ulcers require particularly close nutritional monitoring.

Improving clients' nutritional status requires a multidisciplinary effort. Assess their intake, and help them meet nutritional needs. One way to help clients choose nutritious meals is to assist them in filling out the dietary menu. Also consult a dietitian, as appropriate, to help determine a client's minimal caloric intake required to promote wound healing. The dietitian may request a calorie count to monitor intake and determine whether nutritional requirements are being met. As previously mentioned, clients may require dietary supplementation, such as multivitamins or liquid supplements. Vitamins C, A, and B complex, and iron, copper, and zinc are especially important for wound healing. A client who cannot take nutrition orally may require enteral or parenteral feedings.

Table 27-3 Nutrients and Their Roles in Wound Healing

NUTRIENT	ROLE IN WOUND HEALING
Carbohydrates, fats, and calories	Energy for wound regeneration and repair
Copper	Cross-linking of collagen fibers
Iron	Oxygen transport
Protein	Collagen synthesis, epidermal proliferation, and immune response
Vitamin A	Collagen synthesis, epidermal proliferation, and immune response
Vitamin B complex	Protein synthesis and cross-linking of collagen fibers
Vitamin C	Collagen synthesis and capillary wall integrity
Zinc	Collagen synthesis and immune response

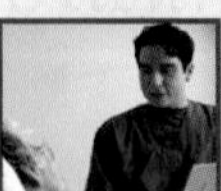

Postoperatively, Mrs. Jacan has little appetite and is not getting adequate nutrition. What effect might Mrs. Jacan's nutrition have on wound healing and development of pressure ulcers? Although Mrs. Jacan tries some nutritional milk shakes, she just cannot eat the solid food on her tray. Keeping in mind Mrs. Jacan's admission history, what foods might the nurse want to include in her diet? How might the nurse involve Mrs. Jacan's daughter in promoting good nutrition for her mother?

Cleansing the Wound. For a wound to heal, the wound bed must be clean and free of infection. Bacteria, devitalized tissue, and exudate must be removed to promote healthy granulation tissue. To cleanse a wound, you will need a wound cleansing solution and a method for applying the solution to the wound. Numerous wound cleansing solutions or antiseptics are available. However, the benefits of a clean wound must be weighed against the potential trauma to the wound bed that could result from cleansing. Povidone-iodine, acetic acid, sodium hypochlorite, and hydrogen peroxide are toxic to fibroblasts. Dakin's solution and some commercial wound cleansers have also been found to be cytotoxic.

Normal saline solution is the preferred cleansing agent because it is physiologically compatible, does not harm tissue, and adequately cleanses most tissues. Irrigate wounds with a device that provides 4 to 15 pounds of pressure per square inch (Table 27-4). Using adequate irrigation pressure enhances wound cleansing without damaging the tissues. An easy way to irrigate a wound is to use a 35-mL syringe with an angiocatheter. This method provides enough force to remove eschar, bacteria, and other debris. Procedure 27-1 outlines the steps of wound irrigation.

Commonly, a physician will order that an incision be cleansed. When cleansing around an incision or drain, always wipe from the cleanest area to the dirtiest (Figure 27-12). Remember that, generally, the wound is cleaner than the surrounding skin. To apply the "clean to dirty"

Table 27-4 Irrigation Pressures by Device

DEVICE	IRRIGATION PRESSURE (PSI)
Spray Bottle-Ultra Klenz (Carrington Laboratories, Inc., Irving, TX)	1.2
Bulb Syringe (Davol Inc., Cranston, RI)	2.0
Piston Irrigation Syringe (60-mL) with catheter tip (Premium Plastics, Inc., Chicago, IL)	4.2
Saline Squeeze Bottle (250-mL) with irrigation cap (Baxter Healthcare Corp., Deerfield, IL)	4.5
Water Pik at lowest setting (#1) (Teledyne Water Pik, Fort Collins, CO)	6.0
Irrijet DS with tip (Ackrad Laboratories, Inc., Cranford, NJ)	7.6
35-mL syringe with 19-gauge needle or angiocatheter	8.0
Water Pik at middle setting (#3) (Teledyne Water Pik, Fort Collins, CO)	42
Water Pik at highest setting (#5) (Teledyne Water Pik, Fort Collins, CO)	>50
Pressurized Cannister-Dey wash (Dey Laboratories, Inc., Napa, CA)	>50

From Beltram, K. A., Thacker, J. G., & Rodeheaver, G. T. *Impact pressures generated by commercial wound irrigation devices.* Unpublished research report, University of Virginia Health Sciences Center, Charlottesville.

rule, clean from the center of the incision and wipe outward. To cleanse around a drain, wipe in a circular direction, changing swabs with each concentric circle.

Maintaining a Moist Wound Bed. Moisture enhances wound reepithelialization, helping a wound heal faster and with less scar tissue. In contrast, a scab that forms when a wound is kept dry does not allow the movement of epidermal cells in the healing process. Moist wound healing does not promote infection. The infection rate for moisture-retentive dressings is 2.5% compared to 9% for dry dressings (Thompson, 2000).

Dressing the Wound. Most surgical wounds heal by primary intention and proceed through the three healing phases previously described. Optimal dressings absorb drainage and provide an aseptic environment that provides a barrier against further trauma (Bryant, in press). To support the "moist wound" concept, numerous wound care products, including transparent films, hydrocolloid dressings, hydrogels, and foams, have been developed (Table 27-5). It may be difficult to determine which type of dressing to apply. Table 27-6, p. 684 suggests specific dressings for each stage of a pressure ulcer.

Action Alert! Always check the physician's dressing orders for the specific site, method, dressing type, frequency of dressing changes, and time frame to evaluate healing.

TIME TO ALLOW: NOVICE: 15 min. EXPERT: 7 min.

PROCEDURE 27-1 IRRIGATING A WOUND

Wound irrigation promotes wound healing by removing exudate, drainage, pus, and slough. Irrigation is a method of cleaning a wound with a gentle flow of a solution. It washes the wound without wiping delicate tissues with a fabric that might cause damage to newly forming granulation tissue. Irrigation also has the advantage of penetrating tunnels or fissures in the wound.

Preventing Possible Complications: Premedicate for pain. The irrigation solution should not be harmful to the tissues and should be injected at a pressure of 4 to 15 psi (pounds per square inch). Newly forming granulated tissue may be damaged if the appropriate psi is not used for irrigation.

DELEGATION GUIDELINES

You may not delegate wound irrigation to a nursing assistant. The complex nature of this type of wound requires your ongoing assessment and careful attention to irrigation technique. The nursing assistant may help with assembling the necessary equipment and positioning the client for your performance of wound care.

EQUIPMENT NEEDED

- Irrigation kit or sterile basin
- 18- or 19-gauge needle or angiocatheter
- 35-mL syringe
- 150 to 500 mL sterile normal saline or other irrigant ordered by physician
- Clean gloves
- Sterile gloves
- Waterproof underpad
- Protective eyewear (if needed)

1 Follow preliminary actions (see inside front cover).

2 Prepare for the procedure.

a. Check the wound care order and the specific order for irrigant. *Wound irrigations are prescribed by a physician or advanced practice nurse.*

b. Premedicate the client for pain if you anticipate discomfort.

c. Perform hand hygiene, and apply protective eyewear and a gown if you anticipate splashing during the irrigation procedure. *Following these steps maintains standard precautions.*

Continued

d. Place the underpad and/or clean basin to catch the irrigant fluid when it drains from the wound.
e. Decide whether the procedure should be clean or sterile. Set up a clean or sterile field by opening the irrigation tray. Add new sterile dressings to the field or open packages where sterile dressings can be accessed once you have donned your sterile gloves.
f. Pour irrigant into the sterile basin.

3 Remove the old dressing using clean gloves.

a. Remove the outer layer. If the dressing is stuck to delicate granulation tissue, moisten it for easier removal.
b. Remove any packing from the wound. Dispose of the dressing according to hospital policy for standard precautions for blood and body fluids.

4 Irrigate the wound.

a. Apply sterile gloves.
b. Fill the syringe with irrigant. With the tip of the needle about 2 inches from the wound bed, flush with slow continuous pressure (see illustration). Repeat as needed. Irrigate the wound thoroughly.

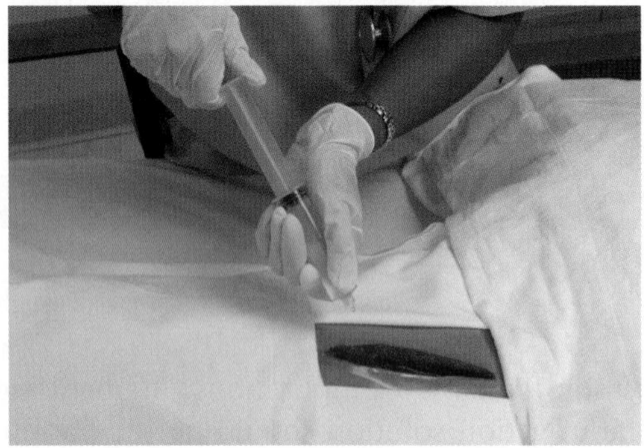

Step 4b. Flushing the wound with slow continuous pressure.

5 Re-dress the wound.

a. Wet-to-moist packing with a dry outer dressing is often used in conjunction with wound irrigations. *Re-dressing the wound with an appropriate dressing promotes healing.*
b. Dispose of used supplies according to standard precautions. If hospital policy dictates that a wound irrigation be a clean procedure, the irrigation kit can be reused for 24 hours. The open bottle of normal saline is good for 24 hours.

6 Document the client's tolerance of the wound irrigation and dressing change, as well as a description of the wound bed. *Documentation of client tolerance and the appearance of the wound bed facilitates communication of the client's condition and allows ongoing assessment of the client plan of care.*

PEDIATRIC CONSIDERATIONS

Consider activity level and developmental stage of the child. Assess the child's pain level, and premedicate if needed. Involve the parents to offer comfort and support if possible. Inform the child and the parent(s) about what will be done. Be sure to use age-appropriate language when describing the procedure. Painful or complex dressing changes should be done in a place other than the child's bed or crib.

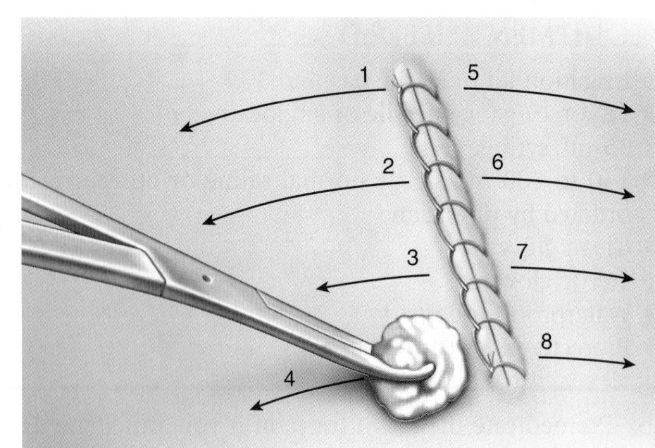

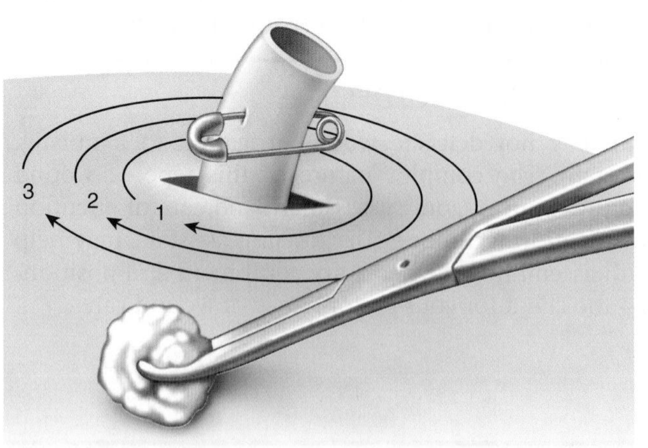

FIGURE 27-12 Cleaning a surgical wound. **A,** Start at the incision, and clean outward. **B,** Start at the drain site, and clean around the drain in a circular fashion. Use a clean, new sterile swab for each stroke to prevent contamination of the wound.

Dry sterile dressings (DSDs) are most commonly used for closed surgical incisions. These dressings protect the incision and absorb drainage or exudate. The initial postoperative dressing is usually left in place for 24 to 48 hours. Some surgeons prefer to change the first postoperative dressing themselves, so check the physician's order and agency policy on initial postoperative dressing changes. Remove the dressing correctly, as described in Procedure 27-2, p. 685. Remember that repeatedly applying and removing a dressing can further impair a client's skin integrity. Montgomery straps are a good choice for clients who need frequent dressing changes or have sensitive skin (Figure 27-13, p. 686). They reduce skin irritation caused by repeated dressing changes.

Table 27-5 Common Wound Care Products

PRODUCT	ACTION	INDICATION	ADVANTAGES	DISADVANTAGES
Gauze dressing	Wound débridement	• Prevent trauma and infection • Wick exudate away from wound • Provide a moist environment for healing (when moistened) • Wounds requiring débridement, packing or management of tunnels and tracts	• Moderately absorptive • Cost-effective • Universally available • Can be combined with other dressings • Can be packed into wounds	• May require frequent changes • May adhere to wound bed and débride healthy tissue
Transparent film	Provides a moist environment that promotes granulation tissue and autolysis of necrotic tissue, allowing oxygen and water vapor to escape while remaining impermeable to bacteria and contaminants	• Superficial wound • Partial-thickness wound • Wound with sloughing or necrosis • Wound with little or no exudate	• Retains moisture • Impermeable to bacteria and other contamination • Promotes autolysis • Allows visualization of wound	• Not recommended for infected wounds or those with heavy exudate • May be difficult to apply • May not stay in place in high-friction area or if exudate is heavy
Hydrocolloid dressing	Provides a moist environment that allows a clean wound to granulate and a necrotic wound to débride autolytically	• Superficial or partial-thickness wound • Wound with necrosis or sloughing • Wound with light to moderate exudate	• Impermeable to bacteria and other contaminants • Promotes débridement • Self-adhesive and molds well • May be left in place for 3 to 5 days, minimizing skin trauma and disruption of healing • May be used under compression • Available in many shapes and sizes	• Not recommended for sinus tracts, infection, fragile skin, exposed bone or tendon, or wounds with heavy exudate • May become dislodged if wound produces heavy exudate • May curl at edges
Hydrogel dressing	Water- or glycerin-based amorphous gel, impregnated gauze, or sheet dressing used to maintain a moist wound	• Partial- and full-thickness wounds • Deep wound with light exudate • Wound with necrosis or sloughing	• Soothes and reduces pain • Rehydrates wound • Promotes débridement • Is easily removed	• Not recommended for wounds with heavy exudate • May be difficult to secure • Becomes dehydrated easily
Alginate dressing	Interacts with exudate to form a soft gel that keeps the environment moist	• Partial- or full-thickness wound with moderate to heavy exudates • Wound with tunneling or sinus tracts • Wound with necrotic tissue and exudate • Infected or noninfected	• Can absorb up to 20 times its weight in exudate • Forms a gel over wound • Promotes débridement • Fills in dead space	• Not recommended for wounds with dry eschar or light exudate • May dry out wound bed • Requires secondary dressings • Contraindicated for dry eschar

Continued

Table 27-5 Common Wound Care Products—cont'd

PRODUCT	ACTION	INDICATION	ADVANTAGES	DISADVANTAGES
Composite dressing (combination of two or more products)	Combines moisture retention with absorption	• Partial- or full-thickness wound with moderate to heavy exudate and with healthy tissue • Necrotic tissue or mixed wounds	• May promote débridement • May be used on infected wounds • Easy to apply and remove	• Not recommended for wounds with minimal or no exudates
Exudate absorber	Conforms to wound surface, eliminates dead space, and absorbs exudate while maintaining a moist environment	• Full-thickness wound with moderate to heavy exudate • Wound that requires packing and absorption • Wound with necrotic tissue	• Absorbs at least 5 times its weight in exudate • Fills in dead space • Promotes débridement • Easy to apply	• Not recommended for wounds with light exudate or dry eschar • May rehydrate wound bed • Requires secondary dressings
Foam	Creates a moist environment and can be removed without trauma	• Partial- or full-thickness wound with minimal to heavy exudates • To absorb drainage around tubes	• Nonadherent • Will not injure surrounding skin • Easy to apply and remove	• Not recommended for wounds with no exudate • May macerate surrounding unprotected skin • Not recommended for dry eschar

Table 27-6 Choosing the Right Dressing for a Pressure Ulcer*

PRESSURE ULCER STAGE	DRESSING OPTIONS
Stage I pressure ulcers	• Hydrocolloids† • Lubricating sprays • Moisturizing lotions • Skin sealants • Transparent films†
Stage II pressure ulcers with light exudate or drainage	• Collagen • Composites • Foams • Hydrocolloids† • Hydrogel wafers • Moist impregnated gauzes • Specialty absorptives • Transparent films† • Contact layers
Stage II pressure ulcers with moderate exudate or drainage	• Alginates • Collagens • Composites • Foam (covers) • Hydrogel wafers • Moist impregnated gauzes • Specialty absorptives • Gelling fibers
Stage III pressure ulcers with light to moderate exudate or drainage; no necrosis	• Collagens • Foam (fillers) • Hydrocolloids (pastes, fillers) • Hydrogels (amorphous, gauze) • Moist impregnated packing gauzes • Wound fillers
Stage III pressure ulcers with moderate to heavy exudate or drainage; necrosis present; tunneling or undermining present	• Alginates • Collagens • Débriding agents • Foams (fillers) • Wound fillers • Gelling fibers
Stage IV pressure ulcers with light to moderate exudate or drainage; no necrosis present	• Collagens • Foams (fillers) • Hydrocolloids† • Hydrogels (amorphous, gauze) • Moist impregnated packing gauzes • Wound fillers
Stage IV pressure ulcers with moderate to heavy exudate or drainage; necrosis present; tunneling or undermining present	• Alginates • Collagens • Débriding agents • Foams (fillers) • Moist impregnated gauzes • Wound fillers • Gelling fibers

Modified from Hess, C. T. (2005). *Clinical guide to wound care* (5th ed.). Philadelphia: Lippincott Williams & Wilkins.
*It remains the responsibility of the nurse to know the actions, indications, and contraindications of wound care products (see Table 27-5) before selecting a dressing.
†Contraindicated for infected wounds.

Occasionally, a dressing will stick to the wound bed. To loosen the dressing easily without disturbing new granulation tissue, moisten it with normal saline solution.

Secure dressings in place using tape, other bandages, or binders, as described in Procedure 27-3. To determine the best method for securing a bandage, assess the wound (including its size), the client's activity level, and the frequency of ordered dressing changes.

Generally, open surgical wounds are managed by keeping the wound clean, moist, free of necrotic tissue,

PROCEDURE 27-2 REMOVING A DRESSING

TIME TO ALLOW: **NOVICE:** 10 min. **EXPERT:** 5 min.

Removal of a dressing allows direct observation of the client's wound and replacement of the contaminated dressing with a clean (or sterile) dressing. The physician will order the frequency of dressing changes.

Preventing possible complications: Remove old dressing, and tape gently to prevent skin tears, further skin breakdown, and reduce pain (see step 3 below).

DELEGATION GUIDELINES

A nursing assistant may be helpful in assisting you in the general performance of wound care. The assembly of necessary equipment and removal of a dressing may be delegated to a nursing assistant who has received specific training in this procedure. You are then responsible for directly assessing and dressing the wound.

EQUIPMENT NEEDED

- Clean gloves
- Red trash bag

1 Follow preliminary actions (see inside front cover).

2 Perform hand hygiene, and apply gloves. *Performing hand hygiene and applying gloves decreases the risk of spreading infection.*

3 Gently begin to remove old dressing by pulling the tape toward the dressing and parallel to the skin (see illustration). Simultaneously apply pressure to the client's skin at the edge of the tape to prevent the skin from being pulled with the tape. *Applying pressure to the client's skin while pulling off the dressing can reduce both the chance of causing further skin breakdown and increasing the client's pain. If the tape has been in place for several days, use of an acetone-free adhesive remover may help you remove the tape. Do not use acetone if the skin is irritated or broken.*

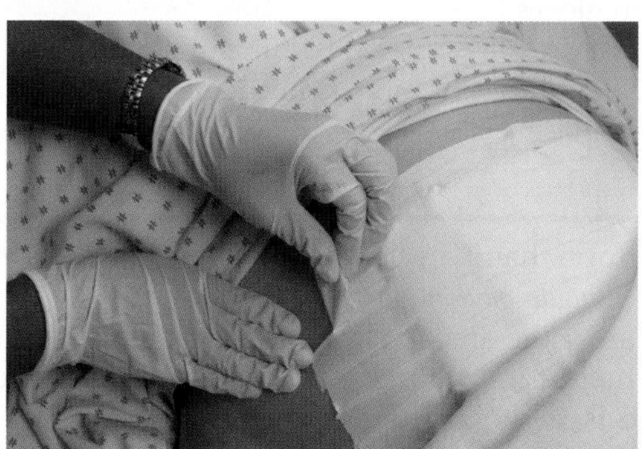

Step 3. Pulling the tape toward the dressing and parallel to the skin.

4 Observe the removed dressing for drainage, especially noting the amount, color, and odor (if any) of the drainage. *Thorough assessment of the dressing can assist with evaluation of the client's treatment plan.*

5 Dispose of the dressing according to agency policy and government regulations. If the dressing is heavily soiled with body fluids or bloody drainage, dispose of it in a red (biohazard) trash bag.

6 Document the odor, color, amount, and consistency of the drainage. Describe the appearance of the wound.

GERIATRIC CONSIDERATIONS

Be careful when removing tape from the skin of an older adult; the skin is more friable and more easily damaged. If the older adult has an abdominal dressing, put the head of the bed as flat as tolerated for easier dressing removal. Be aware, however, that older adults may have respiratory disorders that do not allow them to breathe easily with the head of the bed flat.

HOME HEALTH CARE CONSIDERATIONS

For a nondraining surgical wound, before sutures or staples are removed, the client may wish to use a light dressing to protect the wound under clothes. Clothes should fit loosely and comfortably over the wound without binding. A dressing is not essential, however.

PEDIATRIC CONSIDERATIONS

Consider activity level and developmental stage of the child. Assess the child's pain level, and premedicate if needed. Involve the parents to offer comfort and support if possible. Inform the child and the parent(s) about what will be done. Be sure to use age-appropriate language when describing the procedure. Painful or complex dressing changes should be done in a place other than the child's bed or crib.

and protected with dressings. When caring for an open surgical wound, follow principles for providing pressure ulcer care.

Keep in mind that all pressure ulcers are colonized with bacteria; on occasion, you may need to culture a wound to assess the bacteria growing in it (Procedure 27-4, p. 688). The Agency for Healthcare Research and Quality (AHRQ) recommends effective wound cleansing to minimize wound colonization. When culturing a wound, do not use swab cultures because they detect only surface colonization. The Centers for Disease and Control and Prevention (CDC) recommends obtaining fluid through needle aspiration or through tissue ulcer biopsy.

Topical antibiotics can be used on a clean ulcer that is not healing. Local pressure ulcer infections do not require systemic antibiotics.

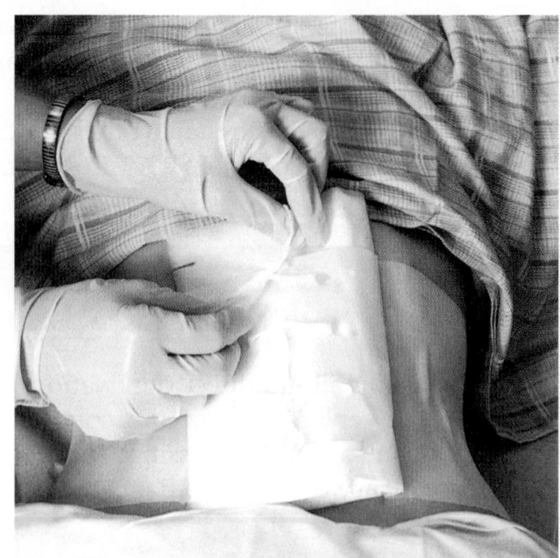

FIGURE 27-13 Montgomery straps are useful for clients with sensitive skin who cannot tolerate tape or for those clients who require frequent dressing changes.

PROCEDURE 27-3

DRESSING A SIMPLE WOUND

Nursing Skills Online: Wound Care, Lesson 3

TIME TO ALLOW: **NOVICE:** 10 min. **EXPERT:** 5 min.

Wounds are covered with dressings to protect them from contamination and injury, to provide compression, to absorb drainage, to débride necrotic tissue, and to apply medication. A simple nondraining wound is covered for protection, and in most cases the dressing is optional.

Preventing possible complications: To prevent infection, dressing changes should be done in a sterile fashion.

DELEGATION GUIDELINES

Institutional policies regarding delegation of this procedure vary widely. In many institutions, the performance of simple, clean dressing changes may be delegated to nursing assistants who have received specialized training in this skill. However, application of new postoperative dressings should not be delegated, nor should dressing changes to open wounds that are known to contain fistulas, that contain draining sinus tracts, or that require packing. The ongoing assessment of the wound and the effectiveness of the dressing technique lie with you; you may therefore determine not to delegate this procedure. A nursing assistant may assemble the necessary equipment and assist in positioning the client for the dressing change.

EQUIPMENT NEEDED

- Clean gloves
- Type of dressing ordered by the physician
- Tape, bandages, or binders needed to secure the dressing in place

1 Follow preliminary actions (see inside front cover).

2 Answer any questions client may have. *Allowing the client to ask questions sets the stage for the client to provide self-care at home. If the client or a caregiver will be changing dressings at home, practicing in the hospital will be helpful.*

3 Confirm the dressing change order. *Dressing changes are commonly ordered by a physician, so you will need to verify the specific order.*

4 Assemble the supplies needed for the dressing change.

5 Perform hand hygiene, and apply gloves. *Dressing changes should be done in sterile fashion.*

6 Remove the dressing from its package, and apply it to the center of the wound (see illustration). The dressing change is sterile as long as the surface of the dressing placed next to the client is sterile. The wound and 1 inch beyond should be covered with the dressing. *A sterile field may be used to hold all dressings, or individual packages may be opened and left in their original packaging.*

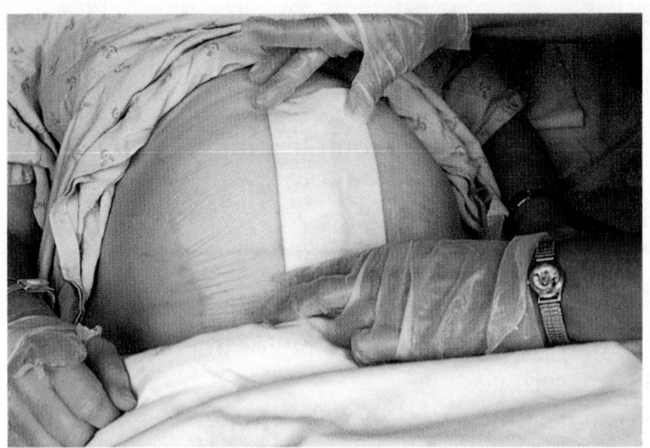

Step 6. Applying the dressing to the center of the wound.

7 Secure the edges of the dressing to the client's skin with tape. Use the least amount of tape necessary to hold the dressing in place.

8 If the dressing will be changed frequently or the client has sensitive or impaired skin, consider using Montgomery straps rather than tape. Montgomery straps will allow you to change the dressing repeatedly without having to pull tape from the client's skin each time.

HOME HEALTH CARE CONSIDERATIONS

If the client or family will need to change a dressing at home, ensure that they have the necessary clean or sterile supplies. An array of sterile dressing supplies can generally be purchased at a pharmacy. If special dressings are needed, determine whether the hospital can supply the needed items on discharge.

PEDIATRIC CONSIDERATIONS

Consider activity level and developmental stage of the child. Involve the parents to offer comfort and support if possible. Inform the child and the parent(s) about what will be done. Be sure to use age-appropriate language when describing the procedure.

Action Alert! Check with the physician about obtaining a wound culture if a pungent, foul, fecal, or musty odor is detected from a wound or pressure ulcer These symptoms suggest infection.

Draining the Wound. Drains are placed in some wounds before the surgical incision is closed to prevent fluid from collecting between the surfaces of the wound, which would separate wound surfaces and prevent them from growing together to heal the wound. Drains are commonly left in place for 3 to 7 days, depending on the type of incision and the surgeon's preference. Common drains include the Penrose, Hemovac, and Jackson-Pratt. A Penrose drain is a small, pliable, flat latex tube placed in the wound to promote drainage (Figure 27-14, *A*, p. 689). Although sometimes sutured in, this drain may simply be placed in the wound. Use caution when changing a dressing with a Penrose drain in place to avoid dislodging it. Hemovac and Jackson-Pratt drains are closed drainage systems that perform self-suction and collection of drainage. Both are opened to air, compressed, and held compressed while closed, thus creating a vacuum. A Jackson-Pratt drain (Figure 27-14, *B*) has a bulb, and a Hemovac drain (Figure 27-14, *C*) has a cartridge, either of which creates its own suction. As the bulb or cartridge fills with drainage, less suction is placed on the wound.

Your responsibilities in caring for a drain include the following:

- Maintaining its patency
- Emptying fluid from the drain, usually once a shift when intake and output are measured
- Maintaining accurate measurements of wound drainage and documenting accurately
- Maintaining the dressing around the drain
- Checking the wound for signs that drainage is incomplete
- Describing the drainage
- Securing the drain to prevent tension on the wound

Débriding the Wound. Débridement is the removal of dirt, foreign matter, and dead or devitalized tissue from a wound. Moist, devitalized tissue supports the growth of organisms. Thus removing this tissue promotes wound healing. Débridement methods include sharp, mechanical, enzymatic, and autolytic. Always use the method most appropriate to the client's condition and wound care goals.

Sharp Débridement. Sharp débridement is the removal of necrotic tissue using a scalpel, scissors, or laser. This method is rapid and efficient but should be performed only by persons skilled at and specially trained to perform this technique. Check your state's nurse practice act for details.

PROCEDURE 27-4

CULTURING A WOUND

Time to Allow: Novice: 15 min. Expert: 5 min.

Wounds are cultured to determine the type of bacteria that may be present in them. Swab cultures are used to detect surface colonization.

Preventing potential complications: To provide for an accurate culture, cleanse the wound before culturing to remove surface bacteria.

DELEGATION GUIDELINES

The sterile nature of this procedure generally precludes the delegation of wound culturing. However, nursing assistants in specialized burn and wound care units, having received specialty training, may perform wound cultures under your direct supervision.

EQUIPMENT NEEDED

- 18- or 19-gauge needle or angiocatheter
- 35-mL syringe
- Normal saline solution
- Sterile swab
- Sterile culture tube
- Gloves

1 Follow preliminary actions (see inside front cover).
2 Rinse or irrigate wound thoroughly with sterile normal saline before obtaining a culture. *Cleansing the wound before culturing it will remove any surface bacteria.*
3 Swab the entire wound bed using a zigzag technique and rotating the swab starting at the top of the wound and proceeding to the bottom of the wound. Swab the wound edges using 10-point coverage. *Using this technique will cover the entire wound bed* (see illustration).

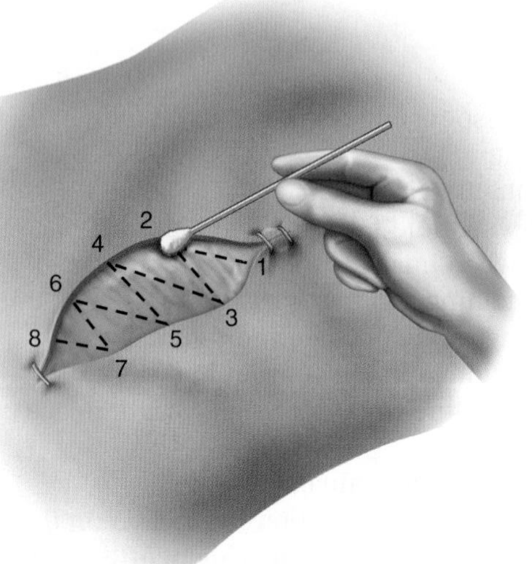

Step 3. Swabbing the wound bed in a zigzag pattern.

4 Place the swab in the culture tube, and send the labeled specimen to the laboratory. *Prompt delivery of the swab specimen will facilitate prompt culturing of the swab.*

Note: Swab cultures generally should not be used because they detect only surface bacteria, and a diagnosis should not be based solely on a swab culture. The Centers for Disease Control and Prevention recommends that fluid be obtained through needle aspiration or tissue ulcer biopsy by a trained provider.

PEDIATRIC CONSIDERATIONS

Consider activity level and developmental stage of the child. Involve the parents to offer comfort and support if possible. Inform the child and the parent(s) about what will be done. Be sure to use age-appropriate language when describing the procedure.

Mechanical Débridement. Mechanical débridement removes dead tissue by applying a mechanical force, such as scrubbing, whirlpool therapy, or a wet-to-moist dressing. The latter is a gauze dressing that is applied wet and removed after it has partially dried (Procedure 27-5, p. 692). As the dressing dries in the wound, the gauze adheres to the wound bed. Removing the dressing removes necrotic tissue. Be aware that mechanical débridement is nonselective and can lead to removal of healthy as well as dead tissue.

Enzymatic Débridement. Enzymatic débridement is a form of chemical débridement in which enzymes are used to break down necrotic tissue without targeting viable tissue. This method must be monitored closely because it can cause erythema around the wound perimeter.

Autolytic Débridement. Autolytic débridement uses the body's ability to digest devitalized tissue. It is most often performed by applying a moisture-retentive dressing (such as a hydrocolloid dressing) to the wound bed (Procedure 27-6, p. 693). The dressing creates an occlusive seal, and then macrophages and neutrophils eliminate the necrotic tissue. Using an occlusive dressing does not promote infection. In fact, such a dressing has many benefits, including less pain at rest, during ambulation, and during dressing changes.

> ***Action Alert!*** Do not use hydrocolloid dressings for immunocompromised clients.

Figure 27-15 summarizes the treatment of pressure ulcers.

Removing Sutures and Staples. Sutures and staples are typically removed 7 to 10 days after surgery by the physician's order. The physician may order only a certain number of sutures or staples to be removed. For example, removing every other suture may allow continued wound healing. Check agency policy to determine which personnel are permitted to remove sutures.

Before removing sutures, determine the type of sutures in place. When removing sutures, avoid pulling sutures that have been on the skin surface through the incision. Doing so may transmit microorganisms into the incision and lead to infection. Use suture scissors designed specifically for suture removal. Cut the suture material as close to the skin as possible, and pull the suture material through the other side of the incision (Figure 27-16, p. 691).

To remove staples, obtain a staple remover and insert the two lower prongs of the staple remover beneath the staple and the middle upper prong on top of the staple. Then squeeze the staple remover closed. The staple should separate from the skin (Figure 27-17, p. 691). Avoid pulling the skin with the staple as it is removed. Remove the staple with a smooth steady hand, and quickly squeeze the staple remover to cause less dragging of the skin. It is common practice to spray the wound edges with tincture of benzoin and apply Steri-Strips at 1-inch intervals across the wound. Teach the client to shower with Steri-Strips in place and discontinue their use when they fall off.

Negative Pressure Therapy. Some chronic wounds may require vacuum-assisted closure (V.A.C.) therapy, also known as negative pressure wound therapy. The vacuum-assisted closure system includes the application of a special foam dressing and the insertion of a collection tube from the wound that attaches to a canister where the wound effluence is collected. The wound is covered with a special adhesive drape that creates an airtight seal when negative pressure is applied. Negative pressure contributes to wound healing by removing excess interstitial fluid and by mechanically drawing the wound edges together, pro-

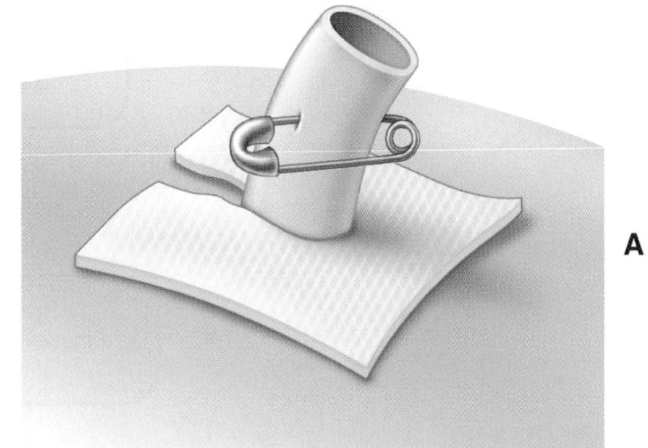

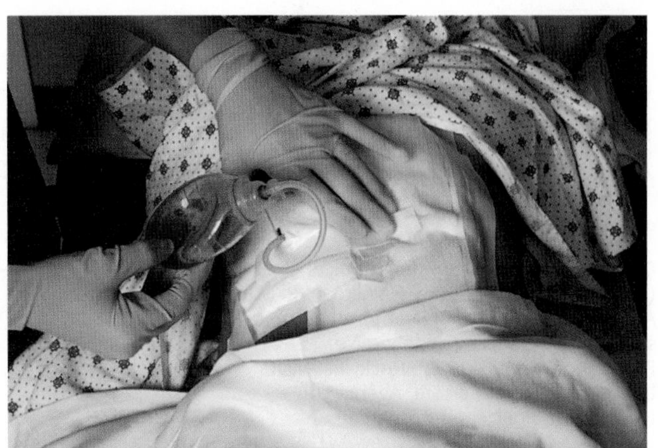

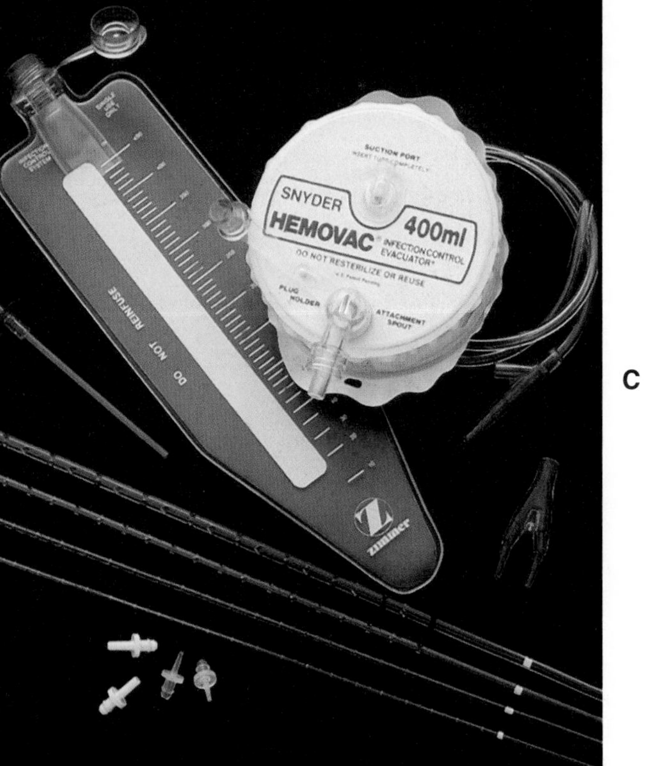

FIGURE 27-14 Common drainage systems. **A,** Penrose drain. **B,** Jackson-Pratt drain (shown in use on a client). **C,** Hemovac drain. (**C** courtesy Zimmer, Inc., Warsaw, IN.)

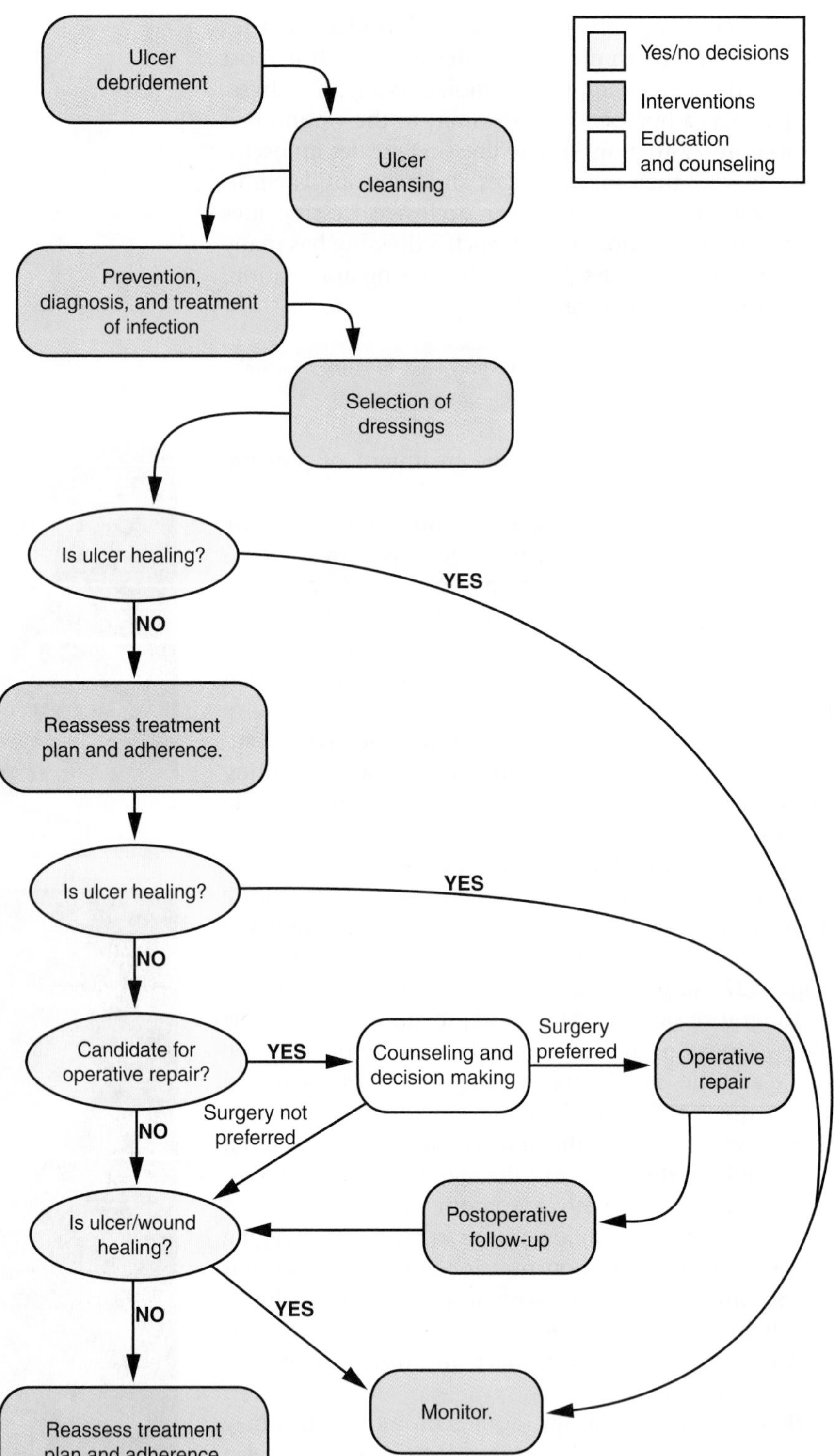

FIGURE 27-15 Decision tree for ulcer care. (Modified from Bergstrom, N., Allman, R. M., Alvarez, Q., et al. [1994]. *Treatment of pressure ulcers* [Practice Guideline No. 15, Publication No. 95-0652]. Rockville, MD: U.S. Public Health Service, Agency for Health Care Policy and Research.)

moting the formation of granulation tissue in the wound bed and wound healing. Stage III and IV pressure ulcers, surgical wounds with dehiscence, and open chronic wounds are appropriate for vacuum-assisted closure therapy. This type of therapy should not be used on a wound with untreated osteomyelitis, wound malignancy, and wounds with eschar (KCI, 2003).

Applying Heat and Cold. The local application of heat and cold to injured body parts can be beneficial. Both heat and cold therapies relieve pain and muscle spasms; however, these therapies work differently at the cellular level. Nurses are responsible for the safe application of heat and cold therapies and therefore need to understand the physiological effects of heat and cold therapies

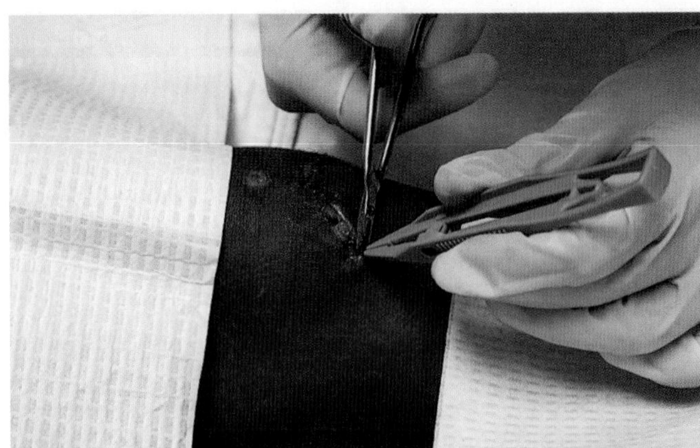

FIGURE 27-16 Removing sutures.

and when to use them. Several factors influence the body's response to heat and cold therapy. These factors include the duration and degree of heat and cold applied, general condition and age of the person, and the body surface area covered by the by the application.

Heat Therapies. The local application of heat raises tissue temperature, producing vasodilatation resulting in an increase in blood flow to the area and tissue metabolism. With an increase in blood flow the viscosity of the blood is decreased and capillary permeability is increased, delivering leukocytes, oxygen, and nutrients to the area and taking waste away more effectively. Heat application decreases muscle spasms and joint stiffness, thus promoting ease and better range of motion and reducing pain.

Heat therapy is generally used for chronic injuries that have no inflammation or in the later stages of rehabilitation of an injury. Heat therapy is ideal for stiff, nagging muscles or joint pain. Athletes often use heat therapy to warm up muscles and joints before exercise.

Heat can be applied in a variety of dry or moist methods. Moist heat penetrates the skin and reaches ligaments, muscles, and joints, whereas dry heat does not penetrate past the skin. One method for applying either dry or moist heat is with a disposable Aquathermia pad (Kpad). A small electrical unit heats water-filled tubes. Aquathermia pads are moldable and can be used on limbs (Figure 27-18).

Another method for applying constant, even heat is with a heating pad molded to the client's body. Use care when applying a heating pad because it can cause serious burns if set too high. Some institutions allow the use of heating pads only with preset limits to prevent burns.

Heat should be applied for 15 to 20 minutes at a time. To prevent burns, never leave a heating pad on for more than 20 minutes or while sleeping and never apply directly to skin without a protective layer such as a towel between the heat source and the skin. Heat should not be used if the injured areas are prone to swelling or show

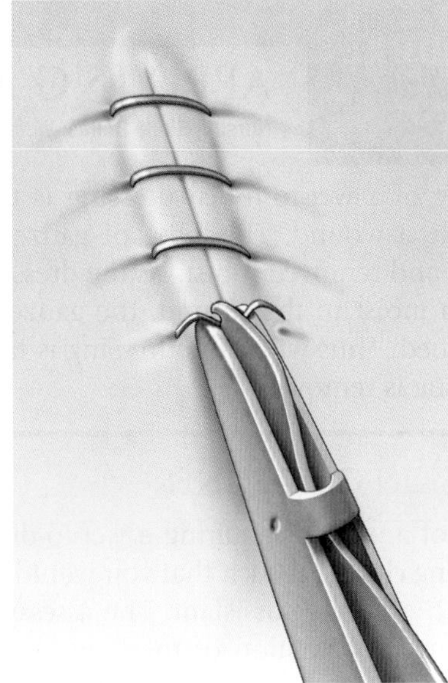

FIGURE 27-17 Removing staples.

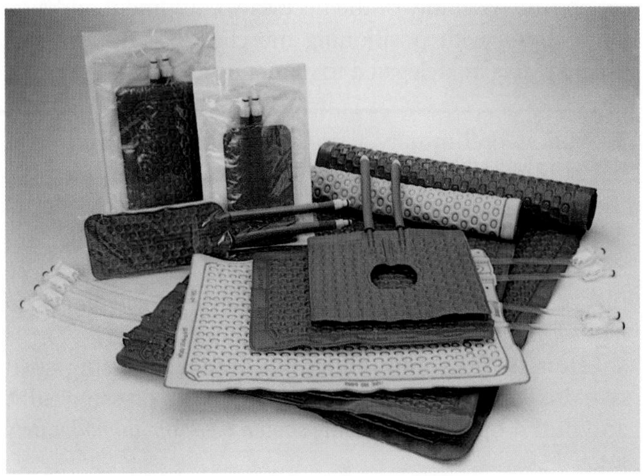

FIGURE 27-18 Aquathermia pads. (Courtesy Zimmer, Inc., Warsaw, IN.)

signs of inflammation or active bleeding because heat increases circulation and would cause further swelling and has the potential for causing continued bleeding.

> ***Action Alert!*** Avoid using heat therapy immediately after surgery to prevent bleeding into the incision or wound bed.

Cold Therapies. The local application of cold reduces the temperature of tissues at the site of injury, reducing blood flow, capillary permeability, and metabolic demand, inducing vasoconstriction. It thus limits bleeding, decreases inflammation and swelling, and limits secondary injury from trauma. Cold therapy has also been found to decrease nerve conduction speed by decreasing the local release of histamine, serotonin, and bradykinin, promoting pain reduction and comfort (Knight, 1989). Further effects from ice include a decrease in

PROCEDURE 27-5

Time to Allow: **Novice:** 15 min. **Expert:** 5 min.

APPLYING A WET-TO-MOIST DRESSING

Nursing Skills Online: Wound Care, Lesson 3

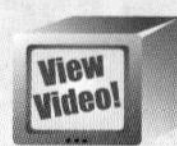

The purpose of a wet-to-moist dressing is to mechanically débride a wound. This type of gauze dressing is applied wet and removed moist. As the dressing changes from wet to moist in the wound, the gauze adheres to the wound bed. Thus when the dressing is taken off the necrotic tissue is removed.

Preventing possible complications: The dressing should not be allowed to become dry. This type of débridement is nonselective and can result in the removal of healthy tissue as well as dead tissue.

DELEGATION GUIDELINES

The nature of a wound requiring a wet-to-dry or wet-to-moist dressing change is such that you would not want to delegate it to a nursing assistant. The assessment, sterile procedure, and intervention of mechanical débridement require your expertise. Within a burn or wound care unit, some unlicensed personnel receive specialized training to perform such dressing changes; these are generally the exception. Assembly of the necessary equipment and supplies, along with positioning the client for the dressing change, may be delegated to a nursing assistant.

EQUIPMENT NEEDED

- Sterile gauze dressing or type ordered by physician
- Sterile dressing to cover wet dressing as ordered by physician
- Tape or Montgomery straps
- Sterile normal saline or other solution as ordered by physician
- Sterile gloves
- Sterile cotton swabs

1 Follow preliminary actions (see inside front cover).

2 Confirm the physician's dressing order, and assemble the needed supplies.

3 Use sterile normal saline solution (or another ordered solution) to dampen the dressing that will be placed into the wound. *Wetting the dressing will promote a moist healing environment.*

4 Don sterile gloves, and twist the wet dressing so it remains wet but is not dripping. Open the dressing fully, and fluff it open. *The dressing should be damp to moderately wet.*

5 Gently place the dressing into the wound (see illustration). Do not pack the wound tightly. *Packing the dressing tightly will block air from entering the wound and will keep the dressing from partially drying.*

6 Cover the damp dressing with a dry sterile dressing, and secure it with tape. If the client is allergic to tape, has sensitive skin, or needs repeated dressing changes, consider using Montgomery straps to affix the top dressing.

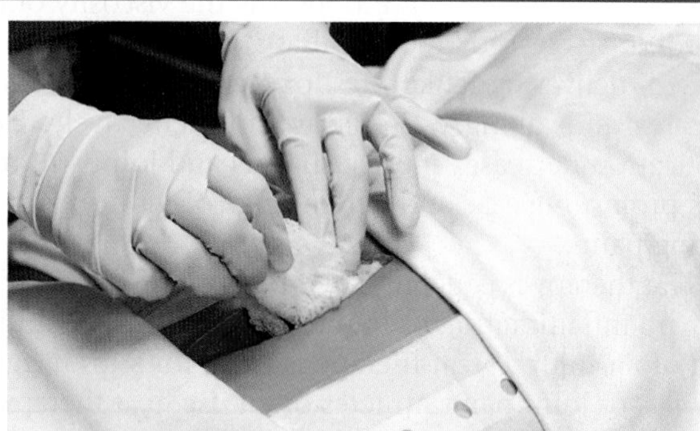

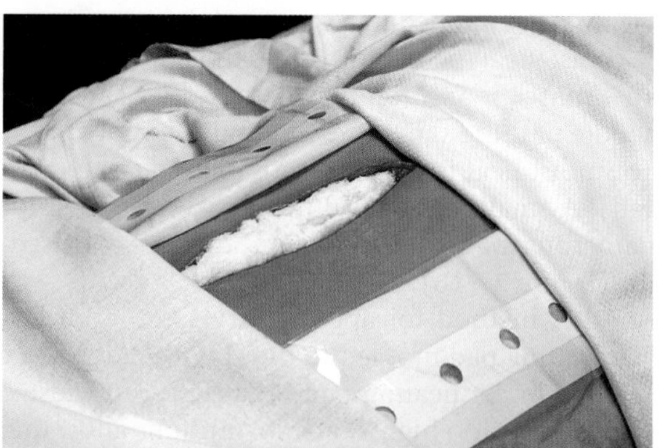

Step 5. **A,** Packing the wound. **B,** Packed wound with the wound edges free.

PROCEDURE 27-6 APPLYING A HYDROCOLLOID DRESSING

TIME TO ALLOW: NOVICE: 15 min. EXPERT: 5 min.

Hydrocolloid dressing is a type of autolytic débridement. This type of dressing causes an occlusive seal, then uses the body's own macrophages and neutrophils to eliminate necrotic tissue. Instead of drying out a wound, this treatment aims at maintaining the moisture in a wound bed.

Possible potential complications: Proper application requires that the dressing be applied larger than the actual wound. Hydrocolloid dressings may have a noticeable odor when removed and should not be confused with infection.

DELEGATION GUIDELINES

The application of a hydrocolloid dressing requires your assessment and expertise and should not be delegated to a nursing assistant. However, assembly of the necessary equipment and supplies may be delegated to a nursing assistant. You may also need the help of a nursing assistant in positioning a client for dressing application.

EQUIPMENT NEEDED

- Sterile gauze dressing or other dressing according to physician's order
- Sterile normal saline or other solution as ordered by physician
- Sterile gloves
- Sterile cotton swabs
- Hydrocolloid dressing; size will depend on the size of the wound
- Hypoallergenic tape

1 Follow preliminary actions (see inside front cover).

2 Confirm physician order.

3 Clean the wound by irrigating it or lightly swabbing it with a gauze dressing soaked in sterile normal saline solution. *The wound bed must be cleansed and debris removed before applying the hydrocolloid dressing. Do not use a hydrocolloid dressings on clinically infected wounds.*

4 Select a hydrocolloid dressing of an appropriate size. It should extend past the wound margins by at least 1 inch. *If the dressing is too small, it will not adhere to the wound bed and, consequently, will not function properly.*

5 Apply the dressing from one side of the wound to the other side. Use hand pressure to hold the dressing in place for a minimum of 1 minute (see illustration). *Applying pressure and warmth with your hands will make the dressing adhere better to the wound.*

6 Depending on the location of the wound and the hydrocolloid dressing used, you may need to place hypoallergenic tape around the edges of the dressing to secure it. *Applying tape will help prevent the edges of the dressing from rolling back.*

7 Leave the dressing in place for 3 to 5 days. Remove the dressing if it is leaking or peeling off, and apply another one. *Leaving the dressing in place will allow moist wound healing to occur.*

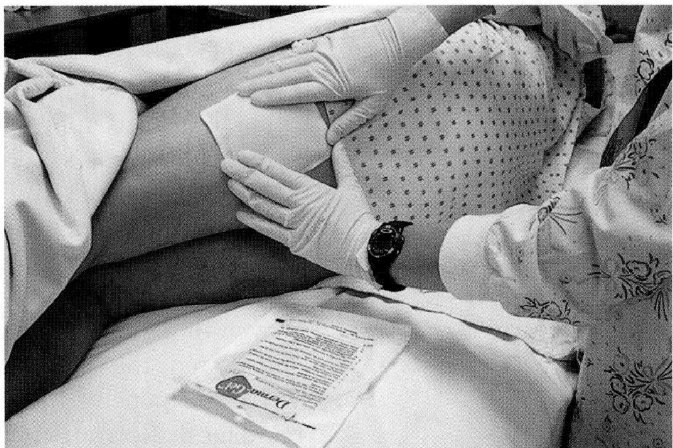

Step 5. Applying a hydrocolloid dressing. Apply pressure with your hands over the dressing for at least 1 minute to ensure good adherence of the dressing.

muscle spasms by making muscles less sensitive to being stretched. Therefore, cold therapy is appropriate to use directly after an injury such as a sprain or strain, muscle spasms, or migraine headaches and to treat some common chronic musculoskeletal or tissue injuries. When in doubt, use cold therapy rather than heat.

Ice is the most common form of cold therapy. Cold therapy is often used immediately after an injury to the musculoskeletal system and for the first 6 weeks following the injury. Common forms of cold therapy include moist cool compress, ice pack, gel pack, or ice bag. Commercially purchased ice packs come as a single-use bag or a reusable pack. Reusable cold packs come in a variety of shapes and sizes. Single-use cold packs are activated by striking or twisting the pack (Figure 27-19). To prepare an ice bag, place crushed ice into a small or large plastic bag, depending on the size of the area to be covered. For a small area, such as a finger, consider filling a glove with ice. For a larger area, such as a fractured ankle, fill a plastic bag. Always cover an ice bag with a barrier such as a towel before placing it on a client's skin to avoid a cold injury. Care must be taken when applying cold over superficial nerves (ulnar nerve at the wrist, and the common peroneal nerve at the knee) and areas with little subcutaneous fat because there is a risk of nerve damage if cold therapy is prolonged (Covington & Basset, 1993). The most effective application of cold therapy is 15 to 20 minutes applied every 2 hours (Knight, 1989). Cold therapy should not be used on people with cold sensitivity, such as individuals with Raynaud's syndrome, and is contraindicated over areas of poor circulation. For example, you would not use cold therapy on clients with diabetes or peripheral vascular disease because circulation in these individuals may already be decreased. It would not be safe to further decrease blood flow to an area that already has compromised blood flow.

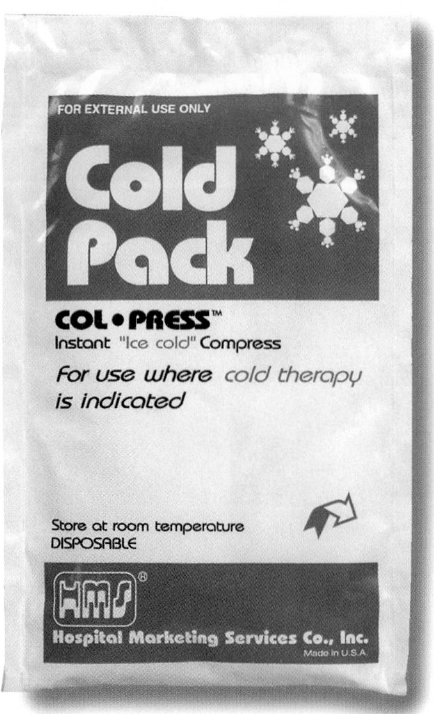

FIGURE 27-19 Cold pack. (Courtesy Hospital Marketing Services, Naugatuck, CT.)

> ***Action Alert!*** Do not use heat or cold therapies for a client with neurological impairment, impaired mental status, or impaired circulation.

Therapeutic Effects of Heat and Cold Therapy. The rebound phenomenon is important to consider when utilizing heat and cold therapies. The therapeutic benefits of cold are due to vasoconstriction. After 30 minutes of cold therapy, blood vessels will dilate rather than constrict, causing inflammation to worsen (also known as Hunting's response) (Kowal, 1983). The therapeutic effects of heat are produced by vasodilatation. If heat is applied for more than 30 minutes, vasoconstriction and tissue congestion occur, for reasons unknown. Be sure to teach clients and families the importance of the appropriate use of hot and cold therapies and the potential for serious injury if not used properly.

Bandaging the Wound. Bandages and binders secure dressings in difficult-to-secure areas (such as the elbow) or provide support to a wound. They may also be used for other purposes, such as the following:

- Apply pressure (e.g., after central line removal or postoperative incision)
- Immobilize a body part (e.g., an elastic bandage wrapped around a sprained wrist)
- Maintain splint placement (e.g., in an elastic bandage placed over an ankle splint)

Before applying a bandage or binder, be sure to use the following assessment strategies:

- Inspect the area for swelling, wounds, and wound drainage.
- Assess the client for pain, and provide prescribed medication as appropriate.
- Assess the client's ability to apply the bandage.
- Assess the client's ability to perform activities of daily living with the bandage in place.
- Assess circulatory function in the bandaged area.

Several types and sizes of bandages are available. Woven or gauze dressings, the most common type, are considered the gold standard in dressing supplies. These inexpensive bandages provide support to other bandages, allow air circulation to the skin, and can be used on many different body parts, including extremities. Gauze also wicks away moisture and exudate from the skin, preventing **maceration** (softening of epidermis), and can assist in débridement. This type of dressing is used in wound packing.

Nonwoven dressings are made of synthetic fibers (most often rayon or polyester). These dressings are soft and most often are used for skin preparation and cleansing. They are not ideal for absorbing drainage. Elasticized bandages are used to provide support or pressure to a specific area.

Choose a dressing type and size on the basis of the area to be bandaged. Generally, a narrow bandage is suitable for smaller areas (such as hand or wrist), whereas a larger bandage is more suitable for a leg. Applying a bandage of the wrong width may cause constriction or excessive pressure on the skin.

Five basic methods or turns can be used to start a bandage, wrap it evenly, and secure the dressing (Figure 27-20). Circular turns are used to anchor the beginning and end of the bandage (Figure 27-20, *A*). Spiral turns are used to bandage extremities by ascending up the extremity (Figure 27-20, *B*). Each turn overlaps the previous turn by half or a third. Spiral reverse turns are used to bandage oblong body parts (such as the forearm, thigh, or calf) (Figure 27-20, *C*). Recurrent turns are used to cover distal body parts (for instance, a stump, skull, or finger). The bandage is first secured with two circular turns and then folded back on itself and brought to cover the distal end. Again, each turn covers the affected body part and overlaps the previous turn by half or a third (Figure 27-20, *D*). The figure-eight turn is most often used to bandage joints because it allows mobility after application. Apply this bandage over the joint in a figure-eight motion above and below the joint (Figure 27-20, *E*).

Binders are used to provide support and protection to larger areas, such as the abdomen or chest (Figure 27-21). A Velcro attachment secures the binder around the client. Apply the binder snugly to provide support, but not so snugly that it creates excessive compression. T-binders are used to provide support for dressings in the perineal area. Use a single T-binder for a female client and a double T-binder for a male client (Figure 27-22).

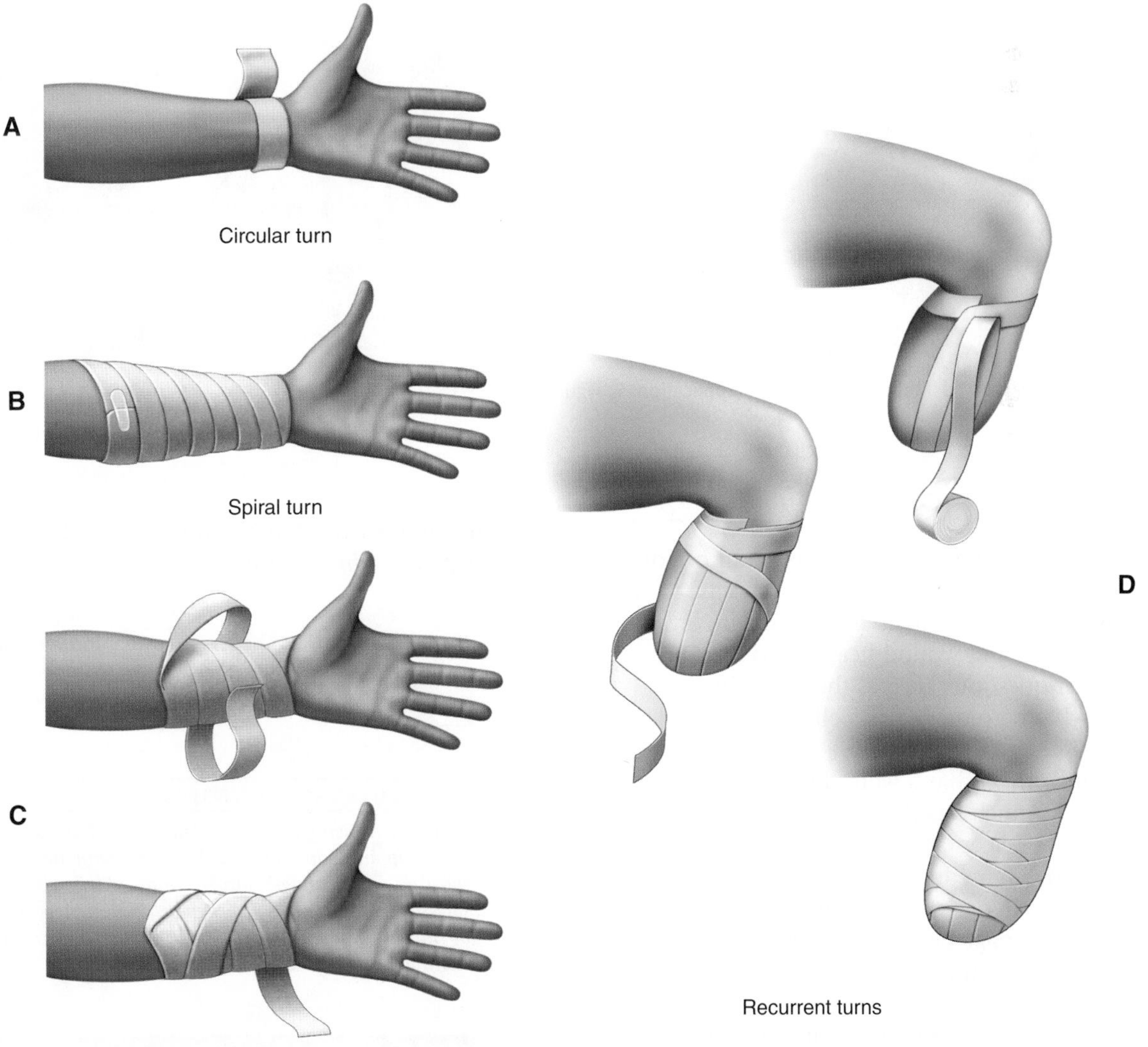

FIGURE 27-20 Methods of bandage application. **A,** Circular turn. **B,** Spiral turn. **C,** Spiral reverse turns. **D,** Recurrent turns.

Continued

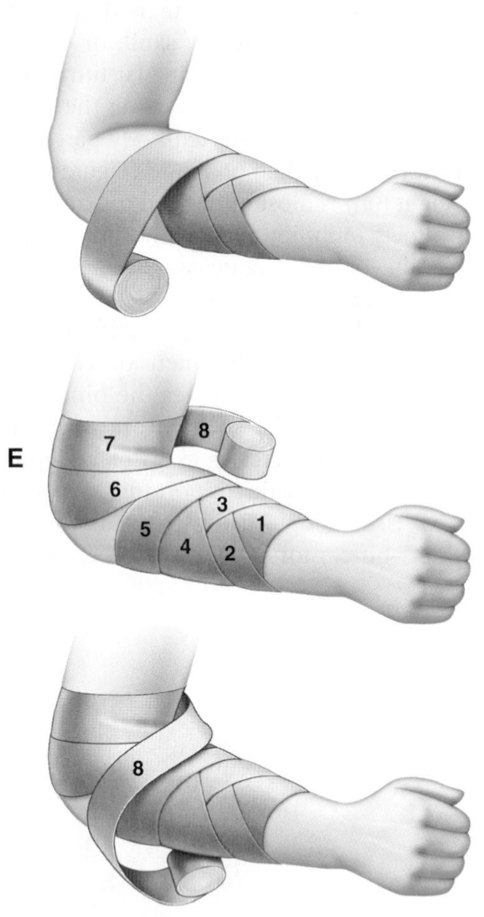

FIGURE 27-20, cont'd Methods of bandage application. **E,** Figure-eight turns.

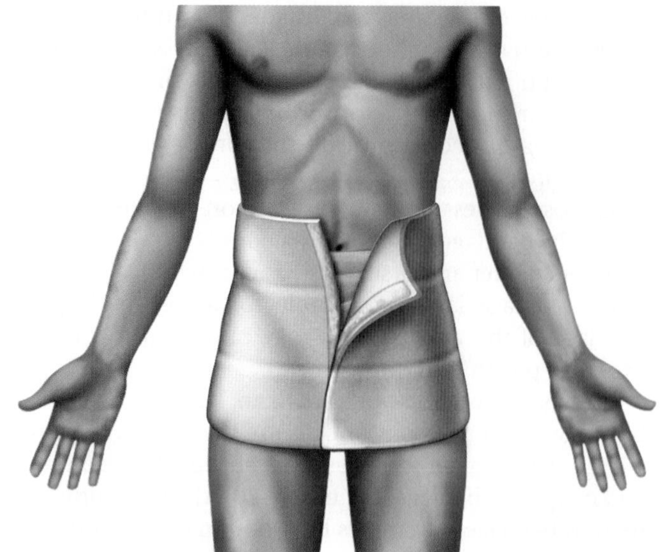

FIGURE 27-21 Abdominal binder.

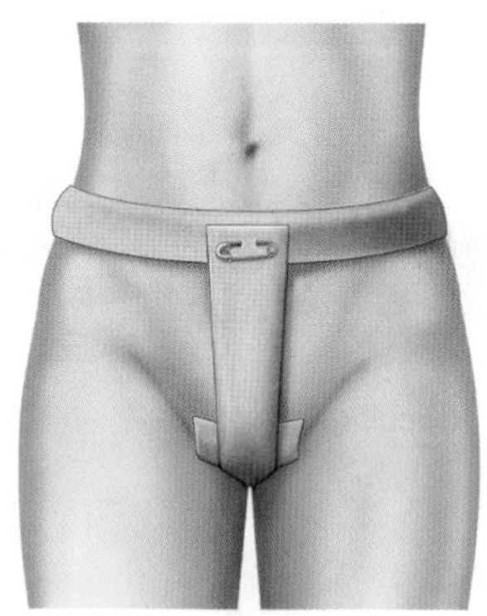
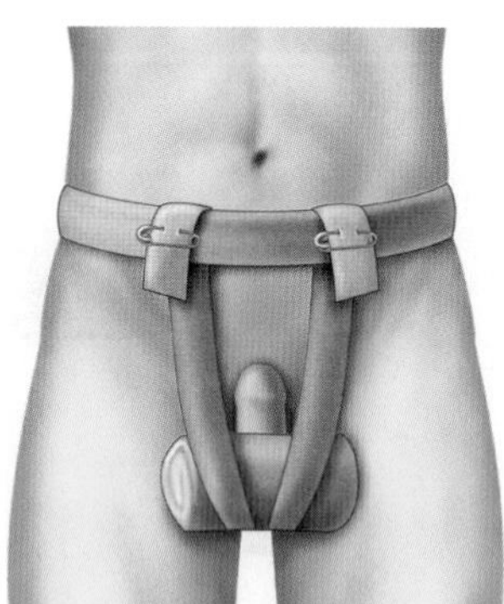

FIGURE 27-22 Female and male T-binders.

EVALUATION

Evaluation of the plan of care is in an ongoing part of the nursing process (Box 27-5). Outcome measurement in wound management is essential to evaluating the plan of care and wound healing. To measure outcomes, consider questions such as the following:

- By what percentage has a client's wound decreased in size?
- By how much has a wound been reduced in depth?
- By how much has the client's pain been reduced?
- By what percentage has necrotic tissue covering the wound been reduced?
- Was the client's wound kept free of infection?
- Is the drainage being managed appropriately?
- To what extent has the client returned to normal activities?

Naturally, in the largest sense, the desired outcome is that the client has an intact integumentary system that serves its normal functions. If the client has *Impaired skin integrity,* the expected outcome is wound healing without infection and further prevention of *Impaired skin integrity.*

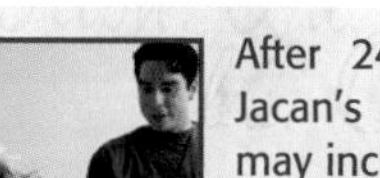

After 24 hours of care, documentation for Mrs. Jacan's nursing diagnosis of *Impaired skin integrity* may include the data shown below.

SAMPLE DOCUMENTATION NOTE FOR MRS. JACAN

Right hip dressing clean, dry, and intact. During dressing change, right hip incision noted to be clean with no areas of redness, swelling, or drainage; sutures intact. Hydrocolloid dressings on sacrum and heels are intact with no drainage. No further areas of skin breakdown noted. Client assists with turning and repositioning every 2 hours.

▼ KEY PRINCIPLES

- The functions of the skin are protection, sensation, thermoregulation, and excretion.

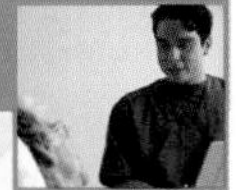

BOX 27-5

Nursing Care Plan

A Client With a Hip Fracture

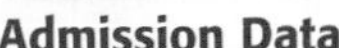

Admission Data

Mrs. Jacan was admitted through the emergency department to an orthopedic unit, where she was prepared for surgery. Phone report from the postanesthesia recovery unit is as follows: "72-year-old woman who fell at home in bathroom 2 days earlier sustained a right femoral neck fracture. She lay on the bathroom floor for 2 days before being discovered by her daughter and had a reddened area to her sacrum and bilateral heels. Underwent pinning of right hip."

Physician's Orders

Turn every 2 hours to unaffected side only
Keep heels elevated off bed at all times
Out of bed (OOB) bid with physical therapy starting tomorrow

Nursing Assessment

Quiet, cooperative older adult woman after hip surgery with stage II pressure ulcer formation on sacrum and bilateral heels. Right hip dressing intact, no drainage on dressing. Slow to progress in physical therapy as well as positioning in bed because of postoperative pain.

NANDA-I Nursing Diagnosis	NOC Expected Outcomes With Indicators	NIC Interventions With Selected Activities	Evaluation Data
Impaired Skin Integrity	***Primary Healing***	***Wound Management***	***After 24 Hours of Care***
Related factors: • Surgical incision on hip • Stage II pressure ulcer on hip and heels; effects of pressure from immobility	**Incision:** • Right hip incision will heal by primary intention and be free from infection.	• Assess for drainage from right hip incision. • Change hip dressing per physician order maintaining sterile technique.	• Right hip dressing clean, dry, and intact. • Dressing changed qd by RN using sterile technique.
	Dressing: • Dressing to sacrum and heels will prevent further breakdown and will promote wound healing.	• Apply hydrocolloid dressing to sacrum.	• Hydrocolloid dressing intact.
	Skin: • No further skin breakdown.	• Turn and reposition q2h. • Apply air mattress to bed. • Teach importance of repositioning and need to be OOB.	• No further skin breakdown noted.

Critical Thinking Questions

1. Before falling at home, Mrs. Jacan was living independently. Her daughter is concerned about her mother's future ability to care for herself and asks you about nursing home placement for her mother. How would you respond?
2. Mrs. Jacan's daughter thinks that she can care for her mother at her home. With which members of the multidisciplinary team would you consult regarding the appropriateness of the plan? What information would you teach the client and her daughter?
3. Mrs. Jacan prefers to lie only on her back while in bed. What rationale would you give her daughter for the need to reposition and turn her mother onto her side?

Nursing outcome and intervention labels from Johnson, M., Bulechek, G., Butcher, H., Dochterman, J. M., Maas, M., Moorhead, S., et al. (Eds.). (2006). *NANDA, NOC, and NIC linkages: Nursing diagnoses, outcomes, & interventions.* St. Louis, MO: Mosby.

- There are four stages of pressure ulcers.
- Wounds can be classified into different categories. Intentional wounds are those caused by surgical procedures or treatments (operations, intravenous therapy). Unintentional wounds are accidental in cause (abrasion or laceration from a fall).
- Although not all pressure wounds can be prevented, the nurse plays an important role in the care of the client in assessing for risk, providing care to a surgical wound, or participating in the treatment of a pressure ulcer.
- A multidisciplinary effort is required to maintain and facilitate intact skin of clients. Members of the multidisciplinary team include physicians, nurses, rehabilitation therapists, certified WOC nurses, social workers, and home health care providers.
- The skin diagnoses are *Risk for impaired skin integrity, Impaired skin integrity,* and *Impaired tissue integrity.*
- The goals of wound healing include keeping the wound and wound bed clean, moist, and free from infection.
- Moisture was once thought to be harmful in the wound healing process. Through research, we now know that moisture facilitates wound healing.
- When the client has an impairment of skin integrity, the expected outcome is wound healing without infection and further prevention of *Impaired skin integrity.*

■ REVIEW QUESTIONS

1. The visiting nurse assesses a client's abdominal incision on the sixth postoperative day. The nurse notes a 2-inch–wide area of redness, heat, and warmth around the incision site. The nurse's first action should be to:

1. Do nothing because this is part of the normal healing
2. Tell the client to elevate the legs to prevent wound dehiscence
3. Notify the physician because the symptoms indicate a wound infection
4. Take the client's vital signs

2. The nurse assesses for which of the following when trying to determine that a client's chronic wound has developed a wound infection?

1. Pain, erythema, swelling, heat, and purulent drainage
2. Pain, erythema, swelling, heat, serous drainage, delayed wound healing
3. Erythema, serous drainage, healthy granulation tissue, elevated white blood cell (WBC) count
4. Healthy granulation tissue, scant serous drainage, decreased wound size

3. A client has a 4 × 3 cm sacral pressure ulcer with 70% necrotic tissue. How would the nurse document the pressure ulcer?

1. Stage II
2. Stage III
3. Stage IV
4. Unable to stage

4. Which of the following statements best represents the purpose of using a zigzag technique to obtain a specimen for culture of an open wound bed?

1. It will ensure obtaining bacteria from the entire wound bed.
2. It will evenly distribute the bacteria on the swab.
3. It will pick up sufficient bacteria to grow a culture.
4. It prevents the absorption of excess exudate by the swab.

5. Which of the following clients would be a good candidate to benefit from vacuum-assisted wound care system?

1. A postsurgical client whose incision has opened 1 inch on the lower edge and is draining
2. A client with a 10 × 14 cm open wound with a large amount of drainage
3. A client with a necrotic great toe with black eschar
4. A client with a venous stasis ulcer on the right malleolus 3 cm in diameter, with no drainage

Bibliography

Baranoski, S., & Ayello, E. A. (2004). *Wound care essentials: Practice principles.* Philadelphia: Lippincott Williams & Wilkins

*Basset, F. H., Kirpatick, J. S., Engelhardt, D. L., & Malone, T. R. (1992). Cryotherapy-induced nerve injury. *The American Journal of Sports Medicine, 20*(5), 516-516.

Beltram, K. A., Thacker, J. G., & Rodeheaver, G. T. *Impact pressures generated by commercial wound irrigation devices.* Unpublished research report, University of Virginia Health Sciences Center, Charlottesville.

*Bergstrom, N., Allman, R. M., & Carlson, C. E. (1992). *Pressure ulcers in adults: Prediction and prevention* (Clinical Practice Guideline No. 3, AHCPR Publication No. 92-0047). Rockville, MD: Agency for Health Care Policy and Research, U.S. Public Health Service.

*Bergstrom, N., Allman, R., Alvarez, O., Bennett, M. A., et al. (1994). *Treatment of pressure ulcers* (Clinical Practice Guideline No. 15, Publication No. 95-0652). Rockville, MD: U.S. Public Health Service, Agency for Health Care Policy and Research.

Bryant, R. A. (in press). *Acute and chronic wounds: Nursing management* (3rd ed.). St. Louis, MO: Mosby.

Carson, S., Overall, K., Lee-Jahshan, S., & Travis, E. (2004). Vacuum assisted closure used for healing chronic wounds and skin grafts in the lower extremities. *Ostomy Wound Management, 50*(3), 52-58.

*Covington, D. B., & Basset, F. H. (1993). When cryotherapy injures. *The Physician and Sports Medicine, 21*(3), 78, 82, 84, 95.

D'Avanzo, C., & Geissler, E. M. (2003). *Pocket guide to cultural assessment* (3rd ed). St. Louis, MO: Mosby.

*Geyer, M. J., Brienza, D. M., Karge, P., Trefler, E., & Kelsey, S. (2001). A randomized control trail to evaluate pressure-reducing seat cushion for elderly wheelchair user. *Advances in Skin & Wound Care, 14*(3), 120-129.

Hess, C. T. (2005). *Clinical guide to wound care* (5th ed.). Philadelphia: Lippincott Williams & Wilkins.

Ignatavicius, D., & Workman, M. L. (2006). *Medical-surgical nursing: Critical thinking for collaborative care* (5th ed.). Philadelphia: Saunders.

Johnson, M., Bulechek, G., Butcher, H., Dochterman, J. M., Maas, M., Moorhead, S., et al. (Eds.). (2006). *NANDA, NOC, and NIC linkages: Nursing diagnoses, outcomes, & interventions.* St. Louis, MO: Mosby.

KCI USA. (2003). *The V.A.C.: Vacuum Assisted Closure: Guidelines for use, physician and caregiver manual, product information.* San Antonio, TX: Author.

*Knight, K. L. (1989). Cryotherapy in sports injury management. *International Perspectives in Physiotherapy, 4,* 163-185.

*Kowal, M. A. (1983). Review of physiological effects of cryotherapy. *The Journal of Orthopedics and Sports Physical Therapy, 5*(3), 66-73.

*Leininger, M. M. (2001). *Cultural care diversity and universality: A theory of nursing.* Boston, MA: Jones & Bartlett Publishing.

Lewis, M., Pearson, A., & Ward, C. (2003). Pressure ulcer prevention and treatment: Transforming research findings into consensus based clinical guidelines. *International Journal of Nursing Practice 9,* 92-102.

NANDA International. (2007). *Nursing diagnoses: Definitions and classification, 2006-2007* (7th ed.). Philadelphia: Author.

*National Pressure Ulcer Advisory Panel. (1998). *Proceedings of the Fifth National NPUAP Conference.* February, 1997. The NPUAP Task Force on Darkly Pigmented Skin and Stage I Pressure Ulcers. Washington, D.C.: Author.

National Pressure Ulcer Advisory Panel. (2003). *NPUAP staging report.* Available at http:/www./npuap.org.

National Pressure Ulcer Advisory Panel. (2003, April). *NPUAP's support surface standards initiative* (S31). Washington, D.C.: Author.

National Pressure Ulcer Advisory Panel. (2005). *Pressure ulcer staging.* Available at http://www.npuap.org.potin4.html.

Thompson, J. (2000). A practical guide to wound care. *RN, 63*(1), 48-52.

*Asterisk indicates a classic or definitive work on this subject.

Chapter 28

Managing Body Temperature

Media Resources

- evolve Evolve Website http://evolve.elsevier.com/Harkreader/
- Companion CD

Learning Objectives

After studying this chapter, you should be able to do the following:

- Describe fever, hyperthermia, and hypothermia
- Identify characteristics of clients with fever, hyperthermia, or hypothermia
- Describe the assessment of the client with fever, hyperthermia, or hypothermia
- Write a nursing diagnosis for the person with fever, hyperthermia, or hypothermia
- Plan for nursing interventions for clients experiencing fever, hyperthermia, or hypothermia
- Evaluate the effectiveness of interventions for clients with fever, hyperthermia, or hypothermia

Key Terms

heat exhaustion
heat stroke
hyperthermia
hypothermia
malaise
pyrogen
set-point

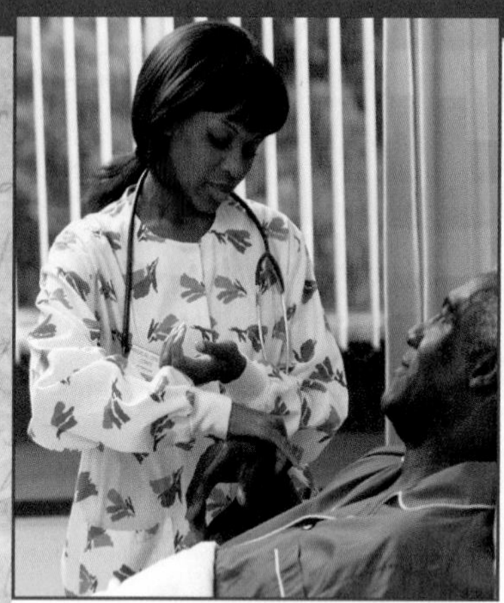

© Fotosearch Stock Photography/Corbis.

Andrew Stephen is a 64-year-old African American man transferred to the cardiac step down unit 36 hours after having coronary artery bypass surgery. His vital signs after transfer include a heart rate of 120 beats per minute, a temperature of 38.9° C (102° F), a blood pressure of 140/82 mm Hg, and a respiratory rate of 16. Mr. Stephen is complaining of feeling cold and has asked for additional blankets. The nurse's physical examination indicates decreased breath sounds on the left posterior side of his chest. The most likely cause of Mr. Stephen's fever is atelectasis, which could lead to pneumonia if unresolved. Less likely causes are wound infection, respiratory infection, or urinary tract infection.

Treatment of fever in Mr. Stephen may include administration of an antipyretic to decrease core body temperature. Considerations when treating fever in Mr. Stephen include that an elevated body temperature contributes to host defense and that an elevated body temperature increases metabolic demands. The report regarding Mr. Stephen's cardiac function is also important to consider. If he has diminished cardiac function, his fever should be treated to decrease the demands on his heart. The nurse considers the diagnosis of *Fever* from the list of possible nursing diagnoses related to thermoregulation (see the key nursing diagnoses box).

Fever presents significant problems to the nurse, whose role is to manage the individual client's response and provide education to the public about evaluating and interpreting the meaning of a fever. Fever, resulting from infection or inflammation, is the most common change in body temperature requiring nursing care.

Fever is a host defense response that frequently occurs in hospitalized people from either the primary diagnosis or from complications. Therefore you are likely to encounter this phenomenon while caring for clients in an acute care setting. In outpatient and home health care settings, you will be responsible for providing information to clients and families to help them evaluate and manage a fever.

Fever can be caused by a wide variety of processes, including infection, inflammation, autoimmune diseases, vascular diseases, neoplasia, and drug reactions.

KEY NURSING DIAGNOSES FOR THERMOREGULATION

Hyperthermia: Body temperature elevated to above normal range

***Fever:** A regulated rise in body temperature (hyperthermia) that is mediated by a rise in temperature set-point

Hypothermia: Body temperature reduced to below normal range

*Diagnoses with an asterisk are not NANDA International (NANDA-I) approved.

The most frequent causes of fever are infection and inflammation. Nurses who understand fever and its management can (1) assist parents who are anxious about children with fever to make good decisions about seeking health care, (2) prevent complications in the hospitalized client through early detection, and (3) impact health care costs.

CONCEPTS OF THERMOREGULATION

Understanding fever is enhanced by a brief introduction to problems in thermoregulation. It helps to understand that body temperature is the balance between heat production and heat loss (Figure 28-1).

PHYSIOLOGY OF THERMOREGULATION

The thermoregulatory system consists of a control center, a sensory component, and effector mechanisms. The temperature of the body is regulated almost entirely by nervous system feedback mechanisms in the hypothalamus. Temperature sensation occurs in the skin, with the face and hands having the greatest concentration of thermoreceptors for hot and cold sensation. Deeper structures, especially the spinal cord and abdominal viscera, are also thought to have the ability to sense temperature. A combination of sensory neuron activity from the periphery and the central nervous system (CNS) provides sensory input. The temperature control center interprets the sensory signals and activates effector mechanisms that raise or lower the body's temperature.

These effector mechanisms are activated when body temperature is above the person's **set-point**—the temperature that thermoregulatory mechanisms attempt to maintain. The resultant actions, such as sweating, dilation of the blood vessels in the skin, and decrease in heat production, promote heat loss into the surrounding environment by the mechanisms of evaporation, conduction, radiation, and convection (Figure 28-2). Effector mechanisms activated when body temperature is below the set-point include shivering, piloerection (muscle contraction at the hair follicles or "goose flesh"), constriction

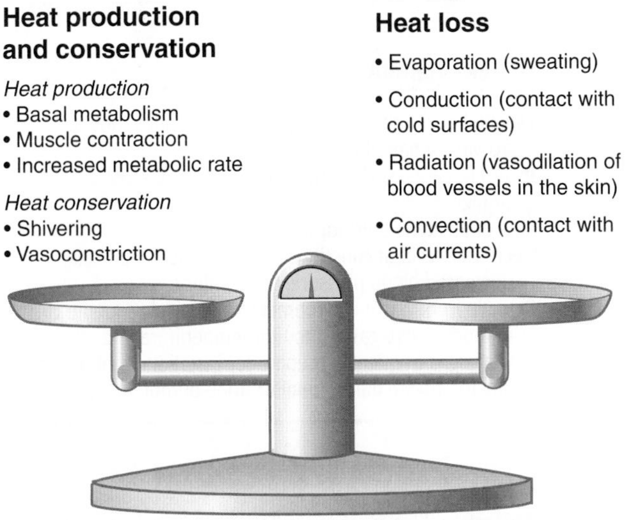

Heat production and conservation

Heat production
- Basal metabolism
- Muscle contraction
- Increased metabolic rate

Heat conservation
- Shivering
- Vasoconstriction

Heat loss
- Evaporation (sweating)
- Conduction (contact with cold surfaces)
- Radiation (vasodilation of blood vessels in the skin)
- Convection (contact with air currents)

FIGURE 28-1 Body temperature is the balance between the production of heat and the loss of heat.

of blood vessels in the skin, and increase in heat production. Shivering generates heat by causing muscle contraction and increases heat production up to four to five times normal (Guyton & Hall, 2006). Vasoconstriction of the skin decreases the amount of heat that would have been lost by radiation, convection, and conduction.

DEFINITIONS OF THERMOREGULATORY STATES

Regulated Rise in Temperature. **Fever** is a regulated rise in body temperature that is mediated by a rise in the temperature set-point. Mediators released in response to a pathophysiological process, such as infection or inflammation, facilitate the rise in the temperature set-point in the CNS. Physiological effector mechanisms are activated by the CNS in an attempt to attain this new elevated temperature set-point.

Nonregulated Changes in Temperature. Although the term **hyperthermia** means elevated temperature, it is generally used to refer to elevation in body temperature related to an imbalance between heat gain and heat loss. In contrast to the temperature elevation that occurs during fever, the temperature set-point during hyperthermia does not change. Instead, the body temperature rises above normal because of excessive heat production, an inadequacy of cooling mechanisms, or a combination of the two.

The most common example of hyperthermia is **heat stroke,** which is an extreme elevation of body temperature, usually above 40.6° C (105° F), resulting in altered CNS function and shock. Heat stroke results from failure of the temperature-regulating capacity of the body, caused by prolonged exposure to sun or high temperature. Heat loss cannot keep up with heat gain; therefore the body temperature increases.

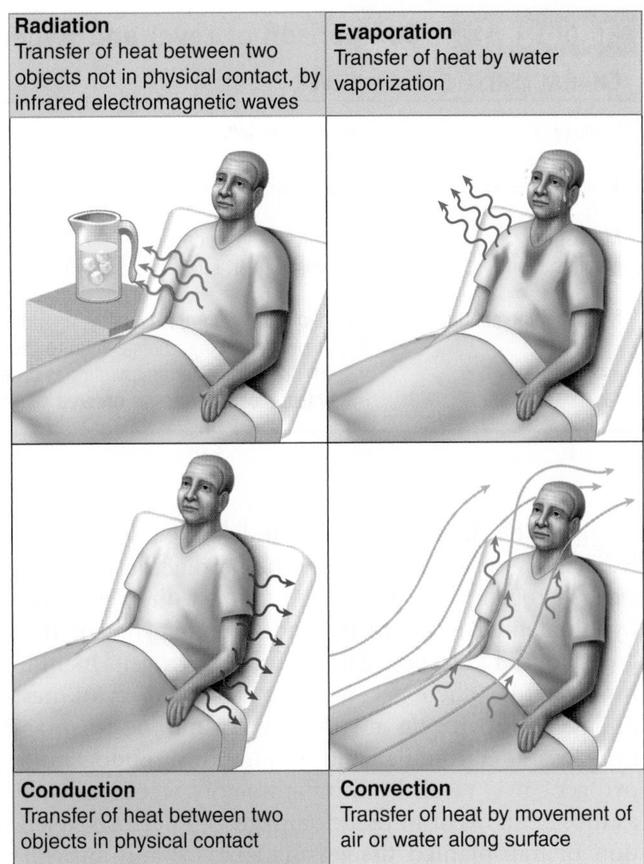

FIGURE 28-2 Mechanisms of heat loss.

Hypothermia is a state in which body temperature is reduced to below normal. It too is a problem of imbalance between heat gain and heat loss. In this case, heat production cannot keep up with heat loss; therefore body temperature decreases. For example, hypothermia occurs when a person is exposed to cold environmental temperatures for a prolonged period of time.

FEVER

Differentiating between fever and hyperthermia is important for properly diagnosing and treating a rise in body temperature (Table 28-1). Fever is often associated with infection and requires additional diagnostic evaluation based on localizing signs and symptoms. It is, however, an adaptive response of the body (Thompson, 2005). Antipyretic medications reduce the fever by decreasing the elevation in temperature set-point. Other therapies promote heat loss rather than decreasing the set-point.

Pyrogens. A **pyrogen** is any agent that causes or stimulates a fever. The initial stimulus for fever is often an exogenous pyrogen. The word *exogenous* indicates an outside stimulus that is introduced into the body. Exogenous pyrogens include bacteria, viruses, fungi, allergens,

Table 28-1 Comparison of Fever and Hyperthermia

CHARACTERISTIC	FEVER	HYPERTHERMIA
Etiology	Infection or inflammation	Elevated environmental temperature, humidity, physical activity, impaired heat loss
Temperature range	Usually less than 40.6° C (105° F)	In severe cases, such as heat stroke, 40.6° C (105° F) or higher
Mechanism	Host defense response	Loss of ability to thermoregulate
Manifestations	Increased heart rate, chills, sleepiness, anorexia	Decreased level of consciousness, increased heart rate, decreased blood pressure, tissue injury
Nursing interventions	Monitor temperature frequently, provide fluids, prevent shivering, change linen to keep client dry, administer antipyretics as ordered, obtain blood cultures as ordered	Remove from warm environment and actively cool the client in more severe cases, monitor temperature and other vital signs frequently, prepare for insertion of intravenous line to provide fluids, monitor urine output

incompatible blood products, and foreign substances. Exogenous pyrogens stimulate the production of *endogenous* pyrogens, internal stimuli that act directly on the hypothalamus. Some of the endogenous pyrogens that are produced in response to exogenous pyrogens include hormonelike chemical messengers called cytokines. Endogenous pyrogens are produced by monocytes, macrophages, neutrophils, and eosinophils. Endogenous pyrogens may result from inflammatory reactions, such as those that occur in tissue damage, cell necrosis, rejection of transplanted tissues, malignancy, and antigen-antibody reactions.

Phases of a Fever. There are three phases of fever: initiation, plateau, and defervescence (Figure 28-3). Thermoregulation during these phases involves activation of the effector mechanisms discussed earlier, as well as initiation of behavioral and experiential responses.

During the initiation phase of fever, pyrogens act on the hypothalamus to reset the temperature set-point to higher than body temperature. Activation of effector mechanisms, such as shivering and decreased blood flow to the skin, increases body temperature to attempt to reach the set-point. In addition, the feverish client exhibits behaviors to decrease heat loss, such as putting skin surfaces together in a fetal position and increasing insulation by adding blankets or clothing. The client will feel cold and may have chills.

During the plateau phase of fever, the body temperature has risen and is maintained at the new elevated set-point. The client may feel quite warm because of this elevation in core body temperature.

During the defervescent phase of fever, the body's effector mechanisms are activated to promote heat loss because of the lowering of the temperature set-point. The client will feel warm and may sweat and appear flushed. Behaviors include shedding of clothing and blankets and requests for ice and fluids. Fever may resolve by a rapid return to normal over a period of a few hours (resolution by crisis) or resolve slowly (resolution by lysis).

Fever Patterns. The pattern of the rise and fall of body temperature is occasionally useful for the diagnosis of a particular causative organism. *Continuous* or *sustained fever* remains elevated above normal with minimal variation and is sometimes characteristic of drug-induced fever (Cuddy, 2004). *Remittent fever* is defined as an elevation and fall in temperature each day, with the baseline temperature remaining above normal for the entire day. Malaria is one example of a disorder that causes remittent fever. *Intermittent fever* is defined as an elevation and fall in temperature to normal each day. Some forms of infection may present with intermittent fever, although this finding is not necessarily helpful in determining the causative organism. With many infections, fever is most likely to be elevated in the late afternoon.

Physiological Responses. Associated physiological responses that occur during fever include increased cardiovascular demands and altered metabolism and immune system function. Cardiovascular responses include increased heart rate and increased cardiac output. Metabolic rate during fever increases 10% per 1.0° C (1.8° F) of elevation in body temperature; if the client shivers, the rise in metabolic rate is approximately 100% to 200% above baseline. Other changes in metabolism include the production of acute-phase proteins that assist with host defense. Effects of fever on immune system function have not been fully determined. The signs of increased metabolic need do not accompany drug reaction fevers.

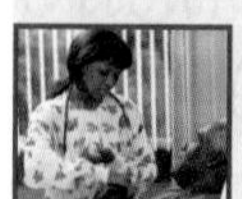

Recall Mr. Stephen, the client in the case study. His fever is in the initiation phase. What behaviors would Mr. Stephen display next?

Action Alert! Observe for fever that occurs without associated metabolic changes or an increase in heart rate—the cause may be a drug reaction.

Additional behavioral responses that occur as part of fever include malaise, anorexia, drowsiness, and altered sleep patterns. **Malaise,** a feeling of discomfort or mild

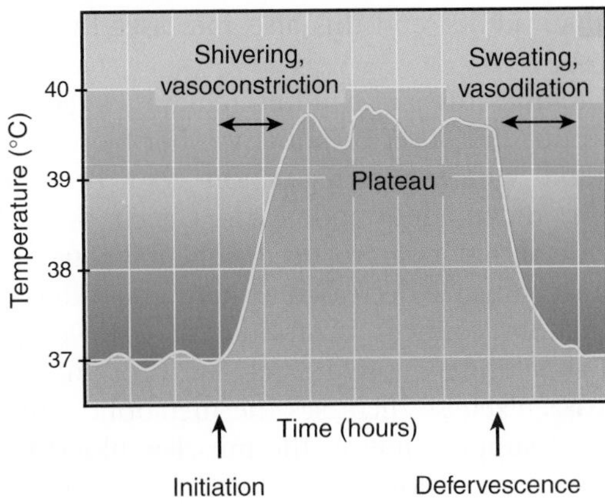

FIGURE 28-3 The three phases of fever: initiation, plateau, and defervescence.

illness, is thought to be an adaptive response that decreases most daily activities, thereby maintaining energy stores for fever generation.

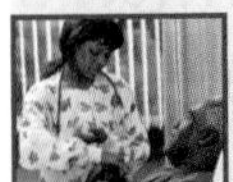

Because Mr. Stephen has had cardiac surgery, his caregivers should be concerned about the effect of fever on the workload of his heart. What changes in vital signs might be attributed to his fever?

Another consequence of fever is a change in the metabolic absorption and distribution of medications in the gastrointestinal tract. Acid secretion decreases, and transit time decreases, altering the absorption of medications. The increase in cardiac output that occurs with fever also alters the distribution of medications.

HYPERTHERMIA

A person who develops hyperthermia does so either by generating too much heat, as during sports activities in hot weather, or by failing to lose heat while in a warm environment (more common in older adults and children).

Sweating is an effective mechanism of heat loss, unless the environment is humid. Increased water saturation in the air prevents evaporation of sweat from the skin, thus decreasing heat loss. Therefore hyperthermia is more likely to occur in humid environments. The amount of fluid loss attributed to sweating varies with the environmental humidity but can be more than a liter per hour with intense exercise. Fluid balance always needs to be monitored in clients at risk for hyperthermia. Maintenance of fluid balance is necessary to maintain perfusion of body systems and perfusion of the skin. Inadequate hydration will reduce blood flow to the skin, thus reducing heat loss.

Increased blood flow to the skin in response to temperature elevation may be impaired in older adults and in some clients with autonomic nervous system dysfunction, such as those with diabetes. The autonomic nervous system controls vasoconstriction and vasodilation in the skin. Problems with nervous system control of blood flow to the skin predispose clients to hyperthermia.

Another population at risk for hyperthermia consists of clients with CNS injury, such as head injury, cerebrovascular accident (stroke), or subarachnoid hemorrhage. Hyperthermia in this group is thought to result from interference with thermoregulation in the hypothalamus.

Heat exhaustion is a rise in body temperature (greater than normal but less than 40.6° C, or 105° F) that is usually related to inadequate fluid and electrolyte replacement during physical activity in intense heat, or the inability to acclimatize to intense heat (Yeo, 2004). Physiological responses associated with heat exhaustion from physical exertion include an increase in cardiac output, release of antidiuretic hormone, increased production of aldosterone, and increased release of norepinephrine. Serum sodium levels usually become concentrated because perspiration represents a relatively greater loss of water than sodium.

In heat stroke, in which the body temperature exceeds 40.6° C (105° F), the client develops alterations in CNS function, such as confusion, convulsions, or a coma. Physiological responses associated with heat stroke include dry skin, hypotension, tachycardia, vomiting, and diarrhea. (Veronesi, 2005). Heat stroke is a life-threatening condition that can lead to cellular damage and multiple organ failure if it is not recognized and treated early (Porth, 2005).

HYPOTHERMIA

Accidental hypothermia occurs because of decreased heat production, increased heat loss, or impaired thermoregulation. Hypothermia is often associated with clinical conditions or factors that predispose clients to a decrease in core body temperature.

Circumstances related to hypothermia (temperature 35° C [95° F] or lower) include drowning, serious illness, systemic infection, trauma, frostbite, overdose, and exposure to persistent cold environment (such as homeless individuals). A common finding in hypothermic clients is the incidence of high alcohol or other drug intake. Alcohol ingestion affects thermoregulation in a number of different ways. It provides a false sense of warmth, inhibits shivering, and causes the skin to vasodilate, thus promoting heat loss. Alcohol also impairs judgment and decisions, raising the person's risk of making inappropriate decisions about exposure.

Hypothermia that occurs in hospitalized clients may be related to treatment (intentional) used to decrease the metabolic rate. This might occur in clients with head injuries (Zeitzer, 2005). Or hypothermia may be associated with therapies implemented in the hospital (Panagiotis, Maria, Argiri, & Panagiotis, 2005). Medications, particularly anesthetic agents, inhibit shivering and vasoconstriction, therefore promoting heat loss. In the operating room, not only do anesthetics contribute to heat loss, but surgical incisions contribute significantly

BOX 28-1 *Physiological Responses to Hypothermia*

CENTRAL NERVOUS SYSTEM
- Apathy
- Poor judgment
- Paradoxical undressing
- Dilated pupils

CARDIOVASCULAR SYSTEM
- Decreased heart rate at temperatures <32° C (89.6° F)
- Decreased cardiac output at temperatures <32° C
- Ventricular fibrillation at temperatures <28° C (82.4° F)

RENAL SYSTEM
- Cold diuresis
- Decreased glomerular filtration rate at temperatures

ENDOCRINE SYSTEM
- Increased aldosterone
- Increased T_4 and T_3

From Granberg, P. (1991). Human physiology under cold exposure. *Arctic Medical Research, 50* (Suppl. 6), 23-27.

to evaporative heat loss. Hypothermia is also associated with rapid infusion of large volumes of fluid, known as fluid resuscitation.

Classification of hypothermia and physiological responses are based on the level of body temperature. Mild hypothermia is a temperature between 35° C and 32° C (95° F and 89.6° F); moderate hypothermia is a temperature between 32° C and 28° C (89.6° F and 82.4° F); and severe hypothermia is a temperature below 28° C (82.4° F). Physiological responses associated with hypothermia affect the cardiovascular, respiratory, renal, nervous, and endocrine systems (Box 28-1).

FACTORS AFFECTING THERMOREGULATION

FACTORS THAT AFFECT NORMAL BODY TEMPERATURE

Various factors can lead to normal or expected variations in body temperature. These variations occur when physiological or behavioral factors influence the balance between heat production and heat loss from the body. It is important to understand these variations so that you can accurately interpret the significance of body temperature measurements and make appropriate clinical decisions for nursing care.

Age. A newborn has an immature temperature control mechanism and requires a carefully controlled environmental temperature for protection, especially against hypothermia. Ensure that clothing is adequate and room temperature is sufficiently warm. Nurses place caps on newborns to prevent heat loss from the head, which could account for as much as 30% of the newborn's heat loss. Infants have a larger body surface area in relation to mass than adults, and this also increases their risk for heat loss.

The temperatures of children remain less stable than adults until the onset of puberty. After being stable in adulthood, temperature regulation again becomes less stable in older adulthood. Factors such as declining basal metabolic rate, reduced subcutaneous fat and sweat mechanisms, decreased activity, and reduced thermoregulatory controls contribute to a lower average body temperature, approximately 36° C or 96.8° F.

Exercise. Exercise increases the metabolic rate of the body as it supplies fuel to the muscles. Blood flow increases to muscles for the purpose of carbohydrate and fat breakdown for energy, and the entire process results in heat production. Strenuous exercise can temporarily increase the body temperature to as high as 40° C (104° F), which explains why the body may sweat profusely during exercise and why it is so essential to drink sufficient fluids during exercise.

Circadian Rhythm. The body temperature normally fluctuates during a 24-hour period by as much as 0.5° to 1.0° C (0.9° to 1.8° F). It is usually lowest during the early morning hours (1 AM to 4 AM) and highest in the evening, sometime between 6 PM and 10 PM. Knowledge of this variation is quite useful when monitoring temperature trends in clients with fever or hypothermia.

Stress. Physical or emotional stress is a trigger to the sympathetic nervous system, which releases epinephrine and norepinephrine and stimulates metabolic activity and heat production. For this reason, clients who are under stress may exhibit a mild rise in body temperature.

Hormones. Reproductive hormones in women may cause greater temperature fluctuations than in men. Just before ovulation, progesterone levels are low, which is associated with a lower basal body temperature. When ovulation occurs, progesterone levels increase, which in turn raises body temperature. The variation between high and low temperatures across the menstrual cycle can be 0.3° to 0.6° C, or 0.5° to 1.0° F.

Environment. Changes in environmental temperatures can affect body temperature in expected ways if the change is too rapid or too great for the body to fully compensate. Environmental heat can cause a rise in body temperature, and cold can cause a decline in body temperature. Infants and older adults are at greatest risk for experiencing effects of environmental changes, for reasons previously described. Proper dress and adequate hydration can help compensate for these changes.

FACTORS THAT PLACE CLIENTS AT RISK FOR FEVER

Clients most likely to develop acute fever are those at risk for infection or inflammation. Bacterial infection accounts for as much as 50% of nosocomial fevers in hospitalized clients. The most likely site of infection is the respiratory system.

Immunosuppressed people are at particular risk for fever because of their high incidence of infection. An immunosuppressed person is still able to generate a fever. Examples of causes of immunosuppression include neoplasms, infection with human immunodeficiency virus, and medications received after an organ transplant.

FACTORS THAT PLACE CLIENTS AT RISK FOR HYPERTHERMIA

There are two classifications of hyperthermia: classic and exertional. Classic heat stroke is most likely to occur in people who have problems with thermoregulation, such as children, older adults, and people with chronic diseases. Additional risk factors include alcoholism, an urban residence, poverty, the use of major tranquilizers, and living on higher floors of multistory buildings. People with classic heat stroke typically have a limited ability to lose heat.

Exertional heat stroke occurs in people who have been physically active in hot, humid conditions. Examples of people at risk for exertional hyperthermia are marathon runners, football players, and military recruits. Heat gain is typically the problem in people with exertional heat stroke. Heat stroke is more common in the humid southern climates. Heat-related deaths occur in prolonged periods of high temperature and humidity.

FACTORS THAT PLACE CLIENTS AT RISK FOR HYPOTHERMIA

People at risk for hypothermia have an altered ability to thermoregulate, or they have experienced excessive exposure to a cold environment. Ineffective thermoregulation occurs in infants, older adults, and in people who have diseases that alter autonomic nervous system function, such as diabetes mellitus. A decreased ability to vasoconstrict in response to cold promotes inappropriate heat loss. Children are at increased risk for hypothermia because of their high ratio of body surface to mass, which promotes rapid heat loss. Hypothermia occurs not only in community settings but also in hospitalized clients after surgery.

ASSESSMENT

Temperature is measured as part of the vital signs during a general health screening or when the client presents with evidence suggesting a fever or is at risk for developing either fever or hypothermia.

GENERAL ASSESSMENT

For a client with altered body temperature, either high or low, perform a complete history and physical examination. As you take the health history, listen for risk factors for infection, environmental considerations, and other causes of altered body temperature. Look also for signs and symptoms that suggest the presence of an infection. Assess the client's general condition and other health problems that might affect the course of the illness. Age and general health status are often important factors in an individual's response to infection.

DIAGNOSTIC TESTS

Temperature Measurement. A thermometer is the instrument used to measure body temperature. Thermometers measure temperatures via many routes: oral, rectal, axillary, and tympanic membrane. The most common type of thermometer used today is an electronic device, although glass thermometers may still be used occasionally. (See Procedure 7-1 in Chapter 7 for measuring body temperature.)

Blood Cultures. A blood culture is a frequently ordered diagnostic test in a febrile client (one who has a fever), particularly when the fever is persistent or the etiology is unknown. Blood cultures can indicate to the clinician the etiology of a fever. Most blood cultures are used to identify bacteria in the blood (bacteremia), but they can also be used to identify viruses in the blood (viremia). It is important to realize that in bacterial pneumonia, urinary tract infection, and wound infection, bacteria may not be present in the blood even though the client has developed an infectious process.

Blood cultures are ordered when body temperature reaches a specific threshold. This threshold varies, depending on characteristics of the client and on practitioner preference. Blood cultures are sometimes drawn at lower temperature levels in immunosuppressed clients because of the likelihood of a life-threatening infection.

When drawing blood cultures, the blood should not be drawn through an intravascular device, such as a central line or intravenous catheter. Instead, the blood should be drawn from a peripheral vein to prevent contamination of the culture. Drawing blood cultures through the intravascular device may be appropriate, however, when trying to determine whether the device itself is the source of the infection.

> ***Action Alert!*** If a blood culture is ordered at the same time as an antibiotic, draw the blood culture before giving the antibiotic. Administration of an antibiotic will alter the results.

FOCUSED ASSESSMENT FOR FEVER

Most hospitalized clients are at risk for an elevated temperature. Inflammation and infection commonly affect the hospitalized client. (See Chapter 22 for a discussion of *Risk for infection.*)

Defining Characteristics. The definition of fever is an elevation of set-point manifested as a rise in body temperature and usually associated with chills. Acute fever is considered a temperature rise to higher than 37.8° C (100° F), but circadian variation must be taken into consideration when assessing fever. A temperature of 37.8° C

(100° F) at 5:00 AM is more of a rise above normal than a temperature of 37.8° C at 6:00 PM in a client with a normal circadian rhythm.

Chronic fever or fever of unknown origin is defined as fever of 3 weeks' duration with evaluation by a medical team for 1 week. Chronic fever is most likely to occur in people with neoplasia, autoimmune disease, and vascular disease. A person with underlying cardiac problems may not tolerate the additional cardiovascular stress associated with fever.

In some clients, fever may not be present during infection. Older adults can have bacteremia without a fever. In older adults, fever does not develop as readily and diagnosis of infection may be delayed, leading to serious consequences. Fever is also a poor indicator of infection in clients receiving nonsteroidal antiinflammatory medications for conditions such as rheumatoid arthritis.

BOX 28-2 *Etiologies of Fever*

INFLAMMATION
- Pancreatitis
- Cholecystitis
- Thrombophlebitis

BURNS

TRAUMA

INFECTION
- Bacterial
- Viral
- Parasitic
- Fungal

DRUG FEVER

NEOPLASTIC DISEASE

VASCULAR OCCLUSION
- Myocardial infarction
- Stroke

Related Factors. Fever is related to a variety of etiologies, including infection, inflammation, neoplasia, autoimmune disease, vascular disease, drug reaction, and miscellaneous causes (Box 28-2).

Assessment of Responses. Responses associated with fever that require monitoring include increased cardiac demand (such as increased heart rate), increased metabolic rate, altered drug metabolism, and altered comfort. Treatment will be based on the client's ability to tolerate fever and the discomfort associated with it. Children who develop fever at high temperatures, usually 103° F or greater, may experience febrile convulsions. Table 28-2 summarizes decision making in the assessment of temperature for different age-groups. Box 28-3 lists teaching points to help parents prevent or manage febrile convulsions in their small children.

FOCUSED ASSESSMENT FOR HYPERTHERMIA

Hyperthermia includes heat exhaustion and heat stroke. At both of these levels of hyperthermia, heat gain occurs at a greater rate than heat loss.

Defining Characteristics. *Heat exhaustion* is more severe than simple heat-related symptoms, which could be relieved by resting in a cool environment and replacing fluids. Symptoms associated with heat exhaustion include weakness, fatigue, headache, giddiness, anorexia, nausea, vomiting, diarrhea, and skeletal muscle cramps. *Heat stroke* is a severe and sometimes fatal condition. It is characterized by hot, dry skin and the absence of sweating, although a person with *exertional heat stroke* still produces sweat. Other manifestations are neurological changes such as confusion, seizures, and coma.

Table 28-2 Decision Making in Assessing Temperature for Different Age-Groups

AGE	ASSESSMENT DATA	DECISION CONSIDERATIONS
Infant	• Infants have immature thermoregulation.	• Protect from environmental changes; keep dry and appropriately clothed.
	• A temperature of >38° C (>100.4° F) in the first 12 months of life is considered significant.	• The parent is often advised to see the primary care provider for temperature above 100.4° F.
	• Convulsions and delirium may occur.	• Tympanic or axillary site is preferred.
Child	• Risk for febrile convulsions and delirium lasts up to 7 years.	• Risk for febrile convulsions begins at 3 months and lasts to 7 years. Febrile convulsions generally occur as the temperature is elevating. Tell the child experiencing hallucinations that the image is not real and will go away when the fever is down.
	• May experience temperature elevation after exercise.	• Educate parents about the risk for convulsions and appropriate actions.
Adult	• 37.1° to 38.2° C (98.8° to 100.6° F) low grade. • >38.2° C (>100.6° F) significant fever. • >40.5° C (>104.9° F) hyperpyrexia.	• Drinking fluids will help maintain hydration with fever at any level. • Temperature regulation is still labile.
Older adult	• Body temperature drops to an average of 36° C (96.8° F) in the older adult.	• Older adults may have decreased sensitivity to temperature changes. • Confusion may be a sign of impending infection with fever.

Sinus tachycardia and hypotension are common. Electrolyte abnormalities include increased serum sodium and decreased serum potassium levels. Heat stroke can lead to acute renal failure and liver damage.

Related Factors. Various factors may be involved in heat-related illness.

Age. Several factors contribute to an increased risk for heat exhaustion or heat stroke in older adults. The size, number, and activity of the sweat glands diminish, making the body less efficient at losing excess heat. Decreased mobility may affect the ability of older adults to get water, and they may also have decreased thirst sensation. Diminished cognitive capacity in an older adult client may also affect decision making related to heat exposure and water intake. Table 28-3 lists other factors that can affect thermoregulation.

Socioeconomic Conditions. Prevention of heat stroke is a public health issue, particularly in crowded urban areas where it may be difficult to maintain cool, well-ventilated housing. In conditions of prolonged

BOX 28-3 *Teaching for Wellness*

Managing Febrile Convulsions

Purpose: To provide parents of small children information about febrile convulsions.

Expected Outcome: Parents will express confidence that febrile convulsions can be prevented or safely managed.

Client Instructions

General Information

- Febrile convulsions are associated with a fever of 38.9° C to 40° C (102° F to 104° F).
- They occur as early as 3 months of age and as late as 7 years of age; 95% of febrile convulsions occur before the age of 5 years, and they are most likely to occur before the age of 24 months.
- Febrile convulsions occur in only 3% to 4% of children, but the risk is greater if the child has had a previous febrile convulsion.
- The child's electroencephalogram remains normal during a febrile convulsion; the child will have little of the confusion that occurs after other types of convulsions; and most importantly, febrile convulsions do not cause brain damage.
- The height of the child's fever does not seem to trigger febrile convulsions as much as a sudden spike in body temperature.
- You can treat your child at home with the specific dosage of medication that the physician prescribes.
- Dress the child with a fever in lightweight clothing; infants should be dressed only in diapers.
- Febrile convulsions occur mostly at night, when parents are not aware of temperature elevations until the temperature is quite high.
- If your child has had one episode of a high fever, try to prevent a second high fever to reduce the risk of febrile convulsions.
- Make sure you take the child with a high fever to the doctor.

Treatment of Febrile Convulsions

- Remain calm, and protect the child from injury.
- Following the convulsion, put a cool cloth to the child's head, and call the physician to determine where the child can be checked (physician's office, emergency department).
- Do not put the child in a tub of cold water; extreme cooling is a shock to the nervous system.
- Do not use alcohol to cool the child; the skin will absorb it, and the fumes are toxic.
- Do not give the child any medications by mouth.
- Do not use an oral thermometer to measure the child's body temperature.

Table 28-3 **Factors Affecting Thermoregulation**

FACTOR	EFFECT
Age	Children have a greater body-surface-to-mass ratio, and children also have a higher metabolic rate. Older adult clients have a lower average body temperature.
Percent body fat	Increased body fat prevents heat loss. This can be beneficial in cold environments or detrimental in warm environments.
Gender	Women have changes in body temperature that are related to the menstrual cycle.
Chronic illness	Some chronic illnesses, such as diabetes mellitus and renal failure, interfere with thermoregulation.
Medications	Neuroleptic medications affect thermoregulation by impairing thirst. Fever may not occur in clients taking nonsteroidal antiinflammatory agents.
Environment	Living areas that have poor ventilation because of windows that cannot be opened or materials that hold heat, such as concrete, may impact thermoregulation in clients.
Occupation	Work that requires exposure to cold environments or physical labor in warm, humid environments affects thermoregulation.
Recreation	Activities such as running, football, etc., generate heat and may be of concern in warm, humid environments.

heat and humidity, ventilation and air conditioning become important. The cost of electricity and air conditioning units may be prohibitive for the poor or older adults on fixed incomes.

Occupation. Heat-related illness, a concern for an occupational health nurse, may occur where a significant number of employees work in conditions of extreme heat. Laborers who do heavy physical work in the hot sun or in metal foundries, mines, or closed shops are vulnerable. Regular breaks, ventilation, lightweight clothing, and plenty of liquids may be helpful in preventing heat-related problems.

Medications. Hyperthermia can also occur as a side effect of medications (Cuddy, 2004). Malignant hyperthermia can occur in response to general anesthetic agents, such as halothane. This increase in body temperature is the result of a genetic abnormality that causes muscle rigidity, leading to a rise in body temperature (Ward, 2005). Neuroleptic malignant syndrome can occur in clients receiving antipsychotic medications such as clozapine. Neuroleptic malignant syndrome is a potentially fatal complication consisting of hypertonicity, pallor, dyskinesia, hyperthermia, incontinence, unstable blood pressure, and pulmonary congestion. Other medications can make the person vulnerable to heat stroke. Diuretics reduce the amount of total body fluid. Beta-blockers, phenothiazines, and anticholinergics decrease the ability to sweat.

Assessment of Responses. In addition to treating the manifestations of hyperthermia, you will be involved in assessing and managing its complications. Complications associated with hyperthermia include altered perfusion to the CNS and kidneys and breakdown of muscle. Clients with a family history of malignant hyperthermia may have anxiety before surgical procedures. Clients with neuroleptic malignant syndrome often have decreased thirst, which contributes to the development of hyperthermia. Nursing diagnoses that may be appropriate are *Anxiety, Deficient fluid volume, Acute confusion,* and *Ineffective tissue perfusion.*

FOCUSED ASSESSMENT FOR HYPOTHERMIA

In clients with hypothermia, heat gain is at a lower rate than heat loss. Because of the higher heat loss, body temperature decreases.

Defining Characteristics. Hypothermia has been categorized as mild (35° C to 32° C [95° F to 89.6° F]), moderate (32° C to 28° C [89.6° F to 82.4° F]), and severe (less than 28° C [82.4° F]).

Thermometers normally used in clinical practice do not provide a scale low enough to assess hypothermia. A thermometer with a lower range should be available, particularly in emergency departments, for accurate assessment of body temperature in clients with hypothermia.

Manifestations associated with hypothermia depend on temperature level (see Box 28-1). Shivering caused by hypothermia will become progressively more intense to the point at which the hypothermic person will have trouble performing voluntary motor functions. Level of consciousness will also decrease as body temperature decreases. Hyporeflexia occurs with severe hypothermia. Life-threatening sequelae, such as ventricular fibrillation, are associated with severe hypothermia.

Initially during hypothermia, cold diuresis occurs, which is an increase in urine production. This occurs possibly because of a reduction in antidiuretic hormone or because of peripheral vasoconstriction and subsequent increased blood flow to major organs such as the kidneys. The hematocrit level then increases because of the fluid loss. As body temperature decreases, cold diuresis slows, renal blood flow decreases, and urine output decreases.

Cardiovascular responses also depend on temperature level. Sinus tachycardia occurs with mild hypothermia. Sinus bradycardia occurs with moderate and severe hypothermia, which could lead to life-threatening ventricular dysrhythmias.

Related Factors. The primary related factors are exposure and medical procedures.

Exposure. People exposed to the cold—for example, hikers, hunters, and others who spend time outdoors—are at risk for hypothermia, particularly if some unforeseen injury occurs and assistance is at a distance. Heat loss, and thus death, occurs at a much faster rate in people accidentally submerged in cold water than in those exposed to cold air. In the southern United States, a case of hypothermia is less common than in northern regions.

Medical Procedures. Hypothermia is also a consequence of procedures performed in the hospital (Panagiotis et al., 2005; Zeitzer, 2005). Clients undergoing surgery and clients receiving fluid resuscitation may be hypothermic after these procedures.

DIAGNOSIS

An elevation in body temperature is due to either hyperthermia or fever. To differentiate fever from hyperthermia, it is useful to consider client history and setting, and this is most difficult in clients admitted to the hospital with neurological injury. The elevation in temperature could be due to the underlying injury or to an infectious process. You need to assess for signs of infection to make the final determination. Table 28-4 shows examples of clustering data used to support thermoregulatory nursing diagnoses.

Determining the cause of fever can be difficult because of the many possible etiologies. It requires examining for localizing signs, such as increased sputum production, abdominal pain, or cloudy urine. Without

Table 28-4 Clustering Data to Make a Nursing Diagnosis

Problems of Body Temperature

DATA CLUSTER	DIAGNOSIS
A mother calls the pediatrician's office, concerned that her 4-year-old has a temperature of 37.5° C (99.6° F). The child is active, does not appear ill, and does not have any gastrointestinal symptoms or respiratory symptoms. Further assessment reveals that the child has a sunburn after swimming yesterday.	*Low-grade fever* related to inflammation*
A 90-year-old woman is admitted to the hospital with a temperature of 40.6° C (105° F). The city is experiencing a heat wave, and the woman lives in a high-rise apartment without air conditioning or adequate ventilation. She has no signs of infection.	*Hyperthermia* related to environmental conditions
A first-day postsurgical client has a temperature of 39° C (102.2° F). Respirations are 10 per minute, breath sounds diminished, and the person is unable to cough.	*Fever* related to postoperative hypoventilation*

*Diagnoses with asterisk are not NANDA-I approved.

localizing signs, the fever may have to be classified as fever of unknown origin.

The age and other demographic data about the client may be useful in knowing what questions to ask when you are looking for the cause of an elevated body temperature. As an example, assessment for causes of fever in children is illustrated in Figure 28-4. A pattern of body temperature change during fever in some cases is related to particular diseases.

One of the clues that an elevation in body temperature is a drug-related fever is that there is no change in heart rate with the rise in body temperature. Generally during fever, there is an associated elevation in heart rate; during drug fever, this may not occur.

PLANNING

EXPECTED OUTCOMES FOR THE CLIENT WITH FEVER

Fever is a component of the host defenses and should be treated only in clients who cannot tolerate the additional physiological or experiential stress caused by the fever. In these clients, body temperature can be brought within normal range using therapies that do not induce shivering. Therefore the goal may be to make the client comfortable rather than to reduce the fever. Sometimes the goal is to teach the client self-care. Possible outcomes are that the client can do the following:

- Maintain a body temperature that is normal for the client
- Maintain dry skin, clothes, and linens
- Maintain comfort
- Maintain fluid intake sufficient to prevent dehydration
- Demonstrate the correct method for measuring a temperature
- Identify when a nurse or physician should be consulted for a fever

EXPECTED OUTCOMES FOR THE CLIENT WITH HYPERTHERMIA

The expected outcomes include that body temperature will be brought to within normal limits to prevent complications related to hyperthermia, such as muscle breakdown. Ideally, there will be no neurological deficits present after cooling. Fluid balance as assessed by serum sodium and urine output will be within normal limits. Precipitating causes of hyperthermia will be evaluated to determine etiology and to prevent future episodes of hyperthermia. Box 28-4 is a guide to teaching preventive measures.

When the diagnosis is *Risk for hyperthermia,* the goal is to prevent heat-related problems. Possible outcomes are that the client can do the following:

- Modify the environment to prevent hyperthermia, such as by repairing an air-conditioning unit or increasing ventilation with fans or open windows
- Identify appropriate dress for a hot, humid environment
- Identify precautions to take when exercising or working in a hot environment

EXPECTED OUTCOMES FOR THE CLIENT WITH HYPOTHERMIA

The expected outcome with hypothermia is to return temperature to normal without complications. Therapies should be monitored closely to prevent the afterdrop that may occur during peripheral warming. Possible outcomes include that the client has the following:

- Normal heart rate and rhythm
- Urinary output within normal limits
- Blood pressure and pulse within normal limits

When the diagnosis is *Risk for hypothermia,* the goal is prevention. Possible outcomes include that the client can do the following:

- Recall safety precautions for walking or skating on frozen ponds
- Demonstrate appropriate dress for cold weather

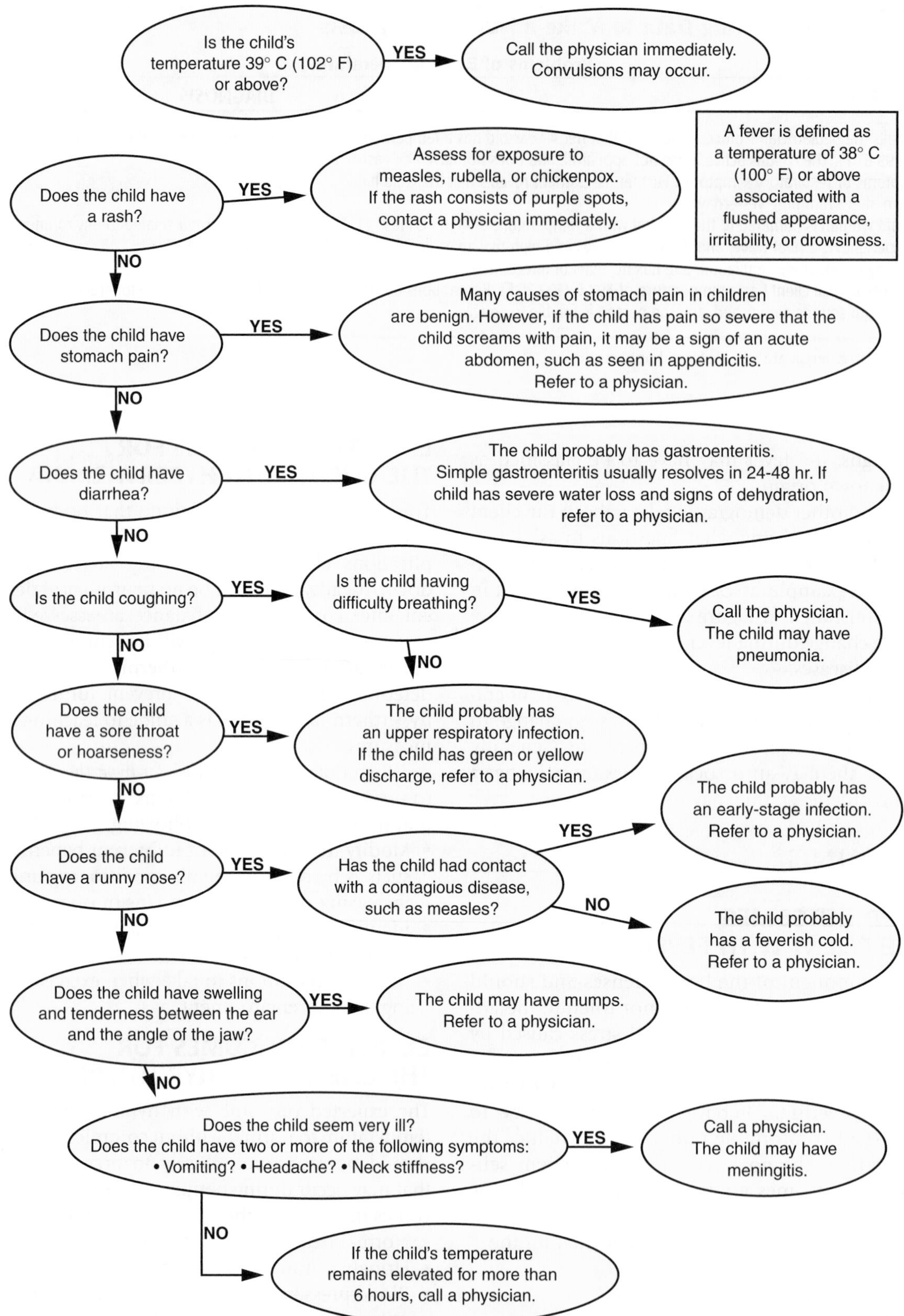

FIGURE 28-4 Decision tree for screening fever in children.

BOX 28-4 *Teaching for Wellness*

Preventing Hypothermia and Hyperthermia

Purpose: To prevent an unbalanced state of heat loss and heat gain.

Expected Outcome: The client will maintain a balanced state of thermoregulation.

Client Instructions

To Prevent Hypothermia

- In cold weather, dress warmly, keep the environment warm, and drink warm fluids.
- Wear a cap to prevent heat loss through the head; children and older people in particular need to conserve body heat in cold weather.
- In extremely cold climates, wear a muffler or a long scarf to protect your face, gloves or mittens to protect your hands and fingers, and insulated boots to protect your feet. All of these articles of clothing prevent exposure to extreme cold that can cause frostbite.
- If necessary, seek help from local community agencies that can help you pay your utility bills to keep your home warm.

To Prevent Hyperthermia

- In warm, humid weather, dress lightly, keep the environment cool with air-conditioning (if possible), circulate air with fans, and drink cool fluids.
- Avoid exercising in hot, humid weather (indoors or outdoors).
- Use a swimming pool or sprinkler on hot, humid days.
- If you need to, seek help from local community agencies that can help you pay your utility bills and that may help you obtain an air conditioner.
- Recognize that heat stroke may manifest itself with hot, dry skin; an absence of sweating; and vomiting, diarrhea, and seizures.
- Recognize that heat exhaustion may manifest itself with weakness, fatigue, headache, giddiness, loss of appetite, nausea, vomiting, diarrhea, and muscle cramps.
- If you or someone you know has been exposed to extreme heat or cold, seek medical attention promptly.

- Modify the environment to maintain heat in the home, such as by repairing the furnace, seeking public assistance for utility bills, or insulating the home
- Implement a plan for checking on the welfare of older adults in the family

INTERVENTION

INTERVENTIONS TO MONITOR TEMPERATURE

Temperature is monitored as part of routine vital signs. The scheduling of routine vital signs varies for an outpatient clinic, a general nursing unit in a hospital, a long-term care facility, or the client's home. On a general hospital unit, the routine depends on institutional policy; it may specify two, three, or four times a day. For the low-risk client, twice a day has a high probability of detecting a rise in temperature.

Frequency of monitoring must be adjusted on the basis of the client's risk for changes in body temperature.

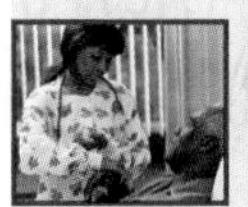

For Mr. Stephen, what schedule of vital signs would be appropriate, given his postoperative status and present vital signs?

Action Alert! The temperature of clients at risk for infection should be measured every 4 hours. If temperature is monitored every 8 hours, a febrile episode may occur between temperature measurements.

If the client has an elevated temperature, monitoring every 4 hours is usually sufficient. However, you should be aware of signs of possible fever and take the client's temperature more often if needed. Clients with severe alterations in thermoregulation, such as hyperthermia or hypothermia, should be monitored as often as every 15 minutes in severe cases.

Temperature is reported in either centigrade or Fahrenheit units; both units continue to be used clinically. Record the temperature according to agency charting format (see Chapter 7).

INTERVENTIONS TO MANAGE A FEVER

Because fever is considered a host defense response, treatment is somewhat controversial. Decisions to treat fever should be made after weighing the benefits of host defense associated with fever versus the host's ability to tolerate the cardiopulmonary demands created by the fever.

Covering the Client. The first sign of the onset of fever may be a chill. The client complains of being cold and requests additional covering. The temperature may be collected as a baseline measurement, but it is not elevated until the chill phase has passed. Chills last from 10 to 30 minutes. Cover the person with a light blanket, but avoid heavy covering. Covers will aid in the body's attempt to maintain heat and may actually increase the impending elevation of temperature.

Administering Antipyretics. The two classes of interventions used for treating fever include antipyretics and physical cooling. Antipyretics (medications that are effective against fever) include acetaminophen, aspirin, and other nonsteroidal antiinflammatory medications (NSAIDs), such as ibuprofen. These medications are effective for treating fever because they act directly on the hypothalamus to decrease the temperature set-point. Aspirin and other salicylates should not be used in children because of the increased risk of Reye's syndrome.

Because treating a fever masks the symptoms of an illness, it is important to know if the absence of fever is a sign of recovery or simply a result of the use of an antipyretic. Knowing the half-life of the medication will help. The half-life of acetaminophen, one of the more commonly used antipyretics, is 2 hours. It will influence temperature for about 4 to 6 hours.

Treatment with an antipyretic agent, such as aspirin or acetaminophen, is relatively safe. However, serious effects can occur in high-risk clients. One of the adverse effects of acetaminophen is hepatic toxicity. This usually occurs only when acetaminophen is taken in very large doses or when the client has preexisting liver disease. Common adverse effects of aspirin include bruising of the skin as a result of its anticoagulant effect and tinnitus (ringing in the ears).

Action Alert! Teach clients to avoid overdose of acetaminophen, especially if they have a history of liver disease. Instruct persons with a history of gastrointestinal bleeding or who are taking an anticoagulant medication to avoid aspirin and NSAIDs. Teach parents that aspirin is contraindicated in children and teenagers, especially with chickenpox or flu, because of the risk of developing Reye's syndrome.

Providing Physical Cooling. Remove blankets and excess clothing. Methods used for cooling include cooling blankets, cool packs, fans, and tepid baths. Physical cooling does not alter the set-point; therefore use of these interventions to decrease temperature is controversial. Physical cooling decreases body temperature by increasing the temperature difference between the skin and the environment. Subsequently, the difference between the skin and the core of the body increases heat loss.

Various physical cooling methods are available. Cooling blankets promote conductive heat loss (Loke, Chan, & Chan, 2005). Fans promote convective heat loss by moving air closest to the skin away from the client. The body warms air that is close to the skin. When the fan moves this air away, colder air moves next to the skin, increasing the difference between the skin and air temperature. Tepid baths used on febrile clients promote evaporative heat loss. Heat can be lost through evaporation of water on the skin in a manner similar to sweating.

One of the more recent innovations in cooling is the convective cooling blanket. This system blows cool air by the client to increase convective heat loss. This system is very similar to one of the mechanisms of heat loss. Remember, however, that cooling systems that blow air by a client who has a wound infection may promote movement of infectious agents into the air.

Action Alert! The decrease in skin blood flow caused by cooling measures increases vascular resistance and may increase the work of the heart. The decreased skin blood flow may also lead to skin breakdown, particularly if the cooling blanket is placed under the client.

Another consequence of using physical cooling is shivering. Because physical cooling does not affect set-point, the thermoregulatory response to cooling will be to maintain the current body temperature. This increase in metabolic rate may add stress to the client who is already physiologically compromised (Holtzclaw, 2004).

Providing Nutrition and Fluids. Anorexia (loss of appetite) is often associated with fever. In an otherwise healthy person, not eating for a short time will not change the course of the illness or result in nutritional deficits. If the person is compromised, however, maintaining nutrition is important. Assess the likelihood of the person tolerating food. Decreased bowel sounds, a distended abdomen, or nausea would suggest the person may not tolerate eating. As soon as the person is able, provide a well-balanced diet that includes proteins, minerals, and vitamins. Carbohydrates may be the food of choice because they are easily digested and provide energy.

Action Alert! Maintain fluid volume, which is essential for maintaining the balance between heat loss and heat gain. Inadequate circulating blood volume impairs an individual's ability to eliminate heat because there is less blood transferring heat to the skin.

Dehydration often contributes to the development of hyperthermia. Clients with fever often lose fluid because of the sweating that occurs when set-point decreases. They sweat to decrease body temperature to attain this lower set-point. Fluid replacement should take these losses into consideration.

Providing Comfort and Rest. Treatment of fever often affects client comfort. If fever is treated with antipyretics on a regular schedule, the client will avoid the cycle of chills and defervescence. Treatment with antipyretics on a less frequent schedule leads to defervescence when the antipyretics are administered and chills when the effects of antipyretics end. This may be more uncomfortable than not being treated for fever at all.

INTERVENTIONS TO MANAGE HYPERTHERMIA

The treatment of hyperthermia is considerably different from treatment of fever because hyperthermia is not a rise in set-point but an alteration in thermoregulation. Appropriate treatment of hyperthermia depends on the etiology, but the goal of therapy in most cases is to promote heat loss. Therefore physical cooling measures that promote heat loss are the standard treatment.

Methods of physical cooling for individuals with hyperthermia include warm air spray, cooling blankets, cool packs, cool gastric lavage, and convective cooling blankets. Warm air spray is an effective means for heat loss because water is sprayed on the client to promote heat loss by evaporation, and air is blown on the client to promote convective heat loss. Although the person is hyperthermic, the warmth of the spray prevents vasoconstriction of the skin, which would impair heat loss. Warm air spray systems can be seen on the sidelines of football games in warm, humid environments to prevent hyperthermia in football players.

Cooling blankets increase the gradient between core and shell temperature by cooling the skin temperature. However, cold applied to the skin also causes vasoconstriction of the vessels in the skin, decreasing heat loss. Methods that avoid cooling the skin, such as cool saline gastric lavage, do not directly stimulate vasoconstriction in the skin and may be more effective at decreasing body temperature.

Managing Malignant Hyperthermia. Malignant hyperthermia is an autosomal dominant genetic disorder that affects calcium levels within the skeletal muscle. Treatment of malignant hyperthermia caused by general anesthesia focuses on decreasing heat production.

Action Alert! Monitor clients during and after surgery with general anesthesia for rapid rise in temperature. Increased calcium levels in the skeletal muscle in response to general anesthetic agents such as halothane lead to skeletal muscle hyperactivity, which increases body temperature to life-threatening levels.

Treatment of malignant hyperthermia is based on decreasing heat production by skeletal muscle. The most effective medication for treating malignant hyperthermia is dantrolene, which decreases the calcium available for excitation in skeletal muscle cells. Physical cooling measures are also applied to promote heat loss and decrease body temperature.

Managing Neuroleptic Malignant Syndrome. Treatment of neuroleptic malignant syndrome is similar to that for malignant hyperthermia, although the underlying mechanisms causing neuroleptic malignant syndrome are not well understood. Treatment of neuroleptic malignant syndrome includes withholding the causative medication, administration of dantrolene, physical cooling, and hydration. Dehydration is thought to be a contributing factor because many neuroleptic medications inhibit thirst. Decreased fluid volume will impair the person's ability to lose heat because less heat can be transferred to the skin through the blood.

INTERVENTIONS TO MANAGE HYPOTHERMIA

Treatment of hypothermia varies according to the level of body temperature. Passive warming methods—such as blankets and increased ambient temperature—are used to decrease heat loss if hypothermia is mild. Active warming methods may be incorporated in more severe cases.

Peripheral methods of active warming, such as warm blankets and radiant warmers, have more of an effect on the shell of the person. Central methods of warming are more invasive and include administration of warmed intravenous fluid. If hypothermia is severe, active methods such as extracorporeal warming of blood by means of a device similar to a cardiac bypass machine may be utilized to warm the client. Other invasive methods of warming include instillation of warm fluid into the peritoneum. Box 28-5 provides evidence-based guidelines supporting the treatment of hypothermia during client resuscitation.

One of the consequences that may occur during peripheral rewarming is a decrease in body temperature termed afterdrop. As warming of the skin increases skin blood flow, the blood becomes cooler than usual because of the coldness of the peripheral tissues. Blood returning to the core will then decrease core temperature. Therefore, during attempts to warm a client peripherally, one of the consequences may be an even lower core temperature.

BOX 28-5 *Evidence-Based Practice*

Treatment of Hypothermia During Client Resuscitation

Problem: According to Mizushima, Wang, Cioffi, Bland, & Chaudry (2000), most experimental studies do not take into consideration the change in body temperature after hemorrhage and resuscitation, and it remains unclear whether hypothermia or normothermia during resuscitation after hemorrhage affects organ function.

Evidence

This study (from the Center for Surgical Research and Department of Surgery, Brown University School of Medicine and Rhode Island Hospital, Providence, Rhode Island) addresses the research question "Should normothermia be restored and maintained during resuscitation after trauma and hemorrhage?" The statistical analysis: One-way analysis of variance (ANOVA) and Tukey's test were used, and the differences were considered significant at $p < 0.05$.

Application to Practice

According to this study, restoration of normothermia during resuscitation improves cardiac contractility, cardiac output, and organ blood flow compared with hypothermia. Restoring the body temperature to normothermia during resuscitation should be performed to optimize the effects of fluid resuscitation on cardiovascular responses and tissue perfusion.

Reference

Mizushima, Y., Wang, P., Cioffi, W., Bland, K., & Chaudry, I. (2000). Should normothermia be restored and maintained during resuscitation after trauma and hemorrhage? *The Journal of Trauma: Injury, Infection and Critical Care, 48*(1), 58 [39 references].

BOX 28-6

Nursing Care Plan

A Client With a Wound Infection and Fever

Admission Data

On the twelfth postoperative day, Mr. Stephen had a follow-up visit from a home health care nurse. She took his temperature: 39° C (102.2° F). Further assessment revealed the following about Mr. Stephen: feeling hot for 2 days, with no chills for 24 hours; malaise; lack of appetite; unwilling to drink adequate fluids even though the mucous membranes are dry; lung sounds are clear, blood pressure is 138/84, pulse 130, and respirations 20. The incisions were healing except one suture line that was oozing a foul-smelling butter-yellow discharge that was enough to saturate a 2 × 4 inch gauze in about 2 hours.

The nurse suggested to the family that the physician should be notified. The family asked the nurse to call the physician and report her observations.

Following the report of client status to the physician, the client was transported to the hospital for admission.

Physician's Orders

Admitting diagnosis: wound infection
Vital signs every 4 hours
Acetaminophen 650 mg PO or rectally every 4 hours, now and prn if temperatures over 39° C (102.2° F)
Culture and sensitivity of wound
IV of 1000 mL $D_5$1/2NS at 100 mL/hr
Cefoxitin sodium (Mefoxin) 2 g every 8 hours IV
Dressing change as needed
Diet as tolerated
Up ad lib
Laxative of choice

Nursing Assessment

Color pale, diaphoretic, vital signs: BP 136/82, T 39° C (102.2° F), P 126, R 20. Reports feeling weak and tired. Incision draining thick, yellow, foul-smelling drainage, edges are red and not approximated distally for about 1 inch. Mucous membranes dry, lips cracked, skin flushed and warm to touch. Sleeping, easily aroused.

NANDA-I Nursing Diagnosis	NOC Expected Outcomes With Indicators	NIC Interventions With Selected Activities	Evaluation Data
Hyperthermia: Fever Related to Postoperative Wound Infection	***Thermoregulation***	***Fever Treatment (and Wound Care)***	
	• Body temperature WNL	• Monitor temperature q4h.	
	• Is free of complications	• Administer acetaminophen as ordered.	• Acetaminophen administered; temperature 99.2° F in 4 hours.
		• Control environmental temperature and amount of clothing and blankets.	• States environment is comfortable.
		• Assess neurological signs (level of consciousness, orientation, pupils) during fever prn.	• Oriented × 3 PERL
		• Monitor WBC, Hgb, and Hct.	• WBC 8000/mm^3, Hgb 13.5 g/100 mL, Hct 35%.
	• Hydration adequate	• Monitor for insensible water loss.	
	• Skin color changes not present		• Skin pink, warm, and dry.
	• Reports thermal comfort	• Monitor intake and output.	• For 8 hours intake (including IV fluids) 1600 mL and output 800 mL.
		• Offer fluids of choice 240 mL by mouth every hour while awake.	
		• Use cool facecloths on forehead or other cooling measures as needed.	

Critical Thinking Questions

1. What factors related to aging might be contributing to the client's impaired immune status?
2. What difference in treatment would there be if the client were a 3-year-old child?
3. What part of the ordered treatment could be carried out in the home?

Action Alert! Monitor the temperature of a client being treated for hypothermia using peripheral warming methods for an afterdrop caused by this treatment method.

Client education should focus on preventing episodes of hypothermia. Teach clients to wear sufficient clothing in cool weather and appropriate coats, hats, scarves, and gloves or mittens in cold or winter weather, especially when wind chill lowers environmental temperature further. Clients should also monitor and limit the amount of time spent out of doors in very cold weather.

EVALUATION

To evaluate the care provided for a client with an altered body temperature, ask yourself the following four questions. Was the client's comfort maintained? Was the body temperature controlled in a timely manner? Are there any residual effects? Are appropriate measures in place to prevent future occurrences?

Fever is uncomfortable and commonly produces a feeling of drowsiness. Appropriate care includes relieving discomfort and providing a quiet environment conducive to rest. Usually, fever is relatively easy to control. Evaluation data include the client's level of satisfaction with the care. Evaluation of prevention measures includes the effectiveness of client teaching to avoid infections. Box 28-6 demonstrates the nursing process for Mr. Stephen.

In hyperthermia, evaluation includes assessment for residual effects. If a hypothermia blanket was used, inspect the client's skin for damage. Assess also the client's neurological status to determine that no neurological damage has occurred.

Assess the hypothermic client for comfort during the course of treatment. In severe hypothermic states, skin damage and sloughing of tissue can occur. Inspect the skin carefully, especially the toes, fingers, and earlobes, for damage from frostbite.

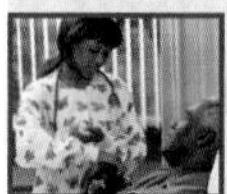

Mr. Stephen's atelectasis resolves, and his recovery from heart surgery proceeds as desired. He is discharged on the seventh postoperative day. The nurse includes the following in a discharge note to address the infection.

Sample Documentation for Mr. Stephen

Lungs clear, temperature 98.0° F. Instructed to notify physician if he has difficulty breathing, pain with respiration, temperature 101° F. Avoid contact with individuals with respiratory infections. Given a prescription for a 7-day course of antibiotics. Instructed to take all of his prescription as directed even if he is not currently experiencing symptoms. Has an appointment with the cardiologist in 1 week. Instructed to call primary care physician for follow-up appointment.

▼ KEY PRINCIPLES

- Fever is a regulated rise in temperature mediated by a rise in temperature set-point.
- Fever is a host defense response and may have a beneficial effect; therefore treatment of fever is controversial.
- The etiology of a fever can be a wide variety of processes, including infection, inflammation, autoimmune disease, vascular disease, neoplasia, and drug reaction.
- A chill may be the first sign of a fever; the temperature rises after the onset of the chill.
- Hyperthermia is a nonregulated rise in body temperature that occurs when a person is unable to lose sufficient heat or is generating more heat than can be lost.
- Hypothermia is often associated with clinical conditions or factors that predispose clients to a decrease in core body temperature, such as severe illness, trauma, immersion, and prolonged exposure to cold environmental temperatures.
- Temperature should be monitored frequently enough to detect elevations in temperature.
- Fever is treated with antipyretics to lower the set-point or with physical cooling to increase the temperature difference between the environment and the skin. Although the most common antipyretics (aspirin and acetaminophen) are relatively safe medications, serious side effects can occur in high-risk clients.
- When a client has a fever, management should include measures aimed at nutrition, fluid and electrolytes, and physical comfort.

■ REVIEW QUESTIONS

1. A client who has been experiencing intermittent fever is shivering. The nurse interprets that the client is in which of the following phases of fever?

1. Initiation
2. Plateau
3. Effervescence
4. Defervescence

2. The nurse is assigned to the care of four hospitalized clients. The nurse would assess which client as being at the least risk of developing fever caused by infection?

1. The client who had a kidney transplant
2. The client with cancer receiving chemotherapy
3. The client with chronic symptomatic human immunodeficiency virus infection
4. The client who had laparoscopic surgery to remove the gallbladder

3. The nurse is caring for a client admitted with hypothermia. Which of the following indicates that the client has not fully met the expected outcomes of care?

1. Urinary output 250 mL in 8 hours
2. Mild skin damage in the exposed area
3. Heart rate 92 beats per minute
4. Blood pressure 124/86 mm Hg

4. Which of the following interventions would the nurse expect to implement only when the client with fever develops a very high temperature?

1. Cover the client with a light blanket
2. Administer a prescribed antipyretic
3. Obtain and set up a cooling blanket
4. Provide increased fluids

Continued

5. The nurse working a 12-hour shift is assigned to the care of a client who is at risk for infection. After noting that the temperature at 8 AM is 98.8° F, the nurse should instruct the nursing assistant to recheck the temperature at what time?

1. 10 AM
2. 12 PM
3. 4 PM
4. 6 PM

Bibliography

*Arbo, M., Fine, M., Hanusa, B., Sefeik, T., & Kapoor, W. (1993). Fever of nosocomial origin: Etiology, risk factors, and outcomes. *American Journal of Medicine, 95*(5), 505-512.

Bradbury-Golas, K., & Washart, C. (2005). A 56-year-old woman with fever, generalized body aches, and anemia after a tick bite. *Journal of Emergency Nursing, 31*(2), 137-138.

*Creechan, T., Vollman, K., & Kravutske, M. E. (2001). Cooling by convection vs. cooling by conduction for treatment of fever in critically ill adults. *American Journal of Critical Care, 10*(1), 52-59.

Cuddy, M. L. (2004). The effects of drugs on thermoregulation. *AACN Clinical Issues, 15*(2), 238-253.

Fallis, W. M., Brunsdon-Clark, B., Andries, A., & Gilbert, E. A. (2005). A parent's response prompts a search for current trends in taking the temperature of pediatric ED patients. *Journal of Emergency Nursing, 31*(5), 462-464.

Gilboy, N., Tanabe, P., & Travers, D. A. (2005). The Emergency Severity Index Version 4: Changes to ESI level 1 and pediatric fever criteria. *Journal of Emergency Nursing, 31*(4), 357-362.

*Granberg, P. (1991). Human physiology under cold exposure. *Arctic Medical Research, 50*(Suppl. 6), 23-27.

Guyton, A. C., & Hall, J. E. (2006). *Textbook of medical physiology* (11th ed.). Philadelphia: Saunders.

*Henker, R. (1999). Evidence-based practice: Fever-related interventions. *American Journal of Critical Care, 8*(1), 481-489.

Hoffmann, K. J. (2001). Letter to the editor re: Creechan, T., Vollman, K., & Kravutske, M. E. (2001). Cooling by convection vs. cooling by conduction for treatment of fever in critically ill adults (in *American Journal of Critical Care, 10*[1], 52-59). *American Journal of Critical Care, 10*(4), 294-295.

Holtzclaw, B. J. (2004). Shivering in acutely ill vulnerable populations. *AACN Clinical Issues, 15*(2), 267-279.

*Johnson, M., Bulechek, G., Butcher, H., Dochterman, J. M., Maas, M., Moorhead, S., et al. (Eds.). (2006). *NANDA, NOC, and NIC linkages: Nursing diagnoses, outcomes, & interventions.* St. Louis, MO: Mosby.

Light, P. A., Hupcey, J. E., & Clark, M. B. (2005). Nursing telephone triage and its influence on parents' choice of care for febrile children. *Journal of Pediatric Nursing, 20*(6), 424-429.

Loke, A.Y., Chan, H. C., & Chan, T. M. (2005). Comparing the effectiveness of two types of cooling blankets for febrile patients. *Nursing in Critical Care, 10*(5), 247-254.

Mennick, F. (2004). Ibuprofen or acetaminophen in children? As the debate continues, the evidence may favor ibuprofen. *American Journal of Nursing, 104*(9), 20.

Miller, K. C. (2005). What's wrong with this patient? *RN, 68*(6), 53-56.

NANDA International. (2007). *Nursing diagnoses: Definitions and classification, 2006-2007* (7th ed.). Philadelphia: Author.

Neno, R. (2005). Hypothermia: Assessment, treatment and prevention. *Nursing Standard, 19*(20), 47-52, quiz 54, 56.

Panagiotis, K., Maria, P., Argiri, P., & Panagiotis, S. (2005). Is postanesthesia care unit length of stay increased in hypothermic patients? *AORN Journal, 81*(2), 379-380, 382, 385-388.

Porth, C. M. (2005). *Pathophysiology concepts of altered health states* (7th ed.). Philadelphia: Lippincott Williams & Wilkins.

Prewitt, E. M. (2005). Fever: Facts, fiction, physiology. *Critical Care Nurse*, February (Suppl.), 8-10, 12, 14 passim, quiz 18-19.

Ross, J. L. (2005). Summer injuries: Near drowning. *RN, 68*(7), 36-38, 40-41, quiz 42.

Snyder, M. L. (2005). Learn the chilling facts about hypothermia. *Nursing, 35*(2), 1-4.

Thompson, H. J. (2005). Fever: A concept analysis. *Journal of Advanced Nursing, 51*(5), 484-492.

Veronesi, J. F. (2005). Heat emergencies. *RN, 68*(6), 46-52.

Walsh, A. M., Edwards, H. E., Courtney, M. D., Wilson, J. E., & Monaghan, S. J. (2006). Paediatric fever management: Continuing education for clinical nurses. *Nursing Education Today, 26*(1), 71-77.

Ward, C. (2005). Neuroleptic malignant syndrome in a patient with Parkinson's disease: A case study. *Journal of Neuroscience Nursing, 37*(3), 160-162.

Yeo, T. P. (2004). Heat stroke: A comprehensive review. *AACN Clinical Issues: Advanced Practice in Acute and Critical Care, 15*(2), 280-293, 299-301.

Zeitzer, M. B. (2005). Inducing hypothermia to decrease neurological deficit: Literature review. *Journal of Advanced Nursing, 52*(2), 189-199.

*Asterisk indicates a classic or definitive work on this subject.

Chapter 29

MANAGING BOWEL ELIMINATION

Media Resources

- Nursing Skills Online
- evolve Evolve Website http://evolve.elsevier.com/Harkreader/
- 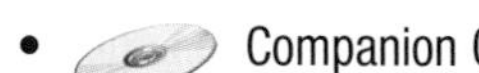 Companion CD

Learning Objectives

After studying this chapter, you should be able to do the following:

- Describe the structure and function of the lower gastrointestinal tract
- Discuss problems of bowel elimination, including constipation, diarrhea, and bowel incontinence
- Explain the effect on bowel elimination of the client's diet and exercise, personal habits, cultural background, age, and physiological and psychosocial factors
- Assess the client for manifestations of and responses to problems of bowel elimination
- Distinguish among the variety of nursing diagnoses for problems of bowel elimination
- Plan for goal-directed interventions to prevent or correct problems of bowel elimination
- Evaluate the outcomes that describe progress toward the goals of bowel elimination

Key Terms

bowel incontinence
cathartic
colostomy
constipation
diarrhea
fecal impaction
feces
flatulence
flatus
guaiac
ileostomy
laxative
occult blood
ostomy
paralytic ileus
peristalsis
steatorrhea
stoma

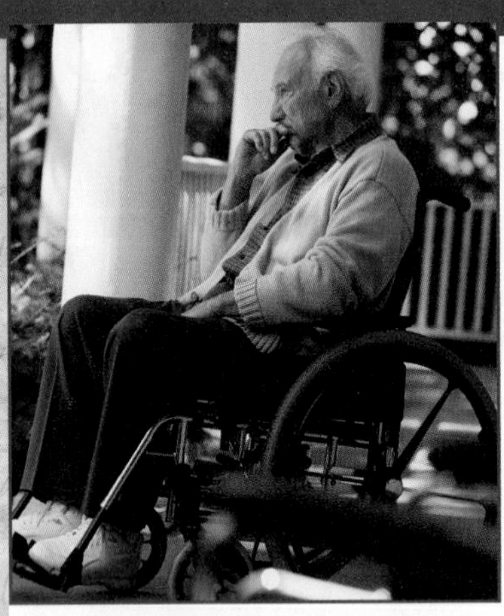

Ninety-two-year-old John Daly lives in a private room in a long-term care facility. He lived alone in his apartment in independent living as long as he could, until bone cancer and declining functional abilities required him to move. Dr. Daly is a retired neurosurgeon. He knows the consequences of immobility and decreased dietary intake and the side effects of pain medications. He called the nurse to report lower abdominal pain and difficulty having a bowel movement that morning. He reported that he had had a small bowel movement the day before, but it was not his usual pattern. Questioning the client further, the nurse ascertained that Dr. Daly's usual pattern of elimination was daily after intake of a high-fiber breakfast. When his routine was regular, the stool was usually formed and soft. The nurse considers the diagnosis of *Constipation* from the list of nursing diagnoses for bowel elimination (see the key nursing diagnoses box).

KEY NURSING DIAGNOSES FOR ELIMINATION

Constipation: A decrease in normal frequency of defecation accompanied by difficult or incomplete passage of stool and/or passage of excessively hard, dry stool
Perceived constipation: Self-diagnosis of constipation and abuse of laxatives, enemas, and suppositories to ensure a daily bowel movement
Diarrhea: Passage of loose, unformed stool
Bowel incontinence: A change in normal bowel habits characterized by involuntary passage of stool
Risk for constipation: At risk for a decrease in normal frequency of defecation accompanied by difficult or incomplete passage of stool and/or passage of excessively hard, dry stool
***Fecal impaction:** Hardened feces in the sigmoid colon and/or rectum that cannot be passed voluntarily
***Flatulence:** The presence of an excessive amount of air or gas in the stomach and intestinal tract, causing distention of the organs and in some cases mild to moderate pain

*Diagnoses with an asterisk are not NANDA International (NANDA-I) approved.

CONCEPTS OF BOWEL ELIMINATION

The nurse's role in helping a client with bowel elimination involves both independent and dependent actions. As a nurse, you may be responsible for assessing the client's bowel status, helping the client maintain a normal bowel pattern, collecting stool specimens, performing diagnostic tests, and intervening in collaboration with the physician to meet the client's bowel elimination needs. A number of bowel elimination needs can be met through independent nursing measures that do not require a physician's order.

STRUCTURE AND FUNCTION OF THE LOWER GASTROINTESTINAL TRACT

To successfully manage bowel elimination problems, you will need to understand the structure and function of the gastrointestinal (GI) tract. Naturally, any change in the GI tract can affect the elimination process.

Organs of Bowel Elimination. The GI tract, or alimentary canal, is a hollow, muscular tube that extends from the mouth to the anus (Figure 29-1). Food is broken down in the stomach into a semiliquid absorbable mass called chyme. Chyme leaves the stomach and enters the small intestine, which is divided into the duodenum, jejunum, and ileum. The 10-inch-long duodenum plays a role in digestion because it receives bile and pancreatic enzymes from the common bile duct. In the jejunum, chyme mixes with digestive enzymes and most of the nutrients are absorbed. Unabsorbed chyme enters the large intestine through the ileocecal valve in a semiliquid state. The large intestine, or colon, is the primary organ of bowel elimination. The four segments of the colon are the ascending, the transverse, the descending, and the sigmoid.

Formation of Feces. The colon absorbs water and electrolytes, leaving approximately 150 mL of water per day to be excreted with body waste materials. These processes require a number of ancillary organs and anatomical structures, chemical substances, and physiological processes. As digested, unabsorbed food travels through the colon, it changes from a liquid to a solid as the colon absorbs water from it.

Feces are the body waste discharged from the intestine. This waste is also called stool, excreta, or excrement. It moves through the large intestine propelled by peristaltic waves and segmental contractions (Figure 29-2). **Peristalsis** is the rhythmic smooth-muscle contractions of the intestinal wall that propel the intestinal contents forward. Although the force could propel intestinal contents in either direction, movement in the GI tract is toward the anus. In segmental contractions, circular muscles in a segment of the colon mix the contents of the colon.

In addition to constant peristalsis, periods of mass peristalsis occur two or three times a day, usually following meals, and are facilitated by the gastrocolic reflex. The gastrocolic reflex occurs when the bolus of food enters the stomach and stimulates peristalsis throughout the entire GI tract. The duodenocolic reflex acts in a similar but less forceful manner. The gastrocolic and duodenocolic reflexes are strongest when a person eats after a period of fasting—for example, at breakfast after a night's sleep.

Eventually, fecal material enters the sigmoid colon, where it collects until it passes into the rectum and is eliminated through the anus. The time required for food to move through the entire GI tract, called transit time, is affected by the rate of motility, amount of residue, and the presence or absence of irritating substances in the colon. However, it may take up to 4 hours for gastric emptying and 3 to 10 hours for food to move through the small intestine.

Flatus is swallowed air and gases (especially carbon dioxide, hydrogen, and methane) produced through the digestive process. The GI tract removes this flatus through the anus.

Defecation. Defecation, or "having a bowel movement," is the process of feces and flatus moving through the rectum, anal canal, and anus and is under both voluntary and involuntary control. Defecation is initiated by reflexes mediated by local enteric nerves and by the parasympathetic nerve center in the sacral segments of the spinal cord.

The rectum usually remains empty until just before and during defecation. When the fecal mass or flatus moves from the sigmoid colon into the rectum, the defecation reflex begins. Feces enter the rectum either from an involuntary mass propulsive movement in the colon or from a voluntary increase in intraabdominal pressure caused by contraction of the abdominal muscles and increased intrathoracic pressure against a closed glottis. This straining or bearing-down action against a closed glottis is called *Valsalva maneuver.* It forces the diaphragm downward, thus increasing pressure. Rectal distention then causes increased intrarectal pressure and the urge to evacuate the bowel. Voluntarily forcing feces into the rectum to stimulate the defecation reflex is less efficient than the involuntary mass propulsive movement.

The anal canal has two sphincters, as shown in Figure 29-1. The internal sphincter is made up of smooth muscle and is innervated through the autonomic nervous system. Distention of the rectum by feces causes

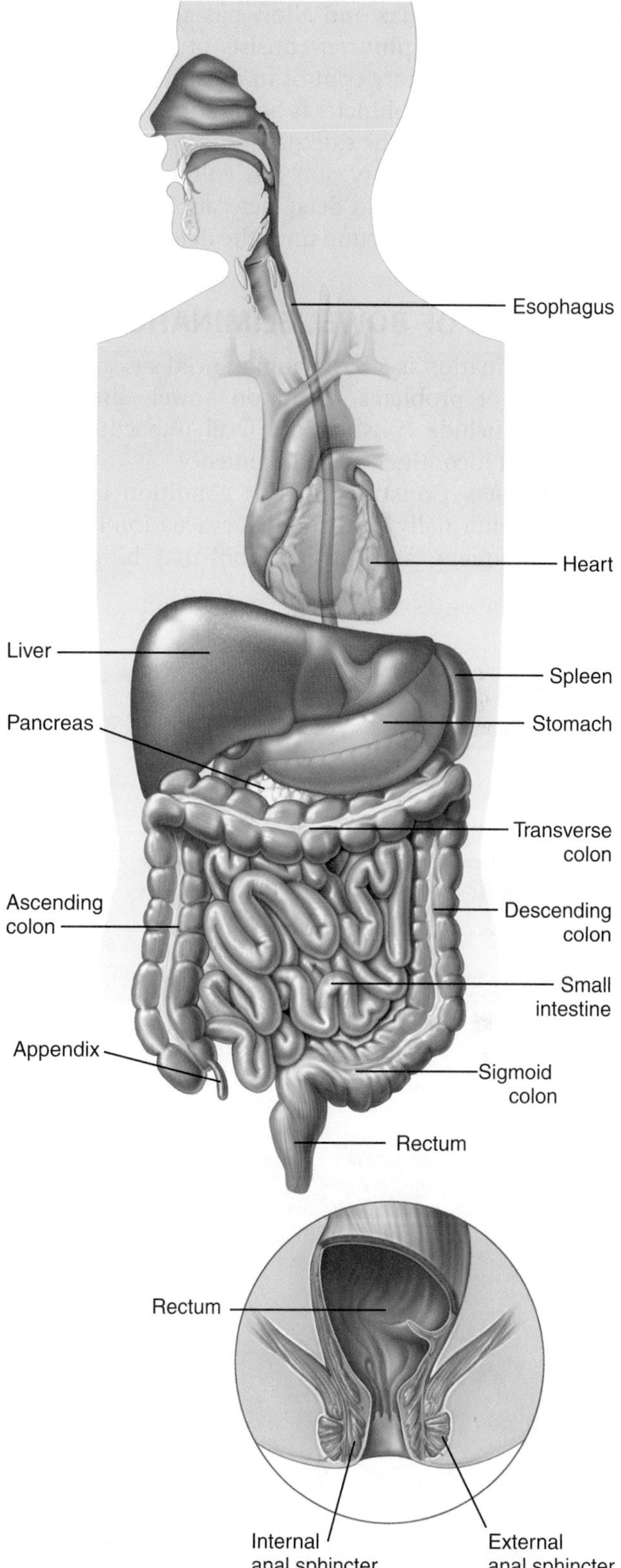

FIGURE 29-1 Organs of the gastrointestinal tract. (The heart is shown for reference.) **Inset:** Detailed anatomy of the rectum.

this sphincter to relax and allow passage of the feces. The external anal sphincter consists of striated muscle and is under voluntary control in most healthy people. When the internal sphincter is being stimulated to relax by descending feces, the external sphincter is stimulated as well. However, the person can voluntarily constrict the external sphincter to delay defecation. In that case, stool remains in the rectum until the defecation reflex is again stimulated.

PROBLEMS OF BOWEL ELIMINATION

Bowel elimination is a basic human need susceptible to a number of problems. Common bowel elimination problems include constipation, fecal impaction, diarrhea, bowel incontinence, and flatulence.

Constipation. **Constipation** is a condition in which feces are abnormally hard and dry, evacuation is abnormally infrequent, and passing stool may be difficult. Discomfort created by constipation may interfere with daily activities and a sense of well-being. Constipation includes any or all of the following: character of stool, frequency of defecation, time required for passage of the stool through the intestinal tract (intestinal transit time), and difficulty expelling rectal contents through the anal sphincter.

Considering the popularity of over-the-counter aids for elimination, constipation appears to be a common worry. In fact, some people feel constipated if they have not had a daily bowel movement. Constipation is a frequent complaint among older adults; about 30% use laxatives at least once a week.

Besides being uncomfortable, constipation can be hazardous. The hazard exists when the constipated person uses Valsalva's maneuver in an effort to pass feces. This action can cause angina pectoris (chest pain) or even cardiac arrest if the person has underlying cardiac disease. It may also be detrimental to a person with head injuries (by increasing intracranial pressure), respiratory disease (by increasing intrathoracic pressure), or thromboembolic disorders (by causing thrombi to dislodge). Exhaling through the mouth during straining reduces the chance of increasing intrathoracic pressure. The best precaution, however, is to avoid constipation.

Straining to pass a stool is detrimental in other ways. Over time, it may contribute to the development of hemorrhoids. If the person has had recent bowel surgery, straining might disrupt the suture line.

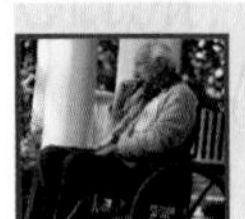

What evidence do you see in this description to suggest that *Constipation* is the correct diagnosis for Dr. Daly?

Fecal Impaction. A **fecal impaction** is a collection of puttylike or hardened feces in the rectum or sigmoid colon that prevents the passage of a normal stool and becomes harder as the colon continues to absorb water. As the fecal mass moves down from the sigmoid colon, additional fecal material may be added to it. Eventually, the mass becomes too hard and large to pass through the anal canal. It is essentially a lower intestinal obstruction; stool can accumulate the entire length of the colon.

Diarrhea. **Diarrhea** is the rapid movement of fecal matter through the intestine, resulting in diminished absorption of water, nutrients, and electrolytes and producing abnormally frequent evacuation of watery stools. As with constipation, some people consider the frequency of defecation as part of the definition, but stool consistency is the primary component.

In general, diarrhea indicates increased intestinal motility, which causes GI contents to move rapidly through the tract. In addition, irritation of the mucosal walls may stimulate increased secretions, which add moisture to the fecal mass. Therefore, when the feces reach the rectum and anus, they are still liquid.

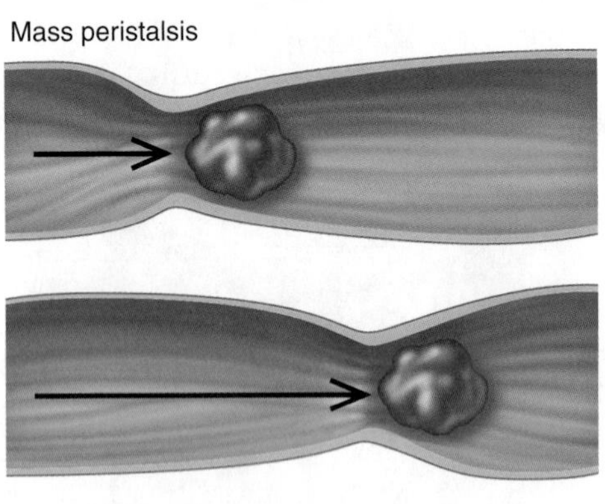

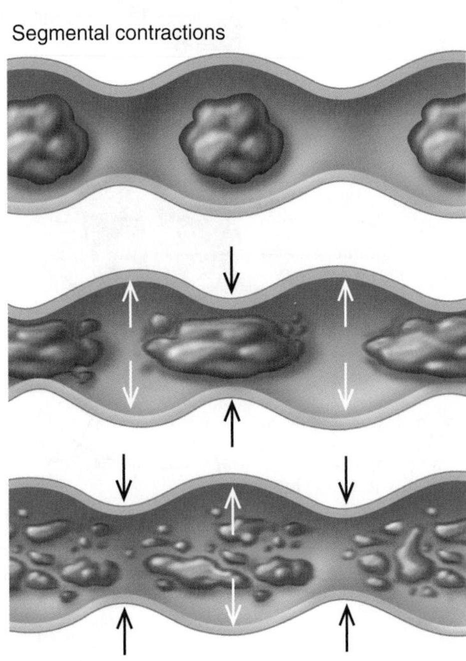

FIGURE 29-2 Movement of feces through the large intestine by mass peristalsis; segmental contractions break up chyme.

Bowel Incontinence. **Bowel incontinence** is the inability to voluntarily control the passage of feces and gas. Bowel evacuation usually occurs voluntarily in response to defecation reflex stimulation. Lack of control is accepted through the first 3 years of life. However, following toilet training, the embarrassment of incontinence causes people to arrange their lives to conceal the problem.

Flatulence. A certain amount of gas occurs normally in the GI tract—usually about 150 mL. Most of it is swallowed air, some of it is produced by fermentation in the intestine, and some of it comes from diffusion of gases from the bloodstream. **Flatulence** refers to the presence of abnormal amounts of gas in the GI tract, causing abdominal distention and discomfort. Belching is the expulsion of gas from the upper GI tract. Flatus is the gas expelled from the lower GI tract. Because it may be painful, noisy, and malodorous, flatulence can be distressing to the client.

FACTORS AFFECTING BOWEL ELIMINATION

The bowel elimination process can be affected by many factors, such as a person's lifestyle, culture, and developmental level. Physiological and psychological factors can influence the bowel elimination process as well.

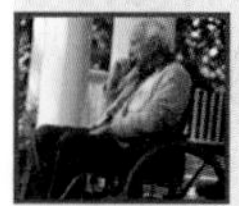

As you read about the factors affecting bowel elimination, can you relate the information to Dr. Daly? What factors may have influenced his bowel elimination problem?

LIFESTYLE FACTORS

The client's lifestyle affects bowel elimination through personal habits of elimination, fluid intake, diet, and exercise. Healthy bowel function is maintained through regular patterns of elimination.

Personal Habits. Personal habits of bowel elimination are important to health. Following a regular pattern of sleeping and eating produces a regular pattern of elimination in most people which can range from daily to every several days. On the other hand, if a person continually ignores the urge to defecate, no rhythmic pattern is established. Travel, which usually disrupts a person's normal schedule, often leads to constipation and sometimes to diarrhea.

Along with timing, many people have other established habits related to bowel elimination, such as drinking warm or cold water, eating prunes, having a cup of coffee, or reading. These activities coupled with the time of day stimulate of the defecation reflex.

Nutrition and Fluids. Diet strongly influences bowel habits. Fiber is the indigestible carbohydrate found in plant cell walls and is either soluble (carrots, oranges, apples, beans, peas) or insoluble (whole-wheat products, corn bran, flax seed, vegetables). Soluble fiber attracts water to form a gel, and insoluble fiber passes through the intestine unchanged, thus adding bulk. Both soluble and insoluble fiber aid defecation: water softens the stool, and bulk assists peristalsis by increasing stimulation of the defecation reflex. A low-fiber, high-carbohydrate diet tends to diminish the reflex. Generally, a person should consume 1 g of fiber for every 100 calories or approximately 25 g of fiber daily.

The amount of water in the fecal mass affects stool consistency. The lower the water content, the harder the mass, and the more difficult it is to pass the mass through the anus. If the person is fluid depleted, more fluid is absorbed from the GI tract to maintain adequate hydration. Thus dehydration can result in constipation.

Various foods can also adversely affect defecation patterns and act as irritants. How the GI tract reacts to a particular food depends on the individual (Box 29-1). For instance, chocolate has no effect on many people but

BOX 29-1 *Foods That Alter Gastrointestinal Function*

Foods That May Cause Gas
- Beans
- Beer
- Cabbage-family vegetables
- Carbonated beverages
- Cucumbers
- Dairy products
- Onions
- Radishes

Foods That Cause Odor
- Beans
- Cabbage family
- Cheese
- Eggs
- Fish
- Garlic
- Onions

Foods That Thicken Stool
- Applesauce
- Bananas
- Bread
- Cheese
- High-fiber foods
- Marshmallows
- Pasta
- Peanut butter
- Rice
- Tapioca

Foods That Loosen Stool
- Alcohol
- Beans
- Beer
- Chocolate
- Coffee
- Fried foods
- Prune or grape juice
- Raw fruits and vegetables
- Spicy foods
- Spinach

Foods That May Block an Ileostomy
- Celery
- Coconut
- Coleslaw
- Mushrooms
- Corn
- Nuts
- Popcorn
- Raisins
- Raw vegetables and fruits
- Seeds
- Stringy meats

causes constipation in some and diarrhea in others. Likewise, milk and milk products constipate some people and cause diarrhea in others. Fatty foods can slow peristalsis and contribute to constipation. Gas-producing foods may stimulate peristalsis by distending the intestinal walls. Irritants, such as spicy foods, within the GI tract usually stimulate peristalsis by local reflex stimulation. Reduction of overall food and fluid intake also directly reduces the amount of bulk present.

Exercise. Muscle tone affects not only the activity of the intestinal musculature itself but also the ability of the supporting skeletal muscles to aid the process of defecation. Weak or atrophied muscles in the abdomen or pelvic floor are ineffective in increasing intraabdominal pressure or assisting the anus in controlling defecation. This inadequate musculature may result from lack of exercise, immobility, neurological impairment, or multiple pregnancies.

CULTURAL FACTORS

Cultural teachings significantly influence a person's defecation habits. In Western society, we are taught strict rules about when and under what conditions defecation can take place. Failure to follow these rules results in social censure and even isolation. Defecation is a private matter, and people go to great lengths to ensure this privacy. Many people avoid any discussion of bowel activity. Therefore some people feel highly anxious or embarrassed when forced to seek out a health professional about problems with bowel elimination. Although people in some cultures tend to be very bowel conscious, not all people are embarrassed or reluctant to discuss bowel habits. Assess the client's lifeways for information pertinent to bowel elimination (Box 29-2).

DEVELOPMENTAL FACTORS

Age plays a role in establishing bowel patterns. Before a child acquires bowel control through toilet training, defecation occurs whenever stool stimulates the rectum. In infancy, the stomach is small and secretes a smaller amount of digestive enzymes. Rapid peristalsis propels food quickly through the GI system, and, because the neuromuscular system is not developed, the infant cannot control defecation.

Bowel elimination usually is not a problem in the adolescent unless the person has a health problem. However, adolescents can experience changes in bowel habits associated with growth, menses, and irregular patterns of eating and sleeping. During adolescence, the large intestine grows rapidly. At the same time, adolescents tend to eat more. Adolescent eating habits vary from very good to poor, with the person's self-concept influencing the intake.

Among older adults, vulnerability to GI disturbances rises. Cancer occurs more frequently, and motor and neurological disturbances are more prevalent. Box 29-3 addresses screening for colon cancer. In addition, diverticulosis (an outpouching in the intestinal wall) occurs almost exclusively after age 40.

The amount of water and fiber in the diet may be inadequate. Cavities, broken or missing teeth, or other problems with dentition impair mastication, allowing inadequately chewed food to enter the GI tract. Furthermore, the amount of digestive enzymes in saliva and gastric acids in the stomach declines, reducing the ability to break down foods. Muscle atrophy and hemorrhoids can decrease control of the internal and external sphincters. In addition, slowing of nerve impulses to the rec-

BOX 29-2 *Cross-Cultural Care*

Caring for a Rural Client of English Descent

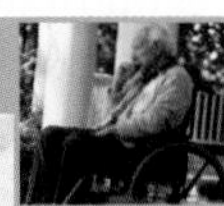

As many rural Americans did, Dr. Daly lived on a farm when he was a boy. He recounts memories of tending a garden, keeping beehives, and raising chickens, cows, pigs, ducks, and other livestock. All of the family's meals were cooked at home, and Dr. Daly's mother commonly used home remedies and medications made from plants to treat illness and injuries. Laxatives were not a choice for constipation problems, but instead a high-fiber diet was provided.

Dr. Daly's family believed in living from the land and using all of its products as fully as possible. In addition, Dr. Daly may have been exposed to the following traditionally Anglo-Saxon beliefs (Leininger, 1991):

- Strength in individualism and self-reliance.
- Competition and achievement.
- Health is achievable through science.
- Helping others is more likely in times of crisis.
- Better life through technology.

He also may have embraced the following values commonly held by farming families (Fish, 1995):

- The best things are those that we work for.
- God gave man dominion over the earth and the responsibility to care for the earth.
- "She did not send me to Sunday School but instead went with me."
- A person has a right to own property, a responsibility to work, and an obligation to take care of his property for his own sake and the sake of his children and the community.
- A person should do his best to take care of himself and not be a burden to others.
- It is possible to love wealth too much, but a greater danger is to be careless of it.

tum may cause some people to be less conscious of the need to defecate.

PHYSIOLOGICAL FACTORS

Bowel elimination problems can be caused by such physiological factors as pregnancy, motor and sensory disturbances, intestinal pathological processes, medications, surgical procedures, and diagnostic procedures.

Pregnancy. Pregnancy itself and medications taken during pregnancy can influence a woman's normal bowel elimination pattern. As the fetus grows, pressure may be exerted on the rectum, slowing the passage of feces through the intestine. Exertion for defecation can cause other elimination problems, such as hemorrhoids. Iron and vitamin supplements prescribed for many women during pregnancy are constipating, which can cause additional problems.

Motor and Sensory Disturbances. Motor or sensory disturbances may result from spinal cord injury, head injury, cerebrovascular accident (stroke), neurological disease, or any condition that causes immobility or otherwise interferes with motor or sensory function. Immobility hinders the person's ability to respond to the urge to defecate. For instance, the person who is unable to walk to the bathroom or reach a call bell to summon help may (1) suppress the urge to defecate, which could eventually lead to constipation, or (2) suffer fecal incontinence.

Intestinal Pathological Processes. Pathological conditions in the intestine itself can be heralded by constipation or diarrhea. These conditions can result from obstruction, inflammation, infection, or cancer.

- *Bowel obstruction:* Partial or complete blockage caused by a tumor, inflammation, strangulation, or adhesion that prevents the movement of chyme through the intestine. Bowel obstruction may initially present with constipation or diarrhea associated with abdominal distention, pain, and hyperactive bowel sounds in one quadrant.
- *Crohn's disease:* A chronic inflammatory bowel disease of unknown origin, usually affecting the ileum, the colon, or another part of the gastrointestinal tract. It is characterized by frequent attacks of diarrhea, severe abdominal pain, nausea, fever, chills, weakness, anorexia, and weight loss.
- *Ulcerative colitis:* A chronic, episodic, inflammatory disease of the large intestine and rectum. It is characterized by profuse watery diarrhea containing varying amounts of blood, mucus, and pus.
- *Irritable bowel syndrome*: A chronic functional disorder of the bowel characterized by motor abnormalities within the gastrointestinal tract, causing variable symptoms including cramping, abdominal pain, constipation, or diarrhea. It does not result in permanent damage to the intestine. Affecting 15% of the population, it can often be managed with alternative therapies (Box 29-4).
- *Cancer:* Signs and symptoms that may indicate referral are a change in bowel habits and blood in the stool. Encourage clients to obtain routine screening tests for colon and rectal cancer.
- *Infectious diarrhea:* Sudden onset of watery diarrhea that can signal acute viral, bacterial, and protozoal infections. Most bacterial or viral diarrhea will resolve in 1 to 7 days. However, severe fluid and electrolyte disturbances can be life threatening, especially to the very young and very old.

Medications. Common side effects of medications are constipation or diarrhea. Medications administered for bowel regulation, antibiotics, narcotics, sympathomimetics, antidepressants, and anticholinergics are examples. The parasympathetic nervous system (cholinergic) stimulates the GI tract; the sympathetic system slows it. A drug given to prevent constipation may cause diarrhea, and a drug given to prevent diarrhea may cause constipation. The overuse of laxatives can lead to physiological and psychological dependence on them. In addition, some medications may affect the color and odor of the feces.

Surgical Procedures. Surgical procedures commonly result in constipation for several reasons. For one, direct handling of the bowel during abdominal surgery can temporarily stop peristalsis; when the absence of peristalsis persists beyond 3 days, the condition is called **paralytic ileus.** For another, any procedure involving the pelvis or perineum, such as rectal, hip, or gynecological surgery, can affect defecation patterns through the effects

BOX 29-3 *Teaching for Wellness*

Screening for Colon Cancer

Purpose: To provide the client information about screening for colon cancer.

Expected Outcome: The client will verbalize correct information about appropriate recommendations for screening for colon cancer, based on age and symptoms.

Client Instructions

Keep in mind the following risk factors, which can place you at higher risk for colon cancer:

- Age over 50
- A family history of polyps or colorectal cancer
- A history of inflammatory bowel disease, such as ulcerative colitis or Crohn's disease
- Living in an urban area
- A diet high in fat and low in fiber

Notify your health care provider if you notice any of the following warning signs of colon cancer:

- Change in bowel habits
- Rectal bleeding

Ask your health care provider about the following recommended screening tests:

- Digital rectal examination every year after age 40
- Guaiac test for occult blood every year after age 50
- Proctoscopy every 3 to 5 years after age 50, after two annual examinations show no evidence of colon cancer

BOX 29-4

Considering the Alternatives

Alterative Therapies for Irritable Bowel Syndrome

Hypnotherapy

Advantages

- Improvement of physical symptoms is statistically verified (Smith, 2006).
- Improvements may last up to 5 years (Gonsalkorale, Miller, Afzal, & Whorwell, 2003).
- Side benefits include improvements in quality-of-life domains, anxiety, and depression.

Disadvantages

- Requires training to administer.
- Requires willing participation by clients.
- As a nontraditional approach, may not be covered by insurance.

Peppermint Oil

Advantages

- Statistically significant improvement compared with anticholinergics (Grigoleit & Grigoleit, 2005).
- Perceived as more natural than other medication.
- Easy administration and dosage because enteric-coated formulations can target the colon through timed release.

Disadvantages

- Gastrointestinal side effects include heartburn and anal/perianal burning.
- Requires continued administration.
- May not be acceptable for clients who do not want to take "pills."

Probiotics

Probiotics are mixtures containing live bacteria, usually those species normally found in the gut.

Advantages

- Effective in alleviating symptoms (Kajander, Hatakka, Poussa, Farkkila, & Korpela, 2005).
- Fewer side effects than medication.
- May suppress the low-grade inflammation that accompanies irritable bowel syndrome.

Disadvantages

- Which species and subspecies are most effective is still being established.
- Not appropriate intervention in immune-suppressed individuals.
- May decrease the action of warfarin (Skidmore-Roth, 2006).

Gonsalkorale, W. M., Miller, V., Afzal, A., & Whorwell, P. J. (2003). Long term benefits of hypnotherapy for irritable bowel syndrome, *Gut, 52*(11), 1623-1629.

Grigoleit, H. G., & Grigoleit, P. (2005). Peppermint oil in irritable bowel syndrome. *Phytomedicine, 12*(8), 601-606.

Kajander, K., Hatakka, K., Poussa, T., Farkkila, M., & Korpela, R. (2005). A probiotic mixture alleviates symptoms in irritable bowel syndrome patients: A controlled 6-month intervention. aliment. *Pharmacology and Therapeutics, 22*(5), 387-394.

Skidmore-Roth, L. (2006). *Mosby's handbook of herbs & natural supplements* (3rd ed.). St. Louis, MO: Mosby.

Smith, G. D. (2006). Effect of nurse-led gut-directed hypnotherapy upon health-related quality of life in patients with irritable bowel syndrome. *Journal of Clinical Nursing, 15*(6), 678-684.

of postoperative edema and discomfort. Operative and postoperative medications can contribute to constipation as well.

In addition, bowel function can be altered permanently by surgical intervention. Fecal diversion involves channeling intestinal contents out of the body at a site other than the anus. The surgical procedure used to create an opening through the abdominal wall and into the intestine is called an **ostomy** procedure. An **ileostomy** is a surgical procedure involving the creation of an opening between the ileum and the abdominal wall. Because water is not reabsorbed until feces reach the colon, the feces from an ileostomy are liquid. A **colostomy** is a surgical procedure involving the creation of an opening between the colon and the abdominal wall. Feces from this area of the colon are semisolid or solid, depending on the segment of the colon that is resected. Each of these surgical procedures establishes a **stoma,** which is an opening between the abdominal wall and the intestine through which fecal material passes.

An ileostomy may be performed because of cancer, a congenital defect, or trauma. However, the most frequent reason stems from ulcerative colitis or regional ileitis (Crohn's disease). Because of the placement of the stoma in the small intestine, the flow of fecal material in most cases is constant and cannot be regulated. Surgical techniques do exist in which a continent ileostomy is formed by creating an internal pouch with a nipple valve that can be emptied with a catheter at the person's convenience.

A colostomy may be performed because of trauma, intestinal obstruction, birth defect, or cancer. It may involve the ascending (rarely), transverse, descending, or sigmoid portion of the colon. The farther down the intestine the stoma is placed, the better are the chances of regulating the bowel. Some people develop such reliable bowel control that they wear no fecal collection bag and only a small dressing to protect the stoma from irritation by clothing. However, most people with ostomies wear a collection pouch or bag that is changed periodically (Figure 29-3).

PSYCHOSOCIAL FACTORS

Clinical evidence suggests a relationship between bowel elimination patterns and stress, although the relationship is not completely clear. Agitation and nervousness can cause diarrhea, usually in the form of frequent small stools without a large-volume fluid loss. Some

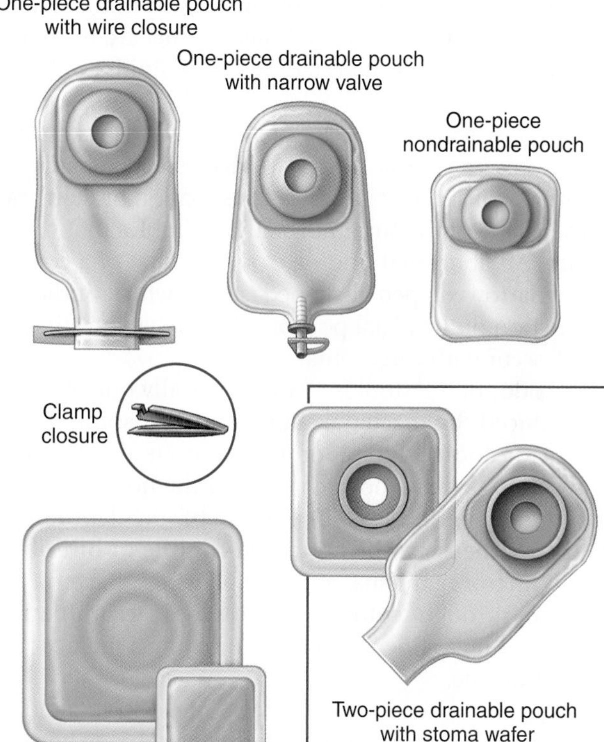

FIGURE 29-3 Examples of ostomy pouches, closures, and stoma wafers.

disease processes that cause diarrhea, gaseous distention, and ulcer formation may have psychological elements either as cause or effect. On the other hand, mental depression can contribute to constipation by slowing all bodily activities.

ASSESSMENT

The need for assessment of bowel elimination problems commonly arises after a client reports a problem. However, it should also be a routine part of any health assessment because bowel elimination is frequently disrupted by illness, surgery, or other treatment.

GENERAL ASSESSMENT OF BOWEL ELIMINATION

The general assessment of bowel elimination should include the usual pattern of elimination, history pertinent to bowel elimination, abdomen assessment, observation of feces, and review of diagnostic tests.

Health History. The health history should include questions regarding the client's normal elimination pattern, health habits, and any psychological or physiological alterations pertinent to bowel elimination. The following are pertinent historical questions:

- What is your normal bowel elimination pattern, including time of day, frequency, and associated stimuli?
- How often do you use laxatives or bowel elimination aids?
- What is your normal dietary intake for a day? Has it changed recently?
- What is your normal fluid intake for a day? Has it changed recently?
- What kind of exercise or physical activity do you get? Has it changed recently?
- Are you unusually anxious or do you have excess stress in you life?
- What medications do you take?
- What do your feces look like, including amount, color, consistency, constituents, frequency, odor, and shape?
- Have you noticed any changes in your bowel elimination pattern?
- Has your use of bowel elimination aids changed recently?
- Have you had any gastrointestinal surgery?
- Do you have a history of stomach or bowel problems?
- How is your current emotional state? Is it different from your normal?
- Have you experienced recent weight gain or loss?

Analyze symptoms (abdominal pain, nausea, vomiting, constipation, diarrhea, incontinence) for onset, duration, frequency, severity, associated symptoms. Elicit a history of other, possibly related, health problems: thyroid disease, diabetes, lactose intolerance, gastroesophageal reflux disease, peptic ulcer, gallbladder disease, pancreatitis, diverticulitis, or ulcerative colitis.

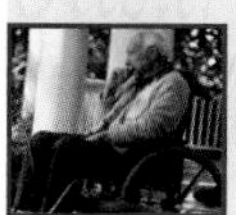
What questions would you ask Dr. Daly to determine the best course of action to assist with his bowel elimination problem?

Physical Examination. Physical assessment of the bowel system should include inspection, auscultation, percussion, and palpation of the abdomen. It may also include inspection and palpation of the anus. With the client in the supine position, inspect the abdomen for peristalsis, contour, symmetry, scars, distention, and masses. Look for signs of hernia, dehydration, striae, or engorged veins. Auscultate the client's bowel sounds, noting their frequency and character. Use percussion to elicit tympani, which indicate the presence of gas, or dullness (indicating fluid and feces) in the GI tract. Use palpation to assess for areas of tenderness, guarding, rebound tenderness, or palpable masses in the abdomen. Turn the client to the side, and inspect and palpate the anus to assess for lumps, ulcers, inflammation, rashes, or excoriations.

Diagnostic Tests. Review the results of diagnostic tests. Prepare the client for and assist with additional diagnostic tests that have been ordered to help identify problems with bowel elimination. Common tests include observation of fecal characteristics and laboratory analysis of feces, radiographic examination of the bowel, and direct endoscopic visualization of the bowel.

Stool Analysis

Specimen collection. Stool specimens are collected in a clean, dry container. If the client uses a toilet, place a receptacle under the seat. If the specimen is collected at home, the client can drape a piece of plastic wrap over the toilet seat so it droops in the middle to catch the feces. After depositing the specimen, the client then finishes the collection process by bringing the corners and edges of the wrap together and twisting them to form a sealed package.

To perform a test on the specimen, use a tongue blade to transfer a portion of it to a smaller, covered specimen container for transport to a lab. Visible blood or mucus should be included in the sample. Avoid mixing urine, soap, or detergent with the specimen.

If the client cannot produce any feces, gently pass a rectal swab beyond the internal sphincter and rotate it carefully to collect fecal material. Then place the specimen in a suitable container for transport to the laboratory.

When collecting stool specimens, make sure you maintain the conditions needed for accurate test results. For example, collect specimens for culture in a clean, dry container, and send them to the laboratory immediately. A specimen to be tested for ova and parasites should be examined immediately because the organisms die if they cool below body temperature. On the other hand, you can refrigerate specimens not needing microscopic examination if you are unable to deliver them to the laboratory right away.

> ***Action Alert!*** Take care in collecting specimens. Urine, soap, detergent, and drying of the specimen destroy bacteria.

To check for pinworms, you will need to collect a specimen from the perianal area. To do so, press the sticky side of a strip of nonfrosted cellophane tape over and around the client's anus. Remove it immediately, place it on a glass slide (sticky side down), and send it to the laboratory for examination. Because the female worm deposits eggs on the perianal area during the night, you will want to collect the specimen early in the morning, before the person has bathed or had a bowel movement.

Characteristics of feces. Fecal material is composed of food residues, bacteria, some white blood cells, epithelial cells, intestinal secretions, and water. Assessing frequency, amount, color, consistency, shape, and odor can help to identify GI problems (Table 29-1).

Bile pigments produce the normal brown color of stool. Absence of bile causes the stool to be white, gray, or clay colored and may indicate biliary obstruction or lack of bile production (acholia). Light-colored stools also can result from barium or antacid ingestion. A gray stool mixed with observable fat and mucus is called **steatorrhea** and results from the malabsorption of fat. In infants, the first stools (called meconium) are normally black and tarry from ingested amniotic fluid, epithelial cells, and bile.

The consistency of stool is a reflection of its water content. Stools can be liquid, unformed, soft, or hard. An abnormal consistency indicates constipation or diarrhea.

The shape of the stool normally resembles that of the rectum. An abnormal finding would be that of a consistently narrowed, pencil-shaped stool, which indicates obstruction of the distal portion of the large intestine, as might occur with carcinoma.

The odor of the stool is characteristically pungent and is produced by bacterial flora and by some foods and medications. Blood or infection in the GI tract causes detectable noxious changes in the normal odor.

Laboratory Analysis of Feces. In the laboratory, stool specimens can be examined for bile or bilirubin, blood, microorganisms, ova, and parasites. Bacteria are detected through cultures. Microscopic examination may reveal meat fibers and fat, indicating a malabsorption syndrome.

A test used to detect **occult blood** in feces (an amount too small to be seen without a microscope) may be your responsibility. You will perform the test in the clinical setting, or teach the client to collect the specimen in the home setting. The instructions in Procedure 29-1 are for the Hemoccult test, which uses **guaiac** as a reagent. Other brands may have slightly different instructions.

Besides supplying information about a current bowel disorder, this test also can be used as a screening procedure for colorectal cancer. The American Cancer Society recommends that people over age 50 have annual tests for occult blood in the stool.

Radiographic Examination of Bowel. Radiographic examination reveals the location and contour of the bowel and supporting structures, as well as the presence and distribution of fecal material and gas in the bowel. A flat plate of the abdomen is taken without contrast material and therefore requires no special preparation. It shows shadows, fluid levels, and gas.

More specific information can be obtained from a barium radiographic study, usually called a "lower GI series." Barium is instilled as an enema to provide a contrast medium to outline the bowel. For maximum visualization, the bowel should be thoroughly cleansed before a barium enema. After the study, a laxative is administered to ensure its complete evacuation. Barium left in the colon can cause impaction (a stool mass too large and hard to pass through the anus) and even obstruction. Although a barium enema is relatively safe, it can produce an anaphylactic reaction in about 1 in 750,000 examinations.

> ***Action Alert!*** Be prepared to manage an anaphylactic reaction in a client who has a barium enema.

Table 29-1 Characteristics of Feces

CHARACTERISTIC	NORMAL	ABNORMAL	POSSIBLE CAUSE
Amount	150 g (varies with diet)		
Color	Adult: brown Infant: yellow	Black or tarry	• Iron ingestion • Bismuth ingestion • Charcoal ingestion
		Black and tarry (melena)	• Upper GI bleeding
		Pale	• Malabsorption of fat • Diet high in milk and low in meat
		Red	• Lower GI bleeding • Ingestion of beets • Ingestion of pyrvinium pamoate, an antiparasitic agent • Hemorrhoids, if the red is smeared on the surface of feces
		Red orange	• Ingestion of rifampin, an antibiotic
		Green or orange	• Large amounts of ingested chlorophyll • Intestinal infection
		White or clay colored	• Absence of bile
Consistency	Formed, soft	Liquid	• Diarrhea • Increased intestinal motility
		Hard	• Constipation
Constituents	Cells lining intestinal mucosa, dead bacteria, bile pigment, fat, protein, undigested food, water	Blood	• GI bleeding
		Fat	• Malabsorption
		Foreign objects	• Accidental ingestion
		Mucus	• Inflammatory condition
		Pus	• Bacterial infection
Odor	Pungent (affected by client's own bacterial flora)	Noxious change	• Blood in feces • Infection
Shape	Appearance of diameter of rectum, about 2.5 cm (1 inch) for adults	Narrow, pencil shaped, or stringlike	• Obstructive condition

PROCEDURE 29-1

Time to Allow: Novice: 5 min. **Expert:** 5 min.

TESTING FECES FOR OCCULT BLOOD

Nursing Skills Online: Specimen Collection, Lesson 4

The Hemoccult test is one of many commercial products used as a screening test for blood in the feces that is not visible to the naked eye. The test is used to detect gastrointestinal bleeding and to screen for colorectal cancer. Testing three separate specimens reduces the incidence of false-negative results. Restricting red meat for 2 to 3 days before the test reduces false-positive results.

Hospital policy may require that the specimen be sent to the laboratory for testing.

DELEGATION GUIDELINES

The test for occult blood is a simple test that may be delegated to a nursing assistant. Review of the instructions for collecting the specimen and test performance can ensure uniform test results.

EQUIPMENT NEEDED

- Hemoccult test slide folder
- Clean gloves
- Wooden applicator
- Hemoccult developing solution

1 Follow preliminary actions (see inside front cover).

2 Instruct the client about the purpose of the test, and have the client defecate into a collection container. Tell the client to avoid urinating in the container. *Urine may contaminate the stool sample. If the client has to urinate, he or she can do so before collecting the stool sample.*

3 Put on clean gloves. *Clean gloves help to prevent transmission of microorganisms from the client's feces.*

Continued

4 With the applicator, obtain a small specimen of feces and smear a thin layer in the first box of the cardboard Hemoccult slide. While obtaining the specimen, observe and document its characteristics. *A small specimen is sufficient to perform the test accurately.*

5 With the opposite tip of the applicator, obtain a second specimen of feces from another location and smear it thinly in the second box of the cardboard Hemoccult slide. *Using the opposite end of the applicator prevents contamination of the second sample with the first.*

6 Close the cardboard Hemoccult slide cover, and turn it over to the reverse side. Open the cardboard flap on the reverse side, and apply *two* drops of Hemoccult developing solution to the guaiac paper. Apply the exact amount of solution specified (two drops) to ensure the accuracy of the test.

7 As soon as you apply the developing solution, start keeping track of the time. If you notice a bluish discoloration on the guaiac paper 30 to 60 seconds after applying the solution, the sample contained occult blood. Consider the result positive if both samples show a positive result (see illustration).

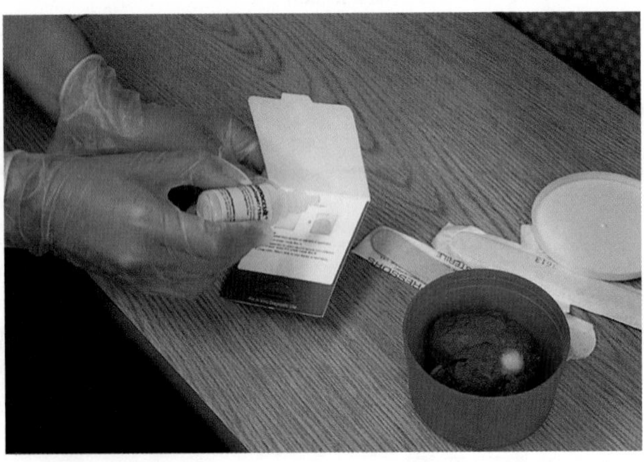

Step 7. Applying Hemoccult developing solution to the guaiac paper.

8 Dispose of the Hemoccult slide in a biohazard waste container, discard your gloves, and wash your hands. *Standard precautions dictate that human excrement be treated as hazardous waste.*

9 Document the characteristics of the client's feces and the results of the guaiac test in the client's chart. *Charting both objective findings and test results gives a complete picture of the specimen.*

HOME HEALTH CARE CONSIDERATIONS

Clients are often taught to collect a specimen for screening for occult blood in the home. Supply the person with the Hemoccult slide, a tongue blade, mailing pouch for returning slides, and the Hemoccult product instructions. Some laboratories may supply the developer or reagent for testing at home.

You may give the client the following instructions:

- Read and carefully follow the instructions included in the package.
- Wait 3 days after the end of a menstrual period; do not collect when you have blood in your urine or from hemorrhoids.
- Collect from a toilet bowl only if it is clean and free of chemicals; flush three times before collecting.
- Collect samples and test (if instructed) from three different bowel movements.
- Protect Hemoccult slides from heat, light, and chemicals.
- Seven days before the test, stop taking aspirin or nonsteroidal antiinflammatory drugs. Acetaminophen is allowed.
- Three days before the test, stop eating vitamin C, red meat, and raw broccoli, cauliflower, horseradish, parsnips, radishes, turnips, and melons.

Direct Visualization of Bowel. A fiberoptic endoscope inserted through the anus and advanced through the bowel allows direct visualization of the lower GI tract. The physician may perform a proctoscopy, sigmoidoscopy, or colonoscopy, depending on the area of the colon to be examined.

The endoscopes used to observe the bowel are hollow tubes through which the examiner can see GI structures. They also allow suction and collection of tissue for biopsy.

Before an endoscopic procedure, explain the test to the client to allay any anxiety. Also, make sure that bowel preparation is complete. If the person's bowel has not been thoroughly cleansed, feces can obscure the fiberoptic examination. Typically, preparation begins 24 to 48 hours before the procedure and includes dietary and fluid restrictions, laxatives, enemas, or a combination of laxatives and saline enema.

A common method of emptying the bowel uses a solution called GoLYTELY (pronounced "go-lightly"). GoLYTELY cleanses the bowel without causing the excretion or absorption of fluid and electrolytes by the body that often occurs with traditional purgatives and enemas. This method is safer for people with congestive heart disease, chronic obstructive pulmonary disease, or controlled renal failure. The solution is consumed cold at a rate of 1.2 to 1.8 L/hr. The client soon develops diarrhea and, within 2 to 4 hours, the rectal output is clear. Because the solution works so quickly, make sure the client has ready access to toilet facilities. However, not all clients can consume the large volume of liquid, and other bowel preparations may be used.

Throughout the endoscopic procedure, provide emotional support. Before the procedure, administer a relaxant medication, as prescribed. Then help the client into the position chosen by the physician, often a side-lying position with one knee pulled up to the chest. Assess the client throughout the procedure because of the awkward position and the effects of the medication. Monitor the vital signs regularly during the procedure. Assist the physician with equipment and specimens, as necessary.

After the procedure, continue to monitor the client's vital signs. Inspect often for fresh anal bleeding, which may indicate continued oozing at a biopsy site. Severe abdominal pain could indicate a bowel perforation.

Action Alert! Monitor for circulatory and respiratory problems during endoscopy examination.

FOCUSED ASSESSMENT FOR *CONSTIPATION*

Assessment for *Constipation* is initiated from a client complaint or your observation that the client has been 3 days without a bowel movement. Assess for signs and symptoms and the probable cause.

Defining Characteristics. The client usually recognizes or suspects constipation when the frequency of bowel movements is less than usual and the abdomen feels full and distended. In addition, the client may report a feeling of fullness or pressure in the rectum, straining to evacuate the stool, abdominal pain, appetite impairment, back pain, headache, interference with daily living, and the use of laxatives. Sometimes the fecal mass can be palpated in the abdomen (NANDA-I, 2007). Hard, dry stool or difficulty passing stool confirms the diagnosis of *Constipation.*

Clients sometimes complain of constipation when digestive signs are absent. The diagnosis of *Perceived constipation* should be made only after ruling out actual constipation. The diagnosis is made when the client expects a daily bowel movement and uses laxatives, enemas, and suppositories to make it happen. The expectation may include passage of stool at the same time every day. Perceived constipation is common among older adults who have health practices ingrained from another era.

Related Factors. To select appropriate nursing actions, you need to identify the cause or causes and determine if the problem is expected to be acute or chronic. An acute problem would need immediate, definitive intervention, whereas a chronic problem would demand long-term lifestyle management. Common causative lifestyle factors include a lack of established bowel pattern; inadequate diet, fluids, and exercise; emotional depression; and weak pelvic floor muscles.

Other, less obvious lifestyle factors may contribute to constipation. Inconvenience is frequently a factor. When the urge to defecate is repeatedly ignored, stool remaining in the rectum continues to lose water and stops stimulating normal reflexes. Overuse of laxatives, suppositories, and enemas contribute to the problem primarily through the resulting loss of intrinsic innervation and atrophy of the smooth muscle necessary for defecation. Constipation frequently accompanies pregnancy, both because of hormonal changes and because of external pressure on the intestine.

Constipation is often associated with an acute illness because of the change in routine, diet, fluid intake, and mobility. Immobility alone is sufficient cause. Constipation may be a symptom of intestinal pathological conditions, including neoplasm, stricture, hernia, megacolon (excessive dilation or stretching of the colon), diverticular disease, and painful anal lesions, in which case the underlying pathological process must be considered in developing a plan of intervention.

Constipation may be associated with chronic health problems. Besides the lifestyle changes required to manage a chronic health problem, medications for pain, hypertension, depression, and gastric hyperacidity contribute to constipation. Additional examples include anesthetics, anticholinergics, and iron supplements.

FOCUSED ASSESSMENT FOR *DIARRHEA*

Defining Characteristics. To assess the client with *Diarrhea,* analyze the symptom with particular attention to fluid and electrolyte loss. Question the client carefully about the frequency and characteristics of the stool. In diarrhea the stool is described as loose, liquid, or unformed. It may contain blood or mucus. Ask the client to describe the nature of the diarrhea. Diarrhea may involve frequent, small stools, or it may represent the loss of a large volume of water. In the latter case, the person may become dehydrated and deficient in important electrolytes. Estimate the amount of water loss on the basis of the number and volume of stools. Is the person able to replace the fluid loss? Look for signs of dehydration—sluggish skin turgor, sunken eyes, low urine output. In the pediatric client, you may notice an absence of tears.

Ask about associated systemic symptoms such as fever, myalgia, malaise, anorexia, and headache. Also ask about associated abdominal symptoms, such as urgency, flatus, pain, abdominal cramping, nausea, and vomiting. Diarrhea is usually alkaline, because it contains digestive enzymes. Assess for skin breakdown or irritation in the perianal area.

Related Factors. Also ask questions that will help determine the cause of the diarrhea. Ask about the duration of the problem; recent exposure to infected people; recent travel; dietary; and medication intake; and the existence of anxiety, stress, or systemic disease that might contribute to a change in elimination patterns.

The causes of diarrhea are numerous and different for acute and chronic diarrhea. Acute diarrhea may be caused by emotional states, especially anxiety; infectious organisms, such as bacteria, viruses, and parasites; alterations in diet, such as increased greasy or spicy foods, or food to which the person is allergic; and medications, such as iron supplements, thyroid agents, magnesium-containing antacids, antibiotics, lactulose, cimetidine, antihypertensives, colchicine, digitalis, and laxatives.

Causes of chronic diarrhea have been identified as lactose-containing or hyperosmolar nutritional supplements; sorbitol and mannitol (ingredients); such diseases as hyperthyroidism, diabetes mellitus, adrenal insufficiency, hyperparathyroidism, inflammatory bowel diseases, and cancer of the colon; GI surgery; radiation enterocolitis; laxative abuse; alcohol abuse; and chemotherapeutic agents.

FOCUSED ASSESSMENT FOR *BOWEL INCONTINENCE*

The risk for *Bowel incontinence* is associated with physical and mental disabilities. An older adult with decreased mobility or cognitive impairment is the most likely to have bowel incontinence. Developmentally disabled people with physical handicaps and mental retardation are the second largest group in whom incontinence is seen.

> ***Action Alert!*** Investigate any fecal odor that arises near a person or a source of soiled clothes or linens.

Defining Characteristics. Fecal incontinence is almost always involuntary and can occur at any age. A primary question to ask is whether or not the person is aware of the incontinence. Then you need to determine if the client is able to assist in the solution or if the nurse needs to assume responsibility for managing the problem. Determine if the client recognizes the incontinence but cannot control it because of the explosive nature of the diarrhea, an inability to move to the toilet in a timely manner, a loss of rectal sphincter control, or the presence of a colostomy or an ileostomy. The focus of the assessment then becomes to determine if the problem is correctable or manageable. Determine the frequency, the duration of the problem, and the presence of associated symptoms such as abdominal cramps.

Related Factors. Related factors for *Bowel incontinence* are the following:

- Gastrointestinal disorder with explosive diarrhea (urge to defecate too overwhelming to control)
- Neuromuscular disorders in which the person lacks the sensation to recognize the urge to defecate
- Loss of anal sphincter control, ileostomy, colostomy; may be secondary to hemorrhoids, tumors, lacerations, rectal prolapse, fistulas, and loss of sensory innervation
- Impaired cognition

Psychologically, incontinence may be secondary to mental illness, as well as being itself the cause of various emotional problems. *Encopresis* is the socially inappropriate passage of a stool when no physical reason exists to account for the behavior. It is thought to occur because of an emotional disturbance or delay in the maturation process. Sometimes a formerly continent child or adult becomes incontinent as a means to gain attention or to express anger.

Probably the most important consequence of incontinence is the loss of self-respect, which is intensified by the reactions of significant others in the person's environment, including nurses, physicians, friends, and relatives. Also, incontinence causes skin irritation and breakdown, and soiling of clothes and linen.

FOCUSED ASSESSMENT FOR *FLATULENCE*

Flatulence is recognized from a swollen feeling, abdominal distention, cramping, and eructation from the anus (flatus). Respiratory distress may also occur if the distended abdomen pushes against the diaphragm. Abdominal percussion produces a tympanic sound.

Probably the most common predisposing factor in flatulence is excessive air swallowing, which results from chewing gum, drinking carbonated beverages, eating rapidly, or sucking through straws. Anxiety and postnasal drip can also lead to excessive air swallowing.

Other causes of gaseous distention include constipation; slowed intestinal motility, as may occur after abdominal surgery; bowel obstruction; medications that decrease peristalsis; decreased physical activity; and eating such foods as beans, cabbage, radishes, onions, cauliflower, and cucumbers.

FOCUSED ASSESSMENT FOR *FECAL IMPACTION*

Impaction consists of hardened feces that a person cannot pass voluntarily or involuntarily. Probably the most common predisposing factor is immobility. Other predisposing factors are nutritional intake, abuse of laxatives, and poor fluid intake.

> ***Action Alert!*** Assess for fecal impaction when there is a continuous seepage of loose feces.

Suspect a fecal impaction when the client has abdominal distention, small amounts of liquid stool, and the absence of a bowel movement over several days. However, a fecal impaction can be present even if the client has had small regular bowel movements that have not emptied the colon. The impaction is confirmed by abdominal palpation, digital examination for the presence of hardened stool in the rectum, or radiographic confirmation. Inquire about the date of the client's last known bowel movement, any previous impaction problems, dietary and medication intake, and immobility that might contribute to the problem. Previous bowel surgery, decreased bowel sounds, immobility, and chronic use of suppositories are risk factors. It is usually associated with decreased mental status.

Often the first symptom of a fecal impaction is the inability to pass a normal stool. However, probably the most definitive symptom is the seepage of liquid stool from the anus. Liquefaction provides the only way that fecal material can get around the impaction. Usually the liquid appears in small amounts, which helps to differentiate it from diarrhea. However, bacterial action on the fecal mass sometimes causes the production of copious amounts of liquid stool. Also, the seepage of stool is usually uncontrolled, since the anal sphincters have become less competent, secondary to prolonged stimulation of the defecation reflex by the hardened mass. Other symptoms indicating impaction include an almost continuous urge to defecate, rectal pain, abdominal fullness, nausea and vomiting, shortness of breath, hypertension, and abdominal distention.

Confirm the presence of an impaction by performing a digital rectal examination. With a gloved hand, insert a well-lubricated forefinger through the anus into the rectum. If you feel a hard fecal mass, an impaction probably exists. If you do not feel a mass but symptoms are present, the mass may be higher up in the colon, out of reach.

DIAGNOSIS

The use of a "risk for" diagnosis is based on the philosophy of early detection and prevention of health problems. For example, a postoperative client is at risk for constipation. Once the diagnosis is actual, it could be written as *Constipation related to immobility and anesthesia.* Figure 29-4 offers more information.

When considering a nursing diagnosis, be sure that the focus of care and interventions are appropriate to the client. Examples of nursing diagnoses that are pertinent to bowel elimination are *Diarrhea related to excessive use of laxatives, Bowel incontinence related to cognitive impairment, Perceived constipation related to impaired thought process,* and *Bowel incontinence related to effects of medication.* Clustering appropriate data can help you arrive at the most appropriate nursing diagnoses (Table 29-2).

Disturbed body image may be present in the client who has had a fecal diversion procedure, such as an ileostomy or a colostomy. The presence of an ostomy is an actual change in body image and may result in the client being reluctant to learn to manage the ostomy care. Bowel incontinence also can produce a body image

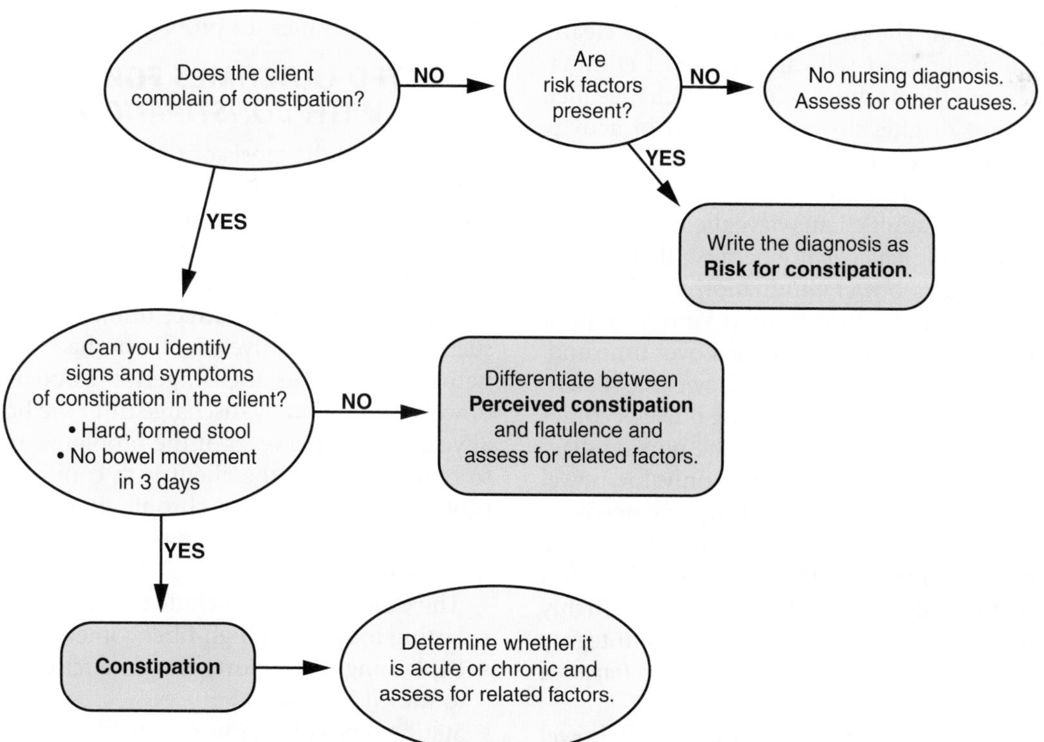

FIGURE 29-4 Decision tree for constipation. Diagnoses are shown in rectangles. Within these rectangles, diagnoses shown in **bold** type are NANDA-I–approved nursing diagnoses; diagnoses shown in regular type are not NANDA-I–approved nursing diagnoses.

Table 29-2 Clustering Data to Make a Nursing Diagnosis

Bowel Elimination Problems

DATA CLUSTER	DIAGNOSIS
An 84-year-old ambulatory woman with Alzheimer's disease has an incontinent bowel movement every morning after breakfast. She cannot find her room in the nursing home; it is not clear if she feels the urge to defecate.	*Bowel incontinence* related to impaired cognition and sensory perception
The third day after gallbladder surgery, a 50-year-old woman calls the doctor's office complaining of abdominal distention and cramping. She reports that she has not had a bowel movement since the surgery. She has been taking acetaminophen with codeine for pain.	*Constipation* related to decreased physical activity and use of pain medication
A 70-year-old woman has been admitted to the hospital with leukemia. She tells you that she must have milk of magnesia every morning before breakfast. She reports that her stool is unformed and a small amount.	*Perceived constipation* related to possible inaccurate health belief
After returning home from traveling in a foreign country, parents report that their 18-month-old infant has developed loose stools that have occurred about seven times a day for more than 2 days.	*Diarrhea* related to possible infectious processes
A 47-year-old man had abdominal exploratory surgery. On the second postoperative day, he complained of abdominal cramping and gas pains.	**Flatulence* related to slowed peristalsis secondary to surgery and decreased mobility
A resident of a long-term care facility has been unable to ambulate or move herself for about 2 years. She recently began losing weight, about 2 to 3 pounds per month, because she was refusing her meals. She also began refusing to take her laxatives on a regular basis. A nurse's aide reported to the charge nurse that she was constantly cleaning up loose, seeping stool for this resident.	**Fecal impaction* related to decreased mobility, decreased nutritional intake, and refusal of laxative medications

*Diagnoses with an asterisk are not NANDA-I approved.

disturbance because it represents a socially unacceptable activity. Embarrassment is often a major factor in managing incontinence.

Ineffective health maintenance is present any time a client has to undergo a lifestyle change to manage a bowel elimination problem. The client with an ostomy clearly has to change methods of self-care for bowel elimination. However, any client who is required to change diet, take medications, or alter the usual pattern of activity and exercise will have to manage the effect of those changes on bowel elimination.

Many times, older adult clients have the nursing diagnosis *Ineffective health maintenance* because they cannot identify and manage a bowel elimination problem. For example, a client may be homebound with very poor nutritional intake. Mobility has declined over time and, as a result, the usual routine of a daily bowel movement after a high-fiber diet is gone. The visiting nurse becomes involved with the client and identifies the nursing diagnosis *Ineffective health maintenance* not only for bowel elimination but for dietary intake and hygiene needs.

Risk for impaired skin integrity is appropriate when the client has bowel incontinence. The contents of the colon are alkaline compared to the skin and, therefore, highly irritable to the skin. The risk for impaired skin integrity is especially high when other risk factors for *Impaired skin integrity* exist.

Toileting self-care deficit is highly associated with bowel elimination problems. The client may be unable to independently perform toileting activities because of immobility, lack of full range of motion, weakness, or intolerance for activity.

PLANNING

After performing a thorough bowel history and assessment, you will plan care to address the nursing diagnoses. During the planning phase of the nursing process, nursing interventions are identified to assist the client in achieving outcomes for problem resolution.

EXPECTED OUTCOMES FOR THE CLIENT WITH *CONSTIPATION*

The goal for a diagnosis of *Constipation* is that the client resumes a normal bowel elimination pattern. Most of the time, a positive outcome is inferred from observation of frequency and the client's subjective experience and report that bowel elimination is normal.

If the problem is a direct result of an acute illness, such as a postoperative client who had no bowel elimination for 72 hours after surgery, the outcome of normal bowel elimination by discharge from the hospital is usually sufficient. However, if the problem can be expected to return—that is, the client is at continued risk or the problem is the result of chronic illness—the outcomes need to include evidence that the person is prepared to manage the risk.

The outcomes may include the following:

- Listing foods with high-fiber content
- Explaining the importance of exercise in relationship to the GI system
- Stating types of laxatives available
- Identifying side effects and contraindications of bowel laxatives
- Administering appropriate laxatives to maintain normal bowel elimination

EXPECTED OUTCOMES FOR THE CLIENT WITH *DIARRHEA*

The expected outcome for the diagnosis *Diarrhea* is also that the client resumes a normal bowel elimination pattern. No evidence of diarrhea will be present, as manifested by a soft, medium-size to large bowel movement every day or every few days, as is the client's routine. The client with diarrhea should be evaluated for risk for reoccurrence. The outcomes may include that the client will achieve the following:

- Be clean and dry
- Avoid foods that contribute to diarrhea
- Note the frequency and amount of diarrhea

EXPECTED OUTCOMES FOR THE CLIENT WITH *BOWEL INCONTINENCE*

The expected outcome for a diagnosis of *Bowel incontinence* depends on the illness that has caused the problem. If the bowel incontinence is a permanent problem, the appropriate outcome is that the client's skin integrity remains intact. If the bowel incontinence is not permanent or can be minimized by intervention, then outcomes could be that the client will do the following:

- Have a daily bowel elimination on a commode or bedpan
- Alter diet and fluids to control elimination
- Establish a set routine for elimination
- Decrease episodes of incontinence

EXPECTED OUTCOMES FOR THE CLIENT WITH *FECAL IMPACTION*

Outcomes for the client with *Fecal impaction* could be that the client will do the following:

- Experience manual removal of feces without pain or other side effects
- Initiate or be placed on a preventive bowel program

EXPECTED OUTCOMES FOR THE CLIENT WITH *FLATULENCE*

Outcomes for the client with *Flatulence* could be that the client will do the following:

- Decrease the production of flatus by modifying diet and/or air swallowing
- Expel excess flatus
- Experience a decrease in symptoms of flatulence

INTERVENTION

INTERVENTIONS TO PROMOTE HEALTHFUL ELIMINATION

You can help clients meet the goal of healthy defecation habits through learning activities. Support normal bowel habits through adjustments in diet, fluids, exercise, and positioning and by providing relaxation and privacy.

Developing a Plan for Lifestyle Management. Even clients who you assume are knowledgeable may have misconceptions about defecation. For example, many people incorrectly believe that it is necessary to defecate every day. If they fail to have a daily bowel movement, they may use laxatives, suppositories, or enemas to induce one. As described later, continued use of such measures begins a cycle that may lead to physical dependence. Because there are many other misunderstandings about defecation, you must give clients accurate information about this normal body function. With appropriate teaching, a client who needs intervention is more likely to be compliant.

Toilet Habits. Many factors influence the timing of bowel movements, such as availability of a bathroom and the demands of personal and professional responsibilities. Consequently, you will need to assess each client's daily routine before planning a bowel program. However, keep in mind that, although defecation can occur at any time, it is best to encourage bowel movements during stimulation of the gastrocolic reflex. As described earlier, this reflex is usually strongest after breakfast. Therefore attempts to have a bowel movement at this time are likely to be the most successful.

Frequency of bowel movements varies from person to person. The normal range for an adult is from three times per week to three times per day. Infants often have three to five stools per day, but for adults and older children, passing stools more than three times a day or less than once a week may indicate a problem. Because many people worry needlessly about the frequency of their bowel movements, emphasize to your clients that the frequency of bowel movements varies among individuals.

> ***Action Alert!*** Stress that the frequency of bowel movements is individualized and that it is not necessary to have a bowel movement every day.

The amount of stool varies according to the amount and type of food ingested, fluid intake, and frequency of bowel evacuation. It is normally about 150 g per day. Because much fecal material is not dietary in origin, people with no oral intake still pass stool. Also, it may take several days for food to move through the entire GI tract. The colon therefore is not empty even if the person has not eaten for several days. Inform people of these facts to motivate them to take measures to prevent constipation.

Help people select a time during the day when they can take time to attend to bowel needs. As indicated, timing depends on lifestyle and daily activities. Once it is decided, encourage clients to make this habit a daily routine. If the time selected is inappropriate, alter it until a suitable one is found. People who have little routine in their lives are a particular challenge.

In addition, hospitalization often alters established routines. During this time, determine the client's normal routine, and then help him to maintain it.

Diet. Dietary fiber is one of the most important elements in maintaining normal bowel function. Dietary fiber increases the weight and water content of feces. It also speeds the progress of feces through the GI tract. Fiber may be soluble or insoluble. The digestive system cannot break down insoluble fiber from a plant. Likewise, fiber does not break down in water but rather retains water. Water retained by fiber softens the stool and promotes regularity. Thus supplementing diets with bran, whole-grain cereals, nuts, and raw fruits and vegetables is effective in promoting normal bowel elimination.

A high-fiber diet can also prevent diverticular disease. A diverticulum is an outpouching of the colon wall that results from weakened muscles in the intestinal wall. This condition can cause problems if the diverticula fill with feces. Perforation, ulceration, and infection can also develop. Diverticular disease is commonly asymptomatic when the client eats a high-fiber diet.

The National Cancer Institute recommends a daily intake of 25 to 35 g of fiber. To increase a client's intake of fiber, add high-fiber foods slowly to allow time for the GI tract to adapt. Large amounts of dietary fiber added abruptly can cause abdominal cramps, gaseous distention, and diarrhea. The client's fiber consumption should include both insoluble and soluble fiber. It should come from foods rather than from supplements, which may not contain needed vitamins and minerals.

In addition to adding fiber, help the client identify and avoid foods that disrupt bowel function. If there are several suspect foods, urge the client to eliminate all of them from the diet and then add them back, one at a time. Tell the client to wait for several days, longer if necessary, between introductions, to see which foods cause the problem.

Fluids. Hydration helps maintain normal bowel function by keeping stools soft. Although experts recommend different amounts of fluid to maintain adequate hydration, most consider about 1200 to 1500 mL per day to be a reasonable minimum for adults. A client with significant fluid replacement needs (such as from increased sweating caused by activity or fever) should consume more. Immobility also requires increased fluid intake because one of the normal aids to defecation—exercise—is limited. However, before increasing a client's fluid intake, make sure that the person has no contraindications, such as cardiac disease, renal disease, or head injury. Fluid requirements for infants and children are based on kilograms of body weight. Infants and children are more vulnerable to changing fluid needs related to ambient temperature and exercise.

Although the amount of fluid intake is critical, the type of fluids consumed may also be important. For example, milk constipates some people. Prune juice is a natural laxative for most people. Other fruit juices, such as apricot, lemonade, cranberry, and orange, can also stimulate bowel activity.

Exercise. Encourage and assist clients, as necessary, to take part in daily physical activity, because exercise improves muscle tone and strengthens the muscles used in defecation. Walking, for example, is an excellent body toner.

Also, teach exercises specifically designed to strengthen the abdominal and pelvic floor muscles. Probably the most effective are isometric exercises in which the client contracts or tightens muscles as strongly as possible for about 10 seconds, and then relaxes them. Instruct the client to repeat each exercise 5 to 10 times, four times a day. Remember that isometric exercises raise blood pressure and may cause coronary ischemia (deficient blood flow to the cardiac muscle) in a client with cardiac disease. Therefore you may need to consult a physician about the client's health status before instituting an exercise program.

Use of Laxatives. Laxatives are short-acting medications that cause defecation. Healthy people should not use them on a routine basis. For clients who cannot defecate because of constipation or fecal impaction, laxatives are used to aid in the bowel elimination process.

Positioning the Client. Proper positioning for elimination promotes comfort and aids defecation in several ways. For one, it makes use of the force of gravity. For another, good positioning facilitates contraction of the abdominal muscles, thereby increasing intraabdominal pressure. Because squatting is the best position for defecation, position the client as near to this posture as possible. The commode and toilet promote this position. You can increase external pressure on the abdomen by having the client lean forward.

If the person is short, place a footstool or other appropriate device under the feet at the toilet to increase hip flexion. Exercise caution, however, with a client who has had hip surgery, especially total hip replacement. This client must avoid flexing the hips beyond 90 degrees to prevent dislocation of the prosthesis. Some clients can use the toilet only with the aid of a device that raises the seat height to decrease hip flexion. Instruct these clients not to lean forward.

If the client must use a bedpan, raise the head of the bed into a high-Fowler's position, if not contraindicated. If head elevation is contraindicated, use a fracture bedpan instead.

Promoting Relaxation and Privacy. Relaxation is critical to normal bowel function. Probably the most important factor in achieving relaxation is privacy. Clients may become anxious if they feel that the odors and sounds that naturally accompany this body function may be communicated to others. Anxiety causes tension in the voluntary musculature, which in turn can suppress defecation. Provide as private an environment as possible to facilitate normal defecation.

For example, if the client is using the bathroom, make sure that other people know the room is occupied. This is especially important when the bathroom has two doors opening into adjacent rooms. If the client must use a bedpan or commode in the room, pull the bed curtains around the bed, ask all visitors or staff to leave the room, open the window if appropriate, and turn on the television or radio. Use room deodorizers to reduce odors.

Make sure that clients have a way to call you when they are finished or need help. In addition to providing a call light, assure them that there is no hurry. Communicate this fact by your actions as well as your words. For example, avoid interrupting them simply to see if they are finished. On the other hand, do keep careful watch on any client who is at risk for accidents, such as fainting or falling. In fact, fainting in bathrooms is a rather frequent occurrence. Bathrooms are notoriously warm and stuffy and, when a weakened person strains to have a bowel movement, the cardiovascular system may not be able to maintain sufficient blood flow to the brain.

Some clients may need pain relief before trying to defecate. If you must administer a narcotic pain reliever, time its administration carefully because these drugs depress central nervous system function. Time the administration so that the client can attempt defecation when pain has been relieved but before drowsiness and sleep set in.

INTERVENTIONS TO MANAGE CONSTIPATION

The treatment of typical constipation requires all the preventive measures mentioned: learning and teaching activities; changes in diet, fluid intake, and exercise; and development of healthy bowel habits. Sometimes, additional intervention is needed.

Administering Medications. **Laxatives** are agents that stimulate defecation, and **cathartics** are strong laxatives that produce a watery stool. Laxatives come in four categories: bulk forming, lubricant, saline, and stimulant. Besides these oral medications, laxatives are also available as medicated suppositories. When inserted into the rectum, they stimulate defecation.

Bulk-forming laxatives are the most natural and least irritating laxative preparations and are frequently used to wean laxative-dependent people from medication misuse. They use synthetic or natural polysaccharides and cellulose derivatives to absorb water and add bulk. This increased volume stretches the intestinal wall, thus stimulating peristalsis. Common examples are bran, psyllium, karaya gum, agar, and methylcellulose. Mix bulk-forming agents with water, and follow the dose with additional fluid to make sure that it has been cleared from the esophagus. Results usually occur in 12 to 24 hours, but they may take up to 72 hours. Encourage high fluid intake to improve the action of the laxative and to avoid GI tract obstruction.

Lubricant laxatives include mineral oil and the docusates. They coat the outside of the fecal mass, making it slippery and inhibiting fluid absorption from it. Mineral oil is a classic example of a lubricant laxative. It is not very palatable, but you can mask the oily aftertaste by mixing it with orange juice or root beer. Administer mineral oil when the client's stomach is empty to keep it from interfering with the absorption of fat-soluble vitamins. Watch carefully if the client has trouble swallowing, because mineral oil aspiration can cause pneumonia. The docusates act as wetting and dispersing agents. Common examples are Dialose, Colace, Doxidan, and Surfak. Poloxamer 188, a nonionic surfactant, is a stool softener.

Saline laxatives, or osmotic agents, contain poorly absorbed salts and sugars, which, through osmotic activity, draw water into the intestine to increase bulk and lubricate feces. These drugs usually act within 1 to 3 hours. Many are purgatives that empty the bowel completely. Magnesium sulfate (Epsom salts), magnesium hydroxide (milk of magnesia), magnesium citrate, and lactulose are osmotic agents. Lactulose causes a severe osmotic reaction and, unless the dose is calculated carefully, causes intestinal rumbling, colic, and flatulence. Because of the salts used and the severity of their action, osmotic agents are usually contraindicated in people with renal, cardiac, or inflammatory bowel disease.

Stimulants (also called irritants) increase peristalsis by stimulating sensory nerve endings of the colonic epithelium or by directly irritating the GI mucosa. In addition, some (such as bisacodyl) may increase GI secretory activity, thus producing bulkier feces. Examples of stimulants include cascara, castor oil, senna, glycerin, and bisacodyl. Be aware that these medications are transmitted through breast milk, causing diarrhea in the nursing infant.

Laxatives are one of the most widely used and misused over-the-counter drugs. Most laxative abuse results from advertising that supports the public's misconceptions about the need for a daily bowel movement. In addition to teaching clients about the proper use of laxatives, warn them never to take these drugs in the presence of undiagnosed abdominal pain or cramps, nausea, vomiting, or diarrhea. These symptoms may indicate appendicitis, inflammatory bowel disease, or obstruction.

Action Alert! Daily laxative administration is detrimental to normal bowel elimination.

Suppositories are semisolid, cone-shaped, or oval-shaped masses that melt at body temperature. To stimulate defecation, medicated suppositories are inserted into the rectum, where they release their active ingredients as they melt. Many types of suppositories are refrigerated because it is easier to insert a cold, firm suppository than a warm, soft one.

The suppositories used most often are glycerin and bisacodyl. Each acts as a local irritant to stimulate GI mucosal secretion. Fecal softeners may also be given by suppository to moisten and lubricate the fecal mass. After administering the suppository, cleanse the client's anal area to remove excess lubricant. Instruct the client to retain the suppository as long as possible—at least 20 to 30 minutes. If appropriate, teach the client how to self-administer the suppository.

Administering Enemas. An enema involves the instillation of fluid into the rectum to stimulate defecation. People who have had no formal instruction in the procedure commonly administer this treatment in the home. Indeed, some people use a daily enema to prevent constipation. Consequently, most people consider enemas to be a harmless, necessary treatment for constipation. This is a misconception. To achieve the safest and most effective results, it is necessary to understand and apply the scientific principles underlying enema administration.

Purpose. Enemas are given for several purposes. The *cleansing enema* is used to treat constipation or fecal impaction, to clean out the bowel before diagnostic procedures or surgery, and to help establish regular bowel function during a bowel-training program. A *retention enema* is retained in the bowel over a prolonged period. It is usually administered to lubricate or soften a hard fecal mass with oil, thus facilitating its expulsion through the anus. Less frequently, a retention enema is used to administer medications, to protect and soothe the mucous membrane of the intestine, to destroy intestinal parasites (anthelmintic), to relieve distention (carminative), or to administer fluids and nutrition (nutritive).

Enemas stimulate peristalsis through bowel distention, irritation of the mucosal wall, or both. Bowel distention results from filling the colon with fluid, either via a large-volume enema, which injects large amounts of fluid into the colon from an external source, or via a small-volume enema, which draws internal fluid into the bowel.

The concepts of osmosis and concentration gradient are important to an understanding of how some enemas work. Briefly, osmosis is the movement of water through a semipermeable membrane to equalize the concentration of particles on both sides of the membrane. Although water continuously flows back and forth across the membrane, the major net flow of water is toward the solution with a higher concentration of molecules.

Types of Enemas. A cleansing enema may use a hypotonic, isotonic, or hypertonic solution. Hypotonic solutions (such as tap water) have a lower osmotic pressure than the fluid in the interstitial tissues, so the net flow of water is out of the bowel into the tissues. The net flow occurs slowly, however, and defecation is usually stimulated before any appreciable fluid is absorbed into the body. Significant absorption can occur if the client is fluid depleted or receives multiple enemas. Isotonic solutions (such as normal saline solution) produce equal concentrations on both sides of the semipermeable membrane. Consequently, no net water flow occurs. Hypertonic solutions are of higher concentration than the interstitial fluid. Thus the net water flow is into the colon, leading to distention and stimulating the defecation reflex.

Hypotonic and isotonic enema solutions are used for large-volume enemas (500 to 750 mL) that result in immediate colonic emptying. The large volumes, however, may present a danger to people with weakened colon walls. In addition, these enemas often require special preparation and equipment. On the other hand, hypertonic small-volume enemas (120 to 250 mL) are available commercially and are easier to administer. A commonly used over-the-counter product is the prepackaged enema, such as the Fleet brand (Figure 29-5). These commercially packaged enemas are available as normal saline enemas or as mineral oil enemas. People who have problems with sodium retention should avoid using hypertonic solutions.

One common enema additive is Castile soap. Added to either tap water or saline solution, it causes mucosal irritation. Other enema solutions, such as milk and molasses, vegetable oils, hydrogen peroxide, and champagne, are reported in the literature. However, these types are rarely used. Various medicated and nutritive formulas, such as sucralfate enemas, are also used, depending on the person's needs.

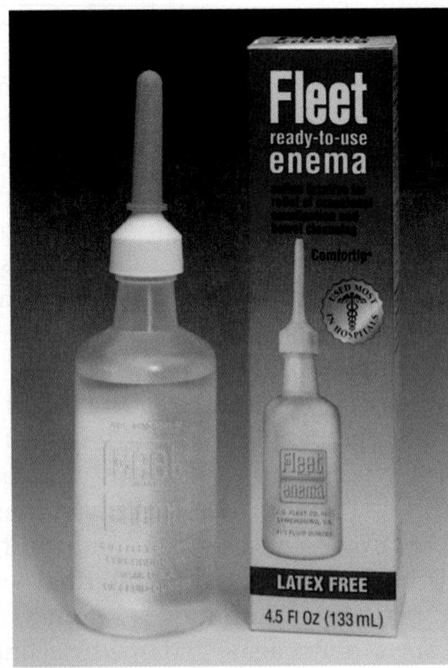

FIGURE 29-5 A Fleet enema. (Courtesy C. B. Fleet Company, Lynchburg, VA.)

Procedure 29-2 describes the techniques for preparing and administering a large-volume enema. Use these methods for enemas of any volume, but make any necessary changes when preparing the solution.

Administration of a hypertonic enema requires several variations in the procedure for an enema, mainly because the solution comes prepackaged and ready to inject. You do not need to warm the solution, but make sure that it is at room temperature to prevent intestinal cramps. The client may be in any position to receive this enema; however, the left lateral position with right leg flexed is recommended to distribute the solution throughout the colon.

PROCEDURE 29-2

TIME TO ALLOW: NOVICE: 15 min. EXPERT: 10 min.

PREPARING AND ADMINISTERING A LARGE-VOLUME ENEMA

A large-volume enema is defined as 500 to 1000 mL of fluid to stimulate the colon to empty. It is unpleasant at best, may have some hazardous consequences for the client, and is seldom used in the health care environment. A large-volume enema is useful when rapid cleansing or evacuation of the bowel is needed. It may also be useful when the gentler forms of bowel cleansing are not effective.

Possible complications: damage to the rectum, loss of fluid and electrolytes, bradycardia from vagal stimulation, discomfort

DELEGATION GUIDELINES

An enema requires a physician's order. Administration of a large-volume enema may be delegated to a nursing assistant. First, however, you must assess the client for risk factors associated with receipt of an enema and instruct the nursing assistant in safety precautions. If the client has diverticular disease or another disorder of the colon, you may instruct the nursing assistant to use a smaller volume of solution or choose to administer the enema yourself.

EQUIPMENT NEEDED

- Enema solution container
- 36 inches of tubing with rectal tip (adult, No. 22 to No. 30 Fr; child, No. 12 to No. 18 Fr)
- Solution: tap water or normal saline, with 1 teaspoon mild liquid soap without additives. (Normal saline solution is the safest option for an enema solution, and tap water requires the least preparation. If the client has severe constipation or needs a thorough cleansing of the bowel, soapsuds may be most useful because they irritate the colonic mucosa.)
- Water-soluble lubricating jelly
- Clean gloves
- Waterproof pad
- Bedside commode or bedpan

1 Follow preliminary actions (see inside front cover).

2 Set up the equipment, and close the door or draw the curtain. Position the client on the left (or most comfortable) side. Drape the client so only the buttocks are exposed. If you expect that the client will be unable to retain the enema solution, position him or her on a bedpan or commode instead. Positioning the client on the left side allows gravity to help the enema solution flow into the rectum. Exposing only the buttocks will help to give the client a sense of privacy. Allowing the client to face the door may help as well.

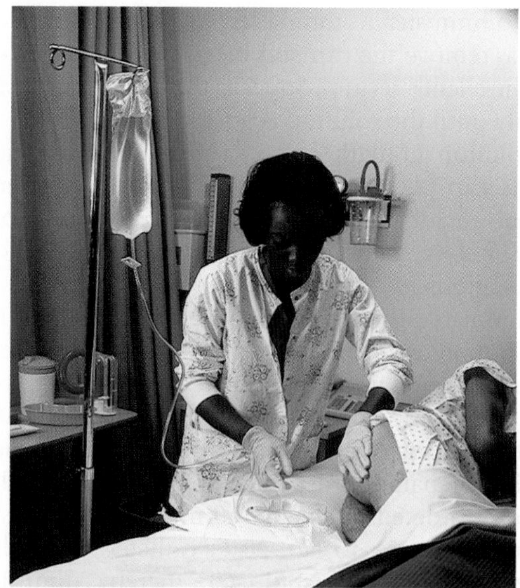

Step 2. Positioning and equipment for administering a large-volume enema.

Continued

3 Make sure the enema solution is lukewarm, about 40.5° C (105° F). Coat the tip of the enema tube with water-soluble lubricant, and gently insert it 2 to 3 inches into the client's rectum. *If the client has hemorrhoids, consider using extra lubricant. Insert the tip gently, with a twisting motion, to pass the hemorrhoids.*

4 Allow 500 to 750 mL of the enema solution to flow slowly into the client's rectum, over about 10 minutes. The enema bag should be approximately 18 inches above the rectum. Keep the flow rate slow enough to prevent cramping and an uncontrollable urge to evacuate the bowel. If the client develops an uncontrollable urge, stop the flow until the urge passes.

5 Encourage the client to retain the solution in the bowel for up to 15 minutes. *With a large-volume enema, most clients will need to expel the solution quickly.*

6 Help the client to the toilet, or assist the client with the bedpan or commode, as needed. *If the client has mobility problems, you may be able to place him or her more quickly on a bedpan than on the toilet. However, the best position for bowel evacuation is on the toilet or bedside commode.*

7 After bowel evacuation, cleanse the client's perianal skin, control odors, and make the client comfortable. *Cleanse the skin thoroughly and gently. Controlling odors promptly can help to minimize the client's embarrassment.*

8 If the physician has ordered enemas until clear, you may need to administer up to three large-volume enemas as described here. If three enemas fail to produce clear results, consult the physician. *Remember that a large-volume enema may produce more than one bowel movement. Allow time between enemas for maximum results.*

PEDIATRIC CONSIDERATIONS

Hospitalized children are prone to constipation and should be carefully observed for this problem. Isotonic saline is often the preferred solution for a large-volume enema in a child. The amount of fluid and the position varies with the age of the child:

- Infant, 150 to 250 mL
- Young child, 250 to 300 mL
- Older child, 300 to 350 mL
- Adolescent, 500 to 750 mL

GERIATRIC CONSIDERATIONS

Enemas in older adults with mobility problems can be challenging. An enema can be given on a bedpan for the person who cannot hold the solution or cannot move to the toilet easily. You may be able to insert the catheter and then turn the client onto the bedpan. Large-volume enemas should not be routinely used to manage chronic constipation. Avoid giving an enema more frequently than every 3 days to prevent dependence on enemas and to prevent the excess loss of electrolytes.

HOME HEALTH CARE CONSIDERATIONS

Enemas should not be used with any frequency in the home setting. Teach the family that cleansing enemas and laxatives should not be used any more often than once every 3 days. Once the bowel is thoroughly cleansed, the client may not need another bowel movement for 3 days. If the client is in the habit of managing constipation with enemas, help family caregivers with an overall bowel management program designed to reduce the need for enemas.

To administer a commercially prepared hypertonic enema, remove the cap and insert the prelubricated tip into the client's rectum. Squeeze the collapsible reservoir steadily until the solution is gone. Have the client retain the solution until the urge to defecate is very strong. Clients can be taught to self-administer a hypertonic enema, and they may be asked to administer one at home before radiographic studies or proctological examinations.

Administration of a retention enema is similar to administration of a hypertonic enema except that the solution must be retained over a prolonged period, usually for at least an hour. Some enemas (such as medicated or nutritive enemas) are never evacuated. The method of solution preparation depends on what type of solution has been ordered. A smaller administration tip is used (usually a No. 14 to No. 20 Fr catheter for adults) to avoid stretching the sphincter, thereby diminishing stimulation of the defecation reflex. Make sure you elevate the reservoir only high enough to allow the solution to run slowly into the rectum. Administration under higher pressure distends the rectum, causing defecation. Finally, protect the bed linen in case the client cannot retain the fluid.

Complications. Enema administration is not without its hazards. Complications include fluid and electrolyte imbalances, tissue trauma, vagal nerve stimulation, and dependence. Fluid imbalances usually occur because of the tonicity of the enema solution. Remember that the body absorbs water from hypotonic solutions. Use caution when administering enemas to people who are susceptible to fluid imbalance (such as infants or clients with decompensated cardiac or kidney reserve). Water intoxication can occur. Symptoms of this condition include weakness, dizziness, pallor, sweating, and respiratory difficulties. Signs of congestive heart failure or cerebral edema may also be present. On the other hand, hypertonic solutions draw fluid from the interstitial tissues and can lead to fluid depletion, especially in children and other people susceptible to dehydration.

Table 29-3 Agents Used to Relieve Constipation

TYPE	ACTION	EXAMPLES
LAXATIVES		
Bulk-forming	Increases the fluid, gaseous, or solid bulk in the intestines and absorbs water into the intestine	• Methylcellulose • Hydrolose • Psyllium (Metamucil)
Lubricant	Softens and delays the drying of feces	• Mineral oil
Saline	Draws water into the intestine to increase bulk and lubricate feces	• Docusate sodium (Colace, Dialose) • Magnesium sulfate (Epsom salts) • Magnesium hydroxide (milk of magnesia) • Magnesium citrate
Stimulant	Irritates the intestinal mucosa, increasing peristalsis	• Bisacodyl (Dulcolax) • Castor oil • Cascara sagrada
ENEMAS		
Hypertonic	Distends colon and irritates mucosa	• Sodium phosphate • Fleet enema
Hypotonic	Distends colon, stimulates peristalsis, and softens feces	• Tap water
Isotonic	Distends colon, stimulates peristalsis, and softens feces	• Normal saline solution
Soap	Irritates mucosa and distends colon	• Castile soap
Oil	Lubricates the feces and the colonic mucosa	• Mineral oil • Olive oil • Cottonseed oil

Electrolyte imbalances also occur. Usually, normal saline is the safest enema solution because of its isotonicity. However, in clients who have problems with sodium retention (such as those with congestive heart failure or cirrhosis of the liver), the body absorbs sodium, which leads to fluid retention. Therefore these clients should not receive saline solutions. Depending on the contents of the enema solution used, other electrolyte imbalances may also occur, such as hypokalemia, hypocalcemia, or hyperphosphatemia.

Action Alert! Avoid giving an enema to a person with inflammatory bowel disease.

Enemas can also cause tissue trauma. The four major sources of trauma are the administration tip, solution delivered under high pressure, a soapsuds solution, and increased peristalsis. If the enema tip has any chips or broken areas, it may lacerate or abrade the rectal mucosa. High fluid pressures can rupture the intestinal wall without causing pain at the time of perforation. In fact, the first indication of rupture may be signs of peritonitis (inflammation of the peritoneum). Do not use a bulb syringe to administer an enema, because you will not be able to control the pressure. Tissue trauma from peristalsis can occur in clients with inflammatory bowel disease. Increased bowel motility enhances cramping and bleeding.

Although the use of soapsuds enemas is questionable, they are still sometimes ordered. As stated, the soapsuds solution chemically irritates the mucosa. This irritation commonly leads to rectal inflammation and colitis, sometimes lasting up to 3 weeks after administration. The higher the concentration of soap in the solution, the greater is the chance of inflammation. Thus the practice of swirling a bar of soap or soap pieces in the enema reservoir is extremely dangerous, because it is impossible to determine the concentration. A soapsuds solution is somewhat safer if you use standardized packages of soap.

As is true of laxatives and suppositories, people can develop physical and psychological dependence on enemas. The underlying mechanism is the same: the enema cleans the bowel so that it takes 2 or more days for enough fecal mass to collect again to stimulate defecation. In the meantime, the person becomes anxious because he or she has not had a bowel movement. Thus the person self-administers another enema. Gradually, the bowel becomes less sensitive to normal defecation reflex stimuli, and the person becomes physically dependent on bowel aids. Table 29-3 summarizes agents used to relieve constipation.

Removing an Impaction. The goal of treatment for a fecal impaction is removal of the mass from the rectum. Oral laxatives or cathartics may be used to moisten and lubricate the fecal mass, although their action may be too slow. A program of enemas may be instituted, starting with the administration of an oil-retention enema and followed by a cleansing enema. These two enemas may need to be repeated.

If the fecal mass is extremely large or the enemas are ineffective in expelling it, you will have to remove the impaction digitally. To do this, insert a gloved, heavily lubricated finger into the client's rectum (Figure 29-6). Remove pieces of the mass manually with a bedpan close at hand. Even though you can use a topical anesthetic agent such as lidocaine, this intervention is uncomfortable and embarrassing for the client. Gentleness may help, but prevention is the best treatment. Sometimes, a fecal impaction must be removed surgically.

INTERVENTIONS TO ALLEVIATE DIARRHEA

The usual intervention for diarrhea is to inhibit peristalsis. However, because this action may slow the expulsion of pathogenic organisms or irritants, it may actually prolong the problem. Consequently, treatment involves removing the precipitating factors, then stopping the diarrhea itself. For example, a client with a GI infection typically receives antibiotics and possibly antidiarrheals.

Administering Medications. Commonly used antidiarrheal drugs, such as kaolin and pectin, may be used. These medications bind and remove irritants from the GI tract and form a soothing, protective coating on the mucosa. In severe diarrhea, the physician may prescribe opiates (such as paregoric or codeine) or anticholinergic drugs (such as diphenoxylate/atropine sulfate [Lomotil]) to inhibit peristalsis. As stated, antibiotics can be used to eliminate the cause of the diarrhea. Normal intestinal bacterial flora can be reestablished by giving the client yogurt, buttermilk, or bacillus-containing medications such as Bacid or Lactinex.

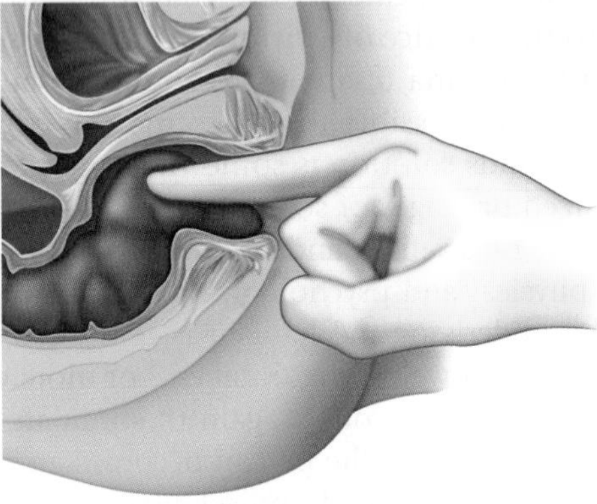

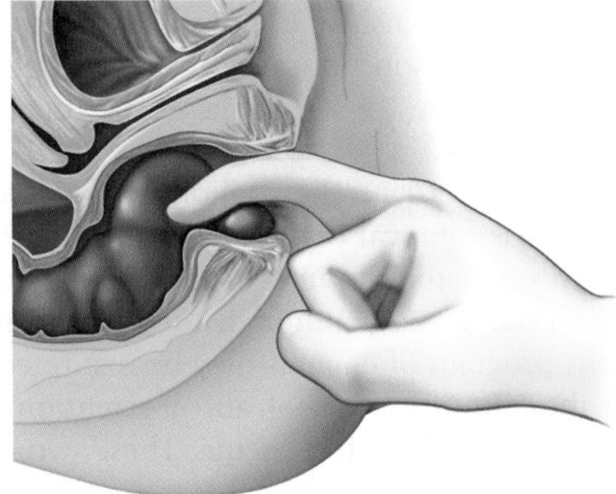

FIGURE 29-6 Digital removal of a fecal impaction.

Limiting Food Intake. Good nutrition and prevention of dehydration are important during episodes of diarrhea. Diet modification may be necessary to counteract the decreased absorption. For mild to moderate diarrhea, short-term therapy involves decreasing or eliminating food intake to reduce stimulation of peristalsis. For severe diarrhea, dietary modification may include a diet low in residue and high in calories and vitamins.

Food may be withheld and fluids restricted to clear liquids, followed by a soft diet in frequent small amounts. Drinking small but frequent amounts of clear liquids, preferably without carbonation, for at least 24 hours will replace fluids while minimizing peristalsis. As the diarrhea slows or after 24 hours, the client may try to eat a bland diet, but if diarrhea worsens, return to clear liquids. Suggested food might include plain toast, bread or crackers, mashed potatoes, rice, apples peeled, noncitrus fruit juices, and cooked vegetables. Raw fruits, vegetables, whole grains, and concentrated sweets should be avoided and added to the diet later. Dairy products and gas formers like cabbage, beans, and broccoli during episode of diarrhea may worsen symptoms for some people. Alcohol, spicy or highly seasoned foods (such as pizza, pepper, chili, tacos, onions, lasagna), greasy fried foods, hot dogs, lunch meats, caffeine, chocolate, raw fruits and vegetables will stimulate peristalsis. Warm liquids may be more soothing than cold liquids. Rest and relaxation may help slow peristaltic activity. If the diarrhea does not improve after 24 hours of clear liquids or if it is accompanied by fever, vomiting, persistent pain in the abdomen (especially the lower right side) or severe cramping, the client should contact the doctor.

The BRATY diet is recommended for children and adults with nausea and vomiting associated with gastroenteritis. The diet can be used for up to 24 hours. The initials stand for bananas (mashed or whole), rice, apples (or applesauce), toast (or crackers—preferably dry), and yogurt (plain).

Restoring Fluids and Electrolytes. Fluid and electrolyte losses are a common complication of diarrhea. Infants and debilitated clients are especially susceptible to this complication. In fact, age is a significant factor when a person has diarrhea. A young infant can soon have a serious depletion of electrolytes, water, and nutrients unless the disorder is promptly corrected. Fluids and electrolytes must be replaced by either oral or parenteral (intravenous) therapy. Emphasize to the client that decreasing fluid intake will not stop the diarrhea.

Using a Bedpan. Many clients need to use a bedpan for elimination, including those restricted to bed rest because of a fracture, recent surgery, or illness (Box 29-5). A client receiving an enema or who has diarrhea may need to use a bedpan as well.

Bedpans, made of metal or plastic, come in two styles: a regular bedpan and a fracture bedpan. The regular and fracture bedpans shown in Figure 29-7 are made of plastic. Fracture bedpans were developed for clients with fractures of the lower limbs who could not elevate easily to have a regular bedpan placed. Because of the ease of use of the fracture bedpans, it has become a common practice to use fracture bedpans with all clients. A metal bedpan of any style is cold; if possible, warm it before use by running warm water over its edges. This is not necessary for plastic bedpans.

You can place a bedpan by having the client lift the hips and sliding it under him or her. Or you can have the client roll onto his or her side, place the bedpan against the buttocks, and have the client roll back onto his or her back. You will need to judge the best method for each client. Either way, the closed-lip end of the bedpan should be placed under the buttocks, making sure that it is positioned to collect the waste (Figure 29-8).

BOX 29-5 *Tips for Putting a Client On a Bedpan*

(See Figure 29-8, *A* and *B*.)

- A bedpan is the least desirable method of elimination. Explore alternatives before deciding to use a bedpan.
- Provide privacy by pulling a curtain and keeping your client covered while using the bedpan.
- Simulate the client's natural position as much as possible. It is difficult to have a bowel movement without getting in a sitting or squatting position.
- Some clients can raise their hips high enough to slide a bedpan under the hips; most clients who need a bedpan rather than a bedside commode cannot raise their hips while lying in bed.
- A fracture pan can be placed in the correct position without raising the hips; with the client flat in bed, bend one or both legs and slide the narrow angled end just under the hips. Then elevate the head of the bed.
- If the larger bedpan is needed, turn the client on one side; place the bedpan in the correct position; push downward and inward on the bedpan as you turn the client onto the bedpan. Be sure the client's hips are in a position to bend at the same place the head of the bed breaks when it is elevated.

Preventing Skin Breakdown. Skin care is especially important for the client with diarrhea. Provide the client with soft material for wiping after each stool to help reduce the irritation. Also, washing the client's perianal area with soap and water after each stool reduces the time that irritating diarrhea stays in contact with the skin.

Ensuring Privacy. The frequency and urgency of bowel movements causes fatigue and embarrassment. Therefore make sure that the client has quick and easy access to the bathroom, commode, or bedpan. Place the call bell nearby at all times. Provide privacy and odor control.

INTERVENTIONS TO RESTORE BOWEL CONTINENCE

Interventions for bowel incontinence include promoting continence through bowel training and maintenance of skin integrity. Caring for the skin of an incontinent person may be a time-consuming task. The main goal is to prevent prolonged contact between the skin and fecal material, which leads to excoriation and breakdown.

Maintaining Skin Integrity. Washing the perianal area with soap and water and drying it thoroughly after each stool keeps the skin in good condition and controls fecal odor. Nonionic detergent preparations (such as Peri-Wash) are even more effective than regular soap. Use powders and creams with caution because they may contribute to skin breakdown.

Application of a rectal incontinence pouch for a client with bowel incontinence protects the skin and the bed linens (Figure 29-9). The rectal pouch has a circular paper adhesive backing that adheres to the perianal skin. An attached plastic bag collects the feces. The adhesive opening can be altered in size to facilitate individual fitting. Perianal hair should be shaved to allow a tight fit of the adhesive back.

If a rectal pouch is not in use, the bed and clothing of the incontinent person must be kept clean. When using plastic or rubber sheeting to protect bed linens, make sure that it does not contact the skin, thus causing irritation. A client with severe incontinence may need to wear

A

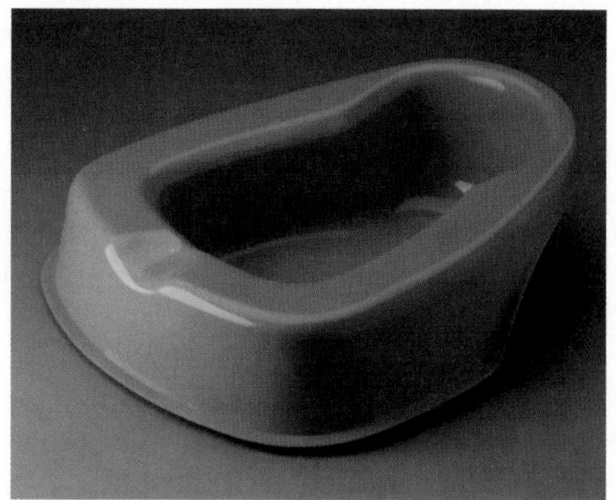

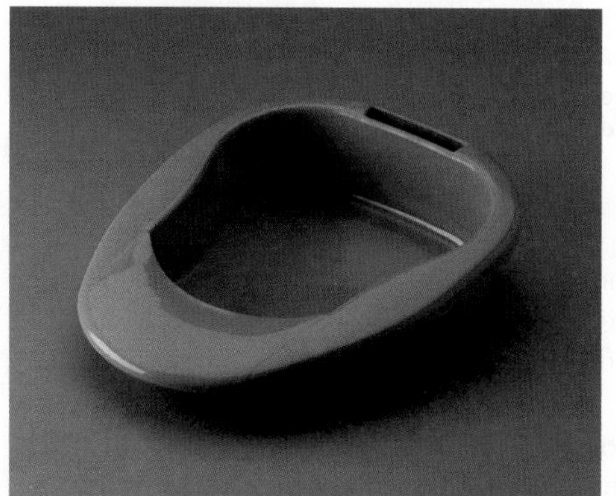

B

FIGURE 29-7 Types of bedpans. **A,** Regular bedpan—plastic. **B,** Fracture bedpan. (Courtesy Bemis Health Care, Sheboygan Falls, WI.)

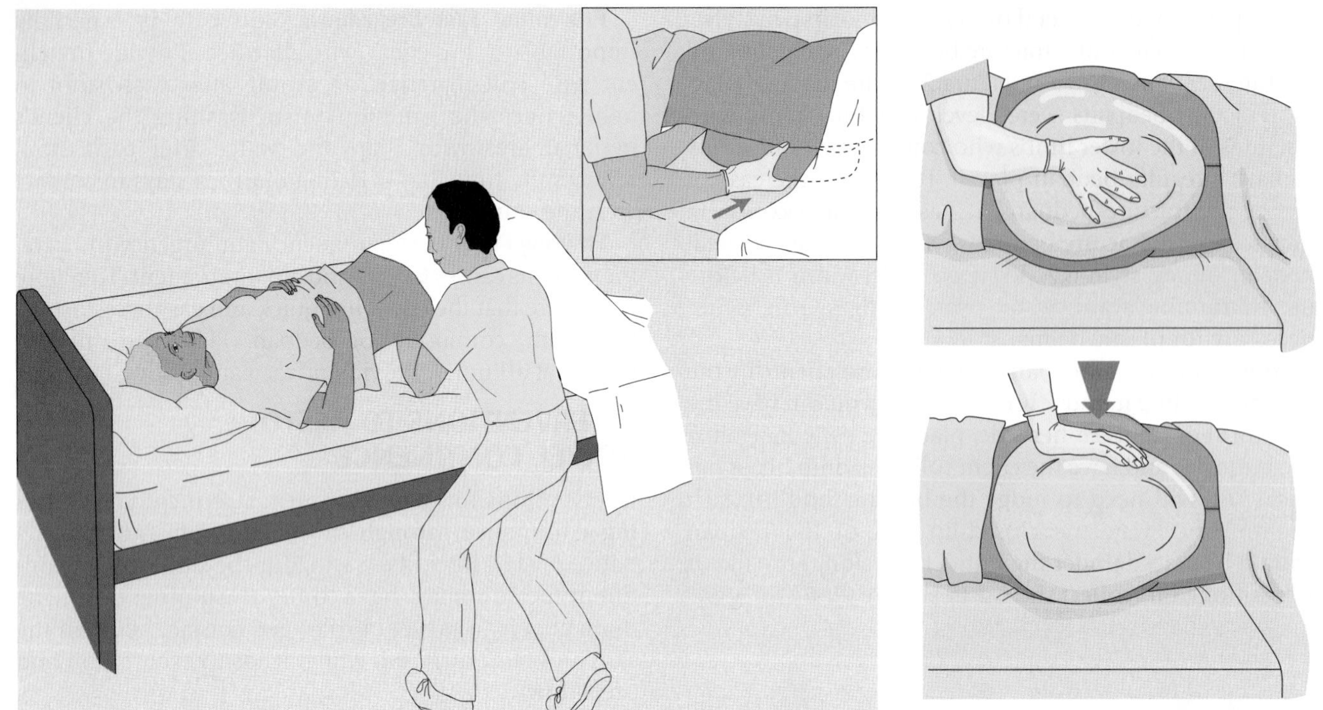

FIGURE 29-8 A, Privacy should not be compromised as the bedpan is placed under the client's raised hips. **B,** The bedpan should be placed with the inner rim encompassing the gluteal fold.

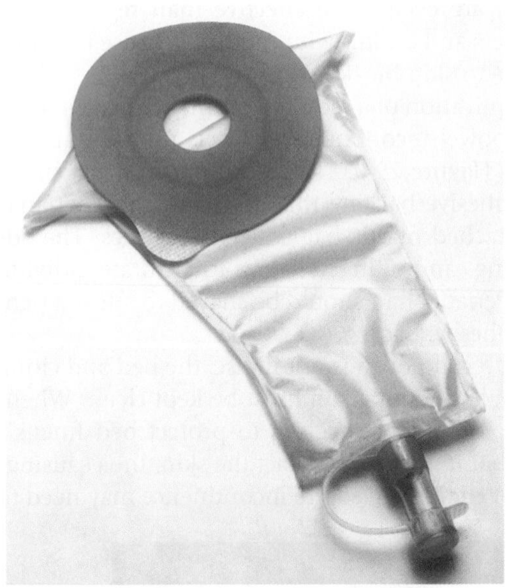

FIGURE 29-9 A rectal incontinence pouch. (Reproduced with permission of Hollister Inc., Libertyville, IL.)

waterproof undergarments to protect clothing. Adult-size disposable briefs are available with cellulose padding to draw fluid away from the skin by capillary action. However, they may make the person feel infantile and appear to give "permission" to be incontinent. Avoid using them whenever possible. The best way to reduce the physiological and psychological effects of incontinence is to reestablish bowel control.

Providing Bowel Training. Bowel training programs are effective for regaining bowel control. They require time, patience, and commitment from nurses and the client, but the results are well worth the effort.

First, assess and diagnose the factors causing the incontinence. Then, discuss bowel training with the client and significant others. Together, decide on a routine for bowel elimination. Base the routine on the person's previous bowel habits and on alterations in bowel habits that have resulted from illness or trauma. In addition, note when the client is most likely to be incontinent during the day.

All bowel training programs include independent nursing measures used to aid normal defecation: diet, fluids, exercise, and maintenance of defecation patterns. Probably the most crucial element of the program is timing. The schedule for defecation should be carefully determined and then strictly followed. If possible, position the client on the commode or toilet at the designated time to take advantage of gravity.

Bowel programming is individualized, although there are many common factors. Habit training, control of diarrhea, and biofeedback are possible strategies for bowel programming. Most programs include stool softeners to facilitate passage of feces. This intervention is especially important for clients with spinal cord injuries or extreme debilitation, because they frequently cannot bear down. Suppositories may be used every 1 to 3 days to stimulate evacuation. In people with spinal cord injuries, the suppository is usually followed in 20 to 30 minutes by digital stimulation of the anal sphincter to augment stimulation of the defecation reflex. In some programs, enemas are used in place of the suppositories. Suppository or enema administration is usually discontinued as soon as bowel elimination can be maintained without them.

Modify the training program as needed until a successful routine is found. Generally, a person is kept on a particular program for at least 3 days before it is changed. This period allows you to be sure that changes are indeed necessary.

Other methods of treating incontinence are available. For example, biofeedback therapy works for some people. This method helps the client modify the incontinence using feedback from instruments. Surgical intervention to create new tissue sphincters has been tried. Electrical stimulation of sphincter control has also been successful in some cases.

INTERVENTIONS TO REDUCE FLATULENCE

The goal of therapy is to remove gas from the GI tract. The most effective and natural way to expel the flatus is by exercise. Exercise stimulates peristalsis, which speeds the transit time of the gas through the colon. Walking is the best method; however, if this is not possible, moving around in bed will help. Prevention is also important. Teach clients to avoid situations and substances that cause flatulence.

If simple, natural methods fail, you may need to use a rectal tube to allow gas to escape from the body. To insert a rectal tube into an adult, lubricate a No. 22 to No. 32 Fr rubber or plastic rectal tube and insert it about 10 cm (4 inches) into the rectum. Place the distal end of the tube into a collecting receptacle to catch any feces that may be expelled. Tape the tube in place and leave it there for 20 minutes or less. Longer periods may cause sphincter damage. Reinsert the tube every 2 or 3 hours if necessary.

Several medications may help to relieve flatulence. Simethicone-containing medications cause gas bubbles to coalesce, making them easier to expel. Some physicians order neostigmine to be given intramuscularly about 20 minutes before a rectal tube or return-flow enema is administered. Neostigmine increases GI motility and facilitates downward movement of the gas. However, this practice is controversial because of the drug's numerous side effects, such as dizziness, severe abdominal cramping, respiratory depression, and nausea and vomiting. If postnasal drip causes excessive air swallowing, a decongestant or antihistamine may eliminate the problem.

INTERVENTIONS TO MANAGE FECAL DIVERSIONS

As with any condition, fecal diversions must be assessed to detect problems and determine appropriate nursing interventions. Physiological problems vary depending on whether the type of ostomy is an ileostomy or colostomy (Figure 29-10).

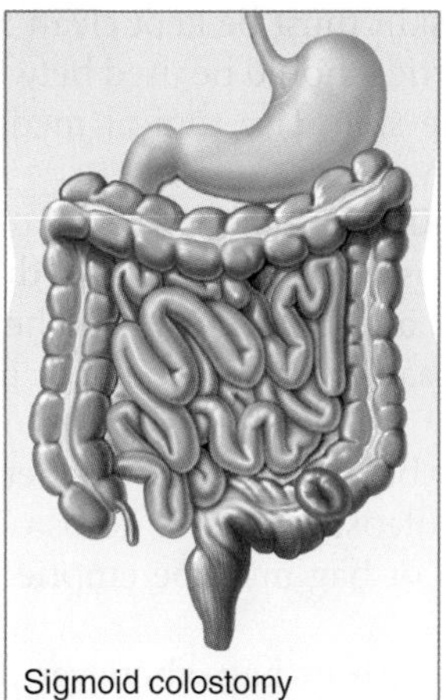

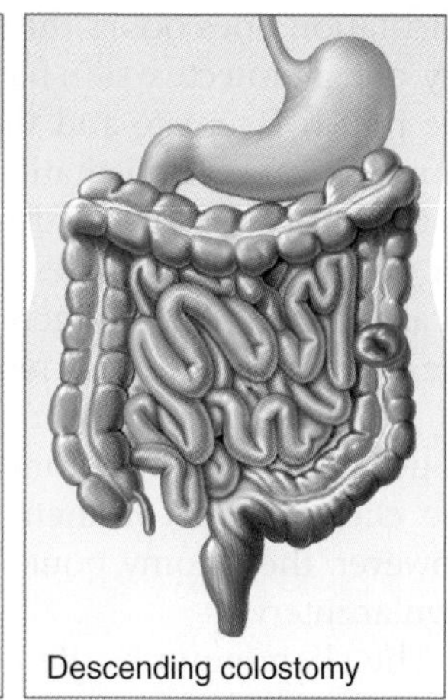

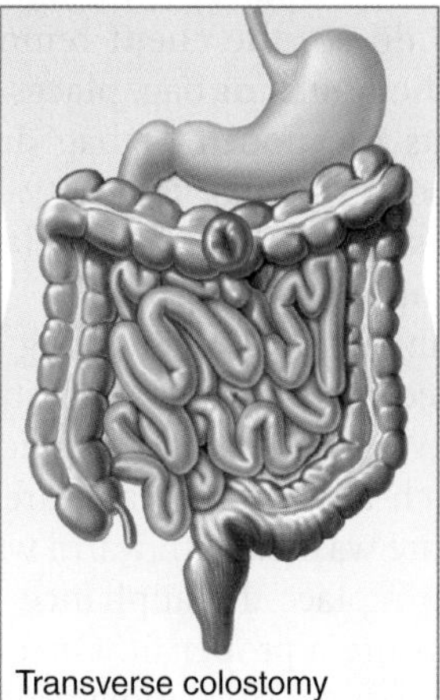

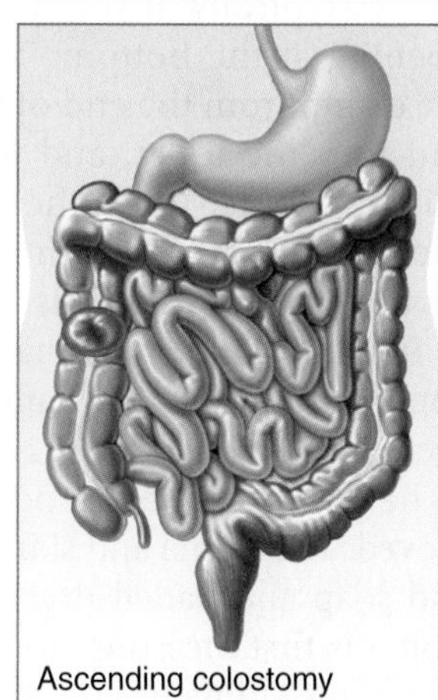

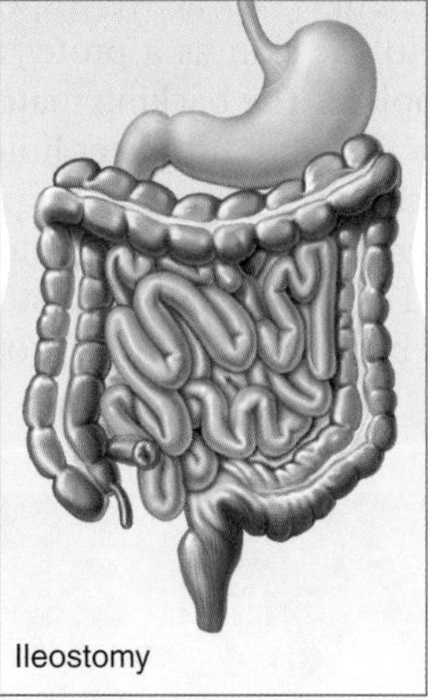

FIGURE 29-10 Locations of ileostomies and colostomies.

The major problems with ileostomies are obstruction, diarrhea, and skin irritation. Obstruction is prevented by chewing food thoroughly, and it can usually be relieved by massaging the abdomen around the stoma or by gentle lavage (washing out) of the stoma with a catheter. Diarrhea is treated as described earlier. The client with an ileostomy is particularly susceptible to fluid and electrolyte imbalances. Therefore diarrhea must be quickly controlled.

Skin irritation is best treated by preventive measures, such as proper fitting and fixation of the collection bag.

If irritation does occur, the skin must be kept clean and dry, and a protective skin barrier should be used between the pouch faceplate and the skin. Use topical medications to treat severe irritation.

Emptying and Changing the Ostomy Pouch or Bag. Except for continent ileostomies, ostomies continually drain fecal material. After surgery, and after the stoma heals, the client is fitted with a reusable ostomy pouch or bag. (A client with a colostomy usually wears an ostomy pouch rather than an ostomy bag.) Regardless of whether the client has a continent ileostomy or a colostomy, however, the ostomy pouch or bag must be emptied at regular intervals.

The client empties the pouch or bag whenever necessary (typically at the time of urination) through an opening at the bottom. To do so, the client removes the clamp from the end of the pouch or bag, places the end into the toilet, and lets the pouch or bag drain (Figure 29-11). Once the pouch or bag is empty, the client wipes the end with tissue and replaces the clamp on the end until it needs emptying again.

In addition to emptying an ostomy pouch or bag, the appliance needs to be changed when it is loose, or about every 3 days (Figure 29-12). When an ostomy bag needs to be changed, the old pouch and stoma wafer are removed. The stoma and skin are washed with warm water and soap and patted dry. To replace the appliance, the stoma is first measured to ensure a proper fit. Once the size of the stoma has been measured, the stoma wafer is cut to the proper size. If the client is very active, a special skin preparation is applied to the skin as a protectant. Next, an adhesive paste is applied. The backing material is removed from the stoma wafer, and the center hole of the stoma wafer is placed over the stoma with light pressure applied to ensure adherence to the skin. The ostomy pouch or bag is then snapped onto the ring of the stoma wafer. The ostomy pouch or bag may be closed or open at the end, depending on the location of the stoma and the client's preference.

Irrigating the Bowel. A colostomy can function adequately without irrigation, but irrigation helps to avoid fecal spillage during the day. Most clients are taught to care for their stomas and irrigate the bowel if necessary. Clients with a stoma who come into the hospital may prefer to continue their own care, or you may temporarily assume these tasks.

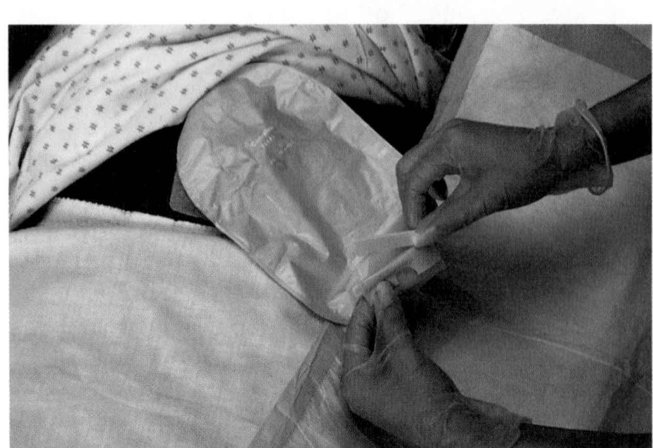

FIGURE 29-11 Emptying an ostomy pouch or bag.

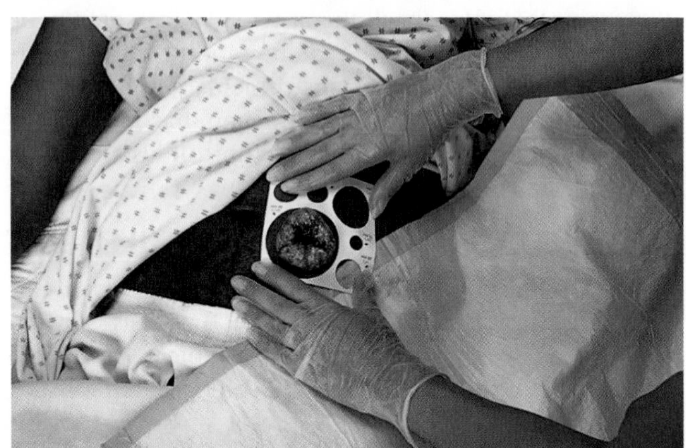

A

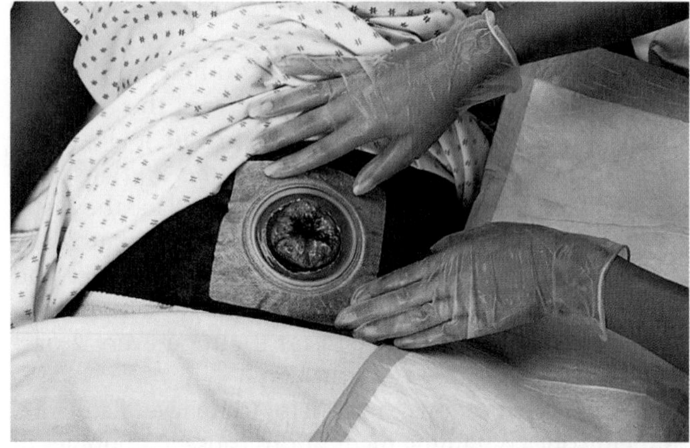

B

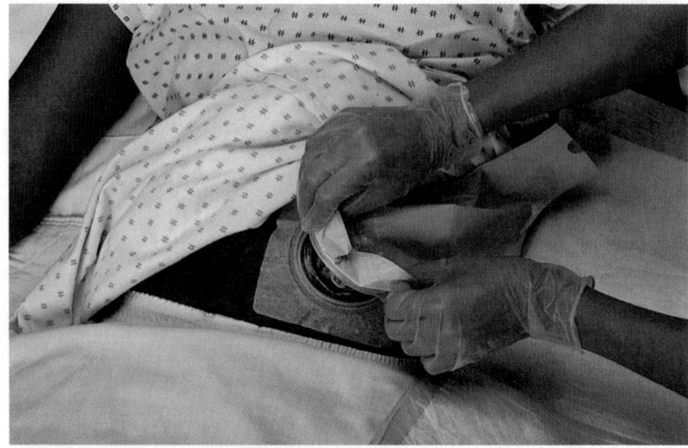

C

FIGURE 29-12 Changing an ostomy pouch or bag. **A,** Measure the stoma size to ensure a proper fit. **B,** Place the center hole of the stoma wafer over the stoma. **C,** Snap the ostomy pouch or bag onto the ring of the stoma wafer.

Irrigation of a colostomy is very similar to administration of a normal saline enema. The major differences are the insertion site and the client's inability to control the expulsion of solution and fecal material. Consequently, some variation in equipment and technique is necessary. An irrigation sleeve channels the expelled contents into the toilet or bedpan. This is a plastic tunnel that fits around the stoma and is held in place by a belt around the waist (Figure 29-13). The irrigating solution and enema equipment are prepared as for a volume enema. Cone-shaped irrigation tips are preferred to catheters because they reduce the danger of bowel perforation. The nipple cone also seals off the stoma so that the irrigating fluid cannot leak. Make sure of the location of the stoma before inserting the cone. If using a catheter, gently insert it about 7.5 to 10 cm (3 to 4 inches) and infuse the solution.

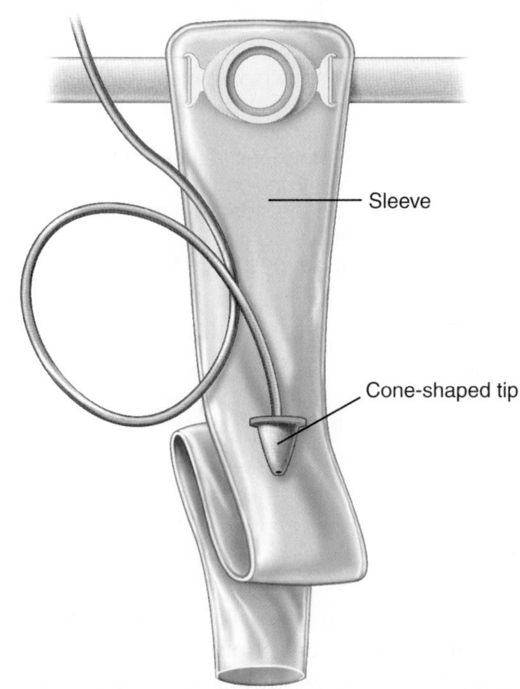

FIGURE 29-13 Sleeve and cone-shaped tip for colostomy irrigation.

When you are ready to remove the administration tip, be sure the irrigating sleeve is well in front of the stoma, because the initial drainage may gush out. Close the top of the sleeve with clips, and allow most of the contents to be expelled. This usually takes about 10 to 15 minutes. Control odor by occasionally rinsing the sleeve with water and flushing the toilet. When the client is sure that the irrigation returns have finished, the irrigation sleeve may be removed, the peristomal skin cleaned, and either a clean pouch or dressing applied.

Teaching the Client Ostomy Self-Care. Clients with ostomies should be taught to live independently and care for their ostomy needs on their own, if possible. Changing the ostomy pouch or bag is the first step in learning and is the same as the procedure just described. If the client will be irrigating the colostomy, the irrigation procedure needs to be taught. Odor control and medication use are other topics of concern (Box 29-6).

For the ostomate who wears a pouch, odor control can be a problem. Careful washing, pouch deodorizers, and medications are possible solutions. The client should also avoid gas-forming foods. Cabbage, cauli-

BOX 29-6 *Teaching for Self-Care*

Ostomy Care

Purpose: To make the client independent in the management of bowel elimination in the presence of an ostomy.
Expected Outcome: The client will demonstrate the ability to manage bowel elimination through an ostomy, prevent complications, and manage lifestyle changes.

Client Instructions

Maintain a regular bowel elimination pattern by following these steps

- Plan for daily elimination at a time most consistent with the urge to defecate.
- Keep in mind that regular patterns of meals and activity may be helpful.

Maintain the necessary supplies

- Skin barriers
- Ostomy pouches
- A pouch belt, if needed
- Clamps or closing devices
- Hypoallergenic tape
- Towel and washcloths
- A mild skin cleanser

Use a pouching system to collect waste from the bowel

- Ensure a proper fit of the pouch to prevent leaks and protect your skin.
- Measure the stoma diameter, and prepare a skin barrier/pouch with each pouch change. The opening should be no more than 1/8 inch larger than your stoma. Measure the stoma weekly for at least 8 weeks or until the stoma has stopped shrinking.
- Apply the skin barrier first. Then ensure that there are no wrinkles in the barrier.
- Apply the pouch to the barrier. Center and apply the pouch. Practice applying the pouch while sitting and standing.
- Change the appliance any time it leaks or is not intact.
- To remove the ostomy appliance, support the skin of your abdomen and gently loosen the seal.
- Cleanse the skin around the stoma. Waste from an ileostomy is especially irritating to the skin.
- Use a mild soap, and carefully dry the area with a clean cloth or towel.

Continued

BOX 29-6 *Teaching for Self-Care—cont'd*

Ostomy Care—cont'd

Use a pouching system to collect waste from the bowel, cont'd
- Choose an ostomy pouch with an open end or a closed end. An open-ended pouch is best for liquid wastes, and the bag can be emptied without changing it.
- Use a clamp that you can manage easily, given your eyesight and manual dexterity.
- Empty an ileostomy pouch when it is one third full. Empty a colostomy pouch as needed.
- To close the pouch, fold the tail up once around the bar of the clamp and fasten the clamp.

Keep in mind the following lifestyle tips
- Avoid foods that cause odor and gas.
- Do whatever you need to do to avoid constipation.
- Treat diarrhea promptly.
- Check periodically to make sure that your ostomy is not blocked.
- Drink 6 to 8 glasses of water daily, 10 to 12 if you have an ileostomy.
- Exercise regularly, especially to strengthen abdominal muscles.
- You can bathe and shower with or without the pouch.
- You can swim with the pouch, but use waterproof tape around edges of the pouch in a picture-frame fashion.
- You can continue to wear your normal wardrobe after an ostomy. No change in clothing is necessary.

Manage skin irritation
- Assess for irregularities in the skin that might cause leaks.
- Use a skin barrier to protect the skin.
- Use a skin barrier paste, if needed, to fill in any abdominal creases or irregular contours.
- Change pouching systems to maintain or create a well-functioning appliance.
- Add an ostomy belt, if needed.
- Notify your health care provider if you detect the following signs and symptoms of a *Candida* (yeast) infection: itching, burning, pain around the stoma, redness of the skin, or whiteheads (pustules).
- Apply an antifungal powder or spray, such as Mycostatin, to the skin around the stoma.

Follow a dietary plan
- Follow a well-balanced diet.
- Watch for foods that cause gas or changes in the consistency of your stool.
- Avoid foods that tend to block your stoma.

flower, onions, and turnips often increase fecal odor. Yogurt, buttermilk, parsley, and green leafy vegetables may reduce fecal odor. Odor control, which can be very distressing, can be managed by the following:
- Carefully washing the appliance after use
- Placing a deodorizing agent in the pouch
- Using internal medications, such as bismuth subgallate
- Ingesting yogurt, buttermilk, parsley, or orange juice
- Placing a few drops of Dispatch in the collection receptacle to mask the odor while emptying the pouch

Review of the new ostomate's medication regimen can help eliminate contraindicated medications. Diuretics, laxatives, enteric-coated medications, and sustained-release oral medications are usually not administered for the ileostomate and some colostomates.

EVALUATION

Evaluation of nursing care for the management of bowel elimination problems involves making decisions about the expected time frame for the intervention to be successful, ongoing monitoring, and measuring the parameters of the outcome criteria. Decision making is centered on whether the problem is acute or chronic. Look for data that suggest the problem is improving, the client is participating in care, and the problem is resolving.

Evaluation of the effectiveness of interventions for constipation is based on ongoing assessment to determine that the problem is resolving. When the problem is constipation, the client should have a bowel movement usually within 24 hours of the onset of treatment. Collect data to determine that the signs and symptoms of constipation are not persistent. When the problem is chronic, data are collected over time to determine that the client establishes a regular pattern of elimination without the signs and symptoms of constipation (Box 29-7).

Evaluation of the effectiveness of interventions for diarrhea requires ongoing monitoring to determine that the diarrhea is resolving, usually within the first 24 hours. Monitor for signs of dehydration and electrolyte loss. Intake and output measurements should be taken. The time frame for diarrhea resolution is directly related to the cause of the diarrhea. For example, some viral infections may have a natural course of 24 to 48 hours. On the other hand, a client with inflammatory bowel disease will have outcome criteria that suggest the problem is controlled rather than cured.

For the problem of fecal impaction, the initial outcome criterion is that the impaction has been removed. Long-term goals are set to prevent the problem from recurring. The client's bowel management program must be modified on an ongoing basis.

For the problem of bowel incontinence, the time frame for evaluation depends on the cause of the problem. If the cause is a medication combined with weakness from an acute illness, the problem can often be resolved quickly. If

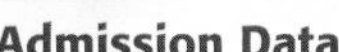

BOX 29-7

Nursing Care Plan

A Client With Constipation

Admission Data

Dr. Daly reported that yesterday he consumed only one fourth of his usual intake of prune juice and bran flakes for breakfast. He consumed only half of his other two meals because of severe pain from bone cancer. He reported that he was concerned about increasing his morphine for fear of falling and other side effects.

Because Mr. Daly is having difficulty with his bowel elimination this morning, the nurse realizes that his nursing diagnosis of *Constipation* may lead to impaction.

Physician's Orders

Diet as desired
Laxative of choice

Nursing Assessment

Dr. Daly has not had his usual bowel movement in 3 days, his bowel sounds are hypoactive, and a fecal mass can be palpated in his lower abdomen. Therefore the nurse considers the possibility of an impaction.

NANDA-I Nursing Diagnosis	NOC Expected Outcomes With Indicators	NIC Interventions With Selected Activities	Evaluation Data
Constipation	***Bowel Elimination***	***Bowel Management***	***After 24 Hours of Care***
Related Factors: • Decreased mobility and morphine use	• Elimination pattern in expected range • Stool soft and formed • Constipation not present • Ease of stool passage • Comfort of stool passage	• Note date of last bowel movement (BM).	• Laxative administered at client's request. Large, hard, formed BM today.
		• Monitor BM frequency, consistency, shape, volume, and color.	• Passage was difficult.
		• Monitor bowel sounds.	• Will continue his usual routine of a high-fiber breakfast.
		• Report diminished bowel sounds.	• Bowel sounds are active.
		• Monitor for signs and symptoms of constipation and impaction.	
		• Teach about alternative foods that help in promoting bowel regularity. • Instruct in foods that are high in fiber.	• Dr. Daly verbalizes foods that promote bowel regularity, including high-fiber food.
		• Give warm liquids after meals as appropriate.	• Dr. Daly drinks warm liquids according to preference.
		• Evaluate medication profile for gastrointestinal side effects.	• Continued monitoring of side effects of morphine is indicated.
		• Allow client choices in bowel management.	• Dr. Daly reports satisfaction with choices in bowel management.

Critical Thinking Questions

1. How would you prevent further constipation in Dr. Daly?
2. Is reducing the dose of morphine an acceptable method of preventing constipation in this client?
3. The client prefers to use fiber as a means of managing constipation. What would you say to him about continuing to use this method?

Nursing outcome and intervention labels from Johnson, M., Bulechek, G., Butcher, H., Dochterman, J. M., Maas, M., Moorhead, S., et al. (Eds.). (2006). *NANDA, NOC, and NIC linkages: Nursing diagnoses, outcomes, & interventions.* St. Louis, MO: Mosby.

the problem is a permanent change in mental status combined with immobility, management will be ongoing. It may take several weeks to determine the best schedule of toileting to prevent bowel incontinence.

The nurse enters the following note into the chart about Dr. Daly's constipation.

SAMPLE DOCUMENTATION FOR DR. DALY

Reports relief of constipation. Will resume his usual routine of a high-fiber breakfast and a warm drink with breakfast.

▼ KEY PRINCIPLES

- The lower GI tract is the main organ system responsible for the elimination of the body's solid waste. It consists of the ascending, transverse, descending, and sigmoid portions of the colon, and the rectum.
- Physiological and psychosocial factors have a strong influence on the act of defecation.
- Assessment of bowel elimination needs includes noting the history of psychological and physiological factors affecting elimination; completing a physical assessment of the abdomen and observing fecal characteristics; and noting the outcome of diagnostic tests completed by radiographic examination, direct visualization, and laboratory analysis.

Continued

- The current NANDA-I list of nursing diagnoses relevant to bowel elimination needs includes *Bowel incontinence, Constipation, Perceived constipation,* and *Diarrhea.*
- The nurse does not order diagnostic tests but, along with assessment findings, does use the results in diagnosing nursing problems.
- Interventions to treat acute constipation would meet the goals of rapid relief from the acute problem and reestablishing a regular bowel elimination pattern; for chronic constipation, the goal is to help the client establish a long-term plan of management.
- Interventions to treat diarrhea would meet the goals of no loose stools and a return of regular bowel elimination pattern.
- Interventions to treat bowel incontinence would meet the goals of maintaining skin integrity and promoting normal bowel elimination.
- Evaluation of outcomes should show that the fecal contents and bowel movements are as near to normal as possible for the client, or that the client has adapted successfully to elimination changes.

REVIEW QUESTIONS

1. You are giving instructions about using GoLYTELY as a preparation for a colonoscopy. The advantage of GoLYTELY over traditional laxatives is that GoLYTELY:

1. Is less likely to change the fluid and electrolyte balance of the body
2. Tastes better than traditional laxatives
3. Is easier for the client to take than traditional laxatives
4. Is less time consuming for the client than traditional laxatives

2. Which is the most important information to determine when assessing a client's complaint of diarrhea?

1. Whether the stool is dark brown, green, or light brown
2. Whether the client also complains of malaise, anorexia, and headache
3. Whether the client complains of flatus, pain, and urgency
4. Whether the client has lost a large volume of fluid

3. Which of the following is the most characteristic sign of a fecal impaction?

1. Abdominal distention and absence of a bowel movement for 3 days
2. Passing a small amount of loose stool six or more times during a day
3. Passing a small hard mass of stool
4. Complaint of distention, abdominal discomfort, and flatus

4. Which type of enema is indicated specifically for passing a hard mass of stool?

1. Cleansing normal saline enema
2. Oil retention enema
3. Tap water enema
4. Hypertonic saline enema

5. Which of the following menus would be most effective in preventing constipation?

1. Spaghetti with meat sauce, white bread, and 6 ounces of apple juice
2. A medium apple, a sandwich with whole grain bread, fresh vegetable salad
3. Turkey breast with gravy over white rice, and tomato soup
4. Corn flakes with a small amount of milk and a boiled egg

Bibliography

Arora, R., & Srinivasan, R. (2005). Is polyethylene glycol safe and effective for chronic constipation in children? *Archives of Disease in Childhood, 90*(6), 643-646.

Birmingham, K. (2005). Debunking constipation myths. *Gastrointestinal Nursing, 3*(1), 6.

Debunking 12 myths of constipation. (2005). *Geriatrics, 60*(3), 18.

*Fish, C. (1995). *In good hands: The keeping of a family farm.* New York: Farrar, Straus & Giroux.

Fletcher, K. (2005). Elimination: Geriatric self-learning module. *MEDSURG Nursing, 14*(2), 127-131.

Gardiner, P., & Kemper, K. J. (2005). For GI complaints: which herbs and supplements spell relief? *Contemporary Pediatrics, 22*(8), 50-55.

Hunter, M. (2004). When antibiotics go wrong. *Gastrointestinal Nursing, 2*(3), 14-17.

Johnson, M., Bulechek, G., Butcher, H., Dochterman, J. M., Maas, M., Moorhead, S., et al. (Eds.). (2006). *NANDA, NOC, and NIC linkages: Nursing diagnoses, outcomes, & interventions.* St. Louis, MO: Mosby.

Kyle, G., Prynn, P., & Oliver, H. (2005). A procedure for the digital removal of faeces. *Nursing Standard, 19*(20), 33-39.

Laxatives: Dealing with irregularity. (2005). *Mayo Clinic Health Letter, 23*(6), 4-5.

*Leininger, M. M. (1991). *Culture care diversity and universality: A theory of nursing.* New York: National League for Nursing Press.

Lu, N., Samuels, M. E., Shi, L., Baker, S. L., Glover, S. H., & Sanders, J. M. (2004). Child day care risks of common infectious diseases revisited. *Child: Care, Health and Development, 30*(4), 361-368.

Mardini, H. E., & de Villiers, W. J. S. (2005). Preventing outbreaks of *Clostridium difficile*–associated diarrhea in LTC facilities. *Long-Term Care Interface, 6*(3), 48-56.

Mauk, K. L. (2005). Healthier aging. Preventing constipation in older adults. *Nursing, 35*(6), 22-23.

NANDA International. (2007). *Nursing diagnoses: Definitions & classification, 2006-2007* (7th ed.). Philadelphia: Author.

Picker, L. (2005). Constipation cures. *Parents, 80*(9), 105-107.

Rogers, J. (2005). Reducing the misery of constipation in children. *Practice Nursing, 16*(1), 12, 14-16.

Rudy, C. (2005). Case studies: Primary care—I have a tummy ache. *Journal of Pediatric Health Care, 19*(5), 314-315, 339-341.

Symeou, H. (2005). Current thinking and practice in healthcare for older people. *Geriatric Medicine, 35*(9), 70, 72.

Vesta, K. S., Wells, P. G., Gentry, C. A., & Stipek, W. J. (2005). Specific risk factors for *Clostridium difficile*–associated diarrhea: A prospective, multicenter, case control evaluation. *American Journal of Infection Control, 33*(8), 469-472.

Walker, B. W. (2004). Assessing gastrointestinal infections. *Nursing, 34*(5), 48-52.

Williams, L. (2005). Liability landscape. Handling constipation and fecal impaction. *Nursing Homes/Long Term Care Management, 54*(4), 64, 66-67.

Wondergem, F. (2005). Relieving constipation. *Journal of Community Nursing, 19*(5), 12-14, 16.

*Asterisk indicates a classic or definitive work on this subject.

Chapter 30

Managing Urinary Elimination

Media Resources

- Nursing Skills Online
- evolve Evolve Website http://evolve.elsevier.com/Harkreader/
- Companion CD
- 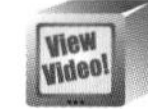 Skills Video Clips

Learning Objectives

After studying this chapter, you should be able to do the following:

- Describe the normal structure and function of the urinary system
- Identify common problems of urinary elimination
- Discuss factors affecting urinary elimination
- Assess urinary function, and identify a client experiencing urinary elimination problems
- Diagnose problems of urinary elimination that can be managed with nursing care
- Plan expected outcomes for goal-directed nursing interventions for managing problems in urinary elimination
- Implement basic nursing care for a client experiencing problems with urinary elimination
- Evaluate care for a person experiencing problems with urinary elimination

Key Terms

anuria
bacteriuria
diuresis
dysuria
enuresis
functional urinary incontinence
hematuria
Kegel exercises
micturition
nocturia
oliguria
polyuria
reflex urinary incontinence
residual urine
stress urinary incontinence
total urinary incontinence
urge urinary incontinence
urinalysis
urinary frequency
urinary hesitancy
urinary incontinence
urinary retention
urinary urgency
urination
void

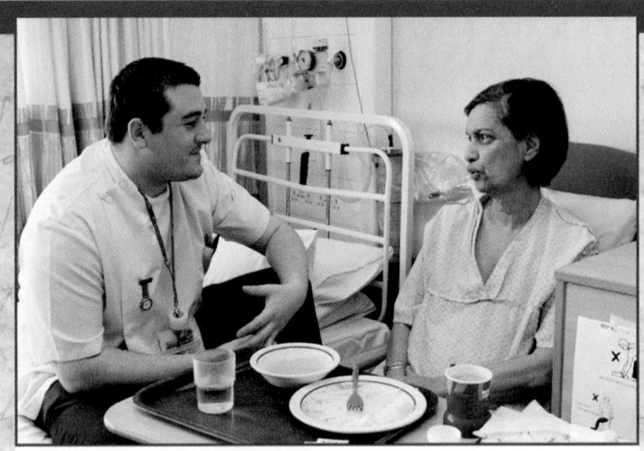

Mrs. Alia Al-Kandari is a 60-year-old who came to the United States from her home in Kuwait. She and her husband are here on a temporary visa with her husband. She developed painless vaginal bleeding and was diagnosed with cancer of the uterus. She is 2 days post vaginal hysterectomy and has a Foley catheter. The nurse knows Mrs. Al-Kandari will likely need assistance reestablishing a normal pattern of urinary elimination after removal of the catheter, and considers the diagnosis of *Risk for urinary retention* from the list of possible urinary elimination nursing diagnoses. She is also concerned about providing privacy during this highly personal aspect of nursing care.

KEY NURSING DIAGNOSES FOR URINARY ELIMINATION

Stress urinary incontinence: A loss of urine of less than 50 mL occurring with increased abdominal pressure

Reflex urinary incontinence: An involuntary loss of urine, occurring at somewhat predictable intervals when a specific bladder volume is reached

Urge urinary incontinence: Involuntary passage of urine occurring soon after a strong sense of urgency to void

Functional urinary incontinence: Inability of a usually continent person to reach toilet in time to avoid unintentional loss of urine

Total urinary incontinence: A continuous and unpredictable loss of urine

Urinary retention: Incomplete emptying of the bladder

CONCEPTS OF URINARY ELIMINATION

As a nurse, you will assess urinary elimination in a wide variety of clients to determine their health practices and to identify any urinary problems they may be having. For example, your client may be an outpatient who needs teaching to manage urinary dysfunction; the family of a homebound, disabled, incontinent person; or an older adult who has undergone a surgical procedure for cancer of the bladder. Community health nurses are also involved with screening and health teaching to manage urinary elimination. Nursing diagnoses involve either incontinence or retention, but you also will assist clients with problems associated with infection, obstruction, and urinary diversion.

Normal urination depends on the production of urine, adequate function of the lower urinary tract, cognitive function, physical mobility, and access to toilet facilities. Personal habits and health practices may enhance or impede normal urinary elimination. Some urinary problems are associated with particular age-groups.

STRUCTURE AND FUNCTION OF THE URINARY SYSTEM

The structures of the urinary system are the kidneys, ureters, bladder, and urethra (Figure 30-1). The kidneys filter the blood to remove waste products from the body and to regulate water, electrolyte, and acid-base balance; this results in the formation of urine. The ureters are two small muscular tubes that carry the urine from the kidneys to the bladder, where the urine is stored until the bladder fills enough to produce an urge to urinate. Then urine is allowed to pass out of the body through the urethra.

Kidneys. The two bean-shaped kidneys are anatomically located for maximum protection of these vital organs. They are retroperitoneal, positioned on the upper, posterior wall of the abdomen outside the peritoneal cavity. They are protected posteriorly by the eleventh and twelfth ribs and anteriorly by the abdominal cavity.

The kidneys form and excrete urine through a process of filtering the blood and concentrating waste products for excretion. The waste products are urea (from metabolism of amino acids), creatinine (from muscle creatine), uric acid (from nucleic acids), the products of hemoglobin breakdown (such as bilirubin), and metabolites of various hormones (Guyton & Hall, 2006).

The kidneys also control the electrolyte composition of the blood and body fluids. Most of the potassium that passes through the kidneys is excreted. Although the kidneys excrete or conserve sodium in response to blood levels of sodium, they are a poor conservator of potassium. They maintain the proper acid-base balance primarily by excreting or conserving bicarbonate ions and by excreting acids produced by the metabolism of proteins.

Adequate blood flow and oxygen are essential to renal function. Although each kidney is only about the size of

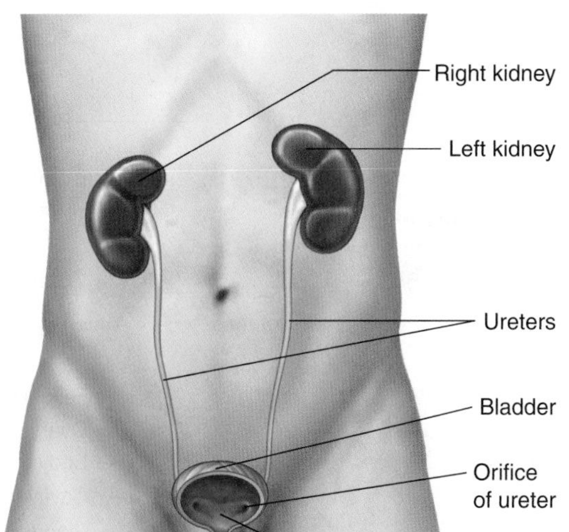

FIGURE 30-1 Structures of the urinary system.

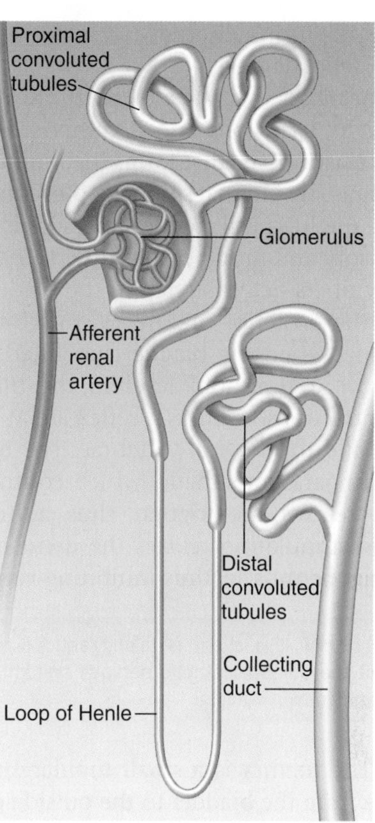

FIGURE 30-2 The renal nephron is a complex system consisting of the glomerulus, where the arterial blood is filtered, and the convoluted tubules and loop of Henle, where reabsorption controls acid-base and electrolyte balance.

an orange and weighs only about 150 g, the two together receive a blood flow equal to about 21% of the cardiac output. The kidneys play a role in maintaining this blood flow through their ability to control arterial pressure. One mechanism by which the kidneys control arterial pressure is through the excretion of water and sodium. Another is through the excretion of renin from the juxtaglomerular cells. Renin contributes to the formation of vasoactive substances such as angiotensin II. The kidney is also self-protective through the production of erythropoietin in response to hypoxia, which in turn stimulates the production of red blood cells.

> ***Action Alert!*** Monitor urinary output as an indicator of renal function, especially when cardiac output is diminished—for example, when the client is in a state of shock.

The nephron is the functional unit of the kidney and consists of a glomerulus and a tubule system. The glomerulus filters water, electrolytes, and waste products from the plasma, and the tubule system controls reabsorption to maintain a balance of electrolytes, buffers, and acids in the body. Glucose and amino acids are completely reabsorbed by the tubules. Water and electrolytes are selectively reabsorbed, depending on the body's need. Waste products, such as creatinine, are almost completely excreted, with little reabsorption. Once urine enters the pelvis of the kidney, it passes unchanged through the ureters to the bladder. Urine is about 95% water. In the renal nephron shown in Figure 30-2, notice the glomerulus, where the arterial blood is filtered, and the system of tubules that controls the resorption of water and electrolytes.

Ureters. The ureters are smooth, muscular tubes of small diameter that connect the kidneys to the bladder. Urine is propelled through the ureters by peristaltic waves. These peristaltic contractions are enhanced by parasympathetic stimulation and inhibited by sympathetic stimulation. The ureters are well supplied with nerve endings, and obstruction usually results in severe pain.

Bladder. The urinary bladder is a body cavity composed primarily of a smooth muscle known as the detrusor muscle. The mucosal surface of the detrusor lies in folds, or rugae, that allow for expansion of the bladder. The trigone muscle is a triangle-shaped muscle at the base of the posterior side of the bladder. The apex of the trigone is in the bladder neck at the posterior opening of the urethra. The ureters enter the bladder through the detrusor at the upper angles of the trigone.

Each ureter enters the bladder obliquely through the detrusor muscle and passes 1 to 2 cm through the detrusor before entering the body of the bladder at the upper trigone angle. The placement of the ureters through the detrusor muscle creates a vesicoureteral valve. The tone of the detrusor muscle collapses the ureter and prevents backflow of the urine into the ureters and renal pelvis. Incompetence of this valve allows urine reflux, or backward flow, into the renal pelvis, thus creating pressure on the nephrons. Excessive or prolonged pressure could cause renal damage.

The funnel-shaped bladder neck at the base of the bladder is 2 to 3 cm long and is composed of detrusor muscle and elastic tissue that forms the internal sphincter for the urethra. The internal sphincter prevents urine from entering the urethra until a critical pressure is reached.

Both sensory and motor nerves innervate the bladder. The sensory fibers detect stretch in the bladder wall, especially in the posterior urethra. A conscious desire to urinate occurs when the bladder has filled, producing tension above a threshold level in the bladder wall. Bladder contractions occur as a reflex arc at the level of the second and third sacral vertebrae. The motor fibers are primarily parasympathetic, which contracts the detrusor and relaxes the trigone, thus aiding voiding. Sympathetic stimulation relaxes the detrusor and contracts the trigone muscle, thus inhibiting voiding.

Action Alert! If a client is taking anticholinergic drugs, which inhibit the parasympathetic nervous system, you should observe for difficulty in voiding.

Urethra. The urethra is a small tubular structure that drains urine from the bladder to the outside of the body. Its mucous membrane is continuous with that of the bladder. Contraction of the detrusor muscle increases pressure in the bladder to produce the urge to urinate and to aid in emptying of the bladder. The urge to urinate is experienced when pressure in the bladder overcomes the internal sphincter and urine enters the urethra.

The urethra also has an external sphincter composed of voluntary skeletal muscle in the floor of the pelvis. It can be contracted consciously to prevent urination. Urination requires relaxation of the external sphincter. When the person is ready to urinate, the external sphincter is consciously relaxed and the abdominal muscles are contracted to assist in **micturition**, the process of emptying the bladder.

The urethra in females is about 3 cm (1½ inches) long. It curves obliquely downward and forward. In males, the urethra is about 20 cm (8 to 9 inches) long. It has a double curve when the penis is flaccid and a single curve when the penis is erect. The male urethra also serves as a passageway for semen to exit the body. The male prostate gland lies at the neck of the bladder, about 1½ inches from where the ureters enter the bladder, and it surrounds the urethra. Figure 30-3 illustrates the male and female genitourinary tracts.

Physiology of Urination. **Urination** is the term commonly used for the act of micturition. **Void** is synonymous with micturition and urination, and it is the term that you will hear most often in clinical settings. Clients may or may not be familiar with these terms and may instead use slang or vernacular expressions to refer to urination.

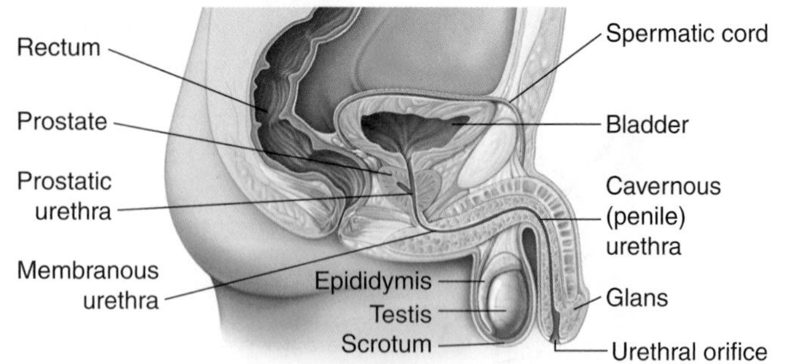

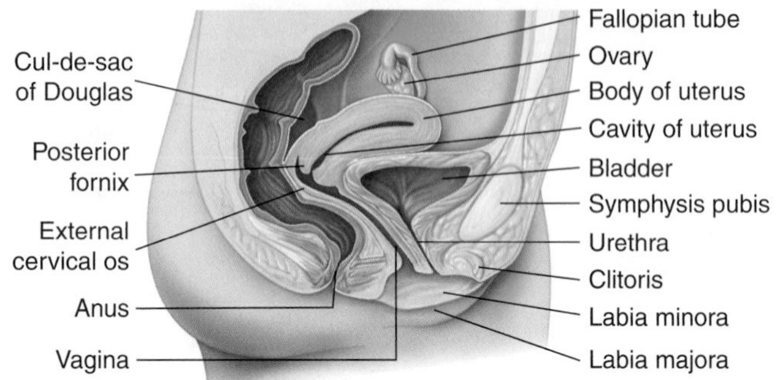

FIGURE 30-3. The male **(A)** and female **(B)** genitourinary tracts. In the female, the bladder is anterior and inferior to the uterus. The urethra opens immediately anterior to the vagina.

As the bladder fills, waves of contractions begin. They occur every 5 to 60 seconds. With each contraction, the pressure rises and the person may feel an urge to void. At this point, however, voiding can easily be delayed. If a person waits less than a minute, the urge usually passes. When the bladder reaches a volume of 300 to 400 mL of urine, pressure rises rapidly and the urge to void becomes strong. Keep in mind, however, that bladder size is an important component of the urge to void. For example, very young and very old people may have small bladders. The urge to void may be strong when the bladder size reaches only about 150 mL.

The cerebral cortex exerts final control over voiding. Normally, all the urine is emptied from the bladder, but 5 to 10 mL may remain.

PROBLEMS WITH URINARY ELIMINATION

As a nurse, you will encounter clients with various problems of urinary elimination, such as dysuria, altered amounts of urine, enuresis, incontinence, retention, urinary tract infection (UTI), obstruction, or diversion.

Dysuria. **Dysuria** refers to difficult or painful urination. It may be accompanied by frequency, hesitancy, or urgency of urination. **Urinary frequency** refers to urination that occurs at shorter-than-usual intervals without an increase in daily urine output. **Urinary hesitancy** refers to a delay in starting the urine stream, commonly with a decreased force of the stream. **Urinary urgency** is a sudden, forceful urge to urinate. Further assessment is needed to determine the cause of these problems.

Often, dysuria is related to irritation, inflammation, or obstruction of the lower urinary tract, where sensory nerve endings are plentiful. Pain immediately before voiding may be related to an irritated or distended bladder. Pain at the start of the stream indicates an irritated bladder neck. Pain at the end of voiding is usually associated with bladder spasms.

Action Alert! Ask questions to determine the specific timing and nature of pain associated with dysuria.

Altered Amount. The amount of urine varies normally with the amount of fluid ingested and the amount lost through the skin, lungs, and bowels. However, altered amounts of urine can also indicate health problems. **Oliguria** is a diminished, scanty amount of urine. It can result from dehydration, a lower-than-normal volume of body water that in turn reduces urine output. Production of less than 30 mL of urine per hour may reflect a blood flow that is inadequate to maintain renal function. This can result in permanent kidney damage.

Anuria is the absence of urine, usually clinically defined as less than 100 mL in 24 hours. It occurs in renal failure, shock, or dehydration.

Polyuria is an excess amount of urine; it is usually associated with diabetes mellitus (a disturbance in the utilization of glucose secondary to inadequate production of insulin) or diabetes insipidus (caused by failure of the pituitary gland to secrete the antidiuretic hormone). Polyuria also may be caused by excess intake. It is sometimes seen with head injuries. Although any amount over the intake might be called polyuria, the term usually refers to amounts greatly in excess of intake, or to amounts greater than 2000 mL in 24 hours.

Enuresis. Enuresis is recurrent involuntary urination that occurs during sleep. Bed-wetting during sleep is not considered a problem until a child has reached the age when bladder control can reasonably be expected. For example, only about 30% of 4-year-olds and 7% of 8-year-olds wet the bed during sleep.

However, bed-wetting without a functional disorder does occur in a small percentage of older children, even as late as adolescence. Functional nocturnal enuresis typically runs in families and is sometimes associated with stage IV sleep, a small bladder capacity, allergy attacks, and urinary tract infections. It may be related to the maturity of the brain and the production of antidiuretic hormone during the night. All children without underlying medical problems grow out of enuresis.

Action Alert! When a parent expresses concerns about enuresis, provide information and instructions about whether to see a physician for an evaluation. Although only a small number of children have physical problems underlying enuresis, a thorough physical examination is important to rule out underlying causes.

Urinary Incontinence. Urinary incontinence is the involuntary passage of urine. It can be transient (acute) or persistent (chronic). Transient incontinence can be associated with a medical or surgical condition and resolves when the underlying cause is removed. Persistent incontinence continues over time and may become worse. However, it is often treatable.

Persistent incontinence is highly associated with the cognitive and physical impairments occurring with advanced age. Identifying the specific type of persistent incontinence experienced by a client (stress, urge, overflow, reflex, and functional) may be useful in selecting interventions, but incontinence commonly results from a mix of problems and may respond only to a comprehensive treatment approach.

Urinary incontinence affects about 13 million Americans. The prevalence of incontinence increases with age, but it should not be considered a normal part of the aging process. Approximately 42% of community-dwelling older women report symptoms of urinary incontinence (Goode, 2005) Among adults more than 60 years of age, women usually have a likelihood of urinary incontinence at least twice that of men. Among residents of nursing homes, the prevalence is generally above 40%, and in some facilities approaches 80% (Merkelj, 2001). Incontinence is strongly associated with factors leading to institutionalization, such as dementia and immobility. In the noninstitutionalized, incontinence interferes with excursions outside the home, social interactions, and sexual activity. It may threaten self-esteem and independent living. Often, minor incontinence is managed independently to the person's satisfaction and never reported to a health care provider. Correctable causes of incontinence include infection, cystocele, rectocele, vaginitis, and uterine prolapse.

Urinary Retention. Urinary retention is the inability to pass all or part of the urine that has accumulated in the bladder. It should not be confused with failure of the kidneys to produce urine. The person may or may not detect this fullness in the bladder. Urinary retention is common in older men because of the increased incidence of benign prostatic hyperplasia (BPH), which can partially or totally obstruct urine outflow.

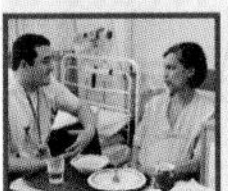

Think about Mrs. Al-Kandari, the client introduced at the beginning of the chaopter. Can you think of any reason she might have urinary retention after a vaginal hysterectomy?

Urinary Tract Infection. A urinary tract infection can occur in any portion of the urinary tract. The infection is termed cystitis if it affects the bladder, urethritis if it affects the urethra, and ureteritis if it affects the ureters. Pyelonephritis is an infection of the kidney. Urinary tract infections are more common in women than in men.

Urinary Obstruction. Urinary obstruction can occur from stones, strictures, tumors, prostatic hypertrophy, or edema.

Stones, or calculi, cause symptoms when the kidneys, ureters, or bladder are blocked or partially blocked or the stone is moving. You may hear the condition called urolithiasis. Most renal calculi are composed of calcium, but they may also contain magnesium, uric acid, and cystine.

Urinary Diversion. Urine can be diverted from its normal pathway, either by congenital malformation or by surgical creation. Hypospadias, in which the urethra opens on the underside of the penis or inside the vagina, is an example of a congenital malformation.

Various types of urinary diversions can be created surgically to treat cancer, a birth defect, an obstruction, or a neurogenic dysfunctional bladder (Figure 30-4). Although the principles of care for urinary diversions are similar, understanding the nature of the following surgical procedures may help you anticipate normal findings in the function of the diversion.

- An *ileal conduit* connects the distal ureters to a resected portion of the terminal ileum, which is used to form a stoma, or opening, onto the surface of the abdomen.
- A *Kock pouch* is a special type of ileal conduit in which a surgeon uses a segment of ileum to create a pouch for holding urine. Nipple valves created from intussuscepted portions of the ileal segment help keep the pouch continent. The client drains the pouch by inserting a catheter through the stoma.
- A *ureterosigmoidostomy* procedure connects the ureters to the sigmoid colon, which allows urine to drain through the colon. The procedure (not shown in Figure 30-4) is a variation of the Kock pouch procedure.
- In a *cutaneous ureterostomy*, the distal end of the ureter is brought to the surface of the skin to create a stoma.
- In a *vesicostomy* (also called cystostomy), an opening is made directly into the bladder.

Unless the client has a Kock pouch, attach a bag to the skin around the stoma to collect urine as it drains from the stoma. The client must be taught to manage drainage from the stoma, to care for the skin, to recognize signs and symptoms of abnormal function, and to manage the feelings associated with a change in body image.

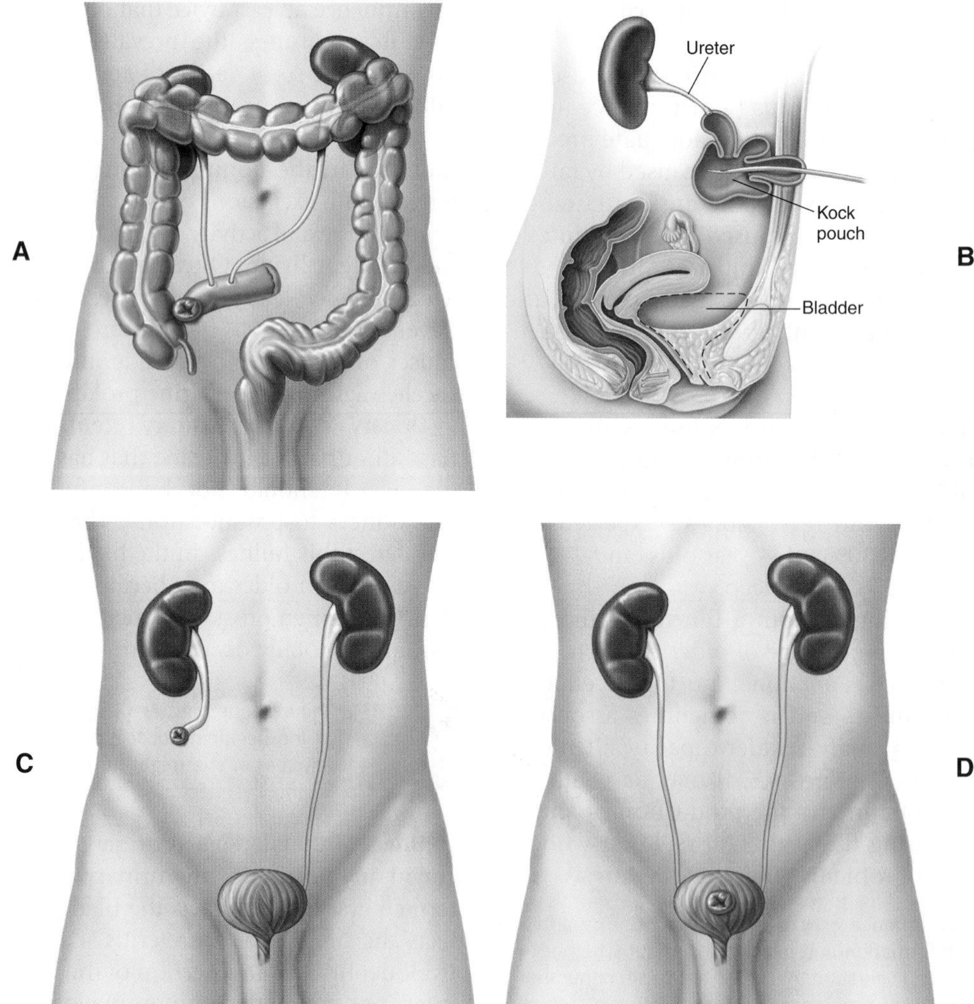

FIGURE 30-4 Types of urinary diversions. **A,** Ileal conduit. **B,** Kock pouch. **C,** Cutaneous ureterostomy. **D,** Vesicostomy.

FACTORS AFFECTING URINARY ELIMINATION

Most people do not give much thought or planning to maintaining a normal pattern of urinary elimination. Voiding typically occurs five or six times daily, although the actual number may vary widely with the volume of fluid intake, the size of the person's bladder, and the availability of toilet facilities.

Urinary output has diurnal variation. The action of antidiuretic hormone and decreased renal blood flow in the recumbent position decrease the volume of urine produced at night. However, some people need to urinate at night, possibly because of a small bladder capacity, increased fluid intake before bed, habit, or certain health problems. **Nocturia** is the term used for nighttime urination. Many factors can affect urination, both at night and during the day.

LIFESTYLE FACTORS

Nutrition and Fluids. The amount of urine produced in a 24-hour period is directly related to the amount of fluid consumed in the same period. The kidneys function to maintain a balance of body water by excreting excess fluids that the body does not need. Six to eight glasses (1500 to 2000 mL) of water daily is the recommended amount to maintain optimal renal function. Because fluid is also lost through perspiration and respiration, any activity that increases these functions also increases the body's need for water. Diarrhea and vomiting may lead to excessive loss of fluids from the gastrointestinal tract.

The water taken in through foods balances the water lost through perspiration and respiration. Foods contain various amounts of water. Fruits, especially watermelon, will add to the fluid intake and increase the production of urine. **Diuresis** is the increased formation and excretion of urine. Watermelon may actually have a diuretic effect. Drinks with caffeine (coffee, tea, some carbonated beverages) and alcoholic beverages (especially beer) cause diuresis and increase the urge to urinate. Artichokes may have some diuretic effect. Foods high in sodium encourage fluid retention.

Psychosocial. Privacy is probably the most important psychosocial issue and may relate to larger cultural issues (Box 30-1). Most people consider urination to be a private matter; some people have difficulty initiating urination in the presence of others. Both men and women may have difficulty voiding in the presence of a person of the opposite sex.

Stressful life events can interfere with complete emptying of the bladder or cause a person to urinate more frequently even though the amount is small. The urge to urinate can occur in response to fear, nervousness, cold, wind, running water, or other stimuli.

Activity and Exercise. During exercise urine production diminishes because water is lost through perspiration. In addition, blood is shunted to muscles to sustain the exercise; thus blood flow to the kidney is diminished. The sympathetic nervous system activity during activity reduces the urge to urinate. When the person goes into a resting state, these mechanisms are reversed and the urge to urinate is felt.

DEVELOPMENTAL FACTORS

Childhood. Given an average intake of fluid, a 6-month-old infant produces about 500 mL of urine, an amount that increases gradually until about age 14, when the average adult volume of 1500 mL is produced.

Adolescents and Young Adults. In the adolescent and young adult, urinary tract problems are likely to be infections associated with sexual intercourse or sexually transmitted diseases.

For some women from puberty throughout the childbearing years, the period preceding menses is marked by fluid retention and weight gain. There may be a temporary decrease in urinary output from extrarenal causes, but it has no significance in terms of normal urinary function.

Pregnancy may also be a period of fluid retention, commonly relieved by reducing sodium in the diet. Pregnant women frequently complain of frequent urination, especially during the first and last trimesters.

Middle and Older Adults. With the onset of menopause, the incidence of incontinence increases and continues to increase as age advances. The decrease of estrogen causes relaxation of the pelvic floor muscles, and this and atrophic changes in the urethra lead to incontinence. In some cases, the changes are associated with multiple births.

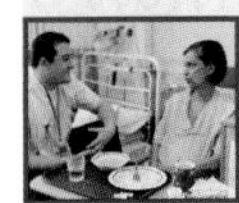

What risk factors for incontinence does Mrs. Al-Kandari have?

Aging is associated with a gradual decrease in the number of nephrons. After age 40, nephrons decrease in number until around age 80, when a person may have 40% fewer functioning nephrons.

The weight and size of the kidneys decrease with age as well. Interstitial tissue increases, the number of glomeruli decreases, and the membranes thicken. However, old age and renal failure are not synonymous; adequate renal function is possible with a loss of 70% of the normal number of nephrons (Guyton & Hall, 2006). Under conditions of good health, renal function is not compromised, but older adults are more vulnerable to renal failure that may occur secondary to serious illness.

As a person ages, bladder capacity decreases, involuntary contractions increase, and the antidiuretic hormone is less active at night. Thus the older adult voids more frequently. The majority have some nocturia, and some older adults need to urinate more than once during the night.

BOX 30-1

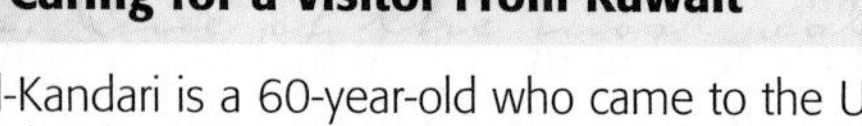

Caring for a Visitor From Kuwait

Mrs. Alia Al-Kandari is a 60-year-old who came to the United States from her home in Kuwait, with her husband. He is on temporary assignment with an oil company. She is a highly independent woman who has been active in the campaign for the women of Kuwait to have the vote. Like many people in Kuwait she speaks both English and Arabic.

It might be easy for Mrs. Al-Kandari's nurse to assume she is Mulsim because 85% of Kuwait is Muslim and 15% Christian and other religions. It may be helpful to ask if she has any religious practices she would like the health care team to honor while she is in the hospital. The nurse would also like to know more about her health care beliefs and practices, food preferences, family role in hospital care, and reaction to pain.

Women in Kuwait range from very traditional Muslim women to highly independent career-oriented women. In conversation with Mrs. Al-Kandari we would want to listen for needs specific to her culture. Although every client is unique, social pattern and beliefs of a person from Kuwait may include:

- All Muslims are brothers and sisters in Islam; they must not treat unjustly or let each other down.
- Family is the nucleus of the Islamic society.
- The human soul is invaluable and honored by God; to sustain it is to sustain humankind.
- Caring for the aged, the weak, and the sick and disabled is a collective obligation on the entire society.
- Person may be actively involved in health promotion activities and seeking health care.
- Person may have a desire for a physician from a similar cultural background.
- Health history question of a personal nature may not be answered.
- Practice of medicine is male dominated.
- Women may use passive-aggressive means rather than confrontation to solve problems in a male-dominated society.
- Family and friends are often present with the client in the hospital. They may be assertive in seeking care and attention from health care personnel.
- Touch is limited to persons of the same sex.
- Immediate pain relief is expected by some, whereas others may only express pain privately with close relatives and friends.
- Hope is valued. Only God knows the true prognosis. Therefore the client may not wish to discuss the possibility of death.
- Pork, carrion, and blood are forbidden in the diet of Muslims.
- While nursing is a low-status job, nurses and pharmacists have the right to prescribe medication.
- Self-medication is practiced.
- The person may be reluctant to go to the health care providers who do not speak their language or are not of Arab descent because they say there is a lack of sensitivity to their needs.
- Modesty demands that Muslim women to be fully clothed when in the presence of another man.
- Women do not want to be touched by a man, not even a handshake.

Data from Geissler, E. M. (1998). *Pocket guide to cultural assessment.* St. Louis: Mosby.

PHYSIOLOGICAL FACTORS

Cognitive Impairment. Because urination is cognitively controlled, a person with cognitive impairment is vulnerable to uncontrolled urination. Cognition is one of the reasons for lack of control over urination in Alzheimer's disease. A client with Alzheimer's disease may initially have incontinence because the client forgets to go to the bathroom or forgets where the bathroom is located. Eventually, however, the client will have no neurological control over the bladder.

Neuromuscular Disease. Any disease that interferes with neurological control of the bladder can cause a problem with the control of urination. A person with a spinal cord injury may or may not have damage to the nerves that innervate the bladder and, thus, may or may not have difficulty controlling urination. A client with multiple sclerosis has intermittent control over bladder function. The detrusor loses tone, and the person may find it difficult to relax the external sphincter to begin the urine stream.

Impaired Mobility. Physical mobility is necessary to move to a toilet and to do so in a timely manner. If a person is physically compromised and otherwise cognitively intact, episodes of uncontrolled urination will be particularly embarrassing.

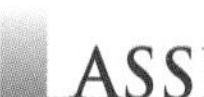

ASSESSMENT

GENERAL ASSESSMENT OF URINARY ELIMINATION

Health History. Begin the nursing history with a review of the client's pattern of urinary elimination. Ask the person to describe the duration and frequency of urination, and the characteristics of urine. Most people void every 3 to 4 hours. However, the normal range varies widely depending on personal habits that have trained the bladder to accommodate more or less urine. If the person reports an increased amount of urine, consider diabetes or the use of diuretics. Decreases in the amount may be associated with dehydration or renal failure. Ask about any pain or difficulties with voiding, unusual color or odor to the urine, and variations in amount. Remember that anticholinergic drugs can decrease the ability to empty the bladder (Table 30-1).

Table 30-1 Medications for Urinary Problems

MEDICATION	ACTION	SIDE EFFECTS
Pyridium (phenazopyridine)	Provides a local analgesic effect to the bladder mucosa to relieve burning; used when an infection is localized to the bladder	Contains azo dye that turns the urine reddish orange
B&O suppository (belladonna and opium)	Has anticholinergic effects to relieve bladder spasms, and opium to relieve the pain in an acute situation	A controlled substance; has anticholinergic side effects
Ditropan (oxybutynin) Detrol (tolterodine) Pro-Banthine (propantheline)	Produce anticholinergic effects, which relax the detrusor muscle; used to treat hyperreflexic bladders by suppressing the unwanted contractions that occur when the bladder has only a small volume of urine; also used to treat bladder spasms	Dry mouth, constipation, tachycardia, urinary hesitancy and retention, impotence, and other anticholinergic effects
Antibiotics sulfamethoxazole/trimethoprim	Treatment of urinary tract infections; needs to be excreted unchanged in the urinary tract; the combination reduces the possibility of resistant strains	Hypersensitivity to sulfa
Minipress (prazosin) Cardura (doxazosin) Flomax (tamsulosin)	Alpha-adrenergic receptor blockers relax the smooth muscle in the bladder neck, thus facilitating urinary flow through the prostatic urethra	Side effects related to blocking the adrenergic receptors could include dizziness, postural hypotension, urinary frequency, impotence, dry mouth, blurred vision

Data from Nissan, D. (Ed.). (2003). *Mosby drug consult.* St. Louis, MO: Mosby.

Ask about any history of difficulty with urination or medical problems that have affected urination, and analyze the symptoms. It may be useful to learn the frequency, timing, and amount of urination, including incontinent episodes. Estimate the amount of incontinent urine by asking how many absorbent pads the person needs a day. If the client reports urinary retention or difficulty starting the flow of urine, ask about associated symptoms and events. If the client reports incontinence, ask if it is associated with coughing, sneezing, or other activities that contract the abdominal muscles. Has there been a history of genitourinary surgery?

To investigate the client's past medical history, ask about a family history of incontinence, injury to the urinary tract, surgery, pelvic radiation therapy, trauma, onset of illness, and use of medications. Ask about a history of previous urinary tract problems, renal failure, calculi, or urinary tract infections. Chronic illness, such as multiple sclerosis or diabetes mellitus, may impair bladder function.

Your history pertaining to the presenting problem should include at least the following topics:

- Signs and symptoms involving the urinary tract, such as nocturia, dysuria, hesitancy, a poor or interrupted urine stream, straining, hematuria, suprapubic or perineal pain, urgency, frequency, enuresis, dribbling, bladder distention, incontinence, and large residual urine volumes
- Fluid intake pattern, including caffeine-containing or other diuretic fluids
- Alterations in bowel habits or sexual function
- Previous treatments for urinary tract infections, and their apparent effects
- Expectations for outcomes of treatment
- A bladder record (time and amount of urination)
- Amount and types of pads, briefs, and protective devices used
- The client's mental status
- The client's mobility status, living environment, and social factors (especially older adults)

Assess for the presence of pain. Kidney pain is dull, aching, and steady, located at or below the posterior costal margin (flank pain). Ureteral pain begins in the costovertebral angle and radiates anteriorly into the lower abdomen, groin, and perineum. It is often a severe, colicky pain. Bladder pain may be felt over the symphysis pubis. Urethral pain can usually be pinpointed as pressure or burning with urination.

Physical Examination. Perform a thorough physical examination to detect conditions that have a potential effect on urinary elimination. Because the production of urine is a reflection of total health status, many problems can affect the urinary system. The assessment may include collecting a sample of urine for urinalysis.

Assess the client's skin. You are primarily looking for signs of dehydration or edema. Edema contributes to nocturia and nocturnal urinary incontinence because the fluid shifts when the person assumes a recumbent position to sleep, improving blood flow to the kidneys and increasing urine production. Dehydration is associated with oliguria and concentrated urine.

Assess for neuromuscular problems that may affect the person's ability to empty the bladder or control urination. Mobility, cognition, and manual dexterity are related to toileting skills among frail and functionally impaired clients.

Assess the abdomen for separation of the abdominal muscles, enlarged organs, masses, inflammation, and the collection of fluid. Changes in the ability to increase intraabdominal pressure or the function of the detrusor muscle may be a factor in emptying the bladder.

Assess for urinary retention by palpating the bladder to determine whether it is distended above the symphysis pubis. When the bladder is filled to about 150 mL, palpation of the bladder may produce the urge to urinate. Remember, however, that an adult's bladder may contain 500 to 700 mL before it is distended enough to be palpated over the symphysis pubis. If you cannot feel the distended bladder but the client reports discomfort or an urge to urinate during palpation, the bladder most likely does contain urine. Percussion of the abdomen reveals a dull sound over a full bladder.

Ask about bowel elimination, and feel for a mass that indicates the presence of feces. Pressure from a fecal impaction may be a factor in urinary incontinence.

The physical examination may include inspection of the perineum. Observe for inflammation, edema, and abnormal discharge. It is normal to find an accumulation of smegma—a white, cheesy discharge from sebaceous glands.

Although nurses do not routinely perform a rectal examination, in some settings it may be part of the nurse's examination. Rectal examination allows you to test for perineal sensation, sphincter tone (both resting and active), fecal impaction, or a rectal mass, and to evaluate the consistency and contour of the prostate gland in men. The pelvic examination in women is used to assess for genital atrophy, pelvic organ prolapse (cystocele, rectocele, uterine prolapse), pelvic masses, paravaginal muscle tone, and other abnormalities.

Diagnostic Tests. Diagnostic tests for urinary disorders involve blood studies to determine renal function, radiological and imaging studies, and direct examination of the urine. When diagnostic testing involves examination of the urine, the nurse often has the responsibility for collecting urine specimens and making observations about the characteristics of the urine.

Urinalysis. **Urinalysis** is a physical, chemical, and microscopic examination of the urine (Table 30-2). It is performed to screen for urinary tract disorders, renal disorders, and other medical conditions that produce changes in the urine. It is economical, produces rapid results, and usually is noninvasive. Although a laboratory technician usually performs it, some analyses of urine can be done with simple procedures not requiring a laboratory.

Urine characteristics. Urine is primarily water, but it also contains various amounts of waste products: urea, creatinine, ammonia, and purine bodies. Sodium and potassium are the principal electrolytes excreted by the kidneys. The excretion of phosphoric acid, sulfuric acid, uric acid, hippuric acid, and ammonia along with the bicarbonate ion help regulate the acid-base balance of the body. The bicarbonate ion is a buffer that can take on hydrogen ions.

Color. Urine is normally pale, straw colored, and clear. Changes in the color of urine may have diagnostic significance:

- Amber-colored urine results from the concentration of urine caused by decreased fluid intake or excretion of water. Urine darkens as it stands outside the body.
- Dark amber urine can also mean bilirubin in the urine.
- Blood appears in various shades of red in urine. It may be occult (not visible to the naked eye), or it may cause the urine to become pink tinged or frankly bloody. Remember, however, that red urine is not always caused by blood. Foods can turn the urine red as well, including rhubarb, beets, blackberries, and red food dyes.
- Bright yellow urine comes from large amounts of carotene in the diet or vitamin therapy.
- Medications can also change the color of urine to red, orange, blue, or green.

Clarity. Freshly voided urine should be clear. Cloudiness indicates the presence of bacteria **(bacteriuria)**, inflammation, or the presence of sperm or prostate fluid. Urine can also become cloudy when it stands.

Odor. Freshly voided urine is aromatic. When it stands, it develops a characteristic pungent odor of ammonia because it quickly becomes contaminated with bacteria. The odor of urine may be affected by foods. A sweet, fruity odor is associated with ketone bodies produced by diabetic ketoacidosis.

Acid-base balance. The body's acid-base balance is reflected by its pH, a measure of hydrogen ion concentration. The normal pH range for urine is 4.5 to 7.8, depending on the body's need for excretion of acids. Abnormal pH measures can indicate systemic acid-

Table 30-2 Normal Values for Urinalysis

CHARACTERISTIC	NORMAL VALUE
Color	Yellow
Clarity	Clear
Specific gravity	1.003-1.030
pH	4.5-7.8
Protein	Negative
Bilirubin	Negative
Urobilinogen	Normal in small amounts
Glucose	Negative
Ketones	Negative
Occult blood	Negative
Red blood cells	No more than three (males) to five (females) per high-power field
White blood cells	No more than five per high-power field
Bacteria	Negative
Leukocyte esterase	Negative
Casts	No more than four hyaline casts per low-power field
Crystals	Few

base imbalances. Some foods and medications can change urine pH. A diet high in meats, eggs, cheese, whole grains, plums, prunes, and cranberries may decrease pH (to more acidic). Vegetables, citrus fruits, and milk increase pH (to more alkaline). You can readily measure urine pH by using a multiagent dipstick and comparing it to a standardized color chart after waiting a specified period.

Specific gravity. Specific gravity is a measure of the concentration of dissolved solids in urine, thus gauging the ability of the kidneys to concentrate and excrete urine. Urine specific gravity normally ranges from 1.003 to 1.030. If the client's kidneys are functioning normally, specific gravity indicates fluid status; in other words, dehydration raises the specific gravity, and overhydration lowers it.

Proteins and glucose. Proteins and glucose are large molecules and are normally not excreted by the kidneys. Laboratory findings should be negative for glucosuria (glucose in the urine) and proteinuria (protein in the urine). In people who have diabetes, glucose spills into the urine when the blood glucose levels become too high. If cells are deprived of glucose long enough, the body metabolizes fat to provide energy, a process that also produces ketones. Ketones in the urine indicate ketoacidosis of diabetes or may be present from exercise and dieting. Glucose sticks can be used for screening in healthy populations but are not sufficiently sensitive for monitoring people with type 1 diabetes. The presence of protein in the urine can indicate glomerular disease.

Bilirubin and urobilinogen. Bilirubin normally does not appear in urine, and urobilinogen normally appears only in small amounts. If the biliary tract becomes obstructed, the bilirubin level rises in the blood and eventually spills into the urine. Urine urobilinogen levels rise in liver disease.

Blood. Blood in the urine **(hematuria)** is an abnormal finding. Blood at the start of urination indicates the urethra as the source. Blood at the end of urination indicates pathological process of the bladder neck, posterior urethra, or prostate. Blood throughout urination indicates pathological condition above the bladder neck. Usually, dark blood comes from the upper urinary tract, and bright red blood comes from the bladder neck or urethra. Occult blood is detected using reagent strips dipped into the urine specimen and compared to the color chart on the bottle of reagent strips.

Urine Culture. A culture can be grown from a sample of urine to determine the specific organism causing a urinary tract infection and to monitor the number of organisms in the urine. The urine and urinary tract are sterile except for normal flora in the distal urethra and urinary meatus.

As with any culture, the specimen should be collected in a manner that prevents contamination from other sources of bacteria. A clean specimen caught in midstream or a specimen from a catheterization procedure is needed. Culture results with no growth are available after 24 hours. Positive cultures require 24 to 48 hours to complete.

When the organism is identified, a test is performed to determine which antibiotics will be effective against the specific organism. The results will report a list of antibiotics to which the organism is sensitive or resistant. The physician may then modify the prescription if a change in antibiotic is warranted.

Collecting urine specimens. Depending on the test planned for the specimen, you may collect a urine specimen in either a clean or a sterile container. Figure 30-5 shows commonly used containers for collecting and measuring urine. When a bedpan, urinal, or specimen hat is used, warn the client that the specimen will need

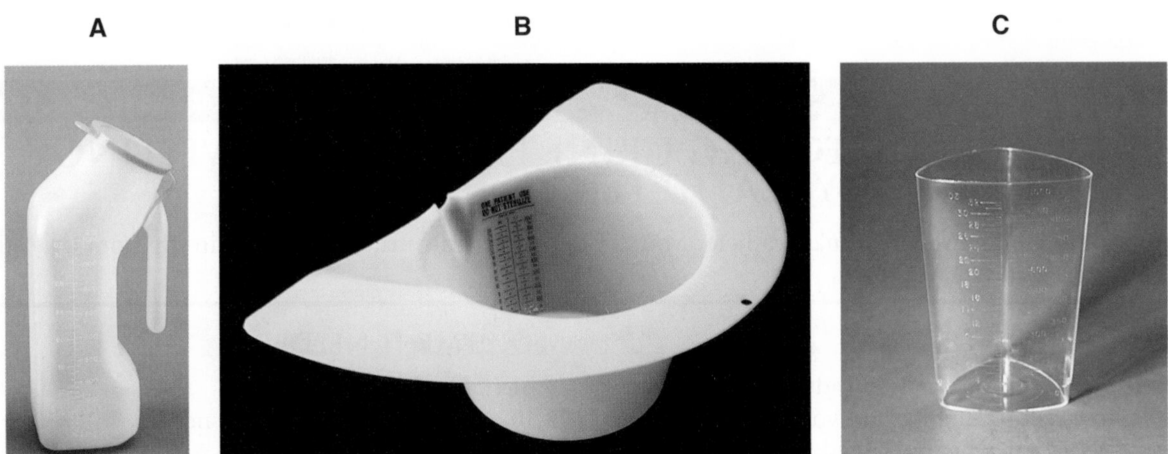

FIGURE 30-5 Devices for collecting and measuring urine (see also Figure 30-7). **A,** Urinal, which is curved to allow placement parallel to the body when the client is recumbent. **B,** Specimen hat, which fits onto the rim of a toilet under the seat, thus allowing the client to sit to void. **C,** Calibrated urine-measuring device. (**A** courtesy Bemis Healthcare, Sheboygan Falls, WI; **B** courtesy Kendall Healthcare, Mansfield, MA.)

to be free of feces or toilet paper. To measure the urine, it must be poured into a calibrated measuring device. The calibrations on the urinal or specimen hat are accurate only for estimation purposes.

If you will be evaluating urine for bacteria, you will need to use a sterile container to avoid contaminating the specimen. Or you will need to obtain the specimen from the client's indwelling urinary catheter or give instructions about obtaining a clean-catch, midstream specimen.

Midstream urine collection. Instruct the client to perform hand hygiene before collecting the specimen. A male client should clean the urinary meatus with three soapy sponges (Figure 30-6, *A*). If uncircumcised, he should retract the foreskin and clean the glans penis. The minimum recommended amount for a urine specimen is 15 mL.

A female client should spread the labia and clean the perineum, vulva, and urinary meatus with three soapy sponges or wipes using one front-to-back stroke for each sponge (Figure 30-6, *B*). Tell her to discard each sponge after using it for one stroke. She should wipe each side of the labia and down the center over the meatus. Ideally, the labia should stay separated until the urine is collected.

Catheterization. If the client already has a catheter in place, you can obtain a urine specimen from a port located on the proximal end of the collecting tubing. Clean the port with alcohol, and insert a needle to collect at least 4 mL of urine that is fresh from the bladder. (Inserting the needle directly into the catheter is a less desirable method of collection.) You may need to clamp the tubing below the port for 10 to 30 minutes to allow urine to collect in the catheter (Procedure 30-1).

A

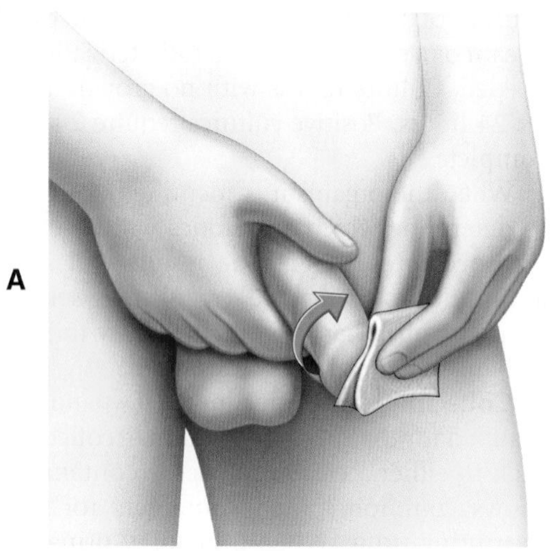

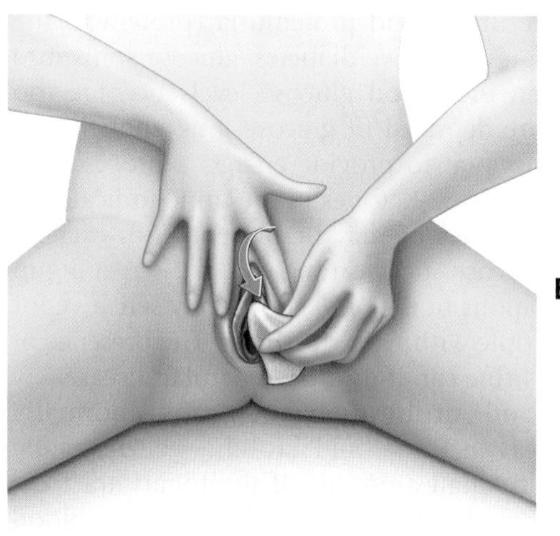

B

FIGURE 30-6 Cleaning the urinary meatus for collection of a midstream urine specimen. **A,** Instruct male clients to clean in a circular motion around the urinary meatus. **B,** Instruct female clients to clean the meatus from front to back.

TIME TO ALLOW: NOVICE: 6 min. **EXPERT:** 3 min.

PROCEDURE 30-1 COLLECTING URINE FROM AN INDWELLING (FOLEY) CATHETER

If your client has an indwelling urinary catheter, you can obtain a sterile urine specimen directly from the catheter's closed drainage system.

DELEGATION GUIDELINES

The collection of urine from an indwelling catheter is a simple, low-risk procedure that you may delegate to a nursing assistant who is trained in this collection technique.

EQUIPMENT NEEDED

- Alcohol wipes
- 10-mL syringe with attached needle
- Sterile container
- Marking pen
- Catheter clamp

1 Follow preliminary actions (see inside front cover).
2 Observe for the presence of urine at the port site. If needed, clamp the catheter distal to the port for 30 minutes or until urine has collected at the port site.
3 Clean the collection port with an alcohol wipe (see illustration).

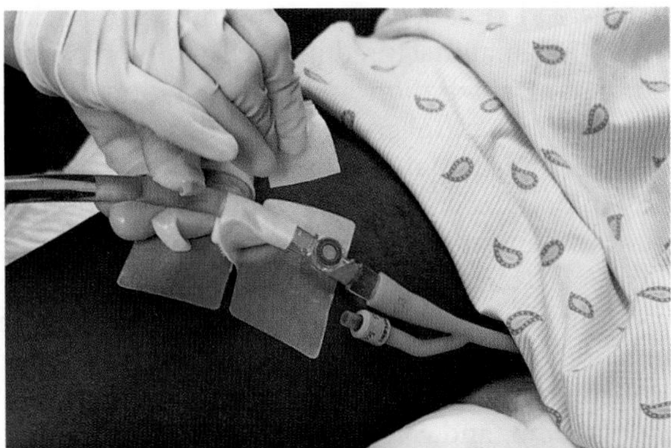

Step 3. Cleaning the collection port.

4 Using a 10-mL syringe and attached needle, insert the needle into the port and withdraw 10 mL of urine (see illustration).

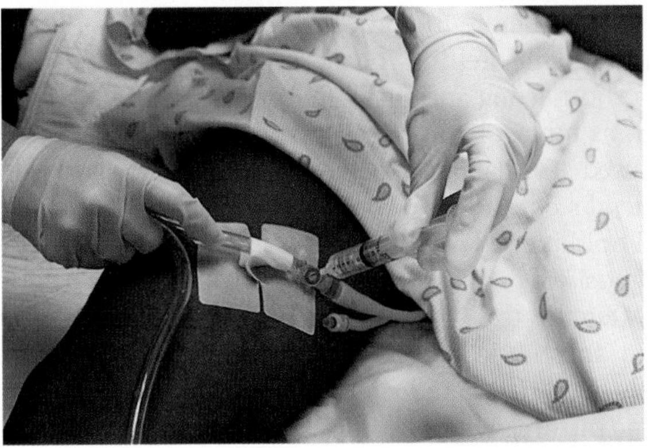

Step 4. Inserting the needle and withdrawing urine.

5 Inject the urine into a sterile container (see illustration). Discard the needle in a sharps container.

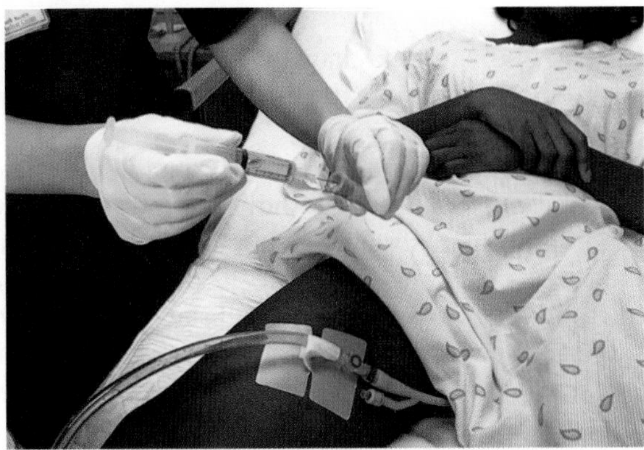

Step 5. Injecting the urine into a sterile container.

6 Label the container with the client's name and the date and time of collection. Immediately send the container to the laboratory. Remove equipment, and make client comfortable.
7 Document the method of collection, amount and characteristics of urine, and time sent to the laboratory.

Sometimes you may need to catheterize a client to collect a urine specimen. A small-diameter catheter attached to a collection bag is recommended because it has the advantage of being a closed system. The catheter is inserted using sterile technique, and urine fills the bag. As soon as the specimen is collected in the bag, the catheter is removed.

Urine collection from infants and young children. Infants and young children who cannot cooperate with collection of a midstream urine specimen will require a special device to collect the specimen. A disposable plastic bag with adhesive attachment is available to collect urine. The bag is attached to the external genitalia and the child voids directly into the bag (Figure 30-7). For a nonsterile specimen, four to five cotton balls can be placed in the diaper; the urine is then squeezed into the collection container.

Twenty-four-hour collection. Collection of all the urine produced in 24 hours is necessary to test for the excretion of creatinine, total urine protein, or electrolytes, because the excretion rate of these substances is not constant over a 24-hour period.

For accurate results, all urine produced in a 24-hour period needs to be collected.

Action Alert! At the start of the collection period, discard the first voided specimen. At the end of 24 hours, have the client void and save the last voided specimen. For accurate results, all urine produced in a 24-hour period needs to be collected.

The end of the test may vary by 15 to 30 minutes from exactly 24 hours, but note the time precisely on the laboratory request.

Store the collected urine in a large container in the client's bathroom until the 24-hour period has ended. Depending on the substance being tested, the container may have a preservative added to it, or it may be iced. Instruct the client, the family, and all staff members who care for the client to carefully save all of the client's urine in the appropriate container. If a specimen is accidentally discarded, the collection procedure must be restarted. Make sure the client and family know that the specimen must not be contaminated with toilet paper or feces.

Blood Chemistry

Creatinine. Creatine is an intermediate product of protein metabolism that is synthesized in the liver, kidneys, and pancreas and is stored in muscle tissue. Creatinine is the end product of the metabolism of creatine. The kidneys filter creatinine from the blood. When renal function is impaired, the serum creatinine level rises. Thus serum creatinine levels can be used to evaluate renal function and to estimate the effectiveness of glomerular filtration.

Creatinine can also be measured in the urine. Creatinine clearance measures the total amount of creatinine excreted in the urine. The meaning of the results is improved by simultaneous measurement of serum creatinine. Urine is collected in an iced or refrigerated container for a 24-hour period as described previously. The client should avoid excessive intake of meat the day before the test and should drink adequate fluids before and during the collection period. At the end of the test, the specimen should be promptly transported to the laboratory.

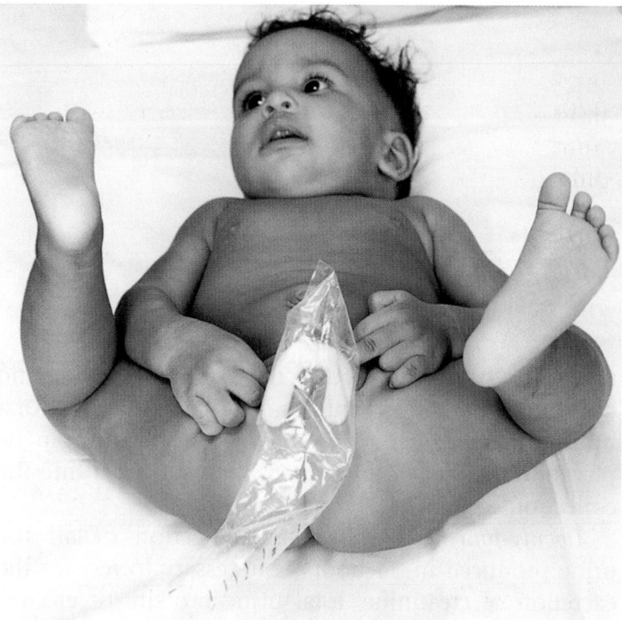

FIGURE 30-7 To collect a urine specimen from an infant or toddler who is not toilet trained, apply an adhesive pouch over the perineum.

Blood urea nitrogen. Urea nitrogen is the major nitrogenous end product of protein and amino acid catabolism. It is manufactured in the liver and excreted by the kidneys. Dehydration and overhydration affect the excretion of urea nitrogen. Increased dietary protein, increased catabolism, and muscle-wasting diseases will increase blood urea nitrogen, as will prerenal (decreased blood flow), intrarenal (damage to renal parenchyma), or postrenal (obstruction to outflow of urine) kidney failure. Therefore the test is less specific than serum creatinine in the diagnosis of renal failure.

Electrolytes. Abnormal excretion of sodium, chloride, potassium, and calcium may indicate renal disease or other problems. The test results must be considered together with related symptoms and diagnostic tests.

Cystoscopy. Cystoscopy is a procedure using a metal or fiberoptic endoscope passed through the urethra for direct visualization of the bladder. The procedure is performed in a urologist's office or in an operating room under local, spinal, or general anesthesia. A sedative is sometimes administered before the procedure, and a local anesthetic is applied to the urethra. The tranquilizer diazepam (Valium) or a short-acting anesthetic that produces a twilight sleep, such as midazolam (Versed), is used. The procedure may be used to dilate strictures, implant radium, or place a ureteral stent (a thin wire to support the wall of the tube and hold it open). A common reason for cystoscopy is the diagnosis of painless hematuria.

After the test, you will monitor the client's recovery from anesthesia and the ability to void normally. The client may need medication for pain or bladder spasm. Some burning with urination and blood-tinged urine are normal for the first three voids. Warm tub baths or sitz baths may help relieve the discomfort. Prophylactic antibiotics are sometimes prescribed for 1 to 3 days. Drinking extra fluids may help the client begin to void normally and relieve some of the discomfort.

The outpatient client should be instructed to report the following problems:

- Persistent, painless hematuria; bright red urine; blood clots in the urine
- Inability to urinate within 8 hours despite a full bladder and the urge to urinate
- Signs of infection, such as flank or abdominal pain, chills, fever, or cloudy urine (an indication of pus)

Urodynamic Tests. Urodynamic tests measure the function of the bladder and urethra by measuring the flow rate of urine passing through the urethra. They produce a graphic record of pressures in the bladder and urethra during voiding. They also show variations in the volume of urine and allow visualization of the bladder with contrast media during voiding. Information obtained from this test is used to evaluate the client for vesicoureteral reflux (backflow of urine into the ureter) and for problems associated with residual urine and incontinence.

Imaging. Computed tomography and magnetic resonance imaging are used to evaluate urinary lesions. Bladder tumors can be detected and evaluated. Malignant tumors can be distinguished from benign growths. If contrast media will be used, make sure to question the client about any allergies to shellfish or iodine, or any reactions to dye or contrast material used in previous radiographic studies. Sedatives are used to assist children under age 3 with the prolonged period of immobilization.

FOCUSED ASSESSMENT FOR URINARY INCONTINENCE

Defining Characteristics. For a client who has evidence of incontinence, ask questions to determine the nature of the problem. The type of incontinence and the extent of the problem are factors in determining the appropriate interventions (Box 30-2).

Stress Urinary Incontinence. **Stress urinary incontinence** is a reported or observed involuntary loss of urine with increased abdominal pressure. This sudden loss of urine occurs with coughing, sneezing, laughing, bending, lifting, sudden exposure to cold air, and climbing stairs. Urgency and frequency may be associated with stress incontinence. Inquire about the type of and the frequency of changing the protective undergarment or pads.

Urge Urinary Incontinence. **Urge urinary incontinence** is a reported or observed sudden desire to urinate and immediate need of toileting facilities. If you are helping such a client to the toilet, you may notice that the person's clothing becomes wet by the time the toilet has been reached. Urge incontinence is associated with a sudden, overwhelming urge to urinate that cannot be controlled long enough to reach a toilet. Urination occurs frequently and in small amounts. Uncontrollable contractions of the detrusor muscle may be the cause.

Functional Urinary Incontinence. **Functional urinary incontinence** occurs as an unpredictable, involuntary passage of urine in the presence of normal bladder and urethral function. At times the person is cognitively unaware of the need to void. Usually, it is associated with cognitive impairment, some types of dementia, depression, or neurological damage. The diagnosis is made by ruling out other causes of incontinence. It is associated with environmental barriers and decreased mobility. The client is unable to get to the toilet or remove clothing quickly enough to respond to the need to void.

Reflex Urinary Incontinence. **Reflex urinary incontinence** is unexpected, involuntary voiding without awareness of the need to void and is specific to the client with a spinal cord injury. It is associated with neurological damage to the spinal cord above the level of the third sacral vertebra. The person is unaware that the bladder is full and voids in response to the spinal reflex. The overfilling of the bladder is often referred to as overflow incontinence, and the intervals between voiding can be predictable. The person maintains a full bladder and is cognitively aware of wetness after reflex voiding has occurred.

Total Urinary Incontinence. **Total urinary incontinence** is the continuous, involuntary, and unpredictable loss of urine. The person is unaware of the urge to void, does not experience bladder distention, and may be unaware of the incontinence. The undergarments or bed is almost continually wet and the client is described as "dribbling" urine. The etiology is usually cognitive impairment and may include a nonfunctional urinary sphincter.

Related Factors

Incompetent or Decreased Muscle Function. The muscles involved in urinary elimination must have good tone and be functional for urination to proceed normally. The periurethral striated muscle (external sphincter) is part of the pelvic floor muscles. The tone of the muscles of the pelvic floor can affect the person's ability to maintain voluntary control over urination.

Stress urinary incontinence is associated with weakness of the pelvic floor muscles or postmenopausal atrophic changes of the urethra, cystocele, and rectocele. The muscles of the pelvic floor may be weak secondary to obesity, aging, childbirth, or recent substantial weight loss.

Decreased bladder capacity results in increased difficulty in holding the urine. Decreased bladder muscle tone can occur secondary to habitual frequency of urination or

BOX 30-2 *Diagnostic Cues for Urinary Incontinence and Urinary Retention*

Assess a client for urinary incontinence in the presence of the following:

- A wet bed or wet undergarments
- An odor of urine
- Report of incontinence
- Membership in a group at high risk for incontinence, such as women after menopause, older adults, or the neurologically impaired

Assess a client for urinary retention in the presence of the following:

- Complaint of a full bladder but inability to void
- Complaint of difficulty starting the urine stream
- Risk factors for acute retention and absence of voiding in 6 to 8 hours
- Membership in a group at high risk for retention, such as those with recent pelvic surgery, difficulty voiding, or anticholinergic use

any other reason that causes the bladder size to never be challenged. An incompetent bladder outlet can occur secondary to congenital urinary tract anomalies.

Bladder Infection or Irritation. Infection or inflammation can cause urge incontinence. Stasis or pooling of urine contributes to bacterial growth. The client who is on bed rest or who has bladder outlet obstruction is at risk for stasis of urine that can lead to urinary tract infection. Symptoms of urinary tract infections include pain or burning on urination, frequency, and sometimes blood in the urine. Trauma to the urethra causes pain and edema that can interfere with voiding. Urethritis can be caused by vaginal infections, use of harsh soaps, or bubble baths. Other causes of irritation are glucosuria and cancer.

Impaired Ability to Recognize Bladder Cues. Neurological injury or disease can affect the person's ability to recognize the need to urinate or to control urination. Injury, tumor, or infection of the spinal cord or brain may be the underlying cause. A cerebrovascular accident (stroke) can make the person cognitively unaware of the need to urinate. Multiple sclerosis and other demyelinating diseases can make the person unable to recognize the need to urinate. Diabetic neuropathy that affects the smooth muscle of the bladder can result in the inability to control the bladder.

Decreased attention to bladder cues can result in incontinence. The person may ignore the urge to urinate secondary to depression, confusion, or an inability to communicate needs.

Invasive Procedures/Medications. Clients may experience transient incontinence after surgery or any procedure that invades the bladder. An example is a transurethral resection of the prostate that may affect the bladder sphincter. Transient incontinence may occur after a cystoscopy or a procedure requiring general or spinal anesthesia. Drugs that reduce control of urinary elimination include sedatives, immunosuppressants, and diuretics.

Environmental Barriers. A major feature of incontinence for older adults is the need to walk a distance to the toilet, poor lighting, unfamiliar surroundings, or a bed that is too high or has side rails. These barriers can make getting to the bathroom difficult. Inability to access the bathroom on time can be secondary to caffeine, alcohol, or impaired mobility.

FOCUSED ASSESSMENT FOR *URINARY RETENTION*

Defining Characteristics. A client with urinary retention typically complains of an inability to void despite a feeling of bladder fullness. Overflow incontinence occurs when the person cannot empty the bladder. When the bladder reaches a critical volume, urine passes involuntarily to relieve the distention. Assess for complications of retention including renal damage from reflux, overstretched bladder, and infection.

Action Alert! Monitor the voiding patterns of any client at risk for urinary retention.

Assess the client who voids frequently in small amounts for urinary retention. A postvoid residual of less than 50 mL is considered normal; more than 100 mL indicates inadequate emptying. **Residual urine** is the amount of urine remaining in the bladder after voiding. To measure residual urine, have the client urinate, and immediately use a portable ultrasound scanner device that measures residual urine volume. Alternatively, insert an in-and-out catheter, and measure the volume of postvoid urine obtained.

Related Factors. Postsurgical clients are at risk for a variety of reasons, including the use of anticholinergic, sympathomimetic, or muscle relaxant medications given with anesthesia. Clients who had surgery in the pelvic region, particularly gynecological surgery or procedures involving the bladder, are at risk for urethral obstruction from edema or blood clots. Discomfort associated with surgery in the pelvic region may make the person reluctant to void. Clients who have had hip surgery have limited mobility, pain, and edema that may lessen their control over urination. Clients who have indwelling catheters removed may temporarily experience problems of retention as well.

The primary reason for retention is bladder outlet obstruction caused by an enlarged prostate, stricture, or edema. It can also be secondary to fecal impaction or chronic constipation. When the bladder or bladder neck bleeds, blood clots can obstruct the urethra. Urinary calculi are more likely to obstruct the ureters than the bladder outlet.

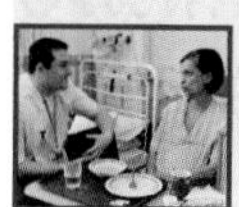

What related factors for urinary retention could Mrs. Al-Kandari experience?

Obstruction is a second leading cause of urinary retention. Men over age 50 have a high risk for benign prostatic hyperplasia. Because the prostate gland encircles the urethra, the incidence of retention is high in this group. Tumors, bladder stones, and blood clots are other causes of obstruction.

FOCUSED ASSESSMENT FOR *RISK FOR INFECTION*

Assess for factors that increase the risk for urinary tract infections. Ask what the client does to prevent urinary tract infections. Usually, infections can be easily managed with low-cost antibiotics. For a person with allergies to the usual antibiotics, more expensive alternatives are required. For clients who must manage an indwelling catheter, intermittent catheterization, or urinary diversion on a long-term basis, consider also the possibility that an antibiotic-resistant strain of the infecting

BOX 30-3

Teaching for Wellness

Methods to Prevent Urinary Tract Infections

Purpose: To minimize the risk for urinary tract infections.
Expected Outcome: The client will not have, or will reduce, the frequency of urinary tract infections.

Client Instructions

For Women

- Maintain perineal hygiene by wiping from front to back after defecating.
- Wear cotton-crotch rather than synthetic-crotch underpants, because synthetic fabrics tend to increase perineal moisture.
- Do not wear tight slacks or pantyhose.
- Do not wear a damp swimsuit for extended periods of time.
- Avoid the use of bubble bath, perfumed soaps, feminine hygiene sprays, or hexachlorophene.
- Urinate before and after intercourse.
- If a lubricant is needed during intercourse, use a water-soluble lubricant.
- Women who use diaphragms are twice as likely to contract urinary tract infections as women who do not use them. Check with your physician if you use a diaphragm and are experiencing frequent urinary tract infections.

For Men and Women

- Take showers instead of baths because bacteria in the bath water can gain access to the urethra.
- Immediately obtain treatment if you develop symptoms of a urinary tract infection, such as painful urination, increased urgency or frequency of urination, fever, and malaise.
- Take medications prescribed to treat a urinary tract infection exactly as ordered. Take all of the prescription, even if you feel better before the prescription is finished.
- If you have a cardiac condition that causes frequent urination, learn to tell the difference between that condition and the frequency associated with a urinary tract infection.

organism may emerge. The best course of action is to prevent the infection (Box 30-3).

DIAGNOSIS

The diagnosis of *Impaired urinary elimination* may be used when you know that a client has a problem with urinary elimination but you have not yet narrowed the focus to a precise problem. Some nurses prefer to use this general diagnosis when the problem is related to a medical procedure, such as a stent, or to the potential complications from a medical procedure. An alternative method is to simply write the diagnosis as *Potential complication*: (name the complication) or as *Risk for* (name the complication). Table 30-3 shows examples of specific diagnoses.

Urinary incontinence should be evaluated to distinguish the type of incontinence so that you can plan interventions appropriate to the specific problem. Usually, you can identify the type of incontinence without specialized testing. The use of an incontinence diagnosis is ideally accompanied by a plan to restore continence. Many times, incontinence responds to treatments that are within the practice of nursing. Indeed, because the least invasive methods are tried first, the management of incontinence often falls to a nurse.

The absence of urine requires that you differentiate renal failure from the inability to urinate. If your client has not voided for 8 hours, you need to decide whether the evidence points to a failure to produce urine or to the retention of urine in the bladder. Often, the client's history will give you some idea of what problems to anticipate. The nursing diagnosis in renal failure is *Excess fluid volume* (see Chapter 26). Other nursing diagnoses include the following:

- *Situational low self-esteem:* Urinary elimination problems are embarrassing to many people because managing the problem involves discussing private body functions with a health care provider. Incontinence is particularly disturbing because one learns in early childhood the importance of controlling urination. Lack of control decreases self-esteem; therefore you should ask about feelings about incontinence and how the person perceives incontinence.
- *Social isolation:* The initial response to urinary incontinence, urinary diversion, or the need for self-catheterization is to avoid social situations that would require modifications in the management of elimination or where odor could become embarrassing. Ask if the urinary problem interferes with socialization. Most people are concerned about controlling the odor of urine or having their clothes wet and soiled with urine. People with urinary diversions who must wear a collection bag have a need to conceal the bag and manage the odor. The client needs to become familiar with modifications that can help to maintain a normal pattern of social interaction.
- *Toilet self-care deficit:* This diagnosis is appropriate until the person has learned the necessary self-care practices. Ask whether the client requires any assistance in managing urination. The presence of an indwelling catheter or a urinary diversion requires a different approach to managing urinary elimination.
- *Impaired skin integrity:* Urinary incontinence is highly associated with skin breakdown and the formation of pressure ulcers. An incontinent client requires special care to prevent irritation or maceration of the skin. Careful assessment of the skin is a high priority. If the client has a problem with incontinence, inspect the skin or ask about irritation or maceration of the skin.

Table 30-3 Clustering Data to Make a Nursing Diagnosis

Urinary Elimination Problems	
DATA CLUSTER	**DIAGNOSIS**
A 60-year-old male client complains of frequent dribbling and a feeling of bladder fullness even after he urinates. He has been diagnosed with prostatic hypertrophy.	*Urinary retention* related to bladder outlet obstruction or *Overflow incontinence* related to bladder outlet obstruction
A 25-year-old woman with multiple sclerosis has occasional episodes of difficulty in urinating. She has made several trips to the emergency department to have a catheter inserted.	*Urinary retention* related to episodic voluntary muscle dysfunction secondary to demyelinization
A 20-year-old woman has come to a clinic for premarital sexual counseling. She has no previous experience with sexual intercourse.	*Risk for infection* related to need for information about risk factors and prevention measures
A 50-year-old menopausal woman has recently been experiencing incontinence when she sneezes, laughs, or suddenly encounters cold air.	*Stress urinary incontinence* related to changes in pelvic floor muscles secondary to hormonal changes
A 75-year-old woman had a total hip replacement yesterday. She has called for the bedpan, but each time she has called too late and has urinated in bed. She did not previously have a problem with incontinence.	*Functional urinary incontinence* related to immobility, first day after total hip replacement, and use of pain medication
A 90-year-old woman with stage 4 Alzheimer's disease continuously dribbles urine, has no apparent awareness of urination, does not have a bladder infection, and does not have residual urine.	*Total urinary incontinence* related to cognitive and neuromuscular limitations

PLANNING

To obtain a complete picture of the effects of nursing care, take into consideration the expectation that the client will take the desired action, the client's ability to take the desired action, measurements of progress, and the actual results of the actions taken. Outcomes include measurements in the following areas: motivation, knowledge, taking action, sustaining consistent action, and obtaining and measuring results.

For example, expected outcomes for a client with incontinence are affected by the following client variables:

- Is the client mentally able to participate in the treatment plan?
- Does the client have the knowledge needed to make choices about managing incontinence?
- Does the client have the motivation to follow a systematic daily regimen for an extended period of time?

Some clients may be only able to reduce the number of incontinent episodes, using incontinence aids to manage the remaining episodes. Other clients may be satisfied with managing infrequent, small-volume incontinence with incontinence aids. Therefore the goal will be learning to manage incontinence with protective pads. Naturally, goals vary for each client and each situation.

EXPECTED OUTCOMES FOR THE CLIENT WITH *STRESS* OR *URGE URINARY INCONTINENCE*

Expected outcomes for a client with *Stress urinary incontinence* or *Urge urinary incontinence* could include that the client will be able to do the following:

- Manage small-volume, infrequent episodes of incontinence with incontinence aids
- Seek medical evaluation for incontinence
- Recognize the signs of bladder infection
- List measures to prevent urinary tract infection
- Verbalize knowledge of possible medical and surgical treatments for incontinence
- Make a commitment to a management regimen
- Report extended periods between urination to increase the bladder capacity
- Correctly perform Kegel exercises

EXPECTED OUTCOMES FOR THE CLIENT WITH *FUNCTIONAL URINARY INCONTINENCE*

Functional urinary incontinence is frequently associated with older adult or disabled clients who are physically or mentally unable to toilet without assistance. A caregiver is usually involved in managing the incontinence. Expected outcomes for a client with *Functional urinary incontinence* could include that the client will be able to do the following:

- Not be embarrassed by the need for assistance to manage toileting
- Be treated with compassion and understanding
- Initiate or ask for assistance to toilet
- Be assisted to the toilet before incontinence occurs
- Have no skin breakdown
- Remain clean and dry
- Have no odor of urine
- Have a reduced number of episodes of incontinence over a 24-hour period

EXPECTED OUTCOMES FOR THE CLIENT WITH *REFLEX URINARY INCONTINENCE*

Expected outcomes for the client with *Reflex urinary incontinence* could include that the client will be able to do the following:

- Develop a method of controlling urination
- Remain dry and odor free
- Maintain intact skin

Table 30-4 Interventions for Urinary Incontinence

INTERVENTION	APPLICATION
Basic evaluation	• Obtain history, physical examination, postvoid residual volume, and urinalysis on all clients with urinary incontinence. • After basic evaluation and initial treatment, clients who fail or are not appropriate for treatment based on presumptive diagnosis should undergo further evaluation.
Routine or scheduled toileting	• Offer to incontinent clients on a consistent schedule. • This technique is recommended for clients who cannot participate in independent toileting.
Habit training	• Use for clients in whom a natural voiding pattern can be determined.
Prompted voiding	• Recommended for clients who can learn to recognize some degree of bladder fullness or the need to void, or who can ask for assistance or respond when prompted to toilet. • Clients who are candidates for prompted voiding may not have sufficient cognitive ability to participate in other, more complex behavioral therapies.
Bladder training	• Use to manage urge incontinence, mixed incontinence, and stress incontinence.
Exercises to strengthen pelvic muscles	• Use to decrease the incidence of urinary incontinence. • Pelvic muscle exercises are strongly recommended for women with stress incontinence, men and women with urge incontinence who also receive bladder training, and men who develop urinary incontinence after prostatectomy. • Pelvic muscle rehabilitation and bladder inhibition using biofeedback therapy are recommended for clients with stress, urge, and mixed incontinence.
Vaginal weight training	• Recommended for premenopausal woman who have stress incontinence. • Use to decrease incontinence in women with stress incontinence.
Pelvic floor electrical stimulation	• Use to decrease incontinence in women with stress incontinence. • May be useful for urge and mixed incontinence.
Medications	• Stress incontinence: Alpha-adrenergic agonists are the first line of therapy when not contraindicated; estrogen may be recommended as adjunct therapy. • Urge incontinence: anticholinergic agents (especially oxybutynin [Ditropan]), antispasmodics, or tricyclic antidepressants.
Surgery	• Correction of prolapsed uterus, removal of large fibroid uterine tumors, and tightening of the pelvic floor may relieve stress incontinence; used uncommonly for urge incontinence. • Surgery to relieve the obstruction is used for overflow incontinence.

From Urinary Incontinence Guideline Panel. (1982). *Urinary incontinence in adults.* (AHCPR Publication No. 92-0038 and 92-0041). Rockville, MD: Agency for Health Care Policy and Research.

EXPECTED OUTCOMES FOR THE CLIENT WITH *URINARY RETENTION*

For a client with a diagnosis of *Urinary retention* as a result of overflow incontinence caused by a neurogenic bladder, expected outcomes could include that the client will be able to do the following:

- Express motivation to perform self-catheterization
- Master self-catheterization
- Maintain clean technique
- Have no urinary tract infections

For other causes of *Urinary retention,* the expected outcomes could include that the client will be able to do the following:

- Establish a normal pattern of voiding without residual urine
- Void within 8 hours of removal of an indwelling (Foley) catheter
- Report no discomfort with voiding
- Recognize the signs of bladder distention
- Have no signs or symptoms of reflux, bladder damage, or renal damage

INTERVENTION

INTERVENTIONS TO PROMOTE URINARY CONTINENCE

Many interventions are available to help control urinary incontinence, as summarized here and in Table 30-4. Box 30-4 discusses evidence-based practice guidelines for preventing and managing urinary incontinence. Box 30-5 presents alternative therapies for incontinence and urinary symptoms.

Establishing Continence

Pelvic Muscle Exercises. **Kegel exercises** are exercises performed to strengthen the pelvic and vaginal muscles to help control stress incontinence in women. They are named for Dr. Arnold H. Kegel, the gynecologist who first developed them. Performed correctly, Kegel exercises can reduce or eliminate incontinence in approximately 60% of cognitively intact, cooperative women (AHCPR, 1996). The exercises are described in Box 30-6. Although used primarily for stress incontinence, they sometimes can be beneficial for reducing urge incontinence.

BOX 30-4

Evidence-Based Practice

Preventing Urinary Incontinence in Older Adults

Problem: Evidence-based information is critical when counseling and treating older adults with urinary incontinence (UI) because quality of life is directly related to the frequency, volume of urine loss, and the degree of urinary urgency that clients may experience.

Evidence

Medline, CINAHL, and MDConsult were the databases used to develop guidelines that were developed by a group of nursing experts from across the country as part of the Nurses Improving Care for Health System Elders (NICHE) project, under sponsorship of The John A. Hartford Foundation Institute for Geriatric Nursing.

Application to Practice

These guidelines present a nursing standard of practice protocol for UI, including the following:

- Assess for the presence of incontinence, etiology, and use of urinary catheter on admission.
- Implement major treatment strategies for UI specific to the type of incontinence.
- Indwelling catheter is appropriate for severely ill clients, client with stage III to IV pressure ulcers of the trunk, or urinary retention unresolved by other interventions.
- Provide the client/caregiver discharge teaching regarding outpatient referral and management.

The level of evidence for recommendations is not given. A complete summary can be found at *http://www.guideline.gov/summary/summary.aspx?=15&doc_id=3507&nbr=2733.*

Read the complete reference below for a more comprehensive summary.

Reference

Dowling-Castronovo, A., & Bradway, C. (2003). Urinary incontinence. In M. Mezey, T. Fulmer, I. Abraham, & D. A. Zwicker (Eds.), *Geriatric nursing protocols for best practice* (2nd ed., pp. 83-98). New York: Springer Publishing [26 references].

BOX 30-5

Considering the Alternatives

Alterative Therapies for Incontinence and Urinary Symptoms

Biofeedback-Assisted Behavioral Training

Advantages

- Preoperative training can decrease the severity of incontinence following radical prostatectomy (Burgio et al., 2006)
- Hastens the recovery of urine control
- No side effects

Disadvantages

- Requires biofeedback availability for behavioral training
- Requires effort and time by clients and practitioners
- May not be available in all areas

Acupuncture

Advantages

- Provides significant improvement in bladder capacity, urgency, frequency, and quality-of-life scores for overactive bladder with urge incontinence (Emmons & Otto, 2005)
- Avoids the risks of surgery
- Fewer side effects than medications
- May be attractive to clients who prefer to stimulate their body's innate responses

Disadvantages

- Some clients may fear the use of acupuncture needles
- May postpone traditional therapies
- May be difficult to find a local practitioner

Myofascial Trigger Point Release and Relaxation Training

Advantages

- Relief from pain and urinary symptoms superior to traditional therapy (Anderson, Wise, Sawyer, & Chan, 2005)
- Avoids the risks of surgery
- Benefits of relaxation training may extend to other systems

Disadvantages

- Requires practitioners trained in myofascial trigger point release and relaxation
- Requires effort and time by clients and practitioners
- May not be available in all areas

Anderson, R. U., Wise, D., Sawyer, T., & Chan, C. (2005). Integration of myofascial trigger point release and paradoxical relaxation training treatment of chronic pelvic pain in men. *Journal of Urology, 174*(1),155-160.

Burgio, K. L., Goode, P. S., Urban, D. A., Umlauf, M. G., Locher, J L., & Bueschen, A., et al. (2006). Preoperative biofeedback-assisted behavioral training to decrease post-prostatectomy incontinence: A randomized, controlled trial. *Journal of Urology, 175*(1),196-201.

Emmons, S. L., & Otto, L. (2005). Acupuncture for overactive bladder: A randomized controlled trial. *Obstetrics and Gynecology, 106*(1):138-143.

Performing the exercises correctly depends on the woman's ability to selectively contract the muscles of the pelvic floor. The initial tendency is to contract the abdominal muscles or the muscles of the buttocks. The correct muscle can be located by starting the stream of urine, then contracting the muscles to stop the flow. Another method is to place one finger in the vagina and contract the pelvic floor muscles around the finger. Biofeedback training is useful for some women to become familiar with the contraction of the correct muscle.

BOX 30-6 *Teaching for Wellness*

Exercises for the Pelvic Floor Muscles

Purpose: To help control stress incontinence in women.
Expected Outcome: The client will experience no urine leakage with an increase in abdominal pressure.

Client Instructions

- To perform Kegel exercises correctly, you must first locate the proper muscles. To do so, sit on the toilet, begin urinating, and try to stop the urine in midstream. The muscles used to stop the urine stream are the ones you need to exercise. Another way to locate the proper muscles is to insert one finger into your vagina and contract the muscles of your pelvic floor around your finger.
- Strengthen your pelvic floor muscles by contracting them for 5 to 10 seconds, relaxing for 5 to 10 seconds, and repeating.
- Perform this exercise three times daily, contracting the muscles 15 times during each exercise period. For example, perform 15 contractions in the morning before rising from bed. Perform 15 more contractions in the afternoon while doing a task that requires you to stand up without moving around. Finally, perform 15 more contractions in the evening while sitting, such as while watching television or reading a book.
- Make these exercises a part of your daily routine. You will begin to see results in about 2 weeks, and you will continue to improve for about 6 weeks.

A vaginal or rectal probe may be used to provide visual feedback when the correct muscle has been contracted. Two thirds of women will need some practice to find the correct muscles.

Bladder Retraining. For the person with urge incontinence associated with a small bladder capacity, training is designed to increase the bladder capacity by having the client adopt a gradually lengthening voiding schedule. Strategies to control the urge to urinate are practiced.

For the cognitively competent person, a bladder diary may be useful for selecting the most useful training protocol. A daily record is kept of the time of urination, whether the person was incontinent, whether the incontinence involved a small or large amount, and associated events or the reason for the incontinence. For the cognitively impaired person, training is different, and a scheduled toileting regimen may be successful. The client's voiding pattern should be recorded for several days to determine whether a pattern exists. Electronic devices to monitor for wetness are sometimes useful in establishing the pattern.

People often need to urinate on arising in the morning, after meals, and at bedtime. However, for some older clients, the schedule may need to be as frequent as every 2 hours. Patience is required. Over time, the regimen becomes habitual and incontinence will improve. Success is partially related to a consistent daily schedule of meals and fluid intake.

For clients with some ability to recognize the need to urinate, a schedule of prompted voiding may be successful, as described later in the chapter.

Maintaining Dry and Intact Skin

External Catheters. External catheters are devices that can be attached to the skin to collect urine. External collecting devices for women are not widely available and have tended to leak and cause skin abrasions. Condom catheters are used successfully for men, however. The condom is a heavy rubber sheath that fits over the penis and is secured with a soft, flexible band (Procedure 30-2). The end of the condom is molded into a drainage tube that can be attached to bedside drainage or leg bag drainage (Figure 30-8).

The risk for urinary tract infection is reduced with an external catheter. The advantages of using a condom catheter are keeping the skin dry and controlling odor. The disadvantages are the difficulty in securing the catheter adequately to control leakage of urine and to keep the catheter in place without causing edema to the penis and excoriation to the skin. The catheter should be removed at least daily to inspect and clean the skin.

Complications include abrasion, dermatitis, ischemia, necrosis, edema, and maceration of the penis. The incidence of urinary tract infection is less than with an indwelling catheter but is still a factor in using condom catheters. An alternative to a condom catheter for men is a retracted penis pouch (Figure 30-9). This device is sometimes successful if the man has a retracted penis that cannot support a condom catheter.

Action Alert! Avoid constricting the penis with a condom catheter, because doing so will cause edema. Remove the condom and inspect the skin daily.

Absorbent Products. Protective garments and absorbent products are highly useful in managing urinary incontinence. Both washable and disposable products may be used. Cost, absorbency, and skin protection should be considered in selecting a product. Underpads may be convenient when the client is in bed. Adult diapers (briefs) allow protection when the client is moving from bed to chair or using a wheelchair. For a female client with incontinence of small amounts of urine, a feminine protection pad may be sufficient. Many people adopt this intervention on their own rather than consulting a health care professional about minor incontinence. Disposable products are widely used for institutional care, often because the cost of laundry makes the disposable products less expensive. The protective lining in disposable products may have some benefit in pulling moisture away from the skin, but the client should have the pad changed immediately after voiding.

Urine that has remained for a period of time has a characteristic foul odor that is associated with poor nursing care and is unpleasant to the client, family, and staff.

PROCEDURE 30-2

TIME TO ALLOW: NOVICE: 5 min. EXPERT: 10 min.

APPLYING A CONDOM CATHETER

Nursing Skills Online: Urinary Catheterization, Lesson 3

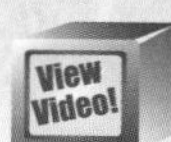

The purpose of applying a condom catheter is to control incontinence in a male client without the risk for urinary tract infection and with greater comfort to the client than an indwelling catheter.

DELEGATION GUIDELINES

The application of a condom catheter is a noninvasive procedure that you may delegate to a nursing assistant who has received specific instruction in this skill. Instruction should include safety and skin care considerations.

EQUIPMENT NEEDED

- Commercially packaged condom catheter
- Soap and water
- Disposable clean gloves
- Drainage bag and tubing

1 Follow preliminary actions (see inside front cover).

2 Position the client on his back, and drape him to expose only his penis.

3 Clean his genitals with soap and water, and dry thoroughly.

4 Apply skin-protecting cream packaged with the catheter to the client's penis. Allow it to dry.

5 Wrap the adhesive spirally around the shaft of the penis (see illustration). *Be careful not to apply the adhesive too tightly. Severe edema can result if the adhesive strip constricts the shaft of the penis, and the client will develop pain and difficulty urinating.*

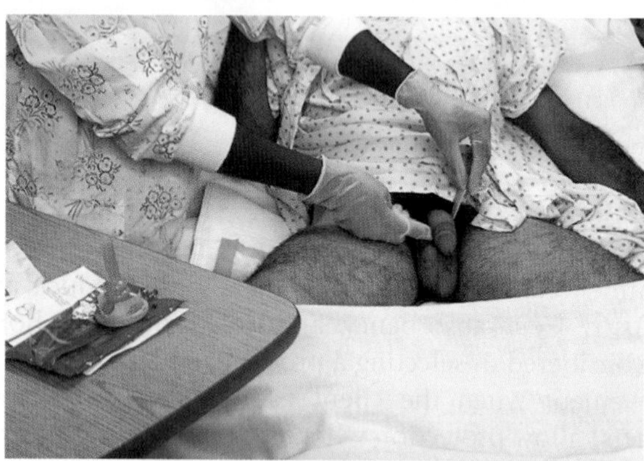

Step 5. Wrapping the adhesive spirally around the penis.

6 Place the rolled condom over the client's glans penis, and unroll the condom over the adhesive liner and the shaft of the penis (see illustration). *If the client is uncircumcised, make sure his foreskin remains in place over the glans penis as you unroll the condom. If retracted, the foreskin may be tight enough to constrict the penis and cause edema of the glans penis.*

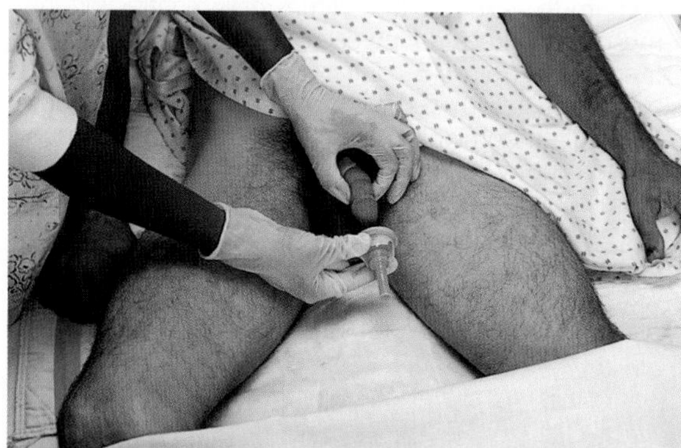

Step 6. Placing the rolled condom over the client's glans penis.

7 Attach the catheter to a collecting system and tape the tubing to the client's leg (see illustration).

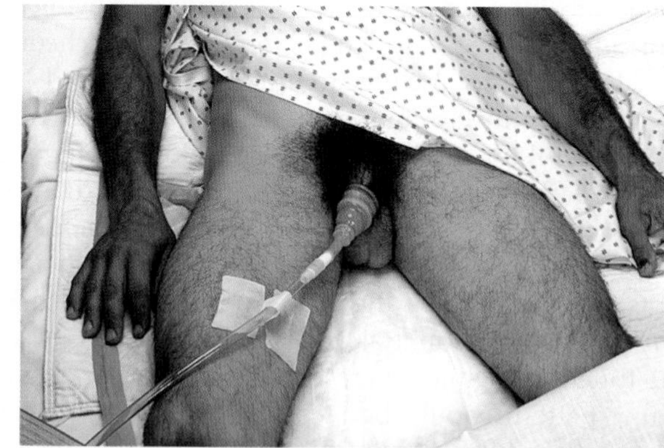

Step 7. Catheter attached to a collecting system and taped to the client's leg.

8 Document date and time of application and assessment of shaft of penis, glans, and foreskin. Observe the client's penis after applying the condom catheter to detect such problems as urine leakage, edema, and changes in skin color.

PEDIATRIC CONSIDERATIONS

For infants and toddlers, diapers or training pants are more appropriate. Change them frequently to prevent skin irritation. Condom catheters are probably not effective until the penis reaches adult size.

GERIATRIC CONSIDERATIONS

The size of the penis may shrink with age and make it difficult to effectively use a condom catheter in some men. Skin may be more fragile.

HOME HEALTH CARE CONSIDERATIONS

Teach family caregivers to apply the catheter and care for the skin. The family should remove the condom and clean the skin daily.

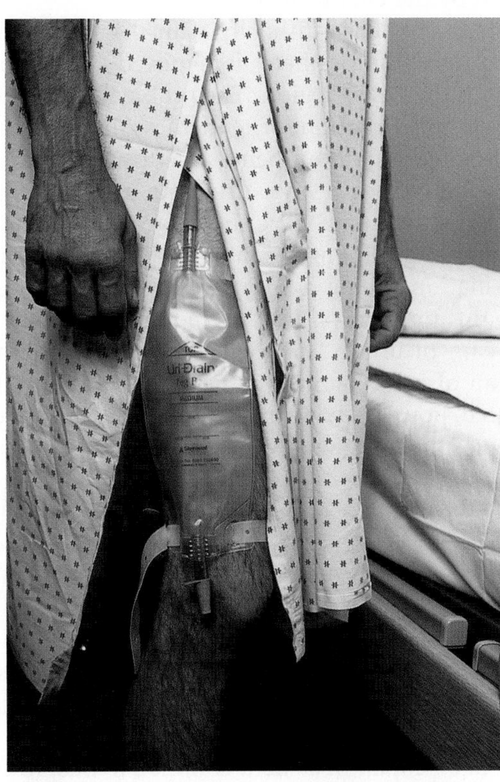

FIGURE 30-8 For the ambulatory client with an indwelling catheter, a drainage bag can be attached to the leg and hidden by the client's clothes.

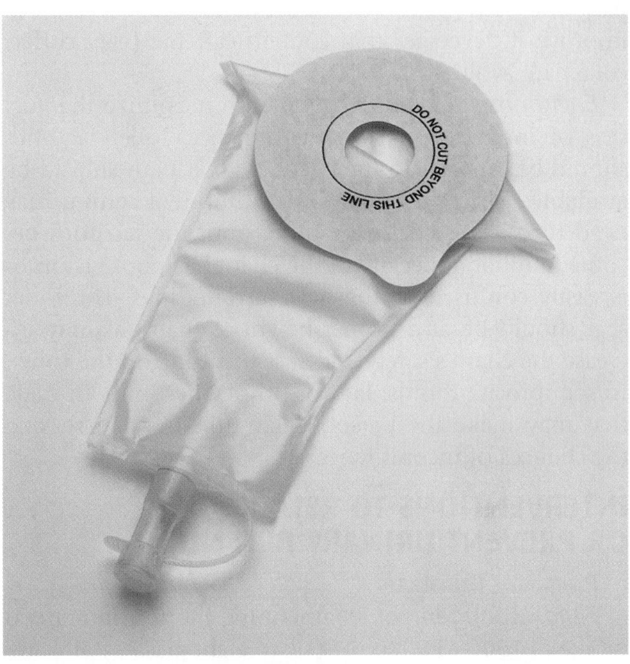

FIGURE 30-9 A retracted penis pouch is available as an alternative to a condom catheter for a male client with a retracted penis. (Courtesy Hollister, Inc., Libertyville, Ill.)

Besides the problem of odor, the skin can quickly develop a rash or excoriation from prolonged wetness, and the client becomes more vulnerable to pressure ulcers.

Managing Bowel Elimination. Urinary incontinence can be reduced by preventing constipation. Hydration is an important component of preventing constipation, so reducing fluid intake is not recommended for the management of urinary incontinence.

Establishing Continence in the Cognitively Impaired Client

Scheduled Toileting and Prompted Voiding. Prompted voiding and regularly scheduled toileting are effective for preventing episodes of incontinence in some clients who are homebound or need long-term care. In a prompted-voiding program, the client should be checked on an hourly basis, offered the opportunity to void, and given a dry protective pad (Box 30-7). The time can be extended as the caregiver becomes familiar with the client's pattern. An electronic monitoring device can be used to determine the pattern of wetness and construct an individualized toileting schedule. Clients are given positive reinforcement for successful toileting. Clients with greater mental impairment are expected to have higher failure rates.

Patterned Urge Response Training. In this intervention, you help the client develop strategies to control the urge to urinate. For example, if there is an urge to urinate, instruct the client to stand still, take a slow, deep breath, and relax. Instruct the client to then quickly

BOX 30-7 *The Steps of Prompted Voiding*

To perform prompted voiding, follow these steps:
- At scheduled times (usually every 2 hours), elicit subjective data about wetness.
- Check for objective evidence of wetness.
- If the client correctly identified being dry, give positive feedback.
- Ask the client about the subjective sensation of the need to use the toilet.
- If the client responds positively, assist to the toilet as needed. If the client responds negatively, encourage to try using the toilet. Never force a client to toilet.
- Give positive feedback for appropriate toileting; never give negative feedback.

squeeze the muscles of the pelvic floor three or four times without holding the squeeze, wait for the urge to pass, and then walk slowly to the bathroom. Success will improve if beverages that contain caffeine (e.g., coffee, colas) are avoided.

Environmental Modifications. To maximize the success of interventions for incontinence, toilet facilities should be familiar to the client. A clear path should be available. A new client in an institutional setting may need to be assisted to the toilet until the facilities become familiar, especially if the client has poor vision or is easily confused by the new surroundings. The toilet seat should be at a proper height. A grab bar may increase the client's safety and ease of sitting on the toilet. In semiprivate rooms, lack of privacy becomes an issue that may make the person delay urination, increasing the chances of incontinence.

INTERVENTIONS TO RELIEVE OR PREVENT URINARY RETENTION

Promoting Urination

Fluid Management. Maintaining the recommended intake of 1500 to 2000 mL (six to eight glasses) of water daily will assist the bladder to fill and stimulate the urge to urinate. Water lost through profuse perspiration should be replaced in addition to the usual amount. Water is preferred to fluids that contain sodium, sugar, or caffeine. Adequate fluid intake will flush the bladder and urethra of bacteria and help prevent urinary tract infections.

Enhancing the Stimulus to Void. For the client who is having difficulty urinating, you may need to provide assistance to stimulate urination. The postsurgical client may initially have difficulty urinating, especially if the procedure involved the use of an indwelling catheter or manipulation of the bladder. Provide privacy to help the person stay comfortable and relaxed. Allow adequate time, and avoid making the person feel a need to hurry.

You will aid urination by helping the person to the position usually used for voiding. A man may be more able to void in a standing position rather than sitting on a toilet or lying in bed. A man with prostatic hypertrophy may not be able to use a urinal lying in bed. A woman may be better able to void when sitting on a toilet rather than lying in bed. If a woman cannot walk to the bathroom, consider using a bedside commode.

The Credé maneuver is sometimes helpful for the client with a neurogenic bladder or BPH. The client presses firmly downward and inward directly into the lower abdomen over the bladder, with one hand (or both hands). Increased intravesical pressure causes the bladder neck to open and allow emptying of the bladder as long as compression is continued. However, prolonged use of this technique may not be recommended by the client's urologist.

Some clients have difficulty with the initial voiding after an indwelling catheter is removed or after having surgery in the pelvic region. The problem can be the result of edema, irritation, or tenderness. It is exacerbated by feeling tension about being able to urinate or about the possibility of pain when urinating. You can try methods to help the person relax, such as relaxation breathing techniques. Running water in a nearby sink may stimulate urination. Using a spray of warm water over the perineum may relax the perineum and help start the stream of urine. The client's sitting in a warm sitz bath can also be helpful. If the client's urine must be measured, however, you will not be able to use a method that mixes the urine with water.

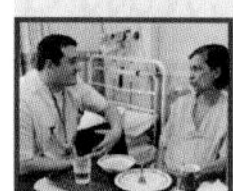

Remember Mrs. Al-Kandari, our case study client? On the second day after surgery, she can walk to the bathroom. What methods would be the most appropriate to help her urinate for the first time?

Using Catheters. A urinary catheter is a tube inserted into the bladder to drain urine. Urinary catheters can be used to prevent incontinence, to avoid the inconvenience of a bedpan in a client confined to bed, to collect urine specimens, and to drain urine from a person unable to void. However, using a catheter as the means to manage incontinence should only done when the risk of not using a catheter outweighs the risk of using one. The primary purpose of a urinary catheter is to prevent urinary retention.

Catheterization. Catheterization refers to inserting a tube into the bladder through the urethra for the purpose of draining urine from the bladder. It may have various indications (Box 30-8). For one-time relief of retention, the catheter is passed, urine is drained, and the catheter is removed. Sometimes referred to as straight catheterization or in-and-out catheterization, intermittent catheterization is also used by clients who need self-catheterization.

When a problem is expected to persist, an indwelling (Foley) catheter is used. This type of catheter has two or three lumens. One drains urine, the second allows inflation of a balloon in the client's bladder, and a third can

BOX 30-8 *Indications for Catheterization*

SHORT-TERM INDWELLING CATHETERIZATION

- After surgical procedures known to interfere with normal urination, such as bladder surgery, pelvic surgery, some types of hip surgery
- When the client's kidney function must be monitored, as when renal function is compromised or the client has a critical illness and a high risk for shock
- After surgical procedures involving the urinary tract, when a catheter can help prevent obstruction from blood clots
- When an orthopedic client cannot be safely turned and repositioned
- When frequent moving causes pain
- To empty the bladder during childbirth (labor and delivery)

INTERMITTENT CATHETERIZATION

- For relief of discomfort from an overdistended bladder when the client cannot initiate urination
- When obtaining a sterile urine specimen for culture
- When assessing residual urine volume after the client voids
- For long-term management of urination in spinal cord injuries, multiple sclerosis, or other causes of incompetent bladder

LONG-TERM CATHETERIZATION

- For irreversible incontinence, when skin rash, ulcers, or wound management is negatively affected by urine on the skin
- For a terminally ill client (especially one in severe pain) whose comfort is improved by minimizing the amount of turning and cleaning needed
- For irreversible, severe urinary retention, especially when the client develops frequent urinary tract infections

be used to irrigate the bladder with fluids or medications (Figure 30-10).

Action Alert! Check an indwelling catheter regularly for patency to prevent urinary retention. Crusts formed with long-term use, blood clots when bleeding is present, or kinking and incorrect positioning of the tube can obstruct catheters.

Indwelling catheters are used for short-term problems that will benefit from catheterization to relieve or prevent urinary retention that cannot be corrected medically or surgically, that cannot be managed practically by intermittent catheterization, and, occasionally, to manage the incontinent client. A client with chronic retention may benefit from a catheter if bothered by persistent overflow incontinence, symptomatic urinary tract infections, or an increased risk for renal dysfunction. If an incontinent client has pressure ulcers, skin lesions, or surgical wounds that are being contaminated by urine, an indwelling catheter may be beneficial as well. Indwelling catheters are sometimes used for short-term management of elimination in the severely ill, in clients undergoing major surgery, and in the terminally ill (Procedure 30-3).

Action Alert! Maintaining straight, gravity drainage from an indwelling catheter will prevent backflow of possibly contaminated urine into the bladder.

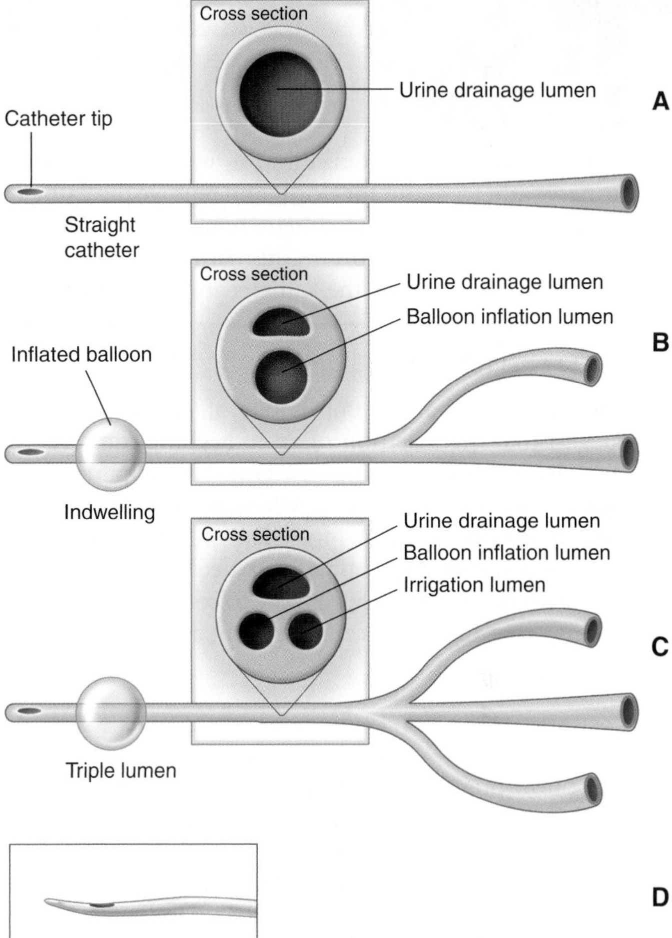

FIGURE 30-10 Types of catheters. **A,** A straight catheter is inserted to drain the bladder and then immediately removed. **B,** An indwelling (Foley) catheter has a second lumen, used to inflate a balloon that holds the catheter in place in the bladder. **C,** A triple-lumen indwelling catheter has a third lumen for instillation of fluid into the bladder for irrigation. **D,** A Coudé tip.

Urinary catheterization carries a high risk for urinary tract infection and should be avoided unless the potential benefits outweigh the potential risks. After a single catheterization (not indwelling), 1% of ambulatory clients will develop infection. With an open drainage system, most clients will develop an infection in 4 to 7 days.

Suprapubic catheters are sometimes placed to reduce the incidence of infection. A puncture wound is made through the abdominal wall into the bladder and a catheter is inserted (Figure 30-11, p. 777). The incidence of infection is less than with a typical indwelling catheter because the abdominal skin has a lower bacterial count than the urethra.

Managing Urethral Catheters

Maintaining comfort. The client with an indwelling catheter should be physically and mentally comfortable. Probably the greatest discomfort for most people is embarrassment and invasion of privacy.

Text continued on p. 777

PROCEDURE 30-3

TIME TO ALLOW: NOVICE: 20 min. EXPERT: 10 min.

INSERTING AN INDWELLING CATHETER

Nursing Skills Online: Urinary Catheterization, Lesson 2

Unlike a straight catheterization, in which you insert a urinary catheter, drain the urine, and remove the catheter right away, an indwelling catheter remains in the client's bladder to provide continuous urine drainage. An inflated balloon holds the catheter in place in the urinary bladder. Besides providing continuous urine drainage, an indwelling catheter can be used to prevent bladder distention, obtain sterile urine specimens, and irrigate the bladder with fluids or medications.

DELEGATION GUIDELINES

The assessment and complexities of sterile technique suggest that the insertion of an indwelling catheter not be delegated to a nursing assistant. This is particularly true in an acute care setting, where the risk for nosocomial infection exists, or in a client in whom difficulty passing a catheter may be anticipated. In a long-term-care setting, it may be appropriate to consider delegation of this procedure after a careful client assessment.

EQUIPMENT NEEDED

- Bottom drape
- Sterile gloves
- Fenestrated drape
- Catheter, connecting tubing, and collection bag
- Syringe prefilled with sterile water
- Antiseptic cleaning solution
- Cotton balls
- Forceps
- Water-soluble lubricant
- Gooseneck lamp or flashlight, especially for a female client

1 Follow preliminary actions (see inside front cover).

2 Select a catheter of appropriate size and material, with a balloon of appropriate size. *Catheters range from No. 6 Fr (the smallest) to No. 24 Fr (the largest). For a child, you probably will use a No. 8 to 10 Fr. Most adult women need a No. 14 to 16 Fr. Most men need a No. 16 to 18 Fr. A client who has had an indwelling catheter for a long time will need a larger catheter to prevent urine leakage from the stretched urethra.*

For short-term catheterization, you probably will use a plastic catheter. It can be inserted easily when well lubricated but may be less comfortable because it is stiff and inflexible. For catheterization lasting up to 3 weeks, you may use a latex or rubber catheter, which is softer than plastic. For catheterization lasting 4 to 6 weeks, you may use a polyvinylchloride catheter, which softens at body temperatures. For catheterization lasting 2 to 3 months, you may use a silicone or Teflon catheter, on which secretions are less likely to adhere and form crusts that could irritate the urethra or obstruct the catheter.

Pediatric catheters usually come with a 3-mL balloon; adult catheters have either a 5-mL or a 30-mL balloon. You may need to use the 30-mL balloon if the client has had an indwelling catheter for a long time or if a male client has had a transurethral resection of the prostate. The larger balloon is thought to provide some hemostasis at the neck of the bladder after prostate resection.

3 Position the client for catheterization.

a. If the client is female, have her lie in a supine position with her knees flexed and separated. *This position allows access to the urinary meatus and typically is comfortable for the client. If the client cannot hold her knees open, ask a colleague to hold them for you; do not spread the client's knees if doing so causes her pain. If the client cannot lie on her back or open her knees, place her in Sims' position with her upper leg flexed at the hip and knee.*

b. If the client is male, have him lie in a supine position.

4 Drape the client for privacy.

a. If the client is female, expose only her labia. To do so, place one corner of a sheet between her legs so that two corners cover her legs and the remaining corner covers her abdomen. Leave the drape fully in place over the client's labia until you are ready to perform the catheterization. You can then lift the corner of the drape that covers her labia and fold it back.

b. If the client is male, use his gown or a bath blanket to cover his upper body down to his penis. Use a bed sheet to cover his lower body up to his penis. *Draping should make the client feel covered and as private as possible but should be simple and not add significantly to the length of the procedure.*

5 Establish a sterile field.

a. Open the prepackaged catheter tray, and place it in a convenient location. If your client is female, consider placing the opened tray on the bed near her perineum. If your client is male, consider placing the opened tray on an over-bed table.

b. Place the bottom drape adjacent to a female client's buttocks (see illustration). Hold the drape only by a corner, allow it to fall open, and place it under her buttocks, still touching only the corners. Place the drape so it overlaps the outer wrapper of the open catheter tray. This will form a continuous sterile field from the tray to the client's buttocks. *This procedure is not practical for female clients who are likely to move their legs during the catheterization procedure.*

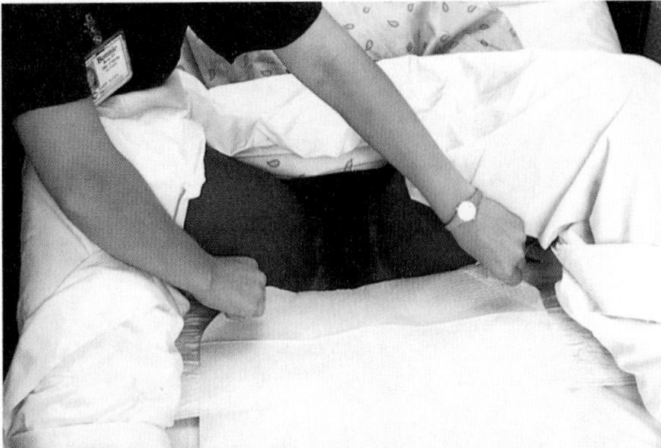

Step 5b. Placing the bottom drape. Touch only the corners to avoid contamination. (The edge of a sterile field is never considered to be sterile.)

c. Put on sterile gloves. If you wish, or according to your facility's policy, use a fenestrated drape (see illustration) to create a sterile field that encircles a female client's labia or a male client's penis.

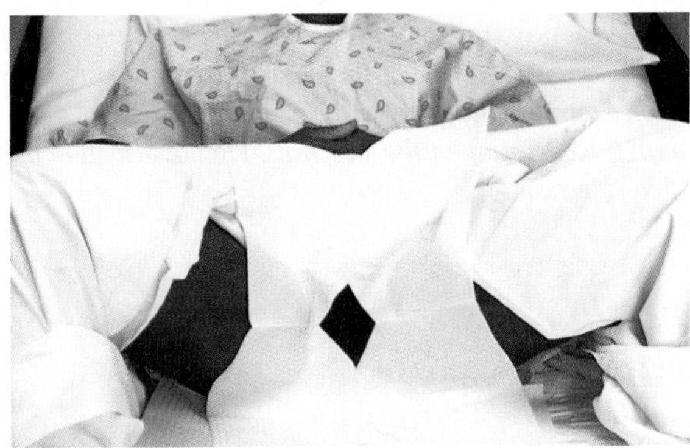

Step 5c. Fenestrated top drape in place.

d. Inflate the catheter balloon to test it for leaks (see illustration).

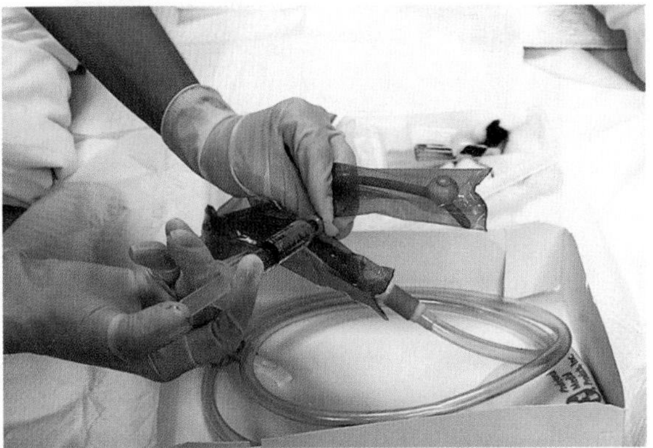

Step 5d. Testing the catheter balloon for leaks.

6 Clean the area around the urinary meatus

a. Pour antiseptic on all three cotton balls.
b. If the client is female, spread her labia with your nondominant hand (see illustration) while using forceps to hold a cotton ball in your dominant hand. *Remember that the hand used to spread the labia is no longer sterile.*

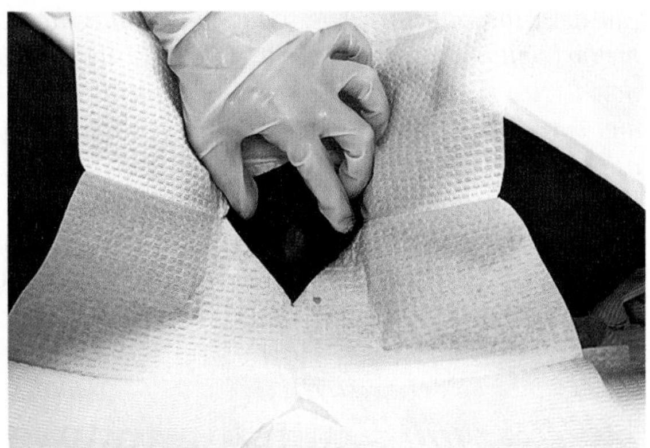

Step 6b. Spreading the labia.

c. With the first cotton ball, clean to the right of the client's urinary meatus. Make one stroke from top to bottom and discard the cotton ball (see illustration). With the second cotton ball, clean to the left of the client's urinary meatus, again making one stroke from top to bottom before discarding the cotton ball. With the third cotton ball, clean down the middle of the client's perineum, directly over the urinary meatus. Then discard the cotton ball. Keep the client's labia spread until the catheter is inserted.

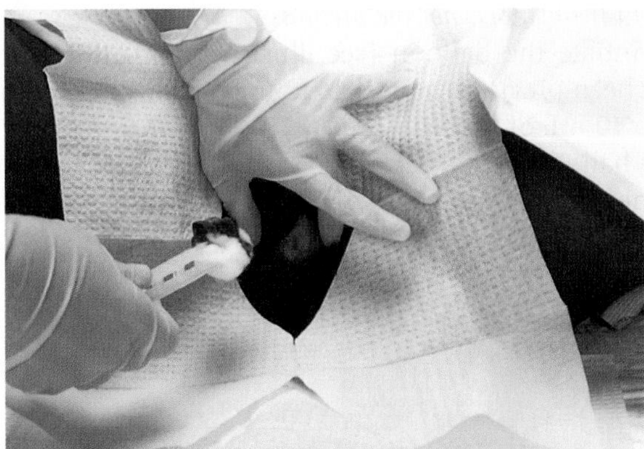

Step 6c. Cleaning the labia and meatus from top to bottom.

d. If the client is male, use at least two cotton balls soaked in antiseptic. Use the first to clean around the glans penis. Use the second to clean over the meatus. Make sure to retract the foreskin if the client has not been circumcised. *Remember to replace the foreskin to avoid edema of the glans penis.*

Continued

7. Lubricate and insert the catheter.

a. Holding the catheter 2.5 to 5 cm (1 to 2 inches) from its tip, lubricate it and insert it into the urinary meatus. If the client is male, use your nondominant hand to hold his penis perpendicular to his body, using your fingers to gently encircle and stabilize the shaft. *If you meet resistance when inserting a catheter, do not force it. Instead, have the client take a deep breath as you twist the catheter while trying to pass it. Often this method will allow the catheter to slide in easily. If it does not, try using a catheter with a Coudé tip; it is smaller and curved to help the catheter pass an obstruction, such as prostatic hypertrophy.*

b. Insert the catheter until urine begins to flow (see illustration). *The catheter should enter a female client 5 to 7.6 cm (2 to 3 inches) or a male client 15.2 to 20.3 cm (6 to 8 inches).*

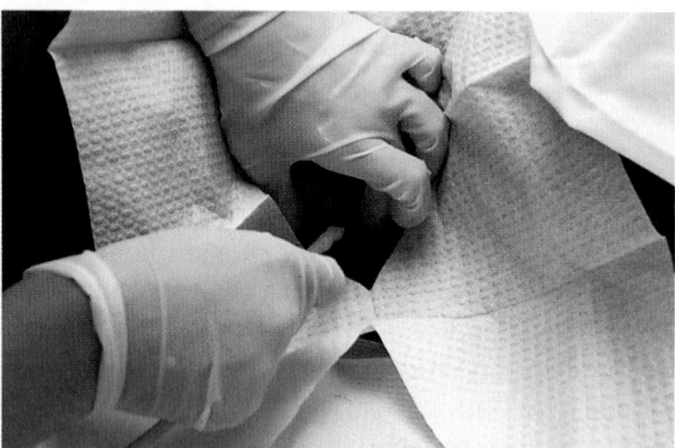

Step 7b. Inserting the catheter.

c. After urine begins to flow, insert the catheter 2.5 cm (1 inch) more. *Doing so will ensure that the balloon is in the bladder, not the urethra.*

8 Inflate the balloon (see illustration). If the syringe has been previously attached to the pigtail, simply inject 8 to 10 mL of water (30 mL +3 if the catheter has a 30-mL balloon). This recommendation is based on most catheters' needing 3 mL more than the amount that fills the balloon, to fill the lumen of the catheter. *You should check the recommendations of the manufacturer.*

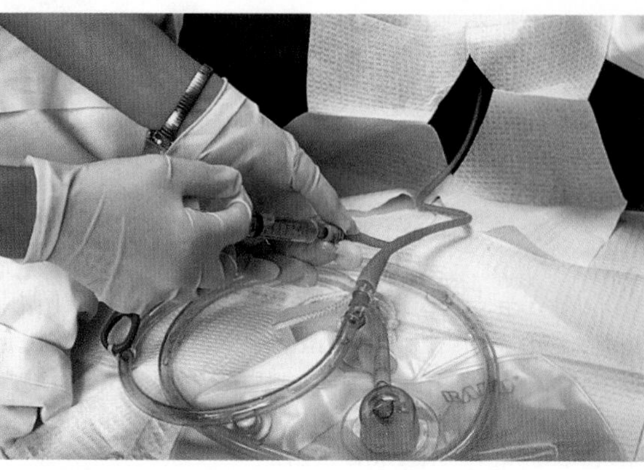

Step 8. Inflating the balloon.

9 Tape catheter to the inner aspect of the thigh (see illustration). Allow enough slack in the catheter tubing to avoid tugging on the catheter when the client's leg moves.

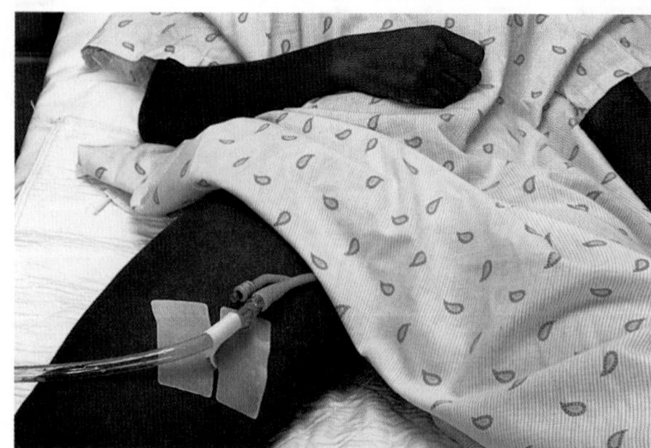

Step 9. Catheter taped to the inner thigh.

10 Establish the drainage system.

a. If the client will use a leg bag to collect urine, attach the catheter to the inner thigh.

b. If the client will use gravity drainage, attach the bag to the bed frame below the level of the client's bladder (see illustration). *In a hospital bed, the bag and tubing should go under the side rails in a position that allows for straight gravity drainage and does not interfere with the operation of the side rails. Do not attach to moveable side rails.*

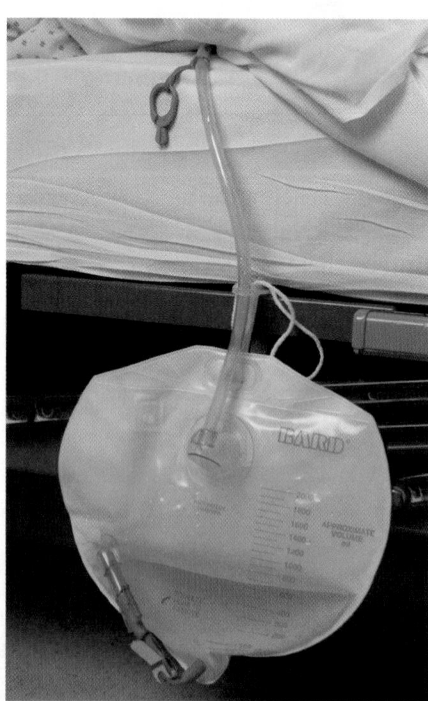

Step 10b. Bag attached to bed frame for gravity drainage.

11 Complete the procedure

a. Discard all trash.

b. Make the client comfortable. Blot or rinse excess solution from the perineum.

c. Document the time the catheter was inserted, the amount and characteristics of the urine that drained from the bladder, and the size of the catheter and balloon.

PEDIATRIC CONSIDERATIONS

When you catheterize a child, you should take time to enlist the child's cooperation. Prepare the child for the sensations associated with cleansing and inserting the catheter. Demonstrating on a doll may be helpful. Encourage the parents to comfort and assist the child with remaining still. Praise the child for cooperation.

GERIATRIC CONSIDERATIONS

Assess for the ability to abduct the thighs. It may be helpful to have an assistant help the person to maintain the position for catheterization. Do not attempt to abduct the thighs beyond a comfortable angle. Privacy is sometimes more important for older adult female clients than for younger clients.

HOME HEALTH CARE CONSIDERATIONS

In the home setting, you will need to be creative in positioning yourself, setting up the sterile field, and establishing adequate lighting to insert the catheter. Provide perineal hygiene before catheterizing. Teach any family caregivers about maintenance of the catheter.

Maintaining a patent catheter. The catheter should be taped to the leg (women) or abdomen (men) to prevent it from pulling on the urethra and to ensure the free flow of urine. Disposable anchoring devices are available, but nonallergenic tape can be used as well. Keep enough slack in the catheter to allow the client to move about without having the catheter pull on the urethra. Taping a male catheter laterally to the side or to the abdomen more naturally follows the normal anatomical direction of the male urethra and avoids the possibility of abscess formation at the penoscrotal junction.

When the client is in bed, the connecting tubing can be placed under the leg or over the leg. Under-the-leg placement may use gravity more effectively for drainage, but the tubing is made of hard plastic and may cause discomfort or pressure on the skin. Coil any excess tubing on the bed to prevent stagnation of urine in dangling loops of tubing. Keep the drainage bag below the level of the bladder, even when moving the person in and out of bed or to a stretcher. Urine in the collection tubing is not sterile and, because bacteria growing in the collection bag could travel up the tubing, urine should not be allowed to flow back into the bladder.

Relieving bladder spasms. Bladder spasms are involuntary, sudden, violent contractions of the muscles of the bladder that can be prolonged and painful. Spasms can occur as a side effect of catheterization or secondary to surgery on the bladder or urethra. Even though the client has a catheter, the urge to urinate is often strong.

Manipulating the catheter to move the balloon away from the neck of the bladder may alleviate the spasms. Increasing fluid intake may be helpful as well. Anticholinergic medications may be prescribed to reduce bladder tone and relieve the spasms. Narcotics will relieve the pain.

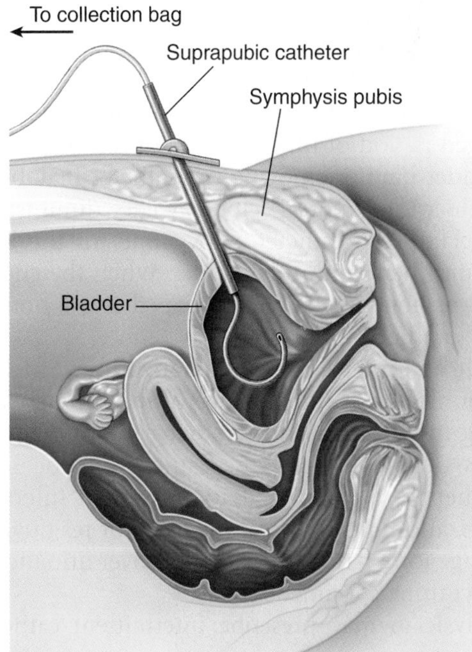

FIGURE 30-11 A suprapubic catheter is surgically placed through a puncture wound to drain urine until the client can void normally through the urethra.

Reestablishing urination after catheterization. Because of the high incidence of infection, an indwelling catheter should be removed as soon as possible. The criterion may be that the person is able to ambulate to the bathroom, the edema has subsided, or the initial inflammatory stage of healing of a surgical wound has passed.

To remove the catheter, select a syringe appropriate to the amount of water in the balloon (usually 5 mL), insert the syringe into the pigtail used to inflate the balloon, aspirate the water from the balloon, and pinch and withdraw the catheter (Figure 30-12). The client may feel a pulling sensation as the catheter is removed. For clients who have urethral irritation, the procedure may be momentarily uncomfortable. Ask the client to take a deep breath, and remove the catheter slowly. A small amount of urine may escape, so it is useful to have a towel under the catheter as it comes out. Empty the bag, and measure the urine in a graduated container; discard the bag. The marks for measuring on the bag are for estimation only. Removing a catheter is a clean procedure employing standard precautions.

Following removal of the catheter, monitor the client for the return of a normal pattern of urination. The client should drink extra liquid to fill the bladder and relieve irritation. Most people void after 2 to 4 hours. Sometimes, measures to help the person relax and initiate the stream are needed for the first voiding. The time to the first voiding should be 4 to 6 hours (a maximum of 8) depending on the person's bladder capacity and fluid intake. If the bladder becomes overdistended, it may be more difficult to void the first time. If the client has had surgery on the bladder or urethra, the urine should be monitored for diminishing amounts of blood.

For a client who has had an indwelling catheter for a prolonged period of time, training or reconditioning of the bladder before removing the catheter may be helpful. Bladder tone and capacity may have diminished. To do so, clamp the catheter, allow time for the bladder to fill, and then drain the bladder. When the client can tolerate having the catheter clamped for 4 hours, the catheter can be removed.

Single and intermittent catheterization. Single catheterization refers to the practice of inserting a catheter, draining the bladder, and removing the catheter. If the client is unable to void, the catheter can be inserted again when the bladder needs to be emptied. Intermittent catheterization is performed to check for residual urine, to manage long-term lack of control over urination, and to collect urine specimens.

A physician may prescribe intermittent catheterization after a surgical procedure that produces a high risk for urinary retention. The order is often written as "catheterize prn" or "in-and-out catheter prn." You must make judgments about the need for catheterization and the frequency of catheterization. This judgment is based on the client's report of fullness, the interval since the last voiding, and an examination for bladder distention. Before inserting the catheter, have the client attempt to urinate. Then immediately insert the catheter. If the client has just emptied the bladder, the amount of urine remaining in the bladder represents retention and is referred to as residual urine.

Ultrasonography is sometimes used to detect the presence of residual urine. It is a noninvasive bedside test.

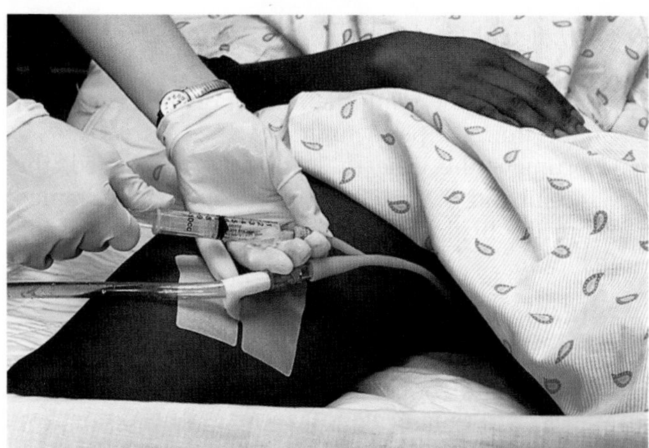

FIGURE 30-12 To remove an indwelling catheter, attach a 10-mL syringe (without a needle) to the pigtail port, and withdraw the normal saline from the catheter balloon.

Catheterization can be avoided for the client who does not have residual urine in the bladder.

Intermittent self-catheterization is a procedure that can be taught to clients who are unable to spontaneously empty the bladder and have chronic urinary retention with overflow incontinence. These clients are usually relatively young, cognitively intact victims of spinal cord injury with permanent paralysis from the waist down. The procedure may also be used for a client with an underactive or a partially obstructed bladder. It is easier for a male to perform self-catheterization than for a female.

Before teaching self-catheterization, determine the reason that the client needs the procedure. The way the procedure can be performed by a client with a neurogenic bladder is different from the way a client who is paraplegic will perform it. Also assess the client's ability and motivation to learn. The client may need a period of adjustment before deciding to master self-catheterization. Assess the client's usual health practices to determine the likelihood of safe management of the procedure.

If the client's immune system is not impaired, you most likely will teach self-catheterization as a clean procedure (Box 30-9). Clean technique has not been shown to result in a higher incidence of urinary tract infection than sterile technique. Long-term use of intermittent catheterization may be preferable to indwelling catheterization from the standpoint of preventing infections and formation of stones.

Teaching at-home use of urinary catheters. If necessary, the client and family will need to know how to manage a catheter safely at home (Box 30-10). The client and family caregivers should learn the functions and purpose of the catheter. Preventing urinary tract infection is probably the most important concept to teach.

BOX 30-9 *Teaching for Self-Care*

Self-Catheterization

Purpose: To help the client manage bladder elimination and establish skills for independent living.

Expected Outcome: The client will be able to self-catheterize successfully to minimize incontinence and the risk for urinary tract infection.

Client Instructions

Establishing a Schedule for Catheterization

- Together with your health care providers, determine an optimal schedule for self-catheterization. It will depend in part on how often you experience incontinence, which may relate directly to your bladder capacity and fluid intake. Consider your work and social schedules as well.
- Seek to maintain a routine catheterization schedule, such as three or four times daily or after a certain number of hours have passed. Some people need self-catheterization every 4 hours.

Performing Catheterization

- Plan to drain the urine into a receptacle or directly into the toilet. If you drain it into a receptacle, you may want to have a towel on hand to catch any spills.
- Assume a position that allows access to your urinary meatus. If you are female and find it helpful, you can use a mirror to locate the meatus. Many women locate it by feel.
- Clean your urinary meatus with warm, soapy water, and rinse.
- If you are male, retract your foreskin, if necessary, and hold your penis erect or at a right angle to your body. If you are female, spread your labia.
- Holding the catheter about ½ inch from the tip, insert it into your urinary meatus. This should not hurt, and you should feel no resistance. The first time you perform self-catheterization, you may feel some pressure as your urethra stretches.
- Advance the catheter until urine begins to flow (about 2 to 3 inches for a woman and 6 to 8 inches for a man). Then advance the catheter 1 to 2 inches farther to make sure it is in your bladder.
- When the urine has stopped flowing, lean forward, and use your abdominal muscles to remove any residual urine.

Maintaining Safety Measures

- Wash your hands vigorously before and after self-catheterization.
- Clean the catheter with warm, soapy water, and rinse it thoroughly after each use.
- Once the catheter is clean and dry, store it in a clean plastic bag or towel.
- Immediately report any signs and symptoms of urinary tract infection to your doctor, such as burning or pain on urination, increased incontinence, malodorous or cloudy urine, or swelling or redness at your urinary meatus.

Clean technique and adequate fluid intake should be included in the teaching. The caregiver should have the knowledge to monitor for the signs and symptoms of urinary tract infections.

INTERVENTIONS TO IRRIGATE THE BLADDER

Surgery on the bladder or prostate may result in bleeding into the bladder. Therefore, when a client has had surgery on the bladder or a transurethral resection of the prostate, the indwelling catheter will need to be irrigated to maintain its patency by preventing the formation of blood clots or removing those that do form.

Irrigation can be accomplished using a closed-bladder irrigation system or by opening the system and using an irrigation syringe attached to the indwelling catheter. Because the urine and bladder are normally free of bacteria, either method should be used with sterile technique.

Action Alert! In high-risk populations, such as hospitalized clients, you will need to maintain sterile technique for catheterization or irrigation of a catheter.

A closed irrigation system uses a three-lumen indwelling catheter (Figure 30-13). The advantage of this closed irrigation system is a reduced risk for infection. The disadvantage is that the client is attached to multiple tubes and the bag of irrigation fluid. The physician's order usually specifies irrigation of the bladder to maintain patency. The fluid can be run continuously through the bladder or instilled intermittently. You will use a sliding clamp to regulate the flow of irrigant to keep the urine pink. If the urine becomes burgundy or red, you will need to increase the flow rate of the irrigant. If the urine stops flowing, the catheter may need to be irrigated with an irrigation syringe, which applies more force to remove clots. Preventing clots is preferable to irrigating forcefully, because forceful irrigation increases the risk for bleeding.

The catheter also may be irrigated to remove sediment, to reduce the number of microorganisms in the bladder, and to instill medications. When catheters are used for the long-term management of urinary incontinence, sediment is formed from minerals excreted in the urine, and it may solidify in and around the catheter. Keep in mind that irrigation for the purpose of removing sediment is controversial because it increases the chance of urinary tract infection.

BOX 30-10

Teaching for Self-Care

Maintaining an Indwelling (Foley) Catheter at Home

Purpose: To maintain the function of the catheter, maximize comfort, and prevent complications from the use of an indwelling catheter.
Expected Outcome: The client will not experience a urinary tract infection as a result of the use of an indwelling catheter.

Client Instructions

Care of the Catheter

- Cleanse the area around the catheter's exit site with mild soap and water. Some people prefer to clean the area around the catheter while showering. Afterward, rinse thoroughly. If you are not bathing in the shower, use a squeeze bottle filled with warm water to rinse the area while sitting on the toilet. Do not soak in the bathtub.
- Use nonallergenic tape to secure the catheter to your thigh. Allow enough slack in the tube to avoid pulling on the catheter when you move in bed or walk.
- Keep the drainage bag below your bladder at all times.
- Avoid using powders and sprays on your perineal area.
- Call your doctor if your temperature goes above 38.3° C (101° F).

Care of the Drainage Bag

- Empty the drainage bag often.
- To drain urine, open the port at the bottom of the bag and allow the urine to drain into the toilet or into a receptacle that you can easily empty into the toilet. When urine stops flowing, reclamp the drainage tube.
- If you use a receptacle, rinse it after emptying it to prevent odor and bacterial growth.

Removing the Catheter

- If your physician prescribes it, schedule an appointment to check for residual urine in your bladder.
- Before you leave the hospital, review the instructions for removing the catheter.
- As instructed, remove the catheter 2 hours before your office visit. To do so, first perform thorough hand hygiene with soap and warm water.
- Sit on the toilet. Insert a 10-mL syringe (without a needle) into the pigtail on the catheter and withdraw all the water from the pigtail. It should be about 5 mL.
- Gently pull the catheter out of your urinary meatus. It should slide out easily.
- Drink 32 ounces of water, and urinate when you feel the urge. If you have trouble starting your urine stream, try running water or rinsing your perineum with warm water from a squeeze bottle. Do not panic if you are unable to urinate.
- At the doctor's office, you will be asked to urinate and your urine will be measured. You will then have a catheter inserted to check for residual urine. If you have more than 3 ounces of residual urine, the indwelling catheter will need to remain in place.
- If you are not ready to have the catheter out, you will be given another appointment and will repeat the same procedure. It is not uncommon to need the catheter for an additional period of time. It does not mean that anything is wrong.
- If you have any questions, always feel free to ask a doctor or nurse.

A

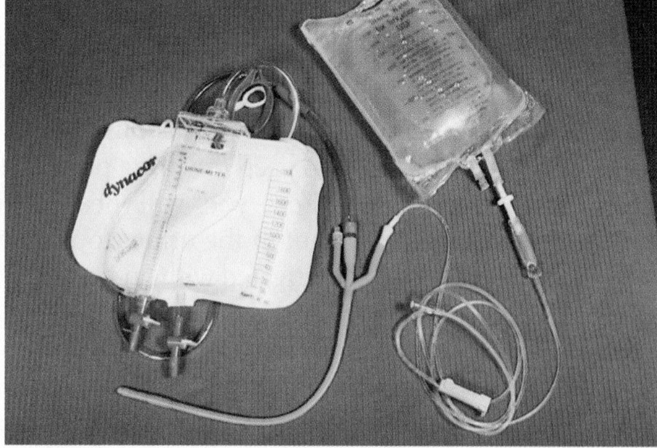

B

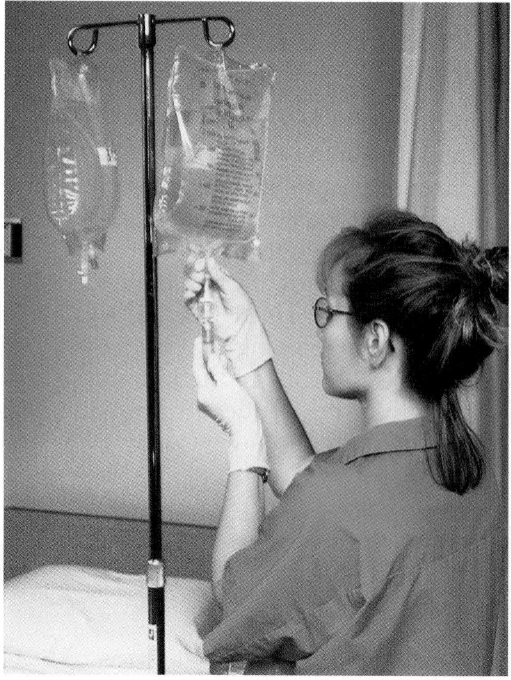

FIGURE 30-13 Closed bladder irrigation. **A,** The setup for closed bladder irrigation consists of a three-way indwelling catheter, a bag of irrigant with tubing, and a gravity drainage system. **B,** The irrigant is hung on an IV pole and is regulated with a sliding clamp on the tubing.

INTERVENTIONS TO MANAGE A URINARY DIVERSION

In the initial postoperative period, you will monitor the client for postoperative complications. This involves tracking the flow of urine and watching for signs of peritonitis, hemorrhage, and a decrease in vital signs. The newly created stoma may have a stent to maintain its patency. If urine leaks from the operative site into the peritoneum, the client will report pain and you will note abdominal distention, guarding, and tenderness.

The goal for the client is to learn to manage life with a urinary diversion. If the person does not have a continent stoma, an appliance will be attached to the skin around the stoma and urine will drain into a bag either at the site or attached to the client's leg. The person with a continent stoma must learn self-catheterization.

Because of the absence of the normal protective mechanisms of the urinary tract, a urinary diversion is prone to infection. So the client must learn to maintain clean technique and must know the signs and symptoms of infection. The skin around the stoma must remain dry and must be monitored for irritation.

INTERVENTIONS TO MANAGE URINARY TRACT INFECTIONS

Urinary tract infections usually are treated with specific or nonspecific antibiotics. When a client has a urinary tract infection, increased fluid intake keeps urine dilute and promotes rapid reduction of the bacterial count in the urinary tract. On the other hand, it can hinder therapy by producing increased urine output, thus lowering urinary concentrations of antimicrobial agents. Therefore the client should drink six to eight glasses of fluid per day but should not force fluids when taking most urinary antibiotics. Encourage clients to void when they feel the urge.

Changing the pH of urine has been recommended as an adjunct to therapy. Lowering the pH enhances the antibacterial activity of urine by increasing the concentration of organic acids normally found in urine. The pH of urine also affects the activity of some chemotherapeutic agents. The activity of methenamine mandelate, methenamine hippurate, and nitrofurantoin (all urinary antibacterials) is increased at a low urinary pH, whereas aminoglycoside antibiotics are more effective at an alkaline pH.

Acidification can be achieved by the use of ascorbic acid or methionine, by a modification of the diet, and by restricting milk, sodium bicarbonate, and fruit juices (except for cranberry juice). However, urinary acidification can be difficult to achieve and can cause precipitation of urate stones. Lowering the pH of the urine with a special diet or with ordered medications is advised. For the client with frequent urinary tract infections, preventive measures should be taught.

EVALUATION

Evaluation of urinary tract problems should be specific to the nature of the problem. Ask yourself if the problem is resolvable or expected to be ongoing. Examine the outcomes, the methods to achieve the outcomes, and the client's level of satisfaction with care (Box 30-11).

Urinary incontinence in immobile, neurologically impaired older adult clients often cannot be resolved. Evaluation seeks to ensure that the client is clean, dry, and comfortable. Equally important is determining that the skin remains intact. The diet should be free of foods or fluids that irritate the bladder. The client should be well hydrated, and the environment should be free of the odor of stale urine. Measures to prevent and detect urinary tract infection should be in place. If the client develops a urinary tract infection, ask what measures should be added to prevent future occurrences.

Urinary incontinence in many cases can be resolved with exercises or other treatment methods. If the problem is not resolved, evaluation includes asking whether the client has been given all available options and is satisfied with the level of resolution. Management may be considered successful if the number of episodes or the severity of each episode is reduced. Consider the client's ability to participate in the treatment regimen and the level of participation observed.

Evaluation also includes examining nursing care. Were the methods of teaching appropriate to the client's ability to learn and to the client's value system? Was the immobile client checked for dryness at sufficiently frequent intervals to detect incontinence? How frequently was the client offered a bedpan or assisted to the toilet? What measures were used to control odor? If odor is present, additional measures should be included in the care plan. Was the client offered a sufficient amount of appropriate fluids? Were measures included to ensure the client's privacy and avoid embarrassment over incontinence?

Evaluation of the care of the client with a urinary diversion considers the same parameters for skin care, diet, fluids, odor control, privacy, and embarrassment. However, a major part of the evaluation examines the client's level of self-care and whether the care is managed in a manner that minimally disrupts the client's preferred lifestyle.

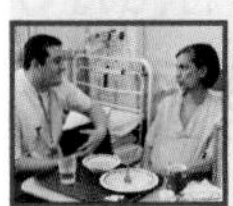

Mrs. Al-Kandari is discharged on the third postoperative day. The nurse writes the discharge note below.

SAMPLE DOCUMENTATION NOTE FOR MRS. AL-KANDARI

Discharged to automobile with husband. Is able to void without difficulty; knows to monitor self for signs and symptoms of UTI and maintain fluid intake of 6-8 glasses of water a day. Has spots of serosanguineous drainage on vaginal pad. Will report increase to physician. Scheduled for physician's office visit in 1 week.

BOX 30-11

Nursing Care Plan

A Postoperative Client at Risk for Urinary Tract Infection

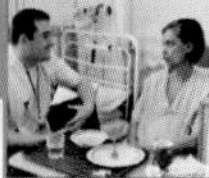

Nursing History
Mrs. Al-Kandari is in the second postoperative day following a vaginal hysterectomy. She has no history of difficulty with urination.

Physician's Orders
Clear liquids; advance diet as tolerated
Activity as tolerated
Demerol 50-100 mg q4h prn for pain
Vicodin 1 or 2 tablets q4h prn for pain
Tylenol 650 mg q4h prn for temperature over 38.8° C (102° F)
D_5½NS at 100 mL/hr
Discontinue IV fluid when able to take fluids by mouth
Discontinue Foley catheter
Laxative of choice

Nursing Assessment
(Morning change-of-shift report) The physician removed the vaginal pack this morning. Client's vital signs are within normal limits. Her temperature is 37.2° C (99° F). She was able to eat a soft diet for breakfast, including 600 mL of fluids. She was out of bed for two brief periods yesterday. Her pain has been controlled with 75 mg of Demerol used every 4 to 6 hours since surgery, but she took two Vicodin this morning. Skin turgor is brisk.

NANDA-I Nursing Diagnosis	NOC Expected Outcomes With Indicators	NIC Interventions With Selected Activities	Evaluation Data
Risk for urinary Retention **Related Factors:**	***Urinary Elimination***	***Urinary Retention Care***	
• Edema, interruption in normal stimulus to void	• Urinary elimination pattern in expected range of 4-6 voidings in waking hours	• Urinary assessment including voiding pattern, intake, and output per shift	• Voided three times in 2 hours after Foley removed without burning or hesitancy
	• Urine passes without hesitancy	• Provide privacy for elimination	• After 8 hours, has voided five times
	• Urine passes without urgency	• Make use of power of suggestion by running water or flushing toilet.	• Reported feeling like bladder empty
	• Empties bladder completely	• Insert urinary catheter as appropriate.	• Intake 900 mL; output 800 mL • Urine clear, yellow

Nursing outcome and intervention labels from Johnson, M., Bulechek, G., Butcher, H., Dochterman, J. M., Maas, M., Moorhead, S., et al. (Eds.). (2006). *NANDA, NOC, and NIC linkages: Nursing diagnoses, outcomes, & interventions.* St. Louis, MO: Mosby.

▼ KEY PRINCIPLES

- Understanding problems of urinary dysfunction involves an understanding of the structure and function of the kidneys, ureters, bladder, and urethra.
- Examination of urine provides information relevant to the function of the urinary tract and to the general health and function of the body.
- Substances in the urine are a result of the filtration, reabsorption, and secretion functions of the kidney as an organ of homeostatic balance.
- Dysuria can result from obstruction, infection, neurological injury, or decreased muscle tone.
- Low urine volumes can result from dehydration, hypotension, antidiuretic hormone, renal failure, or urinary retention.
- The diagnosis of *Impaired urinary elimination* requires differentiation between stress, urge, reflex, functional, and total urinary incontinence.
- Urinary tract infection is not a nursing diagnosis because the nurse cannot prescribe definitive therapy, but the nurse can treat the risk for urinary tract infection by instituting measures to prevent the problem and to educate the client about healthy practices.
- A nurse can assist a client in avoiding urinary tract infections by teaching about hygiene, fluid intake, and measures to change the pH of the urine.
- The bladder is a sterile body cavity but is at risk for infection because the entrance to the bladder is in close proximity to the anus. Women have higher risk than men because their urethra is short.
- The concept of cleaning the perineum from clean to dirty, front to back, is key to preventing urinary tract infection, especially in women.
- The bladder feels full when it contains an average of 300 mL, after which it is emptied completely with each voiding.
- An indwelling catheter should be the treatment of last resort for urinary incontinence.
- Urinary tract infections are highly associated with the use of indwelling catheters.
- Incontinence often results from a correctable cause. A medical evaluation may be appropriate before deciding on nursing care to manage incontinence.

Bibliography

*Agency for Health Care Policy and Research. (1996). *Urinary incontinence in adults:* Acute and chronic management—Clinical practice guideline No. 2. (AHCPR Publication No 96-0682) Rockville, MD: Author.

Baztan, J. J., Arias, E., Gonzalez, N., & Rodriguez de Prada, M. I. (2005). New-onset urinary incontinence and rehabilitation outcomes in frail older patients. *Age and Ageing, 34*(2), 172-175.

Berry, A. (2005). A child with daytime wetting: Three case studies. *Urologic Nursing, 25*(3), 202-205.

Dowling-Castronovo, A. (2004). Try this: Best practices in nursing care to older adults from the Hartford Institute for Geriatric Nursing. Urinary incontinence assessment. *Dermatology Nursing, 16*(1), 97-98.

Dulczak, S., & Kirk, J. (2005). Overview of the evaluation, diagnosis, and management of urinary tract infections in infants and children. *Urologic Nursing, 25*(3), 185-192.

Fletcher, K. (2005). Elimination: Geriatric self-learning module. *MEDSURG Nursing, 14*(2), 127-131.

Giger, J. N., & Davidhizar, R. E. (2004). *Transcultural nursing: Assessment and intervention.* St. Louis, MO: Mosby.

Goldrick, B. A. (2005). Emerging infections. Infection in the older adult: Long-term care poses particular risk. *American Journal of Nursing, 105*(6), 31, 33-34.

Goode, P. S. (2005, September). *Population-based study of incidence and predictors of urinary incontinence in older women.* Poster session presented at the American Urogynecologic Society Twenty-Sixth Annual Scientific Meeting.

Guyton, A. C., & Hall, J. E. (2006). *Textbook of medical physiology.* St. Louis, MO: Elsevier.

Heard, L., & Buhrer, R. (2005). Clinical consultation. How do we prevent UTI in people who perform intermittent catheterization? *Rehabilitation Nursing, 30*(2), 44-55, 61.

Johnson, M. (2005). Draining advice . . . "Urinary tract infection: draining question" (Advice, p.r.n., March 2005). *Nursing, 35*(5), 8.

Johnson, M., Bulechek, G., Butcher, H., Dochterman, J. M., Maas, M., Moorhead, S., et al. (Eds.). (2006). *NANDA, NOC, and NIC linkages: Nursing diagnoses, outcomes, & interventions.* St. Louis, MO: Mosby.

Klay, M., & Marfyak, K. (2005). Use of a continence nurse specialist in an extended care facility. *Urologic Nursing, 25*(2), 101-102, 107-108.

Linsenmeyer, T. A., Harrison, B., Oakley, A., Kirshblum, S., Stock, J. A., & Millis, S. R. (2005). Evaluation of cranberry supplement for reduction of urinary tract infections in individuals with neurogenic bladders secondary to spinal cord injury. *SCI Nursing, 22*(1), 20-25.

Maloney-Monaghan, C., & Cafiero, M. (2004). Male bladder control problems: A guide to assessment. *Ostomy/Wound Management, 50*(12), 42-44, 46-48.

McIntosh, L. (2005). The role of the nurse in the use of vaginal pessaries to treat pelvic organ prolapse and/or urinary incontinence: A literature review. *Urologic Nursing, 25*(1), 41-48.

*Merkelj, I. (2001). Urinary incontinence in the elderly. *Southern Medical Journal, 94*(10), 952-957

Midthun, S., Paur, R., Bruce, A. W., & Midthun, P. (2005). Urinary tract infections in the elderly: A survey of physicians and nurses. *Geriatric Nursing, 26*(4), 245-251.

Moninger, J. (2005). As they grow. 6-8 years: Accidents happen. *Parents,* 80(1), 151-152.

NANDA International. (2007). *Nursing diagnoses: Definitions and classification, 2006-2007* (7th ed.). Philadelphia: Author.

Nissan, D. (Ed.). (2003). *Mosby drug consult.* St. Louis, MO: Mosby.

Perrin, L., Dauphinee, S. W., Corcos, J., Hanley, J. A., & Kuchel, G. A. (2005). Continence care. Pelvic floor muscle training with biofeedback and bladder training in elderly women: A feasibility study. *Journal of WOCN, 32*(3), 186-199.

Specht, J. K. P. (2005). Nine myths of incontinence in older adults: Both clinicians and the over-65 set need to know more. *American Journal of Nursing, 105*(6), 58-69.

Stevens, E. (2005). Bladder ultrasound: Avoiding unnecessary catheterizations. *MEDSURG Nursing, 14*(4), 249-253.

Toughill, E. (2005). Bladder matters. Indwelling urinary catheters: Common mechanical and pathogenic problems. *American Journal of Nursing, 105*(5), 35-37.

Turnbull, G. B. (2004). The ostomy files. The power of knowledge. *Ostomy/Wound Management, 50*(6), 14, 16.

Ward, B. P. (2005). Don't make me laugh—please! Understanding female urinary incontinence. *Nursing Spectrum* (New York/New Jersey Metro Edition), *17*(1), 20-22.

Williams, M. E. (2005). Clinical consultation. How do we teach clean intermittent self-catheterization using touch technique? *Rehabilitation Nursing, 30*(5), 171-172.

*Asterisk indicates a classic or definitive work on this subject.

Chapter 31

Managing Self-Care Deficit

Media Resources

- Nursing Skills Online
- Evolve Website http://evolve.elsevier.com/Harkreader/
- 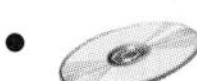 Companion CD
- 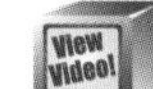 Skills Video Clips

Learning Objectives

After studying this chapter, you should be able to do the following:

- Describe the structure and function of the skin, hair, nails, and oral cavity
- Discuss problems associated with personal hygiene
- Discuss the life span, physiological, and cultural or lifestyle factors that influence hygiene practices
- Assess the client who is at risk for or has an actual self-care deficit in managing personal hygiene, feeding, toileting, or dressing related to physical, psychological, or cognitive impairment
- Choose appropriate nursing diagnoses related to the client's ability to engage in self-care
- Plan client-centered outcomes to assist the client with meeting self-care deficits
- Describe nursing interventions to promote hygiene of the skin, mouth, hair, feeding, toileting, and dressing/grooming
- Evaluate outcomes of nursing care in assisting the client to meet self-care needs

Key Terms

alopecia
caries
cerumen
dentures
gingivitis
perineum
plaque
tartar

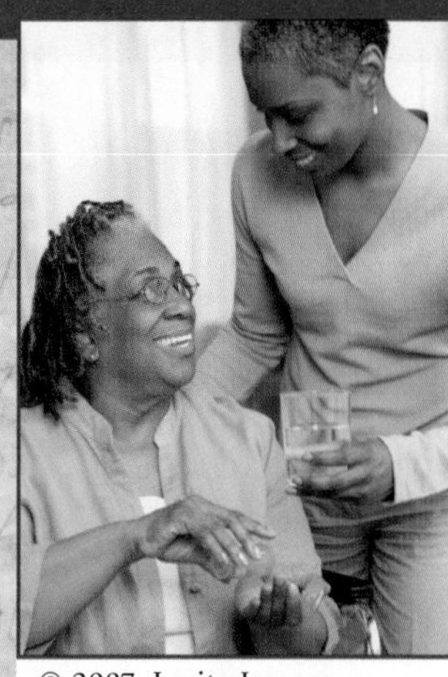

Joy Wilson, age 78, resides with her daughter and son-in-law. Mrs. Wilson is of African American ancestry. She was admitted to the hospital 2 weeks ago after a sudden onset of weakness, nausea, and left hemiplegia. A stroke (cerebrovascular accident) was diagnosed. Her hospital stay is ending, and she is being prepared for discharge to her daughter's home. Her progress in physical therapy has been only fair. Her left side is dominant, so she is being required to adapt by using only her right arm and hand for motor skills that she had previously mastered using her left or both hands. She has a great desire to learn to care for herself, but she is weak and able to tolerate only minimal activity before becoming extremely fatigued. Her cognitive status is slightly impaired because of a short-term memory deficit, as well as some emotional lability. Her frustration at not being able to care for her hygiene needs is evidenced by tears and anger when she cannot achieve a goal.

Mrs. Wilson's daughter is devoted to her mother and desires to provide home health care. Both mother and daughter are opposed to considering nursing home placement at this time. Her daughter is eager to learn to care for her mother and asks pertinent questions that reflect interest in her mother's welfare. Although she plans to be the primary caregiver for Mrs. Wilson, she will use community resources to assist in providing the best possible care. Because Mrs. Wilson has related problems of cognitive impairment, exercise intolerance, and frustration with her altered state of wellness, the nurse assesses that in addition to *Bathing/hygiene self-care deficit* there are other nursing diagnoses that must be addressed (see key nursing diagnoses box).

CONCEPTS OF SELF-CARE DEFICIT

Self-care is the ability to meet one's own needs related to hygiene, dressing, toileting, and feeding without the assistance of another person. These activities are generally independent functions that an individual performs daily. For that reason, they are called activities of daily living (ADLs). Usually acquired in early childhood, these skills and abilities become an integral part of adult behavior (Box 31-1).

KEY NURSING DIAGNOSES FOR SELF-CARE DEFICIT

Bathing/hygiene self-care deficit: Impaired ability to perform or complete bathing/hygiene activities for oneself
Dressing/grooming self-care deficit: Impaired ability to perform or complete dressing or grooming activities for oneself
Feeding self-care deficit: Impaired ability to perform or complete feeding activities for oneself
Toileting self-care deficit: Impaired ability to perform or complete toileting activities for oneself

Personal hygiene consists of those activities that an individual undertakes to maintain body cleanliness and freedom from disease—namely bathing, oral hygiene, and hair care. It is essential to both physical and psychological well-being that hygiene needs be adequately met. If the body is not kept clean, the skin is compromised and the body can be threatened by infection or disease. The individual's comfort, self-esteem, and body image are also enhanced by cleanliness of the body. When illness or injury prevents the client from meeting self-care needs, it is your responsibility to assist clients in meeting these needs, to assist clients in a culturally sensitive manner to be as independent as possible, and to provide clients with information and resources needed to resume self-care abilities to the extent that physical and mental capacities allow.

SKIN

The skin is an organ with highly specialized functions that are essential for human survival. Without skin, adaptation to the environment would be impossible because the intricate functions of this vital organ serve to maintain biological integrity and homeostasis. The surface area of the skin makes it one of the larger organs in the body, covering approximately 20 square feet, or 3000 square inches in the average-size adult.

Strata of the Skin. The skin is composed structurally of three layers (Figure 31-1). The outer portion, the epidermis, is composed of stratified squamous epithelium and contains four kinds of cells. Most of these cells are keratinocytes; they produce keratin, a substance that protects skin and underlying tissues and plays a part in immune function. Melanocytes, which are located at the base of the epidermis, produce melanin, a pigment responsible for skin color and tanning. Melanin also assumes a protective function by absorbing ultraviolet rays, thereby lessening their harmful effects on the skin. Other epidermal cells, the nonpigmented granular dendrocytes, are made up of two distinct cell types: Langerhans' cells and

BOX 31-1

Evidence-Based Practice

Health in Nursing Students

Problem: "While learning to care for others, undergraduate nursing students often fail to care for themselves" (Stark, Manning-Walsh, & Vliem, 2005, p. 266). Self-care is usually associated with health promotion resulting in a healthier lifestyle. Although health promotion is introduced in the nursing curricula for client care, students do not always practice healthy lifestyles.

Evidence

Descriptive statistics were used, and reliability was determined for all scales and variables of interest. A pretest, posttest design was used to test whether 67 students increased their self-care activities after completing a course requiring self-care. The instrument used to collect data, the Health-Promoting Lifestyle Profile-II, has been widely used in nursing research as a measure of the major components of a healthy lifestyle.

Application to Practice

"Introducing a health-promoting lifestyle and self-care strategies during the course of nursing education may allow students to practice self-care and develop healthy lifestyles prior to their entry into practice" (Stark, Manning-Walsh, & Vliem, 2005, p. 266).

Reference

Stark, M. A., Manning-Walsh, J., & Vliem, S. (2005). Caring for self while learning to care for others: A challenge for nursing students. *Journal of Nursing Education, 44*(6), 266-270 [23 references].

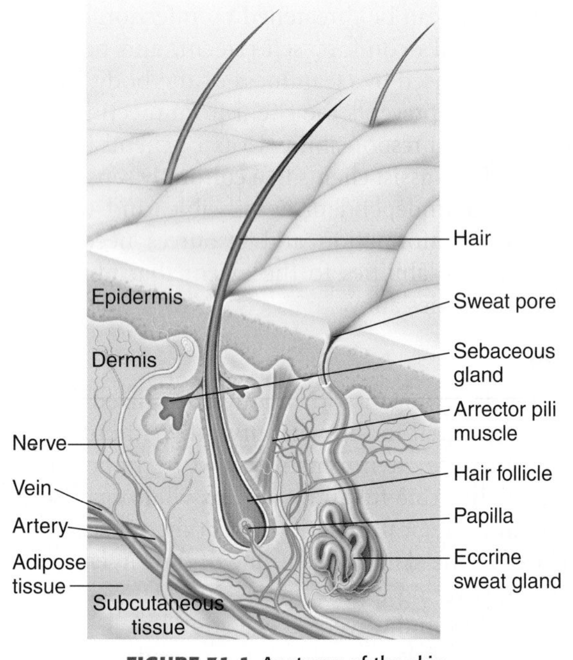

FIGURE 31-1 Anatomy of the skin.

Granstein cells. These cells interact with T cells to assist in the immune process.

The second layer of skin is the dermis, which is composed of connective tissue containing collagenous and elastic fibers. Numerous blood vessels, nerves, glands, and hair follicles are embedded in this stratum of the skin.

The third layer of skin, the subcutaneous tissue, lies underneath the dermis and is also known as the superficial fascia or the hypodermis. This subcutaneous layer consists of loose connective and fatty tissues and provides support and blood supply to the dermis. The strata that make up the skin are connected by fibers that extend from the dermis to the underlying tissues and organs.

Glands of the Skin. Three kinds of glands are associated with the skin. They are the sebaceous glands, sudoriferous glands, and ceruminous glands.

Most sebaceous glands are connected to hair follicles. The secreting portions of these glands lie within the dermis and open into the necks of hair follicles. Those not associated with hair follicles open directly onto the surface of the skin. Their size and shape vary throughout the body, being small in much of the trunk and extremities and larger in the breasts, face, neck, and upper chest. They are absent in the palms and soles.

The sebaceous glands secrete an oily substance called sebum, made up of a mixture of fats, cholesterol, proteins, and inorganic salts. Sebum serves to protect hair from drying and forms a protective film on the skin that prevents excessive evaporation of water. It also helps to keep the skin soft and supple and inhibits the growth of certain bacteria on the skin.

Sudoriferous, or sweat, glands are identified according to their structure and function. The two types of sweat glands are eccrine and apocrine sweat glands. Most of the sudoriferous glands are eccrine sweat glands, which are distributed throughout the skin. They are most numerous in the skin of the palms and soles and their activity is easily observed by the wetness of palms when a person is anxious or under stress. The secretory portion of the gland is located in the subcutaneous layer, and the excretory duct projects upward to terminate at a pore on the surface of the epidermis. Eccrine sweat glands function throughout life and produce a watery secretion known as perspiration or sweat, in which small amounts of waste products are excreted. The primary purpose of perspiration is to regulate body temperature.

Apocrine sweat glands are simple, branched, tubular glands that are distributed primarily in the skin of the axilla and of the pubic region. The secretory portion of this gland is located in the dermis and the excretory duct opens into hair follicles. Apocrine glands begin to function at puberty and produce a more oily secretion than eccrine sweat glands. When the secretions of apocrine glands mix with bacteria on the skin surface, body odors are produced.

Ceruminous glands secrete a thick, heavily pigmented, oily substance called cerumen. **Cerumen** is a waxy secretion of the glands of the external ear canal or external acoustic meatus; it is commonly known as earwax.

Functions of the Skin. The skin is the body's first line of defense. It hosts a large contingent of resident bacteria that serve a useful function. On intact skin, these resident organisms prevent excess growth of fungi. Sebum, secreted into the hair follicles by the sebaceous glands, has antibacterial and antifungal properties. Skin acidity also inhibits growth of pathogenic organisms.

Perspiration, or sweat, is a mixture of water, salts (mostly sodium chloride), urea, uric acid, amino acids, ammonia, sugar, lactic acid, and ascorbic acid. The skin assists in regulating body temperature through production of perspiration by the sudoriferous glands. The evaporation of the water in perspiration carries off large quantities of heat energy from the body surface, thereby decreasing body temperature.

The skin helps screen out harmful ultraviolet (UV) rays from the sun, but it also lets in necessary UV rays that convert 7-dehydrocholesterol (a chemical in the skin) into vitamin D for normal growth of bones and teeth. A lack of UV light and vitamin D impairs absorption of calcium from the intestine into the bloodstream.

The skin is an important sensory organ containing sensory receptors that respond to heat, cold, touch, pressure, and pain. Skin offers protection through its many nerve endings, which warn of environmental sources of harm such as hot coals or sharp blades. The nerve endings also help in sensing the outside world so that physiological adjustments can be made to maintain homeostasis.

HAIR

Hair is considered to be an appendage of the skin because it arises from the skin. It covers the entire body with the exception of the palms, soles, lips, tip of penis, inner lips of vulva, and nipples. Hair consists of two major parts: the shaft (the portion protruding from the skin) and the root (embedded in the skin).

About halfway up the length of the hair follicle is an oil gland, which is located between the follicle and the arrector pili muscle. When this muscle contracts, it pulls the follicle and its hair upright, elevating the skin above the follicle and producing what is commonly called gooseflesh.

Rate of hair growth appears to depend on several factors, of which age, seasonal changes, and hair texture are prominent. Rate of hair growth slows with advancing age. Hair grows faster at night than during the day, and faster in warm weather than in cold. Coarse black hairs grow faster than fine blonde hair. Location of the hair is also a determining factor. Scalp hairs may last 3 to 5 years, whereas eyebrow and eyelash hairs may last only 10 weeks. The average scalp contains about 125,000 hairs.

Although humans do not have as much of a need for the protective covering of hair as many other mammals have, hair does serve some protective functions in humans. Scalp hair serves to insulate against cold air and external heat from the sun and provide a cushion for the cranium.

Eyebrows and eyelashes are cushions for protecting the eyes. Eyelashes serve to screen the entry of foreign particles or objects into the eyes. Nostril hairs trap dust particles and foreign matter that are present in inhaled air to prevent their passage down the respiratory tract to the lungs.

NAILS

The nails are composed of hard, keratinized cells of the epidermis that form a clear, solid covering over the dorsal surfaces of the terminal tips of the fingers and toes. Each nail consists of three basic parts: the nail body, which is the visible portion; the free edge, which projects beyond the tip of the digit; and the nail root, which is hidden in the proximal nail groove.

Most of the nail body is pink because of the underlying vascular system. The semilunar area at the base (lunula) appears white because the vascular tissue is hidden by the thick stratum there. The eponychium (or cuticle) is a narrow band of epidermis that extends from the margin of the nail bed (lateral border) and is the proximal border of the nail. The epithelium of the proximal part of the nail bed is known as the nail matrix. Its function is to bring about the growth of nails by transforming superficial cells of the matrix into nail cells. Functionally, nails help with grasping and manipulating small objects in various ways. They also provide protection against trauma to the ends of the digits.

ORAL CAVITY

The oral cavity is composed of the teeth, the tongue, and the oral mucosa. Eruption of deciduous teeth (baby teeth) begins at approximately 6 months of age. These deciduous teeth are lost in childhood and are replaced by a set of 32 permanent teeth (16 in each jaw), composed of four incisors, two canines or cuspids, four premolars or bicuspids, and six molars (see Chapter 16). All teeth consist of three parts: a root embedded in a socket (alveolus) in the alveolar process of the jaw bone; a crown projecting upward from the gum; and a neck between the root and the crown, which is surrounded by the gum (Figure 31-2).

Each tooth is composed of dentin, enamel, cementum, and pulp. The dentin is the sensitive portion surrounding the pulp cavity, and it forms the bulk of the tooth. The enamel is the white covering of the tooth. The cementum is the bonelike covering of the neck and root. The pulp is the soft core of connective tissue that contains the nerves and blood vessels of the tooth.

The teeth are held in their sockets by connective tissue called periodontal ligaments. The collagenous fibers of each ligament extend from the alveolar bone into the cement of each tooth, allowing some tooth movement during the process of chewing.

The mouth and teeth play vital roles in mastication (chewing) and digestion, which begins in the mouth as food is mixed with saliva for food breakdown and for further digestion. The muscles in the cheeks aid in chewing. The tongue has taste buds for discerning different tastes of food, and it helps mix saliva with food. The tongue also aids in swallowing by moving the food toward the pharynx. Phonation (the forming of words) is also a function of the tongue.

PROBLEMS OF SELF-CARE

Problems of the Skin. Skin types, textures, and conditions are influenced by overall health status, age, nutritional status, and activity level. Infants have skin that is delicate and sensitive because it has yet to be exposed to the environmental influences that alter skin texture. They cannot usually tolerate harsh soaps and extremes of water temperature. Their skin is particularly prone to trauma in the form of abrasions, which may lead to infection.

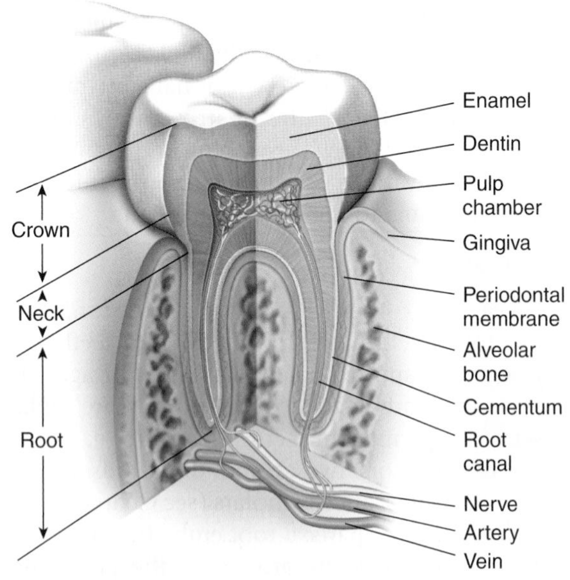

FIGURE 31-2 Anatomy of a tooth.

Adolescents are prone to developing enlarged sebaceous glands of the face because of accumulated sebum, which may take the form of blackheads, pimples, or boils, which is referred to as regular acne. At puberty, the sebaceous glands, under the influence of androgens (male hormones), grow in size and increase production of sebum. Although testosterone, a male hormone, appears to be the most potent circulating androgen for sebaceous cell stimulation, adrenal and ovarian androgens can stimulate sebaceous secretions as well.

Acne occurs predominantly in sebaceous follicles that are rapidly colonized by bacteria that thrive in the lipid-rich sebum. When this occurs, the cyst, or sac of connective tissue cells, can destroy and displace epidermal cells, resulting in permanent scarring, a condition called cystic acne.

Skin of older people is also prone to breakdown due to pressure, shearing forces, poor circulation, and cleanliness. Abrasions may be slow to heal or may become infected. Dry skin is a problem common to aging. Older adults cannot tolerate harsh soaps because of their delicate skin.

Skin rashes or dermatitis are common skin problems. They may be due to an allergic or nonallergic contact. It is important to identify the source irritant and to prevent secondary infection from scratching with resultant destruction of the body's first line of defense, the intact skin. Table 31-1 lists some common skin problems and their causes and treatments.

Problems of the Hair. Normal hair loss in an adult scalp is about 70 to 100 hairs per day. The rate of growth and the replacement cycle may be altered by illness, diet, and other factors. High fever, major illness, major surgery, blood loss, nutritional deficits, such as rapid weight-loss diets, or severe emotional stress may increase the rate of shedding and may result in **alopecia,** which is loss of hair and resulting baldness. Certain drugs and radiation therapy are also factors that increase hair loss.

Dandruff is a chronic, diffuse scaling of the epidermis of the scalp and is characterized by itching and flaking of whitish scales, which are annoying and embarrassing to the client.

Infestation with lice is called pediculosis. Lice may be found on any part of the body that has hair. Lice may be found in the hair of the head, eyebrows, eyelashes, and beard (pediculosis capitis), on the body (pediculosis corporis), and in the pubic hair (pediculosis pubis). Head lice and pubic lice attach their eggs (nits) to the hair shaft with a sticky substance that makes them hard to remove. They may be visible to the naked eye or seen through a magnifying glass as shiny ovals. They may look to the naked eye like dandruff. They live on the skin, and their bites cause itching. Inflamed sores may be visible along the hairline. Body lice suck blood from the skin and live in clothing, making them hard to detect. Scratching and hemorrhagic lesions of the skin are clues that should alert the caregiver to the possibility of infestation. Table 31-2 identifies common problems of the hair.

Problems of the Nails and Feet. The accumulation of dirt and debris around the cuticle and underneath the fingernail is a potential source of infection, especially if the nail should become torn. Hangnails, ragged cuticles, and long untrimmed nails are hazardous to the client. Confused clients sometimes injure themselves by scratching or abrading the skin when they have long, untrimmed or jagged nails.

The nails are affected by aging and disease. Nails become more dry and brittle with age. Fungal infections of the nails are a common problem of adults, primarily because of dehydrated epidermal cells and decreased sebaceous gland secretion. If nails are thickened and yellow, this may indicate a fungal infection. Increased brittleness and angulation between the nail and the nail bed and changes in the thickness or texture of the nails can indicate illness. Clubbing of the nails or marked curvature and lines in the nails may be indicative of serious health problems, such as cardiac or respiratory disorders.

The health of the toenails is vital for good ambulation. Assessment of the client's gait indicate sore feet, ingrown toenails, hammer toes, corns, and calluses, which are uncomfortable for the client. Diabetic clients are at high risk for infection from breaks in skin integrity. They may not have adequate circulation to the extremities, especially their feet and toes due to changes in microcirculation in peripheral tissues, and they may have decreased sensation to pain because of peripheral neuropathies. Renal disease, congestive heart failure, peripheral vascular disease, or other conditions that interfere with blood flow to surrounding tissues may also create problems related to circulation to and from the lower extremities. Clients with circulatory impairment or diabetes who have ingrown toenails may develop an infection or gangrene. Table 31-3 lists common problems of the nails and feet.

Table 31-1 Common Problems of the Skin

PROBLEM	DESCRIPTION	NURSING IMPLICATION
Abrasion	Broken skin that may be weeping or bleeding; may be noted on elbows, heels, sacrum, and other areas that are subject to rubbing motions	Remove source of irritation. Prevent secondary infection; keep wound clean; avoid wearing rings or jewelry when caring for client; lift client when moving rather than pulling across the bed (shearing factor); keep nails short and smooth.
Acne	Oversecretion of sebum, which enlarges the gland and plugs the pore with pus; often occurs on face, chest, and back; most common in adolescence	Prevent secondary infection; instruct client to avoid squeezing and causing additional trauma to tissue; treatment may vary depending on severity of the problem; encourage meticulous skin cleanliness.
Dryness	Flaking and rough skin (generalized or patchy)	Prone to infection if the skin cracks; skin should be kept lubricated; reduce frequency of bathing and hot showers or tub baths; rinse skin thoroughly because soap residue promotes dryness; avoid irritating soaps and alcohol-based lotions; encourage increased fluid intake.
Dermatitis	Inflammation of skin with itching, redness, and blisters; may be allergic reaction to external chemical irritants (fabrics, solutions, plants) or internal (foods or medications)	Identify and remove source of irritation if possible; provide comfort for client with treatment for itching; discourage scratching to prevent breaking of skin and secondary infection.

Table 31-2 Common Problems of the Hair

PROBLEM	DESCRIPTION	NURSING IMPLICATION
Alopecia	Absence of body hair; may be sudden onset of patchy scalp and beard hair loss without any inflammation and usually reversible or sudden loss of all scalp hair or total loss of all body hair including scalp and face	Be aware of client's history and treatment to know if condition is likely to be reversible (chemotherapy) or irreversible; recognize significance of hair to client's self-esteem and body image.
Dandruff	A scaly collection of dried sebum and flakes of dried skin on the scalp; characterized by itching of the scalp	Daily brushing and shampooing; medicated shampoos may help; instruct client to avoid scratching scalp.
Pediculosis	Infestation with lice; characterized by itching and scratching	Removal of nits (eggs) from hair shaft; bathing and shampooing with topical medications; careful treatment of clothing and bed linens to prevent reinfestation with lice.

Problems of the Oral Cavity. Table 31-4 lists some common problems of the oral cavity. Halitosis may be an early indicator of either poor oral hygiene or a health problem, such as a gastrointestinal (GI) tract disorder, tonsillitis, or sinusitis. An offensive breath odor caused by inadequate oral hygiene can be alleviated with cleansing of the teeth and oral mucosa. If the origin of the halitosis is systemic, oral hygiene will not remove the odor.

Dental **caries** are a destructive process causing decalcification of the tooth enamel and leading to continued destruction of the enamel and dentin with resulting cavitation of the tooth. When the enamel barrier is breached, cavities develop. The agent responsible for dental caries is dental plaque. Dental **plaque** is a soft, thin film of food debris, mucin, and dead epithelial cells that is deposited on the teeth and provides a medium for the growth of bacteria. Freshly deposited plaque is transparent unless stained brown by tobacco, coffee or tea. When old dental plaque is present, the teeth appear dull with a dingy, yellowish cast. Cavity formation results when bacterial enzymes combine with the dental plaque and ferment the dietary carbohydrates and organic acids that can remain in the mouth after eating or drinking. These acids initiate the decalcification of tooth enamel. Once the bacteria have gained access to the tissue substance of the tooth, the next step is the development of caries.

Dental plaque can be removed by brushing and flossing at least daily. Food remnants left trapped between the teeth set the stage for the beginning of decay and periodontal disease. **Tartar** is a yellowish film of calcium phosphate, carbonate, food particles, and other organic matter deposited on the teeth by saliva.

Sound nutrition provides some resistance to dental decay. Dietary needs vary with such factors as age and general physical condition. In infants, dental caries can be caused by allowing the infant to go to bed with a bottle filled with a liquid other than water, sometimes referred to as bottle mouth syndrome. A large number of young people have dental caries and mouth and gum disease because of excessive dietary sugar and insufficient oral hygiene.

Table 31-3 Common Problems of the Feet and Nails

PROBLEM	DESCRIPTION	NURSING IMPLICATION
Athlete's foot	Fungal infection of the foot characterized by weeping, itching, excoriated lesions, usually located between the toes	Medicated antifungal medications may be used; regular washing and drying of feet is important; instruct client to wear white cotton socks during treatment to prevent potential infection from dyes in colored socks and to alternate shoes each day.
Corn/callus	A hardened area on the foot, usually caused by pressure or friction	Instruct client to avoid attempting to remove by cutting; use pumice stone to soften; encourage wearing of well-fitting shoes.
Fungal infection of nails	Nails may be yellow or black and thickened	Observe for signs of side effects of treatment regimen, which consists of oral or topical antifungal medication.

Table 31-4 Common Problems of the Oral Cavity

PROBLEM	DESCRIPTION	NURSING IMPLICATION
Halitosis	Offensive odor of breath.	Provide regular oral hygiene, or teach client to perform regular oral hygiene; assess for cause of halitosis.
Caries	Teeth may be dark in carious areas; may be painful.	Advise client to seek dental intervention. Encourage client to perform regular oral care and avoid foods/beverages known to promote caries.
Gingivitis	Gums may be pale and spongy; bleeding may occur with brushing and flossing or may occur spontaneously.	Provide regular oral care or teach client; dental intervention may be necessary.
Periodontal disease	Gums may bleed easily; teeth may be loose.	Advise client to seek dental care.
Stomatitis	Inflammation of oral mucosa; occurs in clients who are in a state of immunosuppression.	Rinse and cleanse mouth at least every 2 hours and after eating; local anesthetic rinses may provide some comfort.
Dryness	Lips and oral mucosa dry and cracked and may bleed; noted in clients who are dehydrated, who are on oxygen therapy, or who are mouth breathers.	Increase fluid intake as appropriate; petroleum jelly to lips; for clients on oxygen use water-based lubricants.

Diet is important because both deficiencies and excesses can contribute to decay. Dietary fats provide a barrier to acid penetration by forming an oily film on the surface of the tooth. The consumption of whole-grain foods that contain phosphorus inhibits caries. The use of a nonabrasive dentifrice (toothpaste or toothpowder) containing fluoride helps to strengthen the tooth enamel against decay.

The gums are also known as the gingiva. It is the firm connective tissue covered with mucous membrane that surrounds the alveolar processes of the teeth. **Gingivitis** is an inflammation of the gums usually manifested by the primary symptom of bleeding of the gums. It is an early stage of periodontal disease. Gingivitis may result from waste products and toxins from organisms in the mouth, which may cause initial injury. When dental plaque remains on teeth, it becomes hardened (calcified) and forms calculus or tartar. The presence of calculus contributes further to gingivitis. Calculus must be removed by dental instruments.

Those at increased risk for gingivitis include people who breathe through their mouths, diabetics, people who use orthodontic supplies (e.g., braces), and people experiencing hormonal fluctuations (adolescents, pregnant women, and those taking oral contraceptives). During pregnancy, the increased circulating levels of hormones cause gingival hypertrophy, which can increase the incidence of periodontal disease if good oral hygiene is not consistently practiced.

Chronic gingivitis causes the inflammation to spread and destroy the underlying bone, causing periodontitis. In an advanced stage of periodontal disease, the periodontium atrophies so that the gums appear to have receded completely away from the tooth. Without adequate supporting structure, the tooth becomes very loosely attached or falls out. Periodontal disease is common among young adults and may be precipitated by emotional stress, which aggravates the inflammatory process.

Tooth loss is not inevitable in older adults; however, it is not uncommon for persons over age 65 to have no teeth. With age, the gums tend to recede and to develop a brownish pigmentation along the tooth edge. Salivation decreases and many older people complain of a dry mouth. Older adults who have few permanent teeth left will have partial or full dentures. **Dentures** are a complement of teeth, either natural or artificial; the term is ordinarily used to indicate an artificial replacement for the natural teeth.

Alterations in the oral mucosa may have several causes. Healthy mucosa is moist and pink without ulceration, dryness, or bleeding. Dryness of the lips and mucosa may occur in the client who is dehydrated or who is breathing through the mouth. Clients receiving oxygen therapy are prone to this because oxygen tends to dry out the mucosa. Irritated, reddened, or excoriated mucosa may also result from ill-fitting dentures. Clients who have experienced rapid weight loss or who have sustained significant changes in facial features may have dentures that are loose, which may cause irritation and pain when eating. Stomatitis is a common problem with certain clients. This condition is an inflammation of the oral mucosa and may occur in clients with the following:

- Receiving drugs such as anticholinergics that cause decreased salivation with resultant mouth dryness
- Poor oral hygiene
- Treatment with chemotherapy or radiotherapy for cancer
- An immune deficiency
- Anemias due to dietary deficiencies
- Mouth breathing

FACTORS AFFECTING SELF-CARE

Self-care practices vary among individuals, groups, and cultures. It is a mistake to assume that all clients will adhere to similar practices of hygiene or that all have similar beliefs about hygiene and methods of practicing it. Variations in self-care practices also may result from life span factors, physiological factors, or cultural and lifestyle factors.

RISK FACTORS ACROSS THE LIFE SPAN

The age of an individual usually provides some expectation of what that person should be able to achieve in self-care. However, nursing interventions should be in accordance with the identified needs and abilities of the individual client, whether or not they are congruent with chronological age and stage of development.

A need for independence in self-care is manifested early in childhood as the child takes pride in eating, grooming, dressing, and caring for hygiene needs. The loss of this ability in adulthood can be stressful, even if the loss is temporary.

Self-concept and the feeling of being in control of the body are threatened by the loss of self-care abilities. It is important to be sensitive to the client's emotional needs when providing hygiene and other assistive care. Being bathed and dressed by a caregiver may be equated with regression to an infantile state. For some individuals, this feeling is not acceptable, particularly if the individual has a strong need for independence. A sense of powerlessness may result from this loss.

Newborns and Infants. The infant is totally dependent on the caregiver to meet self-care needs. Crying to signal need for feeding and diapering is the only action the infant can take in the interest of self-care. Bathing, dressing, and grooming, including oral care, are the total responsibility of the caregiver. Frequency of urine and stool elimination may vary, but infants usually urinate about 20 times a day (250 to 500 mL per day). Stools may vary according to amount and consistency; they may be soft or liquid and may occur frequently.

Meticulous cleaning is essential because the infant's tender skin is susceptible to breakdown. Keep the skin as dry and clean as possible. Never leave infants in wet or soiled diapers for extended periods. The infant's skin and mucous membranes are easily injured and are susceptible to injury and infection.

> ***Action Alert!*** Remind parents to meticulously clean their infant's skin and keep it dry to prevent infection and injury. The use of skin protectants may be warranted to prevent skin irritation and breakdown.

Toddlers and Preschoolers. During the toddler/preschool years, the child develops gross and fine motor skills so that some independent grooming and toileting are possible. Bowel and bladder control is usually achieved by the age of 3 years even though some assistance may still be needed with wiping after toileting. Nighttime dryness may not be complete until a few years later. The preschooler is usually eager to help with dressing and derives great satisfaction with learning to master buttons and zippers.

Toddlers and preschoolers may regress in times of illness or stress and resume infantile behaviors related to toileting and self-care. Bed-wetting may occur again during this period of stress. This is a primary infantile means of coping and for securing the comfort needed at this time of crisis. The child will regain the skills previously learned when the child no longer needs to use this coping mechanism.

School-Age Children and Adolescents. The school-age child may be independent in self-care activities but may need occasional adult supervision to see that skin care and oral hygiene are being done completely and correctly. As the child approaches adolescence, assistance with self-care is no longer necessary, but because of the many physical changes that are occurring, a different kind of assistance, supervision, and teaching may be needed. This is a time when hormonal changes bring about the emergence of axillary and pubic hair in both sexes and facial hair in boys. The skin may become more oily because of increased activity of the sebaceous glands. Skin problems such as acne may occur during this period and can be a source of great distress to the adolescent who is becoming increasingly aware of the importance of appearance in being accepted by peers and attractive to the opposite sex. The apocrine sweat glands also become functional during adolescence, and the presence of body odor becomes an incentive for daily bathing and shampooing, as well as wearing clean clothes and/or deodorant.

Adults and Older Adults. During early and middle adult life, self-care is usually an independent function unless some temporary or permanent physical or mental impairment prevents the individual from performing self-care. Patterns of hygiene practices are well established by this time to meet the individual's goals for personal appearance and health.

Developmental considerations related to aging may affect clients' hygiene practices. This is particularly true in older adults because the aging process may limit agility and endurance, which can therefore alter the ability to perform safely and capably some aspects of good hygiene. Some older adults who were previously meticulous in their grooming may be noted by family members to be less attentive or even totally negligent in bathing and changing clothing. This could be related to mental or physical changes and requires attention from a caregiver because the client is no longer able to meet hygiene needs independently. Assistance in the way of providing prompts or clues, as well as the use of adaptive equipment, may be necessary (Box 31-2).

As physiological changes occur with aging, some hygiene needs and practices must change accordingly. For example, the skin becomes thinner and less elastic with breaks in the skin occurring more readily. Because less oil is being produced, the skin becomes drier. The appearance of the skin also changes with wrinkling and discoloration in the form of age spots, which occur particularly on the face and the dorsal surface of the hands. The incidence of skin carcinomas also increases in aging skin.

The hair changes with aging, becoming thinner and growing more slowly. Baldness in both men and women may occur. Hair color changes to gray or white as the pigment in the hair is lost.

The oral mucosa changes and becomes drier with decreased production of saliva. The teeth may become loose or may even be lost if there is periodontal disease. Many older adults wear dentures.

Care of the nails may be difficult. Nails become thickened and harder to maintain. The older adult may have difficulty with this psychomotor task because of decreased visual acuity and agility, as well as decreased hand strength and coordination.

The feet of the older client are of special concern because many older adults cannot see well enough to inspect or care for their feet. Decreased circulation in the

BOX 31-2 *Factors Affecting Older Adults' Hygiene Practices*

- Pain or discomfort
- Fatigue
- Cognitive impairment
- Lack of motivation
- Perception impairment
- Muscular impairment
- Emotions, such as anxiety, fear, apathy
- Medical restrictions
- Medical intervention/procedure restraining mobility

extremities due to reduced peripheral blood flow from arteriosclerosis or poor circulation, as well as diabetes, puts them at risk for infection. Many older adults, especially diabetics, use the skills of a podiatrist because of the danger inherent in accidentally traumatizing the feet with manicure tools. Some hospitals and nursing homes prohibit foot care by nurses and require clients to secure the services of a podiatrist because the danger caused by inadvertent foot trauma.

Action Alert? Advise older clients, or thier caregivers, to take special care to prevent trauma or infection to the client's extremities because poor circulation puts them at risk.

Older adults frequently have to use at least one assistive tool to support sensory function. Hearing aids, glasses, and dentures are common assistive devices. The care of these devices may be a problem for those older adults who have reduced vision and hearing acuity, as well as psychomotor skills. Your role is to assist in the care of these devices, which are useful in enhancing their quality of life and safety.

PHYSIOLOGICAL FACTORS

An individual's state of health is a major influence in the practice of self-care. Regardless of the motivation to maintain good hygiene and other ADLs, the client may be so ill or weak that there is insufficient energy to perform self-care activities.

Physical Illness. Clients may be temporarily weakened by ordinary health problems, such as the flu. Others may have long-term paralysis or weakness and loss of physical mobility from a cerebrovascular accident, a neuromuscular disorder, a spinal cord injury, or other catastrophic event.

The degree of assistance needed varies according to the nature of the neuromuscular involvement and which muscle groups are affected. Muscular movements are classified as either fine motor or gross motor. Fine motor movement involves precise movements, such as applying toothpaste to a toothbrush, whereas gross motor movement involves the coordination of large muscle groups, such as getting in and out of the bathtub or on and off the toilet. These tasks require intact nervous and musculoskeletal system for their performance. The pathways from brain to muscle and the muscle fibers themselves must be open and able to give and receive impulses. Neuromuscular diseases, such as muscular dystrophy and myasthenia gravis, may affect any level of this pathway.

Action Alert! Teach caregivers to assist clients who have neurological changes with activities such as applying toothpaste, getting in and out of the bathtub, or getting on and off the toilet.

Physicians or nurse practitioners sometimes place clients on bed rest or impose other activity restrictions to help them conserve energy, which is a factor in self-care. Pathological conditions that often deplete one's energy level and cause fatigue are cardiovascular and respiratory diseases. Pain is another physiological factor that limits the ability to perform self-care. Careful pain assessment and management is needed to enable the client to participate as fully as possible in ADLs (see Chapter 37). In some clients, pain is a short-term, acute problem that is easily treated, whereas in others it is so severe that simple movements trigger intense pain and prevent self-care such as arthritis, in which the joints are painful. It is important to plan for self-care activities while medications or other pain management strategies are exerting their peak effect.

Clients with cognitive dysfunction may need either simple assistance or total care depending upon the level of dysfunction. It is important to accurately assess the client's potential for self-care and encourage the client to maintain as much independence as possible.

Sensoriperceptual problems, such as blindness or deafness, may limit the client's ability to participate in self-care, particularly when placed in an unfamiliar environment such as a hospital. Visually impaired clients may need assistance with eating or getting to the bathroom. Hearing-impaired clients may not be able to follow instructions. Specific strategies, such as verbal cuing for visually impaired clients or using gestures or picture boards for hearing-impaired clients, can be employed to help counteract these problems (see Chapter 38).

Medical or Surgical Procedures. Medical or surgical procedures may alter the client's ability to perform self-care. An acutely ill client usually needs a great deal of help with care due to the medical or surgical problem and weakness or pain associated with the treatments or medications.

The use of opioid analgesics for pain relief or sedatives to aid sleep/rest may make the client drowsy or sedated and unable to perform self-care. In addition, a general anesthetic will cause weakness. The client may also have decreased mobility because of problems such as fluid and electrolyte imbalances, hypoxia, or hypovolemia. Equipment that encumbers the client, such as an intravenous (IV) line, monitoring equipment, central lines, oxygen, and catheters, may also interfere with self-care and require assistance from the nurse or other health care provider.

CULTURAL AND LIFESTYLE FACTORS

Cultural and Religious Factors. Culture has an important influence on self-care practices (Box 31-3). Cultural and social norms, as well as the teachings of family, create different perspectives on cleanliness and hygiene. There may be wide variation among groups with regard

BOX 31-3 *Cross-Cultural Care*

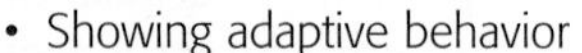
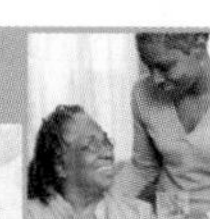

Caring for an African American Client

Mrs. Wilson, the client discussed in this chapter, is of African American ancestry. She grew up in the Deep South as the daughter of sharecroppers who struggled to feed and clothe their 10 children. Mrs. Wilson is the fifth child and the only surviving sibling. She has never lived more than 50 miles from the place of her birth.

Poverty was a reality of her early life, but she says that the difficulties were made bearable by the intensity of love within the family, and she feels that this has been a blessing in her life. She has been a widow for 10 years. Her daughter is her only child, and two granddaughters live nearby.

Several characteristics have been identified in the African American culture that demonstrate their values, beliefs, and worldviews. Attributing specific characteristics to groups is not without risks and is not intended to stereotype individuals. In general, African Americans tend to value the following:

- Having a strong will to survive
- Being steeped in a particular culture and tradition
- Showing adaptive behavior
- Showing strong belief in self-reliance
- Avoiding self-blame for failures
- Having major concern for health and ability to maintain activities of daily living
- Tending to overestimate health status
- Seeing trouble as a "cross one must bear"
- Believing that avoidance of worry and tension is the same as problem solving
- Relying on kinship and family networks to cope with health concerns

to common bathing rituals and the application of preparations to the skin. In some cultures, bathing is done daily or even more often. In other cultural groups, bathing may not occur daily because it is not deemed necessary or for reasons such as the reduced availability of an adequate water supply or provisions for bathing. Some groups apply oils and other preparations to the skin and hair. Shaving of leg and axillary hair, which is practiced by most women in the United States, is not necessarily a standard hygiene practice around the world, particularly in some parts of Europe. It is important to understand these individual differences in caring for clients of diverse ethnic and cultural backgrounds. Some personal hygiene practices may be unfamiliar to you, but their significance to the client should be respected.

Religious rituals may also influence the client's hygiene habits. Some religions have prohibitions against the exposure of body parts, the cutting and care of hair, and bathing during menses or immediately after delivery of a child. In some groups, it is forbidden for a male to attend to the hygiene needs of a female. Be aware of and respect these beliefs and practices that vary from those in traditional Western culture.

Psychosocial Factors. Psychological factors that accompany physical illness may cause the client to need help with self-care, even if it is only in the form of a reminder or encouragement to take a bath or shampoo. If clients are dealing with the stress of a serious diagnosis for themselves or a loved one, encouraging them to participate in hygiene activities may help them exert control over some facet of their daily life.

Emotional disturbances may cause disruptions in the ability to perform self-care. The client with active psychosis is likely to need assistance because of the break with reality and the resultant inattention to hygiene and other self-care needs. Sometimes a change in grooming is an early indicator of mental illness or cognitive changes such as dementia or Alzheimer's disease. Depression can slow a person down because of the lack of psychic energy and therefore physical energy. Poor grooming, lack of interest in appearance, or inappropriate dressing may reflect a need for assistance.

Knowledge Level. Take into account the client's knowledge level in regard to self-care practices. The frequency of bathing, shampooing, and oral care (including flossing and brushing) are usually taught by significant others during childhood. These teachings are not always incorporated into the client's behavior and indicate an opportunity for health teaching about self-care.

Health teaching may be done informally by pointing out to the client ways in which overall health might be improved through specific actions. If family members are present with the client during hospitalization, health teaching is essential if they are to care for the client at home after hospitalization. They need to know principles of aseptic technique, as well as specific procedures that will be necessary at home. All of these can be incorporated into teaching and are most easily taught while care is being given.

Territoriality. Institutions tend to be very depersonalizing. One of the first events that a hospitalized client encounters is the removal of clothing and personal belongings. Provide an identified space for personal belongings, and encourage the inclusion of personal and familiar objects in the client's hospital environment to help make the space psychologically comforting to the client. Pictures, cards, and flowers not only bring a cheerful look to the client's room but also make the space unique for the client. It is a way of defining who that person is as an individual.

Caring for the most intimate needs of ill persons requires that you operate within the personal space of each client. Each client has a sense of "space" in which he or she feels comfortable. This space includes not only the physical area surrounding the person but also the emotional possession of the body and personal self-knowledge. Research has been conducted about clients' needs for physical personal space, and the results have been incorporated into design and allocation of square footage for rooms in hospitals and other health care facilities.

Intrusion into this personal space or territory without permission often causes discomfort. Nursing has implicit permission from society to move into an individual's space as necessary to give care, after obtaining permission whenever possible. This is a rare opportunity not offered to other disciplines and should be considered a privilege. It is important to be aware, however, that some clients may be uncomfortable with this physical and emotional closeness. Assess the client's comfort level so that care can be taken to reduce discomfort and anxiety.

Privacy in an institutional setting is difficult to achieve at times. Respect for the client's privacy is important in preserving dignity and feeling of worth. Carefully drape and screen the client during care, avoid intrusion when the client has visitors or is talking on the telephone, and knock before entering the room to show concern for the right to privacy. Respect the client's personal space also by providing privacy when sensitive matters are to be discussed.

Socioeconomic Factors. Socioeconomic factors influence self-care habits and practices in a number of ways. Financial resources to purchase the necessary tools for hygiene may be limited. An environment that is dreary and unclean does not encourage the individual toward meticulous hygiene. Bathing may assume a low priority in an environment with inadequate heat or a lack of privacy for hygiene practices. When a significant amount of physical and emotional energy is required to meet daily subsistence needs for food and shelter, grooming and hygiene may be neglected. This does not imply that the individual no longer values them; it is simply that basic human needs for physical survival become paramount. An example of this may be seen in the homeless person who is hospitalized and finds comfort from being in a warm and comfortable environment where hygiene needs can be met.

ASSESSMENT

GENERAL ASSESSMENT OF SELF-CARE

Self-care depends on the client's physical and emotional ability to perform feeding, bathing, hair care, oral care, dressing, and toileting. An accurate assessment allows you and the client to mutually determine how much assistance is needed and to what extent the client can participate. If the client has a deficit in self-care ability, it may range from total inability to participate in any self-care activities to a partial deficit, in which case the client may be able to assist to a greater or lesser degree in these activities. If you presuppose lack of ability when some ability may be present, it can further reinforce a client's sense of dependence and helplessness. If you expect participation in self-care activities when the client is physically or emotionally exhausted, the client may feel frustrated or anxious.

> ***Action Alert!*** Assess the client's physical and emotional ability to participate in self-care activities as a safeguard for creating a therapeutic environment for recovery or healing.

Health History. The health history is important in that it will give you information on which to base current self-care status. What are the client's main concerns? Why was the client admitted for home health care services, to an acute care facility, or to a skilled nursing facility? How long has this problem existed? Is it new or long-standing? What was the lifestyle before? What is the history of the illness? What was the previous activity level? What are the hygiene habits? The health history provides information about the client's present and past health and illness experiences. The health history interview should include a review of functional health patterns; question the status of and change in patterns. When did the ability to manage ADLs change? Is this a recent change or has it been coming over time? Is the alteration in functional ability of sudden or slow onset?

Note the client's physical status. An assessment of cognitive function will provide you with clues about how to approach the client and how to proceed. Assess the acuity of the client's vision and hearing. Determine the ability to follow your directions. Look at the client's skin for existing problems such as skin breakdown. Note the presence of neuromuscular weakness or neuromuscular impairment (tics, spasticity, rigidity, palsy, paralysis). If the client's mobility is severely impaired, you may need to involve more than one caregiver. An assessment of the client's energy level is important so that care can be provided while minimizing the client's expenditure of energy. Observe for the presence of pain or discomfort and whether these are aggravated by movement.

Assess for factors that place the client at risk for self-care deficit. Risk factors include developmental stage, current health status, mobility, cognitive status, emotional status, and medical plan of care.

Be aware of the client's age. The very young and the very old have special needs for assistance. Infants have no capacity to perform self-care, whereas older adults may have some need for dependency on caregivers when self-care abilities are affected by physical or psychological impairments.

Mobility may be a risk factor if there is any impairment due to neuromuscular weakness or sensory deficits. Some clients may have limited mobility because of the weakness of one or more extremities.

The client's ability to recognize the need for hygiene measures and the ability to implement this knowledge are necessary to prevent a deficit in self-care. A cognitively impaired individual may not be able to focus well enough to plan the essential steps necessary for self-care or to carry them out.

> ***Action Alert!*** Assess the client's cognitive status; even if the client appears to be well oriented and capable of self-care, your more careful observation may reveal short-term memory loss or other deficits.

The client who is exceptionally stressed or emotionally unstable may outwardly appear to have self-care skills, but because of the intense focus on the emotional stressor, the client may simply not have enough energy to meet these needs. Therapeutic management of illness or trauma, surgical or medical procedures that cause weakness, or pain or nausea may necessitate bed rest and interfere with the client's ability to perform self-care activities.

> ***Action Alert!*** Anticipate the client's risk for self-care deficit by anticipatory planning for the client's therapies and treatment.

Gather subjective assessment data by interacting with both the client and family. Functional health pattern assessment provides valuable information about the client's perceived self-care abilities and difficulties and associated feelings about adequacy. It includes such things as the normal routine for feeding, bathing, grooming, and toileting, and the personal satisfaction with this routine. Ask the client what causes problems and what has been done to deal with these problems. Is the client satisfied with the current state of daily self-care activities? What is the client's level of motivation to regain self-care activities? What are the client's goals and expectations? Is there hope for improvement in self-care status? What level of dependence on family caregivers is necessary?

FOCUSED ASSESSMENT FOR *SELF-CARE DEFICIT*

Defining Characteristics. Assess the client's abilities and deficits in the following areas.

Bathing/Hygiene Self-Care Deficit. Assess the client's ability to wash the body or body parts, to obtain water or regulate the temperature and flow of water, to get bathing supplies, to sit or stand while bathing, and to get to the bathroom (NANDA International [NANDA-I], 2005).

Dressing/Grooming Self-Care Deficit. Assess the client's ability to choose or replace clothing, put on or take off pieces of clothing including socks and shoes, fasten clothing using zippers and buttons, use assistive devices for dressing, and maintain a satisfactory appearance (NANDA-I, 2005).

Feeding Self-Care Deficit. Assess the client's ability to open containers, prepare food, place food onto utensils, bring food to mouth, chew, and swallow, and maintain adequate nutrition (NANDA-I, 2005).

Toileting Self-Care Deficit. Assess the client's ability to get to the toilet or commode, to sit on and rise from it, move clothing to carry out toileting, to flush the toilet, and to use proper hygiene after toileting (NANDA-I, 2005).

Related Factors. The related factors for all of these nursing diagnoses are similar and include fatigue, inadequate or lack of motivation, pain or severe anxiety, perceptual or cognitive impairment, neuromuscular or musculoskeletal impairment, or environmental barriers (NANDA-I, 2005).

DIAGNOSIS

Use the physical assessment database and your observations to determine the appropriate nursing diagnoses (Table 31-5). When the client presents with a self-care deficit problem, it may be total or partial. If it is total, it includes deficits in feeding, bathing/hygiene, dressing/grooming, and toileting. If it is partial, one or more deficits may be present. The client may have a diagnosis that begins with *Risk for* if there is potential for loss of self-care ability.

RELATED NURSING DIAGNOSES

Impaired skin integrity is a potential problem for the client who cannot manage self-care and hygiene. A good time to assess the skin is during the client's bath. Assess the color and temperature, particularly in the extremities. Note areas that are different from other areas (cooler, warmer, paler, reddened); the texture (dry, smooth, rough, scaly, or oily); any lesions, blisters, or impaired integrity; excoriation of the perineal or perianal regions; and pain or sensitivity in any area as it is bathed or moved. Note the client's sense of touch (temperature of water, pressure with rubbing), limitation of motion, stiffness, or pain during range-of-motion (ROM) exercises, emotional state, and ability to communicate.

Impaired oral mucous membranes may apply to clients who are unable to manage oral hygiene, such as persons who have altered states of consciousness or have difficulty getting to the sink or bathroom (e.g., a client with arthritic hands may have difficulty in picking up and holding small items).

Impaired physical mobility may be caused by acute or chronic illness, trauma, psychological impairment, or the need to conserve energy as with bed rest or reduced activity.

Table 31-5 Clustering Data to Make a Nursing Diagnosis: Self-Care Deficit

DATA CLUSTER	DIAGNOSIS
A 65-year-old, poorly nourished, fatigued, and listless woman was diagnosed with Alzheimer's disease 5 years ago. She has shown rapid deterioration and now is unable to care for any of her basic hygiene needs.	*Self-care deficit* related to loss of memory and neuromuscular function
A young man, age 30, has metastatic brain tumor secondary to progressive bronchogenic carcinoma. He is totally blind in his right eye. He also has right hemiplegia and is very limited in his self-care abilities.	*Self-care deficit* related to decreased visual and motor ability
A 55-year-old woman has a history of chronic obstructive pulmonary disease and is now in acute congestive heart failure. She has extreme dyspnea and is able to ambulate only to the bathroom and back to recliner.	*Self-care deficit* related to activity intolerance
A 40-year-old woman has had severe rheumatoid arthritis for 20 years. She has severe limitations of the lower and upper extremities. She has difficulty grasping objects because of the malformation of hands and fingers.	*Self-care deficit* related to limited range of motion and pain
A 20-year-old man was hospitalized after a motor vehicle accident; his pelvis, left tibia, and fibula were fractured. He refuses to move because of the intense pain caused by any movement.	*Self-care deficit* related to pain and limited mobility from fractures

Activity intolerance occurs when the physical or psychological demands of the activity are more than the client can tolerate without manifestations of distress, which may take the form of dyspnea, muscle weakness, fatigue, or tachycardia.

Powerlessness may apply to a client who is dependent on others for activities of daily living. Assess the client's behavior for attempts at establishing control. The client who is demanding and manipulative may be feeling out of control. On the other hand, powerlessness may be expressed as apathy or fastidiousness.

PLANNING

Planning for outcomes should be a collaborative effort between you, the client, and, when appropriate, the client's family. Setting mutually acceptable and attainable goals is essential in assisting the client to attain some degree of independence.

EXPECTED OUTCOMES FOR THE CLIENT WITH *SELF-CARE DEFICIT*

Planning is essential to help the client meet personal care needs when there is a self-care deficit. For the client who has a total self-care deficit, the goal is to provide measures that will prevent complications. For the client with partial self-care deficit, the goal is to assist the client as needed and to encourage as much independence as possible. The goal is always to encourage independence and to return the client to a state of independent self-care. Take the following factors into account when planning:

- The client's general physical condition and functional status
- Individual specific self-care requirements
- Personal preferences and wishes

EXPECTED OUTCOMES FOR THE CLIENT AND FAMILY WITH *SELF-CARE DEFICIT*

Planning with the client and family is important because the desired outcomes may vary with the client's level of illness or with priorities that are different from those you believe to be necessary for the client. Expected outcomes for the client and family with self-care deficit might be the following:

- Client's self-care needs are met.
- Complications are avoided and minimized.
- Client and family members participate in self-care to maximum extent of ability.
- Client and family communicate feelings and concerns.
- Client and family identify resources to help cope with problems after discharge.

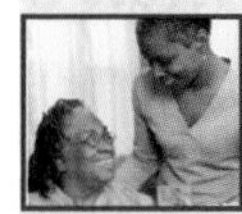

Mrs. Wilson, the subject of our case study, is ready for discharge after 2 weeks of hospitalization following a cerebrovascular accident. What expected outcomes might be appropriate for her and her family?

INTERVENTION

INTERVENTIONS TO PROMOTE SKIN HYGIENE

Principles of Skin Care. Because the skin is the first line of defense against microbes and other harmful substances, healthy intact skin is important to a client's overall health. Bathing is an infection control measure. It provides cleaning and conditioning of the skin as a defense against disease. You need to keep the client's skin clean and dry to protect it from getting diseased and damaged. Remember to bathe the client from cleaner to less-clean areas, working from the head and upper body toward the feet. Keep in mind that hygiene and grooming are directly related to self-esteem.

Bathing the Client. Bathing is an important intervention to promote hygiene. Choice of the method of bathing depends on your judgment, as well as the medical plan of care, in regard to the client's activity level and mental and physical capabilities to perform self-care (Box 31-4). Consider the client's preferences for type of bath and time of day for bathing to allow some degree of control. This may not always be possible because of the client's condition and other factors.

Bathing may be accomplished with a bed bath, a tub or shower, or the client's bathing at a sink or lavatory. Bed baths are less commonly used than in the past as recognition of the need for mobility has assumed precedence over bed rest. Assistive devices, such as shower chairs that can be rolled into the shower, and lifting devices that can lift a client in and out of a tub allow tub and shower bathing for clients who previously would have received bed baths.

BOX 31-4 *Guidelines for Bathing Clients*

- Promote safety and prevent falls.
- Assess psychological and physical needs.
- Determine self-care abilities and limitations.
- Encourage self-help except when contraindicated.
- Allow as much control and involvement as possible; let the client make some choices.
- Provide privacy and warmth at time of bathing; cover and drape sufficiently.
- Use good body mechanics for yourself by keeping a wide base of support, keeping back straight, and using leg and abdominal muscles to move and lift clients.

Action Alert! When possible, bathe the client in a tub or shower. Even if it is more difficult and time consuming for you, it will enhance the physical and emotional well-being of the client.

Some of the goals of hygiene care are the following:

- Comfort and relaxation
- Stimulation of circulation through friction and massage
- Assessment of the skin
- Cleanliness from removal of body waste products and secretions

BOX 31-5 *Teaching for Wellness*

Skin Care

Purpose: To teach client about the care of dry skin, which is susceptible to breaking, and causes itching and roughness.
Expected Outcomes: Client will follow prescribed regimen for skin to alleviate dryness.

Client Instructions

- Sometimes your skin can become dry because you have not taken in enough fluids. Make sure you drink eight glasses of water a day. Avoid dehydrating fluids, such as alcohol and caffeine-containing drinks. These are not substitutes for water.
- Bathing can dry your skin as well. Use a gentle bath lotion or mild soap. No soap is sometimes the best answer.
- Too-frequent bathing may dry the skin. It may be wise to reduce baths from daily to every other day or even twice a week. When bathing, use warm rather than hot water.
- Use bath oils or lubricants immediately after bathing to prevent immediate loss of moisture.
- Pay attention to the way your linens and clothing are being laundered. Harsh detergents and bleaches are irritating to already dry skin. Use mild nondetergent cleaning products rather than harsh detergents. Avoid perfumed fabric softeners.
- Dry skin tends to itch, and you may want to rub or scratch it. Try not to do this because you can hurt your skin. Also avoid rubbing your skin roughly with a towel after bathing. Patting dry is much less harmful to the skin.

Table 31-6 Types of Therapeutic Baths

TYPE OF BATH	PURPOSE
Sitz bath	To decrease pain and inflammation after rectal or perineal surgery, vaginal childbirth, or for pain relief from hemorrhoids. Water should be warm to client's comfort level.
Hot-water bath	To relieve muscle spasm and muscle tension. Water should be deep enough for immersion. Warm to client's comfort level.
Warm-water bath	To relax and soothe. Client's comfort will dictate water temperature. Caution client about time limits for soaking (20 minutes) because of vasodilation.
Cool-water bath	To decrease fever and to reduce muscle tension. Avoid chilling. Water should be cool but not cold.
Oatmeal	To soothe irritated skin. Softens and lubricates dry scaly skin. Place 3 cups cooked oatmeal in a cheesecloth bag and place in tub of water.
Cornstarch	To soothe skin irritation. Dissolve 1 pound of cornstarch in cold water, then add boiling water until mixture is thick and add to tub water.

Bathing a client is a time of close contact that provides you with an opportunity to communicate with the client, as well as assess the client's physical and mental status. The client may appreciate your undivided attention for a concentrated period of time and may feel free to express concern that otherwise would not be expressed. It is a time to provide special skin care and teach the client and family about skin care (Box 31-5).

Several types of baths can be used depending on the client's need. Baths may be used for cleansing or as therapeutic measures related to some skin problem (Table 31-6).

Bathing the client in bed. Procedure 31-1 provides detailed steps for bathing a client in bed. The bed bath is given for the purpose of providing cleanliness for a client who is unable to be out of bed and who is unable to care for hygiene needs because of physical or mental limitations. It is indicated primarily for clients with restricted mobility (people with casts, traction, or back problems), those who have heart and respiratory problems and thus limited exercise tolerance, or those who are at the first postoperative day and thus may be too weak to get out of bed to bathe.

Methods include the following:

- Complete bed bath: giving the complete bath without any assistance from the client
- Partial bed bath: assisting with key areas such as axilla, back, and perineum
- Self-help: giving the client help with hard-to-reach areas, such as the back, legs, and feet

A bed bath may be given using premoistened, disposable washcloths, which come prepackaged. Each package contains eight fragrance-free, hypoallergenic, alcohol-free, antibacterial washcloths with aloe and vitamin E.

Text continued on p. 803

Time to Allow: **Novice:** 45 min. **Expert:** 20 min.

PROCEDURE 31-1 GIVING THE CLIENT A BATH

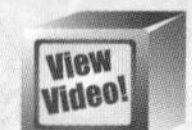

The bed bath is given to provide cleanliness and comfort to a client who is unable to be out of bed because of physical or mental limitations. The client who is unable to perform any of the bath is given a complete bed bath. Most clients can perform some of the bath and in most circumstances should be encouraged to do so. The bed bath is an opportunity to perform range-of-motion (ROM) exercises and skin assessment.

Standard precautions are followed for all bathing procedures. The nurse wears clean gloves for any contact with blood, body fluids, secretions, excretions, and contaminated items. Put on clean gloves just before touching the client's mucous membranes and nonintact skin, and change gloves between tasks and procedures, particularly, after contact with material that may contain a high concentration of microorganisms. Remove gloves promptly after use, before touching noncontaminated items and environmental surfaces. Before going to another client, perform hand hygiene to avoid transfer of microorganisms to other clients or environments.

Safety Issues: Bathing is important to reduce the number of microorganisms in the environment. All devices, including thromboembolic device (TED) hose, must be removed for skin inspection. Use side rails to provide safety during the bath. Avoid chilling or excessively hot water. Assistance with bathing is essential if the client has an IV line or drainage tubes.

DELEGATION GUIDELINES

Once you have assessed your client, you may delegate the performance of a bed bath to assistive personnel. Remember that although the assistive personnel is instructed to observe for changes in the client's skin, such as irritation or discoloration, and report any changes to you, you as the nurse maintain the professional responsibility for assessment and for appropriate action based on assessment. You are responsible for reestablishing any disruption in intravenous (IV) infusions or drainage devices at the completion of the bath.

EQUIPMENT NEEDED

- Washbasin
- Soap or cleansing lotion
- Two washcloths
- Two towels
- Bath blanket
- Clean gown or pajamas
- Toiletry items, such as deodorant, skin lotion
- Oral-care items, if oral care is to be done with bed bath
- Hair-care items, if shampooing is to be done with bed bath
- Shaving items, if shaving is to be done with bed bath
- Disposable gloves (essential for perineal and oral care; otherwise, as needed)
- Laundry bag or cart
- Bedpan or urinal

Continued

1 Follow preliminary actions (see inside front cover).

2 Check physician's orders for activity and any special positioning needs or contraindications. Assess for ability to participate in the bath even if on a limited scale. Evaluate client's need for teaching about skin care, and plan to incorporate teaching into the procedure. Assess for presence of IV lines, catheters, tubes, casts, and dressings. Assess client's ROM. *Cleansing of skin and teaching about skin care and ROM movements can be smoothly integrated so that time and energy are conserved for you and client. If assessment indicates that the bath can be done more efficiently or safely with two people, it is advisable to secure this help. Allowing the client to participate in the bath provides a source of exercise and ROM movement, as well as providing for enhancement of self-worth and feelings of independence.*

3 Prepare the environment.

a. Perform hand hygiene, and apply gloves if needed. Change gloves after oral care, perineal care, or washing nonintact skin. *Some agencies adopt a policy of using gloves for the bath without regard to assessing for intact skin. Other agencies leave it to the nurse's judgment.*

b. Gather equipment, and take to the bedside. Have all necessary supplies and equipment ready for use. *Having necessary supplies readily at hand enhances organization and efficiency in bathing the client.*

c. Raise bed to a comfortable working height, ensure privacy by closing door or curtains, and regulate temperature of the room for comfort. Keep the side rail up on the side of the bed opposite to where you are working. *Applying principles of body mechanics allows you to work comfortably and efficiently without muscle strain. Privacy, comfort, and safety are prerequisites for making the bed bath a positive experience for the client.*

d. Place articles on over-bed table, within easy reach. *Organization of supplies conserves energy and increases efficiency of movement. Having supplies within reach also promotes client's safety because it eliminates the necessity for your turning away from the client or moving away from the bedside to reach for supplies.*

4 Prepare the client.

a. Assist client with using bedpan, commode, or urinal. *Bathing, turning, and placement of extremities in warm water may stimulate the need to void.*

b. Place bath blanket over the client, covering the top linen (see illustration). *The bath blanket is warmer and more absorbent than a sheet. If a bath blanket is not available, the top sheet may be used to cover the client.*

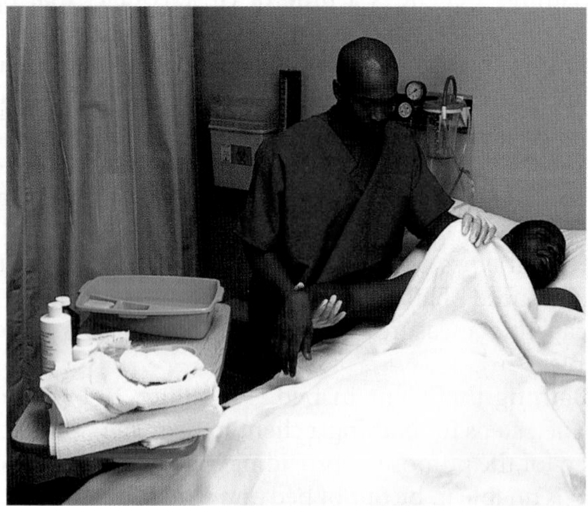

Step 4b. Placing the bath blanket over the client, covering the top linen.

c. Loosen top linen at the foot of the bed, and remove from under the bath blanket. To do so, ask the client to grasp the top of the bath blanket. If client is unable to grasp the blanket, grip it with one hand while removing the linen with the other. The client remains covered with the bath blanket while the soiled sheet is pulled out. Refold any linen that is to be reused and place on a chair. Place dirty linen in a laundry hamper or laundry bag.

d. Place bath towel under head. Remove pillow if the client can tolerate it. If removal of pillow causes any discomfort, leave it in place and place the towel over the pillow. *Removal of the pillow allows better access to the back of the neck and skin surfaces. It also prevents the pillow from becoming damp while the face and neck are being washed.*

e. Help client move to the side of the bed nearest you. Be sure that the side rail on the opposite side of the bed is raised. *Having the client close to you lowers your center of gravity and enhances efficiency of movement and energy, and it protects your back muscles from being stretched.*

f. Remove client's gown or pajamas. If an IV is in place, remove the gown from the arm without the IV first; then, from the arm with the IV—slide the sleeve down, lower the IV, and slide the IV through the sleeve opening. Do not disconnect the tubing. Rehang the IV and assess the rate of flow. If available, clients should wear a gown with snap or tie sleeves if they have an IV or upper extremity injury to have easy access to upper extremities during hygiene.

5 Wash the client's face and neck. *In general, bathe from head to toe (cleanest to dirtiest). Wash, rinse, and dry before moving to the next area.*

a. Fill washbasin one-half to two-thirds full of warm water. Test the temperature of the water with a bath thermometer, or have the client test the water with his or her fingers for temperature tolerance. It should be comfortably warm, between 109.4° and 114.8° F (43° to 46° C). *If the pan is too full, the basin is difficult to handle and spilling is likely. Too little water cools very quickly and is not sufficient for adequate bathing and rinsing.*
b. Put on clean gloves if there is a possibility of exposure to body fluids during the bath. *Standard precautions should be maintained when any exposure to body fluids is anticipated.*
c. Make a mitt with the washcloth. Use either the triangular or the rectangular method of folding (see illustration). Place your hand in the center of the washcloth. Fold the edges over your hand. Tuck the edges in to make a mitt. *Using the mitt prevents the loose ends of the washcloth from dragging across the client's skin and chilling or irritating the skin.*

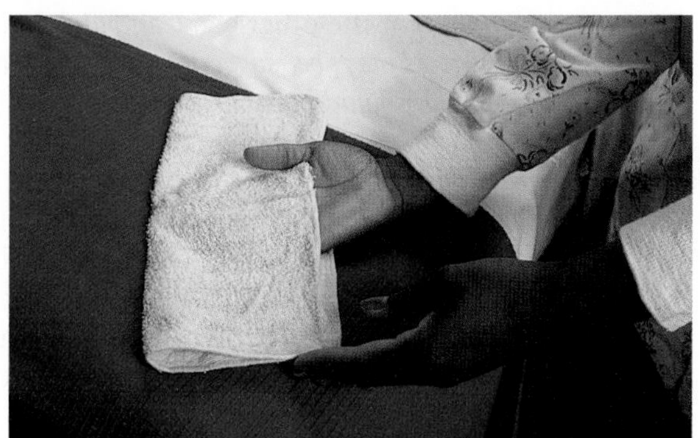

Step 5c. Folding the edges of the washcloth over the hand to make a mitt (rectangular method).

d. Wash the client's eyes with clear water. With one corner of the mitt, begin washing the eye at the inner canthus and work toward the outside (see illustration). Change the placement of your hand in the mitt, and repeat with the other eye. Dry thoroughly. If crusted secretions are present, place warm washcloth or cotton ball over the eye for 2 to 3 minutes until secretions are moist enough to be easily removed. *Using different points on the washcloth prevents cross contamination of the eyes if there is any infection. Infectious secretions are prevented from entering the lacrimal ducts. Moistening dried secretions prevents trauma to the eye on removal of the secretions.*

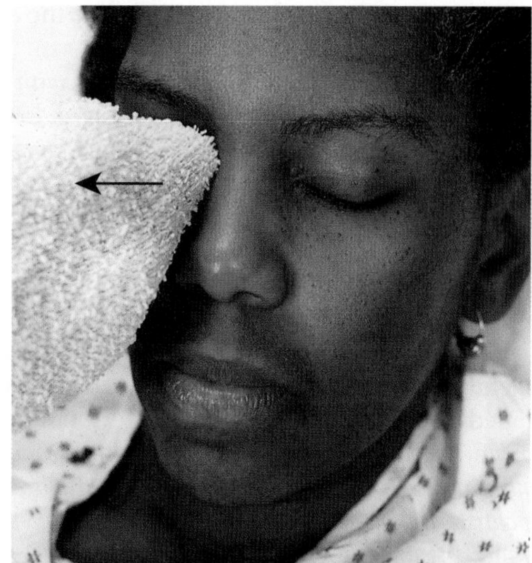

Step 5d. Washing the eye from the inner canthus outward.

e. Wash and dry the client's face using clear water or a mild soap. Soap is sometimes drying to the skin, especially in older people. Many people do not want soap on their face. Ask client for preference before using soap.
f. Wash forehead, cheeks, nose, and perioral areas.
g. Wash the postauricular area. Clean the anterior and posterior ear with the tip of the washcloth.
h. Wash the front and back of the neck.
i. Remove the towel from beneath client's neck.

6 Wash the client's arms. As you move down the body you can wash larger areas at a time. Wash small to moderate-size sections of the body at a time. The size of the area is determined by the likelihood of the person experiencing the discomfort of chilling.

a. Place a towel lengthwise under upper arm and axilla. Wash the upper surface of the arm. Use long, firm strokes, proceeding from the distal to the proximal area (fingers to axilla) (see illustration).

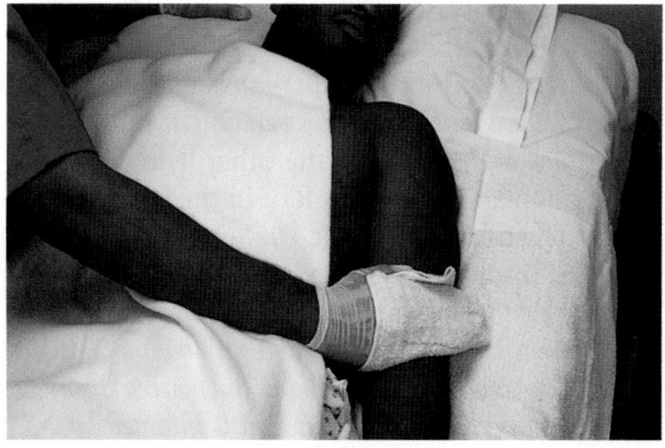

Step 6a. Washing the client's arm.

Continued

b. Grasp the client's wrist firmly, and elevate the arm to wash its lower surface.
c. Wash the axilla. *Elevating the arm helps with ROM movement, and distal-to-proximal stroking aids venous return. Extremities should be grasped at the joint rather than by the body of the muscle when they are being elevated. Gripping the muscle body may cause great discomfort.*
d. Wash the client's hands. Support the wrist joint, and immerse the hand in warm water. Allow it to soak for a few minutes. Do ROM movements with the client's fingers. Dry the hand thoroughly. Nails may be cleaned now or after the bath. Apply lotion if desired. *Moving the joints provides ROM exercise. Soaking the hand is relaxing and pleasant for the client. It also softens the cuticle and makes it easier to clean the nails by loosening any dirt under the nails.*

7 Wash the client's chest.
a. Fold the bath blanket down to the umbilicus.
b. Cover a female client's chest with a towel. Then lift up one side to wash her chest. Wash the skinfolds under female client's breasts. Dry under the breasts and in any skinfolds. Assess breasts, and teach breast self-examination if appropriate. Palpate for axillary node enlargement. *Keeping the client covered protects privacy and prevents unnecessary exposure.*

8 Wash the client's abdomen.
a. Expose only the areas being washed. Keep remaining areas covered with a towel. Fold the bath blanket down to the symphysis pubis.
b. Use firm strokes to wash the abdomen from side to side. Carefully inspect and clean the umbilicus. *Firm strokes decrease the sensation of tickling, which some people have on light abdominal touching.*
c. Observe for signs of distention or visible peristalsis.
d. Re-cover the client with the bath blanket.

9 Wash the client's legs.
a. Expose one leg at a time. Keep the other leg covered with the bath blanket. Keep the rest of the body covered. Remove bath blanket from the farther leg first.
b. Lift leg, and wash it using firm distal-to-proximal strokes. Rinse and dry client's leg from ankle to knee and knee to groin. *Distal-to-proximal stroking stimulates circulation and promotes venous return.* Reverse the coverings, and repeat for the other leg.
c. Carefully place the client's foot in the basin, and leave it for a few minutes to soak. Do ROM movements with the toes. Inspect the feet and nails. *Although it is not essential, soaking the feet can be comforting, especially if the client has been in bed for several days. Soaking aids circulation and softens nails and calluses. Supporting the extremity at the joint prevents discomfort that is initiated by grasping the body of a muscle.*
d. Dry the feet thoroughly, especially between the toes (see illustration).

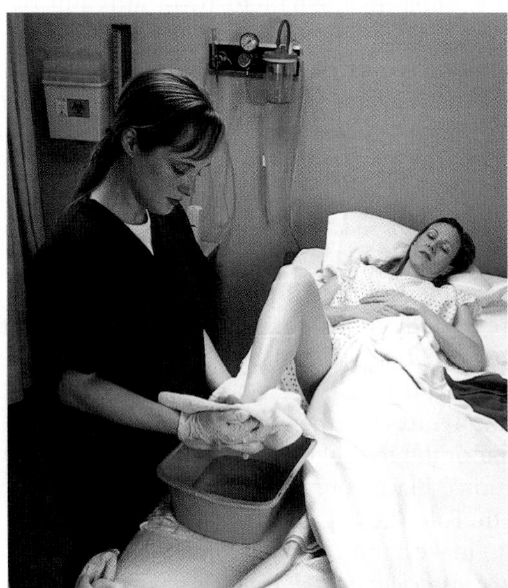

Step 9d. Drying the feet thoroughly.

e. Repeat this process for the other leg. *Calf pain on dorsiflexion of the foot may be suggestive of a positive Homans' sign, which should be reported to the physician immediately.*

10 Provide perineal care.
a. Place the client in a supine position. If the client is able to wash genitalia without assistance, place a basin of warm water, washcloth, and towel within reach and provide privacy. If the client cannot wash the perineal area, drape the area with the bath blanket so that only the genitalia are exposed.
b. Wash the perineal area, as explained in Procedure 31-2.
c. Change the bath water and washcloth.

11 Wash the back, buttocks, and perianal area.
a. Place the client in a side-lying position. Facing away from you.
b. Place a towel lengthwise along the client's back and buttocks while keeping the client covered with bath blanket as much as possible. This provides warmth and undue exposure.
c. Wash, rinse, and dry the client's back and buttocks (see illustration) moving from the shoulders to the buttocks and upper thighs, paying attention to the gluteal folds. *The perianal area is considered the dirtiest area of the body and is bathed last to prevent microorganisms from being transferred to cleaner parts of the body.*

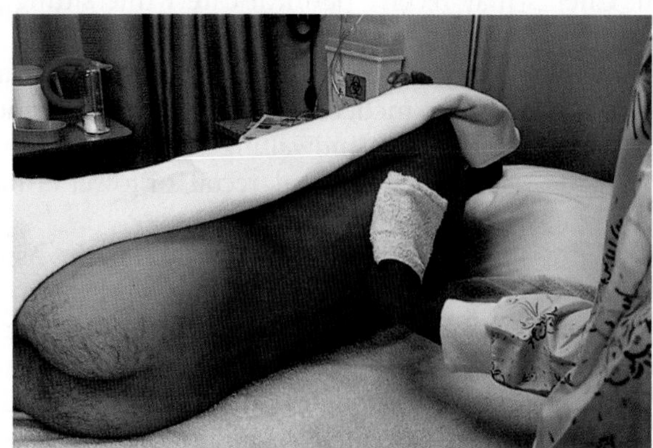

Step 11c. Washing the back and buttocks.

d. A back massage with lotion may be done at this time, or it may be done at the completion of the bath.

12 Help the client don a clean gown or pajamas.

a. While the client is still on one side, place one arm in the sleeve of the gown. (If an IV is in place, place the IV arm in the sleeve of the gown first, after the IV bag and tubing.)

b. Turn the client to the back, and place the other arm in the sleeve.

13 Assist with hair care.

14 Assist with oral care, as explained in Procedure 31-6 (p. 813).

15 Make the bed with clean linens, as explained in Procedures 31-4 (p. 807) and 31-5 (p. 810).

16 Leave the client's environment clean and uncluttered.

17 Document significant observations and assessment findings.

PEDIATRIC CONSIDERATIONS

Regulate the temperature of bath water carefully to avoid burns. Newborn infants do not require tub baths; rather, they should be given sponge baths. Infants should be dried and wrapped immediately after a bath to conserve body heat, because they have an incompletely developed temperature regulating center. Avoid powder, which can be hazardous if inhaled. Children should participate in bathing according to their developmental level; for safety, they should never be left unattended in the bath. Adolescents may need assistance in choosing deodorants to reduce odor from perspiration caused by the reaction of bacteria with secretions from newly active sweat glands. Be sensitive to children's/adolescents' modesty and body image.

GERIATRIC CONSIDERATIONS

Regulate the temperature of bath water carefully to avoid burns. Avoid excessive use of soap to prevent excessively dry skin. Use moisturizers on the skin immediately after bathing while skin is still slightly damp. Avoid the use of powder, which causes moisture loss and could be hazardous if inhaled. Avoid the use of cornstarch in moist areas because it breaks down into glucose and enhances the growth of microorganisms.

HOME HEALTH CARE CONSIDERATIONS

In giving a bed bath in the home, follow the same general guidelines for body mechanics, cleaning from clean to dirty, maintaining physical comfort, and working efficiently. However, the typical home environment requires some modification to meet these guidelines. If the client will need bed baths on a long-term basis, obtaining a hospital bed may be a helpful solution. Some modifications to teach the family caregiver include the following:

- Place a worktable at the bedside.
- Sit on the side of the bed instead of bending over.
- Use a minimum amount of soap.
- Use a no-rinse cleansing product only if there are no contraindications.
- Give a complete bath only every 3 days, with axillary and perineal care in between.
- Check and massage the skin daily.

The packages are warmed in the microwave or warmer for a minute. They are insulated and resealable, so the washcloths can be kept warm during the bath. Clients are bathed, or bathe themselves, using a separate washcloth for each body area, which minimizes cross contamination. There is no rinsing or drying of the client after their use. You must remember not to flush the disposable wash cloths down the toilet but throw them away in the trash.

A bed bath may also be given using a "bag" bath or a towel bath. The client is cleansed with a warm cloth or towel saturated with a quick-drying solution containing a disinfectant, a cleaning agent, and a softening agent mixed with water, such as Septi-Soft. The oil in the solution softens the skin, and clients report a refreshed feeling from this kind of bath.

Advantages of both of these types of baths are that they are brief (10 minutes) and can be used for the client who is easily fatigued and who has limited tolerance for any activity. There is no splashing or spilling of water during the bath, and potential contamination from dirty basins and dumping contaminated water into sinks is eliminated.

Providing perineal care. The **perineum** includes the pelvic floor and associated structures occupying the pelvic outlet, bounded anteriorly by the symphysis pubis, laterally by the ischial tuberosities, and posteriorly by the coccyx. Cleaning the genitalia is usually a part of the bath, but it also may be needed after urinary or bowel elimination. If the client is unable to maintain adequate perineal care, this part of the care is your responsibility (Procedure 31-2).

Perineal care for women involves washing the labia majora and the labia minora, the inner thighs, the perineum, and the anal area. For men, perineal care involves cleaning the upper inner thighs, penis, scrotum and anal area. In both sexes, the perianal area is cleaned last with the client in a side-lying position. Professional behavior helps to reduce anxiety and embarrassment in the client. It is essential to wear gloves to provide perineal care because of the direct contact with body fluids and exudates and because any open wounds or sores on your hands are portals of entry for transmission of infection. Clients may receive perineal care while sitting on the bedpan or toilet.

Clients at risk for skin breakdown, and who may have particular needs for meticulous and frequent perineal care, include those with indwelling catheters, postpartum clients, clients with perineal, rectal, or lower urinary tract surgery, and incontinent clients.

Assisting the client with a shower or tub bath. Assess the client to determine the degree of independence to allow in bathing. Safety becomes a priority because injuries caused by falls in a bathtub or shower are common and often have serious consequences. Assess the client for dizziness; weakness in extremities; hypotension; any sensory impairment, particularly visual; mental capacity; degree of judgment; and clarity of thought. You may determine that the client can be left alone for bathing, or you may plan to remain with the client during the bath.

Time to Allow: Novice: 15 min. Expert: 5 min.

PROCEDURE 31-2 PROVIDING PERINEAL CARE

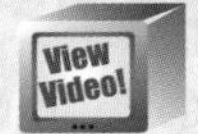

Perineal care is the cleansing of the external genitalia, perineum, and surrounding skin. It is usually part of the bath but is sometimes needed more frequently and is done as a separate procedure. See Procedure 31-1 for standard precautions guidelines and safety issues.

DELEGATION GUIDELINES

You may delegate the performance of perineal care to the assistive personnel who has received specific training in the performance of this task. Instruct the assistive personnel to report if any rash, perineal drainage, or excoriation if observed. You remain responsible and accountable for assessing the client's perineum.

EQUIPMENT NEEDED

- Bedpan
- Two towels
- Two washcloths
- Bath blanket
- Soap
- Cotton balls
- Bottle with warm water or prescribed solution for perineal treatment
- Waterproof pad
- Toilet tissue or premoistened wipes
- Disposable gloves (required) and gown if necessary
- Moisture-resistant bag or receptacle for used cotton swabs

FOR A FEMALE CLIENT

1 Follow preliminary actions (see inside front cover).

2 Prepare for the procedure.

a. Organize necessary equipment. Don clean gloves.

b. Place a protective pad or towel underneath the client before placing her on the bedpan if doing perineal care in bed. *Perineal care may be done with the client on a bedpan or sitting on the toilet or in a commode chair.*

c. Place the client in a comfortable position on bedpan, toilet, or commode chair. She may also sit on a bedpan in a semi-Fowler's position if the dorsal recumbent position is not possible. *Adapting position to the client's needs ensures a more positive outcome of the procedure.*

d. If care is to be given in bed, ask the client to bend her knees and separate her legs.

e. Drape the client with a bath blanket. Cover her legs, and wrap the corners of the bath blanket around her feet so her legs are covered. Leave a flap of drape covering the perineum until you are ready to begin the procedure. *Privacy and respect for the client's dignity are essential; expose as little as possible.*

3 Clean the perineum.

a. Washing from front to back, remove fecal debris with toilet paper and dispose in toilet. Cleanse buttocks and anus. Rinse and dry. Change water. Change gloves and wash hands.

b. Pour warm water or prescribed solution over the perineum.

c. Wash the labia majora. Use nondominant hand to gently retract labia from thigh, and wash carefully in skinfolds with dominant hand. Clean in direction from perineum to rectum. Rinse and dry.

d. Separate the labia with nondominant hand to expose the urethral and vaginal openings. Wash the folds between the labia majora and the labia minora. With your free hand, wipe from front to back in a downward motion with water and soap, washcloth, or cotton balls. Use a new cloth or cotton ball for each downward stroke. *Wiping in this manner prevents cross contamination of areas.*
e. Turn the client to a side-lying position, and wash her anal area. Change gloves.
f. Pat dry with a second towel.

4 Make the client comfortable.
a. Remove equipment and gloves and perform hand hygiene; cover the client.
b. Position her for comfort

FOR A MALE CLIENT

1 Follow preliminary actions (see inside front cover).

2 Prepare for the procedure.
a. Organize necessary equipment. Don clean gloves.
b. Cover the client with a bath blanket. Expose him only as needed to clean the genitalia. *Avoiding unnecessary exposure respects the client's need for privacy.*

3 Clean the perineum.
a. If the client is uncircumcised, retract the foreskin to remove smegma. *Smegma is a cheeselike substance secreted by the sebaceous glands. It collects under the foreskin.*
b. Hold the shaft of the penis firmly but gently with one hand. With the other hand, begin washing at the tip of the penis. Using a circular motion, clean around the head of the penis.
c. Wash down the shaft toward the scrotum. Change to a clean area of the washcloth as needed.
d. After rinsing the penis, replace the foreskin if necessary.
e. Wash around the scrotum; then wash the inner thighs. Turn the client to one side and wash the anal area and buttocks.

4 Make the client comfortable.
a. Remove equipment and gloves and perform hand hygiene.
b. Cover him, and position for comfort.

HOME HEALTH CARE CONSIDERATIONS

For the client who is unable to provide self-care at home, perineal care should be done daily to prevent unpleasant body odor and for comfort. If the client has a Foley catheter, daily perineal care will help prevent urinary tract infection. Gentle cleansing with soap and water is all that is required. Teach the family how to turn and position the client to work efficiently.

Transport the client to the tub or shower in a wheelchair, on a stretcher, or in a rolling shower chair, but use safety precautions such as belt restraints to prevent falling from the chair. Shower chairs are made of metal or plastic so they can be rolled into the shower. Use the hand-held shower nozzle to direct the flow of water. If the person is ambulating, use nonskid slippers. See Procedure 31-3 for details about assisting a client with a tub or shower bath.

Dressings and casts need not always be deterrents to bathing in a tub or shower. Improvised covers and plastic wrap taped over a cast or dressing can afford the person freedom to bathe as desired without damage to cast or dressing. A physician's order may be required for showering or bathing a client with a dressing or cast.

Assisting the client with a sink bath. Sometimes the client is well enough to sit up in a chair and bathe at the sink or can sit on the side of the bed with the bath basin positioned on the over-bed table. Provide privacy by closing the door and using a drape or sheet for cover and warmth. Wash the back, legs, and feet as necessary. If necessary, provide perineal care. Because the client bathes in a seated position, it is wise to stay nearby in case assistance is needed or the client becomes weak or dizzy. If the client is bathing at the sink or in a chair, you may use this opportunity to change the bed linens. If the client is sitting on the side of the bed, you may use this time to prepare for mouth or hair care.

Bed Making. In an acute care facility, the changing of bed linens is often included as part of the routine morning care and is done in conjunction with the bath and grooming. They are changed daily for the client's comfort and to eliminate a reservoir of microorganisms. When linens become wet or soiled, they are changed more frequently. In the home setting, linens may not be changed every day but should be changed when wet or soiled. Care should be taken to smooth the linens and remove crumbs and foreign objects to ensure comfort and safety for the client.

The type of bed making required depends in large measure on the condition and needs of the client. In making an occupied bed, you turn the client to one side, make half the bed, turn the client to the other side, and make the other half of the bed. Procedure 31-4 outlines the steps in making an occupied bed.

TIME TO ALLOW: **NOVICE:** 30 min. **EXPERT:** 15 min.

PROCEDURE 31-3 HELPING THE CLIENT WITH A TUB BATH OR SHOWER

Clients are assisted with a tub bath or shower when they are able to bathe themselves and there is no contraindication to bathing in a tub or shower. Clients who have had medical or surgical treatments may need orders from a physician.

Safety Issues: The client should be carefully monitored for risk of falling and for weakness or dizziness due to change in temperature and exertion. Test water temperature to prevent burns. Follow standard precautions.

DELEGATION GUIDELINES

The assistive personnel may help with the performance of a tub bath or shower. In addition to instruction regarding bathing, the assistive personnel should receive safety and mobility training to appropriately assist the client with this task. You remain responsible for the assessment of the client's independence, skin, gait, mobility, and response to this activity.

EQUIPMENT NEEDED

- Bath towel
- Two washcloths
- Soap or bath lotion
- Skin care products (deodorant, lotion)
- Clean gown or pajamas
- Clean gloves (if indicated)
- Shower chair or bath seat, if needed

1 Follow preliminary actions (see inside front cover).

2 Assess the client's capacity for self-care. Assess tolerance for activity, cognitive state, and musculoskeletal function. *An assessment of the client's ability before initiating the bath procedure is critical to maintaining the client's safety and comfort.*

3 Make sure that the bathroom is prepared and that the tub or shower is clean. Place a disposable bath mat or towel on the floor by the tub or shower. Adjust the room temperature so the client is not chilled during the bath. *Cleanliness and safety are primary responsibilities in caring for the client.*

4 Put on clean gloves.

5 Assess the client's ability to access bathroom. Have client wear robe and slippers. Transport the client in a wheelchair or shower chair if ambulation cannot be done safely without assistance. Accompany the client to the bathroom.

6 Keep the client covered with a bath blanket while preparing the water and while transporting (see illustration). *Chilling occurs quickly when skin is uncovered. Keeping the client covered conserves body heat, preventing chilling.*

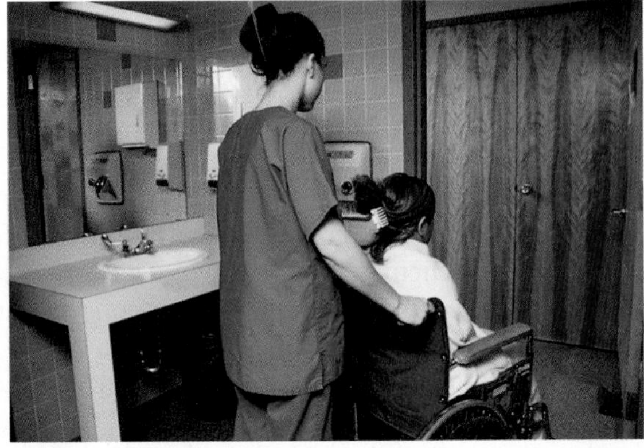

Step 6. Keeping the client covered with a bath blanket during transport to the bathroom.

7 Provide privacy for the client by placing an "occupied" sign on the door. *Bathroom doors are not locked for safety reasons because clients may need unexpected assistance. The need for privacy while bathing is basic to human dignity, and provision for privacy demonstrates respect.*

8 Test the water temperature before the client gets into the tub or shower. Adjust the temperature until it is comfortable. Fill the bathtub no more than half full of warm water (105° F). Caution client not to adjust temperature without assistance. *Testing the temperature before the water is entered prevents burns. Attempts to adjust the water temperature without your assistance can result in scalding.*

9 Provide assistance as the client is entering tub or shower. *Falls in the tub or shower are common accidents and must be prevented by safety measures.*

10 Assess whether the client can safely bathe without assistance. If the client can remain unattended, demonstrate the use of the call signal and the safety bars in the tub or shower. Explain which faucet controls the hot water. The client may wish to sit in a shower chair to conserve energy while bathing. Place all bath supplies within easy reach. *Falls in the tub or shower often occur when client is reaching for an object, such as soap or a towel. Placing everything within easy reach prevents the need to reach.*

11 If the client can be safely left to bathe unattended, check every 5 to 10 minutes to determine if help is needed.

12 If independent bathing is not possible, remain with the client at all times. Assist as needed with bathing. Encourage the client to do as much of the bathing as possible. *This encourages independence as well as motor function.*

13 Wash any areas that the client is unable to reach, such as the back and legs. Assist a female client with shaving her legs or axillae if desired.
14 Watch closely for signs of dizziness or weakness while the client is in the tub or shower and immediately on exiting the tub or shower. *Vasodilation and pooling of blood in the extremities occurs with prolonged exposure to warm water. This may manifest as dizziness, weakness, or faintness.*
15 Help the client out of the tub or shower. First, drain water from tub. Assist with drying.
16 Assist with grooming and dressing in clean pajamas or gown.
17 Help the client return to the room.
18 Assess the client's tolerance for the procedure (level of fatigue, musculoskeletal strength, and sensorium).
19 Leave the bathroom clean. Discard soiled linen. Clean the tub or shower according to agency policy.
20 Document the client's response to the activity.

HOME HEALTH CARE CONSIDERATIONS

The home health care client who can get into the tub or shower will have some concerns about mobility and will need modifications for safety. Be sure the bathroom is equipped with grab bars and that a steady stool or shower chair is available. The bathtub or shower floor should have a nonskid surface. The bath mat should be nonskid, and the floor should not be slippery when wet. For showers in a chair, it may be helpful to install a long, hose-type shower head.

TIME TO ALLOW: NOVICE: 20 min. EXPERT: 10 min.

PROCEDURE 31-4 MAKING AN OCCUPIED BED

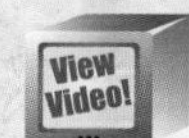

If the client cannot be out of bed, the linens are changed at the end of the bed bath.

> Safety Issues: Clients with neurological or orthopedic injuries may have special positioning restrictions that require your direct supervision of the assistive personnel and assistance while making the bed. To prevent falls, the side rails should be up anytime you leave the bedside.

DELEGATION GUIDELINES

Once you have assessed your client's ability to be turned and positioned in a side-lying fashion, you may delegate the performance of an occupied bed change to the assistive personnel. In the basic training program, the assistive personnel should receive specific instruction in the performance of this task, including safety, client comfort, and infection control.

EQUIPMENT NEEDED

- Bath blanket
- Mattress pad (change if soiled)
- Bottom sheet
- Drawsheet or lift pad (a full-size sheet can be folded for use as a drawsheet)
- Waterproof pads
- Top sheet
- Blanket
- Pillowcases
- Bedspread (change if soiled)

1 Follow preliminary actions (see inside front cover).
2 Organize the environment, and position the client to expose half the bed.
a. Perform hand hygiene.
b. Close the door or curtain for privacy.
c. Be sure that the side rail on the opposite side is up and locked. *This ensures safety as the client rolls to the side of the bed. Upright side rails also allow the client something to grasp to help in turning.*
d. Position the bed at a comfortable working height.
e. Lower the head and knee position to flat if the client can tolerate it. If the client cannot breathe when lying flat, adjust the bed to as near flat as possible. *The flatter the surface of the bed, the more efficiently the sheets can be tucked under the mattress.*
f. Lower the rail on the near side of the bed. Move the client toward the far side of the bed. *Having the bed at waist height and the client at the side of the bed allows the use of correct body mechanics by lowering the center of gravity and avoiding stretching of the lower back muscles.*
g. Loosen the top linens.
h. Place the opened bath blanket on top of the spread. Have client hold the bath blanket. Remove spread, top sheet, and blanket in one movement. If top linens are to be reused, fold and place them in a chair. *Linens should always be folded and not fluffed in the air to prevent the spread of microorganisms.*

Continued

i. Place any linen that is not to be reused in a laundry hamper or linen bag. Avoid contact with your uniform. Hold at arm's length while removing from bed to linen hamper. *The spread of microorganisms from soiled linen to uniform to other clients is prevented by avoiding contact with linen. Any time you leave the bedside be sure the side rail is up.*

j. Loosen bottom sheet on near side of bed. Have the client roll to the opposite side of the bed. Adjust the pillow under the head.

3 Make half of the bed from top to bottom.

a. Fanfold the dirty bottom sheet and drawsheet, and tuck them under the client's back and buttocks as tightly as possible (see illustration). *This allows space for you to place clean linens, and it moves dirty linen close to the other side of the bed for easy removal.*

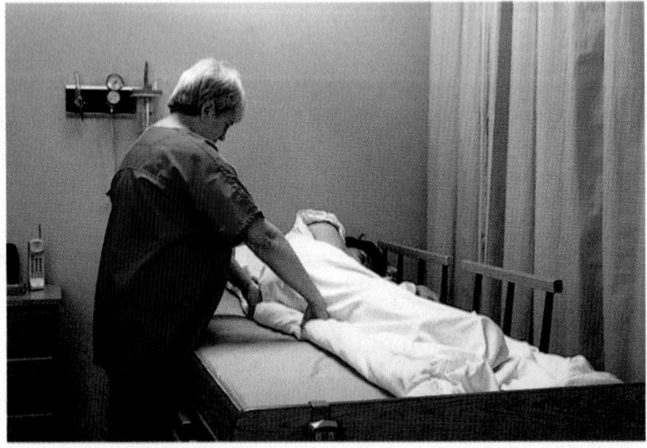

Step 3a. Fanfolding the dirty bottom sheet and drawsheet and tucking them under the client's back and buttocks.

b. Place the clean bottom sheet on the bed. Start with the bottom edge even with foot end of bed and with the center fold in the middle of the bed. Unfold lengthwise to the top of the mattress and allow the extra length to hang over the top. Tuck the top end of the sheet under the mattress. Miter corner by laying a triangular fold of sheet on the bed. Tuck the triangular fold under the mattress. Tuck the sheet well under the mattress, working from top to bottom (see illustrations). If contour sheets are to be used, fit the elastic edges under the top and bottom corners of the mattress.

c. Fanfold the clean sheet to the middle of the bed (see illustration) with the top edge toward the opposite side of the bed. Make the roll of linens as flat as possible. The client will need to roll over the linens gathered in the middle of the bed.

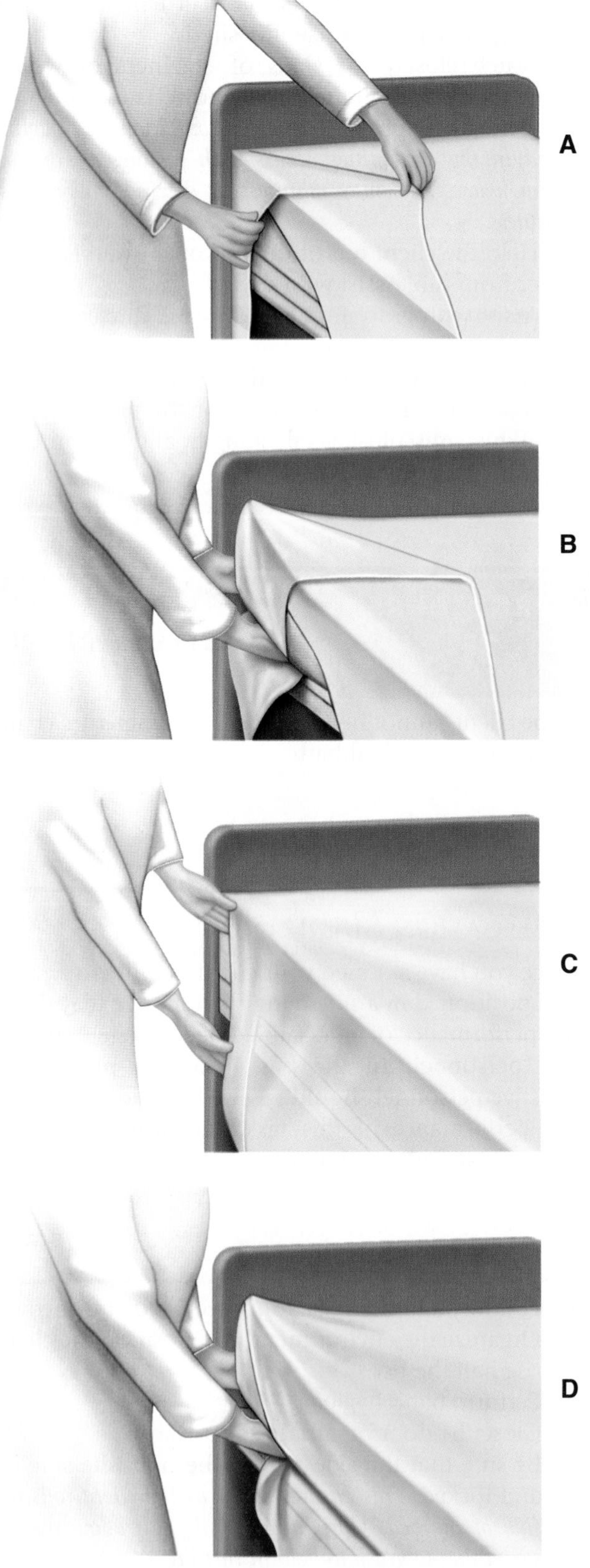

Step 3b. **A,** Beginning a mitered corner by laying a triangular fold of sheet on the bed. **B,** Tucking the end of the sheet under the mattress. **C,** Pulling the triangular fold over the side of the mattress. **D,** Tucking the triangular fold under the mattress.

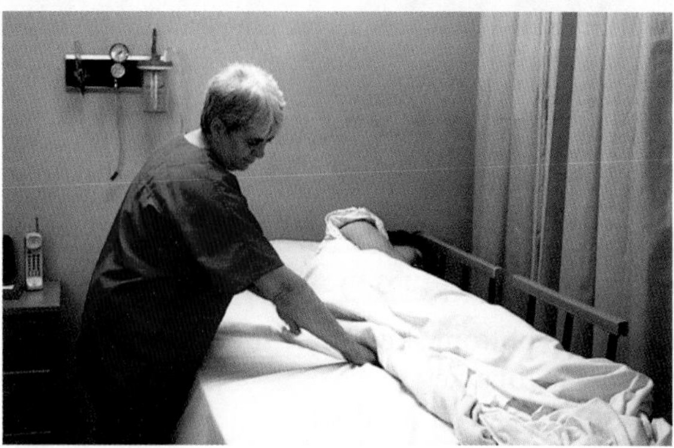

Step 3c. Fanfolding the clean sheet to the middle of the bed.

4 Place a drawsheet on top of the bottom sheet. The folded edge is placed at the top of the client's shoulders. *The drawsheet should cover the bed from the client's shoulders to below the hips.*

a. Place the center fold along the center of the bed.
b. Fanfold the top layer toward the client.
c. Tuck the excess under the mattress along with the bottom sheet.
d. Smooth out the wrinkles.
e. If an incontinence or lift pad is used, fanfold and place it on top of the linens near the client's back.

5 Make the second half of the bed.

a. Raise the side rail, and move to opposite side of the bed. Lower the side rail on that side. Help the client turn onto the clean sheets.
b. Remove the dirty linens, folding toward the center or one end of the bed. Holding the linens away from your body, place them in the dirty linen bag or hamper.
c. Pull the clean linens over the exposed half of the bed.
d. Tuck in the bottom sheet. *As you work from top to bottom, pull the linens tight and tuck one section at a time.*
e. Tuck the drawsheet, moving from the middle to the top to the bottom. Adjust the lift pad.

6 Put on the top sheet and spread.

a. Help the client move back to the center of the bed.
b. Place the top sheet over the client with the seam side up. The center crease should be at the center of the bed. Unfold the sheet from head to toe.
c. Have the client grasp the top sheet while you pull the soiled sheet or bath blanket from under the clean sheet.
d. Place the blanket, and spread evenly over the top sheet. Be sure that they are even on both sides.
e. Make mitered corners at the foot of the bed with the top sheet, blanket, and spread together.
f. Pull the top sheet, blanket, and spread into a pleat over the client's toes. *Pleating removes pressure of bed covers on client's toes.*
g. Cuff the spread, blanket, and top sheet at the head of the bed. Be sure that there is adequate sheet at the head of the bed to cover the client's shoulders.

7 Change the pillowcase.

a. Grasp the closed end of a clean pillowcase at the center point and invert the case (wrong side out) over your hand.
b. Grasp the pillow and the inverted pillowcase in the same hand. Use the other hand to pull the case over the pillow (as you turn the case right side out over the pillow).

8 Return the bed to its low position. Place the call light within the client's reach.

9 Position the client for comfort.

10 Perform hand hygiene, and document your care.

HOME HEALTH CARE CONSIDERATIONS

Help the family make modifications for ease in bed making. Both sides of the bed should be accessible. The client may be using a double bed. To move the client from one side to the other, the family caregiver can get on the bed on the knees. A turn sheet can be used to slide the client across the bed without risking damage to the skin. Teach the family about the importance of a wrinkle-free bed. If soiling is a problem, instruct the family about options for protecting the mattress. A heavy-duty lawn and leaf bag can be used to cover the mattress. Any plastic that is used should be covered with a mattress pad to absorb excess perspiration.

An unoccupied bed can be open or closed. A closed bed has the top covers pulled to the top of the bed, protecting the sheets beneath. An open bed is one that is made when the client is out of the bed. If the client is able to be out of bed because he or she is well enough to sit in a chair or having a procedure or surgery, the bed should be made at this time. An open bed is made with the top covers fanfolded to the foot of the bed, so the client can easily get in bed.

A variation of the open bed is a surgical bed with the sheets being fanfolded to the far side of the bed rather than the foot of the bed. This is done when clients are returning from the operating room on a stretcher. You put the bed in high position, and clear the room of any clutter so that there is no obstruction. Knowing what to anticipate as a result of the surgical procedure is important. If you anticipate that the client will need assistance with turning and moving, place a drawsheet on the bed for use as a lift sheet. Add extra precautions such as incontinent pads if you anticipate vomiting, drainage, bleeding, or incontinence. Procedure 31-5 describes the steps in preparing an unoccupied bed and a surgical bed.

Preparation for bed making is important for the sake of efficiency. Stack clean linen on a chair in the order of

Text continued on p. 812

TIME TO ALLOW: NOVICE: 10 min. EXPERT: 5 min.

PROCEDURE 31-5 MAKING AN UNOCCUPIED BED AND A SURGICAL BED

Bed linens are changed when the client is out of bed. A surgical bed is made when a client is returning from a surgical procedure.

DELEGATION GUIDELINES

You may delegate the full performance of this task to assistive personnel.

EQUIPMENT NEEDED

- Top sheet, bottom sheet, drawsheet (optional)
- Bedspread, blanket
- Waterproof pad (if needed)

MAKING AN UNOCCUPIED BED

1 Follow preliminary actions (see inside front cover).

2 Organize the environment.

a. Raise the bed to a comfortable working height.

b. Lower the side rails.

3 Remove soiled linens. Fold soiled surface inward, and place in the hamper.

a. Remove the bedspread and blanket. Fold and put them in a chair if they will be reused. If they are soiled, place them in the laundry hamper or linen bag. Remove the pillow from its pillowcase.

b. When handling soiled linens, always hold them away from your body. *This prevents the spread of microorganisms from person to person.*

4 Make one side of the bed, and then move to the other side. *This conserves time, energy, and movement and contributes to the smoothness of the sheets.*

a. If the bottom sheet is a contour sheet, place the elastic bands under the top and bottom corners of the mattress. Tuck along the sides. If the bottom sheet is not a contour sheet, unfold it lengthwise and place the vertical crease at the center of the bed (see illustration). Unfold it toward the opposite side of the mattress. Make the bottom edge even with the bottom edge of the mattress. Smooth any wrinkles out of bottom sheet. Make a mitered corner at the head of the bed as explained in Procedure 31-4.

b. Tuck the side in along the mattress.

c. If the client needs a drawsheet, center the drawsheet on the bed and unfold toward the opposite side (see illustration). Tuck under the mattress. If a pull (turn) sheet is needed, fold the drawsheet in halves (a full sheet is folded into four layers), creating a strong sheet to turn and move the client in bed. If an absorbent pad is needed, position at the center of the bed on top of the drawsheet.

d. Move to the other side of the bed. Remove the soiled linen. Fold the soiled side in. Hold the bundle of linen away from your body and place in a linen bag or hamper.

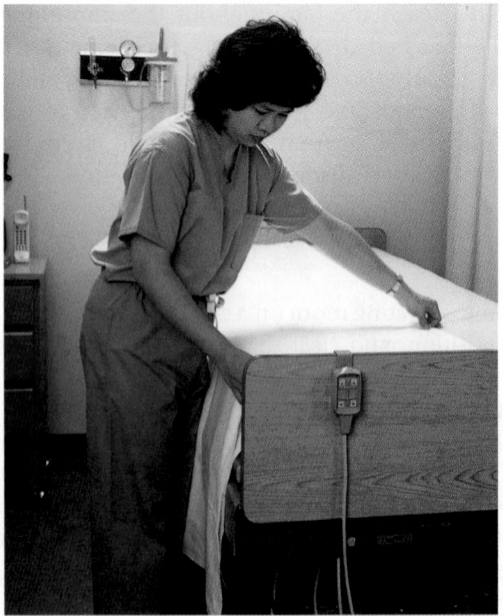

Step 4a. Centering the bottom sheet.

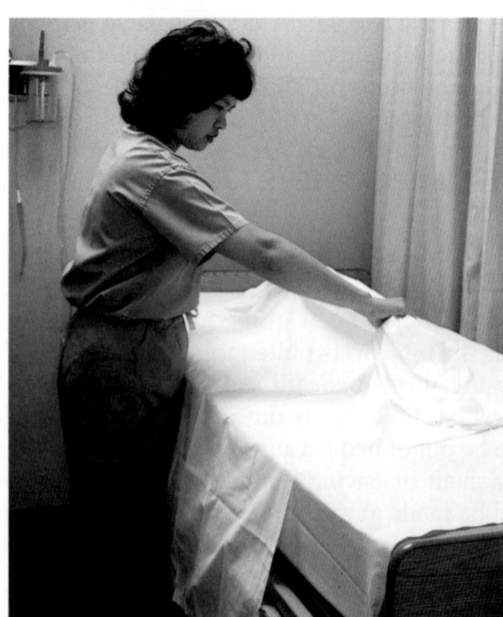

Step 4c. Centering the drawsheet and unfolding toward the opposite side.

e. Pull the linen to your side. Tuck the top of the sheet at the head of the bed. Make a mitered corner at the head of the bed. If a drawsheet is used, pull and tuck it along with the bottom sheet.

5 Place the top sheet, blanket, and spread over the bed.

a. Leave a cuff at the top of the spread.
b. Miter the corners all together at the foot of the bed.

6 Prepare the bed for the client to return.

a. Make a toe pleat (see illustrations).

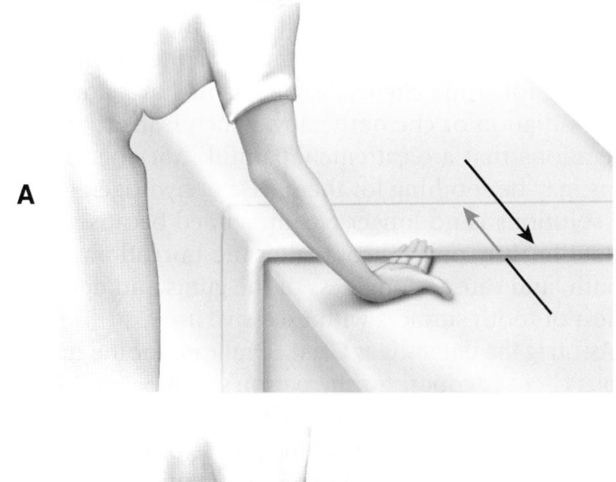

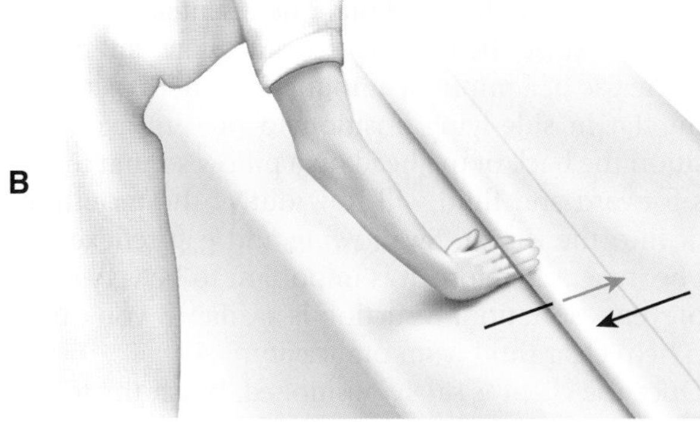

Step 6a. Making a toe pleat. **A,** Vertical toe pleat. **B,** Horizontal toe pleat.

b. Fanfold the linen to the foot of the bed to create an *open bed*.
c. Change the pillowcase.
d. Return the bed to its low position.
e. Position the call light.
f. Dispose of soiled linens.

7 Perform hand hygiene, and document your care.

MAKING A SURGICAL BED

1 Make the bed as in the preceding steps 1 through 5.

2 Fold the bottom and top corners on the near side to the opposite side, making a triangle (see illustration).

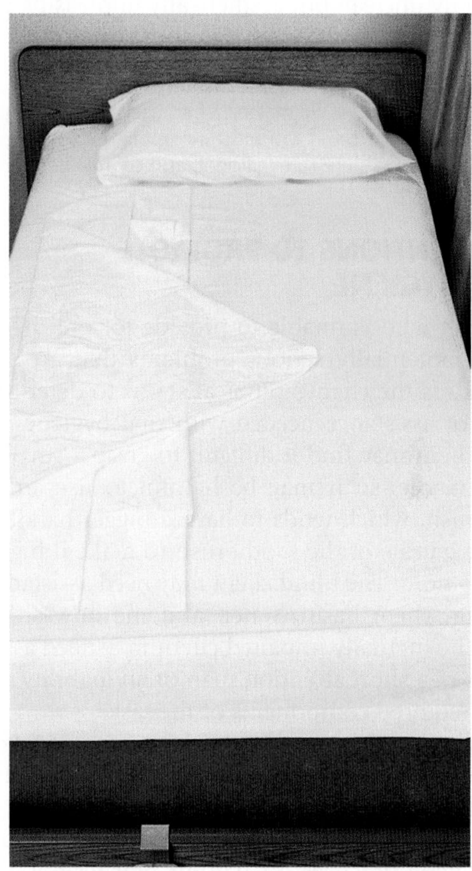

Step 2. Triangle of sheet on surgical bed.

3 Pick up the center point of the triangle, and fanfold the linen to the side of the bed.

4 Leave the bed in high position.

5 Change the pillowcase, and leave the pillow at the foot of the bed or on a chair to be accessible for placement under the client's head after the client is transferred to the bed.

6 Move all objects away from bedside area to leave room for the stretcher.

use so that each item is accessible as needed. Place soiled linens in a hamper as soon as they are removed; *never* place them on the floor. Hold soiled linens away from the uniform at arm's length until they can be placed in the hamper. Do not shake either clean linen or soiled linen because this readily disperses organisms into the air. Do not place soiled linens on the over-bed table. This is not only unclean but aesthetically unpleasing because this is the table from which the client eats.

Action Alert! While making a bed use good body mechanics to protect your back. You must incorporate a variety of skills to make the procedure safe, efficient, and coordinated.

INTERVENTIONS TO PROMOTE ORAL HYGIENE

The client who is unable to provide for oral hygiene is host to potentially serious problems that are preventable. Assess the client's physical status to determine the degree of assistance needed with oral hygiene. The arthritic client may find it difficult to grasp a small toothbrush handle, so it may be helpful to use an electric toothbrush, which tends to have a bigger handle, or to pad the handle of the toothbrush to make it bigger and easier to hold. The blind client may need assistance with knowing where basin, water, and mouthwash are located. The mentally impaired client may need assistance because of a short attention span or an inability to focus on the required components of the task.

The performance of oral hygiene presents an excellent opportunity for teaching (Box 31-6). Inadequate oral hygiene may occur because of lack of knowledge of oral hygiene practices, poor nutritional habits, inadequate oral hygiene practices, or painful oral lesions that are responsible for the neglect. Information about drug interactions, nutrition, and the need for periodic dental assessment can be incorporated into the demonstration of correct oral hygiene measures.

Assisting the Conscious Client. If the client is unable to go to the sink for oral care, it is still possible to provide oral hygiene (Procedure 31-6). Clients with dry mouths or lips may need frequent mouth care, sometimes as often as every 2 hours, to preserve the integrity of the oral mucosa. Dry lips and mucosa tend to crack and fissure, leading to infection and other problems. Rinsing the mouth with water, saline solution, or mouthwash can be helpful for these clients. Mouthwashes come in several varieties. Use bactericidal mouthwashes with caution because they tend to destroy the normal bacterial flora of the mouth, resulting in overgrowth of fungus. Avoid commercial mouthwashes that contain alcohol since they can increase mouth dryness. Saline solution is soothing for some clients. Some clients have stomatitis from radiation or chemotherapy, which leads to mouth ulcerations that are extremely painful. Anesthetic solutions may be soothing for them. Use of hydrogen peroxide solutions is no longer recommended because it can irritate healthy oral mucosa, alter the microflora of the mouth, and cause sponginess of the gums and decalcification of tooth surfaces with excessive use.

Assisting the Unconscious Client. Oral care for the unconscious client is critical for the person's well-being. Clients who have altered sensorium levels often breathe through the mouth, which accentuates the problems related to the mouth and makes frequent oral care essential.

The comatose client can receive adequate oral hygiene with the use of a minimal amount of liquid. Position the client flat in side-lying position to prevent aspiration. Position the back of the head on a pillow so that the face tips forward and fluid will flow out of the mouth, not back into the throat. Swallowing and gag reflexes may not be intact; therefore, it is important to be very careful to prevent aspiration. If suction is available, you can use it to help clear fluid from oral cavity.

Once the client is safely positioned, brush the teeth in the usual manner to clean them. It will be necessary to find a means to keep the mouth open. An easy way is to tape

BOX 31-6 *Teaching for Wellness*

Oral Hygiene

Purpose: To teach the client the importance of good oral hygiene and the need for preventive dentistry to maintain healthy teeth.

Expected Outcomes: Client will perform oral hygiene after each meal, floss daily, and visit the dentist every 6 months for supervision.

Client Instructions

- Brush your teeth thoroughly at least twice a day.
- Floss your teeth once or twice a day.
- Rinse with a commercial dental rinse aimed at prevention of tooth decay and gingivitis.
- Remember that good dental health contributes to your overall well-being.
- Keep in mind that recent studies seem to suggest a relationship between gum disease and heart disease.
- Visit your dentist regularly for preventive care and cleaning. Doing so not only will prevent painful dental problems but also is more cost-effective in the long run.
- Certain foods are best for oral health, such as raw fruits and vegetables. Others are not good for oral health, such as sugary drinks and candy, which you should try to avoid.

tongue blades together and cover them with gauze taped in place. Never place your fingers in the mouth of a person with an altered level of consciousness. Human bites are very painful and potentially dangerous. After brushing the teeth and cleaning the tongue, apply a water-soluble lubricant, lip balm, or petroleum jelly to the lips.

Action Alert! Have the oral suction within reach when you give oral care to an unconscious client in case you need to suction the client to prevent the client from aspirating.

Assisting With Denture Care. Care of dentures becomes your responsibility when the client is unable to care for them. Dentures are expensive, and it is important that you treat them carefully and with respect.

Clients should be encouraged to wear their dentures at all times. This helps with speech, eating, and appearance. Dentures should be cleaned after each meal. Have client brush gums and tongue and rinse mouth. If rinsing and spitting is not possible, clean the mouth with

PROCEDURE 31-6 PROVIDING ORAL HYGIENE

TIME TO ALLOW: NOVICE: 10 min. EXPERT: 5 min.

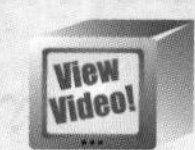

Oral hygiene is provided to maintain the integrity of the client's teeth, gums, mucous membranes, and lips. Oral hygiene ideally means brushing the client's teeth or cleaning the dentures according to the client's usual routine. Moistened toothettes can be used for comfort and moisture in between brushing.

Safety Issues: A client having undergone an oropharyngeal procedure or known to have a bleeding disorder should have a careful assessment before considering delegation of this task to assistive personnel. Have client sit in a high- or semi-Fowler's or side-lying position to prevent choking or aspiration.

DELEGATION GUIDELINES

Generally, you may delegate the performance of providing oral hygiene to assistive personnel. Knowledge of the client's oral anatomy and any necessary precautions related to the performance of this task are your responsibility.

EQUIPMENT NEEDED

- Soft-bristle toothbrush long enough to reach the back teeth
- Toothpaste or dentifrice of client's choice
- Cup of water
- Emesis basin or sink
- Dental floss, regular or fine, waxed or unwaxed
- Tissues
- Face towel
- Antiseptic mouthwash, if desired, or normal saline
- For an unconscious client, petroleum jelly, sponge swab (if desired, instead of a toothbrush), bulb syringe or suction catheter, padded tongue blade
- Disposable gloves

FOR A CONSCIOUS CLIENT

1 Follow preliminary actions (see inside front cover).

2 Prepare for the procedure.

a. Assess the client's ability to participate in procedure.

b. Don clean gloves.

c. Position the client either in high- or semi-Fowler's position or in a lateral side-lying position. *These positions decrease the possibility of aspiration and choking.*

3 Place a towel under the client's chin and over the upper chest. This prevents soiling of the bed linens or the client's gown or pajamas.

4 Moisten the toothbrush with a small amount of water and apply toothpaste.

5 Either give the toothbrush to the client for brushing or brush the client's teeth if necessary.

a. Ask the client to open the mouth wide, and hold an emesis basin under the chin.

b. Position the toothbrush at a 45-degree angle to the gum line (see illustration).

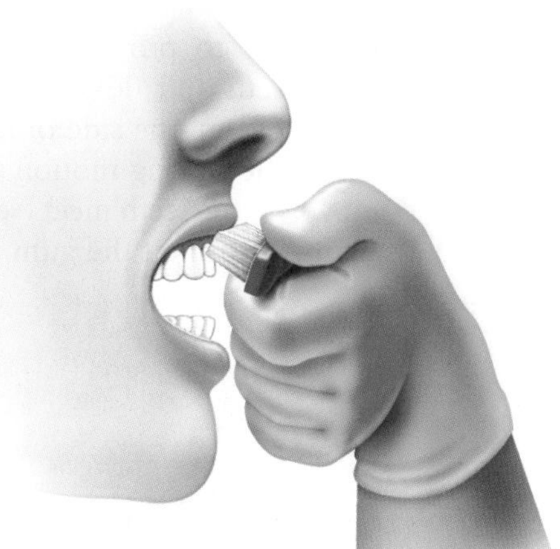

Step 5b. Positioning the toothbrush at a 45-degree angle to the gum line.

Continued

c. Directing the bristles of the toothbrush toward the gum line, brush from the gum line to the crown of each tooth, making sure to clean all surfaces (see illustration). *Brushing action removes food particles from the gum line and stimulates the gums.*

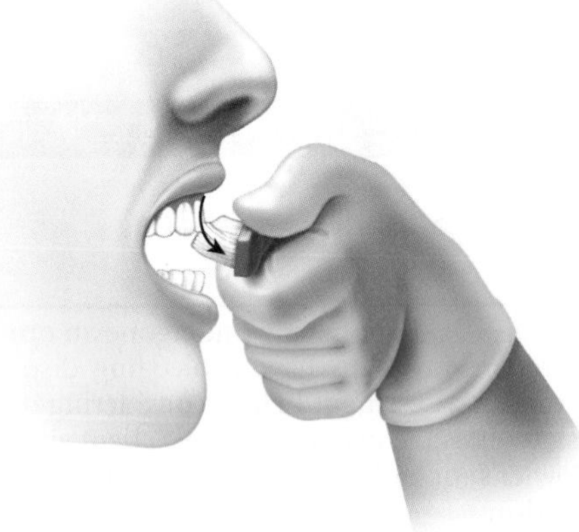

Step 5c. Brushing from the gum line to the crown of the tooth.

d. Using back-and-forth strokes, clean the biting surfaces of the teeth.
e. Gently brush the client's tongue. Do not stimulate the gag reflex by reaching the back surface of tongue. *Bacteria, oral secretions, and food particles accumulate on the tongue and must be removed.*
f. Have the client rinse the mouth with water and expectorate into the emesis basin.

6 Have the client rinse with mouthwash if desired.

7 Floss the client's teeth. *Flossing removes plaque and food particles that collect between teeth and below the gum line and that brushing cannot reach.*

a. Cut a 10-inch piece of floss. Wind the ends of the floss around the middle finger of each of your hands.
b. Holding the floss tightly to provide tension, start with the back lower teeth and floss up and down around the lower teeth from one side of the mouth to the other. Use a gentle sawing motion to get the floss past the point where the teeth meet (see illustration). **Avoid a sawing motion at the gum line.**

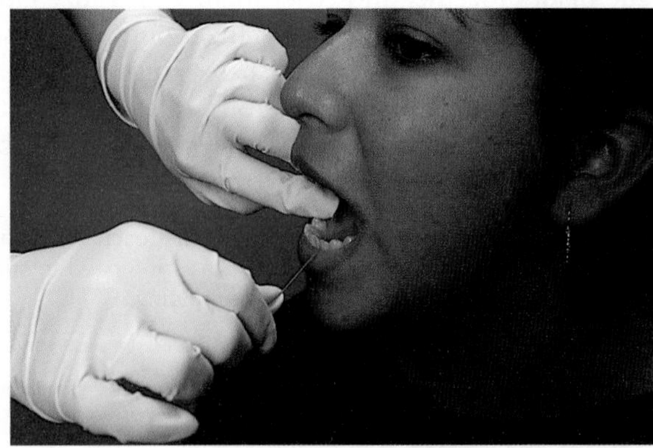

Step 7b. Flossing, using a "sawing" motion to get the floss between the teeth.

c. Cut a fresh piece of floss, and repeat the process on the upper teeth, moving from one side of the mouth to the other.
d. Ask the client to rinse the mouth and expectorate into the emesis basin.
e. Dry the mouth, and help the client to a comfortable position.

8 Remove all equipment, and make the client comfortable.

FOR AN UNCONSCIOUS CLIENT

1 Follow preliminary actions (see inside front cover).

a. Don clean gloves.
b. Place the client in a side-lying position. *The lateral position allows for gravity drainage of fluid and decreases the chance of aspiration. A full lateral position may be preferred for the completely unconscious client.*
c. Place the bulb syringe or suctioning equipment nearby in case the client needs to be suctioned.
d. Place a towel or waterproof pad under the client's chin. Place an emesis basin under the chin as well.

2 Clean the client's teeth and mouth.

a. Use a padded tongue blade to open the client's mouth (see illustration). Never attempt to open an unconscious client's mouth with the fingers. *Oral stimulation often causes the biting-down reflex, and serious injuries can occur.*

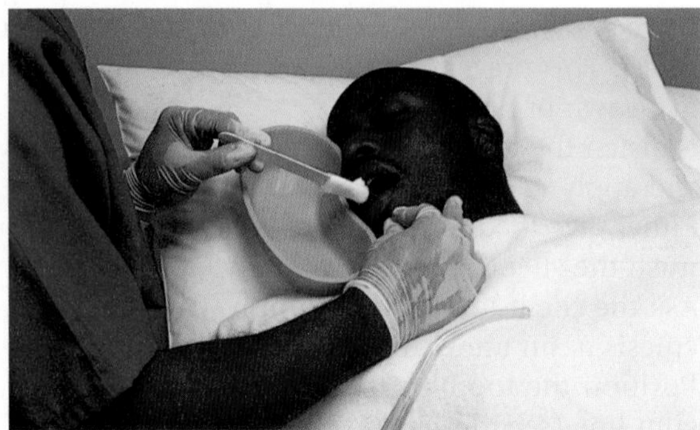

Step 2a. Using a padded tongue blade to open the client's mouth.

b. Swab the inside of the mouth, the tongue, and the teeth with a moist, gauze-covered padded tongue blade or a moistened sponge-tipped swab.
c. Brush the teeth as directed for a conscious client. A toothbrush or sponge swab may be used (see illustration).

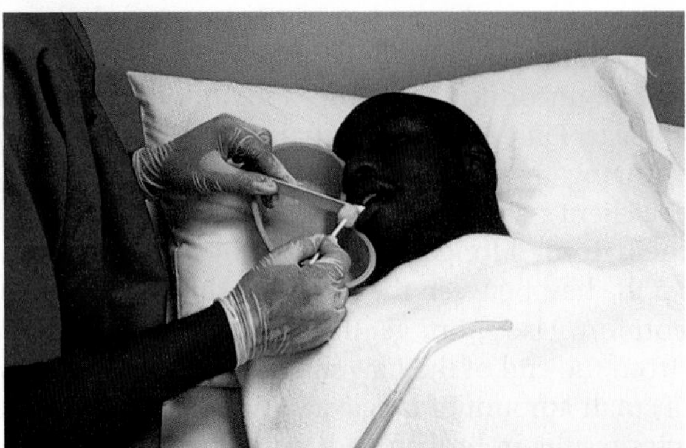

Step 2c. Brushing the client's teeth with a sponge-tipped swab.

d. Rinse the client's mouth using a very small amount of water that can be suctioned readily from the mouth.
e. Lubricate the client's lips with petroleum jelly unless client is on oxygen, then use water-based lubricant. *Petroleum jelly may be applied as often as necessary to prevent drying and cracking of the lips.*

3 Remove the equipment, and document your care.

4 Leave the client dry and comfortable.

FOR DENTURES

1 Prepare for the procedure as in step 1 for a conscious client. Don clean gloves.

a. Ask the client to remove the dentures. If this is not possible, place a gauze square on the front of the upper denture. Grasping the front teeth between your thumb and forefinger, pull down gently until the suction that holds the upper dentures in place is loosened. Loosen lower dentures by lifting up and out. *Use of the gauze square prevents your fingers from slipping. Dentures are slippery and expensive to replace. Hold the dentures firmly until they are secured in a basin or denture cup.*

2 Clean the dentures according to client's usual routine or the instructions on your cleaning product. *It is usually acceptable to clean with any nonabrasive toothpaste.*

a. Soak in a denture cleanser. If unavailable, use warm (not hot) water and a gauze square or toothbrush to clean. *Place washcloth in the sink to pad the basin while you are cleaning the dentures, and work close to the bottom of the sink in case you drop them.*
b. Brush the dentures with a soft-bristle brush (see illustration).

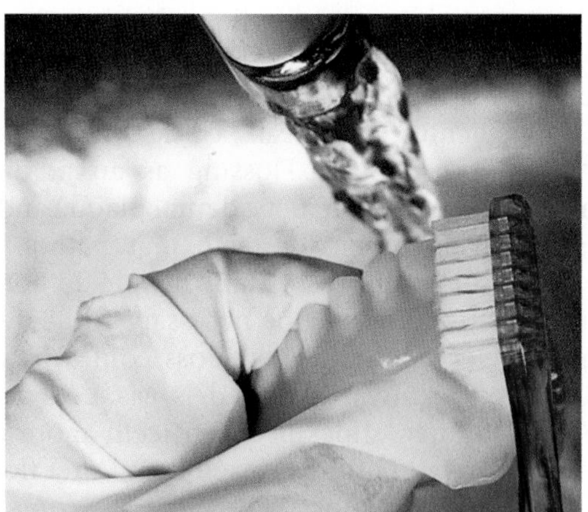

Step 2b. Brushing the dentures with a soft-bristle brush.

c. Rinse under warm water.

3 Brush gums and tongue and rinse mouth before placing dentures.

4 Help the client replace the dentures. *If you need to put the dentures in, start with the molars and use one edge at a 45-degree angle to open the mouth, then turn to a 90-degree angle and stretch the lips to insert the other side.*

5 Use denture adhesive according to the package directions if the client desires.

6 Clean your work area, and make the client comfortable. Document your care.

PEDIATRIC CONSIDERATIONS

Infant dental hygiene should begin when the first tooth erupts. Complete oral hygiene by using a wet washcloth or small gauze square moistened with water. Tooth brushing begins at about 18 months of age using water. Toothpaste is generally introduced later, and dentists recommend using one that contains fluoride.

GERIATRIC CONSIDERATIONS

Promoting good oral hygiene can help relieve the dryness of oral mucosa that accompanies the aging process and can positively affect the older adult's ability to eat. You can assess the integrity of oral mucosa, presence of lesions or sores.

HOME HEALTH CARE CONSIDERATIONS

Teach the family the importance of daily oral hygiene. Help them develop methods to prevent choking and aspiration.

gauze. While the dentures are out of the mouth, assess the oral cavity. Improperly fitting dentures can cause irritation and sometimes make the client vulnerable to cancer of the mouth. Rinse dentures before replacing the dentures. If dentures will not be returned to the client's mouth or are to be stored for the night, they should be placed in a denture cup covered with water so that plastic materials do not dry out, causing the dentures to warp. Assess dentures for breaks, cracks, or food debris.

Assisting With Flossing. Flossing as an adjunct to brushing is essential to remove dental plaque and food debris trapped between the teeth that cannot be removed with the toothbrush. Many people do not floss; therefore, instruction may be necessary while demonstrating the technique. Dental floss comes in waxed and unwaxed textures. Unwaxed is easier to use because it is thinner, slides between teeth more easily, and is more absorbent than waxed floss. After flossing, rinse vigorously to remove debris that has come loose in the mouth.

INTERVENTIONS FOR GROOMING AND DRESSING

Caring for Normal Hair. Grooming includes caring for the client's hair. The appearance of the hair is important because it influences self-image and makes clients feel better. The scalp perspires, oil is secreted, and dirt collects along the hair shaft. Hair care involves daily brushing and combing to remove dead cells and dirt and periodic shampooing to clean the hair shafts and the scalp. Hair care should be a part of daily care, and shampooing should be done at least once a week. Clients with a bathing or hygiene self-care deficit are unable to groom or clean their hair.

When brushing the hair, assess for the presence of scalp lesions and abrasions, dandruff, and the overall quality of hair. The hair itself is an excellent measure of general health. Dull, lifeless hair may indicate problems with nutrition, as well as self-care deficit. Shiny, healthy hair is usually a valid measure of overall health.

A caregiver may comb and brush the hair if the client is unable to do so. However, if the person is able to handle a comb and brush, these activities should be encouraged because they facilitate ROM exercise of upper extremities. If the client is able to sit up in bed or in a chair, styling is facilitated. It is important to learn about caring for hair of various racial and gender groups. Ask the client or family member about grooming preferences, so that the care provided is in keeping with the client's usual routine. Some people prefer oils or other substances to be applied to their hair. Women who are confined to bed for long periods of time may prefer hair to be braided, particularly if the hair is long, so that tangling does not become a problem.

Caring for Hair With Special Needs. Very curly hair requires some additional care and handling, such as a wide-toothed comb. African American clients may prefer to use a large pick comb to prevent damage to their hair (Figure 31-3). An effective way to work with very curly hair is to divide it into small sections then comb and brush it to break up tangles. Using a wide-toothed comb or pick, gently lift hair and smooth it out evenly. Work from the tip of the hair, then from the middle to the tip, then from the scalp to the tip. Be very gentle because some people have an extremely sensitive scalp and this can be an uncomfortable procedure if done roughly and with haste. Patience and adequate time are essential. For cornrowing, make small rows of braids close to the scalp in the client's choice of design. This type of braid is left in the hair for a longer period of time. If hair is tangled, grasp the hair between the head and the tangle to reduce discomfort. Use short, gentle strokes. Work out the tangle from the end of the hair shaft toward the scalp. Work on a small amount of tangle at a time. Working on large tangles results in broken ends and damaged hair shafts. A small amount of vinegar or alcohol may be applied to the hair to make combing of the tangles easier. Style the hair to prevent further tangling.

Excessively Matted or Tangled Hair. If the hair is very matted and tangled, the first impulse is to cut the snarled parts rather than trying to remove the matted hair. This is not acceptable unless the person agrees to have the hair cut. Hair may sometimes be matted with blood in addition to the tangles. First, work with water and/or alcohol. Then, divide the hair into sections and clean one section at a time being careful to prevent injury to the scalp. Avoid brushes and combs with sharp bristles and teeth because they are potentially harmful. Combs and brushes can be cleaned by washing them with hot water and soap

Braiding the Hair. Comb or brush the hair. Before braiding, remove tangles, especially those close to the scalp. Section the hair to equal the number of desired braids. Divide each section into three equal strands.

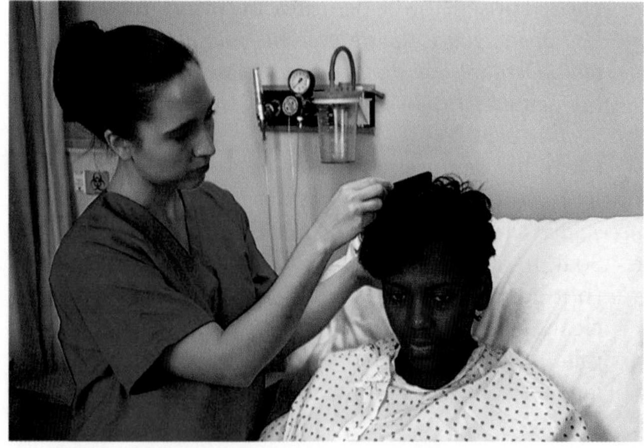

FIGURE 31-3 Combing the hair of an African American client.

Begin the braid so that the base will not be in a pressure area of the head. If the braid is directly at the base of the scalp, it may be uncomfortable for the client who is bedridden. Weave each of the three strands, alternately placing the right strand over the middle strand, then the left strand over the middle one. Work with smooth motions as you move strands from one hand to the other. Keep the strands in your hands at all times. If the tension is released, the strands become loose and you will need to begin braiding again. Continue until the ends of the strands are reached. Fasten the ends of the braid with a barrette or covered elastic to prevent the braid from coming loose. Avoid use of rubber bands because they damage the hair shaft.

Dandruff. Dandruff is usually associated with excessive flaking of the scalp. Brush dry patches loose from the scalp, and work them toward the end of the hair. Shampooing every day helps to reduce dandruff in some people; others require a medicated dandruff shampoo. Some conditioners (e.g., petroleum jelly or various oils) may help decrease itching and flaking.

Pediculosis. Pediculosis is infestation with lice. It is associated with poor hygiene, crowded living conditions, and exposure to others with lice. Pediculosis capitis refers to infestation of the head, eyebrows, eyelashes, and beard. Pediculosis corporis refers to infestation of the body. Pediculosis pubis refers to infestation of the perineal area.

Lice live on the skin, attaching their eggs (nits) to hair, and must be removed. Itching and scratching are a response to lice. Lice nits are difficult to remove because the nits are attached to the hair by an adhesive substance. When lice are discovered, remove and bag clothing and linen to prevent spreading. Lice can be eliminated from clothing and bedding by washing in very hot water. Cloth toys and stuffed animals need to be sealed in a plastic bag for 2 weeks.

Pediculosis is treated by the application of a topical pediculicide. Directions for use will vary according to the particular agent being used and the location of the infestation on the body. Treatment of all contact persons are usually recommended to prevent reinfestation.

Assure the person that lice infestation does not necessarily mean that they are unclean. Explain what must be done to treat the problem and prevent reinfestation. The person may need emotional support.

Shampooing the Client's Hair. Shampooing may be done in a variety of ways even if the client is confined to bed. Unless there are contraindications related to the medical condition, the client may be shampooed in bed, in a chair at the sink, or at the sink on a stretcher (Procedure 31-7).

TIME TO ALLOW: **NOVICE:** 20 min. **EXPERT:** 10 min.

PROCEDURE 31-7 SHAMPOOING THE CLIENT IN BED

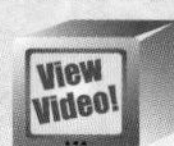

Clients' hair is shampooed in bed if they are bedridden due to prolonged illness or an emergency admission.

Safety Issues: Special precautions may be necessary for the client with a scalp laceration or glass fragments in the hair after a traumatic injury. Use electrical equipment only after the shampoo trough and water have been removed.

DELEGATION GUIDELINES

You may delegate the performance of shampooing to assistive personnel. The requisite skills should be a component of the assistive personnel's basic training program. You should supervise the application of medicated shampoo for the removal of parasites from the hair and scalp.

EQUIPMENT NEEDED

- Gloves
- Shampoo/conditioner
- Two bath towels
- Washcloth
- Bath blanket
- Comb and/or brush
- Shampoo board or inflatable basin
- Water pitcher
- Wastebasket or bucket
- Waterproof pads

1 Follow preliminary actions (see inside front cover).

2 Prepare for the procedure.

a. Place waterproof pads under client's head and shoulders. *This helps keep the bed dry.*

b. Remove pins, clips, or barrettes from client's hair. Undo braids, and brush the hair thoroughly. *Brushing the hair before wetting it reduces tangling and allows even distribution of shampoo.*

c. Place the bed in its flat position.

Continued

d. Place a shampoo board or inflated basin under the client's head. *Pad the client's bed as needed to absorb water leaks.*
e. Drape one towel over the client's shoulders. If using a board, place a folded washcloth to pad the rim where the client's neck touches the board. *The towel prevents the client from becoming damp and provides neck support for comfort.*
f. Uncover the client's upper body by folding the linens down to waist level. Place a bath blanket over the chest.
g. Place a washcloth over the client's eyes. *The eyes should be protected from irritation from shampoo accidentally getting into them.*
h. Place a receptacle such as a bucket, basin, or empty plastic trash can in a position to catch water. *The water receptacle should be at a level lower than the client's head so that water will run away from the head and face. It may need to be emptied several times.*

3 Shampoo the client's hair.

a. Don gloves if appropriate.
b. Using a water pitcher, pour water over the hair until it is thoroughly wet (see illustration). The water should be comfortably warm (110° F). *Water that is too hot may burn the client, and water that is too cold is uncomfortable and chilling.*

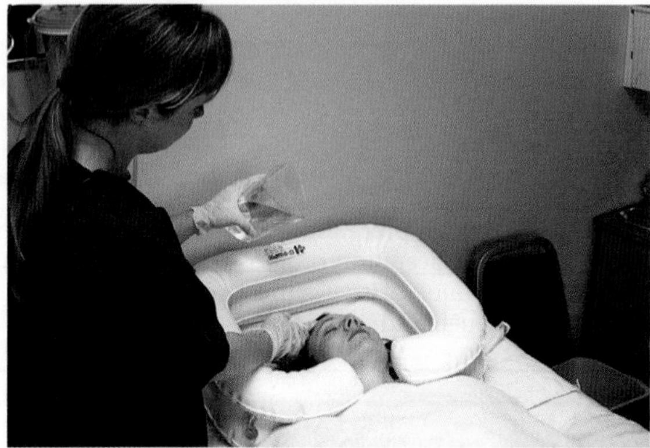

Step 3b. Pouring warm water over the client's hair.

c. Apply a small amount of shampoo (see illustration). Using your fingertips, gently work it into a lather over the entire scalp. Work from the hairline to the neckline. *Massage is beneficial to scalp circulation, and it aids in the cleansing effect of shampoo throughout the hair.*

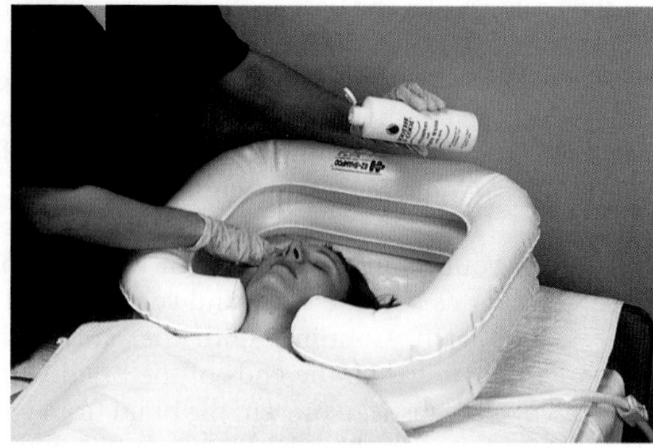

Step 3c. Applying shampoo.

4 Rinse the hair with warm water, and reapply shampoo if needed. Repeat until hair is "squeaky clean" when hair shafts are rubbed. *Thorough rinsing is important because shampoo residue is irritating to the scalp and dulls the hair luster.*

5 Apply a small amount of conditioner if desired. Conditioner serves as a detangler and makes hair easier to comb. Rinse hair according to conditioner instruction.

6 Make a turban by wrapping a towel around the client's head. Pat or towel dry until the hair is free of excess moisture. Avoid rubbing the hair with the towel because this can cause tangling.

7 Change the client's gown and linens if they are wet.

8 Comb, dry, and style the client's hair.

9 Help the client assume a comfortable position.

10 Remove all equipment, and leave the environment clean.

HINTS

If a hair dryer is used to dry hair, avoid the hot setting.

Use electrical equipment only after the shampoo trough and water have been removed.

Special care should be taken with an African American client's hair. It tangles easily, so after shampooing it should be combed while wet. Mineral oil or petroleum jelly can be applied if the hair seems dry. This will make braiding and styling easier.

HOME HEALTH CARE CONSIDERATIONS

Cleansing sprays are acceptable for short-term use. However, the long-term-care client will need to have the hair shampooed periodically. Obtaining a shampoo board may be the easiest option. However, the same can be accomplished by repositioning the client crosswise on a double bed with the head at the edge of the bed. Use plastic garbage bags to protect the bed and to fashion a drainage system to a pan sitting by the bed. Use a minimum amount of water.

It is helpful to know how to improvise if the client is to be shampooed in bed or at the sink. The one item that is necessary is a "trough." This is an item that may be available in the hospital or at home. If no plastic trough is available, you can easily make one from plastic and newspaper or from a rubber sheet and newspaper. Form a trough with raised edges, place the flat portion on the bed, and make a run-off channel that will drain into a waste receptacle that is placed lower than the client's head.

You can also shampoo your client's hair by using a rinse-free shampoo cap with conditioner. This is a microwavable cap into which you tuck the client's hair and then wash the client's hair by gently massaging the client's head and scalp. The client's hair is cleaned and conditioned without the use of water or moving the client to a sink. When finished, remove and dispose of the cap, towel dry if needed, and style hair.

Shaving the Client. Shaving is an important grooming measure for men (Procedure 31-8). Most men shave daily and do not feel well groomed when facial stubble is present. If the client is unable to shave himself, determine his preferences for shaving soap, colognes, and aftershave lotions. Determine also whether the client should use an electric razor instead of a manual razor, such as when taking anticoagulants or other medications that can cause bleeding as a side effect. In such cases, inquire as to whether the family or a friend can bring an electric razor from home, because health care facilities may not routinely supply these. Men who do not shave may require assistance in trimming a mustache or beard.

PROCEDURE 31-8 SHAVING THE CLIENT

Time to Allow: **Novice:** 15 min. **Expert:** 10 min.

Shaving the face is an important grooming measure for men. Most men shave daily and do not feel well groomed when facial stubble is present.

Safety Issues: Clients who are taking anticoagulants should use electric razors because of the prolonged clotting time.

DELEGATION GUIDELINES

The assistive personnel may be assigned to perform or assist with shaving your client. Special precautions may be necessary if the client has undergone a craniofacial procedure. It is your responsibility to assess the safety of shaving the client in this situation. You may choose to shave this client yourself.

EQUIPMENT NEEDED

- Safety razor or electric razor
- Three towels
- Soap or shaving cream
- Aftershave lotion

1 Follow preliminary actions (see inside front cover).

2 Prepare for the procedure.

a. Place the client in a sitting position, either in bed or in a chair.

b. If using a safety razor, apply a warm, wet towel to the client's face to soften the beard before beginning to shave.

c. Apply a thick layer of soap or shaving cream to the client's face.

3 Shave with even strokes in the direction of hair growth to decrease irritation and prevent ingrown hairs (see illustration). If the skin is not taut, use your opposite hand to hold the skin motionless while you shave.

4 Use a damp washcloth to remove excess shaving cream. Inspect for areas that may have been missed. Apply aftershave lotion if desired.

5 Clean the area, make the client comfortable, and document your care.

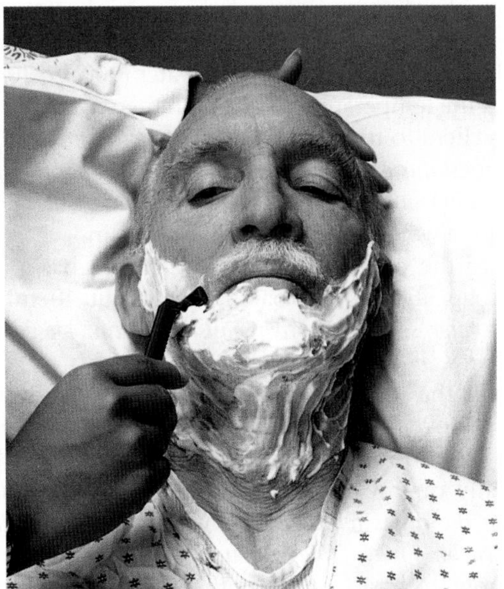

Step 3. Shaving in the direction of hair growth.

INTERVENTIONS FOR FOOT AND NAIL CARE

Nail care is part of personal hygiene and usually includes trimming nails, cleaning under nails, and thoroughly rinsing and drying skin of the hands and feet, especially between the fingers and toes (Procedure 31-9). Filing of nails may be safer than clipping or cutting. Some agencies do not permit you to clip the nails of clients. In this case, families are required to provide a podiatrist for the client or one is supplied by the agency (check agency policy). Clients with peripheral vascular disease or diabetes are particularly prone to injury, and nail care must be done with extreme caution because even a minor cut or abrasion on the foot can lead to serious complications, even gangrene, with resultant amputation.

Problems with nail and foot care may occur because of neglect or abuse. Improper trimming of nails and cuticles, frequent exposure to chemicals, trauma, ill-fitting shoes, and inadequate hygiene can cause problems. Be sure to trim fingernails to a length that is even with the

TIME TO ALLOW: NOVICE: 15 min. EXPERT: 10 min.

PROCEDURE 31-9 PERFORMING FOOT AND NAIL CARE

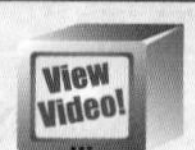

Foot and nail care are given to clients to prevent infection and soft tissue trauma from ingrown or jagged nails and to eliminate odors. Check agency policy before trimming nails.

Safety Issues: Older adult and diabetic clients are the most likely to need special attention to their feet. Trimming straight across prevents nail splitting and tissue injury around nail.

DELEGATION GUIDELINES

Once you have assessed your client's feet, you may choose to delegate routine foot care. Special consideration may be appropriate for your clients with diabetes or vascular insufficiency. You may deem it more appropriate to perform the nail maintenance part of foot care yourself in such cases because of the risk of injury if improperly performed by assistive personnel. For anything other than routine care, refer to a podiatrist.

EQUIPMENT NEEDED

- Nail clippers, file
- Orange stick and/or cotton-tipped applicator
- Waterproof pad
- Washcloth
- Towels
- Washbasin
- Soap
- Lotion

1 Follow preliminary actions (see inside front cover).

2 Prepare for the procedure.

a. Don gloves if necessary.
b. Help the client to sit in a chair if possible. If the client cannot sit in a chair, elevate the head of the bed.
c. Fill a basin half full of warm water (100° to 104° F).
d. Test the temperature with a bath thermometer, or ask the client to test the water. *Clients with impaired circulatory status can be burned if water is too hot. Peripheral sensations may be diminished so that pain is not felt.*
e. Place a waterproof pad under the basin.

3 Place the client's foot or hand in the basin. Wash with soap, and allow soaking for about 10 minutes. *Warm water serves to soften nails and skin, loosen debris under nails, and comfort the client.*

4 Rinse the foot or hand thoroughly with the washcloth, remove from the basin, and place on a towel.

5 Dry the foot or hand thoroughly but gently, being especially careful to dry between the digits. *Moist skin between the digits tends to encourage maceration of tissue. Harsh rubbing may damage tissues.*

6 Empty the basin, refill it with warm water, and repeat with the other foot or hand.

7 While the second foot or hand is soaking, provide nail care for the first hand or foot.

a. Carefully clean under the nails with a cotton-tipped applicator. Use an orange stick to remove debris. Gently push the cuticle back with the orange stick. Be careful to avoid injury to the cuticle and to the skin under the nail rim.
b. Beginning with the large toe or the thumb, clip the nails straight across. Clip small sections at a time, starting with one edge and working across. File and shape each nail with an emery board or a nail file. *Trimming nails straight across or along the slight curve of the nail prevents splitting and the development of ingrown nails. Filing removes rough edges that might produce trauma and injury.*
c. After completing the manicure or pedicure, apply lotion to the client's feet or hands.

8 Help the client to a comfortable position, remove all equipment, perform hand hygiene, and document care.

HOME HEALTH CARE CONSIDERATIONS

Ongoing nail and foot care is especially important for the home health care client. For problem feet, a clinical nurse specialist or a podiatrist may be consulted to develop a plan for care.

fingertips, and cut straight across to prevent the nails from breaking (Figure 31-4).

Some general physical problems, such as diabetes, obesity, and peripheral vascular disease, make a person more prone to nail and foot problems. Poor circulation and altered metabolic function can lead to skin breakdown and infection and alter nail growth and texture. Nails easily grow into soft tissue around them, causing pain, tissue trauma, and infection. Aging also brings about changes in the nails, and older adults often have thick, discolored nails that must be trimmed by a podiatrist. Feet are more susceptible to trauma and prone to infection than other parts of the body. The dark, often moist environment of shoes promotes the growth of bacteria and enhances the chance of infection. Dirty socks or stockings and poorly ventilated shoes also create an environment that encourages bacterial and fungal growth. Box 31-7 provides guidelines for teaching clients about the importance of foot and nail care.

INTERVENTIONS FOR EAR CARE

Unless the client has an ear infection, the ears require minimal care. The external auricles can be cleaned with a washcloth, and excess cerumen can be removed with the tip of a washcloth. Instruct clients to avoid insertion of objects such as Q-tips and bobby pins to remove cerumen because they may traumatize the ear canal or rupture the tympanic membrane. Assess the ear for signs of inflammation, drainage, or external lesions, as well as evidence of discomfort.

INTERVENTIONS FOR EYE CARE

Some clients are unable to maintain their own eye care for a variety of reasons. Those clients who have undergone surgery or who are critically ill or comatose may have lost the blink reflex, which serves to protect the eye from trauma. Assess the eyelids first. Are they encrusted with dried exudate? Are they edematous? Are they inflamed with styes or pustules? Are the lacrimal ducts functioning normally, neither too dry nor tearing excessively? Assess the sclera (the white portion of the eye). It should be white, without redness or jaundice. The conjunctivae should be pink, moist, and not reddened.

If the eyes are draining or if there is crusted exudate, the eyes must be gently cleaned. Take care to avoid transferring infection from one eye to the other.

Clean a client's eyeglasses at least once daily. Cleaning may be done with warm water and a mild soap. If the lenses are plastic, clean them with a plastic lenses cleaning solution. Carefully dry and wipe lenses with a soft nonabrasive cloth or chamois skin because they scratch easily. Label eyeglasses with client's name, and put them in a safe place.

Contact lenses come in two varieties: hard and soft lenses. Hard lenses are worn during waking hours and must be removed while sleeping. Some soft lenses may be worn for extended periods of time and may be worn while sleeping. Contact lenses should be removed from the eyes of comatose clients and stored in an appropriate contact lens solution. The lenses should be placed in separate containers, labeled "left" and "right," and kept in a safe location.

Ocular prosthetics are worn by clients full time and removed only occasionally to clean or as often as directed. Too much handling of the prosthetic can cause irritation to the client's socket and excess drainage. Always wash hands before handling the prosthesis. Remove it, and use warm water to rinse and softly scrub it, removing built-up protein and debris. Dry it with a soft tissue, polishing very lightly in a circular motion. Do not clean or soak the prosthesis in any solvents, disinfectants, or alcohol because

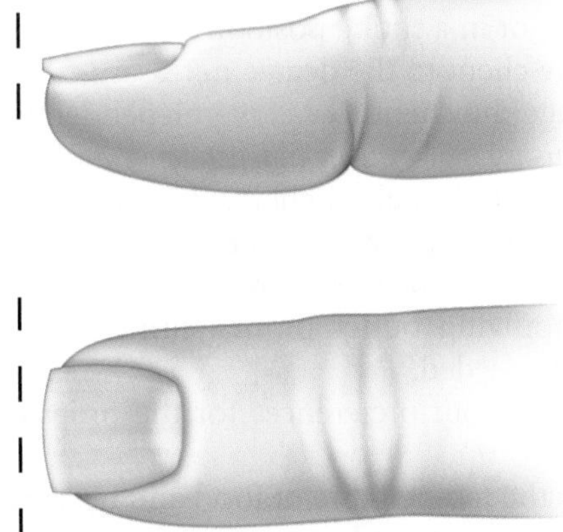

FIGURE 31-4 Fingernails should be trimmed to a length that is even with the fingertips and cut straight across to prevent the nails from breaking.

BOX 31-7 *Teaching for Wellness*

Nail and Foot Care

Purpose: To teach the client the importance of good foot care to prevent foot infection and trauma, which can lead to other serious problems.
Expected Outcomes: Client will avoid habits that are dangerous to foot health, such as trimming calluses and wearing poorly fitting shoes. Client will seek professional help from a podiatrist in trimming nails.

Client Instructions

- Inspect your feet daily, or have someone do it for you.
- Wear white cotton socks, and change them every day.
- Have a podiatrist trim your toenails.
- Wear properly fitted soft shoes.
- Avoid walking barefoot, smoking, and being in extreme cold.
- Avoid garters or stockings that constrict leg circulation.
- Wash your feet with warm, not hot, water.
- Always dry your feet thoroughly, especially between the toes.

they may cause irritation to the client's socket or damage to the prosthesis.

An unconscious client may require frequent eye care, as often as every 4 hours. Eyes must be kept clean, moist, and protected from the drying effects of the air. If the corneal reflex is lost or decreased, the eye has lost a vital protective mechanism. This reflex causes the automatic blinking and tearing that occurs when a foreign object touches the cornea or when the eye begins to dry. In the unconscious client, the eyes may remain open and become dried from the air. Dry eyes can lead to corneal ulceration and possible vision loss. You may need to provide artificial tears or moisture by instilling drops of liquid tear solution or normal saline into the eyes or the conjunctival sac. If the eyes remain completely or partially open, you may need to gently close them and cover them with a protective shield or patch.

INTERVENTIONS TO PROMOTE EATING

The client who is unable to eat independently needs assistance from others to maintain nutrition necessary for healing and to maintain life (Procedure 31-10). Remove bedside care items, and eliminate offensive odors before mealtime. When an adult requires feeding, maintain the client's dignity. Offer food in an unhurried manner, and converse pleasantly. For clients with blindness, describe the food and caution them about hot foods. Allow time for chewing and enjoying the food. Studies show that clients eat more food if you switch from one food to another during feeding.

PROCEDURE 31-10

TIME TO ALLOW: NOVICE: 15 min. **EXPERT:** 10 min.

ASSISTING AN ADULT CLIENT WITH EATING

Nursing Skills Online: Safety, Lesson 4

View Video!

Adequate intake of food is necessary to maintain healthy nutritional status.

Safety Issues: Clients who are weak or have sensorimotor problems may require partial or total assistance with eating. If clients cannot eat in a sitting position, place them in a lateral position to prevent aspirating.

DELEGATION GUIDELINES

The task of feeding or assisting a client to eat may be delegated to assistive personnel. However, as the nurse, you retain the responsibility for assessing the client's ability to eat and any risks to nutritional status and for evaluating the client's actual intake.

EQUIPMENT NEEDED

- Over-bed table and chair
- Meal tray with correct diet and utensils
- Small towel or extra napkin for protection of clothes
- Straw or any adaptive feeding equipment, such as weighted cup, rimmed plate, or special utensils

1 Follow preliminary actions (see inside front cover).

2 Prepare the client and environment.

a. Explain the procedure.

b. Assist the client with urinary or bowel elimination needs before feeding.

c. Help the client to wash hands and possibly complete oral hygiene. *Oral hygiene can improve the taste in the mouth, positively affecting appetite.*

d. Place meal tray on the over-bed table so that the client can see it. *This allows the client to view foods and participate in food choices.*

e. Check the tray for the client's name, diet, and completeness of dietary items. Check the tray against the diet order and the client's identification bracelet. Remove an incorrect tray from the room immediately.

3 Position the client appropriately.

a. Assist the client to a comfortable position, usually sitting in a supported upright position or in a chair.

b. If the client cannot use a sitting position, place the client in a lateral position. *This position enhances swallowing, and the risk of aspiration is less than in the supine position.*

c. Place yourself in a standing position if setting up the meal tray, or in a sitting position if feeding the client.

4 Assist the client to the degree necessary.

a. Encourage the client to eat as independently as possible. *This promotes client independence and self-esteem.*

b. For a visually impaired client, describe the location of foods on the plate using a clock face analogy.

c. Prepare food items by removing food covers, cutting foods, applying butter or margarine, and pouring liquids as needed.

d. Ask client about preferences for the order of eating foods.

e. Monitor the temperature of food and beverages to be sure they are not too hot or too cold.

f. When assistance is necessary, give small amounts at a time, allowing ample time for chewing and swallowing.

g. Provide liquids at client request, or after every three to four mouthfuls of food.
h. Do not hurry the mealtime; create a pleasant environment by conversing according to the client's interests and desire to talk.

5 At the completion of the meal, make the client comfortable.

a. Assist the client with cleaning the mouth and hands.
b. Assist the client to a comfortable semiupright position to prevent regurgitation, if appropriate.
c. Remove the meal tray from the bedside area.

6 Document the client's food and fluid intake, as well as any adverse symptoms experienced (such as nausea or fatigue); report to the nurse if the client does not eat a sufficient diet.

GERIATRIC CONSIDERATIONS

Offer extra seasoning on food unless contraindicated (i.e., low-sodium diet), to compensate for the age-related decline in ability to taste food. Offer sufficient fluids to prevent dry mouth due to decreased saliva production. Allow sufficient time for mealtime if the client has musculoskeletal problems that hinder joint mobility and speed of movement. Observe for dysphagia if the client has neurological or other problems that could affect swallowing. Avoid placing food in the mouth on the affected side.

HOME HEALTH CARE CONSIDERATIONS

Ensure that there are adequate facilities for food storage and preparation (working refrigerator and stove). Assess the client for factors that interfere with proper nutrition, such as oral lesions, ill-fitting dentures, or gastrointestinal disturbances. Teach family members about the importance of a nutritious diet in maintaining health, and, when needed, provide written instructions about dietary needs or restrictions. When appropriate, be sure to include guidelines for special feeding techniques and adaptive equipment if needed.

INTERVENTIONS TO PROMOTE TOILETING

A male client who is unable to toilet himself may need to be given a urinal as a receptacle for voiding. A female client who is unable to toilet herself may need to use a bedpan for voiding. Male and female clients may need to use a bedpan for bowel elimination. Examples of clients who have this need include those restricted to bed rest because of fracture, recent surgery, or other illness. A client receiving an enema or one who has diarrhea may need to use a bedpan as well. If the client is able to get out of bed and sit up, a bedside commode may be anther option.

Refer to Chapter 29 for additional information about choosing and using bedpans for specific clients. Provide perineal care each time the client uses a bedpan.

INTERVENTIONS TO PROMOTE DRESSING

Clients may need assistive devices, such as Velcro in place of button or zippers, to aid them in being able to dress or partially dress themselves. Refer to Chapter 44 for additional information on assisting clients with dressing, grooming, and eating.

EVALUATION

Evaluation of the achievement of self-care outcomes involves determining that the expected outcomes have been met. Safety is an essential outcome. Evaluate both the client and the environment for safety before you leave the room (Figure 31-5).

Typical outcomes that are measured during evaluation are that the client does the following:

- Maintains clean and intact skin
- Maintains intact oral mucosa without gingivitis or caries
- Has clean hair without scalp lesions or abrasions
- Actively participates in feeding activities according to ability
- Actively participates in toileting activities according to ability
- States confidence in caregiver's ability to provide safe care at home

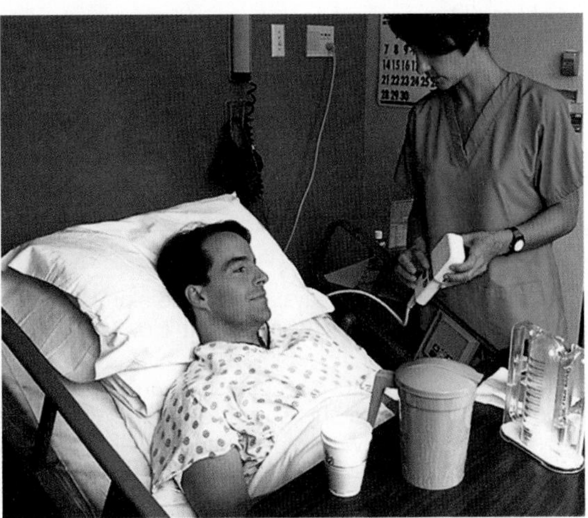

FIGURE 31-5 A minimum standard of safety is an accessible call light and the knowledge of how to use it.

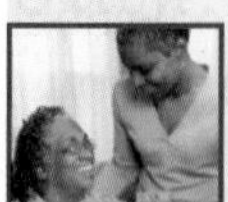

A sample care plan for the client in this chapter's case study, Mrs. Wilson, is outlined in Box 31-8. The expected outcome for Mrs. Wilson's *Bathing/hygiene self-care deficit* is that Mrs. Wilson maintains a satisfactory appearance and that hygiene needs are met. Direct observation will allow you to infer a positive outcome. Mrs. Wilson is well groomed and clean. Her skin and hair are clean and odor free. The oral mucosa is intact with no signs of gingivitis or irritation. Subjectively, she indicates a feeling of comfort and well-being and demonstrates a positive feeling about herself as indicated in verbal interaction.

If the outcomes are not achieved or the client is not making sufficient progress toward achievement of the goals within the expected time, reassessment may reveal an explanation for lack of progress.

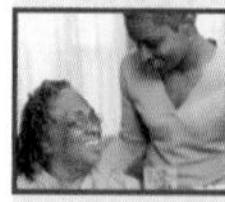

For example, if Mrs. Wilson continues to have halitosis even after adequate brushing, flossing, and rinsing, assessment for other causes of the odor is necessary.

SAMPLE DOCUMENTATION NOTE FOR MRS. WILSON

Participated in bath by using right hand to wash face and brush hair, and attempted to brush teeth without assistance. Assisted with washing of upper body. Asked for shampoo and also for a rest period after bathing was complete.

BOX 31-8 Nursing Care Plan

A Client With a Stroke

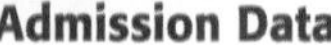

Admission Data

Mrs. Wilson was admitted to the unit from the emergency department. Her daughter and son-in-law accompanied her. She appeared slightly listless and lethargic and allowed her daughter to answer all the questions. Her daughter stated that when Mrs. Wilson awoke after an afternoon nap, she was slightly disoriented and nauseated and had marked left hemiplegia. Her physician advised immediate hospitalization, and she was brought to the hospital by ambulance.

Physician's Orders

Admit to Neurology
Cerebrovascular accident
Regular diet
Skull x-ray stat
MRI in AM
Vital signs qid
Up in chair tid with assistance
Physical therapy consult
Tylenol 650 mg PO q4h prn for headache
Milk of magnesia 30 mL daily prn constipation

Nursing Assessment

6 Days After Admission: Vital signs: BP 170/86, pulse 76, respiration 14, temperature 98.6° F. Skin moist and warm with good turgor. Appetite good but requires assistance with feeding because she is left-handed. Alert and oriented × 3. Responds appropriately to questions. Has some short-term memory deficit. Affect somewhat flat. Speaks in a monotone. Cries easily, especially when frustrated by inability to use left side. Speech clear; no slurring, hesitancy, or stammering. Bowel and bladder control intact; no incontinence. No difficulty swallowing.

NANDA-I Nursing Diagnosis	NOC Expected Outcomes With Indicators	NIC Interventions With Selected Activities	Evaluation Data
Bathing/Hygiene Self-Care Deficit	***Self-Care: Bathing***	***Self-Care Assistance***	
Related Factors: • Inability to wash body parts because of hemiplegia	• Skin is dry and clean.	• Bathe daily. Encourage her to use right hand. Prevent fatigue by allowing her to rest at intervals.	• Used right hand to wash face. Asked for rest period after bath. Assisted with washing of upper body.
	• Hair is clean and free of dandruff.	• Shampoo every week.	• Used right hand to brush hair. Asked for shampoo.
	• Oral mucosa is clean; teeth and gums clean; no halitosis.	• Assist with brushing by putting paste on brush and guiding hand.	• Attempted to brush teeth without assistance.

Critical Thinking Questions

1. On day 2, Mrs. Wilson says, "Leave me alone. I am just too tired to bathe. I just want to rest." How would you respond?
2. Mrs. Wilson's daughter says that she wants to care for her mother at home, but she is unsure whether she can manage all the care. How would you advise her in regard to the availability of community resources and their accessibility?
3. On day 4, Mrs. Wilson was incontinent of urine for the first time since hospitalization. She says that she just "waited too long" because she knew the nurses were busy and she "did not want to bother anyone." How would you respond to this comment?

Nursing outcome and intervention labels from Johnson, M., Bulechek, G., Butcher, H., Dochterman, J. M., Maas, M., Moorhead, S., et al. (Eds.). (2006). *NANDA, NOC, and NIC linkages: Nursing diagnoses, outcomes, & interventions.* St. Louis, MO: Mosby.

In the example given, you have documented that the client has resolved her difficulty with initiating and implementing oral hygiene, one aspect of the self-care regimen. As goals are met, new ones can be established so that the client can emerge from the experience not only with the resumption of previously acquired skills but with new goals.

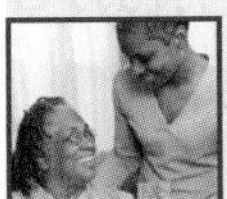

For Mrs. Wilson, new goals are to pay closer attention to oral hygiene and to pursue regular dental assessments, which had not previously been done.

▼ KEY PRINCIPLES

- Self-care and hygiene are important to disease prevention and health promotion.
- *Self-care deficit* may be related to physical or mental factors or a combination of both.
- *Self-care deficit* may include a deficit for bathing/hygiene, dressing/grooming, toileting, and feeding.
- *Self-care deficit* may be partial or total, requiring either total or assisted nursing care. Alterations in functional ability may occur suddenly or over time.
- Inability to bathe oneself, to dress and groom oneself, to feed oneself, or to toilet oneself is validation of *Self-care deficit.*
- Interventions can meet the needs of the client for skin care, hair care, and oral care.
- Interventions can focus on prevention of complications from the inability to maintain adequate self-care.
- Interventions can meet the needs of the client for positive self-image and self-concept.
- Interventions can meet the needs of the client for comfort.
- Evaluation of the achievement of self-care outcomes involves determining that the expected outcomes have been met.

■ REVIEW QUESTIONS

1. This type of gland secretes an oily substance that helps to inhibit the growth of certain bacteria on the client's skin.
1. Sudoriferous glands
2. Apocrine glands
3. Sebaceous glands
4. Ceruminous glands

2. The client's gums are bleeding. The nurse might suspect the client has:
1. Dental caries
2. Dental plaque
3. Dentures
4. Gingivitis

3. This is the first postoperative day for a client who is disoriented, has a fractured tibia, a cast on the right arm, a broken left clavicle, and is unable to get out of bed. The nurse most likely needs to give the client:
1. A complete bed bath
2. A partial bath
3. A self-help bath
4. Perineal care

4. After a client has surgery and returns to the hospital room on a stretcher, the nurse would have prepared the bed as an open bed:
1. With sheets fanfolded top to bottom
2. With sheets fanfolded to one side of the bed
3. By fanfolding the dirty bottom sheet and drawsheet and tucking them under the client's back and buttocks
4. By pulling the top covers to the head of the bed

5. The client has painful hemorrhoids. The nurse can help the client have some relief from the pain by providing the client with a therapeutic:
1. Cool-water bath
2. Warm-water bath
3. Hot-water bath
4. Sitz bath

Bibliography

Ackley, B. J., & Ladwig, G. D. (2006). *Nursing diagnosis handbook: A guide to planning care* (7th ed.). St. Louis, MO: Mosby.

Allasio, D., & Fischer, H. (2005). Experience and reason—briefly recorded. Immersion scald burns and the ability of young children to climb into a bathtub. *Pediatrics, 115*(5), 1419-1421.

Clarfield, A. M. (2005). A warm bath. *Journal of the American Geriatrics Society, 53*(6), 1075-1076.

Cooke, H., & Gutman, G. (2005). Improving the bathing experience for residents with dementia. *Canadian Nursing Home, 16*(2), 13-15.

De Vliegher, K., Paquay, L., Grypdonck, M., Wouters, R., Debaillie, R., & Geys, L. (2005). A study of core interventions in home nursing. *International Journal of Nursing Studies, 42*(5), 513-520.

Garner, J. S., Hospital Infection Control Practices Advisory Committee. (2005). *Guideline for isolation precautions in hospitals.* Atlanta: Centers for Disease Control and Prevention. Retrieved October 19, 2005, from http://www.cdc.gov/ncidod/hip/isolat/isolat.htm.

Hospital Infection Control Advisory Committee. (2005). *Part II: Recommendations for isolation precautions in hospitals.* Atlanta: Centers for Disease Control and Prevention. Retrieved October 19, 2005, from http://www.cdc.gov/ncidod/hip/isolat/isopart2.htm.

Johnson, M., Bulechek, G., Butcher, H., Dochterman, J. M., Maas, M., Moorhead, S., et al. (Eds.). (2006). *NANDA, NOC, and NIC linkages: Nursing diagnoses, outcomes, & interventions.* St. Louis, MO: Mosby.

Kelly, K. (2005). Rub-a-dub-dub. *American Baby: For Expectant and New Parents, 67*(5), 92-94, 96.

Ladwig, G. B., Ackley, B. J. (2006). *Mosby's guide to nursing diagnosis.* St. Louis, MO: Mosby.

Many hospital patients do not receive regular baths. (2005). *NurseWeek* (Mountain West), *6*(2), 6.

Naili, M. (2005). Muslims can take a bath . . . Zeba Arif's . . . *Nursing Standard, 19*(28), 31.

Naili, M. (2005). Starting out: Student experiences in the real world of nursing. Reluctance to interfere should not get in the way of good care. *Nursing Standard, 19*(46), 31.

NANDA International. (2005). *Nursing diagnoses: Definitions and classification, 2005-2006* (6th ed.). Philadelphia: Author.

News for healthy living. Bubble, bubble could cause trouble. (2005). *Alternative Medicine* (Sep), (80), 29.

Olesen, E. M. (2004). Are you "too posh to wash"? *Nursing, 34*(11), 57.

Singh, N., Armstrong, D. G., & Lipsky, B. A. (2005). Preventing foot ulcers in patients with diabetes. *JAMA* 293(2), 217-228.

Smitherman, L. C., Janisse, J., & Mathur, A. (2005). The use of folk remedies among children in an urban black community: Remedies for fever, colic, and teething. *Pediatrics, 115*(Suppl. 3), e297-304.

Vollman, K., Garcia, R., & Miller, L. (2005). Interventional patient hygiene: Proactive (hygiene) strategies to improve patients' outcomes. *AACN News, 22*(8), 12-13, 15-16.

Chapter 32

RESTORING PHYSICAL MOBILITY

Media Resources

- Nursing Skills Online
- Evolve Website http://evolve.elsevier.com/Harkreader/
- Companion CD
- 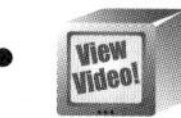 Skills Video Clips

Learning Objectives

After studying this chapter, you should be able to do the following:

- Describe the concepts of the structure and function of the musculoskeletal system pertaining to mobility
- Discuss factors affecting mobility
- Describe the assessment of a client with impaired mobility
- Identify appropriate nursing diagnoses for clients with mobility problems
- Identify expected outcomes for permanent and temporary mobility problems
- Intervene to assist a client with restoring or improving mobility
- Evaluate nursing care for the nursing diagnoses *Impaired physical mobility* and *Activity intolerance*

Key Terms

flaccid
hemiparesis
hemiplegia
isometric exercise
isotonic exercise
kyphosis
paraparesis
paraplegia
PQRST model
proprioception
quadriparesis
quadriplegia
range-of-motion exercises
spastic
synovium

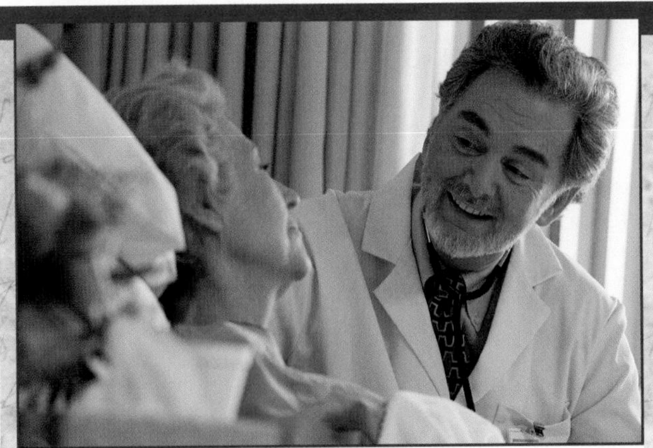

Kristina Lasauskas has been in an assisted living facility since her husband died 5 years ago. Last year she had a stroke, which left her weak on the right side. She ambulates independently with a cane. This morning her neighbor found her on the floor, and she was subsequently diagnosed with a fractured hip. She was admitted to the hospital for emergency surgery to repair the hip.

After the surgery, the nurse assesses her to identify nursing diagnoses and subsequent interventions. Because the client has previous right-sided weakness and has had surgery on her left hip, the nurse considers *Impaired physical mobility* and *Activity intolerance* as potential nursing diagnoses (see key nursing diagnoses box). The nurse also expects the client to have pain.

KEY NURSING DIAGNOSES FOR MOBILITY

Impaired physical mobility: A limitation in independent, purposeful physical movement of the body or of one of the extremities

Activity intolerance: Insufficient physiological or psychological energy to endure or complete required or desired daily activities

CONCEPTS OF PHYSICAL MOBILITY

No matter which health care setting you practice in, you will care for clients with varying limitations in physical mobility. These limitations commonly result from musculoskeletal or neurological injury, disease, or surgery. However, any severe illness or injury may affect a client's physical mobility. For example, congestive heart failure can cause severe fatigue. Complications of long-term impaired mobility, regardless of cause, can lead to serious or life-threatening conditions, such as pneumonia. You will need to understand the structure and function of the musculoskeletal system to assist clients with problems related to mobility.

STRUCTURE OF THE MUSCULOSKELETAL SYSTEM

As a body system, the musculoskeletal system is second in size only to the integumentary system. It includes bones, joints, skeletal muscles, and other soft tissues.

Bones. Bone is a highly vascular and dynamic body tissue. Throughout childhood until puberty, many hormones and other substances influence bone tissue growth. Growth hormone, secreted by the anterior lobe of the pituitary gland, determines bone structure formed before puberty. In adults, the parathyroid hormone, estrogens, and glucocorticoids work together to ensure a balance in calcium, phosphorus, and vitamin D. Over 99% of the body's calcium and 90% of the body's phosphorus are stored in a total of 206 bones.

From puberty through young adulthood, the amount of bone formation (osteoblastic activity) is greater than the amount of bone resorption, or destruction (osteoclastic activity). Beginning at about 35 years, osteoclastic activity becomes greater than osteoblastic activity. The resulting decreased bone mass predisposes middle-age and older adults to bone injury.

Besides forming the skeletal framework and storing vital minerals, bone assists in movement of joints, and it produces red blood cells (RBCs) in its red marrow. Long bones that bear weight, such as the femur, manufacture more RBCs than short bones, such as the phalanges (fingers and toes). Some of the flat bones, especially the sternum and part of the pelvis, also contain blood-forming cells. These sites are commonly used for bone marrow aspiration and analysis to determine the body's ability to produce RBCs.

Joints. A joint is the point of articulation between two or more bones, and it usually allows voluntary movement. The most common type of joint is the freely movable synovial, or diarthrodial, joint (Figure 32-1). The surface of each bone end of a synovial joint is covered with articular cartilage and attached by ligaments. The **synovium** (synovial membrane) is the inner layer of the articular capsule surrounding a freely movable joint. It is loosely attached to the external fibrous capsule and secretes a thick fluid to lubricate the joint and absorb shock.

As adults age, deterioration of cartilage causes pain and possible inflammation. Arthritis, or joint inflammation and degeneration, results from "wear and tear" and can limit mobility.

Some joints are not movable, such as those in the adult skull. They are called synarthrodial joints. In the normal newborn infant, however, the cranial bones are separated by fibrous tissue (sutures) in which growth occurs.

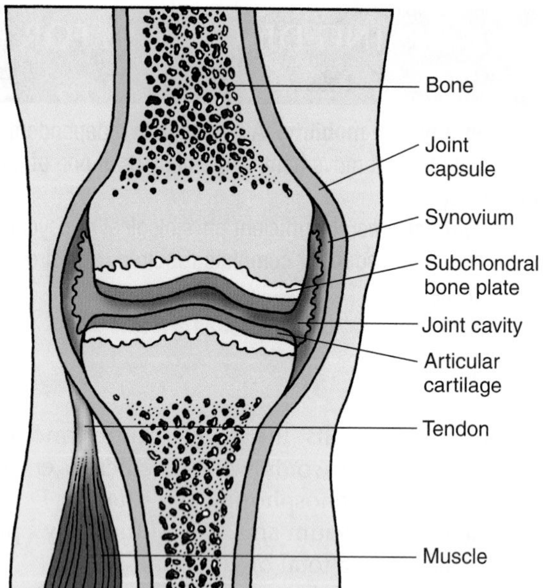

FIGURE 32-1 Structure of a synovial joint. (From Ignatavicius, D. D., Workman, M. L., & Mishler, M. A. [1999]. *Medical-surgical nursing across the health care continuum* [3rd ed.]. Philadelphia: Saunders.)

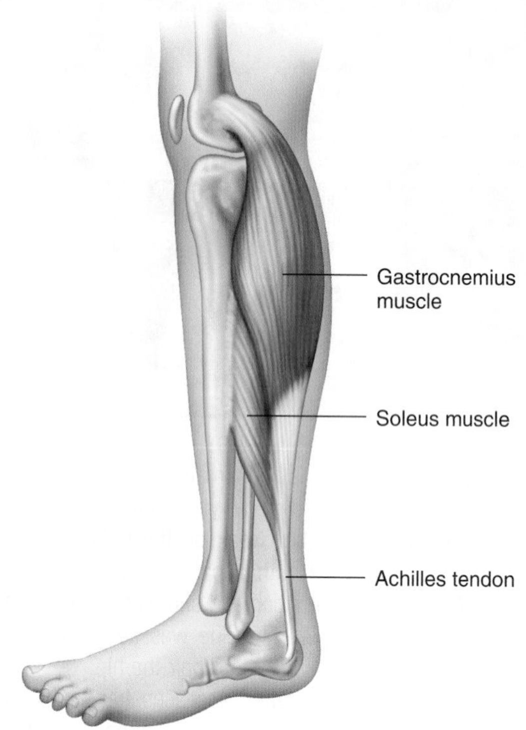

FIGURE 32-2 Tendons attach to muscles and bone.

Other joints, called amphiarthrodial joints, are slightly movable. Joints within the pelvis must be slightly movable to allow for childbirth. Joints between the ribs and sternum are slightly movable to allow the chest to expand with respiration.

Skeletal Muscles. Unlike the smooth, or nonstriated, muscles in organs and the muscle in the heart, skeletal muscles are under voluntary control by the central and peripheral nervous systems. Skeletal muscles are surrounded by dense, fibrous tissue called fascia. Small bundles of muscle tissue, blood vessels, and peripheral nerves make up compartments in the extremities, especially the distal part of each extremity.

As part of aging, muscle fibers decrease in size and number. Exercise helps keep intact fibers from atrophy, a decrease in the size of a normally developed tissue or organ caused by inactivity or diminished function. Muscle atrophy causes weakness that can limit physical mobility.

Soft Tissues. Adjacent fibrous tissues, such as tendons and ligaments, support skeletal muscles and bones. Tendons attach muscles to bone (Figure 32-2); ligaments attach bones to bones at joints. Both of these soft tissue types are prone to injury, especially during contact sports, such as football, or physically demanding activities, such as tennis and skiing.

Cartilage is found on bone ends of synovial joints, the rib-sternum junctions (costal cartilage), nasal septum and trachea (hyaline cartilage), and external ear (yellow cartilage). Cartilage is flexible tissue, but it can withstand enormous tension.

FUNCTION OF THE MUSCULOSKELETAL SYSTEM

Together with the nervous system, the musculoskeletal system enables us to move in a coordinated manner. Muscles are grouped according to the type of movement they allow. For example, *flexors* allow a joint or an extremity to flex or bend; *extensors* allow the joint or extremity to extend or straighten out. The elbow is an example of a synovial joint that can flex and extend. These movements are discussed later under range-of-motion (ROM) exercises.

Regulation of Movement. Movement is regulated by the central and peripheral nervous systems. The primary *motor area* (the motor "strip"), located in the frontal lobe of the cerebrum, is responsible for voluntary muscle contraction of muscle groups. Adjacent to the motor area is the *premotor area,* which directs new movements or movements that have been changed. Motor neurons and premotor neurons, also referred to as upper motor neurons, synapse with the corticospinal tract nerve fibers and descend into the spinal cord. At the level of the medulla, these fibers cross to the opposite side of the body. Thus, the left motor area in the brain controls the right side of the body, and vice versa.

As the nerve fibers descend into the spinal cord, some synapse with peripheral nerves that supply the head, trunk, and limbs (lower motor neurons). Others synapse with interneurons in the cord. The peripheral nerves contain motor, sensory, and sometimes autonomic fibers. The motor fibers stimulate muscles to

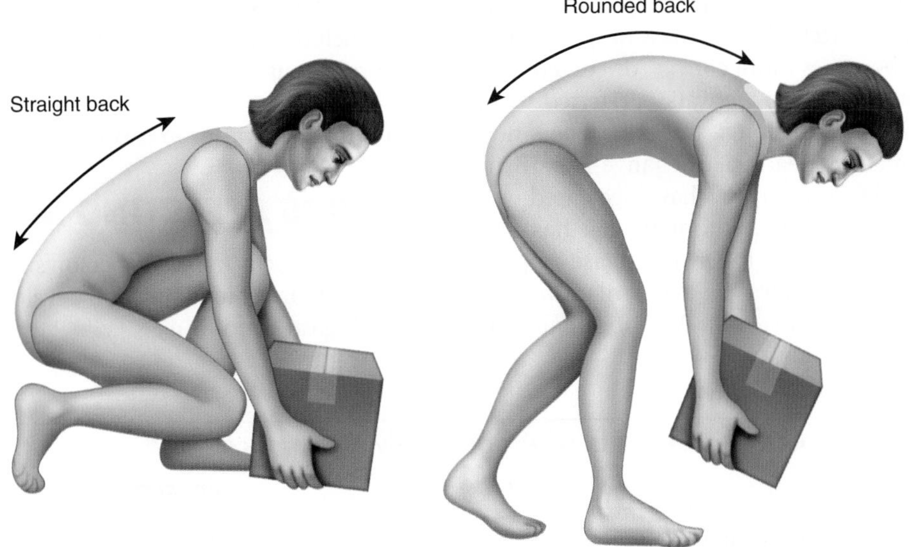

FIGURE 32-3 Lifting an object using proper *(left)* and improper *(right)* body mechanics.

contract. Special chemicals called neurotransmitters, such as acetylcholine, facilitate muscle contraction. After muscle contraction, the muscle then relaxes because certain enzymes destroy the neurotransmitters after muscle contraction.

Proprioception. **Proprioception** is sensation pertaining to stimuli originating from within the body regarding spatial position and muscular activity, or to the sensory receptors that they activate. It is our awareness of body position, posture, and movement. Small receptor cells in skeletal muscle, subcutaneous tissue, and the inner ear respond to stimuli within the body, such as pressure or muscle stretch, promoting this awareness. For example, we know if we are standing or sitting, even if our eyes are closed. In a sense, proprioception is a protective function, enabling us to be aware of our bodies without actually seeing them.

Body Mechanics. Body mechanics describes the use of the body in movement and at rest. Improper use can cause fatigue and injury, such as back strain. Back injury among health care workers and others who perform physical activities is a common and costly health problem that commonly results from poor body mechanics. Health care workers must use proper body mechanics as a baseline effort to prevent injury, maintain balance, and conserve energy.

Components. The *center of gravity,* located within the pelvis, is the point where the body's mass is centered. The body maintains optimal balance and alignment when the *line of gravity* (an imaginary line) passes through the center of gravity. The base of support for the body includes the feet and the distance between the feet.

Principles. While sitting, standing, or lying, the body can easily maintain alignment. However, when lifting, pushing, or pulling an object, the center and line of gravity shift, possibly causing poor body alignment and injury from loss of balance or stress on soft tissues.

Large muscle groups in the legs and arms should perform the work required to lift an object. As seen in Figure 32-3, the proper use of these muscles helps prevent back stress and strain. The back must remain straight during lifting, pulling, or pushing. Moving the feet farther apart broadens the base of support and keeps the body balanced during physical activity. Twisting the body should also be avoided. Pivoting on the ball of one foot keeps the back straight. Table 32-1 summarizes key principles of proper body mechanics.

Body Alignment. When the body is not moving, alignment is also important. When in a standing, sitting, or lying position, the body should be aligned so that the line of gravity passes through the center of gravity and the longer and stronger muscles do the work. Poor positioning changes the center and line of gravity, causing muscle fatigue and stress. When sitting, standing, or walking, good posture allows the least amount of stress on muscles, joints, and soft tissues because the line of gravity passes perfectly through the center of gravity.

Children. When an infant sits, the thoracic spine appears curved or convex because of weak chest and truncal muscles. As the muscles strengthen and the child begins to walk, the back straightens. Normal toddlers and preschool children may actually appear to have an increased lumbar concavity because they have protuberant abdomens. Adolescents who grow quickly may slouch forward, producing a round-shouldered appearance.

Adults. Good posture for adults means that the head is held erect, shoulders are back, and vertebral column is held straight. Poor posture can result in back discomfort from excessive strain. As adults age, especially postmenopausal women, vertebral bone mass decreases and the thoracic spine becomes more convex, or curved.

Gait. The manner in which we walk is referred to as gait. As a person ages, the long, smooth steps often shorten and become less steady. This change is particularly obvious for older women who have decreased vertebral bone mass. The normal, automatic gait has two phases—the stance phase and the swing phase (Figure 32-4). The *stance phase* includes the heel strike through the push-off action of the first foot. An abnormality in the stance phase is called an antalgic gait. The *swing phase* includes the action of the second foot from acceleration through deceleration. An abnormality in this phase is called a lurch. Pain, muscle weakness, and limb shortening are common causes of abnormal gait.

FACTORS AFFECTING MOBILITY

Many factors can affect a person's mobility, including lifestyle, environment, physical development, and pathophysiological conditions.

Table 32-1 Principles and Benefits of Proper Body Mechanics

PRINCIPLE	BENEFIT
• Pull, push, or roll objects rather than lifting them. • Pulling is usually easier than pushing, so pull clients toward you rather than pushing them.	Reduces the workload
• Lower the head of the bed to move a client up in bed.	Decreases opposition from gravity and decreases friction and shear
• Size up your load to determine whether you need help. • Keep your back straight when moving an object. • Use the longest and strongest muscles of your legs and arms rather than the weaker muscles of your back. • Rock your body to use the weight of your body to enhance the force of your arm muscles. • Move your body as a unit when twisting, stretching, or reaching.	Prevents muscle strain
• Lower your center of gravity by bending your knees. • Widen your base of support by moving your feet apart. • Maintain your center of gravity (your pelvis) over your base of support. To support a client, stand close; carry an object close to your body.	Maintains stability

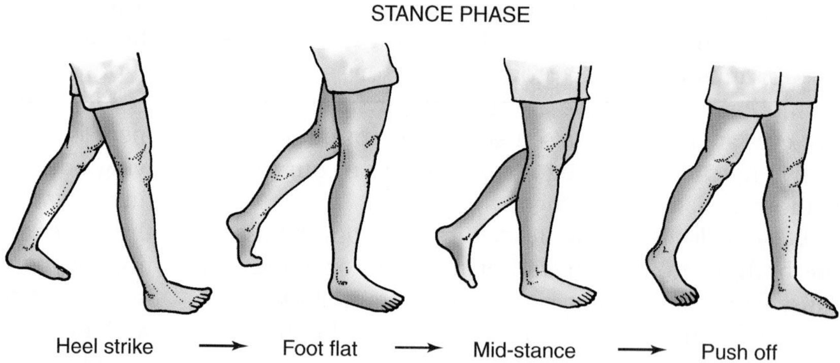

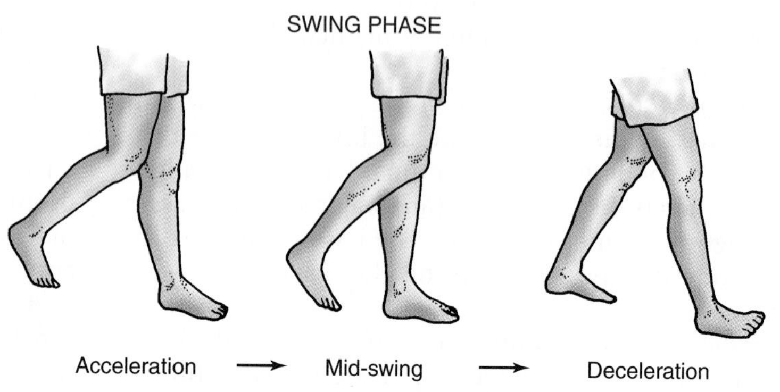

FIGURE 32-4 Normal phases of gait. (From Ignatavicius, D. D., Workman, M. L., & Mishler, M. A. [1999]. *Medical-surgical nursing across the health care continuum* [3rd ed.]. Philadelphia: Saunders.)

LIFESTYLE FACTORS

Some recreational activities place people at a high risk for musculoskeletal injury. For example, physically demanding sports such as skiing, football, and tennis can result in fractures or soft tissue damage. Failure to adequately train or physically prepare for these activities contributes to injuries. Carelessness and unnecessary risk taking also cause accidents, which may be fatal.

Diet and exercise affect mobility. A diet low in calcium, protein, and other vital nutrients prevents bone growth and development in children and contributes to bone loss in older adults. The resulting "brittle" bones are prone to deformity and fracture. Regular exercise helps build strong bones and muscle tissue. Assess your client's cultural beliefs about diet and other lifestyle considerations to determine factors that might affect mobility. Box 32-1 offers one example.

ENVIRONMENTAL FACTORS

Environmental factors can lead to accidents or injury either in the workplace or at home. You can be instrumental in teaching clients about ways to prevent musculoskeletal injury.

Workplace. In the United States, the Occupational Safety and Health Administration (OSHA) establishes standards for workplace safety. The purpose of OSHA is to protect workers from injuries and accidents. The three major causes of worker injury are repetitive motion, poor body mechanics, and accidents.

Lifting and moving clients while using poor body mechanics can cause musculoskeletal injury. Back supports are commonly required for workers who lift objects as part of their jobs. Nurses have an alarming rate of back injury, with 52% of registered nurses (clustered with licensed practical nurses, nurse's aides, and attendants) reporting chronic back pain (Nelson, 2003). The problem is so significant that the American Nurses Association has launched the Handle With Care campaign to promote safe client handling and to prevent musculoskeletal disorders among nurses in the United States (www.NursingWorld.org/handlewithcare/). In 2003, OSHA put forth voluntary ergonomics guidelines to help prevent musculoskeletal disorders in workers in nursing homes.

Effective January 1, 2006, Texas was the first state to legislate that hospitals and nursing homes must implement safe client handling and movement programs. The intent is to reduce the risk of injury to clients and health care workers associated with lifting, transferring, repositioning, and moving clients. The intent is to eliminate manual lifting and mandate the use of assistive devices in routine care. This landmark legislation has spurred similar types of legislation in other states and may be the precursor to a federal initiative for no-lift health care environments (Hudson, 2005).

Home. Accidents from environmental hazards also occur in the home. Because OSHA has no jurisdiction in private residences, the homeowner must ensure that the home structure and equipment are safe. For older adults, reducing environmental hazards is especially important for preventing falls (see Chapter 23).

DEVELOPMENTAL FACTORS

Most age-groups are at risk for decreased mobility, especially children, young adults, and older adults.

Children. Infants may be born with congenital musculoskeletal deformities that decrease their ability to crawl or walk. Abnormal fixed positions of the feet, such as metatarsus varus (pigeon toe, toes pointing in), metatarsus valgus (duck walk, toes pointing out), and talipes equinovarus (clubfoot or twisted foot) can worsen and delay physical development if not corrected.

Congenital dysplasia of the hip is one of the most common musculoskeletal malformations. The femoral

BOX 32-1 *Cross-Cultural Care*

Caring for a Lithuanian American Woman

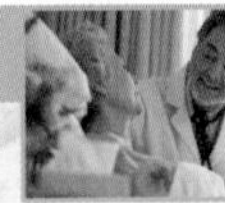

Mrs. Lasauskas is a Lithuanian American who came to the United States when she was 30 years old with her husband and two small children. The family lived with relatives in Boston, where her husband worked as a janitor while he perfected his English. He then received a position as a college professor. Kristina is a devout Catholic and has enjoyed being visited by the young priest from her parish. Her daughter lives nearby and visits her mother daily and sometimes brings the great-grandchildren to play games with "Nana." Although each person is an individual and customs vary, some Lithuanian Americans may share the following values (Leininger, 1991):

- Closeness among extended family members
- Religious beliefs and prayers (Roman Catholic)
- The importance of education
- Hard work and industriousness
- Thriftiness and good use of material resources
- Endurance, persistence, and suffering with economic hardships
- Charity to others
- Helping in times of need
- Hospitality to others
- Sharing with others
- Flexibility
- Cooperation with others
- Praying with others
- Using subtle humor

head is partially displaced from the pelvic acetabulum. If this condition is not diagnosed until after the child walks, the child will have a limp. If both hips are affected, the child will have a waddling gait.

A small number of infants are born without complete extremities, causing marked problems with learning to sit, crawl, and walk. In other infants, toes or fingers may be webbed, ultimately resulting in decreased function.

Congenital spinal deformities may also occur (Figure 32-5). The most common is scoliosis, a lateral deviation of the spine typically diagnosed in preadolescent and adolescent children. If not corrected, this deformity can also affect the cardiopulmonary system.

Young Adults. The highest incidence of musculoskeletal injuries is among young men between ages 18 and 25. Young men often take risks, such as driving at excessive speeds or without a seat belt or operating a motorcycle without a helmet. Alcohol or drug consumption increases the risk associated with these activities.

Older Adults. Aging typically results in muscle weakness and atrophy, decreased coordination and balance, and loss of bone tissue. These physiological changes decrease mobility but should not prevent independent function. Staying active and exercising help keep intact muscle fibers strong and promote coordination and balance. In hospitalized older adults, however, deconditioning can occur in a matter of days (Graf, 2006). This makes it imperative to be concerned with maintaining mobility throughout hospitalization (Fletcher, 2005; Gillis & MacDonald, 2005).

As discussed earlier, after the age of 35, bone breakdown exceeds bone formation. After menopause in women, bone mass decreases (osteoporosis), possibly causing painful fractures of the wrist, vertebral column, and hip. Men have large amounts of testosterone, which results in continued formation of bone until about age 80. After age 80, men also have a high risk of hip fractures. Measures to prevent or slow bone loss include calcium supplements, exercise, and precautions to prevent falls.

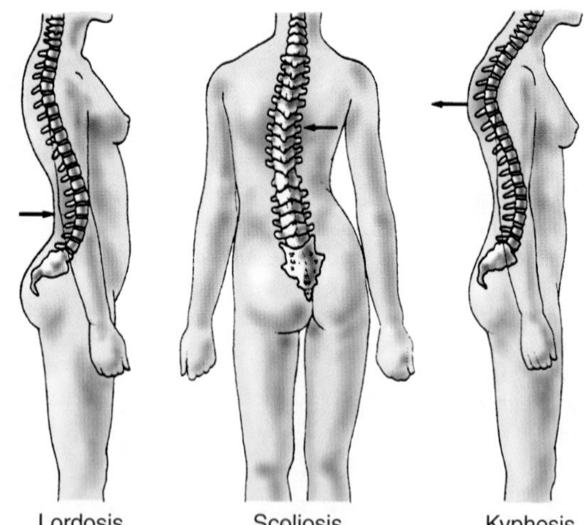

FIGURE 32-5 Common congenital spinal deformities. (From Ignatavicius, D. D., Workman, M. L., & Mishler, M. A. [1999]. *Medical-surgical nursing across the health care continuum* [3rd ed.]. Philadelphia: Saunders.)

PHYSIOLOGICAL FACTORS

Many acute and chronic health problems can decrease mobility; this discussion is limited to common problems affecting the musculoskeletal and nervous systems.

Musculoskeletal Problems. Musculoskeletal problems can be divided into inflammatory, degenerative, traumatic, and congenital problems. Rheumatoid arthritis is one of the most common inflammatory problems occurring at any age and potentially causing joint deformity and chronic pain. This systemic disease also affects major body organs and must be treated aggressively to slow its progress. Degenerative joint disease, or osteoarthritis, is an example of a degenerative process that is seen most often in older adults, but also commonly affects athletes and obese individuals.

Trauma often results in bone fractures or dislocations and soft tissue damage. Fractures occur in any age-group, but they heal most readily in infants and young children. A young, healthy adult heals in 4 to 6 weeks; young children heal in 1 to 2 weeks, and older adults may take up to 3 months for bone healing.

Neurological Problems. Brain or spinal cord damage is a leading cause of immobility. Depending on the level of injury, the person will be weak (paresis) or paralyzed (plegia). When injured at the cerebral or cervical spine level, the client may experience **quadriplegia**—an abnormal condition characterized by paralysis of the arms, legs, and trunk below the level of the injury. Quadriplegia may also be called *tetraplegia.* Alternatively, the client might experience **quadriparesis,** a numbness or other abnormal or impaired sensation in all four limbs and the trunk. Lower-level spinal injuries result in **paraplegia**—paralysis characterized by motor or sensory loss in the legs and trunk. Or the client might experience **paraparesis,** a numbness or other abnormal or impaired sensation in the legs and trunk.

Middle-age and older adults are at risk for degenerative or thrombotic neurological health problems. Parkinson's disease is a common degenerative, progressive process in which the client eventually becomes completely immobile. Cerebrovascular accidents (strokes) are the most costly disability. Part of the brain becomes damaged (infarcted) from hypoxia caused by a thrombus (stationary blood clot), embolus (dislodged blood clot), or hemorrhage. The typical client with a stroke has **hemiplegia** (paralysis of one side of the body) or **hemiparesis** (numbness or other abnormal or impaired sensation on one side of the body), which may limit mobility and activities of daily living (ADLs).

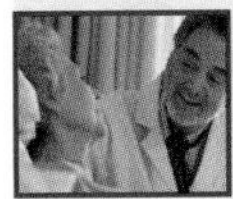

Recall the case study: Kristina Lasauskas's previous stroke had left her with hemiparesis. What concerns should you have about her postoperative rehabilitation program? Might she be at risk for another stroke?

ASSESSMENT

GENERAL ASSESSMENT OF PHYSICAL MOBILITY

Health problems that impair mobility may affect any body system. To assess physical mobility, collect data related to the musculoskeletal system.

Health History. The health history elicits information about the client's chief complaint, risk for musculoskeletal health problems, previous or current treatment plan, and current condition.

Chief Complaint. The most common complaints associated with musculoskeletal health problems are pain, muscle weakness, and inflammation. Pain may be acute or chronic; it may be assessed using the following **PQRST model** of symptom analysis:

P—What was the *provoking incident* that caused the pain, if any?

Q—What is the *quality* of the pain? Is it burning, throbbing, stabbing?

R—Where is the *region* of pain? Does it *radiate*? Does anything *relieve* the pain?

S—How *severe* is the pain?

T—What is the *timing* of the pain? When does it occur and how long does it last?

Also assess any history of muscle weakness or inflammation:

- Have you experienced muscle weakness or fatigue? If so, when does it occur?
- Do you find that you drop items or stumble at times when walking?
- Have you noticed any redness or excessive warmth around your joints or over muscles?
- Have you been unable to carry out any usual daily activity? Have you had to restrict some of your usual activities?

Risk for Musculoskeletal Health Problems. Determine which factors place the client at risk for a musculoskeletal health problem, such as age, work and home environments, lifestyle, and personal and family history of musculoskeletal problems. Some health problems tend to recur. A complete history of previous problems and how they were managed could provide important data that aids in diagnosis and management of the current condition.

Ask the client about treatments that have been or are being received that could contribute to the current health problem. You might use the following questions:

- Have you had any surgery? If so, what and when? (Previous surgery could cause nerve or muscle weakness.)
- What medications are you taking, including both prescription and over-the-counter? (Some medications have side effects that cause weakness, lowered blood pressure, or muscle atrophy. Other medications may be given to prevent musculoskeletal problems, such as calcium and alendronate [Fosamax], to prevent or treat osteoporosis.)
- Are you currently under a physician's care? If so, what for and how is it being treated?

Physical Examination. The musculoskeletal physical examination includes assessing body alignment, gait, joints, and skeletal muscles. For clients who experience musculoskeletal trauma or surgery, you frequently monitor neurovascular function as well.

Body Alignment. If possible, observe the client's posture and positioning while sitting, lying, and standing. Assess for scoliosis and kyphosis. In scoliosis, the vertebral column deviates laterally. In children or adolescents, it may result from habit (functional), muscle weakness, contractures, or a tilted pelvis. Have the client bend forward at the waist. If the deviation disappears when the client bends forward, the problem is functional. If it does not disappear, the problem may require treatment.

Kyphosis is an abnormal condition of the vertebral column characterized by increased convexity in the thoracic spine when viewed from the side. It is common in middle-age and older adults. The client's shoulders are slouched, and the vertebral bones are very prominent. Check to ensure that this problem is not interfering with breathing.

Gait. Observe while the client ambulates if the client can walk. Note the stance and swing phases, looking for limps or other abnormalities in gait. If the lower extremities are not the same length, the client will walk with a limp. Ask the client if there is a congenital abnormality or if surgery was performed on one or both extremities.

Joints. The best method for assessing joints is to use a head-to-toe approach, beginning with joints of the head and neck and progressing to the lower extremities. Inspect the joints for proper alignment, symmetry, redness, and swelling. Then, palpate each joint for tenderness and masses. Finally, put each joint through its ROM to determine function and listen for *crepitus,* a continuous grating sound caused by joint deterioration.

Assessing the extremities is particularly important because the client needs full use of these joints for performing ADLs. For example, clients with shoulder limitations and pain may not be able to perform hair grooming. Clients with hand deformities due to arthritis may have trouble cutting food or opening food containers.

Ask the client to move each joint through its ROM. The normal ROM for each joint is illustrated in Table 32-2. As long as the client can perform ADLs, a slight limitation of ROM is acceptable, especially for older adults.

Text continued on p. 836

Table 32-2 Reviewing Range of Motion

AREA OF BODY/MOTION		AREA OF BODY/MOTION	
NECK Flexion (45 degrees), extension (45 degrees), hyperextension (50 degrees)	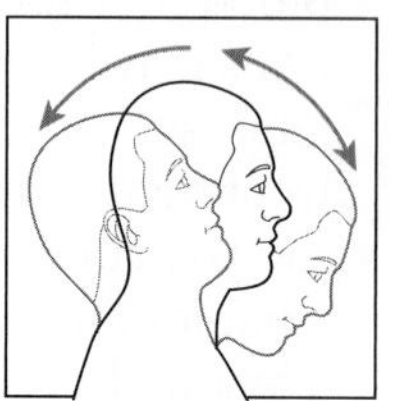	**SHOULDER—CONT'D** Circumduction (360 degrees)	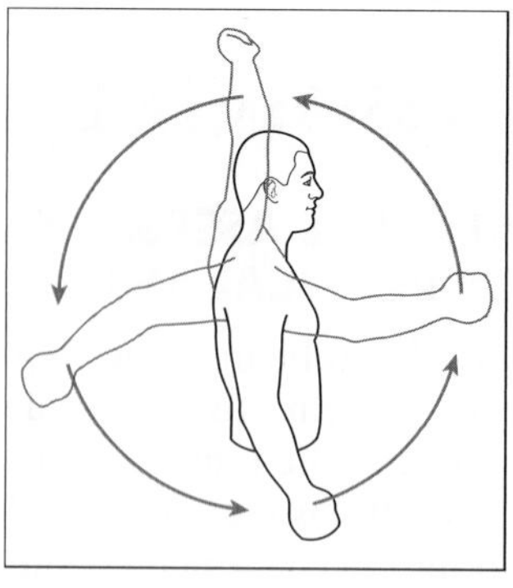
Lateral flexion (40 degrees)	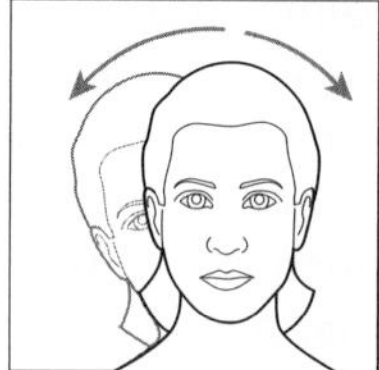	External rotation (90 degrees), internal rotation (90 degrees)	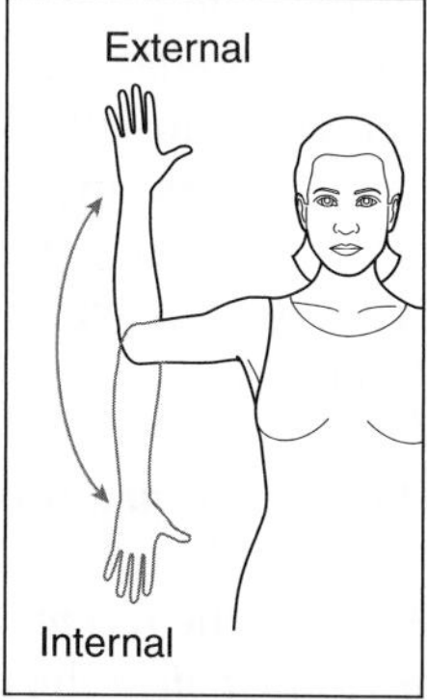
Rotation (70 degrees)	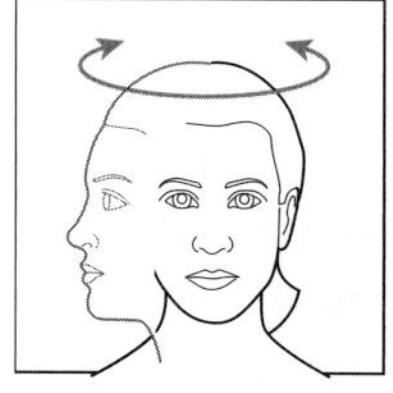	**ELBOW** Flexion (160 degrees), extension (160 degrees)	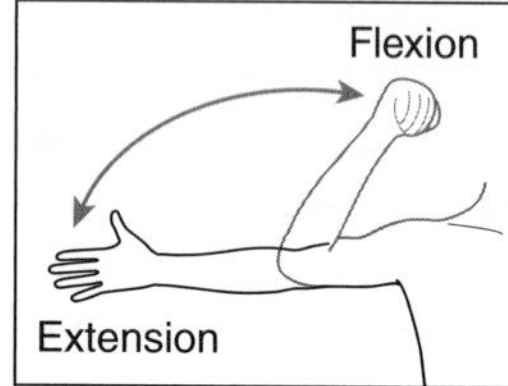
SHOULDER Flexion (180 degrees), extension (180 degrees), hyperextension (50 degrees)	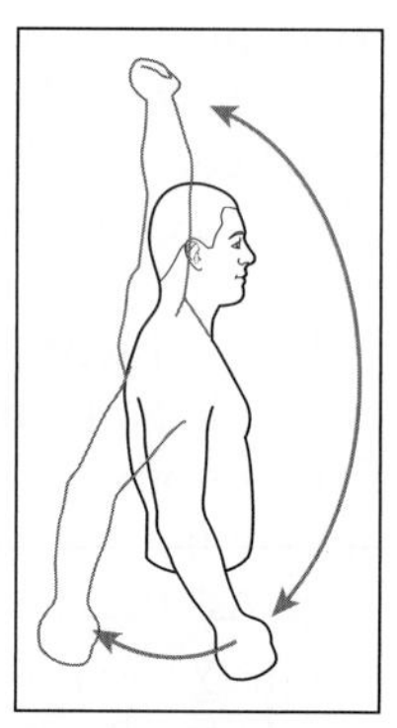	Rotation for supination, rotation for pronation (180 degrees)	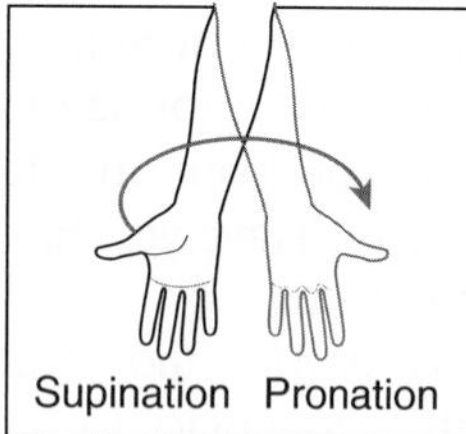
Abduction, adduction	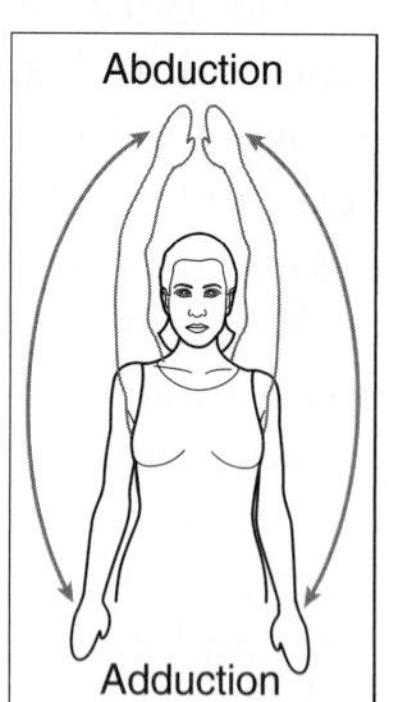	**WRIST** Flexion (90 degrees), extension (90 degrees), hyperextension (70 degrees)	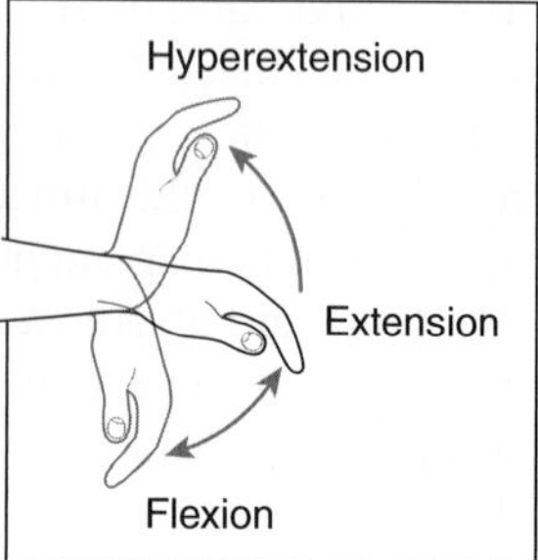

Table 32-2 Reviewing Range of Motion

AREA OF BODY/MOTION		AREA OF BODY/MOTION	
WRIST—CONT'D Ulnar flexion (adduction) (30-50 degrees), radial flexion (abduction) (30 degrees)	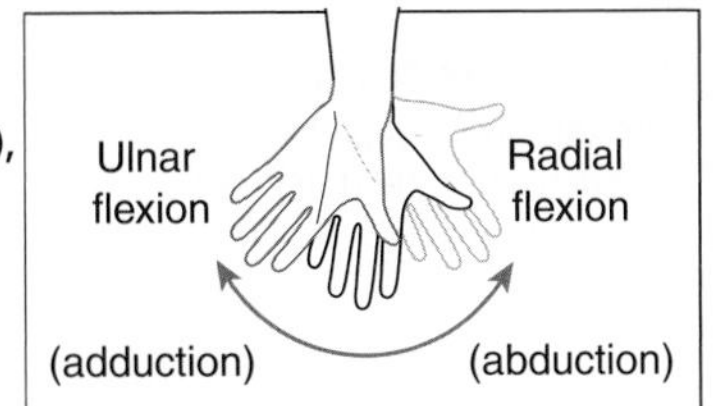	**HIP—CONT'D** Abduction (30-50 degrees), adduction (30-50 degrees)	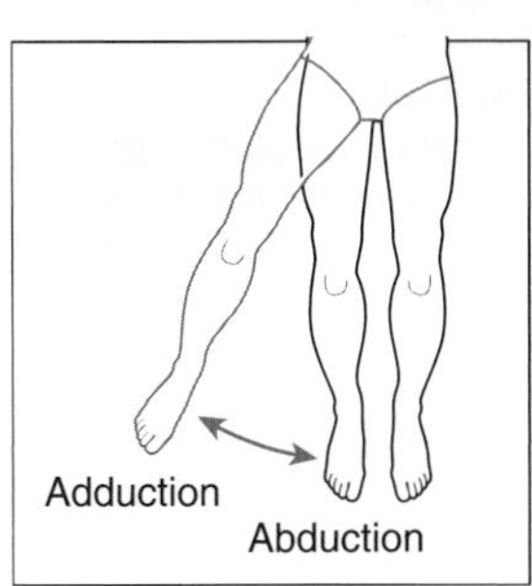
HAND AND FINGERS Flexion (90 degrees), extension (90 degrees), hyperextension (150 degrees)	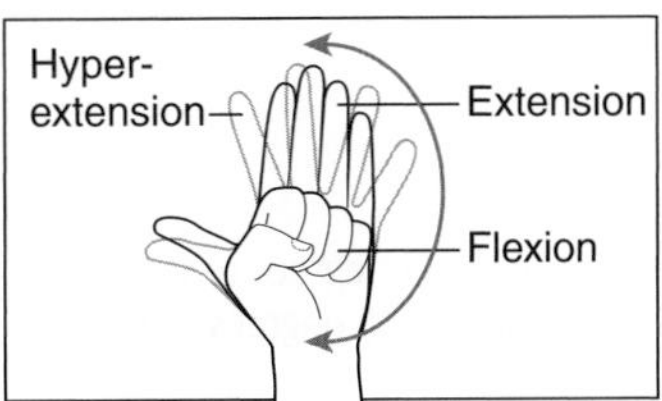	Circumduction (foot makes small circle)	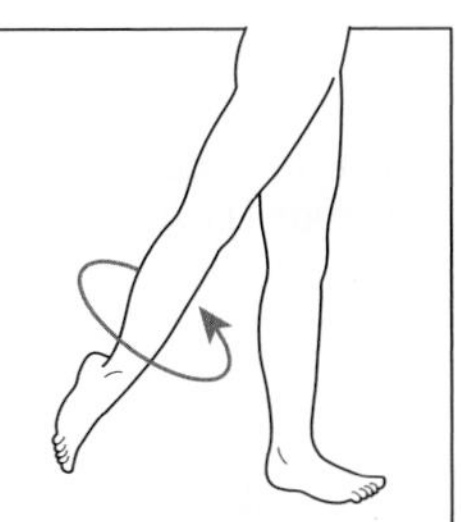
Abduction, adduction (spreads to 90 degrees)	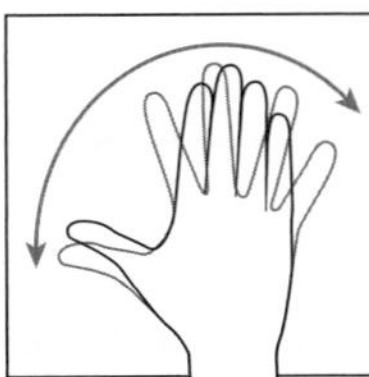	External rotation, internal rotation (90 degrees)	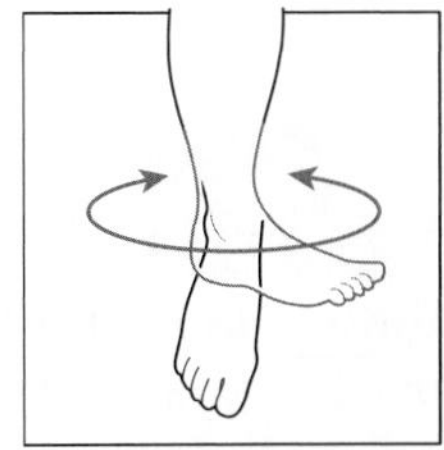
Opposition of thumb (thumb touches each finger)	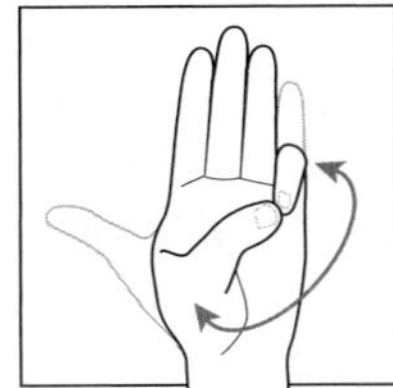	**KNEE** Flexion, extension (120-130 degrees)	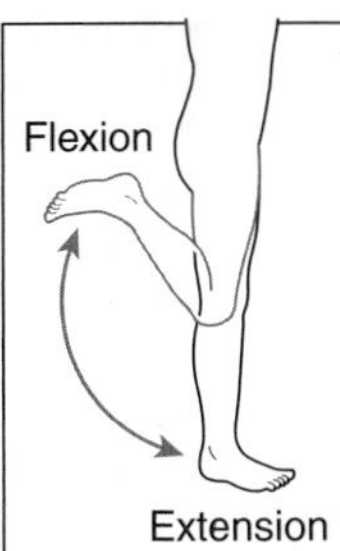
HIP Flexion (90-120 degrees), extension (90-120 degrees), hyperextension (30-50 degrees)	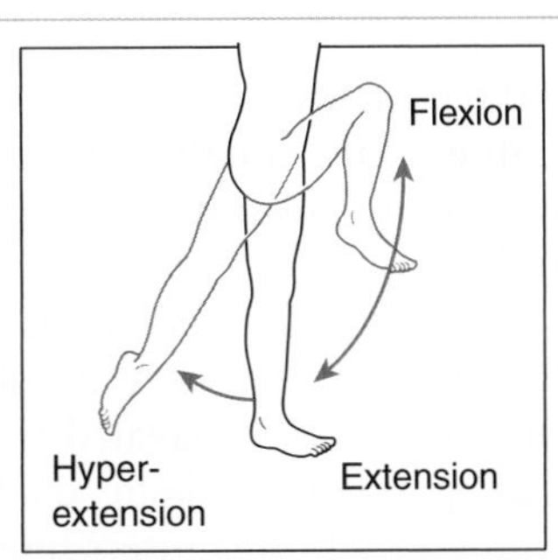		

Flexion: Bending at a joint in the natural direction of movement.
Extension: Moving from the flexed position to a neutral or straight position.
Hyperextension: Moving beyond a straight or neutral position.
Rotation: Pivoting a body part on its axis.
Abduction: Movement of a limb in a direction away from the midline of the body.
Adduction: Movement of a limb in a direction toward the midline of the body.
Circumduction: A combination of movements that causes a body part to move in a circle.
External rotation: Rotation from a joint in the direction away from the midline of the body.
Internal rotation: Rotation from a joint in the direction toward the midline of the body.
Supination: Rotation of the palm of the hand upward or in the anterior direction.
Pronation: Rotation of the palm of the hand downward or in the posterior direction.
Opposition: The relationship of the thumb and fingers for the purpose of grasping objects.
Eversion: Movement of the ankle to turn the sole of the foot laterally (away from the midline).
Inversion: Movement of the ankle to turn the sole of the foot medially (toward the midline).
Dorsal flexion: Flexion of the ankle in the direction of the dorsal surface.
Plantar flexion: Flexion of the ankle in the direction of the plantar surface.

Continued

Table 32-2 Reviewing Range of Motion—cont'd

AREA OF BODY/MOTION		AREA OF BODY/MOTION	
ANKLE Extension (20-30 degrees), flexion (45-50 degrees)	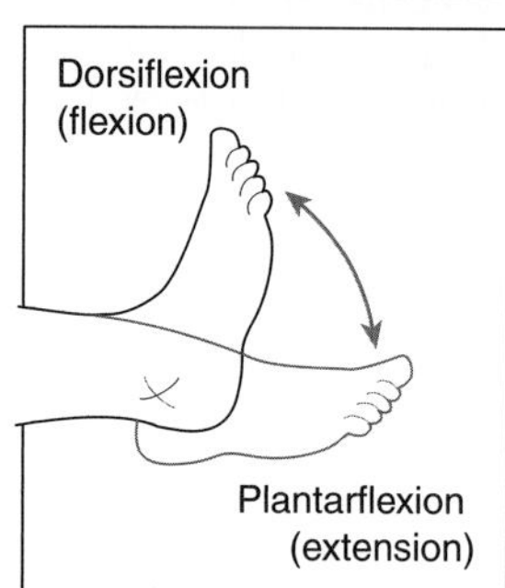 	**FOOT AND TOES** Flexion (30-60 degrees), extension (30-60 degrees)	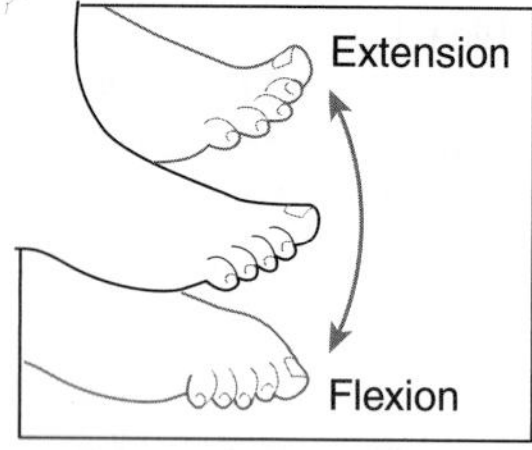
Eversion (10-20 degrees), inversion (10-20 degrees)	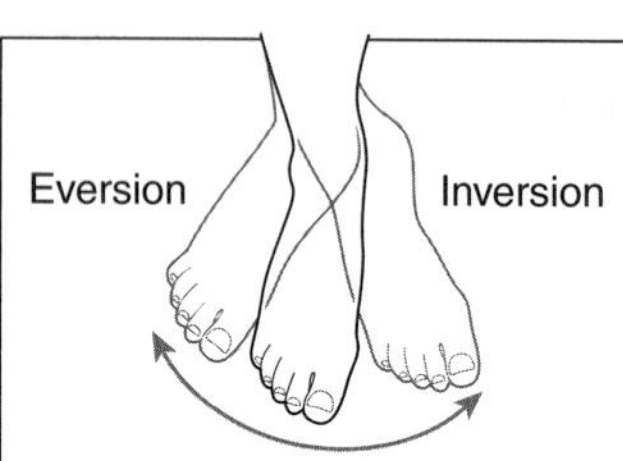 	Abduction (15 degrees or less), adduction (15 degrees or less)	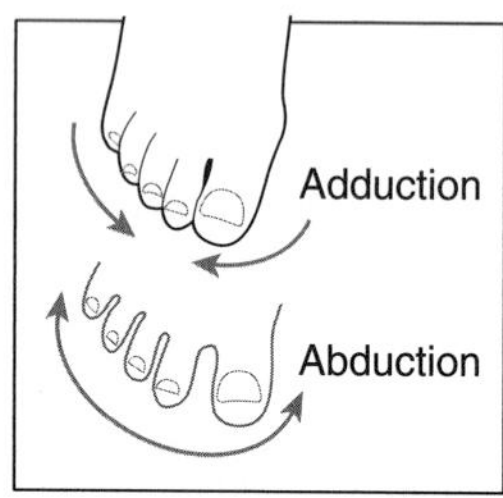

Table 32-3 Lovett's Scale of Muscle Strength

RATING	DESCRIPTION
5	Normal: ROM unimpaired against gravity with full resistance
4	Good: Can complete ROM against gravity with some resistance
3	Fair: Can complete ROM against gravity
2	Poor: Can complete ROM with gravity eliminated
1	Trace: No joint motion and slight evidence of muscle contractility
0	Zero: No evidence of muscle contractility

From Ignatavicius, D. D., & Workman, M. L. (Eds.). (2002) *Medical-surgical nursing: Critical thinking for collaborative care* (4th ed.). Philadelphia: Saunders.
ROM, Range of motion.

Skeletal Muscles. Skeletal muscles can be examined at the same time as joints. Observe each major muscle group for symmetry in size, shape, tone, and strength. Palpate the muscle, and ask the client to demonstrate its strength—for example, by squeezing your hand or a sphygmomanometer. The latter method provides a numerical score that can be used later for comparison. To check for movement against resistance, ask the client to move an extremity while you are trying to prevent that movement.

Physical and occupational therapists perform more detailed assessments of muscle strength using various scales. Table 32-3 describes Lovett's scale for determining muscle strength. Using this scale, the therapist assesses each muscle and scores it as a rating out of a possible 5. For example, if a muscle is rated as a 3/5, the client has fair strength, can complete ROM, but cannot move against resistance. If it is available, review the client's muscle strength evaluation to help determine how much assistance you might need when getting the client out of bed or ambulating.

Neurovascular Status. Your major responsibility is frequent monitoring of neurovascular status, or CMS (circulation, movement, sensation) assessment (Alitzer, 2004). Check for skin color, temperature, movement, sensation, pulses, capillary refill, and pain; document and report adverse changes. Always compare the affected limb with the unaffected one. Table 32-4 describes neurovascular assessment and gives the normally expected findings.

This assessment is especially important when external devices, such as casts and bulky dressings, can compress the compartments created by sheaths of inelastic fascia, causing extensive tissue damage. Excessive tissue fluid from severe burns, insect bites, or infiltration of intravenous fluids can increase compartmental pressure. If this pressure is not relieved, ischemic tissue necrosis can result in 4 to 8 hours. Known as *compartment syndrome*, this phenomenon occurs in the extremities, especially the legs, where a sheath of inelastic fascia partitions blood vessel, nerve, and muscle tissue, and the pressure in this compartment is normally less than capillary pressure.

Action Alert! Notify the physician immediately of signs of compartment syndrome.

Table 32-4 Assessing Neurovascular Status

CHARACTERISTIC	ASSESSMENT TECHNIQUE	NORMAL FINDINGS
Skin color	Inspect the area distal to the injury.	No change in pigmentation compared with other parts of the body.
Skin temperature	Palpate the area distal to the injury (the dorsum of the hands is most sensitive to temperature).	The skin is warm.
Movement	Ask the client to move the affected area or the area distal to the injury (active motion).	The client can move without discomfort.
	Move the area distal to the injury (passive motion).	No difference in comfort compared with active movement.
Sensation	Ask the client if numbness or tingling is present (paresthesia).	No numbness or tingling. No difference in sensation in the affected and unaffected extremities.
	Palpate with a safety pin or paper clip, especially the web space between the first and second toes or the web space between the thumb and forefinger.	Loss of sensation in these areas indicates peroneal nerve or median nerve damage.
Pulses	Palpate the pulses distal to the injury.	Pulses are strong and easily palpated; no difference in the affected and unaffected extremities.
Capillary refill	Press the nail beds distal to the injury until blanching occurs (or the skin near the nail blanches if nails are thick and brittle).	Blood returns (return to usual color) within 3 seconds (5 seconds for older adult clients).
Pain	Ask the client about the location, nature, and frequency of pain.	Pain is usually localized and is often described as stabbing or throbbing.

From Ignatavicius, D. D., & Workman, M. L. (Eds.) (2002). *Medical-surgical nursing: Critical thinking for collaborative care* (4th ed.). Philadelphia: Saunders.

Increased pain on passive motion when compared with active motion, or loss of sensation in the web space between the great and second toes (or between the thumb and second finger on the hand), indicates early compartment syndrome. When the client is in late-stage compartment syndrome and damage is not reversible, the six "Ps" may be present, including the following:

- Pain not relieved
- Paresthesias
- Pallor
- Pulse absent (pulselessness)
- Paralysis
- Palpated tense tissue

Do not wait until these signs and symptoms are present. The earlier compartment syndrome is treated, the better the prognosis is. Compartment syndrome may require amputation of the limb if the neurovascular compromise is not promptly assessed and managed.

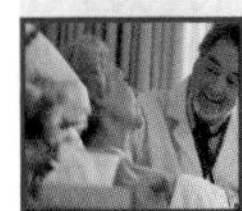

Postoperatively, Mrs. Lasauskas has a physician's order to perform "CMS checks" every 4 hours. Why is this client at risk for neurovascular compromise?

Diagnostic Tests. Diagnostic tests are commonly performed to determine the nature and extent of musculoskeletal health problems that may interfere with mobility.

Radiographs (or x-ray films) detect bone density, swelling, alignment, and continuity. Joint structure can be visualized, but soft tissues are not always clearly differentiated. Remind the client to remain still during the procedure even though the table may feel cold and hard.

The computed tomography (CT) scan provides a better picture of soft tissues and less-dense bone than standard x-rays, especially in the vertebral column. It can also identify problems of the central nervous system, such as strokes and tumors. A CT scan may be done with or without use of a contrast medium to enhance the views. If contrast will be used, check that the client has had nothing by mouth (NPO status) for at least 4 hours, that there is no allergy to iodine or seafood, and that the client has signed an informed consent form.

Magnetic resonance imaging (MRI) is often more accurate than either standard x-rays films or a CT scan for detecting soft tissue damage. The image is produced by the interaction of radio waves and magnetic fields. As with the CT scan, a contrast medium may be used to enhance the view. Ask the client to remove any metal objects, such as clothing with metal fasteners. Metal joint implants are safe, but pacemakers are not.

An arthrogram is an enhanced radiograph of a joint obtained after contrast is injected; it is performed most commonly for knees and shoulders. Inquire about allergies to iodine and seafood. Explain that joint swelling caused by the injection fluid will diminish within a day or two. If the joint injury is not severe, usual activities can typically be resumed within 12 to 24 hours.

A myelogram is a radiograph of the vertebral spine obtained after injecting a contrast medium into the lumbar subarachnoid space. The spinal cord, vertebral bones, intervertebral disks, and surrounding soft tissues can be visualized. The client assumes a fetal position or sits and bends at the waist to open the lumbar intervertebral space before injection.

If a cervical myelogram is done, the client bends the neck forward. The injection site is locally anesthetized. After the contrast medium is injected, the client is moved into various positions while radiographs are taken. After the test, the client must be properly positioned to prevent cerebrospinal fluid (CSF) leakage and subsequent headaches.

Action Alert! To prevent spinal headache or meningeal irritation, the client must remain flat after use of an oil-based contrast or in a semi-Fowler's position after use of a water-based contrast for at least 4 to 8 hours. Check the injection site for CSF leak. Also, frequently monitor the level of consciousness, and the ability to move and feel the limbs, and void spontaneously.

An arthrocentesis may be performed for diagnostic or treatment purposes. A sample of synovial fluid is withdrawn and sent to the laboratory for analysis. Clients with rheumatoid arthritis usually have copious synovial fluid that contains antibodies and white blood cells that are characteristic of inflammatory disease. If the joint swells excessively, some fluid can be removed to alleviate discomfort. Instruct the client that this test is usually done in the physician's office, in a clinic, or at the bedside. The injection site is locally anesthetized before the larger aspirating needle is inserted. After the aspiration, apply pressure until fluid leakage subsides.

In a healthy person, calcium and phosphorus have an inverse relationship, meaning that when the serum calcium level decreases, phosphorus increases, and vice versa. Bone disease and parathyroid dysfunction can cause alterations in this relationship.

Alkaline phosphatase is an enzyme that tends to increase when bone or the liver is damaged. Increases in serum levels reflect an increase in osteoblastic (bone-building) activity.

When skeletal muscles are damaged or diseased, serum muscle enzymes typically increase, including skeletal muscle creatine kinase, lactate dehydrogenase, aspartate aminotransferase, and aldolase. Muscle trauma, polymyositis, and muscular dystrophy commonly cause increased serum muscle enzymes.

FOCUSED ASSESSMENT FOR *IMPAIRED PHYSICAL MOBILITY*

Nursing assessment includes interpreting data to select appropriate nursing diagnoses. A client has *Impaired physical mobility* when there is a limited ability to physically move. If the client has a prolonged impairment, complications of immobility may occur (see Chapter 33).

Defining Characteristics. Defining characteristics for the nursing diagnosis *Impaired physical mobility* include the following:

- Postural instability while performing ADLs
- Limited ability to perform gross or fine motor skills, uncoordinated or jerky movements, limited range of motion, or difficulty turning
- Decreased reaction time
- Slowed movement or movement-induced shortness of breath or tremor
- Gait changes (such as decreased walk speed, difficulty initiating gait, small steps, shuffling of feet, exaggerated lateral postural sway)
- Substitutions for movement (such as increased attention to other's activity, controlling behavior, focus on activities that occurred before the illness or disability)

A client's inability to move includes bed mobility, transfers from bed to chair, and ambulation. Assessing a client's ability to move and perform ADLs is referred to as a *functional assessment.* Several functional assessment tools can be used to determine a client's functional level. A very simple classification system is often used to designate the functional status. This system rates the client's functional ability from a 0 (completely independent) to a 4 (dependent and does not participate in activity). Box 32-2 illustrates the effects of impaired mobility on the life of one person.

Some clients may be able to move but are reluctant to do so because of pain or discomfort, fear of falling, or fear that they will dislodge or disrupt equipment being used in their care, such as intravenous therapy. Reassure the client that the pain can be controlled and should not be tolerated. If equipment and lines are the concern, secure them so they will not kink, become dislodged, or disconnect.

Diseases such as arthritis and trauma such as fractures limit ROM in synovial joints, which reduces the client's ability to move and perform ADLs. ROM is also limited in clients with contractures.

Prolonged immobility can cause muscle atrophy that then worsens the immobility. Neuromuscular diseases, such as Parkinson's disease, muscular dystrophy, and amyotrophic lateral sclerosis, are characterized by muscle atrophy and subsequent decreased muscle strength. Clients with these disorders often experience respiratory failure because of muscle fatigue.

Spinal cord injuries disrupt nervous system communication between the brain and peripheral muscles. A cervical or high thoracic injury (quadriplegia) spares the lower motor neurons, so reflex activity remains intact. The skeletal muscles below the injury are **spastic,** that is, they contract by reflex activity rather than by central nervous system control.

Injuries occurring in the lower thoracic or lumbosacral spine may result in paraplegia. The lower motor neurons, or reflex arcs, are damaged and the client's muscles are **flaccid**—the state of being weak, soft, and flabby, lacking normal muscle tone, or having no ability to contract. Flaccid muscles tend to atrophy and decrease in mass more quickly than spastic muscles.

Related Factors. Factors related to the diagnosis *Impaired physical mobility* include the following:

- Medications

BOX 32-2

A Patient's Perspective

"Fortunately, I Had Nurses and Therapists Who Took Time to Get to Know Me"

As a medic tending the wounded, I saw the ravages of World War II up close. One day I was treating three or four wounded men in a trench when an enemy mortar shell scored a direct hit. My right leg was gone; my left leg and arm were shredded by shrapnel, which also tore through my spine. If the shrapnel hadn't seared the arteries in my legs, I would have bled to death then and there. My first thought was, "There go my dreams: college, a career in professional basketball, marriage, everything I'd hoped for. I was right about basketball but wrong about everything else."

The first year at home was the hardest, like a dark tunnel, wondering what the future had in store, wanting to be as independent as possible—so much to learn. Fortunately, I had nurses and therapists who took time to get to know me before prescribing just how I should achieve maximum independence. They listened. They understood my disability and the limits it imposed. They tried to get me to do as much as possible for myself but didn't push me too hard or too fast. You need to go at your own speed in learning about assisted living. Each person is different. I'm living proof that with the right care and therapy, the body can rebuild itself marvelously.

The beautiful black-haired girl I was engaged to still wanted to marry me, disabilities and all. We've been together 53 years now. She's the greatest thing that ever happened to me. With her love and support, I completed a 2-year business college course in accounting and worked as an accountant for a trucking company until 1948, when the poor circulation in my legs and my spinal problems made it impossible to work at a desk job.

From day one, the VA (Veterans Administration) system has done wonders for me, both in the hospital and out. Whatever I needed for assisted living—wheelchairs, prosthetic legs—they've provided. With the support of the VA, I designed my own house with everything on one level and totally accessible. The sidewalks are 48 inches wide so I can go outside, work in the garden, or do projects in my woodworking shop. I've made furniture, cabinets—you name it, I've made it.

Fifty years with a disability have taught me a lot. Probably the most important lesson is that attitude is everything. How you perceive and respond to your situation has a tremendous influence on your life—your physical, emotional, and spiritual well-being.

I've had a wonderful life: marriage to the woman I love, two sons, eight grandchildren, and, just last week, our first great-grandson. Because I've been so blessed, I enjoy giving to others, especially people who are just learning to live with disabilities. Until 2 years ago, I did chaplaincy work in nursing homes and hospitals.

- Prescribed movement restrictions or lack of knowledge about the value of physical activity
- Discomfort, intolerance to activity, reluctance to initiate movement, limited cardiovascular endurance, or decreased strength and endurance
- Body mass index above the age-appropriate 75th percentile
- Sensoriperceptual, neuromuscular, or musculoskeletal impairments; cognitive impairment; pain
- Depression, anxiety, lack of physical or social environmental supports
- Decreased muscle strength, control, or mass; joint stiffness or contractures
- Sedentary lifestyle, disuse, or deconditioning
- Selective or generalized malnutrition, altered cellular metabolism
- Loss of integrity of bone structures
- Developmental delay
- Cultural beliefs regarding age-appropriate activity

Many chronic diseases, such as coronary artery disease, chronic respiratory disorders, terminal cancer, and neuromuscular diseases, can cause decreased muscle strength and endurance. Assess muscle strength using the Lovett scale, or suggest a physical therapy evaluation to assess individual muscle groups.

Older adults may have decreased muscle strength and impaired mobility because of the combined effects of the aging process, reduced overall activity level, and coexisting health problems that limit mobility. See Box 32-3 for evidence-based guidelines for assessing physical mobility of older adults.

Acute or chronic pain may prevent a person from moving a part or all of the body. Assess the type, nature, duration, and location of pain as discussed in Chapter 37. Repositioning the client, providing massage, or enhancing imagery may help relieve pain and promote mobility. For more severe pain, administer a prescribed analgesic and evaluate its effectiveness.

Action Alert! **For clients who cannot verbalize complaints of pain, especially older adults who have dementia or delirium, use nonverbal cues, such as moaning, crying, or restlessness, to assess their pain level. Anticipate the need for pain relief interventions, including medication.**

Neuromuscular or musculoskeletal impairments may be acute and reversible or chronic and disabling. In addition to the chronic spinal cord injuries, stroke, and neuromuscular diseases described earlier, clients may experience acute problems that temporarily decrease mobility. Fractures or other soft tissue injuries are common examples of acute musculoskeletal impairments. When these injuries heal, the client usually returns to baseline activity level.

Clients with dementia, as in late-stage Alzheimer's disease, experience *Impaired physical mobility* and usually die as a result of complications of immobility. The client forgets how to perform ADLs and ambulate.

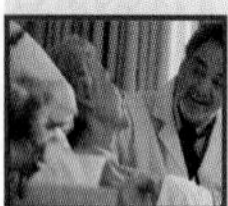

In the case study, Mrs. Lasauskas had been living independently in an assisted living residence. Why might you expect her to be confused immediately after surgery? Did surgery cause her confusion?

FOCUSED ASSESSMENT FOR *ACTIVITY INTOLERANCE*

Activity intolerance results when a client has insufficient physiological or psychological energy to endure or complete a desired activity. It is evidenced when the client reports fatigue, weakness, or dizziness, experiences abnormal vital signs or electrocardiographic (ECG) changes, or has exertional discomfort or dyspnea during or after the activity. If a client has *Activity intolerance,* health care professionals tend to document that the client did not "tolerate" the activity. If the client was able to tolerate the activity without the fatigue or abnormal vital signs or ECG changes, the documentation may be summarized as "tolerated well."

Action Alert! The term *tolerated well* is a vague judgment. Use a more specific description, such as "walked 50 feet without changes in vital signs, shortness of breath, fatigue, or weakness." This provides a clear benchmark against which to compare future activity.

Defining Characteristics. Before asking clients to perform any activity, question whether they are tired or weak. Fatigue or weakness can have a number of causes, including pain, hypoxia, fluid and electrolyte imbalances, and decreased muscle tone and strength. During the activity, major defining characteristics are dizziness or increased fatigue or weakness; discontinue the activity if necessary. At 3 minutes after an activity, defining characteristics are dizziness, dyspnea, exertional fatigue, respirations greater than 24 per minute, and pulse greater than 95 beats per minute (Carpenito-Moyet, 2006).

Some clients with coronary artery disease or respiratory disease are particularly likely to experience changes in heart rate or electrocardiogram recording during ADLs or after a physical therapy plan of care. Other signs of concern would be confusion and pallor or cyanosis.

Clients experiencing pain may have increased discomfort during activity. Evaluate the change in the client's pain level, and discontinue the activity if indicated. Clients with respiratory or coronary artery disease may experience exertional dyspnea during activity. Assess the client before, during, and after the activity for changes in breathing pattern or rate.

Related Factors. Prolonged immobility due to chronic disease or severe injury leads to generalized weakness and subsequent *Activity intolerance.* These clients need to be out of bed and moved as much as possible. Assess changes in muscle tone and joint ROM.

All body tissues require oxygen. When an oxygen deficit occurs or the demand for oxygen exceeds available oxygen, fatigue develops and vital signs change. If the oxygen deficit is severe, ECG changes can occur. For clients with cardiovascular or respiratory problems, use a pulse oximeter to check for oxygen saturation before, during, and after activity. Arterial blood gases provide additional information about oxygenation (see Chapter 34).

BOX 32-3 *Evidence-Based Practice*

Assessing Physical Mobility of Older Adults

Problem: Physical mobility is primarily dependent upon physical strength and endurance, cognitive abilities and motivation, illness, and environment. Sometimes older adults may not have the ability to be physically independent because of alterations in any of these factors. The nurse needs to know how to provide safe, effective, comprehensive care to older clients with deficits affecting alterations in mobility.

Evidence

The guideline *Assessment of function: Of critical importance to acute care of older adults* was developed for nurses by a group of nursing experts from across the country as part of the Nurses Improving Care for Health System Elders (NICHE) project, under sponsorship of The John A. Hartford Foundation Institute for Geriatric Nursing. The method used to collect or select evidence was by searches of Medline, an electronic database. Thirty-seven source documents were used. The method used to assess the quality and strength of the evidence was by expert consensus.

Application to Practice

The objectives of the guideline were the following:

- To identify physical functioning as an important clinical indicator of health/illness, response to treatment, and need for services
- To describe common components of standardized functional assessment instruments
- To identify unique challenges to gathering information from older adults regarding functional assessments
- To assist bedside nurses in monitoring function in elders, preventing decline, and maintaining the function of elders during acute hospitalization

The guideline can be found at http://www.guideline.gov/summary/summary.aspx?ss=15&doc_id=3504&nbr=2730.

Reference

Kresevic, D. M., & Mezey, M. (2003). Assessment of function. In M. Mezey, T. Fulmer, I. Abraham, & D. A. Zwicker (Eds.). *Geriatric nursing protocols for best practice* (2nd ed., pp. 31-46). New York: Springer Publishing [18 references].

DIAGNOSIS

IMPAIRED PHYSICAL MOBILITY AND *ACTIVITY INTOLERANCE*

When caring for a client with musculoskeletal, neuromuscular, or neurological problems, analyze the assessment data to identify which nursing diagnoses will guide your care. If clients are at risk for any of the diagnoses, add *Risk for* at the beginning of the diagnosis—for example, *Risk for activity intolerance.*

Also identify the related factors for actual nursing diagnoses and the risk factors for potential diagnoses. For example, clients with back injury have *Pain related to muscle spasms.* But they may also be at *Risk for impaired physical mobility related to pain,* depending on how severe the back injury is. The related factors or risk factors also aid in goal development and help guide nursing interventions.

RELATED DIAGNOSES

Clients with either *Impaired physical mobility* or *Activity intolerance* often have additional nursing diagnoses. Assess the client comprehensively.

Clients who cannot bathe, dress, groom, toilet, or feed themselves will have *Self-care deficit* in one or more functional areas. Clients experiencing neurological, neuromuscular, or musculoskeletal health problems are often unable to move and therefore cannot perform ADLs independently. Perform functional assessments periodically to determine clients' progress in achieving independence, if possible. Do your best to consider each client's situation with an open mind, no matter how difficult the circumstances.

Immobile clients are at a high risk for pressure ulcers, especially over bony prominences, and the nursing diagnosis *Risk for impaired skin integrity* may apply. Thin, emaciated, and poorly nourished clients are at the highest risk of any group. Assess the skin for reddened areas. Assess nutritional status, especially laboratory indicators such as serum albumin, prealbumin, and transferrin. When these indicators are decreased, the client has inadequate protein stores to prevent or heal tissue breakdown.

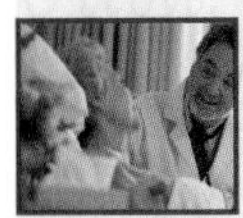

Mrs. Lasauskas is a petite woman, weighing 102 pounds. What preventive measures should you use to help prevent skin breakdown after her surgery?

Exercise, hydration, and fiber are necessary to prevent *Constipation.* Clients who are immobile cannot exercise and often have an inadequate intake of food and water. Assess intake, especially intake of dietary fiber and fluids. Older adult clients are particularly prone to decreased peristalsis and constipation. Monitor bowel habits and the consistency of stools.

The inactive client is at risk for deterioration of all body systems, sometimes referred to as disuse syndrome or complications of immobility. For these clients, the diagnosis *Risk for disuse syndrome* may apply. Assess every body system for possible complications or risk of complications. Chapter 33 discusses disuse syndrome in detail.

The client with osteoporosis may have *Risk for injury* from falls and fractures. Anemia often contributes to the risk. In addition, the client is at risk for thromboembolic complications.

As described earlier, clients with musculoskeletal trauma or conditions that increase peripheral compartment pressure are at high risk for neurovascular compromise, and the nursing diagnosis *Risk for peripheral neurovascular dysfunction* may apply. Monitor clients frequently for this potentially serious complication.

Musculoskeletal injury, surgery, or disease can be very painful, so you will need to assess for acute pain in a client with an injury, such as a fracture, or surgical repair of an injury. For these clients, the nursing diagnosis *Acute pain* may apply. Clients with chronic joint diseases such as degenerative or rheumatoid arthritis experience chronic pain, which is often difficult to control. For these clients, the diagnosis *Chronic pain* may apply.

Clients who have chronic musculoskeletal, neuromuscular, or neurological health problems may feel hopeless when they are unable to move or care for themselves. They depend on others for care and often feel that they are a burden to their families and significant others. This sense of hopelessness can result in clinical depression or suicide. Assess the client's response to illness, and identify clients at risk for *Hopelessness.*

Table 32-5 shows examples of clustering data to arrive at appropriate nursing diagnoses.

PLANNING

Once the nursing diagnoses have been determined, think about what client outcomes can be expected. To the extent possible, outcomes should be individualized, measurable, and realistic. For the client with *Impaired physical mobility,* the overall goal is to improve mobility and prevent complications of immobility. For the client who has *Activity intolerance,* the goal is to improve endurance and tolerance to activities.

EXPECTED OUTCOMES FOR THE CLIENT WITH *IMPAIRED PHYSICAL MOBILITY*

Improvement in mobility depends on several factors. First, try to determine whether the mobility deficit is permanent or temporary. A severed spinal cord results in permanent paralysis below the level of injury. Therefore expecting the client to walk is not likely. However, expecting the client to be able to move about in a wheel-

Table 32-5 Clustering Data to Make a Nursing Diagnosis

DATA CLUSTER	DIAGNOSIS
Mobility Problems	
An older adult woman who fell, resulting in a fractured hip; history of previous stroke with hemiparesis; cries out when moved; degenerative arthritis in both knees	*Impaired physical mobility* related to muscle weakness, severe pain, and joint degeneration
A 12-year-old girl with rheumatoid arthritis; uses a walker to ambulate short distances but relies on wheelchair most of the time; becomes very fatigued when walking; takes two to three naps each day	*Activity intolerance* related to generalized weakness and fatigue
An older adult woman with acute vertebral compression fractures; complains of severe pain when moved; heart rate 120 beats per minute and weak; blood pressure 180/90 mm Hg	*Acute pain* related to muscle spasm and nerve impairment
A 53-year-old woman, first day after total abdominal hysterectomy; requires morphine for pain control; blood pressure low for her	*Activity intolerance* related to pain after surgery and cardiovascular instability

chair may be very realistic. The client with a total knee replacement is expected to walk with a walker or cane within a few days after surgery. This client's physical mobility impairment is temporary.

Second, look at the causes or related factors that could be managed or resolved. For example, if the client cannot move because of pain and discomfort, then interventions directed at pain relief should improve physical mobility.

Third, assess the client's willingness to participate in the treatment plan. If exercises are expected to increase muscle strength and endurance, the client must be willing and able to exercise as prescribed.

The outcomes that might be expected for the client with a permanent impairment in mobility may include the following:

- Moves independently in a wheelchair
- Transfers independently from the bed to chair and vice versa using a sliding board
- Performs ADLs independently using assistive or adaptive devices
- Maintains intact skin, especially over bony prominences
- Drinks at least 2000 mL of fluid daily to prevent constipation and renal or urinary calculi
- Demonstrates passive and active ROM exercise techniques

Possible expected outcomes for a client with a temporary or less severe impairment in mobility may include the following:

- Ambulates independently in home using a walker, crutches, or cane
- Maintains optimal joint function
- Performs ADLs independently
- States that pain is reduced or relieved

Each long-term outcome can be broken into progressive stages. For example, for the postoperative client with a total knee replacement, a realistic intermediate outcome is to walk in the hospital room using a walker. By discharge from the rehabilitation program several weeks later, the client is expected to walk up and down stairs using the walker or cane.

EXPECTED OUTCOMES FOR THE CLIENT WITH *ACTIVITY INTOLERANCE*

The major expected outcome for *Activity intolerance* is that the client tolerates activity without evidence of dizziness, fatigue or weakness, abnormal vital signs, ECG changes, or exertional discomfort or dyspnea.

INTERVENTION

Interventions to promote mobility and improve activity intolerance are interrelated. Mobility skills cannot improve unless the client can tolerate the interventions that are directed toward building tolerance. Therefore interventions for *Activity intolerance* are discussed first.

You will collaborate with members of the interdisciplinary team, including rehabilitation nurses, physical therapists (PTs), occupational therapists (OTs), and physicians, when planning and implementing these interventions. The rehabilitation team is discussed in Chapter 44. Regardless of whether your client is being treated by rehabilitation services, you must still carry out interventions that help the client achieve the expected outcomes.

INTERVENTIONS TO IMPROVE ACTIVITY TOLERANCE

Interventions for improving activity tolerance center around building muscle mass and strength while managing other causes of activity intolerance, such as pain and discomfort.

Building Muscle Mass and Strength. A structured, consistent exercise program is started as soon as the client is medically stable. Several types of exercise may be used to build muscle mass and strength, including isometric, isotonic, and isokinetic exercises.

Isometric exercise (Figure 32-6, *A*) is a form of active exercise that increases muscle tension by applying pressure against stable resistance. Isometric contractions can be accomplished by opposing different muscles in the same person. There is no joint movement and the length of the muscle remains unchanged, but the tone and strength are maintained or increased. They are also called static or setting exercises. Ask the client to tighten certain muscle groups without moving the adjacent joints. These exercises are particularly helpful for strengthening leg, hip, and abdominal muscles. Clients who have lower extremity musculoskeletal surgery, such as hip and knee replacements, are taught how to do "quad setting" exercises. Ask the client to tighten the quadriceps muscles and hold for a few seconds. Then repeat this exercise about 10 times in a set at least twice a day.

Isometric exercises also may increase heart rate and cardiac workload, especially if clients tense the entire body and close the glottis (increasing intrathoracic pressure) during muscle-setting exercises. Supervise clients with cardiac or vascular disease to ensure that they breathe during these exercises; also be aware that blood flow to other parts of the body is not increased with these exercises. In addition, these exercises are not helpful in preventing contractures because joints do not move.

Isotonic exercise (Figure 32-6, *B*) is a form of active exercise in which the muscle contracts and moves. There is no significant change in the resistance, so the force of the contraction remains constant. Isotonic exercise has the advantage of increasing cardiopulmonary function and blood flow, preventing contractures, and building muscle mass and strength. These dynamic exercises involve muscle contraction and muscle shortening. Examples of isotonic exercises performed in a hospital are straight leg raises after hip or knee surgery. Swimming, walking, and cycling are examples of isotonic exercises that the client can do independently to continue the physical conditioning of muscles. These exercises are sometimes referred to as *isokinetic* (Figure 32-6, *C*) because they are dynamic exercises performed at a constant velocity.

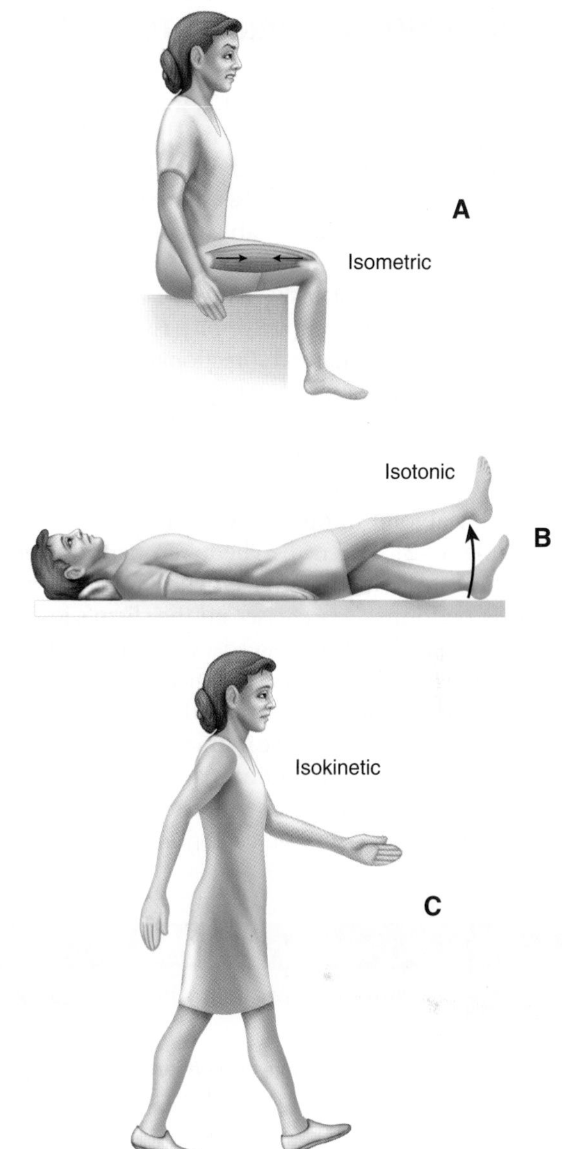

FIGURE 32-6 Three types of exercise: **A,** Isometric. **B,** Isotonic. **C,** Isokinetic.

Mobilizing the Client Progressively. When a client experiences an acute musculoskeletal or neurological health problem, recovery may be gradual. Being confined to bed for more than a day can cause generalized weakness. Anesthesia during surgery also causes weakness and fatigue, sometimes for several weeks after surgery. Infections and other illnesses also deplete the client's energy.

Therefore you will want to slowly build the client's activity tolerance level. For instance, before a client gets out of bed for the first time, raise the head of bed slowly and have him or her sit on the side of the bed with legs dangling. The client may be able to tolerate only this simple activity the first time. Once the client tolerates dangling, help the client transfer from bed to chair. Each time the client gets out of bed, increase the activity, so that eventually the client can walk a few steps.

> ***Action Alert!*** Monitor the client for vital sign changes, fatigue, and exertional discomfort or dyspnea before, during, and after each activity. If the client's heart is monitored, look for ECG changes. Discontinue the activity immediately if any of these changes occur, and notify the physician.

Controlling Pain and Discomfort. If pain occurs before, during, or after an activity, the client may be reluctant to increase the activity level or even perform the same activity again. Before the client gets out of bed or goes for therapy, administer pain medication or provide other appropriate pain-relief measures. Check with your physical therapy department, however, because heavy sedation could prevent client participation in the treatment plan. In some instances, physical therapists do not want clients to have medication because pain is used as an indicator that the client needs to discontinue treatment for that session.

INTERVENTIONS TO PROMOTE MOBILITY

You and the therapist are responsible for promoting mobility, including ADLs. The goal is that the client will be as independent as possible by hospital discharge. Maintaining or improving joint mobility helps with transfer and ambulation skills. Alternative methods for promoting mobility are available to those who can make use of them, as outlined in Box 32-4.

Maintaining Joint Mobility. **Range-of-motion exercises** include any body action (active or passive) involving the muscles, joints, and natural directional movements, such as abduction, extension, flexion, pronation, and rotation. They are the most important interventions to promote and maintain joint mobility. ROM exercises are isotonic exercises in which the client or health care provider moves each synovial joint through its complete range of motion (see Table 32-2). When the client can perform the exercises, they are termed active. When you or the physical therapist performs the exercises on the client's joints, they are termed passive. These exercises also prevent contractures and help build activity tolerance.

If the clients can move, teach them how to perform active ROM exercises. They can move each joint through its range of motion several times a day independently. If they cannot move or exercise their own joints, perform passive ROM exercises for each joint as described in Procedure 32-1. If the clients can assist you, the ROM exercises are called active-assistive.

Action Alert! Follow these safety guidelines when putting a joint through its range of motion:

- Position the bed at an appropriate height to maintain good body mechanics.
- Support the limb being moved, above and below the joint.
- Do not force the joint into any position.
- Move the body part smoothly and slowly, observing the client for discomfort and listening for crepitus.

Assisting With Movement. If clients are strong enough, teach them how to get out of bed independently, as described in Box 32-5. Otherwise you will need to provide assistance. When assisting clients, be sure to use appropriate assistive devices to prevent musculoskeletal injury to yourself, those assisting you, or the client.

Transferring the Client. If clients cannot transfer independently, you will need to assist them. Always remember to use good body mechanics and use a lateral transfer or lift device. At least two people are needed to move a client who cannot help with the transfer. Also, if the client is obese or has multiple pieces of equipment, seek extra help.

Transferring From Bed to Chair. A client may need assistance transferring from the bed to a regular chair, wheelchair, or bedside commode. Transfer belts pro-

BOX 32-4 Considering the Alternatives
Alternatives for Restoring Physical Mobility

Tai Chi

Tai chi is a system of postures linked by elegant and graceful movements, whose purpose is to balance energies within the body.

Advantages

Enhances functional mobility and regulatory T-cell function (Yeh, Chuang, Lin, Hsiao, & Eng, 2006)
As an exercise, has side benefit of improving depression
Potential cardiovascular benefit because it is a form of exercise

Disadvantages

May require weeks to see benefits
Requires instruction to begin
May delay traditional therapy

Trager Therapy

Trager is a type of massage that uses gentle rocking motions.

Advantages

May be perceived as less stressful by client than exercise
Inhibits the evoked stretch responses, allowing increased mobility (Duval et al., 2002)
Can be performed on clients who cannot move themselves

Disadvantages

Does not include strengthening of muscles because it is not an exercise
May delay traditional therapy
Some people may not want to be touched

Exercise Plus Motivation

Advantages

Twice the improvement in disability scores as exercise alone (Friedrich, Gitler, Arendasy, & Friedrich, 2005)
Fewer side effects than medications
Involves clients directly in their recovery

Disadvantages

Requires additional effort by practitioners
May postpone traditional therapies
Requires active participation by clients

Duval, C., Lafontaine, D., Hebert, J., Leroux, A., Panisset, M., & Boucher, J. P. (2002). The effect of Trager therapy on the level of evoked stretch responses in patients with Parkinson's disease and rigidity. *Journal of Manipulative and Physiological Therapeutics, 25*(7), 455-464.
Friedrich, M., Gittler, G., Arendasy, M., & Friedrich, K. M. (2005). Long-term effect of a combined exercise and motivational program on the level of disability of patients with chronic low back pain. *Spine, 30*(9), 995-1000.
Yeh, S. H., Chuang, H., Lin, W. L., Hsiao, C. Y., & Eng, H. L. (2006). Regular tai chi chuan exercise enhances functional mobility and CD4CD25 regulatory T cells. *British Journal of Sports Medicine, 40*(3), 239-243.

TIME TO ALLOW: NOVICE: 15-30 min. EXPERT: 15-30 min.

PROCEDURE 32-1 PERFORMING RANGE-OF-MOTION EXERCISES

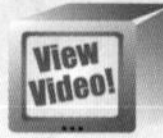

Range-of-motion (ROM) exercises maintain joint flexibility and movement when the client is unable to move or is confined to bed. They also stimulate circulation and relax the body. ROM exercises may be full, which includes all the joints, or for selected joints. ROM will not maintain or improve strength. You need to be familiar with the normal range of motion for each joint. Complications could include pain or joint injury if done too vigorously.

DELEGATION GUIDELINES

Following assessment of your client's functional status and joint mobility, you may delegate the performance of ROM exercises to a nursing assistant who has received special training in the performance of this skill. Provide special instructions outlining those observations and findings that should be reported to you immediately.

EQUIPMENT NEEDED

- Bath blanket to cover the body other than the part being exercised
- Pillows for positioning

1 Perform preliminary actions (see inside front cover).

2 Explain the procedure to the client, and assess the client's ability to assist with the exercises. *If the client can assist or can perform the exercises independently, active-assistive or active ROM can be performed rather than passive ROM.*

3 If moving the joints of the entire body through their ROM, use a head-to-toe approach (see Table 32-2). *This approach helps to organize the intervention so that all joints are moved through their range of motion.*

4 Support the client's body part by cradling or cupping above and below the joint being moved (see illustration). *Supporting the joint prevents injury and stress on the joint and also promotes client comfort.*

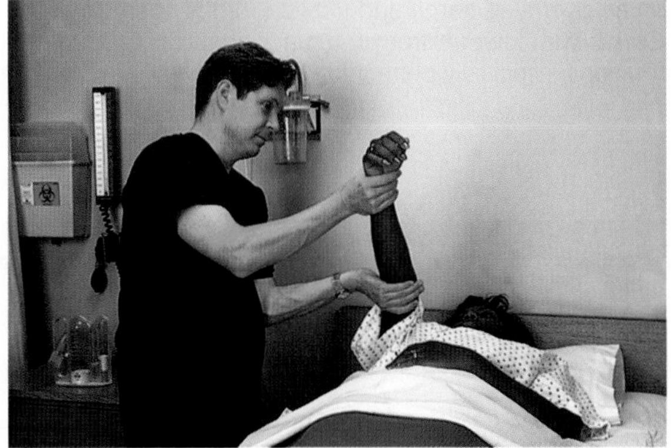

Step 4. Supporting the body part above and below the joint being moved.

5 Put the joint through its complete ROM, but do not force it beyond where it will move comfortably. *Complete ROM of each joint is beneficial in preventing contractures, maintaining joint flexibility, and building muscle tone.*

6 Throughout the exercises, observe the client for tolerance, including pulse rate and discomfort, if any. Do not exercise to the point of producing pain. *If the client cannot tolerate the exercises, discontinue them immediately.*

HINTS

Use slow, smooth movements. Move joint only to the point where you feel resistance. Stop if you reach the point of pain. Assess for fatigue. Finish with the joint in good alignment. Check physician's instructions about the number of sets and repetitions. A typical protocol is four sets daily, with five repetitions for each joint.

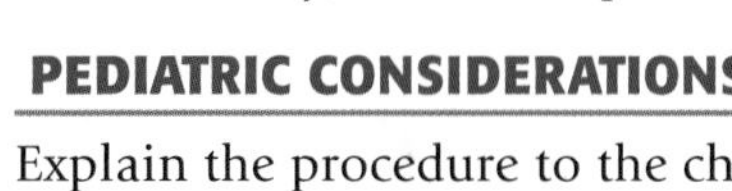

PEDIATRIC CONSIDERATIONS

Explain the procedure to the child using age-appropriate language. Teach ROM exercises to caregivers as part of the routine care for a client who has mobility limitations.

GERIATRIC CONSIDERATIONS

Use caution when performing ROM exercises in older adults to avoid injury. Do not exercise past the point of resistance.

HOME HEALTH CARE CONSIDERATIONS

ROM exercises should be taught to family caregivers as part of the routine care for a client who has mobility limitations. The family may need help to make ROM part of all activities rather than trying to make room in a crowded schedule for several ROM sessions.

vide extra security during a transfer. Procedure 32-2 describes how to help a client from a bed to a chair with or without a transfer belt. This procedure assumes that the client is strong enough to help you with the transfer.

For clients who are totally immobile and unable to assist with the transfer, use a mechanical lift device, as seen in Procedure 32-3. The sling used in the lift remains under the client at all times. Position the client in the chair in proper alignment using pillows and bath blankets for support. Be sure that the client's feet are supported by the footrest and that all necessary items are within reach, including the call light.

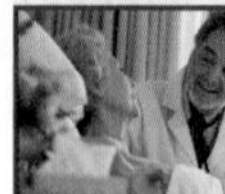

The physician wants Mrs. Lasauskas out of bed in a chair on the first full postoperative day. Given her weakness, hemiparesis, and pain, what transfer technique would you use? How many people should be used to transfer her?

Newer types of lift devices include ceiling-mounted lifts and floor-based air lifts (Nelson et al., 2004). Ceiling mounted lifts increase available floor space during the transfer and allow nurses easier access to the client. Air lifts use separately inflated air chambers to lift a client from the floor to bed or stretcher, such as after a fall.

BOX 32-5

Teaching for Self-Care

Getting Out of Bed Independently

Purpose: To promote client independence in transfer skills, which has the added benefits of increasing mobility, maintaining muscle tone and endurance, and increasing self-esteem.

Expected Outcome: The client will transfer from bed to chair independently.

Client Instructions

- If you have an electric bed, put the bed in its lowest position.
- Raise the head of the bed if needed to decrease the distance to a sitting position.
- Turn onto your side. (If you are stronger on one side than the other, turn toward the stronger side.)

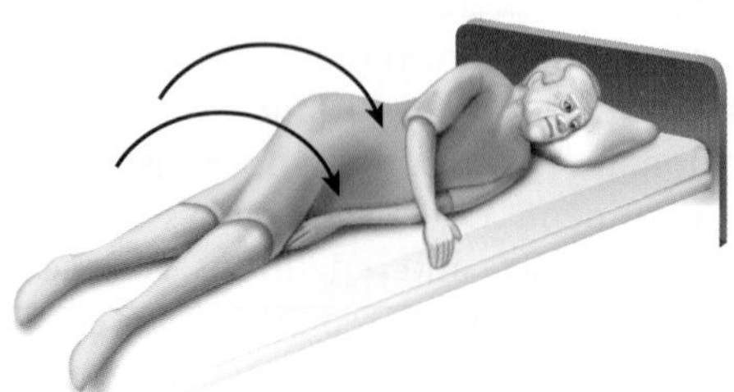

- Push against the mattress with either your elbows or hands to raise your upper body off the bed.

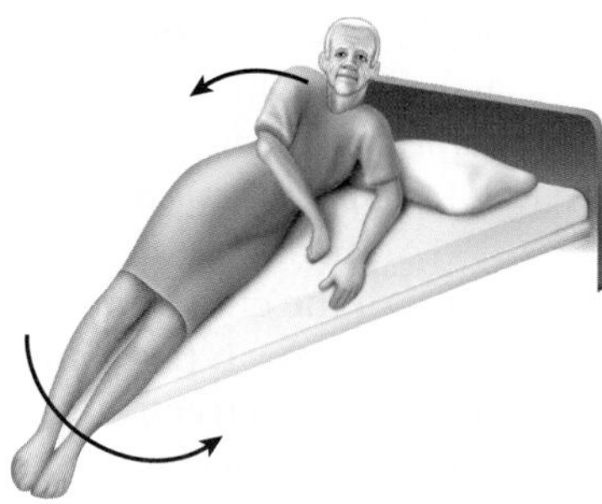

- Once you are in a sitting position, let your legs dangle for a moment over the side of the bed. This will help you get your balance and make sure you are not dizzy.
- If you are not dizzy, go ahead and stand up.

Hint: If the client is too weak to push up from the bed, set up an overhead frame and trapeze for the client to pull on. Clients with lower-extremity trauma or surgery, including amputations, especially benefit from this device.

PROCEDURE 32-2

Time to Allow: Novice: 15 min. **Expert:** 10 min.

HELPING A CLIENT GET OUT OF BED

Nursing Skills Online: Safety, Lesson 3

You can help a client get out of bed with or without a transfer belt. A transfer belt is a woven canvas belt about $2^1/_2$ to 3 inches wide and 6 feet long. It is fastened around the client's waist and secured with a locking device. The belt is used to maintain control of clients when you help them stand, transfer to a chair, or walk. Transferring with a belt is safer and avoids pulling on the arm and shoulder joints.

DELEGATION GUIDELINES

Once you have assessed that the client can stand safely, you may delegate assistance with bed-to-chair transfer to the nursing assistant. The nursing assistant should receive specific instruction in body mechanics and safety concerns related to client mobility. Instruct the nursing assistant to report to you any client complaints of dizziness and any observation of unsteady gait or imbalance.

EQUIPMENT NEEDED

- Transfer belt
- Supportive shoes with rubber soles
- A bathrobe

WITHOUT A TRANSFER BELT

1 Perform preliminary actions (see inside front cover).

2 Place the bed in its lowest position, and raise the head of the bed. *Having the bed in the lowest position is safest in case the client falls. The client can sit up more easily if the head of the bed is up.*

3 Place a chair or wheelchair at a 45-degree angle to the bed. Plan for the client to get out of bed on the stronger side. *Having the client get out of bed on the strong side helps prevent loss of balance and possible falls.*

4 Using good body mechanics, help the client to a full sitting position while swinging the client's legs over the edge of the bed in a single, smooth motion (see illustration). Support the upper body as the client comes to the sitting position. *Moving the client's legs reduces friction or shearing from the sheets while increasing the force of the movement. Supporting the upper body keeps the client from falling backward.*

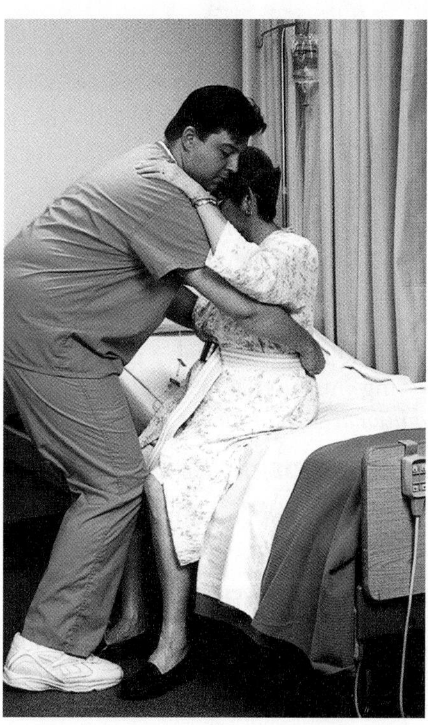

Step 4. Assisting the client to a full sitting position.

5 Support the client in a sitting position on the side of the bed with the feet dangling (see illustration). *Moving from a lying to sitting position can cause postural hypotension, which can lead to dizziness and a subsequent fall unless the client has time to gather equilibrium.*

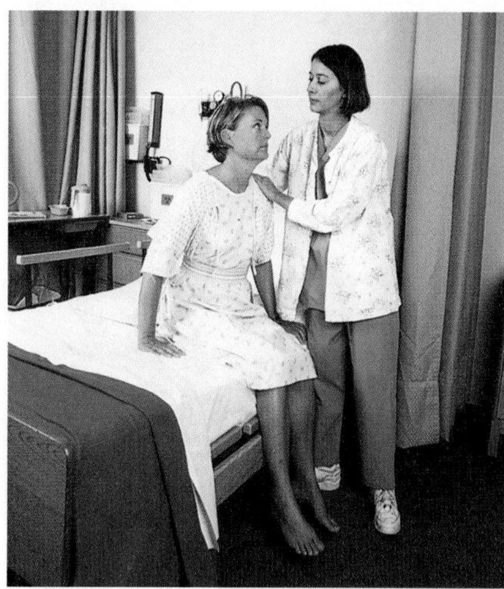

Step 5. Supporting the client in a sitting position.

6 If the client is able, have the client place his or her hands on your shoulders or on the mattress on either side of the body. *When you help the client stand, the client can assist you by balancing against your shoulders while using the leg muscles to stand or by pushing off the mattress with the hands.*

7 Place your hands under the client's arms. Place your knees in front of the client's knees, and help the client rise to a standing position (see illustration). *Keeping your knees against the client's knees prevents them from buckling, thus reducing the risk of a fall. Avoid axillary pressure.*

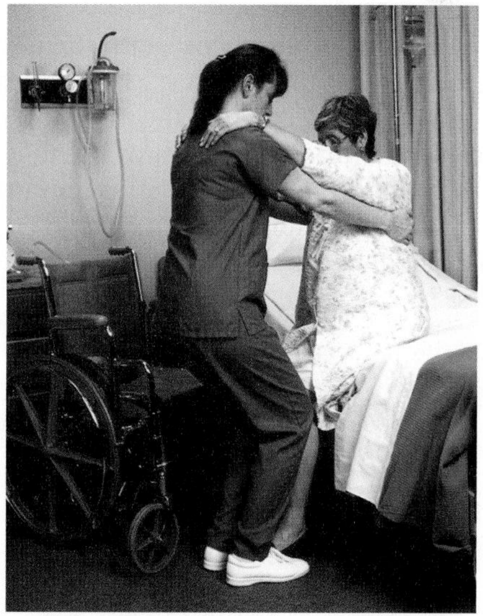

Step 7. Helping the client to a standing position.

8 Pivot with the client toward the chair or wheelchair, being careful not to dislodge equipment or lines (see illustration). *Pivoting prevents twisting your spine and causing injury.*

Continued

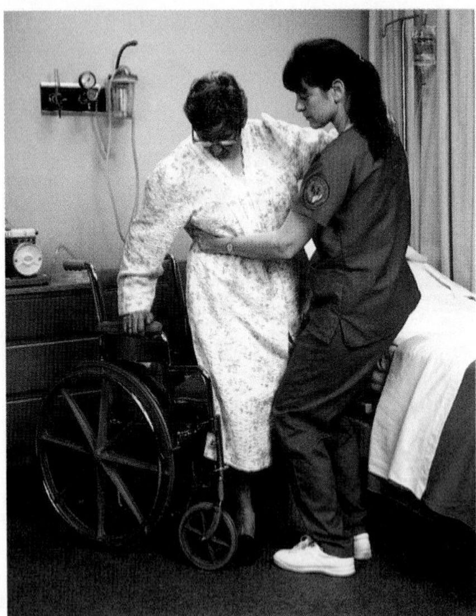

Step 8. Pivoting and turning the client toward the wheelchair.

9 Using good body mechanics, lower the client into the chair or wheelchair slowly and reposition the client in proper body alignment. Make the client as comfortable as possible. *Moving slowly helps prevent dizziness or other discomfort.*

WITH A TRANSFER BELT

1 Place a transfer/gait belt around the client's waist (after completing steps 1 to 5 in the previous section). *The transfer belt allows you to guide the client, and it offers support during the transfer.*

2 Standing in front of the client, grasp the transfer belt on both sides toward the client's back (see illustration). Assess whether the client has the strength to stand. When the client is ready, help him or her to a standing position by rolling your body and arms upward, pulling the client with the transfer belt. *Favoring the client's weaker side helps prevent falls because most clients drift toward, or lose balance on, their weaker side.*

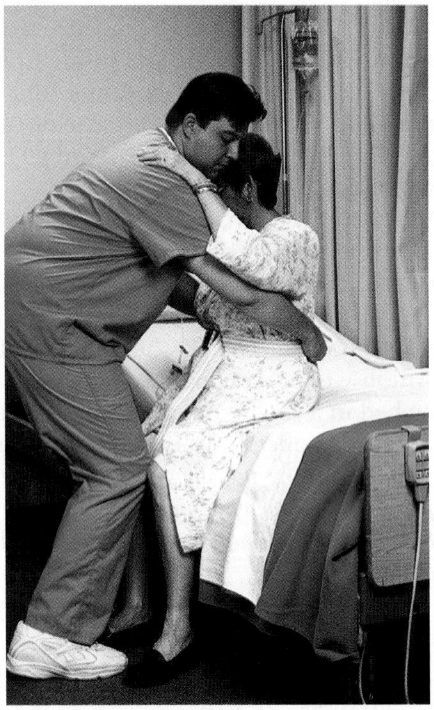

Step 2. Grasping the transfer belt to assist the client to a standing position.

3 Pivot the client toward the chair, and lower the client slowly into it. Ideally, the client will take two or three small steps to get into position to sit. *Pivoting prevents twisting of your spine.*

4 Have the client reach for the armrests, if available, while lowering into the chair. *Holding on to the armrests provides additional support for the client.*

PEDIATRIC CONSIDERATIONS

Use age-appropriate explanations about the procedure. Include family in teaching whenever possible.

GERIATRIC CONSIDERATIONS

Proceed slowly to alleviate any fears related to the procedure. Explain the steps to the client as the procedure progresses.

HOME HEALTH CARE CONSIDERATIONS

Teach family caregivers how to use good body mechanics to prevent back injuries when transferring the client. Most caregivers can be easily taught how to use a transfer belt. If the family cannot transfer the client to a chair, they can rent a mechanical lift or a geriatric chair. The chair reclines, and the feet can be elevated. It also has a tray that fastens on the front for meals and other activities.

PROCEDURE 32-3

TIME TO ALLOW: **NOVICE:** 20 min. **EXPERT:** 15 min.

USING A MECHANICAL LIFT

A mechanical lift uses a hydraulic pump or electric motor to hoist a sling. With the sling around the client, the lift can raise the client off the bed, swing the client into position above a chair, and lower the client while he or she is slowly rolled into the chair. Possible disadvantages are the insecurity clients may feel while suspended in air and the training required to properly use the lift.

DELEGATION GUIDELINES

The use of a mechanical lift for client transfer may be delegated to a nursing assistant who has received training in body mechanics, safety, and the use of this equipment. When reviewing the key aspects of this skill with your assistant, place special emphasis on the client's perception of the experience of being suspended in the air and on protecting the skin from injury.

EQUIPMENT NEEDED

- Mechanical lift
- Bedside chair or wheelchair
- Bath blanket

1 Perform preliminary actions (see inside front cover).

2 Obtain a functioning lift, and move it into the client's room (see illustration). Lock both the bed and chair before beginning. *Make sure that the lift works correctly and safely to prevent accidents. Practice before you take it into the client's room. Locking the bed and chair helps prevents accidents.*

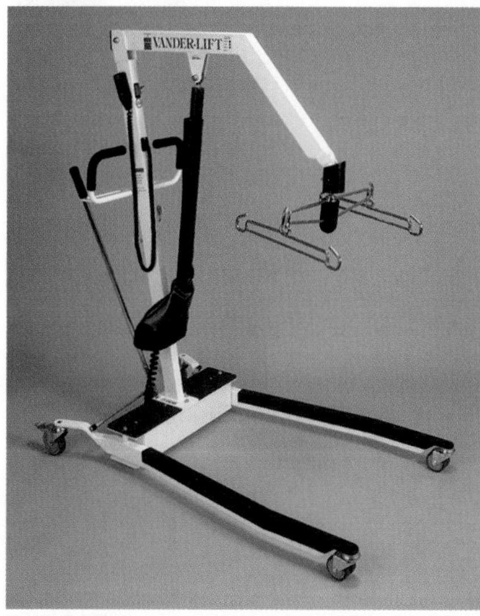

Step 2. Mechanical lift. (Courtesy Vancare, Inc., Aurora, NE.)

3 Place the one- or two-piece sling under the client by turning the client onto the side, placing the sling along the back, and having the client roll onto the sling. Make sure the sling supports the shoulders and buttocks. *Take care not to injure the client's skin with the metal attachments. If the sling is not positioned correctly, the client will not feel secure and may slide out of the sling.*

4 Place the bed in a low position. Securely attach the sling to the lift. Have the client cross the arms across the chest. *Crossing the arms will help prevent injury caused by the client trying to help, thus causing instability of the lift.*

5 Raise the lift to elevate the client enough to clear the bed. *If the client is not completely off the bed, shearing or friction of the skin can result. Promote the client's security by moving slowly and avoiding erratic movements; protect the head if necessary.*

6 Move the lift until the client is aligned with the chair, lock the wheels, release the pressure valve, and lower the client slowly into the chair. *Correct alignment with the chair prevents the client from falling or other injury.*

7 Keep the sling under the client, but position the client into comfortable and functional body alignment. *The sling remains under the client until it is used again to return the client to bed. Disconnect the sling from the lift, and store the lift in a corner out of the way of traffic.*

PEDIATRIC CONSIDERATIONS

This procedure may be unnecessary in very young and lightweight clients. Use age-appropriate explanations about the procedure. Include family in teaching whenever possible.

GERIATRIC CONSIDERATIONS

Proceed slowly to alleviate any fears related to the lift procedure. Explain the steps to the client as the procedure progresses.

HOME HEALTH CARE CONSIDERATIONS

Teach family caregivers how to use the mechanical lift, and help them practice until they are proficient and feel secure before trying to move the client.

Transferring From Bed to Stretcher. Transferring a client from the bed to a stretcher requires at least two people and the use of a lateral transfer device to reduce the risk of harm to both client and health care personnel (Baptiste, Boda, Nelson, Lloyd, & Lee, 2006; Pellino, Owen, Knapp, & Noack, 2006). Lateral transfer devices may be made of a rigid plastic, and the newest ones can be filled with air. Both reduce friction and shear, increasing the safety of the procedure to client and health care personnel. If a lateral transfer device is not available, then you will need to use a turning sheet or drawsheet placed under the client. First, adjust the height of the client's bed to be even with the height of the stretcher. Ensure that the wheels on both the bed and the stretcher are locked. Turn the client, and position the transfer device under the client's sheet or turning sheet. Pull the sheet to slide the client over the transfer device and onto the stretcher in unison. For air transfer devices, follow product literature. Place a pillow under the client's head, pull up the stretcher side rails, fasten the strap around the client, and push the stretcher from the head.

Supporting the Ambulating Client. Some clients cannot ambulate independently and require human or mechanical assistance. The transfer belt serves as the gait or walking belt that you can hold during ambulation. If the client is weaker on one side than the other, stand on the weaker side. The client can also push a portable intravenous pole and use it as an extra support if needed (Procedure 32-4).

If the client starts to fall or faint, support the client and ease him or her to the floor. Make the client as comfortable as possible, and stay with the client until help arrives.

Compensating for Physical Impairments. When human assistance is not available or the client is ready to learn to ambulate independently, assistive devices may be used. If available, a physical therapist will do the initial teaching, but you will need to reinforce the techniques that were taught. Walkers, canes, crutches, and wheelchairs allow independence in ambulation.

Using a Walker. Walkers provide better support than either a cane or crutches (Figure 32-7). They are used most often for older adults who have decreased muscle strength. The standard walker can be adjusted for the client's height so that the hand bar is just below the client's waist and the client's elbows are slightly flexed. The standard walker is used for clients who can bear partial weight, and it must be picked up to be used correctly. Exercises to strengthen the arms are important. For clients who have insufficient arm strength, roller walkers with two or four wheels can be substituted. Some roller walkers have a seat where the client can sit when fatigued.

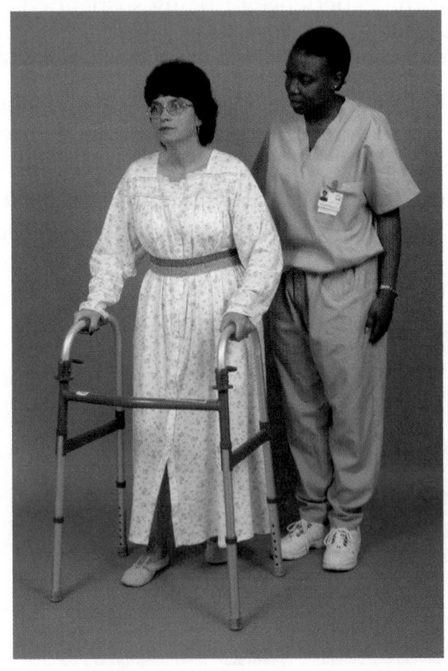

FIGURE 32-7 Client using a walker.

PROCEDURE 32-4

TIME TO ALLOW: NOVICE: 20 min. EXPERT: 10 min.

SUPPORTING THE AMBULATING CLIENT

The first time a client gets out of bed after anesthesia, prolonged illness, or bed rest, assist with ambulation to ensure the client's safety. It is better to be overly cautious by providing assistance than to risk a fall.

DELEGATION GUIDELINES

You may delegate assisting the client with ambulation after your initial assessment of the client's functional status and the client's risk factors for falling. The nursing assistant should receive training in body mechanics, safety, and assisting with mobility.

EQUIPMENT NEEDED

- Comfortable, supportive shoes with rubber soles
- Bathrobe
- Transfer/gait belt

1 Perform preliminary actions (see inside front cover).

2 Apply a gait belt (also called a transfer or walking belt) around the client's waist, and help the client to a standing position as outlined in Procedure 32-2.

3 Stand at the client's side and slightly behind, and walk with the client while holding on to the back of the belt (see illustration). *By holding on to the gait belt while the client is walking, you provide support for the client and you gain some control over ambulation. Grasp the belt from beneath the belt in a manner that will allow you to lift up if the client starts to fall. Your second hand may be used to guide the client's posture to an upright position.*

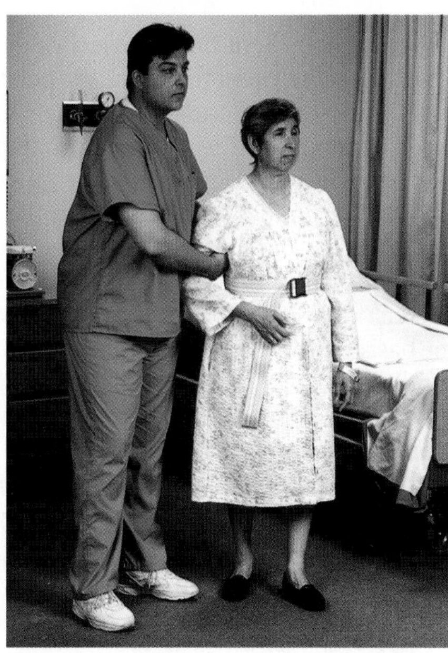

Step 3. Standing at the client's side while holding on to the back of the transfer belt.

4 The client with an intravenous pole can push the pole while walking. *The client with an intravenous line will need a portable rolling pole. However, these poles roll freely and should be used to guide, not to support the client's weight.*

5 If the client is weaker on one side than the other, walk on the weak side while grasping the belt and guiding the client's posture. *The client will tend to lean and could fall toward the weaker side. Remind the client to lean toward the strong side.*

6 If the client is especially weak or this is the first time ambulating, ask another person to walk with you to support the client. If necessary, have another assistant follow with a wheelchair in case the client becomes too weak to stand. *An additional person helps by supporting the client from the opposite side or by moving portable equipment that must go with the client.*

7 If the client starts to fall, do not try to prevent the fall by supporting the weight with your own body. Rather, help the client fall safely, without injury to either of you.

8 As the client starts to fall, move your feet so your stronger leg is somewhat behind you. *This action forms a solid base of support for you and allows you to bear most of the weight on your stronger leg.*

9 At the same time, use the transfer belt to pull the client toward you, allowing the client to slide against you, supported, as you ease him or her to the floor (see illustration).

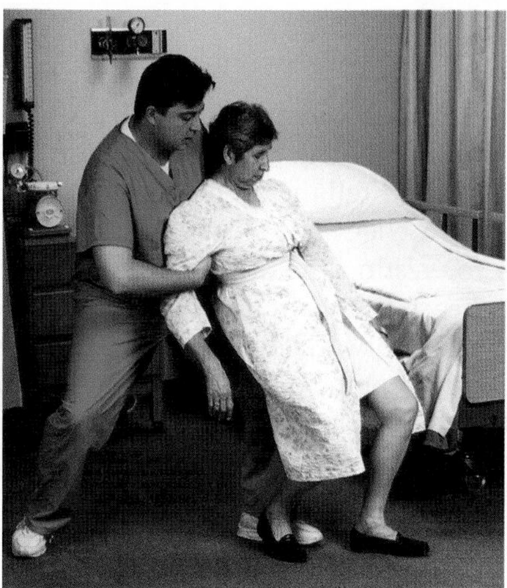

Step 9. Supporting the client and easing her to the floor.

10 Stay with the client until help arrives. Assess the client for injury before trying to move him or her (see illustration). *Even a minor fall can result in a fractured hip for an older adult, especially one who has osteoporosis. Use an air or mechanical lift rather than having the client try to stand. Have the client evaluated by a physician.*

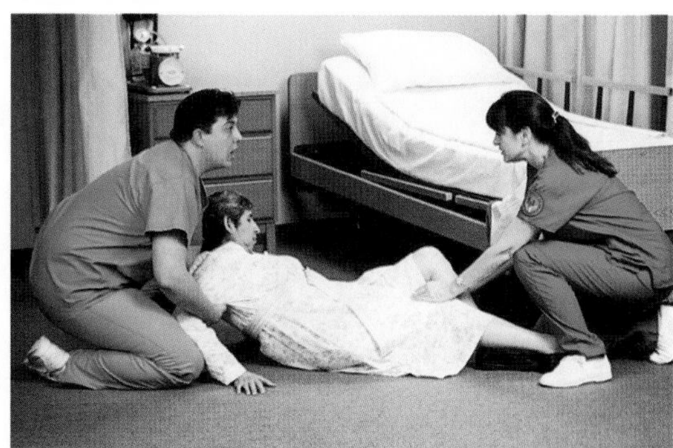

Step 10. Staying with the client until help arrives.

11 Document the events leading up to the fall, your client assessment, notification of the physician, and any action taken.

Continued

PEDIATRIC CONSIDERATIONS

The client's size determines the amount of assistance needed. Encourage family to participate as they are able and interested, but do not relinquish your responsibility for the client's safety.

GERIATRIC CONSIDERATIONS

Recall that reaction times are slower in older adults, so proceed slowly and provide explanations about the procedure.

HOME HEALTH CARE CONSIDERATIONS

Help the family caregivers assess their home environment for hazards, such as throw rugs, slick floors, or obstructed pathways, before getting the client out of bed to walk. A chair should be available that is sturdy, comfortable, and easily accessible. A high-backed chair is preferable to support the client's neck in anatomical alignment.

When teaching a client how to use a walker, place a gait belt around the client and help him or her to a standing position. Tell the client to place both hands on the walker. If a client has severe arthritis in the hands, platforms for resting the arms can be used instead of handgrips. Teach the client to lift the walker and move it about 1 to 2 feet forward, depending on the client's comfort level and strength. While resting on the walker, ask the client to take one or two small steps and check balance. Repeat this procedure while ambulating. You should grasp the gait belt until the client is strong enough to ambulate independently with the walker.

Using a Cane. A variety of canes are available for ambulation, depending on the amount of support the client needs. The quadripod ("quad") and hemicane provide the most support (Figure 32-8). They are used most often for clients who have had strokes. The straight cane provides the least support. All canes should have rubber tips on the end to prevent slipping.

When teaching the client how to use a cane, again use a gait belt and help the client to a standing position. Have the client place the cane in the hand of the stronger side of the body. The length of the cane should permit the elbow to be slightly flexed. Have the client move the cane forward about a foot and about 6 inches to the side, then move the weaker leg one step forward. Then have the client move the stronger leg forward and check the balance.

Like walkers, canes may be used on a temporary or a permanent basis. Some clients learn to ambulate using a walker and then progress to a series of canes as needed.

Using Crutches. For most clients, crutches are used as a temporary measure until they regain full mobility. However, for clients with permanent disability, they may be needed on a permanent basis. Axillary crutches are used most often when temporary support is needed. Lofstrand crutches are used most often for permanent needs (Figure 32-9). Before use, the client

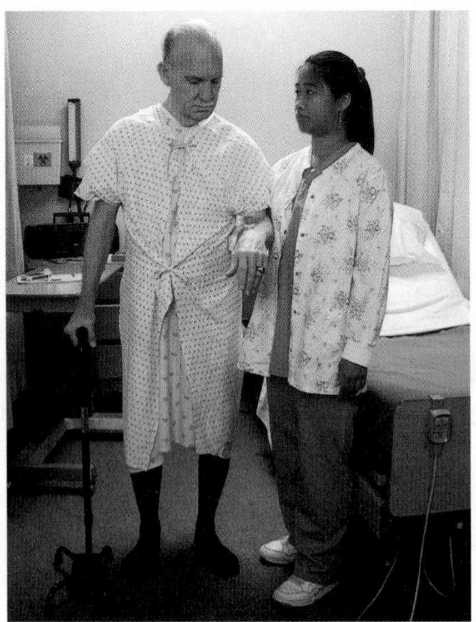

FIGURE 32-8 Client using a "quad" cane.

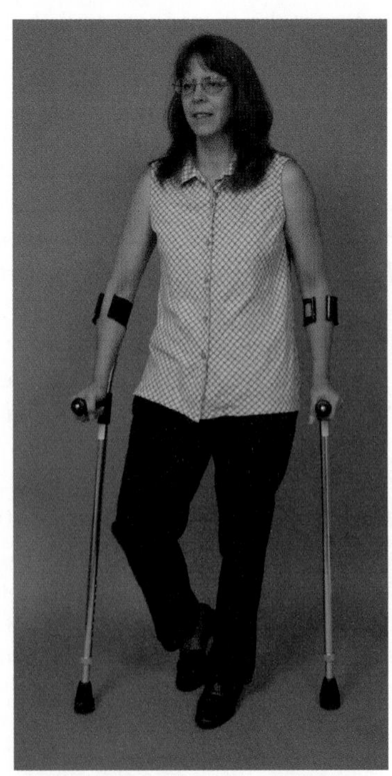

FIGURE 32-9 Client using Lofstrand crutches.

should be measured carefully for adjustments to prevent axillary nerve damage or muscle strain. Each crutch end should have a rubber tip to prevent slipping.

Arm strength needs to be assessed. If needed, the client performs exercises to prepare for the demands of crutch walking. The basic crutch stance is called the *tripod,* or triangle, position. It provides a broad base of support. Several gaits can be used for ambulating, depending on the injury and the client's weight-bearing status. The four-point gait provides the most support, but it requires coordination to maneuver. The three-point gait requires that the client be able to bear full weight on the unaffected leg. The two-point gait is the quickest and requires at least partial weight-bearing ability for both legs. Procedure 32-5 describes these gaits and how to manage stairs and sitting.

Swing-to or swing-through gaits are used for clients who are paralyzed in both legs. Teach the client to move both crutches ahead together by about 2 feet, then lift the body and swing to or past the crutches, whichever is most comfortable and balanced.

PROCEDURE 32-5 WALKING WITH CRUTCHES

TIME TO ALLOW: **NOVICE:** 20-30 min. **EXPERT:** 20-30 min.

Crutches are usually used for clients with orthopedic injuries who are unable to bear weight on one or both legs. Using crutches properly requires good upper body strength and balance. Complications of improper use could include falls and reinjury.

DELEGATION GUIDELINES

The evaluation of the need for crutches and instruction in the use of crutches may not be delegated to a nursing assistant. Assessment and instruction for crutch walking are the domain of a licensed professional, such as you or a physical therapist. Once a client has been instructed and successfully demonstrates crutch walking, you may assign or delegate a nursing assistant to accompany the client, much as you would do with ambulation.

EQUIPMENT NEEDED

- Crutches with rubber tips
- Supportive shoes with rubber soles

1 Perform preliminary actions (see inside front cover).

2 Inspect the prescribed crutch or crutches to make sure that the rubber tips are in place. *Rubber tips prevent slipping and therefore promote safety.*

3 Reinforce the importance of arm exercises, such as flexing and extending the arms, body lifts, and squeezing a rubber ball. *Arm muscles need to be toned to use crutches. Upper body strength is required.*

4 Check that crutches are the correct length (see illustration).

a. First, have the client stand.

b. Next, with the crutch tips and the client in the basic crutch stance (tripod position), check the distance between the axilla and the top of the crutch. It should be at least three finger widths, or 1 to 2 inches (2.5 to 5 cm). If the crutches are not the correct length, the client could sustain axillary nerve damage.

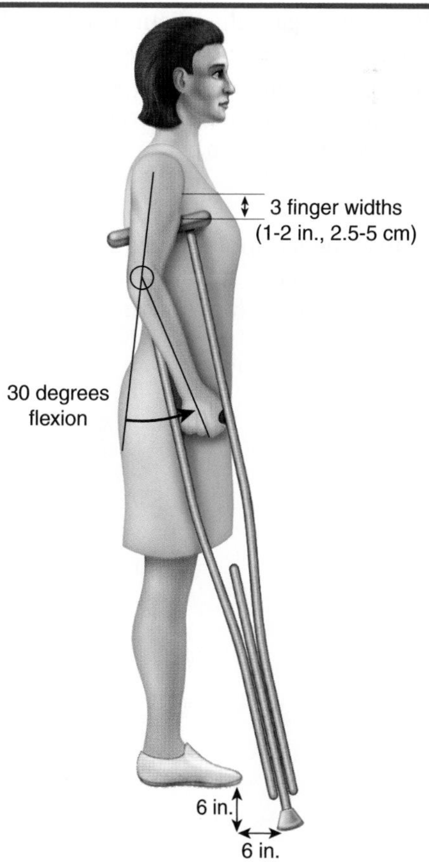

Step 4. Measuring crutch length.

Continued

5 Teach the client how to balance using the tripod (triangle) position by placing the crutches 6 inches (15 cm) in front of the feet and out laterally about the same distance (see illustration). *The tripod position provides a wide base of support and balance to prevent falls.*

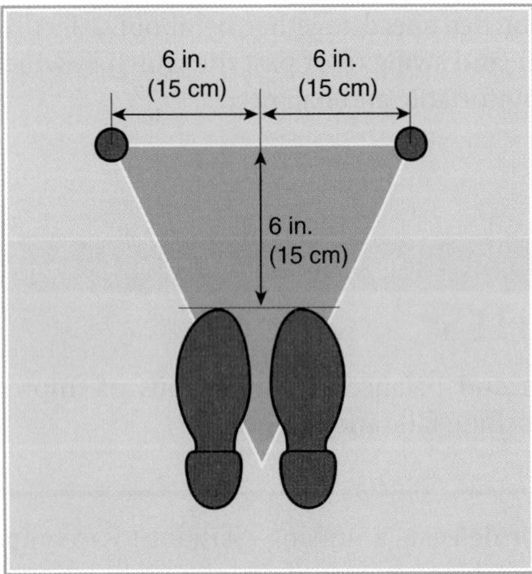

Step 5. Basic crutch stance, tripod position.

6 Check with the physician or physical therapist to determine which gait the client needs: a four-point, three-point, or two-point gait. *The type of injury and the client's balance determine which gait will be recommended.*

a. For a four-point gait, have the client follow this series of steps (see illustration):
   (1) Move the right crutch forward about 6 inches (15 cm).
   (2) Move the left foot forward.
   (3) Move the left crutch forward.
   (4) Move the right foot forward.

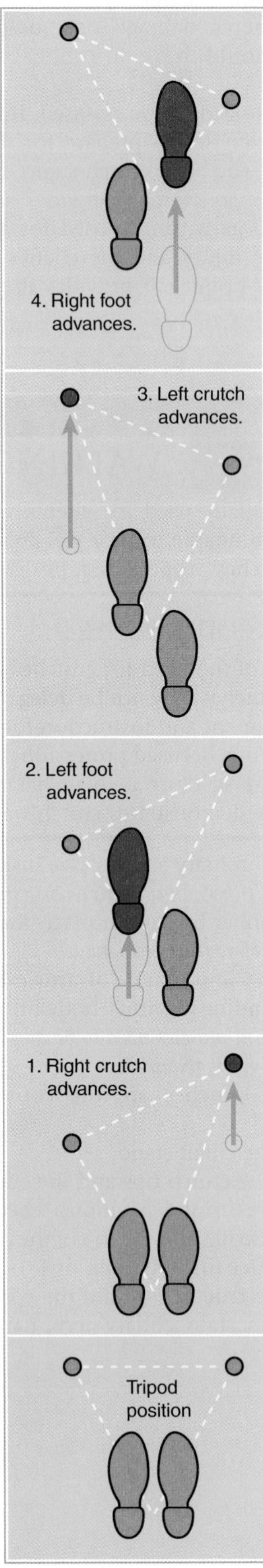

Step 6a. Four-point gait.

b. For a three-point gait, have the client follow this series of steps (see illustration):
   (1) Move both crutches and the weaker leg forward.
   (2) Move the stronger leg forward.

c. For a two-point gait, have the client follow this series of steps (see illustration):
   (1) Move the left crutch and the right foot forward at the same time.
   (2) Move the right crutch and the left foot forward at the same time.

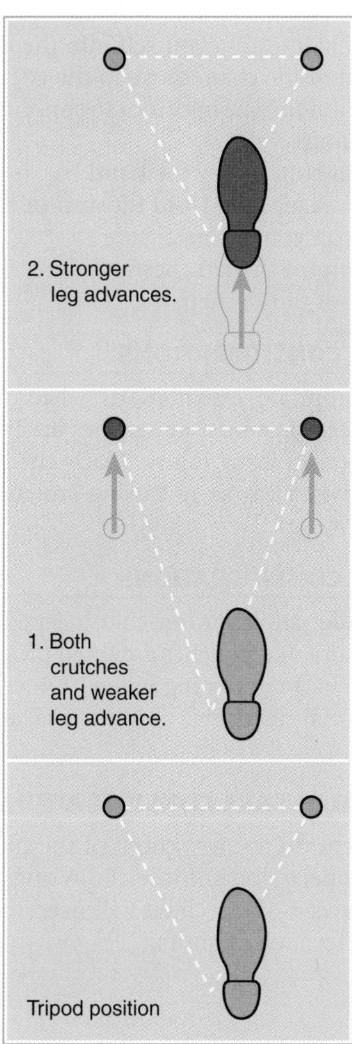

Step 6b. Three-point gait.

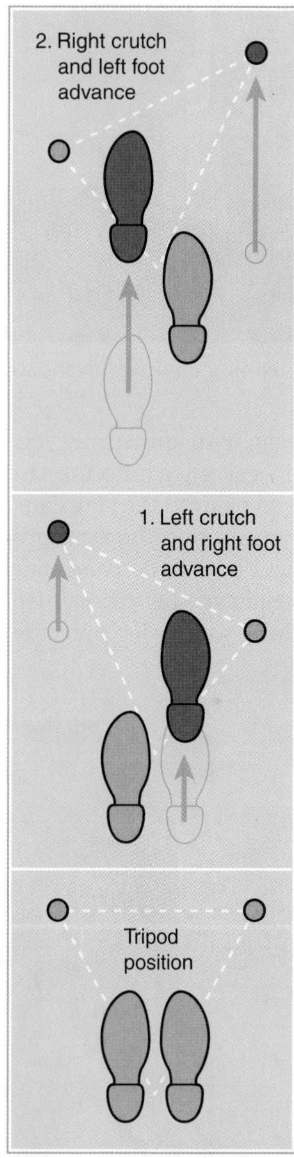

Step 6c. Two-point gait.

Continued

7 Teach the client how to ascend stairs:

a. Step up first with your stronger leg (see illustration).

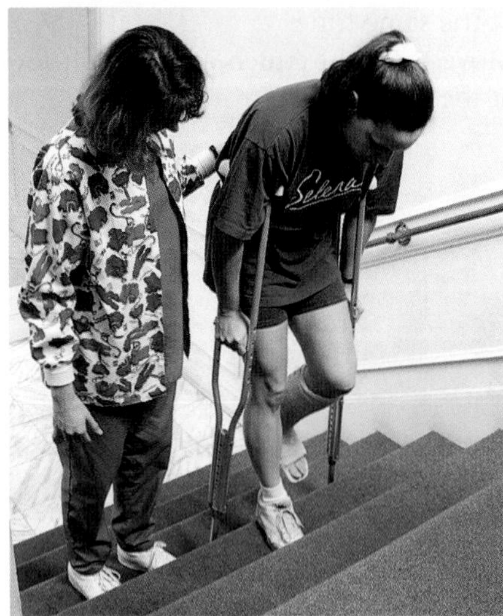

Step 7a. Stepping up first with the stronger leg.

b. Shift your weight to the strong leg, and move the crutches and weaker leg onto the same step.

c. Repeat these steps until the stairs are negotiated. The crutches always support the weaker or affected leg.

8 Teach the client how to descend stairs:

a. Shift your weight to the stronger leg, and move the crutches and the weaker leg onto the lower step (see illustration).

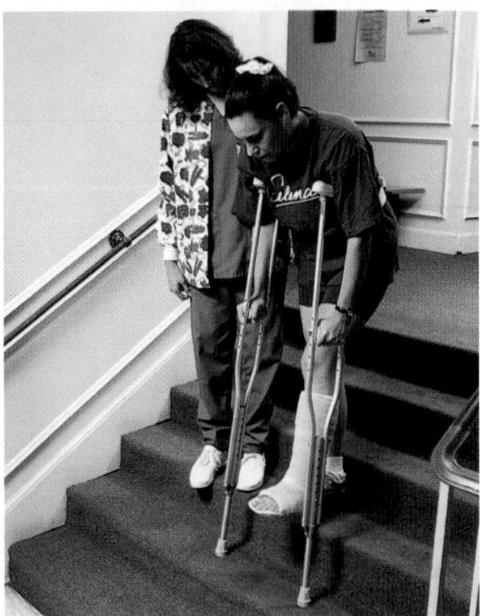
Step 8a. Stepping down first with the weaker leg.

b. Shift your weight to the crutches, and move the strong leg onto that step.

c. Repeat these steps until the stairs are negotiated. The crutches always support the weaker or affected leg.

9 Teach the client how to get in and out of a chair. *The following technique supports the weaker leg and provides the best balance for the client:*

a. Stand with the chair behind you, making sure that the back of your stronger leg is against the chair.

b. Transfer your crutches to your weaker side, and hold them by the hand bar.

c. Grasp the arm of the chair with the hand on your strong side, then lean forward and flex your hips and knees while lowering yourself into the chair.

d. To get out of the chair, move to the edge of the chair and position the stronger foot to support your weight when arising.

e. Hold both crutches by the hand bar, using the hand on your weaker side. Hold the arm of the chair with the hand on your stronger side.

f. Push down on the crutches and the armrest to push yourself out of the chair.

PEDIATRIC CONSIDERATIONS

Use age-appropriate explanations when teaching this skill to children. Ensure that crutches are fitted properly to prevent nerve plexus injury. Teach client and family safety measures, such as not using crutches on wet or slippery floors.

GERIATRIC CONSIDERATIONS

Assess the older adult for musculoskeletal ability to use crutches. Ensure that crutches are fitted properly. Provide teaching about maintaining safety. Older adults may need additional teaching time to master new techniques.

HOME HEALTH CARE CONSIDERATIONS

Help the client do a safety check of the home environment for slippery floors, loose throw rugs, or obstructions in walkways. If the client will need to use stairs, it is preferable to have a handrail.

Using a Wheelchair. For some clients, walking is no longer possible. Clients with complete spinal cord injuries, advanced multiple sclerosis, cerebral palsy, or muscular dystrophy are often confined to a wheelchair. These clients ambulate in their wheelchairs using their arms or other part of the body to propel the chair. Some use electric wheelchairs that can be advanced by a hand control or with a slight head movement.

Clients who are confined to wheelchairs are at risk for skin breakdown and other complications of immobility previously described. Teach the client and family or significant others to inspect skin every day, and have the client perform wheelchair pushups if possible to decrease pressure on the ischial tuberosities. Pushups also build arm strength, which is essential for propelling a manual wheelchair.

As a result of the federal Americans With Disabilities Act, all public places are wheelchair accessible. Ramps, handicapped toilets, and designated parking spaces have allowed wheelchair-bound people access to places they were previously not able to visit.

EVALUATION

Evaluation involves determining whether expected outcomes have been met. If they have not been met, the plan may need modification.

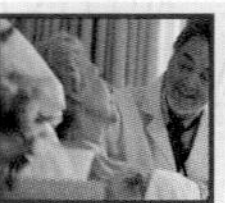

In our case study, Mrs. Lasauskas required rehabilitation for her fractured hip repair. By the fifth postoperative day, she was discharged to the hospital's transitional care unit (TCU). She was able to transfer from her bed to a chair and walk about 15 feet using a walker. Beyond that distance, she became dyspneic and tired. The plan for her continued rehabilitation in the TCU is to increase her ambulation distance and continue to build her tolerance for activity so that she can return to her assisted living apartment.

In this example, the client has progressed slowly but can ambulate with a walker independently for a short distance. The intermediate expected outcomes were met, but the long-term outcomes still need to be achieved before she can be discharged back into the community. Box 32-6 illustrates Mrs. Lasauskas's care after surgery, when she is ready to get out of bed for the first time. When she is discharged to the rehabilitation setting, the nurse writes the following note:

SAMPLE DOCUMENTATION FOR MRS. LASAUSKAS

Discharged to Meridian Rehabilitation per stretcher. Transportation provided by a van from Elderly Assistance, Inc. Vital signs stable. Pain controlled with Vicodin given 30 minutes before getting out of bed. Can feed self and dress with assistance. Physical therapy reports she is ready to begin walking a few steps with a walker. Report called to Meridian.

BOX 32-6

Nursing Care Plan

A Client With a Fractured Hip

Admission Data

Mrs. Kristina Lasauskas is an 80-year-old woman admitted for a fractured left hip. She was taken from the emergency department to the operating room, where she had an open reduction and internal fixation. She was in the recovery room 3 hours and has been admitted to an orthopedic nursing unit.

Physician's Orders

D_5½NS @ 75 mL/hr
Up in a chair tid as tolerated starting in AM
ROM four times daily
Laxative of choice
Lovenox 30 mg subcutaneous q12h
Regular diet, encourage fluids
Plan for discharge to a rehabilitation unit

Nursing Assessment

It is now the morning after her surgery. You receive the following report: Mrs. Lasauskas is 1 day post an open reduction and internal fixation of a fractured left hip. Her vital signs are stable. She is awake, alert, and oriented × 3. Lungs clear. Bowel sounds hypoactive. IV site patent and free of inflammation. She has right-sided weakness from a previous cerebrovascular accident but was able to walk with a cane. She is to be up in a chair today, and physical therapy will start ROM. She is depressed because she believes she will never walk again.

NANDA-I Nursing Diagnosis	NOC Expected Outcomes With Indicators	NIC Interventions With Selected Activities	Evaluation Data
Impaired Physical Mobility **Related Factor:** • Right-sided weakness and healing fracture of left hip	***Joint Movement*** • Active • Transfer performance	***Exercise Promotion*** • Strength training • Joint mobility.	***Data Gathered at Discharge to Rehabilitation Setting***

Continued

BOX 32-6 Nursing Care Plan—cont'd

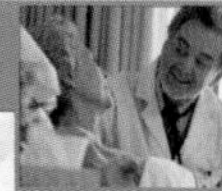

A Client With a Fractured Hip

NANDA-I Nursing Diagnosis	NOC Expected Outcomes With Indicators	NIC Interventions With Selected Activities	Evaluation Data
Impaired Physical Mobility	***Joint Movement*** ***The Client Will*** • Maintain full ROM • Increase upper body strength • Transfer from bed to chair with assistance • Sit in a chair without fatigue or change in vital signs • Perform resistance exercises to right leg and ROM to left leg • Stand at bedside with partial weight bearing to left hip	***Exercise Promotion*** • Full active/passive ROM by physical therapy 0800, 1300 and by nursing 1700, 2100. • Use client's history of self-determination to motivate. • Use 3-pound weights to exercise arms during ROM. • Have great-grandchildren bring colored weights and make a game of exercising. • Pivot to chair 1000, 1500, 1900. • Sit in chair as tolerated, increasing to 30 min. • Use light resistance for ROM to right leg.	***Data Gathered at Discharge to Rehabilitation Setting*** • Has full ROM in upper extremities. • Can perform active ROM. • Performs active ROM on right leg. • Straight leg raising to a 30-degree angle. • Can raise left leg by bending knee to 30-degree hip flexion. • Exercises arms with 3-pound weights. • Tolerates flexion at elbow. Raising weight over her head tires right arm. • Can stand and pivot to chair with assistance. • Can raise right leg against light resistance of nurse's hand on knee. • Puts left leg on floor for balance when standing. • Minimal if any weight bearing.

Critical Thinking Questions

1. Estimate Mrs. Lasauskas's potential for rehabilitation on a scale of 1 to 10, with 10 meaning she will be able to walk as well as she did before she fell.
2. List the criteria you used to make the decision in question 1.
3. Mrs. Lasauskas refuses to do active ROM exercises with her arms. How would you motivate her?

Nursing outcome and intervention labels from Johnson, M., Bulechek, G., Butcher, H., Dochterman, J. M., Maas, M., Moorhead, S., et al. (Eds.). (2006). *NANDA, NOC, and NIC linkages: Nursing diagnoses, outcomes, & interventions.* St. Louis, MO: Mosby.

▼ KEY PRINCIPLES

- Physical mobility requires functional joints, muscles, and bones.
- Factors affecting mobility include lifestyle, environment, growth and development, and pathophysiological factors, especially musculoskeletal and neurological health problems.
- *Impaired physical mobility* occurs when the client experiences limited ability to move within the physical environment.
- *Activity intolerance* results when a client has insufficient physiological or psychological energy to endure or complete a desired activity.
- Physical examination of a client with *Impaired physical mobility* includes assessment of body alignment, gait, joints, skeletal muscles, and neurovascular function.
- Diagnostic tests help you select appropriate nursing diagnoses for clients with musculoskeletal health problems.
- Functional assessment includes determining a client's ability to move and perform activities of daily living.
- Assessment of the client with *Impaired physical mobility* should be holistic and include assessment of all functional health patterns for emotional as well as physiological responses, including hopelessness and pain or chronic pain.
- Expected outcomes for clients with musculoskeletal problems are that the client will experience improved mobility and tolerance to activities.
- Interventions for improving activity tolerance focus on building muscle mass and strength, progressive mobilization, and controlling pain and discomfort.
- Interventions for improving mobility include maintaining joint mobility, assisting with movement, and compensating for physical impairments.
- Evaluation of outcomes for clients with musculoskeletal problems involves promoting ambulation (including wheelchair ambulation), preventing complications of immobility, and building activity tolerance.

REVIEW QUESTIONS

1. The ambulatory care nurse anticipates that which of the following clients should be screened for scoliosis during the routine clinic visit?

1. 4-year-old
2. 13-year-old
3. 27-year-old
4. 45-year-old

2. Which of the following clients assigned to the nurse would be a good candidate for using a walker as a mobility aid?

1. A client who is fully weight bearing and has poor upper body strength
2. A client who is fully weight bearing and has adequate upper body strength
3. A client who is partial weight bearing and has poor upper body strength
4. A client who is partial weight bearing and has adequate upper body strength

3. The nurse is teaching the client to walk using crutches and a four-point gait. The nurse would instruct the client to do which of the following steps first?

1. Move the right crutch forward about 6 inches (15 cm).
2. Move the left foot forward.
3. Move the left crutch forward.
4. Move the right foot forward.

4. You are preparing to use a gait belt when assisting a client, who can stand safely, to get out of bed into a chair. The client asks why you are using the device. What would be the best explanation?

1. "The belt can be used to help pull you up from the bed before sitting in the chair."
2. "The belt can help reassure you that you are not going to fall during the transfer."
3. "The belt can be used to lower you to the floor if you fall."
4. "The belt will allow me to guide you and offer support as you complete the transfer."

5. A client who badly sprained an ankle has been measured for crutches and will begin to ambulate. To ensure proper fit before teaching the client the proper gait, the emergency department nurse checks to see that there is how much room between the axilla and the pad at the top of each crutch?

1. ½ to 1 inch
2. 1 to 2 inches
3. 2 to 3 inches
4. 3 to 4 inches

Bibliography

Alitzer, L. (2004). Compartment syndrome. *Orthopedic Nursing, 23*(6), 391-396.

American Nurses Association. Position statement on elimination of manual patient handling to prevent work-related musculoskeletal disorders. Retrieved July 16, 2006, from http://www.nursingworld.org/readroom/position/workplac/pathand.pdf.

Baptiste, A., Boda, S., Nelson, A., Lloyd, J., & Lee, W. (2006). Friction reducing devices for lateral patient transfers: A clinical evaluation. *American Association of Occupational Health Nurses Journal, 54*(4), 173-180.

Barry, J. (2006). The HoverMatt system for patient transfer: Enhancing productivity, efficiency, and safety. *Journal of Nursing Administration, 36*(3), 114-117.

Carpenito-Moyet, L. (2006). *Handbook of nursing diagnosis* (11th ed.). Philadelphia: Lippincott Williams & Wilkins.

Dabke, H., Gupta, S., Holt, C., O'Callaghan, P., & Dent, C. (2004). How accurate is partial weight-bearing? *Clinical Orthopedic Related Research,* (421), 282-286.

Daniels, C., Huang, G., Feuerstein, M., & Lopez, M. (2005). Self-report measure of low back-related biomechanical exposures: Clinical validation. *Journal of Occupational Rehabilitation, 15*(2), 113-128.

de Castro, A. B. (2004). Handle with care: The American Nurses Association's campaign to address work-related musculoskeletal disorders. *Online Journal of Issues in Nursing, 9*(3), 3.

Fletcher, K. (2005). Immobility: Geriatric self-learning module. *Medsurg Nursing, 14*(1), 35-37.

Gillis, A., & MacDonald, B. (2005). Deconditioning in the hospitalized elderly. *Canadian Nurse, 101*(6), 16-20.

Graf, C. (2006). Functional decline in hospitalized older adults. *American Journal of Nursing, 105*(1), 58-68.

Hudson, M. (2005). Texas passes first law for safe patient handling in America: Landmark legislation protects healthcare workers and patients from injury related to manual patient lifting. *Journal of Long Term Effective Medical Implants, 15*(5), 559-566.

*Ignatavicius, D. D., Workman, M. L., & Mishler, M. A. (1999). *Medical-surgical nursing across the health care continuum* (3rd ed.). Philadelphia: Saunders.

Ignatavicius, D. D., & Workman, M. L. (eds.). (2002). *Medical-surgical nursing: Critical thinking for collaborative care* (4th ed.). Philadelphia: Saunders.

*Johnson, M., Bulechek, G., Butcher, H., Dochterman, J. M., Maas, M., Moorhead, S., et al. (Eds.). (2006). *NANDA, NOC, and NIC linkages: Nursing diagnoses, outcomes, & interventions.* St. Louis, MO: Mosby.

NANDA International. (2007). *Nursing diagnoses: Definitions and classification, 2006-2007* (6th ed.). Philadelphia: Author.

Nelson, A. (2003, March). *State of the science in patient care ergonomics: Lessons learned and gaps in knowledge.* Presented at the Third Annual Safe Patient Handling and Movement Conference, Clearwater Beach, FL.

Nelson, A., Powell-Cope, G., Gavin-Dreschnack, D, Quigley, P., Bulat, T., Baptiste, A., et al. (2004). Technology to promote safe mobility in the elderly. *Nursing Clinics of North America, 39*(3), 649-671.

Pellino, T., Owen, B., Knapp, L., & Noack, J. (2006). The evaluation of mechanical devices for lateral transfers on perceived exertion and patient comfort. *Orthopedic Nursing, 25*(1), 4-12.

*Asterisk indicates a classic or definitive work on this subject.

Chapter 33

Preventing Disuse Syndrome

Media Resources

- Evolve Website http://evolve.elsevier.com/Harkreader/
- Companion CD
- Skills Video Clips

Learning Objectives

After studying this chapter, you will be able to do the following:

- Describe the physiological concepts underlying the diagnosis of Risk for disuse syndrome
- Discuss the factors that may lead to immobility and disuse
- Assess a client who is at risk for complications from disuse
- Diagnose the client at risk for disuse complications
- Plan goal-directed interventions to prevent complications of disuse
- Describe interventions needed to prevent complications of disuse
- Evaluate outcomes that describe progress toward managing immobility and preventing disuse

Key Terms

atrophy
bed rest
contracture
deep vein thrombosis (DVT)
disuse
excoriation
footdrop
friction injury
hypomotility
hypostatic pneumonia
immobility
inactivity
interface pressure
maceration
orthostatic hypotension
orthostatic intolerance
osteoporosis
pressure ulcer
pulmonary embolus
renal calculi
shear
trochanter roll
Valsalva maneuver
wrist drop

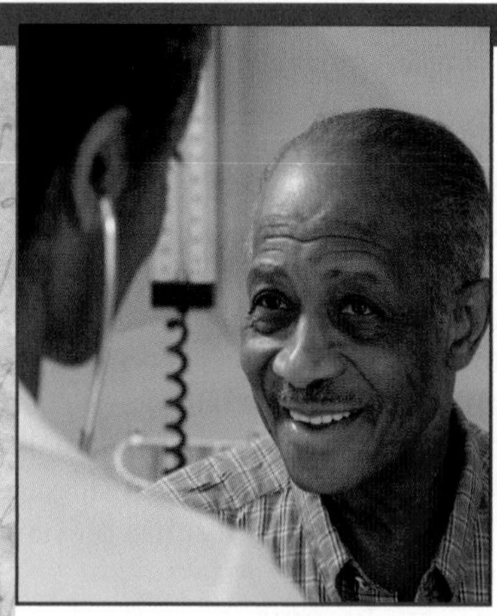

*Mr. Jackson is a 58-year-old African American man who has come to the emergency department after having a cerebrovascular event on the job. The physician diagnoses a ruptured cerebral artery. Mr. Jackson is left paralyzed on the right side. After 1 week in the hospital he has a severe myocardial infarction and is transferred to intensive care. Four days later he is returned to a medical nursing unit. He has recovered some movement in his right side, but his heart is left with a large amount of scar tissue and he is at risk for heart failure. In addition, he is at risk for cardiovascular deconditioning, respiratory infection, urinary tract infection, depression, and skin breakdown. The nurse makes the diagnosis of *Risk for disuse syndrome.*

Activity and movement develop and maintain the normal functioning of all body systems. In contrast, prolonged decreased activity causes physical and mental deterioration. You will care for clients who are inactive from immobility, prescribed bed rest, critical illness, neurological damage, trauma, or pain. Preventing complications of disuse will decrease both suffering and health care costs. Although we generally think of disuse in the client who is completely immobile in bed, functional decline occurs in approximately one third of hospitalized people over the age of 70 across a range of decreased mobility (Brown, Friedkin, & Inouye, 2004; Cornette et al., 2006). Although the length of inactivity is a factor, the effects of decreased mobility can begin within 48 hours of admission. For some of these elders, immobility or low mobility in the hospital is a predictor of institutionalization and even death. Through astute assessment and aggressive interventions, you can prevent many of the complications of disuse.

CONCEPTS OF INACTIVITY AND IMMOBILITY

Disuse is a state (or condition) of decrease or cessation of use of an organ or a body part, restriction of activity, or immobility. Complications of disuse occur in every body system.

Immobility is the inability to move the whole body or a body part. It occurs in clients who are paralyzed or unconscious or who have neuromuscular or orthopedic disorders. Many frail older adults have fewer spontaneous movements because of neurological or musculoskeletal problems. The immobile client is totally dependent on the nurse to maintain safety and body functions.

Bed rest is a prescribed or self-imposed restriction to bed for therapeutic reasons. Complete bed rest is seldom prescribed because of the potential complications of immobility. However, critically ill clients, some orthopedic clients, and clients with severe limitation of movement may be confined to bed. Some clients with prescribed bed rest are able to move about freely in bed, but others require much effort to move or need assistance to move.

Inactivity and immobility have a cyclic relationship with the development of complications. For example, when a client remains inactive, the joints begin to get stiff, and the muscles get weak. The client is less able to participate in activities of daily living (ADLs) and experiences increased risk for disuse. Respiratory and cardiovascular deconditioning occurs, and the client is at risk for skin breakdown. The longer the person is immobile, the higher the risk is for complications of disuse. Preventing complications of immobility requires support of all body systems to break the cycle of disuse.

KEY NURSING DIAGNOSES FOR DISUSE

Risk for disuse syndrome: At risk for deterioration of body systems as the result of prescribed or unavoidable musculoskeletal inactivity

Risk for impaired skin integrity: At risk for skin being adversely altered

PSYCHOSOCIAL EFFECTS OF INACTIVITY AND IMMOBILITY

Initially, most people welcome the brief rest and relief from ADLs that accompanies a brief period of inactivity or immobility. However, long-term or permanent inactivity or immobilization can alter that feeling. Often, the client loses motivation or interest in participating in daily living. Losing contact with friends and work can result in loneliness and social isolation. The client who is forced to rely on others for help feels powerless. Loss of self-esteem is associated with the absence of social roles as caregiver, parent, or breadwinner.

A person's behavior changes in response to a prescribed or unavoidable activity restriction. The client may act out negative feelings of dissatisfaction and frustration in the form of irritation, anger, or aggression. In addition, inactivity can increase mental confusion as a consequence of sensory deprivation. The person is less able to concentrate and focus on learning, memory may be impaired, and problem-solving abilities decline.

Resting in bed 24 hours a day also interferes with the normal circadian rhythm and pattern of sleep. When the client sleeps during the day, the quality of the sleep is not the same as it is during the night. In addition, having slept during the day, the client may be unable to sleep through the night. The psychological manifestations of sleep deprivation may be present.

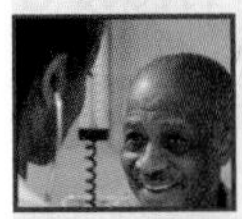

Mr. Jackson is the primary financial support for his family. He has good health insurance but does not have sick leave. What psychosocial manifestations would you predict for him?

MUSCULOSKELETAL EFFECTS OF INACTIVITY AND IMMOBILITY

Active use maintains the strength of bones, strength and tone of muscles, and mobility of joints. Much as the trained athlete becomes deconditioned when not in training, the client who is inactive experiences deterioration of bones, muscles, and joints. Deconditioning is a decline from a previous state of physical fitness.

To maintain their mass and strength, muscles must move against resistance. **Atrophy** is a decrease in the size or physiological activity of a normally developed tissue or organ as a result of inactivity or diminished function. After about 24 to 36 hours of inactivity, a muscle begins to lose its contractile strength. Already, it has begun the process of atrophy.

When a person is immobile, the body breaks down muscle mass to obtain energy, which can result in a negative nitrogen balance. The strength and endurance lost with a brief period of immobility can take several weeks to regain. The client becomes more susceptible to ambulation problems and injury by falling.

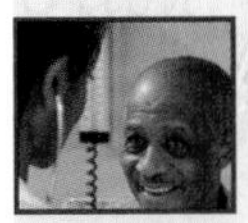

Thinking again about Mr. Jackson, what problems might he experience when he is ready to begin rehabilitation?

After about 5 days of immobility, calcium and fibrotic cells deposit in joints, causing them to become stiff and lose their full range of motion. Reduced range of motion can also be caused by fibrosis of tissues that support the joint or muscles. A joint losing its ability to move and becoming fixated is called ankylosis. Contractures also limit joint movement.

A **contracture** is an abnormal condition of joint flexion resulting from shortening of muscle fibers and associated connective tissue, with resistance to stretching and eventually to flexion and, finally, to permanent fixation. It also can result from loss of normal skin elasticity, as in scar formation. Contractures occur when the longer and/or stronger flexor and adductor muscles overcome the weaker opposing muscles. Often, the most comfortable position or the resting position for a joint is in the flexed position. When muscle flexion occurs for a prolonged period of time without any stretching activity to keep the joint mobile, contractures result.

Fibrosis occurs in the muscle or its supporting structures, causing it to become stiff. A reversible contracture is a shortening of a muscle, which can be corrected by exercise. In a nonreversible contracture, the muscle or tendon becomes permanently fixed or frozen; this can be corrected only by surgery.

A client with a contracture loses functional ability in the affected muscles and joints. For example, a client with a contracture of the wrist or elbow may be unable to hold a spoon or a comb. Other ADLs will be affected as well. Footdrop is a crippling deformity that prevents the person from walking.

Although any joint can become contracted, the wrists and ankles are common—and commonly overlooked—locations. These contractures are particularly disabling when they occur. **Footdrop** is a contracture deformity in which the muscles of the anterior foot lengthen. At the same time, the muscles of plantar flexion and the Achilles tendon shorten, resulting in plantar flexion of the foot (Figure 33-1, *A*). Footdrop can result from the weight of gravity on weakened foot muscles or from damage to the peroneal nerve. **Wrist drop** is a contracture of the wrist in the flexed position (Figure 33-1, *B*). Contractures also commonly occur in the elbows, knees, hips, and hands. Contractures of the neck result in kyphosis.

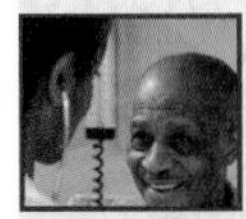

Because Mr. Jackson has recovered some function in his right side, he has good potential for rehabilitation. What nursing care would help maintain that potential until his heart condition is stable enough to begin an active rehabilitation program?

Osteoporosis is a condition in which there is a decreased mass per unit volume of normally mineralized bone (bone density), primarily from a loss of calcium, that makes bones brittle and porous. Osteoporosis can occur when functional (weight bearing) stress on bones

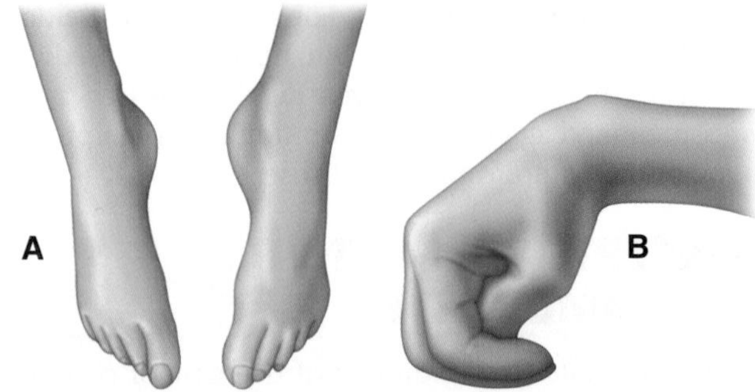

FIGURE 33-1 Two common contractures resulting from immobility. **A,** Footdrop involves plantar flexion, inversion of the ankle, and flexion of the toes. **B,** Wrist drop involves flexion of the wrist and fingers and opposition of the thumb. (**B** redrawn from Bolander, V. B. [1994]. *Sorensen and Luckmann's basic nursing* [3rd ed.]. Philadelphia: Saunders.)

declines. Functional stress is essential to the continuous reformation of bone. Osteoblasts are continually building bone matrix, and osteoclasts are continually breaking down bone matrix. This reformation maintains the tensile strength of bones.

Within about 2 or 3 days of decreased muscle activity and weight bearing, osteoblastic activity slows and interrupts bone reformation. Osteoclastic activity (breakdown) continues, releasing large amounts of calcium from the bone matrix into the blood. The extra calcium is excreted by the kidneys or deposited in the muscles and joints. The bones become brittle and porous, and they fracture easily.

INTEGUMENTARY EFFECTS OF INACTIVITY AND IMMOBILITY

Damage to the skin from prolonged pressure on bony prominences is the major complication of immobility. Additional damage can result from shear, friction, maceration, and infection.

A **pressure ulcer** is any lesion caused by ischemia from unrelieved pressure that leads to necrosis of underlying tissues. When pressure on the skin exceeds capillary pressure, blood flow to the skin is impaired. The supply of oxygen and nutrients is insufficient to maintain the viability of the skin and underlying structures. The cells die and slough, leaving an open crater. Pressure ulcers can range from reddened skin to large, open, deep wounds. Poor nutrition, dehydration, and continued pressure lead to poor wound healing and wound infections. A pressure ulcer can develop in a single day.

The most commonly affected areas are tissues overlying bony prominence (Figure 33-2). The area over the coccyx is probably the most common site of pressure ulcers. However, pressure ulcers also develop over the greater trochanter, shoulder, elbow, back of the skull, heels, ankle, and ear. For a client confined to a wheelchair, the most common sites are the ischial tuberosities and the coccyx. Keep in mind, however, that a pressure ulcer can develop anywhere there is sufficient pressure for a sufficient time.

For a pressure ulcer to occur, the amount of pressure on the capillary bed must exceed the arteriole pressure (the capillary closing pressure is about 35 mm Hg), and the duration of pressure must be long and unrelieved. **Interface pressure** is pressure created in tissues that are compressed between the bones and a support surface by the weight of the body. As the client lies in bed or sits quietly in a chair, interface pressure exerted on tissues by the external surface of the bed or chair interrupts blood flow through the vessels and impairs the delivery of oxygen and nutrients to cells.

Although the development of pressure ulcers has a sole cause (prolonged, unrelieved pressure), additional factors increase the risk for developing a pressure injury. A client who is unable to move independently in bed because of cognitive or musculoskeletal limitations is at high risk. Chronic illnesses, such as renal failure, diabetes, and anemia, further exacerbate the risk. Frail or edematous skin is more likely to sustain damage. Dehydration and poor nutrition (inadequate protein) also decrease the skin's tolerance to injury. Pressure ulcers account for a large proportion of skin injuries that result from bed rest. Because treating these injuries is costly, prevention is always the treatment of choice.

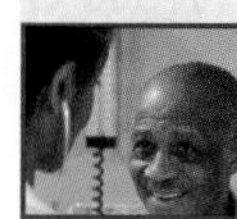

How would you keep Mr. Jackson from developing pressure ulcers? What would be the effect of pressure ulcers on his rehabilitation program?

Shear is a mechanical force that acts on an area of skin in a direction parallel to the body's surface. Shear injuries are a serious form of pressure injury, because they result in necrosis and ulceration, usually over the coccyx. One cause is improper positioning, which can lead to the client sliding down in bed (Figure 33-3). When that happens, blood vessels in the two sacral tissue layers are stretched and torn, which disrupts the blood supply to these cells and causes skin breakdown. Shearing forces cause deep ulcers. Although they may appear small on the skin surface, considerable necrosis may be present in the underlying tissues.

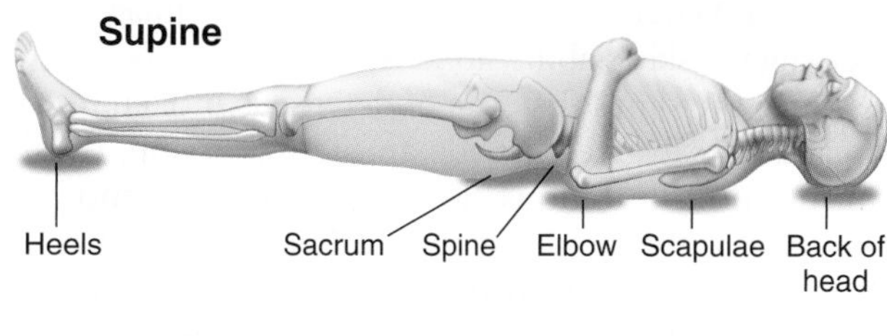

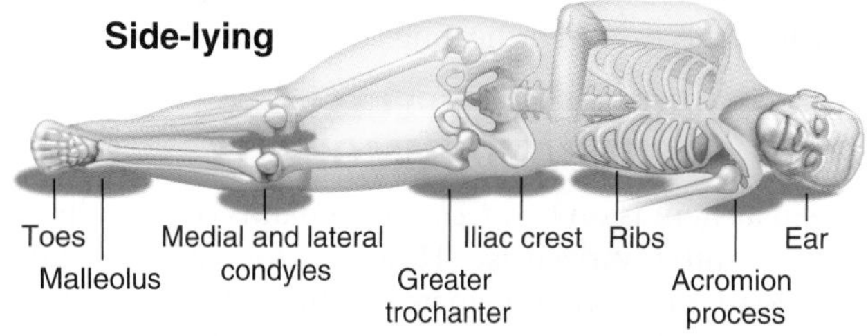

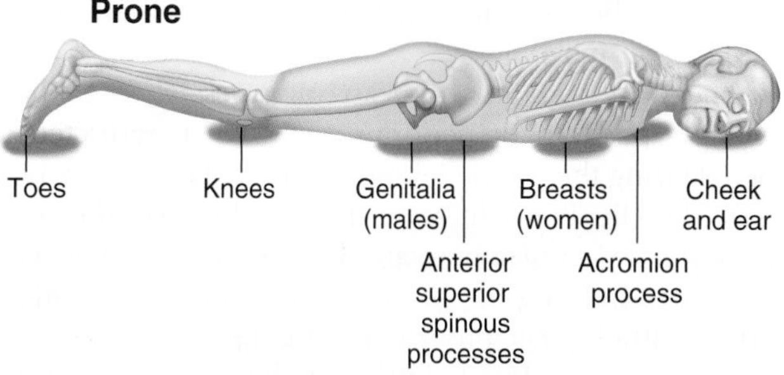

FIGURE 33-2 Bony prominences subject to pressure, ischemia, necrosis, and ulceration in the supine, side-lying, and prone positions.

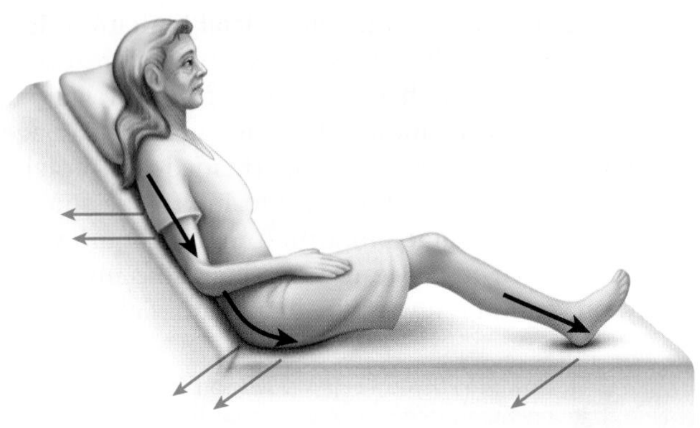

FIGURE 33-3 Shearing forces pull tissue layers in opposite directions. Tissue near the bone slides downward and forward, whereas the skin tends to be held upward and back by friction from the sheets.

Injuries can occur to the superficial layers of the skin. In a **friction injury**, the epidermal layer of skin is rubbed off, possibly from a restraint, a dressing, bed linens, or a tube. Friction injury commonly affects the elbows, which can become irritated as the client moves around in bed. An **excoriation** is an injury to the epidermis caused by abrasion, scratching, a burn, or chemicals, such as sweat, wound drainage, feces, or urine coming in contact with skin. **Maceration** is a softening of the epidermis caused by prolonged contact with moisture, such as from a wet sheet or diaper. Maceration increases the risk for damage by decreasing the skin's ability to resist trauma.

Once the skin's first line of defense is broken, microorganisms can freely invade an ulcer or lesion, causing an infection. Infections slow wound healing and carry the risk for the serious complication of septicemia (infection in the bloodstream). The absence of circulation further decreases the oxygen, immune response, and nutrients necessary for healing.

CARDIOVASCULAR EFFECTS OF INACTIVITY AND IMMOBILITY

When a client is on bed rest, the demands of the cells for oxygen initially decrease. However, the cardiovascular workload may actually increase. In addition, without exercise, cardiac deconditioning begins. These changes in the cardiovascular system lead to decreased energy and further inactivity.

The workload on the heart increases when a client changes position or performs ADLs when restricted to bed. During the "work" of moving in bed or using a bedpan, the client will increase the workload on the heart through the **Valsalva maneuver.** The Valsalva maneuver is the act of holding the breath while performing work; it builds intrathoracic pressure by attempting to force expiration against a closed glottis, usually in preparation for work such as lifting or tightening abdominal muscles to assist a bowel movement. When a breath is finally taken, the intrathoracic pressure suddenly drops, and blood flow increases to the right heart, creating the increased workload. Reflex bradycardia may occur, which can cause syncope or even a heart attack in vulnerable persons.

Unlike arteries, which pump blood forward from the heart, the veins rely on the "squeezing" action of calf muscles to move the venous blood along. In a bedridden client, decreased calf muscle activity and increased external pressure from the bed gradually allow blood to pool in the distal veins. This stasis of blood contributes to three problems: orthostatic intolerance, edema, and thrombus formation.

Orthostatic intolerance is a drop in systolic blood pressure of 20 mm Hg or more and a drop in diastolic blood pressure of 10 mm Hg or more for 1 or 2 minutes after a client moves to a standing position (orthostasis). It is also called **orthostatic hypotension** or postural hypotension, and it commonly results from immobility.

In the supine position (lying flat on the back), blood pools in the legs, and venous return and cardiac output decrease. When the client sits or stands up, blood pressure can drop rapidly. Prolonged supine positioning also decreases the sensitivity of baroreceptors in the aortic arch to positional blood pressure changes. These receptors become sluggish and less responsive in stimulating the sympathetic nervous system to maintain normal blood pressure with changes in position. Dehydration can also contribute to this problem by decreasing the blood volume.

Low blood pressure and orthostatic intolerance increase the client's risk for falling. Signs and symptoms of orthostatic intolerance include dizziness, feeling faint, or feeling light-headed. Orthostatic intolerance is present in about 20% of people over age 65 and in at least 30% of people over age 75.

Stasis of blood in the legs and sacral area increases hydrostatic pressure on vein walls. As the veins dilate in response, the valves open and allow backflow of blood down the veins. Also, this increase in hydrostatic fluid pressure "pushes" more fluid out of the veins into the interstitial spaces, producing edema. Edema constricts blood flow to the tissues and cells, decreasing their oxygen supply.

Stasis of venous blood, viscosity of the blood, and injury to vessel walls predispose the client to thrombus formation in the legs. **Deep vein thrombosis (DVT)** is the condition caused when a blood clot (thrombus) develops in the lumen of a deep leg vein, such as the tibial, popliteal, femoral, or iliac vein. Superficial vein thrombosis is a clot in a superficial vessel.

Deep vein thrombosis can develop when slowed blood flow allows platelets and increased levels of calcium (from the bones) to settle out and come in contact with the intima that lines the vessel. This activates the clotting process, and blood clots form along the vessel wall, particularly if the walls are damaged or if the vessels are tortuous (twisting). Dehydration contributes to thrombus formation by causing the blood to become more viscous.

Signs of deep vein thrombosis are calf tenderness, calf pain with passive dorsiflexion of the foot (Homans' sign), edema that causes one calf to increase in diameter, and slight warmth of the involved leg. The major risk created by DVT is a **pulmonary embolus,** which is a piece of the thrombus that breaks free, is carried by veins to the right heart and the pulmonary circulation, and lodges in a pulmonary blood vessel. As a result, blood flow and oxygen cannot reach the area of lung tissue served by the blocked vessel. This process is also called pulmonary embolism.

Signs and symptoms of pulmonary embolism include the sudden onset of dyspnea, a cough, sudden chest pain, hemoptysis, tachycardia, and tachypnea. A pulmonary embolus can be life threatening and requires immediate emergency action.

RESPIRATORY EFFECTS OF INACTIVITY AND IMMOBILITY

Although bed rest initially decreases the body's metabolic need for oxygen, prolonged bed rest has negative effects on respiratory function. The lungs function at their best in the upright position. The recumbent position (lying flat) compromises respiratory function and predisposes the client to respiratory complications, progressing from hypoventilation, to atelectasis, to stasis of secretions, and eventually to altered gas exchange. When the respiratory rate slows and the depth becomes shallow, atelectasis of some alveoli occurs and secretions stagnate. Eventually, immobility causes the respiratory muscles to weaken, which decreases the bellows effect created by the movement of the chest wall. In addition, pressure of the mattress against the thorax prevents optimal movement of the chest. The abdominal contents push against the diaphragm, decreasing its effectiveness in contracting and expanding the lungs.

Immobility also compromises the client's ability to cough—the normal mechanism for moving secretions out of the lungs. With a diminished cough effort, secretions accumulate and block the airways. Gravity contributes to the stagnation of secretions in the dependent areas of the lungs. If dehydration is present, secretions become thick and tenacious, making them even more difficult to mobilize. **Hypostatic pneumonia** is an inflammation of the lungs caused by stasis of secretions, which become a medium for bacterial growth. Signs of pneumonia are thickened yellow sputum, rhonchi, crackles, wheezes, fever, and rapid, shallow breathing.

GASTROINTESTINAL EFFECTS OF INACTIVITY AND IMMOBILITY

Immobility or inactivity slows the basal metabolic rate and gastrointestinal (GI) motility, and it delays gastric emptying. These effects are manifested as anorexia, constipation, increased storage of fat and carbohydrates, and a negative nitrogen balance.

A client confined to bed may experience a loss of appetite (anorexia) because the metabolic rate slows with rest, thus reducing calorie requirements. With inadequate nutrient intake, the client feels tired and prefers to sit quietly, becoming more and more inactive. If the client does not eat, muscle and subcutaneous tissue are broken down for energy needs. Changes in the client's nutritional status affect endurance and muscle strength. Fatigue and loss of energy lead to further inactivity and immobility.

Anorexia combined with muscle atrophy can produce a negative nitrogen balance when nitrogen excretion exceeds nitrogen intake. The body begins to break down fat for energy, and the client begins to lose adipose tissue and overall weight. The client may become malnourished; effects of malnutrition include anemia, albuminemia, decreased immunity, and dry and cracked skin. Blood cells cannot be synthesized by bone marrow without sufficient protein; lack of adequate protein occurs with poor intake. Without enough white blood cells (leukocytes), there is increased susceptibility to infections—the immune system is less effective. The red blood cells also decrease, which leads to generalized fatigue, anemia, and poor wound healing. The skin, nails, and hair are also affected and become dull, dry, and brittle. Loss of subcutaneous fat affects the ability to effectively conserve heat and protect bony prominences.

Fluid intake may also be affected if the client on bed rest is unable to obtain and drink water. Decreased fluid intake results in dehydration, which causes constipation, decreased blood volume (decreased cardiac output and orthostatic intolerance), decreased tissue perfusion (skin ulceration and poor wound healing), decreased urine output (oliguria and stasis of urine), and stasis of respiratory secretions.

Hypomotility is decreased peristalsis from lack of stimulation of the gastrocolic reflex. Bowel sounds are faint and slowed. With slowed peristalsis, the transit time of food through the GI tract is lengthened, allowing more water to be absorbed. Thus constipation and flatulence often accompany bed rest. This effect can be compounded by an individual's reluctance to use the bedpan to have a bowel movement, leading to further constipation.

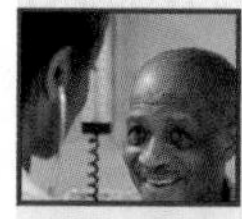

Mr. Jackson is now able to eat a regular diet. However, he spends most of his day in bed. He walks a few steps to a chair four times a day and eats his meals in the chair. How could you prevent constipation for him?

GENITOURINARY EFFECTS OF INACTIVITY AND IMMOBILITY

Immobility diminishes the kidney and bladder function and results in an increased incidence of urinary stasis, retention, renal calculi, and urinary tract infections. Urinary tract infections are the most prevalent hospital-acquired infections in bedridden clients. Signs of a urinary tract infection are dysuria (pain or burning sensation on voiding), urgency, frequency, fever, and voiding frequent, small amounts. In older adults a urinary tract infection can present as confusion.

Residual urine in the immobile client becomes a medium for bacterial growth. The client may also be unable to empty the bladder completely because of an inability to assume a normal voiding position while in bed. The male client with an enlarged prostate gland may be unable to urinate lying flat. Urinary retention results in urine remaining stagnant in the bladder for a prolonged time leading to bladder distention, reflux of urine to the kidneys, growth of bacteria, and urinary tract infections. Placing a client in the supine position can delay drainage of urine from the renal pelvis into the ureters; thus urine accumulate in the kidneys and can result in renal damage.

Inadequate personal hygiene further predisposes the immobile client to urinary tract infections. In addition, personal hygiene and perineal care are difficult for the bedridden client. The accumulation of microorganisms outside the urethra from the anal area encourages bacteria to invade the bladder. Reflux of urine back into the ureters (vesicoureteral reflux) can spread microorganisms from the bladder into the kidneys.

Stasis of urine and infection increase the risk for formation of calculi (stones, lithiasis) in the kidneys, renal pelvis, or urinary bladder. **Renal calculi** are stones formed in the kidney when the excretion rate of calcium or other minerals is high, as when osteoclastic activity releases calcium from the bones during immobility. Stone formation is further exacerbated because the end products of metabolism in an inactive client are generally alkaline because of decreased muscle activity. The high pH of the urine promotes calcium deposits and bacteria growth. Calculi can occur after only 1 or 2 weeks of inactivity.

FACTORS AFFECTING ACTIVITY AND MOBILITY

An optimal level of activity may be altered by a myriad of factors affecting the client's ability or desire for mobility. These factors place a client at risk for the complications of disuse.

PAIN

The immediate response to pain is to reduce activity, such as immobilizing a broken arm. A client with postoperative or cancer pain is reluctant to get up from bed and freely move around.

THERAPEUTIC OR PRESCRIBED INACTIVITY

Although complete bed rest is seldom prescribed, rest does aid healing for a variety of problems. For example, rest reduces the workload to allow the heart to heal. Immobilization allows a broken bone, skin, or nerve tissue to regenerate and grow together.

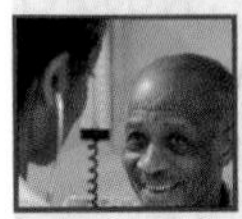

Mr. Jackson, the client in our case study, has limited activity and will be unlikely to return to his previous job. How do you think his cultural values may influence his response to the treatment plan (Box 33-1)?

CHANGE IN LEVEL OF CONSCIOUSNESS

A client who is in a coma or unconscious remains immobile in bed. An automobile accident that causes a head injury may leave the client immobile. The person who experiences a cerebrovascular accident (stroke) may be unable to move.

CHANGE IN MUSCULOSKELETAL FUNCTIONING

The aging process causes skeletal muscles to atrophy and joints to become more rigid and less flexible during the middle and later adult years. In addition, musculoskeletal disorders often limit mobility. Although paralysis is the most obvious cause of illness-related impaired mobility, other causes include amputation, arthritis, and Parkinson's disease. Muscular dystrophy and multiple sclerosis cause the muscles to lose their ability to function.

BOX 33-1 *Cross-Cultural Care*

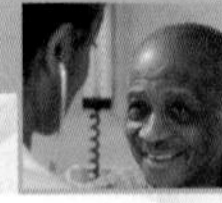

Caring for a Southern African American Man

Mr. Jackson is a 58-year-old African American. He is the head of his household and proud to be its breadwinner. He was employed as a construction worker, but is unlikely to be able to return to this type of work. He enjoys a Southern breakfast of eggs, ham, and buttered grits every morning. His wife does all the cooking in the household. Mr. Jackson is slightly overweight but powerfully built.

When Mr. Jackson leaves the rehabilitation unit, his wife and extended family will take care of him. His wife will "do" everything for him, encouraging him to rest. Although every client is unique, many African Americans from the South tend to value the following:

- Matriarchal family structure
- Male role as decision maker
- Church as center of community life
- "Brother" and "Sister" with other African Americans
- Large, extended family support systems, family get-togethers
- Strong tradition of religious faith; prayer may be an important healing ritual
- May incorporate folk remedies, but also believe in the power of preventive care
- Value and care for older adults

EMOTIONAL OR PSYCHOLOGICAL DISTURBANCES

A depressed client may lack the emotional energy to be active, even to the extent of fixing a meal or getting dressed for the day. Agoraphobia or other fears may prevent a client from leaving the room or even the house, for days.

CHRONIC ILLNESSES

Illnesses can affect the person's ability or energy to move. Either from fatigue or physical inability, the client remains inactive for a period. For example, anemia from blood loss or renal failure decreases the oxygen-carrying capacity of the blood, and the person experiences severe fatigue.

ASSESSMENT

GENERAL ASSESSMENT OF *ACTIVITY AND MOBILITY*

There are two purposes in assessing the immobile client. One is to detect the risk for complications of immobility. The other is to determine how much assistance the client will need to manage ADLs and prevent complications. Whether the client is in the hospital or at home, risk for complications of immobility should be identified and treated early.

Health History. Assessment begins with gathering data about the client's ability and motivation to be active. You should do the following:

- Note any medical or surgical conditions that would limit movement.
- Assess for pain.
- Assess the ability to understand and follow your instructions for self-care.
- Assess any risk factors affecting movement.
- Assess for *Risk for disuse syndrome.*
- Determine the client's previous level of functioning to set appropriate goals for care.

The following client questions may be helpful if the client is able to answer them. Alternatively, you may have some access to information in the medical records and from a family member.

- Describe your usual activities. Are you limited in your exercise or leisure activities because of fatigue, muscle weakness, joint changes, or breathing problems?
- Describe your usual health practices. Nutrition? Elimination? Exercise?
- Have you noticed any lesions on your skin? Do you bruise or injure easily?
- Do you have a history of cardiac, gastrointestinal, respiratory, urinary, or skin problems?

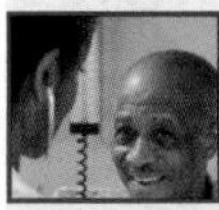

When Mr. Jackson is transferred to a rehabilitation unit, the nurse assesses his ability to perform ADLs and his disuse status. What problems would you anticipate in helping him maintain his ADLs?

Physical Examination. Assess the client's ability to move in bed. Sometimes you can observe the person moving and make a judgment about how much assistance is needed. Other times you may have to ask the client to move his or her arms and legs, squeeze your hands, hold a glass, or perform another activity. You can observe the speed of movement, strength, and coordination. As you perform a complete physical examination, you are assessing the person's ability to move. This is one of the reasons your daily assessment in the hospital or assessment in the home setting includes a physical examination.

Focus especially on the musculoskeletal system, including the client's muscle strength and tone, and ability to move in bed. Check the range of motion in each joint. Assess the skin carefully; this step is a key element of the physical examination for clients with mobility problems. Examine the skin for lesions and frailty.

FOCUSED ASSESSMENT FOR *RISK FOR DISUSE SYNDROME*

Defining Characteristics. *Risk for disuse syndrome* is defined by the presence of its risk factors, and the primary one is immobility. In considering this diagnosis, you will want to assess whether your client is at minimal risk, moderate risk, or high risk for disuse syndrome, as shown in the decision tree (Figure 33-4).

Two important criteria for assessing degree of risk include the client's level of inactivity and the duration of inactivity. The client may experience a combination of these, such as being maximally inactive for a minimal duration. Assessment parameters and interventions should reflect the most aggressive category.

Level of Inactivity. The level of inactivity can be categorized as minimal, moderate, or maximal. A client with minimal inactivity can move about freely within the confines of prescribed rest (in bed or a chair) or in a wheelchair. A client with moderate inactivity can move in the bed or chair but moves slowly, infrequently, or only with assistance. A client with maximal inactivity does not move or is incapable of moving in the bed or chair.

Duration of Inactivity. Duration can also be categorized as minimal, moderate, or maximal. A minimal duration is short and measured in hours. Moderate duration typically means inactivity that lasts for days. Maximal duration typically means inactivity that lasts for weeks, months, or years.

Related Factors. The primary related factors for *Risk for disuse syndrome* are the client's level of inactivity and the duration of inactivity. However, other related factors contribute to the risk as well. If the client has one or more of these factors, you will need to increase the frequency of your assessments and the aggressiveness of your interventions to prevent the complications of disuse syndrome. To help remember these risk factors, use the mnemonic ABCDE, which stands for *a*ge, *b*ody weight, *c*hronic illness, *d*iscomfort, and *e*nvironment.

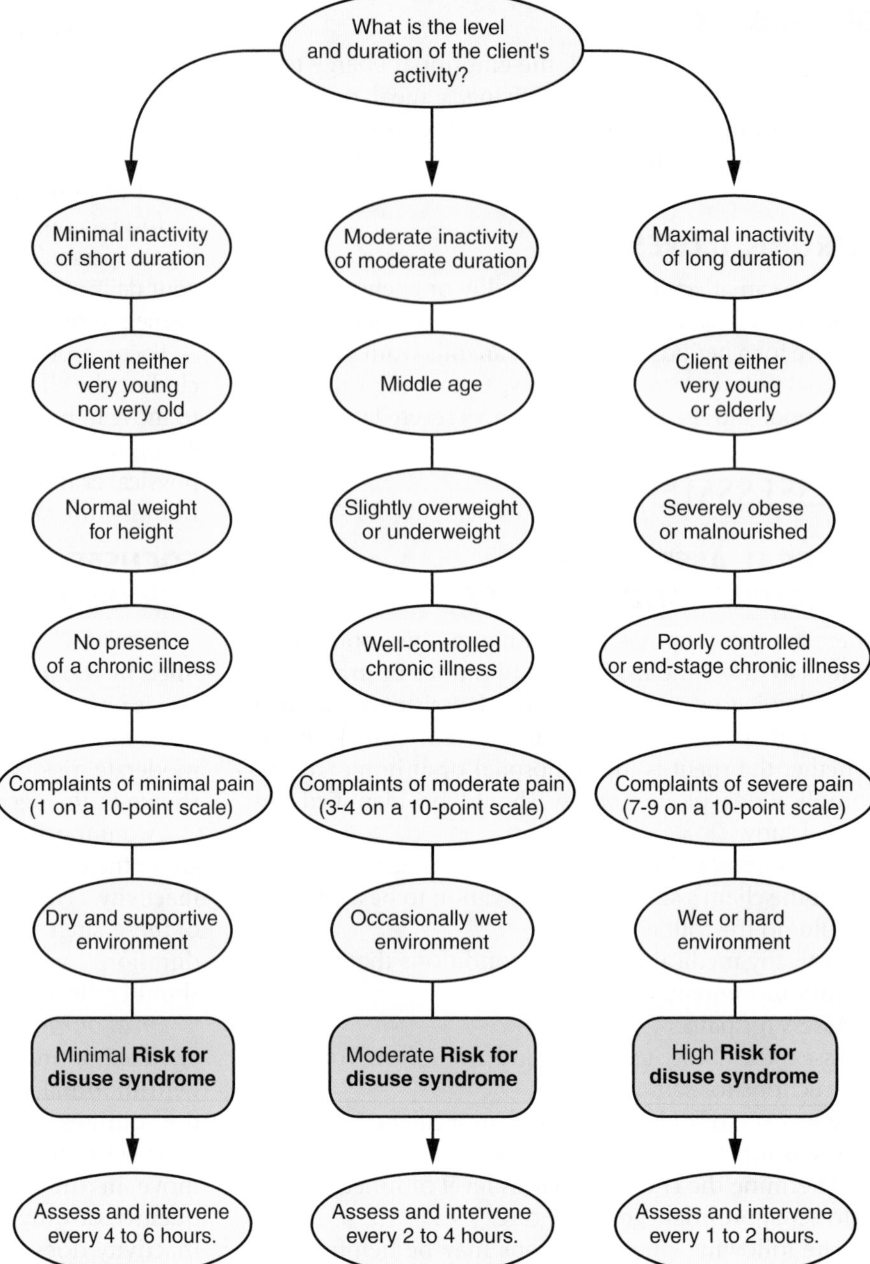

FIGURE 33-4 Decision tree for determining a client's risk for disuse syndrome. Diagnoses are shown in rectangles. Within these rectangles, diagnoses shown in **bold** type are NANDA-I–approved nursing diagnoses; diagnoses shown in regular type are not NANDA-I–approved nursing diagnoses.

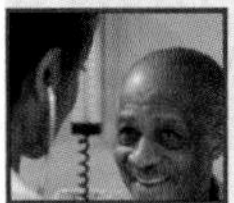

Using this method of risk assessment, how would you assess Mr. Jackson's risk for disuse problems?

Age. Age-related changes occur in all systems, making them more prone to deterioration resulting from disuse. For example, an older adult's skin may become dry, fragile, and more easily damaged by shear or pressure. In addition, the frail older adult may be undernourished from not eating balanced meals because of difficulty obtaining or preparing food.

Body Weight. Being overweight or underweight can be a factor in disuse syndrome. The decreased defenses of a malnourished client raise the risk for complications from disuse. Skin breakdown may occur because the skin is less resistant to pressure and shearing forces. Ulcers form more easily in older adults because of the loss of subcutaneous fat. On the other hand, the weight of an obese client places excessive pressure on bony prominences and may raise the risk for pressure ulcers. Joint changes stem from the increased weight as well, making mobility difficult. The overweight client experiences increased efforts to breathe, which may cause respiratory changes.

Chronic Illness. Chronic illness increases the risk for complications from disuse. For example, diseases such as renal failure, cancer, and diabetes (which interfere with metabolic processes) increase the risk for disuse complications. Diseases such as heart disease, respiratory disease, and anemia must also be considered. Neurological problems must be added to the list because they commonly decrease mobility.

Discomfort. A client with discomfort or pain is typically reluctant to move and instead prefers to lie quietly in bed. This compounds the risk for disuse by creating further inactivity. Adequate pain relief can help offset the effects of this risk factor, especially if relief is attained before a scheduled activity.

Environment. Wrinkled sheets or pillows increase the risk for skin breakdown and ulceration by causing uneven pressure on the skin. Excoriation of the skin occurs when the client is exposed to wound drainage, urine, or feces. The enzymes and altered pH of the drainage irritate and chemically burn the skin. Constant contact with a bed made wet by perspiration causes maceration of the skin. Hard surfaces increase the interface pressure, causing the skin to become ischemic and necrotic.

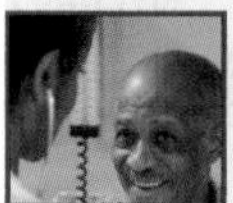

Mr. Jackson is middle-aged, and he has a high level of inactivity of long duration, normal to slightly increased body weight, heart disease, minimal discomfort, and low environment risk. These characteristics yield a moderate *Risk for disuse syndrome.* How often should he receive assessment and intervention?

FOCUSED ASSESSMENT FOR *RISK FOR IMPAIRED SKIN INTEGRITY*

Assessing your client's risk for developing pressure ulcers is an important nursing role. To help determine your client's risk, use a systematic risk assessment tool.

One of the most commonly used and highly reliable tools is the Braden scale for pressure ulcer risk (Figure 33-5). It is based on risk factors for clients in a nursing home population. Using the Braden scale, assess your client in six areas: sensory perception, moisture, activity, mobility, nutrition, and friction and shear. The client's total score may range from 6 to 23. The lower the score, the higher the client's risk for pressure ulcer development: low (23 to 20 points), medium (19 to 16 points), high (15 to 11 points), very high (10 to 6 points). Agency policy usually dictates that a standard of care to prevent skin breakdown be implemented once the score falls below a predetermined level. Other tools include the Norton scale, the Gosnell scale, and the Knoll assessment tool.

Risk factors common to *Risk for impaired skin integrity* may be internal or external. External factors include the following:

- Radiation
- Physical immobilization
- Mechanical factors, such as shear, pressure, and restraints
- Hypothermia or hyperthermia
- Exposure to moisture, including excretions, secretions, and humidity
- Exposure to chemical substances

Internal factors include the following:

- Very young or very old age
- Medications
- Skeletal prominence
- Immunological problems
- Developmental or psychogenic factors
- Altered sensation, circulation, metabolism, skin turgor, nutrition, or pigmentation

A conceptual framework called the *web of causation* helps in understanding the development of a pressure ulcer (Figure 33-6). This framework demonstrates the complex interrelationships of the factors affecting the skin. It considers many factors, including the client's clinical condition, nutrition, incontinence, mobility, activity, motivation, socioeconomic factors, and knowledge.

DIAGNOSIS

The diagnosis of *Risk for disuse syndrome* is a comprehensive way of intervening to prevent deterioration from inactivity. You must differentiate the diagnosis *Risk for disuse syndrome* from *Impaired physical mobility* and *Activity intolerance.* Nursing interventions for *Impaired physical mobility* are directed at increasing the client's ability to move about. Interventions for *Activity intolerance* are focused on the client's endurance in performing activities. However, because immobility and lack of endurance are risk factors for disuse, these two diagnoses are often written with the *related to* phrase.

With inactivity and immobility, the client's list of problems or potential problems may be long. Instead of writing multiple diagnoses to accommodate this list, the diagnosis *Risk for disuse syndrome* ensures a comprehensive approach.

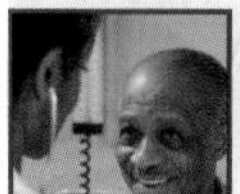

Mr. Jackson would have the nursing diagnosis *Risk for disuse syndrome* related to limited mobility of right side and activity intolerance secondary to heart disease.

RELATED NURSING DIAGNOSES

Powerlessness. A client who is confined to bed, paralyzed, or in traction for a broken bone is helpless. A nurse or caregiver needs to meet all of this person's needs. The mere need to use the bathroom or bedpan requires assistance. The client is unable even to get a glass of water to drink. This feeling of loss of control over the basic functions of life can be frustrating and embarrassing.

Risk for Imbalanced Nutrition: Less Than Body Requirements. With a lack of activity, decreased energy, slowed peristalsis, and abdominal distention, an immobilized client often fails to eat an adequate diet. The client complains of not being hungry or of feeling full too quickly. The person may eat only 20% or 30% of the diet. Fluid intake is decreased.

BRADEN SCALE
For Predicting Pressure Sore Risk

Patient's Name ______________ Evaluator's Name______________ Date of Assessment

SENSORY PERCEPTION ability to respond meaningfully to pressure-related discomfort	**1. Completely Limited** Unresponsive (does not moan, flinch, or grasp) to painful stimuli, due to diminished level of consciousness or sedation OR limited ability to feel pain over most of body.	**2. Very Limited** Responds only to painful stimuli. Cannot communicate discomfort except by moaning or restlessness OR has a sensory impairment which limits the ability to feel pain or discomfort over ½ of body.	**3. Slightly Limited** Responds to verbal commands, but cannot always communicate discomfort or the need to be turned OR has some sensory impairment which limits ability to feel pain or discomfort in 1 or 2 extremities.	**4. No Impairment** Responds to verbal commands. Has no sensory deficit which would limit ability to feel or voice pain or discomfort.				
MOISTURE degree to which skin is exposed to moisture	**1. Constantly Moist** Skin is kept moist almost constantly by perspiration, urine, etc. Dampness is detected every time patient is moved or turned.	**2. Very Moist** Skin is often, but not always moist. Linen must be changed at least once a shift.	**3. Occasionally Moist** Skin is occasionally moist, requiring an extra linen change approximately once a day.	**4. Walks Frequently** Walks outside the room at least twice a day and inside room at least once every 2 hours during waking hours.				
ACTIVITY degree of physical activity	**1. Bedfast** Confined to bed.	**2. Chairfast** Ability to walk severely limited or non-existent. Cannot bear own weight and/or must be assisted into chair or wheelchair.	**3. Walks Occasionally** Walks occasionally during day, but for very short distances, with or without assistance. Spends majority of each shift in bed or chair.	**4. Walks Frequently** Walks outside room at least twice a day and inside room at least once every two hours during waking hours.				
MOBILITY ability to change and control body position	**1. Completely Immobile** Does not make even slight changes in body or extremity position without assistance.	**2. Very Limited** Makes occasional slight changes in body or extremity position but unable to make frequent or significant changes independently.	**3. Slightly Limited** Makes frequent though slight changes in body or extremity position independently.	**4. No Limitation** Makes major and frequent changes in position without assistance.				
NUTRITION usual food intake pattern	**1. Very Poor** Never eats a complete meal. Rarely eats more than ⅓ of any food offered. Eats 2 servings or less of protein (meat or dairy products) per day. Takes fluids poorly. Does not take a liquid dietary supplement OR is NPO and/or maintained on clear liquids or IVs for more than 5 days.	**2. Probably Inadequate** Rarely eats a complete meal and generally eats only about ½ of any food offered. Protein intake includes only 3 servings of meat or dairy products per day. Occasionally will take a dietary supplement OR receives less than optimum amount of liquid diet or tube feeding.	**3. Adequate** Eats over half of most meals. Eats a total of 4 servings of protein (meat, dairy products) per day. Occasionally will refuse a meal, but will usually take a supplement when offered OR is on a tube feeding or TPN regimen which probably meets most of nutritional needs.	**4. Excellent** Eats most of every meal. Never refuses a meal. Usually eats a total of 4 or more servings of meat and dairy products. Occasionally eats between meals. Does not require supplementation.				
FRICTION & SHEAR	**1. Problem** Requires moderate to maximum assistance in moving. Complete lifting without sliding against sheets is impossible. Frequently slides down in bed or chair, requiring frequent repositioning with maximum assistance. Spasticity, contractures or agitation leads to almost constant friction.	**2. Potential Problem** Moves feebly or requires minimum assistance. During a move skin probably slides to some extent against sheets, chair, restraints or other devices. Maintains relatively good position in chair or bed most of the time but occasionally slides down.	**3. No Apparent Problem** Moves in bed and in chair independently and has sufficient muscle strength to lift up completely during move. Maintains good position in bed or chair.					
				Total Score				

FIGURE 33-5 Braden scale for predicting pressure sore risk. (Courtesy Barbara Braden and Nancy Bergstrom, 1988.)

Risk for Deficient Fluid Volume. The inability to obtain fluids or the decreased desire to drink can result in fluid deficits and electrolyte imbalances. A client confined to bed relies on you or another caregiver to provide adequate fluid (see Chapter 26).

Impaired Physical Mobility. Multiple factors affect a client's level of mobility. Assess the degree to which the client can become mobile. The best prevention for disuse syndrome is to maintain activity (see Chapter 32).

Impaired Skin Integrity. With decreased activity, there is more opportunity to develop pressure ulcers if a client's position is not changed at sufficient intervals to prevent excess pressure on bony prominences. Assess for skin breakdown. Do a thorough assessment of the skin daily with the bath and change of linen. In addition, assess the skin each time you change the client's position. Chapter 27 describes the appearance and treatment of pressure ulcers.

PLANNING

Whether a client's period of inactivity is short or long, the expected outcome goal is to prevent complications from inactivity and immobility. Box 33-2 illustrates the complications of disuse in the population of spinal cord injury clients. The primary prevention strategy is to maintain activity. Expected outcomes for *Risk for disuse syndrome* are that the client will do the following:

- Participate in decision making about self-care
- Have intact skin and mucous membranes
- Maintain full range of motion of joints
- Maintain optimum cardiac and respiratory function
- Maintain optimal patterns of elimination
- Maintain orientation to person, place, and time
- Consume calories and nutrients to meet energy requirements and promote healing
- Maintain contact with the outer world consistent with physical ability.

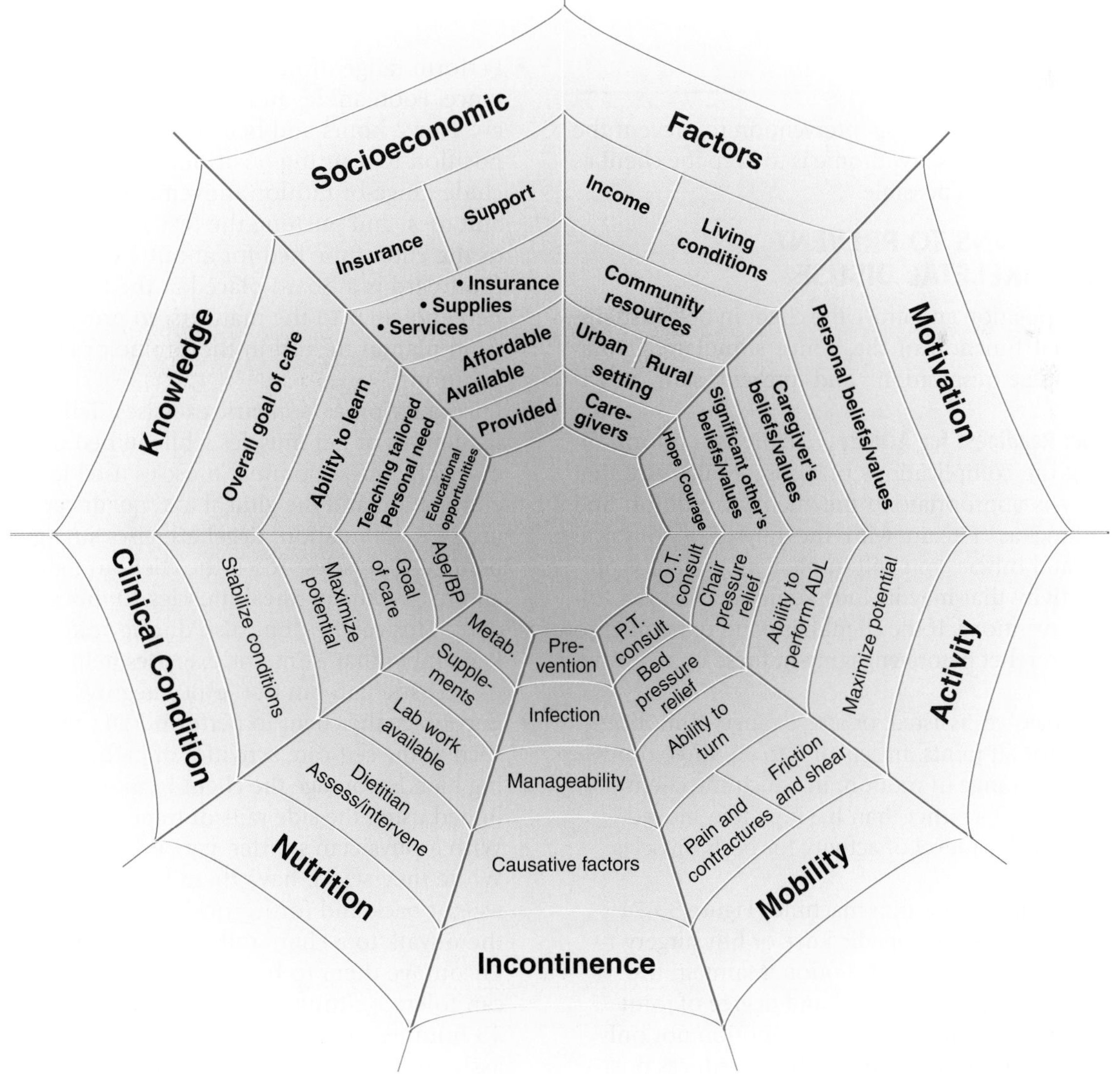

FIGURE 33-6 The web of causation of pressure ulcer development. (Redrawn with permission from Barbara Oot-Giromini, RN, MS, CETN, Binghamton, NY.)

BOX 33-2 *Evidence-Based Practice*

Preventing Complications in Spinal Cord Injury Clients

Problem: Clients with spinal cord injury experience or are at risk for adverse effects of immobility or secondary medical complications (e.g., the decline of body systems, altered functioning) as a result of musculoskeletal inactivity. Knowledge of the incidence of these complications provides a basis for preventative strategies.

Evidence

A study was done to analyze the incidence, risk factors, and trends of long-term adverse complications in immobile clients with spinal cord injury at annual follow-up evaluations. The researchers looked at pneumonia/atelectasis, autonomic dysreflexia, deep venous thrombosis, pulmonary embolism, pressure ulcers, fractures, and renal calculi. The percentage of persons who developed each complication was determined. Annual follow-up in postinjury years 1, 2, 5, 10, 15, and 20 were selected for analysis. Large sample sizes were used for each group. Percentages were compared across groups within each annual evaluation time frame by contingence table analysis and the chi-square statistic.

Application to Practice

This study summarizes significant findings that are important in the recognition of trends throughout the years. For example, the study found that the development of pressure ulcers was the most frequent complication documented at the first annual follow-up year and steadily increased at subsequent evaluations. Autonomic dysreflexia and pneumonia/atelectasis were also found. Risk factors included complete injury, tetraplegia, older age, concomitant illness, and violent injury. This study can assist nurses in prioritizing care and client teaching to prevent adverse effects of immobility.

Reference

McKinley, W. O., Jackson, A. B., Cardenas, D. D., & De Vivo, M. J. (1999). Long-term medical complications after traumatic spinal cord injury: A regional model systems analysis. *Archives of Physical Medicine and Rehabilitation, 80*(11), 1402-1410 [47 references].

INTERVENTION

The most important nursing intervention to prevent the complications of disuse syndrome is to keep the client as active and mobile as possible.

INTERVENTIONS TO PREVENT MUSCULOSKELETAL DISUSE

You should position and move the client in bed to maintain maximal function of the joints, stimulate circulation, maximize respiration, and prevent skin breakdown.

Maintain Readiness for Activity. Activity is a priority in preventing the complications of disuse. Make sure that the activity is appropriate to the client's condition and age. Working as a team with the physician, physical therapist, and others, you will implement a plan of progressive activity that may include some or all of the following interventions. If the client has pain, remember to provide pain relief before engaging in these or any other activities.

- Perform passive, assisted, or active range-of-motion exercises for all joints, in sets of 5 to 10, three times daily. Active range of motion, in which the client moves the limbs rather than having them moved, provides the best level of activity for both muscles and joints.
- A passive range-of-motion machine (Figure 33-7) is prescribed after orthopedic knee or hip surgery to maintain continuous joint motion. Maintain the device at the prescribed speed and degree of joint flexion. Use of continuous passive motion not only maintains range of motion, it actually reduces postsurgical pain.
- Perform range-of-motion exercises against resistance. Foot, ankle, and leg exercises can be done every 1 or 2 hours and before changing from a lying position to a sitting position. These exercises include range-of-motion movements for the ankles and toes, and pushing the feet against a footboard or the end of the bed for about 1 or 2 minutes. A footboard is a board placed at the foot of the bed, perpendicular to the mattress, to prevent the feet from plantar flexion in the supine or Fowler's position.
- Encourage other isometric exercises. Tell the client to tighten his or her muscles while in bed or in a chair, especially the abdominal muscles used for bowel elimination and the gluteal and quadriceps muscles used for ambulation. Kegel exercises strengthen the perineum muscles. Teach the client to tighten, hold, and release the perineal muscles 10 times, three times daily. This can be done also during voiding. Remember that isometric exercises help maintain muscle strength but not joint integrity.
- Encourage the client to perform ADLs independently, such as the self-care activities of bathing and combing hair. Encourage the client to move independently in bed using the side rails or trapeze.
- With a physician's order, get clients out of bed. While they stand, have them begin to shift their weight back and forth, rocking on both feet. Have them walk to a chair and sit, three times daily. Encourage them to be in the chair as long as they can tolerate sitting. An initial goal would be 30 to 45 minutes. As possible, have clients ambulate with assistance or with an assistive device (such as a walker, cane, or quad cane) four times daily or as

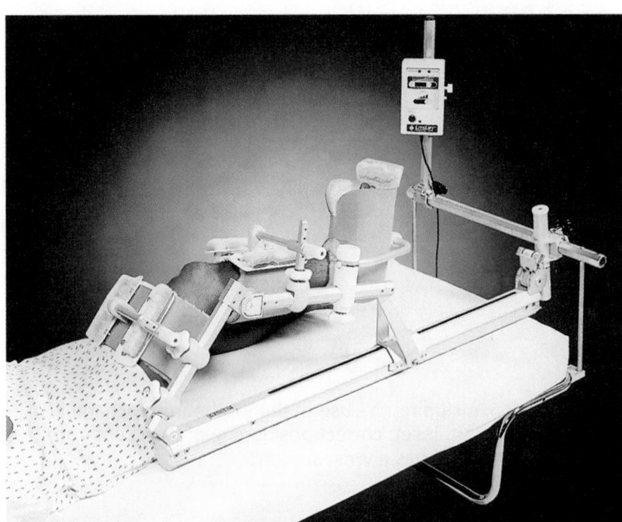

FIGURE 33-7 A passive range-of-motion, or continuous passive motion, device. (From Phipps, W. J., et al. [2003]. *Medical-surgical nursing: Health and illness perspectives* [7th ed.]. St. Louis, MO: Mosby.)

much as possible. As the clients progress, encourage them to be up most of the day with ad lib activity.

> ***Action Alert!*** Prevent the complications of disuse with an aggressive intervention of progressive activity.

Maintain Body Alignment. While in a bed, chair, or wheelchair (or while walking), the client should be positioned in good body alignment. When positioning a client who is unable to move, position the joints in anatomical or functional alignment. Provide support above and below the joints. Alternate the positions frequently, using side-lying, Sims', semisupine, supine, and Fowler's. The prone position is also therapeutic but is rarely used in clinical practice, especially if the client has some type of respiratory impairment (Box 33-3).

> ***Action Alert!*** Perform range-of-motion exercises on each joint to prevent contractures in the client who is immobile. Inactive muscles will contract and become inflexible. The joints will become fixed in a flexed position, making ADLs almost impossible to perform.

Change the client's position every 1 to 2 hours throughout the day and night. Make sure that all joints are positioned in extension (neutral) or in a functional position whenever possible and that you have taken proper precautions (Table 33-1). If a joint is in flexion for a period of time, perform active or passive range-of-motion exercises before the next position change. Use positioning devices such as foam boots or high-top tennis shoes, footboards, hand mitts, hand rolls or supports, eggcrate pads, over-bed cradles, **trochanter rolls,** wrist splints, and heel protectors to keep joints in alignment while the client is in bed (Box 33-4).

When the client is sitting in a chair, the head should be up, and the shoulders should be back. The arms should be supported to prevent pulling on the shoulders. Make sure that the feet are resting comfortably on the floor or are elevated on a footstool. When it is possible, the client should walk with the head up and facing forward, shoulders back, and feet forward.

INTERVENTIONS TO REDUCE THE *RISK FOR IMPAIRED SKIN INTEGRITY*

Skin care is influenced by culture, education, socioeconomic status, religion, and individual preference. You should respect the client's desires while trying to prevent skin complications caused by disuse. Several strategies should be used to prevent skin impairments, including activities to monitor the client, cleanse the skin, provide nutrition, reposition the client, and encourage the client to maintain ADLs. Client teaching is also valuable in preventing development of some skin problems.

Monitor the Client. Skin assessment is essential in identifying the client at risk. Perform skin assessment at least once a day, paying special attention to bony prominences.

One of the most important aspects of preventing *Impaired skin integrity* is recognizing which clients are at risk (Box 33-5). Also consider environmental factors in the at-risk client. For instance, prolonged supine positioning on a stretcher in the emergency department, skin moisture caused by diaphoresis, and wrinkled bed linens can put a client's skin integrity at risk. When caring for a surgical client, monitor all tubes, catheters, and drains because these may cause skin breakdown or exert excessive pressure on the client's skin.

Cleanse the Skin. Keep the client's skin clean. Be sure it is cleansed immediately after soiling and at routine intervals. During cleansing, minimize force and friction to the skin to help prevent skin breakdown. Try to reduce the client's exposure to moisture caused by incontinence, perspiration, and wound drainage. Keep in mind that exposure to moisture may cause skin maceration or breakdown.

If a client is bedridden, a bed bath is indicated. The client can still participate in the bath, however, by performing it as independently as possible. Avoid the use of powder because it may retain moisture and can cause pulmonary damage if inhaled.

Increase Circulation. Increase circulation to the skin to enhance transport of nutrients and oxygen to cells in the skin. Increase the temperature in the room to a comfortable level. Use a bath blanket while bathing the client, and keep the bath water between 105° and 110° F to prevent chilling and vasoconstriction.

> ***Action Alert!*** Do not use hot water and harsh soap to cleanse the client's skin. Tailor the plan for skin cleansing on the basis of the client's preferences and skin care needs.

BOX 33-3 *Common Client Positions*

Lateral, Semiprone, and Semisupine Positions

- In the lateral (side-lying) position, the trunk is at a right angle to the bed. To increase the base of support and comfort, one or both legs are bent, and both arms are extended in front of the body. Because the body weight is borne on the shoulders and hips, the semiprone or the semisupine position is preferred.

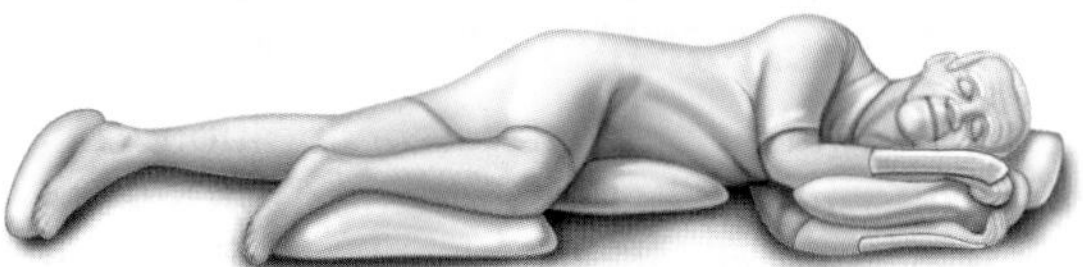

Lateral (side-lying) position.

- In the semiprone position (the Sims' or forward side-lying position), the trunk is rotated 15 to 30 degrees forward from the lateral position, with the superior arm and leg supported in front of the body to form part of the base of support.

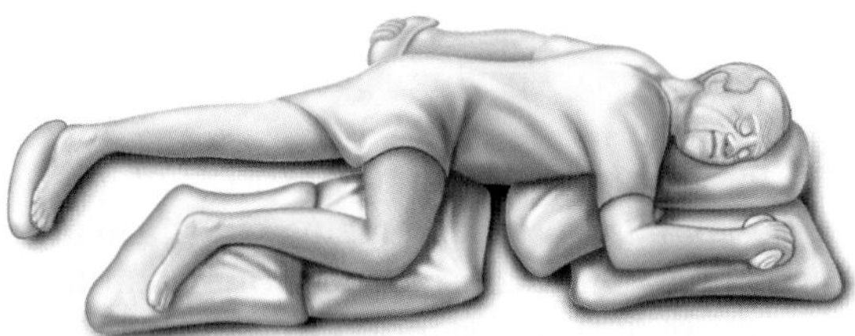

Semiprone (Sims' or forward side-lying) position.

- In the semisupine position (the modified lateral or oblique position), the trunk is rotated 15 to 30 degrees from supine, with the superior arm and leg supported in a comfortable position. The semiprone and semisupine positions minimize pressure on bony prominences of the shoulder and hip.

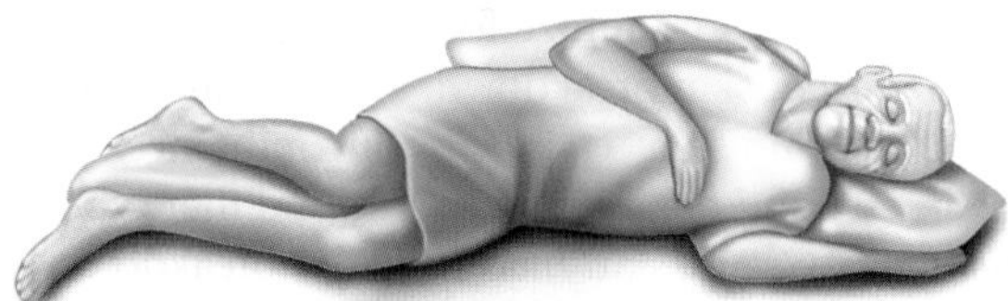

Semisupine (modified lateral or oblique) position, which can be used as a substitute for the side-lying position and results in less pressure on the trochanteric area.

Supine and Fowler's Positions

- Both the supine and Fowler's positions are back-lying positions. Supine is a horizontal position, and Fowler's is a sitting position. The supine position prevents lordosis or kyphosis.
- In high-Fowler's position, the head of the client's bed is elevated to 90 degrees. In semi-Fowler's position, it is elevated to 45 degrees. In low-Fowler's position, it is elevated about 30 degrees. Usually, the client's knees are bent slightly.

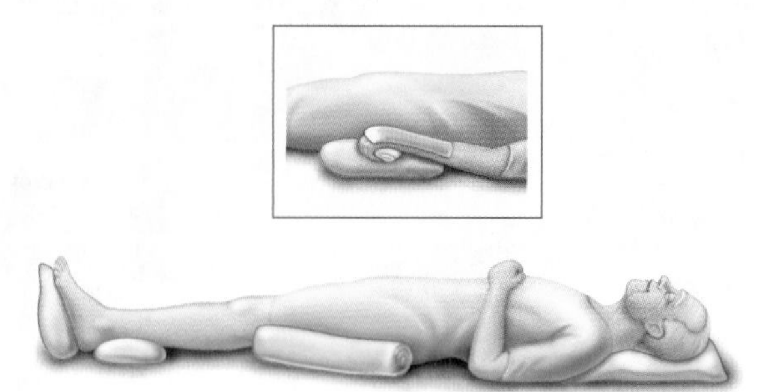

Supine position, including the use of the footboard, trochanter roll, and lumbar support. Inset: correct positioning of the client's arm, which is elevated and has a wrist support.

- Fowler's position concentrates body weight on the sacrum and creates shearing force. Reducing the angle and the time in the position are preventive measures. Prevent hip and knee contractures by instructing the client to shift positions and perform range-of-motion exercises.

Prone Position

- In the prone position, the client lies front down with his or her face turned to the side and one or both arms turned up, as shown. This position may be contraindicated in the presence of abdominal distention or wounds.

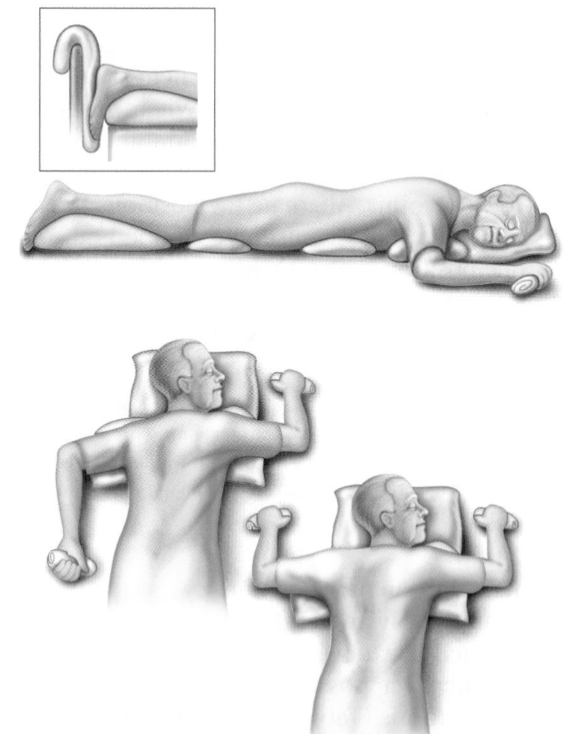

Prone position. The client's arms and shoulders may be positioned in internal or external rotation.

Table 33-1 Precautions for Proper Positioning

LATERAL POSITION, SEMIPRONE POSITION, SEMISUPINE POSITION	SUPINE POSITION, FOWLER'S POSITION	PRONE POSITION
HEAD AND NECK		
• Prevent forward flexion of head, neck, and cervical spine. • Prevent lateral bending of head, neck, and cervical spine.	• Prevent forward flexion of head, neck, and cervical spine. • Prevent lateral bending of head, neck, and cervical spine. • Avoid pressure on back of head.	• Prevent hyperextension, lateral bending, and pressure on cheek and ear.
SHOULDERS • Avoid direct pressure on acromion process. • Prevent adduction of shoulders. • Avoid skin-to-skin contact of axillae.	• Prevent forward flexion. • Avoid pressure on scapulae. • Avoid skin-to-skin contact at axillae by abducting shoulders slightly.	• Prevent forward flexion of neck. • Avoid skin-to-skin contact at axillae.
BREASTS AND MALE GENITALIA	• Prevent skin-to-skin contact in presence of moisture.	• Avoid abdominal pressure.
ELBOWS AND WRISTS • Prevent flexion or hyperextension. • Avoid pressure on thorax and ribs from upper arms. • Avoid pressure on lateral condyle of humerus. • Prevent edema.	• Prevent flexion. • Prevent edema. • Avoid pressure on elbow.	• Prevent flexion by positioning elbows in extension.
FINGERS AND THUMB • Prevent flexion and opposition of fingers and thumb.	• Prevent flexion and opposition of fingers and thumb.	• Prevent flexion and opposition of fingers and thumb.
SPINE • Prevent lateral bending. • Prevent rotation.	• Prevent flexion of lumbar spine. • Prevent lateral bending (shoulders and hips in alignment). • Avoid pressure on lumbosacral area.	• Prevent hyperextension of lumbar spine by using a firm mattress or lumbar support.
HIPS AND KNEES • Prevent adduction, flexion, and internal rotation of upper leg. • Avoid pressure on iliac crest. • Avoid skin-to-skin contact at perineum.	• Prevent adduction, flexion, and internal rotation of upper legs. • Avoid prolonged flexion. • Avoid skin-to-skin contact at perineum. • Avoid compression of popliteal artery.	• Prevent internal rotation. • Avoid pressure on patella and anterior iliac spine. • Avoid skin-to-skin contact at perineum.
ANKLES AND TOES • Prevent inversion and plantar flexion of upper foot. • Avoid pressure on ankle of lower foot.	• Prevent plantar flexion. • Avoid pressure on toes and heels.	• Prevent plantar flexion. • Avoid pressure on toes.

Gently massage the skin, but avoid areas that are reddened or are over bony prominences to avoid additional injury. Use long, firm, strokes, and move from distal to proximal areas during the bath. Encourage the client to participate in ADLs to increase blood circulation.

Action Alert! Avoid massaging over bony prominences where early signs of pressure ulcers are present. Also, do not massage the legs; this could increase the risk for pulmonary embolism if a deep vein thrombosis is forming.

To minimize dry skin, apply topical moisturizing agents and maintain adequate skin hydration. Keep in mind that although the client may find a gentle massage relaxing and soothing, you must use caution when applying creams and lotions to high-risk or reddened skin areas.

Elevate the client's arms on pillows. If the client cannot brush his or her own hair, offer to do so twice a day. If the client is cold, offer extra blankets, socks, and other warm clothing.

Decrease Microorganisms. Removing dead skin cells decreases the growth and accumulation of microorganisms, which can help to prevent skin irritation and infection and reduce body odor. Most clients need to cleanse the skin in some manner each day and any time they

BOX 33-4 Positioning Devices

Foam boots or high-top tennis shoes.

Foam boots or high-top tennis shoes to keep the ankle in dorsiflexion.

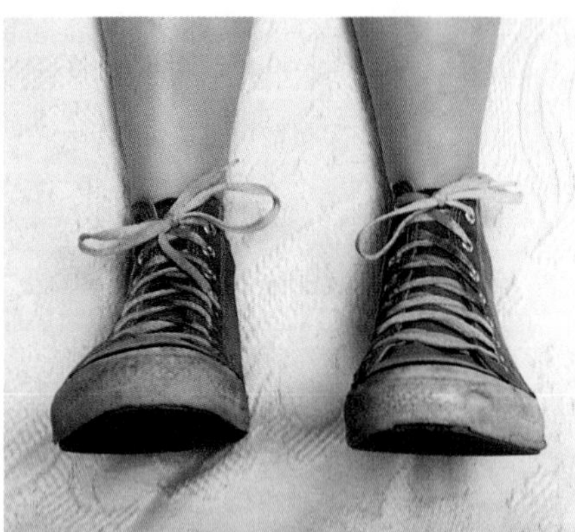

Hand mitt.

Mitten that slides over the fingers to keep the fingers from flexion and the thumb from opposition.

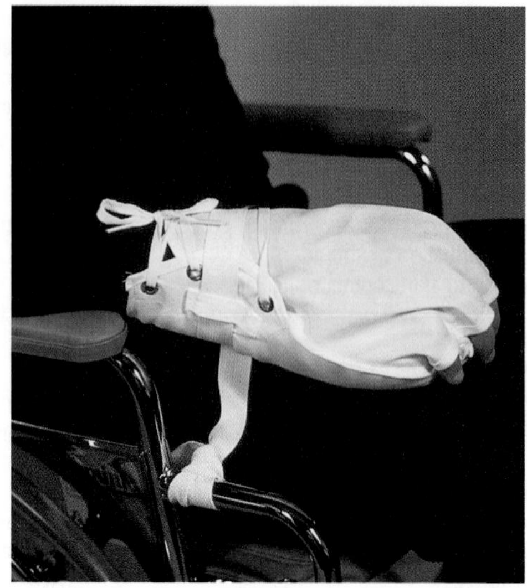

(Courtesy Medline Industries, Mundelein, IL.)

Footboard.

Board placed at the end of bed, perpendicular to the mattress, to prevent the feet from assuming plantar flexion in the supine or Fowler's position. May be used for isometric exercises of the foot and leg to prevent deep vein thrombosis.

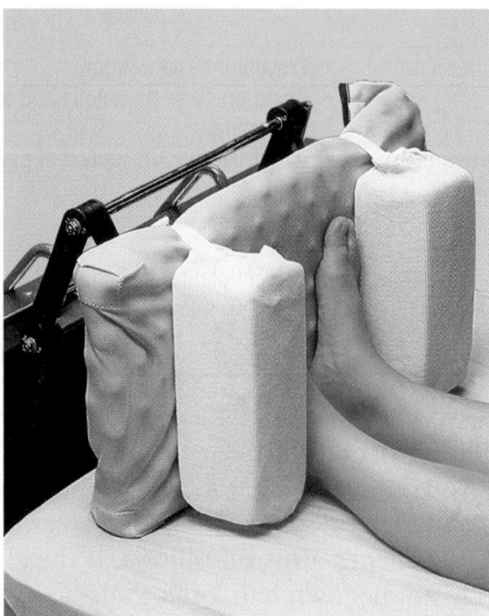

(Courtesy J.T. Posey Co., Arcadia, CA.)

Hand roll/support.

Roll of cloth or manufactured hand grip placed in the palm of the hand used to keep the fingers from flexion and the thumb from opposition.

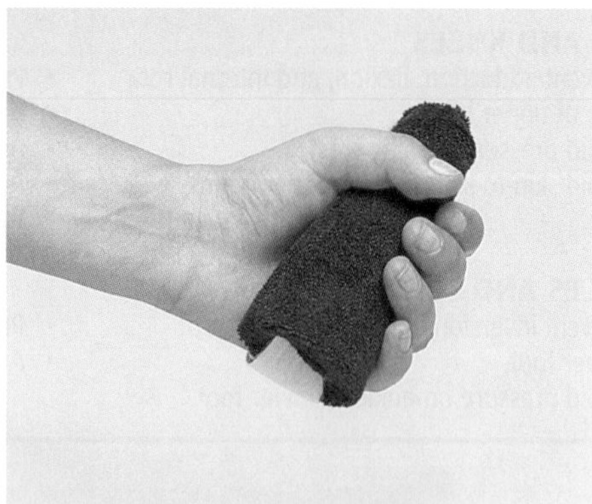

(Courtesy J.T. Posey Co., Arcadia, CA.)

BOX 33-4 *Positioning Devices—cont'd*

Over-bed cradle.	Device placed at the end of the bed to raise the top sheet and thus prevent pressure ulcers on the toes and plantar flexion of the ankles.

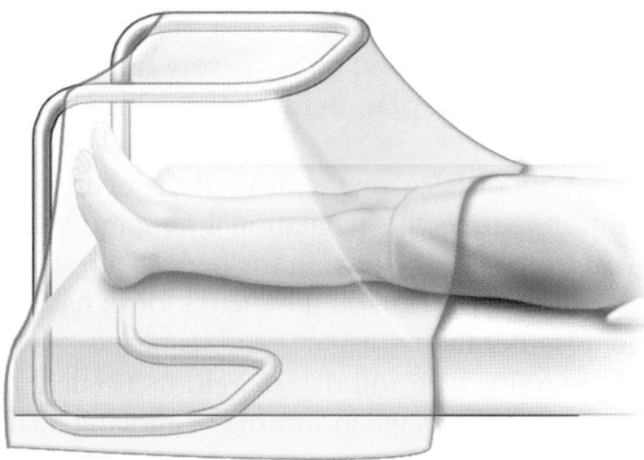

Wrist splint.	Support placed on the client's wrist to prevent flexion.

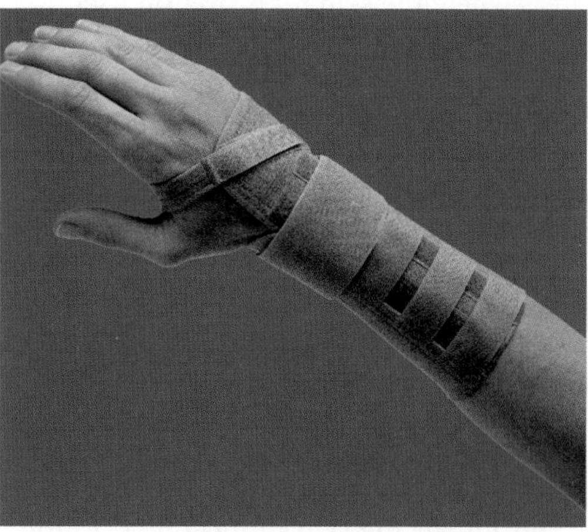

(Courtesy North Coast Medical, San José, CA.)

Trochanter roll.	Sheet placed halfway under a client's hip and rolled snugly against the hip to prevent external rotation of the trochanter (hip joint).

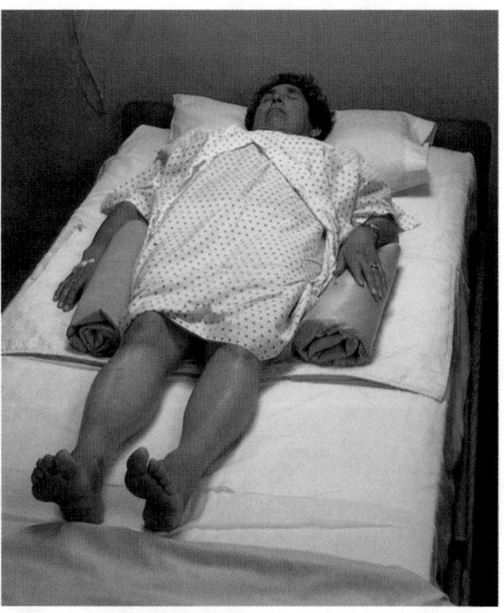

Heel protectors.	Sheepskin or other padded device to prevent skin breakdown at the heels.

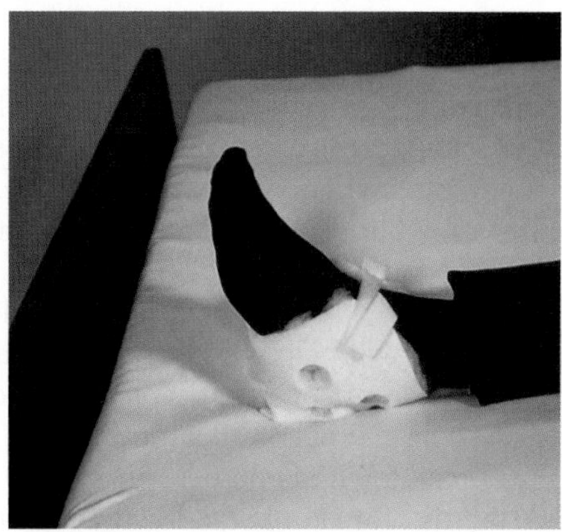

(Courtesy Medline Industries, Mundelein, IL.)

BOX 33-5 *Conditions That Increase the Risk for Impaired Skin Integrity*

- Advanced age
- Altered level of consciousness
- Chronic conditions that limit physical mobility
- Deficient nutrition
- Dehydration
- Diabetes
- Fractures
- Short-term or long-term immobility
- Impaired circulation
- Incontinence
- Multisystem trauma
- Obesity
- Paralysis

become soiled. Older adults may need only a partial bath of the back and perineum.

Remove Excess Moisture. To help keep the skin dry, make sure that bed linens are breathable cotton, not plastic. Dry the client's skin well after bathing, particularly in areas where the skin folds over on itself, such as at the axillae, under the breasts, and in the perineal area. Change the client's bed linens immediately if they become wet from diaphoresis (sweating) or incontinence, and bathe the client. Position the client to allow air to circulate to the axillae and perineal areas.

Remember that, although dry skin discourages the growth of microorganisms, overly dry skin can crack open and form lesions. To help the skin from becoming too dry, use a moisturizing lotion after baths. Do not use soap every day for bathing unless it is very mild; clear water may be used instead. Do not use alcohol on the skin because it has a drying effect and can crack the skin.

Decrease Friction and Excoriation. Friction and excoriation can impair the skin's function as a protective barrier. To decrease the risk for friction and excoriation, gently pat the client's skin dry rather than rubbing with a towel after baths. Use a soft washcloth and soft towels during the bath. Linens should be soft and smooth as well. Use a turning sheet (also called a drawsheet) or trapeze when moving the client in bed. Lift clients, rather than dragging them, when moving them in bed. Use extra help to move clients if needed.

Use protective ointment around wounds or on the client's perineum, as needed. According to the physician's order, change the client's wound dressings frequently. Take care when removing the tape. Place a drainage bag on wounds as needed. Check casts, braces, traction, restraints, and splints for irritation.

Provide Nutrition. Promote nutrition and a well-balanced diet. This will help prevent skin breakdown and pressure ulcer development (see Chapters 24 and 25).

Position the Client Properly. Positioning the client at risk for skin breakdown is one of your major roles. You can reduce the risk for skin breakdown with various positioning strategies, including the following:

- Reposition high-risk clients at least every 2 hours.
- Use positioning devices such as pillows to keep bony prominences from touching one another.
- Raise the client's heels completely off the bed.

> ***Action Alert!*** Do not use doughnut devices to relieve pressure on the client's heels. Instead, suspend the heels off the bed to prevent pressure ulcers there.

- Avoid placing the client's body weight directly on the trochanter when a side-lying position is used. Instead, position the client at a 30-degree angle to reduce pressure on both the trochanter and the sacrum (Figure 33-8).
- Keep the head of the bed as low as the client can tolerate; sacral pressure is reduced when head of bed is 30 degrees or lower.
- When moving the client, use proper positioning, transferring, and turning techniques to minimize friction and shear. For example, use assistive devices such as a trapeze or the bed linens. Consider using lubricants (such as creams and cornstarch), protective films (such as a transparent dressing), and protective devices to help reduce friction.
- Avoid prolonged sitting in a chair or wheelchair by repositioning the client at least every hour.
- Develop a written plan of care for positioning and turning.

Prevent Shear. Placing the head of the bed in a low or flat position reduces the gravitational pull and helps keep the client from sliding down in the bed. As a result, it prevents shearing of the skin on the client's lower back. Lifting the client (rather than dragging) and using a turning sheet helps to prevent shear injuries as well. As needed, ask for help from co-workers when turning or moving a client in bed (Procedure 33-1). Limit the time the client spends in Fowler's position to 30 to 60 minutes. During that time, use a footboard, and support the client's arms on pillows.

Decrease Pressure. To relieve pressure, turn the client to a new position every 1 to 2 hours. To ensure pressure relief, follow a 24-hour turning schedule (side to back to other side to supine). Encourage a client who can sit in a chair to shift position every 15 minutes or to do push-ups on the arms of the chair.

> ***Action Alert!*** Reposition the client on bed rest every 1 to 2 hours, keep the bed dry and wrinkle free, and keep the client dry to help prevent pressure ulcers.

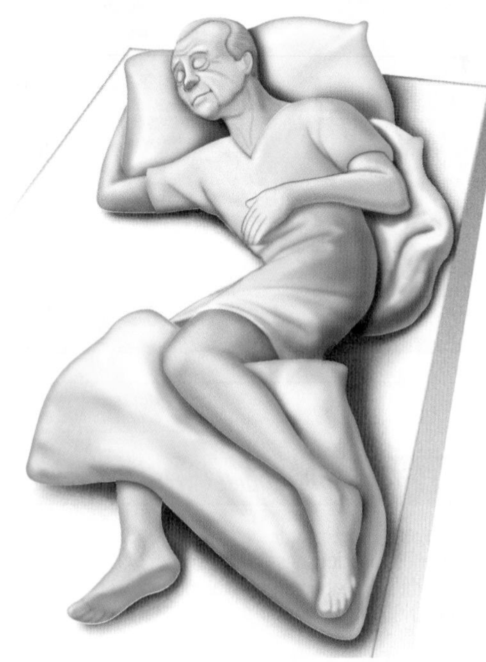

FIGURE 33-8 Position the client on his or her side at a 30-degree angle to prevent pressure on the trochanter and sacrum. To keep the client in this position, provide support with pillows, as shown.

If needed, have the client set a timer to remember to shift weight. Remember that standard mattresses exert considerable pressure against the skin. As needed, use a special mattress to reduce the pressure, such as an eggcrate, foam, sheepskin, gel, flotation, or water bed. Keep the bed linens and pillows free of wrinkles.

Use Support Surfaces When Indicated. Support surfaces are therapeutic devices used to control pressure and protect bony prominences. These devices serve many functions, including reducing pressure, friction, and shear, controlling moisture, and inhibiting bacterial growth. Many support surfaces are available in various sizes and shapes for use on beds and in chairs (Figure 33-9). Use them in conjunction with meticulous turning and repositioning to prevent development of pressure ulcers and, if indicated, to enhance healing of existing pressure ulcers.

Be aware that no single support surface eliminates the effects of pressure on the skin. Assess your client carefully to determine the most appropriate support surface. Keep in mind that *pressure-relieving devices* reduce the interface pressure between the body and the support surface below 32 mm Hg (thus capillary closing pressure). *Pressure-reducing devices* also reduce the interface pressure—but not below the capillary closing pressure. Support surface therapy must be tailored to the client's individual needs. Foam overlays that are 3 to 4 inches thick may also help reduce pressure. Support surface characteristics and cost are important factors to consider. Static air overlays—mattresses that are blown up—also serve to reduce pressure. Low-air-loss beds can benefit a client who needs moisture control and prevention of maceration and friction.

INTERVENTIONS TO MAINTAIN CIRCULATORY FUNCTION

Interventions are needed to maintain the circulatory status and prevent complications.

Decrease Edema Formation. Unless contraindicated, elevate clients' legs to counteract gravity and assist with venous return. This position can prevent dependent edema formation and can reduce edema if present. Keep clients' legs at heart level while they are in bed. Place their feet on a footstool while they sit in a chair. Elevate their arms to prevent edema formation or decrease edema in their hands.

Decrease Blood Stasis. Elastic antiembolism stockings and sequential compression devices can be used to apply external pressure on the client's legs to prevent blood

Text continued on p. 883

TIME TO ALLOW: NOVICE: 10 min. EXPERT: 5 min.

PROCEDURE 33-1 TURNING AND MOVING A CLIENT IN BED

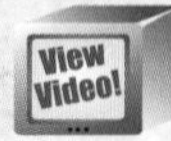

Especially for a client with a *Risk for disuse syndrome*, you will need to pay special attention to proper turning and positioning. Often, you will perform these activities on a schedule tailored to the client's condition and needs. Each time, you must follow appropriate steps to avoid injuring the client or yourself. This procedure describes proper methods for turning a client in bed (alone and with another nurse), moving a client up in bed (alone and with another nurse), and transferring a client from bed to stretcher.

DELEGATION GUIDELINES

The routine positioning and repositioning of a client in bed may be delegated to a nursing assistant. For clients with mobility or positioning restrictions, however, you must first assess the client and then determine the appropriateness of delegation on the basis of risk to the client. For a client requiring multiple personnel for turning and moving, you may perform the procedure together with multiple nursing assistants.

EQUIPMENT NEEDED

- Turning sheet
- Pillows or wedges for positioning
- Trapeze
- Transfer board

1 Follow preliminary actions (see inside front cover).

2 Before turning or moving a client in bed or transferring a client to a stretcher, lock the bed's wheels and assess the client's condition.

a. Can the client assist with turning, moving, or transferring?
b. Do any joints have contractures or need special handling?
c. Can the client tolerate having the head of the bed lowered briefly?
d. Can you turn or move the client alone, or will you need help from colleagues? *Turning or moving a client alone requires that you be sure you can manage the client's weight. If the procedure requires two or three nurses, one nurse should take charge of the procedure.*

Continued

TURNING A CLIENT ALONE

1 Lower the head of the bed and the bed's knee-raising (gatch) device until the bed is flat. Raise the bed to a comfortable working height. *You will be better able to handle the client's weight on a flat surface. Also, the flat position allows you to avoid moving uphill against gravity. Raising the bed height reduces strain on the nurse's back.*

2 Move the client to one side of the bed. *This allows room to turn the client to the opposite side.*

a. First, slide your arms under the client's shoulders and back, and move the client's upper body to one side of the bed (see illustration).

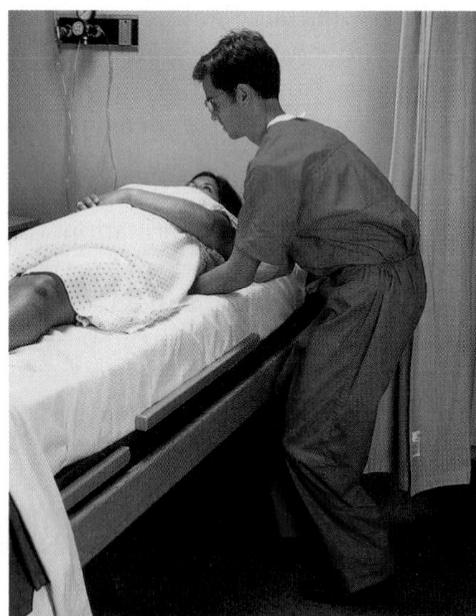

Step 2a. Sliding the arms under the client's shoulders and back.

b. Then, slide your arms under the client's hips, and slide the hips to the side.

c. Finally, move the client's feet and legs to the side of the bed.

3 Cross the client's arms across the chest, and cross the legs at the ankle (see illustration). Position a pillow or wedge at the head or foot of the bed to be used behind the client's back after turning. *Crossing the client's arms and legs helps the body turn as a unit.*

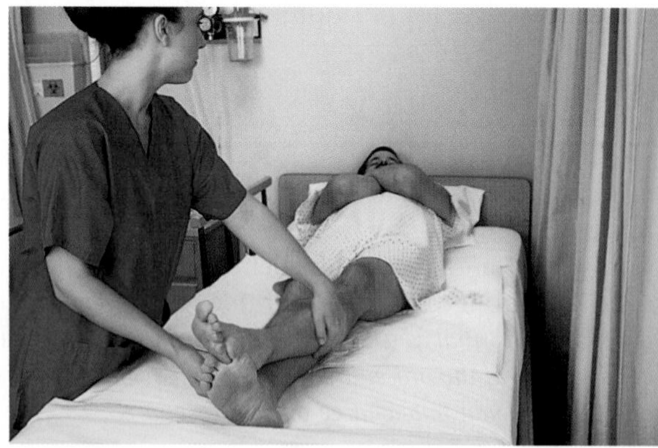

Step 3. Crossing the client's arms and legs.

4 Place one hand on the client's shoulder and the other hand on the client's hip, and roll the client toward you. *Pulling is easier than pushing.*

5 Turn the client far enough forward so that you can release one hand and position a pillow or wedge behind the client's back.

6 You may need to go to the opposite side of the bed and pull the client's hips toward the center of the bed to make the position more stable. Check the position according to Table 33-1, p. 875.

TURNING A CLIENT WITH ANOTHER NURSE

1 Bring the bed to a comfortable working height. With the bed in a flat position, move the client to one side of the bed. *This allows room to turn the client to the opposite side.*

a. If the client is on a turning sheet (a sheet that extends from the shoulders to below the hips), stand on opposite sides of the bed so that each nurse can grasp the top and bottom of the sheet (see illustration).

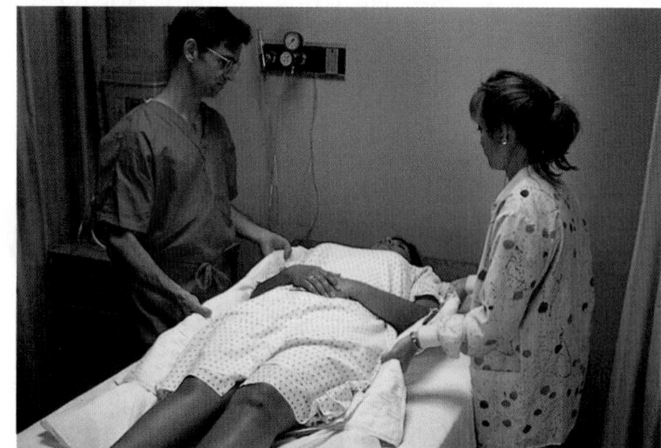

Step 1a. Two nurses grasping the top and bottom of a turning sheet.

b. If the client is not on a turning sheet, both nurses should stand on the same side of the bed. One nurse should slide his or her arms under the client's shoulders while the other slides his or her arms under the client's hips. On the count of three, both nurses should slide the client to one side of the bed. *When turning a client, make sure you stand with your knees somewhat bent and your feet spread so that you have a wide base of support.*

2 Bend the client's knee on the side opposite the one to which you will be turning. Fold the client's arms over the chest. One nurse is positioned on each side of the bed.

3 Turn the client.

a. If you do not have a turning sheet, the nurse positioned on the side of the bed toward which the client will turn should place one hand on the client's shoulder and one hand on the client's hip. The nurse then pulls the shoulder and hip toward himself or herself. At the same time, the nurse on the opposite side of the bed slides his or her hands under the client's bottom hip, pulls the hip toward himself or herself, and places a pillow at the client's back (see illustration).

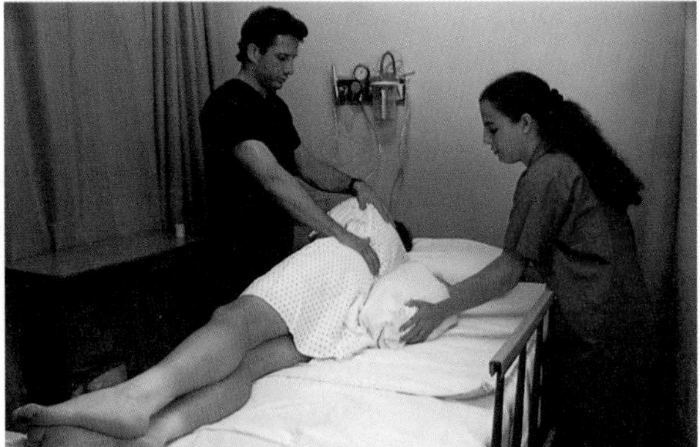

Step 3a. Placing a pillow at the client's back.

b. If you have a turning sheet, use it to pull the client's hips and shoulders in the direction of the turn.

4 Place a pillow between the client's legs (see illustration). *The pillow at the back supports the client in the side-lying position. The pillow between the legs maintains alignment of the spine and hips and prevents skin-to-skin contact.*

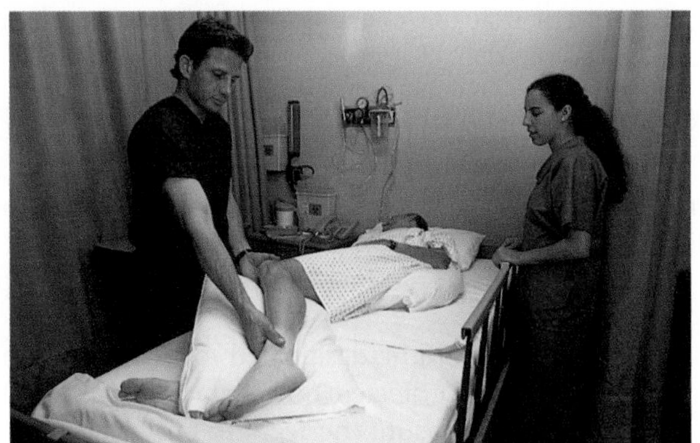

Step 4. Placing a pillow between the client's legs.

5 Check the client's position against Table 33-1, p. 875 to make sure that the client is properly positioned.

6 If the client's condition demands that you maintain anatomical alignment of the spine during turns, you may need three nurses working together to turn the body and head as a unit. The spine is kept straight as the client is turned (see illustration).

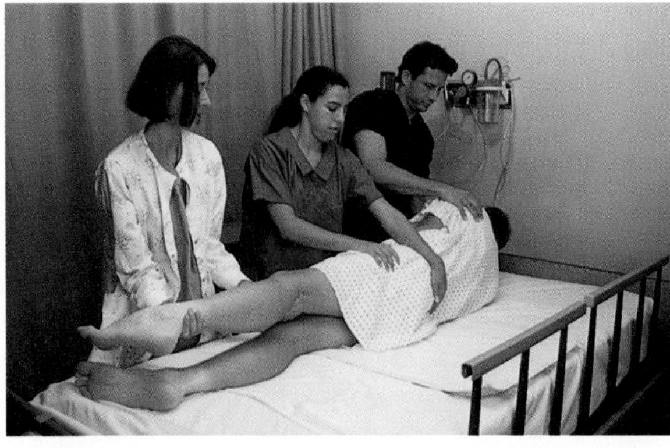

Step 6. Keeping the spine straight as the client is turned.

7 After turning a client, make sure to document that the client was turned. Also document the position assumed. *Proper documentation helps to maintain continuity of care. The next nurses to work with the client will know what positions have been used and the amount of time in the position.*

MOVING A CLIENT UP IN BED

1 Before moving a client up in bed, determine whether you can do it alone or whether you need help from another nurse. If you can do it alone, determine whether to stand at the side of the bed or at the head of the bed. Lower the head of the bed as far as the client can tolerate.

a. For one nurse to assist a client with moving up in bed from the side of the bed, have the client bend the knees and place the feet flat on the bed so he or she can push. Place one hand under the client's back and one under the thighs, close to the hips. Tell the client to push with the legs on a count of three. When the client does, slide him or her up toward the head of the bed (see illustration).

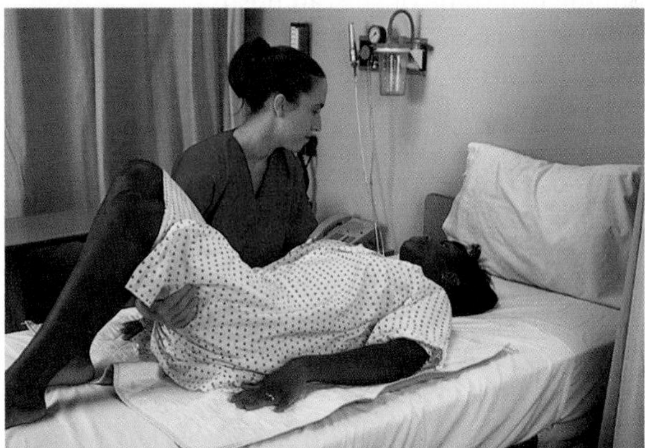

Step 1a. One nurse assisting a client to move up in bed from the side of the bed.

b. For one nurse standing at the head of the bed to move a lightweight client, start by removing the headboard from the bed. Place the bed in a slight Trendelenburg's position (head lower than the feet). When possible, use a turning sheet to move the client; otherwise, slide your hands under the client's shoulders, and pull the client toward you (see illustration).

Continued

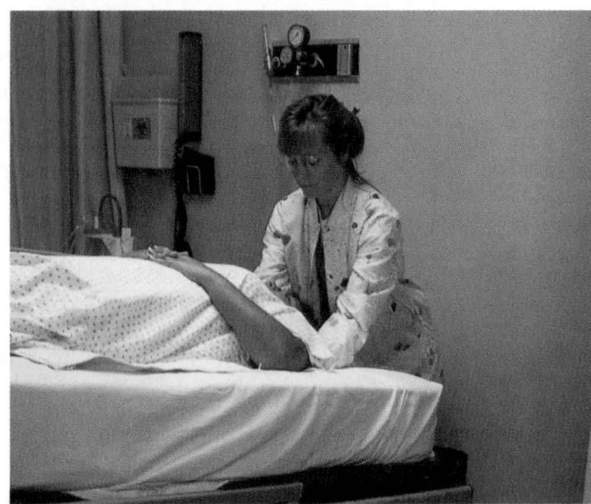

Step 1b. One nurse assisting a client to move up in bed from the head of the bed, using the force of gravity created by a slight Trendelenburg's position.

2 If the client has good upper body strength, use a trapeze to move the client up in bed.

a. Place a trapeze over the bed.
b. Have the client bend the knees and place the feet flat on the bed so he or she can push.
c. Have the client hold on to the trapeze and pull with the arms to lift the hips slightly off the bed (see illustration).

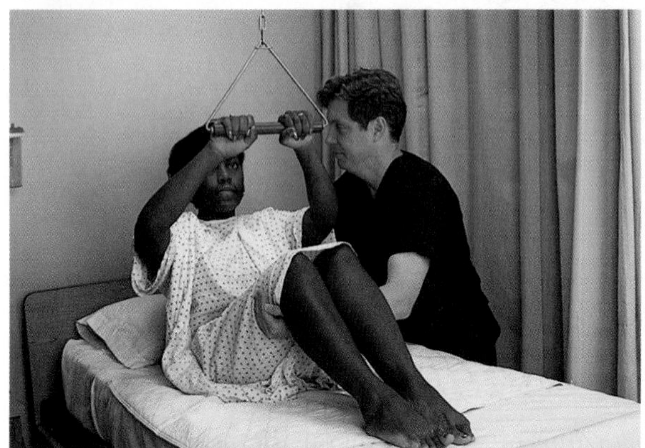

Step 2c. One nurse assisting a client to move up in bed using a trapeze.

d. With hips lifted, have the client push with the legs to move up in bed.
e. You may assist by placing your hands under the client's thighs, close to the hips.

3 If the client is too heavy to move by yourself, get help from a colleague.

a. Stand on opposite sides of the client's bed.
b. With the client's knees bent and feet flat on the bed, each nurse grasps the turn sheet with one hand at the level of the shoulders and the other hand at the level of the hips.
c. On the count of three, the client pushes with the legs as the two nurses slide the torso up in bed (see illustration).

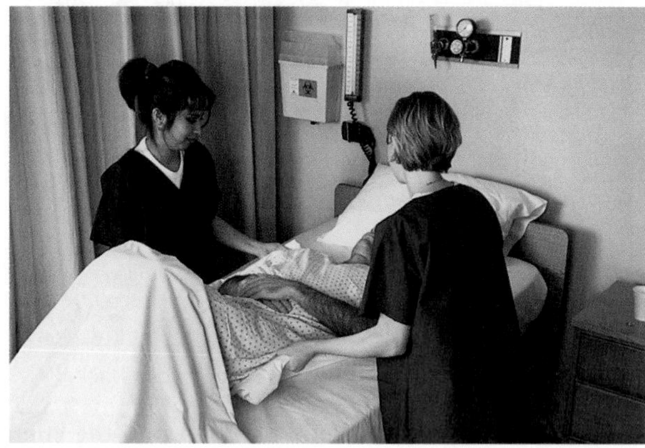

Step 3c. Two nurses assisting a client to move up in bed.

4 After moving the client up, raise the head of the bed, and check the position against Table 33-1.

5 Document that the client was repositioned and the position assumed.

MOVING A CLIENT FROM A BED TO A STRETCHER

1 If a client is unable to move from the bed to a stretcher on his or her own, you will need to move the client.

a. Two caregivers should be positioned on each side of the stretcher.
b. One person should be designated to ensure that the client's head is protected during movement, while another should ensure the feet are protected. Make sure the wheels are locked on both the bed and the stretcher. Position the bed and stretcher next to each other without any gaps in between.

2 Use a sheet to make the transfer easier.

a. Untuck the sheet from the client's bed.
b. Have one nurse grasp the sheet under the client's shoulders while another on the same side grasps it at the client's hips and legs. The nurses on the opposite side of the bed should do the same.
c. On a count of three, the nurses on the stretcher side should lift and pull the client onto the stretcher. The nurses on the opposite side of the bed provide minimal assistance because it is more difficult to push than pull.

3 As an alternative, use a transfer board.

a. Two nurses standing on the same side of the bed turn the client away from the stretcher.

b. Place the transfer board where the client was lying, and turn the client back onto the board (see illustration).

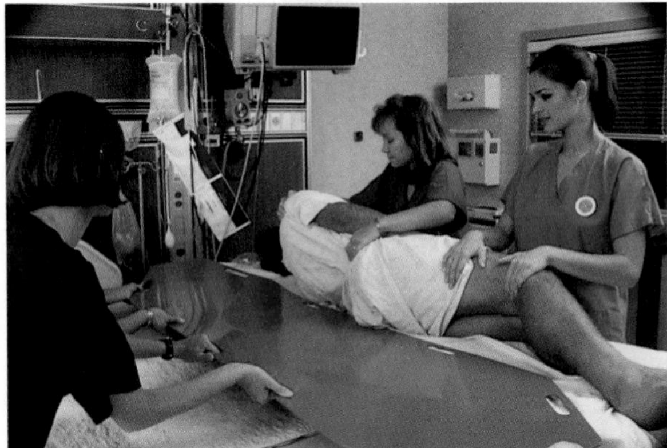

Step 3b. Placing the transfer board where the client was lying.

c. Pull the board onto the stretcher with the client on it.

d. Turn the client again to remove the board.

4 Raise the side rails on the outside of the stretcher, then move between the bed and stretcher and raise the remaining side rails.

5 If the stretcher cannot be positioned adjacent to the bed but can be positioned at a right angle to the bed, use a three-person lift to transfer the client.

a. Position three nurses on the same side of the bed.

b. One nurse slides his or her hands and arms under the client's head and shoulders. The second slides his or her hands under the client's back and buttocks, and the third one slides his or her hands under the legs and thighs. On the count of three, the nurses simultaneously lift the client. *In this procedure, each nurse bears only a third of the client's weight.*

c. The three nurses then move as a unit to rotate and transfer the client to the stretcher (see illustration).

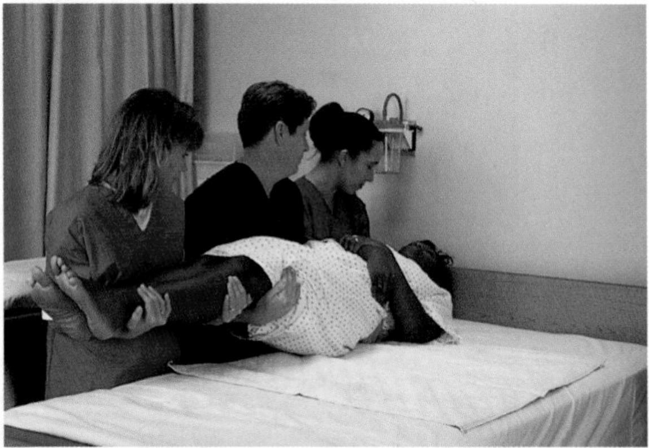

Step 5c. Moving a client from a stretcher to a bed using a three-person lift.

6 Cover the client with a sheet. Supply a pillow, and raise the head of the stretcher if needed for the client's comfort. Fasten a safety strap over the client. It can be fastened loosely if the client is fully alert. Put side rails up.

HOME HEALTH CARE CONSIDERATIONS

Work closely with family caregivers to teach methods of turning and methods of preventing back strain in the caregiver. The family must understand the importance of a regular schedule of turning, even through the night. A single caregiver is not sufficient to provide care around-the-clock to a family member who is unable to turn and move in bed. All family members must understand the importance of skin integrity and agree to participate in maintaining it. Families must also understand that pressure ulcers can form in a chair or wheelchair; the client must periodically shift weight to relieve pressure.

from pooling in the veins. These devices, with the assistance of the calf muscles, "milk" venous blood back up to the heart. They decrease blood stasis and prevent the formation of thrombi and edema.

Antiembolism stockings are elasticized stockings that provide varying degrees of pressures at different areas of the leg. To provide the optimal amount of pressure, the stockings should fit properly and be free of wrinkles. Periodically inspect the feet for evidence of poor circulation, and remove the stockings two to three times daily to inspect the skin (Procedure 33-2).

Leg exercises can supplement the effect of antiembolism stockings in preventing venous stasis. One exercise that can be done by most clients is to flex and extend the foot five times per hour. A second exercise is to bend the knee and draw the foot up to the thigh, then extend the leg again. A third exercise is to raise the leg off the bed, one leg at a time. These exercises can be active or passive.

Sequential compression devices are plastic sleeves that are wrapped around the client's legs. The sleeves have air tubes that are inflated in sequence from the bottom of the leg to the top, helping to move venous blood out of the leg veins and toward the heart (Procedure 33-3). Once the client can ambulate, the device is discontinued.

Maintain Venous Return. Avoiding compression of leg veins maintains blood flow and prevents venous stasis.

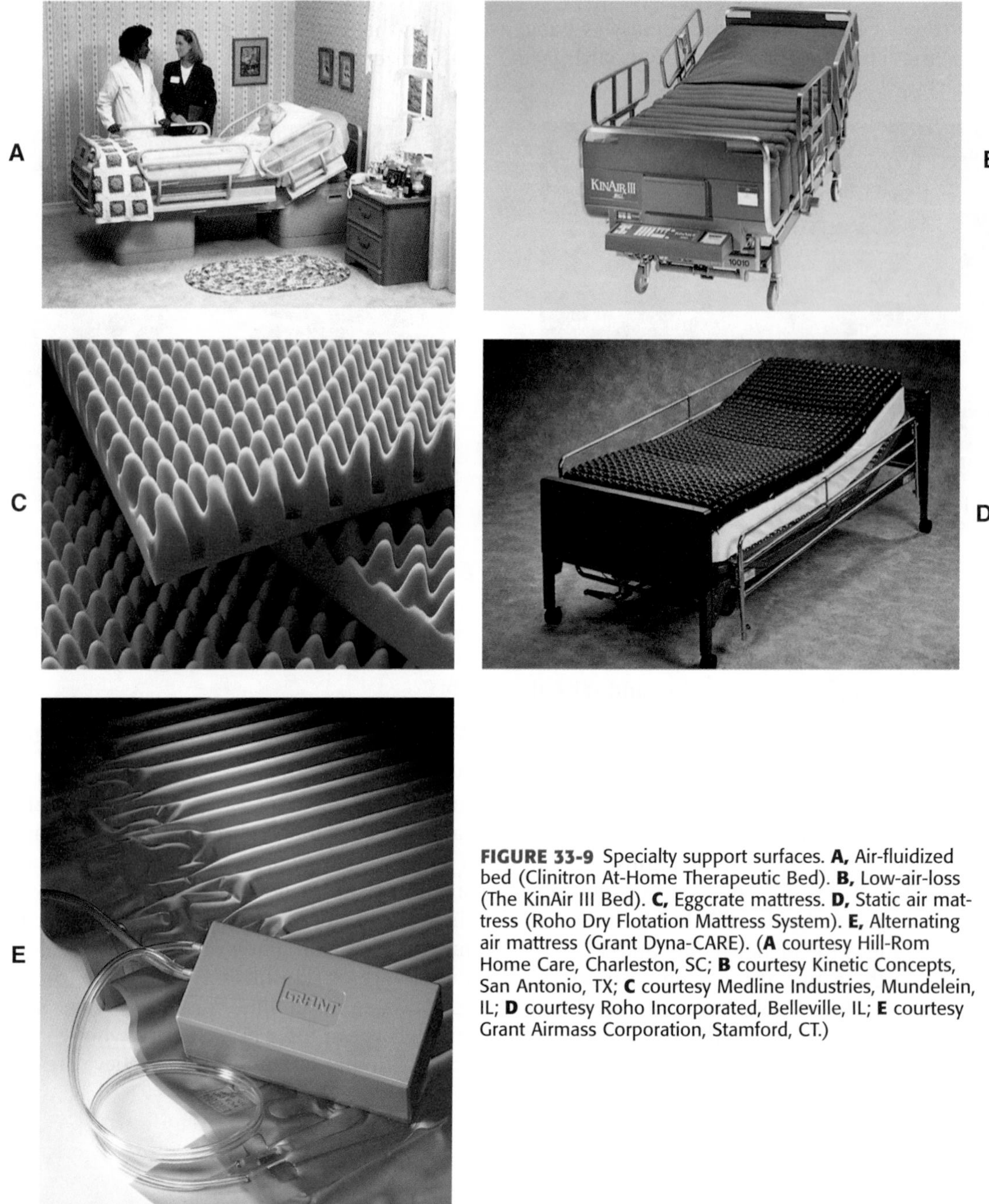

FIGURE 33-9 Specialty support surfaces. **A,** Air-fluidized bed (Clinitron At-Home Therapeutic Bed). **B,** Low-air-loss (The KinAir III Bed). **C,** Eggcrate mattress. **D,** Static air mattress (Roho Dry Flotation Mattress System). **E,** Alternating air mattress (Grant Dyna-CARE). (**A** courtesy Hill-Rom Home Care, Charleston, SC; **B** courtesy Kinetic Concepts, San Antonio, TX; **C** courtesy Medline Industries, Mundelein, IL; **D** courtesy Roho Incorporated, Belleville, IL; **E** courtesy Grant Airmass Corporation, Stamford, CT.)

To avoid compressing the leg vessels, teach the client not to cross the legs at the knee, either while in bed or sitting in a chair. Also teach the client to avoid tight knee socks or garters.

Also, do not routinely use the bed's knee-raising device, or pillows under the client's knees, because they could put pressure on the popliteal artery at the back of the knee. If you use pillows under the client's legs, use them to support the entire length of the leg, not just under the knee. Assess the client's antiembolism stockings frequently to make sure they have not created pressure points.

Encourage Correct Breathing. The change in pressure in the thorax during inspiration pulls blood into the inferior vena cava, thus promoting venous return. If the client holds his or her breath and bears down, blood is unable to return to the heart and can cause decreased blood pressure and cardiac disturbances. When the client moves in bed, instruct the client to breathe out through the mouth rather than holding his or her breath.

The client can also use an over-bed frame, a trapeze, or the bed's side rails when changing positions or moving in bed.

Prevent Orthostatic Intolerance. Provide clients with a planned program of gradual adjustment to vertical positioning in order to recondition the baroreceptors and help stabilize blood pressure. Have clients perform foot and leg exercises for 1 to 2 minutes before beginning any position change. If they have been lying flat for a long time, elevate the head of the bed for 15 minutes before sitting them up or getting them out of bed. When you do sit them up, let their feet dangle over the edge of the bed for a few minutes until they are not dizzy or light-headed before standing. It can take days for a spinal cord injury client to adjust to the upright position.

Action Alert! If a client is experiencing orthostatic intolerance, return the client to the previous position and take his or her blood pressure. Do not leave the client, because he or she may fall. The dizziness, light-headedness, and feeling of fainting experienced on standing usually resolve within a few minutes.

If the client experiences severe hypotension after a prolonged time in the supine position, a physical therapist may need to use a tilt table for position changes.

PROCEDURE 33-2 APPLYING ANTIEMBOLISM STOCKINGS

TIME TO ALLOW: **NOVICE:** 20 min. **EXPERT:** 10 min.

Antiembolism stockings increase venous return, decrease venous stasis, and decrease dependent edema by applying external pressure to the lower legs. They are used to prevent deep vein thrombosis.

DELEGATION GUIDELINES

The application and maintenance of antiembolism stockings may be delegated to a nursing assistant who has been properly trained in this skill. Periodic removal of the stockings and inspection of the skin may be delegated to the nursing assistant, with specific attention to findings that necessitate immediate RN notification.

EQUIPMENT NEEDED

- Measuring tape
- Calf-length or thigh-length antiembolism stockings of correct size

1 Follow preliminary actions (see inside front cover).

2 Check physician's orders.

3 Place client supine in bed with the legs horizontal for 15 minutes. After first use, they should be applied daily before getting out of bed. *This prevents blood from pooling in the legs.*

4 Measure the client's legs to determine the correct stocking size.

a. If the client needs calf-length stockings, measure calf circumference and the distance from the foot to the knee (see illustration).

b. If the client needs thigh-length stockings, measure calf and thigh circumference and the distance from the foot to the thigh (see illustration). *Determining the correct size ensures that the client will receive firm support but no restriction of the circulation.*

A

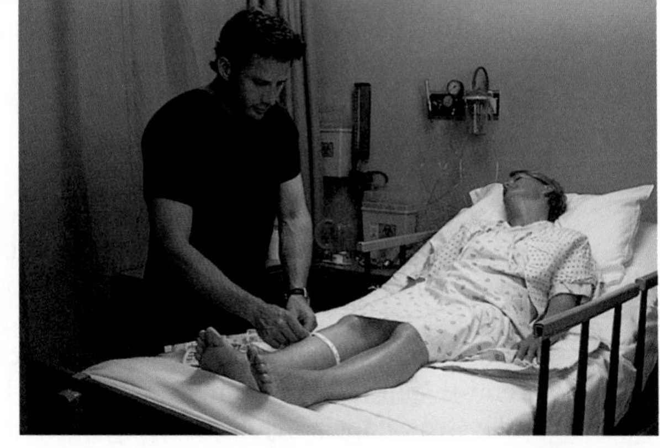

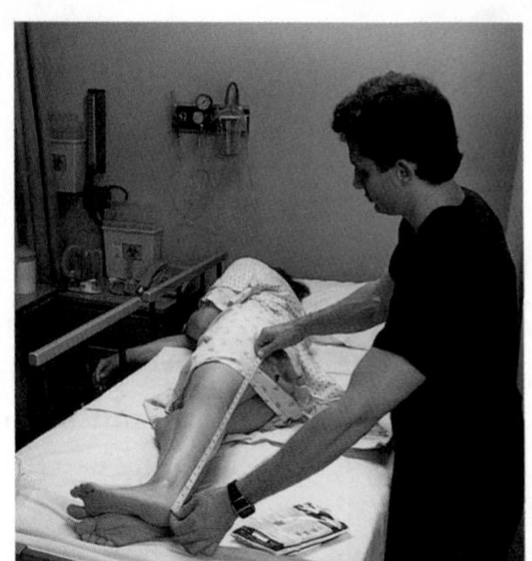

B

Step 4. **A,** Measuring calf circumference. **B,** Measuring foot-to-thigh distance.

Continued

5 Place a stocking on the client's foot.

a. Insert one hand into the top of the stocking, and slide it down as far as the heel pocket.

b. Grasp the center of the heel pocket and turn the stocking inside-out down to the heel area (see illustration).

c. Carefully slide the stocking onto the foot and ankle, making sure that the client's heel is centered in the heel pocket (see illustration).

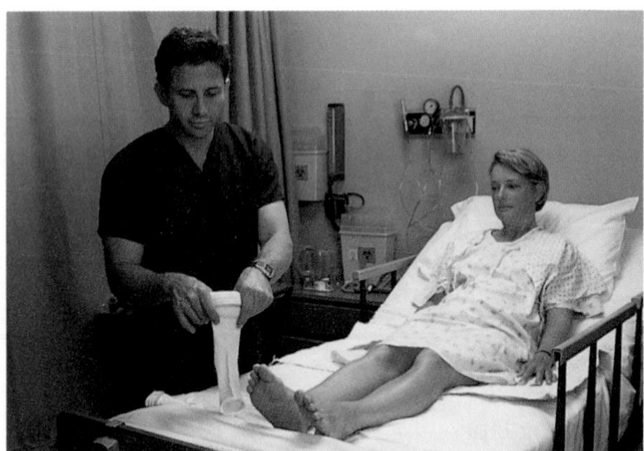

Step 5b. Grasping the center of the heel pocket.

6 Pull the body of the stocking up the client's ankle and calf, making sure as you work that there are no wrinkles that could restrict the circulation (see illustration).

7 Check the client's toes for pressure. Pull the stocking away from the toes to release pressure on them.

8 Repeat with the other leg.

9 Assess the client to make sure the stockings are functioning properly.

a. Make sure the stockings have no wrinkles. *Wrinkles can cause uneven pressure and ulcerations.*

b. Prevent the stockings from rolling down. *Rolls create a tourniquet effect that decreases arterial blood flow and impedes venous return.*

c. Remove the stockings at bath times and before bed to provide skin care and a more complete assessment. Assess the skin for temperature, color, capillary refill, pulses, redness, irritation, and lesions. Ask whether the client feels any tingling or numbness.

10 Document the size and length of the stockings, the time they were applied, the condition of the client's skin, any client complaints, and times the stockings were removed and reapplied.

HOME HEALTH CARE CONSIDERATIONS

For clients at risk for thrombophlebitis, antiembolism stockings should be worn at home. Suggest that the client keep two pairs on hand so one pair can be washed (in mild soap, by hand) while the other pair is being worn.

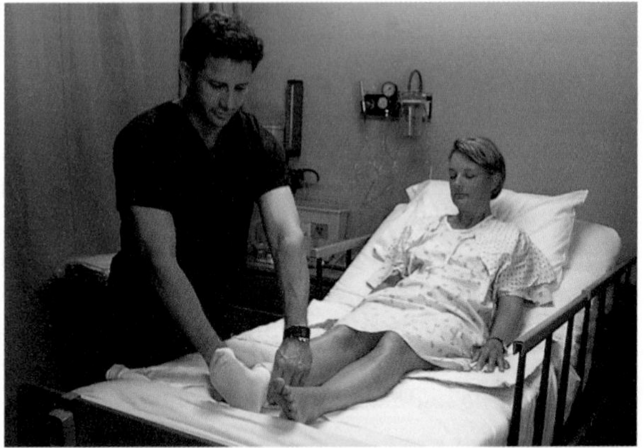

Step 5c. Sliding the stocking onto the foot and ankle.

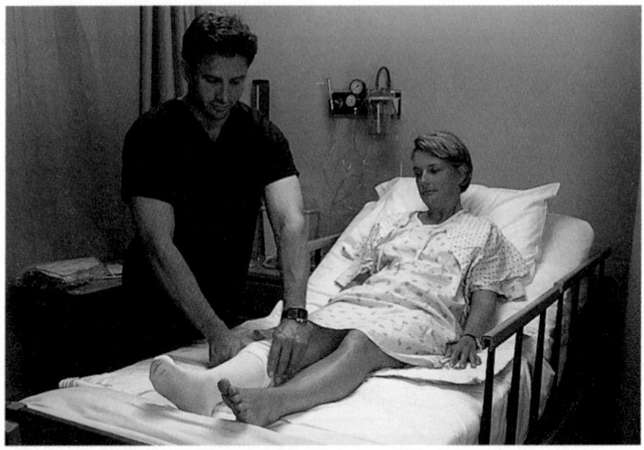

Step 6. Pulling the stocking firmly up the leg.

INTERVENTIONS TO MAINTAIN RESPIRATORY FUNCTION

Without enough oxygen, the client does not have the endurance to be active. Interventions aim to maximize respiratory function by encouraging lung expansion and mobilizing secretions.

Encourage Lung Expansion. To help maximize your client's lung expansion, elevate the head of the bed to 45 or 90 degrees (Fowler's or high Fowler's position) for short intervals. Remember that although this position supports lung expansion, it also increases pressure on the skin over the coccyx. Support the client's arms on pillows. Remind the client to perform deep breathing 10 times every 2 hours while awake. If necessary, have the client use an incentive spirometer 10 times every 1 to 2 hours while awake (see Chapter 34). Reposition the bedridden client every 2 hours. With a physician's order, begin progressive activity and ambulation as soon as possible.

PROCEDURE 33-3

TIME TO ALLOW: NOVICE: 15 min. EXPERT: 7.5 min.

USING A SEQUENTIAL COMPRESSION DEVICE

A sequential compression device creates waves of external pressure that move from distal to proximal areas of the legs. By doing so, the device enhances venous return, decreases venous stasis, and prevents deep vein thrombosis. Typically, you will use a sequential compression device with a bedridden client who is at high risk for thrombosis.

DELEGATION GUIDELINES

The application and maintenance of a sequential compression device may be delegated to a nursing assistant who has been properly trained in this skill. Periodic removal of the device to promote mobility or inspection of the skin may be delegated to the nursing assistant, with specific attention to findings that necessitate immediate RN notification.

EQUIPMENT NEEDED

- Antiembolism stockings of the correct size
- Tape measure
- Sequential compression sleeves
- Compression controller

1 Follow preliminary actions (see inside front cover).

2 Check physician's order.

3 Place the client in a supine position with the legs horizontal. *This keeps blood from pooling in the legs.*

4 Apply antiembolism stockings. *Antiembolism stockings protect the legs from overheating and sustaining skin damage. Cotton also absorbs excess moisture from the skin, helping to prevent maceration.*

5 Measure the circumference of the client's upper thigh. *This ensures that the device is the correct size.*

6 Open the inflatable sleeve on the flat bed, cotton-side up, and place the client's leg on the sleeve (see illustration). Avoid positioning the sleeve so that it places direct pressure on the popliteal artery. Also, avoid positioning it in a manner that could cause skin breakdown on the client's ankle.

7 Wrap the sleeve snugly around the client's leg, beginning with the side that does not contain tubes (see illustration). Fasten the sleeve closed with the Velcro fasteners. Make sure you can fit two fingers between the sleeve and the client's skin. *If the sleeve is too loose, it will function less effectively. If it is too tight, it could cause skin breakdown, compression of the arteries, and neurological changes.*

8 Connect the tubing on the sleeve to the compression controller.

9 Follow the physician's orders in setting the controller to the correct amount and time of compression. After turning it on, observe to make sure the unit is working properly.

10 Remove the client's antiembolism stockings three times daily, and perform skin care during this time. Assess for skin breakdown and pressure ulcers. Examine the toes for arterial changes, such as coolness, pallor, and decreased capillary refill. Ask whether the client feels tingling or numbness.

11 Document the date and time the sleeves were applied or removed. Also, document your assessment findings.

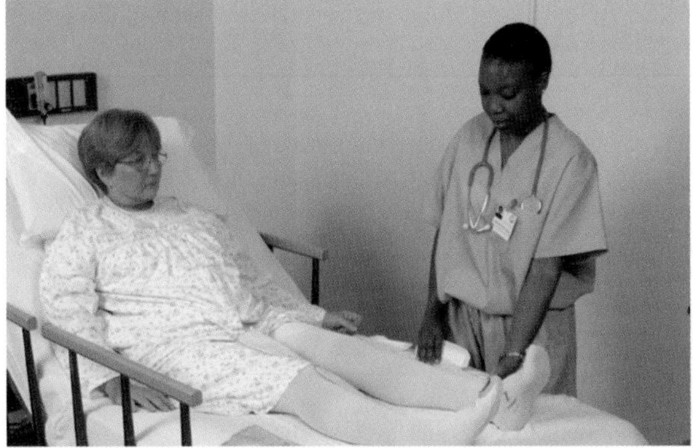

Step 6. Placing the client's leg on the sleeve.

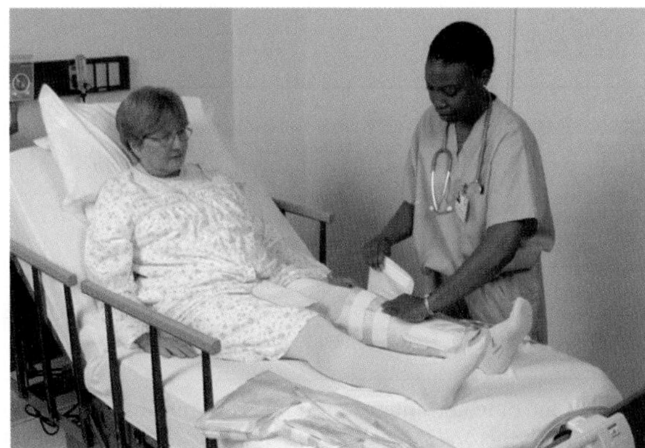

Step 7. Wrapping the sleeve snugly around the client's leg.

BOX 33-6

Nursing Care Plan

A Client With Work-Related Injuries

Admission Data

Mr. Jackson is a 58-year-old African American man who presented to the emergency department following a cerebrovascular event on the job. He was left with right-sided paralysis, and his recovery was complicated by a severe myocardial infarction leaving him with heart failure. He is now in a rehabilitation setting, but he is unable to participate fully in rehabilitation because he has activity intolerance from his heart failure. However, he does not accept that he cannot return to his job and is determined to recover full use of his right side.

Physician's Orders

Occupational therapy to learn to dress and feed himself
Physical therapy: range of motion with resistance qid, out of bed qid with activity to tolerance, over-bed trapeze to assist movement
Accupril 20 mg by mouth daily
Laxative of choice
DASH diet
Daily weights

Nursing Assessment

Vital signs were temperature 98.4° F, pulse 88 and irregular, respiration 16, BP 136/86. After transfer to chair, vital signs were pulse 110 and irregular, respiration 24, BP 148/90. He appears in moderate distress after transfer. Can perform assisted ROM on his right side.

NANDA-I Nursing Diagnosis	NOC Expected Outcomes With Indicators	NIC Interventions With Selected Activities	Evaluation Data
Risk for Disuse Syndrome	***Mobility Level***	***Exercise Therapy: Joint Mobility***	***After 1 Week of Care***
Related Factor: • Reduced mobility to right side and activity intolerance secondary to heart failure	• Muscles will remain flexible, without contractures.	• Encourage right arm and leg exercises against resistance four times daily.	• No evidence of muscle atrophy in upper or lower extremities. Can feed self with an assistive spoon.
	• Unaffected joints will have full ROM.	• Encourage full ROM for left arm and leg at least four times daily. Use trapeze to position self in bed. • Increase number of steps daily to tolerance.	• Mr. Jackson has maintained full ROM in right arm and leg. Uses left arm on trapeze and moves self in bed. • Can walk eight steps with walker; takes less time to bring right leg forward. Tolerates sitting in a chair for 1 hour qid.
Risk for Impaired Skin Integrity	***Skin Integrity*** • Skin will be free of irritation, redness, ulceration, or edema.	***Pressure Ulcer Prevention*** • Inspect skin twice daily. Teach client to shift weight every 15 minutes while sitting in the chair. Support right arm on a pillow while sitting in chair.	• No evidence of skin irritation. No edema present in hands or ankles. States that he does shift his weight every 15 minutes while in a chair.

Critical Thinking Questions

1. What other discharge instructions should have been given to Mr. and Mrs. Jackson? Does he need a home health care referral?
2. Mrs. Jackson calls the clinic stating that Mr. Jackson has a fever, feels warm, and is not feeling well. What do you tell her? Should he come to the clinic or be sent to the hospital? Can Mrs. Jackson drive him safely?
3. What other nursing interventions should be done for Mr. Jackson to prevent the complications of immobility?

Nursing outcome and intervention labels from Johnson, M., Bulechek, G., Butcher, H., Dochterman, J. M., Maas, M., Moorhead, S., et al. (Eds.). (2006). *NANDA, NOC, and NIC linkages: Nursing diagnoses, outcomes, & interventions.* St. Louis, MO: Mosby.

Mobilize Secretions. Thin, watery secretions are easier to expectorate than thick, sticky sputum. Teach the client to drink 2000 to 3000 mL of fluid daily help keep secretions more liquid, unless this is contraindicated by a fluid restriction order to treat a coexisting cardiac or renal disorder. A forceful cough is the most effective method for removing sputum. For a more effective cough, teach the client cascade coughing or huff coughing (see Chapter 34). Coughing should be done five times every 2 hours.

Regular position changes can also help to mobilize secretions by using the pull of gravity. Turn the client every 1 to 2 hours. Also, perform chest physiotherapy and postural drainage two or more times daily (see Chapter 34). Humidify the client's inspired air. As needed, obtain an order for aerosol therapy and a liquefying inhaler medication.

EVALUATION

Risk for disuse syndrome is the nursing diagnosis used to keep the body systems healthy if the client's activity status is suddenly altered. Interventions are implemented to prevent the complications of disuse from occurring, as suggested in Box 33-6. For a more specific and complete list of interventions for each of the nursing diagnoses and correlative problems, consult the appropriate chapter in this book.

Evaluation of outcomes should be done on a daily basis. Because this a *Risk* diagnosis, achievement of the health outcomes occurs if no problems develop. If the outcome is not met because a problem does occur, add the appropriate nursing diagnosis. For example, if the client experiences deterioration of the psychosocial system, the appropriate additional nursing diagnoses might be *Anxiety, Ineffective role performance, Self-care deficit, Powerlessness, Situational low self-esteem, Disturbed sensory perception,* or *Deficient diversional activity.*

If the client experiences deterioration of nutrition and metabolism, you might add *Imbalanced nutrition: less than body requirements, Risk for infection,* or *Risk for deficient fluid volume.* If the client experiences deterioration of the skin, you might add *Impaired skin integrity, Risk for infection,* or *Impaired tissue integrity.* If the client experiences deterioration of the musculoskeletal system, you might add *Impaired physical mobility, Activity intolerance, Self-care deficit,* or *Risk for injury.* If the client experiences deterioration of the cardiovascular system, you might add *Ineffective tissue perfusion, Activity intolerance,* or the collaborative problems orthostatic intolerance, deep vein thrombosis, pulmonary embolism, or decreased cardiac output.

If the client experiences deterioration of the respiratory system, you might add *Ineffective breathing pattern, Ineffective airway clearance, Impaired gas exchange,* or the collaborative problems atelectasis or pneumonia. If the client experiences deterioration of the gastrointestinal system, you might add *Constipation* or *Bowel incontinence.* Finally, if the client experiences deterioration of the genitourinary system, you might add *Impaired urinary elimination, Urinary incontinence,* or *Risk for infection.*

Documenting the outcomes of care is essential. A sample note for Mr. Jackson, the case study client, reads as shown.

SAMPLE DOCUMENTATION NOTE FOR MR. JACKSON

Full ROM present in right arm and leg. Can lift right arm over his head, but lacks fine motor coordination to feed himself. Can bear partial weight on right leg and ambulate three steps with a walker to transfer to a chair. Is short of breath after getting to the chair.

▼ KEY PRINCIPLES

- Disuse syndrome refers to clients at risk for deterioration of body systems from inactivity and immobility.
- Short periods of rest are beneficial.
- Prolonged inactivity causes behavioral changes of anger, hostility, loneliness, and social isolation.
- Independence in performing activities of daily living is lost during immobility.
- Muscle is broken down for energy in states of decreased protein intake.
- Malnutrition causes a decrease in red blood cells, causing anemia, and a decrease in white blood cells, causing infection.
- Lack of activity leads rapidly to muscle weakness and atrophy.
- Bone decalcification causes weak bones and increased serum levels of calcium.
- Immobilization of joints leads to stiffness and limited movement.
- Skin breakdown occurs with increased pressure, shear, friction, excoriation, and maceration.
- Loss of skin integrity allows microorganisms to invade and produce infection.
- Stasis of blood in dependent limbs leads to edema and thrombus formation.
- The development of deep vein thrombosis and subsequent pulmonary embolism can lead to client's death.
- Sudden changes in a client's position can cause blood pressure to drop sharply, a condition known as orthostatic intolerance.
- Hypoventilation and stasis of respiratory secretions can lead to atelectasis and hypostatic pneumonia.
- Hypomotility of the gastrointestinal tract causes abdominal distention, discomfort, constipation, and flatulence.
- Difficulty in voiding leads to urinary retention, residual urine, and urinary tract infections.
- The best treatment for complications from disuse is prevention.
- Increased activity and exercise can prevent most of the complications of disuse.
- When positioning a client who is unable to move, position joints in anatomical alignment or functional alignment. Provide support above and below the joints.

REVIEW QUESTIONS

1. Your client has been unable to move herself in bed since she had a stroke 3 years ago. While you are giving the bath, she suddenly looks frightened and becomes short of breath. Her blood pressure is 160/90 mm Hg, respiration 36 breaths per minute, and pulse 120 beats per minute. Which of the following would you suspect?

1. Pulmonary embolism
2. Pneumonia
3. Thrombophlebitis
4. Fear of falling

2. You and a colleague use a draw sheet to move a client up in bed before elevating the head of her bed to allow her to eat. Risk for which types of injury is most likely in this situation?

1. Spontaneous fracture
2. Maceration
3. Shearing force injury
4. Fall injury

3. Antiembolism stockings are helpful in preventing thrombophlebitis because:

1. External, well-distributed pressure on the legs helps prevent stasis of venous blood
2. These stocking eliminate the need to exercise the legs to increase venous return
3. Simulation of capillary pressure will increase arterial blood flow in the capillary bed.
4. These stocking reduce the flow of venous blood back to the heart, thus reducing cardiac workload

4. Which is the best method of preventing orthostatic hypotension in a client who has been in bed for 24 hours?

1. Get the client out of bed and to a standing position rapidly to stimulate circulation.
2. First raise the head of the bed for 5 minutes, then slowly move the client to a dangling position.
3. Make sure the client has adequate fluid intake before getting out of bed.
4. Have the client take five deep breaths then hold the breath while getting up.

5. You have a client who weighs 120 pounds, cannot move herself in bed, and had abdominal surgery this morning. She can use her arms and hands but has no movement in her legs. To safely turn her in bed, you would need which level of assistance?

1. Have two assistants, one on each side of the bed and you to move the legs.
2. Enlist the client to move her upper torso, while you slide your hands under her hips and turn her.
3. With one assistant logroll her to her side, bend her knees, and place a pillow between her legs.
4. Teach her how to turn herself by moving her legs one at a time with her hands.

Bibliography

An ounce of prevention is worth a pound of cure. (2005). *Senior Care Management, 8*(3), 25-33.

Bates-Jensen, B. M., Alessi, C. A., Cadogan, M., Levy-Storms, L., Jorge, J., Yoshii, J., et al. (2004). The Minimum Data Set bedfast quality indicator: Differences among nursing homes. *Nursing Research, 53*(4), 260-272.

Bhalla, A., Tallis, R. C., & Pomeroy, V. M. (2005). The effects of positioning after stroke on physiological homeostasis: A review. *Age and Ageing, 34*(4), 401-406.

Briggs, D., & Gallimore, D. (2005). Evidence suggests the prone position is safe . . . (art & science June 29). *Nursing Standard, 19*(46), 39.

Brooke, P. S. (2005). Legal questions. Risky patient transfer: Moving mountains. *Nursing, 35*(8), 66.

Brown, C., Friedkin, R. J., & Inouye, S. K. (2004). Prevalence and outcomes of low mobility in hospitalized older adults. *Journal of the American Geriatrics Society, 52*(8), 1263-1270.

Collins, J.W., Wolf, L., Bell, J., & Evanoff, B. (2004). An evaluation of a "best practices" musculoskeletal injury prevention program in nursing homes. *Injury Prevention, 10*(4), 206-211.

Cornette, P., Swine, C., Malhomme, G., Gillet, J., Meert, P., & D'Hoore, W. (2006). Early evaluation of the risk of functional decline following hospitalization of older patients: Development of a predictive tool. *European Journal of Public Health, 16*(2), 203-208.

Dionne, M. (2005). Watch your back: Clinicians need to use good transfer technique when moving a bariatric patient. *Rehab Management: The Interdisciplinary Journal of Rehabilitation, 18*(6), 30, 32-33, 50.

Draw sheets shown to be lateral transfer hazard: Friction-reducing devices work best. (2005). *Hospital Employee Health, 24*(4), 48-50.

FAQs. Preventing heel pressure ulcers in immobilized patients. (2005). *Advances in Skin & Wound Care, 18*(1), 22.

Fletcher, K. (2005). Immobility: Geriatric self-learning module. *Medsurg Nursing, 14*(1), 35-37.

Geraghty, M. (2005). Nursing the unconscious patient. *Nursing Standard, 20*(1), 54-64, 66, 68.

Graf, C. (2006). Functional decline in hospitalized older adults: It's often a consequence of hospitalization, but it doesn't have to be. *American Journal of Nursing, 106*(1), 58-67.

Hanneman, S. K., & Gusick, G. M. (2005). Frequency of oral care and positioning of patients in critical care: A replication study. *American Journal of Critical Care, 14*(5), 378-387.

Jenkins, L., & Egersett, M. (2004). Better lifts and transfers. *Rehab Management: The Interdisciplinary Journal of Rehabilitation,* 17(9), 24-27.

Johnson, M., Bulechek, G., Butcher, H., Dochterman, J. M., Maas, M., Moorhead, S., et al. (Eds.). (2006). *NANDA, NOC, and NIC linkages: Nursing diagnoses, outcomes, & interventions.* St. Louis, MO: Mosby.

Lorio, A. K. (2005). Transfer dependent: Numerous devices and methods are available to therapists who need to move a medically fragile patient. *Rehab Management: The Interdisciplinary Journal of Rehabilitation, 18*(7), 22, 24-26.

Nelson, A., Tracey, C. A., Baxter, M. L., Nathenson, P., Rosario, M., Rockefeller, K., et al. (2005). Current issues. Strategies to improve patient and healthcare provider safety in patient handling and movement tasks. *Rehabilitation Nursing, 30*(3), 80-83.

Schallom, L., Metheny, N. A., Stewart, J., Schnelker, R., Ludwig, J., Sherman, G., et al. (2005). Short communication. Effect of frequency of manual turning on pneumonia. *American Journal of Critical Care, 14*(6), 476-478.

Takamoto, S., Saeki, S., Yabumoto, Y., Masaki, H., Onishi, T., Morimoto, S., et al. (2005). Spontaneous fractures of long bones associated with joint contractures in bedridden elderly inpatients: Clinical features and outcome. *Journal of the American Geriatrics Society, 53*(8), 1439-1441.

Winkelman, C. (2004). Inactivity and inflammation: Selected cytokines as biologic mediators in muscle dysfunction during critical illness. *AACN Clinical Issues: Advanced Practice in Acute and Critical Care, 15*(1), 74-82.

Chapter 34

SUPPORTING RESPIRATORY FUNCTION

Media Resources

- Nursing Skills Online
- evolve Evolve Website http://evolve.elsevier.com/Harkreader/
- Companion CD
-  Skills Video Clips

Learning Objectives

After studying this chapter, you should be able to do the following:

- Describe the physiological concepts underlying the respiratory nursing diagnoses
- Discuss the most common lifestyle, environmental, developmental, and physiological factors affecting respiration, as well as contributing pathological conditions
- Assess the client who has risk for experiencing a respiratory problem and the client's responses to the respiratory problem
- Diagnose the client's respiratory needs that are amenable to nursing care
- Plan goal-directed interventions to prevent or correct the respiratory diagnoses
- Describe and practice key interventions for respiratory care, including positioning, suctioning, providing supplemental oxygen, and maintaining a patent (open) airway
- Evaluate the outcomes that describe progress toward the goals of respiratory nursing care

Key Terms

bronchospasm
chest percussion
chest physiotherapy
cough
cyanosis
diaphragmatic (abdominal) breathing
dyspnea
endotracheal tube
hemoptysis
hypercapnia
hyperventilation
hypoventilation
hypoxemia
hypoxia
incentive spirometer
postural drainage
pulse oximetry
pursed-lip breathing
respiration
sputum
ventilation
vibration

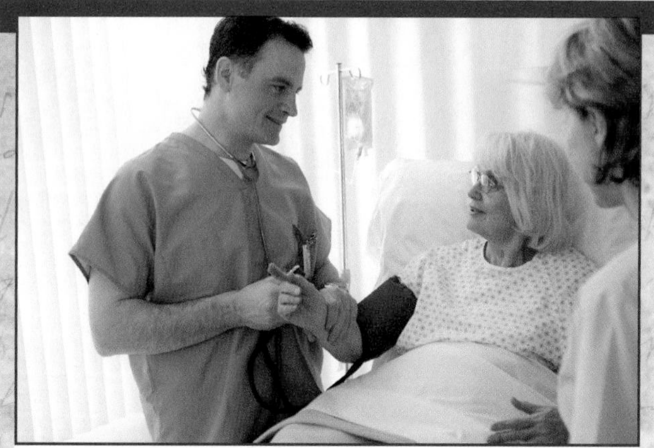

Anna Wilheim is 68 years old and has lived alone since her sister died last year. She called her daughter this morning to say that she did not feel well. Because Mrs. Wilheim had assured her daughter that there was no cause for concern, it was noon before the daughter arrived. Mrs. Wilheim had a temperature of 38.8° C (102° F), and she was pale, cold, and weak. She complained of pain with breathing. Her daughter called the doctor and drove her to the emergency department. She was admitted to the hospital with a diagnosis of pneumonia. Both the daughter and Mrs. Wilheim were frightened.

The nurse makes plans to assist Mrs. Wilheim with managing the effects of her illness and to support her recovery. Because Mrs. Wilheim is having difficulty breathing, the nurse considers the diagnosis of *Ineffective breathing pattern* from the list of nursing diagnoses for respiratory function (see key nursing diagnoses box). Because pneumonia is likely to increase the secretions in her lungs and could interfere with the oxygenation of her blood, the nurse also assesses for *Ineffective airway clearance* and *Impaired gas exchange.*

KEY NURSING DIAGNOSES FOR RESPIRATORY FUNCTION

Ineffective breathing pattern: A state in which the rate, depth, timing, rhythm, or chest/abdominal wall excursion during inspiration, expiration, or both, does not maintain optimum ventilation for the individual

Ineffective airway clearance: A state in which an individual is unable to clear secretions or obstructions from the respiratory tract

Impaired gas exchange: A state in which the individual experiences an excess or deficit in oxygenation and/or carbon dioxide elimination at the alveolar-capillary membrane (specify: hypercapnia or hypoxemia)

CONCEPTS OF RESPIRATION

Nurses encounter clients with respiratory problems in virtually every area of practice and virtually every practice setting. Nursing care of clients with respiratory problems may range from prevention of the spread of the common cold in a school setting to sustaining the life of a client in respiratory failure in the intensive care unit. Respiratory problems are potential or actual problems in the majority of clients admitted to hospitals and nursing homes. Public health and community health nurses screen for respiratory problems and plan community programs for the prevention of respiratory disease. A respiratory diagnosis may be related to a medical diagnosis of respiratory disease or it may be present as a complication of a medical or surgical condition. Regardless of the area of practice or the practice setting, most problems can be described using one, two, or three of the respiratory nursing diagnoses.

PHYSIOLOGY OF BREATHING

As we begin to consider the physiology of breathing, it is important to differentiate between two important concepts: respiration and breathing. The term **respiration** refers to two processes. The first is the exchange of oxygen and carbon dioxide between the atmosphere and the cells of the body. The second process is a series of metabolic activities by which living cells break down carbohydrates, amino acids, and fats to produce energy in the form of adenosine triphosphate.

Air enters the body through the nose or the mouth. The nose is designed to warm and moisten the air as well as to filter debris from the air. The air then passes through the pharynx and trachea before entering the bronchi. The right and left bronchi divide into smaller bronchioles, which in turn branch into millions of tiny air sacs called alveoli. Each alveolus is surrounded by a capillary bed. Gas exchange occurs where the capillary meets the alveolus.

Figure 34-1 illustrates gas exchange in the alveoli. The alveolar wall and the capillary membrane are only a single cell thick. Exchange of oxygen and carbon dioxide between the alveolus and the capillary bed depends on contact between oxygen-laden air in the alveoli and hemoglobin-rich blood in the capillary. The thickness of the capillary membrane is therefore critical to the rate of gas exchange.

Ventilation. Ventilation refers to the cycle of inspiration and expiration of air into and out of the lungs. Air moves into the lungs when the atmospheric pressure is greater than the pressure in the air passages. Two things happen simultaneously to create this pressure gradient:

- Elevation of the ribs and movement of the diaphragm enlarge (expand) the chest cavity. The diaphragm moves downward when it contracts, thus creating more intrathoracic space.
- As the chest wall expands, it pulls away from the lungs, creating negative pressure, which draws the

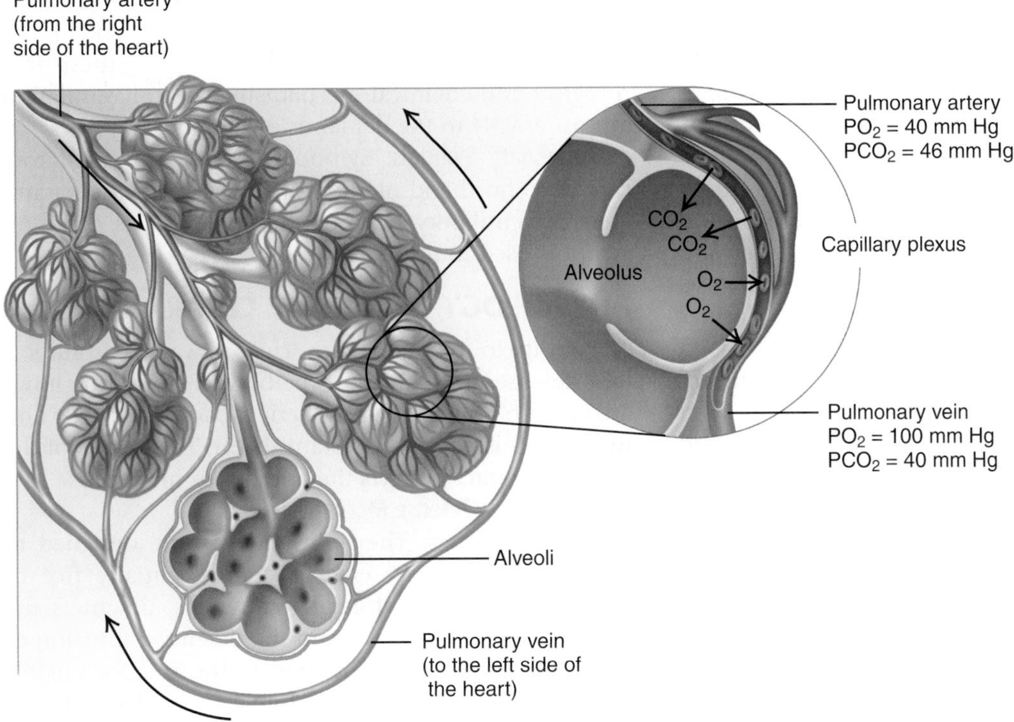

FIGURE 34-1 Millions of alveoli interface with the capillary bed, providing a tremendous surface for gas exchange. Rapid diffusion of oxygen and carbon dioxide saturates the blood with oxygen and removes excess carbon dioxide.

lungs open. As the lungs are pulled open, negative pressure is created in the airways inside the lungs, and the air is drawn into the lungs.

Figure 34-2 illustrates chest wall expansion during inspiration. The chest wall and the lungs must remain intact (no air allowed in the pleural space) for the negative pressure to be created.

Inspiration is a more active process than expiration, because in inspiration the diaphragm contracts, moving downward, and the intercostal muscles contract to elevate the ribs. When the intercostal muscles and the diaphragm relax, the chest cavity becomes smaller and air passively leaves the lungs.

Muscles of Respiration. The primary muscle of respiration is the *diaphragm*. When the diaphragm is relaxed, it assumes a dome shape that ascends into the thorax. As we have seen, when the diaphragm contracts, it flattens along the lower border of the ribs. Again, relaxation of the diaphragm is associated with exhalation, and contraction of the diaphragm is associated with inhalation.

The additional muscles that assist the diaphragm are called the *accessory muscles of respiration*. Three important sets of accessory muscles are the sternocleidomastoid, the scaleni, and the intercostals. During inspiration, the *sternocleidomastoid* muscle raises the sternum, the *scaleni* muscles elevate the first two ribs, and the external *intercostal* muscles elevate the remaining ribs. During quiet respiration, these inspiratory muscles exert little observable activity. The muscles that assist expiration are the internal intercostal muscles and the abdominal muscles. The expiratory muscles become more active during forceful expiration.

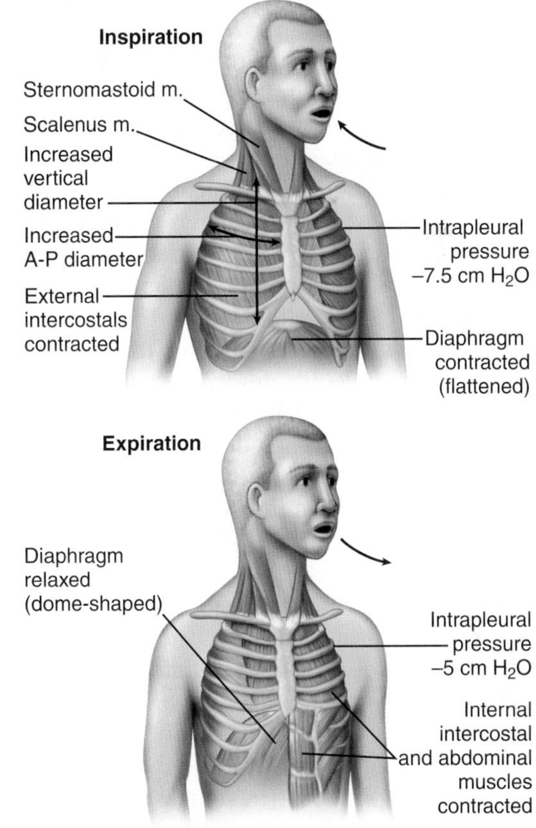

FIGURE 34-2 During inspiration, the diaphragm and the external intercostal muscles contract to increase the intrathoracic space, decreasing the intrapleural pressure to about −7.5 cm H_2O, which expands the lungs. During expiration, the diaphragm relaxes, and the internal intercostal and abdominal muscles contract to reduce the size of the thoracic cavity. A negative intrapleural pressure of about −5 cm H_2O holds the lungs in a somewhat inflated position.

Compliance and Elasticity. Normal ventilation depends on compliance and elastic recoil of the lung tissue. *Compliance* is a measure of the distensibility of the lungs—the degree to which the lungs can stretch. *Elastic recoil* is the tendency of the lungs to return to a nonstretched state. This rebound effect contributes to expiration.

Surface Tension. In the lungs, elastic recoil is produced by elastic fibers in lung tissue and by the surface tension of the fluid that lines the alveoli. This surface tension causes a continuous tendency of the alveoli to collapse. Surface tension is the attraction between the molecules on the surface of a fluid. If you observe various fluids in a glass, you will notice that some have a convex surface (upward curve) created by surface tension. Fluids with less surface tension have a concave surface (downward curve). *Surfactant,* a lipoprotein mixture secreted by the alveolar epithelium, acts likes a detergent to reduce the surface tension and hold the alveoli open. Stretching of the alveoli through periodic deep breaths, known as sighing, stimulates the production of surfactant. For this reason, periodical sighing is an essential physiological mechanism to maintain open alveoli. Surfactant is absent or diminished in premature newborns.

Airway Resistance. The work of breathing is directly related to the amount of *airway resistance,* which is the amount of opposition to airflow within the air passages. The diameter and the length of the airways determine airway resistance. It is normally low; however, any obstruction in the respiratory passages, whether a foreign body, a mass, or mucus, narrows the diameter and increases airway resistance. Contraction of the smooth muscles of the bronchi also decreases the diameter.

Dead Space. *Dead space* is any surface of the airways that contains air but does not participate in gas exchange. On inspiration, a tidal volume of 500 mL of air (in the adult) fills the nose, pharynx, trachea, bronchi, bronchioles, and alveoli. However, only the air that reaches the alveoli is available for gas exchange. The remaining air is said to occupy dead space. Therefore the volume of air that enters the alveoli with each breath is equal to the inhaled air minus the dead space volume. Normal dead space volume in the average adult is approximately 150 mL.

Control of Respiration. Ventilation is controlled by a combination of neurological and chemical mechanisms. Neurological control is in the respiratory centers in the pons and medulla of the brain stem. Several groups of neurons exert different influences on respiration. The medullary rhythmicity area controls the rhythmicity of inspiration and expiration. The apneustic and pneumotaxic areas of the medulla smooth the pattern of respiration into a short inspiration and a longer expiration. These respiratory control centers respond to changes in carbon dioxide (CO_2) and oxygen (O_2) in the blood but are more sensitive to carbon dioxide. Increased carbon dioxide can increase ventilation sevenfold. In addition, chemoreceptors, present primarily in the aortic arch and the carotid artery, respond to changes in CO_2 and O_2 but are more sensitive to oxygen deficit. Together these neurological and chemical mechanisms control ventilation almost exactly to the demands of the body.

Pulmonary Symbols. Symbols are used in respiratory care as a shorthand method of representing the parameters of ventilatory function. Table 34-1 lists common symbols used in respiratory care.

PHYSIOLOGY OF AIRWAY CLEARANCE

The ability to maintain clean, clear airways is an important defense mechanism of the body. Because the lungs are open to polluted atmospheric air, foreign matter and microorganisms are a constant threat. The design of the respiratory tract protects the body from invasion.

Respiratory Defense Mechanisms

Upper Airways. The upper airways are designed to maintain an internal environment essentially free of microorganisms and foreign matter. As air enters the nose, the upper airways begin the defensive function of the respiratory system. The hairs of the anterior nostrils and the mucus remove large foreign particles from the air. The irregular surfaces of the turbinates, septum, and pharynx create obstruction to the passage of smaller particles that escaped the hairs and remained suspended in the air. Figure 34-3 illustrates the structural upper airway defenses.

The upper airways are lined with a mucous membrane that protects the lungs by cleaning, moisturizing, and warming the air. The mucous membrane secretes mucopolysaccharides that trap foreign particles. Its ciliated epithelium, extending from the nose to the bronchioles, propels the mucus into the pharynx, where it can be expelled from the body or swallowed. The mucus

Table 34-1 Common Symbols Used in Respiratory Care

SYMBOL	INTERPRETATION
A	Alveolar
a	Arterial
CO_2	Carbon dioxide
O_2	Oxygen
V	Ventilation
V_T	Tidal volume
$\dot{V}/\dot{Q}$	Ventilation/perfusion ratio
VC	Vital capacity
FEV_1	Forced expiratory volume/time
SaO_2	Percentage hemoglobin oxygen saturation
PAO_2	Partial pressure of alveolar oxygen
PaO_2	Partial pressure of arterial oxygen
$PaCO_2$	Partial pressure of arterial carbon dioxide
pH	Hydrogen ion concentration, acidity or alkalinity
FiO_2	Fraction of inspired oxygen, expressed in decimal form (0.40 = 40% oxygen)

also humidifies the air. Finally, the high vascularity of the mucous membrane contributes to warming of the inspired air.

The sneeze reflex provides added protection against larger particles and more irritating substances. A *sneeze* is stimulated by irritation to the nasal passageway caused by foreign bodies, chemicals, or temperature extremes. During a sneeze, the uvula is depressed, allowing a large volume of air to be forced through the nose and mouth, thus clearing the offending substance. Increased pressure is created in the lungs by taking a deep breath and holding the breath immediately before the sneeze.

Lower Airways. The *glottis* is the opening at the top of the larynx between the resting vocal folds. It divides the upper from the lower respiratory tract. The glottis is open with inspiration, but when we speak, the vocal folds come together, temporarily eliminating the glottis. When we swallow, the epiglottis tips downward to seal off the glottis. This reflex sometimes fails when we try to talk and swallow food or fluids at the same time. However, if foreign particles do pass the glottis, additional protection exists: cilia propel the particles upward, phagocytes engulf the particles, and the cough reflex produces a forceful exhalation to expel the irritating matter.

The cleaning and moisturizing activity of the upper airways continues in the lower respiratory tract. A ciliated epithelium interspersed with mucus-secreting cells lines the lungs down to the level of the bronchioles. Thus the air reaches the alveoli essentially clean, 100% humidified, and at body temperature (Guyton & Hall, 2006).

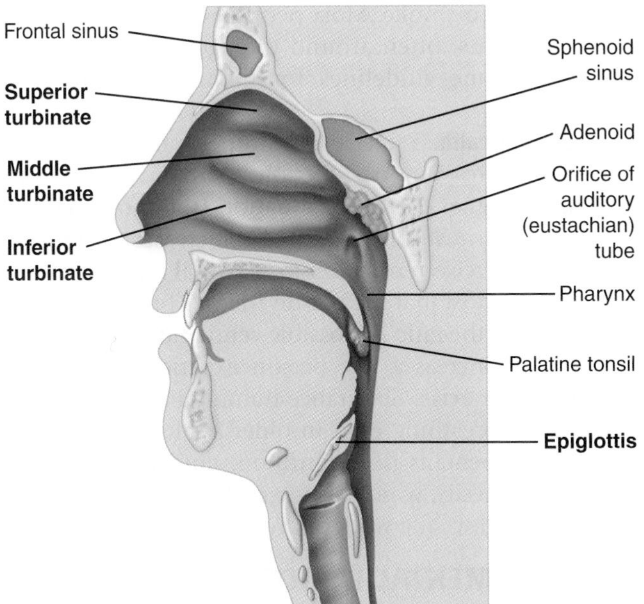

FIGURE 34-3 Upper airway defense mechanisms. The irregular turbinates trap debris that would otherwise fall into the pharynx. The epiglottis protects foreign matter from entering the lower respiratory tract.

The cough reflex is the last line of defense. A **cough** (a sudden, audible, forceful expulsion of air from the lungs, usually an involuntary, reflexive action in response to an irritant) is stimulated when foreign particles or infection irritates the airways. Further down, a cough control center exists in the carina where the bronchus bifurcates into the right and left primary bronchi. If the irritating substance passes the bronchi, the bronchioles and alveoli, which are particularly sensitive to chemical stimulation, will trigger a cough.

The automatic sequence of events in a cough is triggered in the medulla. The person simultaneously takes a deep breath, closes the vocal cords to trap the large volume of air in the lungs, and contracts the abdominal muscles and other accessory muscles of respiration to increase the pressure in the lungs. When the pressure in the lungs rises to an uncomfortable level, the vocal cords and epiglottis are forced open, and the air, with a velocity equivalent to a speeding car, expels foreign particles. The cough reflex is weak or absent in a person with central nervous system depression, such as occurs in comatose clients or in clients on high doses of narcotics for pain management.

Threats to Airway Defenses. The natural defense mechanisms of the airways are vulnerable to damage or destruction from a variety of causes. Box 34-1 lists threats to normal airway clearance. Physical damage that destroys or inflames respiratory cilia or mucus-secreting cells renders these defense mechanisms ineffective. A sudden overwhelming assault or persistent irritants can cause such damage. Although respiratory defense depends on a moist mucous membrane, an overproduction of mucus threatens the ability of the respiratory tract to clear the airways.

PHYSIOLOGY OF GAS EXCHANGE

The exchange of carbon dioxide and oxygen depends on adequate ventilation, which requires not only the movement of air, but a clear air passage. Inefficient patterns of

BOX 34-1 *Threats to Normal Airway Clearance*

CHRONIC PERSISTENT IRRITATION

- Air pollution
- Cigarette smoking

ACUTE TRAUMATIC INJURY

- Endotracheal suction
- Aspiration of vomitus or other foreign body
- Endoscopic examination
- Endotracheal or tracheostomy tubes

OTHER

- Dehydration
- Extreme heat or cold
- Medications that depress the cough reflex
- Pathologic condition that causes increased mucus, irritation, edema

breathing or obstruction of airways can be severe enough to impair gas exchange. *Impaired gas exchange* results in **hypoxemia** (deficient oxygenation of the blood) or **hypercapnia** (high carbon dioxide level in the blood, usually resulting from failure of the lungs to remove carbon dioxide), or both.

Diffusion. Gas exchange depends on efficient transport of oxygen and carbon dioxide across the alveolocapillary membrane by the process of diffusion. Diffusion is a passive process by which molecules move through a cell membrane from an area of higher concentration to an area of lower concentration without the expenditure of energy. For oxygen and carbon dioxide to diffuse across the semipermeable alveolocapillary membrane, there must be both adequate ventilation and adequate blood flow. Oxygen-rich air must reach the alveoli as unoxygenated blood flows into the capillary bed.

The relative concentration of the gases, the thickness of the membrane, and the surface area of the alveoli also affect diffusion. Carbon dioxide is highly concentrated in the blood entering the capillary bed. It crosses the alveolocapillary membrane into the alveoli where the carbon dioxide concentration is lower. Similarly, because the partial pressure of oxygen is greater in the alveoli than in the pulmonary capillaries, oxygen readily diffuses across the membrane from the air sacs into the blood. The thin alveolocapillary membrane and the extremely large surface area across the capillary bed allows rapid, efficient diffusion.

Ventilation/Perfusion Ratio. As we have seen, for optimal transport of oxygen and carbon dioxide, the amount of blood flow *(perfusion)* must be matched to the amount of airflow *(ventilation)*. The upright position is the anatomical position of the body that is optimal for ventilation and perfusion matching. In fact, the overall ventilation/perfusion ratio in the normal upright lung is 0.9, or slightly less than 1:1. This ratio occurs because ventilation is at the maximum in the apices of the lungs and perfusion is at the maximum in the bases of the lung. This phenomenon reflects the relative weights of air and blood in response to gravity. Any condition that upsets this balance may result in a mismatch of ventilation to perfusion and in a less than optimal exchange of oxygen and carbon dioxide.

Oxygen-Carrying Capacity of the Blood. In addition, gas exchange depends on the presence of hemoglobin. Hemoglobin in the red blood cells carries 97% of the oxygen; the remaining 3% is dissolved in plasma. The hemoglobin combines with the oxygen to form oxyhemoglobin. Oxygenation of tissues depends on the perfusion of oxygen-rich blood to those tissues (see Chapter 35).

FACTORS AFFECTING RESPIRATION

A number of factors affect a person's respiratory function. They include lifestyle factors, environmental factors, developmental factors, and physiological factors.

LIFESTYLE FACTORS

Lifestyle factors that affect respiratory function include smoking and the person's general state of health.

Smoking. The primary lifestyle factor affecting respiration is smoking. Inhaling tobacco or marijuana smoke from cigarettes, pipes, or cigars is a chronic irritant to the lungs. Irritation causes increased mucus production. Smokers have varying degrees of reduced ciliary function, bronchoconstriction, and decreased compliance and elasticity. Smoking increases the heart and respiratory rates, constricts blood vessels, and increases blood pressure. Smoking is highly associated with emphysema and lung cancer, as well as other respiratory diseases; 87% of lung cancers occur in people who smoke (National Cancer Institute, 2004).

Smoking is a potential hazard to nonsmokers. Passive smoke in the home has been linked to the incidence of respiratory symptoms, episodes in asthmatics, and acute lower respiratory tract infections in schoolchildren. Breathing in children can be affected through frequent exposure in the homes of friends, in restaurants, and in crowded housing situations that are common among those in low socioeconomic groups.

Nicotine is a highly addictive substance. Once a person starts smoking, quitting is not easy (Box 34-2). In addition to the addiction to nicotine, other barriers to quitting include the following:

- Strong link to habits
- Other smokers in personal environment
- Facing stressful situations without a cigarette

The best defense against the effects of inhaled smoke from tobacco products is to never start smoking in the first place. Adolescents are the highest risk group for starting to smoke. Most people who smoke started as adolescents, often around the age of 12. Box 34-3 provides some guidelines for helping a client stop smoking.

General Health. Exercise and proper nutrition are important to respiratory function. Aerobic exercise increases maximal exercise ventilation (the most that the person can *actually* breathe). It also increases the ratio of maximal exercise ventilation to maximal *voluntary* ventilation (the most that the person *typically* breathes during exercise). As the ratio of possible ventilation to voluntary respiration increases, the person experiences less dyspnea with exercise. Endurance training improves the efficiency of breathing even in older adults. Besides general health benefits from nutrition, nutrition is directly related to obesity, which decreases the ventilatory capacity and increases the work of breathing.

ENVIRONMENTAL FACTORS

Risk for respiratory disease is highly associated with the quality of the air that we breathe. Air pollution increases the incidence of respiratory disease and the exacerbation of respiratory diseases. Additional hazards can occur in the workplace or home.

BOX 34-2

A Patient's Perspective

"I Get Out of Breath Just Walking to the Front Door."

When I moved from the Midwest to Las Vegas, I thought I had found the perfect retirement spot, complete with long-time friends, a couple I had known for years. Before long, however, things began to go sour. Our friends separated and went their separate ways, leaving me a stranger in a strange land. Then, in September 1996, I was diagnosed with lung cancer, and my world turned upside down. Cancer shouldn't have surprised me; I was a smoker, so I have no one to blame but myself. But you always think cancer only happens to other people.

Doctors said the cancer was too close to my heart for surgery. So I had months of chemotherapy, then weeks of radiation. Both left me feeling down and out; I just let myself go. In February 1998, my son came to Las Vegas, took one look at me, and realized I was in trouble. After being hospitalized and treated for dehydration, malnutrition, and anemia, I went back to live with my son and his family. They have a big house, and it's nice to have young people around, especially my three granddaughters and my grandson.

I'm having more radiation treatment now, and the cancer seems to be contained in one lung, but my breathing is severely impaired. I used to be real active. I biked and walked a lot; I walked at least 2 miles several times a week. Now I get out of breath just walking to the front door, and it's worse in humid weather. I'm not totally incapacitated, and I try to help around the house, like loading the dishwasher. It may take me 2 hours, but at least it makes me feel a little bit useful.

In June, I developed another smoking-related problem: blood clots in my legs. Because of the cancer, I couldn't take blood thinners, so I had to have surgery.

My legs are better, but I still have trouble with them. Wearing those heavy elastic stockings helps a lot, and I have a hospital bed that can be elevated at the foot if my legs start to swell.

Since I came to live with my son, I've had wonderful care from visiting nurses. After my surgery, one of the visiting nurses noticed that I was kind of "out of it." When she checked my prescriptions, she saw that the doctor had prescribed a heavy dose of morphine, even though I wasn't in much pain, so she talked to him and got the prescription changed.

Twice a week, a home health care aide comes to help me with my bath. I can still use the shower and the bathtub, but I need someone to help me in and out. Sometimes I wonder if I really need a tub bath, but when it's over, I feel so much better I know it was worth the effort.

Physical therapy has helped me, too. Right after the surgery, my legs felt really wobbly, and I had to use a walker. But the physical therapist had me do exercises with weights, and now I don't have to use the walker.

It was nurses who put us in touch with all of the resources available in the community. If I had known there was so much help available when I was first diagnosed, I wouldn't have ended up in such bad shape.

It's hard being housebound when you've always been independent, especially when you're only 63 years old. But both my sons are here, and we have a lot of other family in the area so there's always someone to take me where I need to go. I'm just glad to be alive and surrounded by people I love. I've already lived longer than the doctors thought I would, and I plan on enjoying life just as long as I can.

Workplace Exposure. The risk for respiratory disease from environmental exposure can be associated with a specific occupation or avocational activities. Acute respiratory injury can occur from exposure to sulfuric acid, ammonia, or hydrochloric acid. Fungal diseases may be associated with a particular occupation, such as "farmer's lung disease" in Midwestern farmers. Often the damage done by environmental exposure does not manifest itself in signs and symptoms for years after the exposure has occurred. The person who has been exposed to asbestos, dust from grinding heavy metals, or caustic chemicals may have no evidence of the disease for years, but the stress of anesthesia or serious illness may precipitate symptoms. Thus a history of exposure is an essential component of assessment of risk for respiratory complications.

Home Exposure. Besides the presence of tobacco smoke, other hazards exist in the home. For people who have allergies, allergens in the home can precipitate asthma attacks. The use of strong chemicals for cleaning, paint fumes, insecticides, and sources of carbon monoxide should be monitored.

DEVELOPMENTAL FACTORS

Risk for respiratory disease is present throughout the life span, with the very young and the very old being the most vulnerable. Exposure to specific respiratory risk factors is related to the age of the person, however.

Infants and Children. Respiratory risk factors in infants and children are generally confined to exposure to common upper respiratory infections. Preschool children who attend day care centers are more likely to be exposed to respiratory infections than children raised at home. School-age children are likely to pick up colds and flu viruses from classmates. Fortunately, respiratory infections in infants and young children are usually not serious, and most children are able to recover quickly without complications.

Certain respiratory conditions are potentially more serious in infants and children. Pneumonia is always a serious infection, but it is especially dangerous in babies under the age of 1 year. It can be fatal for premature infants, especially when surfactant production has not sufficiently developed (hyaline membrane disease).

Other than infections, reactive airway disease (asthma) is the most common respiratory condition in infants and children. It appears as early as 6 months of age, ranges from mild to severe, and can be fatal. The incidence of asthma is on the rise from multiple allergens. For example, dead roaches have been investigated as an allergen in low-income housing.

BOX 34-3

Teaching for Wellness

Helping a Client Stop Smoking

Purpose: To support the client's motivation to stop smoking.
Expected Outcome: The client will develop a plan to stop smoking.

Client Instructions

Nicotine is a highly addictive substance. Although addiction is the primary reason people smoke, smoking is also associated with relaxation, pleasurable activities, relief of boredom, and coping with stress.

Nicotine Replacement: Although nothing delivers nicotine as effectively as a cigarette, about 30% of people receiving nicotine replacement along with support and counseling are able to quit smoking. Nicotine replacement is available as gums, patches, and nasal sprays. Gums and nasal sprays may work better for people who have trouble controlling the immediate urge to smoke, because these forms get nicotine into the bloodstream faster than patches. Nasal sprays have the fastest absorption. However, some people will be more successful with the constant nicotine levels provided by the patches, which keep the craving for nicotine under control. People with gum disease or dentures also may prefer the patches.

Some side effects are associated with the use of nicotine gums, sprays, and patches. Some of these side effects are unique to each form of nicotine replacement; other side effects are related to the nicotine itself. The most common problem with nicotine gum is using the product incorrectly. The user should chew the gum by biting it one or two times and then "parking" it between the cheek and gums. If it is rapidly chewed and the nicotine is swallowed, it causes nausea. The nasal spray can irritate the nose, causing a hot, peppery feeling and sneezing. The patch can irritate the skin. Patches that provide 24 hours of nicotine coverage have been associated with sleep disturbances and strange dreams.

Tips for Helping People Quit Smoking: Most people know that smoking is harmful to health, that it is sometimes offensive to others, and that it is costly. However, because some smokers will use any excuse for not quitting ("My doctor has never told me I should quit"), health professionals should use every opportunity to reinforce the wisdom of quitting. Consider the following gentle reinforcers as part of discharge instructions for a respiratory client:

- "And of course you know you need to quit smoking."
- "I would like to see you quit smoking."
- "Have you thought about quitting?"
- "How can I help you quit smoking?"
- "What methods have you tried to quit smoking?"

The common theme in these statements is that each one places the control with the client and does not make a negative value judgment of the person.

When a client indicates the need for suggestions about how to stop smoking, assess the client's smoking behavior and offer specific suggestions:

- If smoking is strongly associated with specific activities, it may help to change the person's routine. For example, if the strongest urge to smoke comes with morning coffee when the person has just gotten out of bed, suggest a change in routine. On arising, the client might take a bath, brush the teeth, and eat a light breakfast in a different location (on the patio, or in the dining room, rather than in front of the morning news on the couch).
- If smoking is associated with social activities, especially seeking company in a bar or tavern, joining a support group may be a good suggestion. The support group provides an avenue for social interaction that reinforces the client's desire to quit smoking. Eventually, however, the person has to learn to control the urge to smoke in a variety of social situations where others are smoking.
- Increased exercise is an important suggestion. An exercise program may confirm the negative effects of cigarettes, it will give the client something to do rather than smoking, and it will help reverse the cardiovascular and respiratory effects of smoking, thus shortening the time before the client begins to feel a tangible benefit from quitting.
- If the person reports smoking as a response to stress, learning relaxation techniques and coping skills may help.
- Help the smoker find rewards for quitting: reduction of lines in the face, clearer skin, improved taste and smell, reduced stains on the hands and teeth, easier housecleaning, reduced cough, and reduced incidence of respiratory illness. Sometimes living to see grandchildren grown is a motivating force.

BOX 34-4

Cross-Cultural Care

Caring for a German American Client

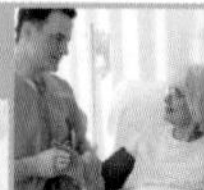

Anna Wilheim, the client whose story we have been following through the chapter, is of German descent. Her family came to Texas in the 1800s through the port of Galveston and settled in central Texas. Leininger (1991) identified a number of values that Americans of German descent, like Mrs. Wilheim, tend to exhibit. Although every client is unique, many German Americans have a tendency to value the following:

- Being orderly, keeping things in the proper place, performing well, being well organized
- Being clean and neat
- Providing direct help to others, giving explicit assistance, getting into action
- Watching the details, following the rules, being punctual
- Protecting others against harm and outsiders
- Controlling oneself and others
- Eating the proper foods and getting rest and fresh air

Adolescents and Middle Adults. The most prominent risk factor in adolescents and adults is smoking. Most people who smoke start smoking in adolescence, and the age of starting to smoke is younger than in previous generations. Inhaling substances, such as glue or paint, to get "high" can cause damage to the lungs. For adults, respiratory risks include smoking and occupational exposure as described earlier.

Older Adults. As a person ages, a decreasing amount of surfactant is produced in the lungs and there is a decrease in compliance, elasticity, and total lung capacity. In addition, the rib cage is less mobile. These physiological changes increase the risk for respiratory dysfunction by reducing the reserve capacity to compensate for increased need for oxygen. Among older adults, exercise tolerance may be compromised by inactivity. The older adult client who is immobilized has a high risk for developing the respiratory complications associated with any illness that requires bed rest. Thus age alone does not produce respiratory dysfunction but does increase the risk.

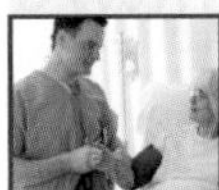

As you prepare for the assessment of Mrs. Wilheim, you should recognize that her health practices may be the product of an earlier era and closely tied to her cultural history. Review the information about Mrs. Wilheim's culture in Box 34-4.

PHYSIOLOGICAL FACTORS

Normal Physiological Variations. Respiration varies to meet the demands of the body for oxygen and elimination of carbon dioxide at different levels of activity. An increased rate and depth of breathing is especially noticed with exercise because exercise increases the demand for oxygen and generates carbon dioxide as a byproduct of metabolism. At rest, breathing becomes slower and quieter.

Body position also affects respiration. As a person assumes different positions throughout the day, ventilation and perfusion shift to maintain the optimal ratio. When a person sits slumped in a comfortable chair, the lungs cannot fully expand, but the oxygen demand is low. When the carbon dioxide level reaches a certain point, the person will sigh or shift position to establish a better balance of ventilation and perfusion. Turning and moving during sleep accomplishes the same physiological purpose.

Respiration changes to compensate for changes in body size and shape. When a person gains weight or is pregnant, the metabolic demand for oxygen increases. In the ninth month of pregnancy, the uterus may displace the diaphragm enough that the woman becomes short of breath with usual activities or lying down in some positions in bed. Severe obesity is associated with shortness of breath with moderate activity and a preference for sleeping with the upper torso elevated. The severely obese person has an increased risk for respiratory infection.

Respiratory Disorders. Physiological factors affecting ventilation generally fall in one of two categories. The problem is either restrictive to lung expansion or obstructive to the movement of air into and out of the lungs. Obstructive disorders produce difficult breathing because reduction in the size of the airway increases airway resistance.

Restriction to chest wall expansion can be from muscle dysfunction, nerve dysfunction, skeletal abnormalities, decreased intrathoracic space, or changes in lung compliance. Paralysis, muscle weakness, and fatigue limit changes in the size of the thoracic cavity. Fractured ribs and thoracic surgery can restrict expansion, particularly when the problem produces pain. Expansion can also be impaired by hemothorax (blood in the pleural space) or pneumothorax (air in the pleural space). The lungs cannot expand because the space in the thorax is diminished and the lungs are atelectatic (collapsed). Pulmonary fibrosis decreases expansion because compliance is decreased by the formation of scar tissue (fibers) as a sequel to any inflammation or irritation.

Restriction to expansion can be from factors other than respiratory disease. Bed rest restricts lung expansion, as does a cast, brace, or rib binder used to treat orthopedic injuries. Abdominal distention, whether from pregnancy, abdominal surgery, or ascites (fluid in the abdominal cavity), inhibits movement of the diaphragm, thus restricting expansion of the lungs. Some examples of restrictive disorders are shown in Box 34-5.

Airway obstruction can be from mucus, inflammation or infection, a tumor, a foreign body, or constriction of the bronchi. Infection or inflammation causes swelling and increased production of **sputum,** the mucus secreted from the lungs, bronchi, and trachea. A tumor or foreign body can partially or totally occlude an airway. Bronchoconstriction is caused by contraction of the smooth muscles of the bronchi or bronchioles in response to an irritant or allergen. Box 34-5 also gives some examples of obstructive disorders.

BOX 34-5 *Common Respiratory Disorders*

RESTRICTIVE DISORDERS

Atelectasis: A collapsed or airless state of the lung or a portion of a lung, caused by obstruction, hypoventilation, restriction to expansion, or absence of surfactant. May be a whole lung, a lobe, or a lobule, or it may be diffuse microatelectasis (scattered microscopic areas of collapse that cumulatively represent significant nonfunctional lung tissue).

Pleural effusion: Accumulation of fluid in the space between the visceral pleura and parietal pleura of the thorax, usually from an inflammatory process secondary to pneumonia, malignancy, or trauma.

Hemothorax: Bleeding into the pleural space secondary to trauma to the chest. May occur in a motor vehicle accident or fall, or it may follow thoracic surgery.

Continued

BOX 34-5 *Common Respiratory Disorders—cont'd*

RESTRICTIVE DISORDERS

Pneumothorax: Air from the lung leaking into the pleural space, or atmospheric air entering the pleural space through a traumatic opening in the chest wall. Spontaneous pneumothorax can occur at high altitudes in depressurized airplane cabins.

Pneumoconiosis: A group of fibrotic lung diseases caused by prolonged inhalation of dust particles, usually from industrial dust (silica, asbestos); eventually develops a chronic obstructive component.

OBSTRUCTIVE DISORDERS

Pneumonia: Inflammation of the lung with consolidation and exudation. May be infectious (viral, bacterial, fungal) or inflammatory (aspiration of vomitus, chemicals, gases, oily substances, foreign bodies). The airways are reduced by consolidation and fill with edema, exudate, and sputum.

Asthma: An inflammatory response that constricts the bronchi and causes edema and increased production of sputum. Asthma can be caused by an allergic response to allergens, such as pollen, dust, smoke, and animal dander, or secondary to chronic infections or heart disease. Marked by recurrent attacks of dyspnea, with wheezing due to spasmodic constriction of the bronchi and increased production of sputum.

Emphysema: Pathological accumulation of air in tissues or organs, usually refers to pulmonary emphysema where air (carbon dioxide) accumulates in the alveoli because of loss of elasticity. Fatigue and dyspnea are the most prominent symptoms.

Tuberculosis: An infectious, inflammatory, reportable disease that is chronic in nature and commonly affects the lungs, although it may occur in almost any part of the body. The causative agent is *Mycobacterium tuberculosis.*

Lung cancer: Malignant growths of the lung tissue. Early symptoms are vague or may not appear at all. The earliest and most common symptom is a dry, hacking cough.

ASSESSMENT

GENERAL ASSESSMENT OF RESPIRATION

As a nurse, you will perform a respiratory assessment as part of a general health screening, as a baseline review of a client just admitted to a hospital or clinic, or in response to cues to possible respiratory problems. The general health screening focuses on risk factors for respiratory disease and evidence of any current problems. For the client being admitted to the hospital, you will be looking for evidence that the client has a risk for the development of a respiratory complication or for the manifestations of respiratory disease. When a cue, such as a cough or shortness of breath, prompts the assessment, you will conduct a focused assessment to determine the nature and extent of the problem.

When assessing respiratory status, you need to be able to determine whether immediate, definitive action is needed. Cues to significant respiratory problems may suggest the need for emergency response to prevent or treat respiratory arrest. You can reduce the need to treat respiratory complications or even respiratory failure by taking preventive action early in the client's illness.

Health History

Chief Complaint. The assessment begins with the chief complaint. Respiratory complaints are difficulty breathing, cough, and pain. Identify the subjective findings by asking the questions necessary to analyze the symptom, such as the following:

- Are you having any difficulty breathing?
- When did it start? How long have you had the problem?
- Is it worse with activity? How much or what kind of activity?
- Is there anything that seems to relieve your difficult breathing?
- Have you tried anything to manage the problem? Medications? Breathing moist air?
- Any pain associated with breathing? Describe the pain. Where is the pain?
- Do you have a cough? Is it productive? Describe the sputum. Color? Amount? Is the cough nonproductive? Hacking? Does it occur at a particular time of day? Does it disturb sleep?

Risk For Respiratory Disease. When the client's problems have not been identified, begin a screening history by assessing for factors that place the client at risk for specific respiratory disorders. Pertinent cues to the risk for respiratory problems in the database would include history of cardiovascular or respiratory disorder, advanced age, anticipated use of anesthetics or narcotics, obesity, inability to cooperate with instructions, and immobility. Risk factors include age, environment, lifestyle, family history, and a history of respiratory problems.

Age. Note the client's age. The very young and the very old have the highest risk for respiratory complications.

Environment. Ask about recent exposure to respiratory infections. Ask about the client's home and work environments. Take an occupational history and a history of travel, particularly to foreign countries, where exposure to uncommon diseases may have occurred.

Lifestyle. Assess for lifestyle factors that contribute to respiratory disorders. Respiratory assessment should include a complete history of smoking behaviors. Not only is smoking associated with lung cancer and emphysema, but it also increases the risk for a person having anesthesia. The smoking history is calculated by multiplying the number of packs per day by the number of years the person has smoked and is expressed as pack-years. For example, someone who has smoked $1\frac{1}{2}$ packs a day for 20 years has smoked 30 pack-years. If you ask about the use of tobacco products rather than smoking, the client may be prompted to give information about cigars and smokeless tobacco. In addition, any history of smoking should include marijuana use, because marijuana is even more harmful to the lungs than tobacco.

Family history. Taking a family history is important because of the possibility of genetically or environmentally transmitted disease. Asthma is an example of a respiratory disease that tends to run in families and may have a genetic component. In addition, family history may suggest the need to screen for infectious diseases like tuberculosis that can be contacted by exposure within the family. Family history may also suggest the need to screen for cystic fibrosis or ciliary defects.

History of respiratory problems. Ask if the client has a history of respiratory problems, especially asthma and emphysema. Particularly, ask about a history of tuberculosis.

Physician's Treatment Plan. Knowledge of the physician's diagnostic and treatment plan will guide the assessment. Interventions that have a risk for respiratory complications include the use of sedatives and narcotics, diagnostic procedures in which an instrument is passed into the gastrointestinal tract or airways, bed rest, and intravenous fluids. Any surgical procedure requiring general or spinal anesthesia has a risk of respiratory complications.

Current Condition. Observe the client's general condition. The person may be described as in excellent or good health, debilitated, or having a high stress level. The general nutritional status may have an impact. It may be sufficient to note that the person appears well developed and well nourished, obese, or undernourished. A history of chronic illness may reveal risk factors. Fatigue and the severity of the current illness can add to the risk. Assess the level of consciousness.

Physical Examination. The physical examination focuses on assessing for abnormal respiratory findings, the effects on vital signs, and signs of oxygen deficit in all body systems. The following help identify objective findings.

Orientation, Level of Consciousness, and Behavior. A sudden or gradual change in the person's level of consciousness or behavior can indicate that the person is not getting enough oxygen.

Vital Signs. An increase or decrease in pulse, respiration, and blood pressure indicates that the client is compensating for an oxygen deficit or can no longer compensate for the deficit.

Skin and Mucous Membranes. Check for color, warmth, turgor, and moisture. Cold, pale, clammy (moist) skin is a compensatory mechanism for oxygen deficit. Decreased skin turgor indicates dehydration.

Breathing Pattern. Check breathing for unusually quiet, labored, noisy, or shallow breathing; shortness of breath; and dyspnea.

Lung Auscultation. Listen for crackles, diminished sounds, rhonchi, and wheezes. Adventitious sounds help identify the cause of the change in breathing pattern.

Abdominal Assessment. Listen to bowel sounds. Assess for abdominal distention. Diminished bowel sounds and distention may be associated with oxygen deficit.

Urine Output. Check the amount and concentration. If the client has a Foley catheter, observe the urine directly. Otherwise, ask when the person last urinated and ask for a description of the amount and color. Diminished urinary output is associated with insufficient oxygenated blood flow to the kidneys.

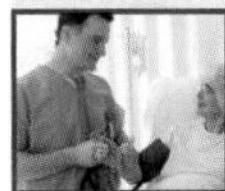

Recall the case of Mrs. Wilheim, introduced at the beginning of the chapter. The nursing assessment for Mrs. Wilheim on admission to the emergency department was as follows: "68-year-old white female in acute respiratory distress. Temperature 38.8° C (102° F), P 100, R 36, BP 106/70. Diminished breath sounds left lower base. Wheezes and rhonchi left lower lobe. Fremitus present. Oxygen saturation 87%. Oxygen started per face mask at 6 L. Oxygen saturation 91%. Skin pale, diaphoretic. Skin turgor sluggish. Complaining of feeling cold. Denies pain. Oriented to person, place, and time. Extremely weak and frightened. Abdomen soft, flat. Hypoactive bowel sounds. Foley catheter inserted. Returned 200 mL concentrated urine. Daughter at bedside. Blood drawn for electrolytes, CBC, chest film, and blood cultures."

Diagnostic Tests. Review the client's chart, and correlate your clinical findings with any available diagnostic data. The physician uses the tests to make a medical diagnosis, whereas you will use the tests to assist in making nursing diagnoses and decisions about nursing interventions.

Complete Blood Count. A *complete blood count* provides information about the oxygen-carrying capacity of the blood expressed as a red blood cell (RBC) count, a hematocrit index (the volume percentage of RBCs in the total plasma), and a hemoglobin concentration. The white blood cell count provides clues to the presence of an infection, which may be the primary cause of the respiratory problem or secondary to the problem.

Chest Radiograph. Chest radiography provides basic diagnostic information about chest disorders and is used for health screening. Pneumonia, pneumothorax, atelectasis, fractured ribs, foreign bodies, and tumors can be distinguished on radiograph. A follow-up chest film may be used to monitor the progress of the disease. Chest radiography is used to screen for tuberculosis when the client has a positive tuberculin skin test.

To prepare the client for a chest film, have the client remove clothing and jewelry from the waist up and don a hospital gown. Advise the client that the quality of the radiograph will depend on the client's ability to take a deep breath and hold it. A portable chest radiograph can be taken with the client in a high-Fowler's position. You may need to assist with placing the x-ray film behind the client, but then you will need to leave the room to avoid exposure to radiation.

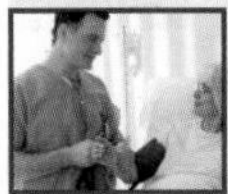

Mrs. Wilheim's chest film shows pneumonia in the left lower lobe. Notice that she had pain with breathing when her daughter found her. Can you correlate the location of her pain with her chest film? How do you think an 68-year-old woman would feel about having pneumonia?

Pulmonary Function Tests. Pulmonary function tests measure lung volumes associated with the mechanics of breathing when the client performs a series of respiratory maneuvers. The volumes are recorded using a spirometer (an instrument for measuring air taken into and expelled from the lungs). Pulmonary function tests may be simple measurements performed at the bedside, in the home, or in a clinic. The full scope of pulmonary function tests requires more sophisticated equipment available only in a pulmonary function laboratory.

The expected lung capacity and volumes are calculated for each client using a formula that includes height, weight, sex, and age. Results are reported as a percentage of the expected value. Table 34-2 describes basic measurements of pulmonary function and illustrates the relationships of lung volumes and capacities. The tests used for bedside monitoring are tidal volume and vital capacity.

Arterial Blood Gases. Arterial blood gases are measured to determine the partial pressures of oxygen and carbon dioxide as an indicator of respiratory function. Full interpretation of arterial blood gases is an advanced skill, but it is possible to quickly learn a beginning level of interpretation.

Drawing arterial blood is an invasive procedure usually performed by respiratory therapists and specially trained nurses. Arteries are deep under the surface of the skin and are located adjacent to nerves; therefore insertion of the needle is highly painful. Use of a heparinized syringe prevents the blood from clotting before the test can be run. A glass syringe may be selected

Table 34-2 Basic Measurements of Pulmonary Function

MEASUREMENT	DESCRIPTION
MEASUREMENT OF LUNG VOLUME	
Tidal volume (V_T)	Volume of air inhaled and exhaled with each normal respiration
Residual volume (RV)	Volume of air remaining in the lungs after a maximum exhalation
MEASUREMENT OF LUNG CAPACITY	
Total lung capacity (TLC)	Volume of air in lungs after maximal inhalation
Vital capacity (VC)	Volume of air that can be exhaled at the normal rate of exhalation after a maximal inhalation
Functional residual volume (FRV)	Volume of air remaining in the lungs at the end of normal expiration
Inspiratory capacity (IC)	Largest volume of air that can be inhaled from the end of a resting exhalation
MEASUREMENTS RELATED TO THE MECHANICS OF BREATHING	
Forced vital capacity (FVC)	Volume of air forcefully (with maximum effort) exhaled after a maximum inhalation
Forced expiratory volume in 1 second (FEV_1)	Amount of air expelled from the lungs during the first second of the FVC

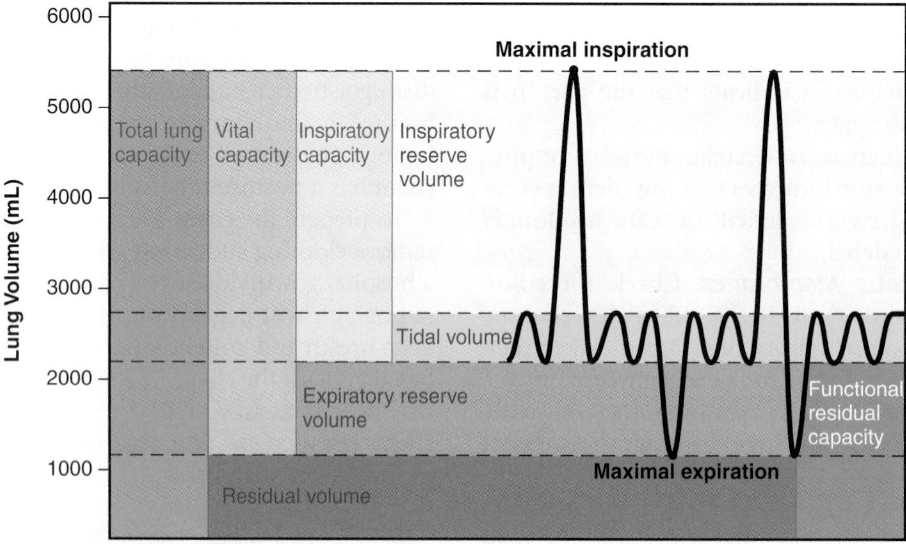

Spirographic representation of the relationship of lung volumes and capacities. Notice that the lungs always have a residual volume of approximately 1000 mL and a vital capacity far in excess of the tidal volume.

because the plunger will move easily, allowing the pressure of the arterial blood to fill the syringe. The needle must be occluded after drawing the blood to prevent the escape of the blood gases; the blood is chilled, especially if the laboratory is a distance from the bedside.

Subcutaneous bleeding is a likely complication even after the needle has been withdrawn. Uninterrupted pressure is applied to the artery for a minimum of 5 minutes to prevent a hematoma from forming.

Blood gas results provide information about oxygenation. The normal value of the arterial partial pressure of oxygen (PaO_2) is based on room air; therefore it can be interpreted only with knowledge of the amount of oxygen the person is breathing. The percentage saturation is the percentage of hemoglobin saturated with oxygen. If the client is on oxygen therapy, the liter flow and delivery device are written on the report. The physician may order the blood gases to be drawn on room air if the client can tolerate having the oxygen removed. It takes about 30 minutes for the arterial oxygen level to become stable on room air.

Blood gas results also provide information about acid-base balance. The arterial partial pressure of carbon dioxide ($PaCO_2$) is directly correlated with the pH, or acidity, of the blood. The respiratory system helps maintain the acid-base balance of the body by controlling the carbon dioxide level in the blood. If the carbon dioxide level is high, indicating acidosis, and the pH is normal, the kidneys have compensated for the acidosis by retaining the bicarbonate ion as a buffer. Renal compensation is observed by an elevation of the bicarbonate level (H_2CO_3) in the reported blood gases. Acidosis or alkalosis can result from metabolic problems, so it is important to distinguish pH changes as having a metabolic or respiratory cause.

Pulse Oximetry. **Pulse oximetry** (SpO_2) is a method of measuring the arterial oxygen saturation of hemoglobin in the blood. It can be used at the hospital bedside, in the home, or in a clinic. A sensing device is clipped to a finger or an earlobe. Within this device, a photoelectrical detector records the amount of light transmitted or reflected by deoxygenated versus oxygenated hemoglobin. Figure 34-4 shows placement of a finger sensor.

Pulse oximetry is a useful clinical tool for monitoring oxygen level. Arterial saturation measured with the pulse oximeter is reliable because it has a close correlation with the saturations obtained from the blood gases when the saturation is above 70%. A saturation of 90% is the critical value for oxygenation to support life. Arterial blood does not develop any significant degree of desaturation until the PaO_2 falls below 60; therefore, when the percentage of saturation falls below 90, the PaO_2 may be below 60.

Pulse oximetry is a helpful tool but should be used only in conjunction with other assessment data. Hypotension, vasoconstriction, hypothermia, reduced blood flow, thick acrylic nails, some dark nail polishes, bright florescent lights, and movement of the finger can interfere with the measurement. Because pulse oximetry does not provide as much information as arterial blood gases, arterial blood is still drawn for analysis in some situations.

Sputum Culture. Sputum culture means growing microorganisms from sputum. When the client has a productive cough, sputum may be collected for a culture and sensitivity test. It takes 24 to 72 hours to grow a culture of the organisms in laboratory conditions. The organism is then identified and tested for sensitivity to a list of antibiotics. In the meantime, the physician makes a judgment of the most likely causative organism on the basis of the presenting signs and symptoms and starts an antibiotic regimen. A Gram stain may be done to narrow the choice of antibiotic within a few hours. Often an appropriate antibiotic has been chosen and the infection is resolving by the time the culture and sensitivity report is available. If the antibiotic needs to be changed, then no further time is lost identifying an appropriate antibiotic.

Any sputum specimen is best collected early in the morning when the sputum has collected in the lungs during the night. For the client who cannot cough deeply enough to obtain sputum rather than pharyngeal mucus, endotracheal suctioning is sometimes requested. Use of a sterile container will prevent cross contamination. The specimen is sent to the laboratory within 30 minutes of collection.

Throat Cultures. Throat cultures are grown from material swabbed from the throat. The most common use of a throat culture is to evaluate a possible streptococcal infection. Because infections with β-hemolytic streptococci can result in rheumatic fever or acute glomerulonephritis, permanent damage to the heart or kidneys can occur. A Gram stain may be used to aid in promptly beginning appropriate therapy. Throat cultures can screen for asymptomatic carriers of organisms.

To obtain a specimen for culture, tilt the head to expose the tonsillar surfaces, and with a sterile cotton-

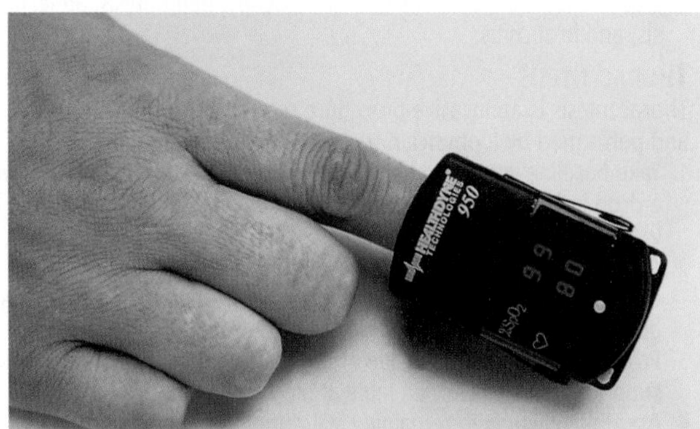

FIGURE 34-4 A pulse oximeter. Before you attach the sensor, clean the client's finger with an alcohol wipe, and remove any nail polish or artificial nails. (Courtesy Respironics, Pittsburgh, PA.)

tipped applicator swab the area from side to side, including any inflamed or purulent sites (Figure 34-5). Return the swab to the culture tube. To ensure that the swab is not cross contaminated by your hands, touch only the cap and the outside of the culture tube, not the swab. Break the ampule of fluid in the bottom of the tube, and send it directly to the laboratory.

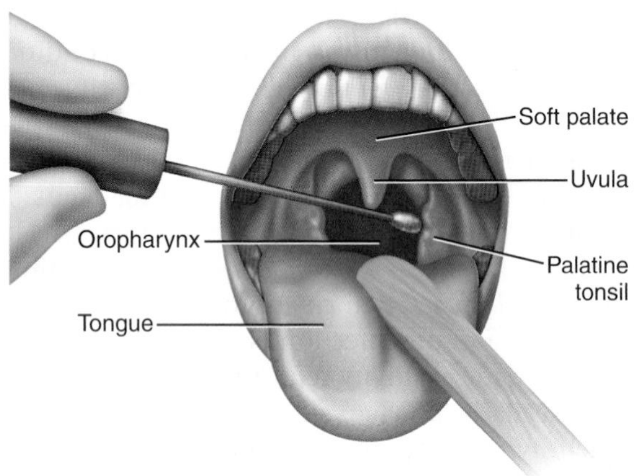

FIGURE 34-5 To collect a specimen for a throat culture, depress the tongue with an applicator, and swab the tonsillar area. Work quickly to prevent gagging.

Bronchoscopy. *Bronchoscopy* is the direct visualization of the larynx, trachea, and large bronchi using a flexible, fiberoptic scope passed into the lungs. It is used to visually guide the physician in obtaining specimens of secretions or tissue for biopsy, removing foreign bodies and mucus plugs, or implanting medications for treating tumors.

After bronchoscopy, the client is positioned for maximum respiratory function (usually in a semi-Fowler's position) and monitored for complications. Vital signs and breath sounds are helpful in detecting problems. Complications are usually minor but may include bleeding, edema, **bronchospasm,** aspiration, and temporary hoarseness. Less often, bronchoscopy can result in pneumothorax. Box 34-6 provides guidelines for assisting the client experiencing a bronchoscopy.

Thoracentesis. In a *thoracentesis,* the physician punctures the chest wall and enters the pleural space. When pleural effusion or blood in the pleural space has been demonstrated on a chest film, thoracentesis drains the fluid and relieves the respiratory distress. Thoracentesis may also be used to obtain a specimen for diagnostic studies. The fluid is examined for abnormal cells, white blood cells, red blood cells, glucose, and microorganisms. Box 34-6 describes the steps for assisting the client undergoing a thoracentesis and shows the most common position for a thoracentesis.

BOX 34-6 *Assisting With Bronchoscopy and Thoracentesis*

BRONCHOSCOPY

Bronchoscopy is an invasive procedure requiring informed consent and performed by a physician.

1. Keep the client on nothing by mouth (NPO) status for 4 to 6 hours before the procedure. Have the client remove any dentures.
2. Administer an analgesic or sedative, if ordered, 30 minutes before the procedure.
3. The physician will apply a local anesthetic to the throat. Keep in mind that the gag and swallowing reflexes will be impaired while the effects of the anesthetic are present.
4. Withhold fluids and food until the swallowing reflex has returned.
5. After the procedure, provide warm saline gargles to relieve a sore throat.
6. Observe for complications of bronchoscopy: hemoptysis, atelectasis, and bronchitis.

THORACENTESIS

Thoracentesis is an invasive procedure requiring informed consent and performed by a physician under sterile conditions.

1. Take baseline vital signs before the procedure. The client may have a drop in blood pressure, especially when a large volume of fluid is withdrawn.
2. Advise the client that a local anesthetic will be injected subcutaneously, but that the client will feel pressure from insertion of a large-bore needle.
3. Position the client on the side of the bed, with the arms folded and supported by an over-bed table at nipple height.
4. Assist the client with remaining still during the puncture to help prevent damage to lung tissue. Coughing or taking a deep breath during the procedure increases the risk of puncturing the lung.
5. If a large amount of fluid is removed from the lungs, observe the client for hemodynamic changes. Take the client's vital signs.
6. Assess the client for atelectasis and pneumothorax.
7. Keep the specimen-filled test tubes upright. Label them, and send them to the laboratory.

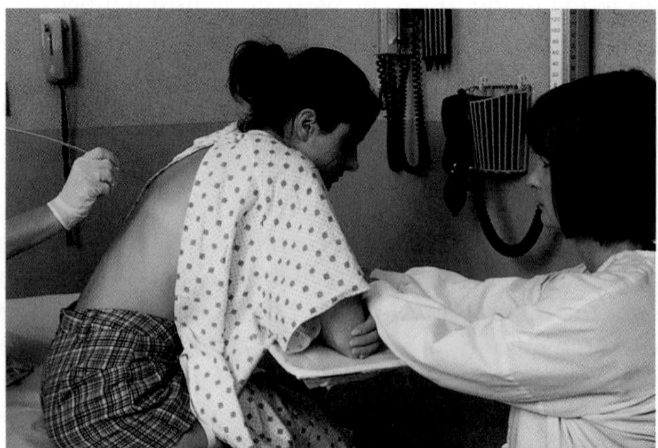

The most common position for a thoracentesis. Gravity allows the fluid to accumulate in the lower thoracic cavity. The spine is slightly curved. The needle must enter the fluid to avoid puncturing the lungs.

FOCUSED ASSESSMENT FOR *INEFFECTIVE BREATHING PATTERN*

Because oxygenation is a high-priority problem, you will need to recognize problems and intervene before the person has an oxygen deficit or before the deficit becomes critical. Keep in mind that the diagnoses are closely interrelated.

Breathing patterns can vary in rate, depth, timing, rhythm, and chest wall and abdominal excursion during inspiration, expiration, or both. Abnormal breathing patterns are those that produce less than optimal ventilation for the individual. *Ineffective airway clearance* describes a client who has difficulty maintaining a clear airway. The airway may be obstructed with secretions, edema, a foreign body, or a tumor or because it has collapsed. *Impaired gas exchange* is a defect in the ability to oxygenate the blood or eliminate carbon dioxide from the blood, or both.

Defining Characteristics

Hypoventilation. When a client is not breathing well, assess for hypoventilation. **Hypoventilation** is a decrease in the rate and depth of breathing, clinically defined as $PaCO_2$ greater than 45 mm Hg. Assessment of the breathing pattern includes rate of breathing, depth of breathing, breath sounds, and sometimes the relationship of inspiration to expiration.

Assess the rate, rhythm, and depth of respiration. The normal pattern of breathing includes inspiration lasting about 2 seconds and expiration lasting about 3 seconds at a rate of 11 to 24 cycles per minute. Normal tidal volume, the amount of air inhaled and exhaled with each breath, is 500 mL. The rhythm should be regular with periodic sighing. The rate that is considered normal varies across the life span. Normal tidal volume is based on age, sex, and body size.

The presence of hypoventilation is inferred at a respiratory rate less than 10 breaths per minute, a depth of respiration that diminishes breath sound, or as a combination of both. Although a rate of less than 10 breaths per minute is generally considered a critical level, the client's baseline rate and associated symptoms should be considered. Rapid, shallow breathing reflects hypoventilation at the alveolar level because the person is poorly inflating the lower two thirds of the lung. Auscultation for breath sounds reveals absent or diminished sounds in the bases.

To be clinically significant, hypoventilation must produce a change in minute ventilation. Minute ventilation is the total amount of air that enters the respiratory passages in 1 minute, and it is calculated as a product of tidal volume and respiratory rate. At a respiratory rate of 12, the minute ventilation would be 500 mL multiplied by 12, or 6 L.

However, even if you could measure the total volume of air moving into and out of the lungs, it would not be sufficient information to decide whether adequate ventilation is occurring throughout the lung fields. Diminished breath sounds are most frequently detected in the bases of the lungs when the person is not taking deep enough breaths to fill the alveoli. Breath sounds could also be diminished in a specific area because of a mucus plug, edema, bronchial constriction, or other obstruction to airflow. Table 34-3 describes the interpretation and management of abnormal breath sounds.

Oxygen deficit and carbon dioxide retention are closely associated with hypoventilation. From a physiological perspective, hypoventilation is defined as a pattern of breathing producing a $PaCO_2$ of more than 45 mm Hg. It is sometimes referred to as alveolar hypoventilation. The carbon dioxide level, rather than the oxygen level, is used because the respiratory control center is more sensitive to carbon dioxide.

> ***Action Alert!*** For the client with rapid, shallow breathing, institute measures to increase ventilation, and assess for oxygen deficit.

Hyperventilation. **Hyperventilation** is an increase in the rate and depth of breathing, clinically defined as $PaCO_2$ less than 35 mm Hg. Under normal conditions, the physiological respiratory control mechanisms return rapid respiration to normal. In some circumstances, however, rapid deep breathing continues to a point that causes a change in the blood gases. Alveolar hyperventilation is defined as deep, rapid respirations sufficient to lower the $PaCO_2$ and produce respiratory alkalosis. The signs and symptoms of alkalosis are feeling light-headed, muscle twitching, numbness, tetany, and, in severe cases, convulsions.

> ***Action Alert!*** The hyperventilating client who has rapid, deep respirations and complains of numbness and tingling in the fingers is in a state of alkalosis. Assist the client to slow the respiration.

Respirations are increased by metabolic need, exercise, fever, acidosis, hypoxemia, or hypercapnia. Hyperventilation can result from any metabolic disease that causes acidosis (increased blood acidity). The body attempts to reduce the acid by elimination of carbon dioxide.

Dyspnea. Rather than being a specific pattern of breathing, **dyspnea** is the subjective sensation of difficulty in breathing and is usually associated with increased rate of breathing. The client reports dyspnea when the work of breathing necessary to meet metabolic demands reaches conscious awareness. Dyspnea is important to consider in a discussion of breathing patterns because it is more closely related to the ventilatory component of pulmonary function than to the gas exchange component. Dyspnea may be acute or chronic. The abnormal breath sounds described in Table 34-3 may be associated with dyspnea.

With normal pulmonary function, the increased work of breathing with exercise will produce dyspnea. Dyspnea

Table 34-3 Interpreting and Managing Abnormal Breath Sounds

ABNORMAL SOUND	ETIOLOGY	MANAGEMENT
Diminished or absent	Hypoventilation, atelectasis, consolidation of lung tissue	Bronchial hygiene, coughing, deep breathing, position changes, ambulation
Abnormal location of bronchial or bronchovesicular sounds	Consolidation or compressed lung tissue	Provide rest to decrease oxygen need. Assist with coughing and deep-breathing until definitive medical therapy reestablishes ventilation.
Crackles (fine): a discontinuous fine crackling sound at the middle or end of inspiration; the sound of alveoli popping open	Atelectasis, mucus in small airways, fluid overload, left ventricular heart failure, or interstitial fibrosis	Diuretics, fluid restriction, a low-sodium diet, or treatment for heart failure
Crackles (coarse): a discontinuous, bubbling sound (sometimes called coarse rales or bubbling rhonchi)	Mucus in the bronchioles	Bronchial hygiene; hydration to loosen mucus; may clear with coughing
Rhonchi: a continuous sonorous or sibilant sound, like air through a hollow tube	A sound in the larger airways (bronchi), produced by vibration of narrowed airways; narrowing could result from edema, bronchospasm, or mucus	Measures to open the airways such as administration of bronchodilators, coughing, or humidification
Wheezes: continuous, high-pitched musical sounds	Bronchoconstriction or bronchospasm, or other obstruction	Bronchodilators; diuretics if the airways are narrowed by edema
Pleural friction rub: the grating, rubbing sound of two inflamed surfaces rubbing together	Inflammation of the pleura	Treatment for the underlying inflammatory process, possibly antibiotics; disappearance may indicate the development of pleural effusion

becomes a symptom when the level of activity necessary to produce dyspnea is a level of activity that would not usually produce it in a given individual. Dyspnea is an important diagnostic cue for the respiratory nursing diagnoses and for the nursing diagnoses *Activity intolerance* (see Chapter 32) and *Decreased cardiac output* (see Chapter 35).

Dyspnea is difficulty in breathing, and it can be acute or chronic. Signs of acute dyspnea are increased rate and depth of breathing, struggling to breathe, use of accessory muscles of respiration, flared nostrils in infants, and, in severe distress, paradoxical respirations. The person may need to sit up to breathe. Assess for pain, and gather information about the pain if present. Chronic dyspnea is evidenced by hypertrophy of accessory muscles, sitting in a forward position with the hands supported on the knees (three-point position), and pursed-lip breathing.

Although dyspnea can occur with or without hypoxemia, the assessment of dyspnea should include assessing for signs and symptoms of diminished tissue oxygenation. Hypoxemia occurs when the compensatory mechanisms that produce dyspnea fail to provide enough oxygen.

Related Factors

Factors Related to Hypoventilation

Immobility. Bed rest or immobility compromises the ventilation/perfusion ratio, decreases the tidal volume, and decreases the total lung capacity. The part of the lung resting against the bed cannot fully expand. Ventilation is best in the upper portion of the lungs. Secretions become stagnant in the lower airways where the alveoli may not be filled by the diminished volume of inspired air.

Pain. Pain or discomfort will prevent the client from taking a deep breath. Pain in the abdomen or thorax causes the client to splint the chest and decrease expansion of the lungs. The presence of abdominal distention, whether from surgery or disease, should prompt assessment of respiratory status. High or lengthy abdominal incisions may compromise respiratory function. Obesity, pregnancy, and severe *ascites* (lymphatic fluid accumulation in the abdomen secondary to cirrhosis of the liver) can compromise respiratory function by exerting pressure on the diaphragm.

Medications. Furthermore, the measures to *treat* pain carry a risk of respiratory depression. Narcotics and anesthetic agents are the most prominent among the central nervous system depressants causing hypoventilation. The first dose or a high dose of central nervous system depressants demands close monitoring of the client during the administration. Older adult clients, clients with liver disease, and clients with respiratory disease also require close monitoring. *Obtundation* describes the client rendered insensitive to painful stimuli because the level of consciousness has been reduced, usually by a narcotic or anesthetic.

Muscle or nerve dysfunction. Muscle or nerve damage may compromise respiratory function. High spinal cord injuries result in paralysis of accessory muscles of respiration or may even affect the medulla to depress respiration. Muscle-weakening diseases such as multiple sclerosis, Guillain-Barré syndrome, and myasthenia gravis result in hypoventilation.

Restrictions to expansion. Trauma to the chest or abdomen should be a cue for assessment. Chest wall damage, hemothorax, pneumothorax, kyphoscoliosis, or fractured ribs can be the cause of hypoventilation. The client is not able to fully expand the lungs or may have a significant portion of the lungs that is collapsed (atelectatic).

Fatigue. The client may be so physically overwhelmed by an illness that decreased energy and fatigue contribute to hypoventilation. This phenomenon is seen in the critically ill, especially when the person has had a prolonged episode of difficulty in breathing.

Factors Related to Hyperventilation. Hyperventilation may be in response to severe anxiety, fear, or metabolic disease, but other causes should be ruled out before deciding that anxiety is the cause. Acidosis resulting from metabolic disease such as renal failure or diabetes can be the underlying cause of hyperventilation. Metabolic acidosis means that excess acids have been produced through a metabolic process. The respiratory system attempts to compensate for the excess acid by eliminating carbonic acid in the form of carbon dioxide. Lactic acid produced by the skeletal muscles during exercise contributes to the increase in respiration with exercise. Head injury, salicylate overdose, and hypoxemia result in increased respiration.

Factors Related to Dyspnea. The underlying causes of dyspnea are a variety of neurological, respiratory, metabolic, and cardiac conditions. Obstructed or restricted breathing can cause dyspnea. Obstructed breathing is discussed next, under *Ineffective airway clearance.*

FOCUSED ASSESSMENT FOR *INEFFECTIVE AIRWAY CLEARANCE*

Defining Characteristics. You may be prompted to assess for clear airways when the person complains of dyspnea, has a change in rate or depth of respiration, complains of feeling "congested," has a cough, or complains of pain. Because the client is not taking deep breaths, fluid may accumulate in the airways. When the fluid remains stagnant, infection may develop, resulting in hypostatic pneumonia. A fever may be present before infection occurs and is a cue that should prompt respiratory assessment. Therefore risk factors for hypoventilation also apply to *Ineffective airway clearance.* In addition, any respiratory disease that results in increased production of sputum carries the risk for *Ineffective airway clearance.*

The most obvious signs of failure to clear the airways are the audible signs of obstructive breathing. *Stridor* is a shrill, harsh sound, especially the respiratory sound heard during inspiration in laryngeal obstruction. Stridor indicates a narrowing of the larynx or trachea, and secretions are probably retained below the obstruction. *Wet respirations* refer to an audible, bubbling sound with inspiration and expiration. *Audible wheezing* also indicates obstructive breathing and is accompanied by retention of secretions.

When the respirations are quiet, you can detect *Ineffective airway clearance* using a stethoscope to auscultate the lung fields.

> ***Action Alert!*** Rhonchi indicate the retention of secretions that can be coughed out. Have the client cough and take deep breaths to reduce rhonchi and an associated fever.

A cough is an attempt to clear the airway; therefore it is a cardinal sign of *Ineffective airway clearance.* A wet- or loose-sounding cough suggests mucus retention. A dry, hacking cough generally indicates airway irritation, but it may result from an obstructive disorder. Sometimes a cough is the only sign of asthma (constricted airways) observable without a stethoscope. A harsh, barky cough suggests upper airway obstruction secondary to subglottic inflammation, especially edema, as in bronchitis. A cough that results in the expectoration of sputum is described as *productive.* A productive cough that does not clear rhonchi, or that clears the rhonchi for only a short period of time, is appropriately described as *Ineffective airway clearance.* Absence of a cough reflex is highly associated with *Ineffective airway clearance.*

Related Factors

Sputum Abnormalities. Pathologic conditions of the lungs carry the risk for *Ineffective airway clearance,* especially when excess sputum is produced. As defined earlier, sputum is the mucus secreted from the lungs, bronchi, and trachea. Interventions are directed at reducing the amount of sputum or helping the client manage expectoration of sputum.

The characteristics of the sputum should be monitored. As sputum is removed from the lungs by ciliary action, the lung is cleared of dead cells and debris. When an infection is present, sputum also contains microorganisms and white blood cells. The volume of the sputum and the tenacity of the sputum are directly related to the ability to clear the airway. The normal daily production of approximately 100 mL of sputum cannot be coughed out. Foreign matter that irritates the respiratory passage increases the production of sputum and stimulates a cough. Detailed observations of sputum help you assess the problem and monitor the course of illness.

Abnormal Quantity. The *quantity of sputum* can be measured as the frequency of the productive cough or directly measured as milliliters produced in a 24-hour period. Clients are more likely to describe the volume of sputum using the more familiar terms of teaspoons, tablespoons, or cups. Intensive care nurses may describe the quantity on the basis of the frequency of the need for suctioning. A reduction in the quantity of sputum indicates progress or, in the case of chronic respiratory disease when excess sputum is always present, may be the desired outcome.

Abnormal Color. The *color of sputum* should be clear or somewhat white. Purulent (yellow or green) mucus indicates infection (e.g., lung abscess or pneumonia). Mucopurulent sputum contains both the increased mucus from an airway disease (e.g., bronchitis, bronchiectasis) and the pus from infection. Blood-streaked sputum indicates airway irritation that can result from excessive coughing with rupture of pulmonary capillaries from high intravascular pressures. Pink, watery, frothy sputum is typical of an acute episode of pulmonary edema. Rusty sputum is from blood that has been in the airways for a period of time. Pneumococcal pneumonia characteristically produces rusty sputum.

Hemoptysis. **Hemoptysis** is defined as coughing and spitting up of blood as a result of bleeding from any part of the lower respiratory tract. It may indicate a potentially life-threatening bleeding problem, cardiopulmonary disease, or irritation of the mucous membrane as occurs with frequent endotracheal suctioning. On the other hand, an overdose of an anticoagulant can result in hemoptysis. A small amount (5 to 10 mL) of frankly bloody sputum may be present in tuberculosis, lung cancer, or pulmonary embolism. Large amounts (60 mL or more) are more likely to be chest trauma with rupture of a larger blood vessel.

Abnormal Consistency. The *consistency of sputum* may help diagnose the client's problem. Thick, tenacious sputum is difficult to cough out. Lack of moisture causes it to stick to the alveoli and the surfaces of airways and predisposes the person to mucus retention. Thick, tenacious sputum is often associated with chronic obstructive pulmonary disease (COPD) or may be caused by dehydration. Thin, watery sputum is associated with allergic responses.

Abnormal Odor. The *odor of the sputum* is an important observation. Normal sputum is odorless. Sputum may have a sweet, foul, or decomposed stench. The odor of sputum may be detected as *halitosis.* Other causes for halitosis (bad breath) are poor oral hygiene, infection in the mouth, or dental caries. A sweet odor to the breath is a reason to suspect diabetic ketoacidosis.

Fatigue or Decreased Energy. When the client's energy level is a related factor, nursing interventions are directed at conserving energy. The prescription for bed rest in the client who is weak or fatigued is sufficient reason to assess for *Ineffective airway clearance.* The client's energy need is a factor in the decision to treat a cough. Recovery is compromised in the client who lacks the energy to cough out sputum or even to take deep breaths. On the other hand, coughing is tiring and may need to be treated to conserve the client's energy. Energy needed for other activities of getting well must be balanced against the need to cough.

Altered Level of Consciousness. When *Ineffective airway clearance* is related to a decreased level of consciousness, more aggressive nursing intervention may be necessary to maintain a clear airway. Both the respiratory control center and the bronchial cough reflex can be suppressed from a neurological cause. A client in a coma, or unconscious from anesthesia or narcotics, does not have a cough reflex. At a higher level of consciousness, the client may be unable to consciously produce a cough but retains the cough reflex and will cough when the epiglottis is stimulated with a suction catheter. A decreased level of consciousness is also associated with the inability to spontaneously change position in bed. Stagnation of secretions is further exacerbated by a reduction in the sighing mechanism.

Pain. Pain can contribute to *Ineffective airway clearance;* therefore pain management may be helpful in maintaining respiratory function. Chest wall or abdominal pain is aggravated by coughing or even by deep breathing. The client attempts to control the pain by splinting the chest and fails to take the deep breaths necessary to clear the airways and prevent atelectasis. In addition, pain is exhausting, depleting the client's energy store and psychological reserves needed for recovery.

FOCUSED ASSESSMENT FOR *IMPAIRED GAS EXCHANGE*

Defining Characteristics. Any factor that predisposes a client to altered respiratory function can be a risk factor for *Impaired gas exchange.* High-risk clients include those who have undergone surgery, have sustained severe trauma, are seriously ill, or have severe respiratory disease. Hypoventilation and *Ineffective airway clearance* are primary risk factors both for the retention of carbon dioxide and for inadequate oxygenation.

Hypoxemia. As indicated, hypoxemia refers to low oxygen levels in the blood. **Hypoxia** refers to inadequate oxygenation at the level of body tissues. Hypoxemia is the usual cause of hypoxia. Hypoxemia is definitively diagnosed with arterial blood gases or pulse oximetry, or it is inferred from signs and symptoms of hypoxia. Holistic assessment is well illustrated in the examination for hypoxemia, because every body system is affected.

Recognize any sign or symptom of hypoxia as a cue to thoroughly assess respiratory status, particularly when the client has multiple predisposing factors. It is easy to think of hypoxemia when the client has multiple signs of oxygen deficiency, but if you are aware of the client's risk, you will consider subtle cues.

Action Alert! If your at-risk client is restless, call the respiratory therapy department for a pulse oximeter if your nursing unit does not have one. Restlessness in a semiconscious or unconscious client suggests the need for a thorough assessment for an oxygen deficit.

Changes in Mental Status. The mental status of the client may be the first cue to diagnosis. Restlessness is the earliest and most often missed sign of hypoxia. A diminishing level of consciousness may progress from difficulty concentrating to confusion, lethargy, and finally coma. The older adult client who becomes restless and confused after surgery should be assessed for hypoxemia.

Changes in Vital Signs. Vital signs change to compensate for hypoxemia. The respiratory rate is initially elevated as a compensatory response to hypoxemia and then may drop as the level of oxygen becomes insufficient to support life. The blood pressure and heart rate will initially increase and then drop. A narrow pulse pressure (i.e., a small difference between the diastolic and systolic pressures) is a warning sign that may be quickly followed by shock. If the client is on a heart monitor, heart block or bradycardia (slow rate) may be seen.

Changes in the Skin. **Cyanosis** is a blue color to the skin that results from the concentration of deoxygenated hemoglobin close to the surface of the skin. It is usually a late sign of hypoxemia. Cyanosis may be absent when the skin is vasoconstricted or if the hemoglobin level is low. Cyanosis may be present without hypoxemia if there is an abnormal elevation of red blood cells (polycythemia vera). Cyanosis is most frequently seen as central cyanosis—that is, in the earlobes, in the mucous membranes of the mouth, or circumorally (around the mouth). A pale skin color is associated with the compensatory mechanism of peripheral vasoconstriction that occurs in the physiological stress response, which shunts blood away from the skin to the vital organs.

Changes in Gastrointestinal Function. Gastrointestinal symptoms are not of immediate concern in identifying hypoxemia but may be considered as secondary symptoms or complications. The gastrointestinal tract slows either from the physiological stress response or from the lack of oxygen. Constipation, abdominal distention, and even paralytic ileus may occur.

Changes in Renal Function. Lack of oxygen to the kidney may be from hypoxemia or from decreased renal blood flow secondary to shock or congestive heart failure. Renal function is assessed by the volume of urinary output. A Foley catheter may be ordered to assist in assessing renal function. Less than 30 mL/hr of urine output suggests renal failure. Blood urea nitrogen (BUN) and blood creatinine levels may be ordered by the physician to determine the effect on the kidneys.

Hypercapnia. Hypercapnia, the retention of carbon dioxide, is synonymous with acidosis from a respiratory cause. In the body fluids, carbon dioxide combines with water to become carbonic acid; therefore the pH immediately drops (respiratory acidosis) when the client hypoventilates or stops breathing. Diminished breath sounds and confusion are cues that alert you to consider the diagnosis.

Hypercapnia is defined as a $PaCO_2$ greater than 45 mm Hg. Clinical signs and symptoms occur in the cardiac, respiratory, and neurological systems. However, the signs and symptoms are not definitive for hypercapnia; therefore the signs and symptoms must be accompanied by a reason to believe carbon dioxide retention has occurred. The cardiovascular signs are increased pulse rate, increased blood pressure, bounding pulse, and palpitations. Cardiac arrhythmias can result from potassium depletion. The respiratory response to hypercapnia is an increased respiratory rate often resulting in a complaint of dyspnea. With persistently elevated levels of carbon dioxide, cerebral edema can cause headache, dizziness, and a feeling of pressure in the head. The client may have lethargy, disorientation, and confusion and may be uncooperative. The result can be convulsions and coma.

Related Factors

Factors Related to Hypoxemia. The factors related to hypoxemia are risk factors that, if left untreated, will result in hypoxemia. Refer to the sections on *Ineffective breathing pattern* and *Ineffective airway clearance.* The client's care is managed as a collaborative problem because the physician must order the definitive treatment to restore oxygenation and to remove the underlying cause. Table 34-4 describes the causes of hypoxemia.

Factors Related to Hypercapnia. Hypercapnia is associated with hypoxemia caused by hypoventilation, apnea, and trapping of air in the alveoli. It is not associated with hypoxemia from other causes. The client with chronic airflow limitation (CAL) is prone to retention of carbon dioxide and may live with chronic hypercapnia.

Table 34-4 Causes of Hypoxemia

CAUSE	EXAMPLE
Inadequate inspiration of oxygen	Airway obstruction with secretions, foreign objects, or tumors; high altitude
Hypoventilation	Impaired ventilation due to disease, injury, medications, or anesthesia
Impaired diffusion	Interstitial lung disease, pulmonary edema, destruction of lung tissue
Impaired perfusion and transport	Anemia, decreased cardiac output, hemorrhage, pulmonary emboli
Altered uptake of oxygen by the tissues	Fever, carbon monoxide poisoning, cyanide poisoning, blood transfusion

FOCUSED ASSESSMENT FOR RESPIRATORY FAILURE

Recognizing the client who should be closely observed to prevent respiratory arrest or respiratory failure requires synthesis of information about the client. Seldom does one factor suggest the need for close monitoring. The severity of the pathologic process, and the client's general condition, medical or surgical treatment (especially medications), and age must be considered together. However, even in an otherwise healthy person, a single factor may be sufficient. For example, a history of allergies may suggest the need to monitor for an anaphylactic reaction that could result in obstructive edema of the airway.

It is crucial that a nurse recognize impending respiratory failure and sudden respiratory arrest. Respiratory failure is a term used to indicate that the respiratory system is unable to exchange enough oxygen and carbon dioxide to sustain life. More technically speaking, *respiratory failure* is a PaO_2 of less than 60 mm Hg or a $PaCO_2$ of greater than 55 mm Hg. *Respiratory arrest* means the absence of spontaneous ventilation. It will result from mechanical obstruction of the airway or from respiratory failure. See Table 34-5 for guidelines for recognizing and managing airway obstruction. Prevention of respiratory failure is a priority in any client with hypoxemia, especially when the person's condition is deteriorating.

The client who cannot exchange air may have no respiratory movement or may have exaggerated chest wall movement with no discernible air movement felt at the nose or mouth. Establishing a patent airway can often start respiration. Lack of a patent airway from upper airway obstruction is a life-threatening emergency. Airway obstruction is defined as any significant interruption in airflow through the nose, mouth, pharynx, or larynx. A partial obstruction may be obvious, or the client may have vague symptoms. Unexplained or persistent symptoms warrant evaluation even if the symptoms are vague.

Respiratory failure is also an emergency, but it is more difficult to identify. Observe for signs of progressive deterioration in the client's condition to anticipate and prevent respiratory failure. Because signs of hypoxia are often subtle, an emergency can exist before hypoxia is detected. To prevent death, respiratory failure must be identified before it is complete.

The related factors are the same as the respiratory problems previously discussed. The *severity of the condition* and *fatigue* are predictive factors. The client who is severely ill and has been struggling to breathe for a prolonged time finally becomes exhausted with the work of breathing and is at risk for respiratory failure. In addition, decreased ventilatory drive, edema, and laryngospasm are especially important.

In particular, consider a decreased ventilatory drive from narcotics, sedatives, anesthetics, and tranquilizers in the client who has multiple risk factors. The client with CAL is vulnerable to decreased ventilatory drive when oxygen is administered. The client who is heavily sedated *(obtunded)* may have relaxation of the muscles of the throat and neck that allow the tongue to drop into the back of the throat and obstruct the airway.

Edema is part of the inflammatory response and therefore can be caused by any condition that produces inflammation. *Laryngeal edema* can result from a burn, smoke inhalation, or an anaphylactic reaction to allergens. Even the client with tracheobronchitis should be observed for severe laryngeal edema. In addition, any irritation to the larynx can cause *laryngospasm,* which tightens the throat and obstructs the airway.

Table 34-5 Recognition and Management of Airway Obstruction

ETIOLOGY	RECOGNITION	MANAGEMENT
Loss of control of the tongue and cricopharyngeal muscles	Noisy, snoring inspiratory sound (partial obstruction) Marked inspiratory effort without ventilation; forceful contraction of the thorax and neck muscles (complete obstruction)	Place the client in a side-lying position with the neck extended. Insert an oral airway. If respiration is not established, initiate the emergency response system.
Retention of mucus	A wet, gurgling noise with respiration or with cough	Assist the client with coughing, or suction the client.
Paralysis, edema, or other obstruction of the vocal cords, larynx, or epiglottis; foreign object	Stridor, inability to produce sound, hoarseness, restlessness, dyspnea, anxiety, respiratory effort without moving air	Call the physician for stat orders: high-Fowler's position, oxygen, and vasoconstrictive or antiinflammatory drugs. Prepare for emergency endotracheal intubation or tracheostomy. The Heimlich maneuver may remove a large foreign object from the upper airway.
Aspiration of stomach contents	Evidence of vomitus in or around the mouth, odor of vomitus, dyspnea, cyanosis, respiratory distress, diminished breath sounds, coarse rales or bubbling rhonchi, crackles	Suction stat; call the physician for stat orders as above. Monitor closely.

DIAGNOSIS

The choice of diagnosis is based on a philosophy of early detection and prevention of health problems. For example, a postoperative client is at risk for hypostatic pneumonia. The diagnosis could be written as *Risk for ineffective breathing pattern: Hypoventilation* related to recovery from anesthesia, narcotic side effects, and immobility. If the client develops hypoventilation with no signs of retention of secretions, the diagnosis would be *Ineffective breathing pattern: Hypoventilation.* If secretions are present, the diagnosis is *Ineffective airway clearance,* and if signs of hypoxemia are present, the diagnosis is *Impaired gas exchange.* See the decision tree in Figure 34-6 for making a nursing diagnosis.

The nursing diagnosis is made with thought to the focus of care and interventions that are appropriate to the stage of the client's illness. For example, the client with COPD lives with a low oxygen level and a high carbon dioxide level. Oxygen therapy is used only in selected cases, particularly those in which oxygen can be expected to increase activity tolerance. In such cases, a diagnosis of *Impaired gas exchange* would be appropriate. However, the goals of treatment are more likely to be aimed at improving ventilation by altering the breathing pattern and clearing the airway.

Sometimes related nursing diagnoses may depict the goals of care more accurately than any of the respiratory diagnoses. Table 34-6 provides examples of clustering data to formulate an appropriate nursing diagnosis.

RELATED DIAGNOSES

Anxiety. Anxiety is an expected response to *Ineffective breathing pattern,* whether that pattern is hypoventilation, hyperventilation, or dyspnea. It is also commonly seen in clients with *Ineffective airway clearance,* especially when caused by asthma, anaphylactic shock, and other conditions of rapid onset. If the client's dyspnea, wheeze, or cough is severe, the level of anxiety can reach panic. Because anxiety can further increase the difficulty in breathing, you must assist the client with constructively managing both the respiratory symptoms and the anxiety.

Anxiety may be the underlying cause of hyperventilation rather than a response. This response is outside the parameters of a normal anxiety response and requires prompt intervention directed toward controlling anxiety (see Chapter 42).

Hopelessness. The client with chronic respiratory disease has no hope for recovery. The best that can be expected is to adapt and to live well with the disease. The ability to live with hope in the face of an incurable illness may be further diminished each time the client is admitted to the hospital

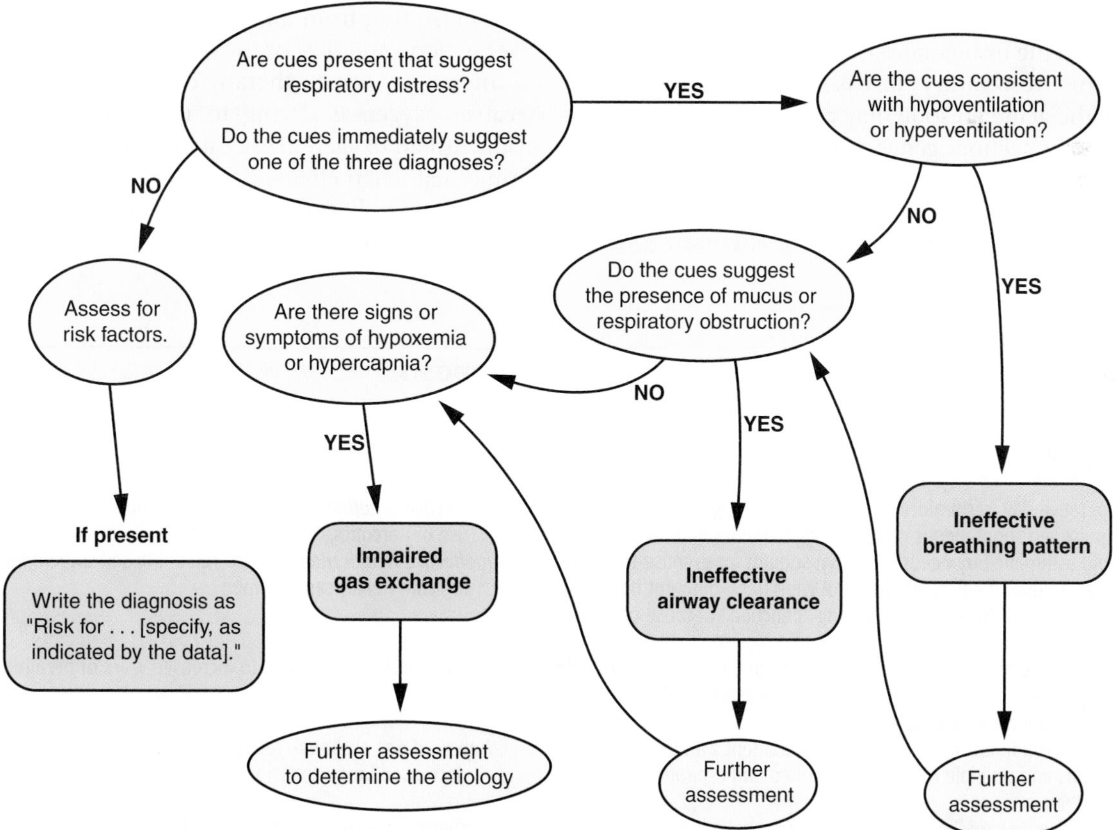

FIGURE 34-6 Decision tree for respiratory nursing diagnoses. Diagnoses are shown in rectangles. Within these rectangles, diagnoses shown in **bold** type are NANDA-I–approved nursing diagnoses; diagnoses shown in regular type are not NANDA-I–approved nursing diagnoses.

for treatment of yet another exacerbation, complication, or episode (see Chapter 49).

In addition, for the client with severe chronic respiratory disease, situational depression is not an unexpected response, and you must be alert to the possibility of depression in these clients. Living with chronic breathlessness and fatigue severe enough to interfere with activities of daily living prohibits the client from gainful employment, an active social life, and even the small pleasures of daily living. Complex, time-consuming daily routines for self-care use up the client's small amount of energy.

Disturbed Thought Processes. Chronic hypoxemia reduces the ability to concentrate and may even produce delusions and hallucinations. Although it has not been objectively demonstrated, the hallucinations and confusion that occur after open-heart surgery or other major surgery, particularly in older adults, may result from an undetected episode of hypoxemia. At the least, hypoxemia may be a contributing factor. These symptoms may be obvious to you and the client's family or may go undetected because the client is reluctant to describe abnormal thoughts and feelings (see Chapter 40).

Powerlessness. The sensation of not being able to breathe, especially if the client is too weak to describe the sensation, is the ultimate feeling of helplessness, of having no control over the body. Although an acute episode of *Ineffective breathing pattern* temporarily produces a situation of powerlessness, this feeling is not expected to last beyond the immediate situation. But for the client with chronic respiratory disease, the powerlessness evoked by the acute episode may continue and be compounded by the feelings generated by recurrent episodes (see Chapter 43).

Ineffective Health Maintenance. As a client recovers from any episode of illness, give extra attention to the need for health maintenance. The client with a single, isolated episode of respiratory disease that resolves without complications or residual effects does not necessarily need interventions to maintain health beyond the period of convalescence. For example, a healthy 30-year-old man who develops a postoperative fever from hypoventilation, is treated with antibiotics and respiratory therapy, and spends 1 extra day in the hospital probably has minimal need for interventions for *Ineffective health maintenance* on discharge. However, if the same man has frequent episodes of asthma, requiring constant adjustment of his lifestyle and medication regimen, he will need assistance to manage the problem of *Ineffective health maintenance* (see Chapter 20).

Imbalanced Nutrition: Less Than Body Requirements. The client with a respiratory problem may need assistance with maintaining nutrition for a number of reasons. First, the physiological stress response to illness suppresses the appetite at a time when energy reserves are already depleted and proper nutrition is especially important. Second, the client with a respiratory problem may find it difficult to breathe while trying to eat. Finally, if the gastrointestinal tract has slowed, the resulting abdominal distention often produces a sensation of fullness that further suppresses the desire to eat.

Deficient Fluid Volume. The client with respiratory problems is at risk for dehydration (a deficit in body water) resulting from an increased insensible water loss from hyperventilation or the diaphoresis associated with an infection. Oxygen therapy compounds the problem because oxygen is drying to the mucous membrane. Also, with an oxygen mask, taking fluids is as difficult as eating. Just when clients need more fluids, they are less likely to remember or to have the energy to obtain them (see Chapter 26).

Table 34-6 Clustering Data to Make a Nursing Diagnosis

Respiratory Problems

DATA CLUSTER	DIAGNOSIS
First postoperative day, respiratory rate 30, shallow, lungs clear, elevated BP and pulse, no spontaneous cough, taking narcotics q4h for pain	*Ineffective breathing pattern: hypoventilation* related to fatigue, use of narcotics, and residual effects of anesthesia
A 10-year-old asthmatic boy needs cromolyn sodium for exercise tolerance to play soccer, refuses medication, does not want to be different from peers. Has dropped out of the team after getting "benched" because of an asthma attack	*Ineffective health maintenance* related to self-esteem interfering with health care regimen
History of COPD, tachypnea, barrel chest, hypertrophy of accessory muscles; unable to prepare own meals because of dyspnea; refuses Meals on Wheels or residential care facility	*Activity intolerance* related to increased work of breathing
Admitted to hospital following a motor vehicle accident with three fractured ribs and multiple contusions; vomited and aspirated; oxygen saturation 85%	*Impaired gas exchange* related to inflammation in the lungs, decreased lung expansion
First postoperative day, midline abdominal incision, splinting chest, refuses to turn, coarse crackles throughout lung fields; temperature 38.8° C (102° F)	*Ineffective airway clearance* related to pain, inability to cough

BP, Blood pressure; *COPD,* chronic obstructive pulmonary disease.

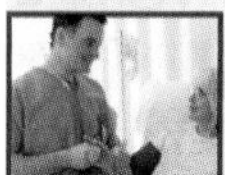

Mrs. Wilheim is started on an intravenous solution of D_5/¼NS at 100 mL/hr. Does this therapy meet her needs for fluid? How much fluid should she have in addition to the IV fluids? Would you anticipate having difficulty meeting her fluid needs?

Fatigue. Because the work of breathing is increased, fatigue often accompanies prolonged ineffective breathing patterns. The fatigue may also result from the illness that underlies the ineffective breathing pattern. Overwhelming, debilitating fatigue is a major finding in chronic respiratory disease. For the client with COPD; fatigue is one of the major contributors to *Activity intolerance* (see Chapter 32).

Constipation. If gastrointestinal function has slowed and dehydration is present, constipation is a likely problem. The risk is increased in the client who does not have the energy for defecation. The exertion required can cause the client to postpone having a bowel movement, thus increasing the likelihood of *Constipation* (see Chapter 29).

PLANNING

The nursing diagnosis selected is an integral part of planning. For the client who has difficult or ineffective breathing, the goal is to improve the breathing. For the client who is unable to maintain clear airways, the goal is to establish clear airways. For the client who has hypoxemia or hypercapnia, the goal is to establish acceptable levels of oxygen and carbon dioxide in the blood.

EXPECTED OUTCOMES FOR THE CLIENT WITH *INEFFECTIVE BREATHING PATTERN*

The overall expected outcome for *Ineffective breathing pattern* is that the client resume normal respiratory rate, rhythm, and depth. Usually, a positive outcome can be inferred from an adequate rate and depth of respiration, an absence of diminished breath sounds, and a subjective experience of comfortable breathing. This outcome is easily achieved when the problem is related to an acute situation and the cause is eliminated in the natural course of recovery.

If the problem is a direct result of an acute illness, such as hypoventilation in the postoperative client during the first 24 hours after surgery, the outcome of normal respiration by discharge from the hospital is usually sufficient. However, if the problem can be expected to return—that is, if the client is at continued risk or the problem is the result of a chronic illness—the outcomes need to include evidence that the person is prepared to manage the risk.

When the problem has a longer duration, intermediate outcomes are used to show progress toward the goal. Improving the efficiency of respiration and managing energy requirements are long-term goals that may result in an improved quality of life for the client with chronic disease. The measures are usually a subjective report from the client that dyspnea has decreased and activity tolerance has improved. Quality of life is measurable only through the subjective report of the client.

Examples of outcomes include the following:

- Demonstrates understanding of benefits of flu and pneumonia vaccines
- States that she will contact an appropriate agency for assistance in weatherproofing home
- Has made an appointment with Meals on Wheels
- States daughter will provide transportation to doctor's appointment next Thursday

EXPECTED OUTCOMES FOR THE CLIENT WITH *INEFFECTIVE AIRWAY CLEARANCE*

The expected outcome for *Ineffective airway clearance* is that the client demonstrates no evidence of airway obstruction or secretion retention as indicated by normal breath sounds. Wheezing, crackles, or rhonchi have disappeared.

A short-term outcome is that the client coughs out sputum without fatigue and vital signs return to normal in 10 minutes. A long-term plan would include the outcome that the client demonstrates regular use of a regimen for maintaining airway clearance.

EXPECTED OUTCOMES FOR THE CLIENT WITH *IMPAIRED GAS EXCHANGE*

The expected outcome for *Impaired gas exchange* is that the client have normal arterial blood gas levels or show no evidence of hypoxia or hypercapnia on room air, or both. An intermediate outcome would be that while on oxygen therapy, the client has an oxygen saturation of greater than 95% by pulse oximetry.

EXPECTED OUTCOMES FOR THE CLIENT WITH RESPIRATORY FAILURE

The expected nursing outcome for respiratory failure is that the client be able to breathe unassisted by an artificial airway or ventilatory support. The short-term outcomes include that the client has a patent airway and breath sounds throughout the lung fields. Normal blood gas levels would be included in the criteria for adequate ventilatory support.

INTERVENTION

The choice of interventions for the respiratory client is derived through a team approach that includes the physician, respiratory therapist, nurse, and dietitian. Many of the interventions that provide definitive therapy are within the medical treatment plan. Respiratory therapy includes a broad range of respiratory interventions, and in many institutions the respiratory therapist provides these interventions. Today's respiratory care practitioners graduate from American Medical Association–accredited programs. They are either certified respiratory therapy technicians or registered respiratory therapists. A person with the registered respiratory therapist credential has passed an advanced national registry test and is the most qualified individual to practice respiratory therapy. Respiratory therapists also provide home health care for persons with chronic illness. The active role of the respiratory therapist in the hospital or home setting, however, does not relieve nurses of responsibility for the client's respiratory needs.

INTERVENTIONS TO CHANGE THE BREATHING PATTERN

Intervention when the client has an ineffective breathing pattern is based on the related or etiological factor. There are also general goals that can be applied to the care of any person with an ineffective breathing pattern.

Positioning for Maximum Respiratory Function. Positioning implies both the position and the frequency of position changes. Maximal chest expansion is possible and the ventilation/perfusion ratio is optimal in the upright unsupported position. Lying down limits lung expansion in the dependent portion (subordinate part) of the lung, but, at the same time, it helps increase ventilation in the nondependent portion of the lung. Perfusion is greatest in the dependent lung. Turning and repositioning redistributes pulmonary blood and airflow, thus compensating for the recumbent position to maintain function throughout the lungs.

The client should be positioned for maximum ventilatory function. Because it is natural to shift positions on the basis of respiratory need, a client who is having difficulty breathing should be allowed to assume the most comfortable position. On the other hand, a weak or debilitated client may not be able to self-reposition. When the client is having difficulty breathing, the first thing to do is raise the head of the bed. Positioning is particularly important in clients with obesity, abdominal distention, or ascites. Elevating the head of the bed for these clients will allow gravity to eliminate the impediment of the abdominal organs on the lungs (Burns, Egolff, Ryan, Carpenter, & Burns, 1994).

A second factor to consider in positioning the client is stagnation of secretions. Drainage of secretions is improved by positioning to allow drainage of all the lobes of the lung over time. For most clients, this is accomplished by turning every 2 hours. Others may need postural drainage (discussed under Chest Physiotherapy, later). Box 34-7 lists possible benefits to be gained from positioning.

In positioning the client, the client's ability to tolerate changing position and different positions should be considered. The best positioning regimen for respiratory function should be determined for each client individually and evaluated on the basis of data indicating respiratory function. The person who is positioned to increase drainage and expectoration may tire from the coughing induced by the drainage of mucus and may need to be repositioned. The person who seeks the position of maximal comfort for pain relief may need to be encouraged to periodically change positions to increase drainage and improve ventilation. For the critically ill client, vital signs may help assess the person's ability to tolerate the repositioning.

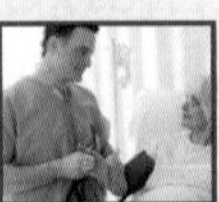

Again consider the case of Mrs. Wilheim. As soon as she arrives on the unit, the nurse elevates Mrs. Wilheim's head 30 degrees. Mrs. Wilheim thanks the nurse, saying that she is more comfortable with her head elevated and is grateful for the nurse's help. You notice that her skin is thin and fragile. How will you plan for preventing skin breakdown?

Stimulating Respiration. Stimulating respiration means increasing the client's rate and depth of breathing to meet the needs of respiratory function. It opens alveoli and distributes the airflow throughout the lungs.

Ambulation. Ambulation is an effective, noninvasive, and inexpensive method of stimulating respiration. While walking, the client is in the optimal physiological position to breathe. In addition, respiration is stimulated by the client's increased metabolic need (Guyton & Hall, 2006). Be careful to confine ambulation to the limits of the client's tolerance (see Chapter 32).

Incentive Spirometry. An **incentive spirometer** is a device that provides a visual goal for and measurement of inspiration, thus encouraging the client to execute and sustain maximal inspiration. Achieving and sustaining a maximal inspiration opens airways, reduces atelectasis, and stimulates coughing. The client benefits from active participation in recovery by developing a feeling of control over the recovery process.

For any of the available incentive spirometers, the goal is to achieve and maintain a maximal inspiration. Correct use requires a slow, voluntary, deep breath. When full or maximal inhalation is reached, the breath

BOX 34-7 *Possible Respiratory Benefits To Be Gained From Positioning*

- The cough reflex may be activated by positioning the client on the right side to encourage sputum to come in contact with the cough control center in the right bronchi at the carina.
- Positioning on a painful affected side may help reduce the pain.
- Positioning with the good lung up may increase ventilatory compensation for a pathological condition.
- Positioning on the unaffected side allows drainage of the area of pathologic process.
- The Sims' position, with the jaw falling forward, is useful for maintaining a patent airway.
- Frequent repositioning will help accomplish multiple purposes.

is held for at least 3 seconds. This sequence is repeated up to 20 times per hour; the client is usually started with five repetitions per session. Incentive exercises are most effective when used every hour while the person is awake. Each device has a means of setting an inspiratory goal derived from a formula based on height, weight, and sex. Lights, balls rising in a column, or other indicators of success provide visual reinforcement. Although the client will initially need instruction and supervision, most people learn the skill quickly. However, occasionally watch the client performing incentive spirometry to ensure continued correct use.

Incentive spirometer therapy is often used postoperatively or when physical mobility is limited. It is most effectively used when people are alert, cooperative, coordinated, and motivated and when they have sufficient strength to generate an inspiratory flow rate that will produce a deep breath and activate the indicator on the incentive device. Repetitions of the deep breaths must be slow to avoid overbreathing, which will lead to dizziness and tremors as a result of sudden hypocapnia. Box 34-8 provides guidelines for teaching the client to use an incentive spirometer.

Medications. Naloxone (Narcan) is used to stimulate respirations in the client whose respirations have been severely depressed by narcotics. The physician's guideline for administering naloxone is usually to administer as necessary (prn) for respiration rates of 10 breaths per minute or below. Before deciding that naloxone is needed, attempt to arouse the client and instruct the client to take deep breaths. If there is no improvement (that is, if the respirations remain fewer than 10 breaths per minute) administer naloxone. If the client does not have a prescription for naloxone, immediately consult the physician.

Intravenous naloxone will immediately reverse the narcotic and result in a deep inspiration. However, the pain-relieving effects of the narcotic are also reversed, so the client may be in pain.

Action Alert! When a narcotic has depressed the client's respirations to less than 10 breaths per minute, the situation may be life threatening. Administer naloxone as ordered to reverse the effects of the narcotic.

Opening the Airways. When airway obstruction is caused by *bronchoconstriction,* bronchodilators are used to dilate the bronchi by relaxing smooth muscles. Airway constriction in clients with asthma or emphysema that responds to bronchodilators is called "reversible airway disease." Sympathomimetic drugs, beta-2-agonists, and theophylline cause bronchodilatation. These medications have varying degrees of the side effects of tachycardia, palpitations, nervousness, excitability, and irritability.

BOX 34-8 *Teaching for Self-Care*

Using an Incentive Spirometer

Purpose: To prevent or treat atelectasis and mobilize secretions.

Expected Outcome: The client will gradually increase the volume of inspiration to reach a predetermined volume based on age, sex, and body size.

Client Instructions

1. Sit up straight.
2. Breathe out normally, and hold the spirometer upright. Holding the spirometer upright is important for correct function and for ease of airflow.
3. Position the mouthpiece between your teeth, and seal your lips around the mouthpiece.
4. Take a slow, deep breath. Rapid, forceful inhalation can collapse your airways.
5. Continue inhaling until the indicator on the device reaches the preset goal. The initial goal is based on your sex, size, and medical condition.
6. When you reach the goal, hold your breath for 2 to 6 seconds. This is your sustained maximal inspiration. Holding your breath at this point opens your alveoli and stimulates the production of surfactant.
7. Exhale slowly. This prevents discomfort and airway collapse.
8. Repeat steps 1 through 7 five to 10 times. Repeat this treatment every hour.

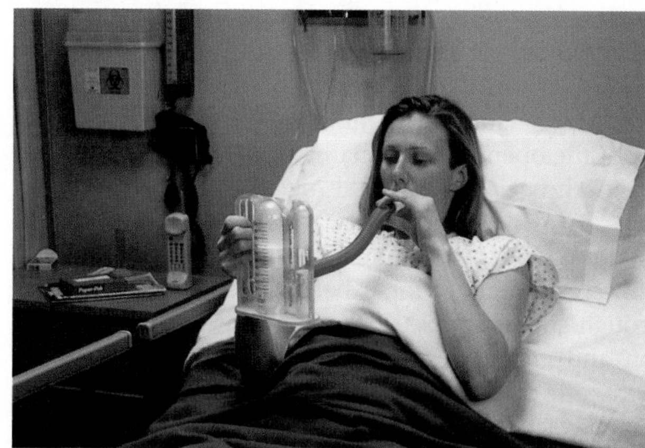

Use of the volume-oriented incentive spirometer. The client inhales slowly. The ball should stay in the "best" area as the client inhales. The setting of the incentive indicator is based on the client's height, weight, age, and sex. The postoperative client may have one-half to one-third the capacity of a preoperative client.

A review of the literature that establishes a research basis for these recommendations is found in Titler, M. G., & Jones, G. A. (1992). Airway management. In G. M. Bulechek & J. C. McCloskey (Eds.), *Nursing interventions: Essential nursing treatments.* Philadelphia: Saunders.

Bronchodilators can be administered orally, intravenously, by nebulizer, or by a *metered-dose inhaler* (which delivers a single dose of medication for inhalation). The oral dose provides a sustained blood level over a long period for the client who has frequent symptoms. The intravenous (IV) route is used for a client with an asthma attack that continues despite more conservative treatment. Topical application by inhalation of a small volume of nebulized medication reduces side effects and is used for the occasional intermittent attack. The metered-dose inhaler is actually the most common type of small-volume nebulizer. Box 34-9 shows how to teach clients to use a metered-dose inhaler. When a metered-dose inhaler is not effective in reversing an acute asthma attack, a nebulizer driven by compressed air (commonly called a hand-held nebulizer) may be more effective in penetrating the airways. It is used for topical administration of bronchodilators, antiinflammatory agents, and antiallergenic medications. See Table 34-7 for examples of respiratory medications.

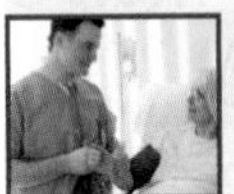

Do you think the inflammation from Mrs. Wilheim's pneumonia could produce wheezes in her chest? What problems would you anticipate in teaching her to use a hand-held nebulizer?

Improving the Efficiency of Respiration. In clients with chronic airflow limitation from emphysema, loss of elasticity causes air to become trapped in the alveoli. Breathing exercises can be effective in strengthening these clients' accessory muscles of respiration and increasing the use of the diaphragm for efficient exhalation of trapped air. The two most common breathing techniques are pursed-lip breathing and diaphragmatic breathing.

Pursed-Lip Breathing. **Pursed-lip breathing** is a technique of mouth breathing that creates slight resistance to exhalation by contracting the lips to reduce the size of the opening, thus maintaining an even reduction of intrathoracic pressure during exhalation. This technique helps prevent the airway collapse that can occur when the functional residual volume rapidly falls below a critical volume during exhalation. By exhaling slowly through slightly pursed lips, the client prolongs expiration and creates resistance that maintains pulmonary pressure to keep the airways open. Box 34-10 describes how to teach pursed-lip breathing.

Once the client has learned pursed-lip breathing, the technique can be used with activities on the borderline of the person's exercise tolerance. Although objective signs of improvement in ventilation have been difficult to demonstrate, individual clients report good results. Some chronic respiratory clients will naturally employ this technique without instruction. An added benefit of teaching the technique may be relaxation and a sense of control over a body function that is out of control.

Diaphragmatic (Abdominal) Breathing. **Diaphragmatic (abdominal) breathing** is breathing in which the majority of ventilatory work is accomplished by the diaphragm and abdominal muscles. It is deliberate use of the diaphragm and abdominal muscles to control breathing, strengthen the accessory muscles of respiration, and provide the client who has chronic respiratory disease with a technique to reduce the high functional residual volume associated with air trapping. First, the client is made aware of the sensations associated with the use of abdominal muscles; then the client learns to use the abdominal muscles to complete the expiratory cycle by contracting the abdominal muscles at the end of expiration. The technique is then used to gain control over dyspneic episodes. Relaxation and a sense of control may contribute to the effectiveness of this technique. Box 34-11 provides guidelines for teaching diaphragmatic breathing.

Additional techniques are aimed at more efficient respirations. General body conditioning and strengthening of respiratory muscles have some usefulness in pulmonary rehabilitation. Severe skeletal muscle deconditioning, commonly associated with chronic respiratory disease, increases the work of breathing. An incentive spirometer resistive breathing device is used to increase respiratory muscle strength and increase exercise tolerance.

Reducing Anxiety. A key to treating the anxiety of acute respiratory distress is recognizing that the client's anxiety is a normal compensatory response to difficulty in breathing. Any verbal or nonverbal suggestion that you believe the client is overreacting can be perceived as a lack of understanding or as a belief that the client is "overly emotional." A positive nurse-client relationship will be jeopardized.

A second key to treatment is to remove the cause of the anxiety—in this case, the difficulty in breathing. No other possible cause is pertinent at the moment. You can gain the client's trust by acting swiftly and assuredly to help the client gain control over respiration. Another effective intervention is reassurance that the client is not in immediate danger. Offer assurance that the client is in a safe place where help will be provided.

Once the acute episode has passed, techniques to prevent and help control anxiety can be taught. For the chronic respiratory client or the client with multiple acute episodes, reducing the general level of anxiety and learning to control episodes of anxiety can be useful in managing respiratory disease and improving the quality of life. Desensitization and guided mastery can assist clients in the management of dyspnea.

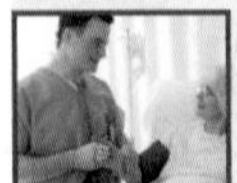

Mrs. Wilheim's anxiety level is high. She knew several people who died of pneumonia, including one of her sisters. Mrs. Wilheim's daughter assumes responsibility for the care of her mother and provides direct practical care to help her feel more comfortable. The daughter also takes responsibility for interacting with the health care team. How would you work with Mrs. Wilheim and her daughter to manage Mrs. Wilheim's anxiety?

BOX 34-9

Teaching for Self-Care

Using a Metered-Dose Inhaler

Purpose: To deliver a specific dose of aerosolized medication to be inhaled into the lungs for a local effect.

Expected Outcome: The client will correctly use an administration technique that results in the medication reaching the lungs.

Client Instructions

1. Insert the medicine canister into the inhaler unit, and remove the cover from the mouthpiece. Shake the unit gently according to the manufacturer's recommendations.

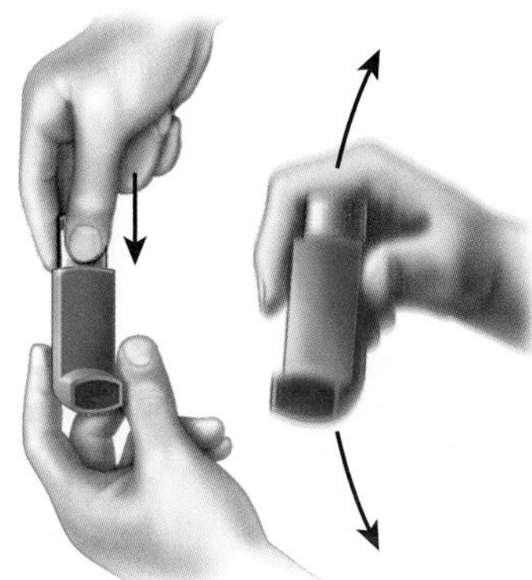

2. Hold the inhaler ready for inspiration. Exhale slowly. (Do not breathe into the inhaler; that could clog the inhaler valve.)

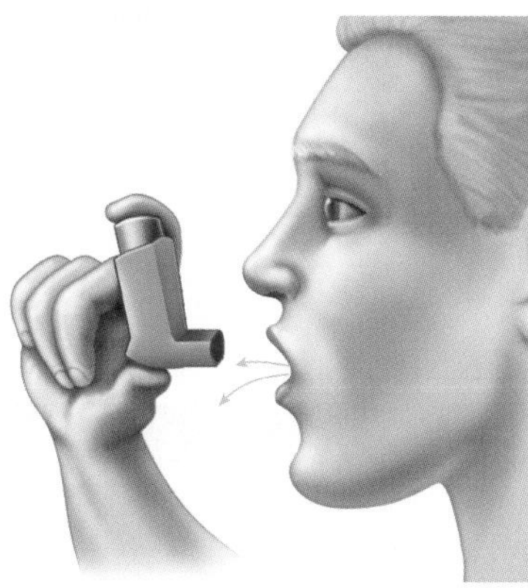

3. Place the mouthpiece into your mouth, and seal it with your lips. Tilt your head slightly back, and keep your tongue away from the mouth of the inhaler. (Alternatively, hold the inhaler 1 to 2 inches in front of your mouth and keep your mouth open. With steroids, do not put the inhaler in your mouth. Ineffective use results from medication bouncing off teeth, tongue, or palate.)

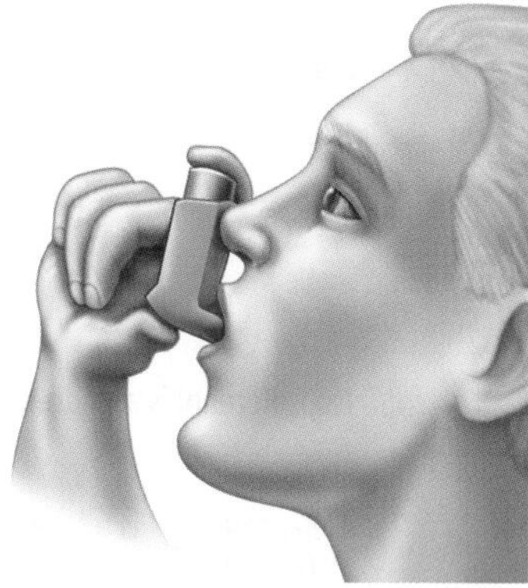

4. Press the top of the canister as you breathe in slowly through your mouth. (Failing to coordinate respiration with inhalation will decrease the amount of medication that reaches your lungs.)

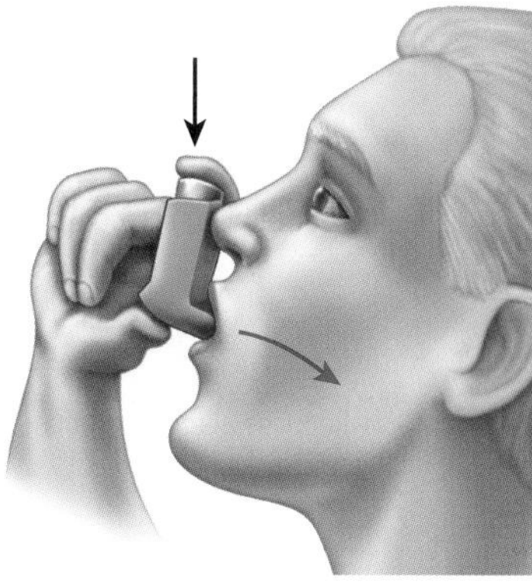

5. Remove the inhaler. Hold your breath for 10 seconds, then breathe out slowly through pursed lips.

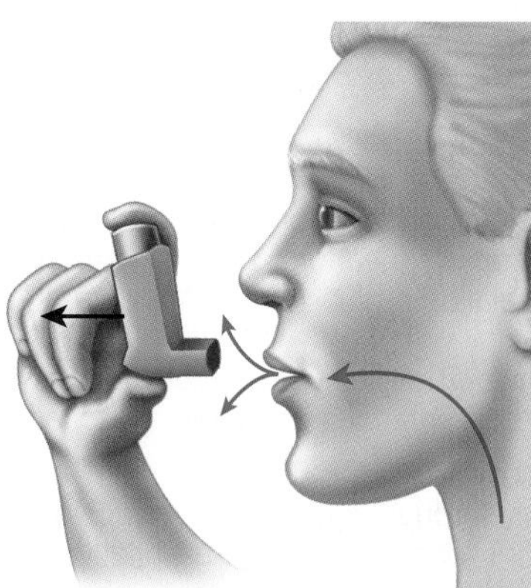

6. Keep the cap in place between uses to prevent dirt from getting into the inhaler. To clean the inhaler, remove the metal canister and rinse the holder in warm water. Dry the holder thoroughly before using it again.

Table 34-7 Examples of Respiratory Medications

MEDICATION	ACTION	SIDE EFFECTS	NURSING IMPLICATIONS
Bronchodilators			
Epinephrine	Epinephrine is for emergency use.	All of these medications have sympathetic nervous system side effects, such as tremors, anxiety, insomnia, headache, palpitations, and elevated blood pressure.	Monitor vital signs. Teach the client to take only as prescribed to avoid overdose. Teach the client that bothersome side effects may decrease with continued use.
Isoproterenol (Isuprel)	Isoproterenol is an adrenergic agent.		Side effects are less common with metered-dose inhalers.
Metaproterenol (Alupent)	Metaproterenol is a later-generation agent (similar to isoproterenol) designed to reduce side effects.		
Theophylline (aminophylline)	Theophylline is the prototype for the group. Aminophylline is used for continuous IV administration in status asthmaticus.		
Corticosteroids	Antiinflammatory.	Fluid retention, hypertension, mood swings, weight gain, gastritis, hyperglycemia Warning: Prolonged use can suppress adrenal function.	Local application by metered-dose inhaler reduces the side effects and the danger of adrenal suppression. Warn diabetic clients that they may need to adjust their insulin.
Antihistamines	Reduce allergic response.	Drowsiness, dry mouth, constipation, blurred vision, urinary retention	Use only with the advice of a physician in asthma; drying effects may increase airway constriction.
Cromolyn sodium (Intal)	Reduces allergic response. Prevents asthma attacks.	Cough, sore throat, dry mouth	Not used to control acute asthma attacks. Takes 2 weeks to become effective.

IV, Intravenous.

BOX 34-10 *Teaching for Self-Care*

Pursed-Lip Breathing

Purpose: To obtain control of breathing and reduce feelings of panic and dyspnea through training the muscles to prolong exhalation and increase airway pressure during exhalation.

Expected Outcome: The client will be able to consciously reduce the rate of breathing and prolong expiration.

Client Instructions

1. Inhale slowly through your nose, keeping your mouth closed. Count "one and two." Pause briefly.
2. Exhale through pursed lips as if gently blowing a candle flame. Count "one, two, three, four." Allow adequate time to empty your lungs and reduce air trapping. Exhalation should take at least twice as long as inhalation.

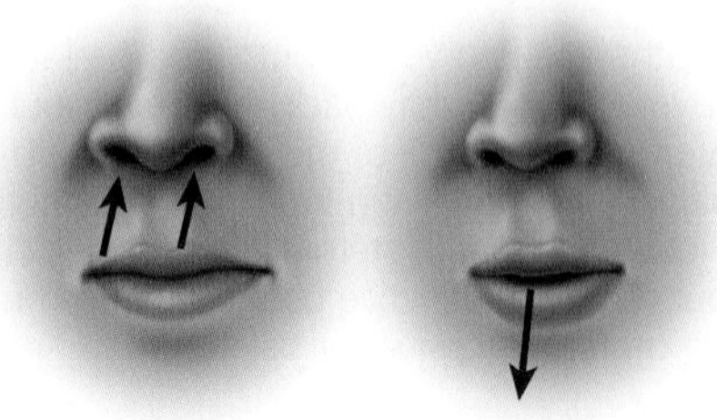

Pursed-lip breathing. The client should inhale through the nose and exhale through pursed lips.

BOX 34-11

Teaching for Self-Care

Diaphragmatic Breathing

Purpose: To reduce the respiratory rate, increase tidal volume, and reduce functional residual capacity.
Expected Outcome: The client will be able to consciously use the diaphragm during respiration.

Client Instructions

1. Assume a comfortable resting position.
2. Place one hand over your upper abdomen so that you will be able to feel the movement of your diaphragm.
3. Place the other hand on your upper chest so that you will be able to feel the movement of your accessory muscles.
4. Exhale through pursed lips. Feel the inward motion of your abdominal muscles.
5. Inhale. During inhalation, your abdomen should expand outward.
6. Avoid overbreathing, which may lead to light-headedness.
7. Repeat this exercise five to six times. Practice several times a day, until the exercise is comfortable and relaxing. Use the technique both to help you relax and to alleviate shortness of breath.

Once the client is comfortable with abdominal breathing, teach him or her to experience the contraction of the lower rib cage and the abdominal muscles at the end of respiration, to push excess residual volume from the lungs. This exercise can be used during periods of dyspnea to gain control over breathing or with activity to increase exercise tolerance.

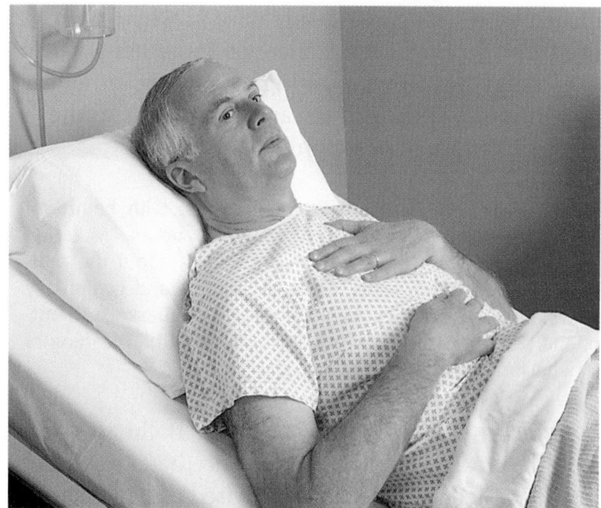

Diaphragmatic breathing is practiced best in a relaxed semirecumbent or recumbent position. Some people require little practice, but others may need several sessions of practice to learn the technique. (From Monahan, F. D., & Neighbors, M. [1998]. *Medical-surgical nursing: Foundations for clinical practice* [2nd ed.]. Philadelphia: Saunders.)

Managing Energy Requirements

Nutrition. Whether the condition is acute or chronic, nutrition intake should, at a minimum, meet the daily requirements for nutrients. In acute illness, more than the minimum daily requirements are needed to meet the increased metabolic demand associated with fever or prostration. However, the severely ill person may not be able to tolerate a normal diet. Small, frequent meals may be helpful in meeting nutritional needs. The foods should be easily digested, easily chewed and swallowed, and palatable to the client.

For the chronic respiratory client who has lost excessive weight, improved nutrition can restore strength and endurance to respiratory and skeletal muscles. This effect is difficult to achieve and maintain, especially in the home, because the problems of activity intolerance, meal preparation, and chronic hypoxemia are closely interrelated.

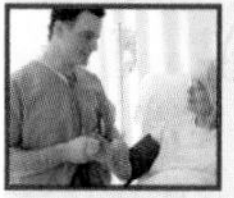

Mrs. Wilheim's daughter expresses concern over how much her mother is eating. Making sure her mother eats properly is her major concern. How would you meet the daughter's need while minimizing the risk for abdominal distention that normal food intake poses for Mrs. Wilheim?

Activity and Rest. The client with respiratory problems needs activity to stimulate respiratory function and needs rest to conserve energy or reduce the metabolic demand. In the hospitalized client, the physician's treatment plan may have specific guidelines for activity, or it may simply call for activity as tolerated. You must make a judgment about the client's needs. Useful parameters may include changes in vital signs and the client's report of fatigue or dyspnea. In planning activities, consider other scheduled treatments and procedures. Activity as routine as a bed bath can adversely affect oxygen saturation.

The chronic respiratory client living at home may need assistance with planning a schedule or with modification of activities to incorporate efficient work habits and conserve energy. Teaching may include the following:

- Prioritize activities. Schedule only part of the day. Plan to accomplish the most important activity on a list. Allow time for rest periods.
- Arrange needed items conveniently. For example, have the coffee pot and all supplies close to the sink. Keep a stool handy to sit at the sink. Keep items needed for paying bills in one location to avoid having to gather supplies to sit down and take care of personal business.

- Simplify everyday life. Uncluttered surfaces are easier to clean. It is easier to find needed items in uncluttered drawers and cabinets. Place most-often-used items within easy reach in closets and shelves.
- Work at a steady pace. As many tasks can be accomplished by working at a steady pace as when hurrying, and it will reduce the energy requirements.
- Save energy by rolling, pushing, or pulling rather than lifting. A small cart to carry items around the house or yard may be helpful.

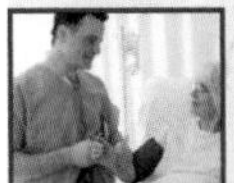

Mrs. Wilheim remains on bed rest with bathroom privileges for the first 48 to 72 hours. While on bed rest, she asks many questions about the bedside stand, lights, and bed controls and continually reviews the location of her glasses, tissues, wastebasket, call button, and personal articles. What do you think is the meaning of her behavior? How can you help her?

Controlling Allergens and Pollutants. Pollutants or allergens in the environment may exacerbate respiratory disease. The client may need to be advised to avoid persons with respiratory infections and areas where smoking is permitted. If the problem in the home environment is severe, the client may need to make some modifications. Carpeted floors can harbor allergens. Installing special air filters, damp dusting the furniture, discarding feather pillows, or even giving away a pet are among the changes that may be needed. The client's personal preferences and values should be considered and changes recommended only if a real benefit can be anticipated. It is sometimes helpful to wear a mask for activities outside the house where the environment cannot be controlled.

Controlling Infection. Infection control includes both protecting the client from infection and preventing the spread of infection when the client is already infected. Always apply universal precautions when working with the person with respiratory disorders. Wear clean gloves if the client has a productive cough or when working with equipment that has been contaminated with the client's sputum. Teach the client to cover the mouth when coughing, and provide a convenient container for disposing of tissues. Wash your hands after each contact with the client. Use all necessary attire including gown and mask, as needed, to protect yourself from contact with airborne respiratory secretions. When working with clients who have a history of copious secretions or those receiving aggressive respiratory interventions, such as coughing or airway suctioning, you may need to wear goggles.

To avoid infection, the client must practice good health habits. A balance of rest and activity, avoiding exposure to extremes of cold or heat, and balanced nutrition are important. Visitors should be screened, and anyone who might expose the person to infection should be asked to leave. A clean environment and personal hygiene will reduce the number of microorganisms to which the client is exposed.

The threat of infection is one of the primary hazards of home respiratory therapy care. Respiratory equipment harbors bacteria; the *Pseudomonas* organism is a major problem. The client needs to be taught hand-washing and cleaning protocols for caring for any equipment being used. Mold growth is also a problem, especially because mold spores are a common allergen. Even though the equipment appears to be clean, periodic cultures may be taken to verify that pathogenic organisms are not present.

Managing Primary Hyperventilation. The treatment for hyperventilation that is not from a metabolic or respiratory cause is rebreathing carbon dioxide. Special equipment is available that can be used with a mask to allow the client to rebreathe carbon dioxide until its level is brought within normal limits. However, a brown paper bag held over the nose and mouth is less expensive and just as effective.

Reexpanding Collapsed Lungs. Atelectasis occurs with any event causing air or fluid to enter the pleural space. Trauma to the chest wall can result in a *hemothorax* or *pneumothorax.* Inflammation of the pleurae from pneumonia or cancer can result in a *pleural effusion* (exudation or transudation of fluid into the pleural space).

A physician inserts a chest tube to remove the trapped fluid or air. The lung can then reexpand. In some cases, the client may continue to bleed or may have an air leak from the lungs. If the fluid or air is expected to continue to enter the pleural cavity, the chest tube is left in place until the lung has reexpanded and it is confirmed that no further problem exists. Placing a chest tube may be done as an emergency procedure or as a planned procedure, depending on the severity of the compromise to ventilation.

Nurses assist with the placement of chest tubes and manage the tube after insertion. Management includes maintaining the placement of the tube, maintaining the patency of the tube, and maintaining the drainage system. The tube is easily dislodged because it is held in place only by the mushroom end of the tube and the occlusive dressing at the tube site. The tube must remain patent to drain the fluid or air. Box 34-12 provides guidelines for managing chest tubes.

Chest tube drainage systems use a tube submerged in water, where atmospheric pressure provides the pressure necessary to counter the negative intrapleural pressure and the water seal prevents air from entering the intrapleural space. The system can use a one-, two-, or three-bottle system. The disposable system is essentially a three-bottle system.

The one-bottle system is the simplest, with the bottle serving to provide both the underwater seal and the drainage collection receptacle. The drainage tubing is connected to a tube that goes through the sealed top of the bottle and is submerged in the water. The water prevents air from entering the connecting tubing, where it could be drawn into the pleural space. The system must

BOX 34-12 *Managing a Closed Chest Tube Drainage System*

Understand the Function of the Components of the System

Closed chest tube drainage systems are designed to maintain negative pressure to assist drainage and to prevent air from entering the pleural space.

The system consists of three main components. The first component, called the *suction control chamber,* is a column of water that acts as a suction control. The level of the water (10 to 20 cm), rather than the amount of suction from the vacuum source, determines the amount of negative pressure created to facilitate drainage. The opening to the atmosphere prevents the buildup of negative pressure in the system. Gentle bubbling should be present in the suction chamber; however, if excess bubbling occurs in this chamber, this may indicate that the suction is too high.

The second component is a dual-compartment *water seal chamber.* One compartment is open to the drainage chamber, and the other compartment is open to a second water seal barrier. The water seal (2 cm) prevents air from entering the chest tube.

The third component is a three-compartment *collection chamber.* It holds up to 3000 mL of drainage. Connecting tubing is attached from the chest tube to the collection chamber. The collection chamber is open to the dual-compartment water seal chamber.

Nursing Responsibilities

Maintain the Integrity of the System

- *Maintain the patency of the tube.* Observe for drainage. Assess the client's breath sounds. Absence of breath sounds indicates collapsed lung.
- *Maintain the occlusive dressing.* The dressing should remain intact.
- *Maintain the water seal.* The water seal must be maintained at all times by avoiding movements that would disturb the water seal, keeping the system upright, and keeping the system below the level of the chest. The tubing should be positioned to maintain a straight line of drainage from the chest to the collection system.
- *Maintain suction.* Suction is regulated by the balance between atmospheric pressure and the height of the column of water. The atmospheric air vent must remain open. Suction pressure of 10 mm Hg to 20 mm Hg is sufficient to create subatmospheric pressure.
- *Observe for air leaks.* Bubbling occurs in the water seal chamber when air is present in the pleural space and is being removed from the chest. When bubbling continues beyond a reasonable time for removing the trapped air, you should consider a possible air leak from the lungs or from the system. Air leaks occur in the system when the connections are not tight. To check for air leaks in the system, use a padded Kelly clamp. Briefly clamp the chest tube as it comes out of the chest wall. If the bubbling stops, the air is coming from the chest. If the bubbling does not stop, move the clamp to below the connection. If the bubbling stops now, air is leaking into the connection. If the bubbling continues now, the leak is at the connection of the connecting tubing to the water seal system.

Monitor the Client's Response to Treatment

- *Respiratory function.* Audible breath sounds throughout the lung fields indicate ventilation. When the chest tube is inserted to relieve atelectasis caused by pneumothorax or hemothorax, the client should experience immediate relief of respiratory distress. Signs of tension pneumothorax include severe respiratory distress, absence of breath sounds on affected side, hyperresonance on affected side, mediastinal shift to affected side, tracheal shift to affected side, hypotension, and tachycardia.
- *Character of drainage.* A chest injury or chest surgery may result in air in the pleural space. Bubbles occur in the drainage compartment until the air is removed. Bloody drainage from a healing wound will change to the straw color of serous drainage in 24 to 48 hours. Continued bloody drainage indicates continued bleeding. Fresh blood would be bright red.
- *Amount of drainage.* Measure the amount of drainage each shift. Because the system must remain intact, do not empty the drainage. Mark the level of drainage on the apparatus and subtract the previous level of drainage.

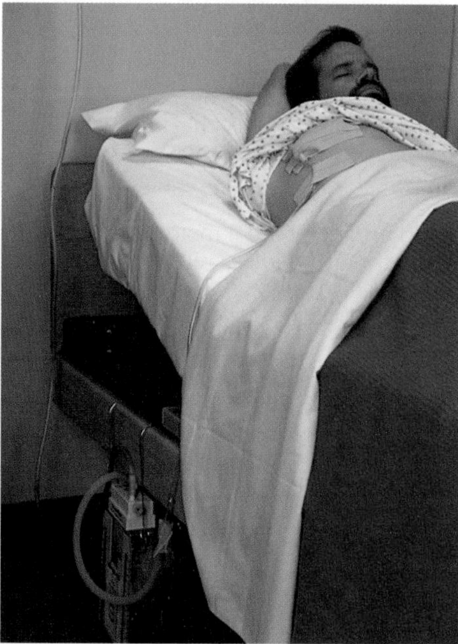

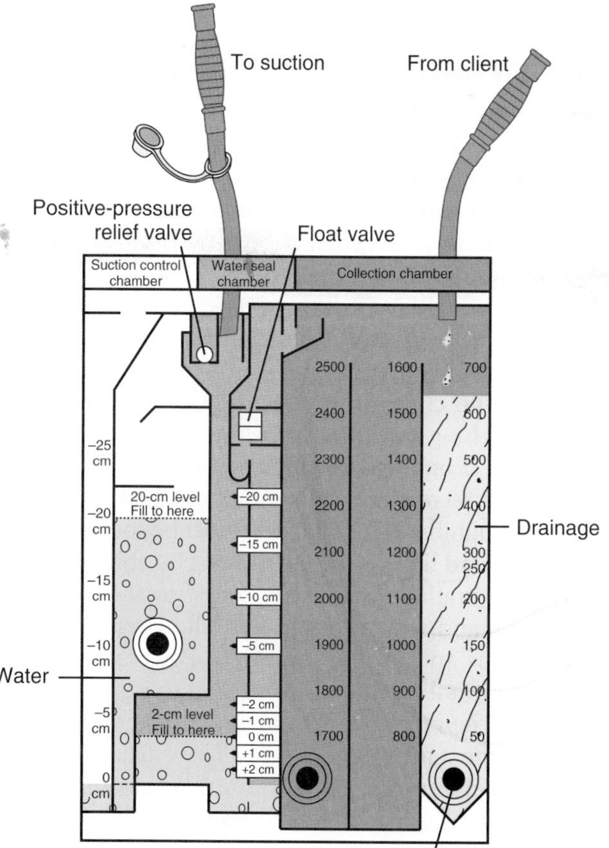

A chest tube attached to a typical drainage device. The chest tube is positioned in the lower thoracic cavity to drain serous fluid or blood. Notice the occlusive pressure dressing at the insertion site.

be airtight. Connections are sometimes taped to ensure that no air leakage occurs. The one-bottle system is appropriate for cases in which the amount of drainage is expected to be small and to drain readily from the intrapleural space. When air is being removed from the lungs it can be seen to bubble in the water seal.

The two-bottle system adds a separate bottle for drainage when larger amounts of drainage are expected. Typically, drainage does not enter the water seal bottle, but if the drainage bottle fills, it could overflow into the water seal bottle. Usually the chest tube would be briefly clamped and the drainage bottle changed before overflow occurs.

The three-bottle system adds a bottle, which is attached to suction to provide negative pressure when more rapid chest drainage is desired. The third bottle is open to the atmosphere with an underwater sealed tube so atmospheric air is drawn into the water and bubbles through the water. The length of the tube that is underwater determines the suction pressure. Pressure is measured in centimeters of the tube that is underwater.

Glass bottles for chest tube drainage are hazardous due to breakage and have given way to the disposable systems. The collection system must be lower than the client's chest at all times. If the bottle breaks, air would be drawn into the client's pleural space and collapse the lung. The disposable systems are economical and convenient. A one-glass bottle chest tube suction device that is mounted on a three-point stand is also commonly used.

INTERVENTIONS TO CLEAR THE AIRWAYS

Assisting the Client With Coughing. As a common symptom of respiratory disease, a cough serves a protective function by clearing the airway of irritants and secretions or by protecting the client from aspiration of irritating or foreign substances. In general, coughing is encouraged as a means of clearing the airways. In the absence of the cough reflex, the client who has a weakened condition or abnormal lung function may need assistance to clear the airways by coughing.

Assisting the client with effectively clearing the airways by coughing out sputum begins before the client attempts to cough. Other interventions to promote movement of secretions may be implemented in preparation for coughing. The secretions must be mobile; that is, nonsticky and liquid. The client must be able to manage deep inspirations before the cough to increase the lung volume and widen the airways, allowing air to get behind mucus and propel it upward. Forceful contraction of the expiratory muscles is needed to expel air at a velocity sufficient to move the mucus. The client must be able to assume a posture that will allow effective use of the abdominal muscles and maximum expansion of the chest. Box 34-13 provides guidelines for teaching an effective cough.

The sudden forceful change in pressure that accompanies a cough can have a deleterious effect, especially for the client with an anatomical pulmonary disease (i.e., a disease that causes a structural change in the alveoli). In rare instances, already weakened alveoli may rupture, causing pneumothorax. A more common though less observable occurrence is collapse of small airways. Clients with anatomical pulmonary diseases like emphysema may benefit from learning a *controlled cough*, or "huff," technique. The client produces a cough by taking small breaths and, with the glottis partially open, coughs two to four times until all the air is exhaled. This process may need to be repeated two to three times before the sputum is actually expectorated.

Suctioning the Airways. If the client is unable to effectively cough sputum from the airways, *oral* or *endotracheal* (into and beyond the trachea) suctioning will clear the airways. Suctioning is a traumatic experience for most clients and should be implemented as a measure of last resort. The benefits should be weighed against the risk of possible complications. Table 34-8 lists indications for suctioning.

Oral suctioning refers to suctioning the mouth and oropharynx. Several types of suctioning tips are available. A Yankauer tip is the least traumatic for oral suctioning, but a whistle tip may also be used (Figure 34-7). Oral suctioning may be helpful when the client is coughing up sputum but cannot get it beyond the oropharynx or when an artificial airway impedes removal of mucus

BOX 34-13 *Teaching for Self-Care*

Effective Coughing

Purpose: To maintain clear airways.
Expected Outcome: The client will produce an effective cough.

Client Instructions

1. Take three slow, relaxed, deep breaths. This will open your alveoli and get air behind the mucus in your respiratory tract.
2. On the last breath, hold your breath for 2 to 3 seconds. Holding your breath increases the pressure in your chest to produce a more forceful cough.
3. Contract your abdominal muscles, and force the air out through your mouth. This contraction produces the forceful exhalation recognized as a cough.

Hints

- Splinting an abdominal incision with a pillow or soft blanket will protect the client from pain caused by uncontrolled movement of the abdomen.
- Having the client sit upright and lean slightly forward will help produce the increased airway pressure that is needed to produce an effective cough.
- Have facial tissues and a waste receptacle close at hand.

from the oropharynx. Suctioning the oropharynx will sometimes stimulate a cough. It is used when swallowing is impaired and aspiration of accumulated oral secretions is a danger. It carries a low risk for complications.

Endotracheal suctioning is accomplished using a whistle-tip catheter attached to a suctioning device. Entering the trachea and branches of the bronchi with minimal trauma to the client requires skill and knowledge of the anatomy of the airways. Because endotracheal suctioning is irritating to the airways, it can actually increase the production of mucus and exacerbate the problems of airway clearance rather than reducing the volume of mucus. Capillary bleeding can further complicate the situation. Procedure 34-1 provides guidelines for endotracheal suctioning. Table 34-9 (p. 927) identifies common complications of suctioning and strategies for prevention. Because of the risk for complications, endotracheal suction should be performed by skilled practitioners under strict guidelines. Box 34-14 (p. 927) discusses the guidelines from the American Association for Respiratory Care.

Suctioning Route. The principle to be followed in clearing the airways is to use the least invasive procedure necessary to produce the desired result. If entering the trachea produces a cough, the sputum can be quickly suctioned without trauma to the lower airways. If no cough is stimulated, the catheter is passed to the carina and an attempt is made to enter both the right and left bronchi. The right bronchus is anatomically easier to enter because the angle is small as it branches off the mainstem bronchus. The left bronchus can sometimes be entered successfully by having the client hyperextend the neck, turning the head to the right. Successful suctioning is confirmed by auscultation of the lungs.

Client Positioning. Position the conscious client to maximize the normal physiological functions, and position the unconscious client to prevent aspiration. If the client can tolerate a semi-Fowler's or high-Fowler's position, airway clearance will be more effective when a reflexive cough is produced when the catheter enters the posterior pharynx or trachea. Administer suction as the client coughs up the secretions; this technique clears the airway with minimal trauma. The unconscious client may be protected from aspiration by use of the lateral position to allow drainage from the mouth by gravity. However, the airway is less accessible for suctioning when the client is in the lateral position. Turning consumes time if the client is not already in the lateral position.

Sterile Versus Clean Technique. Although *sterile* means the absence of any microorganisms, and the airways are not sterile, the airways past the glottis are considered to be sterile. Even though the lungs have protective mechanisms against microorganisms, the principle of preventing infection by not introducing any organisms into a body cavity would suggest the use of sterile technique. Furthermore, the action of suctioning traumatizes the epithelium of the airways, providing a portal for entry of microorganisms.

Hospital protocol generally includes the use of sterile technique for endotracheal suctioning and clean technique for oropharyngeal suctioning or nasopharyngeal suctioning. If both pharyngeal suctioning and endotracheal suctioning are required, you may change catheters after pharyngeal suctioning and before endotracheal suctioning, or you may first suction endotracheally. Sterile technique is believed to have benefits that outweigh the cost in a situation where the risk for nosocomial infection is high.

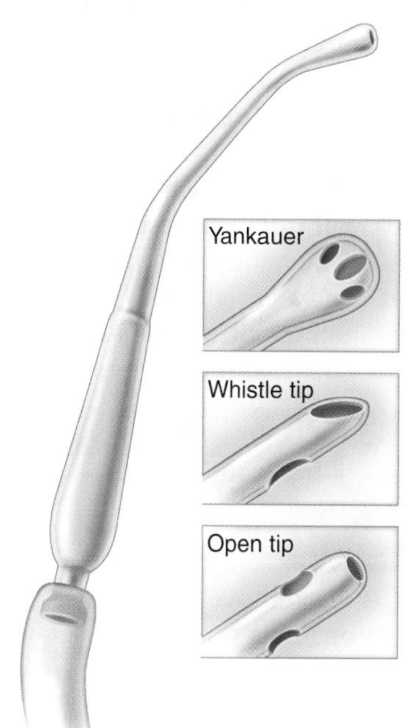

FIGURE 34-7 Types of suction catheter tips: Yankauer tip, whistle tip, and open tip.

Table 34-8 Indications for Suctioning

ASSESSMENT	INDICATIONS FOR SUCTIONING
Visual	Rapid, shallow breathing or difficult, labored breathing suggests need for further assessment.
Auditory	Moist, noisy, or gurgling sounds associated with breathing are definitive if the client cannot cough.
Tactile (fremitus)	Placing a hand flat over the client's chest wall detects vibrations of loose secretions; a more likely finding in an infant.
Auscultation	Coarse crackles (bubbling rhonchi); a loose, continuous, low-pitched rattling sound that disappears after suctioning or coughing.

For the homebound client who requires frequent suctioning on a long-term basis, the cost of sterile technique may outweigh the benefits. Teach family caregivers proper suctioning technique and how to maintain a clean environment. Also, family members may have difficulty maintaining sterile technique. Provide sterile suctioning catheters but explain that the catheters can be reused. Between uses, catheters are immersed in an antiseptic solution of boric acid and 0.4% to 0.5% sodium hypochlorite (Dakin's solution) or washed in warm soapy water. The catheter is rinsed thoroughly before it is introduced into the trachea. Clean rather than sterile gloves reduce the cost of equipment.

Suctioning Frequency. Suction as often as needed to maintain a clear airway without damaging the epithelial lining of the airways. Limiting suctioning to three passes of the catheter for each session of suctioning and 1 to 2 hours between sessions may help reduce trauma and the concurrent increase in mucus production. Bedside judgment must be made to balance the two goals.

Oxygenation. Suctioning removes not only mucus but also oxygen-laden air from the airways. The resulting hypoxemia can be life threatening. Increasing the inspired oxygen concentration to the highest possible safe percentage of oxygen and hyperinflating the lungs with manual or spontaneous breaths before and after suctioning will prevent hypoxemia. The best levels of oxygenation and hyperinflation are achieved with 100% oxygen delivered by a self-inflating resuscitation bag (Ambu bag). Monitor the rate and rhythm of the pulse and respiration to detect adverse effects.

Choose the method of oxygenation appropriate for each client. The client who is able to take deep breaths and does not have other risk factors for oxygen deficit may tolerate suctioning with only deep breaths of room air. The homebound client who is otherwise stable also can usually tolerate suction without supplemental oxygen. The intensive care client is almost always preoxygenated with 100% oxygen before and after suctioning. However, the presence of CAL makes administration of 100% oxygen risky.

Hydration of Secretions. Thick, tenacious sputum is not easily removed by suctioning. Applying the principle of employing the least harmful treatment that will produce the best results, the client's secretions are best hydrated by adequate fluid intake. Sterile normal saline is sometimes instilled into the bronchi in an effort to directly hydrate the secretions. Because this is a controversial procedure, you should check the protocol in your agency. Normal saline may irritate the airways, thus increasing mucus production and bronchospasm.

Vacuum Pressure Control. The maximum pressure setting on the vacuum suction device should be the lowest pressure needed to remove secretions. The gauges on wall-mounted suction units in a piped-in vacuum system are calibrated in millimeters of mercury (mm Hg) vacuum pressure. The safe range for vacuum pressures for adults is 80 to 120 mm Hg. If the catheter is too small or the secretions are too thick, excessive vacuum pressure may be reached—that is, higher than safe limits. Use a larger catheter, and step up measures to reduce the tenacity of the secretions.

Catheter Selection. A suction catheter is selected that will cause the least trauma, minimize occlusion of the airway, and be large enough to remove the secretions. Suction catheters are rubber or plastic tubes approxi-

Time to Allow: **Novice:** 10 min. **Expert:** 5 min.

PROCEDURE 34-1 ENDOTRACHEAL SUCTIONING

The purpose is to remove secretions, thus relieving airway obstruction. This procedure is traumatic to the airways and requires attention to safety to prevent complications.

DELEGATION GUIDELINES

Assessment of the need for airway clearance may not be delegated to a nursing assistant. The potential risks associated with airway clearance by suctioning dictate that this task not be delegated to a nursing assistant in the hospital setting. The assembly of equipment and assistance with suctioning may be delegated to a second person. In this circumstance, the nursing assistant receives direct, immediate supervision. The nursing assistant must receive specialized instruction and demonstrate ongoing competence in the performance of this skill. In long-term care settings, it may be appropriate to delegate clearance of artificial airways to a nursing assistant who has received appropriate training and supervision.

EQUIPMENT NEEDED

- Portable or wall suction unit
- Sterile suction kit (*or* sterile gloves, sterile suction catheter with Y port [thumb-control port], sterile normal saline, sterile cup for normal saline)
- Option: clean supplies
- Towel or waterproof pad

1 Follow preliminary actions (see inside front cover).

2 Recognize the need for suctioning. *Accurate assessment ensures suctioning when needed and prevents unnecessary suctioning.*

a. Wet, gurgling respirations without the strength to cough productively; *or*
b. Auscultation of bubbling rhonchi in the tracheobronchial tree; *or*
c. The presence of a nasotracheal or tracheostomy tube

3 Gather the necessary equipment.

4 Determine whether to use a sterile or a clean procedure. *The choice of using a sterile or clean procedure depends on the client's risk for infection, especially the risk for nosocomial infection. The lungs are not sterile; however, suctioning bypasses normal respiratory defense mechanisms and therefore places the client at risk for infection. Also, the client who needs suctioning is often critically ill. Sterile technique prevents the entry of any microorganisms into the lungs at a time when the client is most vulnerable to infection. On the other hand, clients with permanent tracheostomies or who are on mechanical ventilators at home also need suctioning. There, clean rather than sterile procedures are often used. Clean technique is less expensive and therefore can be used over a longer period.*

5 Get the client's cooperation. *Suctioning will be less traumatic if the client is able to cooperate. When a client needs to be suctioned, the explanation should be brief and to the point. If the client is unable to cooperate fully, a second person may be needed to restrain the client's hands.*

6 Set up the equipment. *You should be ready to suction the client immediately once the client is preoxygenated.*

a. Turn on the suction. Use a vacuum pressure of 80 to 120 mm Hg with wall suction (60 to 100 mm Hg for an infant; 80 to 115 mm Hg for a child).
b. Open the sterile saline; place the cap inverted on a clean surface.
c. Open the suction kit.
d. Pick up the container for the saline, squeeze to open it, and set it aside; keep the inside sterile. Pour water or saline into the container.
e. Then put on sterile gloves.
f. Pick up the sterile catheter with your sterile dominant hand and the unsterile suction connecting tubing with your nondominant hand.
g. Connect the two, keeping your dominant hand and the suction catheter sterile (see illustration). The nondominant hand becomes unsterile when it is used to attach the unsterile connecting tubing to the suction catheter.
h. Test the suction with the sterile water.

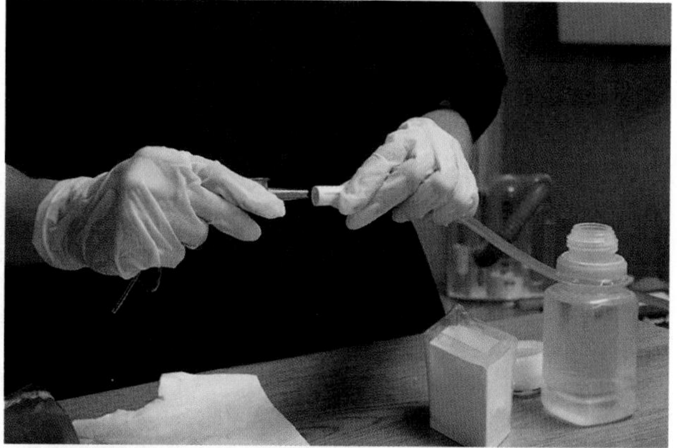

Step 6g. Connecting the sterile suction catheter to the unsterile connecting tubing that leads to the suction unit.

7 When you are ready to suction, have an assistant hyperinflate the lungs with 100% oxygen (see illustration). *Preoxygenation will temporarily increase the PaO_2* and reduce the risk for hypoxemia during suctioning.

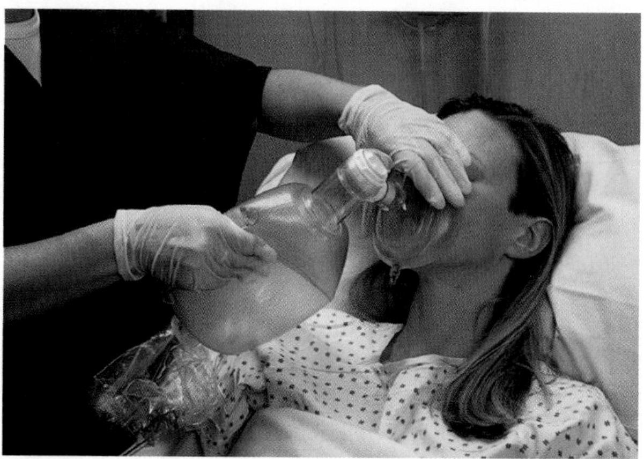

Step 7. Hyperinflating the lungs with an Ambu bag.

a. If the client does not have an artificial airway, have the client take several deep breaths.
b. If the client has an endotracheal tube or tracheostomy, use an Ambu bag to give two to three deep breaths. You have to make a clinical judgment about whether or not to increase the oxygen supply. Usually, you hyperinflate with 100% oxygen.

8 Pass the catheter through the nose into the oropharynx (see illustration). Watch the client's respiration, and pass the catheter into the trachea when the person inhales. Or, pass the catheter directly into the endotracheal or tracheostomy tube. Leave the Y port open while passing the catheter. Pass the catheter until you meet resistance, then close the Y port to apply suction. When you enter the trachea, start counting; you should be out of

Continued

the trachea by the time you reach 10. *Suctioning only while withdrawing the catheter will reduce the degree of trauma to the tracheobronchial tree. Time is a factor in reducing the oxygen deficit with suctioning.*

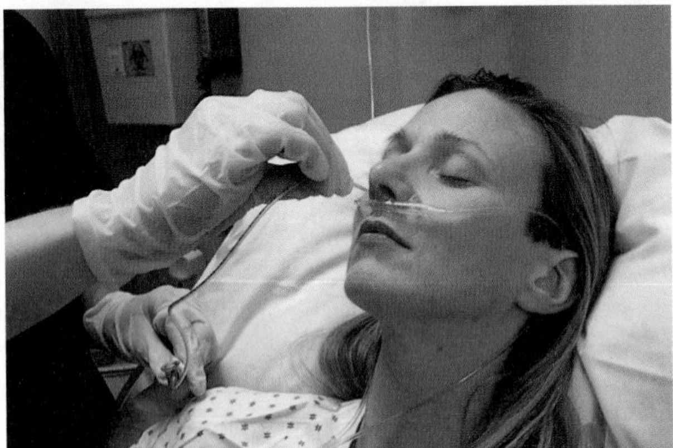

Step 8. Passing the suction catheter through the nose as the client takes a breath.

9 Hyperinflate the lungs to reoxygenate the client. Hyperinflation helps the client restore oxygenation and regain control of breathing.

a. *Client-initiated:* If the client is able or is not intubated, have the client take several slow, deep breaths.
b. *Nurse-initiated:* Use an Ambu bag attached to an endotracheal tube or tracheostomy tube, or use a face mask if the client is not intubated.

10 Assess the results; repeat if needed. Do not withdraw the catheter from the client's nose until you are sure you will not pass the catheter into the trachea again. Clear the catheter by suctioning the normal saline or water before repeating the procedure. Assess the amount and characteristics of the sputum; assess for decreased rhonchi. Suctioning is effective if the rhonchi have cleared or diminished.

HINTS

Having the client in a semi-Fowler's position facilitates passing the catheter and may help the client cough, if a cough reflex is stimulated. If you stimulate a cough reflex when entering the oropharynx or trachea, you can stop passing the catheter and suction the sputum that the client has coughed up into the trachea. You will have accomplished your goal of clearing the airway without having to pass a catheter deep into the tracheobronchial tree. It is helpful for a second person to hyperinflate the lungs, especially when you are inexperienced. Rotate the catheter as you withdraw it, to clear all sides of the airway. Use standard precautions when contact with sputum is likely, especially if blood is present in the sputum. Masks and goggles may be necessary.

HOME HEALTH CARE CONSIDERATIONS

When a client requires suctioning in the home, it is usually suctioning through a tracheostomy. Some clients learn to suction themselves; however, family caregivers most often perform the procedure. The caregiver will need support from the nurse to learn to perform the procedure. Ideally, the caregiver will have an opportunity to practice the procedure before the client is discharged from the hospital. A home health care nurse can then follow up with a home visit to help modify the technique for the home, to plan for the cleaning and storage of supplies, to obtain supplies, and to reinforce the essential elements of the technique. The caregiver will need to be taught to recognize the need for suctioning and to evaluate the results. Some caregivers can learn to use a stethoscope to listen to the lungs.

mately 18 inches long and ending in a whistle tip. The whistle tip is a smooth, rounded, nontraumatic, sealed end with one or more openings on the side. The vents are spaced 1½ to 2 inches on alternate sides of the catheter. This prevents the collapse of the catheter if it becomes occluded or if high vacuum pressures are created. The vents also help reduce mucosal trauma by reducing the pull of the catheter against the mucosa.

You must be able to control the vacuum pressure, turning it off or on. To allow control of suction, the catheters are designed with a Y port, which is attached to the connecting tubing. Occlude the port with your thumb to close the system and produce a vacuum. This feature allows you to enter the trachea without suction on and to apply the suction as the catheter is withdrawn. Entering without suction reduces trauma by allowing the catheter to easily pass through the airway.

Liquefying and Mobilizing Sputum

Expectorants. Expectorants are used to loosen or liquefy the mucus so it can be coughed out more easily. Iodinated glycerol (Organidin), a supersaturated solution of potassium iodide (SSKI), and guaifenesin are thought to stimulate sputum clearance. Guaifenesin is available both over the counter and by prescription. It is available as a single ingredient or in combination, frequently with the antitussive dextromethorphan. If the client is using over-the-counter medications, you may need to teach the difference between antitussives and expectorants. Difficult generic names should be provided in written form. The client should be questioned

Table 34-9 Etiology and Prevention of Complications of Suctioning

COMPLICATION	ETIOLOGY	PREVENTION
Hypoxemia and atelectasis	Suction removes oxygen-laden air.	The PaO_2 can be significantly raised by increasing the FiO_2. Preoxygenate the client with 100% oxygen, and hyperventilate the client at 1½ times the tidal volume is less likely to increase the of the tidal volume. For the client without an artificial airway, you can accomplish this by increasing the liter flow of oxygen and having the client take deep breaths. Hyperinflation and oxygenation after suction are expected to restore the oxygen level and open the alveoli. Avoid vacuum pressure greater than 80 to 120 mm Hg for the adult.
Mucosal trauma	The plastic catheter can damage the mucosa.	Lubricate the catheter. Twist rather than push past minor resistance. Stop when you meet resistance. Apply suction only when withdrawing catheter, and use intermittent suction. If bleeding occurs and frequent suctioning is necessary, consider using a nasal airway.
Vagal stimulation	Suctioning stimulates the parasympathetic vagus nerve, which supplies both the trachea and the heart.	Vagal stimulation shows the heart rate. Bradycardia, ventricular arrhythmias, or cardiac arrest may occur. Suction only when needed, and use preoxygenation and hyperventilation.
Increased mean arterial pressure	Associated with hyperinflation	Hyperinflation by changing the ventilator settings to 1½ times the tidal volume is less likely to increase the mean arterial pressure than is the use of a manual resuscitation bag. This is particularly important for clients with new vascular grafts or with increased intracranial pressure.
Paroxysmal coughing	Irritation of the cough control center at the carina	While stimulating a cough may prevent the need for deeper suctioning in some clients, the uncontrolled cough of others can collapse airways and irritate the tracheobronchial tree, stimulating bronchospasm. Suction only as necessary, and maintain oxygenation.

BOX 34-14 *Evidence-Based Practice*

Clinical Practice Guidelines for Nasotracheal Suctioning

Problem: Clients of all ages and in all settings require maintenance of a patent airway and removal of saliva, pulmonary secretions, blood, vomitus, or foreign material from the trachea and nasopharyngeal area. Some clients have the inability to cough or to clear secretions on their own despite their ability to cough. These clients can have visible secretions, gurgling, adventitious or diminished breath sounds, shortness of breath, hypoxemia, restlessness, or chest radiographic evidence (x-ray films) demonstrating retention of secretions resulting in atelectasis or consolidation.

Evidence

The American Association for Respiratory Care (a professional association) developed a guideline that applies to clients in a wide variety of settings, including critical care, emergency department, inpatient acute care, extended care and skilled nursing care, home health care, and outpatient or ambulatory care. The method used to develop the guideline was a systematic review of searching electronic databases. Both internal and external review was the method used for guideline validation. The method used is as follows: The working group consultants may review the initial draft of the guideline. After completion by the working group, the draft is reviewed by the entire steering committee and then by a review panel (i.e., persons engaged in all facets of the delivery of respiratory care who have volunteered to review drafts of the guideline before publication). The 2004 update was approved by the 2003 Clinical Practice Guideline (CPG) Steering Committee.

Application to Practice

- To improve the consistency and appropriateness of respiratory care and serve as a guide for education and research
- To provide clinical practice guidelines on nasotracheal suctioning

Electronic copies: Available in Portable Document Format (PDF) at http://www.rcjournal.com/contents/09.04/09.04.1080.pdf.

Print copies: Available from the American Association for Respiratory Care (AARC), CPG Desk, 11030 Ables Ln, Dallas, TX 75229-4593; website: www.aarc.org.

Reference

American Association for Respiratory Care. (2004). Nasotracheal suctioning—2004 revision & update. *Respiratory Care, 49*(9),1080-1084 [62 references].

about allergies to iodine before using one of the iodinated compounds.

Guaifenesin and SSKI stimulate sputum clearance but also increase the production of mucus. The overall effectiveness of expectorants has not been clearly defined in careful clinical studies. Clients often report increased ability to cough out sputum.

Mucolytics. *Mucolytics* are medications that alter the viscosity of the mucus so that it is more easily expectorated. Oral mucolytics or expectorants are more effective than topically applied agents. Acetylcysteine (Mucomyst), a once popular mucolytic, is irritating to the tracheobronchial tree and has not been proven to be effective in randomized studies, but it continues to be used on a limited basis. It is administered through a nebulizer. Bronchodilators are recommended in conjunction with mucolytics because the incidence of bronchospasm is high.

Cough Suppressants. *Antitussives,* or cough suppressants, are antithetical to the goal of expectoration of sputum. They are given only for symptomatic relief. It is reasonable to suppress a dry, hacking, nonproductive cough or a cough that is increasing fatigue or disturbing sleep. A productive cough is a means of clearing the airways but might be treated with a cough suppressant when the cough is tiring or is severe enough to cause concern about the complications of rib fracture or pneumothorax.

Humidity. The viscosity of sputum may be directly related to the client's general level of hydration. Assess the client for dehydration, and institute measures to treat or prevent it (see Chapter 25). Systemic hydration is thought to be the most effective means of maintaining moist airways.

Topical hydration of airways may be accomplished by increasing the humidity of the inspired air using room humidifiers and by creating an aerosol. The goal is to provide air with sufficient moisture and in a sufficiently small particle size to carry the moisture to the small airways. Results vary, however, and some practitioners do not believe it is effective.

A *humidifier* is a mechanical device that adds water vapor to the air. Humidification equipment may deliver water at room temperature, heated to body temperature, or slightly above body temperature. Heated air is able to carry more moisture. An *impeller humidifier* produces larger particles of water that may be too large to penetrate deeply into the tracheobronchial tree. Room humidifiers, used in many homes for upper respiratory infections, are the most common examples of impellers. Safe use includes careful cleaning between uses to prevent growth of molds and bacteria. Other, more complex forms of humidification are used with mechanical ventilators.

An *aerosol* is a fine suspension of a liquid or powder carried on a stream of gas. Aerosols may be large in volume (for hydration) or may be produced in small amounts, such as dry aerosols that deliver medications topically into the airway (see more on bronchodilators under Opening the Airways, earlier). To enter the tracheobronchial tree, a particle of liquid produced by an aerosol generator must be 1 to 3 μm in size. Large-volume aerosols can potentially run on a continuous basis. These devices deliver a dense, large volume of water in a large volume of gas (compressed air or oxygen). The large volume of gas plus the dense aerosol significantly helps to hydrate the tracheobronchial tree. Large-volume aerosols are administered via an aerosol face tent, face mask, or tracheostomy tent.

All methods of topical hydration carry a risk of contamination because all devices include a water reservoir. Sterile solutions are used in nebulizers because the warm, moist environment can grow organisms that can be trapped in the particles of moisture and carried to the lungs. Hospitals have protocols for changing equipment regularly to provide sterile mask and tubing.

Chest Physiotherapy. **Chest physiotherapy,** abbreviated CPT or chest PT, is an approach to mobilizing and draining secretions from gravity-dependent areas of the lung; it uses a combination of postural drainage, chest percussion, and vibration. When hydration, aerosol medication, deep breathing, and coughing are not sufficient to clear the airways, chest physiotherapy may be added.

Because secretions are more likely to be retained in gravity-dependent parts of the lungs, chest physiotherapy relies on positioning the person to use gravity to drain the various lobes of the lungs. Chest physiotherapy may cause bronchospasms and hypoxemia in clients with asthma. Other complications can include fractured ribs, bruising, and discomfort.

Postural drainage is a technique in which the client assumes one or more positions that will facilitate the drainage of secretions from the bronchial airways. It is accomplished by placing the client in positions that allow gravity to facilitate drainage of mucus out of the lobes of the lungs and bronchopulmonary segments and into the larger bronchi (Figure 34-8). When secretions reach the upper airways, they may be coughed up spontaneously or removed by tracheobronchial suctioning. Nine or more positions are required to drain all the areas of the lungs. However, the specific location of the pathologic condition may suggest the position that will be the most effective.

It is not clear that postural drainage has more benefit than incentive spirometry, deep breathing, and coughing for most clients with COPD, pneumonia, or postoperative atelectasis. If routine measures are not producing the desired results, postural drainage may be given an empiric trial and discontinued if there is no beneficial response. Clients with COPD and cystic fibrosis who benefit from postural drainage may continue the treatment on a long-term basis at home.

Action Alert! The choice of a time for chest physiotherapy treatments may affect the results. Try to schedule chest physiotherapy as follows: in the early morning, when secretions have accumulated during the night; 1 hour before meals or 2 hours after meals, to avoid aspiration; at bedtime, to clear the lungs and allow sleep free of coughing; or at an appropriate time interval after administration of a bronchodilator when the medication has taken effect.

Percussion and vibration are added to postural drainage to increase the velocity of mucus movement up the tracheobronchial tree. **Chest percussion** is defined as using cupped hands to rhythmically clap on the chest wall over various segments of the lungs to mobilize secretions. It is performed immediately over the portion of the lung where secretions are retained (Figure 34-9, *A*). Cupping the hands in a manner to produce a hollow sound on impact with the chest prevents discomfort to the client. **Vibration** is a technique of chest physiotherapy whereby the chest wall is set in motion by oscillating movements of the hands or a vibrator for the purpose of mobilizing secretions (Fig 34-9, *B*). Vibration theoretically increases the air currents to aid in removing trapped air and mucus.

Clients for chest physiotherapy should be carefully selected. Clients with heart problems, pneumonia, or CAL should be observed for hypoxemia. Rupture of a blood vessel or an abscess can rapidly obstruct the airway. Clients with osteoporosis or on long-term steroid therapy have fragile bones and can fracture a rib.

Action Alert! Some clients become dyspneic or hypoxic with postural drainage. Monitor the client carefully, and discontinue the treatment if problems occur.

Reducing Sputum Production

Corticosteroids. Both antiinflammatory and antiallergenic effects may be achieved with corticosteroids. Aerosolized corticosteroids are available as nasal sprays used to prevent allergic rhinitis or oral inhalers to prevent asthma attacks. Two weeks of use is required before results are experienced. During acute bronchospasm, corticosteroids must be administered systemically (orally or intravenously). Inhalation of steroids may cause an overgrowth of *Candida albicans* in the mouth; therefore the mouth should be rinsed after each administration.

Action Alert! If a client is on a corticosteroid, ask questions about the length of use. Long-term use of corticosteroids can suppress production of corticosteroid by the adrenal gland. Check the physician's orders for supplemental corticosteroids to be given to manage the stress of acute illness or of surgery.

Cromolyn Sodium. Cromolyn sodium has both antiinflammatory and antiallergenic effects. It is used to prevent allergic responses in the airway by preventing the rupture of mast cells and the release of bronchoconstrictive chemicals in the lungs. It is not a steroid, nor is

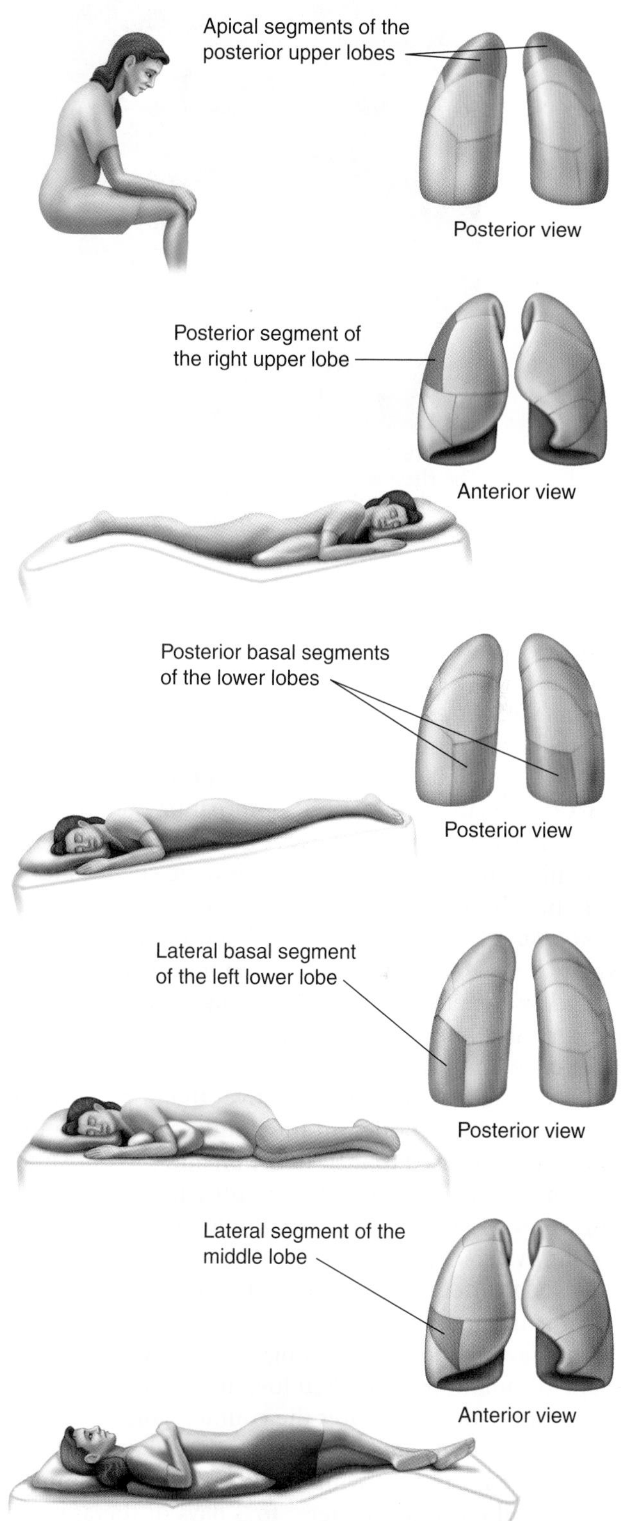

FIGURE 34-8 Examples of positions for postural drainage based on the area of the lung to be drained.

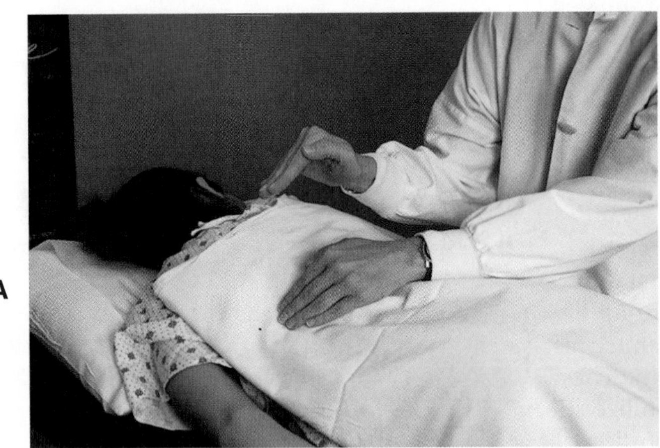

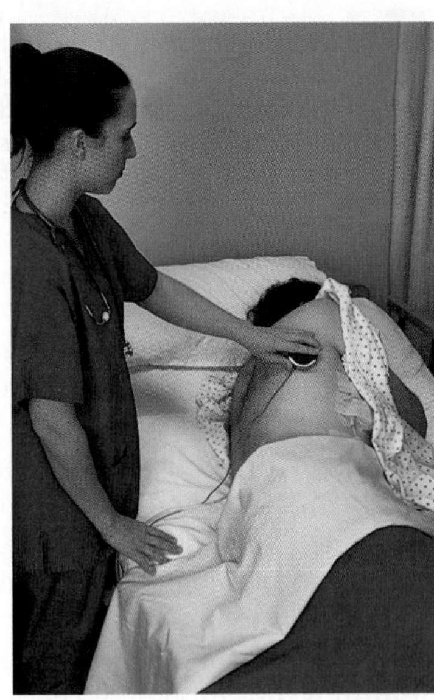

FIGURE 34-9 **A,** Percussion is performed with "cupped" hands. The chest is protected with a towel while the hands rhythmically clap the chest wall. Using the wrist to control the motion ensures a gentle clapping motion. **B,** Use of a vibrator for chest percussion.

it a drug used during acute bronchospastic episodes. It is most effective in asthmatic children and young adults but must be used for 2 weeks before it is effective.

Antihistamines. Antihistamines provide symptomatic relief of rhinitis. Combining them with decongestants is sometimes helpful. Newer antihistamines have less of a sedative side effect. Some antihistamines are more effective after several days of therapy. Because antihistamines have drying effects, asthmatic clients should seek the advice of a physician before using these drugs.

Antibiotics. A broad-spectrum antibiotic is ordered when there is evidence that a respiratory infection is caused by bacteria or when there is high risk for developing an infection. Occasionally, antibiotics are aerosolized to treat pulmonary infections, but topical administration is generally less effective than systemically administered antibiotics. In the home setting, oral antibiotics may be used to treat infection and avert hospitalization. Prophylactic use of antibiotics in the home setting, sometimes prescribed for chronic respiratory clients, is controversial.

Vasoconstrictors. Vasoconstrictors are used as decongestants of the respiratory mucosa. Because they are frequently sympathomimetic drugs, side effects of sympathetic stimulation occur. Pseudoephedrine is an example commonly found in over-the-counter cold remedies. Topically administered nasal sprays should only be used for a limited course of symptomatic relief. Development of rebound congestion after 2 to 3 days of therapy may lead the client to prolonged use.

INTERVENTIONS TO IMPROVE GAS EXCHANGE

Providing Supplemental Oxygen. Oxygen therapy may be prescribed for one of three goals: to maintain the arterial blood oxygen level, to reduce the work of breathing, or to reduce the myocardial workload. For the client with a serious acute illness that results in desaturation because of hypoventilation or a ventilation/perfusion abnormality, the goal is to maintain the arterial blood oxygen level until the cause of the hypoxemia can be corrected. For the chronic respiratory client who has exertional dyspnea directly related to hypoxemia, the goal is to reduce the work of breathing and increase activity tolerance. For the client who has a heart problem (myocardial infarction, heart failure) the goal may be to reduce the myocardial workload. For any specific client, these three benefits often overlap.

Oxygen is a potentially toxic substance and is prescribed by a physician. You will participate in the decision-making process by reporting to the physician findings that indicate a change in the client's condition or the failure to respond to the prescribed oxygen therapy. The goal of oxygen therapy is to achieve an optimal arterial oxygen tension by giving the lowest possible, most effective dose of oxygen while avoiding its toxic effects.

Action Alert! Notify the physician at the earliest sign of hypoxia. Oxygen deficit is life threatening.

Oxygen is given to keep arterial PaO_2 in the normal range of 80 to 100 mm Hg. Oxygen administration should not cause the arterial $PaCO_2$ to rise above 45 mm Hg. Different criteria may be used for a person with COPD who lives with chronically low oxygen and high carbon dioxide levels. In chronic lung disease, the normal drive to breathe from a high carbon dioxide level is suppressed; therefore the only drive to breathe is from a low oxygen level. When oxygen is needed to decrease the work of breathing and increase activity tolerance, low doses are used to avoid bringing the oxygen up to a normal level. Procedure 34-2 provides guidelines for administration of oxygen.

Action Alert! Always ask if the client has COPD before starting oxygen in amounts greater than 2 L/min. Be prepared to recognize the clinical appearance of a client with COPD.

Prolonged exposure to oxygen in high concentrations can cause structural damage to the lung tissue, which can be fatal. Oxygen toxicity is most often seen in the adult or neonatal intensive care unit. Although the exact relationship of long-term high concentrations of oxygen and blindness in premature infants is not clear, oxygen dosage is monitored closely as a preventive measure.

Oxygen Delivery Systems. Oxygen delivery devices are divided into two broad categories: high-flow oxygen systems and low-flow oxygen systems. A high-flow system delivers a flow of gas that exceeds the volume of air required for the person's minute ventilation. Low-flow systems deliver oxygen at variable liter flows designed to supplement the inspired room air to provide airflow equal to the minute ventilation. Because the oxygen is imprecisely mixed with room air, oxygen percentages delivered by low-flow systems are not as consistent as the percentages in high-flow systems.

In a low-flow system, the percentage of oxygen delivered to the tracheobronchial tree is determined by the person's respiratory rate, the tidal volume, and the pattern of ventilation (deep, fast, shallow, irregular). The high-flow system provides a flow rate and reservoir capacity adequate to meet total inspired-air needs. The amount of oxygen to be delivered is ordered as liters of 100% oxygen per minute (LPM), percentage of oxygen in inspired air, or fraction of inspired oxygen (FiO_2). FiO_2 is the preferred method.

The choice of oxygen delivery device and liter flow depends on the client's condition. The principle is to provide the lowest percentage of oxygen that will maintain arterial oxygen saturation within normal range. Arterial blood quickly desaturates below 60 to 70 mm Hg, so the partial pressure of oxygen should be kept above 70. Anything higher is unnecessary. Clinical judgment is needed to decide that the client's condition suggests that a higher FiO_2 may be needed to achieve oxygen saturation. Once the client is stabilized on the prescribed FiO_2, arterial blood gases or pulse oximetry may be used to confirm that the desired results are being achieved.

TIME TO ALLOW: NOVICE: 10 min. **EXPERT:** 5 min.

PROCEDURE 34-2 ADMINISTERING OXYGEN

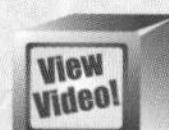

The administration of oxygen requires a physician's prescription. In an emergency, however, a nurse or respiratory therapist can make a decision to initiate oxygen therapy without a physician's order. In many hospitals, the respiratory therapy department initiates oxygen therapy. The respiratory therapist and the nurse work together to monitor the effects of oxygen therapy and to maintain safe, effective administration of oxygen.

DELEGATION GUIDELINES

The decision to initiate oxygen therapy may not be delegated to a nursing assistant. The gathering and assembly of equipment, along with administration of oxygen, may be delegated to a nursing assistant. In this case, specific instructions must be provided to help the nursing assistant monitor the client in any of the following ways: measuring and recording vital signs, observing for evidence of breathing difficulties, noting respiratory rate and depth, color of lips and nail beds, and noting presence of restlessness or irritability. Be sure to provide parameters for immediate RN notification.

EQUIPMENT NEEDED

- Nasal cannula, simple face mask, nonrebreathing mask, or partial rebreathing mask
- Oxygen tubing
- Humidifier
- Sterile distilled water
- Oxygen flowmeter
- Oxygen source
- No-smoking sign

1 Follow preliminary actions (see inside front cover).

2 Assemble the necessary equipment. Check the physician's order for the delivery device and liter flow. *Supplemental oxygen is considered to be a drug and normally requires a physician's prescription. In emergency circumstances, however, you are legally permitted to decide to start oxygen.*

a. No-smoking sign. Also, remove all smoking materials from the room. *Oxygen is not combustible but is necessary to support combustion. Fire from a small spark spreads rapidly in the presence of an oxygen source. A posted sign alerts personnel and visitors to the use of oxygen.*

Continued

b. Humidification device. *Humidity prevents drying of the mucous membranes from dry oxygen gas. An amount greater than 2 L of 100% oxygen per minute (LPM) or for administration longer than 24 hours requires humidification. The use of sterile water for humidification reduces the possibility of growth of organisms in the oxygen-delivery system. The use of distilled water prevents the accumulation of mineral deposits in equipment. Limit the use of humidity to occasions in which the benefit is clearly demonstrated to be cost effective.*

c. Nasal cannula (see illustration). *Flow: 1 to 6 LPM. Percent delivered: Range 22% at 1 LPM to 40% at 6 LPM. The exact amount varies with the minute ventilation. A nasal cannula is the most commonly used device. It is used when a low-liter flow is required or sufficient. It is relatively comfortable and allows the client to eat or drink. However, it is easily dislodged, and it requires patent nasal passages. It is also not comfortable at higher-liter flow.*

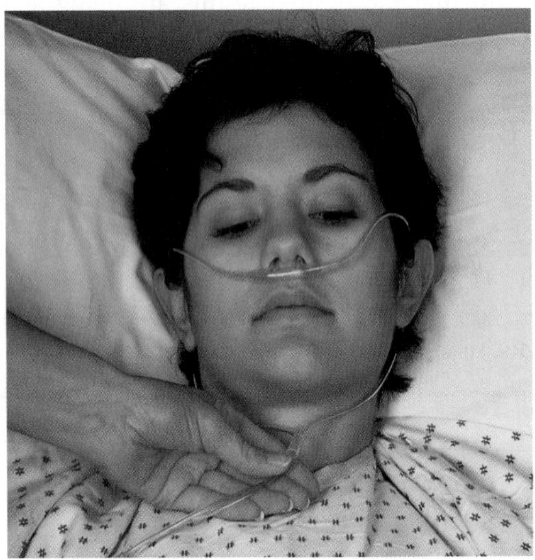

Step 2c. Nasal cannula.

d. Simple face mask (see illustration). Flow: 6 to 12 LPM. Percent delivered: Range 40% at 6 LPM to 65% at 12 LPM. The exact amount varies with the minute ventilation. Caution: Must not be used at flow rates under 6 LPM. A face mask makes it difficult for the client to eat or drink. It may also cause a feeling of confinement or claustrophobia. Use with caution in a client in danger of airway obstruction or aspiration.

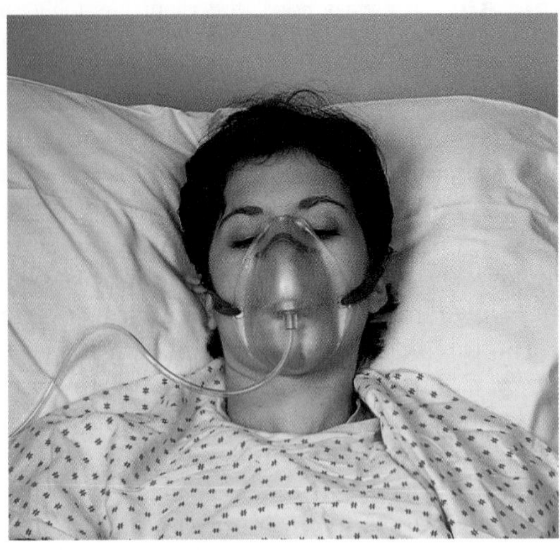

Step 2d. Simple face mask.

e. Face mask with a nonrebreathing oxygen reservoir bag (see illustration). Flow: As required to keep the reservoir bag inflated at least one-third full during inspiration; varies from 6 to 15 LPM. Percent delivered: Range 60% to 90%. A higher percentage requires a well-fitting mask. Useful for short-term administration of high concentrations of oxygen.

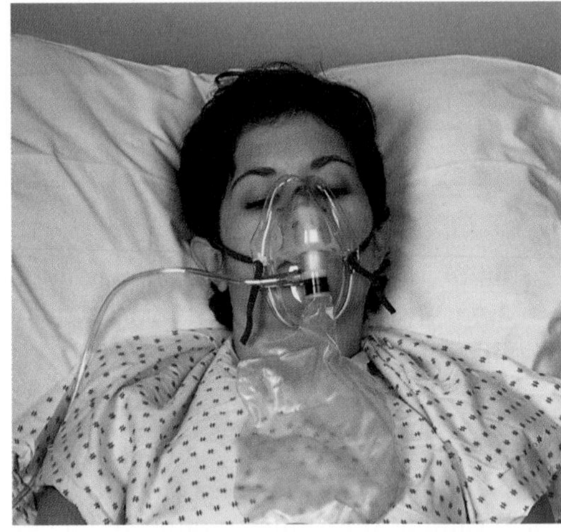

Step 2e. Face mask with a nonrebreathing oxygen reservoir bag.

f. Venturi mask (see illustration). Flow: As recommended by the manufacturer. Percent delivered: Precisely provides 24%, 28%, 31%, and so on up to 50% oxygen. Humidification is not used with a Venturi mask because it interferes with efficient air entrainment. Because a high-liter flow is required and the mask is specialized, the system is expensive and used only when benefits are clearly expected to outweigh costs.

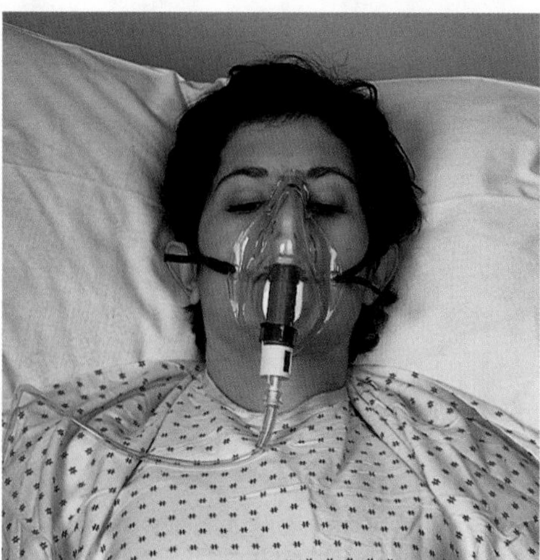

Step 2f. Venturi mask.

g. Face tent (see illustration). Delivers an imprecise amount of oxygen. Can be used with compressed air for humidification only. However, this high humidity is sometimes associated with increased airway resistance.

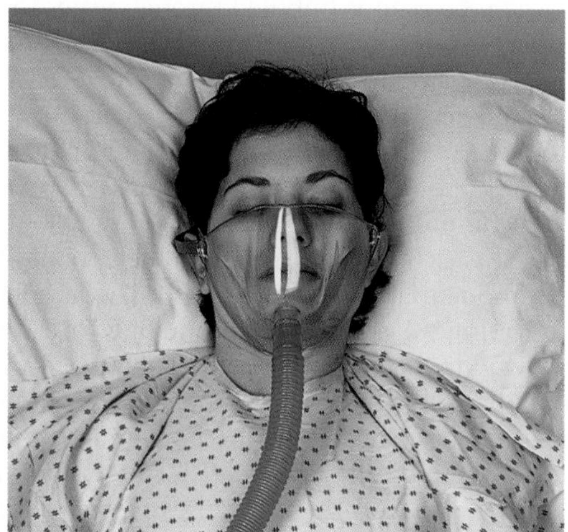

Step 2g. Face tent.

3 Set up the system. Insert the flowmeter into the oxygen source. Attach the connecting tube and delivery device. Add extra connecting tubing if needed. Check the function of the system after establishing the oxygen flow. Observe for bubbling in the water. *The length of the tubing limits the client's movement. This step flushes the system with oxygen and ensures client safety.*

4 Place the delivery device on the client, and make the client comfortable. Relieve the client's concerns about the need for oxygen. Adjust the strap comfortably around the client's head, and prevent pressure behind the ears. Use a water-soluble lubricant to relieve irritation to the external nares. *Explanations about the need for oxygen should convey in a balanced way the importance of ensuring continuous oxygen use against the client's concern that the situation may be life threatening.*

5 Frequently assess the client and the delivery system. Check the liter flow, the humidity, and the position of the device. Monitor for signs and symptoms of oxygen deficit. *This assessment provides information for rapid response if therapy is not effective.*

HINTS

Observe the skin under the elastic band on the cannula or mask. Skin breakdown is common behind the ears. Padding with a gauze pad or cotton ball may increase comfort and prevent skin breakdown. If the client can be out of bed, use extension tubing to allow the person to move to a chair. If the client can ambulate or go to the bathroom, a portable oxygen unit can be used to maintain oxygen therapy. Remember that getting out of bed increases the oxygen need. A pulse oximeter can be used to monitor the effects of activity on oxygenation.

HOME HEALTH CARE CONSIDERATIONS

If a client needs oxygen in the home, a medical supply company will deliver the oxygen to the home and set up the equipment. A respiratory therapist is often sent to provide the initial teaching. The nurse's role is to reinforce teaching and monitor the effectiveness of the therapy. Because of the high risk for infection with oxygen equipment, monitoring the frequency of cleaning and the technique for cleaning the equipment is important.

Consideration is also given to selecting a device that the client will find tolerable for continuous use. For guidelines on administering oxygen see Procedure 34-2.

Low-flow systems. Low-flow systems include a nasal cannula, an oxygen mask, or an oxygen mask with a reservoir. The nasal cannula is the most commonly used oxygen delivery device. It is relatively comfortable and does not interfere with talking or eating. Because the tubing is secured in place by an elastic band placed over the ears and behind the head or by tubing looped behind the ears, you should ensure that prolonged pressure does not cause skin damage. The nasal cannula can be used even if the client is breathing through the mouth. The oropharynx and nasopharynx are natural reservoirs for the 100% oxygen flow. When the client inhales through the nose or the mouth, this accumulated oxygen is drawn into the lungs. Because the nasal cannula can cause the discomfort of dry nasal passages at higher-liter flows, it is usually used when a low FiO_2 is indicated.

The simple face mask is shaped to fit snugly over the nose and mouth. The sides of the mask have holes to allow the exhaled carbon dioxide to escape from the mask and decrease rebreathing of carbon dioxide. Because of the hole and because the mask does not fit to totally occlude airflow, the oxygen is mixed with room air. The simple face mask is used when the client needs a higher FiO_2 than is provided by a nasal cannula to correct hypoxemia. If the mask is removed for meals, the client may need a nasal cannula while eating.

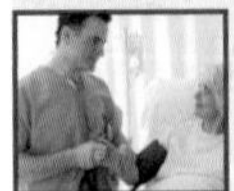

Mrs. Wilheim's oxygen therapy was started with a face mask in the emergency department. Her oxygen saturation was low, and she appeared quite ill. Now, however, you realize that the oxygen mask is frightening to Mrs. Wilheim; she even says that she knows she must be really sick if she needs oxygen. How can you help Mrs. Wilheim? What criteria would you use to request that the physician change the order to a nasal cannula?

To achieve an even higher FiO_2, an oxygen reservoir is added to the face mask. The highest FiO_2 is achieved with the nonrebreathing mask. The bag fills with 100% oxygen from the wall outlet to provide a tidal volume of 100% oxygen. The air holes on the sides of the mask are equipped with a one-way valve to allow escape of exhaled air and to prevent the entrance of room air with inhalation. While most of the tidal volume is supplied from the reservoir, the system does allow some entrance of room air, so the mask with reservoir bag never delivers 100% oxygen. If the bag collapses by more than half its volume with each breath, an adequate tidal volume of oxygen-rich air will not be maintained and the client could suffocate.

A variation of the mask with reservoir bag is the partial rebreathing mask. Part of the exhaled volume enters the reservoir bag. This air is assumed to be mostly from the dead space, and thus is oxygen rich because it has not entered the alveoli where diffusion occurs. The partial rebreathing bag supplies an FiO_2 higher than the simple face mask, but not as high as the nonrebreathing reservoir bag. The partial rebreathing bag has limited usefulness.

High-flow system. The mask with a Venturi device is the only true high-flow system. A higher-liter flow is needed to achieve the same FiO_2 as with a nasal cannula or simple face mask. The Venturi device creates a pressure drop that draws room air in precise amounts to create the desired FiO_2. The fact that small amounts of oxygen can be delivered precisely has been beneficial in treating the client with chronic respiratory disease.

Humidification. Oxygen is a dry gas. Prolonged exposure to the drying effects of oxygen may cause irritation and damage to oral, nasal, and pharyngeal mucous

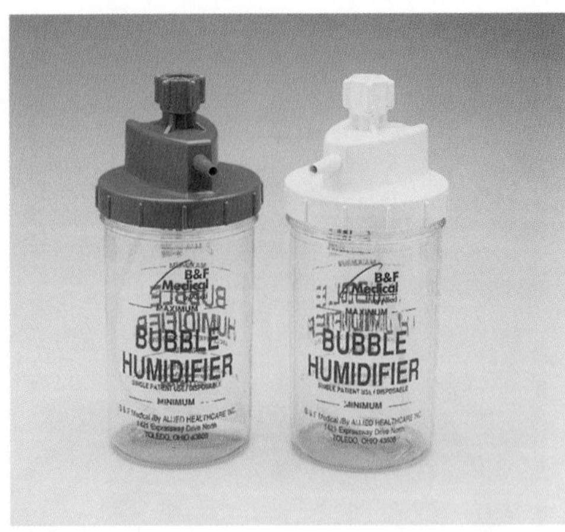

FIGURE 34-10 Bubble-diffusion humidifiers. Oxygen is blown through sterile distilled water in these humidifiers to add moisture to the inspired gas. (Courtesy Allied Health Care, St. Louis, MO.)

membranes. Oxygen is humidified to prevent irritation and drying of the airways and to maintain an optimal environment for the normal function of the cilia. As mentioned previously, humidification is the addition of water vapor to a dry gas.

Bubble-diffusion humidifiers are most often used with oxygen. Oxygen is bubbled through water to allow molecules of water vapor to be mixed with the oxygen. When oxygen is delivered at a low-liter flow for a short time (usually less than 24 hours), the client can usually tolerate oxygen without humidity. Figure 34-10 shows two types of bubble-diffusion humidifiers.

Oxygen humidifiers have limited ability to humidify the inhaled gas. If both oxygen and high humidity are needed, an open face tent can be used. The face tent fits loosely, forming a semicircle around the face. With a properly working face tent, a cloud of vaporized water is seen around the person's face. Condensation accumulates in the large tube that delivers the oxygen and humidity and must be periodically emptied. The water vapor can be either cool or warm. Warm mist carries a larger volume of water, but cool mist is considered to be equally effective in hydrating secretions. The face tent delivers a highly variable amount of oxygen and is not appropriate when the FiO_2 needs to be carefully controlled.

Home Oxygen Systems. The advent of portable (home) oxygen systems (Figure 34-11) has provided selected clients who have chronic respiratory disease with increased exercise tolerance, improved length and quality of life, and reduced hospitalizations. Exercise tolerance and the quality of life are closely related. Oxygen therapy may allow the person to manage activities of daily living, walk a block, or attend a family gathering. Exercise is needed to increase the overall fitness of skeletal muscles, particularly accessory muscles of respiration, which further increases activity tolerance. Oxygen therapy may also improve sleep. Oxygen during sleep is needed if the client has nocturnal hy-

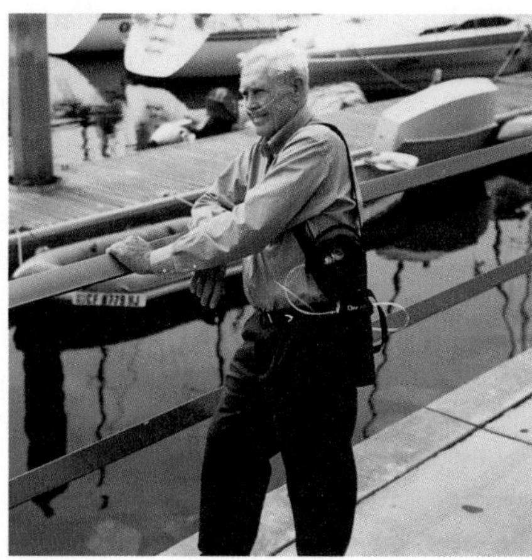

FIGURE 34-11 Portable oxygen systems such as the one worn by this client can enhance the quality of life for clients with chronic respiratory disease. (Courtesy Chad Therapeutics, Chatsworth, CA.)

poxemia. In some clients, improved health and an overall sense of well-being may be a factor in prolonging life. In clients with hypoxemia at rest, continuous oxygen (24 hours a day) is more effective than intermittent use for improving survival time and reducing neuropsychiatric symptoms.

Three methods of oxygen administration suitable for home use are liquid systems, portable cylinders of gaseous oxygen, and oxygen concentrators. Liquid portable oxygen systems are the most versatile and are suitable for people who wish to remain active. Liquid oxygen systems are composed of three parts: a reservoir of liquid oxygen (contained in a Thermos-like container), a flowmeter, and a humidifier. One disadvantage of most liquid oxygen tank systems is that the length of the oxygen tubing limits the client's movement. A portable unit for ambulatory use can be filled with oxygen from the liquid system tank. When filled, the portable unit weighs approximately 9 pounds. It may be carried with a shoulder strap or pulled in a cart. Small portable cylinders of gaseous oxygen, which can be wheeled about on a cart, may also supply oxygen at home. Oxygen concentrators are used when stationary, low-flow oxygen is appropriate. Rather than requiring an oxygen source, room air is concentrated into a higher percentage of oxygen. Liter flow rates are generally limited to 2 to 3 LPM. Medicare has very stringent guidelines for reimbursement for home oxygen. Documentation that demonstrates a clear benefit is important.

INTERVENTIONS TO TREAT RESPIRATORY FAILURE

Whether the situation is one of an acute obstructed airway or a decline in respiratory function, respiratory failure is an emergency. You must swiftly establish an airway and support the client's breathing to prevent death.

Maintaining a Patent Airway. Sudden respiratory arrest is treated by establishing an airway and providing ventilation with mouth-to-mouth technique or with a manual breathing bag (commonly referred to by the trademark name Ambu). When the primary problem is an airway, establishing an airway is often sufficient to reestablish breathing. (See Chapter 35 for the procedure for cardiopulmonary resuscitation [CPR]). If the client continues to be unable to breathe without assistance, mechanical ventilation may be needed.

> ***Action Alert!*** Be prepared to start CPR. Airway obstruction is an emergency. (1) Activate the emergency response system. (2) Lift the client's chin. This action may establish an airway and prevent the need for CPR. *Hint:* Calling for the resuscitation team when you do not need it is better than not calling for the team when you do need it!

Time is often a crucial factor in the prevention of serious and sometimes lethal side effects of a poorly functioning airway. In the case of a totally obstructed airway, an open airway must be established in fewer than 4 minutes to prevent brain damage or death. A partially obstructed airway can cause hypoxemia and may result in irreversible brain damage. Ideally, airway obstruction is corrected before total occlusion occurs.

Oropharyngeal Airway. An *oropharyngeal* airway (Figure 34-12, *A*) is a curved rubber or plastic piece that is inserted into the mouth over the posterior tongue; it maintains a patent airway through the pharynx. The purpose of oropharyngeal airways is to hold the tongue forward. The distal end of the airway is positioned in the mouth between the posterior pharynx and the back of the tongue.

To insert an oral airway, follow this procedure: With the airway turned on its side, slide the airway along the top of the tongue until the tip of the airway reaches the posterior portion of the tongue. Rotate the airway to follow the natural curve of the tongue as it enters the oropharynx. The rotating motion assists in opening the throat to allow correct position of the airway. The curved end will hold the tongue forward. If the airway piece is the correct size, the flat end clears the lips and serves as a "bite block" between the front teeth.

> ***Action Alert!*** When the airway is compromised, work quickly to insert an oral airway.

Oropharyngeal airways are used for unconscious and semiconscious clients. When the client is conscious enough to have a gag reflex, an airway may cause vomiting with aspiration, which is a life-threatening complication. Remove the airway immediately if gagging occurs. Turning an unconscious or semiconscious person into a side-lying position allows the jaw to fall forward and may effectively maintain an open airway without an artificial airway.

Oropharyngeal airways are generally for short-term use with a client who is expected to regain consciousness in a short time. For example, oral airways are frequently placed in the operating room and remain in place until the client has recovered from anesthesia. Mucus may collect in the mouth and can be aspirated into the lungs; therefore the client may need to be suctioned or placed in a side-lying position for drainage, or both. If the client begins to cough and gag on the airway, you will need to remove it.

Oral airways are also used when the client's condition is deteriorating and the airway is becoming obstructed, because with loss of consciousness the muscles of the throat relax and allow the tongue to occlude the airway. Try lifting the jaw or chin. If lifting the chin establishes airflow, an oral airway will maintain an open airway.

Nasal Trumpet Airway. *Nasal trumpet airways* (Figure 34-12, *B*) are cuffless tubes made of soft rubber or plastic and passed through a nostril into the nasopharynx. When inserted into the nares, the tube acts as a guide for the insertion of a suction catheter. The nasal trumpet airway is most commonly used in clients who require frequent nasotracheal suctioning and are developing epistaxis from the traumatic insertion of the suction catheter through the nose.

A nasal trumpet airway extends into the pharynx and is positioned at the base of the tongue. The tongue is separated from the posterior pharyngeal wall, preventing obstruction from the tongue "falling" into the pharynx. The proximal end (nearest the nostrils) of a nasal airway is flared and fits against the external nares. Insertion of a large safety pin through the flared end stops the airway from slipping further into the nose or larynx. Nasal airways are more appropriate and comfortable for conscious and semiconscious clients than oropharyngeal airways.

Select an airway that is slightly smaller than the nares and slightly larger than the suction catheter to be used. Using a penlight, observe the nose for septal deviation that may make one side of the nares more open. Lubricate the airway with a water-soluble lubricant jelly containing a local anesthetic. Petroleum-based lubricants are not acceptable because of the danger of aspiration into the lungs. Insert the tube gently but firmly, following the contour of the nasopharyngeal passageway.

Endotracheal Airway. An **endotracheal tube** (ET tube; Figure 34-12, *C*) is a catheter passed through the nose or mouth into the trachea for the purpose of establishing an airway. Most endotracheal tubes are made of disposable polyvinyl chloride or other synthetic material. A ballooned cuff that is molded into the plastic can be inflated to occlude the main bronchus; thus air passes only through the endotracheal tube. The client can then be ventilated using an Ambu bag or placed on a ventilator.

An endotracheal tube can be passed through the nose or the mouth. In an emergency, or when the nares cannot accommodate the tube, or when the practitioner prefers the oral route, it is passed through the mouth. Passing an endotracheal tube requires special training and practice under supervision. A laryngoscope is used to open the airway and visualize the glottis. The scope then acts as a guide for passing the tube. Air is immediately injected into the balloon by way of a pigtail attached to the cuff. The Ambu bag fits directly to the endotracheal tube, and respiration is immediately established. The whole procedure is completed in seconds, rapidly establishing respiration in the client who is not breathing. Endotracheal tubes are also placed in the operating room, especially when muscle paralysis is needed during the surgical procedure. An endotracheal tube can be left in place for up to 3 weeks, but only if the cuff pressure is carefully monitored to prevent tissue necrosis at the site of the cuff. If mechanical ventilation is needed for an extended period of time, a tracheostomy may be performed.

Tracheostomy. A tracheostomy (an opening made directly into the trachea by surgical incision) is performed when there is obstruction above the trachea or when the client is in respiratory failure and may benefit from reduced airway resistance (length of airway) and dead space. A tracheostomy has the advantages over an endotracheal tube of improved airway suctioning and client comfort. If the need for a tracheostomy is prolonged, the client with a tracheostomy tube can eat soft, well-chewed foods in small bites.

Tracheostomy tubes are inserted through the surgical incision into the trachea. Most tracheotomies are not performed as emergency procedures but under more controlled conditions for the purpose of maintaining long-term mechanical ventilation. A tracheostomy would be performed as an emergency in a case such as that of a burn victim with severe upper airway edema that prevents passing an endotracheal tube. While the tracheostomy wound is fresh and a pathologic condition is present in the lungs, the risk for infection is high.

Tracheostomy tubes (Figure 34-12, *D*) are disposable and made from a polyvinyl chloride or other synthetic material that does not react with human tissue. Cuffed tracheostomy tubes are used when the client may need mechanical ventilation and are the most common. These may be replaced with uncuffed tubes when the risk for respiratory failure has passed. Steel or silver tracheostomy tubes are rarely used today.

Caring for a client with an artificial airway makes use of the nursing diagnosis of *Ineffective airway clearance.* The tube is a foreign object in the airway and increases the production of mucus. In addition, the client is unable to cough to clear the airway. Frequent respiratory assessment and suctioning are required. As the client gains strength and can get in an upright position, it is possible to produce a cough that will clear the tracheostomy tube of mucus. Mouth care is important because it helps the client manage the accumulation of mucus and may prevent infections that could enter the lower airways. The humidifying function of the upper airways is absent; therefore humidification of inspired air is essential. Because mucus accumulates around the tracheostomy tube, frequent cleaning of the site is needed to prevent infection, especially when the wound is fresh (Procedure 34-3).

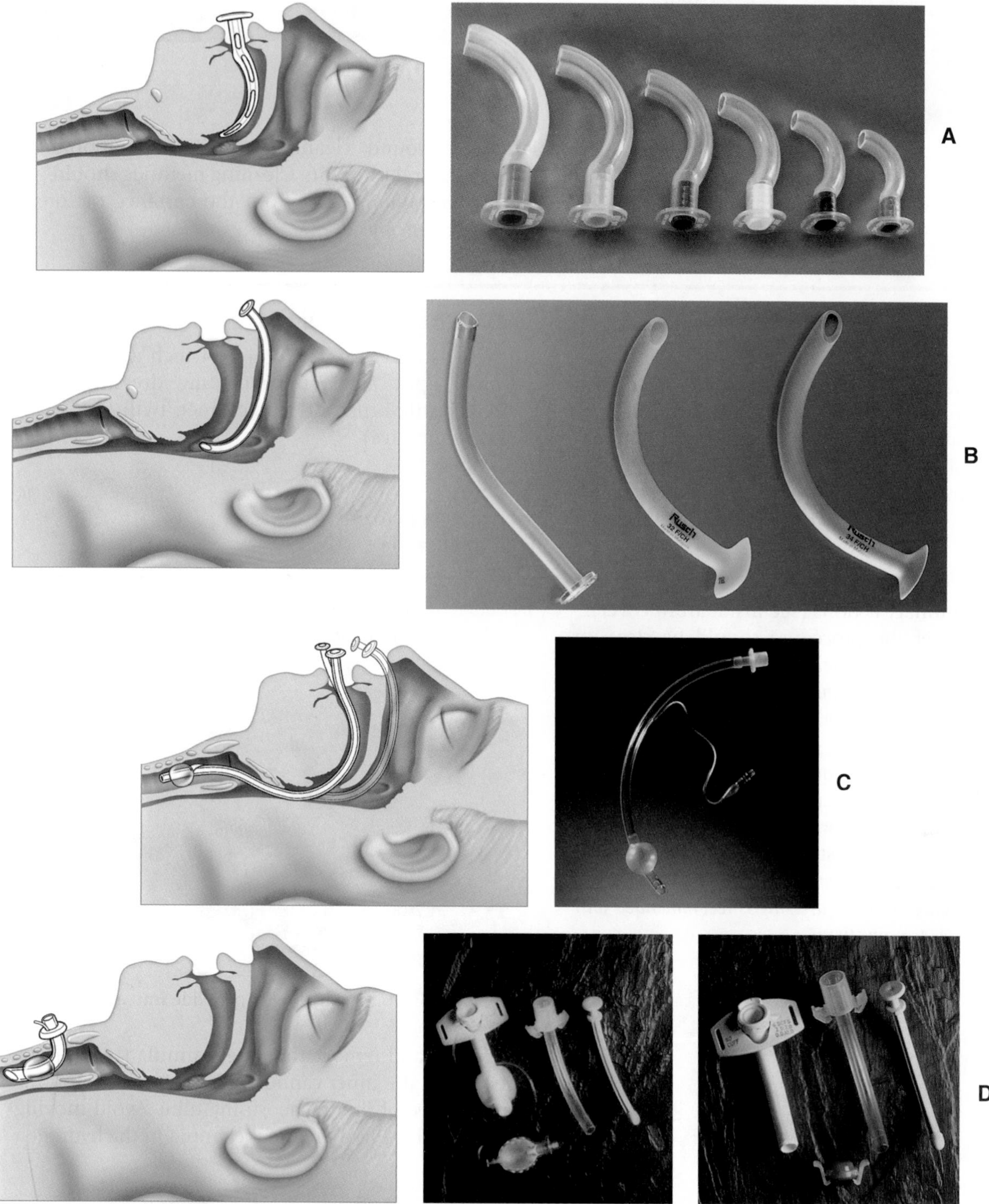

FIGURE 34-12 Types of airways. **A,** Oropharyngeal airway. **B,** Nasal trumpet airway. **C,** Endotracheal airway. **D,** Tracheostomy tube (*left,* cuffed; *center,* cuffed; *right,* uncuffed). (**A** and **B** photos courtesy Rusch, Inc., Duluth, GA; **C** photo courtesy Mallinckrodt, Inc., St. Louis, MO; **D** photo courtesy Mallinckrodt, Inc./Shiley Tracheostomy Products, St. Louis, MO.)

The nursing diagnosis of *Impaired verbal communication* is pertinent because the client with a tracheostomy cannot speak unless equipped with a special tracheostomy tube that is designed to allow speech. These tubes have a one-way valve that closes with exhalation and directs the air across the larynx. The Communitrach is another type of tracheostomy tube with an airflow tube that allows the air to be directed over the larynx when the tracheostomy is covered, thus allowing speech.

For a small group of clients, a tracheostomy becomes permanent. The home health care nurse manages clients with long-term or permanent tracheostomies. Much of the care focuses on teaching the family or other caregiver to manage the client's care and to be prepared to manage

TIME TO ALLOW: NOVICE: 20 min. EXPERT: 10 min.

PROCEDURE 34-3

CLEANING A TRACHEOSTOMY

Nursing Skills Online: Infection Control, Lesson 8

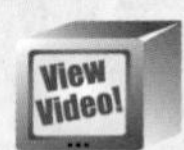

A tracheostomy is an artificial opening into the trachea that bypasses the normal defense mechanisms of the upper respiratory tract. Therefore cleaning the surrounding skin protects the lower respiratory tract from the entrance of bacteria. In addition, when the tracheostomy is a fresh wound, cleaning is especially important to prevent wound infection. Cleaning methods should protect the respiratory tract from the entrance of foreign substances or objects.

DELEGATION GUIDELINES

Care of a new tracheostomy is not generally delegated to a nursing assistant because of the risks associated with inconsistent or improper technique. New tracheostomies are generally present in acute and critically ill clients. However, for clients with long-term, stable tracheostomies, you may be able to delegate tracheostomy care to a nursing assistant who has received appropriate training.

EQUIPMENT NEEDED

- Tracheostomy care kit (*or* 4 × 4 inch gauze, cotton-tipped applicators, tracheostomy dressing, basin, small bottle brush or pipe cleaner, twill tape or tracheostomy ties)
- Scissors
- Gloves
- Hydrogen peroxide
- Normal saline

1 Follow preliminary actions (see inside front cover).

2 Decide whether the procedure should be clean or sterile (supplies should be clean or sterile, depending on this decision). *When the wound is less than 48 hours old or if the client is at high risk for respiratory infection, sterile technique is recommended.*

3 Gather the appropriate equipment.

4 Prepare the client for the procedure. Suction the tracheostomy, or have the client cough. Remove any dressing that is present (see illustration). *You can use sterile gloves to suction the tracheostomy and then remove the dressing without changing gloves. A dressing is recommended only if irritated skin needs protection.*

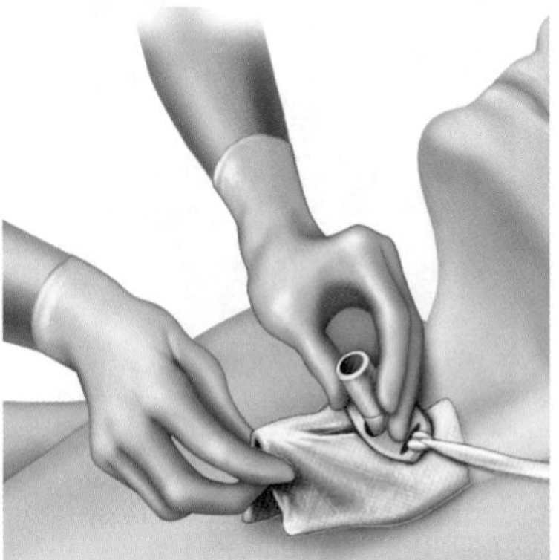

Step 4. Removing the tracheostomy dressing.

5 Select a clear area to set up the equipment, within reach of the client's tracheostomy. Set up a sterile field; the outer wrapper of the kit forms the sterile field. Don sterile gloves. Pour hydrogen peroxide into one basin and normal saline into the other (see illustration). *If the client is on a ventilator, you will need to work quickly: immediately replace the inner cannula because it is needed to attach to the ventilator.*

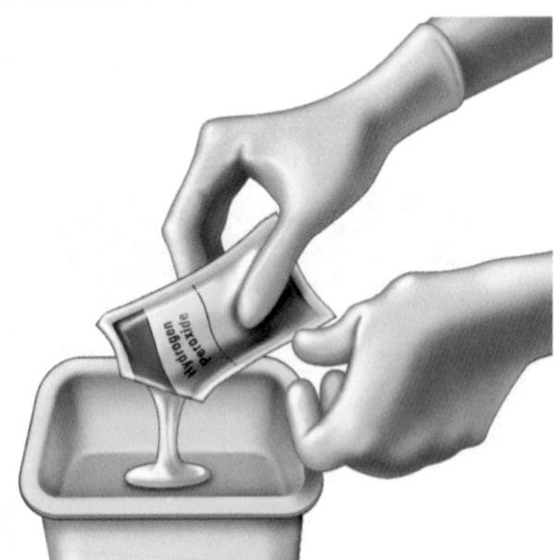

Step 5. Pouring hydrogen peroxide into a basin.

6 Unlock and remove the inner cannula (see illustration). Twist the inner cannula, and pull it out, following the curve of the tracheostomy tube. Avoid moving the outer tube. Place the inner cannula in the hydrogen peroxide.

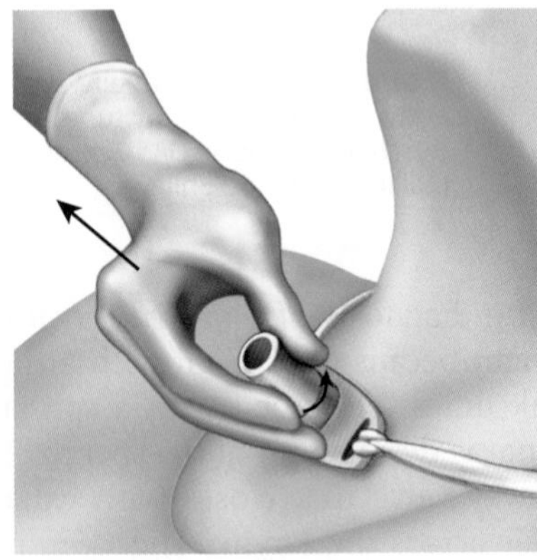

Step 6. Removing the inner cannula.

7 Clean the inner cannula inside and out with a brush or pipe cleaner (see illustration). Frequent cleaning with normal saline prevents accumulation of encrusted secretions that require more vigorous cleaning. Rinse the cannula in normal saline. Replace and lock the inner cannula. *Rinsing in normal saline prevents hydrogen peroxide from entering the tracheostomy.*

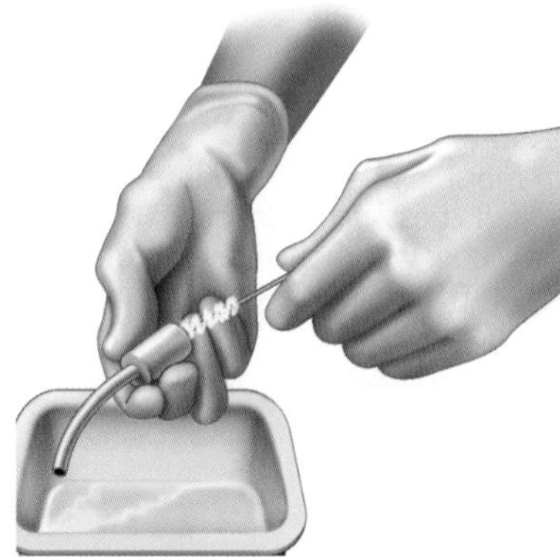

Step 7. Cleaning the inner cannula with a brush.

8 Clean the tracheostomy site (see illustration). Use normal saline to clean the skin, and hydrogen peroxide to clean the external tube. Use gentle pats or strokes. Use either gauze or cotton-tipped applicators, depending on the amount of secretions. *Avoid irritating the wound. The cotton-tipped applicators can be dipped in hydrogen peroxide to clean small crevices of the tracheostomy tube. Absolutely do not get hydrogen peroxide into the trachea, because it will be irritating and will damage the tissue.*

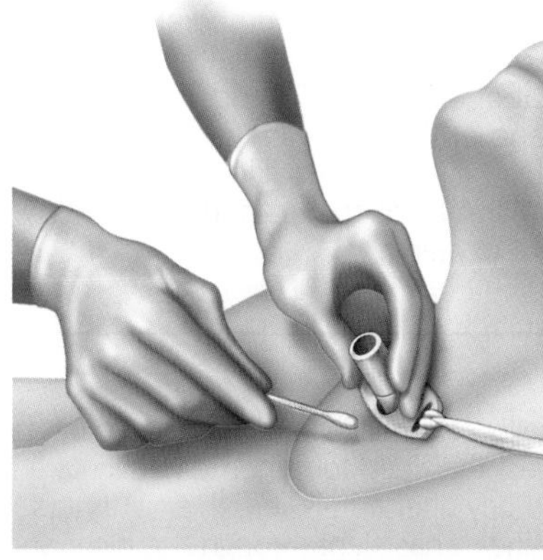

Step 8. Cleaning the tracheostomy site.

9 Change the tracheostomy ties, and apply a dressing, if necessary (see illustration). When the tracheostomy ties are removed, the tube can easily be dislodged, and the airway will quickly close. Use a helper to hold the tracheostomy tube while you remove and replace the ties. The ties should be tight enough that only one finger can be slipped under the tie. *This technique prevents the tracheostomy tube from being dislodged.*

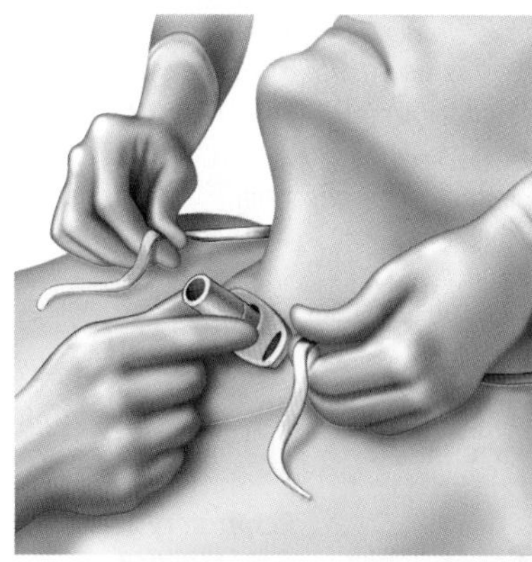

Step 9. Changing the tracheostomy ties with the help of an assistant.

10 Evaluate the results of the procedure. Is the skin clean, dry, and free of inflammation? Is the tube clean and dry? Is the client comfortable?

HINTS

Avoid moving the tracheostomy tube to prevent discomfort to the client and irritation to the trachea. Having an assistant helps the procedure go smoothly. The assistant helps with preoxygenation and holding the tracheostomy tube in place while the ties are changed. Gauze should not be cut to use for a tracheostomy dressing. Frayed, loose ends could enter the tracheostomy. When tying the tube to secure it in the opening, one tie should be longer than the other. Tie the knot to the side of the neck to prevent the client from lying on the knot. Pad the knot, if needed, to prevent pressure. Tracheostomy care is done as often as needed to maintain a clean, dry area. In the hospital, the frequency is usually once a shift. In the home, daily care may be sufficient. Ties are changed daily or more frequently if wet or soiled.

BOX 34-15

Nursing Care Plan

A Client With Pneumonia

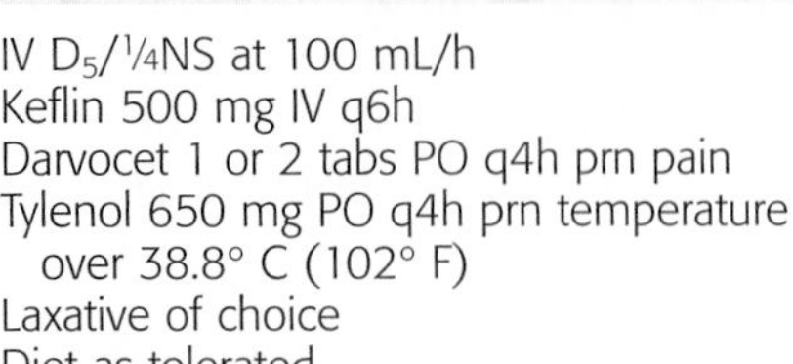

Admission Data

Mrs. Wilheim is admitted through the emergency department to a general medical nursing unit. The emergency department nurse phones the following report: *"Mrs. Wilheim is an 68-year-old German American woman in respiratory distress. We have started oxygen and taken a chest x-ray. Looks as though she has pneumonia. Her oxygen saturation was 85% before we started the oxygen at 4 LPM by face mask. If she is doing all right, she can try a nasal cannula. The saturation is up to 95%, but you will probably need to monitor her. Dr. Anderson is coming up to write orders."*

Physician's Orders

Admitting diagnosis: pneumonia
Oxygen per NC @4L PM
Pulse oximetry
Sputum for culture and sensitivity
IV D_5/¼NS at 100 mL/h
Keflin 500 mg IV q6h
Darvocet 1 or 2 tabs PO q4h prn pain
Tylenol 650 mg PO q4h prn temperature over 38.8° C (102° F)
Laxative of choice
Diet as tolerated
Bed rest with BRP as tolerated

Nursing Assessment

Color pale, skin moist, oxygen saturation 93%, complains of pain in lower left chest with inspiration, diminished breath sounds left lower lobe, wet rhonchi over bronchi, temperature 38.3° C (101° F), pulse 100, respiration 30, BP 118/70. Reports no appetite, appears frightened, moving from wheelchair to bed results in dyspnea.

NANDA-I Nursing Diagnosis	NOC Expected Outcomes With Indicators	NIC Interventions With Selected Activities	Evaluation Data
Impaired Gas Exchange	***Respiratory Status: Gas Exchange***	***Oxygen Therapy***	
Related Factor: • Excess secretions, weakness, and pain secondary to pneumonia	• Mental status in expected range • Ease of breathing • Dyspnea at rest not present • Cyanosis not present • Somnolence not present • O_2 saturation WNL • Chest x-ray findings in expected range	• Clear oral, nasal, and tracheal secretions as appropriate. • Set up oxygen equipment and administer through a heated, humidified system. • Administer supplemental oxygen 4 L per NC. • Monitor the oxygen liter flow. • Monitor position of oxygen delivery device. • Instruct client about the importance of leaving the oxygen device on. • Ensure replacement of oxygen mask/cannula whenever the device is removed. • Monitor for signs of skin breakdown, anxiety about oxygen therapy.	• Diminished breath sounds over left lower lobe; rhonchi diminishing, clear with coughing. • Cough nonproductive and tiring, antitussive given. • Oxygen saturation 97% on continuous 4 L per NC. • Sat in chair 20 minutes; respiration 16, P 88, BP 130/90. • Temperature 99.6° F. • Client states she understands importance of wearing oxgen device. • Skin intact under oxygen cannula.

Critical Thinking Questions

1. Because Mrs. Wilheim lived alone and she was hesitant to call for help, her treatment was delayed. Her daughter asks if you think she needs to move to a protected living situation. How would you respond to the daughter?
2. When Mrs. Wilheim is almost ready for discharge, the nurse begins preparing the discharge teaching plan. What criteria should be used to determine whether Mrs. Wilheim is ready for discharge? What information should be included in the teaching plan? Consider activity restrictions, knowledge of signs and symptoms, diet, medications, and follow-up health care. What possible factors would suggest the need for a home health care referral?
3. On the third day after admission, the night nurse reports that Mrs. Wilheim has slept through the night and that her vital signs are stable. While conducting the morning assessment, you find that Mrs. Wilheim's vital signs are T 37.8° C (100° F), R 30 and shallow, P 100, BP 108/68. Her skin is pale, cold, and clammy. She has diminished breath sounds and bilateral rales. What action would you take? What additional data would you collect?

Nursing outcome and intervention labels from Johnson, M., Bulechek, G., Butcher, H., Dochterman, J. M., Maas, M., Moorhead, S., et al. (Eds.). (2006). *NANDA, NOC, and NIC linkages: Nursing diagnoses, outcomes, & interventions.* St. Louis, MO: Mosby.

emergencies, should any arise. It is also important to plan for assisting the client and family to maintain the quality of life while living with a chronic illness that easily becomes the focus of all the activities in the home.

EVALUATION

Evaluation of the achievement of health outcomes involves reassessing the client to determine that the criteria for evaluation have been met.

If the outcomes are not achieved or the client is not improving within the expected time, reassessment may reveal a reasonable explanation for the lack of progress. For example, a postsurgical client who continues to have fever on the fourth postoperative day, but whose postoperative crackles have cleared, should be assessed for other causes of the fever.

Process evaluation helps connect the outcomes to the nursing care. Connecting outcomes to the interventions requires examining all the process elements that could affect the outcomes. For example, if a client had a physician's order for an incentive spirometer but used it only the two times you actually stayed in the room to provide support, then the outcome of breath sounds throughout the lung fields cannot be attributed to the incentive spirometer. Box 34-15 is an example of the application of the nursing process to Mrs. Wilheim.

The nursing note for Mrs. Wilheim when she is ready for discharge after treatment for respiratory infection might look like the note below:

SAMPLE DOCUMENTATION NOTE FOR MRS. WILHEIM

Lungs clear to auscultation. Breath sounds throughout. Temperature 37° C (98.6° F), P 66, R 14, BP 124/84. No cough. Has verbalized instructions to continue antibiotics at home until the prescription has been completely taken. Will report signs and symptoms of recurrent infection to the physician. Is able to ambulate the length of the hall. Daughter will assist with eating a balanced diet. Home health care nurse will follow up and work with daughter to determine need for protected living.

Notice in this example that the nurse has documented that the respiratory problem has resolved and that she worked with the client to establish new goals. The goals are to maintain health during recovery and to report recurring signs and symptoms.

The nurse helps the client establish new goals through statements such as, "Now that your lungs are clearing, we need to concentrate on being more active and think about going home from the hospital."

▼ KEY PRINCIPLES

- Factors affecting respiration, including smoking, environmental exposure, age, and cardiovascular disease, suggest the need for more intensive monitoring for respiratory complications.
- The nurse does not order diagnostic tests but does use the results in diagnosing nursing problems.
- *Ineffective breathing patterns* are generally hypoventilation, hyperventilation, or dyspnea. A high-priority goal of care is to prevent hypoxemia.
- *Ineffective airway clearance* results from failure of the normal respiratory defense mechanisms or is secondary to hypoventilation. The presence of coarse crackles or rhonchi is sufficient to diagnose *Ineffective airway clearance.*
- *Impaired gas exchange* can be the result of *Ineffective breathing pattern* or *Ineffective airway clearance* or can result from poor perfusion or damage to the alveolar membrane.
- Definitive evidence of *Impaired gas exchange* is abnormal arterial blood gas levels, but the diagnosis can be inferred from signs of hypoxemia.
- Assessment for nursing diagnoses related to respiratory diagnoses includes assessment of all the functional patterns for emotional responses, such as anxiety and hopelessness, as well as for physiological problems, such as fluid volume deficit.
- Because the nursing diagnosis is chosen on the basis of the goal of nursing care, respiratory diagnoses are more commonly used in the acute care setting where the care is associated with physician-initiated interventions aimed directly at managing the respiratory status.
- The outcomes for respiratory diagnoses are a normal breathing pattern, clear lung fields, and normal arterial oxygen and carbon dioxide levels or evidence that the client is making a behavioral change that is expected to improve the respiratory status.
- Interventions to change the pattern of breathing would meet the goals of maximum respiratory function, stimulating respiration, decreasing airway resistance, improving the efficiency of respiration, reducing anxiety, and managing energy requirements.
- Interventions to treat *Ineffective airway clearance* would meet the goals of liquefying and mobilizing secretions and reducing the production of sputum.
- Interventions for *Impaired gas exchange* would meet the goals of compensating for *Impaired gas exchange,* maintaining a patent airway, and providing ventilatory support.
- Evaluation of outcomes for respiratory nursing diagnoses includes evidence that the respiratory status has improved and that the client has a commitment to changing behaviors to prevent future problems.

■ REVIEW QUESTIONS

1. Your client has severe pneumonia. Her blood pressure (BP) has dropped to 100/80 mm Hg, and her pulse rate is 100 beats per minute. Select all the assessment data that should be gathered on this client.

1. Listen for S_1 and S_2 heart sounds.
2. Assess for hypoventilation.
3. Assess pain level.
4. Listen for a pleural friction rub.
5. Assess bowel sounds.
6. Assess for orientation to time, place, and person.
7. Assess pedal pulses.

Continued

2. Your client has a history of asthma. You hear wheezes in his chest, and he complains of dyspnea. Which physiological process is occurring in his lungs?
1. Increased airway resistance
2. Diminished blood flow to the alveoli
3. Limited diffusion across the alveolar membrane
4. Relaxation of the bronchioles

3. Which body position allows optimal or maximal ventilation?
1. Lying in the semi-Fowler's position
2. Standing erect
3. Lying in a semiprone position
4. Sitting in a high-back reclining chair

4. Which of the following is appropriately labeled dyspnea?
1. Rapid, shallow respirations
2. Pursed-lip breathing
3. Complaint of difficulty breathing
4. Using accessory muscles of respiration

5. An RN has just admitted a client from the surgical recovery area. The client was fully awake with BP of 120/80 mm Hg, pulse 80 beats per minute, and respiration 20 breaths per minute on admission. You assign a student nurse to take her vital signs every 15 minutes. An hour later, the student tells you the client is sleeping, BP 100/80 mm Hg, pulse 100 beats per minute, and respiration 28 breaths per minute. You ask the student if she used the pulse oximeter. She says no, because the client does not have cyanosis. What mistake has the student made?
1 She probably does not know how to take a blood pressure correctly.
2. She does not understand what the pulse oximeter measures.
3. She does not understand that cyanosis is a late sign of hypoxemia.
4. No mistake, she should let the client sleep.

6. Your client is restless, has central cyanosis, BP 90/60 mm Hg, and a rapid pulse rate. His pulse oximeter reading is 85%. When you speak to him, he moans, but he does not seem to have the energy to speak. He is breathing through his mouth. The respiratory therapist starts oxygen at 8 LPM with a simple face mask. The daughter asks if he has to have the mask rather than a nasal cannula. Your best response is:
1. The face mask will give him more oxygen and should be used until his condition improves.
2. A face mask is routinely used when a client cannot speak.
3. A nasal cannula cannot be used when a client is breathing through his mouth.
4. The face mask keeps him from breathing room air.

Bibliography

*Ackerman, M. (1993). The effect of saline lavage prior to suctioning. *American Journal of Critical Care, 2*(4), 326-330.

Advice, P.R.N. Pulmonary care: To suction or not? (2003). *Nursing, 33*(2), 12.

Astle, S. M., & Caulfield, E. V. (2003). Bedside tracheostomy: A step by step guide. *RN, 66*(10), 41-46.

Barnett, M. (2005). Tracheostomy management and care. *Journal of Community Nursing, 19*(1), 4, 6-8.

Bennion, K. (2004). AARC clinical practice guideline: Nasotracheal suctioning—2004 revision & update. *Respiratory Care, 49*(9), 1080-1084.

Carroll, P. (2000). Guest editorial. Should suctioning be left to the nurse? *American Journal of Critical Care, 9*(2), 85-86.

Carroll, P. (2003). Improve your suctioning technique. *RN, 66*(5), 30ac2-6, 30ac8.

Considine, J. (2005). The role of nurses in preventing adverse events related to respiratory dysfunction: Literature review. *Journal of Advanced Nursing, 49*(6), 624-633.

Gibbons, D. (2004). Do you have a role in pulmonary rehabilitation? *Practice Nursing, 15*(12), 602, 604, 606-608.

Guyton, A. C., & Hall, J. E. (2006). *Textbook of medical physiology.* Philadelphia: Saunders.

Higgins, D. (2005). Oxygen therapy. *Nursing Times, 101*(4), 30-31.

Johnson, M., Bulechek, G., Butcher, H., Dochterman, J. M., Maas, M., Moorhead, S., et al. (Eds.). (2006). *NANDA, NOC, and NIC linkages: Nursing diagnoses, outcomes, & interventions.* St. Louis, MO: Mosby.

Koschel, M. J. (2004). Emergency. Pulmonary embolism: Quick diagnosis can save a patient's life. *American Journal of Nursing, 104*(6), 46-50, 57.

Leininger, M. (1991). *Culture care diversity and universality: A theory of nursing.* New York: National League for Nursing Press.

MacDonald, S., Yates, J., Lance, R., Giganti, N., & Chepurko, D. (2005). Are you asking the right admission questions when assessing dyspnea? *Heart & Lung, 34*(4), 260-269.

Marvaki, C., Roupa, Z., Pilatis, N., Polikandrioti, M., Melissa, C., Demertzis, B., et al. (2004). Safety during oxygen therapy. *ICUs and Nursing Web Journal,* (20), 5p. Available at http://www.nursing.gr/toc.html.

National Cancer Institute. (2004). *Cigarette smoking and cancer: Questions and answers.* Retrieved December 4, 2006 from http://www.cancer.gov/cancertopics/factsheet/Tobacco/cancer.

Nicholson, C. (2004). A systematic review of the effectiveness of oxygen in reducing acute myocardial ischaemia. *Journal of Clinical Nursing, 13*(8), 996-1007.

Pruitt, B., & Jacobs, M. (2005). Clearing away pulmonary secretions. *Nursing, 35*(7), 36-42.

Roman, M. (2005). Clinical 'how to': Tracheostomy tubes. *Medsurg Nursing, 14*(2), 143-145.

Rumsey, C. H., & Seaberg, D. C. (2004). When the complaint is dyspnea. *Patient Care for the Nurse Practitioner,* 12p.

Simmons, P., & Simmons, M. (2004). Informed nursing practice: The administration of oxygen to patients with COPD. *Medsurg Nursing, 13*(2), 82-86.

Smith, T. (2004). Continuing professional development. Oxygen therapy for older people. *Nursing Older People, 16*(5), 22-28, [30].

Smyth, M. (2005). Acute respiratory failure: Part 2. Failure of ventilation: Exploring the other cause of acute respiratory failure. *American Journal of Nursing, 105*(6), Critical Care Extra, 72AA-DD.

St. John, R. E., & Malen, J. F. (2004). Contemporary issues in adult tracheostomy management. *Critical Care Nursing Clinics of North America, 16*(3), 413-430.

Tubongbanua, N. (2005). Understanding pulse oximetry helps effective assessment. *Nursing Times, 101*(7), 37.

Vollman, K. M. (2004). Prone positioning in the patient who has acute respiratory distress syndrome: The art and science. *Critical Care Nursing Clinics of North America, 16*(3), 319-336.

*Asterisk indicates a classic or definitive work on this subject.

Chapter 35

SUPPORTING CARDIOVASCULAR FUNCTION

Media Resources

- Nursing Skills Online
- evolve Evolve Website http://evolve.elsevier.com/Harkreader/
- 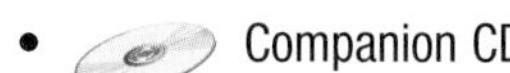 Companion CD

Learning Objectives

After studying this chapter, you will be able to do the following:

- Describe the anatomical and physiological concepts underlying the three tissue perfusion diagnoses
- Discuss some common problems of cardiovascular function
- Identify the life span, physiological, and cultural/ lifestyle factors affecting tissue perfusion and cardiac function
- Assess the client at risk for problems of tissue perfusion or cardiac function, detect the manifestations of an actual problem, and recognize the client's responses to problems
- Differentiate among nursing diagnoses used for clients with cardiovascular problems
- Plan for goal-directed interventions to prevent or correct problems of tissue perfusion and cardiac function
- Evaluate the outcomes of nursing care to promote cardiac function and tissue perfusion

Key Terms

afterload
antidiuretic hormone (ADH)
atherosclerosis
baroreceptors
bradycardia
cardiac output
claudication
diastole
dysrhythmia
edema
inotropic agent
ischemia
necrosis
preload
stroke volume
systole
tachycardia
viscosity

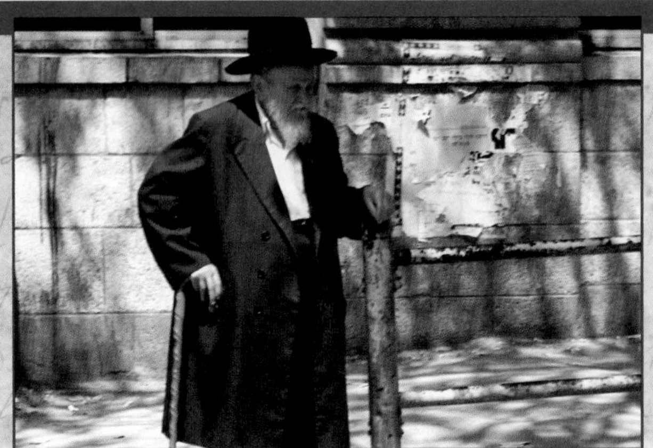

© 2007, JupiterImages Corporation.

Mr. John Yoder, a 74-year-old Amish carpenter, experienced chest pain and light-headedness while moving lumber in his workshop. A neighbor brought Mr. Yoder and his family to the hospital. Mr. Yoder is admitted to the hospital's coronary step-down unit for observation. His wife and son accompany him. The admitting diagnosis is angina pectoris with a possible myocardial infarction.

The initial nursing assessment reveals a moderately anxious man who is currently experiencing chest pain (7 on a 0 to 10 pain scale) that radiates to his left arm. Skin is pale. Vital signs: blood pressure, 150/92 mm Hg; apical pulse, regular 94 beats per minute; respirations, 24 breaths per minute. Admitting orders include bed rest, nitroglycerin for chest pain, cardiac monitor, and a cardiac catheterization in the morning.

After making Mr. Yoder comfortable, the nurse initiates the nursing care plan for this client. On the basis of Mr. Yoder's presenting signs and symptoms, the nurse identifies *Ineffective cardiac tissue perfusion* from the nursing diagnoses for cardiovascular function. Because *Ineffective cardiac tissue perfusion* can adversely affect the function of the heart muscle, the nurse also assesses for *Decreased cardiac output*.

KEY NURSING DIAGNOSES FOR CARDIOVASCULAR FUNCTION

Ineffective tissue perfusion (specify type: renal, cerebral, cardiopulmonary, gastrointestinal, peripheral): A decrease in oxygen resulting in failure to nourish tissues at the cellular level

Decreased cardiac output: Inadequate blood pumped by the heart to meet the metabolic demands of the body

Risk for peripheral neurovascular dysfunction: At risk for a disruption in circulation, sensation, or motion of an extremity

***Shock:** An abnormal condition of inadequate blood flow to the body's tissues, resulting from circulatory collapse; followed by life-threatening cellular dysfunction; associated with decreased cardiac output, hemorrhage, other forms of fluid loss

*Not a NANDA International (NANDA-I)–approved diagnosis.

CONCEPTS OF TISSUE PERFUSION AND CARDIAC FUNCTION

Cardiovascular disease accounted for 39.3% of deaths in the United States and was the leading cause of death in 2003 (American Heart Association [AHA], 2006). In addition, costs of cardiovascular disease can be measured in lost productivity and cost of care. Because of the high incidence of cardiovascular disease, nurses regularly care for clients with problems of tissue perfusion or impaired cardiac function—or who are at risk for these problems.

The need for oxygen and nutrients is met by the cardiovascular system. The heart pumps blood, and the interconnected blood vessels carry it to all parts of the body to deliver oxygen and nutrients while removing the waste products of metabolism. Changes in tissue perfusion range from acute, life-threatening problems, such as heart attacks, to chronic conditions that adversely affect quality of life.

Although all cells require oxygen, demands for oxygen vary among different body tissues. Varying oxygen needs, as well as the degree to which tissue perfusion is impaired, determine the specific interventions indicated for individual clients. Diminished tissue perfusion alters the function of the affected organ or body system. An interrupted blood supply produces tissue **ischemia** (a decreased supply of oxygenated blood to tissues) and **necrosis** (localized death of tissues caused by disease, oxygen deficit, or injury).

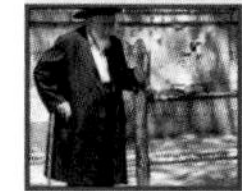

Mr. Yoder's history and symptoms suggest he has diminished circulation to his coronary muscle that is sufficient to cause chest pain. The cardiac catheterization will identify if there is narrowing of his coronary vessels.

Medical intervention is required to correct circulatory problems, and the collaborative role of the nurse in the care of clients with these problems is crucial. Continuous assessment and monitoring allow early detection of potential complications in clients at risk. Early detection and prompt intervention can save a life and prevent disability.

Most cardiovascular problems can be described by three nursing diagnoses: *Ineffective tissue perfusion, Decreased cardiac output,* and, in certain circumstances, *Risk for peripheral neurovascular dysfunction.* Remember that decreased circulation impacts multiple body systems. When caring for clients with circulatory problems, you will need to assess mental, respiratory, gastrointestinal, and renal status in addition to data about circulatory function.

THE CARDIOVASCULAR SYSTEM

A functioning heart to pump the blood and patent systemic blood vessels to transport blood are essential to perfusion of blood to the body's tissues.

Heart. The heart is a muscular organ that acts as a pump to create the pressure that causes the blood to flow throughout the vascular system. It consists of four chambers: two atria and two ventricles. The thin-walled atria contract simultaneously to fill the ventricles. Then the heavily muscled ventricles contract to propel blood to the lungs and the systemic circulation. The right atrium and ventricle transport blood to the lungs. The left atrium and ventricle pump blood to the rest of the body. Figure 35-1 depicts the internal anatomy of the heart.

Blood flow through the heart results from a combination of a pressure gradient, contractions of the heart muscle, and a system of valves (Figure 35-2). Blood flows passively from the vena cava into the right atrium and then the right ventricle because of a pressure gradient across the vena cava, atrium, and ventricle. Then contraction of the right atrium increases atrial pressure and forces additional blood to fill the right ventricle. When the right ventricle contracts, the pressure becomes great enough to exert pressure to close the tricuspid valve; the pulmonic valve opens, allowing blood to flow through the pulmonary artery to the lungs.

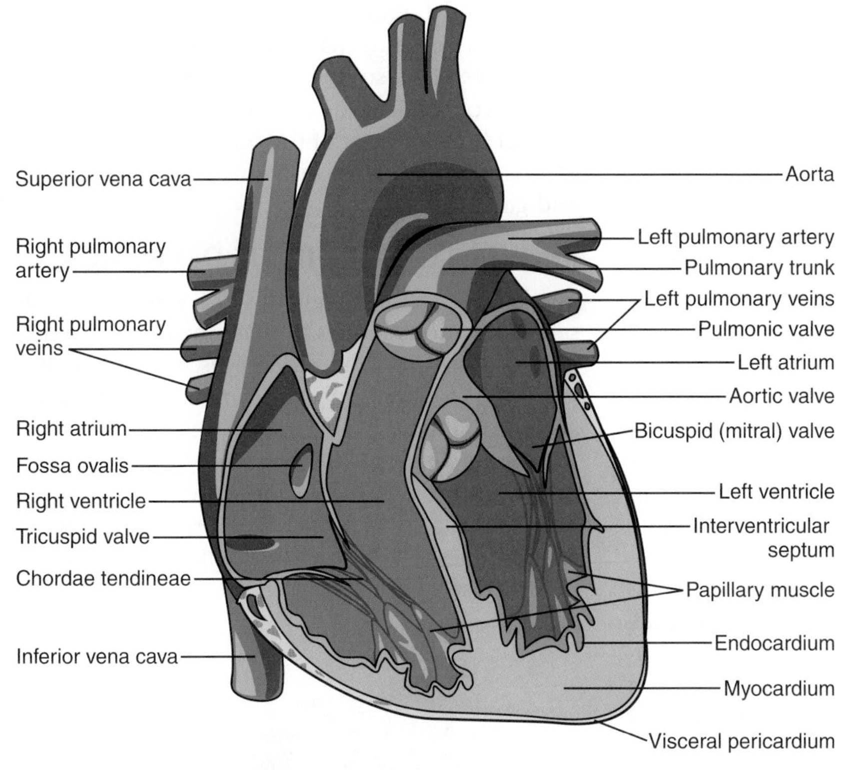

FIGURE 35-1 Internal anatomy of the heart.

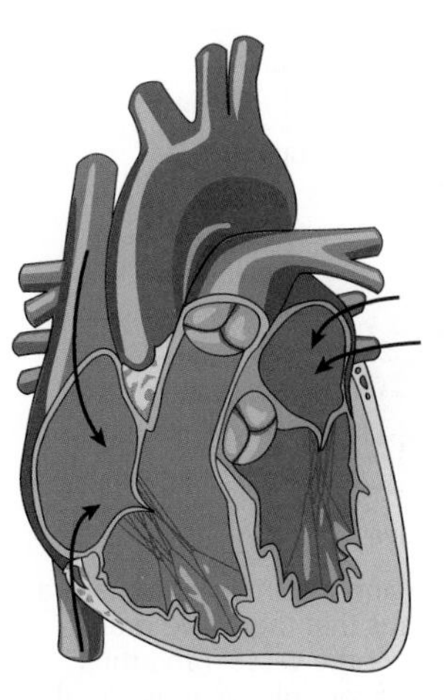

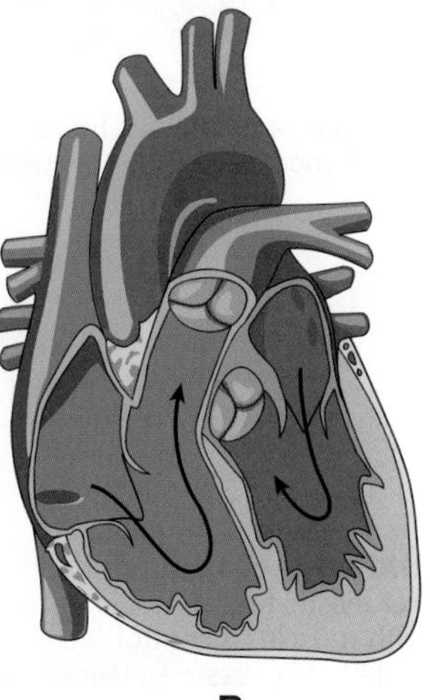

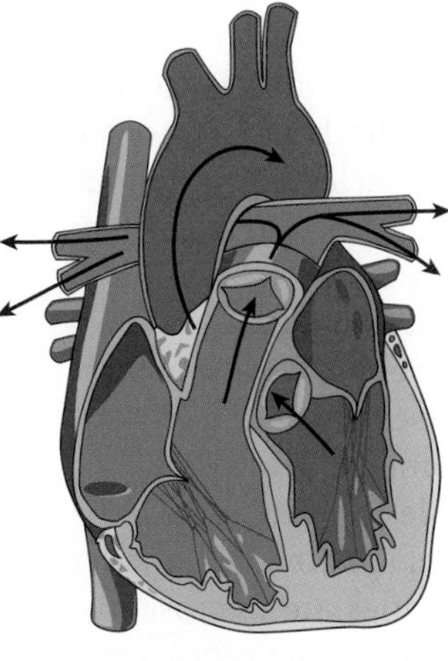

FIGURE 35-2 Dynamics of blood flow through the heart. **A,** During diastole, blood enters the right atrium from the venae cavae and the left atrium and from the pulmonary artery. **B,** At the end of diastole, the atria contract (called atrial systole). **C,** During systole, ventricular contraction propels blood into the lungs and aorta.

From the lungs, blood flows through the pulmonary veins to the left atrium. When the left atrial pressure is higher than left ventricular pressure, the mitral valve opens and blood flows passively into the left ventricle; atrial contraction completes ventricular filling. Contraction of the left ventricle increases pressure in the ventricle, closes the mitral valve, and opens the aortic valve. Because of the thick, strong, muscular wall of the left ventricle, blood entering the aorta is under high pressure.

The time from the beginning of one ventricular contraction to the beginning of the next ventricular contraction is called the cardiac cycle (see Figure 8-35). Because the ventricles perform the work of pumping blood out of the heart, the events of the cardiac cycle are identified in relation to the contraction and relaxation of the ventricles. **Systole** refers to the contraction of the ventricles, and **diastole** refers to the relaxation of the ventricles.

Blood Vessels. Beginning and ending at the heart, the *systemic circulation* consists of a vascular network composed of three types of vessels: arteries (including arterioles) carry oxygenated blood away from the heart; microscopic capillaries allow the exchange between the blood and tissues; and veins (including venules) transport oxygen-depleted blood back to the heart. Blood flow within the circulatory system is dependent on the anatomical characteristics of each of the vessels (Figure 35-3).

Arteries. Arteries carry blood away from the heart. These blood vessels are exposed to fluctuating pressures from the force of heart contractions. A thick middle layer of muscle and elastic tissue in the arteries, called the *tunica media,* enables arteries to expand and contract to regulate the diameter of vessels and thus, the pressure within the vessels.

Veins. In contrast to arteries, the thin-walled veins return blood to the heart in a relatively passive manner. Because of a relatively thin tunica media and large lumen, veins can distend to accommodate a large amount of blood. In fact, up to 64% of the total blood supply of the body can be held within the venous system (Guyton & Hall, 2006). The *tunica adventitia,* or outer layer of the wall of veins, is composed of a thick layer of collagen tissue that provides protection and support.

The walls of veins have little smooth muscle to contract and to propel blood back to the heart. However, contraction of leg and abdominal muscles assists venous blood return. One-way valves inside the veins prevent the backward flow of blood in the venous system. When those valves function ineffectively, the muscles are inactive, or in the presence of varicose veins, blood can stagnates in the venous system. Varicose veins are torturous dilated veins with or without incompetent valves.

Capillaries. Blood leaves the left ventricle via the aorta and travels through a series of smaller and smaller arteries to tissue capillaries. Capillaries are microscopic vessels connecting the arterial system to the venous system and allowing the exchange of nutrients and wastes between the blood and the tissues. This exchange is possible because the thin walls of the capillaries, the smallest vessels of the circulatory system, consist of a single layer of epithelial cells. Capillaries range from 4 to 9 μm in diameter, a size similar to the diameter of a single red blood cell (Guyton & Hall, 2006). The small diameter of capillaries and the proximity of blood cells to the porous epithelium facilitate the exchange of substances between the blood and the tissues. Figure 35-4 shows a schematic view of the systemic circulation.

Blood Components. All cellular components develop from mother cells, known as stem cells, which subsequently differentiate, or specialize, into red cells, white cells, and platelets. Red blood cells transport oxygen to tissues as oxyhemoglobin, a molecule that forms when oxygen and hemoglobin combine. White blood cells fight infection and maintain the body's immune function. Platelets, also known as thrombocytes, are essential for coagulation or clotting of the blood. Plasma is the fluid component of the blood; it carries the cellular elements, electrolytes, protein, glucose, fats, bilirubin, and gases.

REGULATION OF TISSUE PERFUSION

The body precisely regulates the amount of blood it sends to various tissues to meet metabolic needs. Blood flow is determined by differences in pressure and resistance to flow. Resistance is a function of blood viscosity and the diameter of the vessels.

Pressure Gradient. Blood flows from areas of higher pressure to areas of lower pressure. Contractions of the heart produce a high systolic pressure. As blood flows from arteries to arterioles to capillaries to veins, pressure in the vessels decreases until it approaches zero when it

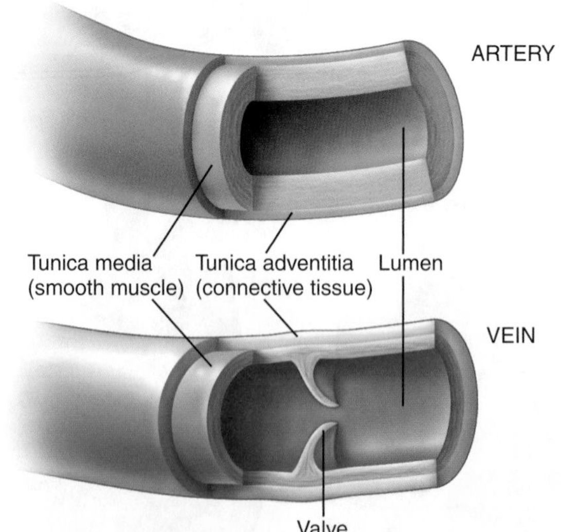

FIGURE 35-3 Comparison of an artery and a vein. Arteries have a thicker elastic tunica media, which means that they have more smooth muscle to control the diameter of the vessel (and thus control blood pressure). Veins are very distensible. Venous blood flow relies on one-way valves and the action of skeletal muscle.

reaches the right atrium. Figure 35-4 illustrates the changes in pressure across the vascular system.

Viscosity of Blood. **Viscosity** is the relative ability of a fluid to flow measured as its resistance to flow. As the viscosity of blood increases, the flow of blood slows. Viscosity is primarily determined by the hematocrit (percentage of red blood cells). Viscosity is also affected by the concentration of protein in the plasma and the tendency of red blood cells to adhere to each other when blood flow is sluggish, but hematocrit is the major determinant.

Vessel Diameter. The larger the vessel diameter, the less resistance there is to blood flow. Arterial diameter is controlled by smooth muscles in the tunica media, which are under the control of the sympathetic and parasympathetic nervous system.

CONTROL OF BLOOD PRESSURE

Adequate blood pressure is needed to maintain tissue perfusion. An increase in blood pressure causes blood to circulate more rapidly, whereas a decrease in blood pressure slows blood flow and decreases tissue perfusion.

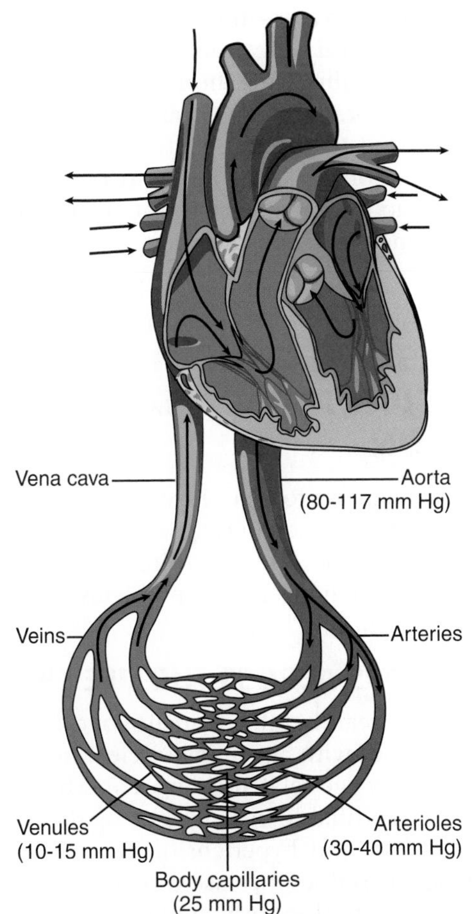

FIGURE 35-4 The systemic circulation. Oxygenated blood exits the left ventricle via the aorta. Exchange of oxygen and carbon dioxide occurs in the systemic tissue capillaries. Veins return deoxygenated blood to the right atrium.

Pressure receptors, the autonomic nervous system, and hormones play important roles in controlling blood flow and blood pressure.

Pressure Receptors. **Baroreceptors** are specialized cells located in the aorta, the carotid, and other large systemic arteries to detect pressure changes in the vascular system. Higher pressure stretches the walls of the arteries, triggering stretch. Low-pressure receptors in the right atrium and the pulmonary artery minimize arterial pressure changes in response to changes in blood volume. Both types of receptors send messages to the central nervous system, which activates the autonomic nervous system to adjust the circulation to changes in pressure and thus maintain a constant flow of blood and a stable blood pressure.

Autonomic Nervous System. The autonomic, or involuntary, nervous system is composed of opposing branches—sympathetic and parasympathetic. Stimulation of the sympathetic branch (adrenergic response) increases the heart rate, strength of myocardial contraction, and constricts peripheral vessels. Stimulation of the parasympathetic branch (cholinergic response) decreases the heart rate and strength of contraction and has no effect on peripheral vessels.

Hormonal Controls. The hormones epinephrine (adrenaline), norepinephrine, and acetylcholine are secreted by the endocrine system for longer cardiovascular control than is achieved by the sympathetic and parasympathetic neurotransmitters—adrenaline and acetylcholine. The adrenal medulla releases epinephrine and norepinephrine when the sympathetic nervous system is stimulated. These hormones have the same effect as the sympathetic and parasympathetic nervous system except the effect lasts 5 to 10 times as long (Guyton & Hall, 2006).

Two other hormonal compensatory mechanisms play a role in tissue perfusion but may take a few hours to show significant response. The renin-angiotensin system and aldosterone help keep the volume and pressure in the circulatory system constant (Figure 35-5). When the juxtaglomerular cells of the kidneys detect a drop in blood pressure, the enzyme renin is released. Renin, in turn, facilitates the formation of angiotensin I, which is a weak vasoconstrictor. Angiotensin I is *then* converted to *angiotensin II* by angiotensin-converting enzyme (ACE), which is found mainly in lung capillaries. The resulting powerful vasoconstriction increases blood pressure. In the final step of the cascade, angiotensin stimulates the adrenal cortex to release aldosterone. This hormone stimulates the kidney to retain sodium and water, which increases plasma volume and circulating blood volume. Expansion of circulating blood volume raises blood pressure. When the kidneys detect a rise in blood pressure, renin secretion decreases, and the cascade is no longer activated; therefore blood pressure subsequently decreases.

Vasopressin is a second hormonal compensatory mechanism, also called **antidiuretic hormone (ADH).** ADH is produced by the hypothalamus and is secreted

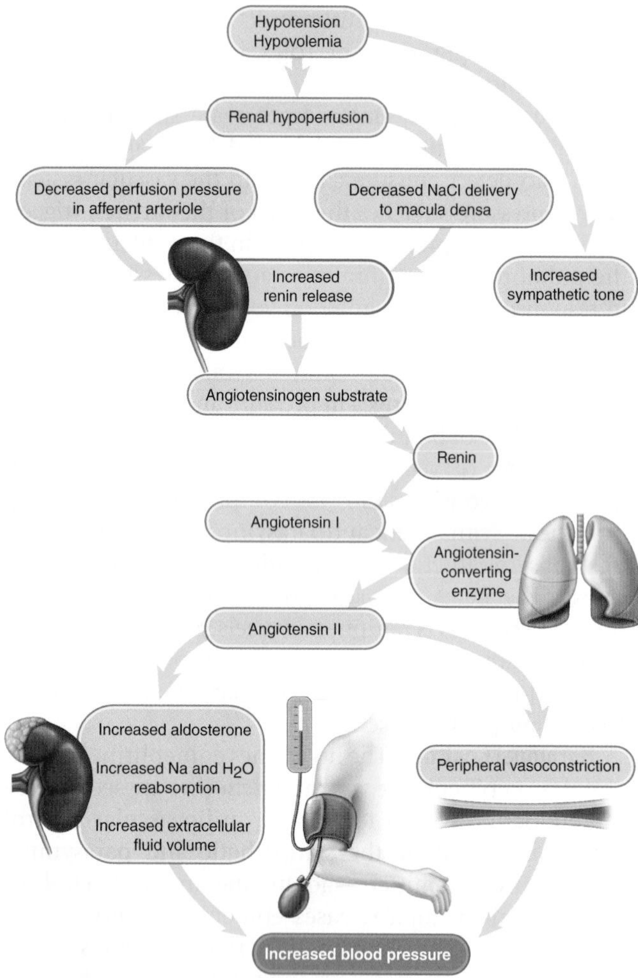

FIGURE 35-5 The renin-angiotensin-aldosterone system, which controls arterial blood pressure. The kidneys play a key role in the control of arterial blood pressure by initiating this chain of reactions in response to decreased renal blood flow.

by the posterior pituitary gland when the sympathetic nervous system is stimulated. It prompts the kidneys to retain water, thereby increasing circulating blood volume and maintaining blood pressure.

REGULATION OF CARDIAC OUTPUT

Cardiac output is the amount of blood pumped by the ventricles in 1 minute. The average cardiac output for an adult is 5 to 6 L/min. Cardiac output is highly variable, however, because it changes to meet metabolic needs. Cardiac output is calculated by using the following equation:

$$\text{Cardiac output} = \text{Stroke volume} \times \text{Heart rate}$$

Stroke Volume. **Stroke volume** is the amount of blood ejected from the heart with each contraction. Normal stroke volume for an adult is about 70 mL. Distensibility (the stretch of the heart's muscle fibers), contractility, and resistance to blood flow affect stroke volume.

Preload, the amount of blood in the left ventricle immediately before contraction, is the main force that stretches cardiac muscle fibers. *Frank-Starling's law* states that the force of contraction of the cardiac muscle is proportional to its length at the beginning of contraction, at least up to the physiological limits to muscle stretching. In other words, the more the muscle is stretched, the stronger the contraction and the greater the cardiac output.

In addition, the strength of the myocardial contraction is affected by epinephrine and norepinephrine, both hormones and sympathetic nervous system neurotransmitters. Chemical imbalances, myocardial ischemia, and parasympathetic stimulation decrease contractility and stroke volume.

Afterload is the final determinant of stroke volume. It is the pressure against which the left ventricle pumps—partly determined by aortic diastolic pressure. Higher aortic pressure forces the heart to work harder, and less blood is ejected from the ventricles with each contraction. Afterload can also be described as the pressure that the chamber of the heart has to generate in order to eject blood out of the chamber.

Heart Rate. There is a direct relationship between heart rate and cardiac output. As heart rate increases, cardiac output increases—up to a point. In very rapid, sustained **tachycardia** (heart rate greater than 100/minute), ventricular filling time shortens, and stroke volume falls. Likewise **bradycardia** (heart rate less than 60/minute) can fail to produce sufficient cardiac output. Just how rapid or how slow the heart rate has to be to reduce cardiac output is dependent on multiple variables including the health and conditioning of the heart muscles.

FACTORS AFFECTING TISSUE PERFUSION AND CARDIAC FUNCTION

The development of problems involving tissue perfusion and cardiovascular function is usually a complex process with multiple factors. Heredity, lifestyle, psychological factors, and underlying health problems all influence circulatory function.

RISK FACTORS ACROSS THE LIFE SPAN

Although it is clear that the incidence of cardiovascular disease increases with age, it is less clear how much of this is primarily age-related changes and how much is related the modifiable risk factors of diet, exercise, smoking, stress, and hypertension. The development of atherosclerosis does increase with age, but it may be preventable by starting early enough in life. However, activity-limiting physical changes associated with aging decrease the aging person's ability to participate in exercise.

Therefore attention has shifted to circulatory risk factors for children and a lifelong prevention. The Bogalusa Heart Study (Hayman, 2004) examined more than 200 children whose parents had coronary artery disease. Children with a positive family history were found to have obesity, hypercholesterolemia, and elevated blood glucose level at younger ages than children without a family history of cardiovascular disease. Because these risk factors correlate with more rapid development of atherosclerosis, the researchers postulate that the overall risk of cardiovascular disease is increased in children with positive family histories.

Although family history is a risk factor that cannot be modified, early interventions with at-risk children may help to slow the atherosclerotic process. Significantly, the particular risk factors detected by this study—namely obesity, hypercholesterolemia, and elevated blood glucose levels—can be modified by weight control and dietary interventions. Researchers continue to follow this population of high-risk children to further evaluate the relationship between age, risk factors, and coronary artery disease.

Certainly, food intake affects the weight, blood glucose, and cholesterol levels of children at all ages. A study involving 55 high schools looked at the types of foods offered in school. Although food served by schools is regulated by federal guidelines and must comply with the Healthy Meals for Americans Act, alternative foods are available to students in vending machines, school stores, and snack bars. Fox, Crepinek, Connor, & Battaglia (2001) reported that the majority of foods sold via alternative sources were high in fat, sugar, and calories. Table 35-1 identifies common foods available in high school stores and vending machines. Healthy options, such as fresh fruit, fruit juices, and pretzels, were less readily available and often more expensive. This study raises interesting questions about food availability and nutritional choices for children.

Table 35-1 Foods Available in High School Stores and Vending Machines

TYPE OF FOOD	PERCENT OF SCHOOLS OFFERING
BEVERAGES	
Juice-based drinks	88
Carbonated drinks	81
Fruit juice	77
Skim or 2% milk	6
SNACKS	
Cheese puffs	54
Chips	54
Pretzels	27
Granola bars	27
Fruit	8
DESSERTS	
Candy bars	60
Cookies	58
Pies	23

PHYSIOLOGICAL FACTORS

Physiological factors also affect circulatory status. In addition to sex and weight, physical circumstances such as pregnancy, health problems, and medications produce circulatory changes.

Sex. Although cardiovascular disease is the leading cause of death in the United States, sex differences create unique risk factors. For example, men are more likely than women to have early heart attacks. Estrogen levels in premenopausal women maintain the elasticity of blood vessels and keep serum cholesterol levels low. However, women have a poorer prognosis for recovery and experience more complications once they develop coronary disease.

Peripheral vascular disease also affects men and women differently. Women have an increased incidence of the peripheral vascular disease *Raynaud's disease,* which involves vasospasms, and men are more likely to have *Buerger's disease,* an occlusive vascular condition.

Weight. Weight control is part of a program for prevention of cardiovascular disease. However, the best choice of diet for weight loss and preventing cardiovascular disease continues to be studied. Box 35-1 illustrates some of the evidence about the most effective diet choice.

Obesity increases the workload on the heart. Excess adipose tissue requires the development of more blood vessels to nourish the tissue. Additional blood vessels lengthen the circulatory network and are associated with hypertension, a condition in which blood pressure is persistently higher than 140/90 mm Hg. Also, the heaviness of adipose tissue resting on blood vessels can compress the vessels.

Pregnancy. The growing fetus and amniotic fluid during pregnancy place considerable pressure on pelvic veins, which flatten easily because of their thin walls. This results in slowed venous return and pooling of blood in the veins of the lower extremities.

Problems of Cardiovascular Function. Cardiovascular dysfunction stems from problems within the heart or blood vessels that can alter tissue perfusion, cardiac output, or peripheral neurovascular function. Diminished heart contractility or blood flow through the chambers of the heart decreases pumping efficiency. Restricted flow through systemic blood vessels lessens perfusion to vital organs.

Disorders of Tissue Perfusion. Patent blood vessels are essential for the delivery of blood to tissues. Conditions that decrease the lumens of blood vessels limit the ability of vessels to carry sufficient blood to meet tissue needs.

Atherosclerosis is a pathological condition in which fat and plaque form deposits on the intimal (inner) surface of the arteries (Figure 35-6). It is the most common disorder that affects the size of blood vessel lumens. These deposits pose a twofold risk to tissue perfusion: they narrow the lumen of the artery, and they break loose, traveling to a distant site where they cause obstruction.

Atherosclerosis particularly targets the heart, brain, kidneys, and peripheral vessels. Diminished function in one or more of the target organs is a consequence of long-standing atherosclerosis.

Disorders of Cardiac Output. Some illnesses and medical treatments put clients at risk for a decrease in cardiac output, which is a way of saying the heart becomes ineffective as a pump. When caring for clients with any of the following conditions, be sure to monitor for a decrease in cardiac output:

- *Angina pectoris* is chest pain resulting from inadequate oxygen supply to the heart muscle, caused by partially occluded coronary arteries.
- *Myocardial infarction* is necrosis of heart muscle resulting from complete occlusion of a coronary artery.
- **Dysrhythmias** are abnormalities of heart rate or rhythm. Dysrhythmias may shorten the time available for the heart to fill with blood. Shortened filling time decreases stroke volume and cardiac output.
- *Bacterial and viral infections* can attack the heart, causing inflammation and scarring of the heart, valves, and pericardial sac. Scarring restricts blood flow through the heart and decreases contractility.
- *Congestive heart failure* is a condition in which the heart has failed as a pump (resulting in a decrease in cardiac output). Swelling of the feet and legs is a prominent symptom of right-sided heart failure. Fluid in the lungs is a prominent symptom of left-sided heart failure.

Peripheral Neurovascular Dysfunction. Conditions that disrupt circulation to an extremity raise the risk of neurovascular damage. Lack of circulation destroys nerves and impairs motor function in the involved extremity. Failure to detect early signs of neurovascular dysfunction can lead to permanent damage. This is a common cause of litigation in the United States.

Examples of situations that can obstruct blood flow include severe tissue edema; excessive pressure on blood vessels from a cast, splint, or tourniquet; clots or occlusions within blood vessels; and trauma to blood vessels, as from invasive procedures involving the vascular system.

CULTURAL AND LIFESTYLE FACTORS

Lifestyle choices are modifiable risk factors for cardiovascular disease. Diet, exercise, and smoking have direct effects on circulation. Some health insurers reward healthy behaviors, such as regular exercise and optimal body weight, with lower insurance premiums. More and more people are experimenting with herbal and other alternative forms of medicine.

BOX 35-1 *Evidence-Based Practice*

Choosing the Best Weight-Loss Diet

Problem: Nurses are always trying to encourage and promote healthy lifestyles. Today, obesity is a major cardiovascular health concern and is one of the causative factors in the development of many chronic health problems. There are many health care professionals and resources such as books, studies, and organizations that promote weight loss as a strategy for improving health outcomes and, as a result, many different types of weight-loss advice and diets offered to help with weight loss. It is popularly believed that a diet with low carbohydrates and high protein will result in greater fat loss and less lean mass loss than the high-carbohydrate, low-fat diet. However, those with high protein may vary in saturated fats, and there may be concern about the effect on serum lipids and subsequent cardiovascular disease.

Evidence

The study sample included 119 females between 20 and 65 years old with other inclusion criteria. They were randomly assigned to one of two diets: (1) the high-protein, low-saturated-fat versus (2) the high-carbohydrate, low-saturated-fat diet. The statistical analysis was performed with the use of SPSS, using the following: univariate analysis of variance, the unpaired *t* test, and Tukey's test.

Application to Practice

In this study a greater fat loss with the high-protein diet was not substantiated. A carbohydrate-restricted, high-protein, low-fat diet provides nutritional and metabolic benefits that are equal to and sometimes greater than those observed with a high-carbohydrate, low-fat diet. Both diets resulted in significant improvements in markers of cardiovascular disease risk, although the high-protein diet from lean red meat and low-fat dairy products resulted in increased satiety and a greater reduction in triacylglycerol concentrations (marker of the metabolic syndrome) and seems to provide a weight-loss advantage in subjects with elevated triacylglycerol concentrations.

It is recommended that the complete article be read for a more comprehensive summary.

Reference

Noakes, M., Keogh, J. B., Foster, P. R., & Clifton, P. M. (2005). Effect of an energy-restricted, high-protein, low-fat diet relative to a conventional high-carbohydrate, low-fat diet on weight loss, body composition, nutritional status, and markers of cardiovascular health in obese women. *American Journal of Clinical Nutrition, 81,* 1298-1306 [32 references].

Nutrition and Fluids. Nutrients, particularly protein and iron, are essential for the formation of blood cells. Diets with inadequate protein are deficient in amino acids needed to build red and white blood cells. Also, if protein intake falls, serum protein levels fall, and the ability to keep fluid in the vascular system is impaired.

Iron is needed to manufacture oxygen-carrying hemoglobin molecules. Iron deficiency anemia develops when the diet lacks adequate iron. Anemia reduces delivery of oxygen to the tissues.

Fat intake also influences circulatory function. Excessive intake of such high-fat foods as red meat, animal fats, and some dairy products raises blood (serum) cholesterol levels. Hypercholesterolemia (high blood cholesterol) is a major risk factor for atherosclerosis.

Fluid balance also affects circulation. Clients on fluid restrictions or those with excessive fluid losses (for example, from diarrhea or vomiting) have the potential to become dehydrated and thus develop more viscous blood. Viscous blood clots more readily and can block blood vessels.

Activity and Exercise. Clients with chronic health problems sometimes must lead more sedentary lives or may be immobile. Many clients without such health problems lead sedentary lives as well. For whatever reason, decreased activity slows venous blood return to the heart.

Changes in activity can be long or short term. For example, heart problems, severe anemia, and debilitating neuromuscular diseases produce long-standing fatigue. On the other hand, travelers on long trips or clients with bone fractures may experience temporary episodes of less dynamic circulation because of activity restrictions. Stagnation of blood in the veins contributes to clot formation.

Smoking. Smoking is a major risk factor that damages circulation in several ways and doubles the risk of heart disease (Bazzano, He, Muntner, Vupputuri, & Whelton, 2003). Nicotine produces vasoconstriction, which restricts blood flow to tissues, lowers the oxygen-carrying capacity of hemoglobin, and causes cellular changes in the intimal lining of arteries. In addition, nicotine lowers blood levels of beneficial, high-density lipoproteins (HDL) and elevates levels of harmful, low-density lipoproteins (LDL); these serum changes hasten the atherosclerotic process. Finally, smoking enhances the detrimental effects of other cardiovascular risk factors, such as blood glucose and cholesterol levels; this is known as a synergistic effect. Box 35-2 summarizes research findings on the synergistic effects of smoking.

Substance Abuse. Substance abuse poses unique hazards to the cardiovascular system. Cocaine and amphetamines are stimulants that increase heart rate and oxygen demand and constrict the coronary arteries. Large amounts of cocaine ultimately have an anesthetic effect on myocardial cells, which decreases cardiac output and produces hypotension. These effects increase the risk for a heart attack (Lai et al., 2005). In contrast, sedatives and opiates depress the central nervous system, causing respiratory depression and hypotension.

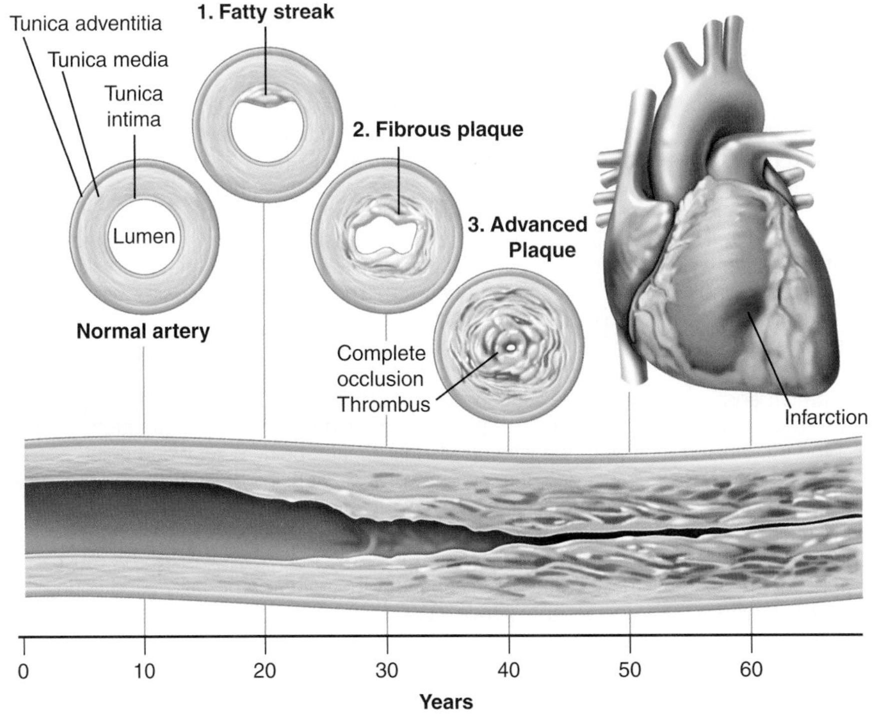

FIGURE 35-6 Formation of an atherosclerotic plaque. *1,* Cholesterol deposits cause fatty streaks. *2,* Fibrin infiltrates the fatty streaks, forming a fibrous plaque. *3,* Platelets aggregate on the irregular endothelial surface, producing what is called a complicated lesion or an advanced plaque. Total vessel occlusion blocks blood flow, eventually killing the tissue cells normally supplied by the blocked vessel. This killing of tissue cells is called infarction.

PSYCHOLOGICAL FACTORS

Emotional stress burdens the circulatory system as well. Stress increases the heart rate and blood pressure, which, in turn, raises the body's oxygen demands.

Many diseases that affect tissue perfusion and cardiovascular function are chronic. The affected person may have to contend with long-term health care issues, changes in quality of life, and complex medication regimens. Living with chronic health care problems requires constant adjustments by clients as their level of wellness fluctuates.

You will need to establish a trusting relationship with long-term clients, assess their motivation, and monitor their compliance. Depression and hopelessness can lessen compliance, and you can be instrumental in recognizing these problems. You can also assist with problem solving as a client's condition changes. Typically, nurses are the client's main source of information and motivation to make life changes and maintain them, as one client describes in Box 35-3.

BOX 35-2 *The Effects of Smoking on Other Risk Factors*

Cigarette smoking affects serum glucose, lipids, blood pressure, and pulse. Well-supported evidence shows that individuals who smoke have a 2 to 9 mg/100 mL reduction in high-density lipoprotein (HDL) levels; less-well-supported evidence shows an increase in low-density lipoprotein (LDL) levels (Gulanick & Cofer, 2000).

Additional effects of smoking include the following (Gulanick & Cofer, 2000):

- Injury to the vascular endothelium
- Promotion of platelet aggregation
- Altered oxygen supply and demand
- Increase in vascular resistance
- Release of catecholamines

ASSESSMENT

A thorough cardiovascular assessment includes a complete history and physical examination. However, ongoing assessment focuses on known and potential problems.

GENERAL ASSESSMENT OF TISSUE PERFUSION AND CARDIAC FUNCTION

Assessment data include both general and specific observations about circulatory status. Overall appearance, condition of the skin, and activity tolerance give general cues about cardiac function. Data about heart sounds, lung sounds, edema, vital signs, weight, peripheral pulses, and pain provide more specific information about cardiac function.

Health History. The health history consists of the duration of the client's chief complaint, past history, and lifestyle data. This information creates a detailed picture of the client's immediate needs as well as the impact of the problem on daily life.

BOX 35-3 *A Patient's Perspective*

"Nurses Do the Real Caring"

To celebrate my sixty-fifth birthday, I planned a 2-month walking tour with friends across my native England. Tickets, passport, and hotel reservations were at the ready when a routine doctor's appointment abruptly changed my destination. A stress test on Tuesday led to an angiogram on Friday. Looking at the x-ray images, I knew England would have to wait. Bypass surgery was scheduled for the following week.

Although disappointed about the change in plans, I spent a pleasant weekend in hospital, telephoning and writing friends. I felt completely comfortable about the surgery, trusting my doctor and the surgeon he recommended, who explained the operation very carefully and thoroughly. That trust proved to be well founded because at no point did things go wrong.

The hours between the chilly wait outside the OR and the tangle of tubes in the ICU are forever lost to me. I only remember the extraordinarily attentive care of the ICU nurses and my own curiosity about what was happening. About the second day, most of the tubes were removed, and soon I was in a regular room. Almost immediately, the nurses got me out of bed and had me walking down the hall (staggering might better describe it), pushing my IV pole. My three incisions—chest, left arm, and right leg (the latter two where veins were removed for grafting to the cardiac vessels)—were held together with amazing adhesive patches: no external stitches.

It took 9 days in hospital to adjust my various medications. Infection developed in the arm incision but was quickly cleaned out and cleared up. Nurse practitioners briefed me on how to care for the chest incision at home, as well giving me tips on medications, diet, and lifestyle changes to aid the healing process. They were outstanding. You could tell they'd been in "the heart business" for years. They were also skilled in pain control. I don't remember any intense pain—just difficulty in finding a comfortable position to sleep.

The nursing care varied from good to excellent. Everyone was terribly nice, but the experienced nurses had a higher energy level than the younger ones and a more intense focus on you and what they were doing. They were more attentive to the little details that matter: being quiet when quiet is needed, turning out the lights at night, being right on time with medications. They were strong, direct, and definite. When they drew blood, plunk! The needle was in. You *knew* they knew what they were doing. The nurses impressed me most. They do the real caring. But there were amazingly good young doctors, too: gentle, considerate, very focused on me.

OR, Operating room; *ICU*, intensive care unit; *IV*, intravenous.

Chief Complaint. Chief complaints related to cardiovascular function range from dramatic to subtle. They include chest pain, palpitations, dyspnea, cough, fatigue, weight gain, edema, syncope, and extremity pain. Because the systemic effects of cardiovascular disease can produce a wide array of signs and symptoms, clear description of the chief complaint can help you prioritize your client's needs. Let HEART guide your assessment of cardiovascular symptoms:

H—Have the client describe the specific location, onset, and duration of the symptom.
E— Explore associated signs and symptoms.
A— Ask about activities that worsen or ease the symptom.
R— Rate the severity of discomfort or incapacity.
T— Talk about treatments or interventions used to alleviate the symptom and their effectiveness.

Ask the client about medications, both prescription and nonprescription, used as treatment for cardiovascular conditions. Keep in mind that over-the-counter medications and herbal supplements (Capriotti, 2004) may interact with prescription medications. For example, the combination of aspirin and Coumadin, an oral anticoagulant, increases the risk of bleeding. Similarly, antihistamines and appetite suppressants are contraindicated for clients with hypertension, because both have vasoconstricting effects. The medication history may help to focus your data collection during the physical examination portion of the assessment.

History. The past health history of the client and the client's family can help to identify genetic tendencies and other risk factors. Assess for the following conditions in the client's past history because they are associated with cardiovascular disease:

- Hypertension
- Diabetes mellitus
- Rheumatic fever
- Elevated blood cholesterol and lipids
- Bleeding tendencies
- Peripheral vascular disease
- Myocardial infarction
- Heart failure
- Renal failure
- Hepatic failure

Lifestyle. Assess for lifestyle behaviors, such as smoking, diet, and exercise. Nicotine, alcohol, and recreational drugs have detrimental effects on the heart and blood vessels. Ask the client about the frequency and the amount of use for each of these substances.

Take a diet history. Note the intake of foods high in fat, which raise serum cholesterol and lipid levels. Also note high-sodium foods, because they contribute to hypertension. Identify food preferences, portion size, snacks, and methods of food preparation.

Investigate the client's exercise habits, because exercise is beneficial for circulation. Ask about the frequency, duration, intensity, and type of exercise the client gets. Also discuss how well the client tolerates exercise.

Finally, explore the client's perceived stress level. Ask about occupation, hobbies, and recreational activities. Identify coping strategies and support systems.

Physical Examination. Use data gathered in the history to focus your physical examination. Although the heart and blood vessels are the primary components of the examination, attention to all body systems is important because of the potential systemic effects of circulatory problems. Assess vital signs, heart sounds, and peripheral circulation. Especially for clients with or at risk for heart failure, be sure to assess for distention of jugular veins (Figure 35-7) and pitting edema (Figure 35-8). See Chapter 8 for a detailed discussion of physical assessment.

Diagnostic Tests. Diagnostic tests provide valuable information about the function of the circulatory system. Some diagnostic tests are used to screen high-risk populations. Periodic diagnostic tests track clients' positive and negative responses to treatment and guide modifications in therapeutic regimens.

Complete Blood Count. A complete blood count provides preliminary data about the cellular components of the blood. The red blood cell count is the number of cells per volume, hemoglobin is the oxygen-carrying pigment in red blood cells, and hematocrit is the percentage of cells to plasma. These components are used to evaluate blood loss, anemia, and hydration. The platelet count is used to evaluate bleeding disorders such as occurs in thrombocytopenia, cirrhosis of the liver, or anticoagulation therapy. Clients with low platelet levels have a tendency to bleed, whereas those with elevated platelet counts are at risk for hypercoagulability.

Coagulation Studies. Coagulation studies provide specific data about the body's ability to form blood clots and are used to monitor drug therapy to prevent the formation of a clot. Prothrombin time (PT) is an evaluation of the extrinsic clotting mechanism or Stage

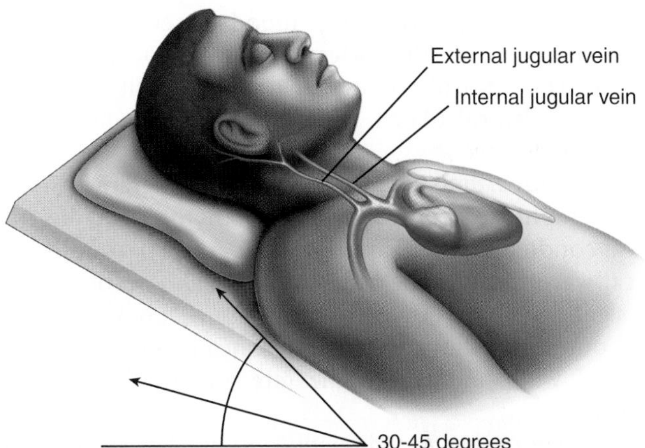

FIGURE 35-7 Measurement of jugular vein distention.

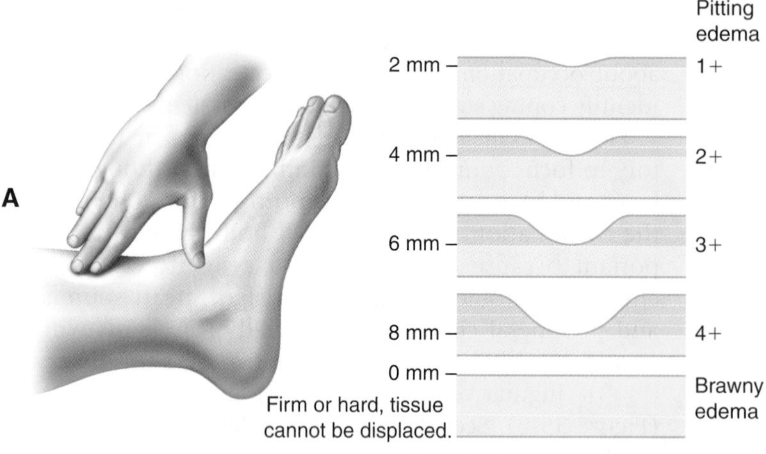

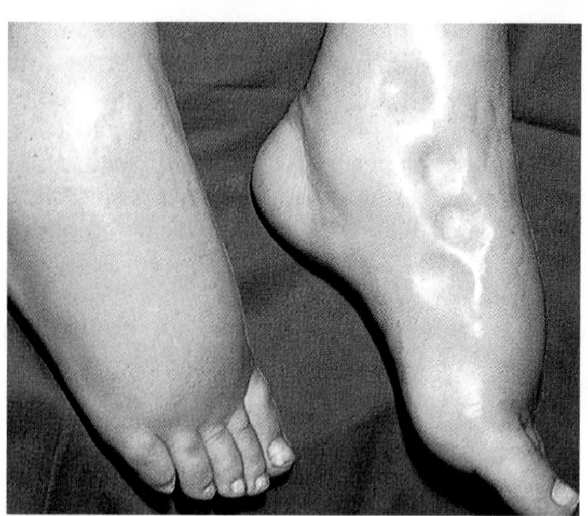

FIGURE 35-8 **A,** Assessment and grading of pitting edema. Pressing on the surface of edematous tissue leaves an indentation that does not immediately rebound once the pressure is released. Pitting edema is graded by the depth of the indentation. **B,** Clinical example of pitting edema. (Photographs from Bloom, A., & Ireland, J. [1992]. *Color atlas of diabetes* [2nd ed.]. London: Mosby-Wolfe.)

II of the clotting mechanism. It is reported as an international normalized ratio (INR) that standardizes the value by comparing it to the control value. A therapeutic level for the administration of the anticoagulant Coumadin is two to three times the control. Activated partial thromboplastin time (aPTT) is an evaluation of the intrinsic clotting mechanism. A therapeutic level for the administration of shorter-acting anticoagulant heparin is 1.5 to 2.5 times the normal value.

Lipid Profile. Cholesterol, triglycerides, and lipids are fatty substances found in the blood. Lipids are further subdivided by laboratory analysis according to density, resulting in percentages of high-density, low-density, and very-low-density lipoproteins. Collectively, the measurement of these substances constitutes a lipid profile.

The lipid profile is used to assess risk for atherosclerosis and vascular disease. Elevations of cholesterol, triglyceride, and low-density and very-low-density lipid levels are associated with atherosclerosis. Conversely, high-density lipoproteins protect blood vessels against the development of atherosclerosis and cardiovascular disease. The ratio of cholesterol to high-density lipoproteins is also calculated. High ratios increase the risk of atherosclerosis.

Electrocardiogram. The electrocardiogram (ECG) is a graphic recording of heart rate, rhythm, and electrical conduction. By examining the pattern of the electrical wave through the atria and ventricles, information is gathered about the efficiency of the heart as a pump, about tissues that are unable to transmit a normal electrical wave, and about the rate and rhythm of the heart.

Angiography. A radiopaque, iodine-based contrast dye is injected into a blood vessel while the heart is viewed under a fluoroscope. Blood is seen flowing through the arteries, providing information about the diameter and patency of vessels. Narrowed or obstructed vessels impede the delivery of blood to tissues.

Before angiography, assess the client for allergies to medications and foods high in iodine, such as shellfish. Nausea, vomiting, difficulty breathing, tachycardia, and chest pain during the angiogram may indicate an allergic reaction to the dye. Report any of these findings to the physician immediately.

Action Alert! Maintain a patent airway if an allergic reaction occurs.

Angiograms are invasive procedures of the circulatory system. Monitor the client's peripheral circulation after the procedure. Adequate circulation is evidenced by strong and equal peripheral pulses; warm, pink skin; and the absence of numbness, tingling, or pain. Inform the physician of any abnormal circulatory findings.

Action Alert! Immediately report pain, pallor, pulselessness, or paresthesia of the client's extremity following angiography. Check the insertion site for bleeding.

This common test can provoke considerable anxiety for a client whose cardiovascular function is already threatened. Thus it is all the more important that you spend time teaching the client about the test and helping to relieve anxiety in addition to providing ordered treatments.

Doppler Blood Flow Studies. Doppler studies use sound waves to evaluate the patency of peripheral blood vessels. Clots in the vessels and diminished blood flow are detected by the Doppler ultrasound probe. This noninvasive test poses few risks for clients.

Table 35-2 Comparison of Peripheral Arterial and Venous Circulatory Dysfunction

DYSFUNCTION	ARTERIAL	VENOUS
Pain	Intermittent and related to activity	Constant aching
Pulses	Decreased or absent	Unchanged
Capillary refill	Less than 3 seconds	Unchanged
Skin color	Pale	Red
Skin temperature	Cool	Warm
Skin appearance	Shiny, with hair loss	Patchy brown discoloration
Edema	Absent	Present
Sensory/motor function	Impaired	Unchanged
Ulcers	Pale ulcer base with even edge	Red ulcer base with uneven edge
Healing	Delayed	Delayed

FOCUSED ASSESSMENT FOR *INEFFECTIVE TISSUE PERFUSION*

Impaired blood flow to an organ reduces the delivery of oxygen and nutrients needed by that organ to function effectively. Pain and impaired organ function are cues to a state of *Ineffective tissue perfusion*. Cerebral, renal, cardiopulmonary, gastrointestinal, or peripheral circulation may be compromised. Use the client history and current clinical manifestations to identify specific areas of compromised perfusion.

Defining Characteristics. Defining characteristics are related to the area of the body affected. Poor renal perfusion is characterized by decreased renal output. Output less than 30 mL/hr is considered to be renal failure. Poor cerebral perfusion manifests as confusion, paralysis, or other neurological symptoms. Gastrointestinal symptoms would include abdominal pain, slowed or absent bowel sounds, and abdominal distention. Cardiac symptoms would be substernal chest pain, often radiating to the right arm or neck, and dysrhythmias.

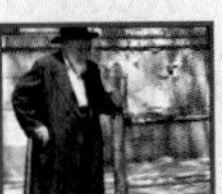

For example, Mr. Yoder, the client introduced at the beginning of this chapter, has altered cardiopulmonary tissue perfusion. Mr. Yoder's admitting diagnosis is angina pectoris. Angina results from a coronary blood supply inadequate to meet myocardial metabolic needs.

In Mr. Yoder's situation, chest pain is the primary manifestation of his cardiac perfusion problem. Myocardial oxygen deprivation can impair the heart's pumping efficiency, which in turn limits oxygen delivery to other parts of the body and produces manifestations of *Ineffective tissue perfusion,* such as pale, clammy skin and light-headedness. On the basis of his signs and symptoms, which other areas of Mr. Yoder's body are also experiencing tissue perfusion deficits?

Peripheral perfusion problems can involve either arteries or veins; the client's signs and symptoms will offer clues to the vessels involved (Table 35-2). Compare the right and left extremity to detect differences. Signs and symptoms of decreased arterial perfusion include decreased or absent pulses, skin that is pale and cool, numbness and tingling of the extremity, claudication, and slow capillary refill. **Claudication** refers to cramplike pains in the calves caused by inadequate blood flow to the leg muscles. Ask the client what level of exercise or activity produces the claudication.

Venous insufficiency, phlebitis, or varicose veins can impair the return of blood to the heart. Pain in the calf of the leg, positive Homans' sign, and edema are suspicious for *deep vein thrombophlebitis*. Redness and warmth may be present in the involved extremity if there is inflammation. **Edema** is an abnormal accumulation of fluid in the interstitial spaces of tissues, commonly known as swelling. *Venous insufficiency* is evidenced by edema, atrophic changes to the hair and nails, and dull, aching pain in the extremity. Eventually venous stasis ulcers may develop.

Related Factors. Occlusion or narrowing of the blood vessels from atherosclerosis, thrombosis, and emboli are the primary causes of arterial *Ineffective tissue perfusion*. Occlusion can occur in blood vessels throughout the body. Myocardial infarction, cerebral vascular accident, and pulmonary embolism are examples of occlusive events.

Venous problems can be related to age, history of deep vein thrombosis (DVT), smoking, a sedentary lifestyle, and obesity. Vocations that involve standing for long periods predispose individuals to increased venous pressure in dependent lower extremities.

FOCUSED ASSESSMENT FOR *DECREASED CARDIAC OUTPUT*

Assess for *Decreased cardiac output* in the presence of any condition that affects the heart's pumping ability or problems that increase the demands placed on the heart. Assessment of cardiac output is assessment of the circulatory system and the whole body.

Defining Characteristics. The clinical characteristics of *Decreased cardiac output* are signs that the cardiac system is no longer able to compensate for a decrease in cardiac output or for increased demands. When compensatory mechanisms fail, hypotension develops; less blood flows to the heart muscle, and bradycardia may develop. Signs of hypoxemia, such as confusion, restlessness, cyanosis, pallor, and decreased urinary output, may be present. Additional clinical manifestations associated with hypoxemia are chest pain and dysrhythmias.

Cardiac output is decreased when the heart is ineffective as a pump—it becomes congested with blood that it cannot expel, and the hydrostatic pressure in the chambers increases. Eventually, because the blood is not being effectively pumped forward, it pools in the form of edema of the lungs or the lower extremities. Signs of heart failure include dyspnea, fatigue, jugular vein distention, pulmonary edema, and peripheral edema.

Other defining characteristics of *Decreased cardiac output* relate to impaired blood (oxygen) supply to vital organs. The brain is especially vulnerable to decreases in blood supply. Restlessness, dizziness, and syncope (fainting) are common manifestations of cerebral hypoxia. Because kidney function depends on adequate blood pressure, urine output drops as a consequence of decreases in cardiac output. In addition, because the body shunts blood to vital organs during periods of decreases in cardiac output, the client's skin will become cold and clammy, cyanosis will appear, and capillary refill will be slow.

Nursing assessment is designed for early detection of impending problems. Tachycardia and elevated blood pressure are short-term compensatory mechanisms to restore stroke volume and maintain tissue perfusion. Look for trends in vital signs, for example, a gradually increasing or decreasing pulse rate. To evaluate tachycardia or bradycardia look for evidence that adequate tissue perfusion is not occurring. Identify changes before the problem becomes serious. Schole and Mininni (2006) identify the following signs and symptoms that indicate the client's condition is seriously deteriorating and that may appear hours before a cardiac arrest:

- Mean arterial pressure less than 70 mm Hg or more than 130 mm Hg (mean arterial pressure is $[(2 \times \text{diastolic}) + \text{systolic}] \div 3$)
- Heart rate less than 45 or more than 125 beats per minute
- Respiratory rate less than 10 or more than 30 breaths per minute
- Complaints of chest pain
- Change in mental status

Related Factors. Underlying cardiovascular disease is the primary factor that affects cardiac output. Disturbances in heart rate or rhythm, medications that decrease contractility, heart surgery, and shock also adversely affect cardiac output. Heart conditions that decrease heart rate or stroke volume result in decreases in cardiac output. Bradycardia, heart failure, myocardial infarction, and cardiogenic shock are examples of problems originating in the heart and diminishing the ability of the heart to pump effectively.

In addition, cardiac output is reduced secondary to conditions outside the heart that place added workload on the heart, such as decreased circulating blood volume. Hemorrhage, burns, and severe dehydration produce hypovolemia (low vascular volume) as a result of a loss of fluid from the vascular space. Although the heart can compensate by increasing the heart rate, stroke volume and cardiac output eventually fall because of decreased venous return and decreased ventricular filling.

FOCUSED ASSESSMENT FOR *RISK FOR PERIPHERAL NEUROVASCULAR DYSFUNCTION*

Neurovascular dysfunction is a preventable complication for most clients. Vigilance on your part is the primary preventive action, starting with identification of clients at risk for neurovascular dysfunction. Frequent assessment will help you detect circulatory compromise promptly and intervene appropriately to relieve pressure on vessels and nerves.

Defining Characteristics. Situations in which pressure is exerted on blood vessels and nerves, particularly pressure in body areas with limited capacity for expansion, constitute risks for peripheral neurovascular dysfunction. Hemorrhage into a muscle or joint, edema secondary to trauma or surgery, or a severe burn increases pressure as a result of local accumulation of blood or fluid. Burns that encircle an extremity are especially dangerous because the circular pattern of edema acts like a tourniquet to block blood flow distal to the injury.

Therapeutic treatments also pose risks for clients. Edema under newly applied casts, an elastic bandage or tourniquet that is applied too tightly, extensive infiltration of intravenous fluids, or misaligned traction leads to neurovascular damage, if undetected.

The signs and symptoms of peripheral neurovascular dysfunction vary with the type of vessel that is occluded. Usually, arterial occlusions present a picture of oxygen deficit, whereas venous occlusions are characterized by venous engorgement.

Arterial Occlusion. Manifestations of arterial occlusion include decreased pulses, pallor, cool skin, slow capillary refill, numbness, tingling, burning, decreased movement of the affected limb, and pain in the affected limb. These signs indicate oxygen deprivation in the tissues and nerves of the involved extremity.

Venous Occlusion. Occlusion of a vein prevents blood from returning to the heart. Venous engorgement in the extremity produces warm skin, red skin, edema, and slow capillary refill in the affected area.

FOCUSED ASSESSMENT FOR *SHOCK*

Shock is a life-threatening circulatory collapse that results from a severe volume deficit, cardiac pump failure, or redistribution of blood. In shock, the heart cannot pump sufficient blood to vital organs. Early manifestations of shock include tachycardia and hypotension, but malfunctions of the heart, brain, and kidney quickly develop. Shock is a medical emergency that requires prompt intervention to prevent permanent damage to vital organs.

Early detection of shock is essential because it is a progressive condition that develops in four stages (Figure 35-9).

Fortunately, shock responds well to treatment in the early stages. Nurses, because of their frequent client contact and ongoing assessment, are instrumental in preventing shock and its devastating consequences. Because of the physiological complexity of shock, the physician and nurse work collaboratively to care for affected clients.

Shock is characterized by signs of impaired tissue perfusion. Changes in vital signs, neurological status, skin, and renal function are evident in roughly the following order:

- *Tachycardia.* In the initial stage of shock, slight tachycardia is the only manifestation. As shock progresses, tachycardia worsens.
- *Hypotension.* When the body can no longer maintain cardiac output by increasing the heart rate, blood pressure falls. Decreases in both systolic and diastolic blood pressure eventually occur.
- *Weakened peripheral pulses.* The heart's inability to deliver blood to peripheral areas of the body progressively weakens peripheral pulses.
- *Changes in neurological status.* Brain cells are very sensitive to oxygen deprivation. Cerebral hypoxia, in early shock, causes restlessness, agitation, and confusion. As shock progresses, the client becomes progressively less alert.
- *Skin changes.* Because blood is shunted away from the skin and sent to vital organs such as the heart and lungs, the client will develop pale, cold, clammy skin characteristic of shock.
- *Decreased urine output.* Hypotension decreases kidney filtration, reducing urine output to less than 30 mL/hr.

As mentioned earlier, heart failure, loss of blood volume, and extensive peripheral vasodilation are critical events that lead to shock. Each of these events triggers shock by altering a component of circulation.

Cardiogenic Shock. Heart failure occurs when contractility or stroke volume falls. When heart failure results in shock, it is called cardiogenic shock.

Hypovolemic Shock. Loss of blood or plasma decreases the circulating blood volume, which results in hypovolemic shock. Hemorrhage, severe burns, and extensive vomiting or diarrhea can trigger hypovolemia.

Distributive Shock. Massive peripheral vasodilation that traps blood in the peripheral microcirculation can result in shock. Although the actual circulating blood volume is unchanged, vasodilation produces a relative state of hypovolemia. Severe allergic reactions, neurological injury, and blood-borne infections from gram-negative organisms are examples of conditions that can cause distributive shock.

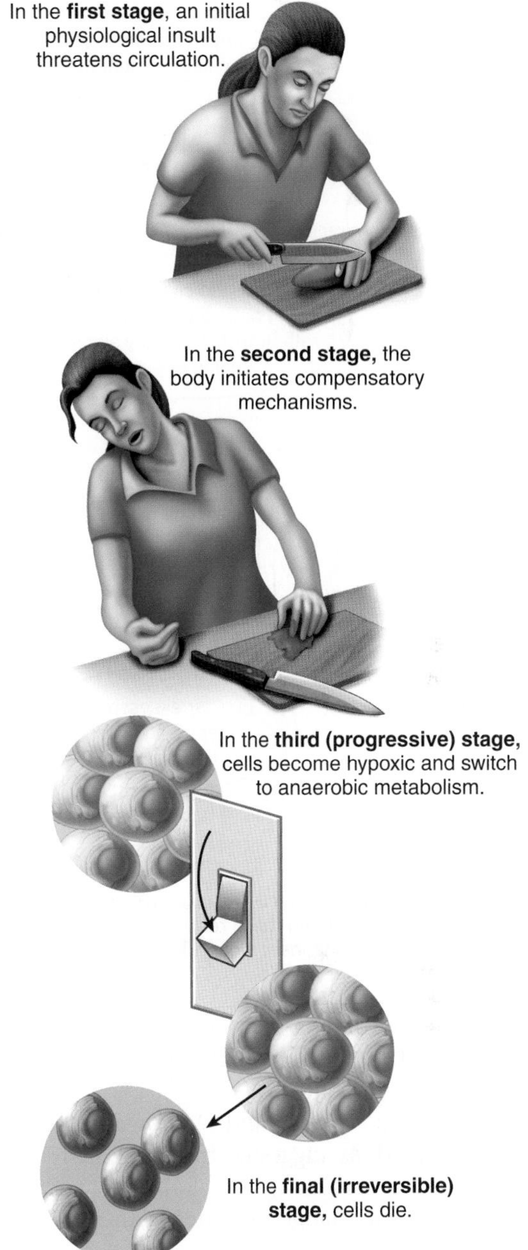

FIGURE 35-9 The four stages of shock.

DIAGNOSIS

Ineffective tissue perfusion, as a nursing diagnosis, addresses a variety of client situations characterized by diminished circulation. Generally, the consequences of tissue perfusion deficits involve decreased or lost organ

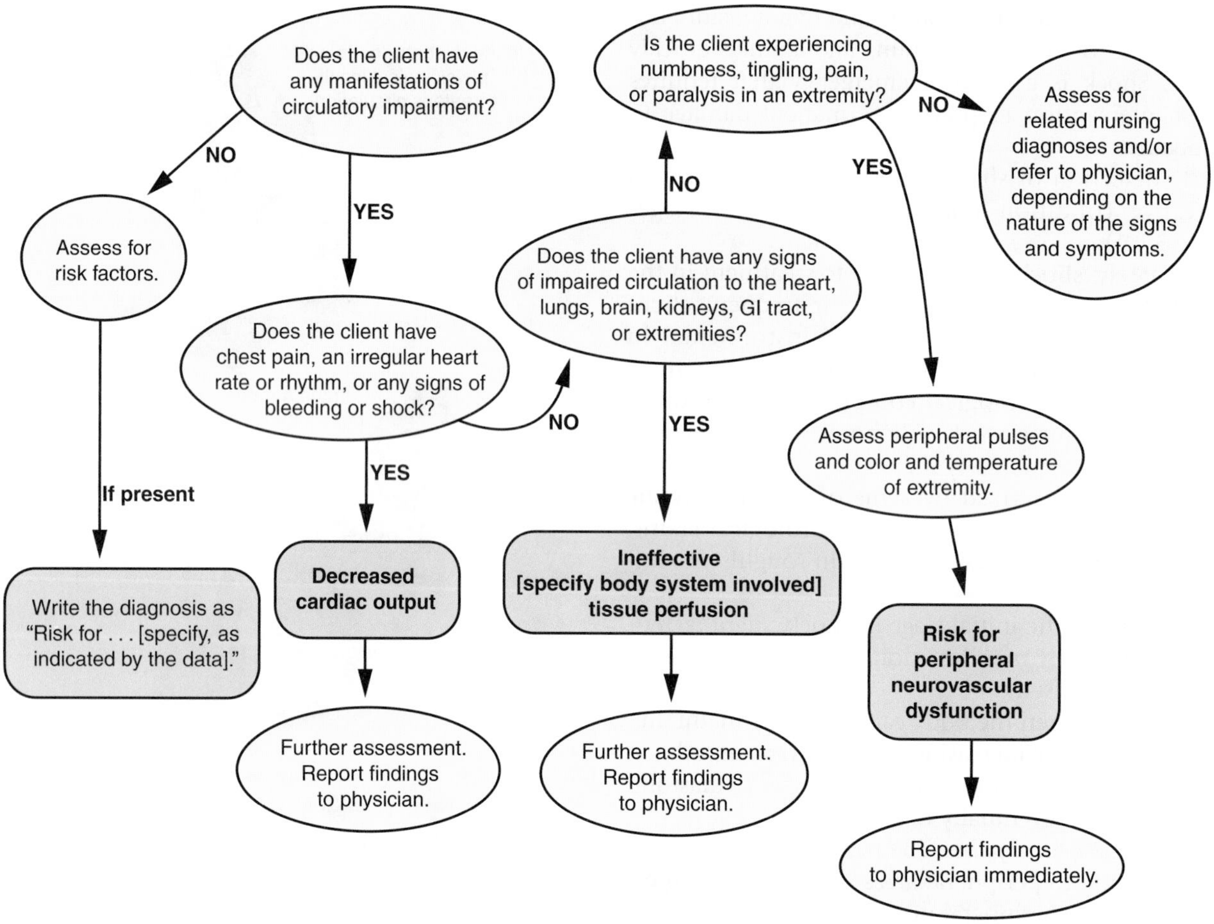

Does the client have any manifestations of circulatory impairment?

NO → Assess for risk factors. → If present → Write the diagnosis as "Risk for . . . [specify, as indicated by the data]."

YES → Does the client have chest pain, an irregular heart rate or rhythm, or any signs of bleeding or shock?

YES → **Decreased cardiac output** → Further assessment. Report findings to physician.

NO → Does the client have any signs of impaired circulation to the heart, lungs, brain, kidneys, GI tract, or extremities?

YES → **Ineffective [specify body system involved] tissue perfusion** → Further assessment. Report findings to physician.

NO → Is the client experiencing numbness, tingling, pain, or paralysis in an extremity?

NO → Assess for related nursing diagnoses and/or refer to physician, depending on the nature of the signs and symptoms.

YES → Assess peripheral pulses and color and temperature of extremity. → **Risk for peripheral neurovascular dysfunction** → Report findings to physician immediately.

FIGURE 35-10 Decision tree for cardiovascular nursing diagnoses. Diagnoses are shown in rectangles. Within these rectangles, diagnoses shown in **bold** type are NANDA-I–approved nursing diagnoses; diagnoses shown in regular type are not NANDA-I–approved nursing diagnoses.

function. Internal organs, such as the heart, brain, and kidneys, as well as peripheral extremities, are common targets of perfusion deficits.

Ineffective tissue perfusion and *Decreased cardiac output* are closely related, as suggested in Figure 35-10. A delicate balance is necessary to maintain circulation. Pathophysiological change in either of these vital components impacts the other.

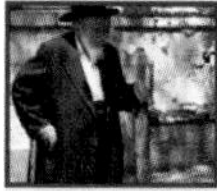

Mr. Yoder is an example of the interrelatedness of these two nursing diagnoses. Mr. Yoder has coronary artery disease, which narrows the blood vessels that nourish the myocardial muscle. When Mr. Yoder's activity increases, as when he works in his carpenter shop, his myocardium has an increased demand for oxygen. An imbalance of supply and demand develops that eventually results in chest pain. If Mr. Yoder stops his activity, the oxygen demand falls, and his chest pain ceases. However, if one or more blood vessels become totally occluded, myocardial cells will die. Mr. Yoder will have a myocardial infarction.

Risk for peripheral neurovascular dysfunction focuses on a smaller cluster of client situations in which circulation to an extremity is jeopardized. Generally, constricting treatment devices, invasive vascular procedures, and occlusive events constitute threats that warrant selection of this nursing diagnosis.

Careful assessment and consideration of underlying health problems will help you to prioritize between *Ineffective tissue perfusion* and *Decreased cardiac output* for individual clients. Goals and interventions that aim to correct the underlying cause of the problem produce the best client outcomes. Table 35-3 gives examples of how to identify the appropriate nursing diagnosis.

RELATED NURSING DIAGNOSES

Problems of tissue perfusion and cardiac dysfunction lead to other problems as well. You will need to prioritize client needs and plan interventions to address problems associated with circulatory dysfunction. The following are nursing diagnoses commonly associated with cardiovascular dysfunction.

Pain. Pain commonly accompanies decreases in circulation. As compensatory mechanisms for inadequate circulation fail, body tissues adapt by switching from aerobic to anaerobic metabolism. The byproduct of anaerobic metabolism is lactic acid. When it accumulates in the tissues, lactic acid irritates nerve endings and produces pain.

Table 35-3 Clustering Data to Make a Nursing Diagnosis

Cardiovascular Problems

DATA CLUSTER	DIAGNOSIS
A 15-year-old boy fractured his arm while playing soccer. A cast has been applied to the arm, and he has just arrived in the nursing unit.	Risk for peripheral neurovascular dysfunction related to tissue trauma and edema formation
An older adult client is admitted with a myocardial infarction. Two hours after admission, she becomes confused and disoriented. Her blood pressure has dropped to 90/50 mm Hg, and her pulse has increased to 120 beats per minute.	Decreased cardiac output related to impaired myocardial contractility
A 48-year-old man is admitted with complaints of periodic leg cramps. Assessment reveals much-diminished pulses and pale, shiny skin on his lower extremities. He has no hair on his shins. The client reports a 20-year history of high blood pressure and diabetes mellitus.	Ineffective peripheral tissue perfusion related to diminished blood flow to the lower extremities, secondary to the effects of hypertension and diabetes

The location of pain caused by decreased circulation depends on the area of the body deprived of blood and oxygen.

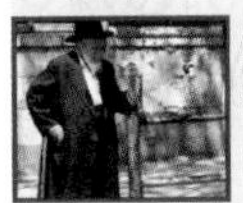

For example, Mr. Yoder, the client introduced at the beginning of the chapter, experienced chest pain from inadequate circulation to the myocardium.

Another example is a client with a newly applied cast who develops swelling of the casted extremity. In this situation, pain in the fractured limb is the expected finding. Restoration of circulation is a priority to prevent damage to tissues and nerves.

Anxiety. Anxiety is a common response both to pain and to the effects of decreased circulation. It also may result from cerebral hypoxia. As mentioned earlier, the brain requires a constant source of oxygenated blood to function properly.

Risk for Impaired Skin Integrity. When circulation is impaired, blood is shunted away from nonessential organs to improve perfusion to vital organs. Diversion of blood from the skin decreases the delivery of nutrients and removal of metabolic waste. Vasoconstriction, which accompanies blood shunting, produces cold, clammy, mottled skin. Chronic circulatory impairment puts clients at risk for pressure ulcers and delayed tissue healing. For example, clients with arterial or venous insufficiency of the lower extremities are likely to develop ulcers and necrotic areas on the legs.

Ineffective Health Maintenance. Clients with cardiovascular problems are frequently advised to change their lifestyle. Assess the client's lifestyle as well as the knowledge and motivation needed to make the changes.

Activity Intolerance. Assess the client with cardiovascular problems for problems in tolerating activities that are essential or desirable for the client. Muscles with inadequate blood supply fatigue quickly, especially with activity that increases their demand for oxygen.

PLANNING

Expected outcomes for clients with cardiovascular problems differ depending on whether the problem is acute or chronic. We will focus now on acute care and the interventions that are aimed at early detection and prevention. Interventions for acute circulatory diagnoses include assessment, monitoring changes in circulatory status, support of circulation, and implementation of medical therapies. Early recognition of impending complications is crucial for successful client outcomes.

However, you must consider multiple factors even when planning care for acute client problems. In addition to physiological factors, you will identify aspects unique to each client. Explore the client's living arrangements, transportation, finances, support systems, and cultural background to help formulate a holistic plan of care that addresses individual client needs.

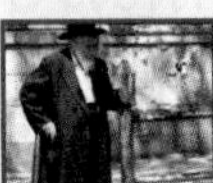

Consider the special needs of Mr. Yoder, the client introduced at the beginning of this chapter. Mr. Yoder's Amish beliefs and lifestyle should be incorporated into the plan for his care. Some cultural needs of Amish clients are summarized in Box 35-4.

EXPECTED OUTCOMES FOR THE CLIENT WITH *INEFFECTIVE TISSUE PERFUSION*

The goal for acute *Ineffective tissue perfusion* is the prevention of permanent tissue damage or even death. Rapid assessment and intervention mean the difference between positive and negative client outcomes. The goals for chronic perfusion problems include improvement of circulation and adaptation to the problem. The role of the nurse in managing a chronic perfusion alteration is to detect subtle signs of circulatory deterioration, teach clients, foster compliance with the treatment regimen, and provide emotional support.

You will evaluate the effects of interventions to maintain or improve tissue perfusion by assessing the client's circulatory status. Examine the overall circulation, as well as the target organs specifically at risk. Expected outcomes that demonstrate adequate tissue perfusion include the following:

- Blood pressure within normal limits for the client
- Palpable peripheral pulses of equal strength and quality
- Skin warm and dry
- Capillary refill in less than 3 seconds
- Absence of pain
- Mental status within normal limits for the client
- Urine output at least 30 mL/hr

Accurate evaluation of tissue perfusion also requires close attention to affected body systems. For example, if you suspect a cerebral perfusion deficit, you would expand your data gathering related to the client's neurological system. If renal perfusion is a concern, you would pay extra attention to urine output and fluid balance.

EXPECTED OUTCOMES FOR THE CLIENT WITH *DECREASED CARDIAC OUTPUT*

The goals for *Decreased cardiac output* are to reduce the cardiac workload, to use prescribed medications effectively to restore or maintain cardiac output, and to control salt and water retention. Short-term or intermediate goals are used to measure progress. Expected outcomes that indicate adequate cardiac output include the following:

- Blood pressure within normal limits for the client
- Absence of abnormal heart sounds
- Lungs clear to auscultation
- Absence of peripheral or dependent edema
- Mental status within normal limits for the client
- Urine output at least 30 mL/hr
- Absence of fatigue and weakness

EXPECTED OUTCOMES FOR THE CLIENT WITH *RISK FOR PERIPHERAL NEUROVASCULAR DYSFUNCTION*

Risk for peripheral neurovascular dysfunction is a narrowly focused diagnosis that addresses impaired circulation to an extremity. Interrupted blood flow or pressure that compresses vessels damages nerves. Immediate intervention is essential to achieve the goal of preserving neurovascular function. Expected outcomes that indicate adequate neurovascular function include the following:

- Palpable peripheral pulses
- Skin warm and pink
- Capillary refill in less than 3 seconds
- Absence of pallor, pain, paresthesia, or paralysis of the extremity

EXPECTED OUTCOMES FOR THE CLIENT WITH *SHOCK*

Expected outcomes for the client with shock include the following:

- Adequate tissue perfusion: client alert and oriented, skin warm and dry, vital signs stable, urine output at least 50 mL/hr
- Blood pressure, pulse, respiration within parameters set by the physician (usually, systolic >100 mm Hg, pulse <100 beats per minute, respiration <30 breaths per minute)
- No complications related to shock; no signs/symptoms of neurological, renal, gastrointestinal, peripheral vascular, or respiratory ischemia or dysfunction

INTERVENTION

Nurses intervene to maximize cardiovascular function and tissue perfusion. Nurses intervene both in prevention and by supporting the client during medical treatment.

BOX 35-4 *Cross-Cultural Care*

Caring for an Amish Client

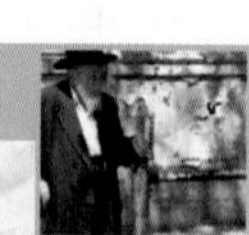

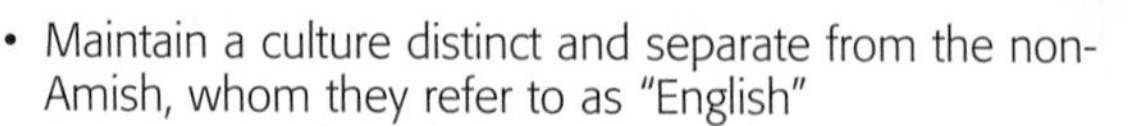

Mr. Yoder is an older man of Amish descent. He still follows the Old Order Amish beliefs and practices of his parents. Mr. Yoder turned over the management of the farm to his sons 5 years ago. He currently works as a cabinetmaker in his carpenter shop in the family barn. Mr. Yoder, his wife, their three sons, and their families all live close by on the farm. Within Amish communities, strict as well as more moderate practices exist. It is important to clarify individual practices of Amish clients. Leininger (1991) and Brewer and Bonalumi (1995) identified the following beliefs and practices as being common to the Old Order Amish:

- Maintain a culture distinct and separate from the non-Amish, whom they refer to as "English"
- Reject materialism and worldliness
- Value living simply; may choose to avoid technology, such as electricity and cars
- Avoid vanity; dress in handmade, unadorned clothing
- Highly value responsibility, generosity, and helping others
- Often work as farmers, builders, quilters, and homemakers
- Use traditional health care and alternative health care, such as healers, herbs, and massage
- Believe that health is a gift from God, but that clean living and a balanced diet help to maintain it
- May choose not to have health insurance

INTERVENTIONS TO MAXIMIZE TISSUE PERFUSION

A functional circulatory system depends on patent blood vessels. Nursing actions that maintain open blood vessels and dynamic blood flow maximize circulation.

Modifying Risk Factors. Preventing problems of tissue perfusion is a primary nursing goal; therefore you will spend time teaching clients how to reduce their risk factors for cardiovascular disease. Although genetic tendencies contribute to the development of atherosclerosis, risk factor modification slows the atherosclerotic process and protects the circulatory system. Clients of all ages benefit from preventive teaching about diet, cholesterol control, weight management, exercise, and controlling concurrent health problems that contribute to atherosclerosis.

Diet. A diet low in cholesterol and saturated fat benefits clients by decreasing the amount of fats available to form atherosclerotic deposits. Box 35-5 gives tips for helping clients decrease their dietary fat intake.

Another benefit of a low-cholesterol diet is better maintenance of optimum body weight. Fats provide 9 kcal/g, whereas carbohydrates and proteins provide only 4 kcal/g. Thus diets high in fat are also high in calories. Excess fat intake is stored as adipose tissue.

BOX 35-5 *Teaching for Wellness*

Decreasing Dietary Fat Intake

Changing ingrained food habits is difficult for most clients. To foster success, identify food preferences, patterns of eating, and commonly used food preparation methods. Stress the value of making small changes in the diet initially; then build on the client's success. Help the client, or the person who prepares the food, to adapt favorite recipes.

Purpose: To educate clients about dietary sources of cholesterol and saturated fat.

Expected Outcome: The client will be able to select low-fat food options.

Client Instructions

Certain foods are high in fat and cholesterol; these substances contribute to the formation of fatty deposits inside blood vessels that can eventually lead to heart and circulatory problems. Offer clients these tips to lower fat intake:

- Avoid visible fats, such as butter and oils, especially coconut oil.
- Use vegetable oil sprays rather than bottled oil when cooking.
- Limit red meats and processed food such as hot dogs and luncheon meats.
- Use skim or 2% milk rather than whole milk.
- Substitute egg whites for whole eggs if possible when baking.
- Limit dairy products made with whole milk or cream, such as cheese and ice cream.
- Remove the skin from poultry before cooking it.
- Eat desserts, such as cakes, pies, and candy, sparingly.

Exercise. Exercise enhances circulatory health in several ways. It helps control weight by increasing caloric expenditure. It also increases the proportion of high-density lipoproteins in the blood; these lipoproteins protect blood vessels. Finally, it stimulates the development of collateral circulation and new blood vessels that supplement tissue perfusion. Box 35-6 describes exercise guidelines for cardiovascular fitness.

Concurrent Health Problems. Underlying health problems, such as hypertension and diabetes mellitus, accelerate atherosclerosis. Teach clients about the relationships between these conditions and circulation, and encourage them to comply with treatment regimens. Careful management and consistent follow-up care keep these problems under better control and may delay the development of circulatory complications.

Preventing Vasoconstriction. Even moderate degrees of vasoconstriction can compromise circulation for clients with already narrowed blood vessels. Improper positioning, cold temperatures, nicotine, and emotional stress are common causes of vasoconstriction.

Positioning. Compression of blood vessels slows and can even obstruct circulation. To help prevent the effects of vessel compression, change the client's position frequently, and limit prolonged sitting. Instruct affected clients not to cross their legs for long periods while in bed. Do not place pillows behind a client's knees, and do not use the knee elevator on the Gatch bed.

Position facilitates circulation. However, optimal positioning depends on the nature of the client's health problem. For a client with arterial insufficiency, place the legs in a dependent position to enhance arterial blood flow. Elevate the legs of a client with venous insufficiency because this position uses gravity to improve

BOX 35-6 *Teaching for Wellness*

Guidelines for Exercise

Purpose: To help the client recognize the cardiovascular benefits of regular exercise.

Expected Outcome: The client will develop and implement an exercise plan.

Client Instructions

- Exercise promotes circulatory health. To be beneficial, it should be done regularly and energetically.
- Check with your physician before beginning any exercise program.
- Ask your physician to establish your target heart rate.
- Select activities that produce rhythmic contractions of large muscles; walking, biking, swimming, and rowing are examples of good choices.
- Participate in exercise three to five times a week.
- Engage in exercise for at least 20 to 30 minutes per session.
- Check your pulse to see that you maintain your target heart rate for 20 minutes.

venous return. Because veins have little elastic tissue, they are very distensible. Elastic stockings provide external support for veins and minimize venous pooling. Active range of motion and ambulation also assist venous return. Muscular contractions of the legs during activity compress veins and drive blood back to the heart.

Cold Temperatures. Peripheral vasoconstriction is a normal physiological response to conserve body heat. However, some underlying circulatory dysfunctions produce more pronounced and prolonged vasoconstriction. For example, Raynaud's disease causes severe arterial spasms when the limbs are exposed to cold temperatures. Teach affected clients to dress warmly, wear mittens, and layer clothing to minimize vasoconstrictive episodes.

Nicotine. Nicotine also causes vasoconstriction. Teach a client with circulatory problems about the effects of nicotine on blood vessels, and encourage smoking cessation. Health care providers have tried a variety of smoking cessation strategies. On an outpatient basis, nicotine gum and patches have been found to help some smokers. Intensive counseling combined with these tools may increase the chances of success.

To maximize a client's success with smoking cessation, offer information about the range of available options. Provide a list of available support groups, and help the client select the support option that will be most effective. Both the American Heart Association and the American Cancer Society sponsor community programs.

Emotional Stress. Emotional stress activates the fight-or-flight response, in which vasoconstriction diverts blood to essential body systems. Teach your client how to reduce stress through deep breathing, progressive relaxation, and imagery. Provide clients with the information they need to maintain their cardiovascular health (Box 35-7).

Administering Medications. For high-risk clients, anticoagulant therapy may prevent occlusion of arteries. You will monitor the client and provide education about medications. Antiplatelet aggregates, anticoagulants, and vasodilators are medications that improve circulation or prevent complications in clients at risk. Antiplatelet aggregates, such as acetylsalicylic acid (aspirin) and clopidogrel (Plavix), reduce the stickiness or adhesiveness of platelets. Clot formation decreases when platelets are less adhesive.

Anticoagulants act directly to increase coagulation time by interrupting a step in the clotting cascade. Examples of anticoagulant medications are warfarin (Coumadin) and heparin. Clients who take an anticoagulant are at risk for bleeding. Observe their gums, skin, urine, and stool carefully for signs of visible bleeding. Using chemical reagents such as Hemoccult and Hemastix, body secretions or excretions can be tested for occult (hidden) blood. Institute safety precautions for all clients who receive anticoagulants. Encourage use of a soft-bristle toothbrush and electric razor to prevent injuries and bleeding.

Monitor serum PT or INR for Coumadin therapy or partial thromboplastin time (PTT) for heparin therapy. Report current coagulation results to the physician before administering an anticoagulant.

Action Alert! Frequently assess clients on anticoagulation therapy for signs of bleeding.

In addition, some clients with impaired circulation receive vasodilating medications. These medications enlarge the lumens of blood vessels to deliver a greater volume of blood to the tissues. These medications produce vasodilation by various pharmacological actions. Table 35-4 reviews vasodilating medications and nursing responsibilities.

Preventing Surgical Complications. All postoperative clients are at risk for developing deep vein thrombosis. Positioning during a surgical procedure and decreased activity afterward slow circulation. Stagnation of blood in the lower extremities favors clot formation. Frequent changes of position and early ambulation help to prevent deep vein thrombosis.

A client with severe circulatory disease unresponsive to medications and other treatments may require surgery to restore circulation and improve tissue perfusion. These procedures include the removal of obstructions and bypassing of diseased vessels.

BOX 35-7 *Teaching for Self-Care*

Maintaining Cardiovascular Health

Purpose: To promote cardiovascular health.
Expected Outcome: The client will implement practices for cardiovascular health

Client Instructions

- Exercise regularly.
- Keep weight within normal limits.
- Eat a balanced diet; avoid fatty foods.
- Have your blood pressure, blood glucose, and cholesterol levels checked by your physician.
- Do not smoke.
- Take time to relax.

INTERVENTIONS TO IMPROVE CARDIAC OUTPUT

Cardiac output changes on the basis of the tissue's needs for oxygen. Therefore, a primary nursing goal for clients with *Decreased cardiac output* is to lessen the need for oxygen at the tissue level. Interventions that decrease oxygen demand ease the heart's workload.

Promoting Rest. Rest is a strategy for conserving a client's energy and decreasing oxygen demand. Remember that the need is for physical and emotional rest because both types of activity boost oxygen demand. Even normal activities, such as turning in bed and coughing, affect cardiac output and oxygen demand for clients with limited cardiac reserves.

Schedule frequent, uninterrupted rest periods for these clients. Help them with activities of daily living. Space activities such as eating, bathing, and ambulating so clients have rest periods in between. Monitor pulse, blood pressure, respirations, and skin color before and after activities to evaluate each client's activity tolerance. Place necessary items, such as water and the call light, within easy reach to conserve the client's energy.

> ***Action Alert!*** Assess vital signs before, during, and after activity. Terminate any activity that provokes hypotension, tachycardia, dyspnea, or chest pain.

A quiet environment promotes rest. In contrast, loud noises, frequent interruptions, and numerous visitors can exhaust clients. Do your best to limit external stimuli to promote a restful environment for a client with impaired cardiovascular function. Involve the client when identifying interventions that contribute to a restful environment. For example, some clients prefer a darkened room for a nap, and others find music relaxing.

Positioning to Improve Cardiac Output. Dilation of the heart with congested blood stretches myocardial fibers beyond the limits of optimum elastic recoil, which further diminishes cardiac contractility. Positioning eases cardiac workload and helps prevent complications. Placing the client in a semi-Fowler's to a high-Fowler's position decreases venous return and preload by pooling blood in the lower extremities. Lowering preload decreases the risk of heart congestion and the development of heart failure. Elevating the head of the bed also optimizes chest expansion and oxygen intake, which in turn reduce the dyspnea and shortness of breath associated with heart failure.

Avoiding Valsalva Maneuver. Teach cardiac clients to avoid the Valsalva maneuver. Instruct them not to hold their breath while moving or turning in bed. Assist clients with position changes by lowering the head of the bed before turning and by helping with the turn.

Bearing down during bowel movements also induces the Valsalva maneuver, especially if the client is constipated. Assess the frequency and consistency of the client's bowel movements. If it is not contraindicated, encourage fluid intake to keep stools soft. Offer foods that increase gastrointestinal motility, such as fruits and fruit juices. Gather input from clients about successful strategies used at home to relieve constipation. Administer stool softeners as ordered.

Avoiding Stimulants. Teach clients to avoid stimulants because these substances increase heart rate and oxygen demand. Some over-the-counter medications, such as

Table 35-4 Vasodilating Medications

MEDICATION	ACTION	SIDE EFFECTS	NURSING RESPONSIBILITIES
NITRATES			
• Nitroglycerin (Nitro-Bid, Transderm-Nitro)	• Relaxes vascular smooth muscles and decreases venous return and preload • Dilates coronary vessels • Dilates systemic vessels, thus decreasing afterload	• Headache • Flushing • Hypotension	• Monitor blood pressure, especially with position change. • Report dizziness, headaches. • Instruct client to avoid alcohol.
CALCIUM CHANNEL BLOCKERS			
• Verapamil (Calan) • Nifedipine (Procardia) • Amlodipine besylate (Norvasc) • Diltiazem (Cardizem)	• Slows movement of calcium into vascular smooth muscle, resulting in relaxation and vasodilation	• Hypotension • Dizziness • Constipation • Peripheral edema	• Monitor vital signs. • Encourage intake of fluids and fiber. • Assess for edema. • Instruct client that medication interacts with digoxin and some gastrointestinal medication; thus should report all current medications to physician.
BETA-ADRENERGIC BLOCKERS			
• Carvedilol (Coreg) • Metoprolol (Lopressor, Toprol) • Atenolol (Tenormin) • Labetalol (Normodyne)	• Competes for norepinephrine binding site, thus blocking beta-1 and/or beta-2 adrenergic actions • Is sometimes added to regimen for heart failure	• Fatigue • Hypotension • Bradycardia • Insomnia • Depression • Heart failure	• Monitor blood pressure, pulse. • Monitor for signs and symptoms of heart failure. • Instruct client to consult physician before beginning an exercise program. • Never discontinue medication abruptly.

appetite suppressants and cold medications, contain stimulants. Advise clients to check with their physician before using these types of medications. Instruct clients to avoid dietary stimulants as well, such as coffee, tea, and chocolate. Offer appropriate dietary substitutes such as decaffeinated beverages and fruits.

Maintaining Fluid Balance. A normal fluid balance prevents circulatory overload, which a weakened heart may be unable to accommodate. Assess your client's fluid status routinely by monitoring intake, output, and daily weights. Assess the client's breath sounds, jugular vein distention, and dependent areas (such as the ankles) for pitting edema. Prompt detection and treatment of fluid overload prevents the life-threatening complication of pulmonary edema.

Action Alert! Monitor for a sudden onset of dyspnea, feelings of suffocation, cyanosis, gurgling respirations, and frothy sputum. Elevate the head of the bed, and notify the physician immediately. Report dyspnea, shortness of breath, and lung crackles immediately.

Fluid and sodium restriction are used to correct fluid overload, along with a low-sodium diet. See Box 35-8 for foods high in sodium. Some clients need more aggressive treatment to maintain their fluid balance. Diuretics, such as furosemide (Lasix), increase urine output and remove excess fluid from the body. Weighing the client daily evaluates the effectiveness of diuretic medication. Diuretic therapy can cause electrolyte imbalances, especially involving potassium. Monitor the client's electrolyte levels, and report abnormal laboratory data to the physician.

Medication Management. Medications are a cornerstone in the treatment of cardiovascular problems. They are used to enhance cardiac output, as well as to manage complications associated with *Decreased cardiac output.*

Inotropic Medications. **Inotropic agents** are medications that increase the contractility of the heart muscle, thereby increasing cardiac output. Digoxin (Lanoxin) is a commonly used inotropic medication. Assess the client's apical heart rate and rhythm for a full minute before administering this drug. Report pulse rates below 60 or above 110 beats per minute to the physician before giving it. The medication dose may need to be adjusted. Also, check the client's serum potassium level; low potassium levels predispose the client to digitalis toxicity. Review the client's serum digoxin level, if ordered, and report a level outside of the therapeutic range (0.5 to 2.0 ng/mL) to the physician.

Antidysrhythmic Medications. Hypoxic myocardium is prone to develop an abnormality of heart rate or rhythm (dysrhythmia). Dysrhythmias pose a serious threat because they further impair cardiac output.

Assess the apical pulse for regularity. If you detect a dysrhythmia, note the pattern and frequency of the irregularity, blood pressure, apical-radial pulse, and skin color. Report hypotension, apical-radial pulse deficit, and pale, moist skin to the physician. Antidysrhythmic medications and other treatments may be needed to correct rhythm disturbances.

BOX 35-8 *Foods High in Sodium: The Six Ss*

The following types of foods are high in sodium:

- Soups
- Sauces
- Salty snacks
- Smoked meat or fish
- Sauerkraut and other pickled food
- Seasonings

Modified from Dudek, S. G. (2005). *Nutrition handbook for nursing practice* (5th ed.). Philadelphia: Lippincott.

Antihypertensive Medications. ACE inhibitors are an important component of treating left ventricular systolic dysfunction; these medications have been found to be superior to digitalis in reducing mortality. Medications that lower blood pressure, such as nitrates (nitroglycerin), captopril (Capoten), and nifedipine (Procardia), ease the workload of the heart and improve cardiac output. Dilation of vessels allows greater blood flow, and a lower blood pressure decreases afterload, thus enabling the heart to eject blood with less effort.

Carefully monitor the blood pressure of any client receiving an antihypertensive medication. Evaluate the response to the medication by checking for orthostatic hypotension—decreases in blood pressure when the client changes from lying to sitting to standing positions. If dizziness or light-headedness occurs, take safety precautions to prevent falls. Instruct clients to call for help before getting out of bed. Teach them to change positions slowly and to sit on the side of the bed for a few minutes before standing.

Increasing Oxygen Supply. Clients with impaired cardiac output deliver less oxygen-rich blood to tissues. Some pathophysiological causes of decreases in cardiac output are irreversible, and others take time to correct. In either instance, interventions may involve strategies to enhance available oxygen. Increasing the oxygen supply helps the client perfuse tissues more easily.

Administering Oxygen. Clients with *Decreased cardiac output* require a careful balance between oxygen demand and supply. Administration of oxygen by nasal cannula increases the supply side of the supply-and-demand equation. Supplemental oxygen increases the oxygen available for use by the circulatory system. Nursing responsibilities for clients receiving oxygen therapy are addressed in Chapter 34.

Avoiding Smoking. Smoking is contraindicated in all situations where circulation is less than optimal because nicotine causes vasoconstriction. The reduced diameter of blood vessels during vasoconstriction lessens the amount of oxygenated blood that can be delivered to body tissues. Teach clients about the physiological effects of nicotine and the relationship between smoking and cardiovascular disease. Provide emotional support to clients who are trying to quit smoking.

Positioning to Facilitate Breathing. Positioning optimizes chest expansion and enhances respiratory effectiveness. Elevating the head of the bed facilitates respirations by shifting the abdominal organs downward in the abdominal cavity and providing maximum space for chest expansion. This position enables the client to breathe deeply and more effectively.

INTERVENTIONS TO PREVENT PERIPHERAL NEUROVASCULAR DYSFUNCTION

Neurovascular dysfunction is a complication that is largely preventable. You can foster prevention by identifying clients at risk and detecting signs and symptoms as early as possible.

Careful assessment is the cornerstone to preventing neurovascular dysfunction. Follow hospital protocol for the frequency of neurovascular assessment after designated procedures, such as cast application or angiography. Use professional judgment to institute more frequent assessments if the client's condition warrants them.

Assess the involved extremity for color, temperature, pulses, numbness, tingling, and pain. Objective findings—such as pale, cold skin and decreased or absent pulses—require immediate intervention. Numbness, tingling, and pain are subjective symptoms of impaired circulation and nerve irritation. Instruct the client to report any of these sensations promptly.

If the client's condition permits, elevate the extremity to decrease edema, which exerts pressure on nerves and blood vessels. Encourage the client to move the fingers and toes of the involved extremity to enhance venous return and reduce edema. Notify the physician promptly whenever you detect abnormal neurovascular findings. The client may need medical interventions, such as cutting a cast or evacuating accumulated blood from a body compartment.

Action Alert! Immediately report absence of pulse, pallor, pain, paresthesia, and paralysis.

INTERVENTIONS TO MANAGE SHOCK

Shock is a complication of serious circulatory dysfunction. It has a number of distinctive clinical manifestations (Table 35-5). For a client at risk for shock, assess vital signs as often as every 15 minutes. Check for tachycardia and hypotension. Monitor changes in skin color, mental status, and urine output. Detection of shock in the early stage improves the client's prognosis.

Table 35-5 Manifestations of Shock

PARAMETER	ALTERATIONS IN SHOCK
Pulse	Rapid, weak, and thready
Respirations	Rapid and shallow
Blood pressure	Systolic blood pressure below 90 mm Hg
Level of consciousness	Restlessness progressing to lethargy
Skin	Pale, cool, and clammy
Urine output	Less than 20 mL/hr
Thirst	Increased

Clients who develop shock have complex physiological needs; most are transferred to an intensive care unit, where a physician directs their care. The nurse works closely with the physician to implement the plan of care and respond promptly to changes in the client's status.

Maintaining Oxygenation. Oxygenation of tissues is essential for survival of clients in shock. A patent airway and supplemental oxygen help correct oxygen deficits at the tissue level. Clients who can breathe on their own receive oxygen via a nasal cannula or mask. Clients who cannot breathe spontaneously require placement of an endotracheal tube and mechanical ventilation.

Positioning for Shock. Positioning the client in shock depends in part on what caused the shock. For example, in hypovolemic shock, you will elevate the client's feet about 15 to 20 inches above the level of the heart. This position uses gravity to increase venous return, thus helping to maintain stroke volume. In cardiogenic shock, the client cannot expel blood effectively from the heart. Thus, when your priority is to decrease venous return to minimize heart congestion, you will place the client in a semi-Fowler's to high-Fowler's position. However, positioning is not always straightforward; use clinical signs and symptoms and the physician's order to determine the best position for clients in cardiogenic shock.

Maintaining Circulating Blood Volume. Fluid replacement during shock also depends on the underlying cause of the problem. Blood, packed red blood cells, volume expanders (dextran, plasma), and intravenous solutions (usually normal saline or lactated Ringer's) are used to restore circulating blood volume for the client in hypovolemic shock. Procedure 35-1 outlines the steps needed to administer blood safely and accurately. Monitor the client closely for transfusion reactions during blood transfusions.

Action Alert! Monitor the client for chills, rash, dyspnea, chest pain, itching, or changes in vital signs during a transfusion. Stop the transfusion immediately if any signs of a reaction occur. Maintain the client's intravenous line, and stay with the client. Notify the physician immediately.

A client in cardiogenic shock requires very cautious fluid replacement. Care will be given in the intensive care unit, where advanced hemodynamic monitoring devices are used to evaluate the client's tolerance for fluid replacement and to monitor for fluid overload. Hemodynamic monitoring usually refers to the placement of one of various types of catheters into the pulmonary artery to monitor various pressures in the vascular system.

Preventing Complications. For a client in shock, it is important to continuously monitor circulatory status and tissue perfusion. You must be able to quickly recognize progression of shock and deteriorating organ function. Promptly report all changes in the client's vital signs, skin color, mental status, respiratory function, and urine output.

INTERVENTION FOR CARDIAC OR RESPIRATORY ARREST

When a client suddenly stops breathing or the heart suddenly stops, the nurse thinks and acts quickly, responding appropriately to this emergent situation by initiating lifesaving techniques. The action could be as simple as opening an airway or as intense as giving cardiopulmonary resuscitation (CPR) with a full arrest procedure (Procedure 35-2, p. 968). Remember, a fully

Text continued on p. 971

PROCEDURE 35-1

ADMINISTERING BLOOD

Nursing Skills Online: Vascular Access, Lesson 2

TIME TO ALLOW: NOVICE: 20 min. **EXPERT:** 15 min.

Blood and blood products are administered to increase the circulating blood volume after blood loss from surgery, trauma, or other causes of hemorrhage. Packed red blood cells are administered in severe anemia. Fresh frozen plasma is administered to provide clotting factors to help control bleeding in clients with hemophilia. You must be absolutely certain to follow hospital policy to ensure that the blood has been properly typed and crossmatched for the specific client. In addition, you must be fully knowledgeable about transfusion reactions and the management of these reactions.

Complications from transfusions: allergic reaction, anaphylactic reaction, infection, cardiac overload.

DELEGATION GUIDELINES

Some aspects of monitoring a client during a blood transfusion may be delegated to a nursing assistant. The nursing assistant may measure and record vital signs. However, you must provide specific parameters for immediate RN notification. The responsibility for ongoing monitoring and assessment, throughout the transfusion, is yours.

EQUIPMENT NEEDED

- Y type of IV tubing with blood filter
- 250- to 500-mL bag 0.9% normal saline (NaCl)
- Intravenous (IV) site with 18-gauge catheter
- Signed consent form (if required by agency)
- Arm band on client for identification
- Type and crossmatch identification on client arm band
- Properly labeled and identified blood or blood products
- Clean gloves

1 Follow preliminary actions (see inside front cover). Check the physician's order to verify the type of blood product and number of units to be administered. *A physician's order is legally required for the administration of blood products.*

2 Verify that the blood is crossmatched and ready in the blood bank. *Blood must be administered within 20 minutes after leaving the blood bank because it provides an excellent medium for bacterial growth. Blood that has been at room temperature for a prolonged period raises the client's risk of infection.*

3 Ask the client about allergies and any previous reactions to blood transfusion. *This step identifies clients at risk for possible transfusion reactions.*

4 Follow your institution's procedures for consent forms. *Most institutions require informed consent before blood can be administered.*

5 Assess and document the client's blood pressure, pulse, respiration, and temperature on the transfusion record. *Baseline vital signs are required before transfusion. Deviations in vital signs during the transfusion indicate an adverse reaction to the blood.*

6 Assemble the necessary equipment.

7 Obtain the blood from the blood bank.

8 Together with another RN, compare the blood and crossmatch slip from the blood bank. Also compare the data with the client's identification band. Verify and document that the following data match: client's name, client's ID number, blood type and Rh factor, donor number on blood container, and expiration date of blood. *The correct blood product must be administered to the correct client to prevent a transfusion reaction.*

9 Don gloves. *Standard precautions mandate gloves in situations in which you could be exposed to blood or body fluids*

10 Prime the Y tubing by following these steps (see illustration):

a. Close all clamps on the Y tubing.
b. Insert one spike of the Y tubing into the bag of normal saline.
c. Open the clamp, and prime the arm of the Y tubing, drip chamber, and tubing below the chamber.
d. Clamp the tubing.
e. Gently rotate the unit of blood.

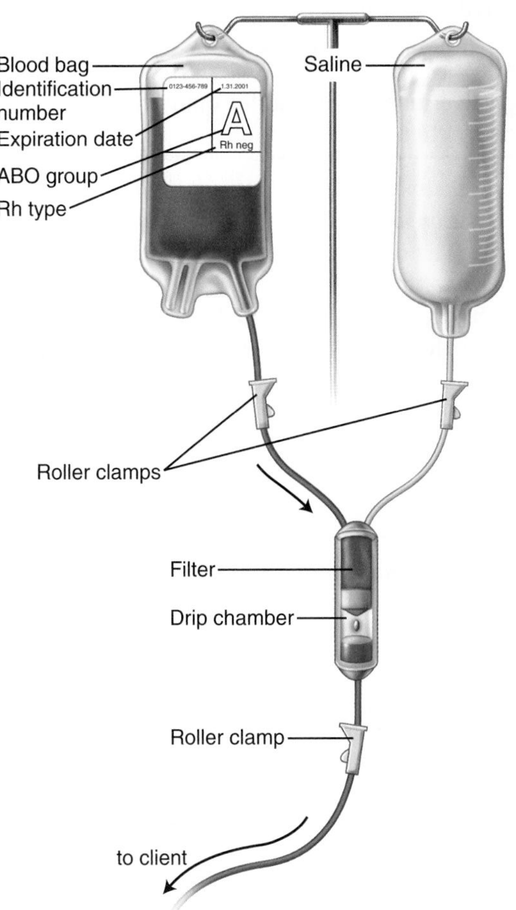

Step 10. Setup for blood administration.

f. Insert the second spike of the Y tubing into the port on the unit of blood.
g. Open the clamp, and prime the arm of the Y tubing to the drip chamber.
h. Close the clamp.

11 If the client does not have an IV line in place, perform a venipuncture with an 18- or 19-gauge catheter. *IV catheters smaller than 18 gauge will damage blood cells and slow the transfusion rate.*

12 Open the clamp on the normal saline, and infuse about 50 mL of saline at a slow rate. *This step verifies patency of the IV line before starting the transfusion.*

13 Close the clamp on the normal saline solution.

14 Open the clamp on the blood, and infuse at a keep-open rate for 15 minutes. Stay with the client throughout this time. *Most transfusion reactions occur within the first 15 minutes of the infusion.*

15 Monitor the client's vital signs, and watch for signs of a transfusion reaction according to your institution's protocol. *Signs of a transfusion reaction include chills, flushing, headache, rash, chest or back pain, nausea, fever, tachycardia, respiratory distress, and hypotension.*

16 If the client has no adverse reactions after 15 minutes, infuse the blood at the prescribed rate.

17 Continue to monitor the client's vital signs and responses according to your institution's protocol. *Most institutions require assessment of vital signs every 15 minutes for the first hour and every 30 minutes thereafter until the transfusion is complete. Ongoing assessment is needed to detect a delayed transfusion reaction.*

18 When the transfusion is complete, flush the IV line with normal saline solution.

19 Complete the transfusion record, and return the designated portion of the form to the blood bank with the empty blood bag. *This step verifies the client's identity and the blood product that was transfused.*

20 Place the designated portion of the transfusion record in the client's chart.

21 Document the following aspects of the transfusion procedure in the client's chart: date, time transfusion started, type and identification number of blood product, time transfusion ended, and client's response to transfusion.

PROCEDURE 35-2

Time to Allow: **Novice:** 4 min. to initiate CPR **Expert:** 4 min. to initiate CPR

ADULT CARDIOPULMONARY RESUSCITATION

If you discover that a client has stopped breathing, that the heart has stopped beating, or both, you will need to "call a code" and start cardiopulmonary resuscitation (CPR) within 4 minutes of the arrest. Done correctly, this procedure helps keep oxygenated blood flowing to the client's brain and other tissues until help arrives and more definitive therapy can be initiated in the form of advanced cardiac life support (ACLS).

DELEGATION GUIDELINES

The nursing assistant may be the first caregiver to discover a client with a cardiopulmonary arrest. Most institutions therefore require assistive personnel to be competent in CPR or basic life support (BLS). The trained nursing assistant may initiate CPR and call for help. Upon arrival of help, the nursing assistant will be relieved of resuscitative duties and employed to gather and assemble the necessary emergency equipment or to summon other expertise as needed. In an institutional setting, the roles of personnel in such emergencies are often delineated in advance of an actual event.

EQUIPMENT NEEDED

- Bag-valve-mask if available; many hospitals have one in every client room.

1 Assess for unresponsiveness. *To see if the person is responsive, tap his shoulder or gently shake him while loudly speaking his name.*

2 If the person fails to respond, call for help by activating the emergency response system according to your facility's policy. *In most facilities you will ask the switchboard operator to announce a certain code along with the client's location. If you are in the community, you will most likely call 911 or a local emergency response system.*

AIRWAY

3 Make sure the person has an open airway.

a. Position the person on his back on a hard, flat surface, if possible. Place his arms at his sides. *This position maximizes the effectiveness of CPR. If you must roll the person over, use a logroll maneuver, in which the person's entire body rolls as a unit. This process minimizes the risk of twisting his spine.*

b. Open the airway using the head tilt–chin lift maneuver or the jaw thrust maneuver (see illustrations for both). *An unconscious person faces a high risk that his tongue and soft tissues of the pharynx will obstruct his airway. If the person might have a neck injury, use the jaw thrust.*

c. Remove visible food or vomitus from the person's mouth. *If the person has liquid in his mouth, cover your index and middle fingers with a cloth and sweep his mouth. If the person has solid material in his mouth, use your index finger to remove it. Use the finger sweep only when you can see solid material obstructing the airway of an unresponsive client. This maneuver has been known to cause injury to the responder and the client.*

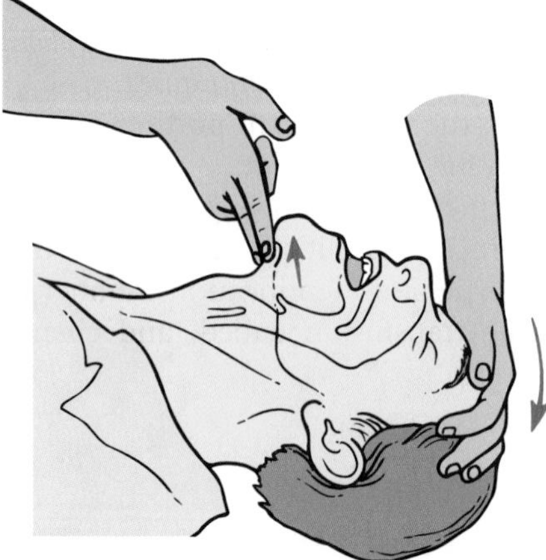

Step 3b. Opening the airway using the head tilt–chin lift maneuver. (From Lewis, S. M., Heitkamper, M. M., & Dirksen, S. R. [2004]. *Medical-surgical nursing: Assessment and management of clinical problems* [6th ed.]. St. Louis: Mosby.

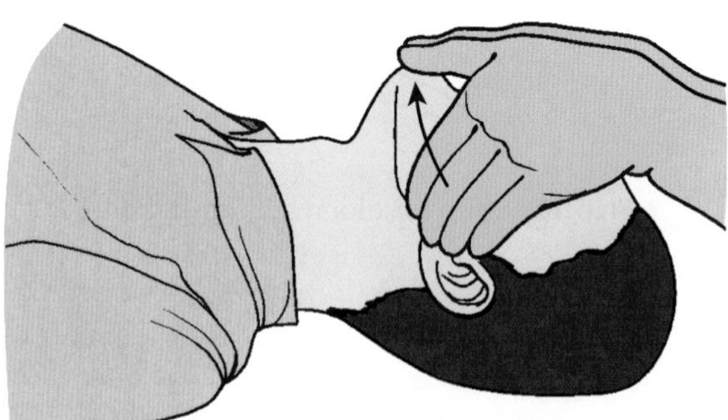

Step 3b. Opening the airway using the jaw thrust maneuver.

Based on American Heart Association. (2005). The American Heart Association 2005 guidelines for cardiopulmonary resuscitation and emergency cardiovascular care. *Circulation, 112*(24, Suppl.). Available at http://www.americanheart.org.

BREATHING

4 Determine whether the person is breathing. Occasional gasps are not adequate breathing; treat the client who has occasional gasps as if he is not breathing.

a. Look to see whether the person's chest rises and falls. If you notice that the person is trying to breathe but cannot, make sure that you have successfully opened the airway. Respiratory effort without exchange of air can mean the victim is trying to breathe against an obstructed airway. Remember that reflex gasping, which occurs early in cardiac arrest, is not adequate to oxygenate the person's blood.
b. Position your ear over the person's mouth and nose. Listen for exhaled air, and see if you can feel air escaping onto your face (see illustration). If you determine that the person is breathing and he has not sustained a traumatic injury, logroll him onto his side (the recovery position), and continue to watch him closely until either he revives or additional help arrives.

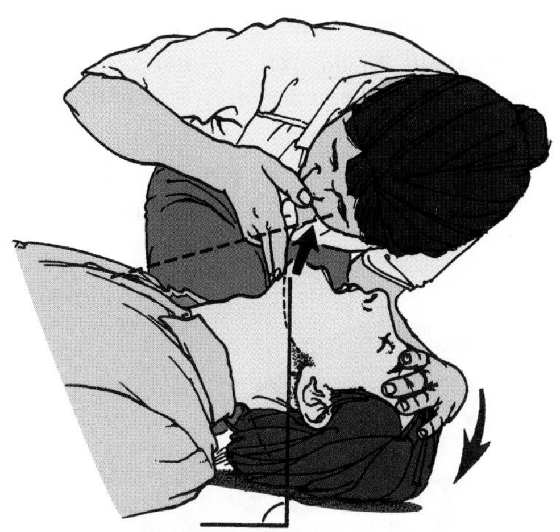

Step 4b. Listening and feeling for exhalation. (From Emergency Cardiac Care Committee and Subcommittees, American Heart Association. [1992]. Guidelines for cardiopulmonary resuscitation and emergency cardiac care. Part 8: Ethical consideration in resuscitation. *Journal of the American Medical Association, 268*[16], 2282-2288.)

5 If you do not detect *adequate* breathing within 10 seconds, give two breaths. Each breath should be only 1 second and only of sufficient volume to raise the chest. *If possible, use a bag-valve-mask or another type of barrier device to administer breaths. If this is not possible, perform mouth to mouth, mouth-to-nose, or mouth-to-stoma breathing. Exhaled air contains enough oxygen to support brain and tissue function. Throughout rescue breathing, remember to keep the airway open.*

a. To administer effective mouth-to-mouth breaths, you will need to keep air from escaping through the person's nose (see illustration). To do so, use the thumb and index finger of the hand resting on the person's forehead to gently pinch his nose closed.

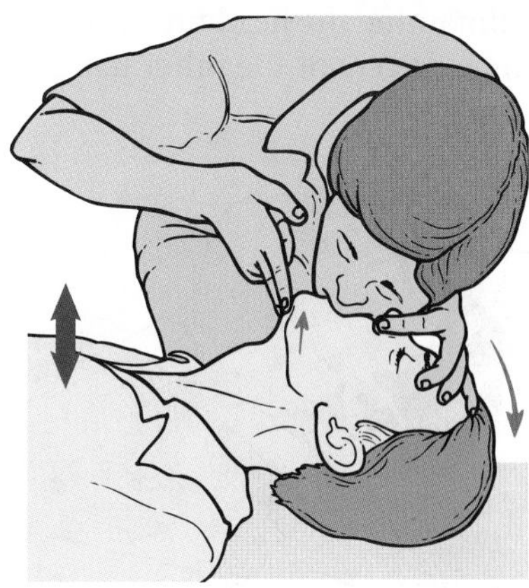

Step 5a. Performing mouth-to-mouth breathing. (From Perry, A. P., & Potter, P. A. [2006]. *Clinical nursing skills and techniques* [6th ed.]. St. Louis: Mosby.)

b. Likewise, to administer effective mouth-to-nose breaths, you will need to keep air from escaping through the person's mouth. Use the hand resting below the person's chin to hold his mouth closed.
c. Take a normal breath, and place your lips around the victim's mouth or nose. *Make sure that your lips have created an airtight seal. If you are using a mouth-to-mouth mask device or bag-valve-mask, hold the edges of the mask against the person's face to make an airtight seal.*
d. Then give two effective breaths. Avoid rapid or forceful breaths. Inhale between breaths if you are not using a bag-valve-mask. *Each breath should last 1 second, long enough to fill the person's lungs. You should see the person's chest rise with each breath (a tidal volume of 500 to 600 mL in an adult). Excessive pressure from rapid, forceful breaths can cause air to enter the person's stomach rather than his lungs and cause regurgitation and aspiration.*
e. After delivering each breath, turn your head so your ear is positioned over the person's mouth and nose. Listen and feel for exhaled air. *If you do not hear or feel the exhalation, reposition the person, make sure his airway is open (by repositioning his head and removing foreign matter as needed), and try again. If you are administering mouth-to-nose breaths, you may need to open the person's mouth to allow exhalation. If you do not get an exchange of air, reposition the victim for a better airway and implement foreign-body airway maneuvers.*

Continued

CIRCULATION

6 Determine pulselessness. Check the pulse at the carotid artery (no more than 10 seconds). *If a pulse is not definitely felt within 10 seconds, proceed with chest compressions.*

a. Locate the carotid artery in the groove between the trachea and the large strap muscles of the neck. While maintaining the head tilt with one hand, place two or three fingers of the other hand in the groove (see illustration).

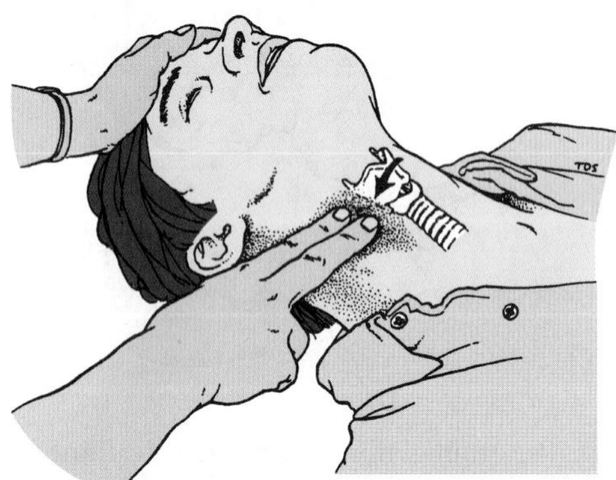

Step 6a. Feeling for the carotid pulse. (From Emergency Cardiac Care Committee and Subcommittees, American Heart Association. [1992]. Guidelines for cardiopulmonary resuscitation and emergency cardiac care. Part 8: Ethical considerations in resuscitation. *Journal of the American Medical Association, 268*[16], 2282-2288.)

b. If there is a pulse but no breathing, initiate rescue breathing at 10 to 12 times a minute.

c. If there is no pulse, begin cardiac compressions.

7 Place hands in the correct position for performing cardiac compressions.

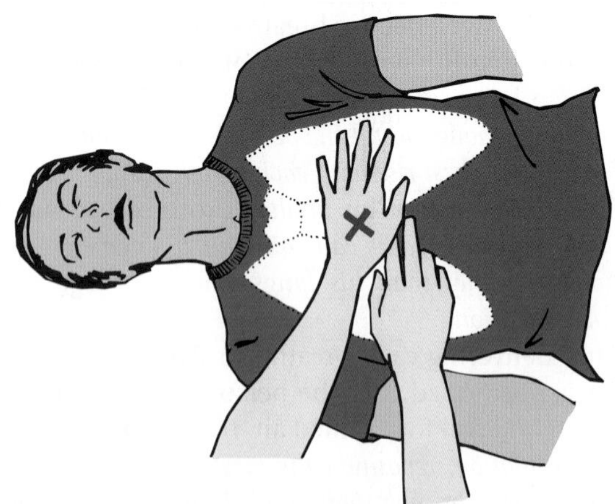

Step 7a. Finding the correct position for external chest compressions. (From Lewis, S. M., Heitkamper, M. M., & Dirksen, S. R. [2004]. *Medical-surgical nursing: Assessment and management of clinical problems* [6th ed.]. St. Louis: Mosby.)

a. Locate the correct hand position on the lower half of the sternum above the xiphoid process. Place the heel of the hand in the center of the chest right between the nipples (see illustration).

b. Place the heel of the second hand on top of the heel of the first hand. Keep your fingers off the chest (see illustration). *If you prefer, you can twine your fingers together to help keep them off the person's chest wall.*

c. Lock your elbows to keep your arms straight. Position your shoulders directly over the sternum, forming a straight line of force from your shoulders through your arms to your hands on the sternum. Apply compression to the chest. Release the compression, and allow the chest to return to its normal position. *The force administered at a right angle (90 degrees) is most effective in compressing the chest. You are using your body weight to aid in compressing the chest. Also, compressing straight down helps keep the person from rolling.*

8 Administer chest compressions. *For effective chest compressions, "push hard and push fast."*

a. With each compression, apply enough force to depress the person's chest by about 1½ to 2 inches. Allow the chest to recoil completely, and allow approximately equal compression and relaxation times. *For a very small person, you may not need this degree of compression. For a large person, you may need more force to create a palpable carotid or femoral pulse. Ideally, a third person will monitor the femoral pulse to determine that the compressions are of sufficient depth to produce a pulse.*

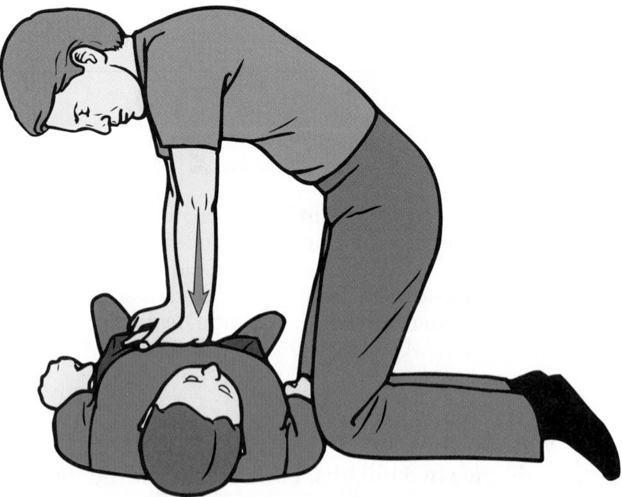

Step 7b. Performing chest compressions. (From Perry, A. P., & Potter, P. A. [2006]. *Clinical nursing skills and techniques* [6th ed.]. St. Louis: Mosby.)

Based on American Heart Association. (2005). The American Heart Association 2005 guidelines for cardiopulmonary resuscitation and emergency cardiovascular care. *Circulation, 112*(24, Suppl.). Available at http://www.americanheart.org.

b. Maintain the recommended rate of 100 compressions per minute. *The rate refers to the speed of compression not the actual number per minute. At this rate, you will actually deliver fewer compressions per minute depending on interruptions for breathing. This rate makes it more likely that the compressions will be effective. Properly performed chest compressions can produce systolic arterial blood pressure peaks of 60 to 80 mm Hg. The person performing chest compressions should be relieved every 2 minutes to prevent fatigue and deterioration in the quality of compressions.*
c. For a one-person or two-person rescue, give two breaths followed by 30 compressions. *Count "one, two, three, four, five, six, seven, eight, nine, ten, eleven, twelve, thirteen, fourteen, fifteen," or "a, b, c, d, e, f, g, h, i, j, k, l, m, n, off." This change in the guidelines for 2005 is based on the belief that less interruption of compressions are needed to maintain blood flow.*
d. Open the airway, and deliver two effective rescue breaths (1 second each).
e. Find the proper hand position, and begin 30 more compressions at a rate of 100 per minute.
f. Perform five complete cycles of 30 compressions and two breaths (or ventilations).
g. Reassess
    - Check for return of the carotid pulse (3 to 5 seconds).
    - If absent, resume CPR with chest compressions.
    - If present, check breathing.
    - If breathing is absent, perform rescue breathing at 10 to 12 breaths per minute and monitor pulse closely.
h. When a second rescuer enters the room, continue through a cycle of compressions. At the end of 30 compressions, open the airway and begin rescue breathing. The second rescuer takes over the chest compressions. At the end of the second breath, the second rescuer begins compressions and counts (out loud) . . . "one, two, three, four, five, ..." Maintain a ratio of 30 compressions to two breaths.
i. When the emergency team arrives, interrupt CPR just long enough for the victim to receive an endotracheal tube, which allows for a well-controlled airway. Connect the bag-valve-mask to 100% oxygen at a high flow rate. *In a hospital CPR procedure, a heart monitor provides direct visual evidence of a heartbeat. The femoral artery pulse is still monitored to determine the effectiveness of the compressions. With an advanced airway, breaths are given without interrupting compressions.*

Based on American Heart Association. (2005). The American Heart Association 2005 guidelines for cardiopulmonary resuscitation and emergency cardiovascular care. *Circulation, 112*(24, Suppl.). Available at http://www.americanheart.org.

trained staff and physician are readily available to assist in the event of a cardiac or respiratory arrest.

CPR is synonymous with the term basic life support (BLS), which consists of the noninvasive assessments and interventions used to treat victims of respiratory or cardiovascular emergencies and stroke. It can include automated external defibrillation. Advanced cardiovascular life support (ACLS) consists of the medical interventions used to treat victims of respiratory or cardiac emergencies and stroke; it includes invasive techniques such as intubation and administration of drugs.

CPR in a health care setting is initiated by the staff member who finds the victim. The plan for initiation includes calling for help by notifying the telephone operator to page for the cardiac arrest response team. You should know the code, and ask the operator to page (give the code) for (give the location). The cardiac arrest or emergency management response team usually includes a respiratory therapist, an intensive care nurse, an experienced general duty nurse, and a physician. Someone to draw blood for the laboratory and a technician with a portable x-ray machine may also respond to the code.

As many as eight people may be on the team to respond to the arrest procedure. Each person has a specific task, assigned in advance, as follows:

- Inserting an endotracheal tube and using an Ambu bag to breathe for the victim
- Performing chest compressions
- Starting an intravenous line
- Setting up intravenous solutions
- Preparing and administering medications
- Attaching a heart monitor, pulse oximeter
- Recording the procedure (legal documentation)
- Caring for the family
- Making contacts with a physician, laboratory, radiology technician, ECG technician

EVALUATION

Evaluation and documentation of a client's status involves comparing current data with the outcome criteria previously established. Box 35-9 gives a nursing care plan for Mr. Yoder at the time of admission.

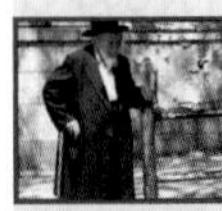

On the third day after admission, Mr. Yoder gets the news that his cardiac catheterization shows moderate atherosclerosis of the coronary arteries. His serum cholesterol and lipid profile are elevated. Mr. Yoder is to be discharged. He is to start taking an antianginal medication and to restrict his activity until he sees his physician for follow-up care in 1 week. In addition, Mr. Yoder is to begin a low-cholesterol diet.

BOX 35-9

Nursing Care Plan

A Client With Angina Pectoris

Admission Data

Mr. Yoder is admitted with chest pain. On arrival in the nursing unit, he reports dull chest pain radiating to the left arm. He rates his pain as 7 on a scale of 0 to 10. The admitting diagnosis is unstable angina pectoris.

Physician's Orders

Bed rest with bathroom privileges
Oxygen 3 LPM per nasal cannula
Stat ECG
Insert saline lock
Nitroglycerin gr 1/150 sublingual prn for chest pain, up to 3 doses
Morphine 3-6 mg IV q5min prn up to 3 doses, for chest pain unrelieved by nitroglycerin
Vital signs q2h
Cardiac monitor
CBC, prothrombin time, and lipid profile in AM
Schedule for cardiac catheterization in AM

Nursing Assessment

Mr. Yoder is lying quietly in bed and appears anxious. His wife is at the bedside. Vital signs: BP 150/92 left arm, lying; P 92 apical, regular; R 24, regular. Color pale.

NANDA-I Nursing Diagnosis	NOC Expected Outcomes With Indicators	NIC Interventions With Selected Activities	Evaluation Data
Ineffective Cardiopulmonary Tissue Perfusion **Related Factor:**	***Tissue Perfusion: Cardiac***	***Cardiac Care***	***Data Collected 2 Hours After Admission***
• Occlusion of coronary artery.	• Vital signs within normal limits (WNL)	• Evaluate chest pain.	• Chest pain relieved by nitroglycerin sublingual ×1; it has not recurred.
	• Angina not present	• Provide means to summon nurse, and let client and family know the call will be answered immediately.	
		• Monitor cardiac rhythm and rate.	• Normal sinus rhythm; BP 120/80, P 80, R 18.
		• Auscultate heart and lung sounds. • Monitor neurological status.	• Reports decreased anxiety; resting quietly; wife is at bedside.
		• Monitor effectiveness of oxygen therapy.	• Is able to describe cardiac catheterization procedure and purpose.
		• Monitor for psychological effects of underlying condition. • Administer nitroglycerin and morphine prn to relieve pain. • Monitor for activity tolerance.	• Has signed consent form.

Critical Thinking Questions

1. How would you help Mrs. Yoder with her anxiety while Mr. Yoder is having his catheterization?
2. Mr. Yoder will probably need an angioplasty to treat his angina. Mrs. Yoder believes that he will not be able to work again, even though the physician has not said this. How would you help Mrs. Yoder?
3. The nurse from the cardiac catheterization laboratory tells you to get ready because Mr. Yoder is returning to his room. How frequently do you think you should take his vital signs?

Nursing outcome and intervention labels from Johnson, M., Bulechek, G., Butcher, H., Dochterman, J. M., Maas, M., Moorhead, S., et al. (Eds.). (2006). *NANDA, NOC, and NIC linkages: Nursing diagnoses, outcomes, & interventions.* St. Louis, MO: Mosby.

A sample of nursing documentation at the time of discharge for Mr. Yoder might include the following.

SAMPLE DOCUMENTATION FOR MR. YODER

Denies chest pain at rest. Skin warm and dry. All peripheral pulses strong and equal bilaterally. Vital signs at rest BP 132/82, P 78 and regular, R 18. Ambulated 75 feet in hall. Vital signs after ambulation BP 138/88, P 82 and regular, R 20 and unlabored. Denies chest pain with activity. Verbalizes medication regimen, "I will take the lisinopril in the morning and at night. If I have chest pain, I will rest and put a nitroglycerin tablet under my tongue. I can take up to three nitroglycerin pills at 5-minute intervals. Then, if I still have chest pain, I need to go to the emergency room." The client and his wife demonstrate comprehension of the low-cholesterol diet by selecting low-fat foods from sample menus. Client states that he will restrict activity to walking to the barn and back for next week. Clinic appointment scheduled for next week; son will transport.

These data identify that Mr. Yoder is no longer experiencing the chest pain that initially brought him to the hospital. His current level of activity tolerance is documented, as well as his activity restriction after discharge. Safety precautions for home management of chest pain and medication regimen are documented. The dietary risk factor modification plan is identified. Because the client's wife is the primary cook, Mrs. Yoder was included in dietary teaching. Peripheral circulation is specifically addressed because Mr. Yoder had a cardiac catheterization 1 day before discharge.

▼ KEY PRINCIPLES

- Circulation is essential for life and optimal function of all body systems.
- Age, genetic predisposition, underlying health problems, and medications can affect circulation.
- Risk-factor modification enhances circulatory health and delays the development of cardiovascular complications.
- Changes in the effectiveness of the heart as a pump, the integrity of blood vessels, or the dynamics of blood flow produce both (1) acute, life-threatening and (2) chronic, long-term manifestations.
- The heart, brain, and kidneys are especially vulnerable to decreased blood supply.
- *Decreased cardiac output* occurs when the heart pumps ineffectively; this threatens blood delivery to body tissues.
- *Ineffective tissue perfusion* results when blood vessels are narrowed by atherosclerosis, vasoconstriction, or obstruction.
- *Risk for neurovascular dysfunction* exists when the nerves are deprived of oxygen.
- Vital signs, peripheral pulses, skin color, level of consciousness, and urine output provide clues about cardiovascular function.
- Early detection and prompt intervention to restore circulation improve client outcomes.
- The health care team works collaboratively to provide acute and long-term care for clients with cardiovascular dysfunction.

■ REVIEW QUESTIONS

1. Your client has had a cardiac angiogram with the catheter passed through his right femoral artery. Which is the highest priority nursing intervention?
1. Decreasing anxiety by having the physician explain the results
2. Allowing his family to visit to know he is recovering well
3. Bilateral comparison of his pedal pulses
4. Taking his vital signs

2. Your client is on a low-fat diet to prevent coronary artery disease. Select the breakfast menu that would be the most consistent with this diet.
1. Two boiled eggs, bacon, 8 ounces whole milk, orange juice
2. Whole wheat toast, two slices Canadian bacon, 8 ounces skim milk, a fresh peach
3. A cheese omelet made with egg substitute, a cinnamon roll, and coffee
4. An egg McMuffin and coffee with cream

3. Your client has a dysrhythmia called atrial fibrillation with a heart rate of 250 beats per minute. Which of the following clusters of data would be consistent with this condition?
1. Decreased blood pressure, pale cool skin, mental confusion, pulse oximetry less than 90%
2. Edema of the feet and legs, fatigue, diminished pedal pulses, brisk skin turgor
3. Claudication, shortness of breath, hemoptysis, elevated blood pressure
4. Hyperalertness, anxiety, cyanosis, and a rising diastolic pressure

4. Your client is on Coumadin. His INR is 3.0. Which of the following would be important to teach him?
1. The signs and symptoms of bleeding and prevention of injury
2. Maintaining a low-sodium diet
3. Monitoring his blood pressure daily
4. The importance of taking the prescription until it is gone

5. Your client has chronic chest pain from partially occluded coronary arteries. He only has episodes once a month. Which of the following medications would most likely be ordered to treat the pain?
1. A beta-adrenergic blocker daily
2. A calcium channel blocker qid
3. Nitroglycerine prn
4. Coumadin daily

Bibliography

American Heart Association. (2006). Heart disease and stroke statistics—2006 update: A report from the American Heart Association Statistics Committee and Stroke Statistics Subcommittee. *Circulation 113*,e85-e15. Available at http://www.circulationaha.org.

American Heart Association. (2005). The American Heart Association 2005 guidelines for cardiopulmonary resuscitation and emergency cardiovascular care. *Circulation, 112*(24, Suppl.). Available at http://www.americanheart.org.

Appel, S. J. (2004). Metabolic syndrome: Broadening the understanding of African-American women's risk for cardiovascular disease. *Journal of National Black Nurses' Association, 15*(1), vii-ix.

Artinian, N. T., Schim, S. M., Vander Wal, J. S., & Nies, M. A. (2004). Eating patterns and cardiovascular disease risk in a Detroit Mexican American population. *Public Health Nursing, 21*(5), 425-434.

Aschenbrenner, D. S. (2004). Drug watch. HRT reconsidered: What should you tell patients about it now? *American Journal of Nursing, 104*(6), 51-54.

Bauer, J. (2005). Clinical highlights. Does aspirin protect women the way it protects men? *RN, 68*(5), [25], 76-77, 33.

Bazzano, L. A., He, J., Muntner, P., Vupputuri, S., & Whelton, P. K. (2003). Relationship between cigarette smoking and novel risk factors for cardiovascular disease in the United States. *Annals of Internal Medicine, 138*(11), 891-897.

*Brewer, J. A., & Bonalumi, N. M. (1995). Cultural diversity in the emergency department: Health care beliefs and practices among Pennsylvania Amish. *Emergency Nursing, 21*(6), 494-497.

Capriotti, T. (2004). Nursing pharmacology. Any science behind the hype of 'natural' dietary supplements? *Medsurg Nursing, 13*(5), 339-345, 350.

CCRN review: Cardiopulmonary system. (2005). *Nursing, 35*(4), 32cc6, [32cc8].

Dudek, S. G. (2005). *Nutrition handbook for nursing practice* (5th ed.). Philadelphia: Lippincott.

Fletcher, B. J., Gulanick, M., & Braun, L. T. (2005). Physical activity and exercise for elders with cardiovascular disease. *Medsurg Nursing, 14*(2), 101-110.

*Fox, M. K., Crepinek, M. K., Connor, P., & Battaglia, M. (2001). *School nutrition dietary assessment study—II.* Final report submitted to the U.S. Department of Agriculture, Food and Nutrition Service. Cambridge, MA: Abt Associates.

*Gulanick, M., & Cofer, L. A. (2000). Coronary risk factors: Influences on the lipid profile. *Journal of Cardiovascular Nursing, 14*(2), 16-29.

Guyton, A. C., & Hall, J. E. (2006). *Textbook of medical physiology* (11th ed.). Philadelphia: Saunders.

Hardy, L. R., Harrell, J. S., & Bell, R. A. (2004). Overweight in children: Definitions, measurements, confounding factors, and health consequences. *Journal of Pediatric Nursing, 19*(6), 376-384.

Hayman, L. L. (2004). Toward evidence-based practice. [Commentary on] Childhood cardiovascular risk factors and carotid vascular changes in adulthood: The Bogalusa Heart Study. *MCN: The American Journal of Maternal/Child Nursing, 29*(4), 268.

Hess, C. T. (2001). Putting the squeeze on venous ulcers. *Nursing 2001, 41*(9), 58-63.

Johnson, M., Bulechek, G., Butcher, H., Dochterman, J. M., Maas, M., Moorhead, S., et al. (Eds.). (2006). *NANDA, NOC, and NIC linkages: Nursing diagnoses, outcomes, & interventions.* St. Louis, MO: Mosby.

Lai, S., Lima, J. A., Lai, H., Vlahov, D., Celentano, D., Tong, W., et al. (2005). Human immunodeficiency virus 1 infection, cocaine, and coronary calcification. *Archives of Internal Medicine, 165*(6):690-695.

*Leininger, M. M. (Ed.). (1991). *Cultural care diversity and universality: A theory of nursing.* New York: National League for Nursing Press.

Martin, B. C., Heuchert, J., Schlitt, C., Barnard, T., & Yeager, A. J. (2005). Healthy People 2010 community partnership. *Chart, 102*(2), 7-8.

Montague, M. C., & Broadnax, P. A. (2004). Health consequences of excess weight and obesity. *Journal of National Black Nurses' Association, 15*(1), 24-31.

NANDA International. (2007). *Nursing diagnoses: Definitions and classification, 2006-2007* (7th ed.). Philadelphia: Author.

Piano, M. R. (2005). Beats & breaths. The cardiovascular effects of alcohol: The good and the bad. *American Journal of Nursing, 105*(7), 87, 89-91.

Prevention in youth: Turning guidelines into interventions. (2005). *Journal of Cardiovascular Nursing, 20*(2), 9A.

Price, J. A. D. (2004). Management and prevention of cardiovascular disease in women. *Nursing Clinics of North America, 39*(4), 873-884.

Quinn, L. (2004). Educating patients with diabetes about cardiovascular disease risk. *Progress in Cardiovascular Nursing, 19*(3), 107-113.

Scholle, C. C., & Mininni, N. C. (2006). How a rapid response team saves lives. *Nursing, 36,* 1, 36-40.

Smith, M. A. (2005). Preface: Cardiopulmonary resuscitation. *Critical Care Nursing Clinics of North America, 17*(1), xv-xvi.

Sol, B. G. M., van der Bijl, J. J., Banga, J., & Visseren, F. L. J. (2005). Vascular risk management through nurse-led self-management programs. *Journal of Vascular Nursing, 23*(1), 20-24.

Staffileno, B. A. (2005). Treating hypertension with cardioprotective therapies: The role of ACE inhibitors, ARBs, and s-blockers. *Journal of Cardiovascular Nursing, 20*(5), 354-364.

Teaching your patient about cardiovascular tests. (2002). *Nursing, 32*(1), 62-64.

U.S. Department of Health and Human Services. (2000). *Healthy People 2010: Understanding and improving health* (2nd ed.). Washington, DC: U.S. Government Printing Office. Available at www.health.gov/healthypeople/About/hpfact.htm.

*Asterisk indicates a classic or definitive work on this subject.

Chapter 36

Managing Sleep and Rest

Media Resources

- evolve Evolve Website http://evolve.elsevier.com/Harkreader/
- Companion CD

Learning Objectives

After studying this chapter, you should be able to do the following:

- Describe the physiological concepts underlying sleep
- Discuss the developmental and lifestyle factors that affect rest and sleep
- Discuss the various sleep disorders
- Describe the general nursing assessment of rest and sleep
- Assess clients for risk for sleep problems
- Discuss nursing diagnoses for problems of rest and sleep
- Plan goal-directed interventions that address sleep pattern disturbances and meet rest needs
- Evaluate outcomes of nursing care for clients with sleep pattern disturbances

Key Terms

bruxism
circadian rhythm
dyssomnia
hypnotic
insomnia
multiple sleep latency test
narcolepsy
nightmare disorder
nocturnal enuresis
non–rapid eye movement (NREM) sleep
obstructive sleep apnea (OSA)
parasomnia
polysomnography
primary hypersomnia
rapid eye movement (REM) sleep
rest
restless legs syndrome
sleep
sleep deprivation
sleep terrors disorder
sleepwalking disorder
sundowning
zeitgeber

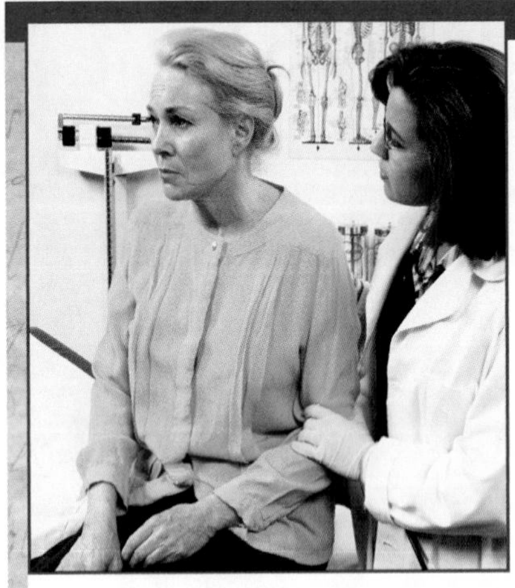

Emma Weiss, a 48-year-old single woman, is seen at the clinic complaining of tension headaches and exhaustion over the past 3 months. Deep circles under her eyes and frequent yawning confirm her statement that she is tired and unable to remember when she last had a good night's sleep. Ms. Weiss feels that her symptoms are closely linked to a recent job promotion, which requires longer work hours. She is currently enrolled in a master's degree program and feels anxious about her upcoming midterm examinations. Ms. Weiss attempted to alleviate her symptoms of insomnia with a glass of wine at bedtime, which has not helped. Ms. Weiss is worried that her exhaustion is beginning to affect her job performance and wants to discuss the possibility of getting a prescription for sleeping pills. The nurse considers the diagnoses of *Insomnia* because the client has identified sleep as her priority and *Fatigue* due to her complaints of physical and mental exhaustion.

KEY NURSING DIAGNOSES FOR SLEEP AND REST

Insomnia: Time-limited disruption of sleep amount and quality
Fatigue: An overwhelming and sustained sense of exhaustion and decreased capacity for physical and mental work at a usual level

CONCEPTS OF REST AND SLEEP

After reading this chapter, you will gain an understanding of the concepts of rest and sleep. Rest and sleep are basic needs to achieve and maintain optimal health. When illness strikes, more metabolic energy is expended, which leads to increased need for rest and sleep; it also may disrupt normal, well-established sleep patterns. By recognizing deviations from the normal sleep patterns, you will better be able to identify and effectively treat clients who have *Insomnia* and/or *Fatigue*.

REST

A person at **rest** is in a state of being physically and mentally relaxed and free from anxiety while being awake and alert. After people rest, they generally feel rejuvenated. The need for rest is highly individualized as are the activities people find restful. For example, a homemaker finds it mentally restful to work in her garden, whereas a bicyclist finds it physically restful to take a break during his 20-mile bike ride. Some of the factors that influence the need for rest include acute or chronic illnesses, stress, anxiety, lifestyle, occupation, medications, conditioning, and age. As a nurse, you will need to assess your clients need for rest and the activities they use to promote it.

PHYSIOLOGY OF SLEEP

Sleep is a state marked by reduced consciousness, diminished activity of the skeletal muscles, and depressed metabolism. Three processes regulate sleep: homeostatic mechanisms, circadian rhythms (a biorhythm), and ultradian rhythms. Of these regulators, homeostatic mechanism is the least understood. Neurons in the brain stem reticular formation and hypothalamus produce neurotransmitters that effect the sleep cycle. Acetylcholine and norepinephrine play an important role in rapid eye movement (REM) sleep; serotonin and gamma-aminobutyric acid (GABA) in non–rapid eye movement (NREM) sleep. Research also indicates that adenosine builds up in our blood while a person is awake and causes drowsiness, and gradually breaks down while sleep occurs (National Institute of Neurological Disorders and Stroke [NINDS], 2005).

Biorhythms (rhythmic biological clocks) are the periodic recurrence of a biological phenomenon that exists in plants, animals, and humans. In humans they control hundreds of physiological processes, including temperature, respiratory rate, and sleep, which are regulated by internal and external factors.

Circadian rhythm is a biorhythm pattern that is regularly repeated at 24-hour intervals. The sleep cycle is a circadian cycle. The mechanisms controlling the circadian nature of the sleep cycle are environmental triggers or synchronizers, or **zeitgebers.** They adjust the human body's internal clock to a 24-hour solar day. Each day's pattern of light and darkness is the most powerful zeitgeber for humans. Melatonin, the "hormone of darkness," regulates the circadian phases of sleep. It is a natural hormone made in the pineal gland. During the day, the pineal is inactive; but when the sun goes down and darkness occurs, the pineal begins to actively produce melatonin, which is released into the blood.

Other zeitgebers that influence sleep-wake patterns include daily routines, social events, noise, and alarm clocks. These can sometimes desynchronize, as may occur in jet lag or shift changes at work, and disrupt the circadian sleep-wake patterns. This in turn can cause a disruption in sleep patterns and fatigue.

Table 36-1 Characteristics of NREM Sleep and REM Sleep

CHARACTERISTIC	NREM SLEEP	REM SLEEP
Synonyms	Slow-wave or delta sleep (stages 3 and 4)	Active or paradoxical sleep
Eye movements	Slow rolling or no eye movements	Episodic bursts of rapid eye movements
Vital signs	Blood pressure, temperature, and heart rate decreased during stages 3 and 4	Heart rate, blood pressure and respirations increased and fluctuate
Muscle tone	Occasional whole body jerk or movement; in slow-wave sleep, muscles are more relaxed	Large-muscle immobility
Manifestations of deprivation	Fatigue, restlessness, decreased pain tolerance, anxiety, increased illness, increased cortisol secretion, increased immunosuppression, delayed healing	Lack of alertness; apathy, irritability, confusion, disorientation, delusions, hallucinations

NREM, Non–rapid eye movement; *REM,* rapid eye movement.

The ultradian rhythms are the regular recurrence in biological rhythms of less than 24 hours. The two ultradian cycles in the sleep cycle are the sleep states, NREM and REM sleep.

SLEEP STATES

Until the 1950s, sleep was thought of as a passive, dormant part of people's daily lives. Since then we have learned that our brains are very active during sleep. It was in the 1950s that researchers first identified two ultradian forms of sleep: NREM and REM sleep (Table 36-1). Research has now proven there are five stages of sleep: stages 1, 2, 3, 4, and REM sleep. These stages progress in a cycle from stage 1 to REM sleep, then the cycle starts over again with stage 2.

NON–RAPID EYE MOVEMENT SLEEP

Non–rapid eye movement (NREM) sleep is a sleeping period without REM. Characteristic physiological changes accompany NREM sleep. These changes include slower metabolic rate, decrease in regional cerebral blood flow, and decrease in blood pressure, temperature, pulse, and respiration. The body moves, especially during transitions from one stage to another.

This sleep state can be further divided into the four stages, during which the brain activity decreases and the person becomes completely relaxed.

- Stage 1 is the lightest sleep. It is the transition from wakefulness to sleep. People are easily awakened in this stage. Their eyes are closed and move very slowly, and muscle activity slows. People awakened from stage 1 sleep often remember fragmented visual images. Polysomnography indicate a 50% reduction in activity between wakefulness and stage 1 sleep. Electroencephalogram (EEG) tracings show low-voltage, nonsynchronous brain activity. This stage lasts for 5 to 10 minutes and is about 5% of time spent asleep in healthy adults.
- Stage 2 is a period of light sleep. The heart rate slows, body temperature decreases, eye movements stop, and our brain waves become slower with occasional bursts of rapid waves called sleep spindles. Polysomnographic readings show intermittent peaks and valleys, or positive and negative waves that indicate spontaneous periods of muscle tone mixed with periods of muscle relaxation. It occupies about 50% of time spent asleep in healthy adults.
- Stage 3 and stage 4 are deep sleep stages, with stage 4 being more intense than stage 3. Stage 3 marks the beginning of bursts of delta waves or slow-wave sleep, interspersed with smaller, faster waves. High-voltage EEG activity and a high arousal threshold, which can make it difficult to arouse the sleeper, characterize slow-wave sleep, also called deep sleep.
- In stage 4 there is no eye movement or muscle activity. The brain produces delta waves almost exclusively and represents the deepest sleep, when resistance to external arousal is greatest. Almost continuous, high-voltage, slow-wave patterns appear on the EEG. There is no eye movement or muscle activity. People awakened during deep sleep do not adjust immediately and often feel groggy and disoriented for several minutes after they wake up. Some children experience bed-wetting, night terrors, or sleepwalking during deep sleep. Collectively, stages 3 and 4 occupy about 10% to 20% of healthy adult sleep time (NINDS, 2005).

RAPID EYE MOVEMENT SLEEP

Rapid eye movement (REM) sleep is the stage of sleep characterized by eyes jerking rapidly in various directions. It is also known as paradoxical sleep because there is high brain activity (EEG activation), respirations becomes more rapid, irregular, and shallow, eyes jerk rapidly in various directions, and limb muscles become temporarily paralyzed, heart rate increases, blood pressure rises, males develop penile erections, and variable arousability. Activity recorded in the brain by EEG during REM sleep is similar to that recorded during wakefulness. Most of the vividly recalled dreams occur during REM sleep. It occupies about 20% to 25% of total adult sleep.

SLEEP CYCLES

Normal adult sleep occurs in four or five cycles each night (Figure 36-1). Each sleep cycle lasts about 80 to 120 minutes. The first sleep cycle contains relatively short REM periods and long periods of deep sleep. As the night progresses, REM sleep periods increase in length while deep sleep decreases. If sleep is interrupted, a new sleep cycle will begin, starting at stage 1 of NREM sleep and progressing to REM sleep. The normal adult sleeps an average of 7 to 8 hours, but the normal range varies from 5 to 10 hours. Each person must determine his or her own sleep needs by paying attention to whether he or she feels rested and alert throughout the day.

Clients who are under anesthesia or in a coma are often said to be asleep. They cannot be awakened and do not produce the complex, active brain wave patterns seen in normal sleep. Instead, their brain waves are very slow and weak, sometimes all but undetectable. In addition, clinical differentiation between sleep and coma is sometimes challenging. Given the proper stimulus, a sleeper can usually be awakened. The comatose client, however, can be awakened by neither painful nor noxious stimuli.

FUNCTIONS OF SLEEP

Although the exact function of sleep is still a mystery, sleep is necessary for survival and is as important as food and water. The two most widely accepted theories about sleep function are energy conservation and restoration.

Energy Conservation. Proponents of the conservation theory argue that sleep is an extension of homeostasis. High energy use during the day must be balanced by decreased energy use at night. The body's metabolic fluctuations offer support for this theory. At night, particularly during slow-wave sleep, the metabolic rate decreases by 5% to 25%. This dip may represent the body's attempt to conserve energy. Activity in parts of the brain that control emotions, decision-making processes, and social interactions is drastically reduced during deep sleep, suggesting that this type of sleep may help people maintain optimal emotional and social functioning while they are awake (NINDS, 2005).

Further evidence for the conservation theory can be found in developmental sleep pattern changes. The amount of slow-wave sleep declines with age. This decline may parallel the decreasing cerebral and body metabolism over the life span. Because energy requirements decrease with age, the need to conserve energy also declines.

Restoration. The most widely accepted view of sleep function by some experts is that sleep gives neurons used while we are awake a chance to shut down and repair themselves. Without sleep, neurons may become so depleted in energy or so polluted with byproducts of normal cellular activities that they begin to malfunction. Sleep appears necessary for our nervous systems to work properly. Too little sleep leaves us drowsy and unable to concentrate the next day and leads to impaired memory and physical performance and reduced ability to carry out math calculations. If sleep deprivation continues, hallucinations and mood swings may develop (NINDS, 2005). **Sleep deprivation** is the state that results from a person not getting enough sleep.

Deep sleep coincides with the release of growth hormone in children and young adults. In addition, sleep also may give the brain a chance to exercise important neuronal connections that might otherwise deteriorate from lack of activity. Many of the body's cells also show increased production and reduced breakdown of proteins during deep sleep. Because proteins are the building blocks needed for cell growth and for repair of damage from factors like stress and ultraviolet rays, deep sleep may truly be "beauty sleep" (NINDS, 2005).

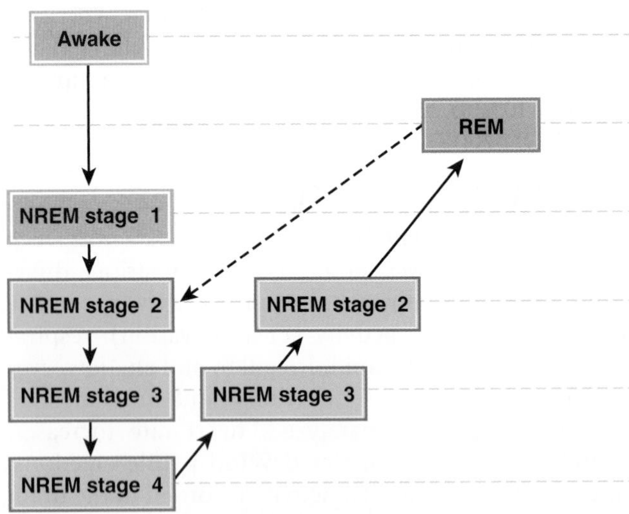

FIGURE 36-1 A normal adult sleep cycle. The stages are typically repeated four to five times during a night's sleep.

FACTORS AFFECTING REST AND SLEEP

FACTORS ACROSS THE LIFE SPAN

To accurately diagnose *Insomnia,* you must first be able to recognize normal, developmental changes in sleep patterns or what specialists call "sleep architecture" (Figure 36-2). Quite simply put, infants and children sleep more, whereas older adults sleep less. Sleep in infants and older adults tends to be more fragmented (Zunkel, 2005).

Infants. In general, sleep patterns stabilize during the first year of life. Normal newborns sleep an average of 16 to 17 hours a day. However, they often alternate between

REM sleep and wakefulness, skipping stages 1 through 4 of NREM. This phenomenon shortens the duration of each sleep period. Their sleep cycle is also shorter, lasting about 40 to 50 minutes instead of 90. If sleep is a time of growth, it is not surprising that newborns spend so much of their time sleeping; their body weight doubles in the first 6 months. By 6 weeks of age, infants are awake more during the day than at night, but more than half are still not sleeping through the night. At the end of the first year, most children are sleeping through the night and nap only once a day. However, sleep needs are individual. As long as infants are active during waking periods and growing normally, they are probably getting enough sleep.

Children. The sleep-wake cycle is fully developed by age 2, and the REM sleep pattern during preschool years is similar to that of an adult. Infants and toddlers seldom have primary sleep disorders. Unless the child is ill, the most common sleep problems at this age are difficulty learning to sleep alone, trouble with bedtime routines, and transitions from wake to sleep.

As children mature, they spend fewer hours sleeping but a greater portion of their sleep time in slow-wave sleep. Infants spend only 50% of their sleep time in deep sleep, whereas older children spend 80% of their sleep time in deep sleep. Although sleep needs by this age are individualized, most school-age children require an average of 8 to 10 hours of sleep. During growth spurts, sleep needs may increase.

Adolescents. During adolescence, total sleep time increases. Teenagers' rapid physical growth, tendency toward overexertion, and overall increased activity levels contribute to fatigue and increased sleep needs. Their increased need for sleep, coupled with their tendency to stay up late, often makes it difficult for teenagers to get up in the morning. These symptoms overlap with those of *delayed sleep phase syndrome,* a common and underdiagnosed circadian rhythm disturbance in this age-group. The internal clocks that regulate the sleep-wake cycles in some teenagers are thought to be exceptionally long. The net result is a sleep cycle shift that causes sleep-onset insomnia and difficulty with early morning rising. The adolescent may be unable to fall asleep until 2:00 or 3:00 AM but may then sleep soundly and feel refreshed if allowed to sleep for 7 to 8 hours.

Adults. Slow-wave sleep declines after adolescence. In fact, it decreases by nearly 40% during the teen years and continues to decline in a linear fashion until age 60, after which there is little remaining delta (slow-wave) sleep.

Female sleep changes are often triggered by hormonal fluctuations. Pregnant women, for example, have an increased need for sleep during the first trimester of pregnancy. Typical symptoms include naps during the day. By the end of pregnancy, the woman's increased body size, as well as the fetus's size and movement, make it hard to sleep. Another shift in hormones for women occurs at midlife with the onset of menopause. Complaints of sleep disturbances occur at this time, which may be an indication of decreasing estrogen levels.

Older Adults. Older adults' sleep includes only a small amount of deep sleep (virtually no stage 4 sleep and scant stage 3 sleep). About half of all people over 65

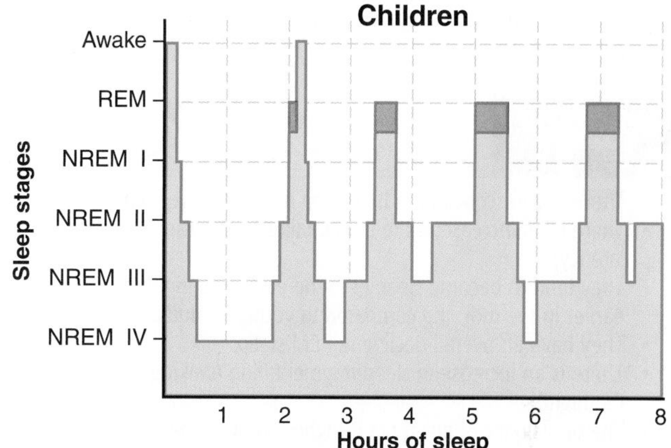

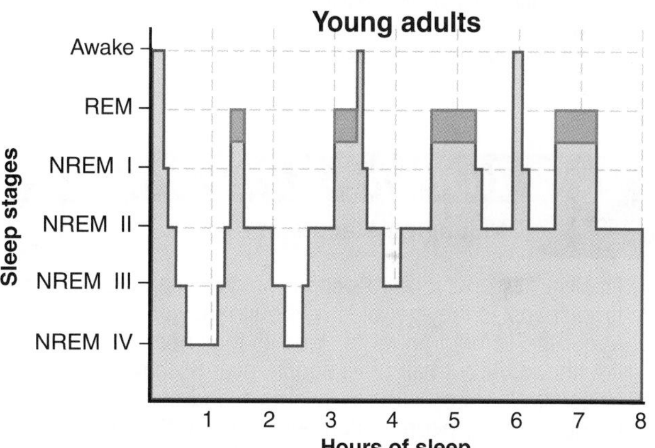

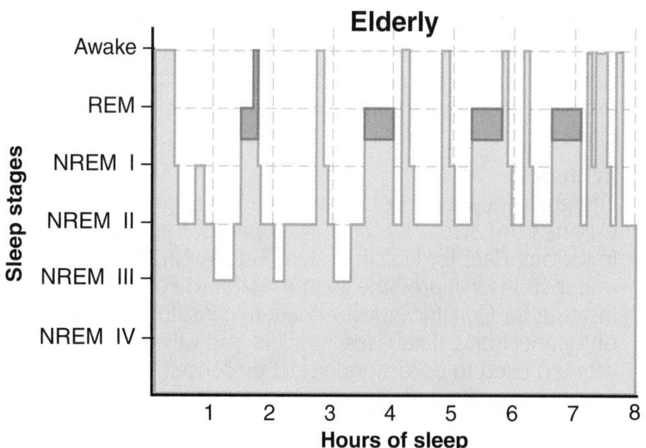

FIGURE 36-2 Sleep architecture over the life span. The amount of slow-wave sleep decreases with age, and the number of awakenings increases with age. (Redrawn from Kales, A., Beall, G. N., Berger, R. J., Heuser, G., Jacobson, A., Kales, J. D., et al. [1968]. Sleep and dreams: Recent research on clinical aspects. *Annals of Internal Medicine, 68* [5], 1078-1104.)

have frequent sleeping problems, such as insomnia, which may result from the changes in sleep patterns, medical problems that are common in older adults, and the medications and other treatments for those problems (NINDS, 2005) (Boxes 36-1 and 36-2).

LIFESTYLE FACTORS

Lifestyle factors, such as sleep patterns ("sleep architecture"), temperature, nutrition, exercise, smoking, and the environment influence sleep and rest.

BOX 36-1 *Factors Affecting Older Adults' Sleep Patterns*

- There is a misconception that sleep needs decline with age.
- There is an increase in the time it takes to fall asleep (sleep latency).
- They tend to become sleepier in the early evening and wake earlier in the morning compared to younger adults.
- They have an overall decline in REM sleep.
- There is an increase in sleep fragmentation (waking up during the night).
- The prevalence of insomnia is higher among older adults.
- The prevalence of sleep disorders tends to increase with age, which can be attributed to physical illnesses, which are often chronic, and psychiatric illnesses and the medications used to treat them.
- Snoring often becomes worse with age.

Sleep Patterns or "Sleep Architecture." People who have a regular sleep-wake pattern are more likely to report beneficial sleep and better performance during the day than people with variable sleep patterns. Anticipated and unanticipated lifestyle modifications can disturb a fixed sleep pattern. Demanding jobs or shift rotations, birth of a baby, and out-of-town visitors are a few examples of potential lifestyle disruptions. Family caregivers may suffer from exhaustion and sleep deprivation. In all cases, chronic sleep deprivation may lead to ineffective and dangerous self-treatment programs, such as abuse of hypnotics or alcohol.

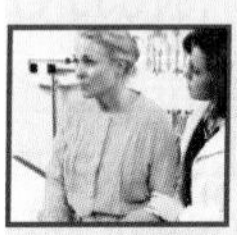

What are some key elements in Ms. Weiss's story that suggest she is having difficulty coping?

Temperature. Body temperature influences sleep-wake patterns; for example, a fever often causes frequent awakenings.

Nutrition. Sleep pattern disturbances may be linked to diet. Hunger or excess food consumption near bedtime can lead to delayed sleep onset, increased arousals, or both. In addition, intake of caffeine and alcohol may influence sleep. Excess caffeine consumption (in

BOX 36-2 *Evidence-Based Practice*

Managing Sleep and Rest

Problem: "People tend to sleep more lightly and for shorter time spans as they get older, although they generally need about the same amount of sleep as they needed in early adulthood. About half of all people over 65 have frequent sleeping problems, such as insomnia, and deep sleep stages in many elderly people often become very short or stop completely" (retrieved June 7, 2006, from http://www.ninds.nih.gov/disorders/brain_basics/understanding_sleep.htm#Sleep%20Disorders). Nurses need to know how to assist the older adult in improving the quality and quantity of sleep, as well as helping them reduce the occurrences of excessive sleepiness during the day, which will improve cognitive functioning, functional status, and performance.

Evidence

The guidelines were developed by a group of nursing experts from across the country as part of the Nurses Improving Care for Health System Elders (NICHE) project, under sponsorship of The John A. Hartford Foundation Institute for Geriatric Nursing-Academic Institution. Searches of the electronic databases, Medline and CINAHL, was the method used to collect and select evidence.

Application to Practice

The guideline was developed for advanced practice nurses, health care providers, nurses and students with the following objectives:

- To identify the signs of excessive sleepiness (ES) and rate these symptoms using a standardized numerical scale
- To describe the signs and symptoms for the most common causes of ES in older adults: obstructive sleep apnea, restless legs syndrome, insomnia, and narcolepsy
- To plan appropriate interventions for the client with ES
- To provide nursing care that incorporates sleep hygiene measures
- To educate clients and families about sleep disorders and sleep hygiene measures
- To modify medical interventions and routines that interfere with sleep maintenance and sleep quality
- To identify and refer clients needing evaluation by sleep medicine specialists
- To support clients in complying with treatment regimens for sleep disorders

The guideline can be found at http://www.guideline.gov/summary/summary.aspx?ss=15&doc_id=3505&nbr=2731.

Reference

Umlauf, M. G., Chasens, E. R., & Weaver, T. E. (2003). Excessive sleepiness. In M. Mezey, T. Fulmer, I. Abraham, & D. A. Zwicker, (Eds.), *Geriatric nursing protocols for best practice* (2nd ed., pp. 47-65). New York: Springer Publishing [35 references].

tea, coffee, chocolate, cocoa, and cola) may be detrimental. Because it has such a long half-life, caffeine taken late in the day may increase insomnia and nighttime arousals. Alcohol, a brain sedative, shortens sleep onset. However, it disturbs sleep patterns late at night because its rapid metabolism causes a rebound arousal. It may also cause early morning awakenings secondary to a full bladder.

Exercise. The person who exercises during the day is more likely to sleep well at night. Increased physical activity increases both REM and NREM sleep. Moderate fatigue, brought on by exercise, is thought to promote restful sleep. Increased exercise increases fatigue, which, in turn, produces a soporific or sleep-inducing effect. However, activity must be carefully timed. Exercise within 2 hours of retiring or excessive exercise in an individual unused to exercise can lead to difficulty getting to sleep.

Smoking. High levels of nicotine cause feelings of arousal and agitation. Because the half-life of nicotine is 1 to 2 hours, the person who smokes more than one cigarette within an hour of bedtime may delay sleep onset. Long-term smoking can eventually contribute to a need for increased physical rest. Permanent lung damage caused by chronic smoke inhalation commonly leads to hypoxia. Hypoxia, in turn, is associated with increased fatigue and a need to intersperse activities with rest. The hypoxia associated with sleep apnea causes excess morning fatigue.

Environment. Most people are accustomed to their home sleep environment. The familiar ambiance provides comfort and security. Without this supportive environment, a person may not be able to relax, and insomnia may result. Many sleepers experience difficulty sleeping in a strange bed and are used to certain sights, sounds, lights, and temperatures, and the absence of these or the presence of novel disruptions can disturb sleep. City dwellers may find the darkness and quiet of the country disconcerting and perceive the early morning crowing of the rooster as an unwelcome alarm clock. By contrast, the urban environment may overstimulate rural travelers.

The hospital, an unfamiliar setting to most clients, can wreak havoc with normal sleep patterns. Strange, loud noises, bright lights, uncomfortable beds and temperatures, restraints in uncomfortable positions, lack of privacy, lack of control, anxiety or personal worry, separation from loved ones, and sleep deprivation can lead to sleep problems. Noises are particularly bothersome and may lead to the need for hypnotics while in the hospital.

The acute care setting, in which clients are monitored around the clock, can be conducive to relaxation and sleep if clients feel protected. However, clients may be frightened by the fact that they require such intensive observation, and their fears may contribute to difficulty falling asleep. The constant interruption of around-the-clock care can hinder the sleep cycle.

Nowhere are sleep stressors more acute than in intensive care units (ICUs). Critical care nurses tend to provide continual care with no regard to the time of day. This oversight can have significant, adverse consequences. *ICU psychosis* is a well-documented iatrogenic complication strongly correlated with REM sleep deprivation in ICUs. This syndrome is characterized by restlessness, loss of reality perception, transient paranoia, hallucinations, and delusions. It occurs after 3 to 5 days in a critical care unit and typically disappears after transfer to another unit.

SLEEP DISORDERS

At least 40 million Americans each year suffer from chronic, long-term sleep disorders, and an additional 20 million experience occasional sleeping problems (NINDS, 2005). The sleep disorders or pathologic conditions are classified based on their epidemiology (Box 36-3).

Primary Sleep Disorders. Primary sleep disorders include **dyssomnias,** which are primary sleep disorders in initiating or maintaining sleep or excessive sleep, and **parasomnias,** which are abnormal behavioral or physiological events that occur during sleep.

Dyssomnias.

Circadian rhythm sleep disorders. Circadian sleep disorders are characterized by a mismatch between the person's sleep schedule and normal circadian sleep patterns. Such persons cannot sleep when sleep is wanted, needed, or expected. In addition, they may be sleepy at undesirable times. The two most common transient circadian rhythm disorders are shift-work sleep disorder and time zone change (jet lag) syndrome.

BOX 36-3 *Sleep Disorder Classifications*

DYSSOMNIAS
- Insomnia, hypersomnia, narcolepsy, sleep apnea, restless legs syndrome
- Circadian rhythm disorders, including shift-work sleep disorder and jet lag disorder

PARASOMNIAS
- *Arousal disorders,* including sleepwalking and sleep terrors
- *Associated with REM sleep,* including nightmares
- Other: bruxism (grinding of teeth) and sleep enuresis

SLEEP DISORDERS ASSOCIATED WITH MEDICAL OR PSYCHIATRIC ILLNESS
- *Mental disorders,* including psychoses, mood disorders, panic disorders, and alcoholism
- *Neurologic disorders,* including dementia, Parkinsonism, familial insomnia, and sleep-related epilepsy
- *Other medical disorders,* including asthma, chronic obstructive pulmonary disease, sleep-related gastroesophageal reflux, and peptic ulcer disease

Some employees, such as nurses and firefighters, must periodically change the shift (time) they work. For these workers, short-term sleeping medications may be necessary during adjustment to shift rotations. However, these drugs only partially solve the problem. Although they promote sleep, they do not reset circadian clocks. Thus shift workers who change to another work schedule must ultimately reset their internal clocks to maintain their work performance and sleep at appropriate times. Shift rotation in a forward direction (nights, mornings, then evenings) rather than a backward direction (evenings, mornings, then nights) facilitates circadian realignment.

The term *jet lag* describes a constellation of symptoms that develops as the result of rapid travel across several time zones. Symptoms include malaise, headache, loss of appetite, irregular bowel movements, difficulty concentrating, fatigue during the new daytime, and an inability to sleep well at night. The symptoms reflect the circadian system's failure to rapidly adjust to sudden shifts. Although both physical cues (nighttime, daylight) and social cues (mealtimes, noise) encourage adaptation to the new circadian system, readjustment may still take several days, particularly if the person has taken an eastward flight.

The consequences of these disorders range from annoying to life threatening. They include depression, sexual dysfunction, learning and memory difficulties, falling asleep while at work, and other medical problems, such as high blood pressure, heart attack and stroke, and obesity. Poor sleep also leads to accidents.

Insomnia. Insomnia is characterized by difficulty initiating or maintaining sleep, sleeping too lightly, easily disrupted sleep with many spontaneous arousals, or early-morning awakenings and the subjective sense that sleep quality is poor and inadequate. It is by far the most common dyssomnia; nearly everyone suffers from it at some point during his or her life. Its occurrence increases with age and affects more women than men (NINDS, 2005; Thobaben, Fossett, & Nadler-Moodie, 2004).

Short-term insomnia is usually self-limiting and can often be traced to acute stress or lifestyle changes, such as disruption of the sleep schedule, unfamiliar environments, or environments not conducive to sleep. If not resolved within 2 weeks, such transient sleep disruption is considered primary insomnia. It is more difficult to cure because of its self-perpetuating nature.

Insomnia can lead to symptoms of sleep deprivation. Awakenings during the first few hours of sleep usually result in the total NREM sleep time being shortened. The disturbance is associated with daytime fatigue, which causes significant distress or impairs the person's occupational, social, and/or other areas of functioning (DSM-IV-TR, 2000; Thobaben et al., 2004).

Primary hypersomnia. Primary hypersomnia is excessive sleepiness that is severe enough to cause clinically significant distress or impairment in occupational, social, and/or other areas of functioning that lasts at least 1 month as evidenced either by prolonged sleep episodes or by daytime sleep that occurs almost daily (DMS-IV-TR, 2000; Thobaben et al., 2004). The person sleeps from 8 to 12 hours and has difficulty awakening in the morning (sometimes referred to as sleep drunkenness). Unintentional daytime sleep episodes can be embarrassing and even dangerous, and the low level of alertness that occurs while an individual fights sleepiness can lead to poor efficiency, poor concentration, and poor memory during daytime activities (DMS-IV-TR, 2000). Sleep tends to be continuous but nonrestorative. It typically begins between ages 15 and 30 years.

Narcolepsy. Narcolepsy is characterized by abnormal sleep tendencies, as well as by pathological REM sleep, manifested as excessive daytime sleepiness (EDS), daytime sleep attacks usually last 20 to 30 minutes, disturbed nighttime sleep, cataplexy, sleep paralysis, and hypnagogic hallucinations. Cataplexy results from the abrupt bilateral loss of muscle tone and paralysis of voluntary muscles. Sleep paralysis is the inability to move during the onset of sleep or awakening. Hypnagogic hallucinations are vivid, bizarre, dreamlike experiences that last from 1 to 15 minutes.

Narcolepsy occurs in both men and women at any age, although its symptoms are usually first noticed in teenagers or young adults. There is no cure for narcolepsy. Clients are often treated with stimulants and antidepressants to help control the symptoms. They are often encouraged to nap at certain times of the day to help reduce the excessive daytime sleepiness (NINDS, 2005; Thobaben et al., 2004).

Obstructive sleep apnea syndrome. The most common form of breathing-related sleep disorder is **obstructive sleep apnea (OSA) syndrome,** a sleep disorder manifested by periodic cessation of airflow at the nose and mouth during inspiration, which arouses the person from sleep. It occurs when air cannot flow into or out of the person's nose or mouth although efforts to breathe continue (DSM-IV-TR, 2000; Thobaben et al., 2004). The airway obstruction is commonly created when the back of the throat is sucked closed or narrowed as the sleeper inhales (Figure 36-3). This airway collapse results from a sleep-induced loss of upper airway muscle tone. It is characterized by loud snores or brief gasps that alternate with episodes of silence that usually last 20 to 30 seconds. In adults, flailing arms and legs or a total body spasm may accompany the snort. Restlessness and bedwetting may be observed in children. It occurs in 1% to 4% of the population, with increased incidence in middle-age and older adults. It is a serious, potentially life-threatening condition (DSM-IV-TR, 2000; Thobaben et al., 2004). Treatment may involve the surgical resection of the palatopharynx or the use of continuous positive airway pressure (CPAP). Untreated sleep apnea puts a client at risk for cardiovascular disease, headaches, memory loss, and depression.

Restless legs syndrome. Restless legs syndrome is a familial sleep disorder characterized by intense, abnormal, lower extremity sensations and irresistible leg movements that delay sleep onset. The sleeper describes an uncomfortable, deep, creeping, crawling sensation in the calf or thigh muscles that leads to an irresistible urge to move the legs when sitting or lying down. It is emerging as one of the most common sleep disorders. This disorder, which affects as many as 12 million Americans, leads to constant leg movement during the day and insomnia at night. Severe restless legs syndrome is most common in older adults, though symptoms may develop at any age. In some cases, it may be linked to other conditions such as anemia, pregnancy, or diabetes (NINDS, 2005; Thobaben et al., 2004).

Parasomnias. In contrast to the dyssomnias, parasomnias are not difficulties with sleep itself but rather with abnormal movements and behaviors that occur during sleep. They involve the activation of the autonomic nervous system, motor system, or cognitive processes during sleep or sleep-wake transitions.

Bruxism is characterized by violent, repetitive grinding of the teeth that occurs during the lighter stages of sleep or during partial arousals. It produces a loud and unpleasant sound that commonly awakens the bed partner or even someone sleeping 10 or 20 feet away. Episodes of bruxism generally last 4 to 5 seconds and can damage teeth and cause jaw pain. The afflicted sleeper may be treated with a rubber mouth guard over the teeth at night.

Nocturnal enuresis, bed-wetting, is repeated urination during nighttime sleep that disrupts the sleep cycle. The enuresis is not due exclusively to a medical condition or the physiological effect of a substance (DSM-IV-TR, 2000). It occurs during the first one third of the night. It limits the child's social activities (spending the night at a friend's house) and affects the child's self-esteem because of the social ostracism of peers and anger and rejection by the child's caregivers. It often coexists with development delays, such as speech, language, and motor skills. Treatment may include low doses of antidepressants, behavioral techniques (such as bladder training or the use of a pad and buzzer), and fluid restriction in the evening.

Nightmare disorder is the repeated occurrence of frightening dreams that lead to awakenings from sleep that occurs primarily during REM sleep and may occur every 90 to 110 minutes. The nightmares can be vividly recalled and often correlate with increased stress, depression, painful life events, insecurity, anxiety, guilt, fever, or abrupt discontinuation of drugs that affect REM sleep. Children ages 3 to 5 years have nightmares of sufficient intensity to disturb their parents' sleep (DSM-IV-TR, 2000).

Sleep terrors disorder is the repeated occurrence of sleep terrors, abrupt awakenings from sleep usually beginning with a panicky screen or cry (DSM-IV-TR, 2000). They begin during the first third of the major sleep episodes and last for 1 to 10 minutes. The client is relatively unresponsive to efforts of comfort during the episode and does not remember it. They are seen in children and typically resolve in adolescents, though adult-onset sleep terrors may occur.

Sleepwalking disorder is a slow-wave sleep parasomnia associated with stereotypical "sleepwalking" behaviors. Sleepers may sit up with glassy eyes, make body

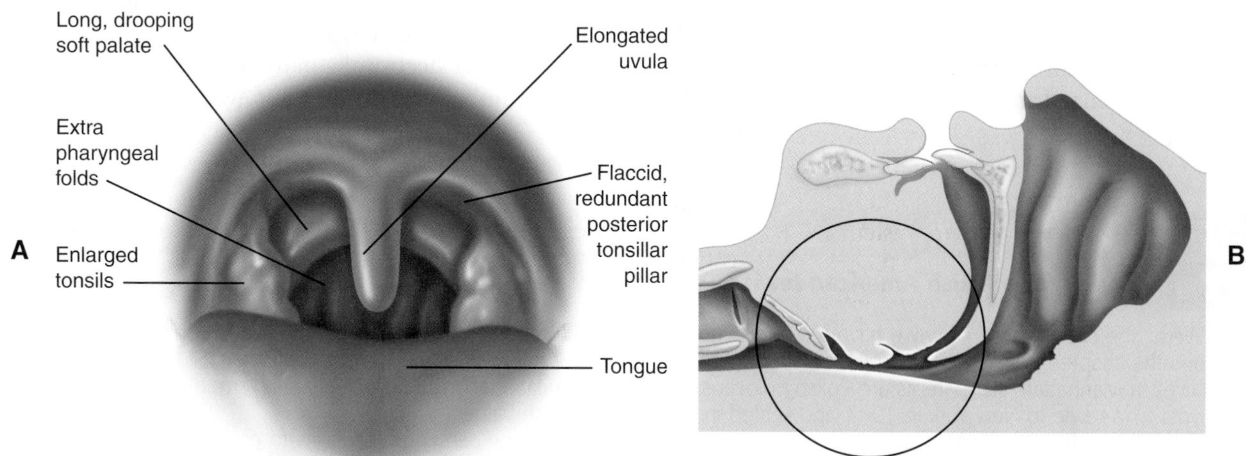

FIGURE 36-3 Anatomy of obstructive sleep apnea. **A,** The collapsible anatomical structures that can obstruct the airway. **B,** Obstruction of the upper airway as the sleeper inhales. (Redrawn from Shemwell, A., & Wilson, P. [1994]. Rest and respiration during obstructive sleep apnea. *Nursing Times, 90*[19], 31.)

movements, get up, and walk around and often avoid or "look through" anyone who attempts to talk to them. It is much more common in children than adults. Although visual intake and coordination of the central nervous system (CNS) is maintained to some extent during sleepwalking, safety is an important consideration.

Secondary Sleep Disorders. Secondary sleep disorders are often a major disabling symptom of underlying psychiatric and medical conditions. When clients have a mental disorder, the pathophysiological mechanism responsible for the mental disorder also affects the sleep-wake regulation. Ninety percent of clients with mood disorders (depression) complain of disturbed sleep. Anxiety commonly causes sleep problems and is frequently experienced by clients who are hospitalized, receiving radiation and chemotherapy, have a life-threatening illness, etc. Prolonged sleep onset and decreased stage 4 and REM sleep mark these disorders. In addition, prescribed medications and other substances such as alcohol can cause sleep disturbance.

The physiological effect of medical conditions can affect the sleep-wake system. Examples include congestive heart failure, chronic obstructive pulmonary disease, gastroesophageal reflux disease, and pain. Problems for clients with Alzheimer's disease includes sundown syndrome, in which clients have delirium, agitation, combativeness, wandering, and vocalization without ostensible purpose occurring during the early evening or nighttime hours (DSM-IV-TR, 2000).

ASSESSMENT

Guided by a theoretical knowledge of normal and abnormal sleep-wake patterns, you can apply the nursing process to better identify individual clients who have or are at risk for developing these problems. A culturally sensitive assessment forms the critical first step in the nursing process. Box 36-4 offers tips that relate to Ms. Weiss, the client described at the beginning of the chapter.

If your assessment is incomplete, sleep problems may remain unrecognized and unaddressed. Assessment must include a sleep history and a physical examination. The sleep history should help identify specific problems accurately. Physical assessment may yield nonspecific findings of fatigue or sleep problems.

GENERAL ASSESSMENT OF SLEEP AND REST

Sleep History. Because most data about sleep pattern disturbances are subjective, the nursing history serves as the primary source of information about sleep problems. To obtain such a history, conduct an interview that identifies normal sleep-wake patterns, bedtime routines, and risk factors that contribute to sleep disturbances. To screen for sleep problems, ask the following questions:

- What time do you usually go to bed?
- Do you have any bedtime routines?
- How long does it take you to get to sleep?
- How easy or difficult is it for you to fall asleep?
- Do you awaken at night? If so, how often, and what is it that most frequently awakens you?
- What do you do when you awaken in the middle of the night?
- How would you describe your sleep?
- Is your sleep restless or restful?
- What time do you awaken in the morning?
- When you awaken, do feel refreshed or tired?
- Is the number of hours you sleep at night about right for you?
- Do you nap during the day? If so, how many naps do you take?
- How long is your usual nap?
- Does your bed partner ever complain about your sleep behaviors?
- Do you regularly take any over-the-counter or prescription drugs?

A weekly sleep diary may provide additional clues about sleep disorders and insomnia (Figure 36-4).

Instruct the client to record the following information (Berrios & Shapiro, 1993):

- Changes in sleep-wake patterns
- The number and duration of awakenings

BOX 36-4 *Cross-Cultural Care*

Caring for a Polish American Jewish Client

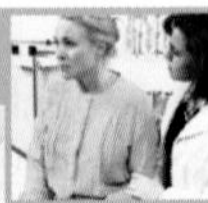

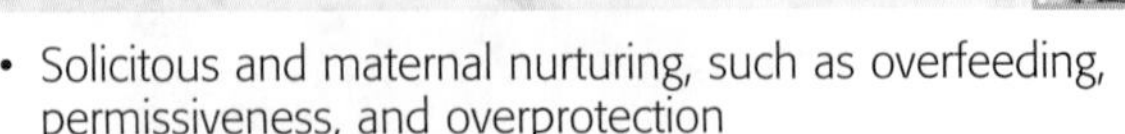

Ms. Weiss, the client whose story we have been following through the chapter, is an American-born Jewish woman who lives in Manhattan. Her parents are Polish holocaust survivors who came to New York in 1944 and settled in Brooklyn. Although every client is unique, Jewish Americans from Poland tend to value the following:

- Open expression of feelings
- Getting the most direct and best help
- Being persistent and persuasive
- Achieving financial and educational success
- Solicitous and maternal nurturing, such as overfeeding, permissiveness, and overprotection
- Educational and intellectual achievements
- Jewish values
- Observing certain precautions to prevent illness, such as not going out with wet hair, getting enough rest, staying in bed when not feeling well

- Sensations just before and during sleep
- The emotional content of dreams
- Alterations in diet, weight, lifestyle
- Alcohol intake
- Menstruation status
- Sexual habits
- Consumption of sleeping pills and other drugs
- Daytime work performance
- Conditions under which the client is unable to fall asleep

Physical Examination. Behavioral manifestations of insufficient or unsatisfactory sleep include agitation, disorientation, mood alterations, restlessness, memory loss, difficulty concentrating, a decreased attention span, lethargy, and apathy. The client also may have mild, fleeting nystagmus (constant involuntary movement of the eyeballs), ptosis (drooping of the eyelids), thickened speech, dark circles under the eyes, frequent yawning, muscle tremors, and a lack of coordination.

Some physical findings in fatigued clients overlap with those found in clients with sleep pattern disturbances. They too may demonstrate memory loss and an inability to concentrate. In addition, fatigued clients often suffer from activity intolerance, manifested as an increased heart rate, blood pressure, and respirations in response to minimal exertion. Their movements may be slow and deliberate, reflecting an attempt to conserve energy. These clients appear lethargic and disinterested in their surroundings.

SLEEP DIARY

Name: ______________ Remember to complete this diary each morning approximately 15-20 minutes after awakening.

Fill in date under each day	YESTERDAY:					THIS MORNING:				
	When I went to sleep last night I felt (circle one)	I went to bed at: (time)	I fell asleep in: (minutes)	During the night, I awoke at: (time)	And stayed awake for: (minutes)	During the night I awoke at: (time)	I slept a total of: (hours)	When I got up this morning, I felt: (circle one)	Overall, my sleep last night was: (circle one)	I use an alarm (yes/no)
Monday	−2 −1 0 +1 +2			— — — — — —	— — — — — —			−2 −1 0 +1 +2	−2 −1 0 +1 +2	
Tuesday	−2 −1 0 +1 +2			— — — — — —	— — — — — —			−2 −1 0 +1 +2	−2 −1 0 +1 +2	
Wednesday	−2 −1 0 +1 +2			— — — — — —	— — — — — —			−2 −1 0 +1 +2	−2 −1 0 +1 +2	
Thursday	−2 −1 0 +1 +2			— — — — — —	— — — — — —			−2 −1 0 +1 +2	−2 −1 0 +1 +2	
Friday	−2 −1 0 +1 +2			— — — — — —	— — — — — —			−2 −1 0 +1 +2	−2 −1 0 +1 +2	
Saturday	−2 −1 0 +1 +2			— — — — — —	— — — — — —			−2 −1 0 +1 +2	−2 −1 0 +1 +2	
Sunday	−2 −1 0 +1 +2			— — —	— — —			−2 −1 0 +1 +2	−2 −1 0 +1 +2	

FIGURE 36-4 A sleep diary. Clients use such diaries to document difficulty falling asleep, interrupted sleep, awakening earlier or later than desired, and not feeling well rested. (Recreated from Berrios, G. E., & Shapiro, C. M. [1993]. ABC of sleep disorders: "I don't get enough sleep, doctor." *British Medical Journal, 306*[6881], 843-846.)

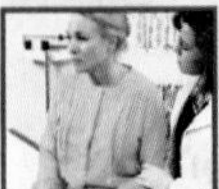

Recall the case of Emma Weiss. The nursing assessment for Ms. Weiss during her visit to the clinic was as follows: Client is a 48-year-old, white, Jewish woman with complaints of transient situational insomnia for 3 months. Wants sleeping pills. Self-medicated with a glass of wine at bedtime, which was unsuccessful in controlling symptoms. Client reports increasing cigarette consumption in response to stress of school and work. Now smokes one pack of cigarettes compared with one-half pack 3 months ago, and she smokes from the minute she awakens until the moment she gets into bed. Drinks up to 10 cups of coffee a day to "stay awake at work." Feels that mood swings and irritability secondary to sleep deprivation are affecting relationships with co-workers. Notes decreased ability to focus on details of work. Reports usual HS is 11:00 PM. For the past 2½ months, cannot fall asleep for at least 2 hours after retiring. Awakens four to five times during the night because of nightmares and once or twice due to nocturia. Sometimes tries to nap during lunch hour. Yawns frequently. Fine intentional tremor present. Eyes have deep circles. BP 120/80, HR 104, R 24, T 98.6° F, orally."

Ms. Weiss's blood pressure, pulse, and respirations are slightly higher than normal. Can you suggest possible reasons for these elevations? Consider what action(s) you might take to validate your hypotheses about the cause of these elevated vital signs.

Diagnostic Tests. People with long-standing unresolved sleep problems may be referred for formal sleep studies. **Polysomnography** is the continuous measurement and recording of physiological activity during sleep by using EEG, electrooculogram (EOG), electrocardiogram (ECG), and electromyogram (EMG) tracings to monitor brain activity, eye movements, heart rate and rhythm, and muscle movements. It may include oral or nasal airflow, respiratory effort, chest and abdominal wall movement, oxyhemoglobin saturation, or exhaled carbon dioxide concentration; these measures monitor respiration during sleep and detect the presence and severity of sleep apnea. The recordings are made synchronously. Polysomnography is usually performed during an overnight stay in a sleep laboratory (DMS-IV-TR, 2000).

The EEG illustrates electrophysiological differences among stages of sleep. It quantifies the brain's electrical activity by means of electrodes placed on the scalp. The EOG measures electrical activity associated with eye movements, helping to identify periods of REM sleep. In the EMG, electrodes are placed on the anterior tibialis and submental muscles (under the chin) to detect muscular electrical activity. An ECG reveals any cardiac arrhythmias that may occur. Analysis of data collected from polysomnography can help diagnose dyssomnias and parasomnias as well as pathologic conditions that might cause disturbed sleep.

The **multiple sleep latency test** is a direct, objective measure of sleepiness used to evaluate excessive somnolence and daytime sleepiness. Another formal sleep study, it is a well-validated instrument designed to quantify daytime sleepiness. The client is given four to five 20-minute nap opportunities at 2-hour intervals. If sleep occurs in less than 7 minutes for three or more tests, an abnormal level of sleepiness is indicated. This test can help establish a definite diagnosis for narcolepsy because narcoleptics will have sleep-onset REM episodes in addition to rapid sleep onset. For the test to be valid, the client must be instructed to discontinue all drugs that are known to affect sleep at least 2 weeks before the day of the test. The client should not take alcohol or caffeine on the day of the test and must discontinue smoking and strenuous activity at least 30 minutes before the test.

Wrist actigraphs are transducers worn on the wrist so that all wrist movements can be recorded during sleep. It is used to study clients' sleep-wake patterns and circadian rhythms and can be used by clients in their homes. Actigraphy can be particularly beneficial when used with sleep diaries.

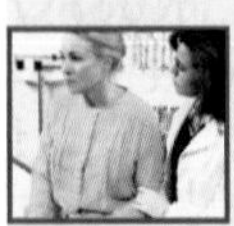

Based on her sleep history and physical findings, is Ms. Weiss a candidate for these diagnostic tests? Justify your answer.

FOCUSED ASSESSMENT FOR *INSOMNIA* AND *FATIGUE*

Defining Characteristics of *Insomnia*. *Insomnia* is a time-limited disruption of sleep amount and quality (NANDA International [NANDA-I], 2005). Clients with such disturbances typically present with at least one of four critical defining characteristics: difficulty falling asleep, interrupted sleep, awakening earlier or later than desired, and not feeling well rested. Data clusters help identify these defining characteristics (Table 36-2).

When a client complains of sleeplessness, increased restlessness, an inability to relax, and racing thoughts at bedtime, it typically indicates difficulty falling asleep. Problems falling asleep may also be linked to a change in the normal sleep schedule.

A client may describe interrupted sleep as awakening at night and being unable to go back to sleep. Excessively rumpled bedding may indicate that increased restlessness has caused brief but unremembered arousals. The client's bed partner may describe frequent leg twitching, jerks, or kicks during the night. If obstructive sleep apnea is causing the interrupted sleep, the partner may mention loud snoring, gasping, or choking.

Action Alert! Refer clients to their physicians for evaluation of possible sleep apnea when they or bed partners complain they have pauses, gasps, choking, or loud respirations during sleep.

A cue that the client is awakening earlier than desired might be the statement, "I woke at 4:00 AM and tossed and turned until the alarm went off." Alternatively, the client awakening later than desired might complain, "I just can't seem to drag myself out of bed to get to work on time."

Clients who do not feel well rested may complain of feeling exhausted or fatigued from lack of sleep. They may doze frequently and need frequent naps or increased caffeine to stay alert during the day. Excessive daytime sleepiness due to insomnia is most frequently associated with sleep deprivation. Sleep deprivation and other sleep problems that result in excessive sleepiness must be differentiated from the excessive sleepiness associated with narcolepsy. The narcoleptic frequently falls asleep while doing tedious tasks, while driving, or during a conversation.

Action Alert! Notify the client's physician if the client complains of excessive sleepiness and makes such statements as "I can fall asleep anytime," for further evaluation for narcolepsy.

Even people who do not suffer from a primary sleep disorder may be at risk for motor vehicle accidents during vulnerable periods of the sleep-wake cycle. Most people are sleepiest and least alert between 2:00 AM and 7:00 AM, and between 2:00 PM and 5:00 PM.

Defining Characteristics of *Fatigue*. *Fatigue* is an overwhelming sustained sense of exhaustion and decreased capacity for physical and mental work at usual levels (NANDA-I, 2005). It is characterized by an incessant and overwhelming lack of energy and an inability to maintain usual routines. Manifestations of physical and mental fatigue differ. Clients often describe physical fatigue as feeling tired, exhausted, or weak. They may also complain of muscle aches, no energy, and a need to lie down to recover. Symptoms of mental fatigue include poor concentration, poor memory, little interest, feelings of sadness, or an inability to get out of bed.

Although fatigue can be a symptom of excessive physical activity and emotional stress, it can also be attributed to lack of sleep. It is nature's warning that rest or sleep is needed. Chronic fatigue is abnormal and commonly associated with illness.

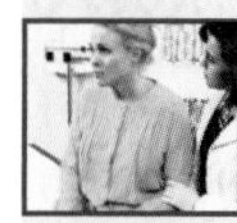

Based on the information collected in the nursing interview with Ms. Weiss, is she experiencing fatigue, insomnia, or both? Justify your answer.

Related Factors. As implied in earlier discussions, insomnia is influenced by changes in internal sensory input and external stimuli. Internal alterations include such variables as hormones, illness, anxiety, and stress. External events such as environmental and occupational changes may also create disturbed sleep patterns.

Fatigue may be experienced after increased or decreased metabolic demands, overwhelming psychological or emotional demands, increased energy needs to carry out activities of daily living, demanding role or social interactions, states of discomfort, and changes in body chemistry (as from medications, drug withdrawal, and chemotherapy).

DIAGNOSIS

To use the nursing diagnosis *Insomnia* accurately, you must determine if the sleep pattern is the problem or if it is an etiologic factor contributing to another problem. For instance, pain and anxiety may contribute to insomnia, but

Table 36-2 Clustering Data to Make a Nursing Diagnosis

Sleep Problems

DATA CLUSTER	DIAGNOSIS
A 76-year-old client was admitted to the hospital from a nursing home with a diagnosis of urosepsis. History of nocturnal confusion and wanderings. Awakens three to four times with nocturia since onset of urinary tract problems.	*Risk for injury* related to nocturnal confusion and nocturia
A 60-year-old client was hospitalized for gastroesophageal reflux. Awakened for the following interventions during the night: 12 midnight and 1:00 AM for IV medication administration, 2:00 AM for vital sign check, and 6:00 AM for hygiene measures. Sleep also interrupted at 3:30 AM by ringing phone and nurses' conversation about phone call. In addition, heartburn disturbed sleep at 3:00 AM. Client complains of feeling poorly rested the following morning.	*Disturbed sleep pattern* related to frequent awakenings and heartburn
A 40-year-old factory worker with a 1-year history of narcolepsy, fired from several jobs after repeatedly falling asleep. Admits to "heavy drinking" after being fired.	*Ineffective coping* related to changes in arousal secondary to narcolepsy
A 50-year-old client 1 week after open-heart surgery refuses to perform AM care or to ambulate as instructed. Complains of inability to sleep at night in such a strange and noisy environment. Reports an average of 0 to1 hour of sleep per night.	*Self-care deficit* related to lack of motivation secondary to sleep deprivation
A 69-year-old man with GI bleeding and multiple complications has been in ICU for 4 days. Requires NG tube suctioning, cardiac and arterial monitoring, multiple medication pump delivery systems, and a ventilator. Lights kept on at all times so staff can monitor him more closely. He has become increasingly irritable and confused about where he is and how long he has been there. He constantly pulls at the IV tubing, the NG tube, and ventilator attachments.	*Risk for disturbed thought processes* (ICU syndrome) related to sensory overload and sleep deprivation
A 64-year-old spouse of a stroke victim confides to the nurse that she is at wits' end with caring for her husband. Feels she could handle daytime caregiver activities if able to get a good night's sleep. Awakens 10 to 12 times a night from her husband's loud snoring and snorting.	(Wife) *Risk for disabled family coping* related to stress associated with spouse's care (Husband) *Impaired gas exchange* related to sleep apnea

GI, Gastrointestinal; *ICU*, intensive care unit; *IV*, intravenous; *NG*, nasogastric.

they are also sometimes nursing problems themselves. Likewise, for a client with symptoms of physical or mental exhaustion, you must decide if the fatigue is a symptom of insomnia or if it is actually a discrete nursing problem.

If *Fatigue* has been ruled out, and you have established that the client has a sleep problem, you must differentiate *Insomnia* from primary and secondary sleep disorders (Figure 36-5).

Sometimes *Insomnia* and *Fatigue* may be accurate diagnoses, but they do not focus on key elements of care as well as other nursing diagnoses might. For example, cardiac clients often have increased rest needs and fatigue as a result of chronic hypoxia. However, if the cardiac client is undergoing rehabilitation, *Activity intolerance* rather than *Fatigue* better focuses on the goals of therapy.

RELATED NURSING DIAGNOSES

The following nursing diagnoses are related to sleep and rest:

- *Risk for injury* related to sleepiness
- *Self-care deficit* related to lack of concentration or motivation
- *Ineffective coping* related to stressful situations leading to poor performance
- *Compromised family coping* related to frequent awakenings of children
- *Disturbed thought processes* related to inability to concentrate

PLANNING

EXPECTED OUTCOMES FOR *INSOMNIA* AND *FATIGUE*

If the identified problem has been difficulty falling asleep, then the client's report of rapid sleep onset is the expected outcome. Additional relevant client behaviors that support this outcome include the following:

- Demonstrates use of bedtime routines
- Exercises 20 to 30 minutes three to four times a week
- Keeps a sleep diary for at least 1 week
- Discontinues use of any prescription or over-the-counter medications that might interfere with sleep onset (such as analgesics that contain caffeine, CNS stimulants)
- Recites the purpose, dose, schedule, and side effects of hypnotics used

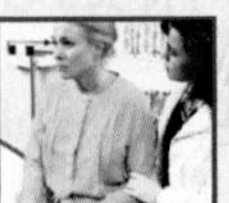

Which of these behavioral outcomes might be appropriate for Ms. Weiss? Justify your answer.

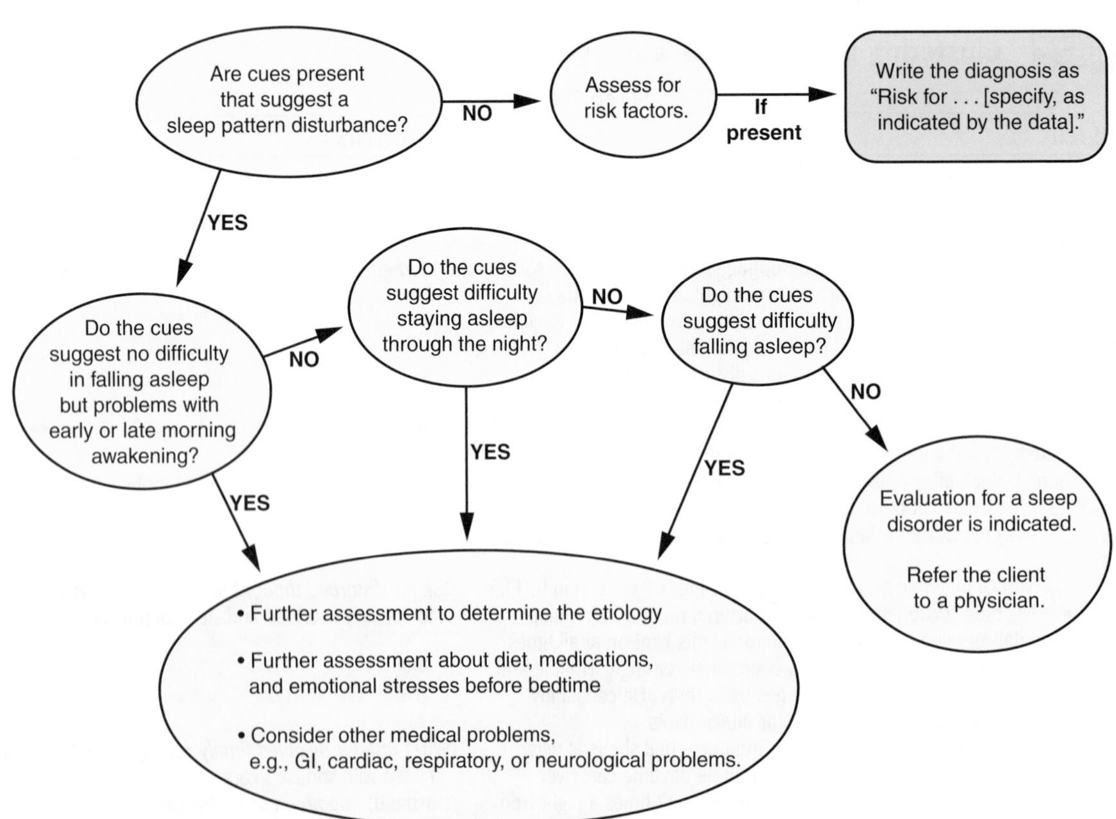

FIGURE 36-5 Decision tree for *Insomnia.* Diagnoses are shown in rectangles. Within these rectangles, diagnoses shown in **bold** type are NANDA-I–approved nursing diagnoses; diagnoses shown in regular type are not NANDA-I–approved nursing diagnoses.

For problems with interrupted sleep, successful management should result in client behaviors to decrease factors that interfere with sleep. Possible outcomes include the following:

- Client does not eat heavy or fat-filled foods just before going to sleep.
- Client eliminates sources of sleep disruption in the home environment (purchases heavy drapes to darken sleep area, for example, or uses white noise or ear plugs to eliminate excess noise).
- Client avoids alcohol for at least 5 hours before going to sleep.

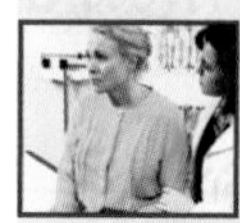

Are any of these behavioral outcomes appropriate for Ms. Weiss? Justify your answer.

If sleep has been interrupted by concomitant medical problems, then expected behaviors would be those that suggest better management of responses to such problems. For example, the client with pain would be expected to do the following:

- Report that pain has decreased to an acceptable level, using a pain scale from 0 to 10 to describe what is acceptable
- Take analgesics as needed 30 to 60 minutes before going to bed

The client with nocturia would be expected to do the following:

- Discontinue fluids 2 hours before bedtime
- Keep a bedpan or commode at the bedside for episodes of nocturia

The client with obstructive sleep apnea would be expected to do the following:

- Demonstrate correct use of the CPAP mask
- Eliminate intake of CNS depressants
- Maintain a patent airway during sleep

In addition, this client's bed partner would report a decrease in the number of snoring, snorting episodes.

The client with depression or anxiety would do the following:

- Describe the purpose, dose, schedule, and side effects of antidepressant or anxiolytic medications
- Report fewer early morning awakenings

If the client can fall asleep quickly, sleep undisturbed, and awaken feeling well rested, then excessive daytime sleepiness should not occur. The only client who might continue to experience such daytime symptoms is the narcoleptic. Appropriate expected outcomes for this client include the following:

- Client recites the purpose, dose, side effects, and schedule of medications.
- Client discusses the illness and its implications with employer and significant other(s).
- Client takes daytime naps, when needed, to maintain alertness.
- Client reports decreased number of sleep attacks, hypnagogic hallucinations, and cataplexy.

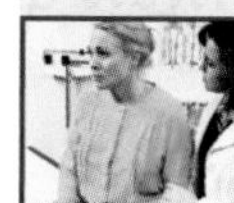

Given Ms. Weiss's sleep history, what statements would be appropriate subjective measures that her sleep has improved? What objective parameters could serve as sleep-improvement outcome criteria?

INTERVENTION

To better plan and implement strategies that promote sleep among hospitalized clients, you must consider factors that clients find disruptive and those they find conducive to sleep. Clients with sleep problems may find the following helpful: staying up later than lights out, back rubs, sleeping medications, position changes, supportive communication, snacks or drinks, turning the lights down, and ensuring quiet.

INTERVENTIONS TO PROMOTE SLEEP ONSET

Helping the Client Relax. A client with insomnia has increased sympathetic nervous system tone. Relaxation may help decrease this tone and thus promote sleep. Progressive muscle relaxation and deep breathing may prove beneficial. The client can be taught to tense and relax voluntary muscles in the feet, legs, back, stomach, arms, shoulders, neck, face, and eyes.

These exercises can be practiced for 20 minutes after going to bed and at other times of protracted waking during the night. In adults, hot baths taken in the early evening may also promote relaxation.

Position changes and extra pillows provide support and comfort. In addition, a back rub—the purposeful manipulation of back, neck, shoulder, and upper buttock muscles—provides physiological and psychological benefits (Procedure 36-1).

For the client who has pain, premedicate with analgesics as needed about 30 minutes before bedtime. If the client complains of constant pain, consider suggesting that the physician order round-the-clock analgesics for the client. Warm or cold compresses may also help alleviate pain.

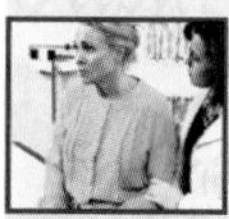

Which of the foregoing interventions might help Ms. Weiss meet her goal of a more rapid sleep onset?

Teaching Behavioral Strategies. To help a client better manage a sleep problem; teach about the function, benefits, and patterns of sleep. You should also work with the client to establish a regular, reliable 24-hour sleep-wake pattern. The Bootzin technique involves behavioral modification strategies that may help meet this goal. Box 36-5 (p. 992) provides guidelines for teaching these behavioral techniques.

Although the role of naps remains somewhat controversial, most clinicians agree that naps can lead to desynchronization of the circadian sleep-wake cycle and thus contribute to sleep problems.

Action Alert! Be aware of the client's medical diagnosis when considering backrubs. A backrub is contraindicated, for example, if the client has fractured ribs.

At home, the client should maintain a regular exercise program. Even though 20 to 30 minutes of exercise three to four times a week is helpful, you should discourage the client from exercising within 2 hours of sleep because such physical exertion increases mental activity and physical functioning. Encourage an older adult client who cannot exercise to engage in a stimulating daytime schedule and increased social interaction.

PROCEDURE 36-1 BACK MASSAGE

TIME TO ALLOW: **NOVICE:** 20 min. **EXPERT:** 20 min.

A therapeutic massage is given for the purpose of relaxing tense muscles, relieving muscle spasms, inducing rest or sleep, or stimulating circulation to maintain skin integrity. It may be given as part of a bed bath, as part of a bedtime ritual, or at any time when the client needs a period of quiet rest.

SAFETY ISSUES: Possible contraindications for back rubs include clients with skin impairment, wounds, and position intolerance and clients with back problems.

DELEGATION GUIDELINES

Back massage may be delegated to a nursing assistant after RN assessment of the appropriateness of massage for the individual client. Assistive personnel should receive training in massage techniques and be instructed to observe skin integrity, especially overlying bony structures.

EQUIPMENT NEEDED

- Soft towel
- Extra covering or blanket
- Body lotion of client's choice

1 Follow preliminary actions (see inside front cover).

2 Decide if the client needs or can tolerate a back massage. *Back massage promotes relaxation and comfort, which can help induce sleep. Rib or vertebral fractures, burns, or open wounds may be contraindications.*

3 Prepare the client for the procedure.

a. Raise the bed to a comfortable working height.

b. Lower the side rail, and help the client into a prone or semiprone position. The client's position should be relaxed and comfortable.

c. Expose the client's back, shoulders, upper arms, and sacral area, covering the rest of the body with the extra covering or blanket. *A raised bed and proper client positioning help ensure proper body mechanics while you apply pressure to the client's back muscles. Consider the client's cultural norms and personal preferences. For example, administer a modified massage if the client does not wish to disrobe during the procedure.*

4 Apply a generous amount of prewarmed lotion to the area or provider's hands. *Prewarm lotion by placing it in a basin of warm water for a few minutes before giving the back massage.*

5 Administer the back rub.

TYPE OF STROKE

a. *Effleurage:* Long, smooth stroke sliding over the skin; relaxing and soothing (see illustration).

b. *Pétrissage:* Kneading of skin and underlying muscles; induces relaxation in tight or tense muscles and promotes circulation (see illustration).

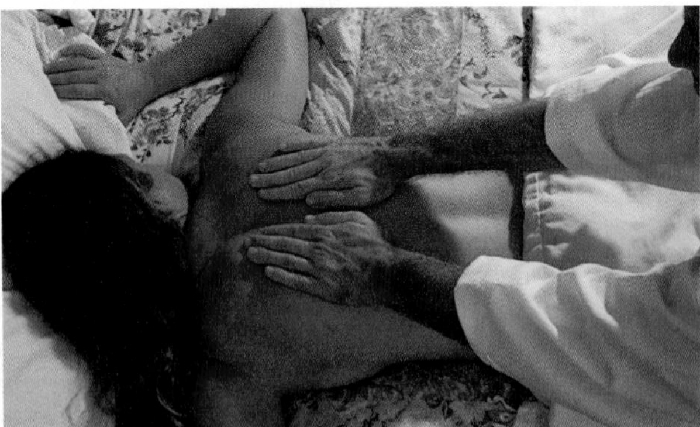

Step 5a. Effleurage: long, smooth strokes from the small of the back to the shoulders.

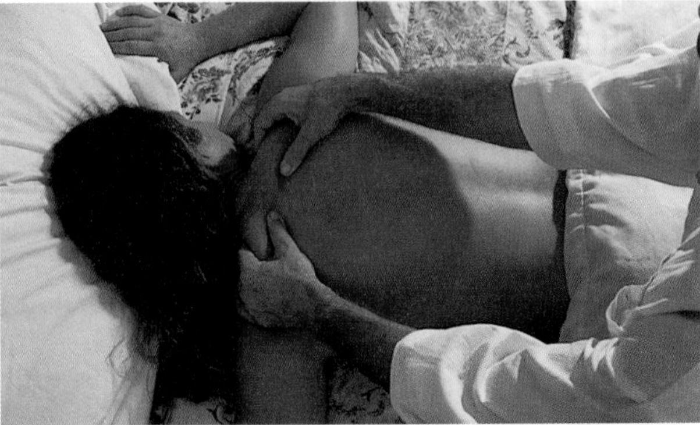

Step 5b. Pétrissage: kneading the shoulder muscles.

c. *Tapotement:* Rhythmic percussion or tapping; used particularly over tense muscles; should be done gently.

d. *Friction:* Use of small circular strokes—movement of the hands also moves the underlying tissue (see illustration). While massaging, keep continuous contact with the client's skin. Most clients find this contact soothing and are less likely to be startled by your hand movements.

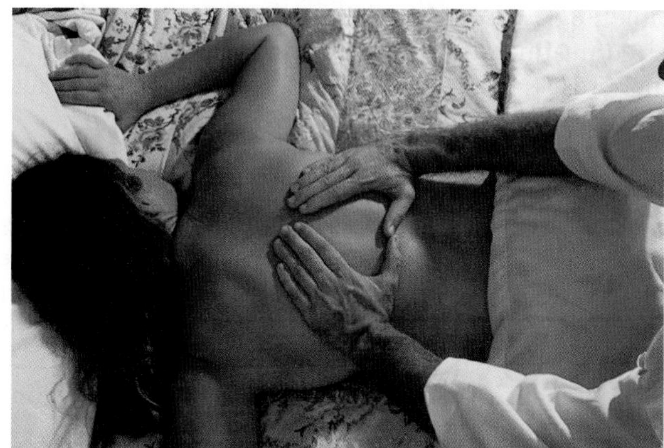

Step 5d. Friction: small circular strokes moving down both sides of the vertebral column.

PATTERN OF STROKE

a. Begin with effleurage. Start in the small of the back, using both hands (one on each side, close to the vertebral column), and stroke gently but firmly to the shoulders. Leave the hands on the skin and return to the small of the back, tracing the lateral aspects of the back. *This technique begins the relaxation process and allows you to assess for tension in particular muscles.* Repeat 8 to 10 times.

b. Focus on the neck and shoulders. Use friction strokes at the base of the skull. Knead the shoulder (trapezius) muscles. Repeat 8 to 10 times.

c. Focus on the muscles, moving down both sides of the vertebral column. Use circular friction strokes. Repeat 3 to 5 circles in each area, ending with the lumbar region. *Concentrate on areas of tension.*

d. Focus on the small of the back. Use effleurage from the center of the spine and out in all directions.

e. Repeat steps a to d with tapotement, if desired.

f. Use effleurage from side to side. Start at the top, and move down the back. Repeat 1 to 3 times.

g. Finish with effleurage as in step a. *This is the most relaxing stroke and will induce sleep in some clients if the massage has been well done.*

h. As a final step, gradually slow the strokes and decrease the pressure until your hands are no longer touching the client. Gentle firm pressure applied to all muscle groups facilitates muscle relaxation. Kneading increases circulation to the back muscles.

6 Wipe off the extra lotion, and help the client put on a gown or pajamas, if needed. *Some clients find wet lotion too irritating and bedclothes too confining.*

PEDIATRIC CONSIDERATIONS

Children may feel uncomfortable undressing in front of a stranger. Health care providers can teach the parent the various types of strokes.

GERIATRIC CONSIDERATIONS

Encourage the client to provide feedback as to the amount of friction being used (to prevent discomfort) and the length of the procedure (to prevent fatigue or overstimulation).

HOME HEALTH CARE CONSIDERATIONS

Just like a nurse in an institutional setting, a busy family caregiver may find that giving a massage is one activity that is tempting to skip. However, if a massage helps prevent pressure ulcers or helps the client sleep through the night, it may be worthwhile. Encourage the family to use the time as a means of maintaining a bond with the client through a pleasurable activity. Teach skin assessment techniques as part of the massage.

Such activities tend to decrease napping, which can interfere with nighttime sleep.

Bedtime routines will shorten sleep-onset time and nocturnal awakenings in children and older adults. Hygiene measures, prayer, light snacks, reading, or listening to music may be part of such rituals. If the client has an established routine, you should honor it to the extent possible. For the client who has not yet recognized the importance of a bedtime ritual, identify and offer suggestions for activities that can be used at bedtime to enhance sleep.

While such behavioral techniques may be successful in alleviating insomnia, they cannot be expected to compensate for lack of discipline or an overtaxing daytime

BOX 36-5 *Teaching for Wellness*

The Bootzin Technique

Purpose: To improve sleep hygiene through behavioral modification techniques.
Expected Outcome: The client will fall asleep within 20 minutes after going to bed.

Client Instructions

- Go to bed only when you are sleepy.
- Use the bed only for sleeping and sex. Do not read, eat, or watch television in bed.
- If you cannot go to sleep after 30 minutes, get up and go to another room. Stay up until you are really sleepy, then return to bed. If sleep does not come easily, get out of bed again. The goal is to associate the bed not with frustration and sleeplessness, but with falling asleep easily and quickly.
- Repeat previous steps as often as necessary throughout the night.
- Set the alarm, and get up at the same time every morning, regardless of how much or how little you slept during the night. This helps the body acquire a constant sleep-wake rhythm.
- Do not nap during the day.

lifestyle. Some insomniacs may need to learn more about time, people, and stress management than about sleep management.

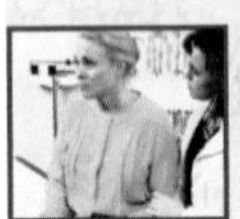

Which of the preceding intervention strategies would be appropriate for Ms. Weiss? What would you counsel her about naps?

Teaching Cognitive Strategies. Because insomnia is often precipitated by reflection or intrusive thoughts, you can help insomniacs by teaching them strategies to forestall such cognition. Remind the client that reflective thoughts may occur at bedtime only because bedtime is often the first opportunity to review the day's events. Preventing such bedtime ruminations can occur by setting aside 20 minutes in the early evening after dinner to reflect on the day's events and consider achievements relative to objectives. Once problem areas and loose ends have been identified, scheduled times to deal with the issues should be set but no actual work should be done that evening.

Administering Medications. Pharmacological treatment for sleeping problems or disorders has two main classes of hypnotics: benzodiazepines and nonbenzodiazepines. A **hypnotic** is a drug that acts on the CNS to shorten sleep onset, reduce nighttime wakefulness, or decrease anxiety when insomnia is associated with increased anxiety. The benzodiazepines drug family includes triazolam, lorazepam, temazepam, clonazepam, flurazepam, and alprazolam (Table 36-3). These drugs suppress REM sleep to various degrees as well as stages 3 and 4 of NREM sleep. Until a few years ago, they were the mainstay for treatment, but they can cause psychological and physical dependence. Their abrupt discontinuation can lead to withdrawal symptoms. Withdrawal increases insomnia for 1 to 2 weeks, but it may take up to 2 months for the drug-associated insomnia to resolve completely. To avoid such symptoms, insomniacs should take these medications for short intervals and only if absolutely necessary.

The new generation of hypnotic drugs, the nonbenzodiazepines (zolpidem, buspirone, and zaleplon) appear safer and are generally as efficient for sleep disorders (see Table 36-3) as the benzodiazepines. They are the preferred treatment for transient and short-term insomnia. They are less likely to change sleep patterns and to cause adverse psychomotor or cognitive effects. There have a risk for dependence.

Chloral hydrate (Noctec), one of the oldest hypnotics, is a sedative with a long history of use. It is only prescribed if the person cannot take benzodiazepines or the newer hypnotics. Chronic use is associated with liver damage and a severe withdrawal syndrome. Older adults are usually more sensitive to the effects of this medication. Diphenhydramine (Benadryl) is an antihistamine that is sometimes used for sleep. It is quick acting, usually between 15 and 30 minutes. It has a half-life of 3 to 12 hours, which is why it may produce some sleepiness the following day. It does not cause dependence or withdrawal symptoms with long-term use. However, it can quickly lose its effectiveness and interfere with normal sleep architecture, in particular the REM cycle.

A client taking a hypnotic needs to be monitored and taught about the potential side effects, as outlined in Table 36-3. Instruct the client to take a sleeping medication shortly before going to bed. Remember that many clients take their medication hours after retiring, when they have finally become frustrated by an inability to sleep. Consequently, their sleep will be out of phase with their normal sleep-wake circadian pattern, and they may experience increased daytime residual effects. Some of these drugs affect memory; thus more verbal and written reinforcements may be necessary. In addition, safety is an important issue in the sedated or less-coordinated clients, because they are at risk for falling when getting out of bed. Older adult clients or seriously ill clients may have a stronger reaction to sleeping medicines and need smaller doses.

Action Alert! Monitor the sleep of an older adult client taking a hypnotic very closely. If the client tries to get out of bed, a fall or injury may occur.

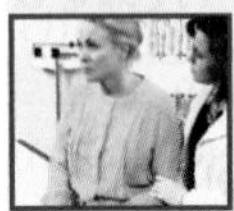

Do you think the physician should give Ms. Weiss a prescription for hypnotics on the first visit? Justify your answer.

Table 36-3 Commonly Prescribed Benzodiazepine and Nonbenzodiazepine Hypnotics

DRUG NAME	HALF-LIFE	DOSE (mg)	POSSIBLE EFFECTS	DEA SCHEDULE
BENZODIAZEPINES				
Triazolam (Halcion)	1.6-5.4 hr (short-acting)	0.125-0.25	• Rebound insomnia (early morning awakening), especially in high doses in older adults • Amnesia, confusion, daytime anxiety, memory changes • Daytime alertness after use	IV
Lorazepam (Ativan)	10-20 hr (intermediate)	1-4	• Morning sedation, lethargy • Memory changes, anger • Mild paradoxical excitation during first 2 weeks of treatment	IV
Temazepam (Restoril)	10-20 hr (intermediate)	15-30	• Sleep-onset insomnia may continue • Rebound insomnia with discontinuation • Daytime alertness after use	IV
Alprazolam (Xanax)	12-15 hr (intermediate)	0.25-0.5	• Drowsiness, depression • Insomnia, fatigue • Paradoxical excitement	IV
Clonazepam (Klonopin)	18-50 hr (long-acting)	0.75-16	• Useful in treatment of restless legs syndrome • Possible daytime sedation and poor coordination	IV
Flurazepam (Dalmane)	50-240 hr (long-acting)	15-30	• Possible daytime sedation and poor coordination • Suppresses daytime anxiety • Relative lack of withdrawal effects	IV
NONBENZODIAZEPINES				
Buspirone (BuSpar)	2-3 hr (short-acting)	15-30	• Dizziness, nausea, headache, nervousness, light-headedness, and dream disturbances	IV
Zolpidem (Ambien)	2.5 hr (short-acting)	5-10	• Drowsiness, dizziness, and diarrhea	IV
Zaleplon (Sonata)	1 hr (short-acting)	5-10	• Dizziness, nausea, headache, nervousness, light-headedness, amnesia, stomach ache, and muscle pain	IV

DEA, Drug Enforcement Agency.

Preparing the Environment for Sleep. The sleep environment should be dark, uncluttered, comfortable, and as free of noise as possible. To darken the room, pull down window shades and draw heavy drapes closed. In addition, shut the client's door and dim the lights. Check equipment and door hinges regularly to decrease noise from these sources. Telephones and intercom systems should be equipped with flashing lights for nighttime use. If possible, place the client away from the nurses' station and housekeeping closets. If necessary, provide the client with earplugs to dampen excessive environmental noise.

Institutions should make noise or disturbance audits part of ongoing nursing quality assurance, and provide in-service education about normal sleep patterns and primary and secondary sleep disorders for nurses.

In the intensive care unit, with its heavy reliance on equipment and intensive monitoring, noise is a particularly acute problem. When intravenous controllers and ventilator alarms are routed away from the bed at night, sleep pattern disturbances may be reduced. Prepare needles and syringes away from the bedside, and turn suction and oxygen off after use if they are unnecessary. You should also consider the meaning of noise to each individual. If you explain the necessity and significance of unfamiliar sounds, the client is less likely to perceive the noise as a threat.

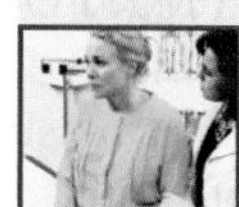

Do you have all the information you need to counsel Ms. Weiss about how to make her home environment more conducive to sleep? What other data might be helpful?

INTERVENTIONS TO FACILITATE UNINTERRUPTED SLEEP

Promoting Dietary Changes. Because diet may play a role in sleep induction and maintenance, counsel clients about specific dietary measures. Instruct them to avoid alcohol, nicotine, and caffeine, because all of these substances have been associated with an increased frequency of arousals. A light bedtime snack may be helpful. Some clients respond well to foods high in tryptophan, such as bananas and milk. Spicy foods should be avoided because they can cause gastrointestinal (GI) discomfort and increased awakenings. Heavy meals and too much liquid in the evening can lead to increased arousals from digestive actions and bladder distention.

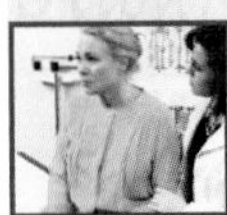

What dietary changes would you encourage Ms. Weiss to make?

Scheduling Nighttime Care. Traditional hospital routines violate many chronobiological findings about human activity and rest cycles. Most people have an early morning deep sleep cycle associated with a low body temperature, yet they are often awakened at this period while in the hospital. They also experience a postprandial dip in energy and alertness between 1:00 and 3:00 PM, a period when therapy is often scheduled. To the extent possible, hospital routines should be adapted to more closely parallel client circadian rhythms.

Minimize the number of times you awaken clients during the night, and be certain that the benefits of the intervention outweigh those of undisturbed sleep. Consolidate tasks to avoid unnecessary nighttime interruptions. Make sure that daytime turning schedules are modified at night. Most people turn spontaneously 30 to 40 times during a typical night's sleep. If you observe the client turning adequately, do not use prompted turning. In addition, post a "Do Not Disturb" sign on the client's door to alert family members and caregivers to check at the nurses' station before entering. Finally, report and chart the amount of uninterrupted sleep a client gets per shift to help the oncoming nurse better plan client care.

To minimize the effects of arousals when they do occur, anticipate each client's nocturnal needs. For a client with angina or asthma, intervention may mean placing nitroglycerin or bronchodilators within easy reach at the bedside. Help the client with nocturia or a chronic disabling condition by putting a commode at the bedside.

Managing Dyssomnias. Interrupted sleep also marks two primary sleep disorders: sleep apnea and narcolepsy. A client with sleep apnea may have little trouble falling asleep but may be awakened up to 100 times a night by apneic episodes. Clients who require nightly nasal CPAP to manage their symptoms are fitted with a nasal mask to deliver it. CPAP pressure is set to meet individualized needs (Figure 36-6).

Teach the client undergoing this treatment about the operation, long-term use, and maintenance of the device. Instruct the client that the underlying disease will recur if the apparatus is not used, even for short periods. Nasal stuffiness, one of the most common side effects of CPAP, can be managed with nasal sprays. The sleep partner and the client may need earplugs to obliterate CPAP sounds. Teach the client to avoid sleeping in the supine position. Encourage the use of pillows to help elevate the head. An obese client with obstructive sleep apnea should be given a weight-reduction diet. Caution the individual that nosebleeds may occur because of the drying effect of oxygen on the nasal mucosa. These should be reported to the physician.

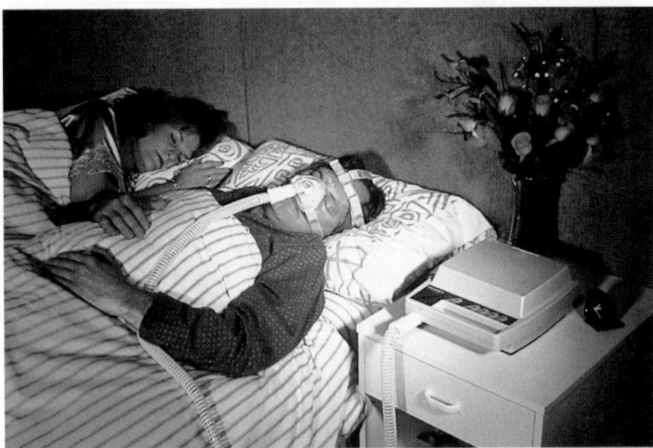

FIGURE 36-6 A client with obstructive sleep apnea wearing a CPAP mask. The CPAP mask provides positive pressure to maintain an open airway. (Courtesy ResMed, San Diego, CA.)

If a client with OSA fails to respond to CPAP treatments, an uvulopalatopharyngoplasty may be necessary. This surgery corrects the apnea by removing tissue from the soft palate, uvula, and pharynx to increase the diameter of the upper airway. Provide preoperative instruction to a client undergoing such surgery. Children with obstructive apnea caused by enlarged adenoids or tonsils benefit from an adenotonsillectomy.

Narcolepsy causes markedly disturbed sleep patterns and is characterized by EDS. Modafinil, a CNS stimulant, is used for the treatment of EDS. It works by changing the amounts of certain natural substances in the area of the brain that controls sleep and wakefulness. It may decrease sleepiness but does not cure the sleep disorder. Tricyclics and selective serotonin reuptake inhibitors are antidepressant medications that have proved effective in controlling cataplexy, a sudden episode of bilateral skeletal muscle weakness triggered by intense emotions, and hypnagogic hallucinations, but tolerance to these drugs may also develop. In addition to medication instructions, counsel a narcoleptic about lifestyle changes. Instruct the client that relaxation and the avoidance of intrinsic stimulation just before scheduled sleep may help extend nighttime sleep. Encourage a healthy diet and avoidance of alcohol and sedatives, both of which may increase daytime drowsiness. Even a well-managed narcoleptic may need additional daytime sleep and may benefit from 10- to 60-minute naps.

Managing Parasomnias. Teach parents of children who have nightmare, sleep terrors, or sleepwalking disorders about safety. If a child has nightmares, teach parents that the child needs comfort and reassurance. Environmental triggers, such as horror stories at bedtime, should be avoided. Recurrent nightmares, a parasomnia seen in both children and adults, may resolve if you help clients verbalize their feelings and resolve their psychic conflicts. If such interventions fail to solve the problem, the client may require psychotherapy and medications that suppress REM sleep.

The child with sleep terrors may need to be restrained during an episode, and breakable objects must be placed out of reach. Parents should not attempt to awaken the child. In addition, the child with sleep terrors may need to be referred for psychotherapy and hypnosis. For the sleepwalker, stair guards, bars on the upstairs windows, and combination locks on outside doors need to be installed. Teach parents of children with either problem about the importance of maintaining the child's routines and ensuring that the child gets enough sleep to prevent an exacerbation of the symptoms.

MANAGING SYMPTOMS THAT DISTURB SLEEP

Nocturnal enuresis may distress both the parents and the child. Provide parents with reassurance that the symptoms usually resolve with age, as the child gains better bladder control. Explaining to children that their sleep patterns are different from adults' sleep patterns, and that children do not always sense the need to urinate, may help alleviate some of the shame and guilt associated with the disorder. You may also provide instructions about bladder training and encourage the parents to restrict fluids before bedtime.

Bruxism, which is highly correlated with stress, can be treated with biofeedback. If a rubber mouth guard is prescribed to protect the teeth at night, you may need to instruct the client about proper cleaning, maintenance, and insertion.

Both GI and respiratory disorders may interrupt sleep. Nursing interventions directed at improving symptoms can help the client maintain unbroken sleep. Teach a client with gastroesophageal reflux to sleep propped up by pillows or to place a foam wedge under the head of the mattress to help prevent regurgitation of gastric contents.

Giving the client with ulcers an antiulcer medication at bedtime will help decrease nocturnal acid secretion and promote more rapid healing of ulcers. Better management of this condition should also lead to fewer nocturnal awakenings from burning gastric pain.

Make sure the client keeps GI and respiratory medications within easy reach at night. Extra pillows may also help the client with dyspnea. Oxygen therapy may be required for a client with hypoxia, which worsens during REM sleep, causing restlessness and arousals.

Managing Bedtime Agitation. Any dementia may severely disrupt sleep. In fact, a reduced ability to sleep typically accompanies the cognitive decline. **Sundowning** (also called sundown syndrome) is a sleep disruption involving the nocturnal exacerbation of disruptive behaviors and agitation associated with clients who have dementia. An exact explanation of sundowning remains elusive. The behaviors are apparently caused by, or at least strongly correlated with, darkness. To manage the client, try to distract and calm the client by playing soft music or turning on the television. Using a rocking chair can also be soothing and have a sedative effect. Physical restraints usually make the agitation worse. You may want to institute a "floor bed" program by placing the client's mattress on the floor to avoid restraints and eliminate the risk of the client falling out of bed. The client may also benefit from daily exposure to sunlight.

INTERVENTIONS TO PREVENT EARLY OR LATE AWAKENINGS

The client most susceptible to early or late awakenings is the one with a disturbed circadian rhythm, as from jet lag, shift work, or clinical depression.

When the production of melatonin is out of sync with the new time, jet lag is induced. The direction of travel has an impact on the severity of jet lag as well. To minimize the effects of jet lag, teach the client to adapt to the destination's time zone a few days before the trip. The client should eat lightly and avoid alcohol on the flight, reset the wristwatch on the plane, and adapt to the destination's circadian clock on arrival, even if it seems awkward or difficult at first.

Like the client who is adjusting to jet lag, the shift worker, such as nurses, must make circadian phase shifts as well. People who work the night shift or change time schedules frequently struggle with their performance and are at risk for accidents and depression. If possible, shift workers should be encouraged to make modifications in their environment such as bright lights (similar to the nocturnal workplace) and complete darkness for the 8-hour sleep period at home to expedite the process of circadian realignment.

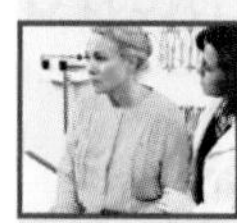

Because sleep deprivation increases the risk for accidents and Ms. Weiss is sleep deprived, what safety issues need to be addressed with her?

INTERVENTIONS TO PROMOTE REST

Remind the client who has an increased need for physical rest about the benefit of prioritizing and pacing activities, as well as alternating activity with frequent rest periods. Naps may be helpful if they do not disrupt usual sleep patterns. Teach the client how to conserve energy while engaging in activities, such as sitting as much as possible when engaged in relatively sedentary activities (food preparation and taking a shower).

Environmental modifications that may help the client conserve energy include replacing steps with ramps, installing grab bars, and raising chairs by 3 to 4 inches. For other energy conservation measures (see Chapter 34).

If the client needs rest but is bored by inactivity, encourage participation in hobbies that do not require high energy expenditures, such as reading, writing, knitting, carving, or model building. If the client complains of mental exhaustion, you may want to teach relaxation techniques, such as meditation or guided imagery. Yoga can help some people to relax muscular tension in a direct fashion. The breathing exercises and meditation can keep some clients from obsessing about sleep. These are helpful in quieting the mind and promoting relaxation.

Alternative Approaches. Herbs thought to have sedative properties include catnip, chamomile, hops, lavender, lemon balm (Melissa officinalis), passion flower, rosemary, willow, and valerian. Most of these substances have not been scientifically investigated, so their interaction with a client's medications would need to be evaluated. Chinese medicine views insomnia as a symptom of excess yang energy. Chronic nightmares or insomnia associated with hysteria and fear may be treated with cinnabar and either magnetic magnetite or "dragon bones". In addition, acupuncture treatments may be used to bring about balance and facilitate sleep (Box 36-6).

BOX 36-6 *Alternatives for Insomnia Treatment*

Tai Chi

Tai chi is a system of postures linked by elegant and graceful movements, whose purpose is to balance energies within the body.

Advantages

Substantial benefits in improved sleep measures
As an exercise, has side benefit of improving depression as well (Li et al., 2004)
Potential cardiovascular benefit because it is a form of exercise

Disadvantages

May require weeks to see benefits
Requires instruction to begin
Mobility issues may limit implementation

Herbs (Kava, Valerian)

Advantages

Effective at decreasing stress-induced insomnia (Wheatley, 2001)
Requires no lifestyle change
May be perceived as less stressful by client than sedatives

Disadvantages

Side effects include dizziness and vivid dreams
May interact with many medications (Skidmore-Roth, 2006)
Not appropriate for use during pregnancy or lactation and not in children

Acupuncture

Advantages

Effective against insomnia in many populations, including older adults (Sok, Erlen, & Kim, 2003)
Fewer side effects than medications
May be attractive to clients who prefer to stimulate their body's natural responses

Disadvantages

Clients may fear needles
May postpone traditional therapies
May be difficult to find a local practitioner

Li, F., Fisher, K. J., Harmer, P., Irbe, D., Tearse, R. G., & Weimer, C. (2004). Tai chi and self-rated quality of sleep and daytime sleepiness in older adults: A randomized controlled trial. *Journal of the American Geriatrics Society, 52*(6), 892-900.
Skidmore-Roth, L. (2006). *Mosby's handbook of herbs & natural supplements* (3rd ed.). St. Louis, MO: Mosby.
Sok, S. R., Erlen, J. A., & Kim, K. B. (2003). Effects of acupuncture therapy on insomnia. *Journal of Advanced Nursing, 44*(4), 375-384.
Wheatley, D. (2001). Kava and valerian in the treatment of stress-induced insomnia. *Phytotherapy Research 15*(6), 549-551.

EVALUATION

Ultimately, nursing interventions directed at alleviating *Insomnia* or *Fatigue* share a common goal: to promote a client's sense of being well rested. Until researchers can identify and quantify events that must occur during sleep for a client to feel well rested, evaluation must be made primarily on the basis of client reports. Refer to Box 36-7 for an example of an application of the nursing process to Ms. Weiss.

A nursing note for Ms. Weiss just after a teaching session might look like the one below.

Sample Documentation Note for Emma Weiss

Agreed to try the Bootzin technique. Plans to purchase and listen to relaxation audiotapes at bedtime. States that she will limit coffee to three cups per day, taken before 5:00 PM. Will consider cutting back on cigarette consumption after her midterm. Will keep a sleep diary, to be reviewed with RN on return to clinic in 1 month. RN will also monitor vital signs, effectiveness of behavioral modification techniques, and dietary changes at that time. If measures to improve sleep prove unsuccessful, will refer client to physician for possible short-term hypnotic prescription.

At 1 month follow-up: *"Reports improved sleep. Sleep diary shows that poor sleep is related to stressful events. Has reduced coffee intake but continues to smoke."*

Notice that the nurse documents that the sleeping problem has been addressed and that the nurse has worked with the client to develop new goals. The goals are to use Bootzin's strategies and audiotapes for sleep induction, to make dietary modifications that will promote sleep onset, and to monitor progress toward meeting those goals through use of a sleep diary.

These are goals in progress; full evaluation of the client's ability to meet these goals must be deferred until the next clinic visit. If outcomes are not achieved, or if the client has not improved by the next scheduled visit, reassess to identify possible explanations for the lack of progress. For example, if Ms. Weiss was not able to incorporate the

BOX 36-7

Nursing Care Plan

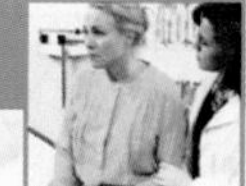

A Client With Situational Insomnia

Admission Data

A 48-year-old white woman with transient situational insomnia for past 3 months. Attributes symptoms to stress of new job and to enrollment in graduate school courses. Usually retires at midnight. Takes her about 2 hours to fall asleep. Describes herself as a light sleeper, but number of arousals has increased in the past 2½ months. Now awakens two to three times because of nightmares and once or twice due to nocturia. Awakens to alarm at 6:30 AM. Often feels "exhausted" on arising. Thinks mood swings and irritability secondary to sleep deprivation are affecting relationships with co-workers. Notes decreased ability to focus on details of work. Rarely naps. Tried eating chicken soup and/or drinking a glass of wine at bedtime to alleviate symptoms, but these remedies did not help. Does not take any OTC or prescription drugs regularly. Drinks up to 10 cups of coffee a day, including 2 cups in the afternoon and 1 cup after dinner. Over the last 3 months, has increased cigarette consumption to one pack per day. Smokes until bedtime. Wants sleeping pills.

Physician's Orders

Counsel for sleep disturbance.

Nursing Assessment

Yawns frequently. Fine international tremors present. Eyes have deep circles. BP 130/90, HR 106, RR 25, afebrile.

NANDA-I Nursing Diagnosis	NOC Expected Outcomes With Indicators	NIC Interventions With Selected Activities	Evaluation Data
Insomnia **Related Factors:**	***Sleep and Rest***	***Sleep Enhancement***	***Home Visit, 48 Hours Later***
• Stress	• Will substitute glass of milk for alcohol at bedtime	• Teach about rebound insomnia associated with alcohol and about sleep inducing properties of foods high in tryptophan, such as milk.	• Reported drinking milk at bedtime.
• Ineffective coping	• Will report falling asleep within 30 minutes of going to bed at night	• Teach about progressive muscle relaxation, Bootzin technique, importance of reviewing the day's events several hours before retiring, establishing a daily bedtime routine.	• Agreed to try the Bootzin technique. • Plans to purchase and listen to relaxation audiotapes at bedtime. • Started a sleep diary; will review with RN in 1 month.
		• Discourage smoking after supper.	• Still unable to cut back on cigarettes; will consider after midterm.
		• Discourage coffee consumption after noon.	• Stopped drinking coffee after 5:00 PM and cut back to 3 cups per day.
	• Will walk briskly for 30 minutes at least four times a week	• Teach about the importance of daily exercise to promote sleep induction. • Encourage exercise as part of ADLs (e.g., walking partway to work).	• Plans to make an appointment with the physician to discuss exercise program and need for testing before exercise, if any.
	• Will report 8 hours of uninterrupted sleep	• Teach to stop drinking beverages at least 2 hours before bedtime. • Refer to physician for possible hypnotic prescription if current measures to induce and maintain sleep fail.	• No further awakenings for nocturia.
	• Will report decreased anxiety	• Discuss possibility of decreasing the number of credits taken while adjusting to new job role. • Review past successful coping strategies that could be used in present situation. • Refer for psychotherapy if needed.	• Spoke with boss about prioritizing and delegating. • Averaging only one nightmare every other night.

Continued

BOX 36-7 *Nursing Care Plan—cont'd*

A Client With Situational Insomnia

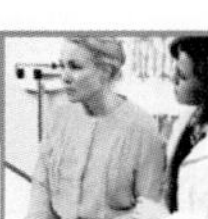

Critical Thinking Questions

1. Can you think of any other measures that might be helpful for Ms. Weiss?
2. After reviewing the evaluation data, do you think that Ms. Weiss needs further follow-up?
3. What criteria would you use to decide whether a referral for psychotherapy would be useful?

Nursing outcome and intervention labels from Johnson, M., Bulechek, G., Butcher, H., Dochterman, J. M., Maas, M., Moorhead, S., et al. (Eds.). (2006). *NANDA, NOC, and NIC linkages: Nursing diagnoses, outcomes, & interventions.* St. Louis, MO: Mosby.

Bootzin technique into her sleep routine, ask her about specific difficulties she encountered and review her sleep diary. Based on her response and any significant findings in the diary, you might want to give her written instructions about the technique, refer her for more intensive counseling services, or teach her additional stress reduction techniques, such as meditation and guided imagery.

As the case study illustrates, evaluation of care should focus on individual client needs. If the plan to improve the client's sleep is not successful after appropriate modifications have been attempted, then the physician may want to consider the next step: referral to a sleep clinic. These sleep disorder centers are often successful in diagnosing and treating severe or less common sleep problems. The American Sleep Disorders Association or the National Sleep Foundation should have a complete listing of local facilities.

▼ KEY PRINCIPLES

- Rest is a state of mental and physical quiet. Lack of rest can lead to fatigue.
- Sleep is a cyclic event that lasts about 8 hours and occurs once every 24 hours.
- Sleep can be subdivided into two categories: REM sleep and NREM sleep.
- During REM sleep, the brain is very active, but the body is quiet, and vital signs fluctuate. In adults, REM sleep lengthens progressively as the night progresses.
- In adults, NREM sleep predominates during the first third of the night. This sleep can be further divided into stages 1 to 4, with stages 3 and 4 representing the deepest or slow-wave sleep. During NREM sleep, the brain's metabolic rate slows, and vital signs are decreased, although the body remains active.
- Zeitgebers (circadian synchronizers) help keep the body's internal 24-hour sleep-wake cycle adjusted to a 24-hour solar clock.
- Developmental and lifestyle factors affect sleep and rest patterns.
- Sleep disorders fall into one of three major categories: dyssomnias, parasomnias, and other medical or psychiatric illnesses.
- Dyssomnias, disorders of initiating and maintaining sleep or excessive sleepiness, include insomnia, narcolepsy, obstructive sleep apnea, restless legs syndrome, and circadian disorders (jet lag and shift-work changes).
- Parasomnias, abnormal behavior or physiological events occurring during sleep, include nightmare disorder, sleep terrors disorder, and sleepwalking disorder.
- When assessing a client for sleep or rest problems, a thorough sleep history is critical.
- Disturbed sleep patterns are sleep problems that nurses can treat independently.
- Disturbed sleep patterns are defined as difficulty falling asleep, interrupted sleep, awakening earlier or later than desired, and not feeling well rested.
- Fatigue can be described as an overwhelming sustained sense of exhaustion and decreased capacity for physical and mental work.
- *Insomnia* and *Fatigue* may increase a client's *Risk for injury* and contribute to *Self-care deficit, Ineffective coping, Compromised family coping,* and *Disturbed thought processes.*
- Expected outcomes of interventions to correct *Insomnia* include client reports of rapid sleep onset, uninterrupted sleep, a satisfactory amount of sleep, and daytime alertness.
- Expected outcomes of interventions to promote rest include reports of feeling well rested and having an increased ability to engage in progressively more demanding activity.
- Interventions that help meet the goal of sleep induction include relaxation and comfort measures, behavioral and cognitive measures, encouraging regular exercise and bedtime routines, and creating an environment conducive to sleep.
- Most measures that promote sleep onset also facilitate sleep maintenance.
- Interventions to help clients cope with jet lag, shift-work adjustment, and depression will assist them in achieving the goal of awakening at a desired time.
- Interventions that promote rest, relaxation, and energy conservation will help alleviate fatigue.

REVIEW QUESTIONS

1. The nurse is aware that the most vivid dreaming occurs during:
1. Stage 1 NREM sleep
2. Stage 2 NREM sleep
3. Stage 3 NREM sleep
4. REM sleep

2. The nurse caring for an older adult who complained of waking up in the middle of the night would recommend the client:
1. Decrease liquids 2 to 4 hours before bedtime.
2. Take a nap mid-afternoon
3. Exercise 30 minutes about 1 hour before bedtime
4. Watch television in bed to relax

3. A client falls asleep while the nurse is interviewing her. The client is most likely suffering from:
1. Sleep apnea
2. Narcolepsy
3. Restless legs syndrome
4. Insomnia

4. The best advice the nurse could give a client to help him get a better night's sleep is:
1. Exercise before going to bed
2. Drink a glass a wine
3. Develop a bedtime routine
4. Take a sleeping pill

5. The nurse is aware that this age-group spends an average of 16 to 17 hours a day sleeping. They often alternate between REM sleep and wakefulness, skipping stages 1 through 4 of NREM. Their sleep cycle is also shorter, lasting about 40 to 50 minutes.
1. Infants
2. Children
3. Adults
4. Older adults

Bibliography

Ackley, B. J., & Ladwig, G. D. (2006). *Nursing diagnosis handbook: A guide to planning care* (7th ed.). St. Louis, MO: Mosby.

*American Psychiatric Association. (2000). *Diagnostic and statistical manual of mental disorders* (4th ed., Text Revision). Washington, DC: Author.

*Berrios, G. E., & Shapiro, C. M. (1993). ABC of sleep disorders: "I don't get enough sleep, doctor." *British Medical Journal, 306*(6881), 843-846.

Black, J. E., Brooks, S. N., & Nishino, S. (2004). Narcolepsy and syndromes of primary excessive daytime somnolence. *Seminars in Neurology, 24*(3), 271-282.

*Bootzin, R. R., & Nicasso, P. (1978). Behavioral treatments for insomnia. In M. Heron et al. (Eds.), *Progress in behavior modification.* New York: Academic Press.

Hilgers, J. (2003). Comforting a confused patient. *Nursing, 33*(1), 48-50.

Johnson, M., Bulechek, G., Butcher, H., Dochterman, J. M., Maas, M., Moorhead, S., et al. (Eds.). (2006). *NANDA, NOC, and NIC linkages: Nursing diagnoses, outcomes, & interventions.* St. Louis, MO.

*Kales, A., Beall, G. N., Berger, R. J., Heuser, G., Jacobson, A., Kales, J. D., et al. (1968). Sleep and dreams: Recent research on clinical aspects. *Annals of Internal Medicine, 68*(5), 1078-1104.

Kennedy, K. (2004). Sharing: A good night's sleep. *Nursing 2004, 34*(12), 51.

Ladwig, G. B., & Ackley, B. J. (2006). *Mosby's guide to nursing diagnosis*. St. Louis, MO: Mosby.

Mosby's medical, nursing, & allied health dictionary (6th ed.). (2002). St Louis, MO: Mosby.

NANDA International. (2005). *Nursing diagnoses: Definitions and classification, 2005-2006* (6th ed.). Philadelphia: Author.

National Institute of Neurological Disorders and Stroke. (2005). *Brain basics: Understanding sleep*. Retrieved June 29, 2006, from http://www.ninds.nih.gov/disorders/brain_basics/understanding_sleep.htm#Sleep%20Disorders.

*Shapiro, C. M., & Dement, W. C. (1993). ABC of sleep disorders: Impact and epidemiology of sleep disorders. *British Medical Journal, 306*(6892), 1604-1607.

*Shemwell, A., & Wilson, P. (1994). Rest and respiration during obstructive sleep apnea. *Nursing Times, 90*(19), 31.

Stringer, H. (2004). The wizards of nod. *NurseWeek*. Retrieved November 24, 2005, from http://www.nurseweek.com/news/features/04-05/sleep.asp.

Suhner, A. G., Murphy, P. J., & Campbell, S. S. (2002). Failure of timed bright light exposure to alleviate age-related sleep maintenance insomnia. *Journal of American Geriatric Society, 50*(4), 617-623.

Thobaben, M. (2003). Culturally competent health care: The national standards on culturally and linguistically appropriate services. *Home Health Care Management & Practice, 15*(5), 454-455.

Thobaben, M. (2003). Insomnia. *Home Health Care Management & Practice, 15*(2), 262-263.

Thobaben, M., Fossett, B., & Nadler-Moodie, M. (2004). *Psychiatric principles and applications for general patient care* (4th ed.). Brockton: MA: Western Schools.

U.S. Drug Enforcement Agency. (2005). Benzodiazepines. Retrieved November 24, 2005, from http://www.usdoj.gov/dea/concern/benzodiazepines.html.

Zunkel, G. M. (2005). Insomnia: Overview of assessment and treatment strategies. *Clinician Reviews, 15*(7), 38-43.

*Asterisk indicates a classic or definitive work on this subject.

Chapter 37

MANAGING PAIN

Media Resources

- Evolve Website http://evolve.elsevier.com/Harkreader/
- Companion CD

Learning Objectives

After studying this chapter, you should be able to do the following:

- Describe the physiological concepts supporting pain-related nursing diagnoses
- Describe the life span, physiological, and cultural or lifestyle factors that affect the pain experience
- Assess the client at risk for or experiencing pain and the client's responses to the experience
- Diagnose the client's pain management needs that will respond to nursing care
- Plan goal-directed interventions to prevent or correct the pain diagnoses
- Describe and practice key nonpharmacological and pharmacological interventions for pain management
- Evaluate outcomes that indicate progress in providing effective pain management

Key Terms

acute pain
adjuvant analgesic
agonist analgesic
analgesia
antagonist
atypical analgesic
breakthrough pain
chronic pain
endorphin
epidural analgesia
equianalgesia
first pass effect
gate-control theory
intrathecal analgesia
mixed agonist-antagonist analgesic
modulation
neuropathic pain
nociception
nociceptive pain
nociceptor
nonopioid analgesic
opioid analgesic
opioid naive
opioid receptor
pain
pain behavior
patient-controlled analgesia (PCA)
physical dependence
pseudoaddiction
psychological dependence
referred pain
rescue dose
somatic pain
suffering
tolerance
visceral pain

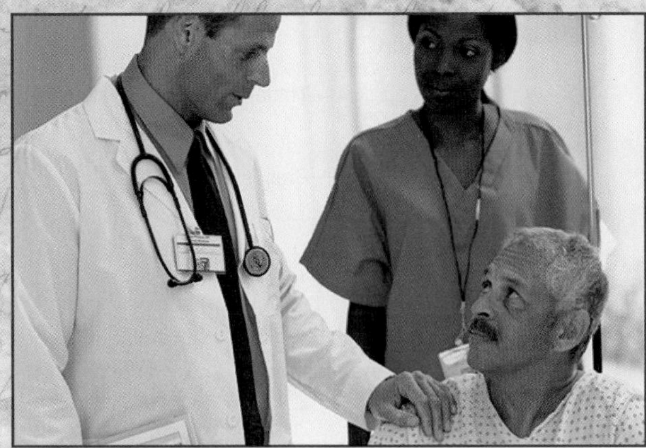

Joseph Valdez is a 54-year-old man who lives with his wife and three children. Two children are in college, and the third, who is 19 years old, has a full-time job. Joseph has worked for the same company since he was 18 years old. His wife, Pamela, raised the children while working part-time. About a year ago, Joseph was diagnosed with adenocarcinoma of the stomach and underwent a partial gastrectomy. After recovering from surgery, he received chemotherapy.

He returned to work, working half days until his determination allowed him to work full-time. In recent weeks, however, he has developed abdominal pain, bloating, and malaise. He refused to see his physician until the discomfort became so severe that he could not work.

Although he has trouble standing, Joseph insisted on driving himself to the physician's office, accompanied by his wife. The physician elicited significant pain on palpation of the abdomen. Joseph was admitted to the hospital for a workup for recurrent malignant disease.

The nurse assigned to Joseph selects *Acute pain* from the list of the NANDA International (NANDA-I) nursing diagnoses for pain (see key nursing diagnoses box) However, given knowledge of recurrent gastric carcinoma, the nurse believes the ultimate diagnosis may be *Chronic pain.*

KEY NURSING DIAGNOSES FOR PAIN

Acute Pain: An unpleasant sensory and emotional experience arising from actual or potential tissue damage or described in terms of such damage (International Association for the Study of Pain); sudden or slow onset of any intensity from mild to severe with an anticipated or predictable end and a duration of less than 6 months

Chronic pain: An unpleasant sensory and emotional experience arising from actual or potential tissue damage or described in terms of such damage (International Association for the Study of Pain); sudden or slow onset of any intensity from mild to severe, constant or recurring, without an anticipated or predictable end and a duration of greater than 6 months

CONCEPTS OF PAIN

According to the International Association for the Study of Pain (IASP), **pain** is an unpleasant sensory and emotional experience associated with actual and potential tissue damage (1994). It is essentially an alert that tissue damage has or is likely to occur in the body. Often, pain is a symptom of an underlying disorder. Pain is primarily a protective mechanism, but it is also a complex biopsychosocial phenomenon.

Pain is common in many illnesses and can last for variable periods. Therapeutically, it functions as a diagnostic tool, an assessment variable, and a measure of response to interventions. Pain may or may not have an easily identified cause, may occur at any time during an illness, may not always respond to conventional interventions, and may change in nature over time. It has several common denominators: all pain has a starting point, clients do not choose to have painful experiences, and clients must interpret and consider pain as significant before they enter the health care system.

Clients experience pain in the diagnostic, acute, ambulatory, home, hospice, extended, and rehabilitative settings. In general, you will find it easier to focus on a client's pain when the person is actually experiencing it. To be most successful in managing pain, however, keep in mind that it has many causes and is best managed by prevention.

McCaffery (1979), a pioneer nursing advocate for clients with pain, defined pain as "whatever the experiencing person says it is and existing whenever he says it does." The IASP acknowledges sensory and emotional components of pain, whereas McCaffery further qualifies the experience as individualized and based on client self-report. People with similar illnesses do not necessarily report similar pain experiences.

The incorporation of client self-report into a working definition of pain acknowledges its highly subjective nature. The client's evaluation of pain is your most important indicator of its nature and intensity. For clients unable to give a verbal self-report, such as newborns, infants, small children, comatose clients, and mentally or verbally impaired clients, you can assess nonverbal, behavioral signs of pain (Young, Siffleet, Nikoletti, & Shaw, 2006).

PAIN AS A PHYSIOLOGICAL RESPONSE

When the body is injured, a nociceptive response is activated. **Nociception** is the process of transmitting a pain signal from a site of tissue damage to areas of the brain where perception occurs. It involves anatomical structures and biochemical neurotransmitters. The initial tissue damage causes the release of biochemical substances (such as potassium, substance P, bradykinin, and prostaglandin) that begin or enhance the nociceptive response. An ascending system of nerve fibers carries the pain signal to the brain, and chemical substances known as neurotransmitters assist in delivering the pain message across synapses.

The Nociceptive Process. This initial injury triggers a series of events: transduction, transmission, and perception (Figure 37-1). Transduction is the process by which a chemical, thermal, or mechanical noxious stimulus is changed into an electrical stimulus by activating nociceptors. **Nociceptors** are the primary afferent nerve fibers that initiate the pain experience when stimulated by tissue damage. These nociceptors have the ability to encode the intensity of the painful stimulus.

Transmission involves a series of events in which the electrical impulse passes from the site of injury to the dorsal horn of the spinal cord and then to the brain. Once the signal enters the dorsal root of the spinal cord, the nerve fibers separate into groups of larger-diameter and smaller-diameter fibers. These fibers synapse with the spinothalamic tract neurons via neurotransmitters, such as substance P. Then the spinothalamic tract nerve fibers cross to the other side of the spinal column and continue upward through the spinal cord, ending in the thalamus. There, the pain signal is transmitted to various areas of the cortex.

In perception, the action potential reaches cortical areas (the somatosensory projections and limbic system) that allow recognition of the pain sensation.

Nociceptive pain is a common type of pain that results from stimulation of nociceptors (pain receptors) when there is tissue trauma, ischemia, or inflammation. This pain may be associated with events such as surgery, a broken bone, a cut, or a headache. The pain is transmitted to higher brain centers along an intact nervous system. Common descriptors of this type of pain are *aching, gnawing, pounding,* and *dull.* Types of nociceptive pain include **somatic pain, visceral pain,** and **referred pain,** as defined in Table 37-1.

Neuropathic pain is the transmission of a pain signal from a site of injury to higher brain centers via a nervous system that has been temporarily or permanently damaged in some way. The nerves themselves are causing the pain. The mechanism of damage may include cutting, crushing, or compression injuries, as well as viral or neurotoxic chemical exposure. These changes in the nervous system can trigger aberrant signal transmissions and may be associated with neural hypersensitivity (Reisman and Pasternak, 2001). Pain in an amputated limb (phantom limb pain) is a dramatic example of neuropathic pain. Examples of other causes are tumor infiltration of a nerve plexus (plexopathy), neuralgia, diabetic neuropathy, and a collapsed vertebra impinging on a spinal nerve root. *Burning, shooting,* and *electrical* are typical verbal descriptors, although the pain differs so markedly from nociceptive pain that clients may find it difficult to describe the sensation accurately.

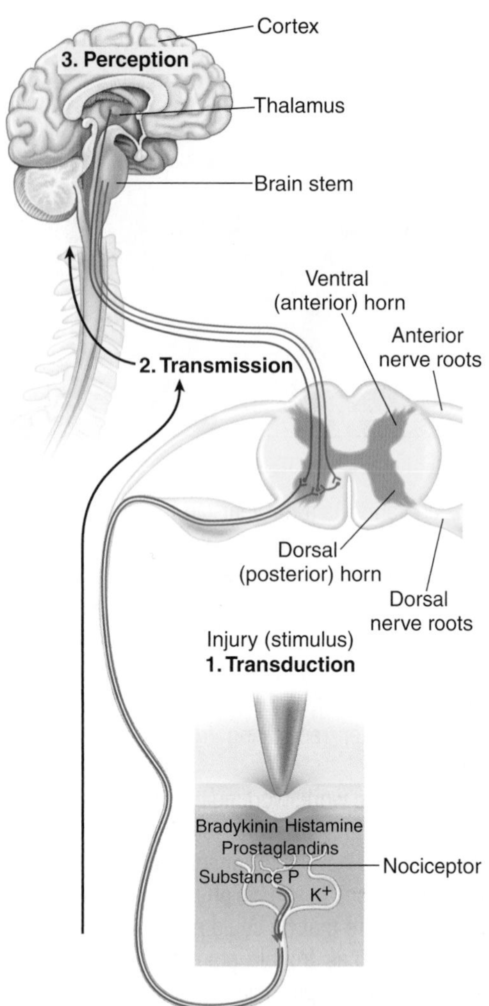

FIGURE 37-1 In the nociceptive process, tissue injury triggers a series of events. *1,* In *transduction,* the injured cells release bradykinin, substance P, prostaglandins, potassium, and histamine, which stimulate the nociceptors to initiate the pain signal. *2,* In *transmission,* the pain signal is sent to the dorsal horn of the spinal cord by A or C fibers, then relayed to the thalamus. *3,* The thalamus relays the pain signal to areas in the cortex where *perception* occurs.

A single disorder may have components of both nociceptive and neuropathic pain. The degree of each can determine the anatomical distribution and characteristics of the pain sensation, effective intervention, and the duration of the pain.

Modulation is an internal or external restraining of the nociceptive process that inhibits transmission of the pain signal at any place along the transmission pathway. An important type of modulation is the inhibition of transmission via descending nerve fibers that originate in the pons and medulla and release biochemicals (such as serotonin, norepinephrine, and noradrenergic substances) that attach to receptors in the dorsal horn. The concept of modulation helps explain why the perception of pain varies widely among clients.

Table 37-1 Types of Pain

PAIN TYPE	DESCRIPTION
NOCICEPTIVE PAIN	
Somatic pain	Well-localized pain, usually from bone or spinal metastases or from injury to cutaneous or deep tissues. Described as achy, throbbing, dull.
Visceral pain	Poorly localized pain. Occurs as a result of nociceptor activation from stretching, distention, or contraction of smooth muscle walls; ischemia of the visceral wall; irritation or inflammation; or torsion or traction on mesenteric attachment organs. Described as squeezing, pressure, cramping, distention, deep stretching.
Referred pain	Pain experienced at a site distant from the injured tissue. Visceral pain is often referred to skin, muscle, and bone. Deep referred pain demonstrates a segmental pattern to sclerotomes (bones supplied by a single spinal segment) and myotomes (muscles supplied by a single spinal segment), whereas superficial referred pain is often felt in a dermatomal distribution (skin supplied by a single spinal segment) related to the affected viscera. Varied descriptors used.
NEUROPATHIC PAIN	
Paresthesia	An abnormal sensation, whether spontaneous or evoked.
Dysesthesia	An unpleasant abnormal sensation, whether spontaneous or evoked.
Allodynia	Pain from a stimulus that does not normally provoke pain (e.g., touching skin with a wisp of cotton; contact with clothing or bed linens).
Hypoalgesia	Diminished pain in response to a normally painful stimulus.
Hyperalgesia	Painful syndrome characterized by an abnormally painful reaction to a stimulus, especially a repetitive stimulus, as well as an increased threshold; explosive onset and greatly exaggerated severity.

From International Association for the Study of Pain. (1994). Pain terms: A current list with definitions and notes on usage. In H. Merskey & N. Bogduk (Eds.), *Classification of chronic pain: Descriptions of chronic pain syndromes and definitions of terms* (2nd ed., pp. 209-213). Seattle, WA: IASP Press.

Certain drugs, such as tricyclic antidepressants, can inhibit transmission of the pain signal as well. Because transmission depends on neurons for transport and on neurotransmitters to carry the signal across synapses, some analgesics reduce pain by interfering with the production or reuptake of a neurotransmitter or by preventing its attachment to the appropriate receptor site. Table 37-2 describes the mechanisms of drugs that affect the nociceptive process. By doing so, they produce **analgesia,** which is a reduction in the perception or experience of pain.

Opioid Receptors. An **opioid receptor** is a portion of a nerve cell to which an opioid or opiate-like substance can bind. These receptors are located throughout the central nervous system (CNS) at the spinal and supraspinal levels as well as in the periphery. There are three primary receptor types (*mu, kappa,* and *delta*) that mediate analgesia, euphoria, sedation, respiratory depression, physical dependence, tolerance, and decreased gastrointestinal (GI) motility. They do this by interacting with an **opioid analgesic,** a morphinelike drug that attaches to an opioid receptor and produces analgesia by blocking substance P. When the opioid locks into the receptor, substance P cannot be released, and analgesia occurs. The strength of the bond between the opioid analgesic and the receptor determines the efficacy and duration of the analgesic effect. A **nonopioid analgesic** is a drug that provides analgesia at the peripheral nervous system level by a mechanism other than the opioid receptor sites.

An **agonist analgesic** is an opioid that stimulates activity at an opioid receptor to produce analgesia. It may also trigger physical dependence, tolerance, decreased GI motility, euphoria, sedation, and respiratory depression. The *mu* receptor mediates analgesia for "full agonist" or "pure agonist" morphinelike analgesics, including codeine, fentanyl, hydrocodone, hydromorphone, levorphanol, meperidine, methadone, morphine, and oxycodone. The *kappa* receptor mediates analgesia and sedation but rarely affects respiratory drive or causes physical dependence. The *delta* receptor primarily mediates analgesia.

The **mixed agonist-antagonist analgesics** (such as butorphanol, buprenorphine, nalbuphine, and pentazocine) are formulations that attach to both *kappa* and *mu* receptor sites. They provide analgesia at the *kappa* receptor site (agonist activity) but can simultaneously block activity (antagonist activity) at the *mu* receptor site if given after the client receives a morphinelike drug.

An **antagonist** blocks activity at *mu* and *kappa* opioid receptors by displacing opioid analgesics that are currently attached. The most common antagonist drug—naloxone (Narcan)—is used to counteract the life-threatening side effects of the agonist opioids attached to the *mu* receptor sites and the agonist-antagonist opioids attached to the *kappa* sites.

The **endorphins** are a group of internally secreted opiate-like substances released by a signal from the cerebral cortex. They attach to opioid receptors and block transmission of the pain signal. Multiple factors affect their release, such as brief pain or stress, physical exercise, massive trauma, some types of acupuncture, some types of transcutaneous electrical nerve stimulation (TENS) units, and sexual activity. Factors that reduce their circulating levels include prolonged pain, recurrent stress, and

Table 37-2 Mechanisms by Which Drugs Relieve Pain

DRUG TYPE	MECHANISM OF PAIN RELIEF
Nonsteroidal antiinflammatory drugs (NSAIDs)	Traumatized cells release prostaglandins that sensitize primary afferent fibers; NSAIDs inhibit prostaglandin synthesis and interrupt the pain signal at the peripheral level.
Opioids (systemic and intraspinal)	Bind to opioid receptors in the dorsal horn, inhibit release of neurotransmitters (such as substance P), and interfere with the relay of the pain signal across the neuronal synapse.
Membrane stabilizers, anesthetics, and anticonvulsants	Block ion channels (exchange of potassium and sodium), preventing generation of the pain signal; primarily indicated for neuropathic pain.
Antidepressants	Inhibit reuptake of serotonin, a neurotransmitter, into neuronal fibers, which makes less serotonin available to relay the pain signal across the synapse; primarily indicated for neuropathic pain.
Noradrenergic agonists	Attach to $alpha_2$-noradrenergic receptors in the dorsal horn of the spinal cord and modulate ascending pain signal.

prolonged use of opioids or alcohol. They seem to have the most benefit for moderate types of pain.

Sources of Pain. Pain can arise from different types of body structures. *Cutaneous (or superficial) pain* arises from the skin surface and is localized fairly easily because the pain is transmitted along defined neurological pathways called dermatomes. A dermatome is the region of the skin served by one spinal nerve and dorsal root.

Deep somatic pain arises from a variety of body tissues, such as tendons, ligaments, joints, muscles, connective tissue, blood vessels, nerves, and the periosteum of bone. Pain is often described as throbbing or aching in quality and is generally well localized, such as when a client sprains an ankle. Stretching and ischemia are frequently the causes of pain in skeletal muscle, such as with vigorous or excessive exercise. Excessive pressure and chemical stimulation are other causes of somatic pain, such as with rheumatoid arthritis.

Visceral pain arises from body organs and their capsules. This type of pain is more likely to be diffuse or poorly localized and to be described as a dull or vague pain. Because the nerves that transmit visceral pain impulses follow the pathway of the sympathetic nerves to the spinal cord, visceral pain is often accompanied by autonomic symptoms such as sweating, diarrhea, cramps, or high blood pressure. Visceral pain may also be sensed as referred pain, which is pain that is felt in an area of the body that is distant from the actual source of pain. An example is the pain of myocardial infarction (heart attack) that is felt in the left jaw, shoulder, back, or arm, instead of the area of the heart. Sometimes pain can be felt in its original location and also in a distant area within that dermatome; this pain is then describing as *radiating* to the second location.

Tolerance, Physical Dependence, and Psychological Dependence. The *mu* receptors mediate tolerance and physical dependence. Both are frequently mistaken for addiction.

Tolerance is an involuntary physiological phenomenon that occurs after repeated exposure to an opioid analgesic; it involves less pain relief despite a stable or escalating opioid dose. It does not occur with short-term use of opioids and is more likely to occur with chronic opioid use for pain caused by malignancy. Usually, the client reports a decreased duration of relief and then a decreased degree of relief. It is not a sign of psychological dependence.

Physical dependence is an involuntary physiological phenomenon that occurs after repeated exposure to an opioid analgesic. The client develops withdrawal symptoms if the opioid is abruptly withdrawn or an opioid antagonist is administered. Physical dependence occurs only after repeated opioid administration. Symptoms of withdrawal may include agitation, insomnia, diarrhea, sweating, and rapid heartbeat. If the source of pain is successfully treated or removed, physical dependence is easily treated by gradually decreasing the opioid dose, for example, by reducing the daily dose by 10% to 25% every 2 days. If opioid exposure is significant and of long duration, a tapering dosage of opioid therapy may be necessary. Withdrawal symptoms are not a sign of psychological dependence but rather of mismanagement of the tapering process.

Psychological dependence (addiction) is a chronic disorder demonstrated by overwhelming involvement with obtaining and using a drug for its mind-altering effects. This kind of dependence can cause great physical, psychological, and social harm to the user. It may be noted by active, compulsive, drug-seeking behaviors (such as seeking prescriptions excessively or from multiple health care providers) and a tendency to relapse even after physical withdrawal subsides. Quality of life is never improved by use of the drug.

Psychological dependence should be differentiated from **pseudoaddiction,** a syndrome of abnormal behavior that develops as a direct consequence of inadequate pain management. It is manifested by behaviors that mimic dependency, namely an overwhelming and compulsive interest in obtaining and using opioid medications. The client may request medication frequently, ask for specific medications by name, and demonstrate behaviors to convince you that pain is both real and severe. These behaviors can develop when the client receives analgesics only when pain develops or increases rather than on a continuous schedule throughout the day, when pain is continuous,

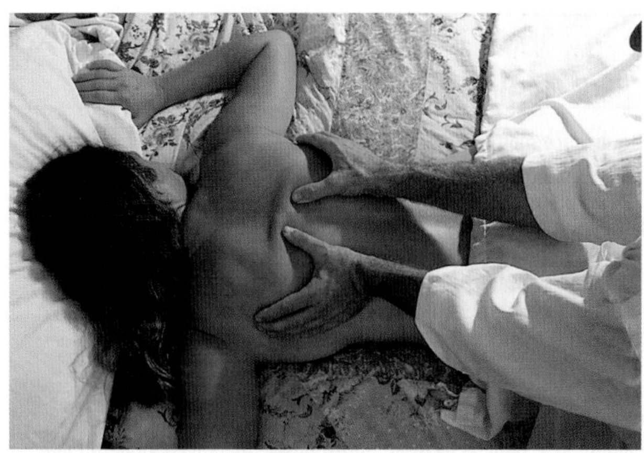

FIGURE 37-2 The gate-control theory provided a basis for a multidisciplinary approach to pain management that integrated physiological and psychological variables.

and when the drug or schedule is inadequate to manage the pain.

Very rarely does the use of opioid therapy during an illness cause psychological dependence. The majority of clients who derive pain relief from opioids experience improved function and better quality of life without harmful consequences.

> ***Action Alert!*** Do not confuse tolerance and physical dependence, which are involuntary physiological behaviors, with psychological dependence (addiction).

Gate-Control Theory. In 1965 Melzack and Wall proposed the gate-control theory of pain. The **gate-control theory** proposed that there is a gating mechanism located in the dorsal horn of the spinal cord, that the pain signal may be inhibited or facilitated by multiple variables, such as competing physiological stimuli, and that the brain could also modulate the pain experience. This theory revolutionized treatment approaches by including attention to psychological factors, as well as physiological factors, into the management of chronic pain. Figure 37-2 illustrates how tactile stimuli, such as massage, may be helpful in reducing pain sensation by causing a competing sensation of pressure.

THE PAIN EXPERIENCE

In 1968 Melzack and Casey proposed three major dimensions of the pain experience: sensory-discriminative, cognitive-evaluative, and motivational-affective. As this framework factored in cognitive and emotional variables, additional physiological structures had to be incorporated into the total pain experience. Somatosensory projections, the limbic system, brain centers that mediated visual and vestibular mechanisms, and cognitive processes were identified as contributors to the overall pain experience.

Sensory Dimensions. The physical sensation of pain can alert a person that tissue injury has occurred. It can serve a useful, diagnostic purpose and trigger a medical plan of care. You can use the client's description of pain and its location to help diagnose the medical problem. Even though pain may be helpful for these purposes, it remains an unpleasant experience for most clients and may take on more importance than its etiology.

Cognitive Dimensions. It is impossible to separate the physical sensation of pain from coexisting intellectual and emotional processes. When a client's attention is focused on pain, the pain is usually perceived to be more intense in nature. Educating a client about what to expect during a painful procedure decreases the pain's intensity and controls pain behaviors.

A **pain behavior** is anything a person says or does that implies the presence of pain. Behavioral expressions of pain are learned from others and may be culturally influenced. Children are particularly susceptible to this kind of learning experience and will imitate the people who are important to them. Some examples of pain behaviors are facial frowns or grimaces, restlessness, slow movements, guarding, lying still with eyes closed, or vocalizations (moaning or crying).

The meaning of pain also affects its intensity, its emotional impact on the client, and sometimes the client's response to medical and nursing interventions. A serious or life-threatening illness that causes the pain can trigger a "why me?" response as the client searches for meaning. If the client believes that the disease and subsequent pain are a well-deserved punishment from a higher being, are inevitable, or are a predetermined learning experience, the person may deny the painful state or fail to comply with analgesic therapy.

Pain can threaten beliefs about control and self-image, largely because most people fear a loss of independence. The feeling that pain cannot be controlled can produce extreme anxiety and a sense of helplessness. For some clients, however, pain may produce secondary gain by eliciting attention and assistance.

Affective Dimensions. Affective or emotional factors can aggravate and be aggravated by the pain experience. Anxiety, fear, apprehension, and depression are affected by the perception of pain. The dimensions of the human personality, such as a predisposition to respond in certain ways to specific circumstances, can influence how a client adapts to or deals with a painful process. Because threat and stress are part of the pain experience, the response to pain is usually consistent with the person's response to any other stressful event. The addition of pain to preexisting psychological stressors may produce a more intense response than might otherwise occur.

Anticipatory anxiety can intensify pain and affect pain behaviors. Many report feeling pain before a procedure begins. If the client has experienced unrelieved pain in the past, the result is a cumulative sense of fear and anxiety.

Pain can also deplete a person's energy. When a client's emotional resources are low, the response to pain is

Table 37-3 Comparing Acute and Chronic Pain

ACUTE PAIN	CHRONIC PAIN
Precipitating event with well-defined pattern of onset.	Occurrence may not be associated with an identified injury or event.
Warning signal that tissue damage has occurred.	No useful purpose after diagnosis is made.
Evidence of tissue damage.	May not have identifiable cause.
Short-term (6 months or less), then pain resolves and normal function returns.	Long-term (longer than 6 months and possibly permanent).
Signs and symptoms reflect hyperactivity of the autonomic nervous system (increased heart rate, blood pressure, respiratory rate, diaphoresis).	Signs and symptoms of acute pain are no longer present, indicating adaptation of the autonomic nervous system.
Behavioral manifestations include groaning, grimacing, guarding, wincing, crying, restlessness, anxiety.	Behavioral manifestations include a blank or normal facial expression, sleeping or resting, and a focus on activities that distract from the pain.
Client reports pain.	Client may not mention pain unless asked.
Pain usually responds to commonly prescribed medical and nursing interventions.	Pain may be difficult to treat, unresponsive to conventional modalities, and ultimately disabling.

more intense. The most inconsequential stressors can trigger pain disproportionate to the circumstances. Whereas pain is the actual physical sensation of discomfort, **suffering** is the unpleasant emotional response to pain (Chapman & Garvin, 1999).

Characteristics of Acute and Chronic Pain. Generic definitions of nociceptive and neuropathic pain are not comprehensive enough to describe the pain experience. Although it is essential to qualify the nature of pain, the chronicity of the experience greatly affects the quality of the client's life.

Acute pain has been defined as a short-term, self-limited pain with a probable duration of less than 6 months. Acute pain may absorb a person's physical and emotional energy for a brief time, but knowing it will disappear as the tissue heals can help a client to cope with the pain. Acute pain does needs to be effectively managed, however, to promote general well-being and to reduce the risk that the client will develop chronic pain.

Chronic pain is long-term, constant or recurring pain without an anticipated or predictable end and is typically defined as having a duration of 6 months or longer. It may be both permanent and permanently disabling. Chronic pain can quickly deplete a person's physical and emotional resources, immobilize the person, lead to physical disability and subsequent loss of employment, significantly impact daily activities, interrupt sleeping habits, and interfere with interpersonal relationships. As the pain experience becomes more complex and seemingly endless, the impact on the client becomes more extensive. See Table 37-3 for a comparison of features of acute and chronic pain.

FACTORS AFFECTING PAIN

Given that pain can be such a complex phenomenon, it is impossible to separate or isolate its impact on any part of the client's experience of living. It can color even trivial everyday affairs as well as the most profound existential issues. Thus the amount of pain a person is willing to endure is a unique response influenced by many physiological and psychological issues.

FACTORS ACROSS THE LIFE SPAN

There is no doubt that the client's developmental stage markedly affects cognitive and behavioral manifestations of pain. Pain behaviors vary in infancy, childhood, adolescence, and clinical assessment, and interventions are based on the client's language skills and ability to understand the circumstances.

However, developmental factors can occur at any age. The client with confusion (D'Arcy, 2006) or dementia or the client with severe learning disabilities may be at greater risk for inadequate assessment and intervention. When complicating factors disrupt communication about pain, the client's inability to communicate may be both frightening and frustrating.

PHYSIOLOGICAL FACTORS

Physiological factors affecting pain necessarily include the underlying health problems that trigger this symptom. These include disorders characterized by injury, inflammation, or irritation of body organs or tissues.

A client may have coexisting morbidities that affect the pain experience. Take, for example, a person with osteoarthritis who falls and breaks an arm. The pain experience is not new, but the additive pain may decrease the person's ability to tolerate what has been an acceptable norm of discomfort.

The gender of the client can influence pain threshold and tolerance, with women having lower pain threshold and tolerance levels to applied pressure (Soetanto, Chung, & Wong, 2006). However, pain in women is more likely to be undertreated because of long-standing myths that women may exaggerate their pain or that pain reported by men is more likely due to physiological causes.

Nurses may also have biases based on the cause of a client's pain or doubts about the client's self-report of

BOX 37-1 **Cross-Cultural Care**

Caring for a Mexican American Client

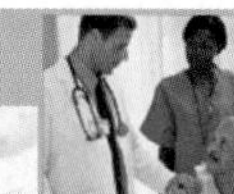

Joseph Valdez, the client who presented with possible recurrent gastric carcinoma, is of Mexican descent. He was born in Mexico City and immigrated to the United States with his parents when he was 14 years old. He became fluent in English very quickly, but his parents continued to speak Spanish, settled into a Spanish-speaking neighborhood, and continued their previous customs. Joe married a classmate from high school who had been born and raised in the United States. This concerned his family for fear he would drift away from their customs. Diversity in the Mexican American population about health beliefs and practices is dependent on the amount of time spent in the United States and the degree of affinity to traditional Mexican culture. Traditional beliefs tend to include the following:

- Avoidance of direct eye contact with health care providers because they are seen as authority figures or of a higher class
- Showing respect when the provider enters the room
- Use of silence to show lack of agreement with the plan of care
- Keeping the most sensitive issues inside the family
- Discussing particularly sensitive issues only with those of the same sex
- Protecting the client from knowledge about the seriousness of the illness
- Strong belief in the mind-body connection and concern that worry will worsen health status
- Traditional belief that health is controlled by environment, by fate, and by the will of God
- Involvement of family members in activities of daily living
- Belief that self-care may adversely affect recovery
- Avoidance of complaints about pain because they show weakness, leading to loss of self-respect
- Respect for inner control and self-endurance
- Embarrassment and secrecy about depression because it is seen as a sign of mental illness and weakness

pain, which can negatively influence the degree to which they treat pain reported by the client. Clients particularly at risk for inadequate pain management include those with sickle cell disease, acquired immunodeficiency syndrome (AIDS), and substance abuse.

CULTURAL AND LIFESTYLE FACTORS

Culture can mold a client's beliefs about pain, its meaning, expected pain behaviors, and the way pain is treated medically. Cultural orientation functions as an experiential filter and a grid for decision making, thus distinctly influencing the pain experience (Box 37-1).

Cultural background can also influence thoughts and attitudes about pain relief. For example, many people believe that older people experience less pain because of a changing pain threshold. Another common myth is that pain is a normal part of aging. The fact is that pain in older adults is the same as for any other population.

RELIGIOUS FACTORS

Religious beliefs can have a profound impact on a client's response to pain. Historically, great significance has been attached to pain and suffering. The pain may be perceived as deserved retribution or as atonement for past behaviors. The client's religious denomination may have belief systems that require certain behaviors (such as stoicism or acceptance) that are independent of cultural orientation.

SOCIAL AND ENVIRONMENTAL FACTORS

The social environment is intricately linked to the pain experience. The way others respond to pain will affect how the client responds. The presence of a strong emotional support system or assistance from others in performing daily tasks may make the pain experience more tolerable. In contrast, the demands of daily life coupled with a lack of understanding or sympathy from others can worsen the pain experience. If the client lives a relatively isolated life, the absence of support may make the pain less tolerable.

A person's ability to perform activities of daily living (ADLs) and to participate in meaningful leisure activities can markedly affect the pain experience. A client accustomed to physical activity at work, at home, or during leisure time may aggravate a painful condition by refusing to change a behavior even when understanding its potential harm. The perception of self as active and strong may be more appealing and emotionally nurturing than acceptance of any kind of disability.

ASSESSMENT

The nature of a client's pain experience will determine the complexity of the assessment required. Although pain is always multifaceted, it is not always complex. A client with temporary, manageable pain secondary to a known cause (e.g., surgery to repair a joint) may require no more than diligent assessment for preanalgesic and postanalgesic pain to ensure adequate pain relief. On the other hand, a client with recurrent cancer accompanied by significant pain requires a thorough assessment that includes both psychosocial and physiological data.

In all cases, assessment determines the appropriate treatment approach. When the disorder cannot be identified, the nature and location of pain may serve as the basis for treatment. Ongoing assessment of pain status allows evaluation of the treatment's efficacy and directs further intervention.

GENERAL ASSESSMENT OF PAIN

Pain assessment may occur in an ambulatory or acute care setting, in the client's home, or in an extended-care or rehabilitation facility. In some cases, the client's detailed health history may already be available for you to consult. In others, you may need to obtain it at your initial visit with the client. In either case, the goals of your assessment are to do the following:

- Determine the current nature and status of the client's pain
- Review the history of the client's pain and its therapies
- Explore psychosocial, religious, and cultural variables that may influence the pain experience
- Collaborate with the client and other health care team members to plan and deliver effective pain management strategies that effect relief

Your pain assessment should focus on both subjective and objective variables. As you interpret the client's pain experience, remember to keep the following basic principles in mind:

- Because pain is a subjective experience, you must use the client's evaluation as your initial standard, even if your attitudes and life experiences make you tend to doubt or disagree with it.

> ***Action Alert!*** Be sure to accept a client's self-evaluation of pain with respect. Failure to do so can trigger an adversarial relationship between the client and health care team and could also ultimately lead to undertreatment.

- The sympathetic nervous system can trigger a number of physiological indicators of acute pain. These include sweating, pallor, and possible increases in pulse, respirations, or blood pressure. Be aware, however, that these signs may only be present for the first few hours of an acute pain episode and then return to baseline, even if the pain has gone untreated.
- Because the nature and duration of the pain experience can activate physiological and psychological adaptation over time, the absence of common pain behaviors in a client with chronic pain does not negate the presence of pain.

> ***Action Alert!*** Expect that as a client adapts to chronic pain, observable signs lessen, although the pain's severity remains unchanged. Do not assess a client who has chronic pain using the acute model, because it produces an inaccurate nursing assessment.

Health History. To obtain a detailed history when pain is involved, avoid expressing any hints of symptoms or diagnoses that could affect the client's report. By allowing the client to explain the pain experience without prompting, you may obtain such a clear picture that the diagnosis can be determined primarily from reported symptoms.

Begin your assessment by addressing the details of the client's chief complaint. The pain may be new, an exacerbation of existing pain, a type of pain different from that previously experienced, or a pain affecting a location other than what was previously reported. The pain's onset can provide etiologic clues. Its duration establishes chronicity, a detail that may offer insight into the client's behaviors. The client's description of the pain experience will help you determine whether to continue the assessment using the acute pain model or the chronic pain model.

Ask questions such as the following:

- Are you having pain or discomfort at the present time?
- Do you have any illnesses at present? Have you ever had pain or discomfort related to this illness?
- When did it start? Did you do something that you normally would not do when it began? When it began, did it come on suddenly? Did it happen over a period of time?
- Is it persistent, or does it come and go?
- Do any other symptoms accompany the pain or discomfort?
- What do you think is causing your pain or discomfort right now?

Characteristics. As you continue to assess the client's pain, you will want to explore the characteristics of the pain. Assessing these will provide you with an overall "photograph" from the client's perspective.

Location. Location is a critical variable. Try to obtain this information while the pain is actually present because the accuracy of the client's report will decrease as the pain diminishes. Have the client point to the areas on the body where he or she feels pain, or have the client make marks on a simple anatomical figure. Many standard pain assessment tools include anatomical renderings for that purpose. Make sure the drawings you use include front, back, left, and right views of the whole body, and right, left, front, and back sides of the head.

When the client indicates an area of pain, inquire whether the pain is new, recurring, or worse than before. Also ask whether it stays at that location or radiates to another location.

Quality. Descriptive words can qualify the pain sensation and give you clues about whether the pain is nociceptive, neuropathic, or both. Words like *dull, aching, gnawing,* and *tender* tend to describe nociceptive pain. Words like *prickly, shooting, electric,* and *burning* are more likely to be used for neuropathic pain.

Clients with neuropathic pain commonly have trouble finding adequate words to describe the sensation. In that case, you may want to give the client a list of descriptors to help the client describe his or her feelings. Many standard pain assessment tools contain descriptor words from which the client can choose. Tell the client to choose as many words as needed, and different words may be chosen for different areas of the body.

Intensity. Intensity is the most subjective of the dimensional characteristics. To measure it, you will use one of several types of pain rating scales. These scales seek to make the client's subjective experience as objective as possible. Once you choose a pain rating scale for a client, continue to use the same scale in ongoing assessments to keep the responses as comparable as possible over time.

Single-dimension self-report tools include the visual analogue scale, numerical rating scale, and verbal descriptor scales. A visual analogue scale is a 10-cm horizontal line (Figure 37-3). At its left endpoint is written *No pain at all.* At its right endpoint is written *Worst pain imaginable.* The client makes a mark at the point along the line that corresponds to the level of pain. Simple and quick, this scale has proven to be reliable and valid. It is abstract in nature, however, and may be difficult for some clients to use.

A numerical rating scale is also quick, simple, and easy to use. The client can point to, mark, or say the number that corresponds to the intensity of the pain (Figure 37-4). Although the numerical scale is relatively easy for most clients to use, it may not reflect subtle changes. When using it, make sure the client can count up to the high end of the scale. The numerical rating scale tends to work best for assessing pain before and after analgesic intervention, the worst pain in a defined period of time, the least pain in a defined period of time, the intensity of continued pain, the intensity of pain that may flare up on occasion, and the amount of pain that the client can tolerate.

A verbal descriptor scale requires the client to choose one word to describe the pain (Figure 37-5). This scale is most effective when the client can see it. Verify the client's understanding of the meaning of each word. The limited choice of words may make the assessment less accurate.

When choosing a scale to use, consider the client's level of comprehension, eyesight, and developmental status. Collaborating with the client is always appropriate. An accurate assessment is more likely if you define the parameters each time you use a scale until the client is comfortable with it.

Regardless of the scale used, clients tend to choose the middle rather than the ends of a scale, a tendency that can alter the accuracy of your assessment. Make sure to query clients closely to clarify the level of pain that they can tolerate or that they consider acceptable. Clients may feel able to tolerate a higher level of rare or brief pain. This kind of clarification helps you set collaborative, reasonable goals with them. Absence of pain is not always attainable. Tolerable relief, increased activity, or improved eating and sleeping habits may be more realistic goals.

Aggravating and Alleviating (Relieving) Variables. Ask clients what, if anything, makes the pain better or worse. Ask whether any specific movements or positions make the pain better or worse. Ask what they think works best to relieve the pain. These and similar questions may provide valuable diagnostic leads, as well as direction for planning analgesic interventions.

Effects of Previous Therapy. Assessing a client's previous treatment can eliminate repetitive interventions that are not helpful or are even harmful. It can also point out interventions that the client believed *were* helpful. Have the client describe both pharmacological and nonpharmacological interventions to give you better insight into past experiences.

Be sure to ask the client questions about specific interventions. For example, ask whether any nonpharmaceutical interventions have relieved the pain, such as heat, cold, a TENS unit, massage, or relaxation techniques. Ask whether any pain medications have been taken and to what extent they relieved the pain. Ask what drug and dosage seemed to work best, what did not work, and whether any pain medications produced nausea or an allergic reaction.

Current Analgesic Therapy. Exploring the client's current therapy can help you manage future regimens. You may find that the current regimen controls the

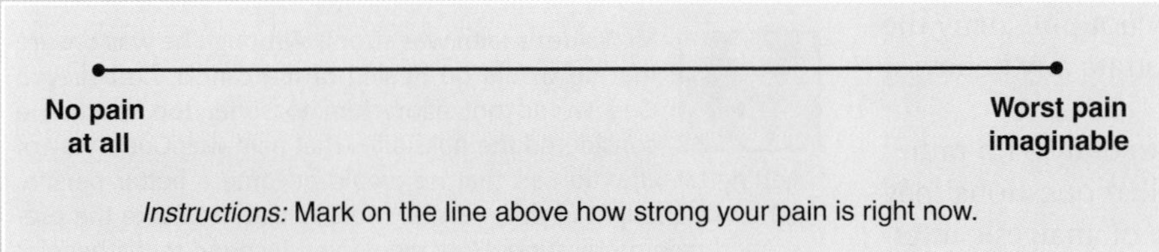

FIGURE 37-3 Visual analogue pain rating scale.

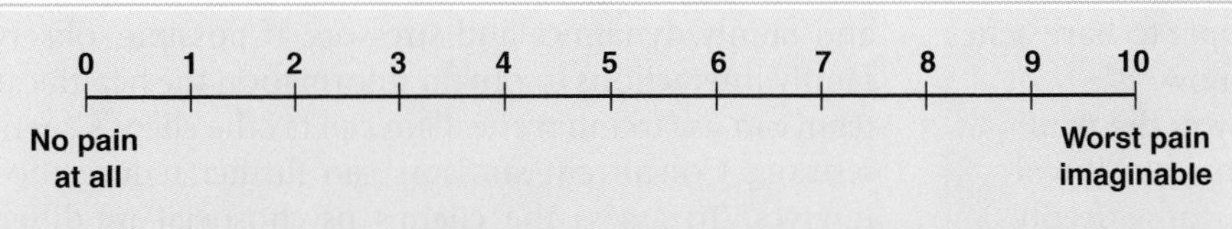

FIGURE 37-4 Numerical pain rating scale.

None / Annoying / Uncomfortable / Dreadful / Horrible / Agonizing

Instructions: Choose the word above that best describes how your pain feels right now.

FIGURE 37-5 Verbal descriptor pain rating scale.

client's pain adequately or that it needs to be changed to enhance analgesic efficacy.

When asking clients to name the medications they take for pain management, also ask the dose or amount they take. Find out how long it takes for the pain to subside after they take a dose. Ask whether they think the medication is working.

Also, make sure to ask what other medications they take, including over-the-counter ones. This allows you to assess any risks from polypharmacy and to identify **atypical analgesics,** which are drugs not primarily indicated for pain but used to treat specific types of pain. For example, an anticonvulsant may be used to treat neuropathic pain. The client may not remember that these medications are used to treat pain. Also ask if anyone other than the client's physician is helping with pain management (e.g., a massage therapist or acupuncturist).

Effects on Activities of Daily Living. Chronic pain and sometimes acute pain can markedly impair ADL. Ask questions about the impact of pain on the client's regular routine. For example, ask whether pain medications cause side effects (such as nausea or fatigue) that interfere with the client's activities. Find out whether the client can go to work every day, has a good appetite, and sleeps normally at night. Ask whether the client feels rested in the morning, and whether he or she needs to take pain medications during the night.

Cultural Variables. Cultural expectations can mold the meaning of pain and the client's subsequent behaviors, and your lack of understanding of those expectations can interfere with an accurate pain assessment. For example, if cultural norms demand stoicism even in the presence of severe pain, the client may not only deny the presence of pain but may not demonstrate any behavior that pain is a problem.

Although every client has the right to deny pain rather than acknowledge it, your tactful, skilled questions may help lead the client toward acceptance of analgesic intervention. For example, ask questions like these:

- You seem to be having difficulty moving around. Are you hurting right now?
- It's not unusual after surgery for people to have aches or sore places. Are you having pain now?
- May I have your permission to give you the pain medicine your doctor has ordered for you? It will probably make it easier for you to breathe deeply and get up and out of bed.
- This particular illness can make people hurt and prevent them from doing things they have always done. Would you like to try the pain medicine the doctor has ordered to see if it can help you to do those things again?

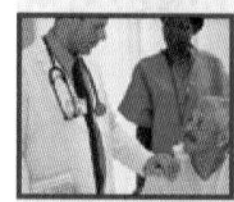

Joseph Valdez was born in Mexico City and came to the United States at age 14 years. His English skills were limited, but through determination and hard work, he became fluent within 1 year. At age 16 he got a part-time job after school at a grocery store, where he met his wife-to-be, Pamela. How might his strong will affect his response to pain? Is your expectation consistent with your stereotype of Latino Americans?

Over the years of their marriage, Joseph was clearly the decision maker. He did not allow Pamela to work, and she raised the children during the early years. When the children were in elementary school, Pamela got a part-time job to put money in a college fund for the children.

When Joseph was diagnosed with gastric carcinoma, he suffered in silence. He did not allow anyone to accompany him to the physician's office or say anything about pain or pain medicine. He underwent surgery and adjuvant therapy without complaint. When he was readmitted to the hospital for recurrence of cancer, the pain was such that he did agree to take some pain medicine. Even though he hurt most of the time, he did not speak of it. His brothers told him to be tough, that he could "beat this thing."

Spiritual Orientation or Beliefs. In addition to asking the client about belief systems, appropriate assessment may include interaction with the client's family members and friends. Their comments about religious beliefs or expectations of conduct may provide important data for your assessment.

For example, ask if the client is affiliated with any religious group. Ask whether the client's church promotes any beliefs about pain and its meaning in life. Ask what pain means to the client.

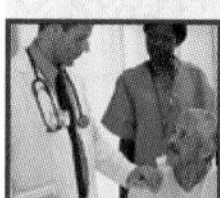

Mr. Valdez's faith was strong. Although he was unsure that he would be healed of the cancer, he believed God would not allow him to suffer too much. He considered the possibility that pain was God's way of getting his attention so that he would become a better person. When he thought of this, he was more reluctant to take the prescribed pain medication. How would you respond to his beliefs?

Psychosocial Modifiers. Your assessment will be more insightful if you understand the client's personal and family dynamics and stressors. If possible, observe family interactions to obtain information the health care team can use to intervene. Pain can tax the client's energy reserves. Concurrent stressors can further reduce those reserves. To assess the client's psychosocial modifiers, consider asking questions like these:

- You seem worried right now. Is there any way I can help you? Can I put you in touch with someone who

might be able to help you deal with these worrisome events?
- Pain can be such an energy-draining experience. Are there other things happening in your life that are also depleting your reserves?
- I've noticed that when you have visitors, you seem to hide your pain from them. Would you like to talk about that?
- You look tired. Is there something besides the pain that is causing your fatigue?
- Has the pain interfered with your enjoyment of others? Have you found it necessary to limit your social activities? Can you participate in family, church, and other social functions as you would like?

Psychological Evaluation. A psychological evaluation can be useful when pain prevents a client from participating in routine activities, adversely affects relationships with others, or causes inappropriate emotional distress. It may also be indicated for clients who use the health care system excessively or demand further assessment or treatment when no obvious reason can be found. Clients who are most likely to benefit from a psychological evaluation are those experiencing chronic, disabling pain. The purpose of the evaluation is to determine which psychological and behavioral treatment strategies are indicated.

Physical Examination. When examining clients who have pain, ask them to identify the location of the pain on their body. This allows you to evaluate the area, check for any signs of infection or damage to the tissue, and gently palpate the area to confirm the source of the discomfort. It is also important to ask the clients about and to palpate any pathological areas that have been documented in previous diagnostic tests. Also assess vital signs, behaviors, and physical appearance.

Vital Signs. Measure the client's blood pressure, pulse, and respiratory rate. A client in acute pain will often show an elevation of some vital signs and may be sweating as well.

If you detect a change in vital signs in clients at risk for pain, ask them if they have pain. As previously mentioned, a client with chronic pain or acute pain that has lasted several hours undergoes an adaptation of the autonomic nervous system and usually will not exhibit any changes in vital signs.

Client Behaviors. Moaning, grimacing, crying, guarding or restricting activity, or refusing to get out of bed or walk are typical behaviors for a client with acute pain. These cues should always elicit queries about the presence of pain.

A client with chronic pain may have adapted behaviorally and have few visible signs despite considerable pain. The person's facial expression may be without affect. Your knowledge that the client has a painful condition should elicit questions about pain status even without behavioral cues.

Physical Appearance. Pain can interfere with ADLs, such as bathing or grooming. Clients who are normally very careful about personal appearance may be unable to perform their normal routines because of pain. A client's focus on chronic pain can absorb available physical and emotional resources and divert the energy needed for personal hygiene and aesthetics.

ASSESSMENT OF PAIN IN SPECIAL POPULATIONS

Infants and Children. Many outdated misconceptions interfere with the accurate assessment of pain in infants and children. These misconceptions should be recognized and dismissed. These biases include the following erroneous beliefs:
- Neonates and infants do not feel pain.
- Children are not as sensitive to pain as adults.
- Children get used to pain and tolerate it very well.
- Children do not remember pain.
- Children will tell you if they have pain.
- Children are always truthful about pain.
- A child is not in pain if he can be distracted or is sleeping.
- Parents exaggerate their child's pain.

In reality, infants may show facial grimacing, vigorous crying, generalized body movements, or chin quivering in response to pain. Physiological responses to pain among children include increases in heart rate, blood pressure, and respiratory rate; restlessness; diaphoresis; and dilation of the pupils. However, children respond in a similar manner when they are anxious, afraid, or angry, so you cannot assume that pain has caused the problem.

Your assessment should be based on the client's developmental level. Whereas cries, screams, behavioral regression, and difficulty being comforted may be appropriate pain behaviors in toddlers, different behaviors are appropriate in preschoolers. Such behaviors include struggling against restraint, aggressiveness, striking out physically and verbally when hurt, and a low frustration level.

As with adults, it is important to obtain a pain history for a child. A child's statements and descriptions of pain are the most important assessment factors. Involving parents provides insight into the child's developmental level and coping strategies.

Many pain assessment tools have been developed for children, using behavioral observation or, for those able to quantify their pain in some manner, self-report. The Wong/Baker FACES Pain Rating scale uses picture faces with expressions that represent varying levels of pain (Figure 37-6). Children choose the face that best represents how they are feeling. This scale also allows for the use of numbers in addition to word descriptors that correspond to each face.

Older Adults. Pain is a significant problem for the older adult. It should not be accepted as a normal part of aging but rather as a sign of disease. Assess pain

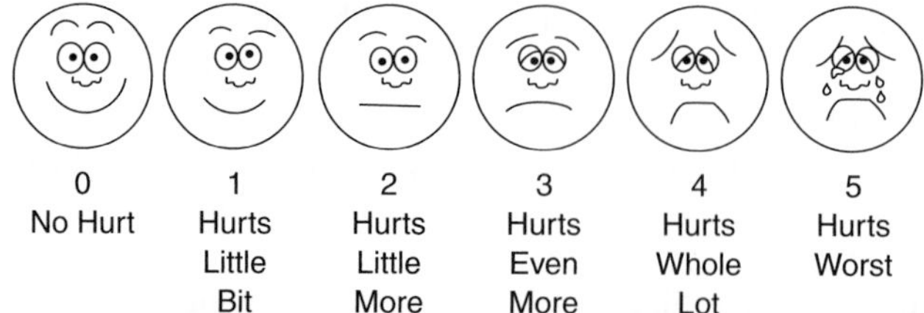

FIGURE 37-6 The Wong/Baker FACES Pain Rating scale uses faces that represent varying levels of pain. Explain to the person that each face is for a person who feels happy because he has no pain (hurt) or sad because he has some or a lot of pain. **Face 0** is very happy because he doesn't hurt at all. **Face 1** hurts just a little bit. **Face 2** hurts a little more. **Face 3** hurts even more. **Face 4** hurts a whole lot. **Face 5** hurts just as much as you can imagine, although you don't have to be crying to feel this bad. Ask the person to choose the face that best describes how he is feeling. Rating scale is recommended for persons age 3 years and older. (From Hockenberry, M., Wilson, D., & Winkelstein, M. L [2005]. *Wong's essentials of pediatric nursing* (7th ed., p. 1259). St. Louis, MO: Mosby.)

every 2 to 4 hours using a standard pain assessment tool in clients who are alert, and every 8 hours only if pain is mild or well controlled (Ardery, Herr, Titler, Sorofman, & Schmidt, 2003). For clients who have confusion or dementia, assess pain using methods for pain assessment in cognitively impaired clients (see next section). Pain may also contribute to confusion in some older adults.

Action Alert! Be aware that confusion or a marked change in behavior may be a sign of pain in the older adult.

To compensate for age-related visual and auditory impairments, use standard communication strategies as outlined in Chapter 38. Face the client when speaking, speak slowly in a normal tone of voice, and remove extraneous noise. Be sure that a visual assessment tool has nonglare paper, simple lettering, 14-point font size, and proper line spacing (American Geriatrics Society, 1998).

Barriers to pain assessment in some older adults include a possible desire to be a "good patient," fears that complaints may affect quality of care, fear of seeming burdensome to family, fear of tests or costs of therapy, and fear of opioid dependence and loss of functioning.

The Cognitively Impaired. Pain assessment may be a special challenge when working with clients who are developmentally delayed, have neurological conditions that alter level of consciousness (LOC), or older adults who have delirium (short-term confusion) or dementia (long- term memory loss); see Chapter 40 for further discussion of delirium and dementia. The client may not be able to remember "past" pain, so it is important to assess the current pain status.

Assess pain in cognitively impaired clients by looking for nonverbal cues, vocalizations, facial expressions of pain, and a change in usual behavior or activity level. Nonverbal cues include such behaviors as restlessness or agitation, bracing, guarding or splinting a painful or surgical site, unusual posture, rocking, withdrawing, repositioning or tense body language, or possibly noisy breathing. Vocalizations include moaning, crying, groaning, sighing, and possible verbal outbursts. Facial expressions include grimacing, wincing, frowning, wrinkling the forehead or brow, closed or narrowed eyes, clenched teeth, and distorted expression. Behavior or activity changes include reduced mobility level, altered appetite or refusal to eat, altered sleep pattern, new-onset or increased confusion, depression, withdrawal, and resistance to or refusal of care (Ardery et al., 2003).

Clients With Communication Barriers. Although neonates, infants, and some older adult clients are included in this population, the main groups at risk for impaired communication are those who speak a different language or have limited language skills, an altered LOC (see preceding section), an endotracheal tube, or possibly mental illness. An interpreter may be needed to assist in obtaining accurate pain assessment data for clients with language issues. Intubated but alert clients may be offered writing materials or asked to use a pain intensity scale for assessment purposes. McCaffrey and Pasero (2001b) warn that some clients with mental illness have higher pain tolerance levels and less frequent reports of pain, making it vital to respond when these clients indicate they are having pain.

Be especially alert for signs of pain in these groups. If any client is known to have a painful condition or undergoes a procedure known to be painful, it is appropriate to pretreat the pain with a trial of analgesic.

Clients at Risk for Substance Abuse. Clients at particular risk for psychological dependence (addiction) include those with a history of alcoholism, drug-related problems and previous treatment, loss of a job due to drug use, regular use of illicit drugs, a history of mental illness or depression, or a history of chronic pain.

Look carefully for physiological causes of pain and be cautious in ruling them out if they are not quickly identified, even if you are convinced that the client has drug-seeking behavior. Interviewing strategies include questioning about drug use in a matter-of-fact manner. Begin with questions about over-the-counter medications (including caffeine and cigarettes) and continue with questions about prescription medications, both current and past. Proceed to questions about alcohol and illicit substances. If you suspect drug use, ask questions that presume normal quantities used such as, "When was your last drink?" "When did you last use cocaine?" or "Do you ever mix drugs?"

In the outpatient setting, look for drug-related behaviors that suggest substance abuse. Prescription abuse, such as forging prescriptions, selling prescription drugs, or obtaining drugs from nonmedical sources, is a typical behavior. Investigate multiple episodes of prescription "loss" and misuse of prescribed medications or therapies. Also, follow up on what seem to be *opioid protection strategies.* These may include requests for a specific brand of analgesic, a history of therapeutic response to opioids only, reports of multiple drug allergies that severely limit the choice of analgesic given, and extreme resistance to multimodal pain therapies. Also watch for deteriorating functional and social skills and frequent missed appointments or late arrivals for appointments. Toxicology screening is essential but requires strict confidentiality.

Working with this client population requires skill, sensitivity, compassion, and patience. Treating the pain, not the addiction, should be your first priority, realizing the client may also be referred for treatment of addiction concurrently or at a later time. Untreated pain could trigger a relapse in a client recovering from addiction or could cause increased substance use in an active user (Compton, 2001).

FOCUSED ASSESSMENT FOR *ACUTE PAIN*

Because of the relatively short-term nature of acute pain, focus your assessment on the nature and intensity of the pain, client behaviors, and response to analgesic interventions. Direct your assessment toward gathering an accurate picture of the client's pain and collaborating with other team members to discern the most appropriate treatment interventions.

Defining Characteristics. Assess the client for the following:

- A verbal or coded report of pain
- Observed evidence of pain, such as a facial mask, sleep disturbance, self-focus or narrowed focus, moaning, crying, restlessness, irritability, sighing, and altered appetite
- Assuming a position or using gestures to counteract or avoid pain, protective behavior, guarding behavior
- Distraction behaviors, such as pacing or repetitive actions
- Autonomic nervous system changes, such as diaphoresis, blood pressure elevation, increased respirations, increased pulse, dilated pupils, altered muscle tone
- Quiet, distracted, or withdrawn behaviors

Related Factors. Factors related to *Acute pain* include biological, chemical, physical, and psychological injury agents. Other related factors that you may notice include the following.

Anxiety. It is common to become anxious when one has sudden or unexpected pain. The anxiety, in turn, aggravates the pain experience. If the prescribed intervention fails to relieve the discomfort, the client may develop even greater anxiety that the pain will not be relieved.

Fear. Clients can become quite fearful in the midst of a pain experience. There are inevitable worries about the cause of the pain, whether the analgesic will be effective and the pain will eventually be gone. Some clients fear becoming dependent on the analgesic.

Nausea and Vomiting. Many of the analgesics can cause nausea or vomiting. Opioid analgesics act on the chemoreceptor trigger zone in the brain, causing an emetic response. Nonsteroidal antiinflammatory drugs (NSAIDs) can cause gastric mucosal irritation, another potential cause of an emetic response.

Immobility. Clients with significant pain are reluctant to move because movement exacerbates the pain. They may refuse to ambulate, breathe deeply (after abdominal surgery, for example), get out of bed, or move in any way that might make the pain more intense.

Impaired Verbal Communication. Because your assessment relies partially on the client's verbal report, impaired communication makes the task of selecting diagnostic and treatment methods much more difficult. It also places the client at greater risk of inadequate pain relief. Neonates, children, mentally challenged or comatose clients, or clients with a language barrier require special approaches.

FOCUSED ASSESSMENT FOR *CHRONIC PAIN*

Chronic pain falls into two major categories: chronic *malignant* pain, which is associated with cancer and other rapidly progressive disorders, and chronic *nonmalignant* pain, which occurs when tissue injury remains stable or is healed. These two types share similarities and differences.

Nonmalignant etiologies includes neuropathic pain, which may be difficult to treat and, at times, more disabling than cancer pain. Other nonmalignant chronic conditions such as osteoarthritis can produce pain, as shown in Box 37-2. The client may be less likely to report chronic pain because it has become a "normal" and unchanging part of life. Box 37-3 offers one client's personal experience with pain.

Components of acute pain assessment are also part of chronic pain assessment; however, assessment of chronic pain may require the addition of a psychological assessment. Physical capabilities, a pain history, role appraisal, a self-esteem and social evaluation, and, most importantly, the client's description of the total experience will help the clinical team to make an appropriate and useful evaluation.

Keep in mind that cancer pain can be acute if treatment cures the disease. It becomes chronic if the disease

BOX 37-2

Evidence-Based Practice

Managing Pain

Problem: Arthritis can be a very painful condition that affects millions of Americans today. There currently is no cure for arthritis, and clients affected with this problem experience both acute and chronic pain that affect their ability to function and diminish their quality of life. Undertreated pain in this client population has prompted the development of an evidence-based clinical practice guideline (American Pain Society [APS], 2002).

Evidence

"The Guideline for the Management of Pain in Osteoarthritis, Rheumatoid Arthritis and Juvenile Chronic Arthritis is based on the best available scientific evidence combined with the expert judgment of the panel, consultants, and peer reviewers." The guideline was developed with the support of many professional organizations, corporations, and consumer groups. "Because of the large amount of evidence reviewed and summarized, it is not possible to include references to all studies. . . . An expanded description of the review processes and the APS reviews are published in a separate report (*Guideline Report for the Management of Pain in Osteoarthritis, Rheumatoid Arthritis and Juvenile Chronic Arthritis,* 2002)" (APS, 2002).

Application to Practice

"The guideline includes information on assessment of pain and functioning in children and adults and takes a comprehensive approach to the use of pain management strategies" (APS, 2002). Some of the topics discussed include the following:

- Pain assessment
- Management of pain, including client and family education, and pharmacological management
- Assessment and treatment of pain in children and older adults

Reference

American Pain Society. (2002). *Guideline for the management of pain in osteoarthritis, rheumatoid arthritis and juvenile chronic arthritis.* Glenview, IL: Author.

is metastatic or rapidly progressive and will most likely intensify as the tumor grows. Chronic cancer pain is very likely to have both nociceptive and neuropathic components and requires attention to the client's verbal descriptors. Pain secondary to a progressive malignant disease is a daily reminder of the illness and limited life expectancy.

Defining Characteristics. In general, the characteristics of chronic pain are more subtle than those of acute pain; the painful area is more difficult to pinpoint; and the intensity is harder to evaluate. The client's suffering is likely to increase over time. The long-term, possibly intractable nature of chronic pain requires assessment of many variables, such as those discussed next.

Verbal Reports. In nonmalignant chronic pain, the client's descriptions of pain may be vague and it may be difficult pinpoint the source. The client may have described the pain to so many different health care professionals that he becomes weary of the effort and provides abbreviated information that is less than helpful. Certainly, your documentation should include the complete pain experience.

In malignant pain, diagnostic testing can usually locate the site of the primary tumor and metastases, if present, to support the client's description of pain. In addition, treatment for the tumor (such as chemotherapy, surgery, and radiation therapy) can itself cause pain. Clients with malignant disease are usually more able to describe the location and particular sensation of the pain than are clients with neuropathic pain.

Observed Behaviors. In nonmalignant chronic pain, clients may have a masklike look of pain, accompanied by a dull affect. Their behavior may be guarded and protective especially around the painful area. Some clients limp or stay very still.

In malignant pain, the facial expressions and guarding behaviors can be similar to those of any person with chronic pain. What may differ somewhat is that a client with advanced disease or undergoing rigorous treatment may feel marked malaise and appear not only tired but also very unwell.

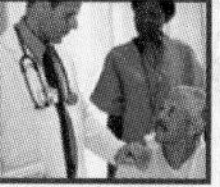

When Mr. Valdez visited his doctor at the office, it was evident he had a significant amount of pain. He was very cautious in his movements, sat rigidly in the chair, was extremely tense during the physical examination, and kept his face very still. He would respond that the pain was "pretty much okay" when questioned. His physician put him on a sustained-release analgesic preparation to be taken two times a day, telling him that although it was a pain medicine, it would also help his breathing, which was becoming more difficult because of the tumor pressing against his diaphragm. Joseph reluctantly agreed to take the medicine for his "breathing."

Weight Changes. In nonmalignant chronic pain, the client may lose weight because of a decreased focus on eating or gain weight if eating becomes a substitute for more active behaviors or a form of self-soothing. Weight loss may further jeopardize clients' health by depleting energy stores and muscle mass. Increased weight can worsen the pain if weight bearing is a contributing variable or if weight gain interferes with prescribed therapeutic exercise or other nonpharmacological interventions.

In malignant pain, weight loss can occur because of tumor growth, cancer therapies and their side effects,

BOX 37-3

A Patient's Perspective

"Sometimes It Even Hurts to Breathe"

I was 19 years old when my first child was born. It was a difficult birth. The doctor tried to deliver the baby using forceps but ended up doing a cesarean. That was December 1955. The following March, I fell and hit my tailbone. In June of that year, I began to have pain in my lower back. Since then I've never been without pain, despite eight spinal operations and two spinal fusions. I'll soon be 62.

Nearly 2 years after my son was born, I became pregnant with my daughter. That was a really hard time. The pain was so intense I had to have injections in my back to give me any relief. A few months after she was born, the pain was just indescribable, not just in my back but a constant headache as well. One look at the myelogram and the surgeon told me he would operate the next day. Scar tissue—probably from the first unsuccessful attempt at forceps delivery of my son—had wrapped around and squeezed my spinal cord. The surgeon said that without that operation I would have been paralyzed. Waking up afterward, I realized that for the first time in months I didn't have a headache.

Each of the surgeries has helped to a degree, but it seems like when one spot gets fixed, another flares up. Fifteen years ago, an MRI showed that I had a disk protruding and bone spurs were pressing on a nerve. By then I'd had seven operations and didn't really want more surgery but the pain was so intense I couldn't walk, so I had no choice. Right now I'm having trouble with my upper back and sometimes it even hurts to breathe. But I've learned to live with the pain. I don't like to take pain medications, other than daily Tylenol and once in a while Darvocet. But I don't like to take any kind of narcotics. I don't want to trade off one problem for another.

Part of living with the pain is learning to relax. Lie down and let your body go limp. That eases the pain, sometimes even without medication. Keeping busy takes my mind off the pain. I hurt worse when I sit down and do nothing. I love to cook, any kind of cooking, but especially Southern dishes and trying new recipes.

I do home health care for older adults. Back in the 1950s, I was trained as a nurse's aide, so I've taken care of people most of my life, including my mother when she was dying. Right now I'm caring for an 86-year-old lady who lives alone. She has to use a walker, and she needs help with her bath, but she's a very "up" person, just a dream to care for. I fix her food, see that she takes her medications, take her to get her hair done or out to dinner. It's a great job.

People in pain need understanding and compassion—tender loving care—but they also need not to feel sorry for themselves; that can make you a total invalid. My father always told us there's no such word as "can't." So I chose to be productive, to fight the pain and not give in to it. And I have a lot of faith. I pray a lot. God gives me the strength I need to go on.

loss of appetite, anxiety, and depression. Some clients who receive corticosteroid medications gain weight.

Affective Disorders. Nonmalignant chronic pain can deplete clients' energy reserves very quickly, and irritability, restlessness, and depression are common. In malignant pain, an existential kind of suffering may be superimposed on the pain state. The threat of loss of life and the loss of control over the disease can contribute to significant sadness and depression.

Changes in Sleeping Patterns. Nonmalignant chronic pain may make it difficult for the client to find a comfortable position at night, may disturb sleep many times during the night, or may prevent sleep altogether. Clients may describe "walking the floor" at night or getting up to watch television if the pain prevents sleep. Sleeping habits may shift to a series of short naps spaced over the 24-hour period. Optimum treatment with opioid analgesics, anxiolytic agents, and sleeping medications may assist the client with sleeping relatively well at night.

Disrupted Social Relationships and Activities. Both nonmalignant and malignant chronic pain can disrupt previously established social relationships with family members and friends. Lack of energy or depression may reduce clients' ability to be with others. An inability to be involved in previous activities, whether social or more functional in nature, is a common occurrence.

A client with malignant pain caused by cancer may find that friends and relatives avoid him. The reasons are varied. Most people "don't know what to say." Others are extremely uncomfortable being around someone with a life-threatening illness. In addition, clients may not want visitors as their level of fatigue rises.

Related Factors. Factors related to *Chronic pain* include chronic physical or psychosocial disability, fatigue, misconceptions about pain and its treatment, and a low tolerance for pain.

Chronic Physical Disability. Intractable pain—malignant or nonmalignant—can cause permanent disability. The client may no longer be able to work, may have to work in a limited capacity, or may have to find employment that does not aggravate the illness.

A client with malignant pain but controlled disease may be able to continue employment and activities of daily living with minor modifications. As the disease advances, the ability to work or pursue ADLs will decline.

Chronic Psychosocial Disability. Chronic, disabling pain—malignant or nonmalignant—also affects clients at an existential level. It is difficult for others to understand how life changing such pain can be. Clients may not be able to verbalize the unappreciated need to grieve for the formerly healthy self. Their self-esteem, if grounded in their ability to be productive and to function in multiple capacities, may be shattered. They may feel ashamed and inadequate that they are not strong enough to endure the discomfort. Ultimately, if the pain is unrelenting and severe, atypical and dysfunctional behaviors may appear.

Clients in the terminal phase of an illness may withdraw from others, even those who are emotionally close. Some turn away from everyone as they face their final days.

Fatigue. Pain depletes energy, and dealing with it on a chronic basis can absorb the client's physical and emotional resources. The fatigue may be compounded by the illness itself or interventions used to treat it.

Misconceptions About Pain and Treatment. Clients with chronic nonmalignant pain are rarely treated with one modality and are best served by a multidisciplinary team. As a result, many clients are confused about which intervention is helping them and whether to seek others to assist in their care. Difficulty in accepting a diagnosis of intractable pain often results in "selective listening." If the source of the pain cannot be identified, the client may continue to hope that the pain will be eliminated once the cause is known.

The management of malignant cancer pain can be extremely effective in most cases if clients comply with the prescribed regimen. A barrier to compliance in these clients may be a fear of addiction. Others may choose to "forget" the discomfort because the pain is a constant reminder of their illness and prognosis.

Low Tolerance for Pain. Many clients with nonmalignant pain have suffered significant and unrelenting pain for so long that their ability to cope with any more or any new pain is impaired. Thus the slightest amount of new or extra pain may produce a disproportionate emotional response.

In malignant pain, the emotional burden of the cancer diagnosis superimposed on significant pain (either new or long-standing) can also trigger a strong emotional response. Anxiety, helplessness, depression, and loss of control deplete the client's ability to tolerate any more pain. Many clients feel not only that it is unjust that they have cancer but also that pain adds indignity and punishment.

DIAGNOSIS

ACUTE PAIN AND CHRONIC PAIN

When a client has either a risk for pain or actual pain, you will base the nursing diagnosis on assessment factors such as the health history, results of diagnostic tests, current vital signs, physical assessment, client self-report of the pain state, anticipated interventions (such as surgery), and an understanding of the expected course of illness. These factors will determine whether *Acute pain* or *Chronic pain* is the more appropriate nursing diagnosis (Table 37-4).

Acute pain or *Chronic pain* can be a primary diagnosis or a related factor. Because pain is a common symptom for many treatable and untreatable illnesses, you must decide whether it is a primary or secondary focus. Even though pain is always worthy of intervention, you may select another nursing diagnosis and provide analgesic treatment as an intervention for managing that diagnosis.

Take, for example, the client who has a total hip replacement. Although significant pain is present during the postoperative period, the client must ambulate and perform the proper range-of-motion exercises as part of the necessary rehabilitative regimen. In this instance, the nursing diagnosis would be *Activity intolerance related to pain.*

In contrast, a client who has intractable pain secondary to breast cancer metastatic to the bone would have a primary nursing diagnosis of *Chronic pain.* When the primary disease cannot be cured, pain becomes the primary illness and the focus of aggressive intervention.

Table 37-4 Clustering Data to Make a Nursing Diagnosis

Pain

DATA CLUSTER	DIAGNOSIS
A 27-year-old man admitted to hospital via the emergency department after a motorcycle accident has a fractured leg, two fractured ribs, multiple contusions. Repeatedly complains of pain and asks for "anything to make this pain better."	*Acute pain* related to extensive tissue damage from multiple trauma and anxiety
Client has history of osteoporosis and steroid use for respiratory disease. Admitted to hospital for hip replacement. Does not want to participate in physical therapy because of hip pain.	*Impaired physical mobility* related to postsurgical tissue trauma, anxiety, and low tolerance for pain
A 38-year-old woman with recurrent breast cancer metastatic to multiple skeletal sites. Rates pain consistently as an 8 (scale 0 to 10) despite maximizing current analgesic regimen.	*Chronic pain* related to malignant disease progression
A 35-year-old man injured in industrial accident. Chronic, intractable back pain has forced him to go on disability. He can no longer help around the house as he did before, and he does not want his buddies to see him in a disabled state.	*Disturbed body image* related to functional loss secondary to pain
Older adult client with severe, escalating pain secondary to metastatic prostate cancer. Disease has progressed despite continued active therapy. Physician referred him to hospice for palliative care. Client believes that the pain will never get better because it is "punishment from God for bad things I've done."	*Hopelessness* related to disease progression, increased pain, and psychological stress

RELATED NURSING DIAGNOSES

Constipation. Constipation is a common side effect of opioid analgesics used to manage many types of acute and chronic pain. Although clients may become tolerant of other opioid side effects, they never develop tolerance to constipation.

Contributing factors for the person in pain may include decreased activity, additional disorders, decreased liquid and oral intake, stress, or grief. A client with acute pain may require temporary intervention for constipation, but the problem resolves when opioid therapy is discontinued if there is no other contributing factor. A client with chronic malignant pain may take significant doses of opioid analgesics but may also have limited oral intake. An aggressive bowel regimen is often necessary for clients receiving chronic or substantial opioid therapy.

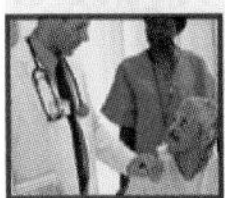

Mr. Valdez did comply with the analgesic regimen and became increasingly constipated. The nurse prescribed a bowel regimen, expecting that he would have a bowel movement at least every 3 days. Joseph did not follow the bowel regimen, however, and went for 10 days without a bowel movement. He did not tell his wife but discussed the matter with his brothers. One of his brothers went to the drugstore and bought over-the-counter enemas for him. Joseph managed to remove the impaction himself and used two small enemas to clear out his lower bowel. He started at that time on the prescribed stool softeners. He never told his wife. Can you think of a teaching approach that might have prevented this problem?

Activity Intolerance. An instinctive response to both acute and chronic pain is to be still and wait until it abates. The client quickly learns what activities to avoid. A client with acute pain understands its time-limited nature and may take analgesics to reduce pain enough to allow some activity. As the tissue heals, activity naturally increases.

In chronic pain, however, clients who begin to consistently decrease their activity levels become weaker and even less tolerant of activity. Sleep disorders, fatigue, and physical deconditioning all further contribute to reduced activity levels.

Ineffective Role Performance. Role performance and role expectations are influenced by social forces, cultural norms, and values. Because performance defines who and what a person is, any disruption can have a significant impact on the sense of self.

Acute pain can temporarily disrupt the ability to perform ADLs and work at full capacity. Some clients may need to use sick leave as they recover from an injury or surgical procedure. Others may continue their jobs in a different capacity until wellness returns. Role expectations may be set aside temporarily because others understand that the person will return to prior functional levels.

Chronic pain can dramatically alter the ability to work, perform ADLs, and interact with others. Because a person's sense of self is closely tied to role performance, low self-esteem can occur in a client who has become even partially disabled. Failure to meet role expectations can threaten life goals, alienate others, and produce extreme stress.

Ineffective Coping. People's ability to cope is reflected in the day-to-day management of their affairs. Although they may at times feel burdened by extra work, temporary crises or problems, the woes of a friend or family member, or changing careers, they can usually use "reserve" physical and emotional resources to deal with and adjust to changing circumstances.

Problems with health can severely reduce these coping resources. When illness and its symptoms (such as pain) become chronic, these resources may become so depleted that clients no longer know how to function effectively. Pessimism, increased anxiety, general unhappiness, self-focus, and defensive behaviors are common. Clients may become unproductive and dependent on others. Support systems may be lost as others turn away from them, no longer seeming to know or like them.

Hopelessness. The term *chronic* conjures up words such as *interminable* and *forever.* Clients who discover that they may live with disabling or severe pain either permanently or for a long time can be overwhelmed by this knowledge. Intertwined are feelings of helplessness, loss of control, and depression. The client with recurrent malignant disease, unresponsive to further therapies, suffers the loss of time in which to complete the business of life.

Hopelessness affects physical, psychological, and spiritual health. Clients may become very passive, withdraw from others, demonstrate a dull affect, refuse to solve problems or make decisions, and lose their spiritual beliefs.

Caregiver Role Strain. As families become more geographically separated and people with chronic illnesses live longer, traditional support systems such as neighborhoods, churches, and social clubs are less prominent in people's lives. It is not uncommon for a client with a chronic illness to rely primarily on a very limited circle of family and friends.

Clients with chronic pain can be extremely demanding, irritable, often angry, and at times very unpleasant. Caring for such a person can be demanding, exhausting, or depressing and can socially isolate the caregiver. Caregivers may find themselves becoming defensive, irritable, and angry, which triggers feelings of guilt. They may become ill themselves while dealing with the needs of the client for whom they are caring.

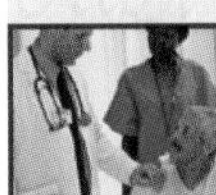

Pamela Valdez did not know what to do. Joseph was becoming increasingly withdrawn and quiet and never told her how he felt about his illness. He muttered that he was "okay" when she asked him about his pain. He did not play with his children as he once had and rarely paid any attention to them. He went to work every day and, when he came home exhausted, he would sit down in front of the television set and not speak to anyone. How could you help Pamela cope?

The caregiver may not feel competent to provide the kind of care required. Clients with chronic malignant pain in the terminal phase of illness often require an array of pain medications and other interventions to manage symptoms. They may take multiple medications scheduled at various times of the day and night. They may have ambulatory infusion pumps for intravenous (IV) or intraspinal opioid delivery. They may need also other medical devices, such as an oxygen delivery system, a nasogastric suction pump or feeding device, or an indwelling urinary catheter. Managing these complex needs can be overwhelming for the layperson.

Ineffective Therapeutic Regimen Management. Acute pain rarely requires a difficult or multifaceted regimen. The client or caregiver can generally manage the short-term nature of the pain and required interventions. Issues may arise if the client or caregiver fears opioid analgesics or if the primary caregiver is forgetful. Even for short-term pain management, provide education to client and family about medications, dosages, schedules, side effects, and the expected outcomes of treatment.

Managing chronic pain requires more complex strategies. Multiple nonpharmacological and pharmacological modalities may be involved. Clients must be motivated and disciplined to devote their energy to adhere to a complex regimen. Feelings of helplessness, hopelessness, and depression, as well as lack of confidence in the outcomes, may predispose the client to miss appointments or to be uncooperative or noncompliant with interventions.

The management of chronic malignant pain may require multiple types of typical and atypical analgesics at scheduled times. Clients and caregivers may struggle to balance the fear of opioid addiction with the need for adequate analgesia. If complex medical equipment is needed to deliver the opioid analgesic, clients and caregivers may give up on this intervention as too bothersome or burdensome.

PLANNING

Developing a plan of care for a client with actual or risk for pain requires collaboration with the client and family. The plan is driven by the nature of the pain, the underlying disorder, cultural and social variables that influence the client, the chronicity of the pain, and any other confounding variables that must be considered when developing the plan of care.

EXPECTED OUTCOMES FOR THE CLIENT AT RISK FOR *ACUTE PAIN*

A client who faces a surgical or diagnostic procedure known to cause acute pain may have *Risk for acute pain.* Your goals should be to prepare the client for the experience and to plan interventions. Clearly explain the expected nature and duration of the pain and planned treatment strategies. Clients should understand that pain medication may not completely eliminate all pain but should reduce it to a satisfactory or tolerable level as reported by that client. Other expected client outcomes include decreased anxiety before the procedure and verbalized understanding of the planned interventions.

EXPECTED OUTCOMES FOR THE CLIENT WITH *ACUTE PAIN*

The goal of care for a client with *Acute pain* is satisfactory pain relief using pharmacological and nonpharmacological interventions. Client education should focus on the rationale for and description of the plan of care. Other expected outcomes are decreased anxiety, client verbalization of planned analgesic interventions, decreased verbal reports of pain and associated pain behaviors, and a decreased need for analgesic interventions as the tissue heals. Usually, the outcome is positive. Pain that is undertreated may result in chronic pain, so it is essential to control the pain.

EXPECTED OUTCOMES FOR THE CLIENT WITH *CHRONIC PAIN*

Desired outcomes for a client with *Chronic pain* (malignant or nonmalignant) are to set realistic goals, to achieve pain reduction to a level that the client can tolerate, to become actively involved (client or caregiver) in the treatment regimen, and to have maximal quality of life. It is imperative that the client understand the rationale for nonpharmacological and pharmacological interventions and be able to verbalize the treatment plan. An additional outcome for the client with chronic nonmalignant pain would be an improved level of functioning or the return to a prior level of functioning.

For the client with chronic malignant pain, additional outcomes would be awareness of myths about opioid analgesic use, to function at highest possible level at any place on the illness continuum, and to obtain the individual and family psychosocial supports needed to cope with chronic pain caused by a terminal illness.

EXPECTED OUTCOMES FOR RELATED NURSING DIAGNOSES

The following list suggests expected outcomes for other nursing diagnoses related to pain:

- *Constipation:* Client has a bowel movement every 2 to 3 days according to the usual pattern prior to admission.
- *Activity intolerance:* Client is able to participate in care activities and ADLs effectively.
- *Ineffective role performance:* Client and family discuss and accept changes needed in family roles during client's illness.
- *Ineffective coping:* Client verbalizes effective coping mechanisms that can be used to deal with current stressors.

- *Hopelessness:* Client expresses feelings of optimism about the present and confidence in attaining goals of therapy.
- *Caregiver role strain:* Caregiver shares frustration about caregiver responsibilities and establishes a plan for support with other family members.
- *Ineffective therapeutic regimen management:* Client and family relate regimen for disease or symptom control and express less anxiety about managing therapy at home.

INTERVENTION

INTERVENTIONS TO MANAGE *ACUTE PAIN*

Because acute pain from surgery, diagnostic procedures, burns, and trauma continues to be underestimated and undertreated, pain management has become a focus of the Joint Commission on Accreditation of Healthcare Organizations. Perform frequent assessments, and evaluate the efficacy of the prescribed intervention. Beware of common misconceptions about treating pain, which can negatively influence how you treat clients in pain (Table 37-5).

Management Principles

Select the Analgesic That Is Effective for the Type and Level of Pain. Acute nociceptive pain usually responds readily to typical analgesics. If pain is mild to moderate, nonopioid analgesics may be effective. They provide analgesia at the peripheral level by physiological mechanisms independent of the opioid receptor sites. Acetaminophen, aspirin, and NSAIDs are likely choices. If the client cannot tolerate anything by mouth, another route is chosen. Nonpharmacological methods may also provide or enhance relief.

If the pain is moderate to severe, an oral or parenteral opioid analgesic is indicated, possibly in combination with an NSAID. Dosage, schedule, incidence and intensity of side effects, and treatment settings are important variables to be considered. Morphine and hydromorphone are typical parenteral opioids used to manage moderate to severe pain. Meperidine has fallen into disfavor because in moderate doses it produces a harmful metabolite, normeperidine. Many other effective oral analgesics are available, and formulations are also available for administration by the transdermal, sublingual, and rectal routes.

Hepatic, renal, or GI dysfunction may influence the selection of appropriate analgesics. Opioid analgesics are metabolized by the liver and are excreted by the kidneys; they may be contraindicated in certain instances of hepatic or renal dysfunction. The nonopioid analgesics, in particular the NSAIDs, interfere with prostaglandin synthesis and can damage the GI mucosa and interfere with renal function. Clients with a GI or renal dysfunction may not be able to receive these medications.

Table 37-5 Common Misconceptions About Pain

MYTH OR MISCONCEPTION	FACT
• Addiction occurs with prolonged use of morphine or morphine derivatives.	• The incidence of addiction is less than 0.1%.
• The nurse or physician is the best judge of a client's pain.	• Only the client can judge the level and distress of the pain; pain management should be a team approach that includes the client.
• Pain is a result, not a cause.	• Unrelieved pain can create problems, such as anger, anxiety, immobility, respiratory problems, and delay in healing.
• It is better to wait until a client has pain before giving medication.	• Playing "catch-up" is not an effective way to manage pain; it is better to routinely administer analgesia, thus maintaining a low pain level.
• Real pain has an identifiable cause.	• There is always a cause of pain, but it may be very obscure and must be assessed carefully. Pain of a psychological origin is just as real as pain of physiological origin.
• The same physical stimulus produces the same pain intensity, duration, and distress in different people.	• Intensity, duration, and distress vary with the individual.
• Some clients lie about the existence or severity of their pain.	• Very few people lie about pain.
• Very young or very old people do not have as much pain.	• All clients with an intact neurological system experience pain; age is not a determinant of pain, but it may influence expression of pain.
• Pain is a part of aging.	• Pain does not accompany aging unless a disease process or ailment is present.
• A person who is asleep is not in pain.	• People in pain become exhausted and may truly be asleep or merely trying to sleep. Some people use sleep as an escape mechanism.
• If the pain is relieved by nonpharmaceutical pain relief techniques, the pain was not real.	• Nonpharmaceutical pain relief methods can be effective. A client's method of relief should be acknowledged as long as it does not harm.
• Nurses should rely on their own definitions of pain and cultural beliefs about pain.	• It is a mistake to impose one's own definitions, cultural beliefs, and values on another person's pain. Let the client tell you what the pain means.

From Black, J., Hawks, J., & Keene, A. (2001). *Medical-surgical nursing: Clinical management for continuity of care* (6th ed.). Philadelphia: Saunders.

Titrate the Dose to Provide Sufficient Pain Relief. A loading dose is the initial analgesic dose required to reduce pain to the client's self-defined level of comfort. Failure to provide an adequate loading dose for severe pain will delay pain relief even though the client may receive several as-needed (prn) or scheduled doses. For the surgical client, a loading dose may be administered in the postanesthesia care unit (PACU). Within the parameters of written medication orders, deliver a loading dose by giving small, frequent doses until the client reports relief or becomes drowsy or by giving a single dose sufficiently large to provide relief.

Continue analgesic dosing until the pain is consistently relieved. If the client requests pain medication before the next dose is scheduled, the dosage is inadequate or the scheduled interval inappropriate. In these cases, consult the prescriber to determine whether the existing order(s) should be changed. A client who has previously received opioid analgesics or who has a history of prior or concurrent substance abuse may require higher initial and maintenance doses. Remember, treating the pain, not the addiction, is your priority at this time.

Choose an Administration Schedule on the Basis of the Drug's Half-Life. Because each analgesic has a limited period of effectiveness, scheduling is driven by the duration of analgesia. When the analgesic schedule keeps the client comfortable between doses, anxiety is decreased. If the pain is expected to be intense or to last for a time, the drug should be given on a scheduled rather than a prn basis for most effective management. This preventive approach also provides the client with increased energy for restorative activity. As the tissue heals and pain decreases, prn dosing is acceptable.

A major barrier to the proper prescribing of opioid analgesics for acute and chronic pain is fear of sedation and respiratory depression. Many clients experience sedation when beginning opioid therapy or when the dose is greatly increased. Respiratory depression as a result of sedation is more common in clients being treated for moderate to severe pain who are **opioid naive** (having minimal or no exposure to opioids), in older adults, or in infants under 6 months of age. Use a sedation scale to detect drowsiness and identify clients at risk for subsequent respiratory depression. You can detect these early by assessing sedation and respiratory status every 1 to 2 hours for 12 to 24 hours in clients for whom there is concern. These clients are often receiving intermittent parenteral doses or continuous infusions by the IV or epidural route.

If the respiratory rate is moderately affected (8 to 10 breaths a minute) or the client is excessively drowsy, withhold the opioid, and reduce subsequent dosages. If the respiratory rate is significantly affected (fewer than 8 breaths a minute), dilute naloxone (Narcan) in normal saline (see product directions) and give 0.2 to 0.4 mg as ordered slowly by the IV push route (see Chapter 21) until adequate respirations return but pain relief remains intact.

> **Action Alert!** Realize that administering significant doses of naloxone (Narcan) to treat respiratory depression restores respiratory function but also removes the opioid analgesic from receptor sites, causing significant pain. Give the smallest dose needed to produce the intended respiratory effect.

Some opioids, such as morphine sulfate, also can decrease blood pressure. Monitor this vital sign to detect decreases after medication administration, especially if ambulation or other activities are planned that could cause orthostatic changes.

Identify the Appropriate Route Needed for Optimal Analgesic Effect. The immediacy of the need for analgesia should determine the route. Outside of spinal analgesia, the IV route produces the most rapid onset of action. Moderate-to-severe pain responds favorably to IV opioids, making it the preferred route if IV access is available. Oral opioids should be used before discharge to be sure they provide adequate relief. Oral and intramuscular (IM) routes have a significant lag time from administration to peak effect. The IM route also has the disadvantages of wide fluctuations in absorption and client discomfort.

There are multiple parenteral opioid preparations for clients who have nothing-by-mouth (NPO) status, intractable nausea and vomiting, inability to swallow, or obstruction of the small bowel. Opioid preparations are available as transdermal patches, rectal suppositories, parenteral solutions, and preservative-free parenteral solutions for intraspinal use.

When changing the route of administration, use equianalgesic conversion data. **Equianalgesia** refers to the dosages of different drugs that provide the same amount of pain relief, independent of route. Table 37-6 lists equianalgesic dosages for commonly prescribed opioids. Oral analgesics are absorbed from the small bowel via the portal circulatory system and travel to the liver, where they undergo significant metabolism. Thus oral opioid analgesics are subject to a **first pass effect:** they are partially metabolized by the liver before they reach the systemic circulation, resulting in decreased opioid bioavailability. Because of the first pass effect, oral dosages need to be greater than comparable parenteral dosages.

Many surgical clients first receive analgesics by the parenteral route and then progress to oral analgesics once the GI tract function resumes postoperatively (positive bowel sounds, flatus, and absence of nausea or vomiting). Use your assessment data and client preferences to help you determine the proper route when orders for either oral or parenteral route are available.

Plan Care Activities at Times of Peak Medication Effect. A client is more likely to cough and deep breathe, ambulate, tolerate dressing changes, or engage in other activities when pain is well controlled. For this reason, plan your care activities and other therapeutic interventions when analgesic medication is at peak effect. It is very helpful to premedicate a client approximately 30 minutes before any procedure or activity that is likely to cause pain and to evaluate its effectiveness as part of the overall plan of care. Be sure to stay with the client who is standing or ambulating to reduce the risk of client injury from sedative or hypotensive side effects.

Treat Procedural Pain Appropriately. Although procedural pain is usually short-term pain, it still requires adequate treatment with the goal of comfort. Describe the procedure to the client and family, and describe what can be done to minimize discomfort. Procedural pain is a significant event that may require the use of local anesthetics and sedatives (such as midazolam) before the procedure and opioid and nonopioid analgesics following the procedure. Children may benefit from the parents' presence during the procedure. Clients using concurrent opioid therapy will require more medication than those who are opioid naive.

Plan for Pain Management Across the Continuum of Care. An increasing number of clients are using patient-controlled analgesia (PCA) or epidural during hospitalization, most often after surgery (see Patient-Controlled Analgesia, later). These therapies require collaboration of the client, nurse, surgeon, anesthesiologist or acute pain service personnel, and others. Specific protocols are often followed when weaning clients from this type of analgesia.

As clients spend less time in the health care system, predischarge assessment of the adequacy of analgesia becomes ever more important. Clients must be prepared to manage their discomfort at home or in an outpatient setting. An analgesic plan should be implemented 24 hours before hospital discharge to assess the efficacy of the drug and route. The intensity of pain determines the approach. If the client has been managed with parenteral opioids and is to be discharged on oral medications, you will need to convert the parenteral analgesic requirement to an equianalgesic oral dosage. Box 37-4 demonstrates a common equianalgesic conversion.

Table 37-6 Equianalgesic Chart for Commonly Prescribed Opioids

DRUG	PARENTERAL DOSAGE	ORAL DOSAGE
Codeine	130 mg	200 mg
Fentanyl (Sublimaze)	100 mcg	NA
Hydromorphone (Dilaudid)	2 mg	7.5 mg
Levorphanol (Levo-Dromoran)	2 mg	4 mg
Meperidine (Demerol)	100 mg	300 mg
Methadone (Dolophine)	10 mg	20 mg
Morphine*	10 mg	30 mg
Oxycodone	NA	15 mg

*Morphine is the gold standard opioid with which all other opioids are compared.

Although oral medications are the simplest to manage, the client may require parenteral opioids subcutaneously or intravenously, using an ambulatory infusion device. The client and family will need the following:

- Instructions on pump management
- Visits by a home health care nurse to check that the device is working and that analgesia is adequate
- Reinforcement of previous client and family teaching

Clinical Accountabilities. You will have more contact with the client than any other health professional. Because of this, implementing an effective pain management strategy requires that you have excellent assessment and advocacy skills. Base your evaluation of treatment on your knowledge of the drug, dosage, duration of effect, and side effects, and report your findings to other members of the health team. Table 37-7 outlines your clinical accountabilities in managing a client with acute pain.

INTERVENTIONS TO MANAGE *CHRONIC PAIN*

Chronic pain has been defined, at its simplest level, as lasting more than 6 months, but it cannot be explained by duration alone. It is a complex problem that affects significant numbers of people and interferes markedly with their quality of life. The symptom ceases to serve a useful diagnostic purpose and becomes a reminder of injury and disability.

Chronic nonmalignant pain requires a multidisciplinary approach that addresses physiological, psychological, emotional, social, and economic variables. Clients may experience social isolation, financial loss, altered self-image, and a continuous search for relief. The pain may be such that it dominates the client's life and has profound effects on physical and mental health.

Action Alert! Remember in your clinical practice that depression does not cause pain, but unrelieved pain can lead to depression.

BOX 37-4 *Equianalgesic Conversion Problem*

EQUIANALGESIC DATA

10 mg of parenteral morphine is equianalgesic to 30 mg of oral morphine.

CURRENT ANALGESIC REGIMEN

Client has required 4 mg of parenteral morphine an hour while hospitalized for trauma from a motorcycle accident. This dosage is expected to be required for 2 more weeks as he participates in the rehabilitative process.

CONVERSION FROM PARENTERAL TO ORAL ROUTE BEFORE DISCHARGE

Step 1: 24 hours × 4 mg = 96 mg parenteral morphine in 24 hours.

Step 2: 96 × 3 (from equianalgesic conversion ratio) = 288 mg *oral morphine in 24 hours.*

Step 3: 288/2 (twice daily dosing) = 145 mg of sustained-release morphine every 12 hours until transition to prn dosing.

Table 37-7 Management of Acute Pain

CLINICAL ACCOUNTABILITY	ELEMENTS
Assess at appropriate intervals.	• Have the client rate the pain intensity before and at an appropriate time after the analgesic is administered. • Consistently use the same rating scale, making sure the client understands its use. • Ensure adequate pain relief. • Monitor for analgesic side effects.
Cultivate knowledge of pharmacology.	• Understand equianalgesic conversion. • Know the efficacy, onset of action, appropriateness of analgesic routes. • Be familiar with the expected duration of effect of commonly used analgesics.
Advocate for the client.	• Treat the client respectfully and appropriately if he or she reports inadequate analgesia. Do not say that nothing else can be done, that the medication should have worked, or that the client must endure the pain. • Assure the client you will communicate with the physician immediately. In the interim, maximize the existing ordered analgesics. • Report the client's status to the physician and other appropriate team members immediately. • Provide an articulate, concise pain assessment based on the client's self-report. Include location, intensity, qualitative descriptors, and response to ordered analgesics, including drug dosage, route, duration of relief, and side effects. • When requesting changes, identify that a particular drug or dosage has been maximized. If necessary, make suggestions for alternative therapy, including drug, route, dosage, and schedule. • Refer to reference or research articles when appropriate. • Address biases and misconceptions of other clinical team members.
Administer ordered analgesics skillfully.	• If more than one drug or route is ordered, select the most effective one for the client's situation. • If there are dosage or titration parameters, use those orders to benefit the client. • Promptly treat analgesic side effects.
Educate the client and family.	• Help client and family to become knowledgeable consumers and effective self-advocates. • Prepare the preoperative client for the location and type of pain, assessment tools that will be used, and expected pain management techniques. • Provide instruction on the importance of preventive intervention, such as asking for or taking the prescribed analgesic when the pain is still mild to moderate in intensity.
Document pertinent data.	• Drug, dosage, route administered. • Pain intensity before and at an appropriate time after analgesic is administered. • Efficacy of nonpharmacological interventions. • Rationale for changes in analgesic regimen.

When you encounter a client with chronic pain, especially from a long-standing problem, barriers can arise. Most likely you have had limited experience with this client population, and misunderstandings are not uncommon. It is difficult to visualize the cause of chronic pain, and you may tend to view the client as a malingerer or drug seeker. The fact that the pain may not be readily amenable to a multitude of interventions can frustrate the health care team and further alienate the client from those providing the interventions.

Action Alert! Remember that the amount of pathological process is not necessarily proportional to the degree of pain.

Management Principles

Develop a Therapeutic Relationship With the Client. A trusting relationship results from listening carefully to the client, without judgment. Acknowledging the existence of pain may markedly reduce client anxiety and establish the foundation for a therapeutic relationship. Although you cannot promise to absolutely relieve the pain, you may bring comfort to the client by your concern and a willingness to mutually attempt to address the problem.

Partner With the Client and Family. The pain is a concern of the client, family and the multidisciplinary team. Any effective strategy requires that all involved be equal partners in assessment, planning, intervention, and evaluation. The client and family must be empowered to manage the pain with the clinical team as partners and facilitators. Realistic outcomes may include improved function, a decrease in pain, and improved quality of life.

Involve a Multidisciplinary Team in Pain Management. The multifaceted nature of chronic pain requires the involvement of a diverse group of health professionals who collaborate to provide the therapies needed for pain relief and improved function. You may provide this client's care alongside physicians, physical therapists, occupational therapists, dietitians, psychologists, and other professionals. Each member of the team must have a clear understanding of the treatment plan and be accountable for supporting or discouraging specific client behaviors.

Use Multiple Modes of Therapy. Although management of acute pain is primarily pharmacological, a key aspect of chronic pain management is nonpharmacological. Medications are often adjunctive rather than primary components of the treatment plan.

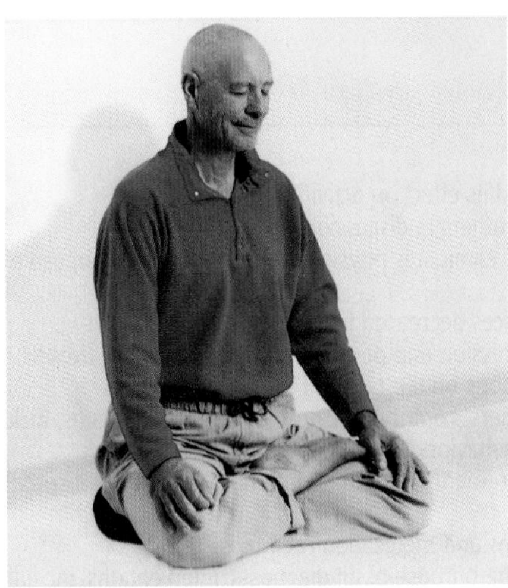

FIGURE 37-7 Yoga is a nonpharmacological approach to pain relief that some clients find helpful.

Selection of nonpharmacological therapies varies according to the underlying disorder and client preference or willingness to use them, but multiple types of intervention generally serve the client well. These therapies, which include both cognitive-behavioral and physical interventions, may consist of client and family education, relaxation, distraction techniques, imagery, biofeedback, and music therapy. Yoga, meditation, and other stress-reducing activities also may be chosen (Figure 37-7). Skilled practitioners may assist with hypnosis in selected cases (Valente, 2006).

Physical agents may include moist or dry heat, diathermy, ultrasound, cold packs, massage, physical therapy, exercise, and TENS units. TENS works in selected cases by modulating the transmission of painful stimuli. Alternatives to conventional therapies may include therapeutic touch, meridian tracing (light massage at points along specific pathways of the body), acupressure, and reflexology.

More invasive treatments may be indicated, such as sympathetic nerve blocks, IV or subcutaneous administration of local anesthetics, and neurosurgical procedures. Acupuncture is a less invasive Eastern therapy that is more popular among many who have traditionally employed the methods of Western medicine.

Pharmacological management of chronic nonmalignant pain remains controversial. A first-line approach typically includes such nonopioids as aspirin, acetaminophen, and NSAIDs. Certain clients may benefit markedly from an opioid. Intractable pain that is unrelieved by other modalities and medications deserves a trial course of opioid analgesics. Criteria for continued opioid use include a stable dosage, increased or improved function, improved analgesic relief, and improved quality of life.

When opioid therapy is used for chronic nonmalignant pain, it is important that it provides pain relief without reinforcing dependency on the medication. Long-acting opioids, either oral or transdermal, may be chosen because they minimize the focus on taking analgesics and have demonstrated markedly good effect without harm in many clients.

Clinical Accountabilities. It is clear that chronic pain management requires a multidisciplinary, multimodal approach. As a nurse with knowledge of pain management, you are a vital and integral part of the health care team. Table 37-8 describes appropriate clinical accountabilities for managing chronic pain that apply to you and other members of the team.

INTERVENTIONS TO MANAGE CANCER PAIN

Pain is one of the most feared consequences of cancer, and it has historically been undertreated. Many clients have known people with cancer who died in pain. Current efforts focus on educating consumers and health professionals and on influencing legislative bodies and regulatory agencies to remove barriers to the appropriate prescribing of opioid analgesics. Unrelieved cancer pain triggers frequent use of the health care system, unscheduled readmissions, and high costs for management of pain.

Cancer pain results from tumor progression, related disorders, and interventions such as chemotherapy, radiation therapy, and surgery. Nearly 75% of clients with advanced cancer have pain; almost half describe it as moderate to severe. Managing cancer pain generally involves multiple treatment options. A combination of nonpharmacological, pharmacological, surgical, neurosurgical, radiological, anesthetic, and psychological interventions may be indicated.

The primary cancer treatment modalities do not generally provide complete pain relief. Surgical and neurosurgical procedures may be used to debulk the tumor, relieve spinal cord compression, stabilize bony structures, and interrupt nerve pathways that transmit pain. Chemotherapy can shrink the tumor and relieve pressure on adjoining tissue and nerves. A short course of radiation therapy can relieve pain from tumor metastases to the bone or alleviate painful nerve compression or infiltration by a tumor.

Anesthetic interventions include temporary and permanent neural blockades and intraspinal catheter placement. Neurosurgical procedures may also be indicated for the rare few for whom less invasive methods have been unsuccessful.

Most cancer pain is relieved pharmacologically. The World Health Organization has formulated an analgesic ladder using nonopioid, opioid, and adjuvant analgesics alone or in combination to treat cancer pain (Figure 37-8). An **adjuvant analgesic** is any medication that may increase analgesic efficacy, thus allowing a smaller opioid dosage. This progressive pharmacological approach begins with nonopioids and advances to the highly effective opioid analgesics as pain increases in intensity.

Table 37-8 Management of Chronic Pain

CLINICAL ACCOUNTABILITY	ELEMENTS
Foster a therapeutic relationship.	• Listen to the client. • Be sensitive to complaints of pain and its effect on activities and emotions. • Ask permission to include significant others in discussion of the issues.
Recognize and respond to the complexity of the pain experience.	• Remember that chronicity reduces or eliminates physiological evidence of pain; use a chronic pain assessment model. • Appreciate that persistent pain produces decreased functioning. • Prolonged discomfort can cause depression and despair. Make sure they are treated. • Identify the impact of physical limitations on lifestyle and role relationships.
Include family and significant others in the plan of care.	• Assess the family's and significant others' contributions to the client's pain status, including role expectations, reinforcement of pain behaviors, and supportive behaviors.
Identify cause of pain.	• Participate in the diagnostic workup, remembering that pain may persist after disorder is eliminated. • Consider preexisting medical problems and medication regimens. • Educate the client and family about the purpose of all diagnostic interventions, including any psychological testing.
Set goals that improve quality of life.	• Minimize pain, anxiety, depression.
Maximize functional level.	• Help client develop realistic expectations. • Be clear that elimination of pain may not be possible, but relief may be feasible. • Outline in a forthright manner that activities may not be fully resumed. • Explore how adaptation to a revised self or new role or identity can be accomplished.
Empower client.	• Use cognitive restructuring to give the client as much control as possible. • Continually reinforce that client ownership of the pain experience is key to pacing activities, setting boundaries, and obtaining pain relief.
Use multimodality, multidisciplinary approach.	• Employ nonpharmacological and pharmacological interventions. • Provide a consistent approach from all health team members, with effective and clear communication among those members. • Include psychological intervention, when appropriate, and social services for financial and social issues.
Use prophylactic approach.	• Medicate on a scheduled basis, preferably using long-acting analgesics to break the pain cycle. • Dispel fears of addiction. Use nonopioids, opioids, and adjunctive medications to relieve pain, then establish a long-term plan. • Educate the client about self-directed pain-relief interventions.

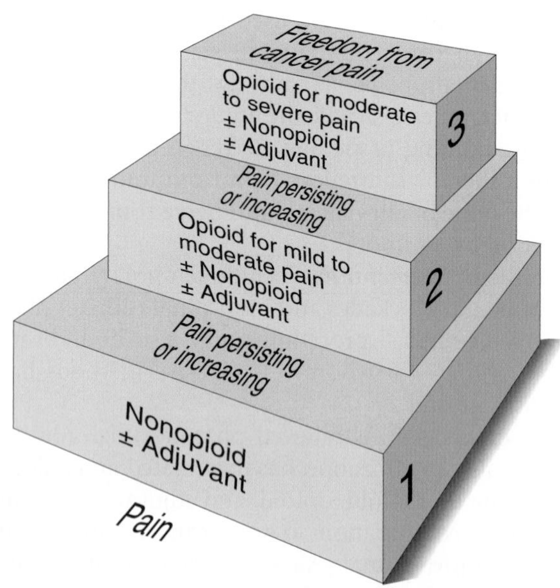

FIGURE 37-8 The World Health Organization analgesic ladder. (Reproduced by permission of WHO, from *Cancer pain relief* [2nd ed.]. Geneva: World Health Organization, 1996.)

Management Principles. Many of these principles may be used to manage acute pain, but the long-term, more complex, and significant degrees of cancer pain require a more intensive approach. The most important principle is to use opioid analgesics in dosages that are adequate to control pain.

Select Appropriate Analgesics. Begin with the mildest agents that control the pain, using a multidrug approach. Even though a stepped approach is recommended, clients may have enough pain to make opioid therapy the initial treatment of choice. Nonopioids and adjuvant analgesics may be used as well and allow a smaller opioid dosage with fewer side effects.

Most traditional NSAIDs (the cyclooxygenase inhibitor type 1, or COX-1 drugs) affect platelet aggregation, the gastric mucosa, and the renal system. Combining them increases the risk of gastric and renal toxicity. Acetaminophen, an exception, may be given safely with NSAIDs. The newer COX-2 drugs, although initially promising, were found to be associated with severe adverse cardiovascular effects. Celecoxib (Celebrex) is the remaining agent of this type on the market, but this drug is often prescribed to treat pain from osteoarthritis.

When the combination of a nonopioid and a mild opioid becomes ineffective at the maximum recommended daily dosage (e.g., eight Vicodin tablets in 24 hours provide the 4000-mg maximum daily dose of acetaminophen), the client should receive a more potent opioid.

Use the agonist opioids as first-line agents, such as oxycodone, hydrocodone, codeine, morphine, methadone, hydromorphone, and fentanyl. Meperidine is not recommended for chronic use because its active metabolite, normeperidine, accumulates and causes central nervous system excitatory effects. Unmanageable side effects require the choice of an alternative opioid. Agonist-antagonist opioids are unsuitable for pain requiring significant and chronic dosages.

Atypical analgesics—those agents that are not primarily indicated for pain management (such as antidepressants and anticonvulsants)—may be useful for clients with neuropathic pain unresponsive or only partially responsive to opioid therapy.

Action Alert! Do not participate in the use of placebos for the control of any cancer pain; this is unethical. Administering a nonanalgesic substance that the client believes to be analgesic constitutes deceitful behavior.

Titrate and Schedule the Dosage Properly. Scheduled dosing is the standard for chronic cancer pain. The administration schedule is based on the analgesic's duration of effect. Maintaining consistent serum (blood) levels of the analgesic provides a baseline of consistent pain relief but does not preclude the need for treating **breakthrough pain,** intermittent episodes of pain that occur despite continuous analgesic use. Breakthrough pain is treated with **rescue dosing,** which involves giving an as-needed rescue doses of an immediate-release analgesic in addition to the scheduled analgesic dosage.

Action Alert! Cancer pain is chronic in nature and requires, with rare exception, both scheduled and rescue dosing.

Scheduled dosing is best accomplished using sustained-release products (every 8 to 12 hours, every 24 hours, or every 72 hours). Rescue dosing requires immediate-release preparations with a short half-life. If possible, use the same analgesic for both scheduled and rescue dosing.

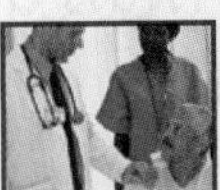

Mr. Valdez reluctantly agreed to take sustained-release morphine twice a day (bid). The physician also prescribed an immediate-release sublingual (SL) morphine tablet every 2 hours as needed for breakthrough pain. Although Joseph did have breakthrough pain, he rarely used the SL tablets. When the physician questioned him about his need for the analgesics, Joseph replied that he did have extra pain "sometimes" but did not want to use the SL tablets. His physician cautiously titrated the sustained-release analgesic upward at each visit. Joseph was compliant with the twice-daily dosing. He did, however, need to take six tablets BID.

Rescue dosing can be used alone when the analgesic dose is uncertain, during initial titration of opioids with a long half-life (such as methadone), or during therapy that may decrease the analgesic dose needed for pain relief (such as radiation therapy for bone metastases).

Frequent rescue dosing requires a change in the scheduled dose. The 24-hour cumulative sums of the scheduled and rescue doses should be added to determine the new 24-hour scheduled dose. This dosage is divided by the number of times in 24 hours that the drug will be given. For example, assume the client's scheduled dose is 800 mg of sustained-release oral morphine every 8 hours (2400 mg in 24 hours) plus 10 rescue doses of 30 mg of sublingual morphine each (300 mg). That equals 2700 mg of morphine in 24 hours. The new scheduled dose would be 2700 divided by 3, or 900 mg of sustained-release morphine every 8 hours.

Taper the opioid analgesic if a client needs a significant decrease in dosage. Chronic opioid exposure produces physical dependence, and sudden cessation will produce signs and symptoms of withdrawal, such as agitation, tremors, insomnia, fear, autonomic nervous system hyperexcitability, and increased pain.

Identify the Appropriate Route. The appropriate route is based on physiological needs, client comfort and preference, and caregiver capacity. It is frequently necessary to change the route as the illness progresses. Choose the route that provides prompt relief. Severe, escalating pain requires IV administration to achieve rapid onset of action. Opioids may be given IV by intermittent dosing, continuous infusion, or a combination of the two. PCA has been used effectively to titrate the analgesic dose to desired effect.

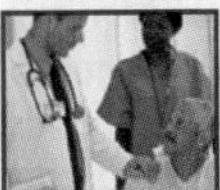

Mr. Valdez's pain became less responsive even with 10 sustained-release morphine tablets bid. His physician talked to him privately and told him that the pain was not going to get better and would probably get worse. He recommended a peripherally inserted central catheter (PICC) and the use of an ambulatory infusion pump to deliver a continuous dosage of morphine, with the capability of rescue dosing for breakthrough pain. Joseph thought about it for a few days and agreed, hoping that the increased pain relief would allow him to continue working. The pump was small and, after the PICC line was inserted, the nurse instructed Joseph how best to place it so that it would not interfere with his job. Do you think the nurse and physician should support Joseph's decision to continue working?

Intramuscular and subcutaneous injections are painful and provide inconsistent absorption. However, low-volume continuous subcutaneous infusions may be very effective when IV access is unavailable or impractical. The epidural or intrathecal route may be appropriate for specified clients when less invasive measures have provided inadequate pain relief.

Manage Side Effects of Therapy. Carefully monitor the client when you begin giving opioid therapy. Respiratory depression can occur in clients who are opioid naive and those with pulmonary disease, but it is uncommon with careful titration. Naloxone (Narcan) is not recommended to reverse non–life-threatening effects, such as confusion or sedation. Hypersensitivity (allergic) reactions are rare. Opioid use routinely causes constipation, and clients do not develop tolerance to this side effect. A prophylactic bowel regimen is recommended.

Clinical Accountabilities. The management of cancer pain requires diligent assessment, a significant pharmacological knowledge base, comfort with the liberal use of opioid analgesics, and ease in the use of multiple administrative routes. The nurse's role incorporates knowledge, skill, compassion, and advocacy to ensure client safety and comfort. Table 37-9 summarizes clinical responsibilities in managing the client with cancer pain.

INTERVENTIONS TO MANAGE PAIN IN OLDER ADULTS

The principles of acute and chronic pain management generally apply to the older population with slight modifications. Polypharmacy, side effects of typical analgesics, comorbidities, declining renal and hepatic function, less lean body mass, and possibly decreasing mental faculties are variables that must be factored into the pain management equation.

Management Principles

Pharmacological Interventions Carry Increased Risk of Toxicity. The use of analgesics in general is not impaired by normal aging, but the older adult is at greater risk for analgesic toxicity. Physiological variables may cause slower metabolism of analgesics, thus increasing their potential for producing harmful side effects.

Nonopioid analgesics, acetaminophen, and NSAIDs are used to provide relatively safe and effective relief for mild-to-moderate pain, generally at a decreased dosage. Opioids can be used for moderate-to-severe pain but are more likely to cause side effects. Constipation, nausea, vomiting, alterations in cognition, and severe agitation may occur. These side effects

Table 37-9 Management of Cancer Pain

CLINICAL ACCOUNTABILITY	ELEMENTS
Understand basic pain management strategies.	• Principles of drug selection and dosing. • Equianalgesic conversion methods. • Advantages and disadvantages of various administrative routes. • Management of nonopioid, opioid, and atypical analgesic side effects.
Assess pain systematically.	• Evaluate effectiveness after each dose until pain is well controlled. • Base assessment on client's report. • Consistently use same rating scale. • Reassess when client's pain has changed or is escalating.
Advocate for the client.	• Communicate with the health care provider when relief is inadequate. • Provide articulate, concise assessment. • Offer suggestions for dosage or medication alternative if appropriate. • Continue collaboration with the health care provider until the client is comfortable. • Question the use of placebos.
Ensure appropriate analgesic intervention.	• Choose appropriate analgesic when more than one is ordered. • Ensure that a multidrug approach is used when appropriate. • Monitor ordered analgesics for incompatibility.
Clarify questionable orders.	• Chronic use of meperidine or an agonist–antagonist opioid. • Scheduled or rescue analgesics not ordered. • Scheduled analgesic does not provide adequate relief because of ordered interval. • Frequent rescue dosing is necessary to maintain adequate pain control. • Conversion to alternative route or drug is not based on equianalgesic conversion principles, resulting in inappropriate dosage. • Route of chronic opioid administration is intramuscular. • Ordered route is or becomes inadequate or inappropriate. • An opioid antagonist is ordered to counteract non–life-threatening sedation.
Anticipate and manage side effects.	• Bowel regimen titrated to effect for all clients on chronic opioid dosing. • Prophylactic antiemetics during initial opioid therapy. • Monitor for central nervous system toxicity as opioid dosage escalates.
Educate client and family.	• Right to and benefits of adequate analgesia. • Client's role in assessment. • Analgesic side effects and their management. • Misconceptions and fears about physical dependence, tolerance, and psychological dependence. • Contractual agreement for opioid use in clients with history of substance abuse.
Document pertinent data.	• Nature, location, and intensity of pain. • Consistent report of results of ordered interventions. • Rationale for changes in analgesic regimen.

can be treated and do not contraindicate the use of opioids for significant pain. As is true with nonopioid analgesics, an older adult may need smaller opioid dosages than a younger person.

Nonpharmacological Interventions Are Useful. Pain can be reduced using common nonpharmacological remedies. Physical and occupational therapists can provide practical advice on ways to reduce physical pain as the older adult goes about the activities of daily living. Some clients may prefer alternative approaches, as shown in Box 37-5.

The older adult is also at risk for emotional problems associated with pain. Older adults who seek emotional support and education seem to hurt less. Adequate analgesia depends, in part, on the extent to which the family and caregiver understand the client's illness and treatment, have supportive and encouraging attitudes, and communicate the client's worth independent of functional status.

Clinical Accountabilities. Your role in responding to the older adult with pain, although grounded in generic analgesic principles, does incorporate some behaviors specific to this special population. Table 37-10 summarizes your accountabilities of pain management in the older adult.

INTERVENTIONS TO MANAGE PAIN IN CLIENTS WITH A HISTORY OF SUBSTANCE ABUSE

Clients with a history of substance abuse experience pain and have the right to effective analgesia. Undertreatment is common in this client population as clinicians try to balance their responsibilities to the client with their ethical concerns. Common barriers to adequate management include reluctance to believe the client's self-reported pain status, reluctance to prescribe opioids or other controlled substances, difficulty in identifying common maladaptive behaviors, moral disapproval of client behaviors, and difficulty in successfully treating these clients.

The plan of care for clients with a substance abuse disorder must include management of acute intoxication and efforts to prevent or minimize withdrawal, followed by establishing an effective analgesic regimen. Problematic behavior must be addressed, and realistic goals must be established. The cause of the pain must be understood in order to intervene successfully. This process occurs within the context of the client's history—whether the substance abuse is current or occurred in the distant past with ongoing participation in a recovery program. If the abuse is current, the

BOX 37-5 Considering the Alternatives

Alternative Treatments for Pain

Chiropractic/Manual Therapy

Advantages

Faster improvement for neck pain than with physiotherapy or general practitioner care

Cost was approximately one third of physiotherapy and general practitioner care (Korthals-de Bos et al., 2003)

Higher client satisfaction than other treatments

Disadvantages

Requires practitioner trained in spinal manipulation

Some clients may not be willing to be touched

More difficult to standardize care than pharmacological interventions

Massage

Advantages

Also improves depression and anxiety (Walach, Guthin, & Konig, 2003)

No negative side effects

Applicable to many types of pain: chronic pain, cancer pain, fibromyalgia, neck pain

Disadvantages

Requires a massage therapist

Some clients may not be willing to be touched

Some types of massage may raise heart rate temporarily

Music

Advantages

Also improves depression and disability (Siedliecki & Good, 2006)

No negative side effects

Applicable to many types of pain: postoperative, procedural, cancer pain, and chronic nonmalignant pain

Disadvantages

May require a device to play the music to the client

Requires ability to hear

Requires active listening by client

Korthals-de Bos, I. B., Hoving, J. L., van Tulder, M. W., Rutten-val Molken, M. P., Ader, H. J., de Vet, H. C., et al. (2003). Cost effectiveness of physiotherapy, manual therapy, and general practitioner care for neck pain: Economic evaluation alongside a randomised controlled trial. *British Medical Journal, 326*(7395), 911.

Siedliecki, S. L., & Good, M. (2006). Effect of music on power, pain, depression and disability. *Journal of Advanced Nursing, 54*(5), 553-562.

Wallach, H., Guthlin, C., & Konig, M. (2003). Efficacy of massage therapy in chronic pain: A pragmatic randomized trial. *Journal of Alternative and Complementary Medicine, 9*(6), 837-846.

Table 37-10 Management of Pain in the Older Adult

CLINICAL ACCOUNTABILITY	ELEMENTS
Set aside misconceptions.	• Understand that pain in the older adult is a sign of disease or impending dysfunction. • Be sensitive to the underreporting of pain, the "good patient" presentation, and the fear of "becoming a burden" to one's family.
Assess systematically.	• Pursue decreased function, slowness of movement as signs of pain. • Be vigilant in assessing for acute pain; it may present in the older adult as atypical or referred pain. • Distinguish between dementia and delirium; search for subtle signs of behavior that are abnormal for that client. • Watch for any behavior change in the confused older client because it may result from pain.
Intervene appropriately.	• Respect client's past experience of "tried and true" remedies. • Maximize relief and improve function through pharmacological and nonpharmacological means. • Manage opioid therapy by adequately treating both the pain and opioid side effects. • Treat anxiety or depression (commonly associated with chronic pain).
Maximize relief and function.	• Respect the older adult's expectations, and support them to the extent possible. • Provide individualized treatment, differentiating between the well and the frail older adult. • Investigate ways the older adult may contribute to the family and others.

client's relationship with medications is markedly different from what it is if the abuse was in the distant past.

Analgesics. General principles of acute and chronic pain management apply to this client population. For chronic pain, scheduled and rescue dosing are appropriate. The client's sense of control may be enhanced when you provide information about the medication, dosage, and schedule. Opioids may be used when they are appropriate for the type of pain the client is experiencing. Withholding analgesics from chemically dependent clients in pain will not enhance recovery from addictive behaviors.

Communication Strategies. Effective communication among clinical team members is essential to ensure consistency and maintain therapeutic direction. The coordinator of care should be identified as soon as possible to keep the team focused and goal directed. The client deserves a clear understanding of the frequency of assessment, treatment goals, and who will be prescribing the analgesics. It is very important to limit negotiations about medications and dosages. Regular team meetings should occur to promote planning for effective pain management, to discuss differences of opinion about interventions, and to collaboratively set limits and identify boundaries.

Action Alert! Setting limits is in the best interest of the client. Never use pain relief as a bargaining tool.

Use of a written contractual agreement can help make the treatment plan explicit. Components of the contractual agreement might include goals of treatment, treatment plan, client and staff expectations, consequences of noncompliance, the staff responsible for the client's care, reevaluation intervals, and consent for random urine screenings.

Outpatient treatment requires additional considerations. There must be policies regarding the replacement of lost or stolen medications, unsanctioned dose escalation, and early refill requests. Clear expectations must be articulated about follow-up appointments; whom to call about medications, analgesic relief, and side effects; and the limited quantity of prescription medications.

The best intentions of the multidisciplinary team may not guarantee success. The client may refuse treatment or fail to comply with the prescribed regimen. The focus must still remain on effective pain management for all clients regardless of any one person's dysfunctional behavior.

INTERVENTIONS FOR RELATED NURSING DIAGNOSES

Constipation. Ensure adequate fluid intake (six to eight glasses of water per day as tolerated) to promote bowel elimination. Provide a stool softener and laxative as ordered. Encourage ambulation and activity, as tolerated, as added measures to prevent constipation caused by side effects of opioid analgesics.

Activity Intolerance. Provide analgesia before any activities known to cause pain, such as repositioning, coughing and deep breathing, ambulating, dressing changes, and many more. Perform these activities during times of peak analgesic effect for greatest effect and client satisfaction.

Ineffective Role Performance. Be aware that the client and family may be stressed by the changing roles that occur during illness. Use therapeutic communication skills when working with clients and families, and explore options for how family members can temporarily assume some of the client's roles. Consult with a medical social worker if the assistance of any outside agencies would be beneficial.

Ineffective Coping. Use your therapeutic communication skills to explore how the client is adapting to the current illness. Assess what coping strategies have worked in the past, and determine if they would be helpful at this time as well. Determine what support systems the client has, such as family and friends. Communicate with other members of the health care team if you believe the client would benefit from a consultation with psychiatric services.

Hopelessness. Listen actively to clients, and encourage expression of feelings. Use reminiscence therapy to help clients explore past life experiences, which can help them find meaning in current life. Encourage clients to participate in decision making and problem solving. Initiate referrals to spiritual or other counselors as indicated.

Caregiver Role Strain. Openly discuss the difficulties of the caregiving responsibilities. Discuss with the caregiver the typical daily and weekly activities, and identify those for which assistance is needed and available (client care and household maintenance). Enlist the assistance of other family members, and initiate referrals to community resources as needed.

Ineffective Therapeutic Regimen Management. Communicate with the client to identify factors that inhibit effective management of the health care regimen. Communicate effectively with the client to promote confidence and positive self-efficacy, reduce barriers to learning, and reduce anxiety. Provide information about the disorder, treatment, helpful lifestyle changes, and support services available. Community nursing services may be indicated.

INTERVENTIONS INVOLVING OPIOID INFUSION DEVICES

Management of pain may incorporate the use of patient-controlled analgesia or intraspinal analgesia at some point during the illness. These approaches to opioid administration are used in multiple settings.

Patient-Controlled Analgesia. **Patient-controlled analgesia (PCA)** is a drug-delivery approach that uses an external infusion pump to deliver an opioid dose on a "client demand" basis (Figure 37-9). This intermittent dosing is driven by the client's need for analgesic relief and the pump's preprogrammed instructions to deliver an identified dosage at specified intervals. The infusion pump's program cannot be overridden by the client. Most pumps also have the capacity to deliver a continuous or background infusion as well.

PCA was developed to manage postoperative pain. Formerly, these clients were commonly managed with *as-needed* IM injections of an opioid, usually in combination with an antiemetic. This approach created a significant delay in pain relief caused by the multistep process from the client's recognition of discomfort to the actual administration of medication. The *as-needed* administration approach also created large swings in serum levels of opioid, which resulted in overmedication and undermedication.

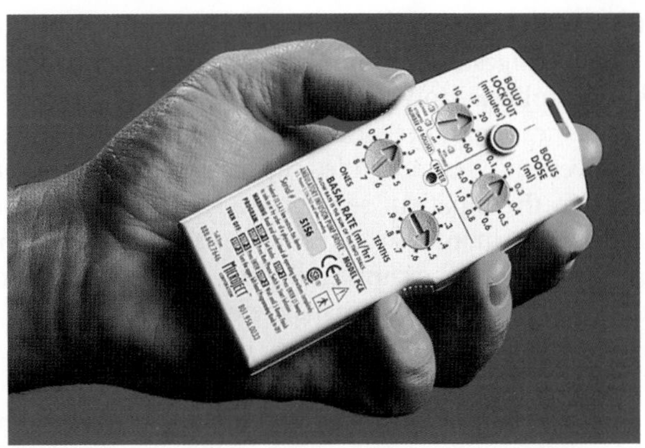

FIGURE 37-9 A patient-controlled analgesia device. (Courtesy Microject Corporation, Salt Lake City, UT.)

Extensive clinical experience with PCA devices has demonstrated that they provide the following:

- Improved pain relief with smaller opioid dosages
- The ability to finely titrate the opioid dosage, with decreased potential for overdosing
- A decreased delay in receiving analgesic relief at the time of need
- Decreased dependency on nursing personnel
- Earlier activity with improved pulmonary status
- Decreased client anxiety resulting from inadequate pain relief

Client Selection. Clients selected for PCA are those who require repeated parenteral opioid doses for moderate-to-severe pain, those who can understand and follow the instructions, and those willing to use this type of therapy. PCA is not appropriate for clients unable to understand the mechanics of its usage or those with insufficient dexterity to self-administer a dose of analgesic.

There continues to be some controversy about the use of PCA in clients with a history of substance abuse. The issue is not one of the need for pain relief but rather a reluctance to place responsibility for opioid dosing in the hands of the client. The clinical team should evaluate this issue before the actual time of need.

Using a PCA Infusion Pump. PCA can be delivered by many routes. Although initially developed for IV use, subcutaneous and intraspinal administrations are growing more common. These allow the client increased access to this modality across care settings.

Intravenous and epidural PCA have been used very effectively in the immediate postoperative period. A client undergoing major thoracic surgery, for instance, may benefit markedly from epidural administration. Adequate analgesia can shorten the client's stay in the intensive care unit and maximize pulmonary function. A client undergoing less invasive surgery does as well with the IV route. Indwelling IV access provides a rapid onset of action and precludes the further discomfort of an IV injection. Analgesics commonly used include morphine, hydromorphone, and meperidine.

The efficacy and practicality of PCA in managing postoperative pain has extended its usage to other client groups in the inpatient setting. Moderate-to-severe pain that decreases in intensity as tissue heals lends itself to this dosing method. For example, clients with burns or trauma pain respond well to this management approach.

On-demand dosing, alone or in combination with continuous infusion, may be used very effectively for analgesic relief. When on-demand dosing is used as single therapy, the pump is typically programmed to provide a modest amount of opioid at intervals of 5 to 15 minutes. A continuous or background infusion typically runs as well. When there is a need for pain relief, the client self-administers a dose using the PCA device.

If the client tries to administer another dose before the programmed time goes by, the device will not deliver it. Once the programmed time has elapsed, the device will once again deliver an opioid dose upon client request.

When on-demand dosing is used concurrently with a continuous or background infusion of opioid, the continuous opioid dosage is generally inadequate to manage the client's total analgesic need. This combined approach allows the client to titrate the remainder of needed analgesic relief with the on-demand dosing.

Both approaches provide clients the ability to titrate the final opioid dosage on the basis of their analgesic needs. As with any other method, it is appropriate and essential to assess the client's response. Dosages may be titrated upward or downward, depending on the level of pain relief obtained.

Clients with chronic pain are also well served by this approach. The on-demand capacity allows rapid titration and determination of the overall analgesic dosage required in a 24-hour period. Chronic cancer pain with episodes of breakthrough pain that is severe, increasing rapidly, or has not responded to less invasive approaches can be effectively managed with PCA. In these circumstances, the IV route with its rapid onset of action is the most efficient and effective way to control the pain and titrate the dosage.

Once the client is maintained on a stable opioid dose with both continuous and on-demand dosing, the clinical team can make an informed decision about the client's discharge needs. Alternatives include the following:

- Converting the parenteral dosage to an equianalgesic oral dosage
- Establishing stable IV access for a client who needs substantial opioid dosages, and discharging him with an IV ambulatory PCA device
- Converting the IV route to subcutaneous PCA. This route requires adequate subcutaneous tissue to handle up to 2 to 3 mL. If analgesic requirements are significant, an opioid must be chosen that is available in a highly concentrated formulation.

Experience in the acute care setting has provided the experience necessary to transfer this method of therapy to the outpatient setting. Home health care and hospice programs now routinely serve clients who have PCA pumps. Although permanent or long-term indwelling IV access devices would support the IV route for ambulatory use, subcutaneous administration is more practical in the home setting and is the route of choice for those without reliable IV access. Reliability and ease of access by a layperson render it both sensible and dependable.

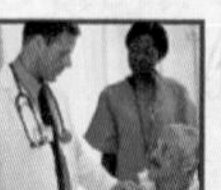

Mr. Valdez continued his PCA therapy with some success. The shoulder strap and carrying bag for the pump allowed him to conceal the system under his jacket when he went to work, and he had the nurse titrate his dosage upward when he needed to use frequent bolus doses. He allowed his wife to help with the dressing changes, because he could not manage it alone. When he could, he preferred to have the office nurse do the dressing change. Do you think the office nurse should accommodate his wishes?

Intraspinal Analgesia. Intraspinal analgesia involves placement of a catheter to deliver medication to the epidural or intrathecal space. This invasive therapy can be temporary or permanent. Temporary catheters are used for short-term postoperative pain relief and to evaluate the efficacy of intraspinal analgesia before placing a permanent catheter. Permanent catheter placement is used for clients unresponsive to less invasive analgesic methods.

Epidural Analgesia. In **epidural analgesia,** a catheter is placed between the spinal vertebrae and the dura mater to allow the diffusion of an analgesic drug across the dura mater into the cerebrospinal fluid (CSF). There, the drug binds with opioid receptors in the dorsal horn of the spinal cord.

Epidural analgesia can be used to manage acute and chronic pain. Indications include the following:

- Short-term pain relief via a temporary catheter for postoperative pain and pain from multiple trauma
- Postoperative pain conditions where mobility and full lung expansion immediately after surgery are especially important
- Chronic cancer pain that does not respond to conventional opioid intervention

Epidural analgesia may be produced by intermittent injections, continuous infusions, or a combination of the two. Patient-controlled epidural analgesia may be used to deliver both continuous and intermittent dosing and is generally reserved for the management of chronic malignant pain.

Benefits of epidural analgesia for the management of acute pain include improved respiratory function, earlier mobilization and return of bowel function after surgery, and heightened alertness. Benefits for the client with cancer pain include improved pain management at a significantly lower opioid dose and the relief of dose-limiting or unmanageable side effects from conventional therapy. Identified risks for both client populations include respiratory depression, catheter tip migration, epidural abscess formation, and epidural hematomas. Box 37-6 gives instructions for the client about changing the dressing on a permanent epidural catheter.

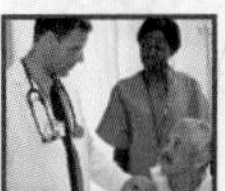

Mr. Valdez's pain has escalated despite consistent upward titration of his parenteral morphine infusion. He reluctantly rates the pain to be a 7 on a scale of 0 to 10 but maintains it "is not too bad." He says the abdominal pain sometimes seems to "shoot" down his leg. He refuses to move in any way that might aggravate the pain and holds his upper abdomen when he moves. He is now unable to work. When in bed, he is very still and sits upright in a rigid position. The morphine infusion has been increased to 300 mg/hr with a 100-mg bolus allowed every 15 minutes prn. He uses at least two boluses every hour. Joseph is developing significant muscle twitching, a side effect of high parenteral opioid dosing. Treatment with anticonvulsants and benzodiazepines has not controlled the twitching, and it is increasing in severity. His physician decides to place an epidural catheter to improve analgesia and minimize the toxicities of treatment.

Intrathecal Analgesia. In **intrathecal analgesia,** a catheter is placed in the subarachnoid space between the dura mater and the spinal cord to allow immediate drug diffusion into the CSF. There, the drug binds with opioid receptors in the dorsal horn of the spinal cord. Intrathecal opioid therapy provides the most rapid onset of analgesic relief.

Intrathecal therapy is traditionally reserved for chronic pain unrelieved by less invasive methods. Selection criteria for cancer pain clients include inadequate pain relief despite escalating doses delivered via conventional routes, intolerable or unmanageable side effects from systemic opioids, and a life expectancy greater than 3 months. Client selection criteria for chronic nonmalignant pain are more controversial and less straightforward. They include therapy of last resort, a baseline neurological examination to identify the causes(s) of pain, and psychometric testing and psychological evaluation documenting that the pain is not primarily of psychological origin.

A "closed" system is typically used to minimize the risk of infection. The system includes a tunneled catheter attached to a surgically implanted infusion pump. The pump is programmed percutaneously via computer, and the pump's drug reservoir is accessed percutaneously. A positive response to a trial of epidural or intrathecal infusion therapy should be documented before the catheter and pump are placed.

Selecting Intraspinal Analgesics. Preservative-free opioids (such as morphine, hydromorphone, fentanyl, and sufentanil), local anesthetics (such as bupivacaine), and alpha$_2$-adrenoreceptor agonists (such as clonidine) are currently used singly or in combination to provide intraspinal analgesia. Opioids are used in significantly decreased dosages because of their proximity to the receptors in the spinal cord. This altered dosage decreases the incidence of central nervous system side effects because very little opioid ascends to the higher brain centers or is absorbed systemically via the blood supply in the epidural space.

Opioids may be used in combination with a local anesthetic when there is a prominent neuropathic component to the pain or when the client has unstable bone pain. Use of local anesthetics may decrease the amount of opioid required. Alpha$_2$-adrenoreceptor agonists provide spinal analgesia that is not reversed by naloxone. This therapy seems to be most effective in clients whose pain is primarily neuropathic in origin.

There are fewer side effects with intraspinal analgesia than with conventional opioid therapy because of the relatively low drug dosages required. Nevertheless, opioid side effects may include GI distress (including nausea, vomiting, or constipation), urinary retention, pruritus on the face or palate, and drowsiness or sedation. Local anesthetics and alpha$_2$-adrenoreceptor agonists have different side effect profiles.

Intraspinal therapy is becoming less rare in the acute care and ambulatory settings. These clients are no longer treated in intensive care units alone. Medical/surgical units and home health care and hospice agencies now routinely care for this client population. Appropriate care requires a thorough knowledge base and skilled clinicians to direct and administer therapy.

EVALUATION

To evaluate a client's outcomes after treatment of pain, reassess the client to ensure that the goals have been met. This forms the basis for revising the plan of care.

Box 37-7 is a sample nursing care plan for Mr. Valdez, who will be undergoing insertion of a permanent epidural catheter.

The nursing note reflects assessment of postsurgical sequelae (catheter placement), signs of infection, analgesic status, functional level, and client/family education. The postoperative goals of decreasing the side effects of opioid therapy, maintaining adequate analgesia, increasing physical mobility, and improving the quality of life have been achieved.

The hospice nursing note for Mr. Valdez after his hospitalization for epidural catheter placement (described in Box 37-7) might look like the one on p. 1034.

BOX 37-6

Teaching for Self-Care

Changing the Dressing Over a Permanent Epidural Catheter

Purpose: To prevent infection during epidural analgesia.
Expected Outcome: The client will remain free of infection at the catheter exit site, the tunneled area, and the epidural space, thus ensuring continued analgesia.

Client Instructions

1. Assemble the required supplies as they appear on the list I have given you.
2. Clean a work surface, and cover it with paper towels.
3. Perform hand hygiene with warm, soapy water. Rinse hands well, and dry with a clean paper towel.
4. Open the supplies, being careful not to touch any sterile supplies or the inside surfaces of their wrappers.
5. Remove the old dressing, starting at the top and working your way downward. Be careful not to pull on the catheter. Discard the old dressing into a plastic bag.
6. Perform hand hygiene again.
7. Look closely at the exit site and the skin around it. If it is hot or red, or if fluid is oozing from it, notify your nurse or doctor after completing this procedure.
8. Take one of the povidone-iodine swab sticks in your dominant hand, and clean the exit site. Starting at the center, wipe the skin in a circular motion, working outward 2 to 3 inches from the catheter (see illustration). *Never touch the exit site with a swab that has touched skin other than at the site itself.*

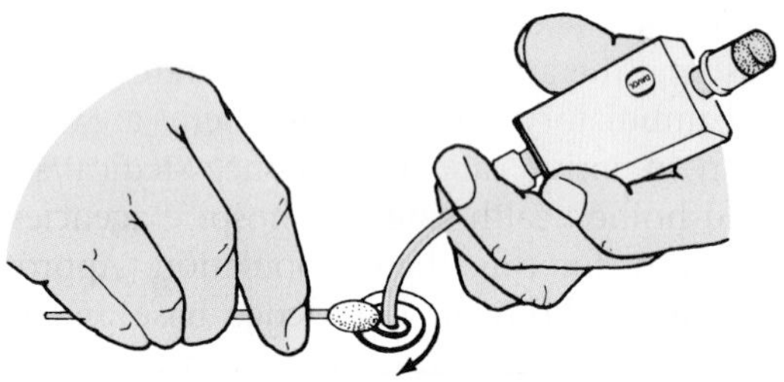

Step 8 Wiping the skin in a circular motion. (Illustration from Bard Access Systems. [1993]. *DuPen long-term epidural catheter: Use and maintenance.* Salt Lake City, UT: Bard Access Systems.)

9. Use a second swab stick to clean the exit site one more time with the same circular motion.
10. Use a third swab stick to clean the catheter itself. Use an upward motion from the exit site to clean about 2 inches of the catheter. Leave the iodine solution on the skin and the catheter, and allow it to completely air-dry. This may take 1 to 3 minutes.
11. Place precut sterile gauze dressing around the catheter (see illustration).

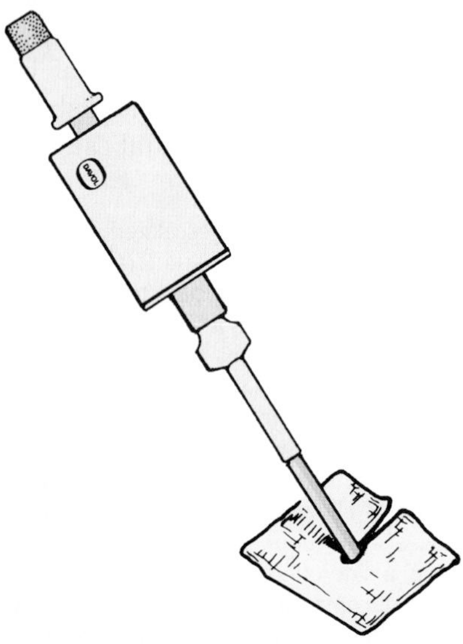

Step 11 Placing the precut sterile gauze dressing around the catheter. (Illustration from Bard Access Systems. [1993]. *DuPen long-term epidural catheter: Use and maintenance.* Salt Lake City, UT: Bard Access Systems.)

12. Place a 3 × 3 inch sterile gauze dressing over the precut dressing and catheter, and tape it in place (see illustration).

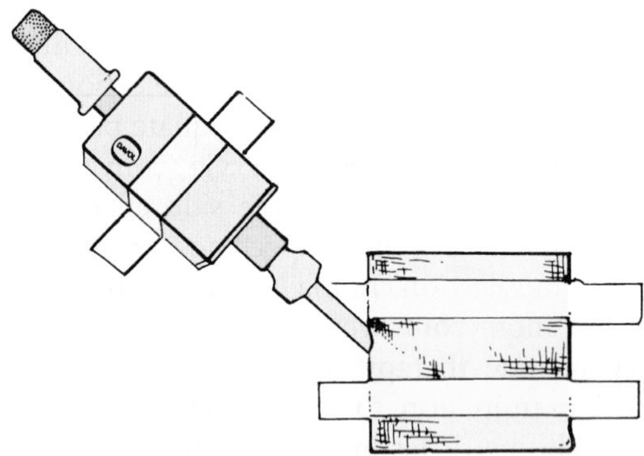

Step 12 A 3 × 3 inch sterile gauze dressing taped over the precut dressing and catheter. (Illustration from Bard Access Systems. [1993]. *DuPen long-term epidural catheter: Use and maintenance.* Salt Lake City, UT: Bard Access Systems.)

13. Make sure the catheter is not kinked or pinched. You may want to tape the catheter to your skin or to the dressing to avoid an extra "tug" on the catheter exit site as you move about.

BOX 37-7

Nursing Care Plan

A Client With Uncontrolled Pain

Admission Data

Mr. Valdez is admitted to the oncology unit for epidural catheter placement. The nurse who will be caring for him understands that he has unrelieved and severe pain and will have a permanent epidural catheter placed. Dr. Terry is on the way to the unit to write orders.

Physician's Orders

Admitting diagnosis: uncontrolled pain secondary to adenocarcinoma of the stomach
Morphine 300 mg/hr via PICC line. Bolus dose 100 mg every 15 min prn. May increase continuous infusion by 100 mg/hr if client uses 2 bolus doses/hr times 4 hours.*
Acetaminophen 650 mg PO for temperature >101° F
Valium 10 mg PO every 4 hours prn for muscle twitching
Elavil 50 mg PO at bedtime
Lactulose 60 mL PO four times/day
Activity as tolerated
Diet as tolerated
PT, PTT, CBC with differential, stat
ECG stat
Chest x-ray stat
Consent for permanent epidural catheter placement
NPO after midnight

Nursing Assessment

Color pale, diaphoretic. Reports pain to be 7 on a 0 to 10 scale, primarily in abdominal area but shoots down leg unexpectedly. Guarding, reduced movement, and wincing when turning in bed. BP 130/90, pulse 100, respiratory rate 14, temperature 98.6° F. Morphine is infusing via PICC line at 300 mg/hr with a 100-mg bolus allowed every 15 minutes prn. He has used 2 bolus doses in the hour since admission.

NANDA-I Nursing Diagnosis	NOC Expected Outcomes With Indicators	NIC Interventions With Selected Activities	Evaluation Data
Chronic Pain	***Pain Control***	***Medication Management***	***After 24 Hours of Care***
Related Factor: • Verbal report of pain	• Verbalizes adequate pain control	• Assess pain level and titrate intravenous analgesics preoperatively and epidural analgesics postoperatively per physician orders. • Provide reassurance that pain relief is the goal.	• Preoperative pain rating of 7. Bolus dose decreased rating to 3. • Postoperative: pain rating of 3 after 24 hours without need to titrate epidural.
		• Assess bowel function, and administer laxative as ordered	• Client had two effective bowel movements before surgery and one movement 36 hours after surgery.
		• Encourage and help client to ambulate after surgery as pain level decreases.	• Walked in room with help 4 hours after surgery. Walked in hallway with help 12 hours after surgery. Went to bathroom without help 18 hours after surgery.

Critical Thinking Questions

1. Given that Mr. Valdez has reluctantly admitted his pain to be at an intensity of 7 and has even demonstrated some behavioral indications that his pain is severe, how will you assess him once the epidural catheter is placed?
2. During the immediate postoperative period, Mr. Valdez's pain is controlled remarkably well as the epidural analgesics are titrated upward. During the night before his morning discharge, he begins to complain of severe pain in his abdomen. What would you look for to explain this sudden change in comfort level?
3. Compare the dose of IV morphine for Mr. Valdez with the usual dose given for a client who is morphine naive. What precautions would you take the first time a client receives morphine or other parenteral opioids?
4. Mr. Valdez is inclined neither to ask his wife for help nor to rely on her for assistance with his care. He would rather not have the care than have someone provide it for him. How will you educate Mr. and Mrs. Valdez regarding epidural catheter care, understanding that Mrs. Valdez must also learn the proper technique?

Nursing outcome and intervention labels from Johnson, M., Bulechek, G., Butcher, H., Dochterman, J. M., Maas, M., Moorhead, S., et al. (Eds.). (2006). *NANDA, NOC, and NIC linkages: Nursing diagnoses, outcomes, & interventions.* St. Louis, MO: Mosby.
*This dose of morphine is in excess of the usual dose for acute pain and would be lethal in the client who has not developed tolerance.

Sample Documentation Note for Mr. Valdez

Epidural exit site without signs of infection. Somewhat tender to palpation; no warmth, exudate, or swelling. Tunneled track without signs of redness or swelling. Posterior incision site dry, no discharge, sutures intact. Temperature 98.6° F. Respiratory rate 12. Alert and oriented. Rates pain in abdomen to be 3 on a scale of 0 to 10. Epidural morphine at 3 mg/hr in 0.15% bupivacaine solution. PCA bolus dose of 1 mg every hour prn used times three in past 24 hours when client bent over. No complaints of nausea, constipation, itching, or numbness in lower extremities. Client reports that he and wife have been out to dinner and a movie on two occasions and that he walks around the house during the day and goes to the table for meals. Client and wife verbalize and demonstrate proper technique for catheter site care and infusion pump maintenance.

▼ KEY PRINCIPLES

- Pain can be a complex, biopsychosocial phenomenon with sensory, affective, and cognitive dimensions. The client and the pain experience may be woven together, making it difficult to separate them into distinct entities.
- The client's self-report of the pain experience is a standard of the assessment process.
- Transmission of the pain signal from the site of injury to the higher brain centers where the sensation is recognized involves multiple anatomical structures and biochemical neurotransmitters. The pain signal may be modulated at various steps along this pathway.
- Tolerance and physical dependence are involuntary, physiological occurrences. They are distinct from psychological dependence (addiction) and should not be considered addiction.
- Psychological dependence (addiction) rarely occurs when clients are using opioid analgesics for the relief of pain. Fears of opioid addiction are exceptionally disproportionate to the reality and are a major barrier to the adequate relief of pain.
- Pain management in clients with substance abuse or addiction requires special collaboration with other members of the health care team. This population is at risk for inadequate pain management, although treatment of addiction may also be necessary.
- Acute pain and chronic pain are markedly different experiences.
- The acute pain model is characterized by increased activity of the autonomic nervous system (increased blood pressure, pulse, respiratory rate, diaphoresis) and typical pain behaviors such as crying, moaning, and grimacing.
- In chronic pain, the client adapts physiologically and psychologically to the pain experience. Changes in vital signs and behavioral clues may not be evident. Assessing a client with chronic pain using the acute model is inadequate and misleading.
- Pain assessment in a client unable to communicate requires particular attention to behavioral clues that indicate discomfort. Neonates, small children, older adults who are delirious or confused, and comatose clients are especially at risk.
- Neonates, children, and older adults experience pain in the same way the younger adult population does. Painful states deserve equal attention.
- Acute pain is short term and generally resolves when the tissue heals. If acute pain is treated inadequately, the client may risk chronic pain.
- Severe acute pain should be treated immediately using an analgesic with a rapid onset of action. The intravenous route provides rapid relief, and the analgesic can be given safely if administered in small increments until the client is comfortable.
- Chronic pain that is intractable, that is difficult to treat, or that leads to disability affects the client physically and emotionally. It is always appropriate to use a multidisciplinary approach that treats all facets of the pain experience.
- Although nonpharmacological interventions and nonopioid analgesics have been given precedence in the treatment of chronic nonmalignant pain, there is increasing evidence that opioid analgesics may be administered to subsets of this client population in a controlled, safe manner.
- Cancer pain is chronic and requires, with rare exception, both scheduled and rescue dosing using nonopioid, opioid, and atypical analgesics.
- Clinicians should include client and family education about pain and its management in the treatment plan, and they should encourage clients to be active participants in the process.

■ REVIEW QUESTIONS

1. When assessing the intensity of acute pain in an assigned client, the nurse should ask which of the following questions?

1. "Where is the pain located?"
2. "Can you rate the pain on a scale of 0 to 10?"
3. "Can you describe how the pain feels to you?"
4. "When did the pain first begin?"

2. Which of the following clients is at risk for experiencing chronic pain?

1. A client who had her gallbladder removed
2. A client who broke an ankle
3. A client who exercises heavily
4. A client with arthritis

3. The nurse would keep in mind which of the following when working with a child who is experiencing pain?

1. Children will not always tell you if they have pain.
2. Children are not as sensitive to pain as adults.
3. Children do not remember pain.
4. A child is not in pain if he can be distracted or is sleeping.

4. The nurse would be most concerned about the risk of excessive dosing in a client who is receiving opioid analgesics for pain and has a history of which of the following health problems?

1. Irritable bowel syndrome
2. Liver disease
3. Headaches
4. Asthma

5. Which of the following clients would be the best candidate for using patient-controlled analgesia (PCA) following a surgical procedure?

1. A client with Down syndrome who is developmentally delayed
2. A client who had vascular surgery and has acute confusion
3. A client with Alzheimer's disease who underwent colon resection for cancer
4. A client who has surgical repair of broken bones after a motorcycle accident

Bibliography

*American Geriatrics Society. (1998). The management of chronic pain in older persons: Clinical practice guidelines. *Journal of the American Geriatrics Society, 46*(5), 635-651.

Ardery, G., Herr, K., Titler, M., Sorofman, B., & Schmidt, M. (2003). Assessing and managing acute pain in older adults: A research base to guide practice. *Medsurg Nursing, 12*(1), 7-18.

*Astor, R. (2001). Detecting pain in people with profound learning disabilities. *Nursing Times, 97*(40), 38-39.

Black, J., Hawks, J., & Keene, A. (2001). *Medical-surgical nursing: Clinical management for continuity of care* (6th ed.). Philadelphia: Saunders.

*Bonica, J. J. (1990). Anatomic and physiologic basis of nociception and pain. In J. J. Bonica (Ed.), *The management of pain* (2nd ed., pp. 400-460). Philadelphia: Lea & Febiger.

*Carr, D. B., & Jacox, A. K. (1992). *Acute pain management: Operative or medical procedures and trauma.* (AHCPR Publication No. 92-0032). Rockville, MD: Agency for Health Care Policy and Research, Public Health Service, U.S. Department of Health and Human Services.

Chapman, R. C., & Garvin, J. (1999). Suffering: The contributions of persistent pain. *Lancet 353*, 2233-2237.

*Compton, P. (2001). Controlling pain: Understanding addictive disease. *Nursing, 31*(9), 28.

*Coughlin, P. (2001). Manual therapies. In M. Micozzi (Ed.), *Fundamentals of complementary and alternative medicine.* New York: Churchill Livingstone.

D'Arcy, Y. (2006). Managing postop pain in a patient who's delirious. *Nursing, 36*(6), 17.

Girdhari, S., & Smith, S. (2006). Assisting older adults with orthopaedic outpatient acute-pain management. *Orthopaedic Nursing, 25*(3), 188-195.

*Hester, N., & Barcus, C. (1986). Assessment and management of pain in children. *Pediatrics: Nursing update.* Princeton, NJ: CPEC.

Hockenberry, M., Wilson, D., & Winkelstein, M. L. (2005). *Wong's essentials of pediatric nursing* (7th ed.). St. Louis, MO: Mosby.

*International Association for the Study of Pain. (1994). Pain terms: A current list with definitions and notes on usage. In H. Merskey & N. Bogduk (Eds.), *Classification of chronic pain: Descriptions of chronic pain syndromes and definitions of terms* (2nd ed., pp. 209-213). Seattle, WA: IASP Press.

*Jacox, A., Carr, D. B., & Payne, R. (1994). *Management of cancer pain: Clinical practice guideline.* (AHCPR Publication No. 94-0592). Rockville, MD: Agency for Health Care Policy and Research, U.S. Department of Health and Human Services.

Johnson, M., Bulechek, G., Butcher, H., Dochterman, J. M., Maas, M., Moorhead, S., et al. (Eds.). (2006). *NANDA, NOC, and NIC linkages: Nursing diagnoses, outcomes, & interventions.* St. Louis, MO: Mosby.

*McCaffrey, M. (1979). *Nursing management of the patient with pain.* New York: Lippincott.

*McCaffrey, M. (2001). Sorting out opioids. *Nursing, 31*(10), 70.

*McCaffrey, M., Ferrell, B. R., & Pasero, C. (2000). Nurses' personal opinions about patients' pain and their effect on recorded assessments and titration of opioid doses. *Pain Management Nursing, 1*(3), 79-87.

*McCaffrey, M., & Pasero, C. (2001a). Assessment and treatment of patients with mental illness. *American Journal of Nursing, 101*(7), 69-70.

*McCaffrey, M., & Pasero, C. (2001b). Using the 0-to-10 pain rating scale. *American Journal of Nursing, 101*(10), 81-82.

*McCaffrey, M., & Pasero, C. (2002). Monitoring sedation. *American Journal of Nursing, 102*(2), 67-68.

*McDonald, D. D., & Weiskopf, C. S. (2001). Adult patients' postoperative pain descriptions and responses to the Short-Form McGill Pain Questionnaire. *Clinical Nursing Research, 10*(4), 442-452.

*Melzack, R., & Casey, K. L. (1968). Sensory, motivational, and central determinants of pain. In D. R. Kenshalo (Ed.), *The skin senses* (pp. 423-439). Springfield, IL: Thomas.

*Melzack, R., & Wall, P. D. (1965). Pain mechanisms: A new theory. *Science, 150*, 971-979.

NANDA International. (2007). *Nursing diagnoses: Definitions and classification, 2006-2007* (7th ed.). Philadelphia: Author.

Pasero, C., & McCaffrey, M. (2005). No self-report means no pain-intensity rating. *American Journal of Nursing, 105*(10), 50-53.

*Reisman, T., & Pasternak, G. (2001). Opioid analgesics and antagonists. In J. G. Hardman & L. E. Limbird (eds.), *Goodman & Gilman's the pharmacological basis of therapeutics* (10th ed.). New York: McGraw-Hill.

Soetanto, A., Chung, J., & Wong, T. (2006). Are there gender differences in pain perception? *Journal of Neuroscience Nursing, 38*(3), 172-176.

Valente, S. (2006). Hypnosis for pain management. *Journal of Psychosocial Nursing and Mental Health Services, 44*(2), 22-30.

Young, J., Siffleet, J., Nikoletti, S., & Shaw, T. (2006). Use of a behavioural pain scale to assess pain in ventilated, unconscious and/or sedated patients. *Intensive Critical Care Nursing, 22*(1), 32-39.

*Asterisk indicates a classic or definitive work on this subject.

Chapter 38

Supporting Sensory/ Perceptual Function

Media Resources

- Evolve Website http://evolve.elsevier.com/Harkreader/
- Companion CD

Learning Objectives

After studying this chapter, you should be able to do the following:

- Describe the normal physiology of sensation and perception
- Differentiate between sensory deficit, sensory deprivation, and sensory overload
- Discuss a variety of factors affecting sensory/ perceptual function
- Describe techniques for assessing a client at risk for *Disturbed sensory perception,* the manifestations of disturbed sensory perception, and the client's response to altered sensory perception
- Identify the related nursing diagnoses of disturbed sensory perception for vision, hearing, movement, taste, smell, and touch
- Plan goal-directed nursing interventions to manage disturbed sensory perception
- Evaluate client outcomes related to disturbed sensory perception

Key Terms

auditory
gustatory
kinesthetic
olfactory
ototoxic
perception
presbycusis
presbyopia
reticular activating system (RAS)
sensation
sensory deprivation
sensory overload
tactile
visual

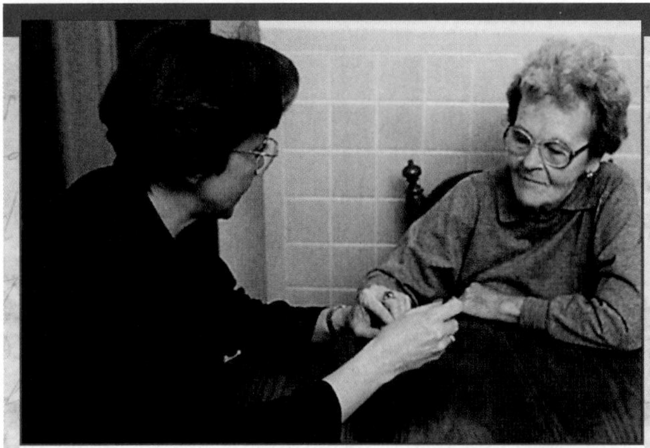

From Elkin, M. K., Perry, A. G., & Potter, P. A. *Nursing interventions and clinical skills* (3rd ed.). St. Louis, MO: Mosby.

Sarah Jane Pfannenstiel is an 82-year-old widow who lives with her only daughter and son-in-law. She has been seeing an ophthalmologist for decreasing visual acuity in the left eye. She describes her vision as "trying to see through a dirty, greasy window." She has difficulty driving at night because of the glare of headlights. She no longer enjoys reading or watching television because her left eye tears and becomes fatigued after short periods of time. She takes frequent afternoon naps because she is "bored." She is anxious and tells her daughter she is afraid of "going blind" and does not want to become a "burden." The daughter reports that her mother no longer goes out socially because she is afraid of falling and breaking an arm or leg.

The ophthalmologist recommends surgical removal of a cataract in the left eye. Mrs. Pfannenstiel is anxious about surgery and having someone "cutting on my eye." The nurse makes the diagnosis of *Disturbed sensory perception: visual* (see key nursing diagnoses box).

KEY NURSING DIAGNOSES FOR SENSORY/PERCEPTUAL ALTERATIONS

Disturbed sensory perception: (specify visual, auditory, kinesthetic, gustatory, tactile, olfactory): A change in the amount or patterning of incoming stimuli, accompanied by a diminished, exaggerated, distorted, or impaired response to stimuli

***Sensory overload:** A state that results from excessive environmental stimuli

***Sensory deprivation:** A state of inadequate reception or perception of environmental stimuli; the cause may be sensory deficit or inadequate variety or amount of stimuli in the environment

*Diagnoses with an asterisk are not NANDA International (NANDA-I) approved.

CONCEPTS OF SENSORY/ PERCEPTUAL FUNCTION

All human beings experience and interact with the environment through their senses. The perception of the world is sensed through taste, touch, smell, sight, hearing, and movement. Most commonly changes in sensory perception begin with the aging process, but they can occur at any stage of development.

Sensory and perceptual dysfunction can impact the independence and functioning status of a client at any age. Nurses in every practice setting should be aware of the potential for disturbed sensory perception in their clients. In the neonatal intensive care unit, there is a high potential for sensory overload related to the immature nervous system of the premature infant. This specialty unit has multiple machines and noises invading the environment of the neonate. The school nurse is concerned with identifying vision and hearing problems that will impact the child's learning and development. In the acute care hospital setting, nurses may have clients with long-term sensory deficits or a new onset of a disease process impacting the client's perception such as a stroke or delirium.

PHYSIOLOGY OF NORMAL SENSORY/ PERCEPTUAL FUNCTIONING

People depend on a continual flow of sensory stimulation from both the internal and external environments. The process of sensory stimulation has three components: sensation, perception, and response. **Sensation** is the reception of stimulation through receptors of the nervous system. **Perception** is the conscious mental recognition or registering of a sensory stimulus, as, for example, when a person smells a sweet fragrance and gets a mental image of a cherry. It is the ability to receive input from the senses, interpret the information in the cerebral cortex, and correlate it in a meaningful way. A *response* is the action a person takes after identifying the sensation, for example, when a person responds to heat by pulling a hand away from the stove.

The human body has six types of receptors that pertain to sensations and sensory structures of the body:

- **Visual:** sensation of sight
- **Auditory:** sensation of hearing
- **Gustatory:** sensation of taste
- **Tactile:** sensation of touch
- **Olfactory:** sensation of smell
- **Kinesthetic:** sensation of body position

Receptors are found in both the central and the peripheral nervous systems. Vision, hearing, smell, and taste are achieved by the central nervous system (CNS). Touch and position senses result from peripheral sensory receptors located throughout the body.

Peripheral sensation involves not only detection of the stimulus but also transmission of information to the CNS. Transmission begins when a peripheral receptor detects a stimulus and sends impulses by means of *afferent (sensory) neurons* from peripheral nerve endings to the posterior horn in the gray matter of the spinal cord. The impulse or sensation may then cause a reflex response, such as withdrawing the hand from a painful stimulus (Figure 38-1). For this to occur, the impulse must travel across *interneurons* to the anterior horn of the gray matter, and then back to the peripheral muscles on *efferent (motor) neurons.* Alternatively, the spinal nerves transmit data to the cerebral cortex, where it will be interpreted and a more complex response formulated.

The cerebral cortex must be alerted or aroused to perceive and produce a conscious act in response to stimuli. The **reticular activating system (RAS),** located in the midbrain and thalamus, keeps the brain aroused. The RAS controls the sleep-wake cycle, level of consciousness, the ability to direct attention to specific tasks, and the perception of sensory input that might alter behavior. When the RAS receives an adequate amount of sensory stimuli from the periphery, the person is aroused and alert; perception and adaptive responses occur. When the RAS receives an inadequate amount of sensory stimulation, the person may experience confusion, boredom, or drowsiness.

ALTERED SENSORY PERCEPTION

Disturbances in sensation, perception, and response may result from deficits in the sense organs, from sensory deprivation, or from sensory overload. Hearing and vision loss are the most common sensory losses.

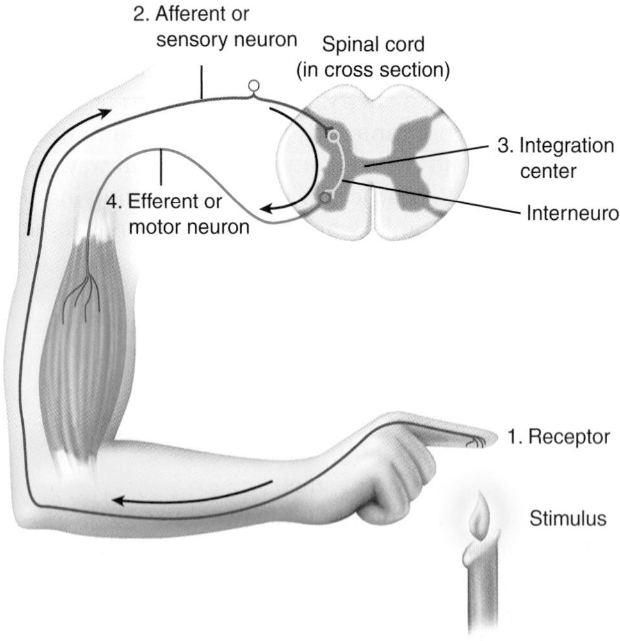

FIGURE 38-1 Reflex response. A sensory stimulus travels via afferent or sensory neurons to the spinal cord. The impulse enters the spinal cord at the posterior horn and travels across interneurons to the anterior horn. The impulse travels back to the peripheral muscle via the efferent or motor neuron.

Sensory Deficits. A *sensory deficit* is any loss in the ability to sense or perceive stimuli. It occurs in the sense organs and is not related to the amount of stimulation in the environment. A person may be born with a sensory deficit (a congenital deficit), or the deficit may be acquired suddenly or gradually. If a sensory function is lost gradually, the person may be able to compensate for the loss. If the loss occurs abruptly, however, compensation becomes much more difficult.

Visual. Because 85% of all information received from the environment is visual, vision impairment is a difficult experience at any age. However, most visual impairments can be corrected.

Uncorrectable visual impairments are relatively uncommon in childhood; however, 1 in 500 school-age children is partially sighted. Partially sighted refers to visual acuity between 20/70 and 20/200. *Strabismus* (an abnormal position of the eye alignment, commonly called crossed eyes) occurs in about 5% of children under age 4 years. If left untreated, it can result in amblyopia—visual loss in the affected eye (Estes, 2006). On a rare occasion, an infant is born blind because of maternal exposure to rubella. The most commonly occurring infant eye disease is retinoblastoma, which is a malignant cancer of the eye.

Although vision loss in adults presents as a wide range of problems, presbyopia and cataracts are among the most common. **Presbyopia** is a loss of near vision in older adults; it develops because the crystalline lens loses elasticity, and the ciliary muscles, which focus the lens by changing its shape, begin to weaken. A cataract results when the lens becomes opacified and cloudy.

In the United States, a person is considered legally blind when the best possible vision in the better eye is 20/200 or less, after correction with glasses. Blindness can also be caused by a constricted field of vision. Legally, a person is considered blind if the field of vision is 20 degrees or less in the better eye (Estes, 2006). See Box 38-1 for terms associated with vision and blindness.

Auditory. Deafness can be partial or complete, and it can be conductive, sensorineural, or mixed. A *conductive loss* results from a problem in the outer and middle ear that reduces sensitivity to tones received by air conduction. A *sensorineural loss* is a weakening of sound produced in some portion of the sensorineural mechanism. Usually, it reduces bone conduction. Mixed conductive and sensorineural hearing loss results from interference with transmission of sound in the middle ear and along neural pathways.

Even though hearing deficits are thought to occur primarily in the older adult population, children may also have hearing impairments. Hearing loss in children is usually genetic, congenital, or a result of trauma. Children with repeated ear infections, usually before age 2, may experience conduction deafness. Other causes of hearing loss in children include meningitis, mumps, and encephalitis.

As people age, they may experience a reduction in their hearing acuity. Hearing of high-pitched tones commonly becomes impaired as older adults lose hair cells in the organ of Corti. Sound transmission may be impaired by sclerosis of the ossicles in the middle ear. Sound perception can be impaired from a loss of ganglion cells in the cochlea and a loss of neurons in the auditory cortex. A common cause of hearing impairment is occupational, caused by loud noises in the workplace. These changes result in sensorineural and conductive hearing loss.

Presbycusis is a sensorineural hearing loss of high-frequency tones that occurs in older adults and may lead to a loss of all hearing frequencies. Consonants become difficult to hear, making the spoken word difficult to discern. Cerumen impaction, which obstructs sound transmission, can cause conductive hearing loss in all ages (Mahoney, 2000).

Kinesthetic. Nerve fibers that conduct information about the body's position (sitting, standing, walking, even on a moving bus) pass directly into the posterior columns of the spinal cord. The nerve response travels up to the medulla and synapses with the secondary sensory neurons. The secondary neurons cross over to the other side of the medulla before continuing on to the thalamus.

BOX 38-1 *Terms Associated With Vision*

Accommodation: Use of contraction of the ciliary muscles to change the focus to an object at a different distance
Ametropia: Abnormal vision
Astigmatism: Uneven curvature of the cornea causing the person to be unable to focus horizontal and vertical rays of light on the retina at the same time
Blurred vision: Objects appear not to have sharp, distinct borders
Color blindness: Inability to detect the difference between some colors
Diplopia: Double vision; objects appear twice in visual field
Emmetropia: The ideal optical condition of having no refractive error of vision
Halos: Appearance of circles of light or color around objects
Hemianopia: Defective vision or blindness in half of the visual field of each eye
Hyperopia, or farsightedness: Near vision is impaired because objects at a distance of 20 feet or more are focused in back of the retina (error of refraction); distance vision is normal; most children are born with hyperopia that disappears by age 8
Myopia, or nearsightedness: Near vision is normal; distance vision is impaired because objects at a distance of 20 feet or more are focused in front of the retina (error of refraction); usually appears before age 8
Partially sighted: Describes person with visual acuity between 20/70 and 20/200
Photophobia: Sensitivity to light
Presbyopia: A decrease in the elasticity of the lens with age that impairs the ability to focus on near objects
Spots: Appearance of dots of various sizes in the visual field

Loss of position sense occurs with diseases of the posterior column, such as multiple sclerosis and vitamin B_6 deficiency. Tumors and vascular malformations in the vertebral column, by compressing the spinal cord, can also keep kinesthetic information from reaching areas of perception in the cerebellum, parietal lobe, or both.

The inner ear also plays a role in maintaining a sense of position and equilibrium. Disorders of the inner ear, such as an infection or Meniere's disease, may cause edema of the labyrinth, impairing a person's sense of balance.

Gustatory. Taste sensations decline normally with age, but a loss of taste may also be associated with damage to the cranial nerves (CN), such as the facial nerve (CN VII) or the glossopharyngeal nerve (CN IX). Also, receptors in the taste buds can be damaged by chemotherapy or radiation to the head or neck. Cigarette smoking inhibits taste sensation. Because the senses of smell and taste work together to enable us to distinguish between foods, people who have permanent tracheostomies or laryngostomies have diminished taste sensations.

Tactile. Disturbances in touch can occur with certain types of damage to the spinal cord. With partial damage, touch is commonly preserved. With a complete transection of the spinal cord, all sensation is lost, and the person develops paralysis and hypoactive reflexes.

Olfactory. The sensation of smell declines with age, nerve damage, or the presence of other odors in the nasal passages. The location of the olfactory nerve, CN I, makes it vulnerable to damage from facial fractures and head injuries. Tumors or atherosclerotic changes at the base of the frontal lobe can also damage the nerve. If one of the two olfactory nerves is intact, the person will still be able to smell. If both olfactory nerves are affected, the sense of smell is permanently lost. This condition is called *anosmia.* Nonneurological factors, such as nasal congestion, sinus infection, zinc deficiency, smoking, or cocaine use, may also result in anosmia.

Sensory Deprivation. **Sensory deprivation** is inadequate reception or perception of environmental stimuli. The cause may be physiological, such as a sensory deficit, or it may stem from an inadequate variety or amount of stimuli in the environment. The situation in which there are too few stimuli results in sensory deprivation and a decreased response to the environment, which could lead to social isolation. Sensory deprivation can occur in the acutely ill when the nurse predominately works with tubes and has minimal direct touch or contact with the client.

An example of inadequate variety in environmental stimuli is a radio tuned to play "elevator music" in a client's otherwise silent room. The same room without any radio at all is an example of an inadequate amount of environmental stimuli.

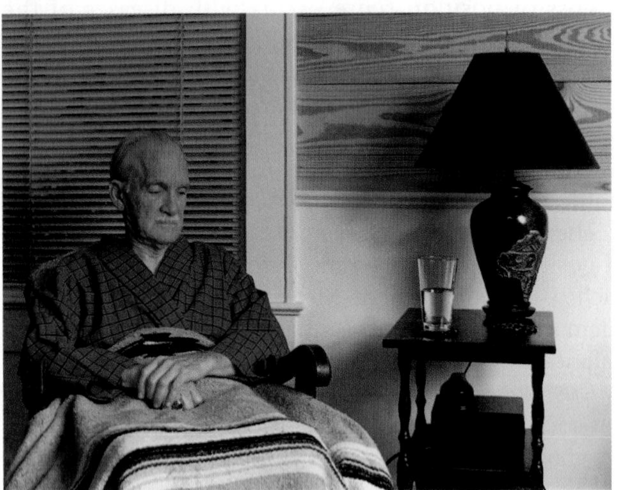

FIGURE 38-2 An older adult who lives alone and has little opportunity to socialize may experience sensory deprivation.

Data on sensory deprivation are derived from experiments involving total sensory deprivation. However, symptoms can be seen in persons who experience little variety in sensory stimulation, such as older adults who live alone and rarely socialize (Figure 38-2). As the sensory deprivation becomes more extreme and prolonged, the symptoms appear more severe. Persons deprived of sensory stimulation may experience central nervous system changes, such as impaired judgment, an inability to solve problems, confusion, disorientation, and even hallucinations and delusions.

Sensory Overload. A problem of increasing proportions in modern society, **sensory overload** results from excessive environmental stimuli, or a level of stimuli beyond the person's ability to absorb or comprehend. The hospital environment, for example, is filled with sights, sounds, smells, and tactile stimuli. These multiple stimuli place clients at risk for sensory overload.

An individual may be admitted to a hospital room located near a busy nurses' station and may have a talkative roommate who is listening to a loud television show. Exposure to such excessive stimuli can result in symptoms of sensory overload, such as anxiety, confusion, disorientation, and an inability to make decisions. Sensory overload can interfere with the person's ability to focus on the important aspects of a situation, such as learning a new skill to regain or maintain health.

FACTORS AFFECTING SENSORY PERCEPTION

People need an adequate amount of sensory stimulation for normal growth and development. There is considerable variation in the amount of stimulation individuals consider optimal. The amount and variety of stimuli are influenced by life span, physiological, cultural and lifestyle, and environmental, socioeconomic, and psychological factors.

FACTORS ACROSS THE LIFE SPAN

The nature and meaning of sensory stimulation changes with age. In the developing infant, sensory stimulation is needed for normal growth and development. As a person ages, there is an alteration in the perception of sensations and in the sensory organs themselves.

Infants and Children. The newborn has immature nerve pathways and cannot discriminate among sensory stimuli. Adequate stimulation is necessary for neural pathways to develop, become refined, and function adequately. Appropriate stimulation includes the following:

- Tactile and kinesthetic sensation, such as holding, rocking, and changing positions
- Auditory sensation, such as singing and talking
- Visual sensation, as from mobiles, color, and bright objects

Adolescents and Middle Adults. Adolescents are at risk for hearing loss if they are exposed to chronic loud noise. Typically, in this age-group, listening to excessively loud music is a popular pastime and may lead to hearing loss.

Sensory changes related to the aging process begin in the middle adult years. Around age 40, adults begin to hold reading material farther from their eyes. When the distance exceeds the length of the arm, the person may decide to have an eye examination and obtain reading glasses. Hearing changes, which also begin in the middle years, include decreased hearing acuity, speech intelligibility, pitch discrimination, and hearing threshold. There is also reduced taste discrimination and sensitivity to odors.

Older Adults. The decline in sensory function that begins in the middle adult years becomes more apparent in the older adult years. However, loss of one sensory function may increase the client's reliance on another. For example, loss of vision may lead the client to rely on the sense of hearing to compensate for the loss. Visual changes include reduced visual fields, increased glare sensitivity, impaired night vision, reduced accommodation, and reduced color discrimination.

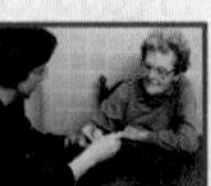

Because Mrs. Pfannenstiel feels that she is trying to see through a dirty, greasy window, she has lost her prior enjoyment of reading and watching television. She also has started to withdraw socially. What nursing concerns would you have regarding Mrs. Pfannenstiel's care? What interventions should be implemented? What are the anticipated outcomes?

The hearing changes experienced by the older adult can vary rather widely. There may be difficulty in discriminating consonants (for example: *f, s, sh,* and *ch* sounds). Speech sounds may be garbled. Reception and reaction to speech may be delayed. Low-pitched sounds may be heard best. The person may have trouble hearing conversations over any background noise.

In addition to visual and hearing changes, the older adult can also experience a loss of balance, spatial orientation, and coordination. Tactile changes develop as well, including reduced sensitivity to pain, pressure, and temperature. These changes place the older client at risk for injury.

PHYSIOLOGICAL FACTORS

A range of physiological factors can affect sensory/perceptual functioning, such as trauma, physical illness, medications, the aging process, and medical procedures.

Trauma. Traumatic injuries may result in a complete loss of sensation, a decrease in sensation (called hypoesthesia), or an increase in sensation (called hyperesthesia). Any of the six senses can be affected by traumatic injury.

Eye trauma is a health concern of all ages. Penetrating eye injuries from firecrackers, slingshots, rocks, fishhooks, sticks, scissors, toy weapons, and other objects are a common cause of blindness in children. Adults are at risk for eye trauma when playing sports or working in an environment that contains chemicals or flying objects. In high-risk work areas, employees are required by the Occupational Safety and Health Administration (OSHA) to use protective eyewear.

Physical Illness. Preexisting illnesses can cause a variety of changes in sensory function. Disorders such as diabetes mellitus, renal failure, and vascular disease can lead to peripheral neuropathy, a disturbance or pathological change in the peripheral nervous system. Other disorders include deficiencies of the vitamins: thiamine, pyridoxine, and folic acid and disorders caused by environmental exposure to heavy metals and industrial solvents. These problems can cause an alteration in pain, touch, smell, temperature, and motor function.

Alteration in visual acuity may result from changes in ocular structure, such as cataracts, glaucoma, macular degeneration, myopia, and hyperopia. Damage to the optic nerve from multiple sclerosis or a cerebrovascular accident also affects visual acuity.

Cataracts are opacities of the lens that cause gradual, painless blurring of the vision. As the cataract progresses, the milky white lens may become visible in the client's eye. Night blindness is one of the most distressing symptoms of cataracts because it interferes with night driving and with seeing in darkened rooms.

Clients with diabetes mellitus also have sensory disturbances secondary to microvascular changes in the retina of the eye. Referred to as *diabetic retinopathy,* this is more likely to occur if the diabetes is poorly controlled and of long duration. Retinal edema and hemorrhage lead to gradual blurring, which can progress to blindness. It is the leading cause of vision loss in adults under age 40.

Macular degeneration is the leading cause of blindness in older adults. It is caused by the deterioration of the macula, which is the area of the retina responsible for fine, detailed vision. There is a painless, gradual loss of central vision. The exact cause of macular degeneration is unknown. Several studies suggest that genetics, smoking and other risk factors associated with atherosclerosis may contribute to the development of this condition. As yet, no treatment has been found to be effective. Recent research points to the use of antioxidants and the mineral zinc to slow the advancement of macular degeneration and possible blindness. Therefore clients are advised to seek early treatment to slow the process (National Eye Institute, 2001; O'Reilly, 2001).

Glaucoma is a disease of the optic nerve resulting from increased pressure inside the eye. Blind spots develop that go undetected until significant damage to the optic nerve occurs. There is a loss of peripheral vision with glaucoma. Left untreated, blindness may result. Once diagnosed, glaucoma may be controlled by lifelong eye medication.

A stroke may cause a loss of sensory function and motor function, depending on the location of the underlying vascular lesion. The person may have a loss of proprioception (coordination and balance). Visual changes may occur as well. *Hemianopia* (loss of one half of the visual field in each eye) results from damage to the optic tract or the occipital lobe.

Sensory disturbances with multiple sclerosis include paresthesias and a diminished sensitivity to pain. Numbness, tingling, burning, loss of coordination, or crawling sensations may also develop. The sensory deficits caused by a spinal cord tumor depend on its location and rate of growth. Clients may present with a slowly progressive numbness, tingling, pain, or temperature loss. They may also have a decreased sense of touch, an inability to sense vibration, and loss of position sense.

Medications. Medications can affect a person's neurosensory system. Sedatives and opioids (narcotics) can alter perception of sensory stimuli. Phenytoin, hydralazine, isoniazid, and amitriptyline can cause peripheral neuropathy, ataxia, and other sensory changes. Captopril, ampicillin, tetracycline, griseofulvin, and carbamazepine can alter taste sensation. Chemotherapy and radiation therapy can affect taste sensation as well. Some medications can be **ototoxic,** having a damaging effect on the auditory nerve (CN VIII) or the organs of hearing and balance. Aminoglycoside antibiotics and furosemide are ototoxic. Aspirin can cause ringing in the ears.

LIFESTYLE FACTORS

Lifestyle choices, such as smoking and the use of recreational drugs, can alter a person's sensation. The senses of taste and smell are diminished by smoking. Overuse of over-the-counter (OTC) nasal preparations, as well as intranasal drug abuse with cocaine or amphetamines, can also alter the sense of smell. A lifestyle characterized by stress can impair a person's tolerance for sensory stimuli and the ability to correctly perceive those stimuli.

ENVIRONMENTAL FACTORS

Environmental factors can affect a person's sensory/perceptual status. Chronic exposure to high levels of noise can affect a person's hearing. People who work around noisy equipment, such as farmers or factory workers, are at risk for hearing loss. Inhalation of irritants, such as chlorine fumes, can decrease the sense of smell. People who live in large cities get used to more noise and may become unaware of the high noise level.

SOCIOECONOMIC FACTORS

Socioeconomic factors can affect a person's ability to manage sensory/perceptual problems. If a person does not have sufficient financial resources, the cost of health care may be prohibitive. A person with decreased vision may not be able to afford an eye examination or eyeglasses. The cost for hearing aids can also be prohibitive.

PSYCHOLOGICAL FACTORS

In addition to physical causes, psychological problems—such as stress—can cause disturbances in sensation and perception. The stress of an illness, hospitalization, or surgery can provide greater stimulation than the person can process without assistance. Pain and fatigue can alter mental status as well, changing the way the person perceives and reacts to stimuli.

A person's mental status affects sensory perception. An agitated client may misinterpret a nurse's touch as aggressive rather than comforting and may respond with aggression. A depressed person has a shaded view of the world and responds to sensory/perceptual stimuli on the basis of this perspective.

Culture also influences response to sensory disturbances. Culturally competent nursing care requires an understanding of these varying responses (Box 38-2).

ASSESSMENT

To detect and define problems in a client's sensory/perceptual status, start by performing a general assessment. On the basis of your general findings, you may then perform a focused assessment of any area of deficit.

GENERAL ASSESSMENT OF SENSORY/ PERCEPTUAL STATUS

When assessing a client for disturbances in sensory perception, obtain a complete health history, and examine the client to determine actual or potential sensory deficits and evidence of sensory deprivation or overload. Make sure to include the client's environment in your assessment.

Health History. Naturally, the chief complaint of a client with disturbed sensory perception will vary depending on the cause of the sensory deficit present. For example, a client with a hearing problem may complain of ringing in the ears. The health history is focused on the sensory system that has the alteration. Use questions such as those that follow to collect data for the health history.

Vision

- Describe the trouble you are having with your vision. Does it affect both eyes? When did it begin? Did it begin suddenly or gradually?
- What have you done to try to correct the problem?
- Do you have yearly eye examinations? When was the last time you had an eye exam?
- Do you use eye medications? What kind? How often? For what reason do you take eye medications? Do you use an over-the-counter eye preparation?
- Do you wear glasses? How often do you clean them?
- Do you wear contact lenses? Are they hard, soft, or extended wear? How do you clean them?
- Do you have difficulty seeing at night?
- Do you see spots (floaters) in front of your eyes?
- Do you see rainbows or colored rings around lights or bright objects?
- Have you ever had an eye injury?

Hearing

- How long have you had the feeling that you do not hear well? Did the change in hearing begin suddenly or gradually?
- What types of sounds do you have trouble hearing?
- Do you have a family history of hearing loss?

BOX 38-2 *Cross-Cultural Care*

Caring for a Volga German American Client

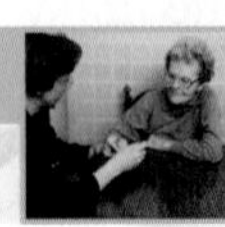

Mrs. Pfannenstiel, the client in the case study in this chapter, is of Volga German descent. Most of these people immigrated to the United States and began farming homesteads. They worked hard to establish a better life for their families. Her family came to Kansas in 1870. Her daughter accompanies her to the eye doctor and is with her at the time of surgery. The Volga German Americans tend to have the following values:

- Very strong work ethic
- Stoic and do not like to ask for assistance
- Skeptical of some health care practices and prefer folk treatments
- Close family ties
- Strong religious values
- Practice primarily the Catholic religion

- Where do you work? In your work or home environment, is there a lot of noise? If so, do you wear protective hearing devices or earplugs? How long have you worked in this area? Has your hearing loss become a problem since working there?
- Does your hearing loss bother you? Does it keep you at home?
- Do you wear a hearing aid? How long have you worn it? Does it help?
- Do you hear noise in your ears? What does it sound like? Ringing, crackling, buzzing? When did it start?
- Has the hearing loss impaired your balance or appetite?
- Are you taking any medications? Does the ringing in the ears have any relationship to the start of the medications?

Gustatory

- Do you add extra salt to your food?
- Does food seem tasteless?
- Do you have increasing difficulty determining that foods are spoiled?

Sensation

- Do you have numbness or tingling? Where is it located? Is it associated with activities? Describe how it feels.

Physical Examination. Physical examination of sensory/perceptual function includes screening for vision, hearing, position sense, taste, touch, and smell.

Visual. Acuity charts are used to check near and distance vision. A distance vision chart is mounted on a wall, and the client reads it from 20 feet away. The Snellen alphabet chart is used most commonly and is appropriate for adults and older children. It contains 11 lines of various letters in graduated sizes. Each eye should be tested separately, and then both together. If the client wears corrective lenses, they should be worn during the test. Figure 38-3 shows a nurse screening for vision using a Snellen chart.

For children under age 4, pictures of common objects are used rather than an alphabet chart. For children ages 4 to 5 and for clients who do not read or speak English, the Snellen E chart is used. It consists of eight Es of graduated size facing in various directions. The examiner can use hand gestures or ask a family member who speaks English to help explain the examination to a client who does not speak English. The client indicates the position of the E by duplicating the position with the fingers.

Near vision can be tested by asking a client to read from a newspaper, Snellen chart, or card held about 14 inches from the client's eyes. As with distance testing, each eye should be tested separately, and then both together.

Color blindness is most commonly tested by asking the client to identify patterns of colored dots on colored plates. A color-blind client will miss the patterns. Early detection allows the child to compensate for the deficit and also alerts teachers to the student's special need.

Auditory. Assessment of hearing loss in infants and children requires attentiveness to subtle signs. The first sign that alerts a parent to a possible hearing loss in an infant may be a failure to respond to loud noises. The infant may not awaken or startle at the sound of a sudden loud noise, for example. Another sign of possible hearing loss is a delay in speech development. The child may respond more to movement than to sound, be afraid of strangers, or avoid interacting with other children.

Older adults should be observed for subtle cues to hearing loss. When the onset is gradual, the person may compensate for the loss and either not be aware of it or be embarrassed to admit to the hearing deficit. One of the early signs is talking louder than usual, asking people to repeat what was said, or turning up the volume on the television or radio. Another sign is turning the "good ear" toward the sounds.

Careful observation sometimes reveals that the person smiles and nods but does not understand what is said, has a blank look, or does not give full attention to the person talking. Learning to lip-read may help the person compensate partially for the hearing loss. The person may have trouble following directions or ask for the directions to be repeated. Again, keep in mind that hearing loss can impair relationships and cause the person to withdraw from social activities or get angry at others, thinking they are talking too softly.

There are three screening tests for hearing acuity: the whisper test, the finger-rubbing test, and the tuning fork test (which includes the Rinne and Weber tests). For the whisper test, instruct the client to cover one ear with a hand. Then stand 1 to 2 feet away from the other ear, in front of or to the side of the client. Shield your mouth while whispering monosyllabic (hat, ball, bat) or disyllabic (baseball, overcoat, highchair) words. A client with normal hearing should be able to repeat at least half of

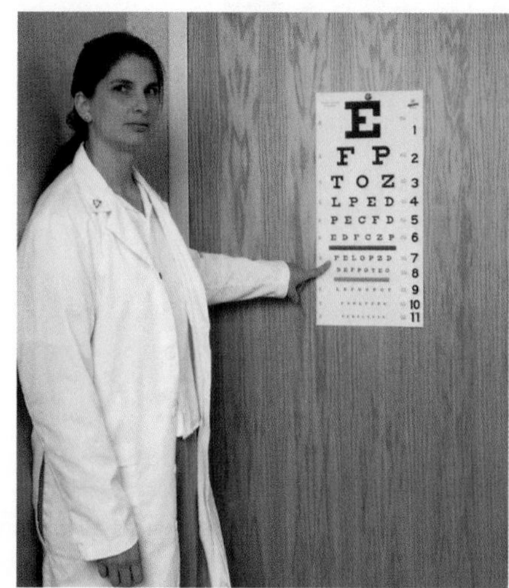

FIGURE 38-3 Vision screening using a Snellen chart.

all the words whispered. After testing one ear, have the client cover it and test the other ear.

High-frequency sounds are evaluated by the finger-rubbing test. Hold your hands 3 to 4 inches from the client's ear and briskly rub your index finger against your thumb. The client should be able to hear the noise produced by rubbing your fingers together. Test the other ear.

The Weber and Rinne tests are auditory screening tests used to evaluate the client for conduction or sensorineural hearing loss. These tests are done with a tuning fork with frequencies of 500 to 1000 cycles per second.

Weber test. The Weber test evaluates transmission of sound through the bones of the skull to the cochlea and acoustic nerve. This transmission is called bone conduction. Perform the test by placing a vibrating tuning fork at the midline of the top of the client's head or in the middle of the forehead (Figure 38-4).

The client should hear the resulting sound equally in both ears. If there is a conductive hearing loss, the client will hear the sound more prominently in the ear with the conductive loss (i.e., the sound will lateralize to that ear). This is because the sound conducts directly through the bone to the ear. If the client has a sensorineural hearing loss in one ear, the sound will lateralize to the unimpaired ear because nerve damage in the impaired ear prevents hearing.

Rinne test. The Rinne test compares bone conduction to air conduction in both ears. Assess bone conduction by placing the base of a vibrating tuning fork on the client's mastoid process and noting how many seconds pass before it can no longer be heard (Figure 38-5). Then, test air conduction by placing the tines of a vibrating tuning fork parallel to the client's auricle, near the ear canal. Hold the tuning fork in this position until the client can no longer hear the tone. Note how many seconds the client can hear it. Repeat with the other ear.

Sound traveling through air normally remains audible twice as long as sound traveling through bone (a 2:1 ratio). Thus sound heard for 10 seconds by bone conduction should be heard for 20 seconds by air conduction. With a conduction hearing loss, the client will report hearing sound longer through bone. If the client reports hearing the sound longer through air, but the ratio is not the normal 2:1, the client may have a sensorineural hearing loss.

Refer to Chapter 8 under Hearing Acuity (under Assessment of the Head and Neck) for the complete procedures for the Weber and Rinne tests.

Gustatory. To test gustatory sense, instruct the client to stick out the tongue. Using a cotton applicator, place sugar, salt, and lemon on the client's tongue, one at a time. The client should be able to correctly identify each taste.

Kinesthetic. To test kinesthetic sensation, the client's eyes must be closed. Grasp the client's finger or toe, and move its position 0.4 inch, or 1 cm, up or down. The client should be able to describe how the position has changed (Figure 38-6, *A*).

Sensory Function. Use light touch, tests of sharp and dull, and vibration sense to assess sensory function. Test

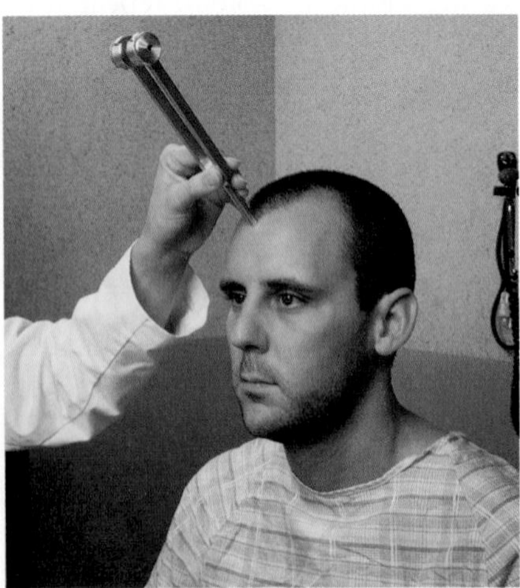

FIGURE 38-4 The Weber test. The nurse places a vibrating tuning fork in the middle of the client's forehead.

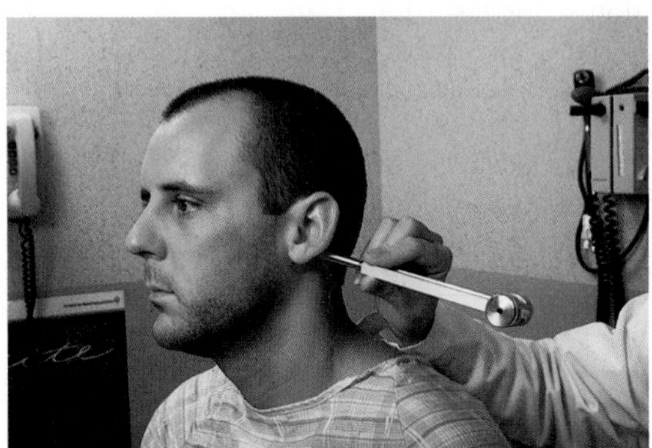

A

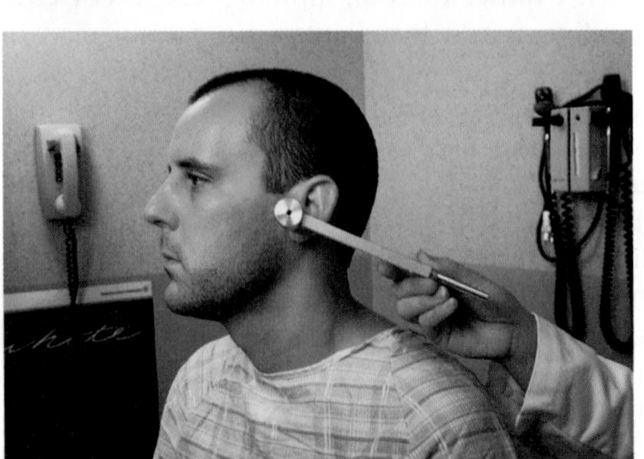

B

FIGURE 38-5 The Rinne test. **A,** The nurse places a vibrating tuning fork on the client's mastoid bone to assess bone conduction. **B,** The nurse then places the vibrating tuning fork parallel to the client's ear to assess air conduction.

the peripheral extremities in several areas. If the sense is intact, no further evaluation is necessary. If it is impaired, move up the extremities until you reach a level or area where sensation exists.

Evaluate light touch by using a cotton wisp. Again, the client's eyes must be closed, and then lightly touch the client with the wisp (Figure 38-6, *B*). The client should be able to correctly identify the spot touched. Test sharp and dull sensations using the sharp tip and the rounded end of a paper clip (Figure 38-6, *C*). Instruct the client to keep eyes closed, and alternately touch the client with the sharp tip and the dull end. The client should be able to identify both the sensation and the location.

Test vibration sense by placing a vibrating tuning fork on a bony area, such as the wrist or ankle (Figure 38-6, *D*). Ask the client to describe the sensation. The client should be able to feel the vibration. Ask the client to tell you when the vibrations are no longer felt, then stop the vibration while the tuning fork is still touching the bony prominence.

Olfactory. Ask the client to identify common aromatic substances, such as coffee, orange, cloves, or tobacco, which are held under the nose while the eyes are closed. Test one nostril at a time. The client should be able to correctly identify the smell.

Diagnostic Tests. The health care provider will order specific diagnostic tests to confirm a sensory/perceptual disorder on the basis of the potential health problem. For example, if a client's chief complaint is decreased hearing, the physician will order audiometry. Either the results of the diagnostic tests will be negative, or they will be positive, indicating a problem.

- *Slit-lamp examination* is a microscopic examination of the anterior ocular structures. A slit lamp allows diagnosis of abnormalities in the cornea, lens, or anterior vitreous.
- *Corneal staining* is indicated for diagnosis of corneal trauma, foreign bodies, corneal abrasions, or corneal ulcers. Fluorescein or another type of topical dye is instilled into the conjunctival sac to stain the cornea. Irregularities of the corneal surface are outlined with the dye.
- *Tonometry* is the measurement of intraocular pressure. A normal range is 10 to 21 mm Hg. Elevated intraocular pressure (>21 mm Hg) reveals glaucoma. Tonometer readings are indicated for all clients over age 40, especially if they have a family history of glaucoma.
- *Audiometry* is the measurement of hearing acuity. There are two types of audiometry: pure tone audiometry and speech audiometry. Pure tone audiometry is performed to determine the threshold of hearing at selected frequencies (the highness or lowness of tones). Speech audiometry determines how well the person understands speech and discriminates between speech sounds.
- *Computed tomography* is a radiographic diagnostic test in which a cross-sectional image is formed by the use of computers. It is helpful in diagnosing tumors, infarctions, and hemorrhage.

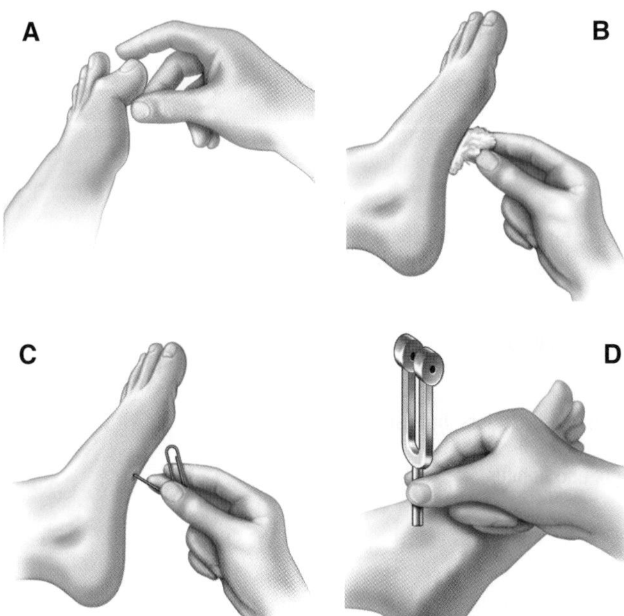

FIGURE 38-6 Peripheral sensory nerve testing. **A,** Position sense. **B,** Light touch. **C,** Pain sensation. **D,** Vibration sense.

FOCUSED ASSESSMENT FOR *DISTURBED SENSORY PERCEPTION: VISUAL*

Defining Characteristics. The critical defining characteristic is impaired visual acuity. The change in visual acuity may lead to visual distortions; disorientation to person, place, and time; and disturbances in the client's response to visual stimuli. In addition, impaired visual acuity may alter the person's ability to conceptualize and to solve problems. The person may respond to the alteration with anger, apathy, anxiety, depression, or restlessness.

Related Factors. Visual loss primarily results from altered sensory perception secondary to damage to the optic nerve, such as occurs with glaucoma, macular degeneration, or diabetic retinopathy. It may also result from damage to ocular structure such as occurs in cataracts.

FOCUSED ASSESSMENT FOR *DISTURBED SENSORY PERCEPTION: AUDITORY*

Defining Characteristics. When people are unable to hear, their ability to communicate is impaired. One of the earliest assessment findings is a decrease in social interaction. This decrease may lead to increasing withdrawal from activities and, eventually, social isolation. The client may respond to changes in hearing with anger, apathy, or depression.

Related Factors. Hearing impairment results from altered sensory reception, transmission, and/or integration. Although hearing impairment is common among older adults, the nurse should be alert to acute causes of hearing loss. Determine whether the client may be taking large doses of aminoglycosides to treat an infection or other medications that may affect the ability to hear (Table 38-1).

Hearing impairment in older adults may be related to cerumen impaction. Risk factors for cerumen impaction include numerous hairs in the ear canal, a hearing aid, bony growths secondary to osteophyte or osteoma, and a history of repeated cerumen impaction.

FOCUSED ASSESSMENT FOR *DISTURBED SENSORY PERCEPTION: KINESTHETIC*

Defining Characteristics. The nurse may first suspect kinesthetic disturbances by observing diminished motor coordination. Closer examination may reveal an inability to identify the position or location of body parts, an inability to perceive changes in angles of joints, muscles weakness, flaccidity, rigidity, atrophy, or paralysis.

Related Factors. Alteration in position sense is primarily related to neurological conditions, such as cerebral palsy, multiple sclerosis, muscular dystrophy, spinal trauma, and spinal tumors. Surgical joint replacement and diseases of the inner ear, such as Meniere's disease, can also alter the position sense.

FOCUSED ASSESSMENT FOR *DISTURBED SENSORY PERCEPTION: GUSTATORY*

Defining Characteristics. A person with altered taste may present with one of the following: a complete loss of taste *(ageusia)*, a distorted sense of taste *(dysgeusia)*, or a partial loss of taste *(hypogeusia)*. Notice the client's interest in food. Usually, a client with a loss of taste will add extra salt or other seasonings, report that the food tastes bland, or both. The decrease in taste may result in a loss of appetite or weight.

Related Factors. Changes in taste may be related to neurological, oncological, nutritional, or viral causes. The specific etiology may be unimportant in deciding how to help the person manage the problem of diminished taste. The result of altered taste can be inadequate nutrition, lack of enjoyment of food, or, in the worst case, ingestion of noxious substances or spoiled food.

FOCUSED ASSESSMENT FOR *DISTURBED SENSORY PERCEPTION: TACTILE*

Defining Characteristics. An altered sense of touch may present as abnormal sensation *(paresthesia)*, decreased sensitivity to stimulation *(hypoesthesia)* or pain *(hypoal-*

Table 38-1 Ototoxic Drugs and Their Effects

DRUG	EFFECTS
ANTIBIOTICS	
Aminoglycosides, such as amikacin, gentamicin, kanamycin, neomycin, and vancomycin	• Can affect both the vestibular (balance) and auditory portion of cranial nerve VIII. • Most drug-induced ototoxicity is associated with aminoglycoside use.
Erythromycin	• Reversible hearing loss with high doses.
Minocycline	• Reversible vestibular toxicity. • Affects women more than men.
DIURETICS	
Ethacrynic acid (Edecrin) Furosemide (Lasix)	• High parenteral dose may cause transient or permanent hearing loss. • Administration of other ototoxic drugs may potentiate hearing loss.
CARDIAC DRUGS	
Quinidine	• Tinnitus, transient hearing loss, and vertigo.
ANALGESICS	
Aspirin	• High doses can cause irreversible hearing loss, but usually transient • May also cause tinnitus and vertigo.
Nonsteroidal antiinflammatory drugs, such as indomethacin (Indocin) and ibuprofen (Motrin)	• Transient hearing loss, vertigo, and tinnitus.
ANTINEOPLASTIC AGENTS	
Bleomycin, cisplatin, dactinomycin, and mechlorethamine	• May be reversible or irreversible. • Usually cause ototoxicity when given in high doses, to people with renal impairment, or to people receiving other ototoxic drugs.

gesia), or an impaired sense of touch *(dysesthesia)*. Abnormal sensation is usually described by the client as numbness, prickling, or tingling.

Related Factors. An alteration in the sense of touch may be related to peripheral vascular disease, such as an acute arterial occlusion, arteriosclerosis obliterans, Buerger's disease, or Raynaud's disease. Clients with a metabolic disorder, such as diabetes mellitus or a vitamin B deficiency, can experience a decreased sensation related to peripheral neuropathy. Paralyzing neurological or neuromuscular diseases, such as a stroke or Guillain-Barré syndrome, will alter the person's ability to perceive touch. The result can be burns, skin breakdown, or injury.

FOCUSED ASSESSMENT FOR *DISTURBED SENSORY PERCEPTION: OLFACTORY*

Defining Characteristics. Changes in olfaction include diminished smell *(hyposmia)* and absence of smell *(anosmia)*. Smell is important to alert the client to danger and to stimulate appetite. Diminished smell may go unnoticed unless the person realizes that smoke or a gas leak was undetected. Sometimes diminished smell is detected as a result of weight loss.

Related Factors. A diminished sense of smell may be related to nasal problems, such as a nasal neoplasm, polyps, sinusitis, rhinitis, or septal fracture. Neurological disorders that cause damage to the vagus nerve (CN X), such as anterior cerebral artery occlusion, brain stem lesion, head trauma, or olfactory meningioma, can alter a person's sense of smell. Altered smell may adversely affect appetite.

FOCUSED ASSESSMENT FOR *SENSORY DEPRIVATION*

Because the aim of assessment for sensory deprivation is to prevent it, assessing the client's level of environmental stimulation is as important as assessing for signs and symptoms of sensory deprivation. Assess the amount of stimulation and its meaningfulness to the client. Determine whether the client can perceive and correctly interpret the environment.

In a situation of sensory deprivation, the usual response is to withdraw and pass the time by sleeping. Symptoms of mild depression are among the early manifestations. As time passes, the client loses track of time and decreases attention to the environment. Thoughts become less organized, and events lose significance. If sensory deprivation is severe and prolonged, symptoms appear that suggest loss of contact with reality. Hallucinations may be present, although they are usually brief and fleeting. Internal and external sensations may become confused; the client is not sure whether something happened or was just a thought. Feelings of disorientation in space and time can become overwhelming.

FOCUSED ASSESSMENT FOR *SENSORY OVERLOAD*

People who are ill, especially those who are seriously ill, are at risk for sensory overload. Factors that contribute to sensory overload include an unfamiliar routine, an environment with excessive noise or light, a disturbed sleep-rest pattern, and pain.

Clients experiencing sensory overload may be disorientated to time, place, and person. They may have an altered ability to think abstractly and to conceptualize and solve problems. They may also have mood swings and exaggerated emotional responses, visual and auditory distortions, or hallucinations.

Sensory overload may occur in a variety of people. The client hospitalized in an intensive care unit after major trauma or surgery is at risk for sensory overload. The intensive care unit has many potential sources of sensory overload, such as equipment noise and alarms. The client experiencing alcohol withdrawal syndrome is also at risk for sensory overload.

DIAGNOSIS

The diagnosis of *Disturbed sensory perception* encompasses all of the sensory deficits. Figure 38-7 illustrates the decision-making process for *Disturbed sensory perception.* It is important to specify the actual cause of the sensory/perceptual disturbance. When writing the diagnostic statement, be sure to specify the sensory disturbance. For example, write "*Disturbed sensory perception: visual* related to lens opacity secondary to cataracts."

A change in the amount of incoming stimuli may result in sensory deprivation or sensory overload. Obtain a history and physical assessment to determine which one a person may be experiencing. If there is a risk rather than an actual experience of a sensory disturbance, write the diagnostic statement like this: "*Risk for Disturbed sensory perception: auditory* related to excessive environmental stimuli, i.e., noise from alarms and equipment in the intensive care unit." A person with a sensory deficit is receiving insufficient environmental stimuli. This places the person at risk for sensory deprivation.

Other diagnoses frequently used with clients who have sensory perceptual disturbances are listed next. Table 38-2 illustrates how to cluster data and provides further assistance in distinguishing among these related nursing diagnoses.

Risk for Injury. Clients with sensory deficits are at *Risk for injury.* People with visual problems may lack compensatory skills to avoid danger in their path, which may cause them to stumble and fall. Older adults with partial visual losses may be at risk for injury in using the stove for cooking, taking medications, walking down the stairs, or driving a car. The hearing-impaired client may be unable to hear noises that would indicate danger, such as fire alarms,

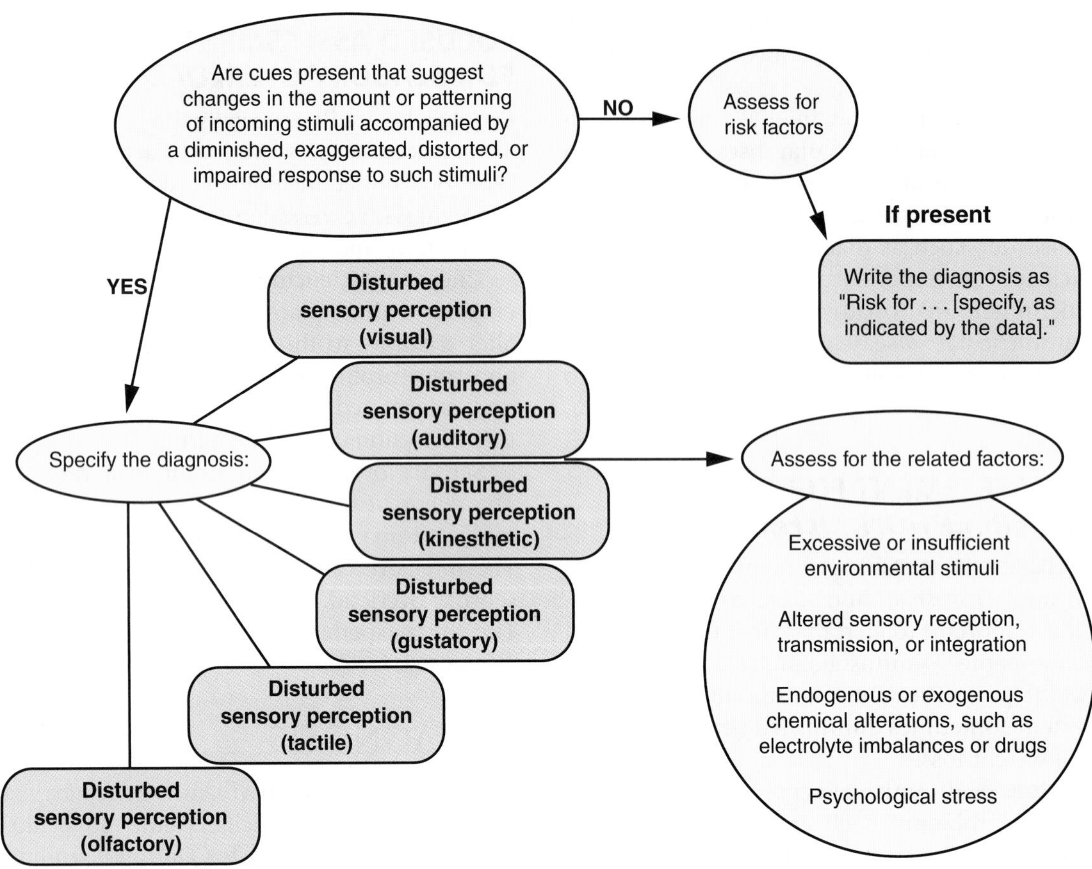

FIGURE 38-7 Decision tree for sensory/perceptual alterations. Diagnoses are shown in rectangles. Within these rectangles, diagnoses shown in **bold** type are NANDA-I–approved nursing diagnoses; diagnoses shown in regular type are not NANDA-I–approved nursing diagnoses.

Table 38-2 Clustering Data to Make a Nursing Diagnosis

Sensory/Perceptual Alterations

DATA CLUSTER	DIAGNOSIS
A 76-year-old man has had progressive hearing loss over the last 6 months, has refused to participate in activities at the extended-care facility, and has often been found sitting alone in his apartment.	*Social isolation* related to inability to communicate secondary to loss of hearing
An 84-year-old woman has a fractured left femur and multiple rib fractures from a motor vehicle accident. At 48 hours after admission, she becomes confused and begins to pull out her indwelling urinary catheter and her intravenous line.	*Disturbed thought processes* related to a change in the environment and an increase in the amount of incoming stimuli
In the first 24 hours after cataract surgery, the client has her left eye patched. She also has a cataract in her right eye.	*Disturbed sensory perception: visual* related to left eye patch and cloudiness of the right lens
A 54-year-old woman receiving chemotherapy and radiation therapy for breast cancer states that food does not taste good any more. She has lost 12 pounds in the last 3 weeks.	*Imbalanced nutrition: less than body requirements* related to loss of taste sensation secondary to the effects of chemotherapy
A 25-year-old man with a spinal cord injury has no movement or sensation below the level of the umbilicus.	*Disturbed sensory perception: tactile* related to severance of nerves in the spinal cord
A 22-month-old child has a history of repeated ear infections. The mother has noted that the child does not look toward noise and has not started to vocalize.	*Disturbed sensory perception: auditory* related to loss of hearing secondary to repeated ear infections

sirens, horns, or oncoming vehicles. Instructions for taking medications may be misunderstood. Being unable to smell odors, such as smoke or leaking gas, may place a person in danger. A person with an alteration in touch may be unable to feel extremes of temperature, pressure, or pain. Impaired position sense places a client at risk for falls. Finally, the person with sensory overload may be so overwhelmed with stimuli that important cues to safety are ignored or missed.

Imbalanced Nutrition: Less Than Body Requirements. Appetite may be diminished as a result of loss of smell and taste. Maintaining an optimal intake of a variety of nutrients may become difficult. If the person has heart disease, hypertension, peptic ulcers, or other health problems that require a special diet, the prescribed diet may alter appetite even more.

Impaired Verbal Communication. The process of communication involves speaking and listening. People with an auditory deficit are at risk for *Impaired verbal communication* because one of the components for communication is missing (see Chapter 39).

Social Isolation. The person with a hearing deficit is at risk for *Social isolation* because interacting with people is difficult when conversations cannot be followed. Clients with vision loss are also at risk for *Social isolation.* They may stay at home, where the environment is familiar. They may be reluctant to leave the house for fear of falling or being unable to find their way.

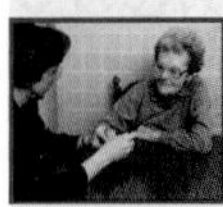

Mrs. Pfannenstiel has been reluctant to leave her daughter's home for fear of falling and breaking a bone. How might Mrs. Pfannenstiel and her daughter increase her social interactions?

Self-Care Deficit. A person who has a visual deficit may find it challenging to perform usual self-care tasks, such as bathing, feeding, dressing, and toileting. The need for protective living may become necessary when hearing or vision loss makes a person unsafe or unable to manage self-care.

Disturbed Thought Processes. An alteration in the characteristics of incoming stimuli, resulting in either too much or too little stimulation, can affect a person's thought processes. The person may have a change in cognitive abilities. Visual or auditory distortions/hallucinations may occur, leading to disorientation to person, place, or time (see Chapter 40). This person may need to be in a protective environment for safety reasons.

PLANNING

EXPECTED OUTCOMES FOR *DISTURBED SENSORY PERCEPTION*

Preventing injury is a high priority for a client experiencing *Disturbed sensory perception.* The expected outcome is that the client does not experience injury. However, because sensory deficits may take many different forms, specific outcomes are necessary. They include the following:

Visual
- Client identifies measures to alter the home environment to prevent injury.
- Client agrees to use adaptive devices.
- Client makes an appointment to have vision evaluated.

Auditory
- Client identifies and uses alternative measures that alert danger.
- Client agrees to use adaptive devices, such as hearing aids.
- Client uses signing, gestures, lipreading, or assistive devices to maintain communication.
- Client uses community resources to help cope with the auditory deficit.
- Client maintains social contacts.
- Client makes an appointment for hearing evaluation.

Kinesthetic
- Client implements safety precautions.
- Skin breakdown is avoided, especially in areas around vulnerable joints.

Tactile
- Client does not experience falls or injury.
- Client does not experience skin breakdown.
- Client describes safety measures to avoid injury.

Olfactory
- Client describes how to identify noxious odors.
- Client can distinguish between safe food items and unsafe ones.
- Client identifies measures to maintain a safe home environment.
- Client consumes 75% to 100% of prescribed diet.
- Client identifies ways to enhance the enjoyment of food.
- Client adheres to proper nutrition, as evidenced by the ability to maintain weight or achieve an ideal body weight.

EXPECTED OUTCOMES FOR *SENSORY DEPRIVATION*

The expected outcome for *Sensory deprivation* is that the client remains oriented to person, place, and time. Short-term outcomes might include the following: using adaptive equipment as needed (such as glasses or a hearing aid), and responding to environmental stimuli.

EXPECTED OUTCOMES FOR *SENSORY OVERLOAD*

The expected outcome for *Sensory overload* would also be that the client remains oriented to person, place, and time. Short-term outcomes might include the following:
- Client voices decreased anxiety and irritability.
- Client communicates in a lucid manner.
- Client recognizes and reports when sensory stimuli are excessive.
- Client reestablishes routine sleep-wake cycle.
- Client demonstrates positive coping behavior when sensory stimulation rises.

INTERVENTION

Interventions for clients with altered sensory perception should promote adaptation to sensory deficits, provide sensory stimulation, and prevent sensory overload, as appropriate.

INTERVENTIONS TO PROMOTE ADAPTATION FOR SENSORY DEFICITS

When a hospitalized client has a vision or hearing impairment, nursing interventions are aimed at helping the person adapt to an unfamiliar environment. Intervene to promote a safe environment, encourage self-care, facilitate communication, prevent injury, teach proper body mechanics, and promote nutrition. A client who is partially sighted or partially deaf may function well in a familiar environment but may need assistance in an unfamiliar one. Other types of sensory/perceptual disturbances will require other interventions. Some examples of interventions for various sensory/perceptual problems are described next.

Promoting a Safe Environment. Providing a safe environment for a client with a vision or hearing impairment is important. Orient the client to the room, and demonstrate how to use the call light. It may take several sessions of orientation to get the client comfortably settled in the room. Remove excess furniture and equipment from the room. However, do not move furniture without letting the client know of its new location. Also, do not leave objects where the client may be walking.

Teach a visually impaired client and significant others about safe illumination, reduction of glare, and use of contrasting colors to assist with visual discrimination. Adequate lighting should be provided in all rooms during the day, and soft lighting should be provided at night. The light switch should be easily accessible. Interventions to reduce glare include avoiding glossy surfaces (such as glass and highly polished floors), using shades to provide diffuse light, wearing sunglasses or a brimmed hat when outside, and avoiding looking at headlights and other bright lights.

Contrasting colors help in visual discrimination and also promote safety. Methods to provide color contrast include marking the edges of steps with colored tape; avoiding white walls, floors, and countertops; using smoked glass instead of clear glass; choosing objects colored black on white; and painting doorknobs a bright color.

> ***Action Alert!*** Orient the client to the surroundings to reduce the risk of injury.

Make sure that all staff members are aware of the client's vision or hearing loss. Record information in the client's care profile, clinical care path, or chart cover, and post the information in the client's room. Respond to the client's call light as quickly as possible.

Glasses and contact lenses are important aids to help the partially sighted person maintain safety in an unfamiliar environment. The client should be able to easily locate these vision aids and know they are safely stored when not in use. Handle glasses carefully to prevent them from becoming misaligned and to keep the lenses clean.

Providing a safe environment for a person with a hearing impairment is important to prevent injury. Visual aids and aids to enhance hearing are helpful. Examples of visual aids include a light that blinks when the doorbell or telephone rings, an alarm clock that flashes a light to awaken the person, flashing lights to warn of fires and carbon monoxide danger, and extra mirrors on a car to enhance vision in several directions. Aids to boost residual hearing include using telephone amplifiers, leaving the car window partly open, and setting the air conditioner, heater, or radio on low so outside noises, such as sirens and other warning signals, can be heard. Hearing aids are helpful but sometimes add to the problem if the level of noise produced by the hearing aid becomes more confusing than helpful. People who use hearing aids sometimes find that they need to limit the number of people in a room and delete extraneous noises like music or television. Even with a hearing aid, the person may need to be in the speaker's direct line of vision to lip-read.

Encouraging Self-Care. Usually, visually impaired clients want to be independent even in a hospital environment. Modify the environment to maximize any vision the client may have. If the client has hemianopia, place the client's personal belongings in an area of the room that maximizes the functional areas of the visual field. Approach the client from the best visual angle, and remind the client to scan the environment to pick up visual cues (Table 38-3).

Safety is also a concern for hearing-impaired clients. Voice responses to call lights may not be effective for these clients. Respond personally to call light as soon as possible.

Facilitating Communication. It is important to develop a means to communicate with a client with a hearing impairment to prevent social isolation. If the client has a hearing aid, encourage its use. Determine how to effectively communicate with the client through the use of gestures, written words, signing, or lipreading. Document the best way to communicate with the client in the care profile or clinical path and on the chart cover.

Interventions to facilitate communication include facing the client when speaking; enunciating words slowly, clearly, and in a normal voice; and avoiding putting your hands to your mouth when speaking. Wearing lipstick helps to define the mouth and facilitates lipreading. Provide sensory stimulation using tactile and visual stimuli to help compensate for the hearing loss. If the client wears a hearing aid, it is important for you to under-

Table 38-3 Nursing Interventions to Promote Self-Care With Visual Disturbances

ACTIVITY OF DAILY LIVING	NURSING INTERVENTIONS
Feeding	• Open up all cartons, packages, and condiments. Cut food into bite-size pieces. • Set up meal tray, and describe the food, liquids, and utensils on the plate using clock-face referents. For example, "Your juice is at 1 o'clock, salad is at 3 o'clock." • Use plain white or light-colored dishes to help client distinguish food items on the plate. • Teach client to scan the area if a visual field loss is present.
Bathing/showering	• When entering the room, announce your presence and introduce yourself. • Speak in a normal tone of voice. *People tend to treat visually challenged individuals as if they also cannot hear.* • Provide privacy, and inform the client what to expect during the procedures. • Arrange bathing equipment within easy reach. • Assess the client's ability to perform hygiene tasks. Watch while brushing hair or shaving, for example. • Leave bed in low position. • Leave call light within reach. Be sure client knows how to use it. • Provide nonskid surfaces for tub or shower.
Dressing and grooming	• Position clothing so that it is within easy reach. • Encourage family to provide clothing that is easily managed by the client—for example, Velcro closures, elasticized waists.
Toileting	• Place call bell within easy reach. • Place bedpan or urinal in client's field of vision. • Place toilet tissue in easy reach. • Provide privacy. • Arrange for grab bars and raised toilet seats in home bathrooms.

stand the proper care and use of the device (Box 38-3). If the client is unable to insert the hearing aid, the nurse may need to do so (Procedure 38-1).

Direct nursing interventions toward promoting communication to increase or maintain social interaction. When communicating with a person who can read lips, face the person and gain attention before speaking. Try not to speak too rapidly, but do not slow the rate of speech below that appropriate for normal conversation. Speak clearly and simply. Do not shout or exaggerate lip movements. Use appropriate gestures to aid in the understanding of what is being said, just as you would with a hearing person. Do not draw letters in the air or make similar gestures.

If the person has residual hearing, try lowering the pitch of your voice. This often helps in communicating with older adults, whose hearing deficit typically involves high-pitched sounds first. Turn off the radio or television so that background noise does not interfere with the person's ability to hear.

For the profoundly deaf person who cannot read lips, supply plenty of paper and pencils for notes. Obtain a sign language interpreter as needed.

Action Alert! Urge a hearing-impaired client to install smoke and carbon monoxide detectors that use flashing lights to signal danger.

To communicate with visually impaired clients, identify yourself when entering the client's room. Explain all actions ahead of time, and help the client anticipate any movements, such as touching the client.

BOX 38-3 *Precautions for Using an External Hearing Aid*

- Do not store in a warm place (such as on a windowsill or in a car). Heat can change the shape of the ear mold, which then does not fit the person's ear.
- Do not twist the cord.
- Do not drop.
- Perform hand hygiene before handling.
- Make sure battery is inserted properly and is in working order.
- Take the battery out of the hearing aid when not in use for a day or longer.
- Remove the hearing aid before radiological examination or therapy to avoid damage from radiation.
- Avoid using an aerosol spray near the hearing aid. Aerosol spray can clog the microphone.

If hearing impairment is caused by cerumen impaction, the impaction may be removed with ceruminolytic agents and lavage of the ear canal (Procedure 38-2). Teach the client the following information:

- Production of earwax is normal.
- Do not place foreign objects, such as cotton-tipped applicators, into the ear canal. Bobby pins and paper clips inserted into the ear can injure the ear and increase the risk for infection.
- Clean the ears with a damp washcloth wrapped around a finger.
- Ceruminolytic agents soften earwax and may allow natural removal.
- See a health care professional if hearing declines or you hear ringing, crackling, or other noise or if you feel pressure.

PROCEDURE 38-1

INSERTING A HEARING AID

TIME TO ALLOW: NOVICE: 10 min. EXPERT: 5 min.

Many clients over the age of 50 use hearing aids. A hearing aid is a delicate, sensitive instrument and requires careful handling and cleaning. Sometimes a client needs assistance with changing the battery or adjusting the volume. You should become familiar with hearing aids.

DELEGATION GUIDELINES

Assisting a client with the care and use of a hearing aid may be delegated to a nursing assistant who is trained in this skill.

EQUIPMENT NEEDED

- Soft, lint-free cotton cloth
- Cleaning solution for ear mold as recommended by manufacturer
- Mild soap and warm water to clean ear canal
- Fresh battery, if needed

1 Perform preliminary actions (see inside front cover).

2 Check that the battery is operating. Hold the hearing aid in your hand, and turn up the volume. If the batteries are working, a "feedback" whistle will be heard. *Feedback is the noise resulting from the sound leaking out and going back through the microphones and becoming amplified.*

3 Inspect the hearing aid. The plastic connecting tubing, present in behind-the-ear aids, should not be cracked or broken. The ear mold should not be cracked or have a rough surface. The ear mold should be free of cerumen.

4 Turn down the volume, insert the ear mold into the ear canal, and secure the rest of the aid in place according to the design. The ear bore or hole should be placed in the ear canal. The ear mold should precisely fit the ear (see illustration). A slight twist may be needed to snugly fit the ear mold into the ear.

5 For a behind-the-ear hearing aid, secure the battery device behind the ear (see illustration). Avoid kinking the connecting tubing.

6 Slowly turn up the volume while speaking to the person in a normal tone of voice. Ask the person to tell you when the volume is comfortable.

7 If feedback occurs, check for a problem. Press on the ear mold. The ear mold may be loose and need to be replaced. Check to make sure the person's ear is not against a pillow, causing the ear mold to be dislodged.

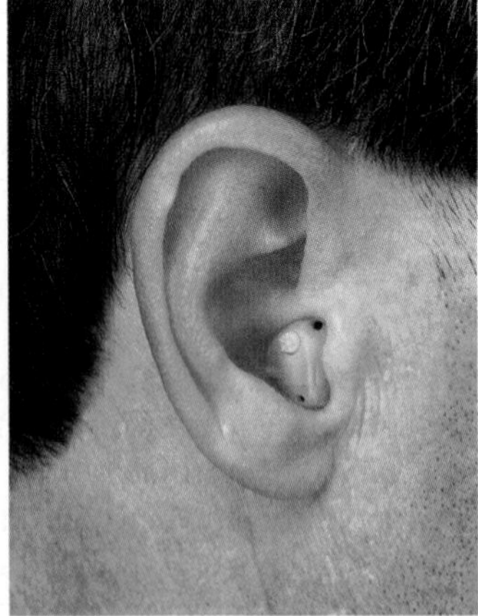

Step 4 An in-the-ear hearing aid in place. (Courtesy Dahlberg, Inc., Golden Valley, MN.)

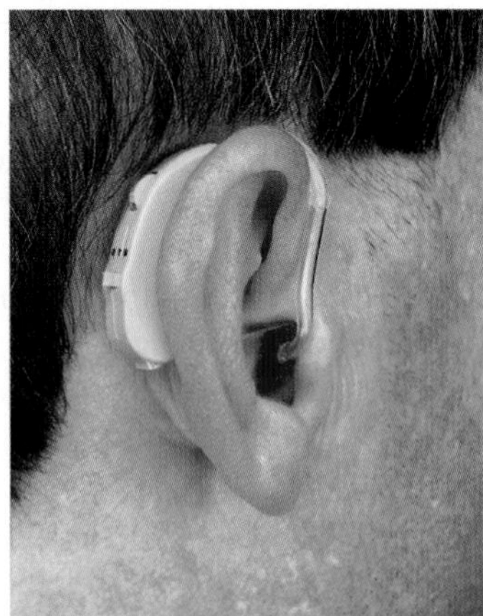

Step 5 A behind-the-ear hearing aid in place. (Courtesy Dahlberg, Inc., Golden Valley, MN.)

PROCEDURE 38-2

TIME TO ALLOW: NOVICE: 10-15 min. EXPERT: 5-10 min.

EAR LAVAGE/IRRIGATION

Ear irrigations are generally performed to remove a foreign body, remove accumulated cerumen, or relieve local irritation. Do not perform ear irrigation if you suspect or detect evidence of rupture of the eardrum. To prevent rupture of the eardrum, do not irrigate the ear canal under pressure.

DELEGATION GUIDELINES

The indications for RN assessment in the performance of ear lavage and the potential risk associated with improperly performed irrigation dictate that this procedure not be delegated to a nursing assistant.

EQUIPMENT NEEDED

- Ear syringe
- Irrigation solution (usually water at body temperature)
- Emesis basin
- Absorbent towel or waterproof pad
- Clean gloves
- Cotton-tipped applicator

1 Perform preliminary actions (see inside front cover).

2 Examine the ear canal with an otoscope. Assess for an intact tympanic membrane and signs of otitis media. *Irrigation is contraindicated in a client with a tympanic membrane perforation or otitis media. However, the usual purpose is to remove cerumen, which may obstruct your vision of the ear canal.*

3 Explain the procedure, and instruct the client to avoid any sudden movements. *Holding still will prevent trauma from the irrigating syringe or catheter.*

4 Check the temperature of the irrigant. A common irrigant is a mixture of water and hydrogen peroxide. Water temperature should be 37° C, or about 98° F.

5 Select the irrigating device. A 20- or 50-mL syringe may be used with a plastic intravenous (IV) catheter on the end. If a 50-mL syringe is used, use caution to avoid exerting excessive pressure, which may damage the tympanic membrane. A dental irrigation device may be used at low settings. *The pulsating action of the dental irrigation device may help to break up the cerumen.*

6 Cover the client's shoulder. Tip the client's head to the side that is being irrigated, and ask the client to hold the emesis basin (see illustration). *The head should be positioned to allow the irrigant to drain into the basin.*

7 Place the tip of the irrigation device just inside the external meatus, with the tip still visible. Straighten the auditory meatus by gently drawing the pinna up and back for an adult. Pull the ear canal down and back for an infant or child.

8 Direct the fluid toward the posterior wall of the ear canal (see illustration). The ear canal can be compared to the face of a clock. Fluid should be directed at 1 o'clock for the left ear and 11 o'clock for the right ear.

9 Irrigation of fluid should be steady. No more than 70 mL of solution should be used at one time. Watch the fluid for signs of cerumen plug removal. If nausea, vomiting, or acute pain occurs, stop the irrigation immediately.

10 Periodically examine the ear canal with an otoscope to determine patency and cerumen removal. If cerumen does not drain out, wait 10 minutes and repeat the irrigation. If debris is not removed after a reasonable time, another method should be considered.

11 Tilt the head to drain excess fluid from the ear. Dry the outer ear canal gently with a cotton-tipped applicator. If cerumen cannot be removed with irrigation, the client may place mineral oil into the ear three times daily for 2 days to soften the dry cerumen. Then the irrigation may be repeated.

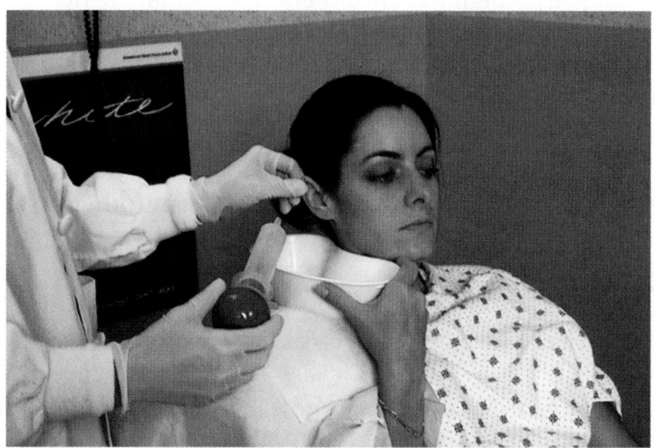

Step 6 Preparation for ear irrigation

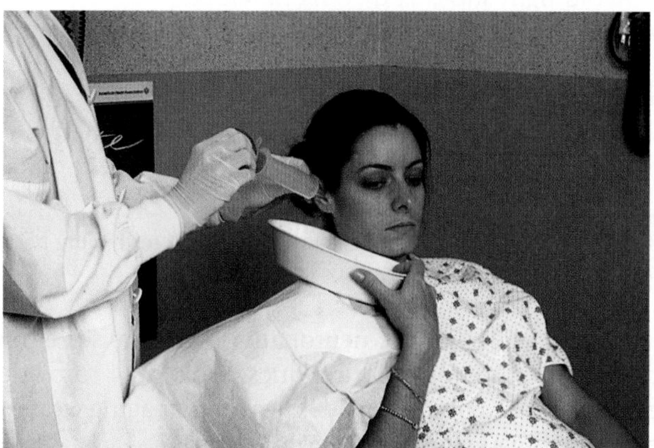

Step 8 Instilling fluid for ear irrigation.

Continued

12 Document the procedure, affected ear, results of irrigation, and client's response to the procedure.

PEDIATRIC CONSIDERATIONS

Children often place tiny objects in their ears. Do not perform ear irrigation if there is reason to think the foreign body may be vegetable material (such as a dried bean) that may swell when wet.

GERIATRIC CONSIDERATIONS

Older adults frequently have dry, impacted cerumen from hearing aid insertion. Ceruminolytic agents may be instilled into the ear canal for a specified time to soften the wax before the irrigation procedure. Have the older adult remain seated for several minutes at the completion of the procedure before standing because of possible alterations in equilibrium.

Action Alert! Warn the client that inserting foreign objects into the ear canal may perforate the tympanic membrane or damage the ear canal.

Preventing Injury. Clients with a diminished ability to perceive the position or location of body parts are at risk for injury. The person with vertigo or dizziness, for example, is experiencing an alteration in position sense and has a potential for injury. Orthostatic hypotension (the decrease of blood pressure on standing) is the most common cause of dizziness. There are numerous contributing factors for dizziness, such as cardiac arrhythmias, dehydration, medication side effects, a prolonged recumbent position, and a sudden change in position.

Teach a client with dizziness to change position slowly and to move from a reclining to an upright position in stages, with a few minutes between stages. Place a chair, walker, cane, or other assistive device nearby to steady the client when getting out of bed. Teach the client to prevent dehydration by increasing fluid intake when excessive fluids are lost during exercise and when perspiring during hot weather.

Teach clients with sensation deficits the following preventive measures to avoid an injury:

- Regularly observe how the hands and feet are placed.
- Inspect skin daily, especially the feet.
- Avoid tight shoes and going barefoot.
- Pad the side rails of the bed, and make any other appropriate environmental modifications.
- Test bath water with a thermometer.
- Protect hands and feet from extremely cold temperatures by wearing gloves and warm socks.

Action Alert! Teach a client with a spinal cord injury how to shift body weight to prevent skin breakdown.

Clients with diabetic neuropathy may have sensation deficits in the lower extremities. Box 38-4 provides evidence-based practice guidelines for managing wounds caused by inadequate sensation.

A loss of smell can also place the person at risk for injury. Home care instructions for the client should include the following:

- Install smoke detectors, and check the batteries regularly.
- If you have gas appliances, contact the utility company about measures to protect against gas leakage.
- Date all foods that spoil quickly; discard them promptly to avoid mistakenly eating spoiled food.

Promoting Nutrition. An alteration in taste and smell places the person at risk for impaired nutrition. It is important that foods be flavorful because appetite is enhanced by smell and taste. The use of spices, such as fresh garlic, onion, and lemon juice, can improve the flavor. Encourage caregivers to prepare foods the client enjoys and to serve them in an attractive manner. A variety of different-colored foods presented at each meal may appeal to the client's visual sense and thus increase appetite. Teach the client that frequent mouth care may increase the taste sensation and improve appetite. Weigh the client weekly to detect weight loss, and monitor for possible malnutrition.

INTERVENTIONS TO PROVIDE SENSORY STIMULATION

Assist or encourage clients to use glasses, hearing aids, or other adaptive devices to help reduce sensory deprivation. Arrange the client's environment to offset any deficit.

- Encourage family to bring in personal items such as photos, cards, and books.
- Provide a night-light.
- Position the client's bed for maximal visualization of the environment.
- Assist the client and family or significant other in planning short trips outside the hospital.

Action Alert! Monitor the environment, and provide sensory stimulation for the at-risk client.

Reality orientation is important for the client with sensory deprivation. Accomplish this by calling the cli-

BOX 38-4
Evidence-Based Practice
Managing Wounds in Neuropathic Disease

Problem: Clients with diabetes frequently suffer from sensory, motor, and autonomic neuropathy due to impaired nerve function from hyperglycemia. The combination of poor perfusion and altered sensation from neuropathy may result in problems leading to pressure on the foot leading to wound development and may eventually lead to infection, gangrene, and limb loss.

Evidence

Searches of electronic databases and hand-searches of published literature were the methods used to collect and select evidence. The primary authors of this guideline independently conducted a literature search of Medline and Cochrane Library databases to identify 174 studies and systematic reviews published from 1980 through 2003. The search targeted meta-analyses, randomized controlled trials (RCTs), prospective clinical trials, retrospective studies, and systematic reviews. Bibliographies of selected articles also were reviewed. Expert consensus was the method used to formulate the recommendations. Each article was assigned a level of evidence rating, for example, Level I was defined as "a randomized controlled trial . . . that demonstrates a statistically significant difference in at least one important outcome defined by $p < .05$." The guideline and rating scheme for the strength of the evidence can be found at: http://www.guideline.gov/summary/summary.aspx?ss=15&doc_id=5912&nbr=3898.

Application to Practice

The guideline was developed to do the following:

- Present an evidence-based guideline for the management of wounds in clients with lower-extremity neuropathic disease (LEND)
- Provide consistent, research-based, clinical information with the goal of improved, cost-effective client outcomes
- Provide increased wound research in the areas where there are gaps between research and practice

Potential benefits of these guidelines:

- Identification of clients with peripheral neuropathy who are at risk for developing wounds
- Identification of clients whose current wounds are caused or complicated by peripheral neuropathy
- Implementation of appropriate strategies and plans to accomplish the following:
  - Attain/maintain intact skin
  - Manage pain and sensory issues
  - Identify/manage complications promptly
  - Optimize potential for wound healing
  - Promote limb preservation
  - Involve client and caregiver in self-management

Reference

Wound, Ostomy, and Continence Nurses Society (WOCN). (2004). *Guideline for management of wounds in patients with lower-extremity neuropathic disease* (WOCN Clinical Practice Guideline No. 3). Glenview, IL: Author [85 references].

ent by name, introducing yourself, and orienting to time, place, and environment. Have a calendar and clock readily visible in the room. Turn on the television and radio for short periods of time, choosing a program on the basis of the client's interest. Discuss other client interests while providing care. Try to be with the client at predetermined times throughout the day to avoid isolation. Encourage family members or significant others to discuss past and present events.

INTERVENTIONS TO PREVENT *SENSORY OVERLOAD*

Hospitalized clients are susceptible to *Sensory overload;* therefore it is important to reorient the client to reality. Call the client by name, and introduce yourself. Orient the client to the environment, including sights, sounds, and smells. Provide information about time, place, and date. Other measures to provide reality orientation include providing clocks and calendars and placing family photos and other personal items at the bedside. Family or significant others should be encouraged to visit frequently.

Measures should be implemented to reduce environmental stimuli by reducing excessive noise, lights, and environmental clutter. Cluster procedures and treatments to avoid disturbing the client unnecessarily. To avoid startling the client, approach in a calm, gentle manner. Teach the client to limit sensory overload by turning off the television, or by reducing or leaving a stimulating environment.

Try to simulate a "normal" environment for the hospitalized client by dimming or turning off lights at night and keeping them on during the day. This should facilitate day/night orientation.

EVALUATION

Evaluate the outcome criteria as specified in the nursing care plan (Box 38-5) to determine whether the nursing diagnosis is resolved. Remember that evaluation requires reassessment of the client. If the outcome criteria are not achieved, reassess the client to determine the reason for lack of progress. The plan of care or outcome criteria may need to be revised on the basis of the assessment.

BOX 38-5

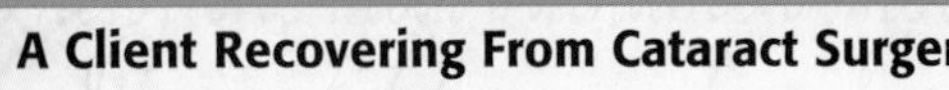

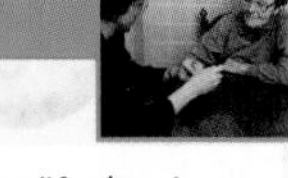

Nursing Care Plan

A Client Recovering From Cataract Surgery

Admission Data

Mrs. Pfannenstiel is admitted to same-day surgery the morning she is scheduled for removal of the cataract in her left eye. She is accompanied by her daughter and appears anxious. She repeatedly tells her daughter, "I really see okay. Maybe this surgery isn't a good idea. I don't like the idea of someone cutting on my eye."

Postoperative Physician's Orders

1. Discontinue IV when taking adequate fluids.
2. May discharge when vital signs are stable and taking adequate fluids without nausea.
3. Please teach client regarding home health care instructions.

Home Health Care Instructions

1. Return to the office the day after surgery with your eye patch in place (if present).
2. DO NOT rub the operated eye.
3. Wear your glasses to protect the operated eye.
4. Wear sunglasses over your glasses for protection from sunlight and wind.
5. Tape the metal shield over the operated eye (if physician ordered) every night before going to bed. This will protect the eye while you sleep.
6. Avoid bending at waist, sneezing, coughing, straining to have a BM, or doing any heavy work.
7. Avoid heavy lifting (greater than 5 pounds) for at least a week.
8. Instill eye drops as ordered.
9. Follow physician's orders regarding resuming activities, driving, and drinking alcohol.
10. Immediately report:
    - Nausea, vomiting
    - Pain that is unrelieved by Tylenol
    - Increased temperature, chills, blurred vision, headache
    - Yellow or green drainage from the eye
11. Avoid aspirin for pain because of its effect on blood clotting.

Nursing Assessment

Upon return to her room, Mrs. Pfannenstiel's left eye is patched. She is awake and immediately recognizes her daughter. Her vital signs are stable, and she denies nausea.

NANDA-I Nursing Diagnosis	NOC Expected Outcomes With Indicators	NIC Interventions With Selected Activities	Evaluation Data
Disturbed Sensory Perception	***Vision Compensation Behavior***	***Environmental Management***	***At the Time of Discharge***
Related Factor: • Left eye patched secondary to cataract surgery	• Implements adaptive strategies to maintain safety and comfort. • Describes the rationale for the use of eye patch.	• Place water and personal articles in line of vision. • Orient client to call light and bed controls. • Provide amount of lighting that client finds most helpful. • Teach daughter safety measures for discharge and modifications for home environment. • Mother and daughter should be treated as though working together for mother's safety and comfort. Tell mother that it is important to let daughter help her.	• Is able to independently take liquids without nausea. • Calls nurse for assistance when needed. • States can see better without bright, glaring overhead lights. • Daughter agreed to walk on affected side; point out stairs and irregular paths. • Will arrange home environment to minimize activity, to have needed items conveniently in place, have a clear path, and avoid sharp objects. Daughter will stay with mother until next physician appointment.

Critical Thinking Questions

1. What feelings would you anticipate in Mrs. Pfannenstiel while she has one eye covered?
2. Knowing that recovery may be more difficult for an 82-year-old woman, what measures would you employ to help Mrs. Pfannenstiel maintain a positive attitude during her recovery?
3. What kinds of problems would you anticipate for Mrs. Pfannenstiel to manage while she is waiting for her eyes to have recovered enough to be fitted for new glasses?
4. How would you deal with Mrs. Pfannenstiel's unrealistic fear that she will not see again?

Nursing outcome and intervention labels from Johnson, M., Bulechek, G., Butcher, H., Dochterman, J. M., Maas, M., Moorhead, S., et al. (Eds.). (2006). *NANDA, NOC, and NIC linkages: Nursing diagnoses, outcomes, & interventions.* St. Louis, MO: Mosby.

A discharge nursing note for Mrs. Pfannenstiel might look like the one below.

SAMPLE DOCUMENTATION FOR MRS. PFANNENSTIEL

Mrs. Pfannenstiel and her daughter verbalize the following measures to prevent injury to the operated eye: (1) Wear glasses. (2) Wear sunglasses to protect eyes from wind and sunlight. (3) Tape a metal shield, if ordered, over the operative eye at night. (4) Do no heavy work, such as moving furniture, working in the garden, mowing the grass, or shoveling snow, for at least a week.

▼ KEY PRINCIPLES

- Sensation and perception are processes that require sensory nerve receptors to convey stimuli to the brain, where they are perceived and interpreted. The person then responds to the stimuli.
- Sensory deficits occur when one of the senses is impaired and stimuli are not conveyed in a normal fashion to the brain.
- Sensory deprivation occurs when the brain receives too few incoming stimuli; sensory overload occurs when the brain receives too many stimuli.
- People at all points along the life span are at risk for sensory/perceptual disturbances. However, older adults are more likely to be affected.
- Assess a client for sensory/perceptual disturbances by taking the client's history, completing a physical assessment of the client's senses, and noting symptoms and responses to sensory deficits or sensory/perceptual disturbances.
- Nursing interventions are aimed at optimizing sensory/perceptual functioning.

■ REVIEW QUESTIONS

1. The nurse would be concerned about the risk of ototoxicity in a client receiving which of the following medications?
1. Phenytoin (Dilantin)
2. Furosemide (Lasix)
3. Acetaminophen (Tylenol)
4. Carbamazepine (Tegretol)

2. The nurse explains to a client that a Snellen chart would be used to assess the client for which of the following?
1. Color blindness
2. Glaucoma
3. Cataract formation
4. Near and distance vision

3. The nurse should do which of the following to enhance communication with a client who has a hearing impairment?
1. Face the client while speaking
2. Speak in a high-pitched voice
3. Overenunciate words
4. Cup the hands around the mouth while speaking

4. The nurse would plan to do which of the following when performing an ear irrigation on an assigned client?
1. Use a 5-mL syringe
2. Direct the fluid toward the posterior wall of the ear canal
3. Tilt the head toward the opposite side of the one being irrigated
4. Stop the procedure if the client has pain lasting more than 15 seconds

5. Which of the following strategies would be least useful in improving safety for a client who is visually impaired?
1. Keep hallways free of clutter.
2. Place a night-light in the bathroom.
3. Place tape on the edges of stair steps.
4. Use bright lights in each room.

Bibliography

*Chen, H. (1994). Hearing in the elderly: Relation of hearing loss, loneliness, and self-esteem. *Journal of Gerontological Nursing, 20*(6), 22-28.

*Das, A. (1999). Prevention of visual loss in older adults. *Clinics in Geriatric Medicine, 15*(1), 131-144.

Estes, M. E. Z. (2006). *Health assessment and physical examination* (3rd ed.). New York: Delmar.

Halle, C. (2002). Achieve new vision screening objectives. *The Nurse Practitioner, 27*(3), 15-35.

Halvorson, P. (2005). The silent thief. *RN, 68*(3), 41-45.

Johnson, M., Bulechek, G., Butcher, H., Dochterman, J. M., Maas, M., Moorhead, S., et al. (Eds.). (2006). *NANDA, NOC, and NIC linkages: Nursing diagnoses, outcomes, & interventions.* St. Louis, MO: Mosby.

Kimel, L. S. (2006). Lack of follow-up exams after failed school vision screenings: an investigation of contributing factors. *Journal of School Nursing, 22*(3), 156-162.

Marcincuk, M., & Roland, P. (2002). Geriatric hearing loss: Understanding the causes and providing appropriate treatment. *Geriatrics, 57*(4), 44-59.

McCullagh, M. C. (2006). Home modification: How to help patients make their homes safer and more accessible as their abilities change. *American Journal of Nursing 106*(10), 54-63.

McGrory, A., & Remington, R. (2004). Optimizing the functionality of clients with age-related macular degeneration. *Rehabilitation Nursing, 29*(3), 90-94.

NANDA International. (2005). *Nursing diagnoses: Definitions and classification, 2005-2006* (6th ed.). Philadelphia: Author.

National Eye Institute. (2004). *Age-Related Eye Disease Study: Results.* Retrieved November 29, 2006, from http://www.nei.nih.gov/amd/index.asp.

Phillips, M. (2003). Genetics of hearing loss. *Medsurg Nursing, 12*(6), 386-390, 411.

Ramos, M. F. (1999). Prevention of work-related injuries: A look at eye protection use and suggested prevention strategies. *Journal of Ophthalmic Nursing and Technology, 18*(3), 117-119.

Slaven, A. (2003). Communication and the hearing impaired client. *Nursing Standard, 18*(12), 39-41.

Spires, R. (2006). How you can help when older eyes fail. *RN, 69*(2), 38-40, 42-44.

Stone, C. (1999). Preventing cerumen impaction in nursing facility residents. *Journal of Gerontological Nursing, 25*(5), 43-45.

Wallhagen, M.I., Pettengill, E., & Whiteside M. (2006). Sensory impairment in older adults: Part 1: Hearing loss. *American Journal of Nursing 06*(10), 40-48; quiz 48-49.

*Walters, G. J. (1993). *Wir wollen Deutsche Bleiben: The story of the Volga Germans.* Kansas City, MO: Halcyon House.

*Asterisk indicates a classic or definitive work on this subject.

Chapter 39

Supporting Verbal Communication

Media Resources

- evolve Evolve Website http://evolve.elsevier.com/Harkreader/
- Companion CD

Learning Objectives

After studying this chapter, you should be able to do the following:

- Describe the concepts of sound production
- Describe the physiological and behavioral concepts underlying impaired verbal communication
- Discuss the most common life span, physiological, cultural, and lifestyle factors affecting communication
- Assess the client who is at risk for impaired communication, who has actual impaired communication, or who has a related nursing diagnosis
- Diagnose the problems of impaired communication that are amenable to nursing intervention
- Plan nursing interventions to prevent or correct impaired verbal communication on the basis of client goals
- Implement key interventions for a client with impaired verbal communication
- Evaluate outcomes for impaired verbal communication to determine the effectiveness of nursing care

Key Terms

aphasia
articulation
Broca's area
communication
dysarthria
dysphagia
dysphonia
neologism
paraphasia
phonation
resonance
telegraphic speech
Wernicke's area

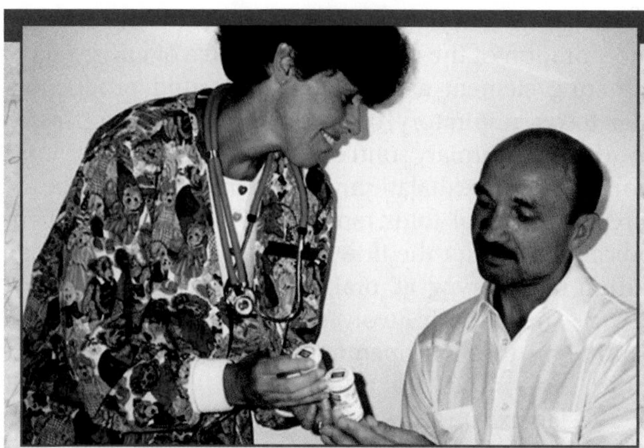

From Kee, J. K., *Pharmacology: A nursing process approach* (5th ed). St. Louis, MO: Mosby.

Señor Juan Martinez, who has a persistent upper respiratory infection, comes to the hospital accompanied by his wife. They are both from Mexico and have been in the United States for only 6 months. Neither Sr. Martinez nor his wife is fluent in English. Sr. Martinez is employed in a beef-packing plant.

His tuberculosis skin test is positive, and he is admitted for further diagnostic workup and is placed on respiratory isolation precautions. The nurse is concerned about being able to communicate verbally with the Martinezes and uses the diagnosis *Impaired verbal communication* related to Spanish as the primary language (see the key nursing diagnosis box) to alert the health care team of the need for an interpreter.

KEY NURSING DIAGNOSIS FOR COMMUNICATION

Impaired verbal communication: Decreased, delayed, or absent ability to receive, process, transmit, and use a system of symbols

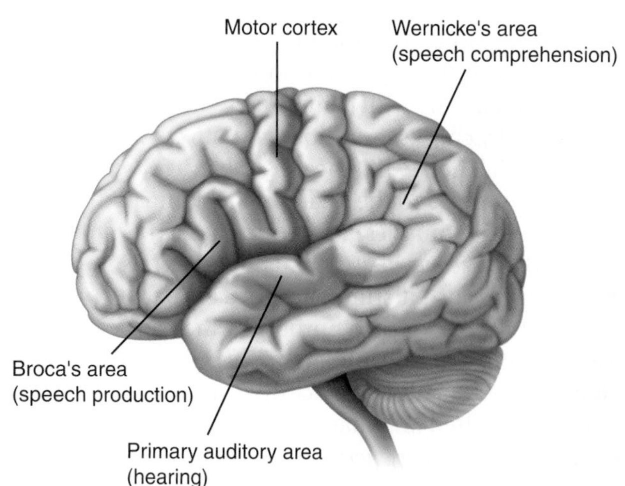

FIGURE 39-1 Major speech-language and hearing areas of the brain.

CONCEPTS OF VERBAL COMMUNICATION

In Chapter 12, **communication** is described as a complex process in which information is exchanged between two or more people. The sender and receiver of the message are unique individuals, with differing perceptions, beliefs, and interpretations of the world. Communication is effective when the message intended by the sender and the message perceived by the receiver are the same.

Communication is an essential part of human interactions, beginning at birth and continuing throughout life. By sharing expressions of physical, social, and emotional needs with other people, we can fulfill those needs while establishing, nurturing, and maintaining relationships with other people. Communication is an important aspect of the nurse-client relationship.

Nurses encounter a variety of situations in which a client cannot communicate verbally. The situations commonly result from a brain injury, dementia, or a cerebrovascular accident (stroke) that impairs the client's ability to understand or to express himself. Impaired communication also can result from anatomical alterations of the vocal structures or the placement of an artificial airway, such as an endotracheal tube or tracheostomy tube. Language barriers, developmental delays, and psychiatric illnesses can impair verbal communication as well. Failure to communicate is frustrating for all involved, especially the client.

NEUROLOGY OF VERBAL COMMUNICATION

Verbal communication depends on an intact, healthy nervous system to form words and sentences and to interpret the meaning of spoken words. Nurses can increase the effectiveness of communication interventions by understanding the neurology of verbal communication.

Brain Centers. The parietal, occipital, and temporal lobes of the brain's dominant hemisphere are involved in analyzing, synthesizing, and interpreting somatic, visual, and auditory information and processing this information into coherent thoughts (Zemlin, 1998). In most people, the major speech-language and hearing areas of the brain are located in the left hemisphere (Figure 39-1). Of these areas, Broca's area and Wernicke's area are crucial to communication; each has its own function.

Broca's Area. Located in the frontal lobe, **Broca's area** is the center of motor speech control. It is responsible for controlling the muscles of the mouth, tongue, and larynx, which are involved in the production of speech (Zemlin, 1998).

Wernicke's Area. Located in the temporal lobe, **Wernicke's area** helps control the content of speech and affects auditory and visual comprehension. It also transmits information to Broca's area. It has an interpretive role in communication that is important for reading and auditory comprehension, spontaneous conversation, and the ability to process sensory information into coherent thoughts (Zemlin, 1998).

Cranial Nerves. Of the 12 cranial nerves, 6 (V, VII, IX, X, XI, and XII) are involved in speech production (Figure 39-2). Cranial nerve V, the *trigeminal nerve,* controls the movements of the lower jaw and the tongue. The *facial nerve* (cranial nerve VII) innervates the muscles of the face (eyelids, cheeks, and lips) and affects facial expression. Cranial nerve IX, the *glossopharyngeal nerve,* provides motor fibers to the pharynx and controls the movement of throat muscles. The recurrent laryngeal nerve, a branch of the *vagus nerve* (cranial nerve X), is important in speech because it stimulates the soft palate, pharynx, and larynx. If the motor portion of the vagus nerve becomes damaged, **dysphagia** (difficulty swallowing), **dysphonia** (difficulty producing vocal sounds), and **dysarthria** (impaired articulation) may result. Cranial nerve XI, the *spinal accessory nerve,* helps control the muscles of the pharynx (throat), the soft palate, and the head and shoulders. The *hypoglossal nerve* (cranial nerve XII) controls tongue movements, which are essential for **articulation,** the process of molding sounds into enunciated words and phrases. Damage to any of the cranial nerves may inhibit speech production (Zemlin, 1998).

SOUND PRODUCTION IN VERBAL COMMUNICATION

Production of speech begins with the production of sound by the lungs and larynx. The sound is modified into speech in the nasal, oral, and pharyngeal cavities through the process of articulation. These structures also control the quality of sound by producing resonance. The structures of speech production are known as the vocal tract (Figure 39-3).

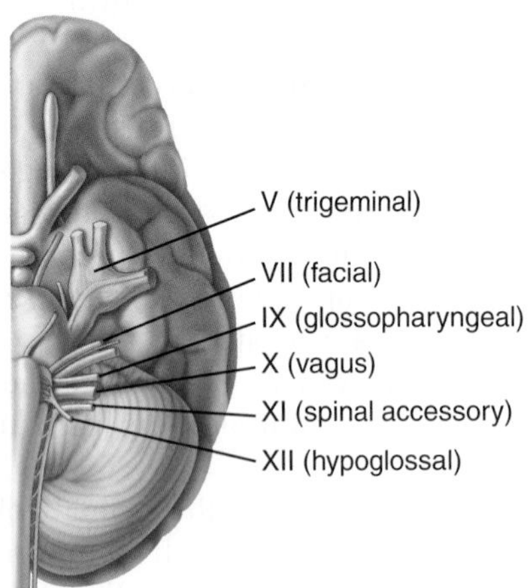

FIGURE 39-2 Cranial nerves involved in speech production.

Phonation. Phonation is the production of sound by the vibration of the vocal folds. A source of energy and a vibrating element are essential for sound production. The lower respiratory tract, especially the lung tissue, provides the primary source of energy for speech production. A smooth exhalation vibrates the vocal folds in the larynx. The vocal folds rapidly open and close to periodically inte rrupt the flow of air to produce vocal tone within the pharyngeal, oral, and nasal cavities (Zemlin, 1998). Thus speech involves the intermittent release of expired air through opening and closing of the glottis, which houses the vocal folds.

The larynx functions as a sound generator or sound producer over a wide range of pitch and loudness. The intrinsic muscles of the larynx are responsible for ordinary speech production. The vocal folds, or vocal cords, are long, round bands of muscle tissue that may be lengthened or shortened, tensed or relaxed, and abducted or adducted to cause varying types of sound production (Zemlin, 1998). The length of the true vocal folds and the size of the glottis are altered by the action of the intrinsic laryngeal muscle, which moves the arytenoid cartilages and the vocal folds that are attached to them.

Singers often describe phonation as voice registers, which are a series of notes with a particular quality or characteristic. They are described as high or low registers, or head or chest registers. The head register is the upper end of the scale. A stereotype of a head register is a person with a light and airy Irish brogue. The chest register is at the lower end of the scale. This is a voice that an actor or actress might use to give the voice carrying power to be

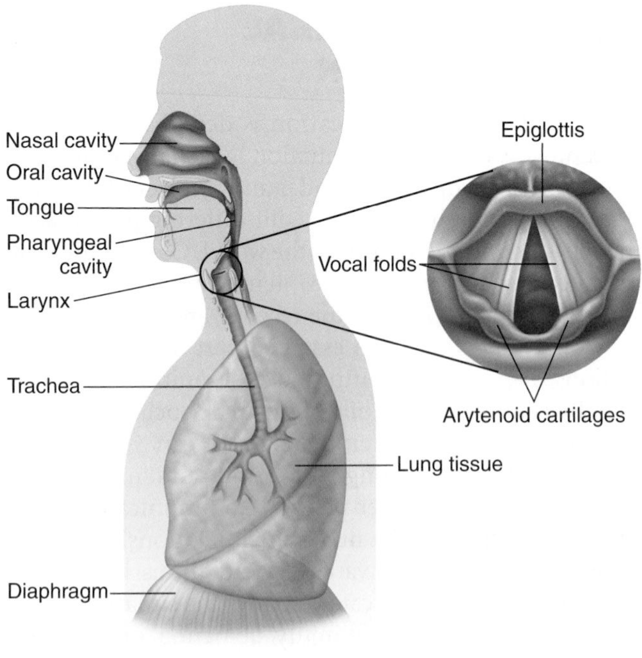

FIGURE 39-3 The structures of speech production (the vocal tract).

heard at the back of the theater. John Wayne was a classic example of an actor who used a chest register.

Head and chest registers are considered the normal range. Falsetto, a very high-pitched voice, is a voice register above the head register. At the other extreme, a depressed person's speech may be very low and slow.

Articulation. The vocal tract not only produces sound but refines it into intelligible speech in a process known as articulation. Movements of the vocal tract mold the sounds of speech produced by the larynx into enunciated words and phrases. **Articulation** is the selective modification of the voiced and unvoiced breath sounds by the tongue, teeth, and lips for the enunciation of words and sentences. It results from adjustments in the shape of the vocal tract that, in turn, change the acoustical properties of the sounds. These structures are known as articulators (Zemlin, 1998).

In speaking, the muscles of the pharynx, tongue, soft palate, and lips are essential for enunciation of sounds into recognizable consonants and vowels for normal speech. Vowel sounds are initiated in the throat and are given their distinctive shapes by movements of the mouth and tongue. Consonants are formed by controlled interruptions of exhaled air.

Voice Quality. **Resonance** is the forced vibration of a structure that is related to a source of sound and results in changes in the quality of the sound. Although the vocal folds actually produce sounds, the quality of the voice depends on the coordinated activity of many other structures. The pharynx acts as a resonating chamber to amplify and enhance the quality of sound. The oral, nasal, and sinus cavities contribute to vocal resonance as well.

Nasality, a voice quality associated with resonance, occurs in the transmission pathway between the mouth cavity and the larynx. Nasality in the voice results from the coupling of the nasal passages and the presence or absence of alternative or additional resonating cavities in the nasal passages, oral cavity, or pharyngeal cavity. Nasality may result from structural alterations, such as excessive adenoid tissue; pathophysiological alterations, such as edema secondary to allergies; or an articulation problem associated with errors in articulation (Zemlin, 1998).

Vocal quality is affected by many other factors as well, such as mass, length, and tension of the vocal folds, the degree of compression between the folds, and the subglottal air pressure. Another factor is asymmetry of the folds. If one fold is thicker than the other, for example, they vibrate at different rates. The most common vocal qualities include breathiness, harshness, and hoarseness (Shames et al., 1998).

When the vocal folds do not close completely, air leakage and friction result. The affected person will have a breathy voice. If the vocal folds do not close completely and there are irregular vibrations present at the same time, the vocal quality is known as hoarseness (Shames et al., 1998). Assignment of these terms is based on individual perception and may vary from person to person.

Variety in Speech. Variety in speech refers to loudness, pitch, rate, and intonation. Variety makes verbal communication interesting and can either enhance or impede the clarity of communication.

Loudness. Loudness of the voice depends on the force with which air rushes across the vocal folds. The greater the force, the stronger is the vibration and the louder the sound. When a person whispers, the vocal folds do not move at all. In contrast, when a person yells, they vibrate vigorously.

Pitch. A person can produce laryngeal tones that vary in range over about two octaves. Pitch is determined by changes in vocal cord length and tension. The more tense the vocal folds, the faster they vibrate and the higher the pitch. The glottis is wide open for deep tones and narrowed to a slit for high-pitched tones (Shames et al., 1998).

Pitch varies between men and women, and it changes with age. Women have an average pitch level about one octave higher than men. There is little apparent difference in pitch between boys and girls until at puberty, when boys' vocal folds grow rapidly while girls' continue to grow at the same rate. This results in a lowering of the pitch by a full octave for boys (Zemlin, 1998).

Rate. Verbal communication is clear when the rate, or pace, matches the intended message. An unintended message may be conveyed if the rate is too rapid or too slow and deliberate. The rate or pace of speech may be related to culture or geographical location.

Intonation. Intonation, or the tone of the speaker's voice, can affect the meaning of the message. Intonation can express enthusiasm, concern, sadness, hostility, or indifference. To communicate most effectively, the message and voice tone should be congruent.

FACTORS AFFECTING VERBAL COMMUNICATION

Many factors can affect a person's ability to communicate verbally. They include life span, physiological, cultural/lifestyle, and psychological factors.

RISK FACTORS ACROSS THE LIFE SPAN

At birth, most children have the physical capacity to develop speech and language. The rate of language development depends on the child's environment and may be hindered by problems in cognitive and neurological development. A stimulating environment aids language acquisition.

Remember that a child's ability to understand spoken words precedes the ability to use words. As speech development proceeds, children learn to use words correctly before they comprehend the full meaning of the words. You must understand the influence of language development and thought processes when communicating with children.

Older adults may have sensory changes in hearing and vision that affect verbal communication. Assessment of hearing and vision is especially important in communicating with older adults. They often can understand lower-pitched voices better than higher-pitched ones.

PHYSIOLOGICAL FACTORS

Gender influences verbal communication. Even within the same cultural group, men and women communicate differently. For example some men may use language to exert influence and power and to resist restrictions that have been imposed. In contrast, some women tend to use language in a relational manner to meet the needs of others and promote a sense of caring.

At any age, the complicated process of language development can be disturbed by other physiological factors such as illness, medications, surgery, and mechanical barriers (such as those that result from a tracheostomy).

For the developing child, disorders such as cerebral palsy, Down syndrome, and autism have varied effects on the development of speech and language. In addition, cleft lip and cleft palate are congenital disorders that affect speech and language development in children by preventing use of the tongue and mouth to correctly form words.

When a loss of hearing affects the child's speech and language acquisition, the child's ability to communicate will be affected. Indeed, a child who is born deaf or becomes deaf at an early age will fail to learn to speak in the usual way. The greater the loss of hearing, the more severe is the impact on speech and language acquisition. Children quickly learn gestures, signs, and other modes of manual communication when hearing is impaired. Hearing loss in the adult usually does not affect speech and language, because the loss occurs after speech and language have been established.

Adult loss of language usually stems from neurological diseases. Damage to speech centers of the brain by cerebrovascular accident (stroke), multiple sclerosis, dementia, or Parkinson's disease may cause speech to be unintelligible, singsong, explosive, mechanical, or slurred. Older adults may experience progressive diseases of the nervous system.

CULTURAL AND LIFESTYLE FACTORS

Culture. The process of communication is universal, but the manner in which information is conveyed varies with different cultures. For example, nurses need to be sensitive to the meaning of nonverbal communication in various cultures. Nonverbal communication, such as facial expression, eye and head movement, body posture, touch, proximity, gestures, tone of voice, and use of silence may have different meanings to different cultures. To give a client a positive signal during a therapy session a nurse may display the American sign of thumbs up. In Iran, however, thumbs extended upward are considered a vulgar gesture.

Verbal expression also varies between cultures. When a health care worker and client are of different cultures, barriers to communication can affect the client's experience and ultimately the client's health.

> ***Action Alert!*** Do not judge competency on the basis of how well the client uses or fails to use Standard English grammar.

Lifestyle. Lifestyle factors can cause problems with the voice. Overuse of the voice, very dry air, bacterial infections, allergies, or inhalation of irritating chemicals can all cause laryngitis. Inflammation of the laryngeal tissues causes swelling and prevents the vocal folds from moving freely. Laryngitis results in hoarseness or the inability to speak above a whisper. Vocal abuse, as from cheerleading, smoking, and alcohol abuse, can lead to laryngeal cancer, which may result in loss of the vocal folds and the ability to communicate verbally. Box 39-1 gives information about care of the voice.

Pharmacological agents, such as prescription drugs, alcohol, and illicit drugs, can interfere with communication by inhibiting or interfering with higher cortical functions. A person may have slow, slurred speech because of impaired motor control in speech centers. Moderate to heavy drug use can cause loss of comprehension and expression by affecting the brain's speech and motor centers. These effects may be temporary or permanent. The use of alcohol or crack cocaine by a pregnant woman may result in speech, language, voice, and fluency problems in her child.

Socioeconomic. Socioeconomic factors, such as education, also affect the communication process. Communication may be more difficult when people have different levels of education; a message will not be

BOX 39-1 *Teaching for Wellness*

Care of the Voice

Purpose: To prevent damage to the vocal folds.
Expected Outcome: The client will establish appropriate vocal behaviors.

Client Instructions

- Do not shout.
- Stay away from noisy places.
- Relax muscle in neck and chest when you talk.
- Keep your throat moist.
- Do not smoke.
- Avoid smoke-filled, noisy, or dusty places.
- Do not drink excessive amounts of alcohol.
- Cough or sneeze as gently and softly as possible.
- Consult a speech-language pathologist about a voice problem.
- Avoid inhaling any irritating chemicals.

clear if the words or phrases used by the nurse are not part of the listener's vocabulary. The same principle applies when providing written instructions or information to clients.

PSYCHOLOGICAL FACTORS

Psychological factors that can affect a person's ability to communicate verbally include self-concept, stress, emotion, mood, and psychiatric illness.

Self-Concept. Self-concept plays a major role in communication patterns with other people. The way people feel about themselves is conveyed in communication with others. If clients are confident and feel in control, their communication will reflect this self-confidence. Conversely, a long series of negative interactions with other people may result in a negative view of the world that affects effective communication.

Stress. Stress may affect a client's pattern or style of communication. A person may communicate aggressive or defensive behaviors in response to stress or may turn inward and become withdrawn or depressed. Consider how stress may be affecting a client's communication when noting such behaviors.

Emotion and Mood. A person's emotions and mood influence communication with others and the ability to receive messages accurately. Emotions and mood can cause a message to be either misinterpreted or not heard at all. If a person is depressed, anxious, sad, or lonely, feelings may not be shared with others.

ASSESSMENT

Assessment cues for impaired verbal communication will arise as baseline data during history taking and physical assessment of a client. Because impaired verbal communication results from a variety of causes, the cues may be varied as well.

GENERAL ASSESSMENT OF VERBAL COMMUNICATION

Assess communication skills throughout the entire interview, health history, and physical examination. When obtaining the history and physical examination, assess the client's ability to respond to questions appropriately and communicate needs clearly. Take note if a significant other speaks for the client, and seek to understand the reason for this.

Health History. While obtaining the heath history, focus your questions to assess the client's ability to speak and comprehend the dominant language. If you see or hear cues that English is not the client's first language, the following questions may be used to elicit information about the client's verbal communication ability:

- What language is usually spoken in your home?
- How well do you speak, read, and write English?
- Is it important to observe any communication patterns in your family? (To whom should questions be directed?)
- Do you understand the meanings of common health terms?

If the client cannot speak or speech is unintelligible, you may have to rely on health records or an informant to obtain information about the client and any health problems. Ask how long the client has had the communication problem and whether its onset was associated with anything specific, such as medication use, illness, or other symptoms. Has the client tried anything to relieve the symptoms? Was it effective? Has speech improved or worsened since the onset of the problem?

If the problem is long term, ask whether the client has seen a physician or speech therapist. Determine whether treatment has been received for the problem. Does the client use any aids to assist speech or hearing?

The amount of information solicited depends on whether you are evaluating the problem to establish communication with the client, to help manage another nursing problem, or to determine the best course of action to correct the problem. Nurses may be interested primarily in determining the client's method of communication.

Physical Examination. If the client can speak, assess whether the communication problem is one of articulation, comprehension, coherence, or voice quality. A normal voice should have inflections and sufficient volume with clear speech. Difficulty in articulation could involve thought processes or functions of the tongue and lips in forming words.

Listen for slurred speech, poorly coordinated or irregular speech, a monotone or weak voice, stuttering, whispering, and a nasal, rasping, or hoarse tone. Pay particular attention to tone, clarity, vocal strength, vocabulary, sentence structure, and pace. Note errors in word choice. These will give clues to potential causes, which can facilitate diagnosis and intervention. For example, if the client's voice is hoarse or soft, it may indicate laryngitis, hypothyroidism, laryngeal cancer, or cranial nerve paralysis. A monotone voice may indicate deafness, depression, or a neurological problem such as multiple sclerosis. The client's vocabulary and word usage may offer clues to level of education or a cultural or language barrier. Slow, garbled speech or hesitant, deliberate speech may indicate a neurological disorder.

The physical examination includes examination of body systems that may be related to the inability to communicate, as well as a detailed mental status examination. For example, examine the client's mouth, nose, pharynx, and lungs to determine any physical cause of impaired communication. The examination should include evaluation of the client's neurological status; including assessment of the cranial nerves (V, VII, IX, X, XI, XII), hearing loss, and cognitive functioning as well.

Diagnostic Tests. Although no specific laboratory or diagnostic tests are available to assess speech or language disorders, the medical examination will include diagnostic tests aimed at detecting the underlying cause. The physician's neurological workup may include an imaging. Neuroimaging, including computed tomography scan (CT scan) and magnetic resonance imaging (MRI), is the mainstay for localizing and diagnosing the underlying cause and to rule out brain tumors or lesions. Because of the potentially serious nature of the underlying causes, the nurse has a role in providing supportive care to the client undergoing diagnosis.

Once the client's physical condition is stable, the physician may request a consult from a speech-language pathologist to assess the client's speech and language function and make recommendations to the health care team to facilitate communication. Assess the client's speech to plan appropriate interventions to facilitate communication.

FOCUSED ASSESSMENT FOR *IMPAIRED VERBAL COMMUNICATION*

Defining Characteristics. Having assessed the client's speech patterns and ability to communicate, you have already identified the defining characteristics. From the multiple factors associated with the diagnosis *Impaired verbal communication*, you can see that the defining characteristics can be grouped on the basis of the underlying cause. Each of these groups requires further assessment.

- The client either speaks no English or speaks English as a second language.
- A child has a delay in the development of language or has developed speech problems.
- An adult or child has lost the use of language because of neurological damage.
- An adult or child has lost the ability to verbally communicate secondary to medical illness or treatment (lacks the strength to speak, surgically altered vocal cords, presence of tracheostomy tube, and so on).
- The client can communicate verbally but lacks skills in communication, vocabulary, or knowledge.
- The client has psychotic thinking.

Related Factors. *Impaired verbal communication* may be related to a variety of factors. Related factors might include neurological injury, anatomical alterations, psychological barriers, developmental problems, or cultural differences. The related factor determines the appropriate nursing interventions.

Neurological Injury. Injury to brain cells may be related to a variety of neurological conditions, such as a cerebrovascular accident (stroke), rupture of an intracranial aneurysm (weakening of an arterial wall in the brain), an arteriovenous malformation in the brain (congenital defect resulting in a tuft of arteries and veins), or brain tumor (malignant or benign). Head trauma may also result in injury to the speech centers in the brain. Blood clots located in other parts of the body (such as the heart or lungs) may dislodge, travel to the brain, and injure brain cells by blocking their blood supply.

Depending on the area of the ischemic injury to the brain, the client may present with different forms of impaired verbal communication, such as aphasia. Such a client may easily become frustrated and withdrawn.

Aphasia. **Aphasia** is a language disorder that results from brain damage or disease that involves speech centers in the brain. It causes a variety of difficulties in formulating, expressing, and understanding language. Aphasia is classified according to the speech area affected. Assessment guidelines for aphasia are presented in Table 39-1. Paraphasia, neologism, or both may be present. **Paraphasia** is a word substitution problem of the aphasic client who speaks fluently. **Neologism,** the creation of new words that are meaningless to the listener, is a common language problem of the aphasic client.

Broca's (expressive) aphasia. Damage to the motor association area of the brain results in Broca's aphasia, also called expressive aphasia. The resulting communication problems may include difficulty with oral expression, especially spontaneous conversation. Speech is slow and monotonous, with short phrases or telegraphic speech. **Telegraphic speech** is telegram-like speech that lacks grammatical elements, such as articles, prepositions, and conjunctions. "Mommy come" for "Mommy is coming" is an example of telegraphic speech. Words may be composed of inappropriate sounds and have inappropriate meaning.

Written deficits usually parallel speech deficits. Clients with Broca's aphasia usually have weakness of the face. They may also have paresis of the right arm because damage may extend into adjacent motor areas of the brain responsible for upper extremity movement on the opposite side of the body.

People with Broca's aphasia typically retain their comprehension of written and spoken language. Usually, the affected client is aware of the deficit in communication ability—an awareness that can lead to frustration and depression.

Wernicke's (receptive) aphasia. Damage in the auditory associations of the brain results in impaired auditory comprehension known as Wernicke's aphasia or receptive aphasia. The client speaks fluently but uses neologisms or made-up words. Paraphasias or word substitutions may be used, such as *spoot* for *spoon*. Often, the client is unaware of the deficit and may become annoyed with other people who, as far as the client knows, should be able to understand what he or she says. Written deficits parallel the speech deficits. The client may write many words, but they make little or no sense.

Global aphasia. Global aphasia is the most severe form of aphasia and results from extensive damage to the dominant hemisphere (both Broca's and Wernicke's areas). Global aphasia results in both expressive and re-

Table 39-1 Assessment Guidelines for Aphasia

ASSESSMENT AREA	ASSESSMENT STEPS	RATIONALE
Word comprehension	Ask the person to point to objects in the room or to body parts as you name them.	Word comprehension is impaired in some but not all kinds of aphasia. Deficiencies in vision, hearing, and intellectual capacity may also affect performance.
	Ask a series of questions that can be answered with "yes" or "no" or with an appropriate head movement, such as, "Are you sitting on a chair?"	
Repetition	Ask the person to repeat items of increasing length and complexity, from monosyllabic words to sentences. Note the fluency and accuracy of the response.	Repetition is impaired in some but not all kinds of aphasia.
Naming	Ask the person to repeat items of increasing length and complexity, from monosyllabic words to sentences. Gradually increase the difficulty–from "hat" and "red" to "belt buckle" and "purple," for example. Note the fluency and accuracy of the response.	Naming is impaired in some but not all kinds of aphasia.
Reading comprehension	Write several simple commands, each on a separate piece of paper in large clear print, such as CLOSE YOUR EYES and RAISE YOUR HAND.	Failure in reading comprehension often accompanies failure in word comprehension, but each may occur independently. Keep in mind that a person's previous reading ability and educational experience affect performance.
Writing	Ask the person to make up and write a sentence about a topic, such as the room or the person's job or family. Note whether the sentence makes sense, has a subject and verb, and contains correctly spelled words.	Writing, like speech, is affected by some forms of aphasia. Motor impairment, such as hemiplegia, may affect performance.

Modified from Bickley, L. S., & Hoekelman, R. A. (2004). *Bates' guide to physical examination and history taking* (8th ed.). Philadelphia: Lippincott Williams & Wilkins.

ceptive aphasia. The client cannot comprehend spoken language or articulate or write words. Table 39-2 compares the different types of aphasia.

Dysarthria. Dysarthria is a speech articulation problem. It results from trauma or neuromuscular disease that impairs neuromuscular control of the muscles of the face, oral cavity, and larynx. The client may have trouble manipulating the tongue, lips, soft palate, jaw, and vocal folds. You may detect this problem as slurred, labored, sluggish, weak, or hypernasal speech. The client may also have trouble chewing or swallowing or may drool. Comprehension of language and ability to select words and form sentences are not affected.

Dysphonia (Aphonia). Dysphonia, also known as aphonia, is a disorder of voice volume, quality, or pitch. The client may be hoarse or speak in a whisper. It results from damage or disease involving the larynx or the vagus nerve (cranial nerve X). Examples include laryngitis, laryngeal tumors, and unilateral vocal cord paralysis. Voice articulation and language are unimpaired.

Anatomical Alterations. Physical barriers—such as an endotracheal tube, tracheostomy, or tumor—commonly impair verbal communication. An endotracheal tube is a temporary physical barrier to communication used to maintain a patent airway or for alteration in breathing patterns. A tracheostomy is a temporary or permanent upper-airway diversion that results in altered speech production. A temporary tracheostomy is a surgical procedure performed to maintain a patent airway for a short period of time. A tracheostomy tube is inserted via a surgical incision into the trachea and secured.

A client who has a *total laryngectomy,* which is the surgical removal of the larynx performed primarily for laryngeal cancer, requires a permanent tracheostomy. The upper airway is diverted and separated from the pharynx and esophagus, and the trachea is brought out through the skin of the neck and sutured in place, creating a permanent stoma (opening). The client has a permanent alteration in speech production.

Action Alert! Establish an alternate means of communication before the client undergoes tracheostomy.

A client with a new, temporary or permanent tracheostomy will not be able to communicate needs verbally and may use hand or facial gestures as a means to communicate. This client may become anxious or frustrated by an inability to communicate and may become depressed and withdraw from social interactions.

Psychological Illness. A client with a psychiatric disorder may have trouble communicating with other people. During assessment, you may notice that the client has loose associations or flights of ideas that make communication difficult. The client may not be able to find the right words, identify objects, name words, or speak in sentences. Furthermore, there may be stuttering or slurring of words.

Clients with psychological barriers to communication may have a history of drug and alcohol abuse and present in a state of alcohol intoxication or drug overdose. Other causes of psychiatric barriers to communication might include bipolar disorder, psychosis, or anxiety states.

Developmental Factors. Language problems in children can be caused by cognitive, environmental, family, or cultural factors. Proper speech patterns and language are best learned in an environment rich in the use of language. Slow cognitive development is associated with language disorders. Speaking a foreign language in the home and the dominant language at school can interfere with learning both languages.

Speech disorders are also associated with physical problems, such as hearing deficits, cleft lip, cleft palate, cerebral palsy, or such psychological disorders as severe deprivation or autism. Speech problems can be idiopathic. The routine well-child examination should include assessment for the development of speech and language problems.

Cultural Differences and Language Barriers. The nurse almost certainly will encounter clients from different cultures who do not speak the same language. A language barrier may occur when the nurse and the client do not speak the same language. Each may be fluent in his or her own language, but they fail to understand each other.

When either the nurse or the client can speak the other's language, but not fluently, a risk is that they think they understand each other when in fact they do not. This problem could cause misunderstanding about possibly crucial information.

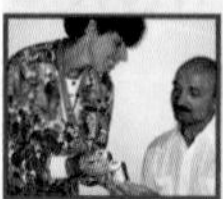

Recall the case study about Señor Martinez and his wife introduced at the beginning of the chapter. Neither Juan nor his wife is fluent in English. The nurse is concerned about their ability to understand information regarding the treatment of tuberculosis. There is a great risk for misunderstanding and failure to adhere to the health care regimen.

Clients who do not speak the dominant language of those in the health care delivery system, or do not speak it fluently, may become anxious or frustrated trying to communicate needs to health care team members. They may give responses that they think the nurse wants to hear. In other words, the clients may express values and beliefs perceived to be the nurse's rather than their own. To help detect language and cultural barriers during assessment, watch carefully for incongruities. For example, notice inconsistencies between verbal and nonverbal communication; clients may nod in agreement while their eyes reflect questioning.

Action Alert! Assess the client's level of understanding regarding condition and care. The risk for misunderstanding is great when the client and the nurse speak each other's languages somewhat, but not fluently. Ask clients to repeat, rephrase, summarize—yes and no responses do not adequately reflect comprehension.

Language differences are not the only communication difficulties for the client and the nurse; there are also dif-

Table 39-2 Comparison of Broca's, Wernicke's, and Global Aphasia

	BROCA'S (EXPRESSIVE) APHASIA	WERNICKE'S (RECEPTIVE) APHASIA	GLOBAL APHASIA
Qualities of spontaneous speech	• Not fluent • Slow; client uses few words and expends great effort to speak. • Inflection and articulation are impaired, but words are meaningful, with nouns, transitive verbs, and important adjectives. Small grammatical words are often dropped.	• Fluent, often rapid, voluble, and effortless • Inflection and articulation are good, but sentences lack meaning and words are malformed (paraphasias) or invented (neologisms). • Speech may be incomprehensible.	• Nonfluent
Comprehension	• Fairly good	• Impaired	• Impaired
Repetition	• Impaired (struggles to speak)	• Impaired due to paraphasia (e.g., saying *pink* for *sink*)	• Impaired
Naming	• Impaired, although the client recognizes objects	• Impaired	• Impaired
Oral reading and reading comprehension	• Good to poor	• Severely impaired	• Severely impaired
Writing	• Paucity of written output	• Severely impaired; meaningless writing	• Severely impaired

Modified from Bickley, L. S. (2004). *Bates' guide to physical examination and history taking* (8th ed.). Philadelphia: Lippincott Williams & Wilkins.

ferences in cultural expression. Cultural expression includes nonverbal mannerisms, values, beliefs, and customs. Box 39-2 provides an example of a Mexican American client's values. An understanding of cultural values can aid in the overall communication process.

DIAGNOSIS

When obtaining the client's history, assess risk factors for impaired communication and the presence of diagnostic cues that might indicate an impaired verbal communication. See the decision tree in Figure 39-4 for making a communication nursing diagnosis.

Clients may present with other nursing diagnoses that are related to the effects of impaired communication. A client who is unable to express thoughts may become depressed and withdraw from social interactions. The focus of care for this client would be the nursing diagnosis of *Impaired social interaction*. For the client with a new laryngectomy, *Anxiety* or *Powerlessness* related to an inability to communicate needs may be a concern, and the nursing care would be directed toward these diagnoses.

BOX 39-2 *Cross-Cultural Care*

Caring for a Mexican American Client and His Family

Señor Martinez and his wife, the client whose story we are following, are Mexican Americans. They immigrated to the United States and settled in western Kansas where other Mexican American families have found work in beef-packing plants. Mexican Americans tend to be a close-knit, family-oriented group. Sr. Martinez and his wife live in a small house with their extended family. They speak primarily Spanish, as do most of their friends and neighbors. Their culture is primarily Roman Catholic in its religious beliefs, which is evident in the religious items in Sr. Martinez's room. The following values tend to be important to the Mexican American client and family:

- Close-knit family relationships, in which the father is the head of the house. Other family members are subordinate to him.
- Social activities revolve around family activities.
- The primary language is Spanish.
- Touch is a common expression among members of the same sex.
- Privacy and confidentiality are valued.
- Religious practices and rituals are maintained during illness, death, or dying.
- Life events are viewed as the "will of God."
- Illness may be viewed as punishment from God.
- Folk medicine may be used.

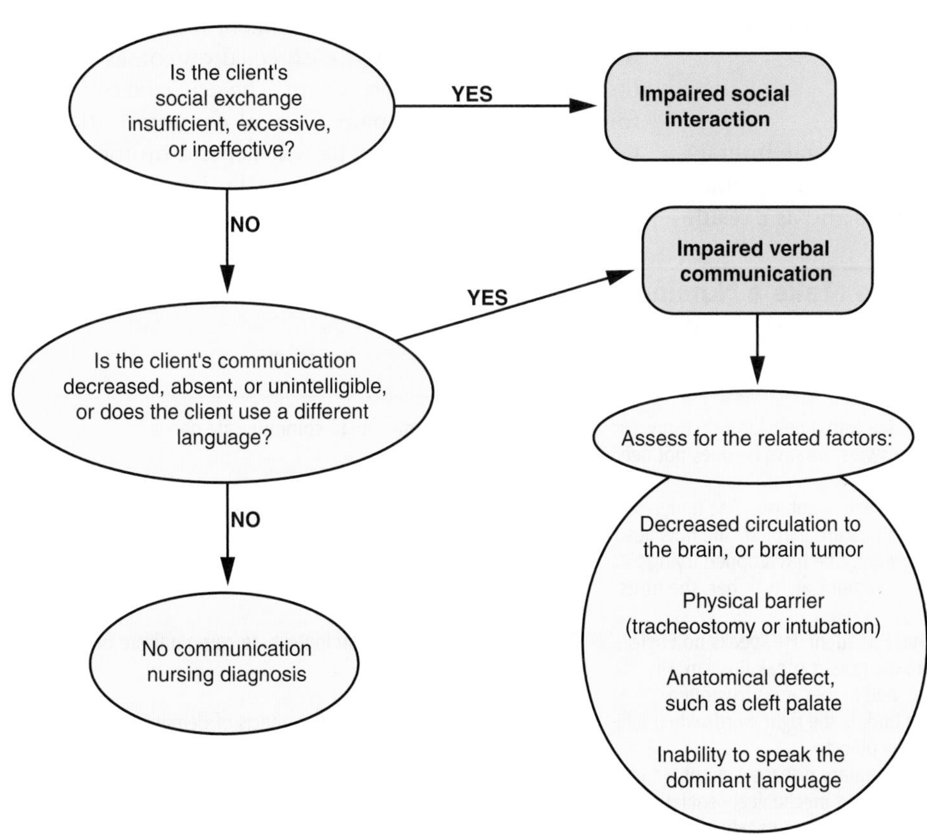

FIGURE 39-4 Decision tree for communication nursing diagnoses. Diagnoses are shown in rectangles. Within these rectangles, diagnoses shown in **bold** type are NANDA International (NANDA-I)–approved nursing diagnoses; diagnoses shown in regular type are not NANDA-I–approved nursing diagnoses.

Be alert to diagnostic cues to accurately diagnose each situation and plan care on the basis of these assessment findings. Table 39-3 provides examples of clustering data to make appropriate nursing diagnoses.

ANXIETY

Anxiety is a common response to an impaired ability to communicate, no matter what the cause. When a client has been able to communicate freely, the sudden loss of that ability is frightening. An alternative method to communicate must be developed to lessen the client's anxiety.

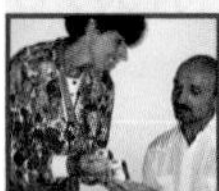

When Juan Martinez arrives on the unit, he is placed on respiratory isolation precautions. He and his wife do not understand the reason why visitors must wear a mask in Juan's room. They become anxious, fearing something terrible has happened to him.

POWERLESSNESS

Powerlessness is not an unusual feeling for a client with *Impaired verbal communication* related to a cerebrovascular accident, a language or cultural barrier, or a tracheostomy. Refusing to eat, to cooperate with care, and to make eye contact are strategies that clients sometimes use to try to gain control in situations in which they feel powerless.

SITUATIONAL LOW SELF-ESTEEM

The client with *Impaired verbal communication* related to aphasia, a tracheostomy, or a language or cultural barrier may also have *Low self-esteem*. Observe the client for direct or indirect expressions of negative feelings about loss of abilities.

IMPAIRED SOCIAL INTERACTION

Assess the client's ability to maintain social interaction. The client may become frustrated and embarrassed about poor communication skills and as a result may decrease social interactions with family and friends. Also assess the degree to which family and friends have the skills to maintain interactions with the client. Friends may feel uncomfortable initiating interactions and may be frustrated by their inability to communicate effectively or help the impaired person. Friends may withdraw and decrease their social interaction with the client.

INEFFECTIVE ROLE PERFORMANCE

Assess the client's ability to maintain usual roles. This includes assessment of the degree to which the spouse or significant other is obliged to take over the client's usual roles and how that change affects the ability of the family unit to function.

PLANNING

After appropriate nursing diagnoses and related factors have been identified for the client with *Impaired verbal communication,* make a plan of care with the client that includes short-term and long-term goals. Short-term goals include establishing an effective communication plan to meet the client's basic needs. Long-term goals include helping the client live with impaired communication or engage in speech therapy to learn to speak.

EXPECTED OUTCOMES FOR *IMPAIRED VERBAL COMMUNICATION*

The causes of *Impaired verbal communication* are varied, so the nurse will need to write expected outcomes to meet the specific needs of each client. The expected outcomes for the client with impaired verbal communication related to injury to brain cells will depend on the client's unique deficits. An appropriate goal might be a return of speech and language to a functional level.

Table 39-3 Clustering Data to Make a Nursing Diagnosis

Impaired Verbal Communication

DATA CLUSTER	DIAGNOSIS
A 52-year-old man is in his first postoperative day with a new laryngectomy. His call light is on frequently. When the nurse answers, he says he does not need anything.	*Anxiety* related to inability to communicate needs
A 66-year-old woman with a new stroke has expressive aphasia. She understands what people are saying, but her responses are garbled. She now lies in bed with her head turned away from the door. She has stopped trying to communicate, and, when someone tries to communicate with her, she turns her head or closes her eyes.	*Impaired social interaction* related to inability to respond understandably
A Russian man is admitted after a motor vehicle accident. He speaks no English and has no relatives living nearby. None of the nurses speak Russian. His attempts to communicate are unsuccessful, and he becomes frustrated.	*Powerlessness* related to an inability to communicate needs
A 78-year-old man with dementia has trouble finding the right words when talking. He also has trouble recognizing everyday objects.	*Impaired memory* related to the effects of dementia
A client with a history of chronic obstructive pulmonary disease is admitted in respiratory distress, which results in intubation and mechanical ventilation. He attempts to speak to the nurse but is unable to communicate his needs.	*Impaired verbal communication* related to anatomical barriers

The client with an anatomical alteration, such as a tracheostomy or endotracheal tube, needs to learn alternative methods to communicate. This could be either a temporary or a permanent means of communication.

For a language barrier, the goal might be that the client communicates needs through an interpreter. If the communication impairment is related to a cultural barrier, the expected outcome would be that the client expresses health beliefs and cultural practices that are of importance.

Other expected outcomes appropriate for impaired verbal communication might include the following:

- Family members and friends learn techniques to promote communication.
- The client communicates needs effectively with minimal frustration.
- The client demonstrates effective use of adaptive equipment.
- The client uses appropriate resources to facilitate learning alternative forms of communication.
- The client uses alternative forms of communication.
- The client explains the relationship of causative factors, such as alcohol, to the inability to communicate.
- The client uses self-help groups and other resources to help with a psychological disorder.
- The client consistently communicates ideas to staff and family.
- The client comprehends written and verbal language.
- The client responds to verbal and auditory stimuli.
- The client uses available resources to help facilitate speech and language abilities.
- The client and family or significant other can communicate at a satisfactory level.

INTERVENTION

Interventions for *Impaired verbal communication* will be aimed at improving verbal communication and assisting in resolution of related nursing diagnoses. The following section describes some general guidelines for intervention in an area that typically requires specialized knowledge and skills.

INTERVENTIONS TO PROMOTE VERBAL COMMUNICATION

Intervening to promote verbal communication requires an individual approach that relates to the cause of the impairment. To intervene appropriately, work both independently and interdependently with others as appropriate.

Using a Team Approach. A team approach is often necessary for impaired verbal communication. Team members might include a speech-language pathologist, interpreter, psychiatric clinical nurse specialist, occupational therapist, physician, psychiatrist, and nurse, depending on the cause of the client's impairment.

If the client has sustained an injury to brain cells or a permanent anatomical alteration, a team approach, involving a speech-language pathologist, physician, and nurse, will be needed. Typically, the speech-language pathologist diagnoses the specific communication disorder. Together, the team then develops a plan of care to help the client communicate. The speech-language pathologist helps the client relearn effective communication patterns and provides guidance and direction to the team for promoting speech and language communication.

Even though the speech-language pathologist works with the client on a daily basis, the nurse will be with the client for extended periods of time and is responsible for the continuity of care. Always follow the speech-language pathologist's instructions when interacting with the client. Also, teach the family and significant other the recommended communication techniques to provide continuity of care.

A team approach is also used for clients with *Impaired verbal communication* related to psychological and cultural barriers. If the communication disorder is related to a cultural barrier, an interpreter may be a part of the team. For a psychological communication disorder, a psychiatrist or psychiatric clinical nurse specialist may be part of the team, as well as an occupational therapist. The nurse is responsible for coordination and ensuring that the plan is implemented and evaluated.

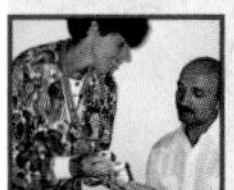

Sr. Martinez's nurse consults an interpreter who speaks Spanish. The interpreter facilitates communication between the client and the nurse. The nurse directs questions to Sr. Martinez and his wife instead of to the interpreter. Through the use of the interpreter, a plan of care is developed for the client and his family. What factors would you consider in selecting a Spanish-speaking interpreter for Sr. Martinez and his family?

Providing a Supportive Atmosphere. Provide a supportive atmosphere to encourage the client to verbalize. Be aware of verbal, *paraverbal*, and nonverbal language. *Paraverbal communication* refers to the manner in which a person speaks; it includes voice tone, pitch, intonation, and body language. It is important to treat the client as an adult and not as a child or someone with poor intelligence. Assume the client can understand. Do not talk about the client in his or her presence. Encourage client verbalization by praising and acknowledging the client's successes. This will help motivate the client to continue efforts at communicating.

Action Alert! Avoid talking down to clients with aphasia.

Listening Actively. Active listening focuses on the feelings of the person speaking as well as nonverbal cues. Take time to listen, and focus total attention on what the client is saying. Pay attention, and keep your mind from wandering. Sit down, face the client, and maintain eye contact. Listen without making judgments. These behaviors facilitate the development of trust between the client and you.

When listening, notice incongruities between the verbal, nonverbal, and paraverbal communication. For example, if the client says, "Oh, I'm fine!" but facial expression is tense and hands are clenched, there is incongruity between behavior and the spoken word that requires further assessment.

> ***Action Alert!*** Listen actively; seek ways to verify that communication has been accurately interpreted.

Helping the Client Practice Speech. Interventions to help the client practice speech are related to the cause of the client's impaired verbal communication. A caring, gentle approach may encourage the client to keep trying.

Broca's (Expressive) Aphasia. The client with Broca's aphasia has difficulty with expression, and your interventions will aim to improve speech. Delay communication when the client is tired or frustrated. In the beginning, to decrease anxiety, ask only questions that require a yes or no answer or a movement of the head.

One method of improving speech is through repeated practice of verbalization. Encourage the client to speak by use of automatic speech or imitation speech. Ask the client to say prayers or engage in social conversation, such as "Hello," "How are you?" and "I am fine."

Speech may also be facilitated by the use of special techniques, such as self-talk, parallel talk, expansion talk, and cueing. Self-talk involves talking about the activity as it is performed. Parallel talk is similar to self-talk and involves describing the activity the client is simultaneously doing with the nurse. Both self-talk and parallel-talk facilitate association of specific words with the activity.

Expansion talk is a technique that increases the complexity of verbalization by adding to the statement. However, it requires the nurse to seek validation that expansion of the client's statement has occurred. Cueing is a technique to help the client verbalize words. Cueing may be done in several ways, such as pronouncing the first syllable of the word, showing a printed version of the word, or presenting sentence completion tasks to fill in the missing word. Cue cards are often used, and repetition greatly improves communication.

Simplifying communication while at the same time providing adequate stimulation will facilitate verbal expression. Introduce ideas one at a time using short sentences that contain simple, common words. Limit choices. Speak slowly but naturally.

Depending on the location and severity of the injury, clients with Broca's aphasia can sometimes communicate in writing. Assess the client's ability to do so.

> ***Action Alert!*** Allow ample time for the client to respond. Do not respond for the client if the client has the ability to respond. Giving the client a chance to respond will increase the client's self-esteem and decrease frustration.

Wernicke's (Receptive) Aphasia. The client with receptive aphasia will have difficulty interpreting auditory, somatic, and visual input, which results in faulty interpretation of stimuli. Speech may be intact but inappropriate. The client may be confused and frustrated. To intervene, control the environment and limit sensory stimuli when communicating. Reducing distractions will improve comprehension. Be sure to get the client's attention before attempting to communicate, for example, touch the client's shoulder, or call the client's name.

> ***Action Alert!*** Limit environmental stimuli and reduce distractions to increase comprehension in the client with receptive aphasia.

Also, limit the use of adjectives, adverbs, and prepositions to increase the clarity of communication. Use short, simple sentences. When repeating a phrase, use the same words, speaking slowly and clearly. Assess the client for clues that indicate understanding. Reinforce appropriate responses. Alternative forms of communication—such as gestures, pictures, and communication boards—may be useful tools for some clients.

Dysarthria. The client with dysarthria may have difficulty with speech articulation. Collaborate with the speech-language pathologist to develop an effective method of communication. Many factors can affect the client's communication, such as fatigue and the rate of the conversation. If the speech is too quick, encourage the client to slow down and use shorter phrases or single words. Ask the client to repeat or rephrase what is not understood. Listen attentively, and provide visual or verbal feedback that indicates comprehension of the client's communication. Encourage the client to use gestures to increase comprehension.

Language and Cultural Barriers. A speech-language pathologist can help the client learn accent modification if the primary language is not the dominant language. This helps modify speech sounds and melodic differences that affect intelligibility.

Developing a Communication Plan. Collaborate with family and other members of the health care team to develop a communication plan. Experiment with different methods of communication to determine which is most effective. Share the plan with the client, family, and other members of the health care team to provide continuity of care.

In communicating with clients of varying educational levels, it is important to use a common language. Assess the client's knowledge by noting responses to questions, the ability to discuss health problems, and questions asked. Use words and phrases congruent with the client's educational level to promote interest, attention, and understanding.

Providing Alternative Forms of Communication. It may be necessary to find an alternative form of communication. For example, teach the client to blink, nod, or tap an appropriate response to a yes or no question. Phrase questions so they can be answered with a yes or no. Consider using an assistive device, such as an alphabet board, picture board, magic slate, computerized communication device such as an intelligent keyboard, or a communication board (Figure 39-5). However, these assistive devices may not be appropriate for a person with neuromuscular disease or with weakened or paralyzed arms. Encourage the use of gestures or pantomime.

Before a client receives a tracheostomy, explain to the client and significant other that speaking ability will be lost after surgery. Develop with the client and significant other an alternative method of communication to lessen anxiety. Again, alternative forms of communication might include a magic slate, an alphabet board, a picture board, or pencil and paper. Demonstrate the chosen techniques to the client and significant other before surgery.

If the change will be long term or permanent, a speech-language pathologist will also meet with the client before surgery to discuss long-term methods of effective speech. Esophageal speech or a mechanical device called an electrolarynx is an effective alternative for clients with a permanent tracheostomy.

Esophageal speech is produced by eructation of swallowed air while the client articulates words with the mouth. Speech rehabilitation should begin as soon as possible after surgery. Clients who cannot master esophageal speech can use an electrolarynx. If a laryngectomy has not been performed, the client may use a tracheostomy plug to facilitate communication, if tolerated.

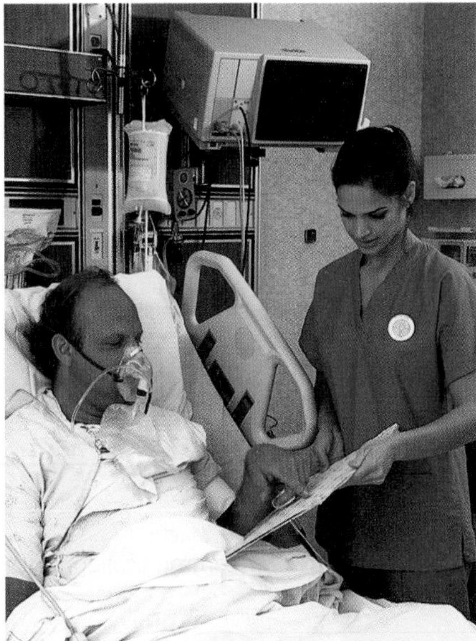

FIGURE 39-5 A nurse and speech-impaired client using a communication board. The client points to the picture that illustrates his need.

After surgery, provide the client with a call light and answer it immediately and in person. Leave a note at the central call-light system that the client is unable to speak. Check the client every 1 to 2 hours. Encourage the client to communicate, and allow adequate time to write words or select pictures. Do not answer questions for the client or finish the client's sentences.

If a laryngectomy has been done, provide the client with information about a laryngectomy club or support group. Before surgery, a visit by a person who has had a laryngectomy may be appropriate. Encourage the client and significant other to attend support meetings.

> ***Action Alert!*** Provide a call light to the client who has had a laryngectomy. Answer the call light immediately to decrease anxiety.

Orienting the Client to Reality. The client who is experiencing impaired verbal communication may also experience confusion related to this unfamiliar state. As needed, orient the client to person, place, and time. Ask orientation questions, such as, "Do you know where you are?" and provide the information factually. Also provide orienting information, such as, "You are in (name the health care facility) because. . . ."

Structure the client's environment and routine. Set a daily schedule. Orient the client to the schedule frequently. Encourage the family to bring in familiar pictures and objects. Provide a clock and calendar large enough for the client to see. Keep the clock and calendar current. Write the shift caregiver names on a wall board in the client's room, if available.

Using an Interpreter. When encountering a client from a different culture, assess for a language or cultural barrier. Observe the client's nonverbal communication. This baseline assessment is critical because language and cultural barriers can obstruct nursing care. If the nurse and the client do not speak the same language, the client may not understand explanations of procedures and treatment. Language barriers also raise an ethical concern for the client who cannot fully understand a consent form or the teaching related to an informed consent that must be solicited before a test, procedure, or surgery. A trained medical interpreter may help the nurse communicate information about tests, procedures, and interventions.

> ***Action Alert!*** When using an interpreter, always direct your questions and attention to the client, not the interpreter.

Use caution when determining whether to use bilingual family, friends, or other institutional employees to interpret. These well-meaning individuals may have different language abilities and may or may not understand medical terms. The request may cause embarrassment to both the client and the potential interpreter and raises potential issues of confidentiality. Become familiar with agency policy regarding use of interpreters to uphold the standard of care for each client. See Box 39-3 for additional information.

Likewise, always consider the client's cultural and health beliefs when planning and implementing care. If interventions do not correspond to health beliefs or culture, the client may not consent to treatment or comply with it after discharge.

INTERVENTIONS FOR RELATED NURSING DIAGNOSES

Impaired verbal communication will affect other aspects of the client and significant other's life. Nursing diagnoses related to impaired communication include *Anxiety, Powerlessness, Low self-esteem, Impaired social interaction, Social isolation,* and *Ineffective role performance.* Interven-

BOX 39-3

Nursing Care Plan

A Client With a Language Barrier

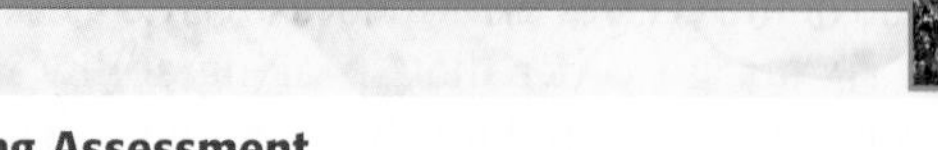

Admission Data

Sr. Martinez is admitted to the respiratory unit and placed under respiratory isolation precautions for tuberculosis. The nurse explains respiratory isolation precautions to him and his wife. As she does so, she points to pictures of the precautions on the isolation card. She then hands Sra. Martinez a mask. During the explanation, they both nod their heads and smile, but afterward they look at each other with questioning eyes. They speak to each other in Spanish and shrug their shoulders. Sra. Martinez obediently places the mask on her face.

Admitting Physician's Orders

Instruct client and wife regarding respiratory precautions.
Sputum culture for acid-fast bacillus (AFB)
Medications: rifampin, 600 mg PO daily; isoniazid, 300 mg PO daily; pyrazinamide, 2000 mg PO daily

Nursing Assessment

When the nurse enters Sr. Martinez's room to obtain the history and physical assessment, she finds Sra. Martinez in the room without the mask. When the nurse asks why Sra. Martinez is not wearing the mask, she looks questioningly back at the nurse. The nurse begins to collect data and asks, "Do you understand English?" Both respond, "si," and nod their heads.

The nurse continues to gather data regarding her ability to communicate with the Martinezes and asks, "Do you speak English?" The wife responds "un pequito." Further questioning leads the nurse to believe that the Martinezes understand enough English to meet their basic needs but not enough to understand medical information. Neither the explanation for respiratory isolation precautions nor the reason for admission to the hospital was understood.

NANDA-I Nursing Diagnosis	NOC Outcomes With Indicators	NIC Interventions With Selected Activities	Evaluation Data
Impaired Verbal Communication	***Communication Ability***	***Communication Enhancement***	***After 24 Hours of Care***
Related Factor: • Cultural language barrier	• Client and wife will express needs through an interpreter.	• Use a Spanish interpreter to explain isolation precautions, the disease, and the treatment plan and to allow the client and wife to express needs and concerns.	• Sra. Martinez agreed to wear the mask. She asked several questions about tuberculosis and the planned treatment.
	• Client and wife will verbalize satisfaction with the communication process. • Client and wife relate feelings of reduced frustration and isolation.	• Allow adequate time for communication. Speak directly and confidentially to the client and wife.	• Sr. Martinez agreed to be treated. The interpreter translated information about isolation. • Sra. Martinez told the nurse, through the interpreter, that she had been frightened when they came to the hospital and that she is grateful for the interpreter and that her husband is being cared for.

Critical Thinking Questions

1. What feelings would you anticipate Sr. and Sra. Martinez to experience in a health care system in a foreign country where they cannot understand or speak the language?
2. How will you provide discharge teaching?
3. Write expected outcomes for communication of discharge teaching.

Nursing outcome and intervention labels from Johnson, M., Bulechek, G., Butcher, H., Dochterman, J. M., Maas, M., Moorhead, S., et al. (Eds.). (2006). *NANDA, NOC, and NIC linkages: Nursing diagnoses, outcomes, & interventions.* St. Louis, MO: Mosby.

tions are directed at helping the client and significant other resolve these diagnoses—or prevent impaired verbal communication in the first place—through teaching, social services, and support.

Teaching the Client and Family. The plan to promote verbal communication is developed by the interdisciplinary team, the client, and the family. Techniques to improve communication are taught to the client and family. These techniques are reinforced until the client and family can perform them.

Referring the Client to Social Services. Referral to social services can facilitate a smooth transition from the acute care facility to home. Social services can find assistance for services that home health care does not provide, such as housekeeping. They can also be helpful in finding financial assistance to pay for needed health care.

Promoting Social Support. A client who is experiencing social isolation or impaired social interaction because of impaired verbal communication will benefit from developing a social support network. As appropriate, refer the client and significant other to a self-help group, such as the Stroke Club, Lost Chords Society, Multiple Sclerosis Society, National Spinal Cord Injury Society, or International Society of Laryngectomies. These self-help groups provide tips and support to ease the role transition and improve the quality of relationships.

EVALUATION

Evaluate the expected outcomes specified in the nursing care plan to determine whether the nursing diagnoses have been resolved. Reassess the client to determine whether the expected outcomes have been met.

Box 39-3 illustrates a sample nursing care plan for Sr. Martinez, who is experiencing *Impaired verbal communication* related to language barrier.

In this example, the expected outcomes for *Impaired verbal communication* have been resolved. If the expected outcomes are not achieved or the client is not making progress toward achieving them, reassessment is essential to obtain additional information to explain the client's lack of progress. Expected outcomes may need to be rewritten to address the cause, and the plan of care may need to be revised to help meet the expected outcome.

Documentation in the nursing notes for the case study in this chapter might look like the one below.

Sample Documentation Note for Señor Martinez

At discharge, Sr. Martinez and his wife verbalize an understanding of respiratory isolation precautions, treatment, and prevention of the spread of disease. Each expresses satisfaction with the care provided and with the interpreter.

▼ KEY PRINCIPLES

- *Impaired verbal communication* may be related to injury to brain cells, anatomical alterations, developmental delays, psychological barriers, or language or cultural barriers.
- Aphasia results from damage to the speech centers in the brain and causes a loss of comprehension, speech production, or both.
- Broca's (expressive) aphasia causes difficulty with oral expression.
- Wernicke's (receptive) aphasia causes impaired auditory comprehension.
- Clients' responses to *Impaired verbal communication* are varied and related to psychosocial aspects of a person's life. Therefore the assessment cues are also varied.
- No specific diagnostic test is used to assess speech or language disorders. A speech-language pathologist may assist in the diagnosis.
- A team approach is used to develop a plan of care for the client with *Impaired verbal communication.*
- Interventions for *Impaired verbal communication* related to injured brain cells aim for a return of speech and language to a functional level and for an increase in social interaction.
- Interventions related to anatomical alterations in communication patterns aim to help the client learn alternative methods of communicating.
- Interventions for *Impaired verbal communication* related to psychological barriers aim to help the client learn to communicate needs to family and friends.
- Interventions to meet language and cultural barriers to communication aim to overcome those barriers through an interpreter and respectful responses to cultural differences.

■ REVIEW QUESTIONS

1. Communication is:

1. Described as a simple process in which information is exchanged between two people
2. An essential part of human interactions, beginning at birth and continuing throughout the life span
3. An exchange of information between and sender and receiver who have the same perceptions, beliefs, and interpretations of the world
4. Not an important aspect of the nurse-client relationship

2. Which of the following would not be involved in sound production in verbal communication?

1. The lungs
2. The larynx
3. The vocal cords
4. Wernicke's area

3. The nurse would assess for which of the following when determining lifestyle factors that affect a client's verbal communication?

1. Voice overuse, smoking, excessive alcohol, and allergies
2. Gender, illness, medications, and surgery
3. Nonverbal communication, facial expression, body posture, and touch
4. Education, self-concept, stress, and mood

4. Which of the following is a priority nursing diagnosis for a client with expressive aphasia?

1. Acute confusion
2. Impaired verbal communication
3. Decisional conflict
4. Impaired environmental interpretation syndrome

Continued

5. The nurse would take which of the following actions when working with a client who has aphasia?

1. Provide instructions to the client in a simplistic manner to ensure understanding.
2. Provide care to the client based on what the client says rather than on nonverbal cues.
3. Complete a client's thought to avoid frustration when the client has difficulty finding or expressing the "correct" word or phrase.
4. Arrange for an alternative form of communication, such as a word or picture board.

Bibliography

Ackley, B. J., Ladwig, G. B. (2006). *Nursing diagnosis handbook: A guide to planning care.* St. Louis, MO: Mosby.

*Adkins, E. R. H. (1991). Nursing care of clients with impaired communications. *Rehabilitation Nursing, 16*(3), 74-76.

Bickley, L. S. (2004). *Bates' guide to physical examination and history taking* (8th ed.). Philadelphia: Lippincott Williams & Wilkins.

*Buckwalter, K. C., Cusack, D., Kruckeberg, T., & Shoemaker, A. (1991). Family involvement with communication-impaired residents in long term care settings. *Applied Nursing Research, 4*(2), 77-84.

*Buckwalter, K. C., Cusack D., Sidles, E., Wadle, K., & Beaver, M. (1989). Increasing communication ability in aphasic/dysarthric patients. *Western Journal of Nursing Research, 11*(6), 736-747.

Dickerson, S. S., Stone, V. I., Panchura, C., & Usiak, D. J. (2002). The meaning of communication: Experiences with augmentative communication devices. *Rehabilitation Nurse, 27*(6), 215.

*Dillard, J. P., & Wilson, B. J. (1993). Communication and affect: Thoughts, feelings, and issues for the future. *Communication Research, 20*(5), 637-645.

*Geissler, E. M. (1991). Nursing diagnoses of culturally diverse patients. *International Nursing Review, 38*(5), 150-152.

*Geissler, E. M. (1992). Nursing diagnoses: A study of cultural relevance. *Journal of Professional Nursing, 8*(5), 301-307.

Greenbaum, M., Flores, G. (2004). Lost in translation. Professional interpreters needed to help hospitals treat immigrant patients. *Modern Healthcare, 34*(18), 21.

Jacobs, E. A., Shepard, D. S., & Suaya, J. A. (2004). Overcoming language barriers in health care: Costs and benefits of interpreter services. *American Journal of Public Health, 94*(5), 866-869.

Lokvig, J. (2004). Effective Alzheimer's communication. *Neurobiology of Aging, 25*(2), S334.

NANDA International. (2007). *Nursing diagnoses: Definitions and classification, 2006-2007* (7th ed.). Philadelphia: Author.

Robinson, M., & Phillips, P. (2003). An investigation into the perceptions of primary care practitioners of their education and developing needs for communicating with patients who may not be fluent in English. *Nurse Education Today, 23*(4), 286-298.

*Shames, G., Wiig, E., & Secord, W. (1998). *Human communication disorders: An introduction* (5th ed.). Boston: Allyn & Bacon.

Stokes, S. A., Gordan, S. E. (2003). Common stressors experienced by the well elderly. Clinical implications. *Journal of Gerontological Nursing, 29*(5), 38-46.

Williams, K., Kemper, S., Hummert, L. (2004). Enhancing communication with older adults: Overcoming elderspeak. *Journal of Gerontological Nursing, 30*(10), 17-25.

Yeo, S. (2004). Language barriers and access to care. *Annual Review of Nursing Research, 22*, 59-73.

Yoshinaga-Itano, C. (2004). Levels of evidence: Universal newborn hearing screening and early hearing detection and intervention system. *Journal of Communication Disorders, 37*(5), 451-465.

*Zemlin, W. R. (1998). *Speech and hearing science: Anatomy and physiology* (4th ed.). Boston: Allyn & Bacon.

*Asterisk indicates a classic or definitive work on this subject.

Chapter 40 MANAGING CONFUSION

Media Resources

- evolve Evolve Website http://evolve.elsevier.com/Harkreader/
- Companion CD

Learning Objectives

After studying this chapter, you should be able to do the following:

- Describe the concepts underlying acute or chronic confusion
- Identify the life span, physiological, cultural and lifestyle, environmental, and psychological factors affecting normal cognition
- Assess a client for risk of confusion, manifestations of confusion, and client responses to confusion
- Diagnose the problems of a confused client that are amenable to nursing care
- Plan goal-directed interventions to prevent, correct, and support a client with confusion
- Evaluate the outcomes of nursing care for the confused client and the client's caretakers

Key Terms

affect
agnosia
apraxia
attention
awareness
cognition
confusion
consciousness
delirium
delusions
dementia
executive function
hallucinations
judgment
memory
neurotransmitter
orientation
pseudodementia
sundown syndrome

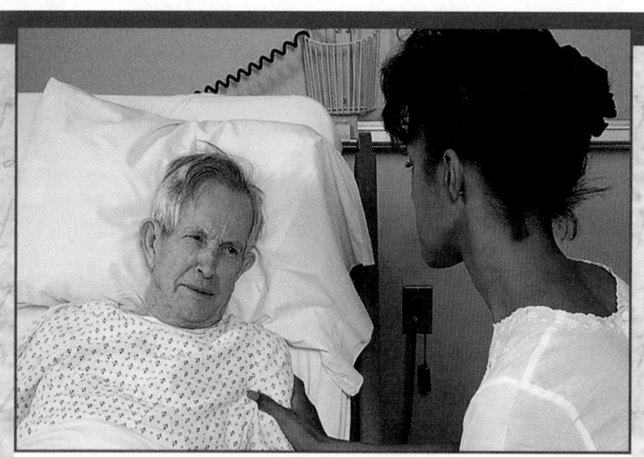

From Elkin M. K., Perry, A. G., & Potter, P. A. (2003). *Nursing interventions and clinical skills* (3rd ed.). St. Louis, MO: Mosby.

Mr. Tellis, an 83-year-old Greek American, was brought to the emergency department by ambulance with his daughter, Mary Appolos, who told the nurse that he had tried to climb out of the ambulance. He talked to the nurse in broken sentences in an incoherent manner. He could not tell the nurse where he was, where he lived, or what had happened to him. He frequently misperceived the door as a person standing nearby. He seemed agitated, terrified, and fearful of being harmed by people he believed were lurking near the door. He was unable to focus on the nurse's instructions. During one lucid moment, he looked at his daughter and said, "Oh, you take control." After saying this, he slumped into a semiconscious doze and was very difficult to arouse.

Mary told the nurse that he lived alone several blocks away from her home and had always been proud of his independence. He had never seen a family physician regularly, although he had had cataract surgery several years ago. Early the night before, Mary had talked to him on the phone. He said he was fine except that he was having "trouble with my water." Then, at about 3:00 AM, a neighbor called Mary to say that her father was "walking around the yard screaming at someone, but nobody's there." Mary came immediately to his house and called an ambulance, which brought her father to the emergency department.

Mary confided to the nurse, "It all happened so fast. He was fine. He wasn't even sick." Within an hour of Mr. Tellis's arrival, four additional family members had crowded into the emergency department requesting information about him.

This case study identifies major clues consistent with confusion. The nurse considers the nursing diagnosis of *Acute confusion* related to unknown etiology from the list of possible nursing diagnoses (see key nursing diagnoses box).

KEY NURSING DIAGNOSES FOR CONFUSION

Acute confusion: The abrupt onset of a cluster of global, transient changes and disturbances in attention, cognition, psychomotor activity, level of consciousness, and/or sleep-wake cycle

Chronic confusion: An irreversible, long-standing, and/or progressive deterioration of intellect and personality characterized by decreased ability to interpret environmental stimuli; decreased capacity for intellectual thought processes; and manifested by disturbances of memory, orientation, and behavior

CONCEPTS OF CONFUSION

Mental confusion is a mental state characterized by a lack of clear and orderly thought and behavior resulting from complex stimuli coupled with high anxiety, a psychiatric disorder, an acute physical illness, or irreversible changes in the brain. Nurses encounter confused clients in virtually all health care settings: acute care, long-term care, and community health care. Recognition of this disorder, initiation of treatment where possible, and administration of care and support to these clients and their families or caregivers is a concern for all professional nurses.

COGNITION

Cognition, or thought, is the process of knowing and interacting with the world. It includes awareness, attention, orientation, judgment, memory, executive function, and learning. Cognition takes place in the cerebral cortex, which is the outer layer or surface of the cerebral hemispheres.

Physiology of Cognition. The cerebral cortex is composed of billions of nerve cells called neurons, which are the primary units of the nervous system. A neuron has three components: a cell body (containing a nucleus), dendrites, and usually a single axon (Figure 40-1). Dendrites carry impulses toward the cell body. Axons carry nerve impulses away from the cell body. Neurons are arranged into networks that are interconnected by miles of axons and dendrites.

Neurons communicate with each other through a process called neurotransmission. Neural information passes between neurons across intercellular gaps—the spaces between neurons where neurotransmitters pass electrical information from neuron to neuron. **Neurotransmitters** are chemical messengers released from the synaptic terminal of a neuron at a chemical synapse that diffuses across the synaptic cleft and binds to and stimulates the postsynaptic membrane. The more than 50 neurotransmitters in the human body include acetylcholine, serotonin, dopamine, epinephrine, and norepinephrine. These chemicals are released from the axon, pass across the intercellular gap, and are received by the dendrite of the adjacent neuron. Each neurotransmitter fits into specific receptor sites embedded in the dendrite's membranes (Figure 40-2).

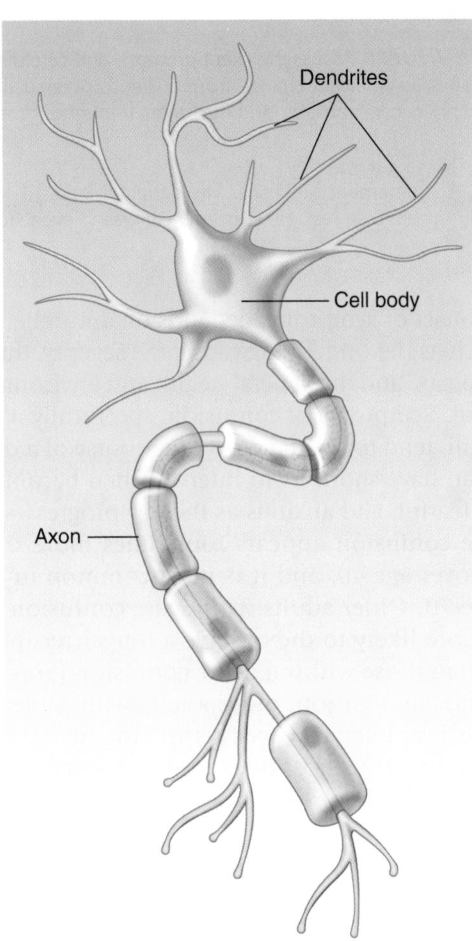

FIGURE 40-1 A neuron. The axon is protected by myelin-producing Schwann cells.

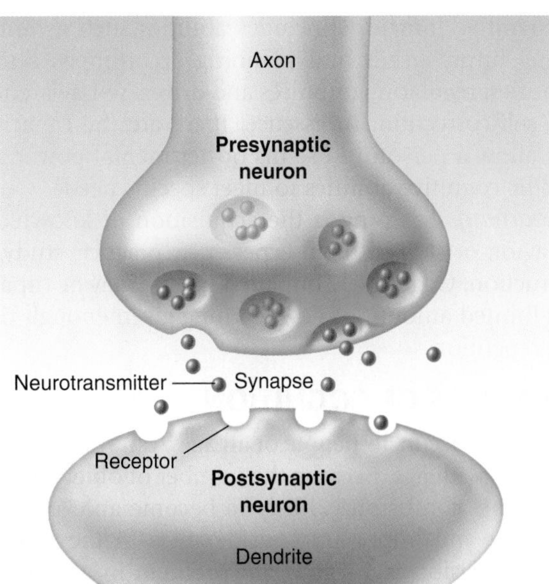

FIGURE 40-2 Neurotransmitters in the synapse make the electrical connection between the axon and the dendrite.

Neurotransmitters can either excite or inhibit action. This communication between brain cells enables human activity, body functions, consciousness, intelligence, creativity, memory, and emotion. The synthesis of neurotransmitters is influenced by the cerebral metabolism, oxygenation, and general health of the person, as well as by diet, drug use, and other factors.

By influencing neural impulses, neurotransmitters play an important role in cognition. Interruption or disruption of cerebral metabolism or cerebral oxygenation affects neurons, transmission of neural information, and, eventually, cognition and is often manifested by the appearance of confusion.

Components of Cognition. Cognition is a group of interrelated activities that begins with conscious awareness and culminates in complex judgments, memory, and learning. The basic components of cognition measured in the mental status examination include awareness, attention, orientation, judgment, memory, executive function, and learning.

Awareness. **Awareness,** or **consciousness,** is the state of being awake and alert enough to *react to environmental stimuli*. Being mentally cloudy, drowsy, lethargic, or unconscious are changes in the continuum of awareness.

Attention. **Attention** is the ability to focus on an object or activity. It involves the ability to maintain sensitivity to important stimuli as opposed to irrelevant stimuli. Attention also includes a person's ability to select or choose a focus or to shift attention at will.

Orientation. **Orientation** refers to an awareness of person, place, and time. An oriented client should be able to say not only who and where he or she is, but also what time it is.

Judgment. **Judgment** involves the ability to make rational decisions. It includes the ability to understand facts and draw inferences from relationships. On a basic level the question is, does the person use "good sense" to look both ways before crossing the street, dress appropriately for the weather, or lock the doors before going to bed. For example, if there is a fire in a wastebasket, a person with judgment makes a rational decision about whether to get out of the way or safely put out the fire.

Memory. **Memory** is the retention or storage of information learned about the world. The triad of memory includes remote (long-term), recent (short-term), and new memory (immediate recall). Long-term memory is memory of the distant past, or at least longer than several days. Short-term memory usually involves minutes or days. Immediate recall typically involves seconds or minutes.

Executive Function. **Executive function** refers to a constellation of cognitive abilities that include the ability to plan, organize, and sequence tasks and manage multiple tasks simultaneously; it includes self-monitoring and self-correcting behaviors. This very large category of cognitive functions includes abilities such as anticipating future needs and planning accordingly, setting priorities, regulating impulses and drives, self-awareness, and self-correction. In essence, these are the capacities that allow a person to use his or her mental power and specific cognitive abilities to meet specific needs.

Learning. Learning is the acquisition of knowledge, behavior, or skill through experience, practice, study, or instruction. Cognitively impaired people may be capable of a limited amount of new learning given enough time and repetition.

PROBLEMS OF COGNITION

Confusion occurs in people of all ages, but the incidence increases with age. Because the number of older adults is increasing, confusion is likely to become an even more prevalent and important consideration in the near future. Confusion is a significant problem in all areas of practice but has special significance in long-term and acute care nursing.

Confusion is a disturbance in one or more of the components of cognition. Confusion is not a disease but rather a syndrome of clinically observable problems. Acute and chronic confusion may appear singly or together. It is often the first or only indicator of serious illness, particularly in the older adult. Because it frequently appears at night, the evening or night nurse is most likely to be the first person to notice this symptom. Along with identifying the underlying cause, safety is a priority nursing concern. The client may try to leave the unit, climb out of bed, or pull out intravenous (IV) lines, sustaining a fall or injury in the process. Clients later identify the intense experience of acute confusion as traumatic.

Acute Confusion. Acute confusion is a medical emergency. It is associated with the medical diagnosis of **delirium,** which is a disturbance in consciousness and a change in cognition that develops over a short period of time (American Psychiatric Association, 2000). Acute confusion or delirium is a major disorder among hospitalized older adults, with occurrence rates estimated at 25% to 50% (Rapp and the Iowa Veteran's Affairs Research Consortium, 2001).

Nature of Acute Confusion. Acute confusion is a syndrome of observable, clinical symptoms, rather than a disease, representing a significant change from the client's previous level of functioning. Usually, acute confusion arises abruptly over hours and is fully developed within 3 days of onset. Family members or caregivers can be helpful in describing the onset of symptoms and previous functioning to establish that the client's confusion is a significant change.

Acute confusion can be a significant sign of many medically treatable disorders. It is sometimes the only early symptom of a serious disorder in older adults. For this reason, identification of the underlying cause or causes is imperative. Comprehensive assessment is important because confusion can have multiple causes.

Action Alert! Assess the client promptly and carefully if the confusion is a significant change from a client's previous level of functioning, occurs abruptly, and fluctuates throughout the day.

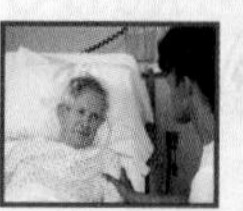

Remember Mr. Tellis? His daughter said, "It all happened so fast. He was fine. He wasn't even sick."

The onset of symptoms depends on a number of factors, such as the underlying cause, the severity, the number of causes, and the general health and environment of the client. Symptoms of confusion, specifically alertness to stimuli, tend to fluctuate over the course of a day. The client can have short, lucid intervals then become incoherent, fearful, and anxious as the day progresses.

Acute confusion appears four times more often in people over age 40, and it is most common in people over age 70. Older adults with acute confusion are six times more likely to die or have a longer recuperation phase than those without acute confusion (Foreman et al., 1999). In addition, older adults with acute confusion are less likely to ever return to their preillness health status. Thus hospitalization is longer, and nursing home admission is more frequently needed after hospitalization.

Acute confusion in hospitalized older adults tends to be a marker of a poor prognosis. If acute confusion is recognized and the underlying factors are treated promptly and appropriately, acute confusion usually disappears. However, if acute confusion is unrecognized and the underlying factors are left untreated, a chronic condition or death can be the result.

Chronic Confusion. Chronic confusion is long-standing, often an irreversible and progressive deterioration of cognition and personality. It is usually associated with the medical diagnosis **dementia,** which involves loss of multiple intellectual functions such as thinking, memory, and judgment severe enough to interfere with social, occupational, and functional activities. There are many forms of dementia; dementia of the Alzheimer's type is the most common.

Chronic confusion is characterized by a slowly progressive deterioration in cognitive ability. Symptoms usually progress in a stable, steady manner. Perceptual disturbances, sleep-wake alterations, and inattention may occur. Although chronic confusion is associated with progressive cognitive decline, sometimes it may be slowed or even halted by treating the underlying causes.

BARRIERS TO IDENTIFYING ACUTE CONFUSION

Acute confusion should be promptly recognized and treated. Beliefs and attitudes can be obstructions to the identification of acute confusion and distinguishing it from chronic confusion, especially in older adults.

The first barrier is the myth that memory loss and confusion is a normal part of aging. Some decline in memory occurs with aging, but acute confusion is a symptom of a serious underlying disorder that requires assessment and treatment. Anytime you see signs of confusion, you need to determine if it is a change from the client's previous level of function and assess for possible causes.

A second barrier can be failure to do a thorough mental status assessment. Assessment of the client's orientation to time, place, and person—in the absence of further assessment—can lead to misdiagnosis because the client may seem oriented but still be confused.

A third barrier is the tendency of the client to mask the early symptoms in chronic confusion. The client may use family or friends to compensate for failing memory and otherwise obscure the full extent of memory loss through pretending or making up information to fill in gaps in memory. This client may be able to hide the cognitive impairment from the nurse during a brief conversation; however, more thorough assessment will reveal the deficits. Failure to fully assess cognitive capacity may result in missed cues—and the opportunity to intervene while the disorder is still mild or even reversible. Only after the disorder borders on debilitating will it likely come to the attention of health care personnel.

A fourth barrier is a deficit in communication about the cognitive status of older adults through shift report and documentation. Mental status assessment must encompass 24 hours to detect changes that occur through the night and follow-up communication to the physician and the day nurse. Document a description of the behavior rather than using overlapping terms, loosely identified symptoms, or inexact descriptions. For example, inattention is not the same as "disoriented" and hypoalert is not the same as "drowsy."

FACTORS AFFECTING COGNITION

When the brain is deprived of oxygen, glucose, or other essential chemicals, the result may be a disruption in cognitive function. A number of factors may affect cognitive status, including life span, physiological, cultural and lifestyle, environmental, and psychological factors. They may be associated with acute confusion, chronic confusion, or both.

FACTORS ACROSS THE LIFE SPAN

Mental disabilities or retardation are leading causes for cognitive disability in childhood and adolescence. Examples of disorders of childhood and adolescence that may be associated with changes in cognition include elective mutism, obsessive-compulsive disorder, Tourette's syndrome, schizophrenia of childhood, conduct disorder, and mental retardation. In infants and small children hallucinations may occur with high fever. Acute confusion can be associated with a concussion or head injury, as well as a wide range of major illnesses. Impaired cognition can occur at any age, but it occurs most often in the older adult because the older brain is more susceptible to insults.

PHYSIOLOGICAL FACTORS

Physiological factors affecting cognition are extensive. They include traumatic injury and a wide range of physical illnesses, such as febrile conditions, hypoxia, metabolic disorders, infections, and fluid and electrolyte disturbances. Cardiovascular and respiratory disorders can affect cognition as well.

Physical Illness

Hypoxia. Hypoxia, or a decrease in oxygen supply, can occur in a number of medical conditions. For example, anemia can result from decreased numbers of red blood cells or a reduction in hemoglobin, causing mental confusion from inadequate cerebral tissue perfusion. Cardiac conditions can also lead to confusion by decreasing cardiac output and, in turn, reducing blood oxygen levels or increasing carbon dioxide levels, or both. When a client becomes acutely confused, hypoxia should be the first thing you rule out.

Infections. Very often, an older adult with a serious infection will have no sign of fever but will instead exhibit a change in mental status. The astute practitioner relies on past history and an understanding of age-related changes to guide assessment.

Fluid and Electrolyte Disturbances. Electrolyte imbalances, specifically involving sodium, can cause mental confusion and delirium. Restoring sodium levels to normal values and preventing further fluid imbalances are the goals of intervention.

Dehydration is a serious health problem, particularly in older adults. Conditions contributing to dehydration, such as heart failure, hypertension, renal disease, infections, and diarrhea, can result in confusion, disorientation, or a change in affect. Environmental conditions, such as hot weather, can lead rapidly to dehydration in the older adult, especially when combined with inadequate ventilation in the living space.

Medications. Prescription medications, over-the-counter (OTC) medications, and herbal preparations may be toxic, particularly to very young children and older adults. Disruptions in cognitive function may occur from taking the wrong drug, from a drug side effect, or from drug-drug or drug-alcohol interactions. Confusion may lead to further difficulty in taking medications properly.

Trauma. Traumatic injury to the brain may damage and change the structure of brain tissue. Specific symptoms depend on the area of the brain affected.

Metabolic Disorders. Metabolic disorders such as hypothyroidism because of decreased thyroid gland functioning may lead to progressive cognitive impairment. Cognitive loss may not be reversible, even after thyroid hormone replacement.

Neurobiological Factors. There are many types of dementia, and although the pathological conditions that cause the degeneration into chronic confusion are varied, the symptoms are similar. Following are some of the more common types of dementia.

Alzheimer's Disease. Alzheimer's dementia is characterized by cognitive deterioration that progresses slowly over months or years. Initially, there is a loss of short-term memory. It is the most prevalent of the dementias and affects about 4 million people in the United States (Progress Report on Alzheimer's Disease, 2000). The incidence and prevalence rise with age. The cause is unknown, but research continues into the roles of acetylcholine (a neurotransmitter) and amyloid (a precursor protein). The risk of developing Alzheimer's disease (AD) rises with a family history of Alzheimer's disease and Down syndrome.

Vascular Dementia. Vascular dementia results from multiple vascular insults (from either hemorrhage or ischemia) to the brain. This type of chronic confusion progresses in a characteristically steplike fashion after each vascular insult. The client's symptoms reflect the brain areas affected.

Parkinson's Disease. Parkinson's disease is a neurological disease characterized by tremors, muscle rigidity, slowed movements, and postural instability. There may be progressive cognitive slowing and impairment in memory retrieval.

Huntington's Disease. Huntington's disease is a hereditary degenerative disease involving a characteristic rhythmic or twitching movement. The chronic confusion associated with this disease is characterized by slowed thinking, poor attention span, and poor judgment. The client becomes hostile, impulsive, and easily frustrated as the stress threshold lessens and deterioration progresses.

Normal-Pressure Hydrocephalus. When excess fluid accumulates in the cranial cavity, the ventricles enlarge and compress the cortex. This can cause symptoms of chronic confusion. A shunt can drain the excess fluid and reverse the symptoms if inserted in time. Early onset of aphasia, ataxia, and incontinence are key characteristics of this disorder.

Creutzfeldt-Jakob Disease. Creutzfeldt-Jakob disease is an infectious form of dementia related to a slow virus. The major symptoms are muscle spasms and deterioration of cognitive abilities or chronic confusion. If this disease is suspected to be the underlying cause of a client's chronic confusion, the client must be placed on blood, secretion, and excretion precautions.

> ***Action Alert!*** Place the client with Creutzfeldt-Jakob disease on body substance precautions immediately.

Pick's Disease. Pick's disease is characterized by the formation of Pick cells in the frontal and temporal lobes. It is rare and usually not reversible. The major symptoms are amnesia, aphasia, and loss of inhibitions.

CULTURAL AND LIFESTYLE FACTORS

Substance Abuse. The ingestion or abuse of harmful substances, such as alcohol, barbiturates, cocaine, amphetamines, and other hallucinogens, can alter cognition.

Nutritional Deficiencies. Deficiencies of thiamine, folate, vitamin B_{12}, iron, niacin, and magnesium also may disrupt brain function. People who chronically ingest large amounts of alcohol may develop vitamin B-complex deficiencies with a resulting encephalopathy and memory loss known as Wernicke-Korsakoff syndrome.

Sleep Disruption. Cognition requires not only enough sleep but also a sleep-wake cycle that corresponds with a normal living environment and situation. Lack of sleep can distort awareness, alertness, attention, thinking, and cognition.

Sexually Transmitted Diseases. Infection with the human immunodeficiency virus (HIV), which causes acquired immunodeficiency syndrome (AIDS), can lead to a syndrome called AIDS dementia complex. Usually, it is a late manifestation of HIV infection, just as neurosyphilis is a late manifestation of tertiary syphilis. HIV infection can stem from the use of contaminated needles, as well as from unprotected sex or any blood-to-blood transfer.

ENVIRONMENTAL FACTORS

Environmental Stimulation. People who are in unfamiliar environments, particularly when they lack sensory stimulation, may become transiently confused (Figure 40-3). For the person with chronic confusion, such as in Alzheimer's disease, any change in environment can lead to complete disorientation. Even moving from one room to another in the same nursing home will take a lengthy period of readjustment. The slightly confused older adult may become very confused when admitted to the hospital, which complicates the nurse's ability to detect acute confusion superimposed on chronic confusion. Furthermore, environments with excessive stimulation—such as noise from a television, radio, intercom, and so on—may worsen chronic confusion, and behavior problems may ensue.

Lead Ingestion. Lead poisoning is a well-known environmental cause of altered cognition. Lead-based paint from old houses and toys/jewelry made in other countries are the most frequent source of lead poisoning in children. The ingestion of lead paint occurs during normal hand-to-mouth activity. Other sources of lead are water pipes contaminated with lead solder, lead-containing pottery being used to serve or store food, and lead-contaminated soil.

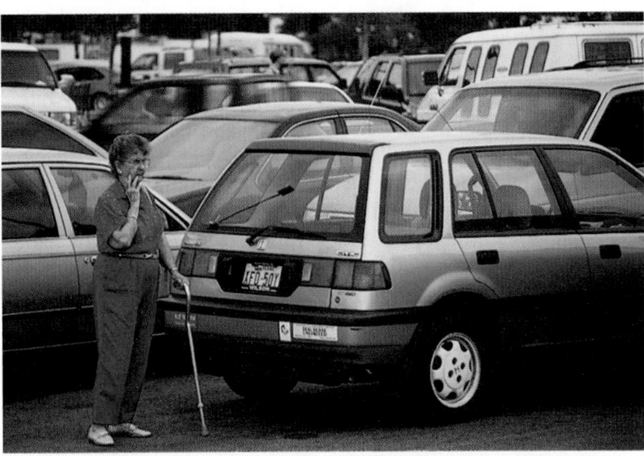

FIGURE 40-3 People who are in unfamiliar environments may become transiently confused. For the person with chronic confusion, complete disorientation can happen.

PSYCHOLOGICAL FACTORS

Depression may affect cognition, particularly in older adults. The reverse is also true: cognitive deterioration can lead to depression in clients who understand that their cognitive ability is declining. **Pseudodementia** is a severe form of depression resulting from a progressive brain disorder in which cognitive changes mimic those of dementia. Clients in the early stages of chronic confusion commonly experience depression. As cognitive and functional abilities fail, the job is lost, and life as previously known is over, the person can feel emotionally flooded with the multitude of losses already experienced, as well as the probable future losses.

Relatively early in the progressive decline of chronic confusion, there is an increased risk of suicide resulting from the twin feelings of powerlessness and hopelessness. As chronic confusion progresses to later stages and memory fails, depression and the risk of suicide lessen.

ASSESSMENT

GENERAL ASSESSMENT OF COGNITION

Assessment consists of a history, physical examination, mental status examination, functional examination, and review of present medical regimen. It involves the appraisal of cognition and identification not only of the impairments but also of the strengths of the person, so that the latter can be used in planning care.

Health History. A good history targets risk factors and defining characteristics that may be present. Determine the time confusion occurred, the mental status changes that occurred, possible precipitating or related factors, recent medication changes, long-term medication use, and history of substance use. Develop a history from the client's family to identify major changes in the person's characteristic behaviors and emotional function. Also check for signs of related factors, such as infection, chronic illness, depression, or previous hospitalization.

If you suspect acute confusion, review the client's medications in detail. Assess prescription, OTC medications, herbal preparations, and any history of long-term medication use or substance abuse. Check to see if the client is sharing medications with a spouse. Assess potential medication intoxication, especially if the client takes a sedative, hypnotic, narcotic, anticholinergic drug, or psychotropic drug.

Assess for both acute and chronic confusion. These types of confusion may exist singly or together. Identification of both types of confusion and underlying causes is necessary to plan treatment appropriately.

The assessment of mental status and cognitive functioning is important to any client with potential confusion but particularly to the older adult. Perform a baseline assessment, and then routinely reassess to detect any changes promptly and systematically. The use of a mental status questionnaire and a behavioral rating scale is recommended to provide a comprehensive assessment.

Assessment Tools. Instruments currently used to detect acute confusion fall into several categories: mental status examinations, rating scales, clinical interviews, and psychomotor tests. All of these tests have positive and negative aspects. The most frequently used tools are mental status questionnaires and rating scales.

Mental Status Examinations. Mental status examinations are questionnaires designed to assess various cognitive functions. Data are collected on such components as consciousness, memory, attention, orientation, and abstract thinking. The most frequently used mental status questionnaires are Pfeiffer's Short Portable Mental Status Questionnaire (SPMSQ) and, more commonly, Folstein's Mini-Mental State Examination (Box 40-1 for sample questions). These tests can help the nurse decide whether a client has a cognitive impairment, but they do not allow finer discrimination. Because these tests require the client to answer questions, adaptations for clients who are deaf, blind, intubated, or otherwise unable to readily participate must be made. For example, the intubated client can be asked to blink eyes, raise a finger, or communicate the answers in some other designated manner (Folstein, Folstein, & McHugh, 1975; Pfeiffer, 1975).

Cultural implications must also be considered when giving a questionnaire. Some experts question the validity of these tests, because age, education, culture, and language can affect the results. It is important to recognize that any questions involving cultural issues can be misleading. For example, the new immigrant may not know answers related to U.S. history that are routinely asked in some mental status examinations. This lack of knowledge about U.S. history does not reflect the person's cognitive ability.

BOX 40-1 *Mini-Mental State Examination: Sample Questions*

ORIENTATION TO TIME

- What is the date?

REGISTRATION

"Listen carefully. I am going to say three words. You say them back after I stop. Ready? Here they are:"
"HOUSE" (pause), "CAR" (pause), "LAKE" (pause)
"Now repeat those words back to me."
[Repeat up to five times, but score only the first trial.]

NAMING

"What is this?"
[Point to a pencil or pen.]

READING

"Please read this, and do what it says."
[Show examinee the words "CLOSE YOUR EYES" on the stimulus form.]

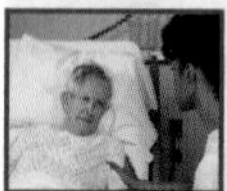

Recall the case of Mr. Tellis, introduced at the beginning of the chapter. The nursing assessment and initial work-up is as follows: "This 83-year-old white man admitted in no acute distress. Temperature is 97.6° F, pulse 90 and regular, respirations 20, BP 140/84 lying, 130/80 sitting, and 110/70 standing. Mr. T. complains of dizziness when standing for BP reading, and increased sway is noted. Neurological exam: pupils equal, round, and reactive to light (PERRL), hand grasps equal and strong, moving all extremities. Able to recall name, but unable to recall place or time. Appears to be anxious at times, and mentation vacillates between lucidity and confusion. Mini-Mental State Examination reveals a score of 24, indicating a mild impairment. Lungs are clear to auscultation throughout all lung fields. O_2 saturation on room air is 94%. Heart sounds S_1 and S_2 heard, no irregularities noted. Skin is dry, and tenting is noted over sternum and forehead. Abdomen is soft, nontender, and bowel sounds are heard in all four quadrants. Bladder percussed and palpated. Findings suggest urine retention. A No. 16 Foley catheter inserted, and 350 mL concentrated cloudy urine is obtained. Specimen sent to lab for urinalysis and culture and sensitivity. Lower extremities reveal dry, scaly skin and dependent rubor relieved by lying down. Palpable pedal, posterior tibial, and popliteal pulses. Blood drawn for CBC, electrolytes, BUN, creatinine. Family remains with client throughout assessment."

From this assessment report, can you see any clues to Mr. Tellis's confusion?

Rating Scales. Because much of the information needed to assess confusion is nonverbal, the use of a rating scale in addition to the mental status examination provides a more comprehensive assessment of client function. When using a rating scale, behavior or symptoms are rated or scored on a predetermined scale. Simply observe the client, and rate what is observed.

A number of behavioral scales have been developed to assess confusion, detect key aspects of acute confusion, differentiate between acute confusion and chronic confusion, and identify differences between confusion and depression. The most common scales are the NEECHAM Confusion scale and the Clinical Assessment of Confusion (CAM). The NEECHAM Confusion scale allows rapid bedside documentation of the client's information-processing defects. It allows you to document key indicators of the development of acute confusion.

The Clinical Assessment of Confusion scale is particularly useful for differentiating between acute confusion, chronic confusion, and depression. It also helps define the severity of the client's problem. These and several other scales are being further researched and developed.

Physical Assessment. The physical examination focuses on assessing cognitive status and identifying possible etiologies for changes in a client's cognition. It includes a head-to-toe assessment, paying particular attention to orientation, basic neurological assessment, level of consciousness, vital signs, skin turgor, lung auscultation, and elimination pattern.

Diagnostic Tests. A number of diagnostic tests may be ordered by a physician or an advanced practice nurse to determine the cause of a client's confusion. These test results help distinguish acute from chronic confusion. Serum (blood) laboratory tests such as a complete blood count and measurement of electrolytes, blood urea nitrogen, creatinine, and glucose may be performed. A chest radiograph, computed tomography scan, electrocardiogram, and urine culture are also often part of the screen done for suspected acute or chronic confusion (Table 40-1).

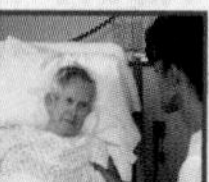

Mr. Tellis's urine culture shows bacteria present in the urine at a level greater than 100,000 per milliliter. Remember that Mr. Tellis complained of "having trouble with my water." Can you correlate the presence of bacteria in his urine with the symptoms of confusion?

FOCUSED ASSESSMENT FOR *ACUTE CONFUSION*

Assessment of *Acute confusion* begins with a baseline study. This will identify whether cognitive symptoms are a change from previous functioning and how abruptly the change developed. Comparing symptoms to a baseline also helps determine current status.

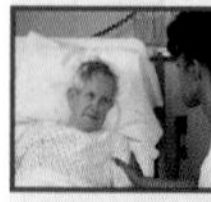

Mr. Tellis's daughter reported that his condition began suddenly. This statement suggests acute confusion and warrants further assessment. If he is found to have acute confusion, the underlying causes will need to be identified and treated.

Table 40-1 Assessing for Underlying Causes of Confusion

AREA TESTED	TEST USED	IMPLICATIONS
Hematological status	• Red blood cell count • White blood cell count • Hematocrit level • Hemoglobin level	• An elevated white blood cell count is consistent with infection. • Decreased oxygen transport or acute infection may be the cause of acute confusion.
Fluid balance	• Electrolyte tests	• Electrolyte changes are useful in determining the body's water balance, which can influence mental status.
Renal function	• Blood urea nitrogen • Creatinine • Urine culture	• Elevation can indicate renal dysfunction, a possible cause of confusion. • Bacteria in urine indicates infection, which can lead to confusion. • Confusion may be the only sign of urinary infection in older adults.
Cardiac function	• Electrocardiogram • Pulse oximetry	• An altered heart rhythm that reduces cardiac output can cause or contribute to confusion. • Reduced blood oxygen saturation may indicate cerebral hypoxia
Respiratory function	• Chest x-ray film	• Infections (such as pneumonia), tumors, or tuberculosis may contribute to acute confusion.
Brain structure	• Computed tomography scan	• Reveals space-occupying lesions (such as tumors), cerebral infarctions, or normal-pressure hydrocephalus.
Metabolic function	• Serum glucose level	• Because the brain requires a steady supply of glucose to function properly, a reduction in blood glucose may affect cognition.
Nutritional status	• Serum vitamin B_{12} • Folic acid (folate)	• Defective B_{12} absorption may lead to pernicious anemia, degeneration in the spinal cord, and associated neurological symptoms, including confusion. • Defective folate absorption may lead to megaloblastic anemia. • This test is especially helpful for assessing an alcoholic client.
Thyroid function	• Thyroxine (T_4) • Triiodothyronine (T_3) • Thyroid-stimulating hormone	• Cognitive impairment may result from either hypothyroidism or hyperthyroidism.
Tertiary syphilis	• FTA-ABS	• Tertiary syphilis can cause chronic confusion.
HIV infection	• Enzyme-linked immunosorbent assay	• Antibodies to indicate infection; AIDS leads to confusion.
Drug levels	• Alcohol • Medications, including digoxin and antiepileptic medications	• Substances abused or taken as prescribed can lead to toxicity, a possible cause of confusion.

FTA-ABS, Fluorescent treponemal antibody absorption test; *HIV,* human immunodeficiency virus; *AIDS,* acquired immunodeficiency syndrome.

When assessing for acute confusion, stay alert to a variety of cues. The client's inattention and inability to follow simple directions should alert you to consider a working diagnosis of *Acute confusion* related to unknown etiology and to pursue further assessment. Other cues may alert you as well. For example, a heavily medicated client may suddenly become incoherent and fearful. A client in the intensive care unit may begin to hallucinate. A newly admitted client may suddenly become incoherent and complain of seeing bugs in the bed when none are present.

As discussed earlier, use a mental status examination, rating scale, or both to help differentiate between acute and chronic confusion and between confusion and other possible conditions. In an emergent situation, in which the safety of the client or others is threatened, act to prevent injury whether or not you have a complete assessment of the client's confusion.

Defining Characteristics of Acute Confusion. Symptoms of acute confusion result from temporary injury to brain tissue. Bouts of acute confusion may last from 1 to 3 weeks if the underlying etiology is identified, or the confusion may resolve on its own. If the injury cannot be reversed, permanent brain injury may result.

The defining characteristics of acute confusion involve disorders in consciousness, attention, perception, memory, orientation, thinking, the sleep-wake cycle, and psychomotor behavior. Impairments of both consciousness and attention are hallmark characteristics of acute confusion (Box 40-2).

Alertness. When considering the client's reduced alertness or lowered ability to react to important stimuli, rule out such factors as pain, fatigue, and infection. In addition, try to differentiate between the altered alertness of acute confusion and boredom or depres-

BOX 40-2 *Characteristics of Acute Confusion*

- Altered consciousness
- Impaired attention
- Altered perception
- Memory loss
- Problems of orientation
- Impaired thinking, judgment, and language
- Sleep-wake disorders
- Psychomotor disturbances

sion. Notice whether alertness tends to lessen when stimuli are boring or meaningless.

Altered Consciousness. Consciousness is significantly reduced in acute confusion. The client may be less able to respond to stimuli and may appear to be in a stupor or may become overly alert, excitable or hyperactive, and hypervigilant.

The fluctuations of consciousness that characterize acute confusion help point out the extent of the client's awareness deficit. This fluctuation is useful because it allows you to see the client in a lucid interval. Unless assessment continues over a 24-hour period, the nurse and health care team may fail to notice this important symptom.

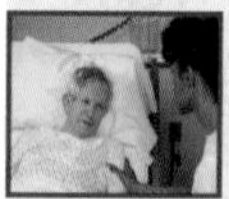

Recall the case of Mr. Tellis. He had a lucid moment where he said to his daughter, "Oh, you take control," before he slumped into a semiconscious daze and became difficult to arouse.

Impaired Attention. Impairment of attention is a major factor in acute confusion. Attention is usually diminished in three operations: focusing, maintaining, and shifting attention. Focusing is the ability to select important points of focus or selectively mobilize attention on some point of choice. The client may be unable to focus, maintain, or sustain attention. Furthermore, the client will be highly distractible, and attention may wander. Extraneous stimuli, such as the hospital intercom or people passing in the hall, may continually cause distraction. Important stimuli, such as rules of safety, may be unattended and ignored.

The ability to shift attention is also reduced. The client may remain focused on a previous topic rather than follow a change of topics as the nurse gives instructions. These disturbances in attention prevent integration and organization of information and disrupt thinking, judgment, communication, and memory. For example, a client who cannot attend to the nurse's instructions may forget how to use the call bell. This client's safety and potential for injury now become important considerations.

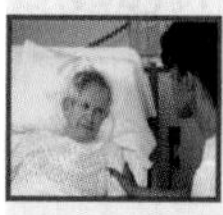

Mr. Tellis illustrated this point when he was unable to focus on the nurse's instructions because of his agitated and fearful state.

Action Alert! Assess for acute confusion if the client seems highly distractible and is unable to focus attention, understand instructions, or shift attention.

Altered Perception. Perceptual difficulties, such as illusions and hallucinations, may occur in acute confusion. The client has a reduced ability to distinguish among dreams, imagery, hallucinations, and reality. Illusions, or mistaken identification of real stimuli, are common. A coat hanging in the closet may be perceived as a person, for example. Perceptual distortions are also prevalent. For example, the client may perceive an object as too large, too small, or too misshapen to resemble real life. Stationary objects may appear to move. Objects may also be perceived as duplicating themselves or flowing into other objects.

Hallucinations are sensory perceptions in the absence of real stimuli. They usually create brightly colored visual hallucinations that seem real. Clients typically see life-size, three-dimensional people or objects moving about. Although visual hallucinations are most common, some people have auditory hallucinations as well, and hallucinations can involve all five senses.

Certain types of hallucinations are characteristic of underlying causes or related factors. For example, typhus has been connected with kinesthetic hallucinations of floating on air or falling. Acute confusion related to alcohol withdrawal (delirium tremens) is usually associated with hallucinations of animals, coffins, hearses, or ghostlike figures. Children under age 3 may hallucinate that they are being attacked by animals or snakes and react with extreme fear. Hallucinations of attacks are common and evoke a defensive response from clients of all ages. They do not, however, constitute psychosis.

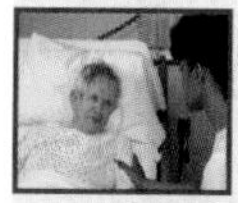

Altered perception was evident in Mr. Tellis's case. He frequently misperceived the door as a person. Furthermore, he was walking around the yard at 3:00 AM screaming at a nonexistent person.

Memory Loss. When considering the client's memory, assess which areas of memory may be affected: immediate, short-term, or long-term memory, or a combination. Consider and cluster these characteristics with other data. If the client displays immediate and recent memory loss, assess further for acute confusion. If there is difficulty with remote and present memory, assess further for chronic confusion.

Short-term or recent memory, as well as immediate recall, is impaired in acute confusion. There is a decreased ability to register, retain, and retrieve information. The decline of short-term memory is often associated with an impaired attention span and possible perceptual distortions of incoming stimuli. Memory simply fails to register correctly.

Because acute confusion can occur in clients with chronic confusion, it is important not to rule out acute confusion based on defects in long-term memory. However, with acute confusion alone, recent memory is usually more affected. The person cannot remember the routine or instructions given. This often affects orientation and causes fearfulness and other emotional reactions.

Problems of Orientation. Orientation to time, place, and other persons may also be affected in serious acute confusion, but rarely will a client forget his or her own identity. A characteristic clue of acute confusion is that clients frequently mistake unknown people as familiar. For example, the client may misidentify the nurse as a family member.

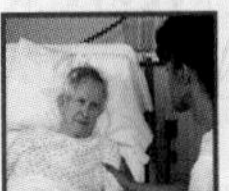

Mr. Tellis demonstrated difficulty with orientation when he was unable to tell the nurse where he was, where he lived, or what had happened to him. If you detected these problems in a client, how would you respond?

Impaired Judgment and Language. The confused client may have a reduced ability to think sequentially, reason logically, grasp or comprehend word meaning, notice important differences and similarities of words or situations, or actively direct thinking. Thus there is a decreased ability to judge, reason, solve problems, plan, or think abstractly. This disturbance in cognition is reflected in language that is disordered, illogical, disjointed, and often incoherent. Conversations become extremely difficult, and safety is a major concern.

Sleep-Wake Disorders. When considering the client's sleep-wake cycle, differentiate between acute confusion and nighttime restlessness that could stem from pain or anxiety. The acutely confused may have hour-by-hour variation in the sleep-wake cycle. A medication (such as a diuretic) may disrupt the normal pattern, or there may be other possible influences on sleeping and waking.

A disrupted circadian rhythm is a classic symptom of acute confusion. Typically, the rhythm is backward; the person will stay awake at night and be less alert and need short naps during the day. The quality of sleep is also affected, and waking is commonly confused, with a dreamlike quality. The person may oscillate continually between waking, dreaming, and perceiving illusions or hallucinations. Lack of sleep can distort awareness, alertness, attention, thinking, and cognition.

Psychomotor Disturbances. When considering the client's psychomotor behavior, notice the type of behavior seen. For example, if the client is hyperactive or hypoactive, is it related to acute confusion or to the possible inability to coordinate motor behaviors (apraxia) that commonly arises in chronic confusion? Also, differentiate between hypervigilance and agitation, a potential indicator of pain or other distress.

Psychomotor disturbances are associated with the underlying cause of confusion and usually are visible as hyperactive or hypoactive behavior. Hyperactive clients tend to be very active or hypervigilant. They may remove IV lines, pick at things in the air, pull at dressings, climb over side rails, call for loved ones, and have such signs as tachycardia, dilated pupils, or a flushed complexion. Hypoactive clients may seem overly fatigued and sleepy. They tend to sleep during the day and seem rather muddled or less alert than usual. Clients with confusion may also have fluctuating symptoms, presenting one clinical picture and then another.

Emotional Reactions to Acute Confusion. A variety of emotions ranging from panic to apathy may result from acute confusion. Commonly, these emotions change as the condition worsens. This is especially true if the person has perceptual distortions, hallucinations, or delusions. Fear and distrust of others are common. The client may try to flee or may become combative if the hallucinations seem dangerous. Depression, powerlessness, apathy, withdrawal, catastrophic behaviors, feelings of loss of control, anger, and fear are all common in acute confusion.

Delusions are false personal beliefs. They are common in a confused client, along with attitudes that differ widely from the client's usual beliefs and attitudes. Suspiciousness, terror, and a fear of persecution or being injured by others are common emotions associated with acute confusion. Paranoid delusions and delusions of persecution may predominate the fragmented thinking already caused by partial memory and inattention. However, unlike the delusions of people with schizophrenia or mania, the delusions of a person with acute confusion are ill defined, unstable, changeable, and usually bound to external stimuli.

Many clients consider acute confusion as traumatizing in itself because of the terrifying perceptions and feelings involved. Clients with febrile conditions and acute confusion report that bright lights and noise are extremely irritating. Simple viral or bacterial infections (e.g., urinary tract infection) can lead to acute confusion in the older adult.

Some clients have aftereffects from the trauma of acute confusion, such as anxiety, sleeplessness, and other symptoms of posttraumatic stress syndrome. Also, clients who recover from acute confusion but receive no education about it may be anxious that it could return without warning.

Thinking and Language. When considering the client's thinking and language, notice whether the client is having trouble finding words or difficulty understanding their meaning. This would suggest chronic confusion. Also notice whether the client is thinking in a disjointed or disorganized manner and speaking incoherently, which would suggest acute confusion.

Early Signs of Acute Confusion in Older Adults. Resnick (2001) reported that early signs of acute confusion in older adults involved forgetfulness, disorientation, fear, misperceptions, insomnia, daytime sleepiness, inattentiveness, easy distraction, and verbal complaints of feeling mixed-up or fuzzy. If the factors underlying the confusion are identified and treated, improvement typically occurs in the client's overall physical condition.

Related Factors. Some of the factors commonly related to acute confusion are alcohol abuse, delirium, and drug abuse. However, a wide range of disorders and conditions can be associated with acute confusion. Indeed, several different factors may be present in a single client.

Acute confusion may be influenced by changes in cerebral metabolism, oxygenation, systemic infections, metabolic disorders (such as hypoxia, hypercarbia, and hypoglycemia), fluid or electrolyte imbalances, hepatic or renal disease, thiamine deficiency, postoperative states, hypertensive encephalopathy, postictal states, and head trauma or brain lesions (American Psychiatric Association, 2000). Other factors include chronic illness, severe illness, fever, polypharmacy, and hospitalization (Foreman et al., 1999).

Populations at risk for acute confusion are young children, older adults, cognitively impaired persons, clients who have just had surgery, or older adults hospitalized for surgery or severe medical illness. Clearly, older adults are more vulnerable to acute confusion because of the altered physiology with aging and the high incidence of risk factors.

Facilitating factors contribute to the development of acute confusion but have not been proven to actually cause acute confusion. The most common facilitating factors are sensory impairment and environmental and personal conditions (Box 40-3).

FOCUSED ASSESSMENT FOR *CHRONIC CONFUSION*

Defining Characteristics. Generally there are three stages for the chronic confusion of Alzheimer's disease that characterize the progressive degeneration found in chronic confusion. In the first stage, the person begins to forget things and becomes concerned about possible loss of memory. Usually the person attempts to hide these deficits. In the second stage, the person loses much of cognitive integrative functioning and becomes unable to handle money, transportation, and cooking. The person may be unable to keep a job. Poor judgment and social isolation become evident. In the third stage, the person loses much of the ability to perform activities of daily living (ADLs). Wandering and combative behaviors often force the family to seek help. By the end of the third stage, the person can no longer attend to personal hygiene, may have urinary and fecal incontinence, and may be unaware of surroundings. Gradually, the client forgets how to eat. Placement in a protective environment may be required.

Characteristically, a client with chronic confusion has a loss of memory and a loss of one or more of the following skills: problem-solving, judgment, or planning skills; abstract thinking; and cognitive or intellectual skills (Box 40-4). There may also be a change in affect or personality, as well as disturbances of higher cortical function, such as language, motor activities, or constructional ability. There may be a progressively lowered stress threshold manifested as purposeful wandering or catastrophic behavior, such as violent, compulsive, or avoidance behaviors. As deterioration progresses, skill loss increases (American Psychiatric Association, 2000).

Memory Loss. Loss of immediate, short-term, and long-term memory is a major defining characteristic of chronic confusion. Initially, the client cannot recall what happened a few moments ago. Assess the client's short-term memory, or ability to learn, by determining whether three objects can be remembered after 5 minutes have passed. Assess long-term memory impairment by determining ability to remember past personal information, such as what happened yesterday, birthplace, occupation, and major life events. Take care to adjust for differences in the person's ability to answer questions based on sensory impairment, culture, educational level, and age.

BOX 40-3 *Factors Related to Acute Confusion*

- Hypoxia
- Infections: respiratory, urinary tract
- Dehydration
- Electrolyte imbalance: hypokalemia, hyponatremia, hypernatremia
- Cardiovascular disorders: congestive heart failure, myocardial infarction, dysrhythmias
- Sleep deprivation
- Medications: anticholinergics, neuroleptics, tricyclic antidepressants, analgesics, histamine-2 blocking agents
- Surgery
- Pain
- Alcohol/drug ingestion or withdrawal
- Environmental changes, sensory deprivation, or sensory overload
- Sensory impairment

BOX 40-4 *Characteristics of Chronic Confusion*

- Loss of memory; progresses from recent to long term
- Progressive loss of executive functions of problem-solving, judgment, or planning skills
- Progressive loss of abstract thinking, cognitive, or intellectual skills
- Change in affect or personality; anger and agitation more likely to occur in the later stages
- Disturbances of higher cortical function
- Progressively lowered stress threshold; may result in catastrophic incidents
- Progressively decreased ability to perform activities of daily living
- Sundown syndrome occurs in about one third of clients

Action Alert! Assess for chronic confusion when a client has a loss of memory and a loss of other abilities, such as problem-solving skills, abstract thinking, and word recall.

Impaired Problem Solving and Judgment. A person with chronic confusion gradually suffers cognitive deterioration to the point that problem-solving ability is lost. The person may not be able to judge safety issues with any degree of insight. To assess problem-solving ability and judgment, consider the client's ability to deal with family and staff interpersonally, to problem solve, and to handle safety issues with insight. Ask the client what to do if a certain event occurred, such as a fire starting in a wastebasket.

Loss of Abstract Thinking. Abstract thinking is characterized by the ability to use concepts and to make and understand generalizations, such as of the properties or pattern shared by a variety of specific items or events. It may be recognized by the ability to find similarities and differences between related words and concepts. Abstract thinking deteriorates as chronic confusion progresses. Also assess the client's ability to recognize and use written symbols, such as those you might use for orientation cues. Keep in mind that some clients are unable to read, not because of chronic confusion but because of illiteracy or inability to see the print size.

Changes in Affect or Personality. **Affect,** or the observable expression of feelings or emotions, changes as chronic confusion progresses, as does the client's personality. Some aspect of the personality may be accentuated, or the personality may change completely. Behavior may change dramatically, which is usually a source of considerable distress to the family.

Disturbances of Higher Cortical Functions. Disturbances of higher cortical functions appear as the syndrome progresses. This includes aphasia, apraxia, and agnosia. Aphasia is a language disorder resulting from brain damage or disease to speech centers in the brain resulting in a variety of difficulties in formulating, expressing, and understanding language (see Chapter 39). Although the client can usually recognize the correct word when it is spoken, the ability to retrieve the word from memory is lost. This problem can create much frustration for the client and the staff. It is important to be aware of the client's needs and develop a method of communication that avoids undue frustration.

Apraxia is the inability to execute or carry out skilled movements and gestures despite the functional ability to perform them. The client may understand the needed action and retain the necessary physical movements, but the cerebral cortex is not connecting with the activity. Apraxia can take the form of the inability to make fine, precise movements with an arm or leg, the inability to make the proper movement in response to a verbal command, the inability to coordinate activities with multiple, sequential movements, such as dressing, eating, and bathing, difficulty coordinating mouth and speech movements, the inability to copy, draw, or construct simple figures, and difficulty moving the eyes on command.

Agnosia is the inability to recognize and identify objects or persons, or know what the object is used for, despite having knowledge of the characteristics of those objects or persons. The client may be unable to recognize the phone or light switch because he cannot recall the object. This problem can be frustrating and frightening.

Lowered Stress Threshold. A decreased ability to withstand stressful situations and adapt to environmental requirements progressively develops with chronic confusion. This lowered stress threshold tends to produce more violent, compulsive, combative, and catastrophic behaviors in response to triggers, stressful situations, or events that exceed the stress threshold. **Sundown syndrome** is a worsening of behavior that occurs as the sun goes down, especially after dark. It may occur with chronic confusion. This worsening can be manifested as restlessness, agitation, disorientation, hallucinations, and a decrease in ability to perform ADLs. Attention span, concentration, and cognition decrease.

Early Signs of Chronic Confusion in Older Adults. The insidious onset of chronic confusion such as in Alzheimer's disease often makes early identification difficult. Initially, the person is successful at compensating for intellectual losses and hiding the loss from family members who are not present 24 hours a day. At first, memory loss is as mild as forgetting where keys or a wallet are kept but progresses to not knowing how to use the key. Eventually, the loss becomes severe and extends into long-term memory. Personality changes and poor judgment may occur. A loss of language ability or aphasia may be exhibited.

Emotional Reactions to Chronic Confusion. Early in chronic confusion, the client typically denies difficulty with memory and blames the forgetfulness on stress, feeling rushed, overworked, or physically ill. Later, as deterioration increases, job performance may suffer and position and functioning may be lost. At this point, anxiety, depression, and frustration may invade the person's awareness.

As deterioration continues, the stress threshold drops and the enormous effort needed to function with problems may overtax the affected client and provoke a catastrophic reaction, such as compulsive, violent, combative, hostile behavior. Sadness, frustration, fear, or simple pleasure may come and go from moment to moment.

Related Factors. More than 60 diseases have been associated with chronic confusion. Alzheimer's disease and vascular dementia are the most common. Because the condition is irreversible, the nurse treats the client's responses to the symptoms or needs rather than the etiology. Some major issues are safety, meeting basic needs, dignity, independence, quality of life, meaningful life, love and belonging, and preventing/managing catastrophic events.

DIAGNOSIS

Arriving at the most appropriate nursing diagnosis for a confused client primarily involves identifying the type of confusion present (acute, chronic, or both). Table 40-2 gives examples of clustering data to derive nursing diagnoses. It is essential to distinguish between acute and chronic confusion because acute confusion is often reversible when it is identified in time (Table 40-3). Identifying the client with chronic confusion who has acute confusion superimposed on an already confused state can be difficult. Using a decision tree (Figure 40-4) can assist with the correct identification of acute or chronic confusion. Multiple nursing diagnoses are often present in the client with chronic confusion.

Impaired Environmental Interpretation Syndrome. *Impaired environmental interpretation syndrome* is defined as a consistent lack of orientation to person, place, time, or circumstances over more than 3 to 6 months, necessitating a protective environment (NANDA International [NANDA-I], 2005). This diagnosis is used with clients in the later stages of chronic confusion. Usually they have irreversible dementia.

Disturbed Thought Processes. *Disturbed thought processes* is a disruption in cognitive operations and activities (NANDA-I, 2007). Problems include lack of contact with reality, memory deficit, hypovigilance, hypervigilance, and inaccurate interpretation of the environment. Thus it may be more clinically useful in psychiatric settings, where the client has difficulty with reality.

Impaired Memory. *Impaired memory* is defined as the state in which an individual experiences an inability to remember or recall bits of information or behavioral skills (NANDA-I, 2007). This diagnosis focuses only on the memory problems and is useful when memory is the primary mental change.

Anxiety. Anxiety is a common response to confusion of all types. Anxiety develops because the client is disoriented, unable to grasp or make sense of what is happening, and usually concerned about safety. When understanding becomes elusive, the client may become severely anxious. A restless, agitated client who pulls at bandages or tries to escape from visual hallucinations may experience terror and injury.

Hopelessness. Hopelessness is frequently seen in early chronic confusion when the person is aware of the

Table 40-2 Clustering Data to Make a Nursing Diagnosis

Confusion

DATA CLUSTER	DIAGNOSIS
An 88-year-old woman takes multiple medications, including those with anticholinergic side effects. She exhibits symptoms of inattention and fluctuations in consciousness.	*Acute confusion* related to disturbance in cerebral metabolism secondary to side effects of multiple drugs taken daily
A 59-year-old man with a history of alcoholism sees animals in the room and insects crawling on his skin.	*Acute confusion* related to disturbance in cerebral metabolism secondary to withdrawal from alcohol
Family reports that a 79-year-old woman has loss of language ability, memory of family members, and ability to recognize body parts. She has gradually deteriorated to this state over a period of 6 years.	*Chronic confusion* related to progressive degeneration of the cerebral cortex secondary to probable Alzheimer's disease

Table 40-3 Differentiating Between Acute and Chronic Confusion

ACUTE CONFUSION	CHRONIC CONFUSION
Occurs abruptly over a few hours or days; often reversible	Usually develops insidiously over a period of years; usually irreversible
Fluctuations in consciousness or alertness, often at night	Progresses steadily with little no diurnal variation in consciousness; sundown syndrome and diurnal mood changes occur; decreased consciousness late in illness
Reduced awareness with lucid intervals	Does not affect consciousness
Reduces the attention span	Does not reduce attention; however, may have selective attention or short attention span; often easy to distract
Disorganized thinking and incoherent language; disorientation	Typically causes aphasia; may substitute words for forgotten words; loss of executive function; disorientation late in illness
Disturbed perception, hallucinations, frightening misperceptions, and dreams	Hallucinations, delusions, and misperceptions, if present, usually late in the course of the illness
Profoundly disturbed, even reversed sleep cycle; hour-by-hour fluctuations	Diurnal reversal and other sleep problems common
May be associated with hyperarousal, hypoarousal, or both	No major changes in arousal until late
Reduces immediate and recent memory	Reduces recent then eventually remote memory

losses, the disabilities, and the expected progression of the disease. As memory fails, hopelessness tends to disappear because the client does not remember the situation and the losses.

Powerlessness. Powerlessness is common in the chronically confused client particularly in the early stages when awareness of the deterioration is associated with loss of control over the person's life. The strain to function despite the deterioration can be overwhelming. Feelings of powerlessness for acutely confused client can be extreme. Perceptual distortions and hallucinations can cause misinterpretation of the nurse's attempt to help as a fearful invasion of personal space.

Chronic Sorrow. Chronic sorrow is a cyclical, recurring, and potentially progressive pattern of pervasive sadness. It is highly associated with clinical depression and may respond to treatment. Remember that severe depression can mimic chronic confusion or coexist with one or both types of confusion.

Risk for Injury. Risk for injury is high with confusion due to lack of judgment and memory impairment. Confused clients can pull out an IV line or catheter, tear or pick at bandages, climb over side rails, wander into dangerous areas, lash out at others, and harm themselves through catastrophic episodes. Frequently, clients in early stages of chronic confusion, who are also depressed, may harm themselves. Clients in later stages may not be aware of actual hazards and may be harmed in numerous ways. In addition, a large number of confused clients are older adults and are at risk for falls. An unsteady gait, failing sight or hearing, and decreased functioning may present hazards and potential injury (see Chapter 23).

Imbalanced Nutrition. Nutrition is an essential aspect of care for the confused client, who may not remember to eat or how to prepare food. As chronic confusion progresses, the person may forget how to use a utensil and finally how to chew and swallow (see Chapter 25).

Deficient Fluid Volume. Dehydration may occur in clients who forget to replenish fluids, sweat profusely, or otherwise suffer from loss of fluid. The aphasic client is unable to express thirst or to indicate need for fluids and may not be able to drink fluids independently (see Chapter 26).

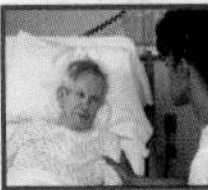

Mr. Tellis has skin tenting on his sternum and forehead, cloudy concentrated urine, and dry scaly skin on his lower legs. These indicate decreased total body water. Did you identify them as factors that could be contributing to his confusion? Fluid intake of 1500 to 1800 mL each day is necessary to ensure adequate hydration and maintain fluid balance.

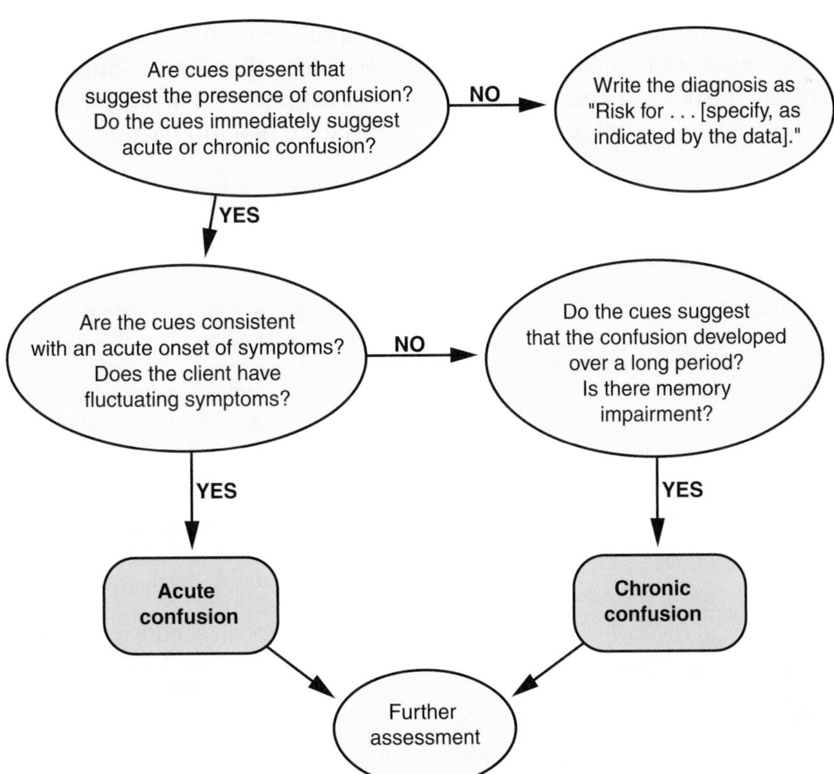

FIGURE 40-4 Decision tree for confusion. Diagnoses are shown in rectangles. Within these rectangles, diagnoses shown in **bold** type are NANDA International (NANDA-I)–approved nursing diagnoses; diagnoses shown in regular type are not NANDA-I–approved nursing diagnoses.

Caregiver Role Strain. Most clients with chronic confusion receive care at home, at least early in the disease. Often, the caretaker goes to great lengths to keep the person at home. Family members, especially those who provide direct client care, are important to consider. The family must be considered as a unit, with needs beyond those specific to the client. Specific suggestions to caregivers about how to provide care to a confused family member are provided in Box 40-5.

PLANNING

EXPECTED OUTCOMES FOR THE CLIENT WITH *ACUTE CONFUSION*

The expected outcome for *Acute confusion* is that the client is free of episodes of confusion. The etiology is identified and treated, and the confusion resolves. Recurrent episodes of acute confusion are avoided by incorporating primary prevention measures into the plan of care. For example, primary prevention is incorporated by setting such goals as "The client at risk will list medications known to influence the development of acute confusion." In this way, the client may avoid future episodes of confusion.

EXPECTED OUTCOMES FOR THE CLIENT WITH *CHRONIC CONFUSION*

The expected outcomes for the client with *Chronic confusion* are varied and depend on the signs and symptoms manifested. A few examples are that the client is in a safe environment, has decreased episodes of combative behavior, recommended body weight is maintained, a fluid intake of 1500 to 1800 mL daily is maintained, and there are no signs of infection. However, the focus of care is on quality of life, dignity, and respect.

INTERVENTION

Numerous supportive interventions can be used to achieve these general goals and outcomes. Some of the most common interventions are highlighted in the following sections. Major goals, client outcomes, and interventions are specifically individualized for the confused client.

INTERVENTIONS TO PREVENT CONFUSION

Interventions for a confused client encompass both primary (recognition and treatment of the conditions that cause acute confusion) and secondary (early intervention to reduce the effects of chronic confusion) prevention strategies. Some causes of chronic disease can be prevented (vascular dementia), but the most common one (Alzheimer's disease) cannot.

Preventing Postoperative Confusion. Postoperative confusion in older adults should be evaluated against the preoperative status. Preadmission education sessions for older adults undergoing surgery are helpful if they identify the possibility of, and the need to report, unusual or strange experiences after surgery. Such preadmission education allows early detection of signs of confusion.

In the postoperative period assess promptly and initiate appropriate treatment for confusion from hypoxia, sepsis, hypothermia, or drug side effects. Confusion is more common for major procedures like cardiac surgery or fixation of a hip fracture.

BOX 40-5 *Teaching for Wellness*

Effective Caregiving for a Confused Client

Purpose: To help a caregiver know how to care for a confused client at home.

Expected Outcome: The caregiver will express satisfaction with the ability to manage the client's care.

Caregiver Instructions

When caring for a confused person, use the following techniques to help keep the person oriented and calm:

- Use simple, clear communication; give only one directive at a time.
- Display easy-to-read calendars and clocks in the person's line of vision.
- Maintain a predictable, consistent routine. Keep personal items consistently in the same place.
- Limit the number of visitors; one at a time is less confusing. Include the confused person in the conversation.
- Limit the number of choices given. Give two choices, both of which are realistic.
- Avoid the use of words such as *don't* or *can't* when communicating. Make suggestions, and let the person "decide" to comply.
- Make mealtime a pleasant experience.
- Place the client in an upright position during meals to prevent aspiration.
- Anticipate toileting needs, and take the client to the toilet frequently. Don't be offended at table manners.
- Keep harmful substances (such as cleaning supplies and medicines) in a locked cabinet.
- Redirect, distract the client who displays inappropriate behaviors.
- If the client wants to pace, provide a safe, secure area for pacing.
- Avoid catastrophic behaviors by recognizing and meeting underlying needs.
- Turn the lights on at dusk to avoid the *sundown syndrome* of increased confusion, agitated or combative behavior.
- Make sure the person carries or wears medical identification in case of wandering.
- Make use of local and national resources, including online services. Resources may include adult day care, a support group, the Alzheimer's Disease and Related Disorders Association (at 800-272-3900), and others.
- Reduce your own stress, and obtain respite when needed.
- Take care of yourself. Laugh often!

Initiating Early Treatment. When Alzheimer's disease is recognized in the early stages, medication is more likely to help. There are four medications approved by the U.S. Food and Drug Administration (FDA) that, if given in the early, or mild, stage of AD, have been shown to augment neurotransmission, thereby improving memory in some and slowing deterioration of cognitive functions in others. These cholinesterase inhibitors are donepezil hydrochloride (Aricept), galantamine hydrobromide (Reminyl), rivastigmine tartrate (Exelon), and tacrine hydrochloride (Cognex). A newer drug, memantine (Namenda) is sometimes helpful in moderate disease. The delay or slowing of disease progression occurs only with continued drug use. If drugs are stopped, progression of the disease or decline of mental state increases. If drugs are begun again, they will not reverse any decline that has already occurred.

Monitoring Medication Use. Attention to medications and possible side effects and interactions should be emphasized, especially for older adult clients (Box 40-6). When the client is admitted, assess for the use of medications known to cause confusion, especially with a person at risk for confusion. Note the types and numbers of medications, both prescription and OTC. In addition, monitor and identify any long-term substance use, including caffeine, nicotine, alcohol, and other drugs. Abrupt withdrawal of alcohol in a person with an established habit commonly causes acute confusion.

Minimizing Sensory Impairment. Minimize sensory impairment by making sure that the client is using all of the aids needed for vision, hearing, and mobility. Frequently, clients are thought to be confused, listless, or hypoalert when they are merely unable to see or hear. Clients should have clean, well-fitting glasses of the proper prescription, hearing aids with working batteries, and canes or walkers that they know how to use.

INTERVENTIONS TO MANAGE CONFUSION

The goal of nursing care is to facilitate optimal functioning to the peak of possible health. Promote respect and self-esteem by helping the client manage confusion through the use of remaining strengths.

Helping the Client Maintain Dignity. Help the client maintain dignity by not equating aging with confusion. Provide care at the level the client needs while creatively taking strengths and abilities into account. It is important to respect the client and provide a sense of self and integrity. Call the client by name, and do not infantilize or embarrass the client by calling attention to deficits. Anticipate the client's needs to enhanced the sense of self or comfort. Provide comfort and a calming atmosphere in an individualized manner. Balance the need for independence to make choices with avoiding unrealistic, overwhelming expectations. To achieve a feeling of control, let confused persons make choices, but only give them two choices, both of which are reasonable.

Orientation is important for the client's sense of integrity and meaningful interpretation of the environment. When providing reality orientation, always do so in a way that promotes dignity. Instead of correcting the disorientation in a way that is embarrassing or frustrating, provide information in a matter-of-fact manner or naturally and subtly as part of the conversation. For example, identify yourself and your reason for approaching the client, because doing so will provide orientation without forcing the client to admit a memory deficit.

Promoting a Safe Environment. Safety is an essential aspect of intervention for the confused client. Provide ongoing orientation to time, place, person, and the environment. Bright, contrasting colors or symbols to identify rooms, bathrooms, or meeting places may help. Notice what tends to orient, calm, or provide comfort to

BOX 40-6 *Client Teaching Tips: Administering Medications Safely*

Especially for older adults, medications and confusion may go hand in hand, in part because of the number of medications taken by older people. Americans over age 65 represent about 12% of the population, but they consume about one third of all prescription drugs and spend billions annually on medications. The average older adult in the community has 11 prescriptions filled yearly; an average of eight drugs is prescribed for each nursing home resident (Eliopoulis, 2001). Polypharmacy increases the likelihood of adverse effects of medications.

Besides taking a larger number of drugs than younger people, older adults tend to see a larger number of doctors, go to multiple pharmacies, have some level of visual impairment, not have enough money to purchase all the medications they need, and be less able to manage the complex dosing schedules required when taking several medications at once.

Points for teaching the client and family about medication administration:

- Make sure clients know the names of all their medications (generic as well as trade names) and the reasons for taking them.
- Explain the dose, route, and duration of each medication.
- Teach the client how to take each medication properly.
- Tell the client what to do if a dose is missed.
- Outline the possible side effects of each medication and which side effects should prompt a call to the doctor.
- Help the client develop a written medication schedule and a method for remembering to take each medication. Use a medication calendar, for example, different-size pill containers, a multichambered medication dispensing box, or even an empty egg carton.
- Advise the client to discard expired medications.
- Warn the client against giving prescription medications to others or taking someone else's prescribed medication.
- Recommend that the client use only one pharmacy to avoid duplicating a medication and to lower the risk of drug interactions.
- Provide information on cost-saving programs if appropriate.
- If necessary, advise clients to wear or carry information that lists the medications they take.
- Reinforce the importance of adequate hydration and nutrition for optimum pharmacokinetics.
- Educate the client about the interactions of alcohol and prescription or over-the-counter medications.

the client. For example, a religious object or picture may calm one client, and holding something comforting may calm another.

Open, uncluttered, well-lit areas tend to promote safety for most confused clients. Cluttered or crowded areas tend to overstimulate. In addition, large areas are commonly needed to safely accommodate the canes, walkers, and wheelchairs clients may require for mobility.

Restlessness and agitation can also be safety hazards. Providing clients with freedom to move while preventing them from wandering off the unit, crawling over side rails, or otherwise being injured is an ongoing challenge. Using a bed with an alarm, a sitter, or a family member in close proximity may be helpful in providing safety. Use restraints as infrequently as possible; they commonly escalate the client's anxiety and combativeness. Providing room for the client to pace or wander may be important for lowering anxiety or restlessness.

Encouraging Independence. Promote independent functioning by helping the client accomplish activities of daily living to the fullest extent possible. Provide needed materials, and encourage independence. Help with the tasks that the client cannot accomplish alone. Divide activities into small steps to avoid overwhelming and frustrating the client. Provide frequent cues of tasks to be done, and allow enough time to accomplish them. Balance the benefit of allowing the client to manage some aspects of care against the client's stress threshold and capability.

Providing Appropriate Stimulation. Meaningful stimulation is important to engage the client in living with dignity and integrity. For chronically confused clients, stimulation must be individualized and balanced with the client's capability, strengths, and interests. Try to identify objects and events that are meaningful to the client. Coordinate emotional bonds, interests, and abilities with activities. Make the health care environment meaningful by allowing family members to bring pictures or objects that are familiar and comforting. Include beliefs that are meaningful to the client in daily life and care. Commonly, religious beliefs and ceremonies provide significant meaning. Encourage family, friends, and pets to visit, and include the client in family news and events to the extent that the client is capable of participating.

Provide a routine and a consistent physical environment. Simple and familiar patterns decrease stress. Limit the number of choices if this tends to overstimulate the client. Use symbols other than written signs to help clients locate bathrooms or dining rooms, especially if they have trouble reading. Also use environmental cues, such as clocks, calendars, and seasonal pictures, to help maintain the sense of orientation to time. Use light to eradicate shadows and minimize misperceptions or perceptual distortions.

Encourage socialization and communication to promote self-esteem and meaning for the client. Use reminiscence and life review to help maintain a sense of worth and integrity. Activities and exercises that are nontaxing can be healthy and invigorating as well. Music therapy tends to have a soothing effect. Often, activities that involve working with the hands provide enjoyment while helping to keep the joints mobile.

Take care to eliminate overstimulation for both acutely and chronically confused clients. Overstimulation can cause frustration or disorientation. Such overstimulation may arise from competing stimuli, such as meaningless noise from the intercom, an unwatched television, and traffic in the hallway. Also, try not to overstimulate the client by expecting and encouraging the client to do more than he or she can. In some cases, the client may need to be moved to another area to reduce stimulation and provide an opportunity for needed rest or sleep. When possible, assign the same staff members to work with the client so that the staff and the environment become familiar.

Promoting Therapeutic Communication. Communication that helps promote dignity and integrity and establish a meaningful environment is especially important for clients with perceptual difficulties. Communication should be clear and simple yet respectful. Wait, and allow the client the time needed to communicate, walk, and perform activities.

Validation therapy is a way of communicating that accepts the personal truth and reality of the person with dementia. Rather than attempt to orient the person to your reality, validate the values, beliefs, and reality of the dementia person—even if it has no basis in your reality. Assume that no matter what illusion the person with AD is living, he or she is right, and nothing you can say or do will convince the person otherwise. For example, if the person is getting ready to "drive to the grocery store," do not tell her she does not have a car; distract her with writing a list of what she will buy. In the process it may become apparent that she is hungry, and you can engage her in getting something to eat. By the time she has eaten, the idea of going to the grocery store may be forgotten.

Validation therapy is based on the idea that all behavior has a logical basis and tries to find the reason behind the behavior or expressed feeling. Paying attention to the concern or message embedded in the communication will help to focus on the true meaning of the communication. Accept and reaffirm the client at whatever place and time he or she is in, regardless of accuracy.

Even when a client is clearly having a hallucination, pay attention to the meaning and concern of the thoughts. This attention to the deeper meaning and concern can do much to maintain self-esteem, calm the client, and provide a more meaningful environment. For example, if the client misperceives a closet door as a dangerous person, attend not only to the need to arrange the room to prevent that misperception, but also to the need to calm the client's concern about safety. Often with acute confusion, the types of hallucinations provide hints of client difficulties. One acutely confused client who hallucinated that her blood was turning to powder later expressed extreme gratitude to the nurse who assessed her for dehydration and provided appropriate intervention.

Validation therapy restores rather than diminishes self-worth, reduces stress and anxiety, and facilitates independent living for as long as possible. The idea is that you cannot restore reality to the client with dementia but can accept them in the reality they understand. The advice regarding delusions and hallucinations for a mentally ill client would be different.

Avoiding Catastrophic Incidents. Catastrophic behaviors are combative, compulsive, angry, or violent behaviors to relatively minor incidents that have been misperceived by the person with dementia. Although the behavior seems inappropriate, the chronically confused client with a lowered stress threshold experiences it as overwhelming stress. Because the stress threshold drops as chronic confusion progresses, catastrophic incidents become more likely as the client's confusion worsens. The stressors that *trigger* catastrophic behaviors are unique for each person but commonly include fatigue, expectations that exceed the person's capabilities, lack of control, confrontation of inability, overstimulation, and changes in routine or environment.

Avoid catastrophic incidents by preventing these triggers. Structure the environment—with soft music, room for wandering freely, activities within the limits of ability, and consistent caregivers—to ensure that the client is not stimulated into violent, compulsive, combative outbursts. In addition, make sure that such outbursts are neither precursors of further illness nor actual signs and symptoms of acute confusion.

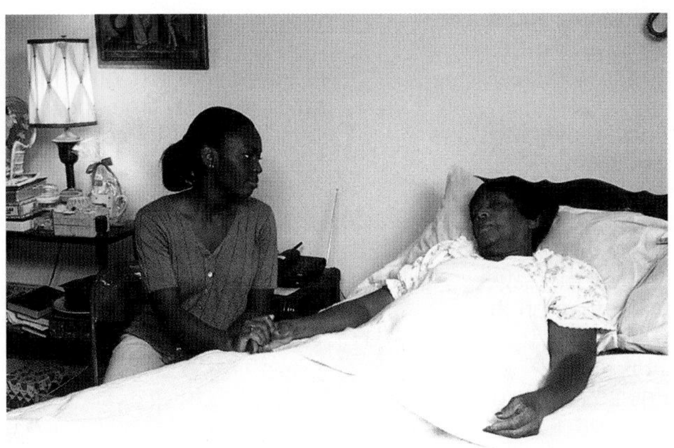

FIGURE 40-5 Considering the needs of supportive caregivers is an essential aspect of caring for a confused client.

INTERVENTIONS TO REDUCE CAREGIVER ROLE STRAIN

Consideration of family members and other caregivers is an essential aspect of caring for a confused client (Figure 40-5). The strain of caring for a confused person while carrying on daily lives and attending to multiple roles can quickly exhaust financial, physical, and emotional resources. When arranging for the care and discharge of the client, take into account not only the needs of the client but also the capabilities of the family and caretakers. Involve family members throughout the continuum of the client's care.

Provide education, resources, information, and support for persons attempting to provide care for the client. Consider the needs and input of all those involved as a necessary part of discharge planning. Help family members consider the need for additional resources to prevent exhaustion. Ongoing education, input into planning, availability to answer questions, and mobilization of needed resources are important supports for families (see Chapter 47). Refer back Box 40-5 for information helpful for caregivers.

A positive attitude about age and culture is important when planning home health care, institutional care, or discharge for the confused client. Family members often take their cues from the expectations and attitudes of health care providers. Examine the cultural beliefs of the client and family. Culture tends to determine how aging and confusion are viewed, how the confused person is treated, and what expectations about the client and family will be used after discharge (Box 40-7).

EVALUATION

Perform evaluation by determining whether client outcomes have been met, as shown in Box 40-8. A confused client may change constantly, which requires ongoing assessment. Characteristics, nursing actions, and client

BOX 40-7 *Cross-Cultural Care*

Caring for a Greek American Client

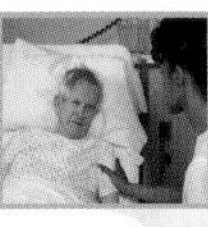

Mr. Tellis, the client whose story we have been following in this chapter, is of Greek descent. He came to the United States as an adolescent in 1929 with his parents and siblings with the hope that America would offer an opportunity to build a rewarding life. He adheres to Greek cultural beliefs and has ties to a large extended family of children, brothers, sisters, and cousins. He is typical of immigrant Greeks of that time, having limited formal education but a strong work ethic, determination, and ethnic pride. Although every client is unique, many Greek Americans have a tendency to hold the following views and values:

- A view of doctors and hospitals as a last resort
- Living independently
- Self-reliance and a sense of freedom and self-worth
- Greater reliance on family for health care and advice than on health care professionals
- Staying with a sick person rather than leaving him or her alone

BOX 40-8

Nursing Care Plan

A Confused Client

Admission Data

Mr. Tellis is admitted from the emergency department to a day unit until the cause of his acute confusion is established. He arrives at the unit with the following summation: *Mr. Tellis is an 83-year-old white man in no acute distress. IV fluid started left antecubital, 1 L D_5LR at 75 mL/hr due to dehydrated status. Monitor for fluid overload every hour. Preliminary urine report suggests urinary tract infection with sepsis. Ampicillin 500 mg q6h started at 0900. Foley catheter in place to closely monitor output. ECG and routine chest x-ray to be done on admission to the unit as these systems seem to be uninvolved. Will be examined by attending MD upon admission to your unit. A decision to proceed with a CT scan to rule out brain pathology will be made then.*

Physician's Orders

Admitting diagnosis: confusion secondary to urinary tract infection
IV 1 L D_5LR at 75 mL/hr
Vital signs q4h
Ampicillin 2 g IVPB q6h
Intake and output q4h
Repeat electrolytes and CBC 4 hours after IV has infused
Chest x-ray, rule out pneumonia
ECG, rule out ischemic changes

Nursing Assessment

No acute distress. Awake and alert. Denies pain, shortness of breath, or difficulty breathing. Mini-Mental State Examination repeated with a score of 24, same as in the emergency department. IV patent and infusing as ordered. Lungs sound clear, no jugular vein distention, and no edema to suggest fluid overload. Temperature is 97.0° F orally, but will continue to monitor frequently because older adults do not always show elevated temperature with infection. BP 140/80 lying, orthostatic BP deferred because client stated he was "dizzy" when he stood an hour ago in emergency department. Foley catheter draining concentrated urine, 350 mL. Oriented to room, call bell given to client with instruction and demonstration on how to use it. Daughter instructed to call for nurse if client becomes confused and tries getting out of bed without nurse.

NANDA-I Nursing Diagnosis	NOC Expected Outcomes With Indicators	NIC Interventions With Selected Activities	Evaluation Data
Acute Confusion	***Cognitive Orientation***	***Delirium Management***	***After 24 Hours of Care***
Related Factors: • Agitation	• Will experience no confusion.	• Provide meaningful communication to maintain reality, orientation, and sense of integrity and dignity and prevent injury.	• No injury occurs.
• Inattention • Fluctuating level of consciousness	• Will have diminished episodes of delirium with less agitation, less inattention, less fluctuating level of consciousness.	• Orient subtly and frequently as needed. • Use simple, concrete directions and break directions into small tasks. • Talk in a calm, quiet manner and allow ample time for client to process information. • Focus on client's real message and concern rather than on the confusion. • Talk about what is real. • Assign the same nurse to provide care when possible. • Provide meaningful stimuli and reduce competing meaningless stimuli (reduce noise: hospital intercom, loud radios, etc.). • Allow client to have personal belongings that aid orientation and calm, such as pictures. • Use environmental cues, such as clock, calendar, bright colors to mark client's door and orient to environment and good lighting to diminish shadows and possible misperceptions.	• Attentive and alert, oriented to place, time and person, except for confused episodes: • "I remember everything except how it happened and how I got here." • Able to perform all tests in neurological tool.
		• Allow presence of familiar person(s), such as family members.	• Family taking turns sitting with client around the clock. • Relies on daughter to make decisions and relaxes when daughter is present. States "She's the boss while I'm in the hospital."

BOX 40-7

Nursing Care Plan—cont'd

A Confused Client

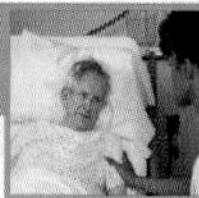

Critical Thinking Questions

1. Mr. Tellis's daughter does not understand how her father can be dehydrated when he drinks eight cups of coffee a day. How would you explain this to her?
2. Mr. Tellis needs a reminder about how much fluid he needs to drink per day. What intervention would you put into place, in his home, to remind him?
3. What community services might be appropriate for Mr. Tellis? Whom would you approach about these suggestions?

Nursing outcome and intervention labels from Johnson, M., Bulechek, G., Butcher, H., Dochterman, J. M., Maas, M., Moorhead, S., et al. (Eds.). (2006). *NANDA, NOC, and NIC linkages: Nursing diagnoses, outcomes, & interventions.* St. Louis, MO: Mosby.

needs change as the client's condition changes. With acute confusion, the client develops the condition relatively abruptly. Rapid, appropriate action and continuous assessment is needed. Recognition and appropriate treatment of underlying factors can often reverse acute confusion. Nursing care of acute confusion is evaluated by the recognition, treatment, and reversal of an underlying etiology that in turn reverses the effects of confusion.

In contrast, chronic confusion gradually changes with the client's progressive deterioration. Evaluation of interventions for chronic confusion involves measuring their ability to halt or slow deterioration, lessen catastrophic episodes, promote dignity and integrity, and enable the client to function at the height of ability. As deterioration progresses, the client's needs tend to increase in number and complexity. In the final stages of chronic confusion, the client requires extensive skilled nursing care. Multiple chronic illnesses are usually apparent as well. Extensive physiological and psychological issues arise. In addition, acute and chronic confusion may appear together and have multiple related factors.

A sample documentation note for Mr. Tellis after 24 hours of care could be like the one below.

SAMPLE DOCUMENTATION NOTE FOR MR. TELLIS

Client attentive and oriented to place, time, and person. No evidence of delusions, misperceptions, or hallucinations. Memory intact except for events during periods of confusion.

▼ KEY PRINCIPLES

- Confusion is a state in which a person experiences or is at risk of experiencing a disturbance in cognition.
- Confusion is not a disease; it is a syndrome of clinically observable phenomena.
- Confusion is profoundly important as a signal of serious neurological difficulty, which can develop into chronic illness and even death if it is undetected and underlying factors are untreated.
- Acute and chronic confusion may occur separately or together.
- *Delirium* is the medical diagnosis associated with acute confusion; *dementia* is the medical diagnosis associated with chronic confusion.
- Acute confusion is often a medical emergency.
- Common barriers to correctly identifying confusion are incorrect beliefs and attitudes about confusion, lack of precise documentation, and mental status assessment that is incomplete or fails to use the proper assessment tools.
- A number of factors can affect cognition, including life span, physiological, cultural and environmental, lifestyle, and psychological factors.
- Assessment of cognition includes a health history, assessment tools, and mental status examination.
- Appropriate treatment depends on differentiation of acute confusion, chronic confusion, and depression.
- In acute confusion, the goals of care focus on prevention, timely recognition, and appropriate treatment of underlying factors.
- In chronic confusion, the goals of care focus on slowing the deterioration process and maintaining quality of life, dignity, and respect.
- Interventions for confusion focus on maintaining the highest level of health, promoting safety, preventing injury, promoting independence without exceeding the client's capacity, providing meaningful and appropriate stimulation and communication, and promoting dignity and integrity.
- Interventions for acute confusion relate to identifying the etiology and treating the cause.
- Interventions for chronic confusion relate to identifying triggers and structuring the environment to minimize catastrophic incidents.
- Preservation of the family unit and support of caregivers are essential focuses when working with the confused client.

REVIEW QUESTIONS

1. You have a client with moderate chronic confusion who has just been transferred to a controlled living environment. You want the client to learn his way around the unit and the routine for meals. Which statement is the best guidance for your plan of care?

1. People with chronic confusion can learn new things but need more time and repetition.
2. People with chronic confusion are unable to learn new things and can only be expected to perform behaviors associated with previous knowledge.
3. Chronic confusion has nothing to do with a person's ability to learn new behaviors.
4. There is no point in trying to teach anything to a person with chronic confusion because the person cannot remember it.

2. Your client has moderate Alzheimer's disease and has just returned to your unit after a surgical procedure. She is swatting at her arms and saying there are bugs on her arms. You do not see any bugs. Which is the best action?

1. Restrain her to prevent injury.
2. Check her oxygen saturation.
3. Orient her to the environment.
4. Ask her family to sit with her.

3. Your older adult client tells you that she saw her husband at the door and wants you to find him. You know that her husband is dead. Which of the following symptoms is the client having?

1. Delusion
2. Hallucination
3. Sundown syndrome
4. Apraxia

4. You assess an older adult client by asking her to state her name, where she is, and the time of the day. She states her name, says she is in the hospital, and that it is morning. You would conclude:

1. She is not confused.
2. She is confused.
3. She is not completely oriented.
4. She is oriented to time, place, and person.

5. Your chronically confused client appears highly anxious. You are trying to find out what is wrong, and she starts screaming for the nurses to get out of her room and leave her alone. Which statement gives the best guidance for developing a plan to prevent future catastrophic events?

1. Catastrophic incidents like this one can be triggered by stressful events unrelated to the behavior.
2. Safety is the first consideration, and restraints may be necessary to control catastrophic behavior.
3. Education will help the client know that the nurses are only trying to help.
4. Calm, nonthreatening actions allow the client to regain control of herself.

Bibliography

*Alzheimer's Association, Massachusetts Chapter. (2002). *Nursing Home Consumer Guide: What to Look for While Evaluating a Nursing Home for Someone With Alzheimer's Disease.* Watertown, MA: Author. Retrieved December 3, 2006, from http://www.alzmass.org/nursinghome_consumerguide/topic_01.htm.

Amella, E. J. (2004). Presentation of illness in older adults: If you think you know what you're looking for, think again. *American Journal of Nursing, 104*(10), 40-52.

American Psychiatric Association. (2000). *Diagnostic and statistical manual of mental disorders* (4th ed., Text Revision). Washington, DC: Author.

Arnold, E. (2005). Sorting out the 3 D's: Delirium, dementia, depression. Learn how to sift through overlapping signs and symptoms so you can help improve an older patient's quality of life. *Holistic Nursing Practice, 19*(3), 99-105.

Beattie, E. R. A., Song, J., & LaGore, S. (2005). A comparison of wandering behavior in nursing homes and assisted living facilities. *Research and Theory for Nursing Practice, 19*(2), 181-196.

Bright, L. (2005). Challenging restraint. *Nursing Older People, 17*(1), 8.

Carpenito, L. J. (2006). *Nursing diagnosis: Application to clinical practice* (10th ed.). Philadelphia: Lippincott Williams & Wilkins.

Confusion, dementia, and mental incapacity are all different. (2005). *Senior Care Management, 8*(4), 42-43.

Dewing, J. (2004). Concerns relating to the application of frameworks to promote person-centredness in nursing with older people. *Journal of Clinical Nursing, 13*(3a), 39-44.

Dunn, D. (2005). Preventing perioperative complications in an older adult: Learn how his advancing age affects his risks so you can take steps to head off trouble. *Holistic Nursing Practice, 19*(2), 54-61.

Eliopoulis, C. (2001). *Gerontological nursing* (5th ed.). Philadelphia: Lippincott Williams, & Wilkins.

Evans, C. (2005). Research digest. Case management for frail older people. *Primary Health Care, 15*(2), 8.

*Folstein, M., Folstein, S., & McHugh, P. (1975). Mini-Mental State: A practical method for grading the cognitive state for the clinician. *Journal Psychiatric Research, 12*(3), 189-198.

Forema, M., Mion, L. Tryostad, L., Fletcher, K., & The NICHE Faculty. (1999). Standard of practice protocol: Acute confusions/delirium. *Geriatric Nursing, 20*(3), 147-152.

*Foreman, M. D. (1993). Acute confusion in the elderly. *Annual Review of Nursing Research, 11*, 3-30.

Johnson, M., Bulechek, G., Butcher, H., Dochterman, J. M., Maas, M., Moorhead, S., et al. (Eds.). (2006). *NANDA, NOC, and NIC linkages: Nursing diagnoses, outcomes, & interventions.* St. Louis, MO: Mosby.

NANDA International. (2007). *Nursing diagnoses: Definitions and classification, 2006-2007* (7th ed.). Philadelphia: Author.

National Institute of Aging. (2006). *Caregiver Guide.* U.S. National Institutes of Health. Retrieved 3/26/06 from http://www.nia.nih.gov/Alzheimers/Publications/caregiverguide.htm#choosing.

Oyama, K. (2005). When delirium takes hold. *RN, 68*(5), 52-6, 76-7, 33 passim.

*Pfeiffer, E. (1975). A short portable mental status questionnaire for assessment of organic brain deficit in the elderly patient. *Journal of the American Geriatric Society, 23*(10), 433-441.

Phinney, A. (1998). Living with dementia from the patient's perspective. *Journal of Gerontological Nursing, 24*(6), 8-15.

Rana, S., & O'Connell, C. B. (2005). Advisor forum. Suspected sundowning in a postoperative elderly patient. *Clinical Advisor, 8*(11), 100-101.

Rapp, C., & The Iowa Veteran's Affair Research Consortium. (2001). Acute confusion/delirium protocol. *Journal of Gerontological Nursing 27*(4), 21-23.

Resnick, B. (2001). Dementia, delirium & depressive in older adults. *Advances for Nurses 3*(22), 15-18.

Stabell, A., Eide, H., Solheim, G. A., Solberg, K. N., & Rustoen, T. (2004). Nursing home residents' dependence and independence. *Journal of Clinical Nursing, 13*(6), 677-686.

Tripp-Reimer, T., & Sorofman, B. (1998). Greek Americans. In L. Purnell & B. Paulanka (Eds.). *Transcultural health care: A culturally competent approach.* Philadelphia: Davis.

Wenborn, J. (2004). The here and now: Making sense of reality orientation. *Nursing & Residential Care, 6*(2), 80-81.

*Asterisk indicates a classic or definitive work on this subject.

Chapter 41

Promoting Self-Concept

Media Resources

- Evolve Website http://evolve.elsevier.com/Harkreader/
- 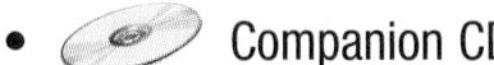 Companion CD

Learning Objectives

After studying this chapter, you should be able to do the following:

- Differentiate among self-concept, self-esteem, personal identity, role performance, and body image
- Discuss factors affecting self-concept
- Assess responses of clients who may be at risk for changes in self-esteem or body image
- Write a nursing diagnosis and develop a care plan for a client experiencing an alteration in the components of self-concept
- Plan goal-directed interventions that address the identified nursing diagnoses
- Describe key interventions for clients who are experiencing alterations in self-esteem and body image
- Evaluate the client's progress toward expected outcomes for alterations in self-esteem and body image

Key Terms

body image
personal identity
role
role performance
self-concept
self-esteem

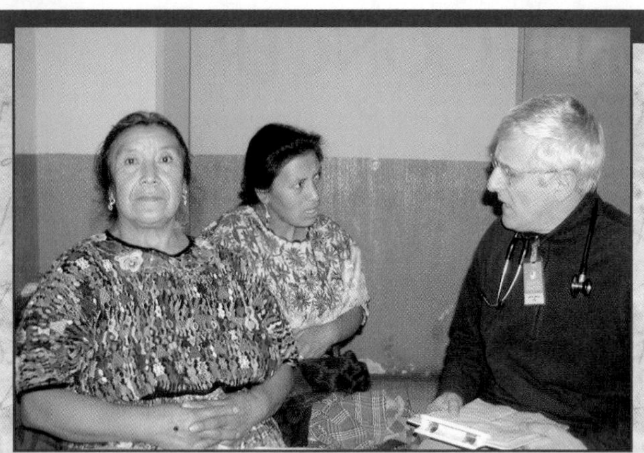

From Jarvis, C. (2003). *Physical examination and health assessment* (4th ed.). St. Louis, MO: Mosby.

Nancy Ward, a 63-year-old Navajo woman, lives with her younger sister, Helen. Nancy's husband of 25 years died 6 months ago from complications of alcohol abuse, diabetes, and coronary artery disease. During the marriage, he was abusive and violent, especially when he was intoxicated. Nancy had been hospitalized twice for physical abuse, and she was also frequently verbally abused. Nancy weighs 285 pounds and is 5 feet 4 inches tall. She was not able to have children because of endometriosis. Two weeks ago, Nancy visited her physician for a routine mammogram. She has returned today because the results indicate a suspicious density that will require a surgical biopsy. The chance that this growth is malignant is of great concern to Nancy. The nurse plans to educate Nancy on the upcoming surgical procedure. Because of Nancy's health history, the nurse considers the diagnoses *Situational low self-esteem* and *Disturbed body image* from the list of nursing diagnoses for self-concept (see key nursing diagnoses box).

KEY NURSING DIAGNOSES FOR SELF-CONCEPT

Chronic low self-esteem: Long-standing negative self-evaluation/feelings about self or self-capabilities
Situational low self-esteem: Development of a negative perception of self-worth in response to a current situation
Disturbed body image: Confusion in mental picture of one's physical self

CONCEPT OF SELF

Self-concept is a relatively enduring set of attitudes and beliefs about both the physical self and the psychological self. It is the totality of ideas that a person holds about the self. Self-concept is not a static state but one that develops and changes over time with life experiences and relationships that influence beliefs about the self. It includes the person's self-knowledge, self-expectations, and self-evaluation. Self-concept guides our actions, motivations, expectations, and goals for the future.

Nurses work with clients who have a wide range of problems involving self-concept. A sound self-concept is important to overall health and may help determine a client's willingness to take action to improve health status. Sometimes a health problem itself has a negative effect on self-concept, and the client may need assistance to accept a change in health status and maintain quality of life. Problems with self-concept are also a major focus for nurses who specialize in mental health nursing.

COMPONENTS OF SELF-CONCEPT

To fully understand self-concept, it is useful to describe the individual elements that make up the mental picture of the self. Self-concept includes four components: self-esteem, personal identity, role performance, and body image (Figure 41-1).

Self-Esteem. The term *self-esteem* is often used interchangeably with the term *self-concept,* but "to esteem" means to regard favorably, with admiration or respect. Therefore, **self-esteem** can be defined as the degree to which one has a positive evaluation of one's self, based on one's perceptions of how one is viewed by others as well as one's views about self.

There are two schools of thought about the development of self-esteem. The first is that self-esteem forms early in life, is based primarily on relationships with early caregivers, and is relatively fixed throughout life. The second is that self-esteem fluctuates whenever life transitions, crises, or illnesses challenge the self-concept or alter the person's status or role (Arnold & Boggs, 2006).

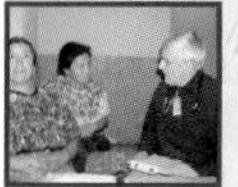

For example, Nancy Ward's self-esteem was probably affected each time her husband abused her; it may be further damaged by the fear of debilitating illness or disfiguring surgery. However, we do not know the level of self-esteem present when Nancy entered into the relationship. Do you think Nancy's self-esteem was formed in early childhood or was shaped by the events of her life? How do you think her past history and view of herself will affect her response to her current health situation?

Having high self-esteem entails having a high level of satisfaction with oneself. It is derived from the internal comparison of the present self to the ideal self. People who possess high self-esteem tend to be more content, in control, confident, accountable, and capable. Low self-esteem can result in a lack of confidence, an inability to act in one's own best interest, feelings of being overwhelmed, having decreased activity or energy, powerlessness, and reduced ability to function.

Men and women base their self-esteem on different things. Men are more likely to base their self-esteem on their personal achievements in life. Women often associate self-esteem with the adequacy of their social support system. Self-esteem in men is often greatly affected by

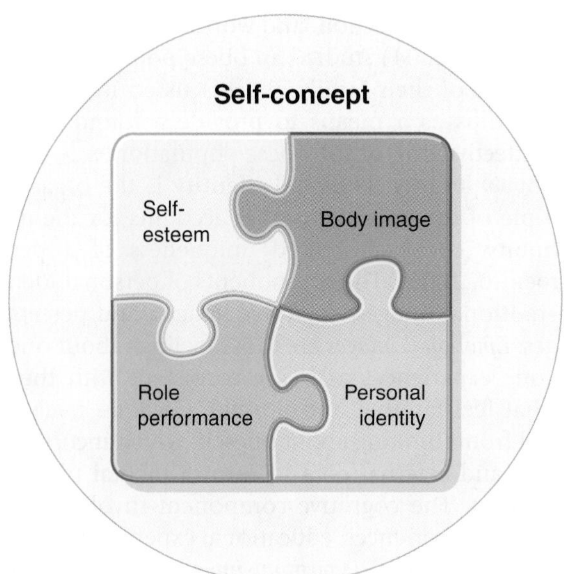

FIGURE 41-1 Self-concept has four interrelated components.

having a sense of well-being, a positive outlook on life, and an ability to perform activities of daily living (ADLs). Self-esteem in women is often affected by whether they are content with their lives and have a feeling that they are needed.

Theories of Development and Self-Esteem. Theories of development are closely interwoven with the concepts of self and self-esteem. In this chapter we will look at two theories of development, those of Abraham Maslow and Erik Erikson, and see how they relate to four components of self-esteem as described by Coopersmith (1981). Elements in each of these theories can be viewed as complementing the others, as seen in Figure 41-2.

Maslow's hierarchy of needs. Maslow (1954) described self-esteem as a requirement for reaching full personal development, which he called "self-actualization." Maslow suggested that people have a "hierarchy of needs," and that physiological needs form the foundation on which safety and security are built. Unless these basic, foundational needs are met, higher-level needs receive less attention and energy. According to Maslow, self-esteem develops after the need for belonging and being loved by others is met and is thus coincidental with the need for esteem from others. In other words, a positive relationship with others leads to the development of a positive self-concept and self-esteem. This theory supports the idea that self-esteem is not fixed but changes in relation to interactions with others.

Erikson's eight stages of man. Erikson (1950) described the development of self-esteem in eight stages, ranging from infancy through old age. According to Erikson, in infancy the child develops *trust* through the concern of caregivers. From ages 1 to 3, the child develops *autonomy* by learning control of the body. Through developing *initiative* and *industry,* the child gradually develops broader control over the environment and finally over his or her own intellect. By age 12, a child has typically developed the ability to derive self-esteem from what is called an "internal locus of control"—that is, from within the self rather than from outside sources. Children with an internal locus of control feel that they have the power to affect what happens to them.

According to Erikson, the adolescent develops *identity.* During this time, an adolescent rebels against parents in an effort to establish personhood, and acceptance by peers dramatically affects self-esteem. Adolescence is also a time when one develops a personal value system and solidifies sexual identity. Adolescents continually vacillate between independence and dependence.

Erikson's last three stages of development—*intimacy, generativity,* and *integrity*—normally occur in adulthood. The tasks to be accomplished in adulthood are the forging of relationships (intimacy), productivity (generativity), and harmony with oneself and with life (integrity). Based on Erikson's theory, self-esteem appears to develop in childhood but could change throughout a lifetime of developmental struggles.

Coopersmith's four components of self-esteem. Coopersmith (1981) identified four important components in the development of positive self-esteem: acceptance/worthiness, power/control, moral worth/virtue, and competence/mastery. According to Coopersmith, it is possible to increase self-esteem by attaining or experiencing success in any of these four areas.

Acceptance/worthiness relates to the perception, attention, and affection of others. It is the amount of concern and care that a person receives from significant others. A person learns to value self through the experience of being valued by others. In infancy, acceptance/worthiness is exemplified by the unconditional love that a parent or caregiver has for the child. Acceptance/worthiness provides toddlers with the freedom to explore further domains of their environment.

Power/control is the ability to influence and control others. Power and control make their first appearance in toddlerhood. Toddlers learn the concept of power and control by exploring their environment and manipulating objects within the environment. They gain an understanding that certain behaviors can bring about certain responses. Power and control over the environment continues to develop in school-age children, further extending the concept into group behaviors in school. Initiative develops within playgroups that have leaders and followers with designated roles. Power and control begins to take on a more realistic viewpoint at this time.

Moral worth/virtue is the adherence to moral and ethical standards. The values and morals of significant others are internalized by the preschool-age and the school-age child. In early childhood, the child adopts behaviors through identification with the same-sex parent and a desire to please that parent. By learning to label these and other behaviors as good or bad, moral development begins.

Competence/mastery refers to successful performance or achievement. It is marked by high levels of performance, with the level and the tasks varying depending on developmental stage. When abilities are sufficient to complete a task, competence/mastery is present, and vice versa. The development of *initiative* and *industry* leads to feelings of competence.

Self-Concept and Health. Research has shown an association between self-concept and health practices across the life span. Kaba, Thompson, Burnard, Edwards, and Theodosopoulou (2005) described concerns of heart transplant recipients about the donor's heart and how receiving somebody else's heart might affect the recipient's own personality; feelings of guilt for the donor's death and feelings of gratitude towards the donor's family; and concerns about the recipient's own heart. Bakewell and Volker (2005) explore the potential side effects of treatment for breast cancer that can affect sexual health and sexual health concerns of young women that can be addressed by nursing. Chao et al. (2006) studied older adult nursing home residents and found that group reminiscence therapy significantly improved self-esteem, although effects on depression and life satisfaction were not significant. Lysaker and Buck (2006) discuss methods to assist the recovery from schizophrenia through development of an integral sense of identity, agency, social connection, and worth. Rogge, Greenwald, and Golden (2004) studied an obese population within the context of their family and discussed interpersonal relationships as a means to provide a foundation for more effective care of the obese population.

Personal Identity. **Personal identity** is the organizing principle of the personality that accounts for the unity, continuity, consistency, and uniqueness of a person (Carpenito, 2005). The components of personal identity are emotional images, cognitive images, and perceptual images. *Emotional images* are those feelings about oneself that one experiences as being consistent with the self and that feel familiar and normal. *Cognitive images* are derived from thinking about oneself, which incorporates internal and external data to form a mental picture of who one is. The cognitive component involves intelligence, past experiences, educational experiences, and the process of thinking. *Perceptual images* are derived from external sensory data and are translated into mental pictures of reality. Two people experiencing the same situation may interpret it in two different ways.

Role Performance. **Role performance** refers to a person's fulfillment of the roles and current responsibilities in that person's life, and it includes the actions, thoughts, and feelings associated with those roles. A **role** is a homogenous set of behaviors, attitudes, beliefs, principles, and values that are normatively defined and expected of someone in a given social position or status in a group.

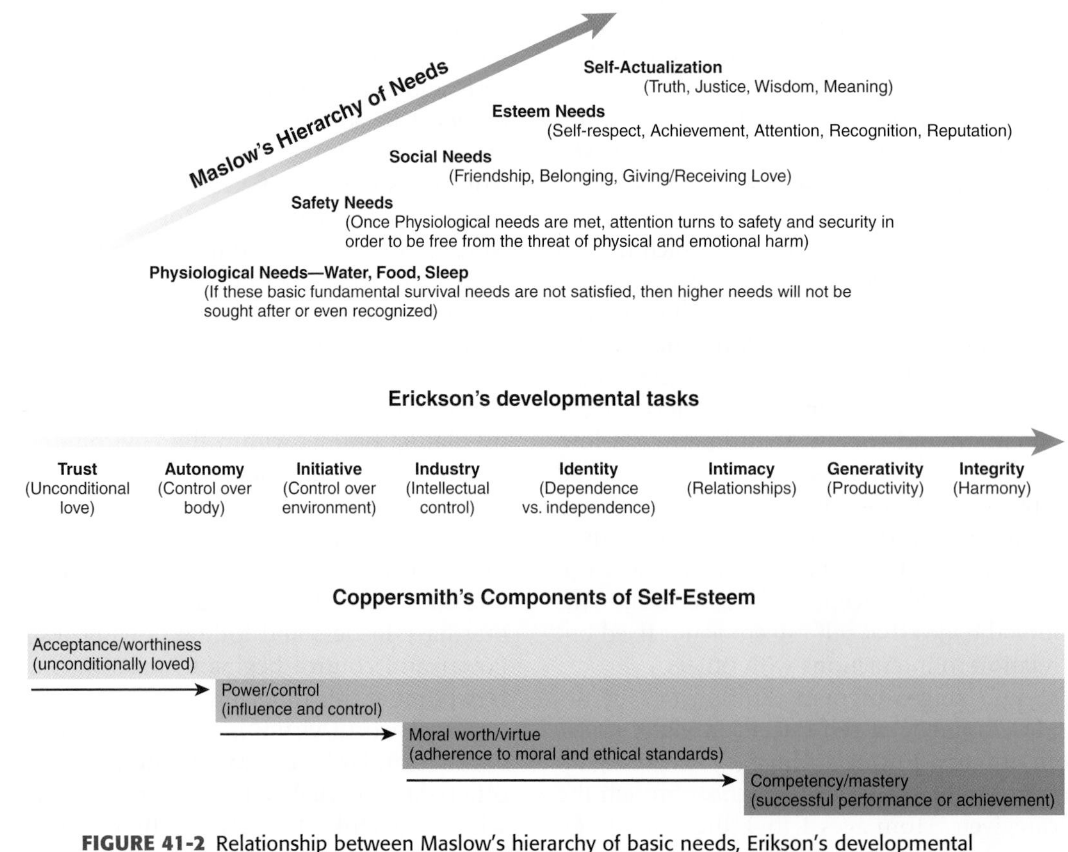

FIGURE 41-2 Relationship between Maslow's hierarchy of basic needs, Erikson's developmental tasks, and Coopersmith's components of self-esteem. (Modified and redrawn from Carson, V. B., & Arnold, E. N. [1996]. *Mental health nursing: The nurse-patient journey.* Philadelphia: Saunders.)

Roles are defined in terms of relationship to others. Some roles are prescribed by age, sex, or position in family, such as mother, father, and daughter. Others are acquired, such as nurse, teacher, or executive. Still others are transitional, such as student (Carpenito, 2005).

An inability to fulfill prescribed role behaviors can affect the other components of self-concept, especially self-esteem. Self-evaluation of how we perform our roles contributes to self-esteem. The evaluations made by others influence it as well.

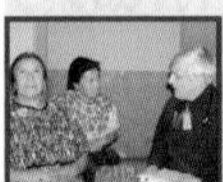

Nancy Ward, introduced at the beginning of this chapter, probably believed that conceiving and bearing children was an integral part of a married woman's role. This may also have been her husband's belief, as well as that of her culture and of society at large. Her low self-esteem was reinforced by her husband's constant negative evaluation of her abilities as a wife. How do you think this part of Nancy's history will affect her present circumstances?

Body Image. **Body image** is the perception of one's own body (Figure 41-3). It is the physical dimension of self-concept, or how one perceives and evaluates one's appearance and function. People can perceive their bodies as male or female, fat or thin, ugly or beautiful, fully functional or disabled, intact or missing some part. Body image changes with physical growth, weight gain or loss, aging, illness, accidents, and social or cultural influences. Body image is closely related to personal identity, role performance, and self-esteem. Self-evaluation of one's body, as well as the evaluations of others, contributes to self-esteem.

The significance of a person's body image varies with the value and intensity attached to that image. Body image is more important when strong emotions are attached to how the body is perceived. The social and cultural influences in American society place a high value on body image, which strongly affects people's personal perceptions.

Body image is dynamic. It develops as a person develops and can change and be changed. However, there is a certain amount of internal consistency to body image throughout life.

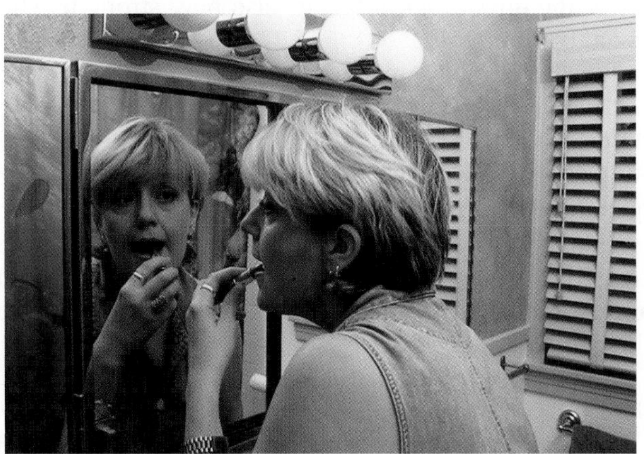

FIGURE 41-3 Body image is an important part of self-concept.

FACTORS AFFECTING SELF-CONCEPT

FACTORS ACROSS THE LIFE SPAN

Infants to Preschoolers. Self-esteem in infants and preschoolers can be related to the type of parenting the child receives. Self esteem is developed in the relationship with parents and siblings. The child learns to value the self through a trusting relationship with a caregiver and mastery of skills. A child who hears a barrage of criticism from parents and cannot count on parents to follow up what they say with consistent actions is at risk for developing a poor self-concept (Lutzen, Dahlqvist, Eriksson, & Norberg, 2006).

School-Age Children. As children leave the preschool period and enter school, the world broadens and there is a threat to self-esteem as they attempt to master the tasks of school and develop relationships with peers. Problems with self-esteem often begin to appear at this time. For example, childhood obesity (Fisher, Lange, Young-Cureton, & Canham, 2005), poor performance in school, and unsuccessful relationships with peers may lead to poor self-esteem in school-age children.

Adolescents. Adolescence, ages 12 to 20 years, is a period of sweeping hormonal changes and rapid physiological growth. It is a very stressful period of major life transition that can threaten self-esteem. In addition, the struggle for self-esteem is part of the search for identity and the transition to adult roles and responsibilities. Perceived rejection, a sense of unworthiness, or feelings of not being trusted are often associated with self-destructive behaviors in adolescence.

Peer relationships—positive or negative—also help to define self-concept in adolescents (Figure 41-4). Body image for teens reflects their peer group's attitude and the desire for acceptance and sameness. Harper and Marshall (1991) identified that teenage girls report more problems with body image than boys. Any event that causes change in a teen's body appearance can positively or negatively alter peer acceptance and lead to a change in body image or self-esteem. Rapid growth spurts and the emergence of acne can cause great discomfort because adolescents perceive that those changes interfere with peer relationships. Acne can cause embarrassment, self-consciousness, and anxiety.

Many factors can contribute to or trigger a persistent state of low self-esteem in teens. Chronic illnesses—such as depression, chronic fatigue, and multiple sclerosis—are associated with low self-esteem. Abusive or violent relationships also can destroy positive feelings about one's capabilities or oneself. Low self-esteem in adolescents has been associated with increased cigarette smoking and substance abuse involving cocaine, marijuana, and alcohol. However, the relationship is frequently circular rather than linear. That is, low self-esteem leads to cigarette smoking and substance abuse, and smoking

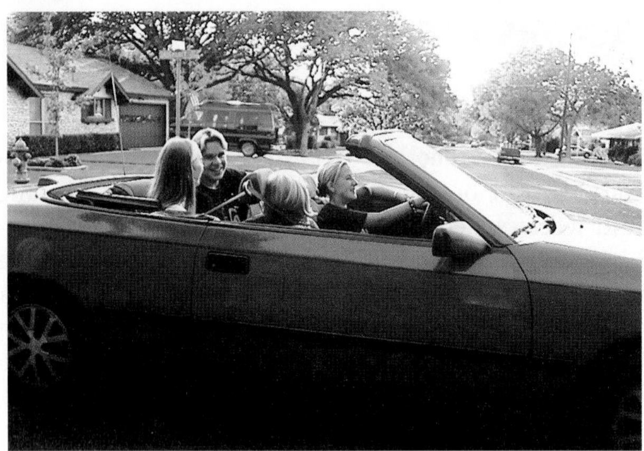

FIGURE 41-4 Peer relationships help define self-concept in adolescents.

and substance abuse lead in turn to low self-esteem (Doswell, Millor, Thompson, & Baxter, 1998).

Three specific categories relevant to self-esteem in teens include home, school, and peers. In one study, home and school were found to have a significant influence on negative self-esteem and the tendency of teens to use or abuse various substances (Young, Werch, & Bakema, 1989). Surprisingly, peers, by contrast, showed no significant influence on self-esteem among teens or on their tendency to use or abuse these substances. Prevention of substance use or abuse may therefore depend on the development of strategies to address problems in the home and school.

Young Adults. Young adults, ages 20 to 30 years, are also vulnerable to altered self-concept. This is a time of decision making about becoming independent, furthering an education, choosing a career, deciding to marry, starting a family, deciding on a place to live, even determining a lifestyle. Decisions about all of these areas can affect self-concept, positively or negatively.

Middle Adults. In middle adulthood, according to Erickson, the task is one of caring for others (elder parents) or guiding the young (children or grandchildren). Multiple life stressors and the beginning of physical decline have a potential to alter the self-concept during this period of life.

Women today lead active lives, typically as mothers, spouses, and workers outside the home. The multiple expectations that women hold for themselves can result in feelings of overwhelming pressure and can lead to role strain or stress and possibly to illness. How well women cope with multiple roles may also provide an indicator of how they can or will manage their overall health.

Women with high appraisal of self-worth may be better able to defend against illness than other women (O'Brien, 1993). Likewise, during stressful events or times of change, positive self-esteem may help women cope with uncertainty (Vera & Wrath, 1995). When a disease or its treatment threatens a woman's health, her security can be shaken, and her confidence can erode. This is especially true if the diagnosis can or will result in an alteration of the body. Role function disturbance or problems with interpersonal relationships may result (Anderson & Johnson, 1994).

The phenomenon of male menopause (andropause) occurs during the late 40s or early 50s. With changing hormonal levels from reduced testosterone production, men may perceive a threat to their masculinity, which could lead to a disruption of a previously stable relationship. Many men begin to lose scalp hair in middle adulthood. These phenomena may affect self-esteem and thus self-concept. During middle adulthood, men may take on the softer attributes of tenderness, caring, and assisting more with domestic tasks, such as cooking, laundry, and gardening.

Many health problems in middle age are the same for both men and women. The risk for cardiac disease equalizes between the two sexes. Diseases (such as cancer and hypertension), alcohol and nicotine use, drug addiction, and accidents affect both women and men during this period.

Older Adults. Older adults have many stresses that can threaten their self-concept. Many must cope with several chronic illnesses while other changes also occur in their lives. Learning to live with a chronic illness can lead to depression. Other contributing factors are loss of loved ones, retirement, reduced financial resources, loss of a body part or functional ability, and reduced independence. If older adults cannot adjust to these changes, they may begin to feel powerless and exhibit negative behaviors as a mechanism of control. They can thus become angry, manipulative, withdrawn, self-destructive, dependent, grieved, or depressed.

PHYSIOLOGICAL FACTORS

We have said that multiple stressors can affect self-esteem. It is often a combination of the specific physical or psychosocial stressor and the associated developmental stressor that has a major impact on self-concept. The following physiological factors also have strong psychosocial components.

Fatigue. The basis of fatigue is not fully understood, but it may be a factor in low self-esteem. Stress, boredom, unhappiness, and depression are related factors. Fatigue is a state in which a person lacks energy to adequately perform ADLs. Not only are energy levels very low, but hormonal and muscle cell activity is also decreased. Fatigue is a common complaint in both men and women, but women are more at risk, especially in the childbearing years.

A condition called chronic fatigue syndrome may be the cause of fatigue in some cases. However, the nature and existence of this syndrome continue to be debated.

Some researchers are able to clearly define the characteristics of this elusive disorder.

Trauma. Trauma or traumatic injuries can cause the loss or change of a major body part or a disfigurement, which can lead to a change in body image. Even when temporary, trauma is still frightening. It forces people to become dependent, even if only for a short time, which may affect self-esteem. Trauma may leave permanent losses or changes, such as crippling, scarring, and unrelieved acute and chronic pain, with consequent impact on self-concept. Visible injuries, such as facial trauma, may be even more difficult for clients to adjust to than other injuries and may have a greater impact on body image.

Chronic Illness. Coping with the burdens of chronic illness can affect one's self-concept. For example, research shows that quality of life and self-esteem are decreased in clients with chronic obstructive pulmonary disease and arthritis (Anderson, 1995). Likewise, Flett, Harcourt, and Alpass (1994) demonstrated that clients who have chronic leg ulcers also tend to suffer from low self-esteem, in part because of problems with independent functioning. During chronic illness, clients are at risk for low self-esteem because they have a sense of loss of control. In older adults, this decreased self-esteem can lead to decreased life satisfaction, increased incidence of depression and other physical illnesses, and medication use (Bensink, Godbey, Marshall, & Yarandle, 1992). When a person with a chronic illness must depend on a family member or other caregiver for care, this dependence can lower self-esteem.

Surgery. Whenever a client undergoes a surgical procedure, particularly for cancer, there is a risk for a change in body image and lowered self-esteem. Self-esteem and postoperative progress are related.

The diagnosis of cancer, especially breast cancer, has the potential to alter a woman's body image and lower self-esteem. Not only is the diagnosis of breast cancer devastating, but the treatment can be disfiguring. Use of chemotherapy and radiation can add to the problem of an altered body image and lower self-esteem because of hair loss, including loss of eyebrows and eyelashes.

Other surgeries can be equally disturbing to self-concept. Procedures that affect the reproductive system can alter body image in a powerful way. Some examples include removal of the ovaries (oophorectomy), hysterectomy, removal of the testes (orchiectomy), breast surgery, circumcision, and prostate surgery. Surgery that disfigures the face, such as removal of skin cancers—particularly the deep excisions for aggressive melanoma skin cancers—can profoundly affect body image. Procedures that drastically alter lifestyle, such as a permanent tracheostomy or a colostomy, can also have a major impact on self-concept.

Disability. The disabled are at risk for a disturbance in body image. For example, Mona, Gardo, and Brown (1994) found that a disabled woman's self-image was directly related to the age at which the disability occurred. Women who were disabled in younger years apparently were better able to master the skills needed to cope.

Body image and self-esteem can be affected by a spinal cord injury. The loss of independence and control associated with spinal cord injury can lead to lowered self-esteem, body image disturbance, loss of personal identity, lessened ideal sexuality, and loss of role function.

Obesity. Being overweight can elicit negative responses in others. Some people believe that obese individuals have poor self-esteem and are lazy, slow, and less competent than thin people. These responses may negatively affect the obese person's self-concept. Also, comparing one's appearance to an unrealistic societal ideal can generate negative thoughts about oneself, resulting in feelings of shame and frustration (Vera & Wrath, 1995).

CULTURAL AND LIFESTYLE FACTORS

Culture. Cultural factors and beliefs may contribute to a client's self-concept (Box 41-1). Be aware, too, that cultural influences can be as diverse as the people within cultures and religions. Sensitivity and understanding are keys to successful communication with all clients and family members. Remember that positive self-esteem consists of these: acceptance/worthiness, power/control, competence/mastery, and moral worth/virtue.

Socioeconomic status has a direct relationship to self-concept. A person's position on the health-illness continuum may in part result from the interrelationship of socioeconomic status, health care practices, and lifestyle. In addition, needing public assistance may have a negative impact on self-concept.

Living conditions are an important factor in the lives of clients who must seek public assistance. Often, public housing does not supply people with much more than the basic needs. The repair and condition of government housing is sometimes poor and does not foster self-esteem. Also, illness is more common when living conditions include rodents and roaches, and illness can contribute to a negative self-concept.

PSYCHOLOGICAL FACTORS

Depression. Depression is associated with low self-esteem. Difficulty finding appropriate, cost-effective treatment for depression may contribute. Other factors that contribute to depression include stress, powerlessness, helplessness, sexual bias, stereotyping, lack of control, single parenthood, multiple role conflicts, and poor educational or career status.

Stress. Stress can overwhelm a person to the point that physical and mental functioning is impaired. Self-concept is affected when a person's ability to function is reduced.

Loss. Loss is a factor that can easily lower self-esteem. Examples include the loss of a spouse, a loss or

BOX 41-1

Cross-Cultural Care

Caring for a Navajo Client

Nancy Ward, the client whose story we have followed throughout this chapter, is a Navajo. She and her husband left the reservation when they married. Her husband was not successful in maintaining employment off the reservation. They returned and lived most of their married life close to their families. Although Navajos follow many different paths, they have a tendency to maintain the following patterns of living:

- Younger Navajos often leave the reservation, voluntarily or involuntarily, to seek employment opportunities.
- The basic social unit is the nuclear family, but members live close to other families, sharing economic and social support. The Navajo family is very flexible in sharing with other families who are in need. Family may be defined in a broader context that includes kinship ties and close friends.
- Older adults are held in high esteem for their material wealth and knowledge wealth. Navajo children are expected to care for grandparents and great-grandparents. Grandparents also play major roles in caring for children.
- Navajos are often initially silent and reserved when meeting strangers. Eye contact is considered disrespectful and is avoided.
- Women are expected not to achieve more than their husbands. Divorce does occur despite the strong belief in maintaining the family.
- Navajos often gather the family for consultation when a clinic or hospital visit is prolonged.
- People of Navajo culture advocate for a balance among body, mind, and spirit.

A risk factor that contributes to a lowered self-esteem in Native Americans is mistrust of the establishment (authority) and of Western health care providers. Other factors include feelings of oppression from the loss of tribal lands, high unemployment rates, lack of acceptance in the mainstream workforce, alcoholism, and a sedentary lifestyle. The average Native American usually lives to be only 45 years old. Alcohol is a big factor in the poor health and death of many Native Americans.

Because of Nancy Ward's Native American culture, she may believe that she is in some disharmony with nature and that her illness may be the result. An interested third party, such as the medicine man, or shaman, may be helpful to fully gain Nancy's participation in the health care plan. This medicine man will be interested in Nancy's spiritual and physical health, and the mutual goal will be the restoration of good health and harmony.

change of employment, or the episodic loss of previous good health. Even temporary losses—such as financial problems, job layoffs, premenstrual syndrome, disharmony in relationships, children in trouble with school or law officials, career changes, incarceration, or institutionalization—may have an impact on self-concept. How these losses are accepted, and how a person moves on in life, depends greatly on the successful use of coping skills.

Abusive Relationships. Women who are involved in violent or abusive relationships often, understandably, have low self-esteem. Of these women, those with a weak sense of self can contribute unwittingly to the ongoing cycle of abuse. The strong, more dominant partner is rarely sensitive to the less powerful one, and it becomes increasingly difficult for the victim to resist the psychological hold of the abuser. Eventually, the victim incorporates the opinions of the dominator into her self-concept and assumes blame for the relationship.

ASSESSMENT

GENERAL ASSESSMENT OF SELF-CONCEPT

Health and illness affect self-concept (Figure 41-5). As a nurse in general practice, however, you will rarely, if ever, conduct an in-depth assessment of a client's self-concept. Nurses do this only when the client has presented with problems that are closely associated with disturbances in self-concept and when the goals of care are likely to include working on problems in self-concept.

Typically, this is the case for a client with a mental health problem.

When taking a health history in any setting, however, do make observations about the person's self-concept and its impact on health. For example, you may note that a client is well groomed, attractively dressed, sits erect, and comfortably enters into the conversation with the nurse. This is a good time to make these observations and to interweave questions that elicit data about the client's self-concept.

Action Alert! Listen and observe for cues to self-concept throughout the health history.

While taking clients' health history, listen for statements that indicate how they feel about themselves. If you have a therapeutic relationship with them, it may be natural to ask direct questions to elicit information about their self-esteem, especially in relation to the current situation. For example, when a woman is being scheduled for a hysterectomy or is being admitted to the hospital for the procedure, you might ask how she feels about having the procedure. You can help her be more specific by making a statement of fact and asking the client for a response. For example, you might say, "Some women have a sense that a hysterectomy changes their femininity or sexuality. How do you feel about that?"

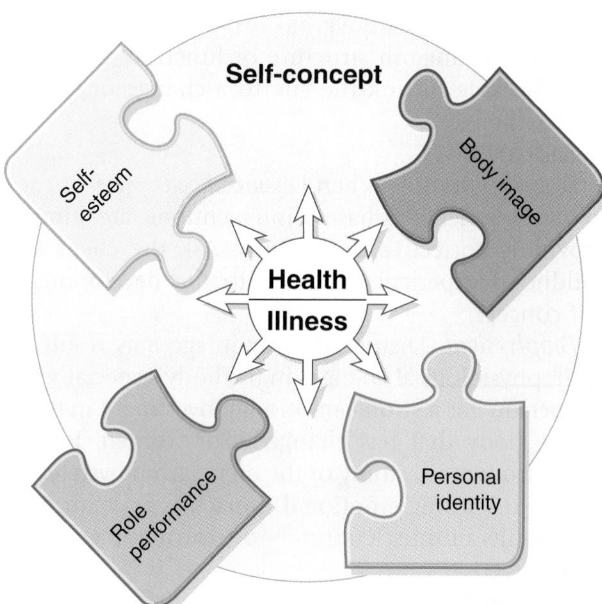

FIGURE 41-5 Health and illness affect self-concept.

When you sense that the client's self-concept is being affected by the health situation, you could follow up with questions about the impact or potential impact of changes in self-concept on the client's life. Using the woman needing a hysterectomy as an example, suppose the client responds to you by saying, "I guess I have to accept that I'll be less interested in sex. I'm getting older, and it's natural that it's less important than it used to be." You now have the opportunity to explore the impact of the procedure on the client's perception of herself and on her relationship with her husband. You also have the opportunity to provide some health teaching.

While listening for cues to the client's self-concept, consider the context in which the self-concept is being assessed. Are there other factors that would explain the person's behavior? In a different context, would the person display a different perception of the self? Even consider *your* influence on the client. As you ask questions and interact with the client, you want to be sure that you do not influence the client's responses. Look for evidence that in other areas of the person's life the self-concept is intact and healthy.

Action Alert! Validate behavioral cues. Behaviors can have many meanings.

Assess the sources of support and information the client has used in managing the feelings associated with the current situation. For example, you might ask the client about to undergo a hysterectomy whether she has discussed with her physician how soon she can engage in sexual intercourse following the hysterectomy.

At times it may be appropriate to do a focused assessment of specific aspects of self-concept. Assessment of self-esteem and body image are included below. See Chapter 44 for a full assessment of role performance.

FOCUSED ASSESSMENT FOR *LOW SELF-ESTEEM*

There are three nursing diagnoses related to self-esteem: *Situational low self-esteem, Chronic low self-esteem,* and *Risk for situational low self-esteem.* Because the first two are actual nursing diagnoses, there are both defining characteristics and related factors for these diagnoses. Because *Risk for situational low self-esteem* reflects a potential rather than an actual problem, it has risk factors but no defining characteristics.

Defining Characteristics. Assess for *Situational low self-esteem* by noting statements consistent with a current situation that poses a challenge to self-esteem, expressions of helplessness or uselessness, or inability to deal with a current event or situation. Also assess for negative statements about the self and indecisive, nonassertive behaviors.

Assess for *Chronic low self-esteem* by noting negative verbalizations about the self or rejection of positive feedback about the self. Assess for frequent negative comments, such as referring to self as stupid, ugly, or incompetent, or similar statements. Single, isolated negative comments about the self may not necessarily indicate low self-esteem unless they are part of a pattern of behavior. Evaluate body language, such as lack of eye contact and tone of voice, which is also important. Notice the pattern of relationships with others. Clients with low self-esteem have difficulty accepting a compliment or may exaggerate negative feedback from others. They are also frequently hypersensitive to criticism or minor rejections by others. The person who continually seeks acceptance, who is boastful, or who appears to have feelings of grandeur has not developed a positive sense of self-worth.

Observe the client's interactions with others to assess feelings about the person's ability to influence others or to have control over the person's own life. A feeling of lack of control can be manifested by a reluctance to ask others for help, to engage in social activities, or to make suggestions or to offer opinions. Assess the extent to which the client indicates an inability to deal with events, a lack of success in work or other aspects of life, or indecisiveness, passivity, or nonassertiveness. Table 41-1 compares characteristics of people with high and low self-esteem.

Assess feelings of competence by observing actions. Low self-esteem can manifest as a reluctance to try new things, to change jobs, or to move to a different residence. Low self-esteem can result in haphazard work or being overly concerned with details and perfection, either of which can result in poor quality of work.

Related Factors. The related factors differ somewhat depending on whether the low self-esteem is situational or chronic. *Situational low self-esteem* can be related to health problems that lead to disturbed body image, functional impairment, or loss. Examples include hysterectomy, amputation, a slow recovery from illness, or other situations that challenge a person's coping resources. *Chronic low self-esteem* may result from a more pervasive problem in unhealthy interpersonal relationships, failure to achieve developmental milestones, failure to achieve life goals, failure to live up to a personal moral code, or a sense of powerlessness.

The risk factors associated with *Risk for situational low self-esteem* are similar to those just listed. They include such factors as physical illness, developmental changes, functional impairments, disturbed body image, loss, social role changes, and a history of abuse, neglect, or abandonment.

FOCUSED ASSESSMENT FOR *DISTURBED BODY IMAGE*

Defining Characteristics. The nursing diagnosis *Disturbed body image* applies when a client has a change in the body and inadequately accepts the change, which then interferes with necessary health practices, abilities, or lifestyle management.

Assess for client statements that indicate a changed view of body appearance, structure, or function. These may range from preoccupation with the change to refusal to acknowledge the change. They may also include negative feelings about the body, or fear of negative reaction from others. Assess for client statements that focus on past strength, function, or appearance, or that emphasize remaining strengths. Assess for objective data such as a missing, nonfunctional, or traumatized body part. Note whether the client avoids looking at part of the body and whether the client either intentionally or unintentionally hides or overexposes that part. As you conduct your assessment, be sure to observe for verbal or nonverbal cues to the client's coping. For this diagnosis to apply, the client must exhibit either a verbal or nonverbal response to an actual or perceived change in structure or function; that is, you must be able to link the cue to a change or to a perceived change.

Related Factors

Developmental. When *Disturbed body image* is rooted in developmental phases, interventions are aimed at providing corrective experiences. Ask the client about childhood experiences related to the development of self-concept.

Biophysical. Disturbed body image may result from pathophysiological changes in the body, especially when the person has a strong emotional investment in the part of the body that has changed. For women, loss of a breast from mastectomy or the uterus from hysterectomy can have a strong emotional impact. For a man, illness that results in muscle atrophy or scarring may have the same effect.

Traumatic injuries that result in disfigurement will require the person to change the self-concept to include the changes in the body's appearance. Injuries that leave the face scarred are particularly difficult to manage. However, scars on any part of the body may have a significant impact on body image. For example, a 55-year-old man who has had coronary artery bypass surgery will have characteristic scars on his chest and leg that many people will recognize.

Changes in body image may be involved even when the change does not affect outward appearance. Less obvious but very real changes in body image can result from the loss of function of any body organ. For example, the person with a kidney transplant may not look different but must cope with a change in body image from that of a healthy, well-functioning body to that of a body vulnerable to infection and incorporating an organ from another person.

Table 41-1 Characteristics of People With High Self-Esteem Versus Low Self-Esteem

PEOPLE WITH HIGH SELF-ESTEEM	PEOPLE WITH LOW SELF-ESTEEM
• Accept responsibility for their own well-being and take charge of their own lives.	• Blame others for their lack of a sense of well-being and failures in life. Their behaviors are passive and obstructive.
• Expect to be valued and accepted by others. They like and value others.	• Expect people to be critical of them and to avoid their company. They are prone to condemn others.
• Have positive perceptions of their skills, appearance, sexuality, and behaviors.	• Have negative perceptions of their skills, appearance, sexuality, and behaviors.
• Perform equally well when being observed as when not watched. Motivation comes primarily from within.	• Perform less well when being observed. Motivation is primarily to avoid punishment.
• Accept criticism, evaluate it accurately, and change behaviors if needed.	• Are unrealistic and passive in response to criticism.
• Can accept compliments easily.	• Have difficulty accepting compliments.
• Evaluate their performance realistically.	• Have unrealistic expectations about their performance.
• Are relatively comfortable relating to authority figures.	• Are uncomfortable relating to authority figures.
• Express general satisfaction with life.	• Are dissatisfied with their lot in life.
• Have a social support system that gives positive feedback and encouragement.	• Have a weak social support system that reinforces resentments, fears, and vices.
• Have primarily an internal locus of control.	• Rely on external locus of control.

Modified from Arnold, E. C., & Boggs. K. U. (2006). *Interpersonal relationships: Professional communication skills for nurse* (3rd ed.). Philadelphia: Saunders.

Medical treatment, too, can affect body image. For example, chemotherapy can result in hair loss that may alter one's body image. Surgery may alter not only appearance but also function, such as in ostomy surgery, radical head/neck surgery, and amputation. Even the onset of a chronic medical condition requiring maintenance medication, such as asthma, hypertension, or diabetes, can affect body image.

Situational. Most people have experienced events that have a negative impact on body image. Usually these feelings are brief and resolve with a good night's sleep or a subsequent positive experience. However, some events are sufficiently traumatic to produce lasting effects. For example, *Disturbed body image* commonly occurs in victims of sexual abuse or rape. Rape victims, in particular, frequently report that they feel dirty and that no amount of bathing will remove the feeling.

Use the decision tree in Figure 41-6 to help determine which of the nursing diagnoses that relate to self-concept best applies to a particular client situation.

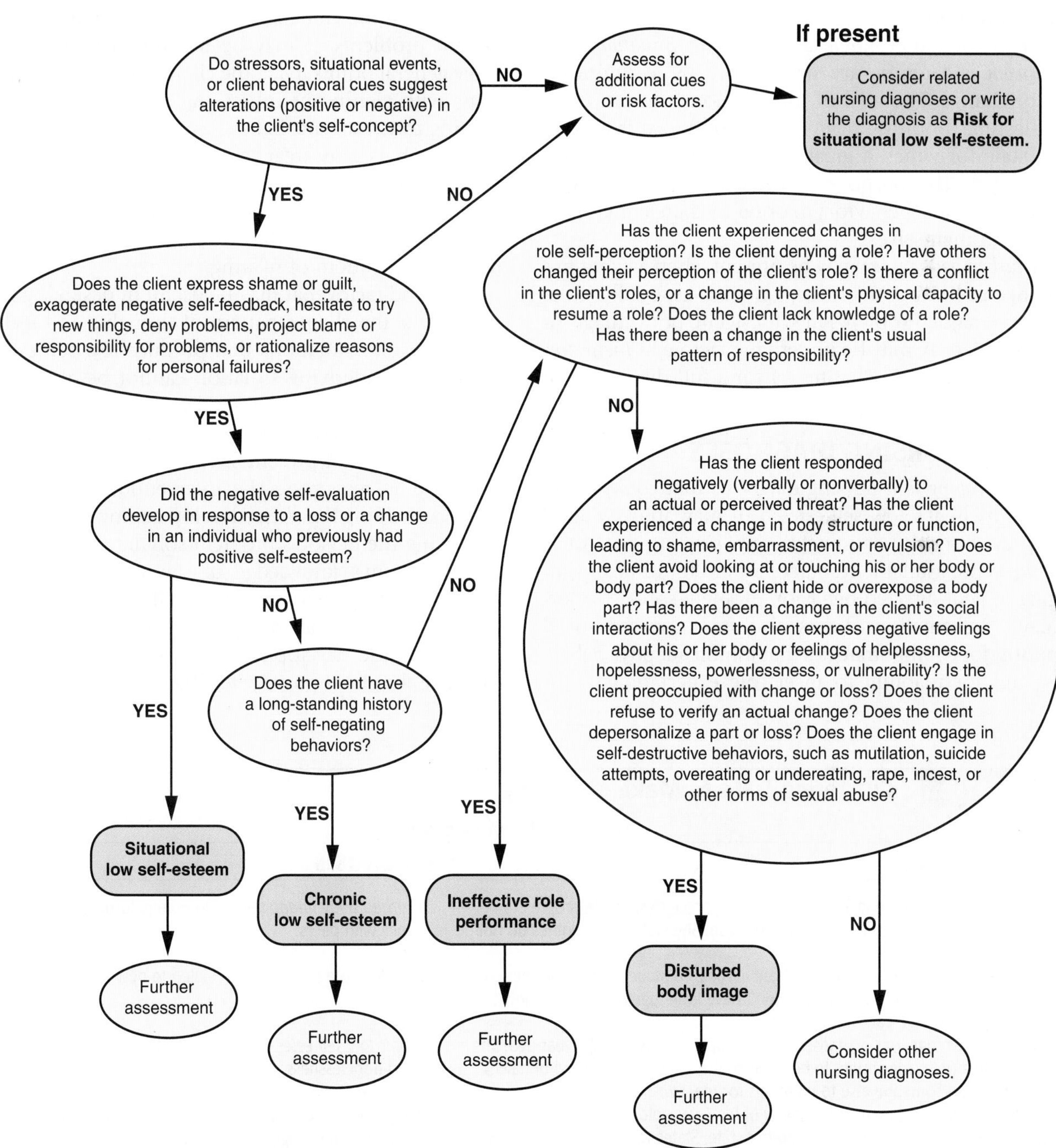

FIGURE 41-6 Decision tree for self-concept nursing diagnoses. Diagnoses are shown in rectangles. Within these rectangles, diagnoses shown in **bold** type are NANDA International (NANDA-I)–approved nursing diagnoses; diagnoses shown in regular type are not NANDA-I–approved nursing diagnoses.

DIAGNOSIS

The self-concept nursing diagnoses are highly interrelated. Often, intervention for any one of them involves intervention for one or more of the others. For example, *Ineffective role performance* (see Chapter 44) and *Disturbed body image* affect self-esteem. Select the appropriate diagnosis on the basis of the predominant feature of the problem, how the client identifies the problem, or the goals of care. Clustering data can help you arrive at the most appropriate nursing diagnoses (Table 41-2).

When making a diagnosis that involves self-esteem, select from *Risk for situational low self-esteem, Situational low self-esteem,* and *Chronic low self-esteem. Situational low self-esteem* is a temporary state caused by a significant loss or change. The goal of intervention is to prevent a long-lasting condition. *Chronic low self-esteem* is a long-term state for which a greater number of interventions are needed. The purpose of these interventions is to teach clients new behaviors in order to change their feelings about themselves.

Disturbed body image may be present when a client has a change in body structure or function, especially if the change is major. Problems in self-esteem, body image, or personal identity may be underlying factors in *Ineffective role performance.* See Chapter 44 for a full discussion of this nursing diagnosis.

RELATED NURSING DIAGNOSES

Ineffective coping is a nursing diagnosis that could be related to a client's low self-esteem. It may apply when a client has difficulty accurately appraising stressors or is unable to use available resources. Assess for difficulty engaging in goal-directed behavior, problem solving, or organizing information. Assess also for decreased social supports, for coping strategies that inhibit adaptive behaviors, and for inability to meet role expectations. Poor concentration, excessive fatigue, high illness rate, and risk-taking or self-destructive behaviors may also be present.

Powerlessness occurs when one perceives a lack of control over a situation or an inability to influence an outcome. Risk factors for this nursing diagnosis are acute or chronic illnesses, hospitalization, aging, inadequate information about a health care problem or the health care system, a dependent lifestyle characterized by ineffective coping patterns, and low self-esteem or body image.

PLANNING

When planning nursing care for clients with low-self-esteem problems, it may be helpful to keep in mind three general points. First, the client's patterns of interactions with significant others can provide direction for nursing care. If clients behave as though their self-worth is low, others may treat them as unworthy. This treatment causes them to feel and behave as though they are unworthy. Low self-esteem may thus be improved by nursing interventions that help the client to interrupt this circular pattern of relating.

A second factor that may be useful in designing interventions is the client's pattern of thoughts and feelings in response to situations that produce low self-esteem. Often, the underlying situation cannot be altered, but the client's perception of the situation can be redefined.

A third factor that is useful in planning interventions is an awareness of present situations that strain the client's coping resources. The interventions are then directed at helping the client develop coping skills, such as increasing the person's problem-solving ability, increasing the client's knowledge of the situation, teaching health care actions to change the situation, helping the client to reduce behaviors that increase the distress, and promoting the development of social support systems that give the client positive feedback.

Table 41-2 Clustering Data to Make a Nursing Diagnosis

Problems of Self-Concept

DATA CLUSTER	DIAGNOSIS
A 15-year-old girl with scoliosis needs to wear a brace to slow the progression of the scoliotic curve, but she refuses to do so. She states, "My clothes do not look right when I wear this thing."	*Disturbed body image* related to nonconformity in appearance with peers
A 24-year-old mother of a 2-day-old infant verbalized inadequacy of her new role, stating, "My husband and I already don't have time together. I don't know how I will be able to take care of this child."	*Ineffective role performance* related to new role of parenting
A 41-year-old woman was diagnosed with multiple sclerosis over a year ago. She has made a poor adjustment to her illness. She states, "I'm so tired of having to depend on someone else to do things for me. I wish I could die."	*Chronic low self-esteem* related to feelings of helplessness and hopelessness
A 32-year-old divorced man with custody of his 3-year-old child. His ex-wife is in a drug rehabilitation program in another state. States that he does not know what to do with the child. "I have to work all day and do not have the skills to care for a child. I couldn't make my marriage work. How can I raise a child?"	*Situational low self-esteem* related to role stress secondary to divorce and change to single-parent status

Because the self-concept nursing diagnoses are so closely interrelated, and because expected outcomes and interventions are so similar, this discussion will focus on just three diagnoses as examples of how to tailor expected outcomes, interventions, and evaluation to the specific client situation: *Situational low self-esteem, Chronic low self-esteem,* and *Disturbed body image.*

EXPECTED OUTCOMES FOR THE CLIENT WITH *LOW SELF-ESTEEM*

The outcome criteria for a client with *Situational low self-esteem* are selected according to the individual needs of the client. Examples of appropriate client outcomes statements are that the client will do the following:

- Identify the precipitating stressors and discuss them openly
- Identify aspects of the self that are positive
- Examine own behavior and its consequences
- Identify actions needed to take control of the situation and influence the outcome
- Return to baseline or improved level of functioning

The outcome criteria for a client with *Chronic low self-esteem* are also selected according to the individual needs of the client. Examples of client outcomes statements are that the client will do the following:

- Identify negative self-talk or reduce the incidence of negative self-talk
- Name the feelings associated with negative self-talk, and tell how it affects behavior
- Appraise the situation in a realistic manner, without distortions
- Identify personal strengths and positive attributes
- Replace negative self-talk with positive self-talk
- Engage in positive behaviors (name the behavior)
- Demonstrate healthy coping patterns (specify)

When working with a client to improve self-esteem, be sure to select behavioral outcomes consistent with the client's developmental stage. When children have a sense of high self-esteem, they play in groups, may be leaders, may be better achievers, and may have positive peer relationships. They will also be better able to make independent judgments, take more initiative, and avoid troublesome situations. When adults have high self-esteem, they are more likely to be satisfied with their lives, their jobs, and their personal relationships. Adults with high self-esteem are more comfortable with themselves and need less approval from others. They better realize their own capabilities, are better able to handle criticisms and failures, and demonstrate positive coping skills.

Increased self-esteem is a long-term expected outcome for clients with *Situational* or *Chronic low self-esteem;* short-term or intermediate outcomes provide important milestones for the client. The short-term outcomes can be as simple as maintaining good personal hygiene and grooming. Rather than setting outcomes that sound unattainable to the client, such as demonstrating self-confidence, making decisions, or showing a belief in self and self-capabilities, help the client identify specific goals and commit to taking small steps. For example, encourage a client to state a short-term goal like this: "I will fill out one job application today."

Increased self-esteem has been shown to influence quality of life positively. Having the client describe what quality of life would mean personally can be helpful in establishing outcomes that will help motivate the client to engage in the work of increasing self-esteem.

EXPECTED OUTCOMES FOR THE CLIENT WITH *DISTURBED BODY IMAGE*

The goal for a client with *Disturbed body image* is that the client will physically and mentally adapt to the changes in body image. You will need to plan interventions to assist the client in the following four stages of adaptation:

1. Experiencing the impact of the change
2. Retreating from the situation
3. Acknowledging the meaning of the change
4. Reconstructing life psychologically and physically

To accomplish the overall goal, you will design interventions to help the client identify and express feelings, identify self-value and strengths, identify the relationship between behavior and self-appraisal, develop support systems, develop successful coping strategies, and implement new coping patterns. Expected outcomes may include that the client will do the following:

- Verbalize and demonstrate acceptance of the client's appearance (grooming, dressing, posture, eating patterns, presentation of self)
- Demonstrate an interest in, and willingness to resume, self-care or responsibilities
- Discuss the impact or meaning of the change
- Initiate new or reestablish existing support

INTERVENTION

You will need to design interventions that assist the client in identifying the source of poor self-esteem, identifying and valuing strengths, exploring the relationship of behavior to self-appraisal, developing a positive support system, and developing coping skills.

INTERVENTIONS TO INCREASE SELF-ESTEEM

Interventions to increase self-esteem are designed to enhance the four components of self-esteem. These interventions are diagrammed in Figure 41-7.

Promote Feelings of Acceptance/Worthiness. One of the most important nursing actions to help clients feel acceptance and worthiness is to establish a trusting relationship with them. Allow them to freely express themselves without your making judgments about their

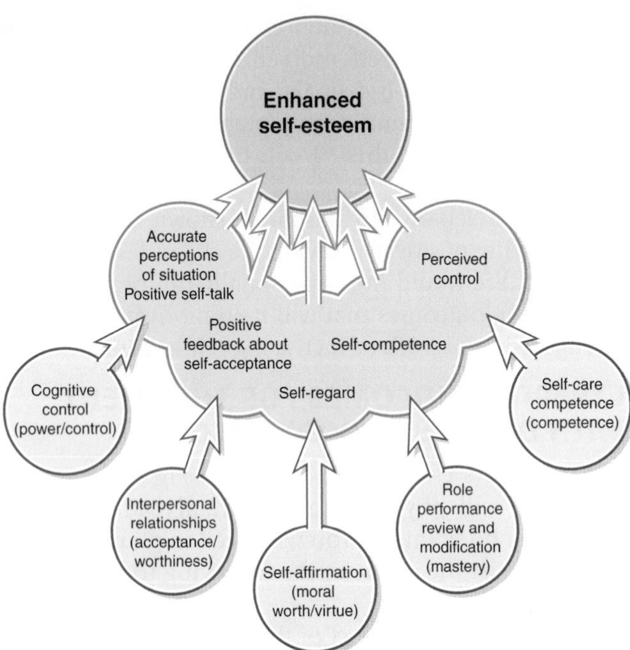

FIGURE 41-7 Interventions to increase self-esteem. (Redrawn from Miller, J. F. [1992]. *Coping with chronic illness: Overcoming powerlessness* [2nd ed.]. Philadelphia: Davis.)

feelings or behaviors. Use touch and maintain eye contact to help establish a relationship that enhances active listening (Figure 41-8). If the client is angry, grieving, or fearful, offer understanding and acceptance of those feelings rather than solutions to the problem or evaluation of the reasonableness of these emotions.

> ***Action Alert!*** To establish a trusting relationship with the client, sit at eye level, conveying a genuine interest.

Asking clients open-ended questions may help them open up to you. The following are some examples of open-ended questions to initiate a dialogue:

- How do you value yourself?
- Tell me what you are most proud of about yourself.
- Tell me what you like about yourself.
- Name at least one of your weaknesses and one of your strengths.

Providing positive reinforcement for steps toward healthy behavior is more effective than negative reinforcement for unhealthy behaviors. High self-esteem develops in the presence of positive feedback, whether that feedback is from others or is in the form of positive self-talk (Figure 41-9).

Hospital-based nurses can provide guidance to clients suffering from *Acute* or *Chronic low self-esteem* by encouraging their acceptance of family members and friends. Visits or contacts with others may provide clients with a chance to share their feelings with significant others and to learn from others with similar experiences. Help the family to help the client by explaining the usual feelings

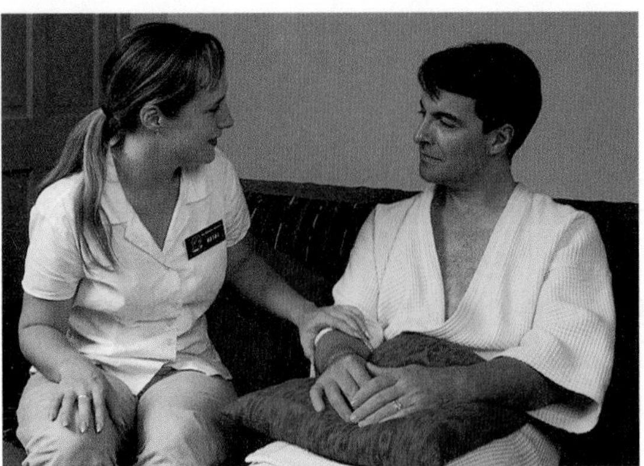

FIGURE 41-8 Touch and eye contact help establish a relationship that enhances active listening.

associated with the client's illness; emphasize that showing understanding of the feelings is more important than trying to talk the client out of those feelings.

Promoting a Sense of Competence/Mastery. For any client, whether a school-age child who is crying because he is routinely excluded from a group of playmates or a 60-year-old man recovering from a colostomy, mastering a skill helps develop a sense of competence. The child can learn to draw or perform gymnastics and gain the confidence to approach other children and make friends. The 60-year-old man can learn to care for his own ostomy, and these self-care skills can promote a sense of competence (Figure 41-10).

Promoting a Sense of Power/Control. Developing feelings of power and control is closely related to developing mastery. The diabetic can develop control over the diabetes and have the knowledge that control comes from mastery of insulin injection. The child who ignores rejection by other children and develops skills in art or gymnastics is also taking charge of his or her own life and enhancing self-esteem through power and control.

Indirectly, reminiscence of life experiences is a form of therapy in older adults and may contribute to a sense of power and control. Assist older adult clients with reminiscing by listening to the stories and life events that have given meaning to their life. Reminiscence is useful because one of the goals in life is to come to terms with the past, often by recognizing the value that life has held. Reminiscence is thus one way to help older adults improve or maintain their self-esteem (Figure 41-11).

Promoting a Sense of Moral Worth/Virtue. Values clarification is a useful tool to gain a sense of moral worth or virtue. A high level of self-esteem is associated with clear personal values and the ability to act in a manner consistent with those values. The first step in values clarification is to help the client identify values that underlie behavior. Approach this discussion of values with a nonjudgmental attitude. Then, help the client identify areas in which values are in conflict. Examples of value conflicts can be found in clients who state that health is a value, yet they

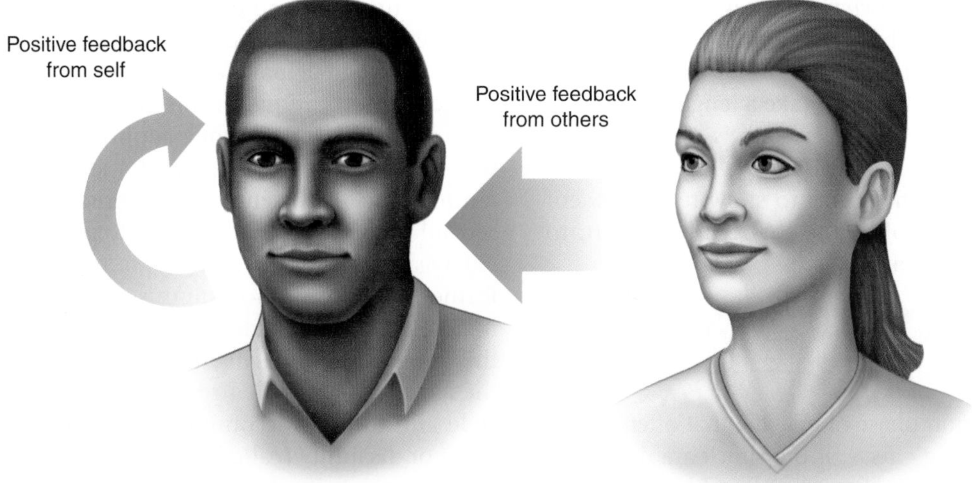

FIGURE 41-9 High self-esteem develops when a person engages in positive self-talk (positive self-feedback) and receives positive feedback from others.

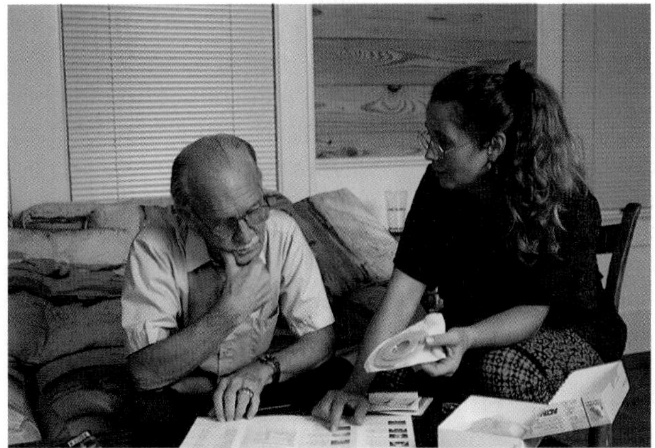

FIGURE 41-10 Learning self-care can help to counteract the loss of self-esteem associated with an illness.

behave in a manner that is not consistent with health-seeking behaviors. Note the following examples:

- A person who has sustained a severe fracture to an ankle, but who is not actively engaging in the exercise needed to regain mobility, may have a conflicting value that states, "I deserve to rest because I have been injured."
- A mother who has had surgery returns to full-time housekeeping against her physician's advice because of a value that it is her responsibility to care for her children.

These clients need assistance in recognizing and naming the conflicting values and making a choice that will promote self-esteem. By considering in turn the consequences of actions consistent with each value, the client is better able to make a choice between conflicting values.

The highest level of clarity about values is acting consistently in a manner that demonstrates the value. Low self-esteem results when a person cannot or will not act in accordance with strongly held values.

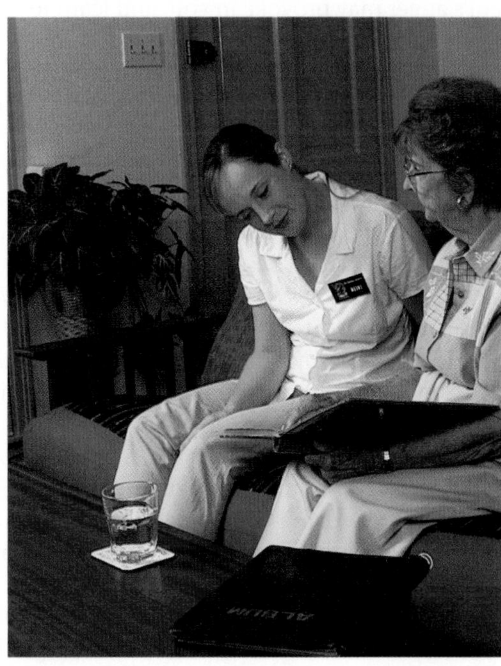

FIGURE 41-11 Reminiscing with the client about family history promotes self-esteem in older adults.

INTERVENTIONS TO INTEGRATE A CHANGE IN BODY IMAGE

When a client loses a body part or function, the loss activates the grieving process. The first stage of grieving is a state of shock and disbelief. The client needs time to experience the impact of the event and allow the meaning of the event to come into conscious awareness. Do not force the client to full awareness of the change in the body; allow the client, instead, to proceed at a natural pace.

As the client gradually shows signs of readiness to discuss what has happened, use active listening to determine the meaning of the loss or change for the client.

The meaning of the loss or change will be affected by the visibility of the loss or change, how much function has been lost, and the emotional significance of the change for the client. Amputations may take a lengthy period of adjustment because the loss of a limb is highly visible, functional loss is high, and the loss has a high emotional component. As the client begins to show readiness, encourage the client to look at the changed body part, to touch it, and to participate in care.

Action Alert! Allow the client sufficient time to express personal feelings openly and honestly.

Anger is a common phase of grieving that often sets in as the initial numbing effects of the shock are declining. Communicate to the client that it is acceptable to be angry. Normalize the response by suggesting that anger is a common response. Assist the person in expressing the anger, frustration, and resentment. Be aware of the anxiety that the client's anger may provoke in you, and learn to control this anxiety in order to continue to be present for the client. Anger can be acted out in many different ways, some of which may be harmful. Do not allow the client to cause harm to self or others in acting out this anger.

As the client becomes exhausted with anger, feelings of helplessness and hopelessness are common. Be ready for depression to become evident. Assess for suicide tendencies, and protect the client from self-harm.

Acceptance of the loss will come gradually. With a therapeutic nurse-client relationship, you will be able to recognize teachable moments when you can provide the client with information that will help with the ultimate adjustment to the change in body image. You may be able to provide the necessary teaching yourself, or the client may need referral to specialized therapists to learn skills in self-care. Become knowledgeable about the services that physical therapists, occupational therapists, enterostomal therapists, and other specialists can offer so that you can share information about available resources and what to expect from them. Encourage clients to use these resources.

Action Alert! Encourage clients to participate in their care to promote acceptance of the loss or change.

Assisting a client through the loss of a body part or body function is best started before the loss, if possible. The client who has the opportunity to plan for the loss can begin to make adjustments in advance. For example, the client who needs colon surgery that will result in the creation of a colostomy can become mentally prepared by talking to others who have had the surgery. Many client fears may be dispelled when the client talks with others who managed the same problems.

Norris and Spelic (2002) state that clients who experience significant changes in appearance or functional abilities undergo a three-stage process called reimaging in order to adapt to body image disruptions. In the first stage, the client actually experiences the body image disruption. Interventions in this stage are similar to those already described, and they support the client through the initial grieving process and support the client's attempts at self-sufficiency and emotional recovery. In the second stage, the wishing for restoration phase, the client wishes to restore, and works toward restoring, the former self. Interventions in this stage include encouraging rehabilitative efforts and screening for depression. In the third stage, reimaging the self, the client fully accepts the changed self (called reconciliation) and adapts lifestyle and roles to accommodate any residual disfigurement or disability (called normalization). Nursing interventions to assist the client in this stage are to assess adaptation, support lifestyle adjustments, and encourage educational and support opportunities for the client and significant others.

EVALUATION

Evaluation of clients with any of the self-concept nursing diagnoses can take several approaches. Three common approaches are the client's subjective report of progress, measurement of expected outcomes, and the use of before-and-after rating scales or instruments, as described in each of the following sections. Each method has advantages and disadvantages; a combination of methods may yield the best results.

SELF-ESTEEM

Because *Acute* or *Chronic low self-esteem* is a subjective experience, the response to intervention logically would be evaluated from a client's subjective report of feeling better about the self. However, several problems could occur with this method of evaluation. The client could report what the nurse wants to hear. Similarly, the client could report feeling better, but that report could be skewed by the fact that the client feels better in the presence of the nurse. A third possibility is that the client's self-esteem has improved, but troublesome behaviors (such as drug abuse) have not.

The second method of evaluation is to compare behavior with expected outcomes. The assumption with this method of evaluation is that changed behaviors indicate a change in self-esteem. Although changed behaviors are a measure of progress, they may not indicate a change in self-esteem.

The third method of evaluation—using a rating scale or instrument—is perhaps the most precise method of measuring progress in improving self-esteem. However, its effectiveness depends on the reliability and validity of the instrument. If the instrument is not sensitive to detecting the particular manifestations of self-esteem that you are trying to measure, it will not be an effective evaluation instrument. In addition, if it relies on a subjective report, it will have the same problems as any subjective report.

Regardless of the evaluation method used, it is essential to document the outcomes of nursing care. The plan of care can then be either terminated, modified, or continued according to need.

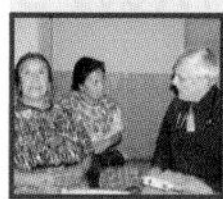

The nurse has formulated a tentative nursing diagnosis of *Situational low self-esteem* for Nancy Ward, the client in the case study at the beginning of this chapter. Box 41-2 identifies a sample plan of care with identified interventions for this client.

A sample documentation note for Nancy Ward, the case study client, could be like the one below.

Sample Documentation Note for Nancy Ward

Client unable to restate information about breast biopsy. Client's sister states she will reinforce this information at home. Client indicates she does not wish to talk about possible treatments if the diagnosis is cancer.

BODY IMAGE

For clients with a major body image change, it may take 6 months to a year to fully integrate the change. Measuring

BOX 41-2 *Nursing Care Plan*

A Client With a Breast Lump

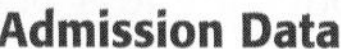

Admission Data
Nancy Ward has come to the clinic to receive preoperative instructions before her breast biopsy in 2 days.

Physician's Orders
Chest x-ray examination

Nursing Assessment
Sister is present. Nancy seems to ignore most of the instructions but repeatedly asks how the breast will appear after the procedure. The physician has told Nancy that there will be several treatment options presented to her after the biopsy. Nancy has a friend who had a mastectomy, and she seems to be focusing on this possibility.

NANDA-I Nursing Diagnosis	NOC Expected Outcomes With Indicators	NIC Interventions With Selected Activities	Evaluation Data
Situational Low Self-Esteem	***Psychological Adjustment: Life Change***	***Anticipation Guidance***	***End of Preoperative Visit***
Related Factor: • Threat of loss of breast as a treatment for cancer		• Repeat the description of the biopsy several times using different words. Emphasize that the scar will be small and that no further treatment will be performed until Nancy agrees to the treatment.	• The first two times the nurse repeats the description of the biopsy, Nancy asks a question like, "Yes, but how much smaller will my breast be?"
		• Answer questions honestly.	• Nancy does not appear to listen to the answers.
		• Encourage the client to restate information about the biopsy.	• Nancy's sister restates the information and says that she will tell Nancy again after they get home.
		• Provide an opportunity for Nancy to talk about her feelings of possible loss.	• Nancy does not want to talk about the possible treatments if the diagnosis is cancer.
		• Ask Nancy about her favorite activities.	• Nancy likes to babysit the children in the area. She is good at making up games for them to play.
		• Notice positive features or attributes about Nancy, and share these with her.	• When the nurse tells Nancy she has beautiful skin, Nancy looks at her blankly.

Critical Thinking Questions

1. What key factors would you consider to ensure that Nancy Ward receives adequate follow-up care after the biopsy?
2. How would you use the four components of self-esteem as you plan to help Nancy accept chemotherapy?
3. Why might Nancy appear relieved upon learning that she will be able to wear her charm to surgery?

Nursing outcome and intervention labels from NANDA International. (2005). *Nursing diagnoses: Definitions and classification, 2005-2006* (6th ed.). Philadelphia: Author.

short-term goals in the form of expected outcomes is important to ensure that the client is making progress. Review the expected outcomes to ensure that they reflect movement through the phases of adaptation.

The client's subjective report of changes in body image may be less reliable than objective measures until the client has reached the stage of acceptance. While the client is in the stages of shock, disbelief, anger, and depression, progress and satisfaction are difficult for the client to recognize.

Instruments are available to measure adaptation. However, before using one of these instruments, be sure to determine whether it is appropriate for the specific population or client. To do this, become familiar with the population that the instrument was designed to evaluate, and decide whether your particular client or population fits within that population.

▼ KEY PRINCIPLES

- Self-concept consists of self-esteem, personal identity, role performance, and body image.
- Self-concept remains relatively enduring throughout life but can change with life experiences.
- Self-esteem is relatively fixed but can change with life transitions or crises.
- The four components of self-esteem are acceptance/worthiness, power/control, moral worth/virtue, and competency/mastery.
- Self-esteem is associated with good health practices.
- There is a difference in the way men and women tend to determine their self-esteem (men with personal achievement; women with social support systems).
- Self-esteem is developed in children by age 12 but can change in adolescence and adulthood.
- Self-esteem in the preschool child is related to interactions with parents and caregivers.
- Self-esteem in the adolescent is strongly influenced by peers.
- Self-esteem may be diminished in the older adult, as a result of losses (physical, social, and mental).
- Body image is related to self-esteem.
- Body image is a critical dimension of adolescence.
- Personal identity is the ability to distinguish between self and nonself.
- Interventions for altered self-esteem are aimed at restoring acceptance/worthiness, power/control, moral worth/virtue, and competence/mastery.
- Interventions for *Disturbed body image* are aimed at helping the client through the four stages of adaptation.

■ REVIEW QUESTIONS

1. The nurse is working with a client who states, "I have nothing good to offer anyone." Using Maslow's hierarchy of needs theory, the nurse interprets that the client's statement is reflective of which level of need?

1. Safety
2. Self-esteem
3. Self-actualization
4. Physiological

2. The pediatric clinic nurse is working with the family of a toddler who is resistant to using the toilet. The nurse concludes that this toddler is experiencing which expected stage of normal growth and development according to Erikson?

1. Trust versus mistrust
2. Autonomy versus shame
3. Initiative versus guilt
4. Intimacy versus isolation

3. The nurse is caring for a client who has sustained trauma during childhood. Which assessment findings in the client would suggest *Low self-esteem?*

1. Can accept compliments easily
2. Accepts responsibility for own well-being and takes charge of own life
3. Has a weak social support system that reinforces resentments, fears, and vices
4. Has primarily an internal locus of control

4. The nurse is caring for a client who has recently lost a limb in a motor vehicle accident. In helping the client adjust to this recent loss the nurse should:

1. Insist that the client begin talking about the loss of the limb
2. Allow the client sufficient time to express personal feelings openly and honestly
3. Tell the client he will be just fine and not to worry
4. Let the client know that he should adjust to the loss within 3 months

5. Select the best method of developing goals/outcomes for the client with low self esteem.

1. Select behavioral outcomes consistent with the client's developmental stage.
2. Ask the clients family how to improve the client's self-esteem.
3. Tell the client that you also have poor self-esteem.
4. Select goals and objectives with the client's input.

Bibliography

*Anderson, K. L. (1995). The effect of chronic obstructive pulmonary disease on quality of life. *Research in Nursing and Health, 18*(6), 547-556.

*Anderson, M. S., & Johnson, J. (1994). Restoration of body image and self-esteem for women after cancer treatment. *Cancer Practice, 2*(5), 345-348.

Arnold, E. C., & Boggs, K. U. (2006). *Interpersonal relationships: Professional communication skills for nurses* (5th ed.). St. Louis, MO: Elsevier Science.

Bakewell, R. T., & Volker, D. L. (2005). Sexual dysfunction related to the treatment of young women with breast cancer. *Clinical Journal of Oncology Nursing, 9*(6), 697-702.

*Bell, R. (1994). Prominence of women in Navajo healing beliefs and values. *Nursing and Health Care, 15*(5), 232-240.

*Bensink, G. W., Godbey, K. L., Marshall, M. J., & Yarandle, A. H. (1992). Institutionalized elderly relaxation, locus of control, self-esteem. *Journal of Gerontological Nursing, 18*(4), 30-36.

Campbell, S. L. (2005). Resident attractiveness: An influential factor in the quality of care in nursing homes. *Journal of Gerontological Nursing, 31*(8), 18-25.

Carpenito, L. J. (2005). *Nursing diagnosis: Application to clinical practice* (11th ed.). Philadelphia: Lippincott.

Chao, S. Y, Liu, H. Y., Wu, C. Y., Jin, S. F., Chu, T. L., Huang, T. S., et al. (2006). The effects of group reminiscence therapy on depression, self esteem, and life satisfaction of elderly nursing home residents. *Journal of Nursing Research, 14*(1), 36-45.

Clarke , J. N. (2006). Mother's home healthcare: Emotion work when a child has cancer. *Cancer Nursing, 29*(1), 58-65.

*Coopersmith, S. (1981). *The antecedents of self-esteem* (Rev. ed.). Novato, CA: Consulting Psychologist Press.

Davidson, M., & Knafl, K. A. (2006). Dimensional analysis of the concept of obesity. *Journal of Advanced Nursing, 54*(3), 342-350.

Devlin, B. (2006). The art of healing and knowing in cancer and palliative care. *International Journal of Palliative Nursing, 12*(1), 16-19.

Dochterman, J., & Bulechek, G. (2004). *Nursing interventions classification (NIC)* (4th ed.). St. Louis, MO: Mosby.

*Doswell, W. M., Millor, G. K., Thompson, H., & Baxter, B. (1998). Self-image and self-esteem in African-American preteen girls: Implications for mental health. *Issues in Mental Health Nursing, 19*(1), 71-94.

*Erikson, E. (1950). *Childhood and society.* New York: Norton.

Fisher, A., Lange, M. A, Young-Cureton, V., & Canham, D. (2005). The relationship between perceived and ideal body size and body mass index in 3rd-grade low socioeconomic Hispanic children. *Journal of School Nursing, 21*(4), 224-228.

*Flett, R., Harcourt, B., & Alpass, F. (1994). Psychosocial aspects of chronic lower leg ulceration in the elderly. *Western Journal of Nursing Research, 16*(2), 183-192.

Franklin, L. L, Ternestedt, B. M, & Nordenfelt, L. (2006). Views on dignity of elderly nursing home residents. *Nursing Ethics, 13*(2), 130-146.

Giger, J. N. (2004). *Transcultural nursing: Assessment and intervention* (4th ed.). St. Louis, MO: Mosby.

*Harper, B. K., & Marshall, E. (1991). Adolescents' problems and their relationship to self-esteem. *Adolescence, 26*(10), 104-107.

Hayter, M. (2006). Productive power and the 'practices of the self' in contraceptive counselling. *Nursing Inquiry, 13*(1), 33-43.

Hildingh, C., Fridlund, B., & Lidell, E. (2006). Access to the world after myocardial infarction: Experiences of the recovery process. *Rehabilitation Nursing, 31*(2), 63-68; discussion 69.

Hill, M. J. (2006). Body dysmorphic disorder: Implications for practice. *Dermatology Nursing, 18*(1), 13.

Hovey, J. K. (2006). Differences in parenting needs of fathers of children with chronic conditions related to family income. *Journal Child Health Care, 10*(1), 43-54.

Johnson, M., Bulechek, G., Butcher, H., Dochterman, J. M., Maas, M., Moorhead, S., et al. (Eds.). (2006). *NANDA, NOC, and NIC linkages: Nursing diagnoses, outcomes, & interventions.* St. Louis, MO: Mosby.

Johnson, M., Maas, M., & Moorhead, S. (2004). *Nursing outcomes classification (NOC)* (3rd ed.). St. Louis, MO: Mosby.

Jurgens, C. Y. (2006). Somatic awareness, uncertainty, and delay in care-seeking in acute heart failure. *Research in Nursing and Health, 29*(2), 74-86.

Kaba, E., Thompson, D. R., Burnard, P., Edwards, D., & Theodosopoulou, E. (2005). Somebody else's heart inside me: A descriptive study of psychological problems after a heart transplantation. *Issues in Mental Health Nursing, 26*(6), 611-625.

Karnick, P. M. (2005). Human becoming theory with children. *Nursing Science Quarterly, 18*(3), 221-226.

*Klyde, B. (1994). The cultural context of Native American health issues. *Journal of American Academy of Physician Assistants, 7*(10), 700-706.

Lutzen, K., Dahlqvist, V., Eriksson, S., & Norberg, A. (2006). Developing the concept of moral sensitivity in health care practice. *Nursing Ethics, 13*(2),187-196.

Lysaker, P., & Buck, K. (2006). Moving toward recovery within clients' personal narratives: Directions for a recovery-focused therapy. *Journal of Psychosocial Nursing and Mental Health Services, 44*(1), 28-35.

*Maslow, A. (1954). *Motivation and personality.* New York: Harper & Row.

Maunder, E. Z. (2006). Emotion work in the palliative nursing care of children and young people. *International Journal of Palliative Nursing, 12*(1), 27-33.

McCaffrey, C. N. (2006). Major stressors and their effects on the well-being of children with cancer. *Journal of Pediatric Nursing, 21*(1), 59-66.

*Mona, L. R., Gardo, P. S., & Brown, R. C. (1994). Sexual self views of women with disabilities: The relationship among age-of-onset, nature of disability, and self esteem. *Sexuality and Disability, 12*(4), 261-277.

NANDA International. (2007). *Nursing diagnoses: Definitions and classification, 2006-2007* (7th ed.). Philadelphia: Author.

Norris, J., & Spelic, S. (2002). Supporting adaptation to body image disruption. *Rehabilitation Nursing, 27*(1), 8-12.

*O'Brien, M. T. (1993). Multiple sclerosis: The relationship among self-esteem, social support, and coping behavior. *Applied Nursing Research, 6*(2), 54-63.

Pelusi, J. (2006). Sexuality and body image. Research on breast cancer survivors documents altered body image and sexuality. *American Journal of Nursing, 106*(3 Suppl.), 32-38.

Prasopkittikun, T., Tilokskulchai, F., Sinsuksai, N., & Sitthimongkol, Y. (2006). Self-Efficacy in Infant Care Scale: Development and psychometric testing. *Nursing and Health Science, 8*(1), 44-50.

Raty, L., & Gustafsson, B. (2006). Emotions in relation to healthcare encounters affecting self-esteem. *Journal of Neuroscience Nursing, 38*(1), 42-50.

Rogge, M. M., Greenwald, M., & Golden, A. (2004). Obesity, stigma, and civilized oppression. *ANS Advances in Nursing Science, 27*(4), 301-315.

Romanek, K. M., McCaul, K. D., & Sandgren, A. K. (2005). Age differences in treatment decision making for breast cancer in a sample of healthy women: The effects of body image and risk framing. *Oncology Nursing Forum, 32*(4), 799-806.

Salloum, M. (2005). Self-esteem disturbance in patients with urinary diversions: Assessing the void. *Ostomy Wound Management, 51*(12), 64-69.

Shu, B. C., Lo, L. H., Lin, L. L., Hsieh, S. C., Li, S. M., & Wu, S. C. (2006). Process of self-identity transformation in women with autistic adolescent. *Journal of Nursing Research, 14*(1), 55-64.

Turnbull, G. B. (2006). Is there a gap in ostomy rehabilitation? *Ostomy Wound Management, 52*(1), 19-20.

*Vera, L., & Wrath, K. (1995). Feelin' groovy. *The Canadian Nurse, 91*(1), 26-30.

Wu, T. Y, Rose, S. E, & Bancroft, J. M. (2006).Gender differences in health risk behaviors and physical activity among middle school students. *Journal of School Nursing, 22*(1), 25-31.

Young, C. V. (2005). The effects of malodorous fungating malignant wounds on body image and quality of life. *Journal of Wound Care, 14*(8), 359-362.

*Young, M., Werch, C., & Bakema, D. (1989). Area-specific self-esteem scales and substance abuse among elementary and middle school children. *Journal of School Health, 59*(6), 251-254.

*Asterisk indicates a classic or definitive work on this subject.

Chapter 42

MANAGING ANXIETY

Media Resources

- evolve Evolve Website http://evolve.elsevier.com/Harkreader/
- Companion CD

Learning Objectives

After studying this chapter, you should be able to do the following:

- Discuss the concepts associated with anxiety
- Describe the three stages of the general adaptation syndrome
- Discuss factors affecting anxiety responses
- Assess clients who are anxious to determine the level of anxiety
- Differentiate diagnoses for anxiety and related nursing diagnoses
- Plan goal-directed interventions to prevent, reduce, or manage anxiety
- Evaluate achievement of the expected outcomes for clients who are experiencing anxiety

Key Terms

adaptation
anxiety
anxiety disorders
anxiolytics
fear
homeostasis
panic
vulnerability

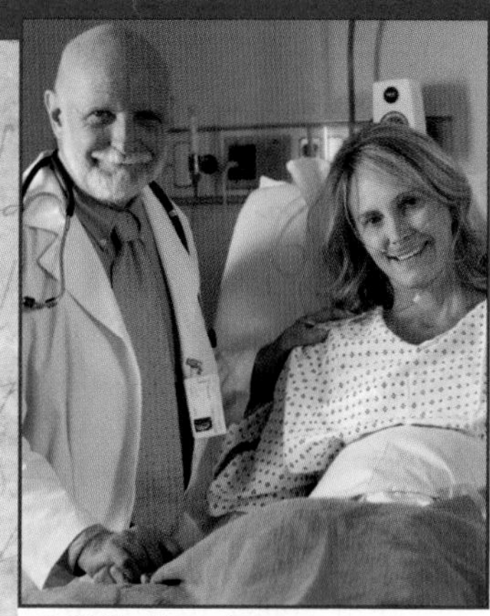
© 2007, Getty Images.

Ida Adkins is a 42-year-old woman of Appalachian descent who grew up in the mountains of West Virginia. Ms. Adkins is the single parent of a 16-year-old son. They live with her parents on a small rural hillside farm.

Ms. Adkins is taken by her mother to the clinic with complaints of chest pain, shortness of breath, nausea, dizziness, numbness and tingling, palpitations, and nervousness. Her mother says that Ida has "a bad heart" and "even badder nerves." When the symptoms began early this morning, her mother treated Ida with tea from bleeding heart leaves. When that had no effect, she gave her daughter garlic to eat and two of the pills she got from the clinic the last time this happened. When Ida still complained of "heart pains" after her mother's treatments, they decided Ida needed to be seen by her physician.

In addition to nursing diagnoses related to cardiac disease, the nurse assesses Ms. Adkins for *Anxiety* from the list of nursing diagnoses for anxiety (see key nursing diagnoses box).

CONCEPTS OF ANXIETY

Anxiety is one of the most commonly observed symptoms in clients. As a nurse, you will be caring for many anxious clients, assessing how anxiety is affecting their health and daily functioning and teaching them new coping strategies.

DEFINING CHARACTERISTICS

Anxiety is a diffuse, highly uncomfortable, sometimes vague sense of apprehension or dread accompanied by one or more physical sensations. It is an alerting signal that warns of potential danger and alerts us to a variety of threats, such as threats of bodily harm, pain, separation from loved ones, and threats to our sense of wholeness. It initiates protective defense mechanisms and survival strategies that have life-preserving qualities and that increase feelings of safety and security. Whether clients perceive an event as stressful or dangerous depends on the nature of the event, their personal resources, and their coping abilities.

Anxiety is a normal, expected, intermittent, and transient response to stress. It also may be chronic and disabling, in which case it can complicate other illnesses by affecting pain perception, decreasing immune function, reducing client compliance with treatment plans, and interfering with client teaching.

The anxious state can vary from edginess and uneasiness to alarm to terror and panic. **Panic** is profound terror experienced with an intense urge to escape or fight. It is accompanied by disintegration of personality organization and inability to control thoughts and actions. The source of this uneasiness is not always known or recognized, which can add to the distress the client perceives.

KEY NURSING DIAGNOSES FOR ANXIETY

Anxiety: A vague, uneasy feeling of discomfort or dread, accompanied by an autonomic response; the source is often nonspecific or unknown to the individual; a feeling of apprehension caused by anticipation of danger

Fear: Response to perceived threat that is consciously recognized as a danger

THEORIES

Psychoanalytic theory proposes that anxiety comes from unconscious conflicts that arose from events and situations (real or symbolic) that were threatening in infancy and childhood. These conflicts often include fears stemming from separation and loss. This theory states that we all face different levels of anxiety and different conflicts at various developmental stages.

Learning theory suggests that anxiety is a learned behavior that is a conditioned response to a specific stimulus. This model states that individuals who have been exposed to intense fear in early life are more likely to develop anxiety in later life. Some of the most effective treatments for anxiety and anxiety disorders have evolved from learning theory. A man who as a child was attacked by a dog is now phobic about all dogs. A technique called desensitization may help reduce his anxiety and fear of dogs, so that he could eventually enjoy petting a dog.

In general, it is helpful to think of anxiety as falling into two primary categories:

- Threat to biological integrity: actual or anticipated hindrance to basic human needs such as food, fluid, warmth, or shelter
- Threat to ego integrity: unmet expectations important to identity and self-integrity, need for status, possible disapproval by significant others, inability to gain or reinforce self-respect or approval from others, and guilt or disparity between self-concept and actual behavior

PHYSIOLOGICAL RESPONSES TO ANXIETY

The body's physiological response to the cognitive appraisal of danger activates a chain of physiological, behavioral, cognitive, and emotional reactions designed to prepare us to face the danger and either fight or flee to safety. The goal of physiological adaptation is to maintain stability, or homeostasis, during internal or external environmental change. **Adaptation** is a process through which individuals accommodate to changes in the internal or external environment to preserve functioning and pursue goals. It also refers to behaviors of change that occur as an individual responds to anxiety and stress. **Homeostasis** is a state of internal stability of our physiology and our emotions. It maintains balance by returning the body to a relaxed state after the stress response.

The autonomic nervous system (ANS) is controlled by the hypothalamus. Two divisions of the ANS are involved in preparing the body to deal with stress or danger and then in restoring homeostasis when the danger has passed. The sympathetic nervous system activates emergency resources, whereas the parasympathetic branch of the ANS induces a relaxed state. Normally, when a person is in a serene, unstimulated state, the "firing" of neurons in the locus ceruleus is minimal. When a stimulus is perceived, it is relayed from the sensory cortex of the brain through the thalamus to the brain stem. That route of signaling increases the rate of noradrenergic activity in the locus ceruleus, which activates the sympathetic nervous system, the part of the ANS that is responsible for initiating the fight-or-flight response, and the person becomes alert and attentive to the environment. The hypothalamus also delivers a message to the endocrine system to initiate the secretion of epinephrine (adrenaline) and norepinephrine (noradrenaline) from the adrenal medulla and cortisol from the adrenal cortex to prepare for fight-or-flight response.

The parasympathetic nervous system, the other branch of the ANS, is designed to return the physiology to a state of homeostasis after the threat or danger is no longer perceived to be imminent. People's breathing, muscle tension, heart rate, and blood pressure decrease, while peristalsis and other digestive processes increase again. The body regenerates and restores for future activity.

GENERAL ADAPTATION SYNDROME

The "acute stress response," or the flight-or-fight response, was first described by Walter Cannon. It was later recognized as the first stage of the general adaptation syndrome (GAS) first identified by Hans Selye (Figure 42-1). In describing the stress response, Selye (1956) identified three physiological stages of what he called the general adaptation syndrome: the alarm reaction stage, the resistance stage, and the exhaustion stage.

In the alarm reaction stage, the sympathetic nervous system initiates the fight-or-flight response and activates defense mechanisms. Adrenaline surges, the heart speeds, and the body prepares for fighting or running away. This fight-or-flight response is sustained by the hypothalamic-pituitary-adrenal axis, which releases cortisone, norepinephrine, and epinephrine into the blood.

In the resistance stage, the body attempts to adapt to the stressor. The parasympathetic nervous system modulates the body's response by opposing the actions of the sympathetic nervous system.

As a consequence of the resistance stage, the person either recovers or becomes exhausted. If the latter occurs, the person enters the exhaustion stage, in which the body cannot function defensively against the stressor, and physiological regulation decreases. If the stress continues in the exhaustion stage, death can result.

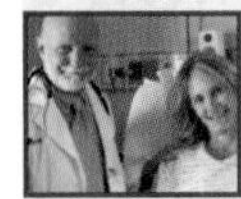

Do you recall what symptoms Ida Adkins was experiencing when she was brought to the clinic? Could those symptoms be related to the general adaptation syndrome just described?

PSYCHOLOGICAL RESPONSES TO ANXIETY

Anxiety is a normal part of life. There are many occasions when anxiety is expected: speaking in public, a musical solo, and anyone facing illness and hospitalization. Only when there is a marked discrepancy between an individual's perception of the environment and its actual characteristics is anxiety considered abnormal.

A core concept of anxiety is a sense of vulnerability. **Vulnerability** is a feeling of helplessness, lack of control, and inadequate resources for defense when faced with threat or danger. Factors that contribute to a sense of vulnerability include feelings of shame or embarrassment, maladaptive personality features, poor coping skills, or a tendency to regress in threatening situations. Sudden onset of the threat, unavailability of significant others, feeling alone, significance of a particular illness, or having to relinquish control to others may leave us feeling unprotected and vulnerable.

Another characteristic of anxiety is its involuntary nature. We may be unaware or only partially aware of anxiety-producing thoughts and beliefs when they begin, and we may remain unaware of these thought patterns until uncomfortable symptoms are noticeable. Even before being aware of anxiety, the ability to reason can be impaired, and repetitive thoughts of danger occur. In addition, when a person recognizes that certain thoughts may not be logical, the thoughts can continue to exert pressure and a loss of perspective occurs.

Because we are not fully aware of anxiety, it is easily self-perpetuated; that is, we can actually create or worsen

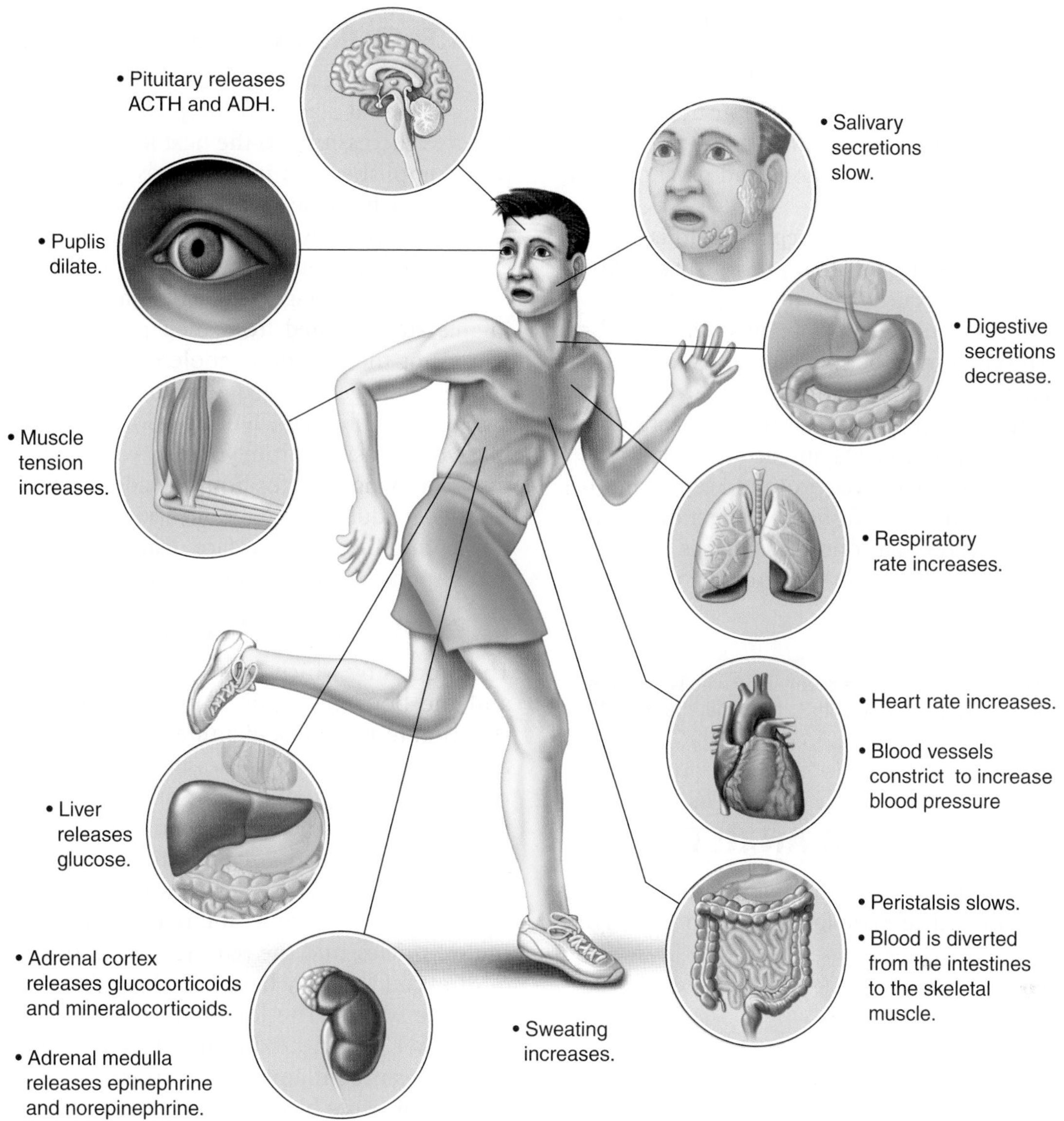

FIGURE 42-1 Physiological responses in the alarm phase of the general adaptation syndrome.

our own anxiety. Negative self-talk can decrease self-confidence and set up a cycle of escalating anxiety (Figure 42-2). Telling ourselves things like "This is awful," "This shouldn't have happened," or "I'll never be able to face anyone again" heightens the effects of anxiety. Often, an anxious person may not even be aware of such thoughts. Making clients aware of personal stresses, self-talk, and the anxiety these evoke is helpful. Just the awareness can decrease the anxiety to a great extent in many people.

In addition, anxiety can change our behavior in a way that creates a self-fulfilling prophecy. People seem to bring on unwittingly the things they fear or detest the most. For example, excessive anxiety about pain in childbirth has been shown to increase the perceived severity of pain.

Anxiety stimulates adaptation and psychosocial coping responses. *Coping* is any effort directed toward management of dangerous, threatening, or challenging situations. People learn to cope with and adapt to stressors by using methods that were successful for them in the past. They adapt psychologically to preserve the self and to maintain self-esteem.

LEVELS OF ANXIETY

Anxiety can vary dramatically in presentation and intensity. It can range from mild tension to terror. The following list describes different levels of anxiety:

- *Mild anxiety:* The person's perceptual field is wide with acuity and alertness enhanced. Observations are sharper. The relationship between events is clear. Potential for learning, growth, and creativity is increased. Symptoms such as irritability, restlessness, insomnia, repetitious questions, and seeking reassurance or attention may be noted.

- *Moderate anxiety:* The perceptual field is constricted. Alertness is intensified and concentration is focused on one specific detail. Anything irrelevant to the immediate issue is blocked from consciousness. The relationship between events is still understandable. An increase in physiological functions and psychomotor movements occur.
- *Severe anxiety:* The person's perceptual field is extremely distorted. Details that previously served as a central focus are exaggerated and misinterpreted. Attempts to communicate may be incoherent to the listener. The client may be extremely hyperactive, with all energy aimed at obtaining relief.
- *Panic:* Disintegration of personality organization and inability to control thoughts and actions occur in panic. The client experiences profound terror and has an intense urge to escape or fight. Danger of harm to self or others becomes a concern. Paralysis of functioning can occur. The client may freeze and even lose consciousness.

Action Alert! Do not leave a client alone who is experiencing panic. At this level of anxiety, the client may harm self or others.

FACTORS AFFECTING ANXIETY

Many factors affect anxiety, including risk factors across the life span, cultural/lifestyle factors, and physiological factors.

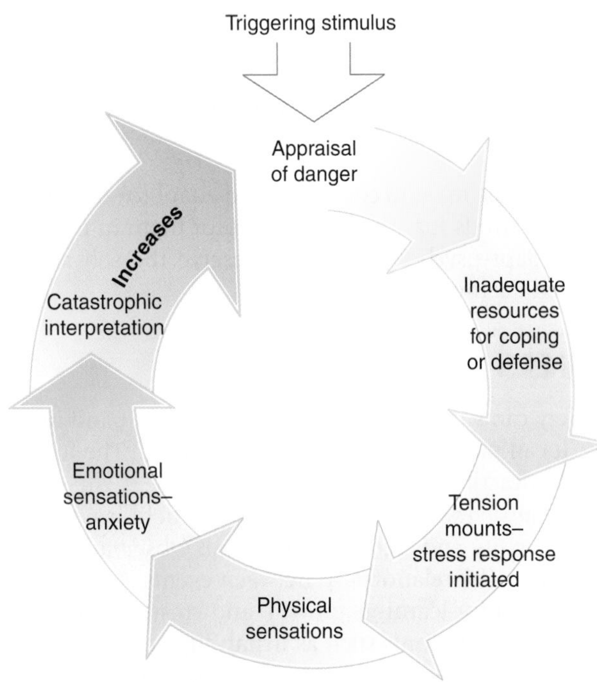

FIGURE 42-2 The vicious cycle of anxiety.

RISK FACTORS ACROSS THE LIFE SPAN

You are aware that people go through various physical and emotional stages in the process of maturation. To progress successfully to the next level, certain tasks must be accomplished. An infant needs to be held and loved and to have basic needs met. Without this, an individual will have difficulty in forming relationships and progressing through other developmental stages.

These tasks or stages can lead to anxiety, such as when infants are separated from their parents, children go to school for the first time, adolescents go on a first date, young adults get married, and older adults contemplate aging and retirement. During adolescence, we strive to make the transition from youth to young adulthood. This can be a trying time for both the adolescent and the parent. Older adults may have blocks to reassessing life experiences and be unable to face death. Increasing demands and responsibilities can also create crisis (Box 42-1).

PHYSIOLOGICAL FACTORS

The process by which an event is perceived as a stressor and the body responds is not fully understood. Biochemical research has identified neurochemical, genetic, and structural abnormalities in anxiety and anxiety disorders. The role of neurotransmitters such as serotonin, norepinephrine, and gamma-aminobutyric acid (GABA) is being investigated. Imaging studies of brain structures and functions have identified some abnormal findings in certain areas, such as the right hemisphere, the cerebral ventricles, and the right temporal lobe.

Stress and anxiety have been linked to changes in the immune system. The long-term presence of high levels of cortisol, which are produced by the stress response, suppresses the inflammatory process, decreases the production of white blood cells, and can lead to atrophy of immune system organs/tissues.

In addition, genetic influences in anxiety are being investigated. Family studies show that anxiety disorders are more prevalent within families having a history of anxiety.

A great number of legal (alcohol, nicotine, caffeine, cold remedies, bronchodilators for asthma, tricyclic antidepressants, attention-deficit/hyperactivity disorder

BOX 42-1 *Factors Affecting Anxiety in Older Adults*

- Changes in health status
- Chronic and/or terminal diseases
- Decreased functional ability and independence
- Difficulty handling new situations
- Need for relocation
- Loss of family and friends
- Blocks to reassessing life experiences
- Unable to face death
- Becoming a caregiver

[ADHD] medications, thyroid medications, and herbal remedies) and illegal substances (cocaine) can cause physical symptoms of anxiety, either from intoxication or withdrawal. Remember that prescription medicine can be abused as well. A careful medication history, including herbal therapies, is an important part of assessing the etiology of anxiety.

Anxiety can frequently resemble symptoms of medical conditions such as asthma, cardiac dysrhythmias, and mitral valve insufficiency. Your client may report feeling nervous, palpitations, shortness of breath, headache, chest pain, and other symptoms that could indicate anxiety. A thorough physical examination may confirm or rule out a physical reason for the symptoms (Table 42-1).

Table 42-1 Medical Conditions That Commonly Resemble or Contribute to Anxiety

CATEGORY	EXAMPLES
Endocrine disorders	• Cushing's disease • Addison's disease • Hyperthyroidism • Premenstrual dysphoric disorder • Hypoglycemia
Cardiovascular disorders	• Dysrhythmias • Myocardial infarction • Angina • Mitral insufficiency
Gastrointestinal disorders	• Colitis • Peptic ulcer
Infectious diseases	• Human immunodeficiency virus • Tuberculosis
Pulmonary disorders	• Asthma • Pneumothorax • Hypoxia • Pulmonary embolus
Neurological disorders	• Stroke • Seizure disorder (especially temporal lobe)

Anxiety has profound effects on pain perception. It intensifies the client's appraisal of physical symptoms, making them seem more sinister and distressing. Anxiety can lower the pain threshold dramatically, causing caregivers to note marked inconsistencies between reports of pain and objective findings. This can be misinterpreted as a dependence on pain medication.

CULTURAL AND LIFESTYLE FACTORS

Culture. The client's cultural background has a major effect on anxiety and illness behavior (Box 42-2). In some cultures, a stoic response to health problems is expected. In other cultures, emotions and feelings are expressed openly and with flair. Some cultures encourage touching, hand holding, and hugging, whereas others may not condone personal touching at all.

Self-Concept. Self-concept is the belief that our abilities will allow us to reach our goals and protect ourselves against failure and devaluation by others. A discrepancy between our expected abilities/achievements and actual abilities can lead to anxiety. Thus unmet expectations can negatively affect our identity and self-concept. Disapproval by significant others, inability to achieve goals, and loss of independence and ability to provide for ourselves change how we see ourselves and can cause intense anxiety.

Individual Integrity. Any threat, whether symbolic or actual, to a client's ability to function in roles in family, career, and other areas vital to identity poses danger to individual integrity. This can range from changes in social position to the inability to control emotions. Threats to self-sufficiency, functioning of mind and body, maintenance of health status, and even survival can affect one's identity, leaving one feeling vulnerable and helpless. In addition, even positive events can cause stress, such as a marriage, the birth of a baby, moving to a new home, or even a vacation. The number and significance of psychosocial stressors in a client's life and the ability to cope with them affect such things as the degree of disability caused

BOX 42-2 *Cross-Cultural Care*

Caring for an Appalachian Client

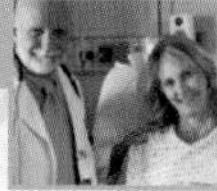

Ida Adkins is of Appalachian descent. She grew up in rural West Virginia and has always lived within sight of her parents' home. Her family has lived in this area for 150 years. She and her husband recently divorced, and their 16-year-old son stayed to live with her. Although each client is unique, many people of the Appalachian culture value the following:

- The ethic of neutrality
- Avoidance of aggression and assertiveness
- Loyalty
- Patriotism
- Avoidance of dominance over others
- Seeking agreement and avoidance of arguments
- Not interfering in others' lives
- Protectiveness over personal business
- Respect for older adults
- Folk healers and herb doctors
- Medicine only when they think they need it

Karla, a nursing student working in the clinic, tries to demonstrate cultural sensitivity during her first interaction with Ida Adkins by observing both physical and psychological symptoms. She inquires about how Mrs. Adkins handles symptoms such as headache at home and incorporates folk healing practices that would not be harmful. Karla also recognizes the importance of family in the Appalachian culture and allows Mrs. Adkins's mother to stay with her in the examination room.

by a health problem and the ability to recover. The more stressors a client experiences at one time, and the more disturbing the stressors are to the client, the greater is the effect on the client's ability to adjust.

Economic. Economic factors also play a major role in anxiety and illness. Third-party payers may limit available treatment options and medications that can be covered. Both public and private health insurance plans tend to provide limited coverage for mental health treatment.

Health Care Settings. Most of us find comfort and security in familiar things and places. Health care settings, with their atmosphere of illness, pain, suffering, death, and separation from loved ones, friends, and familiar surroundings, are stressful and can trigger anxiety. The uncertainty in illness, treatments, surgery, pain, ability to function, loss of independence and identity, and the possibility of death can produce intense anxiety and be extremely stressful.

Those who lead healthy lifestyles are not immune to the effects of stress or to illness, but they may manage them better. A healthy diet, exercise, stress reduction techniques, and a positive outlook can increase our health status and our resistance to stress.

ANXIETY DISORDERS

Anxiety can be a component of almost all psychiatric disorders. Clients with a previous history of psychiatric illness or prolonged reactions to stressors may be at an increased risk for anxiety, especially when facing health problems. Those with depression, substance abuse or dependence, and personality disorders are especially vulnerable.

When anxiety becomes an excessive, irrational dread of everyday situations, it has become a disabling disorder. **Anxiety disorders** are serious medical illnesses that fill clients' lives with overwhelming anxiety and fear. Unlike the brief anxiety caused by a stressful event, anxiety disorders are chronic, relentless, and can grow progressively worse if not treated. The common anxiety disorders are defined in Table 42-2.

Generalized Anxiety Disorder. Generalized anxiety disorder (GAD) is much more than the normal anxiety people experience day to day. It is a chronic disorder in which clients are always anticipating disaster, worrying excessively about health, money, family, or work even though there is little or nothing to provoke it.

Posttraumatic Stress Disorder. Posttraumatic stress disorder (PTSD) is a debilitating condition that can develop following a terrifying event like war, physical or sexual assault, or a natural disaster. The suddenness and severity of a trauma affect our reactions. Symptoms such as nightmares, intrusive thoughts, insomnia, a hyperstartle response, avoidance of stimuli that include memories of the trauma, flashbacks, irritability, avoidance of events that rekindle memories of the trauma, and increased anxiety may be present.

Phobias. Phobias are a type of anxiety disorder. Clients who are phobic experience a persistent irrational fear of an object or a situation in which anxiety develops when they come into contact with the object or situation and a strong desire to avoid it occurs.

ASSESSMENT

All clients in any health care setting are vulnerable to some degree of anxiety. Although anxiety is normal and even useful, you should be aware of levels of anxiety that are not helpful and may even be harmful in some circumstances. Anxiety is usually not difficult to recognize, even

Table 42-2 Common Anxiety Disorders

DISORDER	DESCRIPTION
Acute stress disorder (acute psychological consequences of previous trauma)	Excessive and persistent anxiety that occurs within 1 month after exposure to an extreme traumatic stressor.
Agoraphobia	Fear and avoidance of being in places or circumstances in which help may not be readily available should some disabling or embarrassing event occur. Some agoraphobics are unable to leave their houses or apartments.
Generalized anxiety disorder (nonspecific anxiety)	Chronic, excessive, and exaggerated worry and tension about everyday life events that often are unrealistic or out of proportion for the situation.
Panic disorder with/without agoraphobia (unprovoked panic attacks)	Unexpected, recurrent episodes of intense anxiety occurring in situations that do not usually evoke anxiety.
Obsessive-compulsive disorder (obsessive thoughts and compulsive rituals)	Uncontrollable thoughts, images, or impulses and behavioral rituals that the client cannot dismiss. Obsessions and compulsions typically occur together.
Posttraumatic stress disorder (PTSD)	Reexperiencing a traumatic event, which is characterized by intrusive thoughts, dramatic physiological reactivity, flashbacks, nightmares of the event, behavioral disturbances, and avoidance of stimuli associated with the trauma.
Social phobias (irrational fear of embarrassment)	A persistent, intense dread and avoidance of social or performance situations that evoke fear of humiliation or embarrassment.
Specific phobia (other specific irrational fears)	A specific type of fear that is often exaggerated and incapacitating. A main characteristic of phobias is the appraisal of high risk in a situation that is fairly safe.

when the cues are indirect, such as selective inattention, being distracted, or focusing on problems or issues unrelated to the current situation. A person who is receiving an initial chemotherapy infusion may be chattering about a recent movie while the nurse is trying to give needed information about the treatment. Nurses may recognize that clients have a high level of anxiety that is interfering with their ability to receive the education. In such cases, the care plan will have to be modified to address the anxiety before the education can be continued.

GENERAL ASSESSMENT OF *ANXIETY*

Assess clients for the presence and intensity of anxiety. Gather data from observations of the clients' behavior, what they say about how they are feeling, information from family and friends, and information from medical records, physical examinations, and diagnostic tests related to medical problems. Throughout your contact with clients, continue to assess and reassess their emotional status.

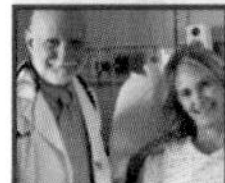

After assessing Ms. Adkins's presenting symptoms, vital signs, and other physical parameters, the nurse in the clinic reviews past chart entries. She sees that Ms. Adkins had a myocardial infarction about 5 years ago and has a history of psychiatric problems. The nurse notes that Ms. Adkins was in the clinic 4 to 5 weeks ago with similar symptoms. Her diagnosis at that time was a panic attack. What factors would you consider in determining how to proceed?

Health History. The nursing history is the arena in which the therapeutic relationship begins. Ask about the client's current life situation, personal relationships, and history of any nonspecific medical ailments or illness behaviors. It is important to understand the client's frame of reference, the reaction to stress and coping measures used (e.g., anger, crying, withdrawal), family history, cultural background, and belief system.

When assessing specifically for anxiety, valuable pieces of the puzzle can be gathered from the client's reported internal state, observation of the client's behavior and ability to function, reports from friends and family, and prior documented medical history. Begin by asking the client to describe thoughts and feelings. Observe the client's behavior for nonverbal clues that suggest that the internal state is different from what the client is reporting. You may use this opportunity to say to the client, "I noticed you are up walking in the halls and can't sleep. What is on your mind?"

Help the client identify stressors, and determine what fears they elicit. Use direct questions to elicit specific details. Open-ended questions can encourage elaboration and exploration of thoughts and feelings. Ask the client, "What scares you the most?" or "How have you dealt with these concerns before?"

Anxiety may be a symptom of a medical or psychiatric problem. Critical issues to assess include medical illness that could present with anxiety-like symptoms, medication-induced anxiety, anxiety associated with use of or withdrawal from substances such as alcohol or illicit drugs, and/or presence of a past or concurrent psychiatric disorder, such as depression or an anxiety disorder.

Talk with the client's family and friends because they are an invaluable source of information. They have known the client over a span of time and are aware of usual behavior in both stressful and nonstressful situations. They may note reactions or symptoms of which you as the nurse, or even the client, are not aware. For example, those close to a client may notice that the client becomes more anxious at night, or a family member may tell you that the client has been getting confused at night for several weeks.

Historical data from prior health records, when available, is extremely helpful as well. Compare this information with that given by the client to develop a more complete picture. One thing to keep in mind is that the client knows best how he or she is feeling.

Many assessment tools are available to evaluate a client's level of anxiety. A fast and simple way to get an idea of the anxiety level is to use a 10-point scale. Ask clients to rate their anxiety on a scale of 1 to 10, with 1 being totally relaxed and 10 being ready to panic and lose control. The level clients report provides clues to the severity of their anxiety. If, for example, they say, "About a 7," recognize that anxiety is a significant problem. Additional questions you might ask include, "Does your anxiety affect your ability to get things done around the house or at work? Are you able to care for your child? Do you find yourself restless or worrying for no reason? Has this affected your ability to relate to others or perform your daily activities?"

Physical Examination. Anxiety causes a variety of symptoms in multiple functional systems and may be observed during the physical examination. Physical symptoms may be found in these domains: physical, behavioral, cognitive, and affective. Individual patterns of anxiety vary widely according to the nature of the problem and the person's frame of reference. These symptoms are both subjectively and objectively recognized.

Physical symptoms of anxiety are numerous and can be found in every major body system (Box 42-3). These symptoms can be extremely unpleasant and range from mild to intense. They can be so severe that clients may interpret physical symptoms as indicating a medical emergency. Severe levels of anxiety and panic can become incapacitating disorders in themselves.

Behavioral symptoms can be observed as restlessness to agitation, avoidance, impaired coordination, speech pattern and enunciation changes, freezing, fighting, or fainting. It is important to identify the source of the client's anxiety and take measures to reduce it; however, if the behaviors are pronounced, you may have to deal with them first before you can actually sit down and talk with the client.

Cognition can be profoundly affected by anxiety. Clients may have difficulty concentrating if they have impairment in information retrieval, especially from short-term memory. They may be unable to focus on a given task or to comprehend what is being said. An important consideration for clients who are very upset is their selectivity. Anxious persons are apt to select certain items in their environment and overlook others in the effort to prove that they are justified in considering the situation frightening and responding accordingly. They will have difficulty with reasoning and decision making. It is also important to remember this concept when talking with family or significant others who are worried about a loved one who is ill.

Anxiety's effects on thinking, perception, and learning are powerful. Anxiety can produce confusion and distortions of perception, which interfere with learning ability by decreasing concentration, impairing recall, and interfering with the capacity to associate one item or idea with another. Cognitive manifestations of anxiety also include a fear of losing control, self-consciousness, and even perceptual distortions to the extremes of hallucinations.

Affective symptoms vary from a vague sense of uneasiness to hysteria. Irritability, crying, hostility, heightened sense of pain, constant attention seeking, uncooperativeness, and catastrophizing are all affective or emotional manifestations of anxiety. Clients tend to describe their symptoms in psychological terms such as "I can't cope" or "I feel nervous."

Many clients attribute their symptoms to physical causes and focus their complaints on a specific body system such as the cardiovascular system. Even clients who suspect an emotional cause for their symptoms may hesitate to say so. They may believe that the health care team is concerned only with physical disorders and see emotional problems as a sign of weakness and lack of control. Box 42-4 suggests circumstances in which the client may need assistance with coping strategies.

FOCUSED ASSESSMENT FOR *ANXIETY*

Anxiety is the body's most common response to stress. It can be observed in situations requiring adaptation to physical, psychological, social, or spiritual stressors. The defining characteristics for the nursing diagnosis *Anxiety* include behavioral, affective, physiological (sympathetic nervous system), and cognitive characteristics:

- Behavioral characteristics such as diminished productivity, poor eye contact, insomnia, and fidgeting
- Affective characteristics such as being distressed, anxious, worried, overexcited, and scared
- Physiological characteristics (see Box 42-3) such as sleep disturbance, abdominal pain, increased pulse, reflexes, and respirations
- Cognitive characteristics such as blocking of thought, impaired attention, decreased perceptual field, and confusion (NANDA International [NANDA-I], 2005)

BOX 42-3 *Physiological Evidence of Anxiety*

Cardiovascular
- Tachycardia, palpitations, or irregular heart rate
- Chest pain
- Sweating
- Flushing, pallor

Respiratory
- Dyspnea
- Smothering sensation
- Hyperventilation

Gastrointestinal
- Dry mouth
- Nausea
- Vomiting
- Diarrhea
- Choking sensation
- Abdominal pain

Neurological
- Tightness of muscles, twitching, tremors
- Headaches
- Dizziness, vertigo
- Numbness around the mouth
- Numbness and tingling in extremities
- Dilated pupils

Genitourinary
- Urinary frequency
- Urinary hesitancy

Reproductive
- Sexual dysfunction

Other
- Itching/hives
- Changes in sleep patterns, sleeping difficulties, and nightmares
- Difficulty concentrating or mind going blank
- Generalized weakness
- Irritability, including loss of temper

BOX 42-4 *Client Education Related to Coping Strategies*

Call your health care provider if you experience the following:
- You are unable to work or function properly at home because of anxiety.
- You do not know the source or cause of your anxiety.
- You have a sudden feeling of panic.
- You have an uncontrollable fear—for example, of getting infected and sick if you are out, or a fear of heights.
- You repeat an action over and over again, like constantly washing your hands.
- You have intolerance to heat, weight loss despite a good appetite, lump or swelling in the front of your neck, or protruding eyes. Your thyroid may be overactive.
- Your anxiety is elicited by the memory of a traumatic event.
- You have tried self-care for several weeks without success, or you feel that your anxiety will not resolve without professional help.

Related Factors. Factors related to the nursing diagnosis *Anxiety* include such things as situational or maturational crises, substance abuse, threat of death, and threat to or change in health status, self-concept, environment, economic status, or stress.

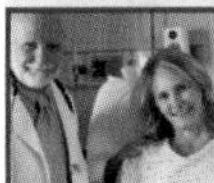

Like many people who suffer from panic attacks, Ida Adkins is afraid she is dying. How would you determine whether Ms. Adkins is experiencing the fear of death that is typical of a panic attack from the sense of impending doom that can accompany a serious cardiac event?

FOCUSED ASSESSMENT FOR *FEAR*

Fear is an intense feeling of dread related to an identifiable source that the person can verify. The source of fear can be a threat of bodily harm or psychological harm. A primary defining characteristic for the nursing diagnosis *Fear* includes the client's ability to identify the specific source of the fear. Separation from sources of support in a potentially threatening situation (such as hospitalization), surgery, and treatments or procedures can evoke fear.

Some behaviors that may indicate fear may be refusal to leave home, refusal to risk coming into contact with the feared object or situation, symptoms of apprehension or even panic or a tendency for flight or fight when exposed to the feared object or situation (NANDA-I, 2005).

Related Factors. Factors related to the nursing diagnosis *Fear* are specific phobias or other mental illnesses, learned responses, sensory or cognitive impairment, threat to self-esteem or ego integrity, loss of a body part or function, pain, and threat of death (actual or perceived).

DIAGNOSIS

Anxiety and fear have similar manifestations and are often difficult to differentiate. Clustering the available data can help (Table 42-3). Fear is derived from a threat that is known, external, and definite, whereas anxiety is said to derive from an unknown internal stimulus, inappropriate to the reality of an external stimulus or concerned with a future stimulus.

The difference between anxiety and fear may also lie in the intensity and duration of symptoms and in the interpretation of an event by the client. Not only do you collect information about your client, but you also make nursing judgments about the meaning of the information and its effect on a client's health and ability to function. This helps you decide on a nursing diagnosis.

From the assessment data gathered, you would choose *Anxiety* as the nursing diagnosis when the client expresses a vague feeling of threat or of an inappropriate threat that persists over time. *Fear* would be the diagnosis of choice if the event occurred suddenly and was brief and/or vivid. The threat can be easily identified, and symptoms usually dissipate quickly once the threat is gone.

Additional diagnoses may be useful in the client who is anxious. *Powerlessness* is a nursing diagnosis common in clients experiencing anxiety. Clients believe that their own abilities are insufficient to affect the outcome of a situation. Passivity, apathy, resignation to their fate (or "giving up") may be noted. Doubt and frustration may be expressed. The clients may refuse to participate in their care or decision making. The related factors for *Powerlessness* can be the health care environment, interpersonal interaction, illness-related regimen, or a lifestyle patterned on helplessness.

Ineffective coping can be used for clients who experience anxiety when they are unable to meet basic needs, the demands of life, or role expectations. This nursing diagnosis can be used when the client responds to stress and anxiety with maladaptive or regressive behaviors such as manipulation or inappropriate anger (see Chapter 47).

Table 42-3 Clustering Data to Make a Nursing Diagnosis

Anxiety	
DATA CLUSTER	**DIAGNOSIS**
A 39-year-old business executive is admitted with a myocardial infarction. "I'm scared. My father died of a heart attack when he was 40. Am I going to die?" He is restless and questions the nurse's every activity.	*Anxiety* related to change in health status and threat of death
A 27-year-old client with alcoholism is admitted for substance abuse detoxification and rehabilitation. He is agitated and hyperventilating. "I don't think I'll make it through this. Will I say things I shouldn't? You won't leave me alone will you?"	*Fear* related to the unknown and to withdrawal from alcohol
A 62-year-old man with metastatic liver cancer reports continuous nausea and a feeling of death being near. He is jaundiced with severe ascites. He says, "Give me enough medicine to stop this misery."	*Powerlessness* related to terminal illness and impending death
Mother of four returns to full-time work after being out of the workforce for 13 years. She says, "I'm so tired since I've gone back to work. I can't sleep, and I have constant headaches. Other women do this. Why can't I?"	*Ineffective coping* related to life changes and unrealistic expectations

PLANNING

The goal of managing anxiety is not a total absence of anxiety but its reduction to a level that is manageable or that allows the person to effectively cope with stressors. Outcomes that are indirectly related to anxiety include behaviors that indicate trust in the health care profession, decrease in pain, and participation in managing the illness. The following expected outcomes for the anxious client are directly related to a reduced state of anxiety:

- Experiences reduction in anxiety level as evidenced by decrease in symptoms of anxiety (reduced tension, fatigue, restlessness, irritability, sweating, tremors); improved sleep, cognitive skills, mood; normal vital signs (pulse, blood pressure, respirations, temperature)
- Identifies own anxiety symptoms and participates in planning care as evidenced by ability to recognize and verbalize signs and symptoms of escalating anxiety; identifies stressors associated with the anxiety; reports own behaviors to nurse; relates feelings and behavior; verbalizes ways to intervene in anxiety escalation
- Develops effective coping and anxiety reduction skills as evidenced by demonstrating relaxation strategies; uses problem-solving skills; participates in decision making related to treatment and discharge planning; uses available resources (e.g., chaplain, psychologist); maintains anxiety level at a tolerable level

INTERVENTION

The heart of nursing practice lies in alleviating mental and emotional suffering, as well as in relieving physical suffering. Caring for the highly anxious or fearful client can be challenging.

INTERVENTIONS TO PREVENT AND MANAGE ANXIETY

Many things can be done to decrease client anxiety, and they range from very simple interventions to complex techniques that require specialized training. Treatment begins with recognition of the client's anxiety. The path to understanding anxiety is clarification of a client's frame of reference or belief system and cognitive interpretation of a set of circumstances. Data collection begins in the assessment phase, during the nursing interview and history taking, but it continues throughout the nursing process as you come to know the client and the significant others better. The more you know about a client's background and point of view, the better you can understand the client's behavior.

Communicating a Sense of Caring. One of your most powerful tools is your presence, or your therapeutic use of self. Communicating a sense of caring, which is the essence of nursing, through respect, listening, and being there is vital to healing. We often underestimate the profound effect of just being there for our clients. The quiet acceptance of our clients as individuals speaks abundantly about how much we value them. Clients rely on nurses to respect and protect them and to watch over them. Knowing the nurse is available if necessary reduces fear and anxiety and gives comfort.

Giving Permission. Give permission or acknowledge clients' right to their own feelings. This in itself can often normalize those feelings and reduce anxiety. Everyone experiences anxiety at various times during contact with the health care system. Tell the client, "It's okay to be nervous about a spinal tap. Many people become nervous. I will be with you during the procedure and will coach you on ways to make it easier. If you get scared or if it hurts, just squeeze my hand."

Listening Actively. Active listening involves more than just hearing what is being said. It involves not only listening to the words but "tuning in" to the feelings behind those words and observing nonverbal cues as well (facial expression, tone of voice, and tension level in the body). During active listening, reflect the client's feeling back with words such as "It sounds as if you are angry that your life was disrupted by a heart attack." Restate or paraphrase what has been said, or use open-ended statements to encourage further exploration and clarify meaning. Encourage clients to explore the cause of their anxiety, because many are able to discover the reasons for it and once they find this, their discomfort often decreases.

Be aware of what you communicate to clients that can raise their anxiety level. Verbal and nonverbal cues communicate feelings, attitudes, and reactions. Being in a hurry and glancing at a watch are often unconscious behaviors. As your behavior can communicate positive messages, it can also decrease rapport and client trust. Through your hurried, preoccupied manner, the client can perceive an attitude of "Let's get this over with" or "I don't have time for you."

You can suggest to your clients that the most effective solution is to find and address the source of their stress or anxiety. Unfortunately, this is not always possible. A first step is to take an inventory of what they think might be making them "stress out":

- What do you worry about most?
- Is something constantly on your mind?
- Does anything in particular make you sad or depressed?

Then, they can find someone they trust (friend, family member, neighbor, clergy) who will listen to them. Often, just talking to a friend or loved one is all that is needed to relieve anxiety. Most communities also have support groups and hotlines that can help. Social workers, psychologists, and other mental health professionals may be needed for therapy and medication.

Modifying the Environment. The environment can contribute to stress and anxiety. Hospital and other health care settings are unfamiliar to most people. Many clinical areas such as intensive care units, surgical suites, and emergency departments are designed for maximum efficiency and high-tech treatment. Some clients and families may see these areas as cold, sterile, and threatening, which can increase anxiety. Give clients simple explanations of what to expect in their particular setting to decrease anxiety. Ask family members to bring in some of the client's articles to personalize the client's space. Many surgical departments allow comfort items such as rosary beads, bibles, small blankets, or stuffed animals to go with clients into surgery.

Noise is another environmental stressor. Major sources of noise in a hospital setting are people and equipment. Nurses often become used to these noises and learn to tune them out, whereas clients do not. Turn down volume on noisy equipment. Explain noises to the client and the family. Attempt to maintain quiet in halls and client rooms during usual sleep hours.

Spiritual Support. Beliefs and values can be challenged as the result of serious illness, suffering, loss, moral and ethical dilemmas, and overwhelming life changes. Spiritual resources and practices can provide a tremendous source of comfort and support for clients experiencing anxiety and fear (see Chapter 49).

Teaching. Cognitive behavioral therapy is treatment that helps clients identify thought patterns and behaviors that contribute to their anxiety and then develop plans to respond to those stimuli with nonanxious responses and by looking at worries more realistically. When clients understand their experience of anxiety, they can recognize the early signs and symptoms and perhaps reduce the level or thwart the episode (Thobaben, Fossett, & Nadler-Moodie, 2004). The unknown can be terrifying. Imagination can make situations far worse than reality. Information and knowledge empower people. Explain the reasons for diagnostic tests, treatment, and medications to help develop trust and reduce anxiety. Using a matter-of-fact and caring manner, explain all procedures before doing them.

Because of its impact on cognitive function, anxiety can interfere with client teaching. An anxious client has difficulty focusing on a specific object or topic for a sustained period of time. The client's cognitive capabilities may be so burdened by coping with the perceived threat that minimal resources are available to manage other stimuli making demands on cognitive processing.

Acknowledge clients' right to be anxious. Take their current level of cognitive functioning into account, and tailor the teaching plan to meet their needs. Initially, a client who is informed of a severe diagnosis may feel devastated and hear little else. Avoid long, involved explanations. Encourage the client to make as many decisions as possible about treatment issues and daily nursing care. However, when a person is highly anxious, it might not be a good time to make major life decisions such as getting a divorce or changing jobs. The client might need to be encouraged to wait before making such decisions. Do not discuss a client's diagnosis and treatment with others within the client's range of hearing. Explain alternative options, because knowing there are choices helps restore the client's sense of control.

Encouraging Family Support. The presence of a family member or significant other can provide comfort and reduce anxiety for many clients. When children are ill, having a parent stay (if at all possible) greatly reduces fear, anxiety, and feelings of abandonment. Encourage family and significant others to call, visit, and be involved with the client's care. However, in some cases the presence of a family member may agitate the client and increase distress. In such instances, limit visiting. Give the client and family a list of resources available to help them cope with anxiety.

Administering Medications. Because anxiety is a normal reaction to stress, most episodes of anxiety do not require medication or require it only on a short-term basis. Furthermore, medication does not solve all problems. Teach clients other methods of dealing with anxiety, such as relaxation and problem-solving techniques. However, if anxiety becomes disabling, medication is often indicated.

Anxiolytics are antianxiety medications that act on the central nervous system to reduce the feelings of anxiety and associated symptoms such as muscle tension and restlessness. They are used to treat both acute anxiety and chronic or long-term anxiety disorders. A common class of antianxiety medications, the benzodiazepines (alprazolam [Xanax], chlordiazepoxide [Librium], diazepam [Valium], and lorazepam [Ativan]), are often used to treat acute anxiety, especially in a hospital setting. They are usually prescribed with caution because of their potential for physical and psychological dependence. Clients can become fearful that they cannot handle their anxiety without taking medication, which can lead them to overuse and abuse of their medication (Thobaben et al., 2004). Buspirone (BuSpar) may be prescribed to treat chronic anxiety, and it does not cause sedation (sleepiness) or lead to dependency. Some of these medications may take several weeks before full onset of therapeutic response is attained. The client needs to understand the delay in onset of therapeutic effect and the use of other methods of controlling anxiety until the therapeutic effects are achieved. The client may need to be reassured or given a concomitant medication during this brief initial phase of treatment. It is also important to remind clients that once they begin to feel better, this means that the medication is working and they should continue to take it as prescribed. You need to encourage clients to take their medications only as prescribed, assess the effectiveness of the drug, and monitor the clients for potential adverse side effects (Thobaben et al., 2004).

Action Alert! Initiate safety measures for any client who receives an anxiolytic, especially an older adult, because most anxiolytic medications cause central nervous system depression and thus sedation.

Providing Complementary Therapies. Complementary therapies, such as touch therapies, relaxation, spiritual support, and music can prevent, reduce, or manage anxiety, as well as enhance the effects of traditional Western medicine and facilitate healing (Box 42-5).

Touch Therapies. Touch therapies have often been associated with spiritual healing, and they convey a blessing or anointing. The main types of touch therapies used by nurses are therapeutic touch (TT) and healing touch (HT). Dolores Kreiger and Dora Kunz introduced TT to nurses in the early 1970s. Kreiger organized the Nurse Healers Professional Associates International in 1979. In 1996 it was organized as Healing Touch International. She integrated additional modalities along with TT. Healing touch is a technique recognized by the American Holistic Nurses Association, and therapeutic touch, also called the Kunz-Kreiger method, is recognized by the Association of Nurse Healers. Certification is available in both techniques for trained practitioners.

The object of touch therapies is to "relax; soothe; stimulate; relieve physical, mental, emotional and/or spiritual discomfort; or aid in transition of the client to a heightened plateau of being" (Dossey, Keegan, & Guzzetta, 2005, p. 641). The techniques involve centering (a state of deep concentration), assessing the state of the energy field, and using appropriate interventions to modulate and balance the energy field. Touch decreases the heart rate, reduces diastolic blood pressure, lowers anxiety, and relieves pain.

Nurses, physicians, other health care professionals, and lay practitioners provide touch therapies. Nurses, however, seem to have taken the lead in the establishment of these modalities into health care settings and into the nursing profession. Many hospitals offer touch therapies to clients who request this service. Touch therapies have been used in many settings, from intensive care units to clients' homes. They have also been used across age-groups.

BOX 42-5 *Considering the Alternatives*

Alterative Therapies for Anxiety

Emotional Freedom Techniques

Emotional Freedom Techniques (EFT) is a meridian-based procedure in which the practitioner taps on acupressure points while the client makes self-validating statements despite their anxiety or phobia.

Advantages

Validated in a randomized controlled trial (Wells, Polglase, Andrews, Carrington, & Baker, 2003)
Client can be taught to self-administer the treatment
Benefits of one treatment endured at 6 to 9 months' follow-up
May provide benefit in posttraumatic stress disorder

Disadvantages

May be difficult to find a local practitioner
May delay standard care

Exercise

Advantages

May also decrease depression (Manger & Motta, 2005) and improve cardiovascular function
Self-determination: Client knows he or she is in charge of progress in this treatment
May work by stimulating the body's own endocannabinoids (Dietrich & McDaniel, 2004)

Disadvantages

Requires more time than pharmacological interventions
Potential for injury if overdone
Preexisting cardiovascular problems may limit implementation

Herbs (*Melissa officinalis* [Lemon Balm] and *Valeriana officinalis* [Valerian])

Advantages

Perceived as more natural than medical sedatives
Supported by randomized controlled trial (Kennedy, Little, Haskell, & Scholey, 2006)
Valerian also shown effective in treating insomnia and angina

Disadvantages (Skidmore-Roth, 2006)

May potentiate the sedative effects of barbiturates and central nervous system depressants
Numerous side effects
Not appropriate for use during pregnancy or lactation or in persons hypersensitive to them; lemon balm should not be used by persons with hypothyroidism

Dietrich, A., & McDaniel, W. F. (2004). Endocannabinoids and exercise. *British Journal of Sports Medicine, 38*(5), 536-541.
Kennedy, D. O., Little, W., Haskell, C. F., & Scholey, A. B. (2006). Anxiolytic effects of a combination of *Melissa officinalis* and *Valeriana officinalis* during laboratory-induced stress. *Phytotherapy Research, 20*(2), 96-102.
Manger, T. A., & Motta, R. W. (2005). The impact of an exercise program on posttraumatic stress disorder, anxiety, and depression. *International Journal of Emergency Mental Health, 7*(1), 49-57.
Skidmore-Roth, L. (2006). *Mosby's handbook of herbs & natural supplements* (3rd ed.). St. Louis, MO: Mosby.
Wells, S., Polglase, K., Andrews, H. B., Carrington, P., & Baker, A. H. (2003). Evaluation of a meridian-based intervention, Emotional Freedom Techniques, for reducing specific phobias of small animals. *Journal of Clinical Psychology, 59*(9), 943-966.

Relaxation. Relaxation techniques can be extremely effective in reducing stress and anxiety. Clients may be unaware of the tension in their bodies and need to learn to monitor it. They are taught relaxation techniques that involve a systematic relaxation of the major muscle groups in the body to help to control the muscle tension. It is especially effective for clients with anxiety and agitation. The nurse at the bedside can use this technique, or clients can be given taped instructions for use at home (Box 42-6). Abdominal breathing (deep breathing exercises) and physical exercise are also effective relaxation techniques nurses can teach clients. Some clients find yoga, meditation, and visualization, such as imaging a peaceful scene, effective techniques to reduce their anxiety (Thobaben et al., 2004).

Music Therapy. Music therapy is defined as a behavioral science that uses specific types of music, such as classical or easy listening, to promote changes in behavior, emotions, and physiology. Music has been used in the treatment of numerous medical and psychological diseases, such as cardiovascular disease, hypertension, pain, gastrointestinal disorders, nausea and vomiting from chemotherapy for cancer, acquired immunodeficiency syndrome (AIDS), dementia, and stress management.

Biofeedback. Biofeedback helps clients to reduce anxiety by providing information about their muscle tension, heart rate, and/or other vital signs in order to gain control over certain body functions that cause tension and physical pain. Therapists use a variety of machines, such as electromyographs (EMGs) that measure muscle tension, and respiration feedback devices that measure the rate, rhythm, and type of breathing. Clients learn exercises that can help them affect the function that is causing a problem (Thobaben et al., 2004).

EVALUATION

You will assess and reassess your clients for anxiety and its level of intensity. When you are sensitive to your clients' emotional needs, you can greatly reduce their suffering and promote healing. Evaluation of the attainment of outcomes previously determined will let you know whether the nursing interventions were effective for the anxious client. If interventions were not effective, you need to reassess the client and determine what revisions to the plan of care are needed.

Box 42-7 provides an example of the application of the nursing process for Ida Adkins, the client experiencing anxiety.

Criteria being met include evaluative statements such as the following:

- The client identifies three personal stressors that induce anxiety.
- The client demonstrates progressive muscle relaxation techniques.

BOX 42-6 *Teaching for Self-Care*

Progressive Muscle Relaxation

Purpose: To promote relaxation by the release of muscle tension in all parts of the body.

Expected Outcome: The client will successfully use progressive muscle relaxation that results in a decreased anxiety state.

Client Instructions

1. Find a quiet, undisturbed place for the relaxation experience, and get comfortable.
2. Keep your legs and arms uncrossed.
3. Close your eyes, and keep them closed throughout the exercise.
4. Become aware of your body. Take notice of any areas that feel especially tense.
5. Breathe in deeply to a count of four.
6. Hold your breath for a count of four.
7. Breathe out to a count of four.
8. Continue to breathe slowly and deeply.
9. Beginning with your feet, tense your muscles for a count of three or four. Curl your toes, and point your feet. Become aware of the feeling of tension. Then relax. Become aware of the feeling of relaxation in your feet.
10. Now tense your feet by bringing them forward toward your head and spreading your toes, again for a count of three or four. Feel the tension, then relax. Feel the relaxation in your feet.
11. Now tense the calves of your legs. Feel the tension. Then relax, and feel the relaxation in your calves.
12. Continue this process with all the muscle groups for the rest of the body, including thighs, buttocks, lower abdomen and pelvis, small of the back, stomach (expand it out and press it in), chest, shoulders, hands, arms, neck (bend your head forward so your chin is trying to touch your chest, then press it back into the pillow), face, forehead, and finally your entire body.
13. Relax and search inwardly for any tension. If you find any tense muscles, relax them.
14. Breathe in deeply to a count of four.
15. Hold your breath for a count of four.
16. Breathe out to a count of four.
17. Continue to breathe slowly and deeply.
18. Notice any sensations of heaviness or relaxation. Observe the changes that have taken place in your body.
19. Allow yourself to remain relaxed for a few minutes. When you feel ready, open your eyes slowly, and slowly stretch.

- The client reports a decrease in anxiety and exhibits no tremors, sweating, or restlessness.

When Ida Adkins is discharged, the nurse writes a final evaluation in her discharge summary as shown in the sample documentation note.

SAMPLE DOCUMENTATION NOTE FOR IDA ADKINS

Discharged to automobile with her mother. States she is feeling calm and believes this episode was related to her son leaving home. However, she is not confident that she can sustain her present state over time. States she will take the antianxiety medication twice a day and report its effects to her doctor. She has a follow-up appointment at the mental health center.

BOX 42-7 *Nursing Care Plan*

A Client With Anxiety

Admission Data

Ida Adkins, a 42-year-old white divorced woman, presented to the Mountain View Clinic with reports of chest pain, shortness of breath, nausea, dizziness, numbness and tingling, racing heart, nervousness, and a feeling of imminent doom. Her mother reports the onset approximately 1 hour before coming to the clinic.

At time of admission, client was afebrile, pulse 120, respirations 32, blood pressure 160/90. Pale, restless, diaphoretic, very anxious, and complaining of intermittent, nonradiating, sharp chest pain, 7 on a scale of 1 to 10. IV started left forearm. Gave 10 mg of morphine sulfate IV and placed on O_2 at 2 LPM per nasal cannula. Cardiac monitor showed sinus tachycardia without ectopy.

Client's medical history includes a myocardial infarction (MI) in 1995 and a psychiatric history of panic attacks. It is significant to note that this afternoon her 16-year-old son informed her he is unhappy with her and wants to live with his father.

At time of transport, vital signs coming down toward normal limits, client rates her chest pain as a 4 on the 1 to 10 scale, but remains restless, slightly queasy, and fearful. Because of her history, we are sending her for admit and observation. Ambulance transport to the County Medical Center with mother in attendance.

Physician's Orders

Admitting diagnosis: rule out MI
Admit to telemetry unit—monitored bed
Oxygen per NC at 2 to 6 LPM prn
Vital signs of shift
Labs—CBC, electrolyte panel, cardiac enzymes/isoenzymes, chest x-ray, and ECG upon admit and per unit protocol
Bed rest with BRP as tolerated
Low NA, low-fat diet
IV D_5NS at 100 mL/h
Nitroglycerin translingual spray—1 to 2 metered doses under the tongue q5 minutes prn
Morphine 10 mg IV q3h prn pain
Phenergan 25 mg PO q4h prn nausea. Give rectally or parenterally if oral dose not tolerated
Ativan 2 mg PO q4h prn anxiety
Notify client's psychiatrist of admission

Nursing Assessment

Color pale, skin cool and dry. Drowsy, but arouses easily and responds appropriately to questions. Reports mild nausea. Cardiac monitor shows normal sinus rhythm at a rate of 80, respirations 20, blood pressure 140/90, temp 98.6° F. Apical heart rate 82. Says heart pain gone. Peripheral pulses palpable with immediate capillary return. Lungs clear. Abdomen soft with active bowel sounds × 4 quadrants. Mother at bedside. Awaiting laboratory work to rule out MI versus anxiety-panic attack.

Nanda-I Nursing Diagnosis	Noc Expected Outcomes With Indicators	NIC Interventions With Selected Activities	Evaluation Data
Anxiety **Related Factors:**	***Anxiety Self-Control***	***Anxiety Reduction***	***After 24 Hours of Care***
• Threat of loss • Feelings of powerlessness	• Eliminate precursors of anxiety. • Monitors intensity of anxiety.	• Acknowledge client's perception of threat/situation.	• Expressed that it helped to have someone who understood what it was like to feel alone.
		• Encourage description of physical and emotional feelings.	• Talked about son wanting to leave and intense feelings of aloneness.
		• Provide privacy to encourage client to talk.	• Cried.
		• Allow feelings of anger, grief, sadness, fear, etc.	• Mother provided comfort and support.
		• Allow mother to be present.	• Mother stayed at bedside during the night; client stated she felt less "alone."
		• Observe for verbal/nonverbal signs of anxiety to determine when anxiety changes.	• Exhibiting mild to moderate anxiety. No further signs of severe to panic level of anxiety.

BOX 42-6

Nursing Care Plan—cont'd

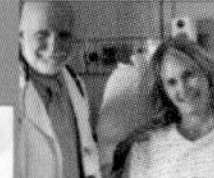

A Client With Anxiety

Nanda-I Nursing Diagnosis	Noc Expected Outcomes With Indicators	NIC Interventions With Selected Activities	Evaluation Data
Anxiety	***Anxiety Self-Control***	***Anxiety Reduction***	***After 24 Hours of Care***
	• Uses (or plans) effective coping strategies.	• Encourage planning activities and meeting with friends.	• Reports "sitting a spell with my mama and sippin' on mama's herb tea" helps calm anxiety.
	• Behavioral manifestations of anxiety absent.	• Teach relaxation techniques, such as progressive muscle relaxation.	• Returned demonstration of relaxation technique.
		• Administer anxiolytic agent as prescribed.	• Visibly relaxed; vital signs WNL. • Verbalizes feeling calm and ready to go home.
		• Initiate referral to Visiting Nurse Association for home monitoring of anxiety management and medication management.	• Referral made and first visit scheduled.

Critical Thinking Questions

1. With a cardiac history and a known anxiety disorder, Ms. Adkins is at high risk for continued admissions just like this one. What other information should be included in Ms. Adkins's teaching plan to prepare her for self-care at home? What are some other complementary therapies that would help her manage anxiety? What cultural factors would you consider?
2. Ms. Adkins denies that her son will leave her, because she feels it would kill her. How would you help her realize the denial and recognize the reality without causing another panic attack?

Nursing outcome and intervention labels from Johnson, M., Bulechek, G., Butcher, H., Dochterman, J. M., Maas, M., Moorhead, S., et al. (Eds.). (2006). *NANDA, NOC, and NIC linkages: Nursing diagnoses, outcomes, & interventions.* St. Louis, MO: Mosby.

▼ KEY PRINCIPLES

- Anxiety is both a universal and a personal experience of daily life. Its purpose is to alert us to possible danger and prepare us for defense and self-preservation.
- The general adaptation syndrome is the body's method of mobilizing its resources to defend against threat or harm.
- The impact of anxiety may be overlooked unless the nurse is sensitive to both the emotional and the physical needs of clients.
- A number of medical conditions, a variety of medications, substance abuse or withdrawal, psychiatric disorders, and stressors can also cause anxiety.
- The symptoms of anxiety can be acute in nature or chronic and disabling and complicate other illnesses by reducing client compliance with treatment plans, increasing perception of pain, and impairing the immune response.
- Without appropriate intervention, anxiety can be self-perpetuating and develop into a vicious cycle.
- Symptoms of anxiety and fear are similar and may be difficult to distinguish.
- There are many interventions for management of anxiety, ranging from simple, basic techniques to complex strategies that require specialized training and certification of the practitioner.
- Evaluation of previously determined outcomes will let you know whether interventions were effective in decreasing anxiety.

■ REVIEW QUESTIONS

1. The nurse would monitor for which of the following as a physical manifestation of stress in a client by:
1. Hyperventilation
2. Decreased heart rate
3. Ability to concentrate
4. Constricted pupils

2. An appropriate nursing intervention for a client who has chronic anxiety is to tell the client to:
1. Never experience anxiety
2. Learn to suppress anxiety
3. Understand that medication is necessary to control anxiety
4. Learn to identify situations that trigger anxiety

3. Two divisions of the autonomic nervous system are:
1. Sympathetic and parasympathetic
2. Platelets and white blood cells
3. Red blood cells and platelets
4. Liver and heart

Continued

4. The client exhibiting the symptoms of insomnia, irritability, restlessness, and attention seeking would be identified by the nurse to be in which level of anxiety?
1. Mild
2. Moderate
3. Severe
4. Panic

5. Anxiety affects clients in all these areas except:
1. Physiological
2. Behavioral
3. Financial
4. Cognitive

Bibliography

Ackley, B. J., & Ladwig, G. D. (2006). *Nursing diagnosis handbook: A guide to planning care* (7th ed.). St. Louis, MO: Mosby.

*American Psychiatric Association. (2000). *Diagnostic and statistical manual of mental disorders* (4th ed., Text Revision). Washington, DC: Author.

Anselmo, J. (2005). Relaxation: The first step to restore, renew and self-heal. In B. M. Dossey, L. Keegan, & C. E. Guzzetta (Eds.), *Holistic nursing: A handbook for practice* (4th ed., pp. 523-564). Sudbury, MA: Jones and Bartlett.

Antai-Otong, D. (2003a). Anxiety disorders: Helping your patient conquer her fears. *Nursing, 33*(12), 36-41.

Antai-Otong, D. (2003b). Anxiety disorders: Treatment considerations. *Nursing Clinics of North America, 38*(1), 35-44.

Antai-Otong, D. (2003c). Current treatment of generalized anxiety disorder. *Journal of Psychosocial Nursing and Mental Health Services, 41*(12), 20-29.

Dossey, B. M., Keegan, L., & Guzzetta, C. E. (2005). Using our healing hands. In B. M. Dossey, L. Keegan, & C. E. Guzzetta (Eds.), *Holistic nursing: A handbook for practice* (4th ed., p. 641). Sudbury, MA: Jones and Bartlett.

Johnson, M., Bulechek, G., Butcher, H., Dochterman, J. M., Maas, M., Moorhead, S., et al. (Eds.). (2006). *NANDA, NOC, and NIC linkages: Nursing diagnoses, outcomes, & interventions.* St. Louis, MO: Mosby.

Kerasiotis, B., & Motta, R. W. (2004). Assessment of PTSD symptoms in emergency room, intensive care unit, and general floor nurses. *International Journal of Emergency Mental Health, 6*(3), 121-133.

*Kreiger, D. (1979). *The therapeutic touch: How to use your hands to help or heal.* Englewood Cliffs, NJ: Prentice Hall.

Ladwig, G. B., & Ackley, B. J. (2006). *Mosby's guide to nursing diagnosis*. St. Louis, MO: Mosby.

NANDA International. (2005). *Nursing diagnoses: Definitions and classification, 2005-2006* (6th ed.). Philadelphia: Author.

Preville, M., Cote, G., Boyer, R., & Hebert, R. (2004). Detection of depression and anxiety disorders by home care nurses. *Aging & Mental Health, 8*(5), 400-409.

*Selye, H. (1956). *The stress of life.* New York: McGraw-Hill.

Swanson, E. (2006). *NANDA, NOC and NIC linkages: Nursing diagnoses, outcomes, & interventions* (2nd ed.). St. Louis, MO: Mosby.

Thobaben, M. (2004a). Alternative approaches to mental health care. *Home Health Care Management & Practice, 16*(6), 528-533.

Thobaben, M. (2004b). Phobias. *Home Health Care Management & Practice, 16*(5), 414-416.

Thobaben, M. (2005a). Defense mechanisms and defense levels. *Home Health Care Management & Practice, 17*(4).

Thobaben, M. (2005b). Generalized anxiety disorder (GAD). *Home Health Care Management & Practice, 17*(2).

Thobaben, M., Fossett, B., & Nadler-Moodie, M. (2004). Nursing management of the patient who is anxious. In *Psychiatric principles and applications for general patient care* (4th ed.). Brockton, MA: Western Schools.

Tyrrell, M. (2005). School phobia. *Journal of School Nursing, 21*(3), 147-151.

U.S. Drug Enforcement Agency, Drug Enforcement Administration. (2005). Depressants. In *Drugs of abuse.* Retrieved December 11, 2005, from http://www.usdoj.gov/dea/pubs/abuse/6-depress.htm.

*Asterisk indicates a classic or definitive work on this subject.

Chapter 43

MANAGING VULNERABILITY

Media Resources

- Evolve Website http://evolve.elsevier.com/Harkreader/
- Companion CD

Learning Objectives

After studying this chapter, you should be able to do the following:

- Describe a conceptual model for understanding the needs of vulnerable populations
- Describe a variety of vulnerable populations
- Identify factors affecting vulnerable populations
- Understand the concept of the community as client
- Assess individuals and groups for factors affecting vulnerability
- Write nursing diagnoses for vulnerable individuals and populations
- Plan goal-directed interventions for vulnerable individuals, groups, and communities
- Evaluate the impact of nursing care on vulnerable populations

Key Terms

community
community forum
community health nursing
environmental resources
epidemiology
focus group
health status
human capital
key informant
opinion survey
parish nurse
participant observation
population
public health nursing
relative risk
resource availability
social integration
social status
vulnerable population
windshield survey

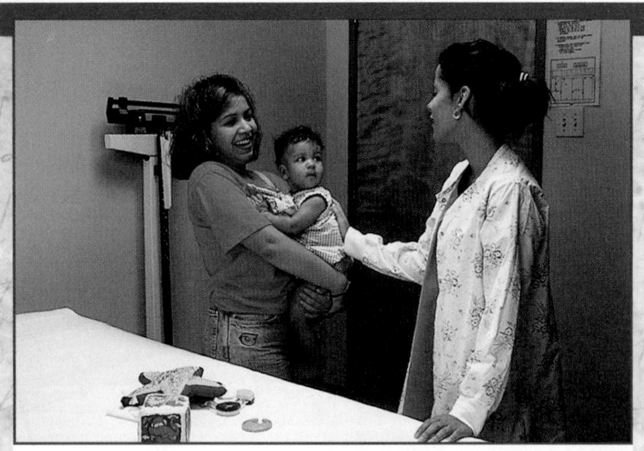

Eighteen-year-old Brenda Carter brought her 2-year-old son to the County Hospital Ambulatory Clinic for his well-child checkup. Brenda, living in poverty and alone with her son, had been unable to adapt to his developing independence:

"I take a lot of time away from him now that he's two 'cause he's got them terrible two's and it's real frustrating to be around him . . . but when he was younger, he used to be my whole life. When he was younger, it was like my face was straight on him, my focus was on him. But now, he's so bad, you know . . . I have to tell him 20 times before—and I won't hit him exactly when I tell him not to do it, but I'll tell him 20 times and then I'll hit him. And then he wants to hit me back."

At the clinic, Brenda described herself as having no control over her life. "I am just stuck here with this baby with no chance to do nothing." Hopelessness had grown out of a series of abusive relationships with men and a lack of resources. Social isolation has afforded Brenda little opportunity to observe the behavior of typical 2-year-old children—behavior not unlike that of her son. The nurse considers the diagnoses *Hopelessness* and *Powerlessness* (see the key nursing diagnoses box).

KEY NURSING DIAGNOSES FOR VULNERABILITY

Hopelessness: Subjective state in which an individual (or a family, a group, a community) sees limited or no alternatives or personal choices available and is unable to mobilize energy on own behalf

Powerlessness: Perception that one's own actions (individual, family, group, community) will not significantly affect an outcome; a perceived lack of control over a current situation or immediate happening

In Chapter 19 you studied a concept of health for the individual, family, and community. Brenda's situation is closely related to health care at all of these levels: she has concerns for her own health, for her family, and she is part of a group of women who are at risk for health problems for both themselves and their children. These women lack the personal resources to change the situation in which they find themselves. They are members of a vulnerable population. The health of the community at large is at risk if the problems of clients like Brenda are not addressed and resources are not made available to prevent the effects of the powerlessness and hopelessness of these groups.

A philosophy of preventive health care requires examination of the groups within a community who are most at risk for health problems. Recognizing the presence of a single factor that is highly associated with a particular disease can define risk. For example, smoking is correlated with an increased incidence of lung cancer. However, some populations within our society are at risk because of multiple interrelated problems. Preventive health care needs to address the factors that make these populations vulnerable.

Vulnerable populations are social groups who have limited resources and consequently are at high risk for myriad health-related problems. Vulnerable social groups include the poor; persons subjected to discrimination, intolerance, subordination, and stigma; and those who are politically marginalized and disenfranchised (Flaskerud & Winslow, 1998). The homeless are an example of one such group (Figure 43-1).

Understanding vulnerable populations will assist nurses in providing services to vulnerable clients that will be acceptable to them. Clients who are on the margins do not always follow the advice of nurses and other health providers. To understand why, health care professionals must look beyond the characteristics of the individual to better understand the characteristics of the group to which the individual belongs. Sometimes nurses need to plan health services specifically designed to meet the unique needs of a particular vulnerable group.

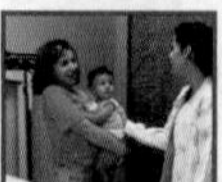

Brenda's problems are multifaceted. The nurse must consider not only Brenda's personal characteristics but also the influences of the social, political, and economic conditions that have contributed to Brenda's problems. There are many clients like Brenda in communities across the nation. Nurses who work with vulnerable groups must understand the concepts of vulnerable populations and community nursing to effectively work with these clients. In this chapter, approaches to working with both the individual and the community as the client will be discussed.

The nurse's client can be an individual, family, aggregate, or entire community. Nurses in all settings plan for the population served by that setting. In a hospital, a nurse working on a gynecology unit plans for the needs of clients who have a gynecological problem as the com-

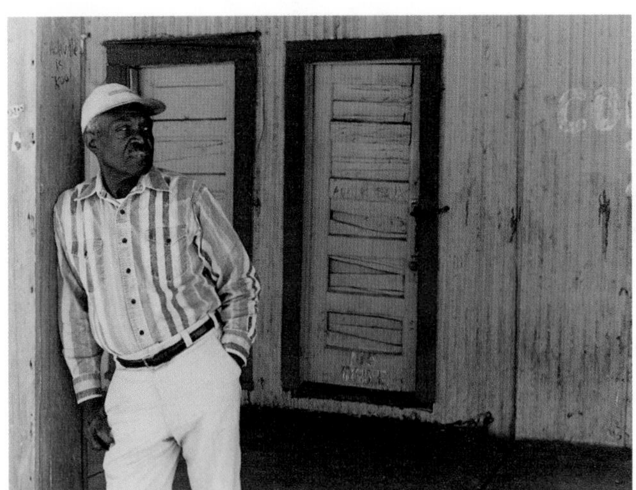

FIGURE 43-1 The homeless are among the groups served by community health nurses.

mon element. The same is true in community settings, where the nurse may plan for outpatient oncology clients, migrant workers, Native Americans living on a reservation, pregnant teenagers, or homeless clients with tuberculosis. Further examples of nurses and their communities include the following:

- A school nurse planning a program for pregnant teenagers
- A public health nurse investigating tuberculosis cases among a homeless population
- A public health nurse serving a population of Cherokees living on a reservation
- A clinic nurse serving a population of clients receiving chemotherapy for cancer
- A home health care nurse caring for frail older adults living in their own homes

A **population** is a group of people who share common characteristics, such as an environment, and common needs. Nurses are involved in planning and providing health services to varied populations. The population is the client to the extent that the nurse plans interventions that affect the whole population. Examples of such interventions follow:

- Posting notices about screening for tuberculosis at sites where large groups of homeless people gather
- Offering classes on parenting for pregnant teenagers within a high school setting
- Providing wheelchairs and assistance to cancer clients to facilitate their visits to the oncology clinic

These groups have certain general characteristics in common—characteristics that may result in difficulty in having their health needs met. Because they share these characteristics, they have been identified as vulnerable populations.

The **community** is the client when the nurse is involved in planning and implementing services that affect the community, which can be at the city, county, or state level. Community nursing can also target a smaller community within a city or county, such as a neighborhood, a particular geographical area, or clients served by a particular clinic.

CONCEPTS OF VULNERABLE POPULATIONS

When problems are complex, a conceptual model is a useful tool for organizing thoughts and developing comprehensive plans. The vulnerable populations conceptual model (Flaskerud & Winslow, 1998) provides a framework for understanding vulnerable populations by examining the relationships among limited resource availability, health-related risk factors, and the health status of the vulnerable populations. The major concepts, or domains, intrinsic to this model include resource availability, relative risk, and health status (Figure 43-2).

Resource Availability. The first domain, **resource availability,** refers to the availability of socioeconomic resources. The dimensions of this domain include human capital, social integration, social status, access to health care, and quality of care.

Human capital includes income, jobs, education, and housing. Poverty, social inequality, poor educational resources, and limited vocational resources are just a few of the socioeconomic constraints found in vulnerable populations. These factors are tied together in a web of cause and effect, creating a maze from which it appears there is no escape. In this maze, rewards and satisfactions in life are often in the immediate present and may be associated with high-risk behaviors.

Social integration means having a harmonious relationship with society in which the person participates as a full member of the society. A lack of social integration is apparent when a person experiences social segregation, marginalization, discrimination, or absence of both formal and informal social supports.

Social status is the position of an individual in relation to others in the society. It is reflected in power to control the political process and the distribution of resources.

Environmental resources include *access to health care* and *quality of health care* (Flaskerud & Winslow, 1998). A lack of socioeconomic and environmental resources is linked to increased risk factors among populations who experience these hardships (Flaskerud & Winslow, 1998).

Relative Risk. **Relative risk,** the second domain of the conceptual model, is considered to be a ratio that compares the risk for poor health among populations who do *not* receive resources and *are* exposed to risk factors, with those populations who *do* receive resources and are *not* exposed to these risk factors. The dimensions of this domain are the following (Flaskerud & Winslow, 1998):

- Lifestyle and behavior choices (e.g., dietary behavior, physical activity, sexual behaviors, and use of tobacco, alcohol, and illicit drugs)

RESOURCE AVAILABILITY
↓Societal and environmental resources

RELATIVE RISK
↑Risk factor

Research practice ethical and policy analysis

HEALTH STATUS
Morbidity and mortality

FIGURE 43-2 The vulnerable populations conceptual model. (From Flaskerud, J. H., & Winslow, B. J. [1998]. Conceptualizing vulnerable populations: Health-related research. *Nursing Research, 47* [2], 69-78).

- Use of screening procedures, immunization programs, and health promotion services (e.g., screening for cancer, tuberculosis, sexually transmitted infections [STIs] including the human immunodeficiency virus [HIV], high blood pressure, prenatal care, and health education)
- Exposure to or participation in stressful life events—in particular, abuse and violence

Health Status. The dimension of **health status,** the third domain of the model, includes age- and gender-specific morbidity and mortality. Socioeconomically disadvantaged groups and those who are discriminated against, subordinated, and stigmatized are exposed to more risk factors and experience increased morbidity and premature mortality (Flaskerud & Winslow, 1998). In addition, vulnerable populations often do not receive the level of health care they require to improve individual and aggregate outcomes (Fiscella & Shin, 2005). This is compounded by the fact that increased morbidity and mortality often exacerbate socioeconomic and environmental disadvantages. Illness and death in a social group may deplete resources, resulting in a decline in human capital, social integration, social status, and access to care (Flaskerud & Winslow, 1998).

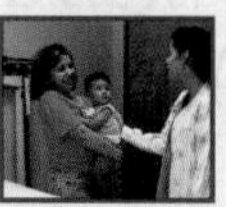

Consider the case of Brenda Carter. Apply the vulnerable populations conceptual model to her story. What aspects of her life characterize her as a member of a vulnerable population?

VULNERABLE POPULATIONS

Vulnerable populations are subgroups of a larger population who are at increased risk for health problems or have greater difficulty obtaining health care. These subgroups include the poor, the homeless, cultural minorities, and those who live in rural communities. This category also includes the uninsured, as well as groups of people stigmatized for their personal situations, their particular illnesses, or both (Fiscella & Shin, 2005; Hunt, 2004). These include individuals who have a mental illness, HIV, or acquired immunodeficiency syndrome (AIDS).

Clients Living in Poverty. Poverty is highly associated with the lack of resources to maintain a healthy lifestyle and prevent illness. The poor are less likely to have access to high-wage employment; safe, affordable housing; and postsecondary education than people at higher income levels. The poor are more likely to require health services because they suffer from a higher rate of chronic illness and diminished physical health, demonstrate markedly higher morbidity and mortality rates, and have a shorter life expectancy than those who do not live in poverty (Seccombe, 2002). Populations most affected by inadequate finances include women, children, older adults, the homeless, the disabled, and those living in rural communities.

The inability to pay for health care services is a major barrier to health care. Although Medicaid insurance has been available to the poor since 1966, only about half the people living below the poverty level qualify. Those who do qualify encounter many providers who have stopped accepting Medicaid because insufficient benefits are paid. The working poor may not be insured or may be underinsured. Copayments and deductibles can be barriers to access at some level of income.

Clients Who Are Homeless. An increasing number of homeless people can be found in both urban and rural areas. The rise in homelessness over the past 15 to 20 years results from a growing shortage of affordable rental housing and a simultaneous increase in poverty. Poor people are frequently unable to pay for housing, food, child care, and health care. They may be forced to make impossible choices between food, shelter, and other basic needs. Housing, which absorbs a high proportion of income, sometimes must be abandoned. Once people have no regular place to live, their vulnerability markedly increases.

Health problems among the homeless include tuberculosis; skin infestations; respiratory infections; and chronic physical disorders such as asthma, anemia, and malnutrition. A prevalence of addictive disorders also exists among homeless populations (National Coalition for the Homeless, 2005). A significant percentage (30% to 50%) of homeless individuals also experience mental health problems (Roche, 2004). In addition, homeless people are more vulnerable to accidental injury and assault and are unable to get adequate rest, exercise, and nutrition. Homeless children may go without immunizations, may be developmentally delayed, and may show signs of behavioral problems.

Migrant Workers. In the United States, it is estimated that there are approximately 3 to 5 million migrant farm workers and their families. They face health problems similar to those of the homeless. Even if they can find health services, the transient nature of their work makes it difficult to provide continuity of care. Their occupation is hazardous because they are exposed to occupational dangers, such as falls and machinery accidents. Migrant workers have a high incidence of respiratory illnesses, including hypersensitivity pneumonitis, or "farmer's lung." Exposure to pesticides and chemicals used to spray crops increases their risk for contracting a variety of malignant and nonmalignant chronic diseases. Many migrant workers are uninsured, unaware of existing health care services, unable to use services due to cultural or communication barriers, and may lack transportation (Clemen-Stone, McGuire, & Eigsti, 2002; Stanhope & Lancaster, 2004).

Ethnic Groups. African Americans, Hispanic Americans, Native Americans, Asian and Pacific Islander Americans, and Native Americans are populations that experience health disparities (Pender, Murdaugh, & Parsons, 2002). Reasons for this vary and include language barriers, as well as limited job opportunities and resources, which adversely affect personal finances and opportunities for health care insurance and transportation (Stanhope & Lancaster, 2004).

Clients in Rural Areas. Barriers to health care for people living in rural communities include poverty, the need to travel long distances, lack of private and public transportation, poor outreach services, lack of knowledge about services, and communication and cultural barriers (Stanhope & Lancaster, 2004). Small rural hospitals that aim to promote health and prevent disease often experience barriers such as inadequate reimbursement, insubstantial local economies, low educational levels, and lack of adequate personnel (Olden & Szydlowski, 2004).

Stigmatized Populations. Certain other aggregates of people have difficulty accessing health care because of "prejudice, discrimination, and lack of status or power" (Hunt, 2004). They may have illnesses that are misunderstood, and therefore feared, such as HIV/AIDS, or severe mental illness. Additional groups of people that may be devalued by the dominant society include pregnant adolescents, individuals with addictive disorders, and older adults, especially older women (Cohen, 2002; Inglehart, 2002; Stanhope & Lancaster, 2004).

Pregnant Adolescents. Every year close to one million adolescents in the United States become pregnant. Although they become pregnant for a variety of reasons, the effects of poverty combined with poor academic achievement and resultant feelings of low self-worth is a major reason. Other reasons range from the belief that having a baby will give them someone that loves them, forgetting or not understanding how to use contraceptives, to getting closer to a boyfriend or rape. The medical complications related to teenage pregnancies include low birth weight, preterm labor and delivery, poor maternal weight gain, anemia, and sexually transmitted diseases. Lack of prenatal care accounts for these poor outcomes. Other factors associated with poor pregnancy outcomes—such as poverty, lack of education, and poor family support—add to the complications caused by inadequate prenatal care (Stanhope & Lancaster, 2004).

For adolescent males, poverty, poor academic performance, and poor school attendance are correlated to teenage pregnancy (Coughlin, 2005). Early parenthood is often deeply imbedded in the context of these young people's lives, and they are making choices from limited options. Impoverished youth who are failing in school need a positive vision for their future, as well as educational and vocational resources if pregnancy is to be delayed until adulthood.

The childbearing adolescent often has multiple risk factors that reflect lifestyle and behavior choices beyond being pregnant and an adolescent. Adolescent mothers have often engaged in impulsive high-risk activities before their pregnancies, such as early initiation of sexual activity, unprotected sexual activity, multiple sexual partners, gang affiliation, school truancy or dropout, and alcohol and other drug use.

Health-related problems of adolescent mothers include both pathophysiological and psychosocial changes that adversely affect the lives of these young women and their children such as a high maternal mortality rate, pregnancy-related hypertension, anemia, sexually transmitted diseases, substance abuse, poor nutrition, disrupted school attendance, ongoing poverty, reduced career opportunities, separation and divorce from the infant's father, and subsequent pregnancies (Coughlin, 2005). Parenting problems such as child neglect and abuse, domestic violence, depression, and suicide attempts are additional concerns. Lastly, health-related problems of infants born to teen mothers include increased mortality and morbidity (Gilbert, Jandial, Field, Bigelow, & Danielson, 2004).

Suicidal Adolescents. One in every eight teens experiences clinical depression, and due to its differing forms of presentation, it can easily be overlooked (Wysong, 2005)

(Figure 43-3). Suicide is the third leading cause of death among adolescents in the United States, and depression is an important risk factor for suicide (Conwell, Duberstein, & Caine, 2002; Murphy, 2005). Risk for suicide in depressed adolescents is compounded by substance abuse (U.S. Department of Health and Human Services, 2005). Depressive disorders evolve from both biological and contextual issues. Risk factors for depression in adolescents include the following (American Academy of Child and Adolescent Psychiatry, 2006; National Youth Violence Prevention Resource Center, 2003):

- Parental psychopathology
- Parental conflicts
- Physical illness
- Poor coping skills
- Stressful events (both large and small)
- Dissatisfaction with scholastic endeavors (grades)
- Behavioral problems (internal and external)
- Substance abuse
- Prior suicide attempt(s)

Feelings of hopelessness, powerlessness, worthlessness, and inappropriate guilt are frequently present with depression and are linked to teen suicide (Murphy, 2005).

Frail Older Adults. Another social group with an increased risk for health-related problems is older adults (Hall & Brown, 2005). Older adults are more likely to be living in poverty than younger adults. Three factors have been identified as associated with this poverty: (1) inadequate retirement income, (2) the high cost of medical care, and (3) financial exploitation and criminal victimization. Social isolation and poor nutrition are well-known risks of older adults that may result in increased susceptibility to illness. Thirty-one percent of older adults who live in the community live alone. Hunger, a severe form of food insecurity, is experienced by 1.7% of older adult households (Hall & Brown, 2005).

Although many older adults live in their own homes and may have adequate financial and health care resources, there is a segment of this population that can be described as vulnerable. They are physically frail, have multiple chronic health problems, and lack the resources to manage without help. After 20 or more years of retirement, the once-adequate fixed retirement income no longer covers the person's needs. These older adults lack preventive and health maintenance services because of decreased finances, lack of transportation and mobility, and inadequate knowledge about prevention (Box 43-1).

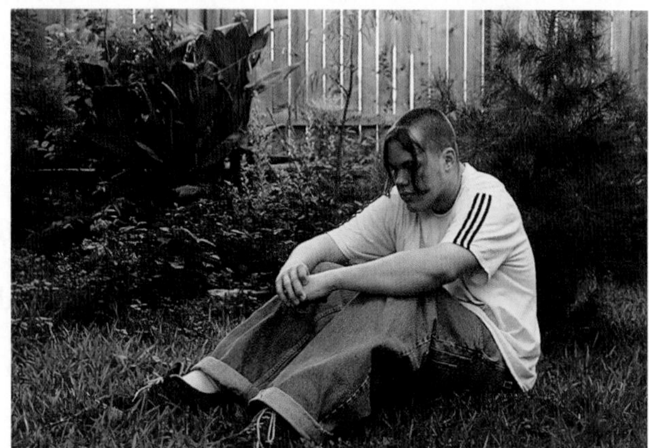
FIGURE 43-3 One in eight adolescents will experience depression by age 18.

Suicidal Older Adults. A high risk for depression exists among older adults. Depression in late life is linked to stressors such as physical illness, hospitalization, and the loss of a loved one. Older adults at increased risk for depression are those suffering from chronic disorders, such as heart disease and arthritis, and those living in nursing homes. The older adult suicide rate exceeds that of all other age-groups, with individuals 85 years old or older at greatest risk (Geriatric Mental Health Foundation, 2005).

Clients With HIV and AIDS. Persons infected with HIV and those living with AIDS are more susceptible to further health and socioeconomic risks and discrimination. They have an increased risk for developing cancer (such as Kaposi's sarcoma) and other opportunistic diseases because of their weakened immune systems. Many individuals living with HIV/AIDS suffer from poverty, homelessness, and lack of family support due to job loss, mental illness, health-related costs, hospitalization(s), substance abuse, addictions, domestic violence, and a lack of reasonably priced housing (National Association of Social Workers, 2003).

THE CONCEPT OF COMMUNITY AS A CLIENT

To understand the concept of the community as a client, we need to define community and community health nursing. A community is a geographical location or an aggregate or population of individuals who have one or more personal or environmental characteristics in common (Hunt, 2004). In other words, location, people, and social systems define a community. As a location, a community is defined by its geographical boundaries (e.g., a city, county, or nation) or by political boundaries (e.g., a precinct or ward). A community can also be defined as a group of people or a population with a common interest, culture, religion, or race. Communities can vary in size, from a small group to the global community.

BOX 43-1 *Older Adults: Potential Barriers to Care*

- Inadequate income
- High cost of medical care and pharmaceuticals
- Financial exploitation
- Increased criminal victimization
- Stereotyping and discrimination
- Social isolation
- Poor nutrition and hunger

Community health nursing is the field of nursing that promotes and preserves the health of populations by (1) understanding and applying concepts of public health and community, (2) working with community organizations to assist in community development, (3) providing generalist care to selected individuals, families, and groups, and (4) providing health promotion, health maintenance, health education, and coordination of care. Community health nursing is a synthesis of nursing theory and public health theory aimed at preserving and promoting the health of communities. In some settings, an individual is the client, and when nursing practice is focused on a group or community, the community is the client. Improving the health of individuals, families, and groups increases the health of the community. Community health nursing is an umbrella term for all nurses who work in a community setting.

The term *community health nursing* is often used interchangeably with *public health nursing*, even though the former is a broader concept. **Public health nursing** is more strictly defined as the practice of promoting and protecting the health of populations through nursing activities to improve the quality of life (including its physical, mental, and social aspects), to prevent disease, and to control communicable diseases consistent with available knowledge and resources using knowledge from nursing, social science, and public health science. It is a synthesis of public health practice and nursing practice. Public health nursing requires specific educational preparation in epidemiology, statistics, and research; it has to do with the health care system itself, application of public health concepts to groups and communities, and the regulations affecting public health practice.

Settings and Agencies for Community Health Nursing. Community health nurses are employed in state and local public health departments, businesses, industrial settings, schools, prisons, day care centers, residential centers, and mental health centers. In addition, community health nurses provide hospice care at home and in acute care settings. They also provide care in long-term care facilities, day clinics, ambulatory settings, and shelters for battered women and homeless people.

Roles of Nurses in Community Health Nursing. In most nursing specialties, nurses' roles include caregiver, educator, manager, researcher, consultant, role model, leader, and client advocate. Community health nurses function in these roles, but the settings and agencies of practice differ from typical acute care settings; these differences influence the roles of the community health nurse.

Home health care nurses provide direct care to clients and families and teach clients and families the "how-to" and "why" of self-care. There has been an increase in home health care visiting because the cost for home visits is lower than for institutional care, fewer family-member caregivers are available to mobile families, many clients are homebound but not ill enough to be hospitalized, and more older adult clients are in need of home health care because of increased life expectancies. Home health care nurses care for the chronically ill, the terminally ill, and those who need "high-tech" care, such as ventilators.

School nurses play a pivotal role in student, family, and faculty health-related activities. They provide immunizations, health screenings (vision, hearing, and so on), counseling, administering of medications, and basic care (first aid) for minor complaints. School nurses are also actively involved in educational opportunities relevant to environmental health, school safety, and communicable diseases. They take part in case finding, case management, and record keeping, as well as in health promotion and preventive health care campaigns, including family education in communicable diseases.

Occupational health nurses promote the health and safety of workers through worksite programs. They provide direct care and treatment for job-related illnesses or injuries. They coordinate health education programs for smoking cessation, healthy diets, exercise, and weight control. They participate in employee assistance programs for substance abuse and coping with personal problems. They act as employee advocates for job safety and maintain records of occupational health histories.

Discharge planning nurses help clients in the process of moving from one health care setting to another. These nurses must know about the resources available to clients so they can coordinate the delivery of those resources (Box 43-2).

Case management nurses coordinate access and utilization of health services. They are responsible for the client's care from entry into the health care system through discharge.

Nurse epidemiologists are detectives of illness and disease. **Epidemiology** is the study of the cause and distribution of disease, disability, and death among groups of people. The nurse epidemiologist uses the epidemiology triangle in solving health care mysteries (Figure 43-4). The triangle represents the relationships among agent, host, and environment necessary for disease to occur. Elimination of any one of these may modify the occurrence of disease.

The nurse epidemiologist uses many sources of information to look for trends in health issues. These include vital statistics reports, morbidity and mortality reports, demographic statistics, and biostatistics. Trends can be seen over time, in a specific geographic area, and affecting a population. This information is helpful in making changes for healthful outcomes.

The nurse epidemiologist may conduct case studies, field investigations, and field surveys and may assist in surveillance or monitoring activities. Through these projects, information is reported to local health authorities and passed on to district, state, provincial, and national officials.

BOX 43-2 *Activities of Discharge Planning Nurses, Case Management Nurses, and Nurse Epidemiologists in the Community*

Discharge Planning Nurses
- High-risk or referral screening
- Assessment for anticipated needs after discharge
- Assessment of resources available, accessible, and affordable for client
- Interdisciplinary, family, client, and provider conferencing
- Goal setting
- Referral and coordination of resources and providers
- Education of client and caregivers
- Monitoring of outcomes
- Documentation of process and outcomes in client records

Case Management Nurses
- Case finding
- Screening
- Assessment
- Identification of problems
- Prioritizing problems and planning
- Advocating in the interest of clients
- Arranging service delivery
- Monitoring of clients during service
- Reassessment
- Evaluating and documenting

Nurse Epidemiologists
- Case studies, in which the nurse assesses a client's environment, including family, community, and health history
- Field investigations, in which the nurse gathers information regarding variables surrounding a problem or disease, then looks for causal relationships
- Field surveys, in which the nurse acts as a part of a team to determine the frequency of a problem or disease at a specified time or the amount of the problem or disease in an entire population group
- Surveillance, in which the nurse monitors the incidence and prevalence of communicable diseases through accurate record keeping and data collection

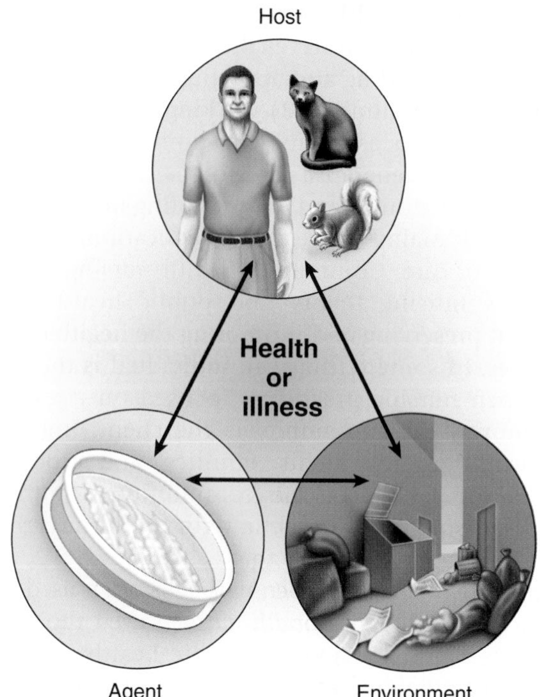

FIGURE 43-4 The epidemiological triangle. The *agent* is an animate or inanimate factor whose presence or absence may lead to disease, disability, or death. It is most often viral, bacterial, fungal, or protozoal. The *host* is a living species—human or animal—susceptible to disease, disability, or death. The *environment* includes all external conditions and influences affecting the living species, which in turn can affect transmission of the disease.

FACTORS AFFECTING VULNERABILITY

Multiple factors are often present that contribute to a group's or individual's vulnerability. Lifestyle, family structure and function, and personal factors are among those factors that affect vulnerability.

LIFESTYLE

Understanding the lifestyle of vulnerable populations goes beyond the physical and social elements of how and with whom a person lives. It includes the values that motivate behavior, the dynamics of making choices, the mechanisms of attaining self-esteem, the effects on hope, and the nature of power in a situation where resources are limited.

These attributes can be linked to the behavioral factors that can be directly related to high-risk behaviors and health risks. Reducing health risks in vulnerable populations requires recognizing the interrelationship of multiple risk factors.

FAMILY STRUCTURE AND FUNCTION

The developmental stage of the family, family dynamics, access to resources, skills in negotiating the health care/social service systems, and other problems in the family constellation can affect the vulnerable client's ability to cope. Families can create a multiproblem situation for vulnerable populations rather than help alleviate the problems. A situation that might be manageable, though difficult, can become more complicated in the context of a multiproblem family situation where limited resources are already stretched.

PERSONAL FACTORS

Taking action to change a life in which problems seem insurmountable requires both a vision of a better future and a belief that one has the power to create that future. Vulnerable populations can easily become overwhelmed by the difficulties of life, making it impossible to envision a better future, much less implement a plan to attain it.

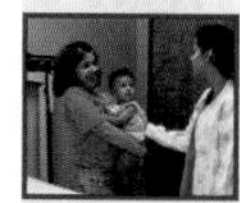
Brenda's nursing diagnoses of *Hopelessness* and *Powerlessness* are common in other members of the vulnerable groups for whom nurses care, both in the community and in acute care settings.

Hope. Plato described hope as the images that man forms for himself about the future. It has to do both with the mental pictures of what the future might be and with the wish that it will be that way. To have hope, there must be a desire and some expectation that the desire will be fulfilled. The expectation that what is wished for will come to be does not have to be absolute; any degree of belief in the future being different, better, or meeting expectations constitutes hope.

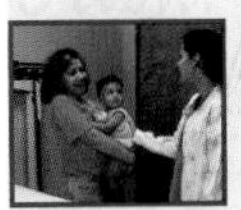

Reflecting back to our case study, what cues does Brenda offer that suggest that she has little hope for change in her life?

Hope exists when a person knows that certain actions will result in predictable consequences. Having inner strength and a belief that the self is efficacious in connection with the outer world comes from the self. Thus hope exists on both a conscious and an unconscious level. On a conscious level, a person can name or describe the expectations for the future and even predict the likelihood that the expectations will be realized. On an unconscious level, hope is a life force that provides the energy to drive the individual forward.

Hope cannot logically exist when a person knows that no known action will result in the desired consequences. However, hope often continues in this circumstance. This hope comes from a belief that forces external to the self can positively influence what happens to a person, so that when the person has done everything he or she knows how to do or is able to do, hope remains. Hope is often derived from religious faith but can be faith in any power greater than the self.

Power. Having power means having control in direct relationship to the self, having power to control the actions of others, or having power to control the environment. The perception of personal control is the belief that through one's own actions, behaviors, or personal characteristics, one can affect outcomes. One who feels in control perceives the ability to make decisions about one's own actions, to control a situation, and to get what is desired from life. Control has to do with preventing bad things from happening and making good things happen.

The concept of power may be viewed in terms of "power over" or "power to" (Hawks, 1991). *Power over* emphasizes strength, control, and competitiveness, whereas *power to* suggests the development and achievement of goals. Assisting a person with having *power to* involves developing trust, caring, knowledge, cooperation, interpersonal skills, respect for the individual's beliefs, communication skills, and decision-making skills.

ASSESSMENT

INDIVIDUAL ASSESSMENT

The complex nature of the relationship between inadequate resources and the many risk factors for health-related problems makes a comprehensive evaluation necessary when making assessments of an individual who is a member of a vulnerable group. This evaluation includes a psychological, social, and physical needs assessment.

Psychological Needs Assessment. Community health nurses assess for psychological needs that may be factors in health-seeking behaviors. For example, routine psychological screening of pregnant adolescents and teen mothers includes screening for symptoms of depression, suicidal ideation, and history of suicide attempts. Other known risk factors for suicide, such as social isolation, substance use, and access to weapons, should be identified. Nurses can identify pregnant teens already suffering with depressive symptoms or suicidal ideation and assist these young mothers in attaining mental health counseling before the birth of their baby, before they experience the added stressors inherent in premature motherhood.

Action Alert! Immediate referrals to drug treatment programs may be indicated for chemically dependent pregnant and parenting youth.

Social Needs Assessment. Social needs involve the client's relationships with others. Social assessments must include screening to identify victims of previous and current violence, as well as the client's perception of current family support. For example, clients with AIDS may have conflict with their parents and with their partners yet still value them as an important source of support.

Social needs are also concerned with the social or environmental structures affecting the client's life. Assessment of the risk of neighborhood violence and neighborhood resources for healthy living is crucial for understanding the risks faced by vulnerable populations. Environmental issues include cleanliness of housing, including presence of rats, roaches, contaminated water, and sewage. However, you need to look beyond the immediate home to the neighborhood (Figure 43-5).

Physical Needs Assessment. In addition, the nurse will assess for physical needs by performing a thorough physical examination and obtaining a thorough history. It is important to be aware of the common medical problems in the population and to include screening measures for these problems. The community health nurse will also include screening for the ability to meet basic human needs such as nutrition, safety, and access to health care.

One of the most important tasks in the general health evaluation of pregnant and parenting teens is to assess their concrete needs. This includes housing needs, nutritional needs, necessary supplies (e.g., diapers), educational needs, and vocational training. To make appropriate referrals, nurses must have extensive knowledge about available services and eligibility requirements for programs such as Medicaid, nutritional services (including the public assistance program for women, infants, and children [WIC] and food stamps), child care subsidies, educational programs, and vocational programs.

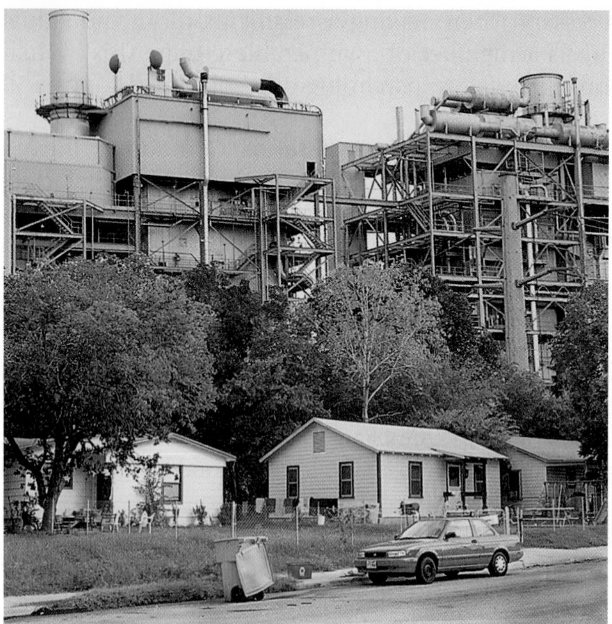

FIGURE 43-5 Many factors affect the health of individuals, families, and communities. In this community, families live with the possible health risks associated with proximity to a chemical plant.

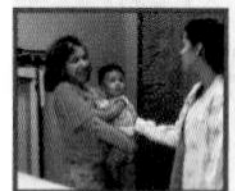

Recall the case of Brenda Carter. What concrete needs does she have that could reduce her sense of helplessness and powerlessness?

In addition, the nurse should assess for problems with known risk factors in the specific population. For example, early prenatal care is essential for all pregnant teens who, with proper health care management, can expect to have normal pregnancies and good birth outcomes. Timely identification of problems is vital for reducing complications of pregnancy. Besides standard prenatal and postpartum health assessments, testing for STIs (including HIV) must be provided. Physiological changes that occur during pregnancy, such as opening of the cervix, increase HIV risk; however, condom use during pregnancy and in young mothers is rare. Intervention programs that include skill building in the areas of sexual negotiation and condom use are imperative so that these young mothers can protect themselves and their unborn babies from HIV and other STIs.

COMMUNITY ASSESSMENT

The vulnerable client is assessed both as an individual and as part of a susceptible population within the community. Thus, nurses, particularly those working in community settings (e.g., community and school-based clinics), are uniquely positioned to be instrumental in the development and implementation of community strategies for health risk reduction.

When assessing the community or group as the client, a broader scheme or framework of assessment must be used. Types of data to be collected include environmental, cultural, socioeconomic, political, and demographic data, as well as health data. Factors that affect the type and scope of the assessment are shown in Box 43-3.

BOX 43-3 *Factors Affecting the Type and Scope of Community Assessment*

- Purpose (will expenditure of time and money accomplish the purpose?)
- Size of community or group (use random sampling, interviews, telephone survey?)
- Location of community or group (geographically accessible?)
- Time to complete the assessment (available?)
- Personnel, and expertise of the person directing the assessment (sufficient?)
- Political environment (if applicable) within community or group (amenable to assessment?)
- Cost/benefit relationship (ratio of assessment cost to benefit of results–sufficiently low?)

Types of Data. Environmental data include location, climate, physical geography, housing, sanitation, water supply, toxic hazards, public utilities, transportation, industrial versus residential areas, public services (such as police and fire departments and emergency services), health care facilities and services available, schools, libraries, grocery stores, and other types of stores (Figure 43-6).

Cultural data include types of ethnic groups and religious groups (including their beliefs and value systems), language barriers, alternative health care practices and use of alternative healers, and dietary customs. Identifying existing priorities and motivations is an important step in assessing a community.

Socioeconomic and political data include income status, educational level, educational resources, employment status, employment availability, unemployment rates, governmental structure, formal and informal community leaders (including distribution and use of power), community history, community harmony and violence, media and communication avenues, community stressors, leisure and recreational activities available, and political processes.

Demographic data include information collected through the census, such as race, age, and number of persons living in specific locations, population growth, and family statistics. Other sources of information include birth and death certificates, crime reports, morbidity and mortality reports, and secondary data from previously collected information.

Methods of Data Collection. Methods of collecting data include windshield surveys, participant observations, focus groups, interviewing key informants, community forums, opinion surveys, and secondary data analysis. In addition, research data and statistics from previous studies on similar health problems can be highly beneficial in assessing, diagnosing, planning, and evaluating.

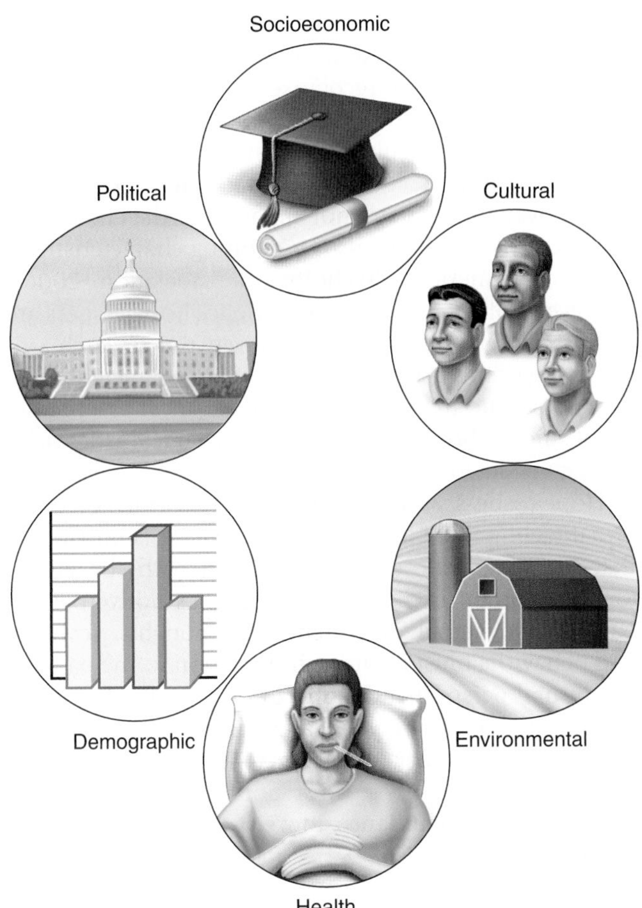

FIGURE 43-6 Types of data to collect when assessing a community or group.

A **windshield survey** is a method of data collection in which the researcher drives through a neighborhood to conduct a general assessment of that neighborhood through observation. It is a quick way to get an objective view of the neighborhood environment and the observable facets of community living conditions.

Participant observation is a method of community assessment that examines formal and informal social systems at work. The researcher (e.g., nurse, social worker) shares in the life activities of the group while observing and collecting data. The data collector takes part in the life of the community and observes how health and health care may be affected by identified conditions.

A **focus group** is a method of data collection in which 6 to 12 people from a group or aggregate are brought together for discussion, guided when necessary by a skilled, nonjudgmental leader. The leader listens carefully and guides the group only when necessary. Through the use of focus groups, the participants' opinions, beliefs, and experiences can be analyzed and used in making health care decisions. Focus groups can stimulate research questions, develop recruitment strategies, validate data from other sources, and evaluate outcomes of interventions.

A **key informant** is a community leader, professional, politician, or business person who possesses knowledge of the needs of the community and who can act as a useful source of data and a supporter of new programs. These persons may have access to important information and may also be influential in persuading certain sectors to make health care changes.

An **opinion survey** is a method of data collection performed through telephone interviews, mailed questionnaires, or door-to-door interviews or at clinic sites. These are more expensive forms of data collection, and they also limit the categories of persons who will respond. Some people have no telephone, some people cannot read (and therefore cannot answer a questionnaire), and some people simply prefer not to take part in a survey.

A **community forum** is an open meeting where members of a community or group may come to share opinions and concerns about a particular issue. Information gathered here may be different from that gathered by other means because these meetings are open to the general public.

Finally, the nurse may access secondary data gathered on previous occasions. This includes data from records of schools, health departments, police and fire departments, or volunteer organizations such as the American Cancer Society, Planned Parenthood, or a community domestic violence hotline.

FOCUSED ASSESSMENT FOR *HOPELESSNESS*

Defining Characteristics. *Hopelessness* is conveyed in the client's communication patterns, behavior, and emotional response. It may be expressed directly or indirectly, verbally or nonverbally (Figure 43-7).

Verbal. Ask questions about the client's expectations for both the immediate and the long-term future. Does the client have plans for the future? Does the client express a belief that the present difficult circumstances can or will change? Is the client able to list several alternative behaviors for managing problems, attaining goals, or otherwise coping with circumstances? Listen for verbal expressions of pessimism, of negative future expectations, and of futile efforts toward meeting desired goals. If the client does not make a direct statement about the future, the nurse could ask, "When you think of your future, say 6 months from now, how do you see yourself compared with now? And how does this make you feel?" Listen for themes that reflect a sense of loss, deprivation, or despair, or feelings such as "I'm a total failure in life" or "Life has no more meaning."

Verbal statements of hopelessness and pessimism may be clear or may require clarification to validate the meaning. Listen for themes of being incompetent, worthless, or a failure in life. Hopelessness is evident when the client describes futile efforts at problem solving or actions

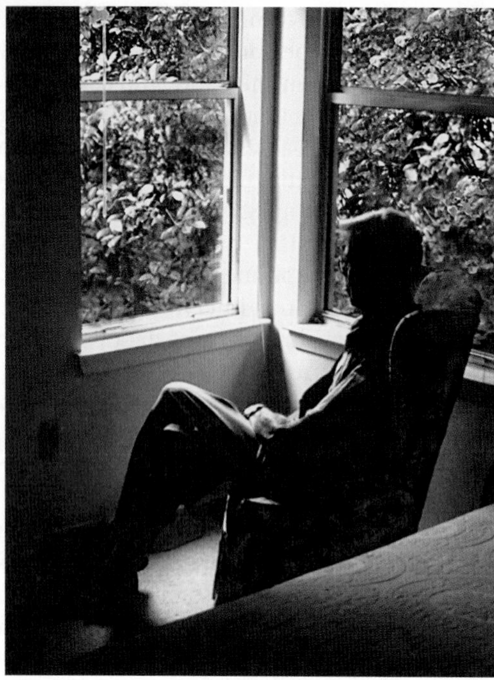

FIGURE 43-7 Hopelessness is conveyed verbally and nonverbally.

that have not produced the desired results. It may be clear that the client has given up.

Nonverbal. Hopelessness is also conveyed nonverbally. Observe the client's appearance. Grooming, body posture, eye contact, and affect (generally showing sadness and marked apathy) can provide cues to *Hopelessness.* Clients experiencing *Hopelessness* actually speak very little, very seldom initiate a conversation, and usually respond to questions with few words in a monotone voice. The nonverbal defining characteristics of turning away from the speaker, shrugging in response to the speaker, and minimal eye contact should be assessed within the context of the client's overall communication pattern. The meaning of these behaviors needs to be validated.

Social. Another defining characteristic of *Hopelessness* pertains to problems with social relationships. These problems include perceived difficulty of interactions with others, loss of gratification from roles and relationships, impaired interpersonal relationships, perceived lack of social support, and possibly social withdrawal.

Hopelessness is also identified through a need for increased sleep and lack of spontaneity. Chronic fatigue, decreased motivation, anorexia, and weight loss contribute to decreased self-care. The client manifests decreased motivation and a general lack of interest or initiative.

Defining characteristics of *Hopelessness* include decreased problem-solving skills and decreased flexibility in thought processes. Thought processes are constricted so that perceptions are narrowed, with evidence of cognitive rigidity and dichotomous thinking. These cognitive characteristics limit the range of problem-solving options. Clients feel overwhelmed by untenable situations that are perceived as affording no relief or way out. The client is unable to recognize any sources of hope.

Assess the reality of the situation. The client may be experiencing a difficult life situation perceived as unbearable with few solutions. The nurse may restate alternatives available that are not apparent to the client.

Affective. Hopelessness is a defining characteristic of *depression* (American Psychological Association, 2006). However, not all clients who experience hopelessness are depressed. On the other hand, given the research evidence regarding hopelessness as a core characteristic of depression and the evidence of hopelessness as a predictor of suicide, both of these defining characteristics need to be considered in assessments.

Hopelessness as a psychological construct or emotional feeling is subjective, and therefore it is imperative that the diagnostic cues be validated with the client. Most important is that all of the client's nonverbal behaviors and verbal descriptions of thoughts, feelings, and behaviors must be viewed in relation to the particular cultural perspectives of the client and what hopelessness means to the client.

Related Factors. Related factors for *Hopelessness* include the following:

- Self-concept disturbance, low self-esteem
- Lack of initiative
- Self-care deficit
- Ineffective problem solving and unrealistic goal setting
- Failing or deteriorating physiological conditions or prolonged pain and discomfort
- Abandonment or separation from significant others or loss of someone or something one values in life
- Loss of belief in transcendent values/God
- Exposure to long-term physiological or psychological stress
- Inability to achieve developmental tasks (e.g., identity, integrity)

FOCUSED ASSESSMENT FOR *POWERLESSNESS*

Defining Characteristics. The most specific defining characteristic of *Powerlessness* is the client's verbal expression of having no control or influence over a situation, an outcome, or self-care. The client may also be observed as not participating in health care decisions. The client's affect is generally apathetic, and the overall appearance may be passive.

Assess the client for participation in general health care or in decision making when opportunities are provided and for reluctance to express feelings out of fear of alienating caregivers. When assessing the client, the nurse needs to ask the client about usual decision-making patterns: "How would you describe your usual method of making decisions (e.g., career, health care)?" Similarly, ask questions about individual and role responsibilities. "What responsibilities did you have at school? . . . At home? . . . At work?"

Assess for indirect expressions of powerlessness, such as anxiety or anger. Dependence on others may result in irritability, resentment, anger, and guilt. In addition, the client may express discomfort or dissatisfaction with the health environment or an inability to perform previous tasks, activities, or roles. Signs of uncertainty include defending self-care practices when challenged and expressing uncertainty regarding fluctuating energy levels. In contrast, signs of taking control in a health situation include monitoring progress and seeking information regarding care.

To assess the client's experience of control, the nurse could ask, "How would you describe your ability (high/poor) to control or alleviate your present health situation (e.g., pregnancy, diabetes, obesity)?" "To what or to whom (e.g., self-preventive measures, other individuals) do you attribute your ability to control fate?" "Do you ever feel like you have no control over life events?"

Powerlessness is a subjective state, and therefore the nurse's assessment must be validated with the client. It is also imperative that all of the client's verbalizations be considered in relation to the particular ethnic and cultural perspectives on the meaning of control and influence to the client.

Related Factors. Related factors for *Powerlessness* include the following:

- Decreased self-esteem
- Lack of knowledge
- Perception of nonsupportive health care environment
- Poorly controlled chronic illness
- Perception of having no control over the health care regimen

DIAGNOSIS

INDIVIDUALS

Hopelessness and *Powerlessness* are closely related concepts. A primary distinction between *Hopelessness* and *Powerlessness* rests in the concept of control. Hope can be present even when the client feels no ability to control a situation. However, *Hopelessness* suggests that the client lacks the psychic energy to change the situation, is unable to perceive alternatives, or has alternatives that are clearly limited. The client who is experiencing *Hopelessness* may also experience *Powerlessness* in a specific situation.

When you have confirmed that the client is experiencing *Hopelessness,* the focus of intervention will be on giving the client hope and facilitating realistic positive and healthy outcomes. Outcomes will be in terms of the client's self-perception, interpersonal relationships, and views of his or her future. Through assisting, encouraging, and teaching in areas that require changes in self-concept, self-care, interpersonal interactions, support systems, problem solving, and developing realistic goals, you will contribute to the client's return to a healthy level of functioning.

The diagnosis of *Powerlessness* clearly deals with the inability of the client to take action, to gain control, or to gain the perception of control. When you have confirmed that the client is experiencing *Powerlessness,* the focus of care will be on relieving the client's powerlessness by selecting interventions that increase the client's feelings of increased control through strategies that empower the client to achieve a healthy level of functioning. The same interventions can be used to prevent *Powerlessness.* To differentiate *Powerlessness* from other closely related diagnoses, consider the focus of care, the client's perception of the problem, and the interventions related to *Powerlessness.*

Individuals who are members of vulnerable populations may have many nursing diagnoses. Assessment of social, psychological, and physical needs leads to focused assessment for a number of problems. Frequently diagnosed problems include the following:

- Chronic or situational low self-esteem
- Impaired parenting
- Social isolation
- Ineffective coping
- Imbalanced nutrition: less than body requirements
- Risk for injury

COMMUNITY

Formulating a diagnosis for a group or a community is somewhat different from formulating a diagnosis for an individual. However, any NANDA International (NANDA-I) nursing diagnosis can be applied to an individual, family, or community and across a spectrum of ages by using the classification system by NANDA-I (2005). The diagnosis can be an actual or a potential problem affecting the specified group or population, with specific etiology and effects.

In keeping with the focus of community health nursing to promote health, community health nurses also use *wellness diagnoses.* A wellness diagnosis describes positive healthful responses, listing related factors that sustain the healthful response. This type of diagnosis directs nurses toward actions that support the promotion and maintenance of health.

Therefore the components of a community nursing diagnosis include (1) the name of the community group and a statement of the problem (actual or potential) or the healthful response, (2) related factors identified for that problem or healthful response, and (3) signs and symptoms that characterize the problem or the positive, healthful actions for promoting or maintaining health.

The purpose of making a diagnosis is not only to identify the problem or healthful actions but also to give direction for planning intervention, encouraging positive actions, and evaluating outcomes.

PLANNING

INDIVIDUAL

The goal for the client with *Hopelessness* is to experience hope. Hope may emerge secondary to improvement in the related factor. *Powerlessness* is perhaps more directly treated. The goal for the client with *Powerlessness* may be that the client actually gains power or gains the perception of power. Because hope and power both have to do with the ability to achieve goals, it is especially important that planning to achieve hope or power be done *with* the client. Expected outcomes for the client with *Hopelessness* and *Powerlessness* are summarized in Box 43-4.

COMMUNITY GROUPS

To identify goals and plan interventions for groups, the community health nurse needs to have certain knowledge, skills, and attitudes. These include the following:

- Ability to identify existing community networks
- Knowledge of subcultures
- Comprehension that the goals, interests, and motivation of the community are the same as those of the health care providers
- Understanding of how to build community consensus and cohesiveness
- Recognition that external factors or determinants have an impact on a group's health
- Acknowledgement of planning and implementation

When working with groups, the nurse must recognize, value, and respect the group's capabilities, strengths, intelligence, uniqueness, and goals. Working successfully with community groups requires measures to ensure community participation. Through community participation come community development and community empowerment.

In community development, health care providers and community groups work together to define problems, identify resources, and use existing community leaders and organizations to carry out interventions toward health goals. Empowering a community assists the group in finding its own strength and taking charge of its destiny through teaching skills, information, and access to community resources. Empowerment provides tools and opportunities, and the group makes change through educated and informed decisions. An empowered community is able to improve the quality of life for its members. Box 43-5 gives an example of planning for a population.

INTERVENTION

Interventions are actions or activities implemented to reach goals or objectives or to solve a problem.

INTERVENTIONS TO RESTORE HOPE

Offering Presence. Because hope is an existential concept, instilling hope may be accomplished through the existential intervention of presence. A nurse cannot necessarily change the situation that has caused feelings of hopelessness. However, you can offer your presence to the client who experiences hopelessness. Through your presence, you can offer the client empathy or understanding of the feelings associated with being in a desolate situation. You can offer positive regard, and sometimes you can offer physical help.

Valuing Feelings. In the therapeutic nurse-client relationship, you can help clients value their own feelings and themselves. Because hopelessness is closely related to the ability to achieve goals and thus related to self-assessed ability, instilling hope can happen as a byproduct of helping a person experience the self as a valued, worthwhile person.

Setting Goals. Setting goals that are realistic, achievable, and based on a well-developed personal system of values can instill hope. Whether the person is dying from cancer or is a pregnant teenage girl, goals are a way

BOX 43-4 *Expected Outcomes for the Client With Hopelessness and Powerlessness*

HOPELESSNESS

- The client identifies choices available to mobilize energy on own behalf.
- The client has improved self-concept.
- The client takes initiative to accomplish achievable goals.
- The client participates in self-care within capabilities.
- The client uses problem-solving strategies to accomplish achievable goals.
- The client achieves a small goal for improved health status.
- The client recognizes personal power to affect outcomes.
- The client participates in spiritual renewal activities.
- The client achieves elements of neglected developmental tasks.

POWERLESSNESS

- The client expresses and demonstrates an increased sense of control over the life situation.
- The client verbalizes positive feelings about own abilities.
- The client engages in problem solving.
- The client demonstrates increased self-esteem.
- The client verbalizes the knowledge needed to accomplish goals.
- The client perceives support from the health care environment.
- The client displays that he or she has the chronic illness under control.
- The client demonstrates control over own health care regimen.

of looking to the future. For the dying person the future is limited, and for the pregnant teenager it is uncertain, but a plan that is achievable takes the client out of the moment to connect to the possibilities of the universe. Small accomplishments increase the belief that the present can be improved.

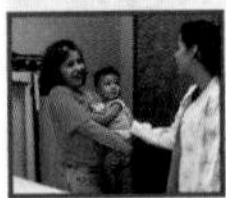

Recall the case of Brenda Carter. Identify three goals that the nurse might want to discuss with Brenda to reduce her sense of hopelessness and powerlessness and foster an improved relationship with her child.

Establishing Relatedness. Helping a person have a sense of relatedness to others, or helping the person in the manner of the relatedness, can instill hope. Through our relationships, we know ourselves to be valued human beings, valued because we are important to others and because we have something to contribute to others. Help the client reach out to others, and help others reach out to the client.

Preventing Self-Harm. When a client feels hopeless, there is a higher probability of self-destructive behavior. At the extreme end, the person may become suicidally depressed.

BOX 43-5

Nursing Care Plan

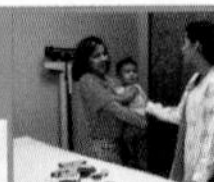

Planning Care for a Population With an Outbreak of Infectious Diarrhea

Notification of Outbreak

ABC Day School is a day care center for children ages 18 months through 11 years. It provides care from 7:00 AM to 6:00 PM Monday through Friday. During the past 2 weeks, many of the children and several of the staff have had diarrhea. A community health nurse from the county health department has been called to assess the situation, identify the cause or causes of the outbreak, and advise on methods of prevention.

Nursing Assessment of Population Group

The children are divided by ABC Day School into the following general age-groups:

18 months	20 children
2 years	21 children
3 years	21 children
3.5 years	23 children
4 years	24 children
5-11 years	34 children

Although the total number of children at this time is 143, not all children are necessarily at day care every day. Also, the children ages 5 to 11 are present only before and after their regular school hours: 7:00 to 8:30 AM and 3:00 to 6:00 PM. Generally, the children come from upper middle-class families. Most live with both parents, although a few are from single-parent homes. Most children are here for care while parents are working.

Each class has a certain amount of structured learning to it, depending on the age-group. Activities vary and may include playtime (indoors and outdoors), arts and crafts, naptime, and lunchtime. Each age-group has its own room (with bathroom included) and playground, where the majority of their time is spent. There is a common lunchroom. All rooms are carpeted except for the lunchroom and the room reserved for 18-month-old children. A total of 20 teachers and other personnel have contact with the children. A total of 20 children and 3 staff members had complaints of diarrhea. No particular age-group was affected more than another.

Identified Risk Factors

Related to the Children

- Forty-one children under 3 years old (the age-group at highest risk for infectious diarrhea)
- Lack of knowledge and practice of proper hygiene (not bowel trained)
- Immature and inexperienced immune system

Related to the Caregivers

- Inadequate training in personal and environmental hygiene
- Breaks in sanitary routines because of frequent, spontaneous, and urgent demands from children
- Cross-coverage of different child age-groups can facilitate transfer of organisms from one group to another.
- Inadequate screening for chronic infectious diseases

Related to the Environment and Economics

- Close physical interactions between children and between children and caregivers
- Less-than-optimal hygiene from use of bowel-training chairs that promote environmental contamination; poorly designed placement of sinks, diaper-changing area, and food handling areas; and common use of moist art supplies and communal water play
- Economic pressure to decrease staff/child ratio to limit the cost of child care
- Work pressures on parents to bring all children to day care facility

Resources and Constraints

Resources or Beneficial Aspects

- Management at the day care center is eager to make it a healthier, safer place for the children.
- Staff is willing to attend in-service programs to increase their knowledge of preventive measures against infectious diseases.
- Children are divided into groups by age and usually have the same two teachers (leaving them less open to cross-infections from other groups).

Constraints or Deterrents

- Enteric pathogens can be spread directly by person-to-person transmission or indirectly by the hands of staff, fomites, environmental contamination, or contaminated food.
- The criteria of an outbreak of diarrheal illness have not been established.
- Many parents send their children to day care not knowing that the diarrhea their child has is infectious.

NANDA-I Nursing Diagnoses

Deficient knowledge related to age of population as evidenced by lack of awareness and ability to practice proper hygiene

Deficient knowledge related to inadequate training in personal and environmental hygiene as evidenced by day care staff not performing hand hygiene after changing infants' diapers

Continued

BOX 43-5

Nursing Care Plan—cont'd

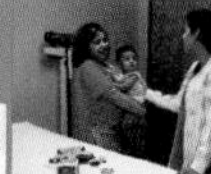

Planning Care for a Population With an Outbreak of Infectious Diarrhea

Omaha Nursing Diagnoses

Domain	Problem	Signs and Symptoms
Environmental	Sanitation: precautions against infection or disease	Personal hygiene: individual practice conducive to health and cleanliness Infectious agent
Psychosocial	Caretaking: providing care for dependent child	Difficulty providing preventive health care
Physiological	Bowel function: ability to evacuate waste	Abnormal frequency/consistency of stool (20 persons with diarrhea in 2 weeks)
Health-related behaviors		Inadequate hand hygiene by children and day care personnel

Interventions

- Conduct weekly in-service program for 4 weeks to educate day care personnel in the principles of general hygiene to reduce the development and spread of infection. In-service will include information on the mode of transmission of infectious agents, the importance and techniques of proper hand hygiene (a videotape is available for viewing), disposal or cleaning of materials and surfaces contaminated with body secretions, food handling and meal service, and diaper changing and toileting.
- Wash, on a regular basis, toys and other objects that children handle or put in their mouths.
- Assign same cots and linens to same children during naptime. These also should be washed on a regular basis.
- Separate any child who becomes ill from the other children until the ill child can be sent home.
- Develop an information letter for parents regarding infectious diarrhea and how to prevent it from spreading.
- Establish criteria for exclusion of ill children by defining what constitutes diarrhea.
- Establish policies for readmission of previously ill children.
- Establish policies for administration of medication to children who have been diagnosed.
- Monitor compliance of preventive hygiene practices taught.
- Monitor outbreaks of infectious diarrhea and other infectious diseases.
- These plans will be put into action over a period of 4 weeks. The daily interventions will continue for the next 3 months with a monthly monitoring.

Evaluation

Four months after inception of the program (1 month to establish interventions and 3 months to use interventions), an outcomes evaluation was completed. The goal of fewer than 3.85 episodes per month of infectious diarrhea was met, with only 2 episodes in the first month, 2 episodes in the second month, and 3 episodes in the third month. The outcomes of knowledge, behavior, and health status all improved.

	Before Interventions	After Interventions
Knowledge	2—Minimal	4—Adequate
Behavior	3—Inconsistently appropriate	5—Consistently appropriate
Health status	2—Severe signs and symptoms	4—Minimal signs and symptoms

Numerical scores range from 1 to 5 in each category.

The ABC Day School will continue with the interventions suggested and offer an annual review of this prevention program for its staff.

Critical Thinking Question

What would you do if the episodes of infectious diarrhea exceeded 3.85 per month?

Action Alert! Pay attention to hints of suicide. Ask, "Have you ever considered harming yourself?" Take all suicide threats seriously. Do not leave the person alone. Remove anything from a hospital room that could be used to inflict self-harm. Refer the client to an appropriate therapist or psychiatrist who can help such clients to manage their feelings.

However, suicide is not the only avenue of self-harm. The person who feels hopeless may engage in harmful behaviors, including alcohol and other drug abuse, or fail to take action to maintain health and safety. Safety may be a concern just because the person is not paying attention to the environment.

Developing Coping Mechanisms. Assess the client's methods of coping with the circumstances surrounding hopelessness. Help the person recall coping methods that have worked in the past. Some helpful coping mechanisms include the following:

- Focus on a small achievable task, away from the seemingly insurmountable problem.
- Prioritize. Accomplish essential activities. Make a list of nice-to-do activities, and do one each day.

- Do something for someone else each day.
- Do something for yourself each day.

Maintaining Energy. Overwhelming fatigue often accompanies hopelessness. The very activities that might relieve the feelings of hopelessness require more energy than the client has. A state of inertia sets in that is hard to overcome. Recognizing that activity is needed to overcome the inertia, you will feel tempted to recommend physical activities. However, the activities must be chosen carefully, and the energy requirements must be within the limits available to the client.

Help the client maintain optimal physical health. Rest, nutrition, exercise, and vitamin supplements may be helpful. Be aware that the client, as a member of a vulnerable population, has limited resources. Help the client include a mentally healthy activity in each day.

INTERVENTIONS TO EMPOWER CLIENTS

To empower another individual you need to respect the individual's capacity for self-determination. Make the assumption that clients have the ability to make decisions and take action on their own behalf. Nurses cannot empower clients; only clients can empower themselves.

The client needs to be actively involved in defining both the problem and the solutions. When the nurse is the major decision maker, dependency is the result. However, clients may make decisions that are different from the decision the nurse might make, or they may reject help altogether. These decisions must be accepted.

Loss of power is often associated with a sense of distrust, a feeling of alienation, and an attitude of self-blame. For the empowerment process to be effective, there needs to be mutual respect, a sharing of power, and trust between the client and the nurse.

Empowerment focuses on promoting and enhancing clients' abilities to meet their own needs, make their own decisions, and mobilize the necessary resources to feel that they are in control of their own lives. However, you can provide information and assistance in engaging in empowering behaviors. Nurses can help the client to develop, obtain, and use resources that will encourage a sense of control and self-efficacy through which individuals can empower themselves.

The personal significance of empowerment varies with the individual and the level of empowerment at which the individual is currently functioning. From the client's perspective, empowerment can mean the following:

- Identifying feelings associated with power and control
- Having knowledge
- Strengthening self-expression of preferences, needs, values, and attitudes
- Participating in family, group, or social life or in decision making
- Choosing among actions, friends, health care alternatives, or activities and taking responsibility for the consequences of choice
- Developing coping skills or methods of managing a problem
- Being of help to others
- Bargaining for what you want
- Expanding the spiritual self

INTERVENTIONS FOR THE INDIVIDUAL AS CLIENT

As described previously, applying the community approach to health risk reduction in individuals who are members of a vulnerable social group is critical. This includes appropriate referrals for needed community resources and services.

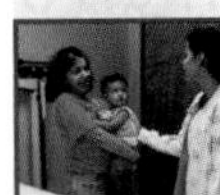

For Brenda, community referrals might include educational and vocational programs, parenting and preschool programs, adolescent mother support groups, and mental health counseling for depression and history of abuse (group and individual). In addition, if Brenda is not already receiving these services, referrals should be made to WIC, Medicaid, and other financial assistance programs that would be appropriate. Individualized care on which the nurse could focus would require that Brenda return to the clinic regularly (at least until she is well connected with these other services) for longer-term intervention.

Arranging for transportation, child care, and home-based interventions may be necessary to ensure that vulnerable populations are provided with necessary services. In addition, interventions must be scheduled so as not to conflict with the person's crucial daily responsibilities such as school, work, and child care.

INTERVENTIONS FOR COMMUNITY GROUPS

Interventions used to promote, improve, or maintain health for communities include community participation, development, and empowerment; community outreach programs; health promotion and education activities; and activities that promote social change.

Community Activation. Community activation emphasizes the involvement and coordination of major community institutions (such as schools, universities, and local health departments) to mobilize community leadership and resources for health promotion and to improve public awareness of health issues. It includes organized efforts to increase community awareness and agreement about health problems, to increase coordinated planning of prevention and environmental change programs, to increase allocation of resources between organizations, and to increase citizen involvement in these processes.

Participatory Action Research. Participatory action research is a research model that relies on local community knowledge and empowers group members to develop their leadership potential. It is a combination of community involvement, research, and action that supports local ability and judgment in solving community problems. It is a flexible and collaborative effort between the researcher and the community.

Community Partnership Primary Care. The community partnership primary care model emphasizes community development and community empowerment as an avenue to improved community health. Health professionals can empower communities to take action on their own behalf by working with the community to identify strengths, problems, and needs in the community and then develop strategies to improve the health of the community.

Parish and Neighborhood Nursing. Parish nursing and neighborhood nursing are forms of community outreach. This type of care is useful in primary prevention and health promotion.

Action Alert! Parish and neighborhood nurses are in key positions in the community to improve accessibility to care.

A **parish nurse** is a registered nurse who is employed by (or volunteers for) a religious or health care organization for the purpose of providing nursing care to members of faith communities. The nurse operates through churches to promote wellness, using a holistic approach. This revival of church-based health care occurred in 1983 with the development of parish nursing by Lutheran chaplain Granger Westberg (Pravecek, 2005).

Parish nurses address not only the physical but also the emotional and spiritual needs of congregational community members. Parish nurses do not provide home health care services or perform invasive nursing procedures. They do provide education, advocacy, counseling, and screening. They also train and coordinate volunteers, make referrals to community resources, and develop and facilitate support groups.

Neighborhood nursing (also referred to as block nursing) is an outgrowth of the idea of district nursing that seeks to promote healthy communities by collaborating with people where they live, work, and go to school. Neighborhood-oriented nursing can provide broad-based case management and care coordination. Neighborhood nurses can detect problems early, before they become crises.

The biggest single factor limiting the growth and success of these innovative approaches to meeting the health needs of community groups is funding procurement. Although many community-based health care projects have received funding through grants and donations (DoBias, 2006), many other worthwhile projects continue to face financial challenges.

CHALLENGES OF COMMUNITY HEALTH NURSING

Health promotion interventions are used to increase the health and well-being of individuals, families, and communities. Health promotion activities include using health appraisals, encouraging healthy lifestyle behaviors, providing healthy environments, developing effective coping skills, and educating to promote healthful decision making. On a broader scale, health promotion activities often require changes involving health policy, economic conditions, legislation, or funding. The goals for these changes may take longer to be accomplished.

Influencing Public Policy. Political influences affect the areas in which federal, state, and local governments carry out health care functions: providing direct health care services, financing health care, collecting and disseminating health care information, and setting health care policy. Providing direct care includes programs for immunization; providing health care to Native Americans, veterans, and members of the military; and running specialized clinics (e.g., for tuberculosis).

The government finances research; direct care through Medicare, Medicaid, and Social Security programs; and special programs, such as the supplementary food programs for WIC. Collection and dissemination of health information by the government includes gathering vital statistics, compiling morbidity and mortality data, taking census reports, and undertaking numerous other topics of surveillance and reporting. The purpose of government policy setting is to prevent problems, solve problems, or both, depending on the policy. An example of policy setting was the passage of amendments to the Social Security Act in 1965 that established Medicare and Medicaid (public health care insurance programs for older adults, the poor, and the disabled). In the ongoing process to decrease the federal government's budget deficit, governmental programs—including those affecting health care—are under scrutiny for elimination or redesign.

Nurses who work with communities and population groups will identify the need for change in social, political, economic, or health care systems. Public policy is one way to make changes to promote health. Public policy is a planned course of action taken to address selected issues or problems through allocation and distribution of resources to meet the health needs of a population. The policy-making process assesses the problem, then plans, finds resources, implements, and evaluates programs.

Interventions to change social, political, economic, or health care systems, as well as the physical environment, often require policy change. These policy changes take time, personnel, energy, and finances. You must carefully assess the situation, work effectively with the community system, and recognize the many variables (such as resistant community officials or scarce funds) that could affect the change process and outcomes. Change is more readily accepted when information is disseminated in ways compatible with the community's norms, values, and customs. Finally, once again, by developing and strengthening community participation and action, health care providers will promote a community's ability and opportunity to take appropriate action to protect and improve the health of its members.

Promoting a Supportive Environment. A supportive environment is essential to changing health care. Steps to build the supportive environment include distributing information to inform as well as to recruit. Nurses can help establish a supportive environment by contacting key persons in the community, especially those persons who have relationships with the targeted groups. Having rapport with these persons helps build a base of support. Most important, maintaining open communication and supplying current and accurate information regarding developments are essential to successful change.

Encouraging Community Participation and Action. Community action is an integral component of making changes to promote health. The community must acknowledge the changes to be made and must then become a part of those changes. These programs are successful when people who are living in the community participate. Community members who are knowledgeable and motivated take part in assessing, planning, implementing, and evaluating health programs.

> ***Action Alert!*** If community members fail to see value or worth in a change, the community will not work as effectively toward the goals.

Collaborating With Other Disciplines. In community health, the focus cannot be limited to physical health. Other aspects of life and lifestyle affecting health must be considered. Interdisciplinary collaboration is needed among health care providers, social services, environmental specialists, and city planners to meet the health needs of a community. People who are influential in areas affecting the environment, industry, housing, sanitation, politics, education, and social services of the community must work together to create change in the total community.

Using Technology Appropriately. The Internet and ever-improving computer technology connect community health nurses and clients to each other and to information resources. The computer is used to support the education of community members and health professionals as well as offering clinical application.

Telehealth is the use of technology to connect the client to a health professional who provides clinical care (Figure 43-8). Telehealth is a mechanism used to reach groups or populations who do not have access to health services in their immediate geographical area. Laboratory work, electrocardiograms, and radiography can be performed at a local site and transmitted to another site where a physician can interpret the information. Privacy and ethical issues concerning high-quality and safe care will need to be addressed as this type of practice develops. Nurses are expected to be highly involved with this type of medical practice, even practicing across state lines.

Environmental Issues. The physical environment of a community influences health. Clean, well-built housing, adequate energy and water supplies, and sanitation services are important to health. Safety services (fire, police, and emergency medical) are essential. Well-maintained roads and transportation services, adequate avenues of communication (radio, television, newspapers, postal service), and accessible educational, religious, and recreational facilities all affect a community's health.

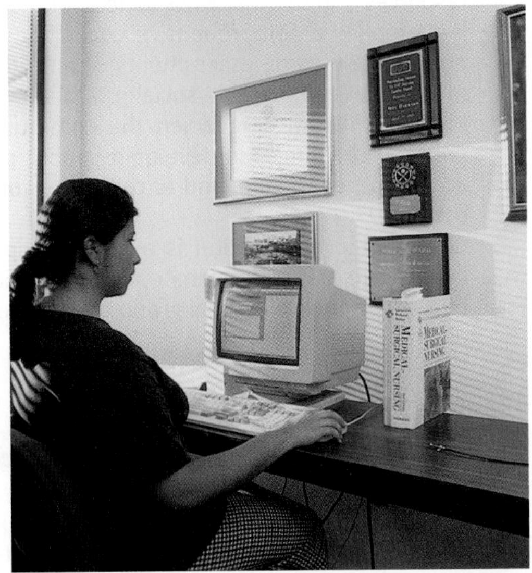

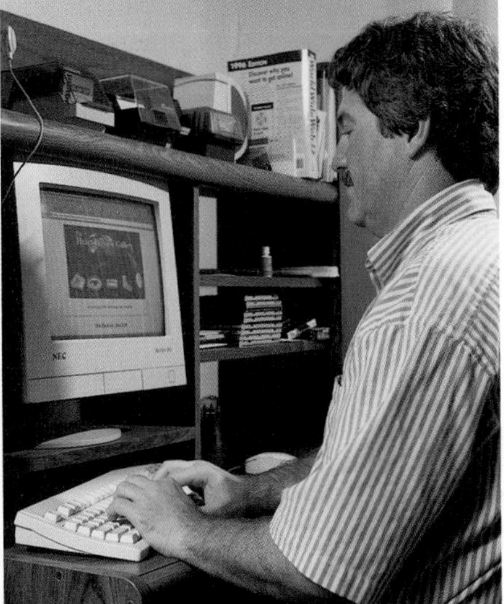

FIGURE 43-8 Through online computer links, clients can connect with community health practitioners in physicians' offices and home health care agencies.

Additional services, such as Meals on Wheels, school nutrition programs, Big Brother/Big Sister programs, crisis intervention programs, and day care programs, add to the improved health and well-being of a community. Lacking essential services can put a community at risk for poor health outcomes.

EVALUATION

Evaluation is the process of determining whether the goals or objectives of a program have been met. To evaluate the outcomes of health interventions, goals or objectives must first be identified. Whether identifying goals for an individual, an aggregate, or a community, the nurse assesses the individual or group and identifies diagnoses and related factors. Evaluations of interventions or programs can be accomplished while in progress. This is called a *formative* or *process evaluation*. Evaluations completed at the end of interventions or programs are called *summative* or *outcomes evaluations*.

A documentation note for Brenda Carter's son might appear as shown below.

SAMPLE DOCUMENTATION NOTE FOR BRENDA CARTER'S SON

Referred to social services for follow-up of self-report of difficulty in disciplining her child and possible abuse and need of mother for support services. Child currently has no signs of physical abuse, but risk is present. Written report sent to social services.

EVALUATING INTERVENTIONS FOR INDIVIDUALS

Evaluation of the interventions for *Hopelessness* and *Powerlessness* requires examination of psychological, social, and physical data. Assess for a change in the way the person thinks about the self in relation to others and the environment. Listen again for the themes in the client's conversation, and compare the frequency of negative statements with what you heard before. Observe the client's interactions with others. Does the client wait for someone else to make decisions or take control? Does the client more frequently initiate a relationship? Assess progress in physical health and the ability to manage health problems. Is the client displaying positive coping skills?

Client satisfaction is a significant element in evaluation of these diagnoses. Does the client feel that progress is being made, feel that life is better, or feel an increased self-control? The evaluation of *Hopelessness* may show that the client has achieved acceptance of a situation that cannot be changed.

EVALUATING INTERVENTIONS FOR COMMUNITIES

Several methods are useful in evaluating community health interventions. A *case study* evaluates a program through observation of program activity, review of reports prepared during the program, and conversations with program personnel. Data collected can be both objective and subjective.

Observational methods are another means to evaluate programs. In *participatory observation*, the observer actually takes part in the program. In *nonparticipatory observation*, the observer remains outside the program, observing only at specified times. *Surveys* are an evaluation tool that can be used to describe and analyze the results of a program. These can be completed through questionnaires or by personal interviews. *Pretest-intervention-posttest* is an evaluation method used to identify whether changes in knowledge, behavior, or attitudes have taken place after an intervention has been applied or a program is completed. A *cost/benefit analysis* and a *cost-effectiveness analysis* are two formal analytic methods used to evaluate the economic costs and benefits of a program. It is important to know and understand how each of these methods can help you evaluate a community health intervention program while planning the program, before it begins.

▼ KEY PRINCIPLES

- Preventive health care must address the factors that make vulnerable populations vulnerable.
- The framework for understanding vulnerable populations recognizes the relationships among the limited resource availability, the health-related risk factors, and the health status of vulnerable populations.
- Poverty, social inequality, and poor educational and vocational resources are among the socioeconomic constraints common in vulnerable populations.
- Community health nursing is a combination of nursing and public health science designed to promote health and prevent illness in vulnerable population groups.
- The complex nature of the relationship between lack of resources and the many risk factors for health-related problems makes a comprehensive evaluation necessary when nurses are making assessments of an individual who is a member of a vulnerable social group.
- Providing health care when the community is the client presents challenges in developing public policy, promoting access to health care, and encouraging community participation.
- Community participation is a key concept of community health care and is concerned with the various ways members of a vulnerable social group are involved in health care planning.

■ REVIEW QUESTIONS

1. A population is:

1. A group of people who share common characteristics
2. A group of people with dissimilar characteristics
3. A random statistical cluster
4. A group of people with physical ailments

2. Vulnerable population groups are those who have:
1. Ample resources
2. A broad assortment of social support networks
3. Limited resources and social support
4. Low risk for myriad health-related problems

3. The age group most at risk for suicide is:
1. Troubled adolescents
2. Nontroubled adolescents
3. Older adults
4. Older adults living in nursing homes

4. Factors such as race, age, number of persons living in specific locations, population growth, and family statistics are an example of:
1. Socioeconomic data
2. Environmental data
3. Cultural data
4. Demographic data

5. Client empowerment is achieved through:
1. Distrust
2. Communication
3. Unequal distribution of power
4. Self-determination

Bibliography

American Academy of Child and Adolescent Psychiatry. (2006). Adolescent psychopathology: IV. Specificity of psychosocial risk factors for depression and substance abuse in older adolescents. Retrieved June 14, 2006, from www.jaacap.com/pt/re/jaacap/abstract.00004583-199509000-00021.htm.

American Psychological Association. (2006). Triggers and signs. *Changing your mind about mental health.* Retrieved January 20, 2006, from www.apahelpcenter.org/featuredtopics/feature.php?id=37+ch=5.

Carter, C. S. (2002). Perinatal care for women who are addicted: Implications for empowerment. *Health and Social Work, 27*(3), 166-174.

Clemen-Stone, S., McGuire, S. L., & Eigsti, D. G. (2002). *Comprehensive community health nursing: Family, aggregate, & community practice* (6th ed.). St. Louis, MO: Mosby.

Cohen, H. L. (2002). Developing media literacy skills to challenge television's portrayal of older women. *Educational Gerontology, 29*(7), 599-620.

Conwell, Y., Duberstein, P. R., & Caine, E. D. (2002). Risk factors for suicide in later life. *Biological Psychiatry, 52*(3), 193-204.

Coughlin, L. (2005). AAP report on pregnancy in adolescents. *American Family Physician, 72*(7), 1398-1400.

DoBias, M. (2006). Mixed blessing: Centers welcome attention, but want more funding. *Modern Healthcare, 36*(13), 12.

Fiscella, K., & Shin, P. (2005). The inverse care law. *Journal of Ambulatory Care Management,* 28(4), 304-312.

*Flaskerud, J. H., & Winslow, B. J. (1998). Conceptualizing vulnerable populations: Health-related research. *Nursing Research, 47*(2), 69-78.

Geriatric Mental Health Foundation. (2005). *Late life depression: A fact sheet.* Retrieved June 19, 2006, from www.gmhfonline.or/gmhf/consumer/factsheets/depression_factsheet.html.

Gilbert, W. M., Jandial, D., Field, N. T., Bigelow, P., Danielson, B. (2004). Birth outcomes in teenage pregnancies. *Journal of Maternal-Fetal & Neonatal Medicine, 16*(5), 265-270.

*Gordon, C. (1996). Adolescent decision-making: A broadly based theory and its application to the prevention of early pregnancy. *Adolescence, 31,* 561-584.

Hall, B., & Brown, J. L. (2005). Food security among older adults in the United States. *Topics in Clinical Nutrition, 20*(4), 329-338.

*Hawks, J. H. (1991). Power: A concept analysis. *Journal of Advanced Nursing, 16*(6), 754-762.

Hunt, R. (2004). *Introduction to community-based nursing* (3rd ed.). Philadelphia: Lippincott Williams & Wilkins.

Inglehart, R. (2002). Gender, aging, and subjective well-being. *International Journal of Comparative Sociology, 43*(3-5), 391-409.

Lesser, J., Oakes, R., & Koniak-Griffin, D. (2003). Vulnerable adolescent mothers' perception of maternal role and HIV risk. *Health Care for Women International, 24*(6), 513-528.

Murphy, K. (2005). What can you do to prevent teen suicide? *Nursing, 35*(12), 43-45.

NANDA International. (2005). *Nursing diagnoses: Definitions and classification, 2005-2006* (6th ed.). Philadelphia: Author.

National Association of Social Workers. (2003). HIV/AIDS and homelessness. *Poverty and Social Justice Practice Update, 1*(1), 1. Retrieved January 9, 2006, from www.naswdc.org/practice/peace/psj0703.pdf.

National Coalition for the Homeless. (2005). *NCH fact sheet #6: Addiction disorders and homelessness.* Retrieved December 30, 2005, from www.nationalhomeless.org/publications/facts/addiction.pdf.

National Youth Violence Prevention Resource Center. (2003). *Youth suicide risk factors.* Retrieved June 14, 2006, from www.safeyouth.org/scripts/faq/suiciderisks.asp.

Olden, P. C., & Szydlowski, S. I. (2004). Health promotion and disease prevention by small rural hospitals: Reasons, obstacles, and enablers. *Journal of Healthcare Management, 49*(2), 89-101.

Pender, N. J., Murdaugh, C. L., & Parsons, M. A. (2002). *Health promotion in nursing practice* (4th ed.). Upper Saddle River, NJ: Prentice Hall.

Pravecek, E. J. (2005). The parish nurse ministry. *Plastic Surgical Nursing, 25*(3), 124-128.

Roche, B. (2004). Multiple health needs and homeless people. *Primary Health Care, 14*(7), 20-22.

Seccombe, K. (2002). 'Beating the odds' versus 'changing the odds': Poverty, resilience, and family policy. *Journal of Marriage and Family, 64*(2), 384-394.

Singh, S., Darroch, J. E., & Frost, J. J. (2001). Socioeconomic disadvantage and adolescent women's sexual and reproductive behavior: The case of five developed countries. *Family Planning Perspectives, 33*(6), 251-258, 289.

Stanhope, M., & Lancaster, J. (2004). *Community & public health nursing* (6th ed.). St. Louis, MO: Mosby.

U.S. Department of Health and Human Services, National Institute of Drug Abuse. (2005). Depression elevates suicide risk in substance-abusing adolescents. *NIDA Notes, 19*(6), n.p. Retrieved June 14, 2006, from http://www.nida.nih.gov/DirReports/DirRep205/DirectorReport20.html.

Wysong, P. (2005). Dark moods. *Current Health 2, 32*(4), 14-17.

*Asterisk indicates a classic or definitive work on this subject.

Chapter 44

Managing Functional Limitations

Media Resources

- evolve Evolve Website http://evolve.elsevier.com/Harkreader/
- 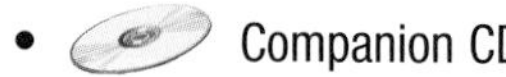 Companion CD

Learning Objectives

After studying this chapter, you should be able to do the following:

- Discuss the concepts of functional limitation and rehabilitation
- Describe factors affecting ability and disability, including the client's developmental stage and physiological, cultural, lifestyle, psychosocial, and environmental factors
- Identify assessment tools used for a person with a functional limitation
- List three major nursing diagnoses for a person with a spinal cord injury
- Implement nursing interventions to provide quality care for people with functional limitations
- State several ways to evaluate whether or not rehabilitation outcomes have been met

Key Terms

activities of daily living (ADLs)
chronic illness
chronicity
community reintegration
functional limitations
instrumental activities of daily living (IADLs)
interdisciplinary team
psychosocial adaptation
rehabilitation
rehabilitation nursing

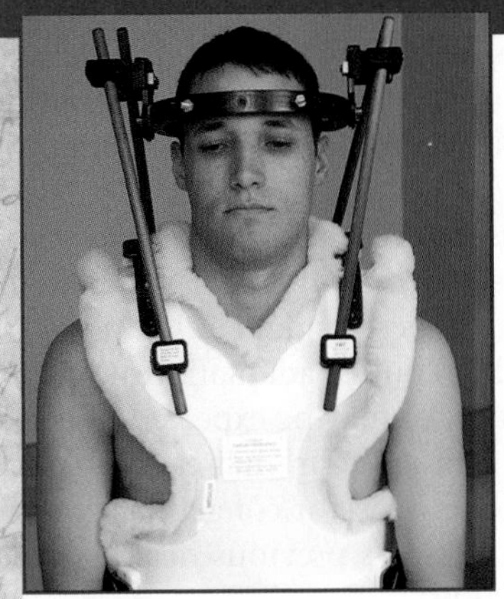

Robert Baldwin, 18 years old, sustained a complete C5-C6 spinal cord injury (SCI) from diving into a shallow swimming pool. After stabilization in an acute care hospital, Robert spent 2 months in a rehabilitation unit, learning to make the adjustments to living required by changes in his functional abilities resulting from tetraplegia. Once an active high school student, Robert now uses an electric wheelchair. He has fair-to-good shoulder movement and biceps activity, along with minimal wrist extension, but otherwise no active movement below his shoulders. He requires 6 to 8 hours of daily attendant care for activities of daily living.

Robert also struggles with feelings of powerlessness related to his inability to control many aspects of his life. He said to one of his friends, "I don't feel like I have control over anything in my life anymore." Robert has experienced a number of losses and is working through the grieving process.

Reintegration into the school environment was challenging. The public school assigned a caregiver to help him during the school day. Air-conditioning was also installed in parts of the building where Robert spends much of his day to accommodate his heat intolerance (common in SCI) during the warmer months. An automatic door opener was installed for Robert to enter the building. These adaptations assisted him with adjusting positively when he returned to school.

The social support from family, friends, teachers, and the community played a significant role in his ability to adapt to his limitations. In addition to *Self-care deficit* and *Impaired physical mobility,* Robert needs assistance with adaptation in the area of *Ineffective role performance* as he finishes high school and plans his adult life with permanent physical limitations.

CONCEPTS OF FUNCTIONAL LIMITATION

The percentage of working-age individuals reporting a disability was 12.1% in 2004 in the United States. Although disabilities are present in about 19% of Americans overall, there is an increased incidence in adults over age 65, of whom approximately 50% have some type of disability (U.S. Census Bureau, 2002). Disabilities include sensory impairments (particularly hearing and vision), physical mobility impairments (from injury, chronic illness, congenital defect, or psychiatric conditions), and emotional/cognitive impairments. Physical conditions that can disable people include a spinal cord injury, cerebrovascular event, amputation of a limb, a severe injury, cancer, cardiorespiratory disease, or a chronic progressive disorder. About 250,000 people in the United States are disabled by a spinal cord injury such as Robert's (Spinal Cord Injury Information Network, 2005). Adaptation to long-term health alterations is influenced by socioeconomic status, psychosocial status, environment, culture, educational level, lifestyle, and resource availability.

KEY NURSING DIAGNOSIS FOR ROLE PERFORMANCE

Ineffective role performance: Patterns of behavior and self-expression that do not match the environmental context, norms, and expectations

Persons with physical or mental limitations do not necessarily like to describe themselves as *disabled or handicapped.* Disability suggests that a person is not able, although many people with physical and mental problems are able to work, take care of themselves, raise children, and enjoy life. The term *handicap* suggests a difficult interaction between the client with a disability and the environment. A handicap is a disadvantage experienced by a person as a result of an impairment that limits the person's "normal" function and environmental impediments. Referring to persons as *disabled* or *handicapped* is a judgment that society places on people when they view them as disadvantaged citizens.

Although people with physical challenges may have difficulty performing some tasks, they are still able to do many other tasks or use adaptive equipment to complete tasks. Thus *limitation* suggests that it is not that the person is disabled but that a limitation in function exists (Figure 44-1). *Impairment* is the physical or physiological cause of the limitation, whether related to disease, trauma, or birth defect that may or may not be associated with limitations. For example, a person with a visual impairment may have the limitation of needing to wear glasses.

Functional limitations refer to difficulties people may experience in performing activities of daily living (ADLs) or instrumental activities of daily living (IADLs). **Activities of daily living** are the basic activities usually performed in the course of a normal day in a person's life, such as eating, toileting, dressing, bathing, or brushing the teeth. **Instrumental activities of daily living** are food preparation, housekeeping, laundry, transportation, using the telephone, shopping, and handling finances.

Rehabilitation is "the process of adaptation, or recovery, through which an individual suffering from a

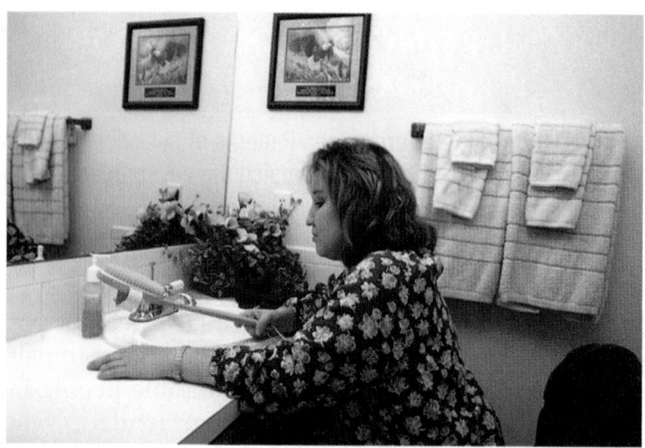

FIGURE 44-1 Although people with physical challenges may have difficulty performing some tasks, they are still able to do many others, sometimes with the use of adaptive equipment. Like this woman in a wheelchair, persons are not "unable" or "disabled"; they have a physical or functional limitation.

disabling condition, whether temporary or irreversible, regains, or attempt to regain, maximum function, independence, and restoration" (Easton, 1999). Adaptation can mean changing the physical environment, changing the methods of managing activities, or psychosocial adaptation to living with a limitation. Rehabilitation is a concept, not a place, and should begin the first day a person is diagnosed with a disorder that can result or has resulted in functional limitation.

Action alert! Begin rehabilitation the day the client is admitted to a hospital, and implement rehabilitation activities from admission to discharge.

Psychosocial adaptation is the process by which a person adjusts, copes, or responds to the functional, psychological, and social changes that occur with the onset and experience of living with a physical/mental limitation or chronic illness. Persons with long-term limitations may require time and assistance to adapt to their situation. Often, life-changing events that result from catastrophic injury or illness will lead to a person feeling that he or she is unable to cope with this new situation and limitations. Rehabilitation assists persons and their families with the psychosocial adaptation process to foster the experience of a satisfactory quality of life and to maximize their ability to be independent.

ETIOLOGICAL CONDITIONS

Disabilities or functional limitations are common in musculoskeletal impairments, neurological impairments, sensory/perceptual deficits, cognitive disorders, mental disorders, and chronic illnesses. Both reversible and irreversible conditions may benefit from rehabilitation.

Musculoskeletal and neurological impairments occur across the life span. Childhood musculoskeletal impairments, such as cerebral palsy, are often congenitally acquired. In the adolescent and young adult, spinal cord or brain injuries may be the cause. In the older adult, the impairment often results from arthritis or a hip fracture. Cerebrovascular events, Parkinson's disease, and multiple sclerosis are additional examples of common neurological impairments.

Functional limitations can result from stable or progressive chronic illnesses. **Chronic illness** is an impairment that is permanent, leaves residual limitations of function, is nonreversible, requires adaptation training, requires changes in lifestyle, or may be expected to last a long time. **Chronicity** is a broad term that encompasses chronic illnesses as well as disease or congenital defects that permanently alter a person's previous health status (Easton, 1999; Lubkin, 2006).

INTERDISCIPLINARY TEAM

An **interdisciplinary team** is a group of people working together with the client to achieve mutually established rehabilitation goals for recovery or adaptation. An array of doctors, nurses, physical and occupational therapists, social workers, psychologists, and nutritionists make up the team. Also, auxiliary personnel contribute to the client's recovery, including pastoral care personnel, recreational therapist, vocational counselor, audiologist, prosthetist, orthotist, and other specialists.

Rehabilitation nursing is a specialty in which nurses with expert knowledge in the care of clients and families affected by chronic illness or disability assist them with goal attainment, prevention of complications, promotion of self-care, and reintegration into the community. "Rehabilitation nursing is a dynamic, creative specialty which promotes the positive adaptation of individuals with disabilities, through a holistic, nurturing environment, by combining your clinical skills, advanced knowledge, and resourcefulness with the perseverance, motivation, and strengths of the client to achieve maximal independence and an acceptable quality of life" (Easton, 1999).

Rehabilitation nurses use specialized knowledge based on scientific restorative principles and the philosophy of rehabilitation to assist clients and their families with mutual goal setting and goal attainment. Rehabilitation nurses also encourage self-care, prevent complications related to persons' disabilities and chronic health problems, help them with reintegration into the community, and strengthen coping strategies to maximize adaptation (Association of Rehabilitation Nurses, 2005).

Nurses who care for those with functional limitations become experts in several areas of assessment and care. These include physical and psychosocial assessment, bowel and bladder management, skin care, nutrition, behavior, teaching, and family participation. Education of clients and families is a key nursing skill when preparing people to reenter the community after experiencing a long-term health alteration. Creating an environment that is conducive to a person's rehabilitation is another special function of the nurse (Pryor, 2000).

Rehabilitation nurses function in the roles of teacher, caregiver, advocate, counselor, consultant, and researcher. Depending on the nurse's education and experience, these roles take on different degrees of emphasis. For example, an advanced practice nurse (APN) in rehabilitation may engage much more in the roles of teacher and consultant than that of direct caregiver, whereas a nurse with a doctorate may focus more on research.

The Association of Rehabilitation Nurses (ARN) is the specialty organization in this field of interest. The ARN was founded in 1974, recognizing rehabilitation nursing as a specialty. Certification in rehabilitation is attained by successfully passing an examination that tests knowledge in the area of rehabilitation. Registered nurses with 2 years of current experience in rehabilitation and who meet other stated requirements may take the examination. The credential CRRN indicates a certified rehabilitation registered nurse.

Physiatrists are physicians specializing in physical medicine and rehabilitation. They help evaluate overall functional progress, prescribe medications and treatments, and give medical direction and guidance to the team.

The *physical therapist* (PT) is a licensed rehabilitative professional who uses specially designed exercises and physical treatment modalities to help clients regain or improve their physical abilities to address problems in range of motion (ROM), mobility, strength, balance, and gait, as well as working with the person on ambulation activities. With expertise in muscle and joints they manage movement disorders, fit clients for adaptive devices, supervise whirlpool treatment for pressure ulcers or wounds, and perform dressing changes after whirlpool treatment. Physical therapists manage pain through the use of hot or cold packs, transcutaneous electrical nerve stimulation (TENS) units, and other modalities.

The *occupational therapist* (OT) is a licensed health care professional who is concerned with restoring useful physical functionality following disabling accidents and sickness. The therapy teaches independent living strategies and develops skills in activities of daily living and instrumental activities of daily living, vocational skills, and home management skills (such as cooking, doing laundry, shopping).

The *speech therapist*, or speech-language pathologist, assesses swallowing, respiration, and phonation and language ability. Speech therapists help clients improve communication using a variety of treatment modalities, including auditory, verbal, visual, and motor processing (Figure 44-2). The speech-language pathologist works with those having difficulty with verbal expression or cognitive problems. Common treatments include exercises of muscles used in speech and swallowing, thermal stimulation, and memory cues. Stroke clients with dysphagia or aphasia often require the services of a speech therapist to help them regain the use of oral-facial muscles needed for speaking and swallowing.

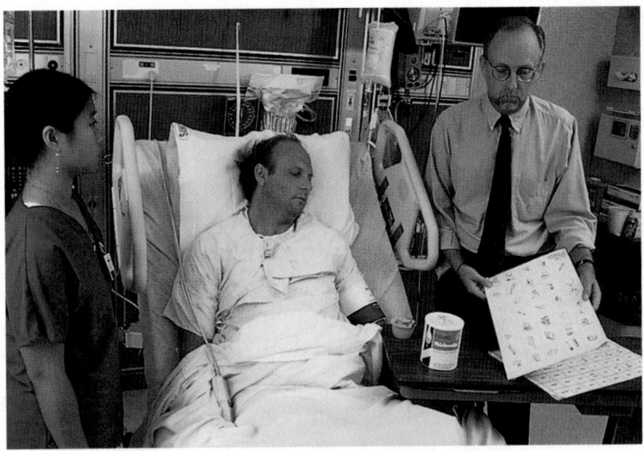

FIGURE 44-2 Speech therapists assist clients in improving communication using a variety of treatment modalities such as auditory, verbal, visual, and motor processing; communication charts or boards may be helpful for the person with difficulty speaking.

The *nutritionist* or dietitian plays an important role on the team for clients who may be receiving tube feedings or those with nutritional deficits. Causes of *Nutrition: less than body requirements* include dysphagia, aspiration, and anorexia. Nutritionists can provide information on the contents of various nutritional supplements. They also educate about dietary modifications or restrictions, whether in a group setting or on a one-to-one basis.

Social workers provide support for the client and family, coordinate discharge planning, and assist with financial problems and family conflicts. The social workers can arrange for adaptive equipment and home modifications, arrange placement to another facility, provide a link to community services, and coordinate insurance benefits. Social workers engage in client and family counseling to develop appropriate coping mechanisms, manage grief, and modify family dynamics. In addition, they assist the team with issues of insurance coverage, including reimbursement protocol and documentation. This *case management role* is sometimes performed by nurses.

Psychologists provide client and family counseling. The focus of the psychologist is on behavior modification and family adaptation. Treatment is supportive and evaluative, helping the client and family utilize appropriate coping mechanisms during crisis situations. Psychologists may also assist the team itself directly by providing insight into group dynamics and the processes through which the team is working.

The *recreational therapist* plans a variety of activities to incorporate therapeutic use of leisure time. Activities such as painting, making party decorations, horticulture, pet therapy, or music therapy are common. Entertainment and socialization are also key elements of a comprehensive recreational therapy program. Recreational therapists may help plan and implement community reentry trips or outings. They arrange for special activities such as birthday parties, holidays, or group events such as the Wheelchair Olympics. Although not all facilities are able to afford the services of a qualified recreational therapist, the notion of this type of therapy should be included in every rehabilitation program and long-term care facility.

The client's *spiritual leader* may be a priest, rabbi, minister, deacon, or layperson. Many facilities have chaplains or other spiritual guides available to sit with people or offer prayer. Some facilities offer religious services. Clients with long-term health alterations often use prayer as a coping mechanism and look to faith in God or another spiritual being for a source of comfort (Mauk & Schmidt, 2004). The client's spiritual leader can help with the experience of spiritual distress.

The *prosthetist* and *orthotist* are team members whose services are required by some clients. The prosthetist works with those needing an artificial device (prosthesis) used to replace a missing body part, such as a limb, tooth, eye, or heart valve (Figure 44-3). The orthotist fits orthoses, an external orthopedic appliance that prevents or assists the movement of the spine or limbs, such as braces and splints.

SETTINGS OF CARE

Rehabilitation care encompasses a variety of services that may be on an outpatient or inpatient basis. The most appropriate care setting for each person is determined by the degree of functional impairment, personal preference, current living arrangements, financial resources, cost of services, and available family or informal caregiver support. All clients with functional limitations should be encouraged to maintain independence as long as possible; therefore outpatient treatment is preferred, but the most appropriate service should be selected for the individual client. The more services the client requires, the more likely institutional care is the better option.

Community-Based Services. *Home delivered meals* or Meals on Wheels is a service available for people unable to prepare adequate meals for themselves. These programs provide at least one nutritionally balanced meal daily, usually at noon. For the person who can manage a simpler meal for breakfast and dinner, this service can help maintain independence while providing balanced nutrition. Some older adults eat part of the meal at noon and save the rest for the evening meal.

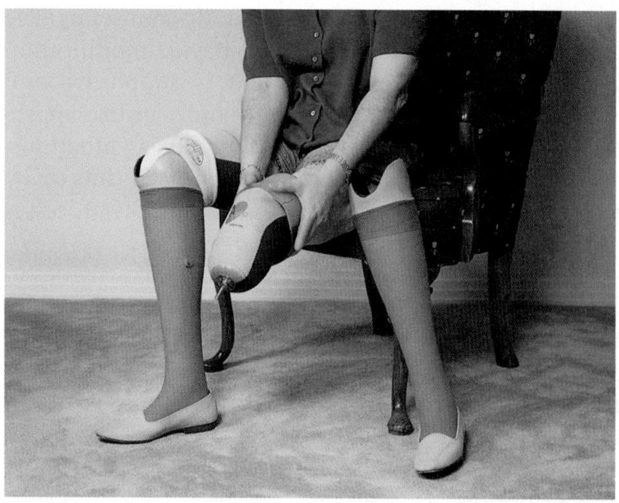

FIGURE 44-3 Prosthetists work with people needing artificial limbs or other prosthetics, like this woman who has had bilateral lower-limb amputations. Her lower-leg prostheses promote ambulation while offering a near-normal cosmetic appearance.

Chore services offer help with home maintenance and include yard work, heavy housecleaning, minor house repairs, and errands and may be a key factor for some people in being able to maintain independent living. Family and friends most often provide chore services. However, limited funding may be available for these services through a home health care agency. Some churches and other service organizations may also offer this type of assistance.

Homemaker services provide assistance with personal care, supervision of self-medication, light housekeeping, shopping, and meal preparation. As with chore services, limited funding may be available.

Home health care programs provide additional services to people requiring medical care that can be managed at home. These services include physical, occupational, and speech therapy; skilled nursing care; and nursing assistant services to assist with personal care. Home health care is warranted when a person is considered homebound.

Respite care is a temporary service enabling family caregivers to take a break from their responsibilities for a few hours to a week or longer. Respite care is provided at home by home health care services or at a day care center or nursing home, and it is believed to reduce subjective caregiver burden, enhance caregiver well-being, and delay or decrease the likelihood of institutional placement (Johnson & Kastner, 2005). To meet the needs of family caregivers, respite care should allow flexibility, choice, and consumer control.

Adult day care centers offer care in a protective setting away from the older adult's home during daytime hours. This care includes health maintenance, restorative measures, and recreational activities. When 24-hour supervision or assistance is required and family caregivers have other daytime obligations, enrollment in an adult day care center makes it possible for a person to continue living in a familiar environment with family and friends. These programs often serve older adults who need supervision because of illness, disability, or the effects of aging. Older adults may attend full- or part-time. Adult day care is cost-effective and allows older adults to interact with others under professional supervision.

Facility-Based Services. Living facilities include adult foster care, board and care homes, group homes, residential care units managed by nursing homes, and assisted living units in retirement communities. These facilities combine shelter with other support services, such as meals, housekeeping, laundry, shopping, and some personal care.

Long-term care facilities, or *nursing homes,* provide interdisciplinary care to people who do not require hospitalization but whose needs for care exceed available informal and formal community resources. Typical long-term care facilities provide several levels of care. Skilled nursing care provides rehabilitative and subacute care services, including measures such as intravenous fluids, medications, wound care, enteral feeding, and therapy. Intermediate care units may offer custodial care. Nursing home placement may be emotionally difficult for both the client and the family member. Having an opportunity to evaluate available facilities helps alleviate the guilt and fear that may be associated with this decision. Questions for families to ask when evaluating a nursing home are suggested in Box 44-1.

AMERICANS WITH DISABILITIES ACT

The Americans With Disabilities Act (ADA) is a significant piece of legislation that advocates for those with disabilities. According to this law, employers must provide "reasonable accommodation" for workers with functional limitations or disabilities. An employee cannot be discriminated against or fired on the basis of physical limitations. The employer must make reasonable efforts to accommodate the special needs of employees. For example, buildings must be accessible. If this means that a ramp needs to be installed for a worker in a wheelchair, then this must be done. If the sinks in the bathrooms must be raised so a wheelchair can go under them, then this is generally reasonable. If an employee cannot climb stairs because of a disability or an injury, then an elevator may need to be installed.

The ADA also provides increased access to public services such as ground transportation and buildings, as well as requiring telephone companies to furnish telecommunication devices if needed to those with hearing and speech impairments (Watson, 2000). Buildings constructed since the enactment of the Americans With Disabilities Act are much more likely to be accessible to those with functional limitations.

FACTORS AFFECTING FUNCTIONAL LIMITATIONS

A wide range of factors influence a person's ability to cope with physical limitations and adjust to long-term health alterations. These include developmental stage,

BOX 44-1 *Questions to Ask When Evaluating a Nursing Home*

Ownership, Licenses, and Certification
- Who owns and manages the facility?
- Is it a for-profit or a not-for-profit facility?
- What levels of care are provided?
- Does the facility have a current state license?
- Does the administrator have a current state license?
- Is the facility currently accredited by the Joint Commission on Accreditation of Healthcare Organizations?
- Is the facility Medicaid/Medicare certified?

Location
- Will the location enable family and friends to visit easily?
- Will the location enable continued use of a personal physician?
- Is there a hospital nearby?
- Is the facility located in a safe neighborhood?

Safety
- Is there evidence of accident prevention measures, such as handrails in the hallways, grab bars in the bathrooms, sturdy chairs, nonskid floors, and ample lighting?
- Is the facility currently in compliance with state and federal fire safety codes?
- What infection control measures are enforced?

Living Environment
- Are private bedrooms available?
- If residents share bedrooms, how are roommates assigned and what is the policy for resident conflict?
- Is storage space for clothing and personal belongings adequate?
- Does each bedroom have a bathroom with a shower and accommodation for a wheelchair? If not, how many people share a communal shower area?
- Are hallways large enough for two wheelchairs to pass easily?

Meals
- Does the staff include an on-site registered dietitian?
- Is attention given to special dietary needs and preferences?
- Is there an attractive, inviting dining room for ambulatory residents?
- Is socialization encouraged at mealtime?
- Is the food adequate, tasty, and attractively served?

Nursing Service
- Is there commitment to individualized care and maintaining resident dignity?
- Is there positive support for restorative and rehabilitative care?
- Are staff well groomed, courteous, and respectful?
- What is the composition and educational preparation of the staff?
- What are the staff-to-resident ratios on day, evening, and night shifts?

Medical and Other Special Services
- Who are the staff physicians? Are they board certified in geriatric medicine?
- Is a physician readily available for emergencies?
- Are physical, occupational, speech, and respiratory therapies available?
- Are there provisions for eye, dental, and foot care?
- Does the staff include an on-site or a consulting social worker?
- Are beautician and barber services available?

Social, Educational, Recreational, and Religious Activities
- Are visiting hours flexible?
- Are there inside and outside common areas for visiting and walking?
- Is there a planned orientation for new admissions and their families?
- Are there family programs such as support groups and educational programs?
- What recreational opportunities are provided?
- What provisions are made to meet religious needs?

Cost
- What is the daily basic rate?
- What services are included in the daily basic rate?
- What additional costs will there be?
- Are billing procedures and payment policies clearly explained?

physiological, cultural, lifestyle, psychosocial, and environmental factors.

FACTORS ACROSS THE LIFE SPAN

A person's stage of growth and development influences the ability to adapt to change. The age at the onset of a functional limitation affects the person's knowledge and personal resources for coping with a change in functional capacity.

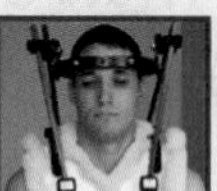

In the case study at the beginning of this chapter, Robert, the teenager with a spinal cord injury, has major adjustments to make. Not only does he have to cope with the usual stresses of teenage life and high school, but after his injury there are many additional factors to deal with. Once an active teen, he is now paralyzed. What issues associated with Robert's developmental stage might the multidisciplinary team need to address? Consider issues related to sexuality and future goals for a career, marriage, and children. How might Robert's level of maturity influence his ability to deal with these life changes?

PHYSIOLOGICAL FACTORS

Many people have multiple coexisting illnesses or problems in addition to a physical limitation. For example, a person may have had an amputation of the lower leg because of diabetes and poor circulation. These chronic problems are generally progressive and can negatively influence a person's ability to adapt to a functional limitation. Similarly, it is difficult for a person who is legally blind from glaucoma to perform activities of daily living.

Physiological changes that occur as a normal part of the aging process contribute to the number of people experiencing a decreased ability for self-care. Also, people with physical limitations are living much longer than in past years. New problems are being discovered that result from the aging process in those who have a disability that occurred decades ago. The probability of having multiple chronic conditions, including arthritis, hypertension, heart disease, hearing impairment, and orthopedic problems, increases with advancing age. The majority of older adults report at least one chronic problem (Eliopoulos, 2005).

As the number of older adults in the population increases, so does the percentage of those needing assistance with daily activities. As life expectancy increases, so does the number of older adults living with disabilities. Older adults (the fastest growing age-group in the United States) and the disabled include people from all racial, cultural, religious, and socioeconomic backgrounds, making the need to address the problems of aging and disability a primary and universal concern for the future in health care.

CULTURAL AND LIFESTYLE FACTORS

Culture. Culture and ethnicity may also influence ability and disability. Some ethnic groups are more likely to have a higher incidence of certain chronic illnesses. For example, older adult minority men have disproportionately higher rates of disease and death as a result of influenza, pneumonia, and chronic respiratory conditions such as bronchitis and emphysema (Eliopoulos, 2005). According to current research, those in ethnic minority groups have more functional limitations, increased medical problems, poorer health, and more work-related disabilities (Lehman & Poindexter, 2006).

In addition, cultural norms may influence how people seek treatment for illnesses. People belonging to ethnic minority groups are more likely to rely on informal health services such as folk cures and may have limited access to professional health care. Even if there is access to health care, certain cultural norms encourage the use of folk medicine and remedies before going to the physician. Persons living in rural communities may face similar barriers to those of ethnic minorities. Also, some cultures do not believe in nursing home use, preferring to care for their relatives at home, so a greater amount of client and family education may be needed. Intergenerational care may lead you to explore a variety of teaching options in working with a vast age range of caregivers.

In summary, cultural norms, including religious beliefs, influence a person's ability to adapt to disability and the support systems needed for best outcomes. It is important to develop cultural sensitivity to provide optimal nursing care to people from ethnic or religious groups different from your own.

Lifestyle Factors. The onset of a health problem resulting in functional limitations often requires lifestyle changes. The person may have to learn a new job, modify the means of transportation, or establish new communication systems. Adjustments may even be as basic as maintaining life functions. Lifestyle changes include adaptations in activities of daily living.

ENVIRONMENTAL FACTORS

Environmental factors that can affect ability and disability are many. They include the person's living situation, the workplace, and the sites of leisure activities. If a living situation is unsafe, either in a physical sense (e.g., if it adds to fall risk) or in a psychological sense (e.g., if it causes additional stress from abuse or neglect), the risk of disability may be increased. Workplaces can pose additional health threats, although employers are required to reveal potentially hazardous materials in the work environment to employees and to provide adequate protective equipment and education to minimize injury. Some individuals engage in high-risk behaviors with regard to leisure activities.

Lack of community resources also affects people with functional limitations. There may be many architectural barriers to overcome. Going out to dinner may require major time in planning and preparation. The person has to consider not only transportation issues but also accessibility to bathroom facilities, dining facilities, walkways, parking lots, and the like. You should know the community resources available for people with physical limitations so that you can encourage community reintegration. **Community reintegration** is the return and acceptance of a person with functional limitations as a participating member of the community.

PSYCHOSOCIAL FACTORS

Many psychosocial factors influence long-term outcomes after a physical limitation is apparent. The client's previous coping patterns and ability to adapt to change and the amount of available social support can positively or negatively affect the situation (Box 44-2).

Socioeconomic status may affect the person's ability to pay for needed health care. Transportation and access to care often present barriers for people with physical limitations.

Some clients may feel that the health care system will not benefit them. They may not believe that the treatment prescribed will help. If clients do not believe that rehabilitation or other care is going to make a difference, they are less likely to participate. Likewise, if clients feel that they have little or no control over their situation or that their actions make little difference, they are less likely to be ready to learn ways to help themselves.

Self-image and self-esteem are affected by long-term physical problems. People may need assistance in adjusting to an altered body image.

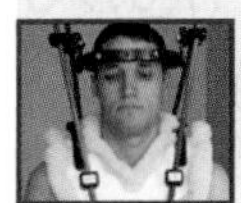

How might Robert's self-image, self-esteem, and body image be affected by his tetraplegia?

BOX 44-2 *A Patient's Perspective*

"I Had No Idea How This Accident Was Going to Change Our Lives"

I was at work when the phone call came. My husband, Mike, had been rushed to the hospital, unconscious. While evaluating the roof of an apartment building, he had fallen through a skylight onto a concrete floor 25 feet below.

The next few hours are a blur. As soon as I got to the hospital, someone gave me Mike's wedding ring. I put it on my hand and kept it there. A hospital volunteer stayed with me for the first couple of hours. I was in shock. I didn't cry, didn't talk much, just prayed a lot. As family members came in, the volunteer explained to them what had happened and that Mike was in a coma.

Then a nurse took me into the emergency department to see Mike. He was almost unrecognizable. His whole head and face were swollen and discolored; his right ear was crumpled and black. He looked like a big plum. His right arm was in a cast because he had fallen on his right side and broken his wrist. He had tubes everywhere. The doctors told me he had a 50-50 chance of living through the night and that they were going to do a CT scan to check for paralysis. That's when I fell apart. I hadn't even thought about the possibility of paralysis. Mike was only 29 years old. I was 22. I had no idea how this accident was going to change our lives; I just wanted him to live.

After he survived the first 24 hours, the ICU nurses told me that the next 3 days would be critical. I stayed at the hospital, but I couldn't sleep until those 3 days were up. He lay in a coma for 21 days, cared for by an amazing, wonderful team of ICU nurses. Most of them took time to explain the how and why of every procedure. I needed that reassurance, needed to trust that he was getting the best possible care. They talked to Mike, not knowing whether he could hear or understand, and they talked with me, asked how I was doing.

Mike spent 99 days in the hospital, and I visited him every day. I stayed with him every night until he was out of the coma—an incredibly difficult time. Our parents were taking turns looking after the children, and it was hard for them to understand just what was going on, especially our daughter, who was just 18 months old.

When Mike came out of the coma, he had episodes of violence, punching at people, trying to run away. He even tried to break out of the restraints, so they assigned one-on-one nurses, most of them male, to be with him so I could get away for a little rest. These nurses were great companions to both of us, very understanding and supportive.

The rehabilitation team was wonderful too. They never gave up on him. They encouraged him, praised his progress—and that helped keep me going. When Mike was in rehab, I took our 6-year-old son and our daughter to see him for the first time. My son seemed relieved to see Mike. I think until then he had believed his dad was dead.

Looking back on that experience, I realize how much I came to depend on the nurses for information and support, and how much I appreciated their patience, honesty, and basic human kindness. Most of them were so gentle with him when they bathed him and shaved his face. And they spent time with me too, asked how I was doing, asked about the children, and talked with me about our life before this happened. One nurse brought in books and articles to help me understand what was happening with Mike. Others told me about patients with similar injuries and how they and their families had coped.

There were a few nurses—just a few—who could have done a better job. Some of them just seemed to give up on Mike and told me I might never get him back. That outright negativity was unacceptable. Once they found out how young I was, they didn't give me credit for being able to handle the situation. One night a nurse came in and told me to go home, didn't introduce herself or anything, but kept repeating "You need to go home and get some rest." I couldn't explain why I couldn't go home, why I needed to be there, and so we got into an argument. That was awful.

It's been almost a year since the accident, and Mike is doing well. He looks the same as ever and is walking and talking fine. He's come a long way. After he came out of the coma, he didn't know me; he thought I was one of the nurses. Telling him over and over about our life together has helped rebuild his memory, especially about the children. He's very sweet, but he didn't remember me, and he's not the person I remember. We've gone from being husband/wife to sister/brother, but it's like starting over in the marriage. With therapy and counseling, he's slowly beginning to remember things. Sometimes he surprises me by remembering something on his own, and it's like getting a present.

Those with disfiguring burns, colostomies, or paralysis or anyone who must use adaptive equipment may feel stigmatized. This is the negative way that society may view people who are different from the norm. Coping with such stigmas is difficult enough for those with adequate coping mechanisms and family support, but for those without many resources, it can be devastating.

ASSESSMENT

GENERAL ASSESSMENT OF FUNCTIONAL LIMITATIONS

When working with people with functional limitations, you need to have excellent assessment skills. Although the entire interdisciplinary team aids in holistically assessing the client, you as a nurse are primarily responsible for documentation in several key areas. One of these is the person's overall health and functional assessment.

> ***Action Alert!*** Be sure to adhere to professional and agency-based standards for documenting a client's overall health status and functional assessment.

Health Assessment. A comprehensive history and current assessment across all functional health patterns is essential to planning holistic care for the person with functional limitations. Ask the client to describe the onset of symptoms and history of the current problem. Focus on any symptoms that may affect the rehabilitation program, such as pain and how it is managed. In addition, the client's previous functional status is important to determining the expectations for the current rehabilitation program. Often rehabilitation can only expect to return a client to the previous level of function. Determine the client's goals and expectations for rehabilitation.

Assessing current functional status is a team effort. Functional status refers to a person's ability to perform self-care activities and other tasks that are necessary for independent living. A systematic approach to assessment of functional status enables objective appraisal to determine the kind of support needed and the client's responses to such support.

A standardized tool is useful for objective comparison of the client's progress from admission to discharge, as well as for setting goals throughout the rehabilitation stay. Such instruments help determine physical functional status, document the need for interventions and services, devise a treatment plan, and assess and monitor progress.

Many tools or scales are used to assess functional status; some of the more commonly used instruments include the Functional Independence Measure (FIM) scale, the Instrumental Activities of Daily Living scale (Table 44-1), the Katz Index of Activities of Daily Living, the PULSES Profile, and the Barthel index (Granger, Albrecht, & Hamilton, 1979).

The FIM scale is one of the most reliable and valid tools for measuring functional status. It measures disability in categories of both cognitive and motor functions. The team member rates the individual from being dependent (1) to being completely independent (7) in several different categories. Scores can be totaled in several ways and compared. Many facilities have each team member complete specific sections. Team members may also keep more detailed FIM scores through separate documentation related specifically to their discipline. Having a quantitative measure is helpful for insurance coverage and can show progress in a numerical way, allowing goals and outcome predictions.

The Katz Index of Activities of Daily Living (Box 44-3) is designed to evaluate six functions: bathing, dressing, toileting, transferring, continence, and feeding. Performance is rated as independent or dependent. This tool is easy to use and offers a quick assessment of the basic tasks needed for self-care.

Physical Examination. The focus of the physical examination will vary depending on the reason for admission to the rehabilitation unit: cardiovascular, respiratory, or neuromuscular. When the admission is for neuromuscular dysfunction, this examination should be thorough, looking for any associated neurological deficits. In addition to ROM, strength, movement, and reflexes of the affected limb(s), a cranial nerve assessment should be done if neurological deficits are suspected. Standard assessments should include orientation, cognition, memory, swallowing, and speech.

> ***Action Alert!*** Note any neurological abnormalities, and convey them to other rehabilitation team members, particularly the physician.

Also assess respiratory function, cardiac function, general nutritional status, condition of the skin, and elimination.

FOCUSED ASSESSMENT FOR *INEFFECTIVE ROLE PERFORMANCE*

Defining Characteristics. Defining characteristics for *Ineffective role performance* (Doenges, Moorhouse, & Geissler-Murr, 2005) include the following:

- Altered perception of role by self or others
- Role strain, conflict, confusion, ambivalence, denial, dissatisfaction, or overload
- Inadequate external support for role enactment
- Inadequate adaptation to change or transition
- Family system conflict, uncertainty, or pessimism
- Change in usual patterns of responsibility; inadequate self-management
- Discrimination, domestic violence, harassment
- Inadequate motivation, confidence, role competency, skills, or knowledge
- Inappropriate developmental expectations

Table 44-1 Instrumental Activities of Daily Living Scale

ACTION	SCORE
A. Ability to use telephone	
1. Operates telephone on own initiative: looks up and dials numbers, etc.	1
2. Dials a few well-known numbers	1
3. Answers telephone but does not dial	1
4. Does not use telephone at all	0
B. Shopping	
1. Takes care of all shopping needs independently	1
2. Shops independently for small purchases	0
3. Needs to be accompanied on any shopping trip	0
4. Completely unable to shop	0
C. Food preparation	
1. Plans, prepares, and serves adequate meals independently	1
2. Prepares adequate meals if supplied with ingredients	0
3. Heats and serves prepared meals, or prepares meals but does not maintain adequate diet	0
4. Needs to have meals prepared and served	0
D. Housekeeping	
1. Maintains home alone or with occasional assistance (e.g., "heavy work–domestic work")	1
2. Performs light daily tasks such dishwashing, bed making	1
3. Performs light daily tasks but cannot maintain acceptable level of cleanliness	1
4. Needs help with all home maintenance tasks	1
5. Does not participate in any housekeeping tasks	0
E. Laundry	
1. Does personal laundry completely	1
2. Launders small items: rinses socks, stockings, etc.	1
3. All laundry must be done by others	0
F. Mode of transportation	
1. Travels independently on public transportation or drives own car	1
2. Arranges own travel via taxi but does not otherwise use public transportation	1
3. Travels on public transportation when assisted or accompanied by another	1
4. Travel limited to taxi or automobile with assistance of another	0
5. Does not travel at all	0
G. Responsibility for own medications	
1. Is responsible for taking medications in correct dosage at correct time	1
2. Takes responsibility if medication is prepared in advance in separate dosages	0
3. Is not capable of dispensing own medication	0
H. Ability to handle finances	
1. Manages financial matters independently (budgets, writes checks, pays rent, bills, goes to bank), collects and keeps track of income	1
2. Manages day-to-day purchases but needs help with banking, major purchases, etc.	1
3. Incapable of handling money	0

From Lawton, M. P., & Brody, E. M. (1969). Assessment of older people: Self-maintaining and instrumental activities of daily living. *Gerontologist, 9*(3), 179-186. Copyright © The Gerontological Society of America. Reproduced by permission of the publisher.

- Powerlessness, inadequate coping, anxiety, or depression
- Change in capacity to resume role
- Inadequate opportunities for role enactment

A client with *Ineffective role performance* is experiencing conflict in the perception or performance of a role. The client may believe that others have changed their expectations. For example, a man who has had a heart attack may say, "My wife won't let me do anything because she's afraid I'll have another heart attack."

Action Alert! When working with an ill client, make sure to elicit concerns about role changes caused by illness or hospitalization.

Related Factors. Factors related to the diagnosis *Ineffective role performance* may be social, knowledge based, or physiological. Social factors may include inadequate or inappropriate linkage with the health care system, job demands, youth or developmental level, conflict or domestic violence, lack of reward, poverty or inadequate support, and inadequate role socialization (expectations or responsibilities, for example). Knowledge-based factors might include inadequate role preparation or knowledge about a role, lack of opportunity for role rehearsal, unrealistic expectations, or lack of education, skills, or a role model. Physiological factors might include illness, cognitive deficits, substance abuse, mental illness, depression, low self-esteem, pain, fatigue, and altered body image.

BOX 44-3 *Katz Index of Activities of Daily Living*

The Index of Independence in Activities of Daily Living is based on an evaluation of the functional independence or dependence of clients in bathing, dressing, toileting, transferring, continence, and feeding. Independence means without supervision, direction, or active personal assistance, except as specifically noted. The evaluation is based on actual status and not on ability. A patient who refuses to perform a function, even though deemed able, is considered as not performing the function.

GRADING INDEX

- A–Independent in feeding, continence, transferring, toileting, dressing, and bathing
- B–Independent in all but one of these functions
- C–Independent in all but bathing and one additional function
- D–Independent in all but bathing, dressing, and one additional function
- E–Independent in all but bathing, dressing, toileting, and one additional function
- F–Independent in all but bathing, dressing, toileting, transferring, and one additional function
- G–Dependent in all six functions
- Other–Dependent in at least two functions, but not classifiable as C, D, E, or F

DEFINITIONS OF INDEPENDENCE AND DEPENDENCE FOR SPECIFIC ACTIVITIES

Bathing (Sponge, Shower, or Tub)

- *Independent:* Assistance only in bathing a single part (such as the back or a disabled extremity) or bathes self completely
- *Dependent:* Assistance in bathing more than one part of body; assistance in getting in or out of tub, or does not bathe self

Dressing

- *Independent:* Gets clothes from closets and drawers; puts on clothes, outer garments, braces; manages fasteners; act of tying shoes is excluded
- *Dependent:* Does not dress self or remains partly undressed

Toileting

- *Independent:* Gets to toilet; gets on and off toilet; arranges clothes; cleans organs of excretion; may manage own bedpan used at night only and may or may not be using mechanical supports
- *Dependent:* Uses bedpan or commode or receives assistance in getting to and using toilet

Transferring

- *Independent:* Moves in and out of bed independently and moves in and out of chair independently (may or may not be using mechanical supports)
- *Dependent:* Assistance needed in moving in or out of bed and/or chair; does not perform one or more transfers

Continence

- *Independent:* Urination and defecation entirely self-controlled
- *Dependent:* Partial or total incontinence in urination or defecation; partial or total control by enemas, catheters, or regulated use of urinals and/or bedpans

Feeding

- *Independent:* Gets food from plate or its equivalent into mouth (precutting of meat and preparation of food, such as buttering bread, are excluded from evaluation)
- *Dependent:* Assistance needed in act of feeding (see preceding); does not eat at all or needs parenteral feeding

From Katz, S., Ford, A. B., Moskowitz, R. W., Jackson, B. A., Jafe, M. W., & Cleveland, M. A. (1963). Studies of illness in the aged. The Index of ADL: A standardized measure of biological and psychosocial function. *Journal of the American Medical Association, 185* (12), 914-919.

DIAGNOSIS

Many NANDA International (NANDA-I) nursing diagnoses are frequently used in the care of those with functional limitations. A few of the more common diagnoses are discussed here.

Ineffective role performance refers to a change in the way a person perceives or enacts a role. This change can occur when the person encounters role transition, role distance, role failure, role conflict, and role strain. Such changes in roles often occur when a person is no longer able to function in previous roles (such as a job) because of a chronic illness or physical limitation.

The initial response to loss of function is feelings of helplessness and powerlessness. The client undergoing rehabilitation may express feelings of powerlessness through anger or apathy. The nursing diagnosis *Powerlessness* may therefore be appropriate for a client with a newly diagnosed functional limitation. *Risk prone health behavior* may be another appropriate nursing diagnosis when a person has difficulty making the lifestyle or behavioral changes necessary to regain or maintain health when an illness or injury occurs.

Self-care deficit is applicable to people experiencing impaired ability to perform any one of the basic self-care activities such as feeding, bathing/hygiene, and toileting. Dressing and grooming are additional activities that those with *Self-care deficit* may have difficulty completing. Be sure to specify which ADLs are affected when using this diagnosis.

The diagnosis *Impaired physical mobility* focuses care on improving the person's mobility. Movement is fundamental to performing ADLs, so it is essential that interventions address maximizing rehabilitation potential, as well as minimizing further loss of physical movement.

Activity intolerance is a relevant diagnosis to supplement *Self-care deficit* when reduced strength and endurance are major factors influencing the ability to perform ADLs. People with stroke, chronic airflow limitation, cardiovascular disease, arthritis, end-stage renal disease, lupus, and multiple sclerosis often experience activity intolerance. Activity intolerance may also be related to deconditioning. Although there is a gradual decline in strength and endurance with advanced age, particularly after the age of 75, this problem is compounded by pathologic conditions.

When a person has impairments in sensory or perceptual areas that interfere with the ability to live independently, the nursing diagnosis *Disturbed sensory perception* may apply. Be sure to identify the specific alteration when using this diagnosis—whether visual, auditory, kinesthetic, gustatory, tactile, or olfactory. For example, people with glaucoma may have visual alterations, and people with hemiplegia as a result of a stroke might have tactile impairments.

Risk for injury is an important nursing diagnosis in managing care for clients with functional limitations, because risk for injury increases as functional ability declines. Falls are a common problem among older adults with reduced functional capacity and a major factor contributing to dependence. Fear of falling or loss of confidence also contributes to dependence because of self-imposed, unwarranted avoidance of activities. Specific preventive strategies are needed to reduce the risk of injury due to falls, as well as measures to restore self-confidence.

Some additional problems and diagnoses related to those already discussed may be present. The reader is encouraged to refer to the chapters in this text listed for each of these related diagnoses for further information: *Imbalanced nutrition* (Chapters 24 and 25), *Powerlessness* (Chapters 42 and 43), *Hopelessness* (Chapters 41 and 43), *Ineffective coping* (Chapter 47), *Chronic low self-esteem or situational low self-esteem* (Chapter 41), and *Insomnia* (Chapter 36).

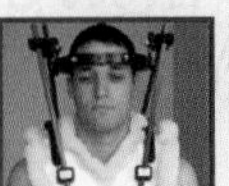

What defining characteristics of *Impaired physical mobility* does Robert evidence? What cues suggest that he might have *Self-care deficit?* What type or types of self-care deficit does he appear to have? What did Robert say to suggest that *Powerlessness* might be an issue? How might *Ineffective role performance* impact Robert's life? What factors might be present if Robert displays *Impaired adjustment?*

PLANNING

GOALS OF THE REHABILITATION PROCESS

The goals of rehabilitation are for the person to achieve maximum possible functional status coupled with a satisfying quality of life and to prevent further complications. Rehabilitation may (1) help persons to remain independent to be able to live on their own and take care of themselves, (2) to help persons become independent, (3) to prevent them from losing the ability to function, or (4) to enable persons to function as well as they did before the problem that prompted rehabilitation.

The desired outcomes for each rehabilitation client are mutually established between team members and the client. Both long-term and short-term goals are essential to the rehabilitation process. Individual team members will assist the client in establishing outcomes for their specialty; the entire team will also set goals that are worked on together, such as those in Box 44-4. Weekly interdisciplinary team meetings allow you to stay current with the expected outcomes of other team members.

BOX 44-4 *General Client Goals of the Interdisciplinary Rehabilitation Team*

- Fostering self-care, self-sufficiency
- Encouraging maximal independence level
- Maintaining function
- Preventing complications
- Restoring optimal function
- Promoting maximal potential of function
- Emphasizing abilities
- Adaptation/adjustment
- Promoting acceptable quality of life
- Maintaining dignity
- Reeducation
- Community reintegration, community reentry
- Promoting optimal wellness

From Easton, K. L. (1999). *Gerontological rehabilitation nursing.* Philadelphia: Saunders.

When planning nursing care, keep in mind the goals of rehabilitation. Expected outcomes should include performing self-care, becoming or remaining independent, preventing complications, and achieving self-esteem. Assist clients in doing everything they can for themselves, thus promoting independence and autonomy. These activities will then promote quality of life and general feelings of well-being.

Typical outcomes for which to plan include improvement in mobility and functional status, as measured by a tool such as the FIM. You would also expect to see increased ability to perform self-care, increased independence, and increased self-esteem. Planning for home discharge is always a goal. You may need to arrange for caregivers. However, independence at home is not always possible, so alternate arrangements should be considered.

EXPECTED OUTCOMES FOR THE CLIENT WITH *INEFFECTIVE ROLE PERFORMANCE*

The following outcome criteria are common for clients with the diagnosis *Ineffective role performance.* As determined in concert with the client, the client will be able to do the following:

- Express feeling or beliefs about roles held within a certain time frame (1 month, for example)
- Name a certain number of factors that contribute to the disturbance in role performance by a specified date
- Describe a certain number of realistic expectations for self in a given role
- Identify behaviors needed for fulfilling a modified role expectation

- Assume certain behaviors in a modified role by a specified date
- Design an alternative role by a specified date
- Seek assistance from selected resources inside and outside the community by a specified date

INTERVENTION

INTERVENTIONS TO PREVENT DISABILITY

The effectiveness of nursing interventions for clients with long-term problems has been well documented (Derstine & Drayton-Hargrove, 2001; Easton, 1999). Nursing care plans that emphasize support and education help clients and family members cope with and adjust to the complications of long-term health problems. Nurses have been shown to make a positive impact on outcomes for those with chronic illness and functional limitations through rehabilitative interventions.

Addressing Factors That Contribute to Functional Limitations. Optimal health will assist the rehabilitation process. Instruct clients and families about how they can modify health practices to achieve a high level of general health. Examples include a diet low in cholesterol, increasing exercise, smoking cessation, maintaining an ideal weight, limiting alcohol consumption, and managing stress.

Psychosocial adjustment will help the person cope with the demands of an altered lifestyle. Social support, including family, friends, and religious support, can help buffer the effects of stress. Learning to use community resources is important to adjustment. Transportation may be a key issue if the person is in a wheelchair, cannot drive, or lives in a rural setting.

Teaching Safety. Teach the client to pay attention to the affected body part and to move safely within the environment. The spinal cord injury client has no or decreased sensation below the level of injury, and the survivor of a cerebrovascular event may lack sensation on one side of the body. Problems in proprioception and unilateral neglect contribute to the risk for injury. *Unilateral Neglect* (also know an hemispatial neglect) is the failure to perceive stimuli coming from the affected side. These stimuli may be auditory, visual, or tactile. In other words, the patient acts as if the affected side of his or her world has ceased to exist and may be largely unaware of the paralyzed side of the body. Proprioception is the sense of the position of parts of the body, relative to other neighboring parts of the body. It is the sense that indicates whether your body is moving with required effort, as well as where the various parts of the body are located in relation to each other.

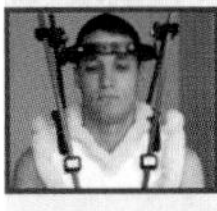

Robert had no feeling from the level of his injury down. Thus he and his family would need to be instructed to avoid extremes in temperature to avoid burns. What specific measures might you teach them to help him avoid sunburn and other burns? Robert would also be in danger of not feeling injuries, such as bumps or bruises caused by adaptive equipment. What would you need to teach him about the use of a wheelchair to help him avoid injury?

Many people with functional impairments, even those with quadriplegia, may be able to drive. Hand controls may be used for people with spinal cord injury. Usually cognition is not a factor, so physical abilities could be developed. However, cognition is a factor for those with stroke and head injury. People with these types of problems may not realize that driving a vehicle would be unsafe. The team must carefully evaluate each client to be sure that driving would be a safe activity.

Teach clients to protect themselves from falls. Psychological responses in the aftermath of a fall, even without serious injury, can cause the older person to make adjustments in lifestyle and living arrangements. Recognizing that serious injury could have occurred, the person responds emotionally to the fall and fears falling again. Anxiety results in loss of confidence. People may become overly cautious and restrict their activities, which results in social withdrawal or isolation. Feelings of vulnerability and fragility carry over into other dimensions of the person's life.

Modifications may need to be made in the home environment for the client's safety. For example, throw rugs should be removed and stairways clearly marked. Handrails may need to be installed. Nonskid shoes should be worn at all times, and the person should be encouraged to call for assistance or supervision at home if needed.

INTERVENTIONS TO PROMOTE SELF-CARE

In working with clients and families in long-term care or those with chronic health alterations, a large proportion of your time will be spent in client and family teaching. All team members focus on assisting the person in performing self-care. This involves helping people find ways to adapt to changes in functional status and abilities. Adapting to the use of splints, braces, adaptive devices, and devices such as halo traction are all part of the rehabilitation process (Figure 44-4). In the following paragraphs, a few of the more common tasks to promote self-care are discussed.

Assisting With ADLs. The OT leads the team to teach the person to perform ADLs. The OT and speech therapist develop the plan for clients with eating and/or swallowing difficulties to learn to feed themselves and safely swallow. However, nurses contribute and reinforce these self-care activities.

The specific technique for dressing and hygiene depends on the person's limitation and uses the remaining ability. For example, people with one-sided weakness or paralysis are taught to put on a shirt or dress by dressing the weaker extremity first. That is, the person uses the stronger arm to put the weaker arm into the sleeve. Likewise, the weaker leg is put into the trousers first, then the stronger.

For some people, especially those with balance problems, dressing in bed may be easier than dressing in a chair. The OT will teach the client additional techniques, such as propping one leg on the knee of the other to put on or take off socks without bending over or using adaptive equipment such as reachers and grabbers to facilitate dressing. Likewise, to make grooming easier, long-handled sponges and one-handed showerheads may help with bathing. Other common adaptations include having the toothpaste held on a suction cup base to keep it from moving or having a Velcro handle for clients with little grip strength. Teach the use of all such tools that promote self-care.

Swallowing difficulties are common among clients with stroke, head injury, Parkinson's disease, and multiple sclerosis. Other clients will have trouble feeding themselves because of impaired use of the upper extremities but may not have swallowing difficulties (e.g., those with spinal cord injury). The speech therapist will suggest guidelines to prevent aspiration when swallowing problems are present. Nurses should also realize that the level of energy and alertness of clients is important in regard to their ability to eat and swallow safely (Westergren, Ohlsson, & Hallberg, 2001).

Remember that all ADLs will take considerably longer when a person is attempting to complete them independently after experiencing a disability. The person may feel exhausted by even simple activities and thus become discouraged. Extra time and patience are essential. Family members need to be encouraged to allow clients to do everything they can for themselves, even though it may be frustrating. Doing things for them encourages dependence on a caregiver and does not promote autonomy.

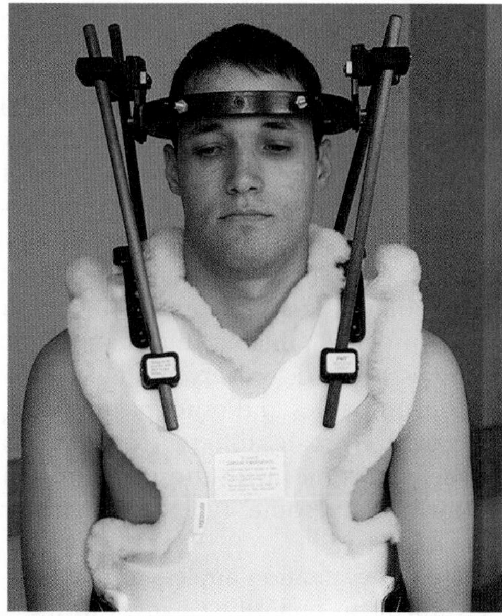

FIGURE 44-4 Adapting to the use of splints, braces, adaptive devices, or temporary traction (such as this man wearing a halo brace for cervical spine stability) may be part of the rehabilitation process.

Action Alert! Allow extra time to encourage clients with functional limitations to do what they can for themselves.

Assisting With Medication Management. One of the most important areas of client teaching is that of medications. Almost all people with long-term health problems take medications. Many clients are able to learn their medication schedule, but some, particularly those with cognitive deficits, may require the assistance of a caregiver. Two of the most useful tools for teaching medication management are the medication schedule and the medication box. When writing out a schedule of the person's daily medications, use large and simple print. The information should include the name of the medication, dosage (number of pills or milligrams, or both), time of self-administration, the drug's action (in simple terms), and medication side effects or other important information.

A medication box can assist the person in organizing daily medications. There are four compartments in most boxes, and seven separate containers, each of which can be removed for the person to take with him or her for the day. Thus if a person cannot set up his or her own medications, the caregiver can set them up for a week at a time. Boxes can be modified for each individual if different time intervals are needed.

When teaching a client or family member to set up a medication box, the first step is to learn the medication schedule and use it as a guide. People soon learn to recognize each pill by its color, shape, and size. Using this information as auditory and visual cues assists with learning. For example, you might say, "This is Lasix, your water pill, the small white one." Likewise, tactile cues may be helpful for those with visual impairments. When placing medications from the package or bottle into the box for setup, the bottle should be checked at least before and after opening. Check each medication with the client and family, and engage in teaching about the medication while setting up the box. In addition, having a routine, such as scheduling medications to be taken at mealtime, helps reduce errors or forgetfulness.

Keeping a journal of blood glucose levels when the person takes daily insulin may be needed. Setting out pills and the needed supplies around a meal, such as breakfast, may help an older person with minor memory problems to recall all that needs to be done. Giving step-by-step instructions may also be needed.

Reducing Unilateral Neglect. The client with unilateral neglect may have minor neglect or may be experiencing a more severe form, in which a body part, most often a paralyzed arm, is not recognized as the client's own.

Unilateral neglect occurs with several conditions but particularly after stroke or brain injury. Those with this problem may benefit from cueing visual attention and planning an action to accomplish ADLs, self-feeding, and positioning. Frequent cues to pay attention to environmental cues on the affected side and the affected body parts may help them accomplish tasks. Cue the person to the presence of persons and objects on the affected side, to food on the affected half of the plate, to dress the affected side, and to move the affected arm or leg.

Set up the environment to maximize performance and success. A general rule to follow is to work especially with the affected extremity during therapy and all interactions, but to place items on the unaffected side when a caregiver is not present, to avoid feelings of isolation. If items such as the water pitcher or call light are placed on the affected side, the person may not see them or may not be able to get to them, thus contributing to a sense of isolation and helplessness.

Referring to Community Resources. An important yet simple way to assist those with functional limitations is to be knowledgeable about community resources. Because people with functional limitations are largely influenced by the external environment, try to become aware of architectural barriers as well as accessible buildings within the community. Know about available support groups and where they meet or key contact people for specific concerns. Provide lists of support groups, mentors, transportation for those in wheelchairs, meal arrangements, or senior centers to help with community reentry and to reduce social isolation. Also use the social worker and chaplain, as well as the local church or synagogue, as resources within the community. It is important to be able to instruct clients in strategies for living alone if that is their life situation (Box 44-5).

> ***Action Alert!*** Remember that the goal for those with functional limitations is to achieve the maximum possible level of independence.

INTERVENTIONS TO ENHANCE ROLE PERFORMANCE

Interventions specific to enhancing role performance center around clarifying roles, developing resources, referrals for job retraining, teaching, and practicing redefined roles.

Clarifying Roles. You will need to provide opportunities in a predetermined time frame (daily, biweekly, weekly) for clients to express their perception of their roles, their responsibilities, and the causes of *Ineffective role performance.* This schedule gives them a chance to see the reality of their abilities and limitations, as well as to look at adjustments to roles or alternative roles. For example, a client may describe the roles in a daily journal.

Another task for clients is to identify how significant others' perceptions of their role differ from their own perception. Sometimes this difference in perception requires negotiation about what role behavior should take priority and what the role is to be.

Developing Resources. You can help clients identify resources needed to fulfill their roles. These resources will vary and should be identified by the client and you. For example, if a client needs child care, you may help the client explore the types of child care facilities available and help narrow the list down to the most acceptable and affordable.

Referrals for Job Retraining. When illness or disability forces a career change, it may be appropriate for the client to receive job testing and counseling from a career counselor. An example of a resource for the client who has become disabled is the state rehabilitation department.

Teaching. You can provide clients with education about a role, you can model the role, or you can help them identify role models. In some cases, role distance can be reduced when clients obtain added knowledge and skill. You may include in your teaching strategies such activities as role clarification, exploration of role expectations, and role modeling where appropriate.

Practicing Redefined Roles. Clients can practice roles and then share their reactions to these roles with you. Roles can be further redefined as practice reveals where clients feel successful and where they feel uncomfortable. Feedback from significant others helps clients to redefine roles as well.

EVALUATION

CLIENTS WITH FUNCTIONAL LIMITATIONS

The evaluation phase of the nursing process with regard to clients with functional limitations or disabilities is generally focused on the outcome. The most objective way to measure progress in functional status is by using scales or tools such as the previously discussed FIM scale. Such tools provide quantifiable data with which to compare initial function to outcomes after completion of therapy. In addition, statistics such as these can provide valuable information about the client's progress toward recovery and help justify costs to insurance companies and other payers. Using a nationally recognized scale, different facilities can also compare their outcomes with those of similar institutions, allowing for some type of quality control measurements.

Other types of evaluation are less formal, and results are more difficult to quantify. Changes in life satisfaction, perceived quality of life, and improved coping and adaptation skills are more difficult to measure, but they are intangible benefits of rehabilitation. Although valid

BOX 44-5

Teaching for Self-Care

Strategies for Living Alone

Purpose: To help the client develop effective coping strategies for living alone.
Expected Outcome: The client will perform adequate self-care and maintain satisfaction with living arrangement.

Client Instructions

- To minimize waste and repetitive leftovers, buy small amounts of food or specially packaged one-person servings. Consider shopping at a store that sells some products by bulk out of large bins. That way, you can buy just the right amount of sugar, flour, beans, cereal, or other staples. Doing so not only will reduce the shopping bill but will also allow you to build more variety into your meals.
- Consider asking the butcher to cut portions of meat suitable for one person and to help you select tender cuts.
- Another way to maintain variety, minimize waste, and have quick meals is to use your freezer strategically. Whenever you make bread, muffins, cookies—almost anything, really—freeze some in small portions. Consider freezing soup, spaghetti sauce, or marinade in ice cube trays; then remove the cubes and keep them frozen in plastic freezer bags. If you make something like a meatloaf, separate the mixture into four loaves and freeze three of them uncooked. That way, you can cook one and have others for future use. Make sure to label bags and wrapped packages with the contents and date.
- To keep meals interesting and tasty, make foods appealing to the senses. Use such flavorings as packaged herb seasoning, lemon pepper, imitation butter, dried onion flakes, minced garlic, dried parsley, and bouillon cubes. (Make sure to consider the sodium content, however.) To build your seasoning collection, consider trading some of your abundant seasonings with a neighbor who has different ones. When serving your meal, try garnishing the plate with a slice of fruit or a colorful vegetable cut decoratively.
- When you eat, set the table with a cloth or special place mat and a colorful napkin. Put a small fresh flower in water to decorate the table. Play music that you enjoy. Try inviting a friend or neighbor over for dinner on a selected night each week.
- When selecting a person to invite over for a meal, look for someone who is positive and upbeat, a problem solver. In fact, whether you invite the person over or not, try to make contact with such a person every day just to chat.
- As possible, plan inexpensive outings, preferably in the company of a friend or neighbor. Friends can help boost your mood and make you feel that you are learning, developing relationships, and participating fully in life. Your local newspaper will list upcoming events. Also consider attending a group for hobbyists, people interested in a certain topic, or people simply interested in social interaction. Plan to dine out or see a movie on a regular basis. Dining out can be easy and relatively inexpensive if researched; many restaurants have early evening specials and senior citizen prices.
- Helping others can make you feel good about yourself and more satisfied with your life in addition to broadening your circle of relationships; consider doing some volunteer work. Call a nursing home, hospital, children's home, library, or other place of interest, and ask about volunteer opportunities. Naturally, you will want to choose something in keeping with your interests, abilities, and available transportation.
- A carefully selected pet can provide a valuable relationship and source of interest and responsibility. A pet may provide physical health benefits as well. Before selecting a pet, consider your interests in various types of animals, the care they require, and your physical and financial ability to provide that care.
- You will be more alert and content during the day if you can establish a satisfactory sleep schedule at night. Set up a sleep routine that you follow every night, such as a special light snack, a shower or bath, toothbrushing, and special sleeping attire. Try to use the bed only for sleeping rather than for reading, watching television, or talking on the phone.
- Take steps to help yourself think positive thoughts and take positive actions. Every day, count up the number of positive thoughts you had and positive things you said or did with others. Do something nice for someone. Try to increase your positive thoughts and behaviors every day. Positive thoughts and deeds decrease stress, increase energy, and improve relationships.

and reliable tools exist to measure such abstract constructs, most facilities lack the time and trained staff to routinely conduct the necessary studies for adequate outcome measures. You and other health care professionals may rely more on observations and clients' statements about their life having improved as a result of interventions to gauge success in meeting emotional, spiritual, and psychosocial needs.

CLIENTS WITH *INEFFECTIVE ROLE PERFORMANCE*

For clients with *Ineffective role performance,* compare newly acquired behaviors against the stated outcomes developed while planning care. Determine the client's satisfaction with the current level of role performance, and seek input from significant others as well. Refine the plan if adaptations need to be made. See Box 44-6 for the plan of care and its evaluation as written by the home health care nurse for Robert, the case study client.

A note documenting progress for the nursing diagnosis *Ineffective role performance* might look like the one below.

Sample Documentation Note for Robert Baldwin

Client states he has adapted well to return to school and his role as high school student. Copes with adjustment issues by talking about them with parents and friends. Is having difficulty identifying a future career consistent with current abilities. The current plan is to meet with high school guidance counselor and vocational rehabilitation counselor. Ineffective role performance not fully resolved.

BOX 44-6

Nursing Care Plan

A Client With Functional Limitations

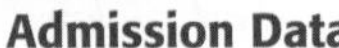

Admission Data

Robert Baldwin, 18 years old, is admitted to the home health care agency after undergoing rehabilitation following a complete C5-C6 spinal cord injury. Robert has tetraplegia and now uses an electric wheelchair. Robert lives with his family, who help care for him. He has returned to the local high school following renovations that made the building wheelchair accessible.

Physician's Orders

Referral to VNA for evaluation of ongoing need for skilled nursing service
Home health care aide referral for assistance with activities of daily living
Referral for evaluation and treatment by physical therapy
Referral for evaluation and treatment by occupational therapy

Nursing Assessment

Client states, "I don't feel like I have control over anything in my life anymore. How will I be able to get a job and take care of myself when I can't even walk around? I just don't know if I can deal with all of this." Client has fair-to-good shoulder movement and biceps activity, along with minimal wrist extension, but otherwise no active movement from just below the shoulders down. Family is supportive and wants to help in any way possible.

NANDA-I Nursing Diagnosis	NOC Expected Outcomes With Indicators	NIC Interventions With Selected Activities	Evaluation Data
Ineffective Role Performance	***Psychosocial Adjustment: Life Changes***	***Coping Enhancement***	***After 6 Weeks of Home Health Care***
Related Factors: • Powerlessness • Inadequate coping • Change in capacity to assume role	• Discusses current roles and area of satisfaction and dissatisfaction with them.	• Appraise the impact of client's current life situation on coping and roles.	• Robert is adapting well to return to school and role as a high school student.
	• Identifies coping skills that may be useful in dealing with current lifestyle changes.	• Encourage client to identify a realistic description of change in role.	• Robert is having difficulty identifying a profession or career consistent with his interests and physical limitations.
		• Explore with client previous methods of dealing with life problems and how they might be used currently.	• Robert has dealt with life problems by talking about them with parents and friends, which he continues to do at this time.
	• Begins to explore options for future professional or career goals.	• Assist client in identifying positive strategies to deal with limitations and manage needed lifestyle and role changes.	• Robert feels that talking with parents and friends continues to be useful, but feels that a specialized counselor is needed to help him select a career.
		• Refer to vocational counselor and other community resources as needed.	• An appointment has been scheduled with the high school guidance counselor and a vocational rehabilitation counselor.

Critical Thinking Questions

1. What follow-up should be done by the home health care nurse to determine the effectiveness of the plan of care?
2. How will the nurse know when or if it is appropriate to discharge Robert from home health care services?

Nursing outcome and intervention labels from Johnson, M., Bulechek, G., Butcher, H., Dochterman, J. M., Maas, M., Moorhead, S., et al. (Eds.). (2006). *NANDA, NOC, and NIC linkages: Nursing diagnoses, outcomes, & interventions.* St. Louis, MO: Mosby.

▼ KEY PRINCIPLES

- Rehabilitation should begin the first day a person is diagnosed with a disorder that can result or has resulted in functional limitation.
- Chronic illness and disability affect every area of a person's life.
- Motivation is important to attaining maximum independence.
- Rehabilitation assists people with achieving the maximal level of independence possible.
- Emphasizing a person's strengths is a key to preventing powerlessness.
- Rehabilitation focuses on working with remaining functions, not lost functions.
- Activity is important in the prevention of the hazards of immobility.
- Care of people with functional limitations must be holistic to be effective.
- Clients who develop functional limitations may find that they also have *Ineffective role performance.*

REVIEW QUESTIONS

1. The nurse wishes to know about a certain client's insurance coverage in rehabilitation. Which of the following is the most appropriate team member to seek information from the client regarding this?

1. Physical therapist
2. Occupational therapist
3. Social worker
4. Physiatrist

2. Which of the following best represents an interdisciplinary client goal for rehabilitation?

1. The client will, with cues from staff, lock his wheelchair brakes 100% of the time to prevent falls.
2. The client will, with cues from staff, lock his wheelchair brakes by discharge to prevent falls.
3. The client will, with cues from staff, lock his wheelchair brakes 100% of the time by discharge to prevent falls.
4. The client will lock his wheelchair brakes 100% of the time to prevent falls.

3. A teenager with a complete spinal cord injury that resulted in tetraplegia may be assessed by the nurse to have which of the following diagnoses?

1. *Self-care deficit*
2. *Impaired nutrition*
3. *Powerlessness*
4. 1, 2, and/or 3

4. The nursing diagnosis of *Ineffective role performance* relates to all but which of the following?

1. Family system conflict, uncertainty, or pessimism
2. Change in usual patterns of responsibility; inadequate self-management
3. Inadequate motivation, confidence, role competency, skills, or knowledge
4. Difficulties with swallowing

5. Which of the following assessment tools would be most appropriate for use when measuring the ability of persons to function by themselves?

1. Barthel index
2. Katz Index of ADLs
3. FIM scale
4. Kenny self-care scale

Bibliography

Association of Rehabilitation Nurses. (2005). *What do rehabilitation nurses do?* Retrieved December 26, 2005, from http://www.rehabnurse.org/about/definition.

Derstine, J., & Drayton-Hargrove, S. (2001). *Comprehensive rehabilitation nursing.* St. Louis, MO: Elsevier Health Sciences.

Doenges, M. E., Moorhouse, M. F., Ceissler-Murr, A. C. (2005). *Nursing diagnosis manual: Planning, individualizing, and documenting client care.* Philadelphia: F.A. Davis.

*Easton, K. L. (1999). *Gerontological rehabilitation nursing.* Philadelphia: Saunders.

Eliopoulos, C. (2005). *Gerontological nursing* (6th ed.). Philadelphia: Lippincott Williams & Wilkins.

*Granger, C. V., Albrecht, G. L., & Hamilton, B. B. (1979). Outcome of comprehensive medical rehabilitation: Measurement by PULSES Profile and the Barthel Index. *Archives of Physical Medicine and Rehabilitation, 60*(4), 145-154.

Johnson, C. P., Kastner, T. A. (2005). Clinical report. Helping families raise children with special health care needs at home. *Pediatrics, 115*(2, Pt. 1), 507-511.

*Johnson, F., Foxall, M. J., Kelleher, E., Kentopp, E., Mannlein, E. A., & Cook, E. (1988). Comparison of mental health and life satisfaction of five elderly ethnic groups. *Western Journal of Nursing Research, 10*(5), 613-628.

Johnson, M., Bulechek, G., Butcher, H., Dochterman, J. M., Maas, M., Moorhead, S., et al. (Eds.). (2006). *NANDA, NOC, and NIC linkages: Nursing diagnoses, outcomes, & interventions.* St. Louis, MO: Mosby.

*Katz, S., Ford, A. B., Moskowitz, R. W., Jackson, B. A., Jafe, M. W., & Cleveland, M. A. (1963). Studies of illness in the aged. The Index of ADL: A standardized measure of biological and psychosocial function. *Journal of the American Medical Association, 185*(12), 914-919.

Lathbury, K. (2000). The road ahead: Managing a spinal cord injury. *Case Manager, 11*(3), 55-57.

*Lawton, M. P., & Brody, E. M. (1969). Assessment of older people: Self-maintaining and instrumental activities of daily living. *Gerontologist, 9*(3), 179-186.

Lehman, C. A., & Poindexter, A. (2006). The aging population. In K. L. Mauk (Ed.), *Gerontological nursing: Competencies for care.* Sudbury, MA: Jones and Bartlett.

Lubkin, I. M., & Larson, P. D. (2006). *Chronic illness: Impact and interventions* (6th ed.). The Jones and Bartlett series in nursing. Boston: Jones and Bartlett.

Mauk, K. L., & Schmidt, N. A. (2004). *Spiritual care in nursing practice.* Philadelphia: Lippincott.

NANDA International. (2007). *Nursing diagnoses: Definitions and classification, 2006-2007* (7th ed.). Philadelphia: Author.

Parker, B. J. (2000). Community and family centered rehabilitation nursing. In P. Edwards (Ed.), *The specialty practice of rehabilitation nursing: A core curriculum* (4th ed., pp. 17-31). Glenview, IL: Association of Rehabilitation Nursing.

Pryor, J. (2000). Creating a rehabilitation milieu. *Rehabilitation Nursing, 25*(4), 141-144.

Rehabilitation Research and Training Center on Disability Demographics and Statistics (StatsRRTC). (2005). *2004 Disability Status Reports.* Ithaca, NY: Cornell University.

Spinal Cord Injury Information Network. (2005). Spinal cord injury facts and figures at a glance. Retrieved December 26, 2005, from http://www.spinalcord.uab.edu.

U.S. Census Bureau. *Census 2000.* Retrieved August 20, 2002, from http://www.census.gov.

Viggian, K. (2000). Health maintenance and management of therapeutic regimen. In P. Edwards (Ed.), *The specialty practice of rehabilitation nursing: A core curriculum* (4th ed., pp. 80-101). Glenview, IL: Association of Rehabilitation Nursing.

Watson, P. G. (2000). The Americans With Disabilities Act: More rights for people with disabilities. *Rehabilitation Nursing, 25*(4), 145-149.

Westergren, A., Ohlsson, O., & Hallberg, I. R. (2001). Eating difficulties, complications and nursing interventions during a period of three months after a stroke. *Journal of Advanced Nursing, 35*(3), 416-426.

*Asterisk indicates a classic or definitive work on this subject.

Chapter 45

MANAGING LOSS

Media Resources

- evolve Evolve Website http://evolve.elsevier.com/Harkreader/
- Companion CD

Learning Objectives

After studying this chapter, you will be able to do the following:

- Define the concepts of loss, grief, mourning and bereavement, death, and thanatology
- Compare and contrast the types of loss and grieving
- Identify a variety of factors affecting the grief response
- Describe the assessment of a client or family member who is experiencing grief
- Describe the focused assessment of a dying client
- Differentiate among nursing diagnoses that describe problems associated with loss
- Plan nursing interventions used in caring for the dying client
- Plan interventions to help the client and family feel understood and to facilitate grief work
- Evaluate the outcomes of caring for a person experiencing grief

Key Terms

anger
anticipatory grief
bereavement
code status
complicated grief
denial
disenfranchised grief
grief
grief attack
grief work
hospice
loss
mourning
normal grief
palliative care
searching
selective attention
sense of presence
thanatology

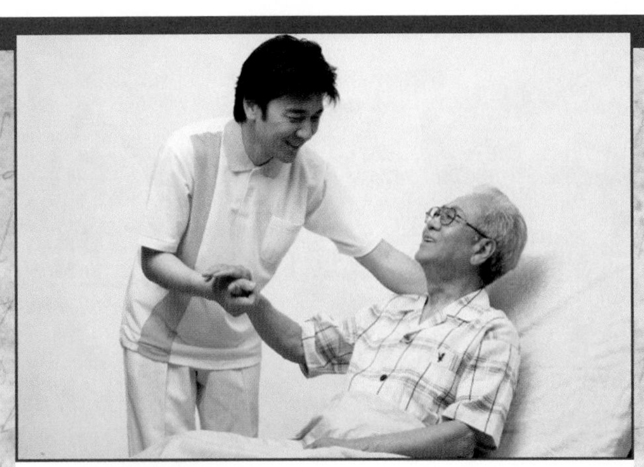

Mr. Hashimoto is a 54-year-old, first-generation Japanese American man who holds an executive position in an international computer manufacturing company. He has been diagnosed with terminal cancer of the stomach. Until recently, the client thought he had an ulcer and had been treating his pain with meditation, prayer, and a special combination of herbs and roots prepared by the local Japanese chemist.

Four days ago, the client experienced generalized pain and vomiting. The vomitus had a fecal odor. He had his son take him to the family doctor because he was too weak to drive himself. The physician admitted him to the medical center for diagnostic tests. Statistically, the client has about 4 to 6 weeks left to live, and he understands that no aggressive treatment will cure his condition. The client's nurse knows that the consulting oncologist has been forthright with Mr. Hashimoto about his diagnosis and prognosis and makes a tentative diagnosis of *Grieving* from the list of nursing diagnoses for loss and grieving.

KEY NURSING DIAGNOSES FOR LOSS AND GRIEVING

Grieving: A normal, complex process that includes emotional, physical, spiritual, social, and intellectual responses and behaviors by which individuals, families, and communities incorporate an actual, anticipated or perceived loss into their daily lives

Complicated grieving: A disorder that occurs after the death of a significant other, in which the experience of distress accompanying bereavement fails to follow normative expectations and manifests in functional impairment

***Imminent death:** The expectation that death will occur in the next few hours or days

*Not NANDA International (NANDA-I) approved.

CONCEPTS OF LOSS AND GRIEF

As a nurse, you will confront loss and grief regularly in all health care settings. For some clients, loss results from changes in health and its effect on lifestyle. For others, loss results from the dying process or from the eventual death either of a loved one or of the self. You must understand the physical and psychological effects of dying and death to provide appropriate care and support to clients and family members as they work through grief and the life changes associated with loss. You must also understand how loss affects you as well, and you must learn to confront not just a client's death but your own death if you are to provide empathic care.

You may provide support to grieving, dying clients and families in settings ranging from acute care, to rehabilitation, to hospice. Currently, most people die in acute care settings. However, nurses are becoming more involved in assisting people who choose to die in their homes or other setting where the focus is on palliative or hospice care. **Palliative care** is "the active total care of patients whose disease is not responsive to curative treatment . . . where control of pain, of other symptoms and of psychological and spiritual distress is paramount" (Ferrell & Coyle, 2001). Palliative care is not limited to the final few months of life. Both palliative and hospice care are tailored to meet the specific needs of clients and their families through a multidisciplinary team approach to utilization of services available from the caring community.

Hospice is a philosophical concept of providing palliative or supportive care to dying persons, in which the goal of care at or near the end of life is to accentuate living and enhance the quality of life (Figure 45-1). A person in hospice care is known to be dying, usually within 6 months or so, and receives palliative or supportive care rather than curative care.

DEFINITIONS

Loss. **Loss** is the removal, change, or reduction in value of something valued or held dear and the feelings that result. Something of value, tangible or intangible, is taken away, rendered unavailable, or rendered less valuable. The loss may involve physical alterations, changes that affect public persona or self-esteem, or separation by death. A loss may be sudden and unexpected or anticipated and predicted.

Losses are encountered daily by each of us. They can be minor or major and are measurable only by the person experiencing the loss. The experience of loss must be defined broadly and with a clear understanding of the personal pain and disruption that can accompany it.

Bereavement. *Bereave* means to rob or to remove something of value, and traditionally it means to deprive through death. **Bereavement** encompasses grief and mourning and denotes emotions and behaviors of a person or a group or community suffering a loss, especially a

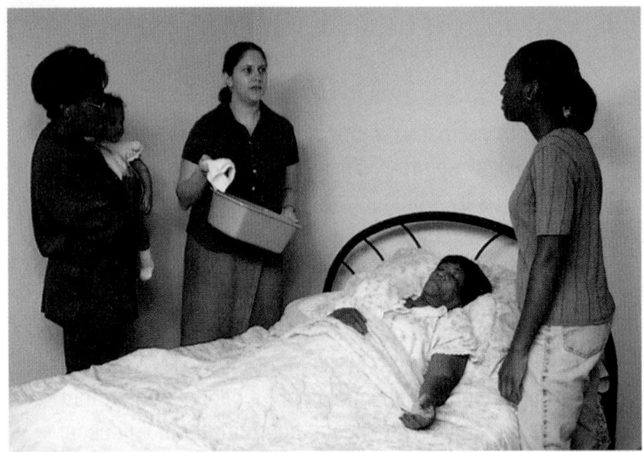

FIGURE 45-1 Hospice is not a place; rather it is a philosophical concept of providing palliative or supportive care to dying people.

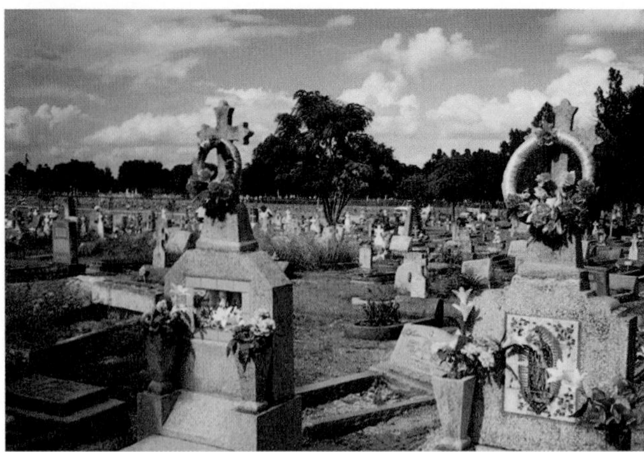

FIGURE 45-2 Mourning practices include individualizing burial sites to memorialize the deceased and comfort the family.

loss associated with death. The concept of a "bereavement period" is the extended time it takes to grieve, process the loss, and to regain a balance in life without the lost other. Bereavement is very specific to the survivor or survivors in the case of community grief (Egan, 2003).

Grief. **Grief** includes emotional, physical, cognitive, and behavioral responses to bereavement, separation, or loss. It is a complex integration of feelings, attitudes, actions, and symptoms elicited by the body and mind at the time of a loss. The intensity of these manifestations changes over time. Grief is an individual, unique experience, not a finite set of experiences or emotions.

Grief influences all elements of a person's life and activities. Severe grief can cause physical illness, exacerbate existing illness, and, in extreme cases, lead to death. Every grieving person does not experience all grief responses, but all persons in grief encounter some of them.

Mourning. **Mourning** is the term used to describe social and cultural acts and expressions used by a bereaved person to convey thoughts and feelings of sorrow. It involves traditions and practices that help people accept the reality of a loss and integrate that reality into their view of their future. Mourning practices evolve, and many cultural mourning practices exist. In all cases, however, mourning honors the dead and helps manage the emptiness after death.

One common mourning practice is the wearing of black clothing to express grief for the deceased. However, a simple black band can express sorrow and respect, such as the black band on the badge of a law enforcement officer to mourn a fellow officer. In some cultures, other colors are traditional; Buddhists, for example, wear white as the color for mourning.

Acts of mourning include religious rituals, expressions of condolence, and burial practices. These acts show respect for the family by conforming to cultural and societal expectations of grieving, Guidelines for the length of time to wear black clothing, to resume social activities, and to return to work have been affected by the accelerating pace of life in the United States. Mourning practices include decorating the burial site to memorialize the deceased and comfort the family (Figure 45-2).

Death. Life ends when the heart stops beating and respiration ceases. However, medical science can stimulate the heart with a pacemaker, use a respirator to breathe for the person, and provide artificial means of nutrition. If treatment is discontinued, the person will be dead. Therefore we need a way to make decisions about discontinuing treatment when there is no hope of recovery, especially when viable organs can be harvested to save another life. The concept of brain death has come to be an alternative way to make decisions about continuing treatment.

Pronouncement of death depends on standard criteria accepted by individuals legally permitted to determine that death has occurred. Current guidelines are often based on the Harvard criteria developed at the Harvard Medical School in 1968, and the 1981 President's Commission on the definition of death. Both definitions agree that death exists when a person is unresponsive to all stimuli and exhibits an absence of reflexes and lack of circulation to all parts of the brain, including the brain stem. The Harvard criteria have five components: unreceptive and unresponsive, no movements and no breathing, no reflexes, a flat electroencephalogram (EEG), and no circulation to or within the brain. The 1981 President's Commission's definition of death specifically states, "Absence of respiration and heart beat, or if mechanical means are being used to maintain these somatic activities, by the irreversible cessation or absence of all brain functions, including brain stem" (Kastenbaum, 1998).

The cessation of brain function is determined, if any doubt about the status exists, through diagnostic evaluations and through determination of the cause of a coma, or through periods of observation, therapy, or both. Complications may invalidate the usual criteria and require special examinations or additional time to establish brain death when certain conditions exist, such as drug and metabolic intoxication, hypothermia, immaturity (especially children under age 2), and shock.

Thanatology. **Thanatology** is the discipline that deals with death and death-related topics. This field of study examines death from the perspective of its definition, as well as attitudes, rituals, and related practices of individuals, groups, cultures, and religions. It encompasses death themes in art and literature, historical perspectives on death, mortality statistics, and factors influencing perceptions of death, dying, grief, and bereavement. It contributes to a better understanding of the effects death and dying have on individuals and groups, including health care practitioners, and the care of persons and families dealing with loss through death. With knowledge from thanatology, you can better assist clients, families, medical staff, and colleagues in understanding death-related events and applying tools to mitigate the impact of death and facilitate grieving.

TYPES OF LOSS

Losses are categorized into two groups: those that are considered concrete or tangible, and those that are psychological, symbolic, or intangible.

Tangible losses are apparent and easily recognized. Examples include death, removal of a body part, and changes in physical health. Tangible losses also include miscarriage; divorce; separation; losses of property or possessions from disasters, theft, or accidents; and changes in lifestyle and reduction of income due to employment layoffs or transfers.

Psychological, or intangible, losses are less obvious. They may be tied to personal perceptions, such as prestige, power, dreams, plans, ambition, confidence, security, and pride. Because these losses are less likely to be acknowledged, admitting to the accompanying feelings of loss can be difficult or embarrassing. Consequently, emotional support may be inadequate.

The death of a child from a terminal disease is a tangible loss for the parents. Society recognizes this loss and supports the parents' grief through various mourning practices. The symbolic or intangible losses associated with the child's death are less obvious and thus less overtly supported within mourning activities. These symbolic losses may include loss of personal and family identity and the loss of eagerly anticipated parental and grandparental roles. The symbolic loss may also include hopes and dreams for the child's success and possibly even the loss of money spent to care for the child over the course of the disease. Intangible losses are often not acknowledged at the time of the death but may be identified at birthdays, holidays, and family events. Support for a parent's grief is often minimal.

Death is a significant and usually traumatic loss, but grief is experienced because of emotional attachments to anything lost. Loss of a job, property, marriage, or body parts is overtly recognized. Losses associated with developmental stages may be taken for granted. For example, older adults may lose independence along with physical or mental health as they reach the later stages of adulthood. Only the person affected, who alone recognizes the nature and magnitude of what is now missing from life, may perceive the nature of a loss. Whether apparent to others or only perceived by the heart, loss is real to those who grieve it.

The loss of self is recognized as the ultimate loss. People who are dying experience physical, emotional, and behavioral responses. Recognition of the end of life and the loss of contact with people and possessions held dear will precipitate many thoughts, feelings, and behaviors in the dying person. These may be components of their survivors' grief as well. The timing of grief and the feelings of the dying person and the dying person's survivors depend on the circumstances of the terminal events.

Action Alert! The meaning of loss is individual. Be alert to the feelings associated with many kinds of loss.

TYPES OF GRIEVING

Grieving is a normal human response to a loss, especially the loss of a significant person or the anticipated loss of one's own life. Natural responses include normal grief and anticipatory grief. Appropriate nursing support can create a therapeutic environment that fosters personal growth for the bereaved. In contrast, complicated grief can lead to lifelong problems and breakdowns in psychological and physical health. Nursing care is especially needed to foresee risks and problems as they evolve and to intervene to reduce or eliminate the negative effects of grief that compromise functioning.

Normal Grieving. Significant interest in grief and grieving began in the health care literature as early as 1917. The concept that grief could be normal as opposed to pathological was introduced by Sigmund Freud, and research continues today to study and identify grief responses. Early research described grief in terms of a syndrome of normal responses after a significant loss. The proposal that "grief work" could assist in resolving grief came from this early research.

In 1969 Elisabeth Kübler-Ross became internationally known through the publication of her book *On Death and Dying.* From interviews she and her students conducted, five stages were outlined that she believed were displayed by persons facing death. The five stages were denial, anger, bargaining, depression, and acceptance.

These stages addressed the prototypical responses associated with many persons engaged in grief reactions at various points during their bereavement. "Denial" addressed the shock, disbelief and feelings of being overwhelmed triggered by traumatic news. This early response (see section on denial in this chapter) reflects our reluctance to accept truth, which initiates the coping and buffering mechanism of denial. Anger grows out of realization that expectations and future goals will not be achieved. Anger (see section on anger in this chapter) additionally manifests itself when we lose control of situations and outcomes and are thus powerless to change the course of events. Bargaining arises when grieving persons attempt to regain some measure of control over a world spinning madly out of control. Bargains can be struck between the griever and many different other entities, such as health care professionals, fate, or, often with God. Promises are made about the griever doing something in return for achieving a specified outcome or reaching a particular point in time, such as a child's wedding day. Depression inevitably arises as complete realization of the truth and facts surrounding the anticipated or experienced loss begin to be clear to the griever. An understanding of the full scope of the loss and all that it will entail brings on anguish and heartache. The depth of depression and reflection of it within daily life will depend upon the perception of what is lost and how irreplaceable that loss is to the griever. Lastly, Kübler-Ross designated a stage she called "acceptance." This last stage is the most controversial. She intended it to reflect the griever reaching some personal peace with events by placing those events psychologically within a personal view of life and death. However, many thanatologists believe that acceptance is not realistic for many people. Grievers may move along with life after the loss and those dying may progress along their trajectory toward death, and in doing so it should be acknowledged that for many individuals acceptance is never encountered or achieved due to complex factors within their life and grief process.

Kübler-Ross's model was easy to remember and understand, and it was widely incorporated into client assessments and plans of care. The understanding of grief responses has expanded beyond these five stages, and nurses now recognize a significantly greater degree of complexity to grief and its manifestations. Within thanatology today, Elisabeth Kübler-Ross is esteemed and credited with bringing the topic of grief, death, and dying into professional practice and for promoting awareness of the needs of the dying. However, research since publication of her seminal work has clarified the complexity of grief, the uniqueness and individuality of bereavement, and the understanding that persons cannot be easily categorized into simplistic emotions or behaviors (Kübler-Ross & Kessler, 2006).

Normal grief encompasses a very diverse and unique set of emotions and responses. Most thanatologists believe that all grief responses are always considered normal within the situation of loss, and thus there are no abnormal grief responses. Each person reacts to loss with responses that are appropriate and individual for him or her.

Grief work is the effort by a grieving person to acknowledge the physical and psychological pain associated with bereavement and to integrate the loss into the future. It is necessary for completing normal grieving and the mourning process, thus preventing complicated grieving. It uses intellectual and emotional responses to direct and guide behaviors or displays of grief. These responses help a person modify the self-concept, identity, and roles in life that have changed because of the reality of a loss. The significance attached to a loss contributes to the nature of the grief work, the length of acute grief, and the outcome of grief. The concept of normal grieving includes a wide range of responses and times.

> ***Action Alert!*** Recognize grief over a loss as normal, and the manifestations of grief as normal, even if they are not consistent with the person's usual pattern of behavior.

Anticipatory Grieving. **Anticipatory grief** involves the intellectual and emotional responses and behaviors by which individuals, families, and communities attempt to work through the process of modifying self-concept on the basis of the perception of potential loss (NANDA-I, 2007). The recognition of an impending loss can trigger realization of other associated losses such as loss of good health, independence, financial stability, cognitive ability, autonomy, and life itself (Egan & Arnold, 2003). Thus anticipation will engender different grief responses depending on the impact of these future losses. This preparatory grieving occurs in terminally ill clients and their families as they deal with the impending death. The extent of anticipatory grieving depends on the length of time between the understanding that a loss will occur and its actual occurrence.

A person who faces the ultimate loss—his or her own death—engages in intellectual, emotional, and behavioral responses spanning a wide variety of reactions and thoughts. A person with a terminal illness may begin to consider a rapidly diminishing future in which previous goals may not be achieved. The person may cognitively and emotionally address the foreseeable changes in the physical body from the terminal illness and the personal losses these changes will bring.

Family members progress through many of the same responses as the dying person. Surviving relatives, however, are faced with continuing daily life after the death of the loved one. Anticipation of such a loss can open opportunities to settle personal and family issues, confirm love and support, seek participation of the loved ones in plans for the burial, and draw families together through the pain of loss. It may be that having time before a loss can help lessen the pain and trauma.

> **Action Alert!** Do not consider plans in anticipation of the loss of a loved one as a sign of not caring about the person. Anticipatory grief normally includes making plans for living after an ill person dies.

Complicated Grieving. Some people encounter difficulty dealing with grief that is unresolved over time. There is no specific time line for the completion of grief and no set series of responses that must occur for successful grieving to take place. **Complicated grief** refers to a disorder that occurs after the death of a significant other, in which the experience of distress accompanying bereavement fails to follow normative expectations and manifests in functional impairment (NANDA International [NANDA-I], 2007).

Sometimes people cannot reconcile their new life with the way life was before the loss. The survivor needs to acknowledge the contribution the deceased made to life and that the deceased is no longer an active part of it. This task may be daunting. The inability to make such a transition may create psychological and physiological consequences detrimental to life. Complicated grieving may be present when daily functioning is compromised or coping strategies are maladaptive and possibly prolonged. Professional counseling becomes an avenue toward resolution.

> **Action Alert!** Be cautious in making the diagnosis of *Complicated grieving.* The time needed for grieving is highly variable.

FACTORS AFFECTING THE GRIEF RESPONSE

Although grief is a highly personal response, certain aspects are common to many grieving people. These responses vary with the person's culture, religion, values and beliefs about life and death, and practices and rituals associated with dying, death, and mourning. Box 45-1 offers one such example.

Developmental factors can also influence the perception and meaning given to the loss and grief responses. Children and adolescents have unique needs when handling a loss. Men and women reflect grief in different ways, partly because of the difference in sex but also because of the perceived roles each plays in society. Men generally display a strong, controlled reaction; women

BOX 45-1 *Cross-Cultural Care*

Caring for a Japanese American Client

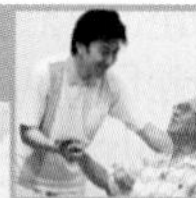

Mr. Hashimoto is a 54-year-old, first-generation Japanese American. He has been a U.S. citizen for the past 23 years and currently works in corporate administration for a large computer company. His wife is 53 and has never worked outside the home. They have three children. The oldest is a 28-year-old son who is married and lives in the same town. They also have two daughters, a 24-year-old who works part-time in a laboratory and will start doctoral work in the fall and a 22-year-old who is completing the last semester of a bachelor's nursing program. Both daughters are single and living at home.

The entire family professes the Catholic faith. Mr. and Mrs. Hashimoto were raised as Buddhists and converted to Catholicism after coming to the United States. Their local parish priest is a second-generation Japanese American and also a converted Buddhist. Although all clients are unique, many Japanese American clients tend to value the following:

- Avoidance of physical contact or, if necessary in the health care setting, contact only after obtaining permission
- Avoidance of direct eye contact, which is considered rude
- Avoidance of questions that begin with "Don't you . . ." because, to be polite, the Japanese person may say "no" three times before giving a true answer
- The belief that a nod or smile does not necessarily mean agreement or understanding
- Strong remnants of Buddhism in the faith practices and rituals of Christian converts
- A view of death as a passage
- Stoicism, especially in men
- Restraint of public expressions of sorrow
- Endurance of pain and suffering without complaint to show strength and avoid worrying family members
- Clearly defined roles for husband (the breadwinner) and wife (the caretaker)
- Hospital care for the terminally ill, with daily visits from family
- Coming home to spend the last days with family, during which the wife, daughter, or daughter-in-law acts as primary caretaker
- Being uninformed about the true nature of a terminal illness to avoid losing strength and hope
- The authority of the physician and dependence of the client
- The belief in psychological interactions with deceased family members giving a greater feeling of peace with death

Data from Hirayama, K. K. (1990). Death and dying in Japanese culture. In J. K. Parry (Ed.), *Social work practice with the terminally ill: A transcultural perspective.* Springfield, IL: Charles C Thomas; McQuay, J. E. (1995). Cross-cultural customs and beliefs related to health crises, death, and organ donation/transplantation: A guide to assist health care professionals to understand different responses and provide cross-cultural assistance. *Critical Care Nursing Clinics of North America, 7*(3), 581-594; Christine Rook, a Japanese American registered nurse (personal communication).

tend to be granted an allowance for weakness and emotionalism. Although these reactions are clearly stereotypical, they are commonly displayed, and guilt may arise if these models are violated.

Situations associated with the nature and timing of death, and perceptions of whether the death could have been avoided, also contribute to the intensity and manifestations of grief. When a death falls outside the perceived natural order, such as a child dying before the parent, it is more difficult to accept. It is also more difficult to pursue grief work when a death is unexpected, particularly when the death involves a child or young person. If the death violates the explicit or implied mores of a society, such as suicide or certain diseases, the client and survivors may be criticized or shunned while being denied needed support.

Psychosocial factors are also varied in nature and sources. Grief can be lessened by factors that link a death to feelings of fairness, rightness, and naturalness. The nature of the relationship between the deceased and the griever and the degree of value accorded the loss by the griever bear significantly on the view of life and living after a loss. When death occurs in defense of others or country, the survivors often perceive the death as heroic and of merit.

Perceptions and personal integration of previous grief experiences contribute to the context within which a recent death is placed. Indeed, cumulative grief can occur when a previous grief experience is not resolved before another loss is added to the psychological burden. The person's ability to effectively address a new loss is then compromised. The person's coping mechanisms and stress management techniques affect the response. Nontherapeutic coping methods, such as those that use alcohol or drugs, and ineffective interpersonal relationships compromise a person's ability to engage in grief work. Depression or mental illness can complicate grief work as well. Stress is multiplied, and existing stress management methods are taxed even more.

Last, a person's physical condition influences grief. Illnesses previously in remission may return, and increased stress may yield physical manifestations. These physiological factors siphon the energy and attention needed to deal with grief. Occasionally, they lead to life-threatening problems.

ASSESSMENT

Grief is a universal human experience, but it has unique personal characteristics and varies with societal mores, the circumstances of a loss, and the value the griever associates with the loss. The responses associated with grief are extensive, complex, and personal, and any response pattern may be normal for an individual in a given time and situation.

It has been suggested that grief is a syndrome that occurs in stages. However, grief is also nonlinear, meaning that it does not occur in a strictly predictable pattern or rigid stages. Grief is multifaceted and complex; thus the individual nature of grief must be acknowledged when interacting with grieving persons.

GENERAL ASSESSMENT OF GRIEVING

Normal grief reactions can be divided into three areas—recognition, reflection, and redirection—each with specific somatic, psychological, and behavioral responses (Jeffery, 2006-2007). Many responses can occur simultaneously, some recur after long periods of time, and others never arise in some people. The areas are not finite in time or in the type of responses displayed but progress throughout grief work. The labels of the three groups reflect the tasks encountered by the griever.

Recognition: Shock and Denial. The initial response to a loss, particularly a death, provides time to emotionally and intellectually absorb its painful reality. It has been called the "listen now, hear later" phase because it grants the griever time to buffer the truth while mobilizing coping resources to face that truth.

This initial reaction period has no clear time frame. Circumstances associated with unexpected news or anticipated news influence the time needed to recognize the reality of the events. However, many similar responses and expressions of grief have been identified at this beginning point in grief work.

> ***Action Alert!*** Offer direct practical help in calling close family, deciding on a funeral home, and gathering the person's belongings (if in the hospital) at the time of a death. During the initial shock just after the death of a loved one, critical thinking may be compromised.

Somatic Responses. These reactions are physical in nature, and many reflect a panic-attack response mediated by the sympathetic nervous system. Somatic responses may include gastrointestinal symptoms, such as nausea, vomiting, abdominal cramping, a perception of hollowness in the stomach, and diarrhea.

Cardiopulmonary reactions may include tachycardia or palpitations, chest pain or tightness, dyspnea, or tachypnea. The person also may have trouble swallowing, a dry mouth, muscle weakness, tremors, dizziness or syncope, lack of energy, and increased sensitivity to noise. Reactions of diaphoresis, flushing, or cold and clammy sensations have also been reported.

Psychological Responses. Initial psychological reactions serve to buffer or delay the awareness of bad news until other coping resources can be identified and mobilized. Here the concepts of shock and disbelief are most obvious. Immediate emotional responses are often feelings of numbness, confusion, and a sense of unreality. Feelings of emotional pain and separation generally replace the numbness when psychological awareness takes place. Anxiety, fear, and panic may be perceived, along with a sense of depersonalization, isolation, or separateness from the environment. The person may sense that a part of the self has been removed or cut out and is missing. The death of a loved one may create the feeling that part of the survivor also died.

A failure to comprehend events and information occurs early in many cases and may continue for some time despite an intellectual acceptance of the reality of the loss. This results from denial. Denial is a complex concept and can take various forms in differing circumstances.

Denial is both a defense mechanism and a cognitive activity. As a defense mechanism, it is primarily responsible for allowing time to assimilate and integrate new information into the cognitive realm. It is an attempt by the mind to alter a person's perception of reality. Statements of disbelief or protestations about mistaken information reflect this. In addition, denial is an intellectual process that does not alter reality but is used to help the person cope with the undesired reality. It can take various forms. Cognitive denial is reflected in the following situations.

Selective attention. Selective attention is the act of choosing when and to whom attention is given regarding a loss and when thoughts and feelings are allowed to enter the conscious mind. The person may choose to avoid talking to staff that the person feels are not receptive to his or her concerns. Or the person may avoid talking to family members in an effort to spare them emotional distress.

Compartmentalization. Compartmentalization is at work when a person appears to completely understand the existing circumstances yet acts in a manner that does not correlate appropriately with reality. For example, a husband may talk about taking his wife home from the hospital, as he has before, despite clear evidence that her condition is grave and prognosis poor.

Deception. In deception, denial is reflected through knowingly altering facts or deliberately giving inaccurate information. Deceptive games are played, and energy is wasted as efforts are expended to protect the other person. In some cultures, withholding negative medical information from dying clients is an accepted practice and is done out of respect for the emotional burdens already carried by the ill person.

True denial. In true denial, the person blocks recognizing reality. True denial can also arise when a person perceives reality as overwhelming. Responses may be bizarre or reflect psychotic thinking. The person may show strong self-protective efforts. For example, a mother who delivers a stillborn, full-term infant may seem to be dealing well with the unexpected event until the morning of discharge, when you find her preparing to take her new baby home from the hospital.

Anger. Anger or even rage is a common characteristic of grief. It occurs as the denial and disbelief are replaced with the growing awareness of reality. Anger and fear appear to be linked as the person faces a life changed by loss, especially death. The comfortable world is disrupted and security threatened.

Anger at unwanted feelings of vulnerability and powerlessness may rise to the surface. It may be displaced onto others in the environment, such as those the person holds responsible for a death or a supreme being for failure to change the outcome (Figure 45-3). Anger may be directed inward as well for perceived failures associated with the loss.

Guilt or remorse is frequently interwoven with anger when the person takes the blame for a real or imagined contribution to the death or when feelings such as relief are deemed unsuitable in the circumstances.

Behavioral Responses. Behavioral responses associated with the recognition phase may include hysteria or crying, the release of anger and rage, or stoic, calm, and resigned behaviors. Cultural and societal mores commonly govern such actions. Hypoactivity or hyperactivity may also be noted, sometimes in conjunction with pointless or repetitive actions. Task-oriented activities may be helpful to the griever as he or she accomplishes necessary tasks associated with the loss. Critical thinking, cognitive functioning, concentration, and attention may be impaired, reducing the person's decision-making ability at a time when it is most needed. Further, hygiene, nutrition, rest, and self-care may be neglected or become an excessive focus.

The initial reaction to a loss may last a brief few minutes to several weeks. The important point is that until the reality of the loss has been acknowledged, further

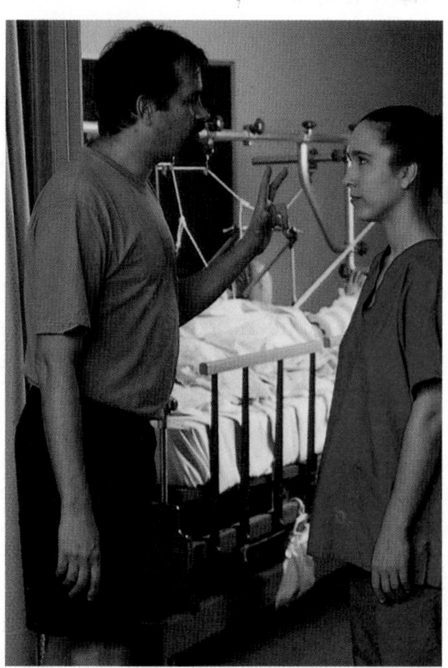

FIGURE 45-3 Grieving people sometimes displace anger onto others in the environment. Nurses sometimes get caught in the cross fire.

grief work is constrained. Responses at this stage generally reflect the griever's attempts to establish the reality in the conscious and unconscious worlds. When that task has been sufficiently addressed, further work will begin in the second broad phase of grief responses.

Reflection: Physical, Emotional, and Spiritual Suffering. During the second broad period of responses, grief work is focused on achieving a sense of stability after instability, control after chaos, and comfort after pain. In these responses, significant efforts are expended to return to a routine daily life without the overwhelming suffering and sorrow attached to the loss. For some, this may never occur, but for many persons the pain does not lessen, it simply gets softer.

Personal growth, with resulting changes in self-concept, occurs as the person confronts, understands, and internalizes a loss. Such reconciliation of the permanency of the loss into the physical and psychological world of the griever takes place over an extended time period.

Somatic Responses. Somatic responses can include continuing somatic distress similar to that experienced early in the grief process, such as weakness, panic attacks, and gastric distress or hollow feelings in the stomach. Depressed immune function has been observed with a correlated increase in physical illness.

Chronic diseases, such as cancer, ulcerative colitis, asthma, rheumatoid arthritis, heart failure, leukemia, and diabetes, occur more often in the newly bereaved. And several studies have shown a major increase in the death rate of both sexes (especially widowers) during the first 6 months of bereavement. Complaints of fatigue are common. Eating and sleep patterns may be disturbed as well, leading to either increased or decreased activity levels.

Psychological Responses. Psychological responses, after the shock dissipates, may be extensions of those begun at the initial time of grieving. This is a period when the mind comes to clearly understand that the loss is irreversible and life has changed irrevocably. The griever is faced with determining and understanding how the loss has impacted life presently and for the future.

Spiritual distress may arise as issues about life and death are examined and questioned. Long-held values and beliefs may be shaken because of the circumstances of the death. This is particularly true in the death of a child or young person, a senseless death, a violent or crime-related death, or an unusually horrific death. These can cause questioning and doubts about a supreme being and about religion. Some persons may abandon lifelong faith practices because of such questions, whereas others discern spiritual renewal and personal growth from such introspections about spiritual beliefs.

Anger resurfaces frequently and unexpectedly. Guilt can lead to remorse or regrets over past events and actions taken or not taken. The person may ruminate over the events preceding the death. Feelings of helplessness and disorganization can be precipitated by the overwhelming nature of the loss and the perceived future after that loss.

Helplessness may then slide into despair, hopelessness, and apathy as the griever succumbs to the sheer magnitude of the impact of the death. Concurrent within these feelings are elements of sadness, self-pity, loneliness, and panic or fears about the future. Clouded thinking, trouble with decision making, and loss of confidence may still be evident at times.

The person may show labile emotional behaviors by crying spontaneously at times not clearly linked to sad events. Indeed, many grievers express surprise at the suddenness of mood swings and emotions associated with grief. These unpredictable emotional responses are a normal part of the grief process.

Keep in mind, however, that many people have feelings of relief or emancipation from burdens after a person's death. These feelings commonly stem from the end of the loved one's suffering or the release of a commitment to care for an ill person. Whatever the motivation, feelings of relief may be unacceptable to the griever or may increase feelings of guilt over this personal reaction to the death. However, especially when a lingering disease has altered life for both the client and the caregiver, feelings of relief are realistic.

Other reactions are unique to this period after the initial responses have passed. The deceased is remembered, and opportunities for reminiscence affect grief in specific ways. There is sometimes identification with the deceased, such as assuming admired traits, mannerisms, interests, goals, and opinions of the loved one. Commonly, memories become selective and filter out negative characteristics. The bereaved person may also experience a sense of presence or grief attacks.

Sense of presence. A **sense of presence** is a nonthreatening, comforting perception by the bereaved of the deceased's presence. These perceptions range from general feelings of somehow being watched to complete sensory experiences. This involves one or more of the senses, or it occurs in dreams, fortuitous events, or conversation. In such experiences, the griever describes the presence of the deceased as a feeling that the deceased is present in visions, in formed and unformed hallucinations, in voices and conversations, in smells and touch, in dreams and signs, or in fortuitous events. These experiences are considered to be part of searching behaviors. In this context, **searching** refers to conscious and unconscious efforts by the bereaved to negate the reality of the loss through finding the deceased alive and well. Such events may be treated as religious experiences in which the deceased communicates a continued presence in the lives of loved ones and is safe, comfortable, and at peace. Research reflects that such experiences do not occur at a specific point within the grief process but often last over a longer period of time throughout grief (Bennett & Bennett, 2000).

Grief attacks. A **grief attack** is an unexpected, involuntary resurgence of acute grief-related emotions and behaviors triggered by routine events and sometimes accompanied by uncontrollable crying or emotional display. An analogy to a grief attack is waves hitting a person standing at the ocean's edge with his or her back to the water. Waves come in at irregular intervals, some small enough to only flow over the feet—the person stands firm. Other waves hit higher on the legs and cause momentary wavering. Still others hit with enough force to knock the person down. The difficulty in withstanding the waves is that the person cannot see when a wave is coming or how large it will be until it hits. Triggering events for grief attacks may include special music, sights, and places shared with the deceased or other events that precipitate feelings of sadness not directly associated with the original loss, such as movies or conversations about the death of another person.

Gradually, over days and weeks, emotions become less labile. The sadness of the loss never completely disappears, but it becomes less disruptive to daily life. Emotions may resurface at anniversaries and special holidays, but in general, emotional equilibrium is achieved and maintained.

Behavioral Responses. Behaviors associated with this roller-coaster period vary widely. Social withdrawal is common because depression and feelings of helplessness make the bereaved reluctant to engage in interpersonal activity in public. Poor hygiene and inadequate self-care may result from depression as well. Crying may continue for extended periods.

Absent-mindedness may be part of the confused and altered critical thinking processes. Seeking control over a world spinning out of control leads to questioning and efforts to clarify events associated with the loss. Searching behaviors extend beyond the emotional context, and the person may feel momentary hope when a face in a crowd resembles the deceased.

Avoidance behaviors may arise as the person tries to minimize the stress of coping with the loss. They may include smoking, drinking, or using drugs to blunt the pain, especially if the person used these forms of coping before the loss. These behaviors are physically and psychologically harmful. Overt risk-taking behaviors that threaten personal safety are infrequent but may occur. They reflect a subconscious belief that life is no longer worth living.

Personal possessions associated with the deceased are usually treasured. Belongings can be preserved by giving them special significance and honor in the home or by giving them to people special to the deceased. Respecting these possessions then perpetuates honoring the memory of the deceased.

Mummification is a term that conveys a symbolic preservation of a deceased person by leaving the physical environment just as it was when the person was alive and well. This behavior is a form of denial. It differs from storing the person's belongings until a time when judgment and decision making return to normal. A person who disperses or disposes of a deceased loved one's belongings quickly after the death may be in denial as well. These actions are efforts to minimize the pain of seeing or dealing with the person's belongings.

Redirection, Reorganization, and Moving Forward. The third phase in grief work may last years. For some, it may never be completed. The responses reflect a griever's return to daily life in a manner that reconciles the past with the present and simultaneously looks toward the future. This subsequent life without the deceased reflects the new directions that have been taken through integration of modified identities and roles. Realistic memories and hopeful planning are integral to successful grieving, and this final series of responses reflects a positive outcome achieved from all the previous grief work. There is optimism about a future without the loved one and willing efforts made to create that future.

Somatic Responses. Somatic responses decline, and the person returns to the quality of health experienced before the loss. Appetite and sleep patterns return to normal. Sex drive returns to normal. Energy and strength last throughout the day. Overall health is again renewed, and the person reports feeling like his or her old self.

Psychological Responses. Although the person continues to have periods of sadness, anger, or regret, they become less frequent and less intense. Feelings of stability, hope, and personal capability begin to override negative emotions. Increasingly, the person has episodes of happiness, joy, and pleasure. Self-confidence and decision making improve. The idealization of memories associated with the loved one decreases, and the person resumes more realistic perceptions. Grief attacks are less frequent. Overall, emotions become less intense and more balanced and realistic.

Behavioral Responses. Behavioral responses mirror the person's improved emotional and physical state.

Seeking behaviors diminish in frequency and seeming realism. Decisions about the disposal of possessions are made without guilt or feelings of abandonment. The person reinvests energy into a life without the deceased and assumes new roles. The ability to look to the days ahead without the deceased is a strong indicator of successfully processing the event both intellectually and emotionally. Behaviors communicate this accomplishment as the person returns to a routine daily lifestyle.

FOCUSED ASSESSMENT FOR *GRIEVING*

Grieving begins when a person faces a potential or expected loss. Grief work before a loss is common among clients and their families when the client has a progressive or terminal disease. It has long been believed that such "preparatory grieving," as Kübler-Ross called it, results in less intense grief after the death. Contemporary thanatologists generally do not hold with this view, and numerous researchers have produced contradictory findings (Kehl, 2005). Many responses are linked with prolonged predeath grieving, particularly in spouses and in parents of children who have extended terminal illnesses.

Defining characteristics for the diagnosis *Grieving* may include the following:

- Actual or potential loss of a significant object
- Expression of distress at actual or potential loss
- Sorrow, guilt, or anger
- Denial of loss or the significance of the loss
- Altered communication patterns, eating habits, sleep patterns, dream patterns, activity levels, or libido
- Bargaining
- Difficulty taking on new or different roles

Grief that begins with an impending loss and has inherent risks. Possible negative outcomes include the potential of distorting and ruining the few remaining months or weeks of a relationship. The emotional and physical pain of grief can cause an emotional distancing at a time when the dying person most needs support. In some instances, psychological detachment leads to physical and emotional withdrawal before the death occurs.

Some cultural groups believe that a critically or terminally ill client should not be told of his or her impending death. Families will go to great lengths to keep this information from their loved one in the belief that the knowledge will add an unnecessary burden and remove hope needed for recovery. Such events result in the illusion of uncaring and callous attitudes, which can lead to public censure and private guilt. The dying person, who is dealing with imminent death, may now have to deal with the belief that family members are not particularly concerned or aggrieved. Physical and psychological isolation can leave the person to die amid high-tech equipment and away from loved ones. These risks may negate the positive outcomes and color the final days with negative emotions and painful memories.

Recognition of an impending loss can help families and friends use the remaining time to reconfirm relationships, settle issues, and build peace. Families that are encouraged to communicate with the dying loved ones and to address the five phases in Box 45-2 often find that these phrases facilitate later grief work. The effective use of time and opportunity during a period of anticipatory mourning can decrease guilt, confirm affection and approval, and counter misinterpretations. The outcome can create positive lifelong memories for survivors.

BOX 45-2 ***Five Phases of Communication With Dying Loved Ones***

Forgive me.	I love you.
I forgive you.	Goodbye.
Thank you.	

From Byock, I. (1997). *Dying well: The prospect for growth at the end of life.* New York: Riverhead Books.

FOCUSED ASSESSMENT FOR *COMPLICATED GRIEVING*

Complicated grieving is a possible outcome of significant or traumatic loss, a loss that overwhelms the coping skills of the bereaved, or when cumulative losses are unable to be managed simultaneously.

Not every person can traverse the grief experience and arrive at a comfortable emotional, physical, and spiritual assimilation of the loss. For some, the loss is perceived as so devastating that self-concept cannot be satisfactorily modified and reconciled with reality. They become overwhelmed and resort to maladaptive and unsuccessful coping strategies, further impairing their ability to function (Egan & Arnold, 2003). Prolonged but unsuccessful efforts to move toward a satisfactory incorporation of the loss into their psychological and physical world result ultimately in marked evidence of dysfunction.

Defining Characteristics. Defining characteristics for the diagnosis *Complicated grieving* may include the following:

- Crying, sadness, anger, guilt, or a labile affect
- Reliving of past experiences with little or no reduction in the intensity of grief
- Expression of unresolved issues, distress at the loss
- Interference with life functioning
- Idealization of the lost object
- Difficulty in expressing loss, or denial of loss
- Alterations in eating habits, sleep patterns, dream patterns, activity level, libido, concentration, or pursuit of tasks
- Developmental regression
- Repetitive use of ineffectual behaviors in attempts to reinvest in relationships
- Onset or exacerbation of somatic or psychosomatic responses
- Prolonged interferences with life functioning

However, many of these behaviors could also represent normal grief. The criterion is whether it interferes with function. Recognition of complicated grief warrants close observations for cues that may demonstrate behaviors and reactions that deviate from responses generally considered to be normal. William Worden (2001) has proposed the following four types of dysfunctional grief. Some people experience two or more simultaneously.

Chronic. In chronic complicated grief, grief has continued for a prolonged or excessive period and does not reach a successful conclusion involving the establishment of a new and different self-concept. In this form of complicated grief, the griever is unaware that the traditional period of mourning has passed and does not recognize the ongoing disruption to life.

Delayed. Delayed complicated grief is characterized by a diminished emotional response at the time of the initial loss and excessive grieving over a later, lesser loss. A correlation between the cumulative effect of two losses is common in complicated grieving.

Exaggerated. Exaggerated complicated grief is evidenced by severe reactions, such as anxiety attacks, phobias, or irrational despair. The person has a significant interruption in daily life, illogical thinking, and an indefinite delay in restructuring a new self-concept.

Masked. Symptoms and behaviors that the griever cannot identify as grief characterize masked complicated grief. The person may develop physical symptoms experienced earlier by the deceased person, especially pain or specific somatic symptoms associated with the cause of death of the deceased.

Complicated grief responses include a wide variety of cognitive and behavioral manifestations. Basically, the griever is trapped in a pathological stress reaction because the griever cannot meld the changes in his or her world and self with the griever's previous environment and identity.

Related Factors. Factors related to the diagnosis *Complicated grieving* include an actual or perceived loss of person, possession, job, status, home, ideals, or body parts and processes.

Factors associated with an increased risk of complicated grief arise from a wide variety of issues and situations (Box 45-3). Some are easily recognized and addressed in supportive ways. Others are not obvious to those who could support the bereaved.

BOX 45-3 *Risk Factors for Complicated Grief*

- Highly ambivalent, narcissistic, or dependent relationships
- Uncertain, sudden, or overcomplicated circumstances surrounding the loss
- History of depression, low self-esteem, guilt, or previous complicated grief reactions
- Conflict between perception of self as strong and feelings of dependency and neediness
- Socially unspeakable, negated, or disenfranchised losses
- History of current or past substance abuse
- Decrease or loss of social support systems
- Cumulative grief over multiple unresolved losses

Factors that can influence a person's risk of complicated grieving include how the event and the context of the event interact with the person's personality and coping style. Personality guides the conscious evaluation of the loss, the choice of coping mechanisms, the duration of each phase of grief work, and the perception of changes in self-concept that accompany grief work. Personality directly affects the adaptive completion of a mourning process.

Another factor that can influence the risk of complicated grieving is the social acceptability or understanding of the loss. **Disenfranchised grief** lacks social acknowledgment, validation, and support for the bereaved. Therefore the grief is not granted merit by society in general. It may arise in response to gay relationships, extramarital relationships, or death of an ex-spouse, for example. Social negation of grief may also arise from society's erroneous beliefs that the grief is not present or that it is inappropriate. Many believe that mentally handicapped people and young children are incapable of grieving, for example.

Another factor in the risk of complicated grieving is the attitude that grieving should occupy a rigid and restricted time frame, after which the person is expected to move forward with few or no backward glances. This usually reflects the belief that grief is a sign of weakness and vulnerability and should be avoided. It can also arise when people are expected to return to roles and responsibilities that require their full attention, such as employment situations or homemaker. Risk factors for complicated grief must be assessed and nursing interventions made early to alleviate or prevent its development.

FOCUSED ASSESSMENT FOR *IMMINENT DEATH*

When death occurs gradually, changes take place throughout the body and are evident in major body systems (Box 45-4). The changes reflect the incremental failure of each system. Assessment of these signs will help you provide appropriate information to families and determine plans of care for the terminally ill client.

BOX 45-4 *Physical Signs of Imminent Death*

Musculoskeletal System

- Generalized weakness and fatigue, with possible surges of energy
- Loss of overall muscle tone and general weakness; a lack of active, independent mobility and an inability to maintain positioning without support
- Relaxed facial muscles, resulting in a sagging jaw and flaccid lips and cheeks
- Bladder and bowel incontinence
- Decreased gag reflex and difficulty swallowing

Gastrointestinal System

- Anorexia and decreased oral intake
- Decreased or lack of swallow reflex
- Dehydration, as evidenced by dry oral mucous membranes and low-grade fever
- Decreased peristalsis, as evidenced by decreased nausea, abdominal distention, and constipation
- Possible diarrhea

Continued

BOX 45-4 *Physical Signs of Imminent Death—cont'd*

Cardiovascular System
- Alterations in vital signs
- Decreased peripheral circulation
- Extremities begin to appear cyanotic and mottled and become cool, cold, or clammy
- May perspire and/or run a fever
- Poor skin turgor
- Edema
- Reduced rate of absorption of medications from tissues
- Diminished kidney perfusion with decreased urine output

Respiratory System
- Altered patterns of respiration, such as slow, labored, irregular, or Cheyne-Stokes pattern
- Increased secretions, adventitious bubbling lung sounds or "death rattle"
- Irritation of tracheobronchial airway, as evidenced by hiccups, chest pain, fatigue, or exhaustion
- Poor gas exchange, as evidenced by hypoxia, dyspnea, or cyanosis

Neurological System
- Altered levels of alertness
- Increased drowsiness, sleeping, and unresponsiveness
- Periods of mental cloudiness, confusion, delirium, or disorientation
- Possible agitation and restlessness
- Variable pain levels
- Possible blurred vision
- Diminished blink reflex with accumulation of secretions over eyes
- Dry conjunctiva
- Intact sense of hearing

BOX 45-5 *Nursing Diagnoses Relevant to Psychosocial Support*

Defensive Coping
- Related to projection of blame or responsibility
- Related to altered family dynamics

Ineffective Coping
- Related to inappropriate implementation of coping strategies
- Related to difficulty expressing emotions (especially anger, guilt, and fear)
- Related to giving up hope and spiritual values

Ineffective Denial
- Related to feelings of increased stress or anxiety
- Related to fear of death, pain, loss of autonomy, separation
- Related to feelings of omnipotence

Social Isolation
- Related to infrequent visits by family, friends, or both

Impaired Social Interaction
- Related to visitors' discomfort about terminal illness

Spiritual Distress
- Related to challenges to belief system
- Related to separation from faith community of support and rituals

DIAGNOSIS

Grieving is a useful diagnosis when working with families and clients as they face medical tests and treatments that could change their lives. Anticipating life changes and possible death can trigger many other, more specific nursing diagnoses as well (Box 45-5). Assess the client and family thoroughly for risk factors and current status to help differentiate between the diagnosis of *Grieving* and other diagnostic labels.

You will use the diagnosis *Complicated grieving* less frequently, but you still must assess and be vigilant about the possible development of this problem. Thanatologists differentiate normal from complicated grief with the following comparison. **Normal grief** is characterized by painful dejection, loss of interest, and inhibition of activities. Complicated grief goes further and adds episodes of panic, hostility toward self, regression to narcissistic self-preoccupation, and signs of deflated self-esteem. The overwhelmed person may use maladaptive coping methods; however, the primary indicator is the inability to use coping methods that would facilitate development of a new self-concept that integrates the reality of the loss and its unique meanings.

A clear understanding of the definitions and defining characteristics of all relevant nursing diagnoses will help you use them accurately when planning care for dying clients and their families. The decision tree in Figure 45-4 will help you distinguish between diagnoses that specifically address grief.

PLANNING

Planning care for a terminally ill client requires you to address widely varying responses from both client and family. You must recognize that you are really caring for two clients: the dying person and the immediate family unit. These two clients have different needs and require separate planning. You can consider anticipatory grief and normal grief together when planning supportive

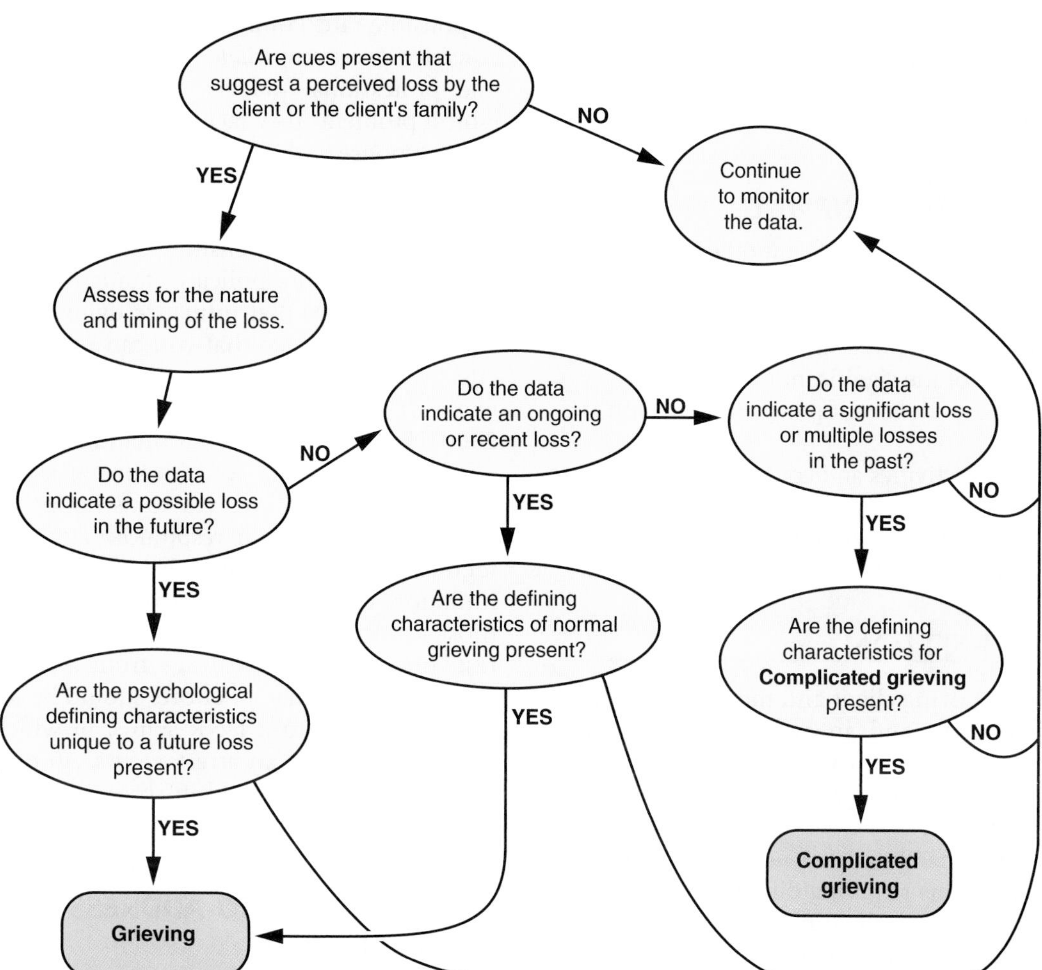

FIGURE 45-4 Decision tree for loss and grieving nursing diagnoses. Diagnoses are shown in rectangles. Within these rectangles, diagnoses shown in **bold** type are NANDA International (NANDA-I)–approved nursing diagnoses; diagnoses shown in regular type are not NANDA-I–approved nursing diagnoses.

interventions for clients and families, because of the similarity in responses.

At some point in the course of the client's disease, the goal of treatment will shift from curative to palliative. Everyone involved in planning the client's treatment must accept this shift. It may be difficult for both the health care team and the family, but it is crucial to recognize when further treatment becomes futile. At that point, comfort priorities become appropriate and will significantly improve the quality of the remaining time, both for the client and for family members.

For many dying clients, you will need to plan daily for the client's care. Be open with the client and family about care goals, and share your expected outcomes with them. Establish priorities for the dying client on the basis of the physical manifestations of the dying process and the accompanying psychosocial needs. Make care goals realistic, accommodating of the client's and the family's perspectives, and make the goals flexible so that they can change as the client's condition changes.

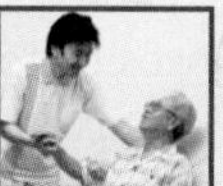

In the past 72 hours, Mr. Hashimoto has had visits with his son to discuss financial affairs and has privately discussed with his son his view that, although he considers himself an American, he would still like to have some Buddhist rituals performed for the benefit of the family and Japanese American friends. The parish priest has visited the client twice and has assured the family that church members have been praying for Mr. Hashimoto and his family. He also says that he will try to accommodate any special requests they may have during this time.

Mrs. Hashimoto and both daughters have arranged their time to make sure someone has always been at the bedside during the client's hospitalization. He has chosen to be treated with comfort measures only, and arrangements have been made for discharge with home health care. He is being transported by ambulance to his home today.

EXPECTED OUTCOMES FOR *GRIEVING*

When the client is dying and the grief process is in anticipation of the loss of the person's own life, the following are examples of expected outcomes:

- Remembrance of satisfying lifetime memories

- Completion of meaningful goals
- Participation in decision making
- Satisfaction that affairs are in order
- Death with dignity

EXPECTED OUTCOMES FOR *COMPLICATED GRIEVING*

When the client has lost a significant other, the expected outcomes are highly individualized. Some examples of expected outcomes are the following:

- Reports a decrease in physical symptoms associated with memories of the significant other
- Reports fewer experiences of preoccupation with the loss
- Increases social activities and contacts with support systems
- Reports plans for the future or intends to engage in future-oriented activities

INTERVENTION

Nursing care of a dying client and the family demands sensitivity, creativity, and an awareness of common grief responses. Remember to consider the client's and the family's cultural background as you encounter these responses.

Also remember that the client's needs and the family's needs may differ, thus requiring differing interventions. Use interventions that are tailored to support both the client and the family; this will allow you to provide excellent nursing care during the client's last days. Supportive interventions will continue for family members after the client's death. It is much more difficult for a grieving person to achieve a healthy, satisfactory, comfortable conclusion to a loss when appropriate support is not received.

Whether for physical or psychological responses or to meet ethical and legal interests, any supportive interventions must be based on a clear understanding of the grief process. If you have a narrow view of what constitutes grief, you may have trouble designing and offering the appropriate interventions to facilitate client and family coping. Your personal attitudes about death, dying, and expressions of grief are also pivotal factors. If you are uncomfortable facing the reality of your own future death, you will find it difficult to provide support to others facing these same circumstances and issues.

INTERVENTIONS FOR ETHICAL AND LEGAL ADVOCACY

Medicine and client care have been tremendously influenced by technology that can extend life or prolong dying. Because of these advances, concerns have arisen among health care professionals about withdrawing or withholding treatments, using heroic measures at the end of life, allocating scarce resources, and providing responsible care. Polling evidence has shown that nurses consider *do not resuscitate* (DNR) orders, clients' rights, and professional practice issues the most important ethical problems they face in their daily practice.

In response to these concerns, ethics committees have developed policies on resuscitation, advance directives, withdrawal of artificial nutrition and fluids, organ donation, and many other sensitive issues. You must be familiar with legislation, policies, standards of practice, and ethical dilemmas that influence dying clients, families, and professionals, so that you can offer support that is effective and within accepted legal and ethical frameworks (Dobbins, 2005; Forbes, Bern-Klug, & Gessert, 2000). For more specific information, see Chapter 2.

One major area of concern for nurses, dying clients, and their families involves resuscitation efforts if the client has a cardiac or respiratory arrest. **Code status** identifies the physician orders for a client regarding initiation of resuscitative actions, and the extent of those actions, at the time of a cardiac or respiratory arrest. Interventions can range from a full code status, which indicates that all efforts should be used to resuscitate a person, to a DNR status, in which no action should be taken if an arrest occurs. An out-of-hospital DNR order is being used in some states to help guide emergency personnel when caring for a dying client who is not in an acute care-hospital setting.

INTERVENTIONS TO ADDRESS PHYSICAL NEEDS

The physical needs of a dying client depend in part on the course and effects of the particular disease. You will need to assess the client's condition routinely and provide physical care to manage these effects as the client's body systems gradually slow down.

Comfort care remains a high priority throughout the dying client's care. Pain control commonly tops the list and should involve both pharmacological and nonpharmacological interventions. The end of a person's life is not the time to delay or withhold narcotic analgesics out of fear of addiction. Also, avoid making judgments about the nature and extent of the client's expressions of pain, because this only delays pain management. Relaxation, distraction, and antianxiety actions should be used to complement and enhance drug therapy. Efforts to reduce emotional tension have been recognized as contributing to physical relaxation and reduction of perceived pain levels.

Interest in and concerns about the comfort of dying clients and other end-of-life issues continue to be the subject of research (Meijburg, 2005; SUPPORT Group, 1995). Many studies focus on withdrawal or withholding of artificial nutrition (tube feeding) and intravenous hydration. The findings repeatedly conclude that prolonged efforts to maintain hydration actually run counter to comfort promotion (Amella, Lawrence, & Gresle, 2005; Post, 2001).

Dealing With Dehydration. The problem underlying the hydration dilemma is the emotional response of the family to starvation and dehydration. Remember, however, that physiology changes in the dying client. Several studies have found that dehydrated dying clients rarely complain of thirst. Other studies reported that many dying people felt no thirst or only slight thirst. This level of thirst can be managed with small sips of water and by moistening the oral mucous membranes during oral care.

The advantages of dehydration in the dying client are many. Decreased urine production means less need for a bedpan, commode, urinal, or catheter. It also reduces incontinence. Decreasing gastrointestinal fluid decreases nausea and vomiting and reduces the need for tubes and suctioning to decompress the bowel. The decrease in respiratory secretions relieves congestion and coughing. Reduced pharyngeal secretions may enhance swallowing while decreasing choking and the sensation of drowning.

Also, the azotemia that contributes to the onset of coma is believed to provide a natural anesthesia and some measure of analgesia, possibly associated with increased production of a natural opioid. The need for narcotics and their risks and side effects can thus be reduced.

Despite what many believe, pain and suffering are not automatic sequelae of dehydration. Studies reflect a high comfort level in severely dehydrated persons nearing death. Many hospice staff believe the natural dehydration that comes with dying is not cruel but palliative and compassionate.

The timing for withdrawal of hydration modalities must be examined carefully. For many clients not yet in the end stage of their disease, correction of fluid and electrolyte imbalances may stabilize their condition, reverse some symptoms, and possibly prolong life. Collaborating with the physician can help you maintain an appropriate critical analysis of the timing and benefits of continuing or withdrawing fluids. Your responsibility in this arena is as client advocate and a resource to the family. Provide them with factual information, and help them converse openly with the client's physician.

Providing Comfort Measures. Families interpret physical care of their loved one as a reflection of the respect given by those implementing the care. Attention to the comfort and dignity of the dying client conveys that respect clearly and will be remembered by the family long after the death (Ufema, 2006).

Nursing care provided routinely for other clients, such as complete bathing, full linen changes, and turning schedules, may need to be reprioritized for the dying client. Maximizing the dying client's comfort may mean leaving the client undisturbed in a comfortable position for longer than usual. Expected outcomes for the dying client no longer focus on skin integrity and prevention of infection through baths, linen changes, and repositioning but shift instead to fostering dignity, providing comfort, and ensuring uninterrupted time with the family.

This change in priorities for routine tasks may be difficult for you at first. Do your best to maintain a realistic appraisal of the client's and the family's end-of-life concerns and needs. Doing so will help you alter the elements of physical care as needed and thus provide for a more individualized and humane death.

INTERVENTIONS TO PROVIDE PSYCHOSOCIAL SUPPORT

Interventions that support the psychosocial needs of client and family stem from recognizing their feelings and emotions. Grief has a tremendous psychological impact. Keep in mind that cultural factors may influence a person's displays of emotion. Society may impose expectations on a person's displays of grief as well, possibly adding the burdens of shame and guilt to a visibly grieving person.

For you, identification of underlying emotions becomes an important assessment activity. Do not assume that obvious behaviors and comments represent all of the feelings being experienced. Emotions can be varied and unpredictable, manifested in different ways throughout the grief period. To help the client and family navigate this period, do your best to use therapeutic communication and help them manage their denial, anger, and spiritual distress.

Promoting Therapeutic Communication. Loss, death, and grief create surprising, conflicting, confusing, often overwhelming emotions. The freedom to express these emotions and to be supported during that expression is pivotal to managing grief successfully. You will need to use therapeutic communication strategies with both the client and the family members to help them cope.

Communicating With a Dying Client. Communicating with a dying client involves personal risks. You will undoubtedly feel uncomfortable emotions and possibly unpleasant memories. You may feel inadequate to discuss your client's serious questions—questions for which you have only incomplete answers at best.

A primary mechanism for supporting dying people is to "be there." Support, in this context, means allowing time when the avenues of communication are open. When you are trusted with personal reactions and feelings, you are invited into a private area that should be honored (Box 45-6).

Elisabeth Kübler-Ross identifies three "languages" used by dying persons: plain English, symbolic nonverbal language, and symbolic verbal language. By plain English, she means conscious, direct articulation of thoughts, feelings, questions, and fears.

In symbolic nonverbal language, concerns, thoughts, and needs are revealed through overt behavior. Needs are communicated through frequent requests of staff, projection of anger, or asking of peripheral questions. These behaviors secure attention but fail to clearly express real needs.

The clients who most need support and attention use symbolic verbal language. The meaning of the message is hidden behind symbols. For example, a client facing extensive testing for cancer may tell a story about a pet that had to be "put to sleep" after a long illness. Symbolic language can also be used when a person seeks validation of self-worth in comments such as "I don't know why you spend so much time on me. There are others who need you so much more." Such statements may arise when the client's physical condition deteriorates and unpleasant sights and odors develop. Caregivers who are attuned to such communication techniques will be able to sense the implied fears and concerns underlying the statements.

Many factors can block your communication with a dying client and the family. If you seem emotionally detached, they may interpret your attitude as a lack of interest or a lack of empathy. Avoiding direct discussion of sensitive topics wastes opportunities for constructive exchanges and may create confusion. Misunderstanding can block communication as well; avoid using euphe-

BOX 45-6 *Communicating With a Dying Client*

PROVIDE FOR PRIVACY

For a client to openly share personal, intimate feelings with you, you must provide privacy. Consider moving to the chapel, asking visitors to leave for a while, or tell the client that you will return when visitors are gone. If the client is in a semiprivate room, draw the dividing curtain and sit close to the bed so the client can talk softly without worrying about being overheard.

LET THE CLIENT SET THE AGENDA

Allow the client to decide when, where, and to whom he will communicate. Do not try to force conversations or direct the topics of conversations. If you are doing most of the talking, you are thwarting the goals of therapeutic communication. Try not to worry that you have failed if a dying client chooses not to confide in you. Remember that not every client will find such conversations helpful. You need only convey a willingness to listen.

AVOID CLICHÉS

Clichés, platitudes, and pat answers are patronizing and discount the uniqueness of the client's situation and the magnitude of the fears or concerns. Avoid such phrases as "I know how you feel," "Don't worry about that now," or even "Everything will be all right." They minimize clients' feelings, fears, and beliefs and will undermine their trust in you.

GIVE ACCURATE, HONEST ANSWERS

If you do not know an answer, say so. Then find the answer, and get back to the person. Do not try to spare clients' feelings by avoiding unpleasant truths; doing so will undermine their trust in you and waste valuable communication time with game playing. Use other health care team members, such as the physician or social worker, to contribute facts to discussions as needed.

CONVEY NONJUDGMENTAL ACCEPTANCE

Leave all personal opinions, judgments, and beliefs out of fact-based discussions so clients can make their own decisions. Convey your acceptance of these decisions with such phrases as "That must be important to you" or "What do you think?" Phrases that reflect your awareness of what the client is coping with might include something like "I imagine that this is hard for you." This example does not presume to know how the person feels but acknowledges a perception of something reasonable under the circumstances. The client is then free to contradict or confirm your empathetic guess. Be alert to the values and beliefs of the client and family, and avoid talking about what you would do if you were in their place.

USE OPEN-ENDED RESPONSES

Open-ended sentences or questions offer opportunities to talk without limiting the client's responses. By using phrases such as "How do you feel about that?" or "What other things are you thinking about?" you allow the client to direct the conversation. Closed-ended statements (such as "Are you afraid of dying?" or "Will you be able to talk to your family about this?") restrict the client's answers.

Use closed-ended questions when you need to gather specific information, to clarify a client's comments, to encourage an anxious or uncommunicative client to talk, to focus the client on a specific point, or to move the conversation from a deep level to a more superficial one (as when closing an interview).

PROVIDE ADEQUATE RESPONSE TIME

A guaranteed way to stifle communication and make your client frustrated and angry is to ask a question and not wait long enough for the answer. This gaffe also leaves you with incomplete assessment data. If you are uneasy waiting for an answer, you are probably uncomfortable with silence. You also may not be recognizing factors that naturally lengthen the dying client's response time. As the client becomes weaker and more easily fatigued, even talking can be an effort. Take time to analyze why you have trouble waiting for adequate responses; then take steps to remedy the problem.

USE SILENCE EFFECTIVELY

Silence can be intimidating if you are unaware of its importance as a communication tool. Too many nurses try to fill periods of silence because they believe them to be an opening to speak. Unfortunately, this tactic can simply cut off or impede the client's communication. Silence can convey acceptance and support, give the client time to gather his or her thoughts, and prompt further discussion. An occasional nod or a single-syllable word can fill some periods of silence and convey that the client still has your attention.

On the other hand, too much silence can produce anxiety and may be interpreted as inattention or lack of interest. Maintain eye contact, and sit quietly during periods of silence. Stay alert for nonverbal cues to messages behind the silence. For example, silence may precede crying. Breaking eye contact with silence may reveal the client's embarrassment or insecurity about something he just said. Sensitivity and awareness of the power of silence can help you build relationships and promote the exchange of even sensitive, intimate thoughts.

CONVEY CARING THROUGH TOUCH

In general, clients give nurses permission to touch them in ways not offered to other acquaintances. Thus touch offers you a special avenue by which to convey caring and acceptance.

As a person dies, he or she may become less physically responsive. The person's condition may make the person's friends, even his or her family, uncomfortable. Visitors may become less frequent. It is therefore even more meaningful when you hold the person's hand, stroke his or her back or cheek, or touch the person's shoulder or arm.

When touch does not cause pain and is used to provide physical care or communicate with the client, it confirms your acceptance of the client and symbolically acknowledges the difficult path he or she is traveling. For confused or disoriented clients, touch can serve to help them maintain reality and confirm they are not alone.

misms, medical terms, analogies, and vague terms, such as *passed on* or *lost* instead of *dying* or *died*. Communication can also be blocked if the staff minimizes or overlooks pain, indignity, fear, or unresolved personal issues.

Effective communication requires that you explore beyond the obvious and seek the hidden elements of behaviors and complaints. Sensitivity, astuteness, and empathy are integral elements that enhance and improve psychosocial support.

Communicating With the Family. The grieving family requires many of the same communication approaches used for the client. Be sensitive to the family's emotions, behaviors, and physical reactions to loss and grief while applying nursing interventions that promote their grief work. Remember that you will have significant influence on the family. Indeed, because they will see you as both a resource and an authority at this time of crisis, your comments will carry tremendous credibility and importance.

Choose your words carefully when talking with family members. Recognize that certain statements may be helpful, whereas others may be harmful (Box 45-7). Remember that families may remember your words, and the decisions your words encouraged, for years after a client's death. Your behaviors and responses will permanently color their memories of the events surrounding their loved one's death. Because of their trust in you and the important role you play in their daily life during this time, therapeutic communication is crucial.

In general, statements that diminish the uniqueness of grief and loss are perceived as not helpful. When you say something like "I understand how you feel," you intimate that grief and loss can be reduced to a common denominator, making one person the same as the next. Statements that criticize grief responses or the feelings of grievers or that dictate appropriate grief responses, such as telling someone to cry, are also not helpful. Finally, attempts to rationalize a loss on the basis of your priorities and alternatives may anger family members and harm their relationship with you. Phrases such as "You wouldn't want him to continue living in this condition" are likely to be met with clear messages that the family would indeed want to keep their loved one in any condition because they love him and do not want to lose him.

You must be mindful of the hidden messages that can be transmitted through seemingly harmless phrases. No one intends to be callous and detrimental to the grief processes. However, forgetting to convey nonjudgmental acceptance of grief can impair your relationship with a client and the family at a time when they need you the most.

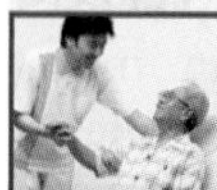

Mr. Hashimoto has been at home 2 weeks and currently is being visited only twice a week by a registered nurse who performs an assessment and confers with Mrs. Hashimoto about care needs. Mrs. Hashimoto has continued her efforts to keep the household intact and has turned to her eldest daughter for advice regarding her husband's immediate care. She also provides most of his physical care while depending on her daughter for support and guidance. She does not communicate with the home health care nurse but has her daughter do this instead. Can you think of anything the home health care nurse can do to facilitate communication with more members of the Hashimoto family? How can the nurse determine the family's needs?

BOX 45-7 ***Facilitative and Nonfacilitative Helping Statements***

Facilitative Helping Statements

- Come be with us now.
- You must be (angry, frustrated, sad, confused, etc.) right now.
- You're being strong.
- It must be hard to accept.
- It's okay to be angry at God.
- Tell me about him.
- You must have been close to him.
- Tell me how you're feeling.
- How can I be of help?
- It's all right to let yourself grieve.
- People really cared for him.
- I'm thinking of/praying for you.

Nonfacilitative Helping Statements

- He (God) had a purpose. It's God's will.
- You wouldn't want to have them back in the condition they were.
- Be thankful you have another (son, parent, child, etc.).
- I know how you feel.
- Time makes it easier.
- You shouldn't question God's will.
- Try not to think about it because it will only upset you.
- You have to get on with your life.
- Everyone has to die sometime.
- You're not the only one who suffers.
- That's over now. Let's not deal with it.
- The living must go on.
- It's too soon to (date, clean out closets, give away deceased's possessions, take a vacation, etc.).

Managing Denial. Denial is a common psychological response for both client and family. Because denial is a protective function, you should support it while the impact of facts and reality comes to the client's and the family's consciousness. Confronting denial directly is neither therapeutic nor effective (Box 45-8). It only increases anxiety and produces more denial. It can also undermine your relationship with the client and family by destroying their trust and removing you from the circle of people with whom they will confide honest feelings.

Sometimes you may become frustrated and concerned that you are being manipulated while caring for a client who is in denial. If you allow yourself these feelings, however, you run the risk of displaying harmful judgmental attitudes and projecting blame onto the client. Do your best to recognize such feelings before they compromise your care or your relationship with the client. Use techniques known to facilitate honest communication without creating a risk of psychological harm to the client during periods of denial.

Managing Anger. If it is not addressed, the anger that arises during grief can become deeply entrenched and interfere with successful grief work. It is rare for a person to have no anger during the grief process. In fact, nurses commonly bear the brunt of this anger. To keep from becoming personally distressed over misplaced anger, consider the situation from this perspective: Clients and family members who speak out in anger tend to think that your professional knowledge will keep you from taking it personally. Consider it a compliment to your professionalism and skill, and try to avoid the defensiveness that you as the caretaker may feel in such situations. Use sound communication techniques to help clients and families manage their anger appropriately (Box 45-9).

Managing Spiritual Distress. A holistic view perceives each person as a balance of mind, body, and spirit. Each dimension affects and is affected by the other. The spiritual element is the spirit, or the soul, as distinguished from the body or material matters. Each person has this spirituality. It is different from religious affiliation or beliefs.

It is important for you, as a nurse, to support your clients' spirituality. This action is grounded in your respect for each person's beliefs, values, and practices. Facilitating the expression of those beliefs is an important intervention, and it both validates your acceptance and helps the client engage coping mechanisms tied to spiritual beliefs. Members of your facility's pastoral care department are integral to this process and can draw on community-wide resources, as well as those within the institution, to meet specific needs (Figure 45-5).

During the period of dying and grieving, clients and families may experience spiritual distress. You can use particular communication skills to help them cope within their own spiritual beliefs (Box 45-10). Spiritual reactions to dying and death vary widely, just as other emotions do. Many people become angry at God or a higher being because of the perceived unjustness of death. Even people who have practiced their beliefs and doctrines faithfully for a lifetime may question how God could allow such unfairness, especially in a distressing death or one that involves a young person.

For others, death completes a cycle that is explained and justified by their faith. Death does not test their beliefs; rather, it validates their faith. Findings have suggested that belief in God seemed to reduce levels of depression and hopelessness, although the degree of Christian knowledge or depth of commitment to Christian beliefs did not.

INTERVENTIONS TO PROMOTE HEALTHY GRIEVING

Your interventions for a grieving person will not be strictly divided by the stage of the person's grief. In general, however, certain types of interventions do provide the most benefit within certain times in the process.

BOX 45-8 *Guidelines for Managing Denial*

RESPECT EXPRESSIONS OF DENIAL

Expressions of denial help to protect a person who must adjust to unpleasant or horrifying news. Even when the person uses selective attention or deception, the goal is to protect the self or others. Respect this phase of the grief process by not challenging the person or making him "face reality."

However, do not lie to foster the denial. You must be honest; hearing the truth will not harm the grieving person. Also, avoid reinforcing denial by agreeing with it. Continue to express truthful facts, and avoid perpetuating denial-induced thinking. When conversing, continue to provide reality-based information that is accurate and current. Correct misinformation in a nonconfrontational manner (Jeffrey, 2001-2002).

USE ALTERNATIVE APPROACHES TO AVOID DIRECT CONFRONTATION

Using a "back door" approach can help a client focus on issues that provoke little anxiety while the client processes higher-anxiety issues. Another technique derived from the assertiveness literature is called fogging or agreeing with the truth. To use this strategy, agree with the part of the denial that reflects reality. For example, say something like "It sounds like you're not sure the test results are accurate" rather than a confrontational statement such as "The test results are accurate, or your doctor wouldn't have told you they were" (Forchuk & Westwell, 1987).

RECOGNIZE AND ACKNOWLEDGE HOPES AND WISHES

As a defense mechanism, denial reflects a desire that the truth not be true.

You can validate the underlying yearning while not reinforcing the denial.

Phrases such as "It would be wonderful if that happened" or "I wish it wasn't true too" leave the client's hope intact without suggesting that the hoped-for event will occur.

ENCOURAGE DISCUSSION OF FEELINGS, CONCERNS, AND FEARS

Talking with clients helps them process information intellectually, validates legitimate fears and concerns, and reinforces their sense of being supported during this stressful period. Sitting at eye level with clients rather than standing creates an atmosphere of conversation rather than of hurried exchanges. Actively listen with undivided attention, allowing the clients to do most of the talking. Remember that touch conveys attention and concern.

PROVIDE SMALL AMOUNTS OF INFORMATION AT A TIME

Stress and denial block the conscious processing of information, so give a client smaller fragments of information at a time. These smaller amounts will be better understood and accepted. Encourage questions and open conversations to clarify and confirm facts. Encourage and facilitate decision making, beginning with self-care and progressing to treatment choices when reality has replaced denial.

From Forchuk, C., & Westwell, J. (1987). Denial. *Journal of Psychosocial Nursing, 25*(6), 9-13; Jeffrey, J. C. (2006-2007). *Course guide for death and dying* (unpublished). Austin, TX: Austin Community College.

Recognition: Shock and Denial. The most important intervention during this phase of grief may be your presence. The events often create a feeling of unreality, and your presence can stabilize the situation. Reinforce the reality of events despite the client's denial. Remember that shock and numbness compromise people's critical thinking, so you will need to let them make decisions at a rate they can fully comprehend. Help to facilitate necessary decisions by clarifying the person's options and sources of assistance. Give small amounts of information at a time, and repeat the information until you know the client has understood it. Encourage questions, and be prepared to repeat answers when the person's memory is fragmented.

Allow the client to cry, and use silence supportively while the client expresses emotions or gathers thoughts. Allow the griever to direct the course of discussions. Stay with bereaved people who are clearly shocked, dazed, hostile, or combative when faced with news of a loss. Activate appropriate resources as needed from nursing administration or the pastoral care department. Box 45-11 offers hints about breaking bad news to family or client.

Reflection: Physical, Emotional, and Spiritual Suffering. Again, your presence is crucial. Acknowledge the client's and the family's grief, and accept the validity and intensity of that grief. Continue to use touch (see Box 45-6) and effective listening skills. Listen more than you talk, and ask for clarification when necessary. Make no assumptions.

Adapt your teaching strategies to accommodate any symptoms of depression. Explain any equipment being used, procedures needed, and care options. Allow family members to help with the client's care as much or as little as they desire. Foster a sense of control and collaboration about decisions. Develop plans of care with their input. Gain trust through honesty and by keeping any promises you make.

Watch for evidence of caregiver role strain and physical stressors on family members who spend a lot of time with the dying person. If possible, provide alternatives or breaks from the bedside vigil. Look beyond overt anger to determine its roots. Act as an advocate to help the client and family navigate the health care system, and facilitate physician and client or family conferences.

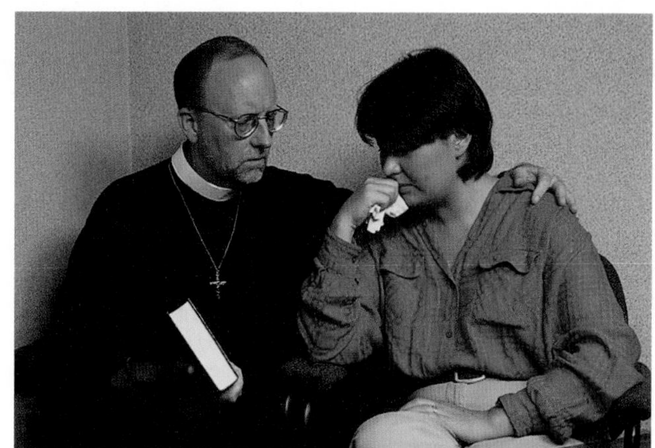

FIGURE 45-5 Members of the pastoral care department are integral team members in the care of people experiencing loss.

BOX 45-9 *Guidelines for Managing Anger*

Recognize the Roots of Anger

Unresolved issues and feelings of frustration, resentment, powerlessness, confusion, fear, and guilt can be the basis for anger. Such emotions may not be apparent to the person who holds them, because they are integrated in the complex emotional upheaval of grief. In some people, the anger is buried and unrecognizable. In others, anger displaced from past events may surface within the context of present situations. You will need to keep your focus while identifying the real issues behind a person's anger and exploring possible solutions.

Respond to the Sources of Anger, Not the Anger Itself

Confronting a client about expressions of anger places the two of you in adversarial roles and may force the client to become defensive. This problem will harm the nurse-client relationship needed for therapeutic interactions to take place. Instead, use such statements as "This must be frustrating for you" or "I imagine I'd be scared if I were in your place" to convey your intuitive understanding of the real reason for the anger. Doing so may help the client open up rather than making the client defensive and closed.

When conveying intuitive understanding, avoid statements that could patronize or presume to speak for the client. Instead, simply indicate an astute perception of what might be going on in the dynamics of grief for this client. The client should feel free to clarify the accuracy–or inaccuracy–of your perception.

Acknowledge the Emotions Behind Rhetorical Questions

Questions such as "Why me?" and "Why did God let this happen?" cannot be answered, and you should not try. Simply recognize that the client is conveying frustration and anger that life is not fair and that the client is unprepared for the reality of his or her mortality.

Set Limits on Inappropriate or Harmful Displays of Anger

Anger that threatens the safety and welfare of clients, staff, or visitors must be addressed in an immediate and forthright manner. Acknowledge the validity of the anger but make clear that certain expressions of anger are not acceptable. Help clients redirect their energy into more beneficial outlets, such as pounding a pillow or pad, strenuous physical activity, yelling, or talking about their feelings to a sympathetic listener.

Provide guidance and accurate information about advance directives and end-of-life decisions in understandable and nonjudgmental terms. Offer spiritual support in nonjudgmental ways as well. Meet the physical needs of the dying client, particularly comfort needs.

Redirection: Reorganization and Moving Forward. Still, your presence is crucial. Do not abandon or neglect the client. Answer call lights, and meet the person's physical needs promptly. Avoid the need for the client or family to request pain medications: deliver them exactly at the scheduled times.

Touch and talk to dying persons. Keep them informed of events and activities, particularly the approach or arrival of loved ones to the bedside. Remember that hearing seems to stay intact longer than the other senses; many clients will linger until family arrives if you tell them that family is on the way.

Avoid using euphemisms or vague terms. Instead, use clear words, such as *die* and *dead.* Act as a role model so family members will understand the importance and appropriateness of speaking to and touching the dying person. Otherwise, they may fear being intrusive or being perceived as silly.

Help family members make arrangements as necessary. Provide privacy for phone calls and, if desired, time alone with the client both before and after death. Call in clergy support when necessary. Crying with a family is acceptable in keeping with a caring and professional im-

BOX 45-10 *Guidelines for Support in Spiritual Distress*

- Provide time to listen to the person's concerns and feelings.
- Help the person explore current and past beliefs and spiritual experiences to help the person put this event into perspective.
- Contact the person's usual spiritual counselor or cleric, if one exists. Encourage visits from members of the client's faith community. If the client's personal cleric is not available, solicit help from the pastoral care chaplain in your facility.
- Provide an uninterrupted few moments for silent prayer, or pray with the person if appropriate. Read from religious material if the person desires it. Make necessary arrangements for important religious rituals, such as communion or anointing of the sick.
- Inform the client and family of available spiritual resources within the facility, such as the location of a meditation area or services held by pastoral care.
- Allow the client to continue to wear religious objects or clothing whenever possible and to keep religious mementos in view.
- At the time of death, allow the family to practice meaningful rituals. Leaving the body undisturbed for a time, saying special prayers over the body, turning the body to a specific direction, or covering the body with special cloths are important rituals for some. Many of these rituals are associated with beliefs about transmigration of the soul.

Data from Hirayama, K. K. (1990). Death and dying in Japanese culture. In J. K. Parry (Ed.), *Social work practice with the terminally ill: A transcultural perspective.* Springfield, IL: Charles C Thomas; McQuay, J. E. (1995). Cross-cultural customs and beliefs related to health crises, death, and organ donation/transplantation: A guide to assist health care professionals to understand different responses and provide cross-cultural assistance. *Critical Care Nursing Clinics of North America, 7*(3), 581-594.

BOX 45-11 *Breaking Bad News*

Generally, it is the physician who delivers unexpected bad news, but occasionally nurses need to give families the news of a death. Accompany the physician who is approaching a family with unexpected or traumatic news, especially when it involves a death, and remain with the family after the physician leaves. When you must deliver bad news, use the following guidelines:

- Determine the relationship of family members to whom you will be talking and their role in the client's care and daily life. Be sensitive to cultural influences within family structure and roles. It is important to ascertain family dynamics so that the appropriate persons receive the information from a health professional.
- Plan your words ahead, organize your thoughts, and have all the facts and the answers to questions that can be predicted.
- Provide privacy, and establish rapport. If other team members have already developed such rapport, include them in the meeting with the family.
- Introduce yourself, and identify your role in the care of the client.
- Create an environment that allows time for the presentation of information and discussion of the meaning and consequences of the information. Turn off your pager or cell phone, sit down, maintain eye contact, and listen attentively.
- Determine what the family already knows, and what the individuals want to know. Do not make assumptions about the extent of information or details desired by family members.
- Use language that is unambiguous; avoid medical terms and acronyms. Use basic terms to discuss medical situations and interventions. Present information at a level commensurate with the educational level of the participating family members. Use medical personnel as interpreters, if needed, rather than having a family member interpret facts and medical information to other family members.
- Assess nonverbal body language and indicators of emotional status.
- Continually assess and reassess family members' understanding of information being presented and discussed. State information repeatedly until it is heard and understood by families who are in shock or numb from the related events.
- Bring in clergy who can support and remain with families after the formal discussion of facts has concluded, if the family desires. Seek nursing supervisor assistance when needed to further assist family members as indicated.
- Confirm that safe transportation is available when the family is ready to leave. Escort them out and up to the car in which they will drive away from the facility. A last measure of respect for the deceased person is conveyed when a staff member accompanies the family as they exit the place where a loved one has died.

age. Never allow yourself to cry so vigorously that the family must turn their energy to comforting you. Attend the funeral, if possible, when a close bond develops between you and the client or family. If you cannot attend the funeral, send a note of condolence.

Agency bereavement protocols should be initiated. Some nursing units maintain a file of client death dates with family names and addresses. Four notes are written at the time of death and signed by all the staff members who interacted with the client and family. These notes are then sent at intervals beginning the week of the death and again at 3, 6, and 12 months from the death date. Such follow-up has been shown to contribute to positive grief work in surviving family members (Fauri & Ettner, 2000).

CARE AT THE TIME OF DEATH

Many institutions no longer require staff to perform structured postmortem care before discharge to the mortuary. However, procedures implemented after death are based on the physiological aspects of dying and death, and most nursing actions are taken because of these specific changes in the body (Box 45-12).

Care of a person's body at the time of death should continue to convey the respect and emphasis on dignity that was evident during the dying process. Awareness of specific cultural practices or rituals further supports the family and facilitates the mourning that begins. These rituals may include specific handling of the body or the presence of clergy or faith leaders. Facilitate family transition into bereavement by allowing privacy and the opportunity to contact other family members. Offer to contact pastoral care support or a clergy of their choice. Recognize that critical thinking may be disrupted, and assess the need for assistance in making mortuary contact or handling other legal matters. Allow time for the family to spend with the body or to help with cleaning of the deceased, if desired. Remember that the memories associated with a death are lifelong, and you can be instrumental in helping create positive memories for the survivors.

INTERVENTIONS TO MAINTAIN YOURSELF AS A CAREGIVER

To maintain your function as a caregiver, you must take care of yourself physically and emotionally. Burnout is a significant risk in nursing, particularly among nurses who work frequently with dying clients. Make use of stress reduction techniques, exercise, and proper eating and sleeping patterns. Recognize and acknowledge the physical effects of the stressors of terminal care so you can care for yourself before burnout sets in. Reaffirm life, and counter the repetition of death by spending time with your own family and close friends.

You will need support from colleagues as well to help you deal with your grief for dying clients in your care (Figure 45-6). The old adage "If you can't take the heat,

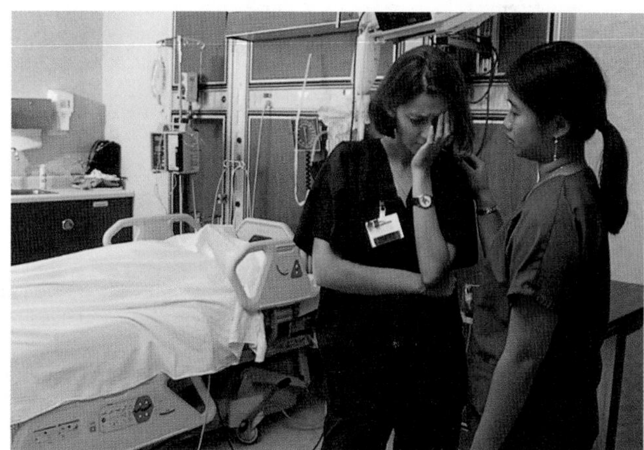

FIGURE 45-6 Collegial support can help nurses deal with their own grief over dying clients and their families.

BOX 45-12 *Guidelines for Postmortem Care*

- Identify legal issues associated with organ donation, autopsies, burial.
- Identify rituals, customs, or faith practices to be implemented at the time of death.
- Remove tubes, medical supplies, and equipment, unless this is contraindicated, as in situations requiring coroner clearance. Agency policy should dictate actions in such circumstance.
- Bathe and dress the body, or facilitate ritual cleaning if done by others.
- Place dressings over leaking wounds.
- Clean up any incontinence.
- Position the body in alignment, close the eyes, and insert dentures if possible. Rolling a towel under the chin may help to close the mouth. Rigor mortis occurs between 2 and 4 hours.
- Prepare the family for what they will see—for example, the coolness and appearance of the skin.
- Allow the family time with the body to say good-bye and initiate closure. Role-model touching the body. If desired, help the family collect a lock of hair as a keepsake. This may be the last time they can touch or hold the loved one before the mortuary takes the person away.
- Dispose of remaining medications according to agency policy and protocols.
- Document details regarding time of death, specific rituals rendered or physical care given to the body, family presence and nursing support extended, clergy or pastoral care presence, disposal of personal effects, and time of mortuary contact and release of body to the mortuary.
- Initiate any agency protocol for bereavement support and follow-up.

BOX 45-13

Nursing Care Plan

A Client With Terminal Cancer

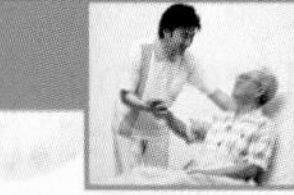

Home Health Care Data

Mr. Hashimoto has resumed meditation and the use of medicinal herbs to combat nausea and pain. He has openly discussed his prognosis with his son and daughters but minimally with the home health care nurse. Mrs. Hashimoto has refused to participate in these discussions, saying that she does not believe he is as sick as the doctors have told him.

The family priest has visited regularly and brought communion to Mr. Hashimoto and his wife and daughters. Further discussions have taken place between the priest and Mr. Hashimoto about his desire for cremation and the use of traditional Japanese-Buddhist mourning rituals after his death. The son has assumed the traditional family role of carrying out his father's wishes and making the necessary funeral arrangements.

Nursing Assessment

Physical: Alert, oriented ×3; skin warm, dry, and pale. Breath sounds diminished in lower lobes, with crackles heard on inspiration. Bowel sounds hypoactive in RUQ and RLQ; abdomen slightly distended and tender to palpation in RUQ. Last BM two days ago: small, formed, dark brown, guaiac-positive. Rates pain at 2/10, refuses Demerol. Vital signs: temperature 99.8° F, pulse 104, respirations 28 and shallow, BP 154/88.

Psychological: States that he can handle the discomfort, saying, "I don't want my wife to worry." His son explained his father's desires that traditional Buddhist rituals of body cleansing and purification rites be observed in preparation for the passage of death. They view this as complementary to Catholic death rituals, not counter to them.

NANDA-I Nursing Diagnosis	NOC Expected Outcomes With Indicators	NIC Interventions With Selected Activities	Evaluation Data
Grieving	***Grief Resolution***	***Grief Work Facilitation***	
Related Factor: • Recognized terminal status	• Client and family will discuss thoughts and feelings about impending death together.	• Allow opportunity for sharing: with the whole family together, individually, and in dyads; role-model open communication.	• Mr. Hashimoto spoke privately with each family member. He was able to tell his wife that he would die soon.
	• Client and family will maintain hope as part of the meaning of death.	• Offer time for meditation or prayer. Assist if needed.	• Meditates daily. Has communion twice a week from priest and from lay Eucharistic minister.
	• Client and family will engage in spiritual activities, both formally with the priest and informally in private.	• Contact priest if requested. Help the family identify when death is near, so that the priest can be called.	• Has not asked for additional visits from priest.
	• Client and family will share expectations and concerns for the future.	• Initiate conversation with husband and wife individually to determine expectations for the future.	• Mrs. Hashimoto shared her future plans; was able to admit that her husband was dying.
		• Facilitate a conservation between them, if appropriate, using therapeutic communication.	• Mr. Hashimoto is reluctant to talk to the nurse about his feelings; says he has provided well for his wife. Open-ended sentences met with no response.

Critical Thinking Questions

1. How would your feelings and beliefs about death affect your care for this family?
2. Mrs. Hashimoto has refused to participate in these discussions and seems to be in denial. What would your nursing interventions be for her?
3. What types of nursing interventions would indicate that you were giving culturally relevant care to this family?

Nursing outcome and intervention labels from Johnson, M., Bulechek, G., Butcher, H., Dochterman, J. M., Maas, M., Moorhead, S., et al. (Eds.). (2006). *NANDA, NOC, and NIC linkages: Nursing diagnoses, outcomes, & interventions.* St. Louis, MO: Mosby.

get out of the kitchen" has no place in the context of terminal care. Condemnation by other nurses or health care team members about attachments and feelings for clients in your care is detrimental both to you and to team dynamics.

Humor needs to be incorporated into daily activities whenever possible. However, it is inappropriate to allow the dark humor often used in health care settings to take place around clients and families. Dark humor or jokes about death can help to reduce stress for professional caregivers, but it is inappropriate and unhelpful for people outside the health care team. General humor can be therapeutic when used within appropriate limits. Some units have an area called the humor center with cartoons, fun reading, and brief humorous or whimsical stories. Laughter is good for both physical and emotional health, and it should be encouraged within the professional setting.

EVALUATION

Evaluation is ongoing throughout your care for a dying client and the client's family. Interventions provided for physical changes, comfort, and psychological support require continuous assessment and evaluation. Compare and analyze these interventions in relation to the client goals you established, and modify the plan of care as needed. Make your nursing approaches individualized and specific. Use your evaluation to help deliver care that focuses on the person rather than on the disease process (Box 45-13).

Your evaluation will also encompass nursing goals. These goals are not included in the formal plan of care, but they do help to motivate your nursing care for a terminal client and the family. Nursing goals include establishing a relationship of trust and confidence between you and the client and family, which you must continually reevaluate to maintain the therapeutic relationship so crucial for this arena of nursing care. The client and family must feel that you and other nursing staff are supporting them and providing the highest quality of care possible to the dying loved one.

The hospice nurse visits the Hashimoto family shortly after the death of Mr. Hashimoto. She documents the visit as shown below.

Sample Documentation Note for the Hashimoto Family

Visited with Mrs. Hashimoto and one daughter. They talked with affection for Mr. Hashimoto and described his last hours in detail. Mrs. Hashimoto described the funeral as being "exactly the way he had planned it." Both women said the support from hospice had made the last months of his life "easier for all of the family."

▼ KEY PRINCIPLES

- Grief is a normal response to loss, whether the loss is a person, an object, or something less tangible.
- The responses that are characteristic of grief are predictable, patterned behaviors, and they are also highly individual.
- Grief has its own time and agenda based on the person involved and the loss experienced.
- Grief is neither linear nor finite. A person can express grief responses in any order, may never have some responses, and may return over and over to a response.
- Projected anger or other feelings caused by the loss of a loved one may be misdirected at nurses. Your recognition of the real source of anger is helpful both to you and to the griever.
- It is not a requirement that the dying person reach the stage of accepting death.
- Families and friends of the dying person typically need help in maintaining a relationship with the dying person and confronting the impending death.
- Care in the last hours of life is usually directed at maintaining comfort for the dying person and helping the family say good-bye.
- The most important concept in caring for a dying or grieving person is that of presence.
- Complicated grieving indicates a person's inability to successfully resume life while still holding memories of the deceased.

■ REVIEW QUESTIONS

1. The phase of "reflection" primarily allows the grieving person to do what?

1. Plan the rituals associated with death and burial in the traditions of the deceased and survivor
2. Realistically perceive both positive and negative characteristics of the deceased
3. Make life changes that will promote future life activities without the deceased
4. Acknowledge the real impact of the death on both present and future life of the survivor

2. Which of the following would be **most likely** to contribute to a survivor's disenfranchised grieving?

1. Encountering complex legal arrangements for the burial of the deceased
2. Being allowed by nursing staff to spend time with the deceased
3. Having friends avoid contact because of judgments about the death of the deceased
4. Failure to be included in the last will and testament of the deceased

3. The bereaved adult daughter tells you that she has clearly smelled her deceased father's favorite aftershave scent as she sat in church recently. She questions that she might be "going crazy." You explain to her she is experiencing:

1. Intrusive memories
2. Sense of presence
3. Complicated grief
4. Grief attacks

Continued

4. Which physiological indicator of an active dying process would be used by the nurse to minimize use of intramuscular injections for pain and go to more direct administration with an intravenous or transdermal route?

1. Reduced peripheral circulation
2. Cheyne-Stokes breathing pattern
3. Diminished swallow reflex
4. Low urinary output secondary to kidney failure

5. When the respiratory system is shutting down during the dying process, which assessment finding is **most** reflective of *Ineffective airway clearance* as a stem for a nursing diagnosis?

1. Secretion accumulation in the lungs, sometimes called "death rattle"
2. Sluggish capillary refill and cyanotic nail beds
3. Cool, pale extremities with mottled coloring at the knees
4. Slow, shallow, irregular respiratory breathing pattern

Bibliography

Ahrens, J. (2003). The positive impact of hospice care on the surviving spouse. *Journal of Health and Social Behavior, 44*(2), 215-232.

Amella, E. J., Lawrence, J. F., & Gresle, S. O. (2005). Tube feeding: Prolonging life or death in vulnerable populations? *Mortality 10*(1), 69-81.

Banja, J. (2005). Talking to the dying. *Case Manager, 16*(1), 37-39.

Bennett, G., & Bennett, K. M. (2000). The presence of the dead: An empirical study. *Mortality, 5*(2), 139-158.

Burkhardt, M. A., & Nathaniel, A. K. (2002). *Ethics and issues in contemporary nursing* (2nd ed.). New York: Delmar-Thompson Learning.

Dobbins, E. H. (2005). Helping your patient to a "good death." *Nursing 5*(2), 43-45.

Egan, K. & Arnold, R. (2003). Grief and bereavement care. *American Journal of Nursing, 103*(9), 42-52.

End-of-Life Nursing Education Consortium (ELNEC). (2004). *Peaceful death: Recommended competencies and curricular guidelines for end-of-life nursing care.* Washington, DC: American Association of Colleges of Nursing & City of Hope.

Fauri, D. P., & Ettner, B. (2000). Bereavement services in acute care settings. *Death Studies, 24*(1), 51-65.

Ferrell, B. R., & Coyle, N. (2001). *Textbook of palliative nursing.* Oxford, England: Oxford University Press.

Forbes, S., Bern-Klug, M., & Gessert, C. (2000). End-of-life decision making for nursing home residents with dementia. *Journal of Nursing Scholarship, 32*(3), 251-258.

Hattori, K., McCubbin, M. A., & Ishida, D. N. (2006). Concept analysis of good death in the Japanese community. *Journal of Nursing Scholarship, 38*(2), 165-170.

Jeffrey, J. C. (2006-2007). *Course guide for death and dying* (unpublished). Austin, TX: Austin Community College.

Johnson, M., Bulechek, G., Butcher, H., Dochterman, J. M., Maas, M., Moorhead, S., et al. (Eds.). (2006). *NANDA, NOC, and NIC linkages: Nursing diagnoses, outcomes, & interventions.* St. Louis, MO: Mosby.

Kastenbaum, R. J. (1998). *Death, society, and human experience.* Boston: Allyn & Bacon.

Kehl, K. A. (2005). Recognition and support of anticipatory mourning. *Journal of Hospice and Palliative Nursing, 7*(4), 206-211.

Kübler-Ross, E., & Kessler, D. (2006). *On grief and grieving: Finding the meaning of grief through the five stages of loss.* New York: Scribner.

Kuebler, K. K., Berry, P. H., & Heidrich, D. E. (2002). *End of life care: Clinical practice guidelines.* Philadelphia: Saunders.

Lammers, W. M. Jr. (2005). Symptom control in end-of-life care: Pain, eating, acute illnesses, panic attacks, and aggressive care. *Journal of Pain & Palliative Care Pharmacotherapy, 19*(4), 71-75.

Long, S. O. (2004). Cultural scripts for a good death in Japan and the United States: Similarities and differences. *Social Science & Medicine, 58,* 913-928.

Meijburg, H. H. K. (2005). The significance of dying well. *Illness, Crisis and Loss, 13*(1), 49-62.

NANDA International. (2007). *Nursing diagnoses: Definitions and classification, 2006-2007* (7th ed.). Philadelphia: Author.

Post, S. G. (2001). Tube feeding and advanced progressive dementia. *Hastings Center Report, 31*(1), 36-42.

Sanz-Ortiz, J. et al. (2005). Spiritual issues: A philosophical consideration of attitudes toward death. *European Journal of Palliative Care, 12*(5), 215-217.

Sherman, D.W., Matzo, M. L., Pitorak, E., Ferrell, B. R., & Malloy, P. (2005). Preparation and care at the time of death: Content of the ELNEC curriculum and teaching strategies. *Journal for Nurses in Staff Development, 21*(3), 93-102.

Ufema, J. (2005a). Insights on death & dying: Impending death—seeing the signs. *Nursing, 35*(9), 65-66.

Ufema, J. (2005b). Insights on death & dying: Sudden Death—leaving a mark. *Nursing, 35*(11), 14.

Ufema, J. (2006). Insights on death & dying: Grieving family—enough analgesia? *Nursing, 36*(4), 66.

Warren, B. J. (2005). The cultural expression of death and dying. *Case Manager, 16*(1), 44-47.

Williams, J. R. (2005). Depression as a mediator between spousal bereavement and mortality from cardiovascular disease: Appreciating and managing the adverse health consequences of depression in an elderly surviving spouse. *Southern Medical Journal, 98*(1), 90-95.

*Worden, J. W. (2001). *Grief counseling and grief therapy: A handbook for the mental health professional.* New York: Springer.

*Asterisk indicates a classic or definitive work on this subject.

Chapter 46

MAINTAINING SEXUAL HEALTH

Media Resources

- evolve Evolve Website http://evolve.elsevier.com/Harkreader/
- Companion CD

Learning Objectives

After studying this chapter, you should be able to do the following:

- Describe the biological, psychological, social, and cultural influences in the development of sexuality
- Discuss concepts related to sexual development
- Assess the client who is at risk for or is experiencing alterations in sexuality patterns or sexual dysfunction
- Identify nursing diagnoses for sexual problems that are amenable to nursing care
- Use a standard model of care to provide goal-directed interventions to prevent or correct sexuality diagnoses
- Evaluate the outcomes that describe progress toward the goals of nursing care for sexuality issues
- Discuss sexual health promotion across the life span
- Describe issues in the health care of gay men and lesbians

Key Terms

androgyny
arousal
bisexual
gender
gender identity
gender role
heterosexual
homophobia
homosexual
libido
orgasm
sexual desire
sexual dysfunction
sexual identity
sexual orientation
sexual patterns
sexual response cycle
sexuality

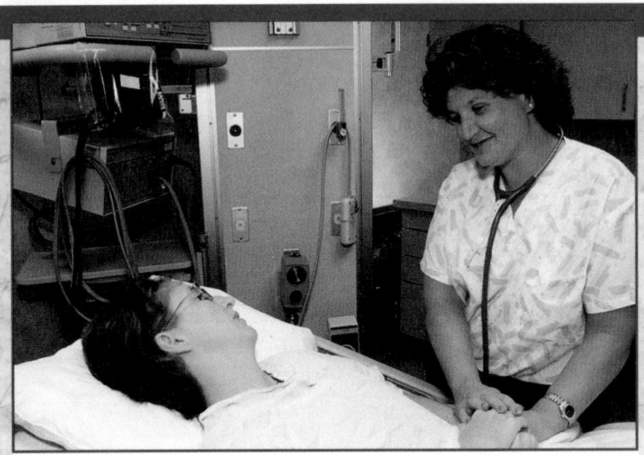

From Black, J. M. (2004). *Medical-surgical nursing: Clinical management for positive outcomes* (7th ed.). St. Louis, MO: Elsevier.

Lisa Simonelli, 46 years old, was diagnosed with breast cancer and lymph node involvement. She had a radical mastectomy 5 years ago. She has now come to the outpatient surgery clinic for a biopsy of a "growth" in her uterus. Even though her physician has indicated that the growth is probably benign, Lisa is very anxious about the outcome, and, because of her history, she is concerned about the possible need for a hysterectomy.

During the initial assessment, the nurse learns that Lisa is an Italian American, is a practicing Catholic, has been married for 11 years to Vincent, and has no children. Lisa indicates that she and her husband have a solid relationship but says she is concerned about their level of intimacy. Over the past 2 years, it has been declining, and the couple has not had intercourse in more than 3 months. She feels unattractive and wonders if her uterine biopsy will make intercourse impossible. Vincent refuses to talk about any of his concerns and seems indifferent to both of their sexual needs.

The nurse schedules some time to talk with Lisa before discharge to address her sexual concerns and to teach her about the effects of the biopsy and postoperative self-care. She assigns two nursing diagnoses from the list of nursing diagnoses for sexuality (see the key nursing diagnoses box). *Ineffective sexuality pattern* is the primary nursing diagnosis because there have been some negative changes in sexual functioning about which Lisa is concerned. *Sexual dysfunction* may also be present. How would you describe Lisa's self-image? What other factors might be contributing to the decreased intimacy she has expressed? As you consider other nursing diagnoses, remember that sexual patterns within a relationship are dynamic and interrelated within a partnership.

CONCEPTS OF SEXUALITY

A person's sexuality is a vital component of health and is influenced by biological, psychological, sociological, and cultural forces. **Sexuality** is the state or quality of being sexual, including the collective characteristics that distinguish male and female. Holistically, sexuality has the following two meanings:

- Awareness and feelings of being male or female
- The pursuit of sexual pleasure, reproduction, and the need for love and personal fulfillment

Beyond the two basic meanings of sexuality are the broad-based meanings sexuality has individually. The pursuit of sexual pleasure should be considered in the broad sense and throughout the life span. An infant who is held, cuddled, kissed, and gently stroked is learning healthy associations with physical contact. Shared affections such as holding hands, hugging, or simply sitting together and sharing conversation among parent and child, siblings, and friends are examples of fulfilling the need for love, acceptance, and personal fulfillment. These healthy actions contribute to the development of a healthy sexual being.

KEY NURSING DIAGNOSES FOR SEXUALITY

Ineffective sexuality pattern: Expressions of concern regarding own sexuality

Sexual dysfunction: A change in sexual function that is viewed as unsatisfying, unrewarding, or inadequate

BIOLOGICAL SEXUAL DEVELOPMENT

Biological sex, or gender, is determined by chromosome structure at the moment of conception. The XX chromosome combination produces a female, and the XY combination produces a male. The male-determining factor in the Y chromosome causes testes to develop from the gonad medulla; without the male factor, ovaries develop from the gonad cortex. Further sexual differentiation occurs when additional internal and external genital organs develop, creating obvious sex characteristics. A combination of hormonal and genetic controls determines which one develops.

The fully developed external structures of the male include the penis and scrotum. Internal structures include the testicles, epididymis, seminal vesicles, and prostate gland. The fully developed external structures of the female, collectively called the vulva, extend from the pubis to the perineum and include the labia majora, labia minora, clitoris, and vaginal orifice. Internal structures include the uterus, fallopian tubes, ovaries, vagina, and various glandular structures (Figure 46-1).

Although all reproductive organs are present at birth, they are immature and nonfunctional. Male spermatogenesis and female ovulation, accompanied by the production of estrogen and progesterone in the female and testosterone in the male, occur during puberty. Adequate nutrition, good hygiene, exercise, and ample rest are important to maintain the body's energy during sexual development.

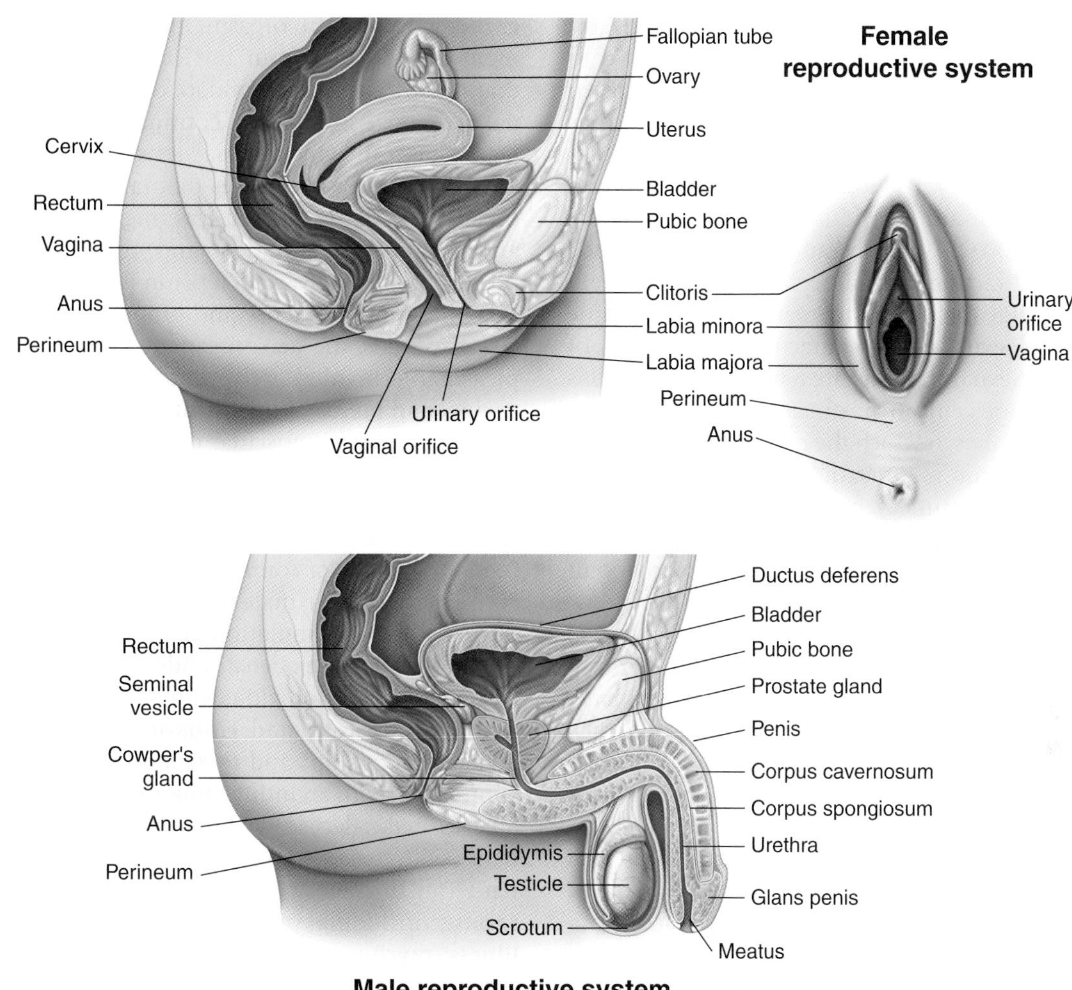

FIGURE 46-1 Anatomy of the male and female reproductive systems.

SEXUAL HEALTH

To understand the range of experiences that you might encounter regarding sexuality, the parameters of sexual health must be defined. The World Health Organization (WHO) describes sexual health as the integration of somatic, emotional, intellectual, and social aspects of sexual being in ways that are enriching and that enhance personality, communication, and love (WHO, 2005). Some characteristics of being sexually healthy are described in the following paragraphs.

Behavior Consistent With Gender Identity. According to the Centers for Disease Control and Prevention (CDC) (2006a), **gender** is defined as identifying the sex of an individual as either male or female. The terms *sex* and *gender* are used interchangeably, although the specific definitions of these terms differ. Usually, a newborn's gender is obvious at birth by external genitalia, which reflect the internal chromosome structure. Sexual anatomy sets the stage for the gender that society believes the child to be and in which the child is raised. Gender refers to responses, meanings, and cues that are socially learned and taken as reflections of society's conceptions of masculinity and femininity.

Gender identity, or **sexual identity,** is the internal belief or sense that one is male or female. This characteristic develops between the ages of 18 months and 3 years. Psychological, social, and cultural influences shape one's gender identity and behavior. One's gender identity is reinforced during adolescence. The child observes and imitates role models to learn cultural and social gender-typical behaviors and to form the basis for interactions among peers and adults.

Gender role refers to the outward appearance, behaviors, attitudes, and feelings deemed appropriate for males and females. These qualities are culturally defined as masculine, feminine, or androgynous. **Androgyny,** an anthropological term, means that a person may display both male and female characteristics and may relate to both male and female gender identity and roles. In general, children learn acceptable role behaviors through praise and criticism. In Western society, however, there is increasing acceptance of a wide variety of roles and behaviors for each gender. For example, husbands are encouraged to take part in the birth experience and to help nurture and rear their children. Women can often be found engaged in work that was once thought of as "men's work."

Sexual orientation refers to a person's emotional and sexual attraction toward individuals who are a potential partner (LeVay, 2003). Types of sexual orientation include **heterosexual** (attraction to members of the opposite gender), **homosexual** (attraction to members of the same gender), and **bisexual** (sexual attraction to members of either gender). **Sexual patterns** are a person's expressions of sexuality and are generally instinctual and tempered by society or the manner in which the person is raised. These patterns may include manner of dress; desired and expressed methods of intimacy, both verbal and nonverbal; and other identified expressions of intimacy.

Awareness of sexual feelings usually does not occur until adolescence, at the onset of mature sexuality; however, it is believed that sexual orientation is established in early childhood and is not changeable. At one time, homosexuality was listed as a disorder in the American Psychiatric Association's *Diagnostic and Statistical Manual of Mental Disorders (DSM),* and it was thought to be curable. In 1993, however, biologists discovered a variation on the X chromosome in 33 out of 40 pairs of brothers who were gay, which was thought to be the basis of their homosexual orientation. No comparable marker was found in lesbians. So far, insufficient data exist related to genetic predisposition as a cause of sexual orientation, but theories suggest an interaction of environmental, biological, and cognitive factors. Today the most current *DSM-IV-TR* (text revision) does not list homosexuality as a disorder.

Most societies adhere to heterosexuality as the norm and therefore may view homosexuality and bisexuality as deviant or not acceptable. The arbitrary ways in which sexual feelings are described as appropriate or inappropriate has been challenged by lesbian, gay, and bisexual populations, with the result that most can now live in heterosexual societies although not yet completely openly or comfortably in many realms of their lives.

Being Knowledgeable About Sexual Phenomena. Basic to understanding all the facets of sexuality are concepts relating to sexual intercourse: sexual desire, arousal, and response. **Sexual desire** is a wish to participate in sexual intimacy that is activated by thoughts, fantasies, emotions, and psychological wants and needs. Sexual desire commonly precedes **arousal,** in which physical and emotional stimuli heighten desire and begin the physiological changes that mark the **sexual response cycle.** Arousal can result from touching, especially in erogenous body areas, viewing provocative material, fantasizing about a partner, and other cognitive and physiological factors.

Masters and Johnson (1966) did classic studies of the bodily responses that occur during sexual arousal. They also defined four phases of the sexual response cycle: excitement, plateau, orgasm, and resolution. The excitement phase results from any form of sexual stimulation that causes a person to initiate or to be receptive to sexual activity. If stimulation continues, it leads to the plateau phase, in which sexual tension continues the intense physiological changes that take place in the sexual organs, as well as sex flush covering the face, neck, chest, and sometimes shoulders and thighs. The orgasmic phase occurs when sexual tension is at its height. During this phase muscles tense and blood vessels engorge. For a few seconds, the person experiences **orgasm,** a highly pleasurable involuntary response in which the clitoris, vagina, and uterus of the female or the penis of the male undergo repeated muscular contractions. Afterward, the person enters the resolution phase, which consists of involutional changes that return the body to the preexcitement phase. During this phase, the female typically remains capable of continued orgasms when adequately stimulated, but the male experiences a refractory period during which restimulation is impossible.

Physical and Emotional Ability to Engage in Sexual Relationships. For individuals to enjoy sexual health, they must be physically and emotionally able to engage in sexual relationships and to experience pleasure in erotic stimulation with an intimate partner. They should also be able to make decisions about sexual behavior in accordance with their values and beliefs. However, many problems can threaten a person's sexual experience and response, including organic problems, such as chronic illness; psychosocial problems, such as alcoholism; and situational stressors, such as the death of a spouse. A person in poor health or who takes certain prescribed or illicit drugs may not have the physical capacity for a sexual response or the emotional capacity to make the experience significant. Emotional health also influences sexual response, especially if the person is fatigued, stressed, depressed, or experiencing relationship conflicts.

Willingness to Make Adjustments in Sexual Functioning. Individuals who enjoy sexual heath are able and willing to make adjustments in sexual functioning when needed. Examples of these situations include, but are not limited to, illness or injury of self or partner, medication effects, and when a partner is unavailable.

Ability to Communicate About Sexual Issues. A sign of sexual health is the ability to communicate with one's sexual partner about sexual issues. This type of communication should occur without embarrassment, conflict, or discomfort and be present at any stage of life (Figure 46-2).

NURSE'S SELF-ASSESSMENT

Many clients will have questions about how their illness may affect their sexual activity. Would you feel comfortable addressing your clients' sexual concerns? Do you feel comfortable with clients asking you about their sexual concerns? Remember that your attitudes, prefer-

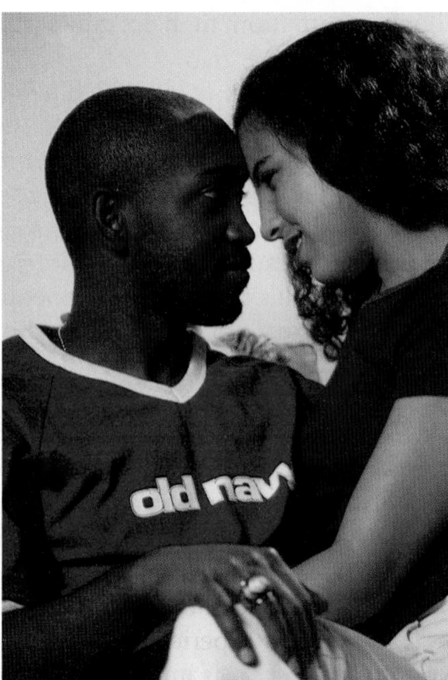

FIGURE 46-2 Sexual health includes the ability to communicate about sexual issues with one's partner.

ences, and prejudices affect all of your interactions with clients. That is why your self-assessment is a necessary part of addressing your clients' sexuality concerns appropriately. You need to be clear about your own values and beliefs about sexuality and to accept those values and beliefs without feeling that they are better or more correct than those of your clients are. Otherwise, you will interfere with the nurse-client interaction about the sensitive topic of sexuality. In discussing sexuality with your clients, you are asking them to disclose the most intimate aspects of their human character. That will happen successfully only if you view your clients' values and beliefs with respect.

Action Alert! Be aware that your anxiety or embarrassment in discussing sexual concerns will be communicated to your client, either overtly or covertly, and will prevent you from sharing information pertinent to sexual health care.

The first step in your self-assessment about sexuality is to determine areas of comfort and discomfort with the topic. Discussing anxieties, biases, and general feelings about sexuality with a trusted colleague or peer can help you detect inappropriate nursing behaviors in the nurse-client relationship. For example, if you feel overly uncomfortable when inspecting a client's genitals, you may need to think and talk about any taboos that you learned about exposing genitals as a part of your socialization. Having a general knowledge about sexuality and sexual beliefs and experiences, and obtaining information specific to a client's concerns, will help you comfortably include sexual health as a regular part of your practice.

FACTORS AFFECTING SEXUALITY

The patterns of expressing oneself sexually can be rewarding and enriching or they can be emotionally and physically distressing. Sexuality can be affected by life span, physiological, and cultural and lifestyle factors.

FACTORS ACROSS THE LIFE SPAN

Developmental factors that affect sexuality include the person's internal and external environments. Overall, good physical health practices aid the physical and sexual maturation of men and women. Externally, an environment that is nurturing and caring and promotes positive human interactions fosters development of healthy sexuality. A person needs to have open communication with role models to learn respect for his or her body and to discuss age-appropriate sexual feelings and behaviors. Every aspect of a person's life experience has the potential to influence sexual development.

Infants and Children. Sexual health begins in infancy with good hygienic practices in the care of external genitalia and protection from disease and injury. Children learn gender behaviors through interactions with adults. The ways in which children are dressed and responded to may promote gender-typical behaviors. Active displays of affection by adults to both sexes promote caring responses. Sexuality is multifaceted and evolving at every stage of life. Culture, self-esteem, emotions, attitudes, religion, sexual identity, experiences, and health or illness contribute to overall sexuality.

Imparting sexual values, such as respect for individual differences and expected ways of behaving toward individuals of the opposite sex, is important at an early age. Role models that teach children to be more androgynous invite more healthy behaviors. Examples are teaching boys not to take advantage of their strength against girls (or each other) and encouraging girls to stand up for themselves and yet be fair in arguments. Development of healthy sexuality in interpersonal interactions is also enhanced by witnessing caring and loving behaviors in adults.

Early childhood is a time when gender differences may become more apparent and curiosity leads children to explore their bodies. Touching genitals is a natural part of this exploration. Educate caretakers that curiosity is natural, discourage negative reactions to it, and teach respect of body. As language develops, children should be taught the proper words for body parts, such as vagina and penis. In working with parents or children, always answer questions truthfully and without embarrassment.

Action Alert! Teach children about good touch and bad touch. Encourage them to tell a parent, teacher, or other trusted adult when a touch is uncomfortable for them. There are many excellent established programs for educators, nurses, and other professionals working with children that may serve as a guide for teaching.

Adolescents. Adolescence is a time of establishing identity and a growing awareness of sexuality related to pubertal changes and social behaviors. The development of secondary sex characteristics tends to focus the adolescent on body image. Teaching girls about menstruation and boys about erections and wet dreams is important. Even though teaching about sexual activity should begin in childhood, reinforcing the nature of sexual intercourse and the risks involved in unprotected sex is a primary concern. Given the incidence of rape in our society, socialization about respect for the bodies of others and ways to interact in sexually appropriate ways should be a part of the education process for adolescents. It is critical to provide information about safe and healthy sexual practices, such as the following:

- Monogamous relationship with a partner who does not have sexually transmitted diseases (STDs) or infection with human immunodeficiency virus (HIV)
- Professional counseling prior to becoming sexually active
- Use of latex nonoxynol-9 condoms for vaginal, anal, and oral sex
- Use of latex rubber dams for oral sex
- Supporting and educating adolescents who are not ready for sex but may experience peer pressure

The adolescent is also in the process of affirming sexual roles and lifestyles. Nurses (and parents) might discuss personal and cultural values regarding sex and sexuality to help adolescents integrate what they have learned into rewarding peer relationships. Role models are also important at this time of life, and discussing sexual issues with a respected adult is a healthy outlet.

Adolescents are usually uncomfortable or hesitant about talking openly about sexual issues, especially if the subject has been taboo in their families. You can be most helpful if you accept whatever the adolescent discloses, reassure the client of confidentiality (unless doing so would jeopardize the client's safety), and discuss sexual issues in a rational, nonthreatening manner.

Adults. Adult sexuality issues are multifaceted and complex. You cannot expect to be completely competent in situations involving sexuality. Being sensitive and responding to specific physical, psychosocial, and relationship issues may help your clients sort out areas in which they lack information, need treatment or counseling, or desire enhancement of a relationship or sexual intimacy. Encouraging good health practices and teaching preventive activities, such as breast and testicular self-examinations, are measures that ensure continued sexual enjoyment. Knowledge about methods of birth control and safer sex may be a need for adults who wish to delay or prevent pregnancy or avoid STDs. Health care providers and other organizations provide excellent literature for the lay public on various aspects of sexuality. For example, the American Heart Association (http://www.amhrt.org) and the Centers for Disease Control and Prevention (http://www.cdc.gov/doc.do/id/0900f3ec802720b8) have excellent information to help guide clients back into a fulfilling sex life.

Older Adults. We are in an era in which people are living longer and healthier lives; sexual health is very much a part of the aging person's existence. Some older adults feel embarrassment or guilt when discussing sexual intimacy, some of which stems from Western society's emphasis on youth and beauty. There are numerous myths surrounding older adult's sexuality. Many people believe older adults to be asexual and not interested in or capable of sexual intercourse. In fact, older adults can be just as sexually active as anyone else can.

Some older adults prefer not to engage in sexual intercourse for a variety of reasons, and sexual abstinence by choice is also normal at any age. As people age, there are some hormonal changes and physiological factors that can affect sexual activity (Box 46-1).

Older adults can express intimacy in a variety of ways (Figure 46-3). Holding hands, embracing, cuddling and even interactive activities such as dinners, dancing, walking, or other activities enjoyed by a couple may fulfill intimacy needs. Encouraging hobbies and activities en-

BOX 46-1 *Older Adults: Factors Affecting Sexuality*

- Pathological factors that affect sexual function include cardiovascular disease, diabetes mellitus, dementia, arthritis, and surgery.
- Pharmacological factors play a role in sexual problems, particularly drugs that affect the autonomic nervous system.
- Changes that occur in sexual physiology of an aging male can affect both erectile function and ejaculation.
- The physiological effects of aging on women's sexual function are primarily caused by decreased amounts of circulating estrogen after menopause.
- Cognitive deterioration relating to dementia disorders may affect sexual behavior.
- Body deformities, wearing medical attire such as special pads or being catheterized, can affect sexual behavior.
- Being sexual inactive during an illness may negatively affect an individual's ability to resume sexual activities when well.

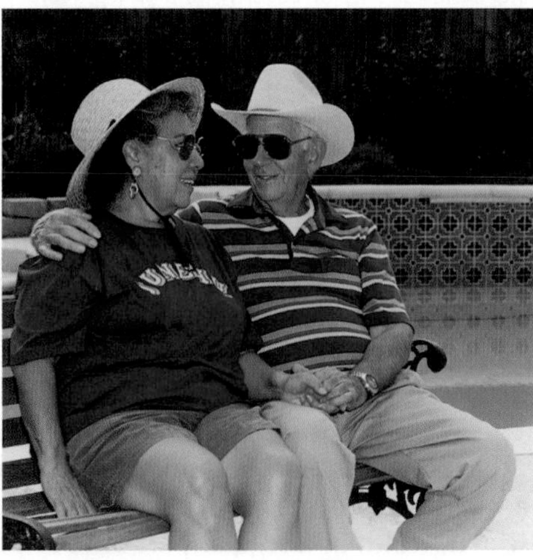

FIGURE 46-3 Older people express intimacy in a variety of ways.

joyed by older couples will help them remain active and interactive.

Action Alert! Older adults may express their sexuality by holding hands, sitting close, embracing, cuddling, dancing, and even relationship activities such as dining together and walking.

You can play an active role in promoting the sexual health promotion of older adults through education, debunking myths, exploring attitudes and values that can inhibit sexual expression, and correcting misinformation about the aging process. You can encourage good physical health practices, such as regular physical checkups, and health promotion activities, such as exercising.

PHYSIOLOGICAL FACTORS

Physiological factors affecting sexuality are illness, infection, surgical procedures, and medications. They may affect a person's sense of worth, body image, attractiveness, and sexual desire. Acute or chronic illnesses contribute significantly to alterations in sexuality patterns. Disease can affect the sexual organs directly, as in uterine or testicular cancer. Other physical illnesses, such as diabetes, may detract from sexual expression because energy is redirected toward recovery or contending with the illness. Some chronic illnesses or medications may directly interfere with or inhibit sexual arousal and response (Table 46-1).

Sexually transmitted diseases typically exert a major physiological influence on a person's sexuality. The more common STDs include chancroid, chlamydia, condylomata, genital herpes, genital warts, gonorrhea, hepatitis B, HIV infection, streptococcal infection, syphilis, pubic lice, scabies, and trichomoniasis. These disorders cause rashes, lesions, itching, pain, and usually a desire to avoid transmission to another person through sexual contact. STDs can be transmitted through sexual intercourse; intimate oral, genital, or anal contact; or contact with the body

Table 46-1 Conditions That May Alter Sexuality Patterns

CATEGORY	EXAMPLE	SEXUAL ALTERATIONS
PATHOPHYSIOLOGICAL		
Endocrine system	Diabetes	Impotence occurs primarily with uncontrolled diabetes; often improved with control of blood sugar; may interfere with orgasm in both sexes.
Genitourinary system	Sexually transmitted diseases	Pain with intercourse; fear of transmitting disease.
Neuromuscular and skeletal system	Parkinsonism	Interferes with male orgasm.
	Arthritis	Difficulty positioning for intercourse; however, the physical activity may actually make arthritis better.
TREATMENT-RELATED		
Medications	Alpha-adrenergic blockers Amphetamines ACE inhibitors Nitrates Tricyclic antidepressants Antihistamines Beta-adrenergic blockers Anticholinergics Thiazide diuretics Estrogen H_2 antagonists Narcotics NSAIDs	These classifications are associated with alterations such as impotence, changes in libido, inhibition of ejaculation, gynecomastia, and menstrual irregularities; the incidence of alterations is usually very small. There is some thought that telling the client about the possibility of alterations increases the likelihood of their occurrence.
Therapeutic procedures	Perineal resection of prostate	Nerve-sparing procedure can prevent impotence.
	Irradiation of pelvis	The prevalence rate of erectile dysfunction with this procedure is 25%.
SITUATIONAL		
Unprotected sex	Fear of pregnancy Fear of sexuality transmitted diseases	Psychological barrier to enjoyment of sexual intercourse.
MATURATIONAL		
Strict religious upbringing	Guilt over sexual activity	Can inhibit sexual response or decrease enjoyment.
Negative sexual teaching	Shame regarding one's body and genitals	Interferes with sexual arousal, including erection in men and orgasm in women.

Medication information from *Drug facts and comparisons.* (2006). St. Louis, MO: Facts and Comparisons.
ACE, Angiotensin-converting enzyme; *NSAID,* nonsteroidal antiinflammatory drug.

fluids (such as blood, urine, or vaginal or penile discharge) of the infected person. Fear of contracting STDs inhibits participation in sexual intimacy (CDC, 2006).

CULTURAL AND LIFESTYLE FACTORS

In an otherwise physically healthy person, socialization that leads to embarrassment and disgust about one's genitals, as well as taboos against openly discussing sexuality, may have a negative effect on the patterns of sexuality the person develops. Even more destructive to healthy sexual expression is exploitation through physical sexual abuse or adherence to sociocultural beliefs and myths that invoke guilt or shame. Infibulation is the practice of surgical closure of the female labia, thus sealing off female genitalia. Only a small hole is left for menstruation and urination. The practice of infibulation may also include female castration or removal of the clitoris.

Culturally dictated sexual practices are very diverse, but most cultures transmit messages regarding the nature of sex and beauty, the acceptability of specific sexual behaviors, the relationship of sex and love, marital sexual behavior, homosexuality, and the appropriateness of specific sex roles (Figure 46-4). The diagnosis of *Ineffective sexuality pattern* must consider the client's socialization and cultural context, as suggested in Box 46-2.

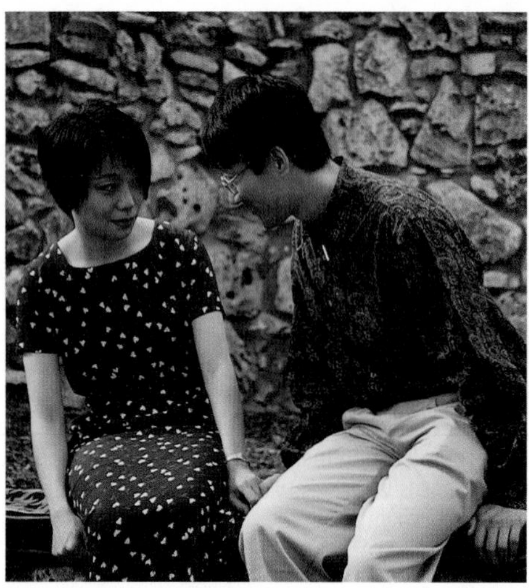

FIGURE 46-4 Most cultures transmit messages about sexuality.

ASSESSMENT

GENERAL ASSESSMENT OF SEXUALITY

Health History. Sexuality assessment is a legitimate aspect of holistic care and may be done as part of the client's basic history (see Chapter 6) or at any time the client, either overtly or covertly, indicates concern about sexual health. You may also initiate a discussion and assessment of sexuality on the basis of your knowledge that an illness, procedure, or medication may influence a client's sexual pleasure and functioning. Assessment may also have therapeutic value because it lets the client know that it is appropriate to discuss concerns about sexuality.

Encourage the client to elaborate on family and work roles to help you assess for typical, atypical, and more flexible, androgynous gender role behaviors. Analyzing these data in the context of the client's developmental level helps you determine whether to further assess for specific sexual issues related to the client's condition.

Action Alert! When engaging the client in a discussion about sexual issues, be sensitive to the environment; a planned time and utmost privacy are necessary to conduct a sexual assessment.

The sexual history may be comprehensive or brief, depending on the client's needs. It should proceed from general to more specific and from comfortable to more sensitive. Make sure to use appropriate language when referring to parts of the client's anatomy, but pay attention to the client's level of knowledge. If the client uses slang terms (such as *dick* for penis), simply acknowledge the client's statement and continue on with the history. If the client has trouble responding to a specific, necessary question, allow time. If the answer is not absolutely necessary, do not press for one.

BOX 46-2 *Cross-Cultural Care*

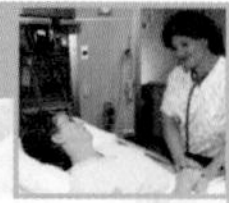

Caring for an Italian American Client

Lisa is an Italian American, and, at the initial interview, the nurse learns that her family came to America four generations back. Her extended family members all live in another state (as does her husband's family). All of her family members have many traditional ethnic customs. Although all clients are unique, Italian Americans have a tendency to hold the following values:

- Family and the church are very important.
- Focus is on the present.
- They may be fatalistic but usually are very resilient.
- Illness is caused by the "evil eye" or "curses"; severe and life-threatening illnesses are caused by more powerful sources.
- Suppressed emotions, stress, anxiety, fear, and grief can cause illness.
- Cure is "in the hands of God," although most seek explanations about care given to them.
- Cooperation with health care providers is valued.
- Discussions of sex and sexuality are avoided out of modesty or shame.

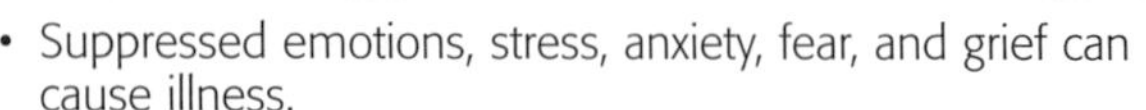

A brief sexual history may include questions such as the following:

- Do you have any concerns or issues about your sexuality or sexual response? (Remember that anything that affects the client's physical status, emotional comfort, interpersonal relationships, sociocultural mores, or moral and religious attitudes may threaten some aspect of sexuality.)
- When did the problem begin, and what were the circumstances surrounding the problem? Specifically, what prompted you to mention this problem?
- What do you think caused the problem?
- Has anything made the problem better? Worse?
- What would you like to do or have happen about the problem at this time?

A comprehensive sexual history should include details of the client's past history and current concerns (Table 46-2). While completing the history, take note of the client's nonverbal cues to help discern attitudes or discomforts about sexuality. Watch for any reluctance to answer questions, for brief answers that are not very informative, for embarrassment or blushing, and for inappropriate acting out of a sexual nature. The client's affect—such as sadness, indifference, anger, elation—or incongruence between words and affect will give you additional information about what the client may be experiencing about sexuality issues.

Action Alert! When taking a comprehensive sexual history, use open-ended questions to allow the client freedom of choice in response. Then ask for elaboration or clarification as necessary to understand the client's answers.

Physical Examination. Carry out physical assessment of the client's sexual anatomy by inspecting genitalia and secondary sexual characteristics (see Chapter 8). Observations that may warrant further questioning, examination, or reporting include the following:

- Deviations in genitalia or breasts
- Lesions on, ulceration on, infections of, or unusual discharge from genitals or nipples
- Evidence of poor hygiene
- Unmet outcomes from medical or surgical interventions

Table 46-2 Elements of a Comprehensive Sexual History

PAST HISTORY	
Sexual knowledge	• From whom and how information about sexuality and sexual response was obtained • Information obtained from classes or formal learning • Information about sexually transmitted diseases
Life cycle influences on sexuality	• Influences from caretakers, role models about being male or female during formative years, development of gender or androgynous role behaviors • Self-views of being male, female, gay, or lesbian • Values and beliefs about sexuality from family, religion, or culture • Initiation of sexual activity • Sexual patterns • Sexual relationships or interactions, and whether they are positive or negative
Physical problems relating to sexuality	• Difficult menstruation or menopause • Development of secondary sex characteristics • Trauma, infection, or disease affecting sexual organs • History of sexual abuse, including rape
CURRENT CONCERNS	
Client's perception and understanding of his or her sexual health status or other physical condition affecting sexuality	• Issues related to body image or self-esteem • Ways in which sexual function or response is affected • Changes in sexual activity or patterns • Unsatisfactory or painful intercourse • Stresses influencing sexual health • Potential or expected changes in sexual health or activity related to illness or injury • Significance to the client of changes in sexual health or activity • Client's outlook or expectations about changes in sexual health
Sexual partners	• Inquire about single or multiple partners • Specific sexual practices, including vaginal, oral, and anal intercourse • Precautions client takes to practice safe sex
Effects of client's current sexual health on significant others	• Influence of alteration in client's sexual health or function on significant other(s) • Anticipation of changes in significant relationship(s)
Changes in sexual function	• Changes in sexual function as a result of illness, medical treatment, surgery, emotional illness, or medications
Client's wants and needs regarding sexual health at this time	• Thoughts about ways in which needs might be met • Expected outcomes • Willingness and comfort of client to discuss sexual needs with an appropriate professional, should that be warranted

While gathering data, form an opinion about the client's body image and self-image as a sexual being (see Chapter 41). You can infer these concepts from the manner in which the client interacts with you. Does the client use appropriate modesty in exposing the genitals for examination? Is the client overly shy and embarrassed? Too bold? Does the client hesitate to use anatomically correct terms when answering your questions? How does the client display gender identity in dress, grooming, and posture? Does the client interact with you in a manner that respects each of you as a sexual being? (For example, does the client call you by name rather than by a derogatory or seductive term?) Finally, does the client practice breast or testicular self-examination? If not, provide appropriate teaching (Box 46-3).

BOX 46-3 *Teaching for Self-Care*

Breast and Testicular Self-Examination

Purpose: To teach female clients about the monthly breast self-examination and male clients about the monthly testicular self-examination according to the American Cancer Society Guidelines.

Expected Outcome: The client will use the breast self-examination or testicular self-examination on a monthly basis and report irregularities to a physician promptly.

Client Instructions

- Set aside about 15 minutes on the same date each month.
- When examining your breasts or testicles, make sure you perform a complete examination with full coverage of the area.
- Follow the same procedure each time.
- Use the top third of your fingers (the pads) for palpation.
- Use enough pressure to feel deep tissues.

Breast Self-Examination

1. Standing before a mirror with your breasts exposed, inspect your breasts with arms at your sides (see illustration).

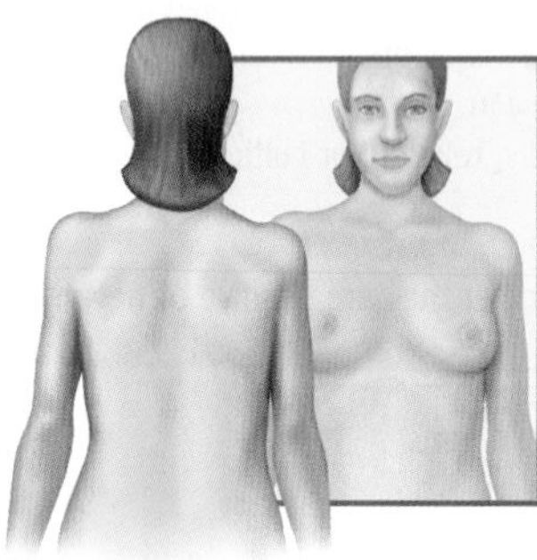

2. Raise your arms overhead, and look for changes (see illustration).

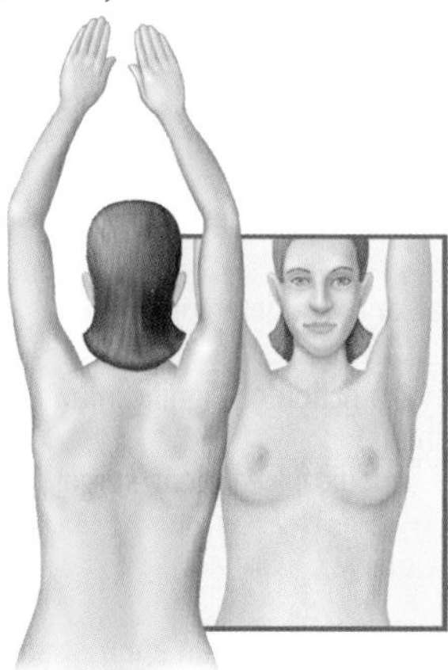

3. With your hands on your hips, flex your chest muscles and look for changes (see illustration).

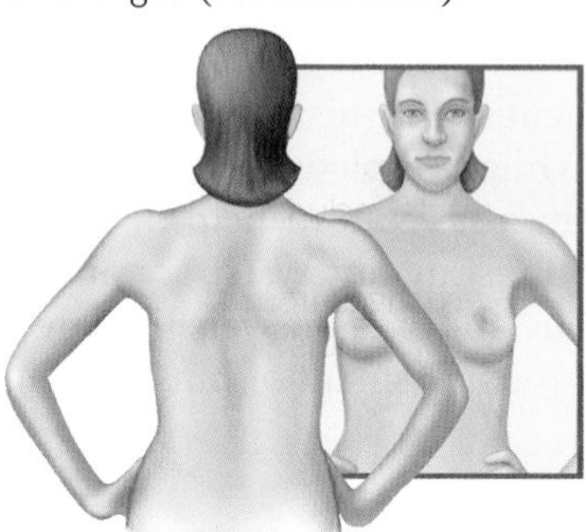

4. Gently squeeze your nipples, and look for discharge (see illustration).

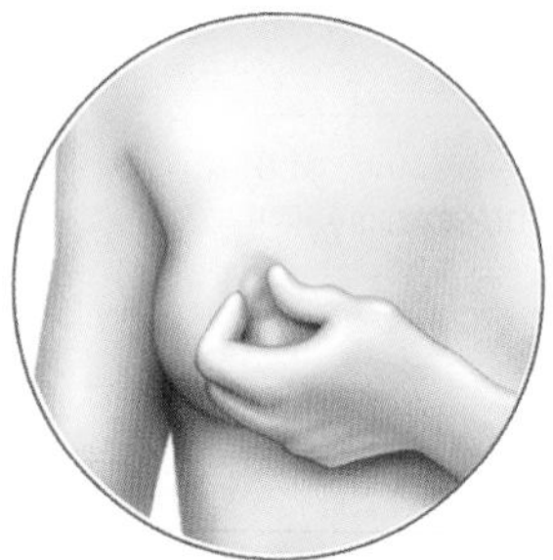

5. Palpating your breasts is easiest in the shower because your fingers will glide easily over the wet skin. With your fingers flat, move gently but firmly over every part of each breast. Use a circular motion starting with the nipple and moving outward. Alternatively, you can use a pattern of vertical parallel lines. Check for any lump, hard knot, or thickening (see illustration).

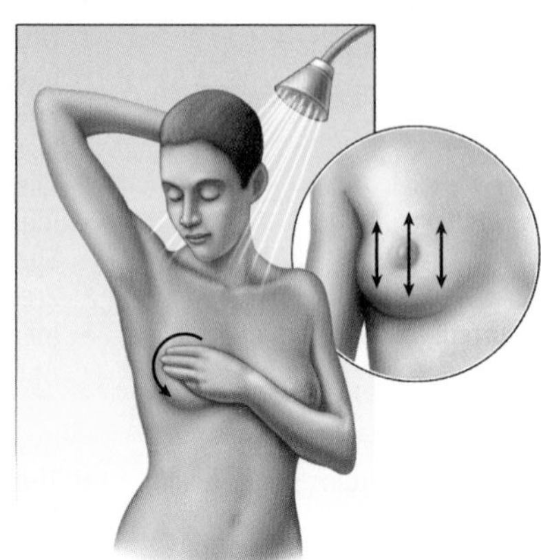

BOX 46-3 *Teaching for Self-Care—cont'd*

Breast and Testicular Self-Examination

6. If you prefer to perform the examination lying down, place a pillow under your shoulder to flatten your breasts. Use the middle three fingers of your opposite hand to feel for lumps or changes in one of the same patterns just described (see illustration).

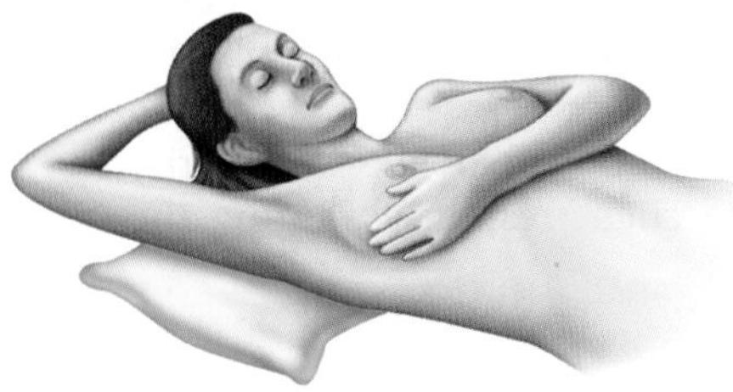

7. Examine both breasts, including your chest area and armpits.
8. If you notice any changes from one month to the next, notify your physician or nurse practitioner.

Testicular Self-Examination

1. The best time to perform this examination is right after a shower when your scrotal skin is moist and relaxed, making the testicles easy to feel.
2. Gently lift each testicle. Each one should feel like an egg, firm but not hard, and smooth with no lumps.
3. Using both hands, place your middle fingers on the underside of each testicle and your thumbs on top.
4. Gently roll the testicle between the thumb and fingers to feel for any lumps, swelling, or mass (see illustration).

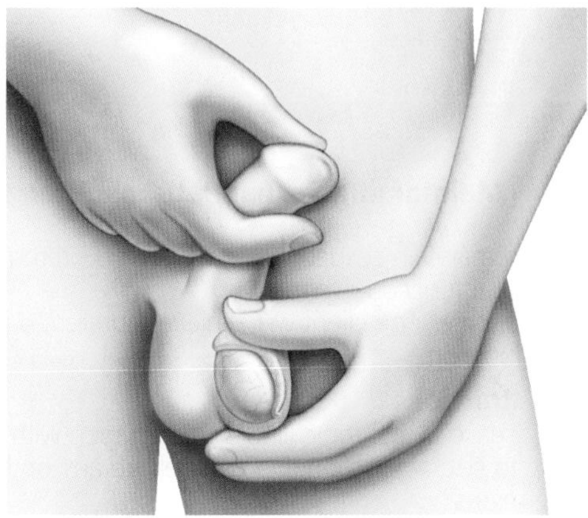

5. If you notice any changes from one month to the next, notify your physician or nurse practitioner.

Data from National Alliance of Breast Cancer Organizations. (2003). *Breast self-exam (BSE)*. Retrieved June 14, 2006, from http://www.mydna.com/health/breast_cancer. Data from The Testicular Cancer Support Center. Retrieved December 12, 2006, from http://crc.acor.org/tcexam.html.

FOCUSED ASSESSMENT FOR *INEFFECTIVE SEXUALITY PATTERN*

Numerous health problems can have a biochemical effect on sexual energy and the ability to engage in sex. These conditions may affect the person's **libido,** which is the conscious or unconscious sex drive or desire to please or satisfy. For example, breast cancer and all its attendant worries and stresses, including financial aspects, can negatively affect all areas of a woman's life.

A vital part of your assessment of a client with *Ineffective sexuality pattern* is to understand the client's sexual knowledge and attitudes. Investigate the client's sources of sexual education, formal and informal, so that you can respond to negative thoughts or misconceptions that contribute to the diagnosis. Consider, for example, the nurse who discovers that her prepubertal male client is intensely embarrassed by nocturnal emissions (wet dreams). Assessment reveals that no one has told him that wet dreams are normal and will not last forever. By teaching him about hormonal changes in puberty and encouraging further discussion in an accepting, matter-of-fact manner, the nurse can reduce his concerns and promote acceptance of his developing sexuality.

Or consider the example of a teenage girl who has unprotected sex but says she gives little thought to her increased risks of pregnancy and STDs or to her lowered self-esteem. While interviewing this teen, the nurse discovers that although the girl says she has had "lots" of teaching about contraception, it was all from pamphlets. The client has virtually no practical knowledge about using contraceptive devices and is uncomfortable suggesting them to her sexual partners. She feels too embarrassed to talk to peers about it, and she simply assumes that all girls her age are "doing it" (engaging in sexual intercourse). Working with this client would provide you with an excellent opportunity to explore her values and beliefs about sexual activity, discuss the emotional aspects of engaging in sex without having other intimate interactions as well, and offer practical teaching about contraceptives, how to use them, the risks of pregnancy, and the option of abstinence. This may be an opportunity to determine if your client wants and needs further counseling. You will need to provide teaching appropriate to each client's needs to help maintain normal sexuality patterns.

Many of the risk factors for *Ineffective sexuality pattern* stem from medical-surgical conditions or the processes of aging. Most clients wonder how such factors will affect their sex lives, but few will be willing to ask you direct questions about it. Therefore you should take the initiative to assess the client and prompt discussion about the influence of illness or aging on sexuality. Even if the client is not ready or willing to talk about it at the time, your initiative leaves the client with the belief that you are ready and willing to talk about this sometimes-difficult topic (Box 46-4).

Defining Characteristics. *Ineffective sexuality pattern* is a broad nursing diagnosis that considers all physical, psychosocial, and cultural aspects of sexuality (Table 46-3). Defining characteristics include reported difficulties, limitations, or changes in sexual behaviors or activities. These may involve actual or anticipated negative changes in sexual behaviors, sexual health, sexual functioning, or sexual identity. In addition, defining characteristics may include expression of concern about inappropriate sexual verbal or nonverbal behavior or changes in primary or secondary sexual characteristics (Carpenito, 2005).

Related Factors. Many factors may be related to alterations in sexual patterns. To assess for related factors, observe for nonverbal cues and clarify any vague or incomplete client responses during the interview.

BOX 46-4 *Teaching for Wellness*

Maintaining Sexual Patterns After a Myocardial Infarction

Purpose: To maintain sexual health, which is a prerequisite for normal sexual function.

Expected Outcome: The client will achieve a preferred pattern of sexual function.

Client Instructions

- Heart disease is a chronic illness that is laden with myths relating to sexual function. Do you believe any of the following myths?
  1. Sex after a heart attack can easily cause sudden death.
  2. It is best for the man to be on the bottom during sex after a heart attack.
  3. Impotence and lack of sex drive always occur after a heart attack.
  4. If angina occurs during sex, you should stop having sex permanently.
- These are myths. They are not correct. The fact is that most men and women can safely resume sex within a few weeks or as soon as they feel ready after a heart attack or heart surgery. However, do not rush into sex just to prove yourself after a heart attack or heart surgery.
- Before resuming sexual activity, you should be able to tolerate physical activity. Specifically, you should be able to climb two flights of steps or walk one city block without shortness of breath or chest pain. If you are not sure you are ready, your physician can administer an exercise test to check your physical capacity for sex.
- You should be able to experience the same desire and arousal after your heart attack that you did before your heart attack.
- Depression is a common response to a heart attack or heart surgery, and it may interfere with your normal level of desire temporarily.
- Some heart medications interfere with the sex drive and sexual function. With some adaptation, however, sexual pleasure and performance need not be worrisome.
- Feel free to discuss any concerns you have about sexuality or sexual function with me. If needed, you may want to talk with a professional sex counselor as well. The American Heart Association (http://www.amhrt.org) and the Centers for Disease Control and Prevention (http://www.cdc.gov/doc.do/id/0900f3ec802720b8) have excellent information to help guide you back into a fulfilling sex life.

Table 46-3 Clustering Data to Make a Nursing Diagnosis

Problems of Sexual Function

DATA CLUSTER	DIAGNOSIS
A 12-year-old boy admits to his friends that he masturbates several times a week. He heard his minister say that masturbation is sinful. The boy is worried he is not normal.	*Ineffective sexuality pattern* related to feelings of guilt, worries about normal functioning, and need to express himself sexually through masturbation
A 30-year-old newly married woman discovers that she does not like sex. Her mother died when she was 4 years old; she was raised by her father who was very strict with her upbringing.	*Sexual dysfunction* related to lack of sexual desire and lack of a female role model as she was developing as a young woman
A couple in their mid-50s is thinking of separate bedrooms because sexual intercourse has become very painful for the wife. She is beginning menopause and is noticing physical changes in her body.	*Sexual dysfunction* related to painful intercourse secondary to dryness of the vagina
A recent widower in his 60s cannot bear to look at women who speak with him at work and church. He is afraid of violating his wife's memory by interacting with any woman, and he does not feel he can ever be sexually intimate again.	*Ineffective sexuality pattern* related to feelings of inadequacy and violation of his wife's memory through pursuit of sexual contact

Client comments during the physical examination may also alert you to the need to inquire about specific related factors or sexual concerns, such as fear of pregnancy or STDs, conflicts with sexual orientation, or impaired relationships.

FOCUSED ASSESSMENT FOR *SEXUAL DYSFUNCTION*

Sexual dysfunction implies a change or disruption in sexual health or function that the affected person views as unrewarding or inadequate. It can be either a disruption of sexual behavior or an extreme variation of sexual behavior, and it may be one of four major types: sexual desire disorders, sexual arousal disorders, orgasmic dysfunction, and sexual pain disorders (Table 46-4).

Defining Characteristics. The defining characteristic of sexual dysfunction is a verbal report of an actual or perceived change in sexual function or limitation on sexual performance, often imposed by disease or therapy. Sexual dysfunction may also include a change of interest in oneself or others, value conflicts, lack of satisfaction, an altered relationship with a partner, a need for confirmation of desirability, and alterations in achieving a perceived sex role.

Related Factors. Factors related to *Sexual dysfunction* are similar to those for *Ineffective sexuality pattern*. In fact, sexual dysfunction can alter sexuality patterns, so it may be difficult for you to differentiate between the two. Related factors for *Sexual dysfunction* include problems such as physical or psychological abuse, conflicting values, or altered body structure or function.

DIAGNOSIS

There is much overlap between *Ineffective sexuality pattern* and *Sexual dysfunction*. In the latter, the client's report of a problem is a key factor. However, interventions related to *Sexual dysfunction* are fairly complex and require the expertise of a nursing specialist (Carpenito, 2005). The generalist nurse typically uses the broader diagnostic category of *Ineffective sexuality pattern*. Use the decision tree in Figure 46-5 to help you choose the nursing diagnosis that best fits your client's situation.

RELATED NURSING DIAGNOSES

Sexuality is a major part of many life processes, and you will need to consider diagnoses in several other areas of nursing care. Additional nursing diagnoses that could relate to sexual concerns are in the areas of self-esteem, body image, coping, adaptation to life changes and family processes, risk for infection (STDs), mental illness (including substance use and abuse), and potential for being taken advantage of (rape or sexual abuse).

One nursing diagnosis, *Ineffective coping*, is illustrated in the following example. A 49-year-old male client was being assessed for psychosocial counseling in an outpatient clinic. He reported as one of his symptoms having no intercourse or any desire for sexual activity with his wife over the past year. This problem had no medical, pharmaceutical, or surgical cause. Lack of sexual desire or activity over a prolonged time is one indication of clinical depression; therefore, the client should receive a nursing diagnosis of *Sexual dysfunction* and appropriate

Table 46-4 Sexual Dysfunction

DYSFUNCTION	DESCRIPTIONS
SEXUAL DESIRE ALTERATIONS	
Hypoactive desire	• Deficiency or absence of desire for sexual activity
Sexual aversion	• Aversion to and active avoidance of genital sexual contact with a partner
SEXUAL AROUSAL ALTERATIONS	
Female	• Inability to attain or maintain sexual activity to completion • May result from inadequate lubrication and swelling response in the excitement phase or from a psychological problem, medical problem, or substance abuse
Male	• Inability to attain or maintain sexual activity to completion • May result from the inability to obtain and maintain an adequate erection or from a psychological problem, medical problem, or substance abuse
ORGASMIC ALTERATIONS	
Female	• Delayed or absent orgasm following a normal sexual excitement phase
Male	• Delayed or absent orgasm following a normal sexual excitement phase • Ejaculation before the client wishes it: before, at, or shortly after penetration
SEXUAL ALTERATIONS CAUSED BY PAIN	
Dyspareunia	• Genital pain associated with intercourse • Occurs in both women and men • May result from organic cause or traumatic event, such as rape, incest, or sexual abuse
Vaginismus	• Involuntary contraction of the perineal muscles surrounding the outer third of the vagina upon penetration of penis, tampon, speculum, etc.

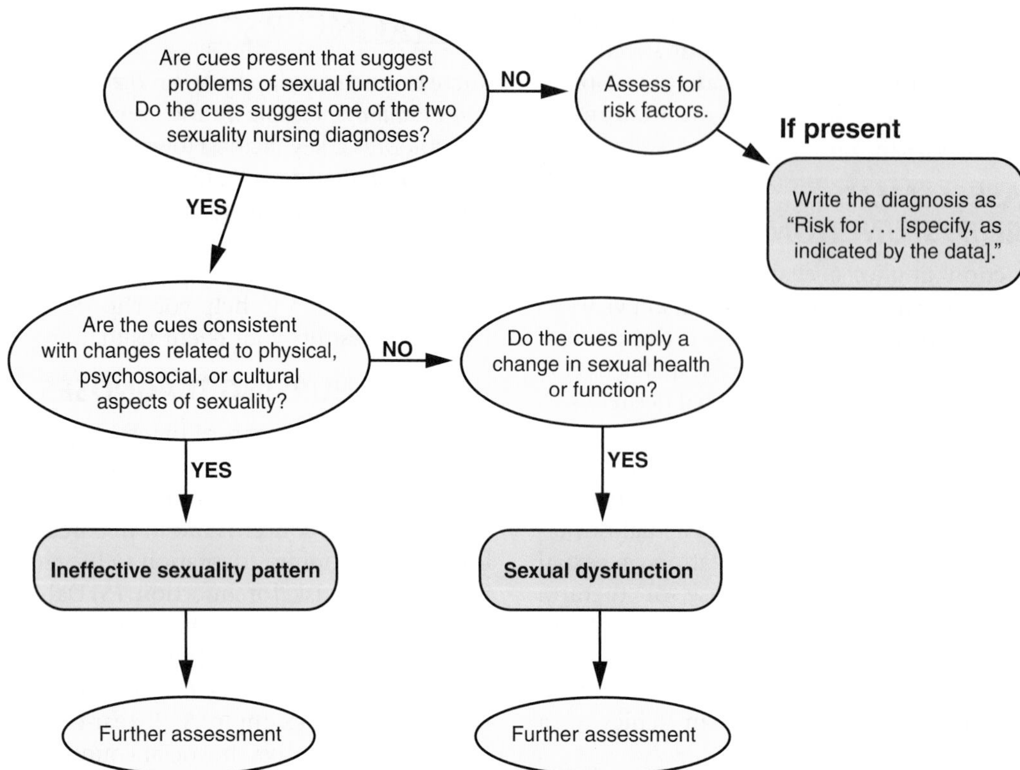

FIGURE 46-5 Decision tree for nursing diagnoses related to sexuality. Diagnoses are shown in rectangles. Within these rectangles, diagnoses shown in **bold** type are NANDA International (NANDA-I)–approved nursing diagnoses; diagnoses shown in regular type are not NANDA-I–approved nursing diagnoses.

nursing diagnoses representing responses to depression, such as *Hopelessness* and *Insomnia.*

Another example is a divorced mother of a young child. She is in a steady relationship but finds it difficult to become more intimate with her partner because her child is anxious about her mother's intimacy with a man who is not her father. This client might receive a nursing diagnosis of *Interrupted family processes* related to insecurity secondary to altered family structure.

PLANNING

Anything that affects a person's physical being, emotional comfort, sociocultural mores, or moral and ethical attitudes may threaten some aspect of sexuality and result in a diagnosis of *Ineffective sexuality pattern.* Planning should consider the client's category of need, such as anatomical disruptions, physiological alterations, pharmacological interference, life cycle issues, emotional alterations, or environmental influences. Classifying the client's need will facilitate planning in accordance with the client's physical skill needs or teaching and counseling needs.

In addition, your plan should consider your own level of expertise, the accuracy and depth of your information about human sexuality, your awareness of your own value system, your level of comfort in communicating about sexuality, and your interpersonal skills. Your plan should demonstrate your respect for the client as a sexual being by ensuring care that minimizes exposure of the client's genitals and the female client's breasts.

EXPECTED OUTCOMES FOR THE CLIENT WITH *INEFFECTIVE SEXUALITY PATTERN*

Expected outcomes for intervening in *Ineffective sexuality pattern* might include the client's being able to do the following:

- Discuss sexual concerns with minimal or no hesitancy
- Express feeling less anxious about sharing private information
- Acknowledge the nurse's professional interest and acceptance of the client's feelings
- Restate factual information received and seek clarification of data presented
- Identify a specific problem or problems to work on
- Establish clear and realistic goals
- Identify stressors that may inhibit resolution of the problem
- Seek further treatment or counseling as needed

EXPECTED OUTCOMES FOR THE CLIENT WITH *SEXUAL DYSFUNCTION*

If you suspect or the client reports symptoms of sexual dysfunction, your plan should include specific information that would indicate a need for referral to a professional with expertise in treating the problem. In addition, planning should include the same considerations stated for *Ineffective sexuality pattern.*

It may be difficult for a client to accept referral to a "sex specialist," whether for physical care or for counseling. Be prepared to help the client understand that, while others may joke about or stigmatize the need for expert sexual care, it may offer the most effective method for reducing the emotional pain of a sexual problem. Outcomes for the client experiencing sexual dysfunction might include that the client will do the following:

- Acknowledge that sexual concerns have been evaluated
- Display nonverbal behavior that indicates increased relaxation or less sadness about the sexual problem
- Express increased physical comfort as a result of nursing care
- State knowledge of resources available and ways to access them

INTERVENTION

Interventions for *Ineffective sexuality pattern* will be related to how the client defines the problem as well as to your assessment. Engaging the client in self-care as much as possible will prevent later resistance toward improved sexual health. Asking what the client would like to have happen here and now as well as in the future is a good place to begin. Making sure the client receives answers to all questions is also crucial, as illustrated in Box 46-5. For outcomes to be successful, interventions must consider the client's knowledge, beliefs, and attitudes.

DEALING WITH CLIENTS EXPRESSING INAPPROPRIATE SEXUAL BEHAVIOR

Inappropriate sexual behavior may be expressed by a wide range of clients. Clients suffering from Alzheimer's disease to clients simply being inappropriate with the nurse may display sexual behaviors that the nurse must deal with. These behaviors may include unwanted sexual advances such as touching or inappropriate comments, lewd commentary, or open masturbation. The nurse must deal with this behavior quickly and clearly. Often a clear statement to stop will suffice. Do not respond in anger; rather give a clear calm statement to stop. If the client is demented, provide redirection to another activity. When providing care to a young client, always

BOX 46-5 *A Client's Perspective*

"Breast Cancer Shattered My Life"

Breast cancer crashed into my life when I was 42. Noticing a lump in my left breast, I wasn't too alarmed; my small breasts were always lumpy-bumpy. But my ob/gyn froze when his fingers touched the lump. "What's this? It wasn't here at your last visit." Four hours later, I was in the surgeon's office. Two days after that, I became a one-breasted woman with a life-threatening illness.

The surgeon wasn't optimistic or pessimistic. He was just what I needed—neutral and honest—so I trusted him. He didn't give me more information than I asked for. (I only ask questions if I know I can deal with the answers.) He said it was serious, one of the fastest growing types, and there was no time to waste.

Life happened at warp speed. A day and a half in the hospital after surgery. Five days later, a meeting with the oncologist. Four days after that, the first in a year of chemotherapy treatments. Then 6 weeks of radiotherapy and 6 more months of chemo.

Because I trusted my surgeon, I never hesitated or agonized over decisions about treatment. I never sought a second opinion. I just wanted the cancer out of my body and out of my life. And I wanted to know: What did I do wrong? Why was this happening to me?

At my first appointment with the oncologist, I couldn't stop crying. He pigeonholed me as "hysterical." He never gave me credit for being intelligent, and he didn't listen. I was 3 months into treatment before he told me that chemo would last not 6 months but a full year!

No doctor warned me about the possibility of lymphedema. When it happened, I was told, "There's no treatment. Just learn to live with it." Living with it has meant two hospitalizations with cellulitis, repeated rounds of heavy-duty antibiotics, and the continuing fear that the tiniest cut or burn will trigger another flare-up. Every day, my swollen arm and hand remind me of breast cancer.

My first postdiagnosis year, I was in treatment. My husband was in denial. He didn't go to doctor's appointments with me, which made me angry. Looking back, I realize that's the only way he could deal with it. He did look after the children on weekends and hired a babysitter for Mondays and Wednesdays. When my treatment ended, he wanted the whole thing to be over. Finished. We've worked on that issue over the years, but the idea that I have cancer and could die is still horrific to him.

Our son was 5 when I was diagnosed, our daughter just 18 months. I asked the pediatrician what to tell my son. "Be factual about what's happening, but don't tell him it's life threatening. If the time comes when that's necessary, tell him then." That seems to have worked. My daughter was too young to understand, but now that she's 10, I know we need to have that conversation before many more years go by.

I had good care, but after surgery and during chemo and radiation, it was sometimes hard to understand what was happening and whether what I was feeling was something to worry about. My contacts were primarily oncologists and med techs, so it was sometimes hard to get my questions answered in a timely way. Having access to a knowledgeable nurse for explanations and answers would have helped a lot. My support group was invaluable in helping to answer my questions and confirm that much of what I was going through was "normal."

Breast cancer shattered my life. Picking up the pieces and rearranging them has been an extraordinarily humbling experience. It's made me more compassionate and less patient. When I talk to women who are going through treatment, getting the same drugs I had nearly a decade ago, I get angry because so little has changed. When I look at my 10-year-old daughter, who now has a family history of breast cancer, I get furious and frightened because there's no sure way to keep it from happening to her.

provide him or her with privacy as needed and provide care with consideration of needed modesty, such as covering, to maintain the professional relationship.

MODEL OF INTERVENTION

The PLISSIT model of intervention (the acronym stands for permission, limited information, specific suggestion, and intensive therapy) is based on a behavioral approach to treatment and incorporates four progressive levels of intervention in sexual problems (Estes, 2002). Each succeeding level requires increasing knowledge and clinical skill on your part.

Permission. Many clients hesitate to bring up sexual issues. Through skillful communication, however, you can give clients *permission* to discuss all their concerns. In giving permission, you assure them that you will give professional attention to anything they wish to share. Permission may also involve assuring clients that they are normal. For example, a single adult woman who is not in a stable relationship may need assurance that masturbation is normal and acceptable.

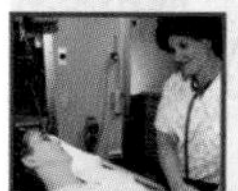

The case study client, Lisa, may be fearful of disclosing her personal anxieties and beliefs about sex. Assure such clients that sometimes sharing personal information is necessary to provide the best possible health care. Emphasize that you will respect her privacy.

Limited Information. Often, permission to talk about sexuality concerns reveals that the client has negative beliefs about aspects of sexuality that are based on cultural or religious upbringing. In response, you can provide factual information and appropriate resources. Giving *limited information* allows you to share knowledge related to the client's concerns and to answer questions directly and clearly. Do not include extraneous information that was not asked for or needed.

For example, when teaching adolescent girls about menstruation and what they might expect, you would initially refrain from overwhelming them with every detail. When conducting a seminar about HIV transmission, you would limit the discussion to relevant knowledge and research. When helping parents teach their children about sexuality, you would advise them to limit their information to what is appropriate for the child's age.

Specific Suggestion. At this level of the PLISSIT model, you help clients change their behavior by giving *specific suggestions.* The change in behavior should help to attain goals that are directly related to a particular problem. Once you and the client have the necessary information, and together have set clear goals, your specific suggestions may include reading appropriate literature, attending support groups (such as a cancer survival group in Lisa's case), role-playing discussions a couple might have about sexuality or sexual intercourse, and referral to professional resources.

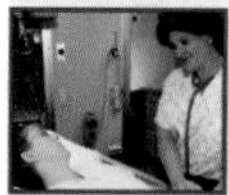

In the case study, Lisa indicates that nonsexual aspects of her relationship with her husband are good. The stress of illness and uncertainty about outcomes in a chronic or life-threatening disease may be inhibiting sexual intimacy in both partners. Perhaps providing her with increased skill in communicating her feelings, needs, and desires to her husband, as well as with ways to elicit the same from him, would facilitate resolution of their altered sexuality pattern. Another intervention would be offering to listen to the husband's thoughts or suggesting resources for him. Box 46-6 gives a sample care plan for Lisa.

Few generalist nurses are prepared to intervene in detail at this level of the model and beyond. Therefore your specific suggestion may be a referral to an expert professional, such as a nurse specialist, a psychologist, a marriage or sex counselor, or another mental health professional. Make sure to tell your client that counseling from an expert is a normal, natural part of treatment. Make every effort to match the client's specific problem to the specific resource.

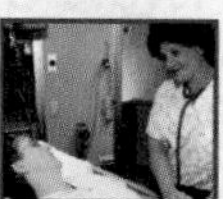

Perhaps Lisa's husband, Vincent, is just as anxious or fearful as she is about what is happening to her. Perhaps he worries constantly about whether her cancer will recur and what her chances of survival are. If he has not heard specific medical information about Lisa's condition, start by suggesting that he talk with Lisa's physician. How else might Vincent be encouraged to share his view of their marital relationship?

Intensive Therapy. The last step in the PLISSIT model is *intensive therapy.* It is recommended for more complex and highly individualized problems of sexual health.

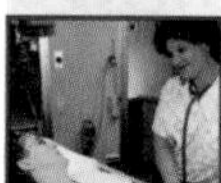

Lisa's problems may need a sex therapist's expertise to be resolved. Before referring Lisa and her husband to counseling, it is optimal to assess the overall health of the couple's relationship, the extent of their knowledge, their fears, the reasons each gives for lack of sexual intimacy, what their past sexual patterns have been, and their willingness to work toward resolution, individually and as a couple.

Using the PLISSIT Model. To understand more about the PLISSIT model and how it is used, consider these examples. A 53-year-old woman who has been menopausal for 2 years is distressed about pain upon penetration during intercourse. Assessment determines that the client has no physical defect. Using the PLISSIT model, give the client permission to discuss her dilemma with her partner and together try to find more comfortable positions for intercourse. Specific suggestions would include a thorough physical assessment to determine the cause of the pain. In addition, suggesting the use of a water-soluble vaginal lubricant before intercourse may be helpful. Dryness is common in menopausal women and may be causing the pain.

An adolescent boy comes to the school nurse with abrasions caused by a fight in the schoolyard. He says that the other boys all brag about "doing it" and ridicule him for not having sex with his girlfriend. He is

BOX 46-6

Nursing Care Plan

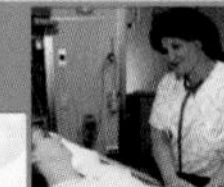

A Client With Ineffective Sexuality Pattern

Admission Data

Client states that she is feeling unattractive and expresses concern about the results of her biopsy. She reports there has been no intercourse with her husband for the past 3 months. She appears sad when discussing her husband's indifference to her.

Physician's Orders

Complete blood count
Sonogram, uterus
Height and weight
Chest radiograph
ECG
Preparation for uterine biopsy

Nursing Assessment

No eye contact. Fidgeting with wedding ring. States she has irregular periods and is afraid of surgery. Believes husband has stopped loving her. Does not wish to discuss problems with her spiritual advisor.

NANDA-I Nursing Diagnosis	NOC Expected Outcomes With Indicators	NIC Interventions With Selected Activities	Evaluation Data
Ineffective Sexuality Pattern **Related Factors:** Loss of breast Stress of anticipated results of surgery	***Body Image*** • Discusses concerns about how the effects of surgery will further affect sexuality.	***Body Image Enhancement*** • Reassure Lisa that her feelings are usual following the loss of a body part. • Use active listening. • Provide accurate information. Inform Lisa when and what results will be available to her. • Contract for time to talk privately before and after procedure. • Provide emotional support.	• Lisa reports sexual concerns on return visit. Facial expression shows relief. Shares more feelings with nurse. • Acknowledges understanding of necessary tests and time to conduct them. • Acknowledges difficulty in discussing sexual concerns. Agrees to talk with nurse. Agrees to talk with spouse.

Nursing outcome and intervention labels from Johnson, M., Bulechek, G., Butcher, H., Dochterman, J. M., Maas, M., Moorhead, S., et al. (Eds.). (2006). *NANDA, NOC, and NIC linkages: Nursing diagnoses, outcomes, & interventions.* St. Louis, MO: Mosby.

not sexually active because of his religious and moral objection to sex outside a committed relationship. Again using the PLISSIT model, give him permission to be different from his friends; stress that his sexual inactivity is just as normal as the other boys' sexual activity. Help him brainstorm assertive responses to use when other boys tease him that would not alienate or provoke them but instead would confirm his choice of abstinence.

INTERVENTIONS TO RESOLVE *SEXUAL DYSFUNCTION*

The PLISSIT model is most appropriate to use in identifying a specific sexual dysfunction and for directing the client toward effective resources. Before referring to counseling, urge the client to have a thorough physical evaluation and diagnostic tests to rule out any physical or physiological abnormalities.

Another intervention is to recognize that anxiety or depression may accompany sexual dysfunction. Acknowledge the client's feelings, and offer support that further assessment will be done through follow-up treatment and referral as needed. Encourage the client to pursue follow-up treatment and any referrals because treatment is offered for many dysfunctions. Be alert for signs of depression that may accompany chronic illness such as cancer, and provide referral in addition to good hygiene practices and physical care that assist the client in achieving physical comfort until further treatment begins.

INTERVENTIONS TO PROMOTE SEXUAL HEALTH

Educating the public on the many facets of sexual growth and development and health is an essential nursing function and an important strategy toward promoting healthy sexuality. The astute nurse will find opportunities for discussing health issues in many arenas, such as with parents whose children are hospitalized or are in home health care, in the schools, at parent-teacher sessions, in community groups, at health fairs, and with children in hospitals and clinics (Figure 46-6). Opportunities arise when working with older adults as well, during hospitalization, in extended-care facilities, and in community health or senior centers.

INTERVENTIONS TO PREVENT SEXUALLY TRANSMITTED DISEASE

A high priority in sexual health promotion is the prevention of sexually transmitted diseases (STDs). STDs affect men and women of all backgrounds and economic levels. Recent statistics suggest that 15.3 million new cases of STDs arise each year in the United States (CDC, 2006b). In addition, women are bearing the brunt of both the risk and the consequences of STDs. The reason is, at least in part, that the warm, moist vaginal environment promotes the growth of flora and that mucosal tears during intercourse provide an entry for infection.

Chlamydial infection is the most common bacterial STD in the United States today. It is more difficult to diagnose in women than in men because it is usually asymptomatic. Untreated, chlamydial infections have serious reproductive tract consequences, which are preventable through treatment. What many people do not realize is that STDs have a latent or subclinical phase in which the person is infected but asymptomatic. Thus the disease may be transmitted without either partner knowing it exists.

In light of this information, and because multipartner sexual contact is accepted in our society, prevention is a formidable task. Publicity aimed at prevention and public education has a great potential to reduce the problem. Just as you must take the initiative in assessing clients for sexual health problems, nurses also must take the initiative to speak out in appropriate public forums (such as parent-teacher meetings, health-related seminars, and high school or public health fairs). Take every opportunity to do individual assessment and teaching, especially with adolescents and young, single adults, and to support social causes that promote awareness of the extent of the STD problem.

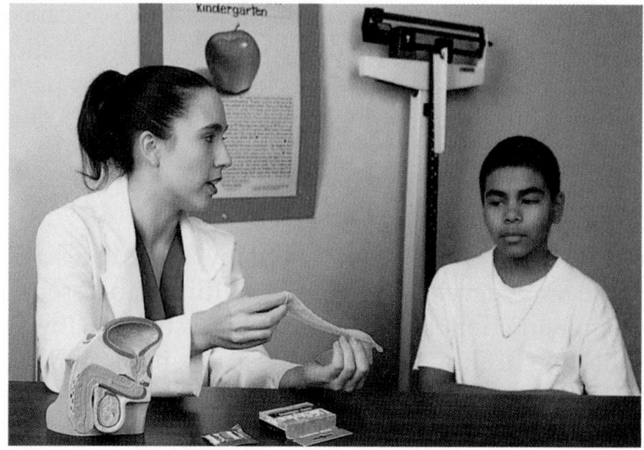

FIGURE 46-6 School nurses can provide sensitive counseling about sexual behavior.

Action Alert! Provide teaching about the prevention of STDs through the use of abstinence or safe sex. Be explicit when explaining that safe sex means always using protection during sexual intimacy. Also explain that even safe sex is not as safe as abstinence.

INTERVENTIONS FOR LESBIANS AND GAY MEN

In interviewing your clients, it is preferable to talk about sexual practices by using the phrase "sexual partner" rather than assuming a male partner for a female client and a female partner for a male client. Some of your clients will be lesbians and gay men. Even though public awareness of the existence of gay men and lesbians has been raised, many people, including nurses, are still uncomfortable or fearful about interacting with these clients. **Homophobia** is a fear of becoming homosexual through contact with lesbians and gay men (a myth) or a fear of having close or intimate feelings toward someone of the same sex.

Research conducted by Bailey, Farquhau, Owen and Whittaker (2002) indicates lesbians and bisexual women may have wide-ranging histories with both male and female partners. Men generally have more positive attitudes about casual sex, and therefore casual sex among gay men is more prevalent than among heterosexuals. This practice raises a number of health-related issues, including knowledge about and prevention of STDs and such medical conditions as rectal and anal infections and trauma.

Lesbian and bisexual women experience significant barriers to health care, partly because of homophobia and heterosexism in the health care system, but also for financial reasons. In general, women make less money than men and are more likely to be in jobs that have no health care benefits. If a woman identifies herself as lesbian or bisexual, attitudes of health care providers vary from acceptance to tolerance to disapproval and even to disgust and hatred. However, if women choose not to disclose their sexual orientation, they risk being treated improperly, especially in relationship to gynecological problems. In fact, lesbian and bisexual women experience similar sexual alterations and dysfunctions as heterosexual women (Chernin & Johnson, 2002).

Both homosexual men and women experience a good deal of stress as a result of being an oppressed and stigmatized minority. Discrimination against homosexuals in health care is unethical, yet it exists. You are obligated to care for a homosexual client just as sensitively as for any other client. You must maintain a nonjudgmental attitude without presumed assumptions. Facilitate more effective care by first examining your own beliefs, fears, and biases about homosexuality; determine to what extent, if any, these will interfere when you encounter homosexual clients. Seeking factual knowledge and exploring attitudes with peers will increase your objectivity in nursing care. Talking with lesbians or gay men who are open to such interaction can help alleviate your anxiety and assure you that, aside from their sexuality, these clients are just like your other clients.

Nurses in a variety of practice settings have excellent opportunities to promote healthy sexuality, including safe sexual practices. People of all ages and sexual orientations are likely to talk more readily with nurses about sexual issues, particularly when the nurse listens for and is comfortable with sexual themes. The caring, nonthreatening, unhurried manner in which nurses engage others in such discussions has the potential to make a marked difference in the ways people view and experience themselves as sexual beings.

EVALUATION

Evaluation of nursing care for sexuality problems includes determining whether the expected outcomes have been met. In addition, you should determine whether the problem has been resolved to the client's satisfaction. Particularly in the sensitive area of sexuality, the client may not have clearly identified the problem. If so, the client may be left with some discomfort, indicating the problem has not truly been resolved.

Evaluation can be based on a review of the PLISSIT model. To evaluate the phase of *permission*, observe the client's level of comfort in discussing sexuality. Ask questions to determine whether the problem has been resolved. Questions might include "Are you satisfied with the sexual aspects of your life?" "Has the work we have done together helped?" "Has it addressed the problem as you perceived it?" To evaluate the client's level of comfort with therapy and with current sexuality, nonverbal observations may be helpful. Notice the client's posture, eye contact, and ease in communicating. Have these changed from your initial contact with the client? Can the client ask questions and discuss sexual concerns freely?

To evaluate the effects of providing *limited information*, determine whether the client has understood and retained the information, whether the information has adequately addressed both spoken and unspoken questions, and whether having the information has been helpful.

To evaluate the *specific suggestions* phase of the model, ask whether the client has been able to try the suggestions and to describe the results. At this point, you would also want to know whether the client thought of other ideas that worked better than the suggestions you gave. You can also reinforce positive behaviors and correct any misperceptions.

To evaluate the last phase, *intensive therapy*, ask whether the client followed up on your referral to seek more intensive therapy and whether the therapy was helpful. Because intensive therapy may be long term, you may be able to evaluate only on the basis of whether the client has begun the process.

In addition, you should evaluate the client's level of self-care. Does the client have the knowledge to maintain sexual health? Is the client aware of resources to obtain further information or to manage the present or future problems?

Sample documentation that includes evaluation of the plan of care for Lisa, the case study client, is shown below.

Sample Documentation Note for Lisa Simonelli

Reports having sexual concerns during this return visit. Acknowledges difficulty in discussing sexual concerns but agrees to talk further with nurse and with husband. States she understands necessity of diagnostic and lab tests and the time frames for obtaining results.

▼ KEY PRINCIPLES

- The biological, psychological, social, and cultural influences one experiences throughout life have a significant impact on human sexuality.
- Physiological, psychosocial, and developmental factors affect sexuality.
- Self-assessment of your attitudes, preferences, and prejudices should precede assessment of the client's sexuality.
- Sexuality is a major part of many life processes.
- Sexual needs vary in health and illness for clients across the life span.
- The PLISSIT model (permission, limited information, specific suggestion, and intensive therapy) is an appropriate model to use for nursing intervention.

■ REVIEW QUESTIONS

1. A staff nurse is assigned a client experiencing sexual dysfunction. Which characteristic or qualification is most important for the nurse to have when working with sexual dysfunction?

1. An understanding that all sexual disorders can be corrected
2. An earnest awareness of personal feelings about sexuality
3. Previous experience working with clients with sexual dysfunction
4. An understanding that most sexual disorders have a poor prognosis

2. A client is newly diagnosed with a sexual dysfunction. What is most important for the nurse to know?

1. All sexual dysfunctions are curable.
2. Most sexual dysfunctions have a poor prognosis.
3. The nurse should understand his or her own personal feelings, thoughts, and biases about sexuality.
4. The client will want to know everything possible about his or her sexual dysfunction.

3. A mother of three children, ages 4 years, 7 years, and 9 years, is scheduled to undergo a double mastectomy. What is the best information she can share with her children?

1. Tell the children that Mommy is going into the hospital for a special check-up and will be back in a few days.

Continued

2. In order to protect the children's security and avoid frightening them, tell them Mommy is going on a short trip.
3. Secure quiet family time and tell the children the truth using simple, calm, and straightforward language.
4. Find a book that speaks about this and read it to the children.

4. A client is receiving discharge education after a hospital stay that was the result of a heart attack. Which of the following would not be included in discharge education?

1. Provide a list of foods that are considered low salt and heart friendly.
2. Establish exercise guidelines in collaboration with cardiologist.
3. Instruct that death can occur during sex after a client has suffered a heart attack.
4. Educate about prescribed medication regimen and side effects that may occur, as well as adverse side effects to report.

5. The appropriate words to use when speaking to a client who is gay about his or her partner is:

1. Male partner for the gay male and female partner for a lesbian
2. Sexual partner
3. Boyfriend for a gay male and girlfriend for a lesbian
4. Husband or wife, either one will be acceptable, because you should treat a gay client as you would a heterosexual client

Bibliography

American Psychiatric Association. (2000). *Diagnostic and statistical manual of mental disorders* (4th ed., Text Revision). Washington, DC: Author.

Anderson, P. B., Spruille, B., Venable, R. H., & Strano, D.A. (2005). The relationships between heavy episodic drinking, sexual assaulting and being sexually assaulted for Southern urban university students. *Electronic Journal of Human Sexuality,* Vol. 8. Retrieved June 28, 2006, from http://www.ejhs.org.

Bailey, J. V., Farquhau, C., Owen, C., & Mangtani, P. (2004). Sexually transmitted infections in women who have sex with women. *Sexually Transmitted Infections, 80*(3), 244-246.

Bailey, J. V., Farquhau, C., Owen, C., Whittaker, D. (2003). Sexual behaviour of lesbians and bisexual women. *Sexually Transmitted Infections, 79,* 147-150. Retrieved June 20, 2006, from http://sti.bmjjournals.com/cgi/content/full/79/2/147.

Blackburn, M. (2002). *Sexuality & Disability* (4th ed.). St. Louis, MO: Elsevier.

Carpenito, L. J. (2005). *Nursing diagnosis: Application to clinical practice* (11th ed.). Philadelphia: Lippincott Williams & Wilkins.

Centers for Disease Control and Prevention. (2004). *Sexually transmitted disease surveillance, 2004: National surveillance data for chlamydia, gonorrhea, and syphilis.* Retrieved June 29, 2006, from http://www.cdc.gov/std/stats/trends2004.htm.

Centers for Disease Control and Prevention. (2006a). *Interactive atlas of reproductive health: Demographic groups.* Retrieved June 14, 2006, from http://www.cdc.gov/reproductivehealth/GISAtlas/Demographics.htm.

Centers for Disease Control and Prevention. (2006b). *STDs today.* Retrieved June 29, 2006, from http://www.cdcnpin.org/scripts/std/std.asp.

Chernin, J. N., & Johnson, M. R. (2002). *Affirmative psychotherapy and counseling for lesbians and gay men.* Thousand Oaks, CA: Sage Publications.

Dixon, K. D., Dixon, P. N. (2006). The PLISSIT Model: Care and management of patients' psychosexual needs following radical surgery. *Lippincott's Case Management, 11*(2), 101-106.

Estes, J. P. (2002). *Beyond basic ADLs.* Retrieved June 28, 2006, from http://www.rehabpub.com/features/42002/7.asp.

Gorman, L. J., Raines, M. L., Sultan, F. S. (2002). *Psychosocial nursing for general patient care.* Philadelphia: F. A. Davis.

Hanser, M. (2005). *Alternative therapies: Growing options in nursing practice.* National Center of Continuing Education. Retrieved June 28, 2006, from http://www.nursece.com/onlinecourses/9017.html.

Johnson, M., Bulechek, G., Butcher, H., Dochterman, J. M., Maas, M., Moorhead, S., et al. (Eds.). (2006). *NANDA, NOC, and NIC linkages: Nursing diagnoses, outcomes, & interventions.* St. Louis, MO: Mosby.

LeVay, S. (2003). *The biology of sexual orientation.* Retrieved June 14, 2006, from http://members.aol.com/slevay/page22.html.

Masters, W., & Johnson, V. (1966). *Human sexual response.* Boston: Little, Brown and Company.

McManus, A. J., Hunter, L. P., Renn, H. (2006). Lesbian experiences and needs during childbirth: Guidance for health care providers. *Journal of Obstetric, Gynecologic, and Neonatal Nursing, 35*(1), 13-23.

Meyer, K., & Laederach-Hofman, K. (2003). Effects of a comprehensive rehabilitation program on quality of life in patients with chronic heart failure. *Progress in Cardiovascular Nursing, 18*(4), 169-176.

NANDA International. (2005). *Nursing diagnoses: Definitions and classification, 2005-2006* (6th ed.). Philadelphia: Author.

National Alliance of Breast Cancer Organizations. (2003). *Breast self-exam (BSE).* Retrieved June 14, 2006, from http://www.mydna.com/health/breast_cancer.

Pelusi, J. (2006). Sexuality and body image. Research on breast cancer survivors documents altered body image and sexuality. *American Journal of Nursing, 106*(3, Suppl.), 32-38.

Ronner, A. D. (2005). *Homophobia and the law.* Washington, DC: American Psychological Association.

Serrant-Green, L.(2005). Breaking traditions: Sexual health and ethnicity in nursing research—a literature review. *Journal of Advanced Nursing, 51*(5), 511-519.

Spector, R. E. (2004). *Cultural diversity in health & illness* (6th ed.). Upper Saddle River, NJ: Pearson/Prentice Hall.

Steinke, E. E. (2005). Intimacy needs and chronic illness: Strategies for sexual counseling and self-management. *Journal of Gerontologic Nursing, 31*(5), 40-50.

Steinke, E. E., Gill-Hopple, K., Valdez, D., & Wooster, M. (2005). Sexual concerns and educational needs after an implantable cardioverter defibrillator. *Heart Lung, 34*(5), 299-308.

Thompson, J., McFarland, G., Hirsch, J., & Tucker, S. (2002). *Mosby's clinical nursing* (5th ed.). St. Louis, MO: Mosby.

Whitman, J. S., & Boyd, C. J. (Eds.). (2003). *The therapist's notebook for lesbian, gay, and bisexual clients: Homework, handouts, and activities for use in psychotherapy.* New York: Haworth.

World Health Organization. (2005). *Gender and reproductive rights.* Retrieved June 28, 2006, from http://www.who.int/reproductive-health/gender/sexual_health.html.

Chapter 47

Supporting Stress Tolerance and Coping

Media Resources

- evolve Evolve Website http://evolve.elsevier.com/Harkreader/
- Companion CD

Learning Objectives

After studying this chapter, you should be able to do the following:

- Describe physiological and psychological concepts of stress
- Identify factors affecting stress tolerance
- Discuss the assessment of a client's stress tolerance and coping skills
- Differentiate stress-related nursing diagnoses from other related nursing diagnoses
- Plan goal-directed interventions to prevent, reduce, or manage stress
- Evaluate achievement of the expected outcomes for clients' progress toward stress tolerance and coping

Key Terms

adaptation
adaptive coping
anxiety
coping
crisis
defense mechanism
developmental crisis
homeostasis
maladaptive coping
psychoneuroimmunology
resilience
situational crisis
stress
stressor

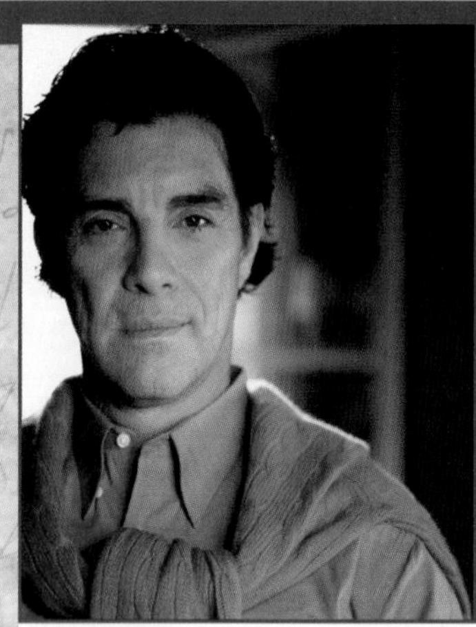
© 2007, Getty Images.

Billy Osceola is a 55-year-old Native American man. He has diabetes and is recovering from a left below-knee amputation performed 10 days ago. During your first home health care nursing visit, you see a liquor bottle open on the table. He raises his voice angrily when you try to talk to him about following a diabetic menu plan. Alcohol is on his breath. When you question him about it, he grunts and angrily asks you to leave, shouting that he does not need any nurse coming to see him. He refuses to let you near him. You go, telling him you will be back to see him the next morning.

The next day, Mr. Osceola is polite and sober but basically noncommunicative. You are concerned when you see him put a stained, damp rag on his stump over the remains of a surgical dressing. When you ask him about it, he says his leg hurts and he is trying to fix it with an herbal potion he got from the shaman. He refuses to talk further about his leg and says there is no need to come see him.

Mr. Osceola is stressed. He is having difficulty accepting his current situation. His behavior has the potential to interfere with wound healing and prevent him from taking positive action to manage his health. In analyzing Mr. Osceola, the nurse considers stress-related nursing diagnoses (see key nursing diagnoses box).

Nurses often encounter clients who are stressed and whose usual patterns of coping with difficult situations are ineffective.

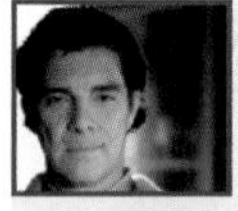

Mr. Osceola has been coping through the use of alcohol and reliance on culturally prescribed health practices. Although the alcohol may have made his life seem bearable and the shaman has helped him manage health problems in the past, he is facing the possibility of a life-threatening infection that could probably be more effectively treated with antibiotics and wound care. In addition to the usual stressors in his life and the loss of his limb, Mr. Osceola has the stressor of the conflict of his culture with the treatment recommendations of his physician.

KEY NURSING DIAGNOSES FOR STRESS

Ineffective coping: Inability to form a valid appraisal of the stressors, inadequate choices of practiced responses, and/or inability to use available resources

Ineffective denial: Conscious or unconscious attempt to disavow the knowledge or meaning of an event, to reduce anxiety or fear, to the detriment of health

CONCEPTS OF STRESS

Stress is a physiological response produced by the normal wear and tear of bodily processes and external and internal demands. It is a normal part of life. It is an elusive concept because it can be acute or chronic, physical or psychological, and mild or severe.

In small quantities, stress is good—it can motivate you and help you be more productive. However, too much stress, or a strong response to stress, is harmful. Persistent and unrelenting stress often leads to anxiety (see Chapter 42) and unhealthy behaviors like overeating and abuse of alcohol or other drugs. To the extent that stress is a causative factor in disease, illness can be thought of as an imbalance that occurs when the body fails to adapt to complex physical and emotional stressors. **Stressors** are a cause of stress, such as extreme hot or cold, an argument, a virus, an examination, cigarette smoke, a death, or any of the countless demands of the environment.

PHYSIOLOGICAL STRESS RESPONSE

General Adaptation Syndrome. **Homeostasis** is a healthy, more or less stable, physiological state in which there is not undue imbalance. It is a state of internal stability of our physiology and our emotions. It maintains balance by returning the body to a relaxed state after the stress response. For example, sympathetic nervous system activity increases heart rate, cardiac output, respiratory rate, muscle tension, mental alertness, and glucose levels during a stressful event. The parasympathetic nervous system returns the body to a relaxed state by slowing heart rate, decreasing blood pressure, and returning other body systems to a normal body condition (see Figure 42-1, in Chapter 42).

As described in Chapter 42, the "acute stress response," or the fight-or-flight response, is the first of three physiological stages called the general adaptation syndrome (GAS): the alarm reaction stage, the resistance stage, and the exhaustion stage.

In the alarm reaction stage, the sympathetic nervous system initiates the fight-or-flight response and activates defense mechanisms. Adrenaline surges, the heart speeds, and the body prepares for fighting or running away. This fight-or-flight response is sustained by the hypothalamic-pituitary-adrenal axis, which releases cortisone, norepinephrine, and epinephrine into the blood.

In the resistance stage, the body attempts to adapt to the stressor. The parasympathetic nervous system modulates the body's response by opposing the actions of the sympathetic nervous system. As a consequence of the resistance stage, the person either recovers or becomes exhausted. If the latter occurs, the person enters the exhaustion stage, in which the body cannot function defensively against the stressor, and physiological regulation decreases. If the stress continues in the exhaustion stage, death can result.

Stress and Illness. Stress has become an important psychological variable in the field of psychoneuroimmunology. **Psychoneuroimmunology** is the study of the interface between the brain and immunology. It provides a framework for examining the relationship between health outcomes and behavioral and physiological phenomena. Research shows that psychological stress can lead to increased susceptibility to disease by suppressing the immune response.

Stress has a significant impact on various bodily organ systems, including the gastrointestinal tract, the endocrine system, female and male reproductive systems, and dental pathologic conditions. It can cause some diseases and exacerbate others, as well as induce cardiovascular disease, arrhythmias, and sudden death.

Likewise, illness can cause stress. When illness occurs, there is an attempt at the physiological and the psychological levels to strike a balance and achieve homeostasis. The ill person attempts to adapt to physical changes, and wellness or additional illness can result. An ill person may not eat, and nutritional imbalances may introduce additional stress.

CONCEPTS OF COPING

PSYCHOSOCIAL COPING

Psychosocial coping is another way to achieve balance or homeostasis. **Coping** is the ability to deal with dangerous, threatening, or challenging situations. It is a major component in the relationship between the experience of stress and health. The concept of coping is similar to that of adaptation. **Adaptation** is a process through which individuals accommodate to changes in the internal or external environment to preserve functioning and pursue goals. They learn to cope with and adapt to stressors by using methods that were successful for them in the past. For example, a client learned from prior experience that she could escape from an unpleasant situation and return to homeostasis by reading a mystery book.

METHODS OF COPING

What is stressful at one time may not be stressful at another. People respond to stress in many ways in an effort to alleviate stress and increase their level of comfort. They use coping devices that are familiar to them, whether those devices are ultimately helpful or not. Coping behaviors can be adaptive or maladaptive. **Adaptive coping** is a process that fosters problem solving, growth and development, and the ability to perceive reality and respond in a way that supports emotional and physical well-being. The devices may simply reduce the perception of stress, thus creating a mental climate that promotes clear thinking. Examples include the following:

- Listening to music
- Talking with a supportive person
- Praying or meditating
- Playing with pets
- Creative activities, such as drawing

Maladaptive coping is the use of methods or efforts directed toward management of dangerous, threatening, or challenging situations and producing feelings and behaviors that decrease the quality of life and lead to unhealthy outcomes. It can cause difficulty with interpersonal relationships and mastery and growth and has the ability to negatively affect treatment outcome. It includes the following:

- Use of drugs and alcohol
- Violence directed at self, others, animals, or property
- Withdrawal from family and friends
- Excessive risk taking
- Increased compulsive behavior (e.g., overeating, gambling, promiscuity)

In a hospital setting, maladaptive coping may be seen as a refusal to participate in treatment, noncompliance, demands for attention, or manipulation of staff or family.

People also respond to stress by using defense mechanisms (Table 47-1). **Defense mechanisms** (or coping styles) are methods used to protect oneself from stress and maintain psychological homeostasis. They operate without individual awareness and are not an attempt to solve a problem but mediate individuals' reactions to emotional conflicts and to internal and external stressors. They lessen uncomfortable feelings of anxiety, prevent pain, and protect individuals by allowing them to deny, distort, or restrict full awareness of unpleasant thoughts, feelings, and feared impulses (American Psychiatric Association [APA], 2000; Thobaben, Fossett, & Nadler-Moodie, 2004).

FACTORS AFFECTING STRESS TOLERANCE

Although every person has a unique response to stress, some people have more reserve or capacity to resist challenges to self-integrity. This is partly because how a person tolerates and copes with stress is influenced by developmental stage, genetics, lifestyle, and culture (Box 47-1).

CRISIS

A **crisis** is an upset in a balanced or stable state for which the usual methods of adaptation and coping are not sufficient. A person in crisis is faced with overwhelming adaptive tasks. As anxiety rises, the person's ability to perceive what is happening declines steadily and internal disorganization and feelings of helplessness occur. Feelings of grief and shame can also be associated with a crisis, as well as disruptive or violent behavior in an effort to regain control.

A crisis has the following characteristics:

- Disturbs homeostasis
- Involves loss
- Does not respond to usual adaptive coping activities
- Is perceived as overwhelming or life threatening
- Is self-limiting
- Is associated with increased affect and decreased communication abilities
- Brings unresolved problems to the foreground
- Demands a relatively immediate response
- Requires intervention to reach equilibrium
- Produces positive or negative change

A crisis usually lasts a brief period of time, from a few days to a few weeks. During the crisis, the person's mind, body, and spirit attempt to return to a balanced state of homeostasis. Being confronted by a crisis event requires new responses to adapt to the situation. These responses may be new internal competencies, such as learning a different way to think through a problem, or they may be external social skills, such as phoning a suicide-prevention center. Either the problem is solved, or the person adapts to the lack of a solution. In either case, a new state of balance is reached. Because of the temporary state of disorganization, the person in crisis is likely to remember old problems related to the present event.

Table 47-1 Defense Mechanisms

MECHANISM	DESCRIPTION
Compensation	Excelling in one area to overcome a real or imagined deficit
Conversion	Converting feelings into a physical disability or symptom
Denial	Avoiding emotional conflicts by refusing to acknowledge anything that might cause intolerable emotional pain
Depersonalization	Losing a sense of identity; having feelings of being someone else
Displacement	Shifting feelings from a less socially acceptable or more threatening object or person to a more acceptable or less threatening one
Identification	Modeling oneself after an admired person
Intellectualization	Denying feelings by answering with detailed impersonal statements
Projection	Attributing unacceptable thoughts, impulses, or feelings to others
Rationalization	Using an excuse to justify behavior while disguising an unconscious motive
Reaction formation	Acting directly opposite to one's unconscious wishes, feelings, or desires
Regression	Behaving in ways that were appropriate at earlier developmental periods
Repression	Placing traumatic situations out of awareness so they cannot be consciously remembered
Sublimation	Unconsciously redirecting an unacceptable tendency to a more acceptable one
Suppression	Deciding consciously to exclude unacceptable thoughts and feelings
Transference	Attributing feelings and attitudes of an early-in-life significant person to a currently significant person, such as a therapist

BOX 47-1 *Cross-Cultural Care*

Caring for a Native American Client

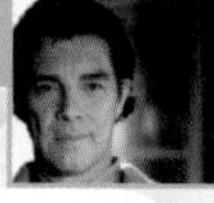

Billy Osceola, the client presented in this chapter, is a Native American of the Seminole tribe. He has always lived on the Big Cypress reservation in Florida. Mr. Osceola runs a smoke shop for the reservation. A number of values and beliefs that Mr. Osceola exhibits tend to be common in Native Americans of the Seminole tribe. Although every client is unique, many members of the Seminole tribe tend to hold the following values and beliefs:

- The shaman relies on a number of medicinal plants and herbs, including St. John's wort, willow, and ginseng. Herbal potions are often used in conjunction with lengthy chants.
- Eating should coincide with hunger rather than being set at three meals a day.
- Family is very important, with extended family the norm.
- Use of silence indicates respect for the other person.
- Eye contact is avoided because it is a sign of disrespect.
- Sacred myths and legends provide spiritual guidance. Religion and healing practices are blended together.
- Illness is caused by disequilibrium with nature. Everything that happens is the result of something else.

RISK FACTORS ACROSS THE LIFE SPAN

Developmental and situational are two major types of crises. An example of normal developmental tasks are the developmental tasks for older adults included in Box 47-2. A **developmental crisis** occurs when a person is unable to complete the tasks needed for a particular developmental level. A developmental crisis can occur at any stage of life and may result from a wide range of stressors. Examples are included in Table 47-2.

LIFESTYLE FACTORS

A **situational crisis** is a physically or psychologically hazardous situation that is not easily anticipated and for which a person is inadequately prepared. Two factors to consider are the person's perception of the stressful event, coping skills, and resilience.

Perception of a Stressful Event. Stressors in themselves are neither positive nor negative but are stressful only if perceived on some level as stressful. Consequently, the stimuli needed to produce stress vary with the individual. As an example of the highly individualized and fluid perceptions of what is stressful, and of the different responses to a situation, consider two people who miss a bus to work. One person starts to worry about being fired; the other pulls out a novel and calmly reads until the next bus appears. Similarly, a person can meet a crisis situation with a state of balance one day and imbalance the next. It all depends on the demands of the internal and external environment and how they are interpreted.

Coping Skills. A person's coping skills are challenged by anxiety-provoking stressors and a crisis situation. The precipitating stressors are different for each person. Having an illness diagnosed or being injured can provoke an identity crisis. In addition to coping with the fear of the disease or injury itself, clients may have to change their view of themselves (Thobaben et al., 2004).

Anxiety is a diffuse, highly uncomfortable, sometimes vague sense of apprehension or dread accompanied by one or more physical sensations (see Chapter 42). The feeling of discomfort ranges from mild apprehension to panic.

BOX 47-2 *Older Adults' Developmental Tasks*

- Adjusting to increased vulnerability to physical and emotional stress
- Finding coping patterns and adapting to change
- Adjusting to physical and physiological changes
- Adjusting to changes in family life cycle, such as adult relationship with children, death of a spouse
- Adjusting to changes in lifestyle, such as retirement, living accommodations, lower and fixed income
- Finding the meaning in life

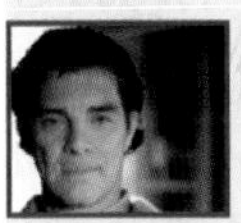

When you discover that he did not have breakfast, Mr. Osceola agrees to let you prepare lunch for him. A proud man, he refuses to use the crutches that lie at his bedside. When he gets out of bed, he gets around in an old wheelchair a neighbor loaned him. While preparing lunch, how would you assess Mr. Osceola further for anxiety and the methods he uses to cope?

Resilience. Resilience is the ability to identify or develop resources and strengths to flexibly manage stressors to gain a positive outcome, a sense of confidence, mastery, and self-esteem. It is the individual's ability to

Table 47-2 Developmental Crises

DEVELOPMENTAL LEVEL	APPROXIMATE AGE	STRESSORS THAT COULD PRECIPITATE A CRISIS
Infancy	Birth to about 2 years	• Lack of unconditional love • Lack of basic needs being met • Lack of ability to make beginning environmental manipulations
Childhood	About 2 to 6 years	• Inability to influence others with verbal communication • Inability to delay satisfaction • Inability to increase motor control • Refusal of others to grant autonomy
Juvenile	6 to 9 years	• Entry into school • Inability to learn appropriate roles • Inability to produce assignments • Difficulty with pal relationship • Inability to compete, compromise, or cooperate • Blocks to increasing motor, social, and/or physiological growth
Preadolescence	9 to 12 years	• Confusion about physiological (sex) changes
Adolescence	12 to 21+ years	• Blocks to evaluation of strengths and limitations
Adulthood	21+ to death	• Inability to produce children • Parenthood, especially firstborn • Blocks to communication with other age-groups • Inability to achieve personal concept of success • Inability to adapt to success
Old age	Varies	• Extreme physical, social, or economic restrictions • Blocks to reassessing life experiences • Inability to face death • Social or sensory deprivation

recover from or successfully cope with both internal and external stresses. It helps to explain individual differences in response to stressors. The quality of resilience is often attributed to people who can adapt and restore equilibrium to their lives in the face of overwhelming adversity. Factors thought to enhance resilience include intelligence, a sense of humor, a supportive family and friends, cultural and spiritual beliefs, hope, autonomy, self-esteem, and a sense of purpose (Figure 47-1).

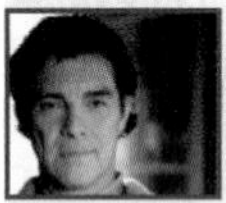

Mr. Osceola is flushed. He picks at his lunch and rubs the rag damp with a herbal potion around and around on his stump. He chants repeatedly under his breath. You ask to see the herbal cloth so you can visualize the stump dressing better. Mr. Osceola holds it out, but he will not let you hold the cloth. You can see drainage on the old dressing, and an odor seems to be coming from the wound. You ask to test his blood for "sugar" and finally touch his hand. Mr. Osceola's skin is burning hot. How would you assess Mr. Osceola's condition at this point? Is this adaptive or maladaptive coping?

ASSESSMENT

Assessment of a client under stress includes obtaining subjective and objective data. A general assessment of the client's coping abilities and stress tolerance can be incorporated into the health history and physical examination.

GENERAL ASSESSMENT OF STRESS TOLERANCE AND COPING

Health History. Gathering health history information to determine stress tolerance and coping is done by interview. To have a successful interview, you must respect the client, provide privacy, and ensure confidentiality. Throughout the interview, you will begin to build a therapeutic relationship with the client and begin to understand the source of stress. During the interview, ask questions designed to assess the client's stress tolerance and coping, such as those in Box 47-3.

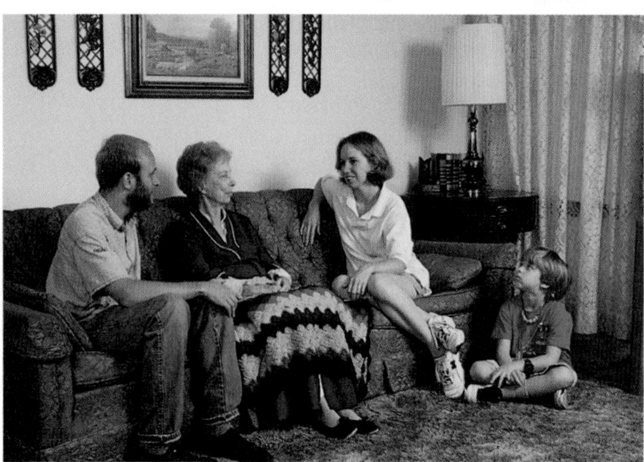

FIGURE 47-1 Family resilience and a caring family are resources that help a person to resist stress.

Physical Examination. This portion of the client assessment provides objective data. Physical signs of stress would be observed during this examination. Cardiovascular signs of the stress response are increased heart rate, increased blood pressure, and palpitations. Also, the client may complain of headaches, muscle tension, gastrointestinal disturbances, disturbed sleep, unusual fatigue, restlessness, and poor cognitive function. However, these physical signs alone cannot justify a conclusion that the client has a stress response.

FOCUSED ASSESSMENT FOR *INEFFECTIVE COPING*

Use the diagnosis *Ineffective coping* when the client demonstrates an inability to form a valid appraisal of the stressors, inadequate choices of practiced responses, or inability to use available resources (NANDA International [NANDA-I], 2005). Conduct a focused assessment by finding out how the client views (or perceives) the situation. Does the situation seem overwhelming to the client? Does it affect the client's occupational, social, or academic functioning? Does the client use too little or too much energy in attempting to adapt? Talk with the client's significant others to determine their perceptions of the stressful event. Answers to these questions may support or refute your diagnosis of *Ineffective coping*.

Defining Characteristics. Assess the client's perception of the situation. When the client expresses an inability to cope, or when you observe the client's inability to ask for help, you need to assess the underlying cause of this behavior. It may result from inadequate problem-solving skills, a narrowed perceptual field in the present circumstances, or a long-standing pattern of coping.

Assess for a change in the usual patterns of behavior. You may need to interview significant others to determine the usual pattern of communication, problem solving, ability to meet role expectations and basic needs, and use of social support.

Assess for signs and symptoms of distress such as tension, unexplained fatigue, sleep disturbance, poor concentration, or a high rate of illness or accidents.

BOX 47-3 *Sample Interview Questions to Assess Stress Tolerance and Coping*

- Are you worrying about anything?
- What worries you the most?
- What has been the most stressful event that has happened to you during this hospitalization/holiday season?
- How do you feel when you are stressed?
- Have you experienced any recent changes in your life (in the last year) related to your health, family, lifestyle habits, daily activities, work, or finances? Have you had any losses?
- How would you rate these life changes on a scale of 1 to 10 (10 being the most stressful)?
- How have you coped with similar stressors before? What do you do to make yourself feel less stressed?
- Have you received treatment for any stress-related problems in the past?

Assess for destructive behaviors. Substance abuse, risk-taking behaviors, withdrawal from possible sources of support, and destructive behavior toward self or others impede adaptive behavior.

Excessive goal-directed behavior that is disconnected to the problem and diverts attention from the problem represents *Ineffective coping*. In addition, lack of goal-directed behavior or the inability to attend to and organize information represents ineffective coping.

Related Factors. In assessing the factors related to *Ineffective coping,* consider the client's usual pattern of coping and if the client has the physical and psychological energy to cope.

Interventions may be aimed at personal characteristics related to the stressor. Clients may be using patterns of thinking that create a lack of confidence in their ability to cope, have an incorrect appraisal of the threat, or feel that accepting help requires giving up control. They may be experiencing a situational crisis when the diagnosis and prognosis are unknown, or they may be experiencing a developmental crisis.

FOCUSED ASSESSMENT FOR *INEFFECTIVE DENIAL*

Denial can be a healthy defense mechanism that permits clients to retain hope at certain stages of coping and/or allows them time to have more effective ways of adapting to a stressful event. Use the diagnosis *Ineffective denial* when your assessment indicates that clients consciously or unconsciously attempt to disavow the knowledge or meaning of an event to reduce their anxiety or fear and that this is detrimental to their health (NANDA-I, 2005).

Defining Characteristics. Focused assessment for *Ineffective denial* starts by evaluating the client's degree of denial and its effectiveness as a coping strategy. Ask yourself questions such as the following: Has the client delayed seeking care to the detriment of health? Does the client refuse treatment even after claiming to understand its benefits? Does the client's nonverbal behavior show fear even though none is expressed in words? Does the client continue to engage in behavior that can exacerbate the condition (e.g., a newly diagnosed diabetic who continues to eat concentrated sweets)? If you find many positive responses to these questions, the client is probably using denial inappropriately with possible untoward health effects.

Related Factors. Factors related to *Ineffective denial* include such things fear of death, loss of control, or loss of autonomy. The client has underlying feelings of hopelessness and helplessness, fear of change of role within the family or community, and/or knowledge deficit.

DIAGNOSIS

After conducting an assessment, cluster the data to help in identifying an appropriate nursing diagnosis (Table 47-3). The defining characteristics and recognition of cues and patterns will assist you in evaluating whether the client's problem can be resolved with nursing care alone. Related factors must be elicited to help define how the problem should be solved.

Use the diagnosis *Ineffective coping* when the client is experiencing a life event that tends to produce crisis. Diagnostic cues include observable anxiety and behavior and language that are disorganized and difficult to understand.

When the client delays seeking health care to the point of harm, refuses treatment after hearing the benefits of care, and shows signs of physiological imbalance, consider using the nursing diagnosis *Ineffective denial.*

The differentiating factor between the two diagnoses is the inappropriate use of denial as a coping behavior. *Ineffective coping* is differentiated from *Anxiety* based on the predominant symptoms.

Table 47-3 Clustering Data to Make a Nursing Diagnosis

Stress-Related Problems

DATA CLUSTER	DIAGNOSIS
A 26-year-old woman is admitted to the emergency department with a foot laceration resulting from accidental injury. History reveals complaints of poor appetite, poor concentration, neck and back pain, and insomnia. She works 32 hours per week and stated that her supervisor has been complaining about her work performance. She attends college full time, and her grades are falling, which is uncharacteristic for her. She is a single mother of two children.	*Ineffective coping* related to situational crisis
A 70-year-old man was diagnosed with prostate cancer 2 weeks after the death of his wife 1 year ago. He has no children, but a cousin lives nearby. He refused cancer therapy because "I don't have any prostate problems." The client's cousin brought him to the physician's office when he complained of not urinating for 2 days.	*Ineffective denial* related to fear of death and personal loss
A 33-year-old woman seeks care in the emergency department. She is pacing, wringing her hands, and crying. She is sweating profusely, her blood pressure and pulse are elevated, and respirations are 32 per minute and shallow. She says that her husband left 2 weeks ago, and she recently lost her job. She states, "I'm afraid I'm going crazy."	*Anxiety* related to stress of lifestyle change

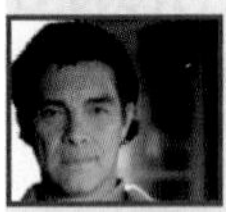

You are unable to test Mr. Osceola's blood glucose level. He says that he did not have any insulin in the house anyway. He wants you to leave, because, he says, "You are trying to do things I don't need." You tell him you will leave, but you have to replace the dressing on his leg first. "Fine, hurry up and do it so you will leave me be!" You recognize that Mr. Osceola is denying the need for your help out of fear of the consequences of infection. How will you address Mr. Osceola's plan of care?

PLANNING

Together, you and the client will need to develop a plan of care that reflects realistic and measurable goals. Interventions will be identified to attain expected outcomes that will help the client better tolerate stressful events. Planning for a client who is experiencing stress would include overall goals that the client will do the following:

- Be able to identify potential stressors
- Demonstrate, both verbally and behaviorally, decreased stress
- Develop effective methods of coping with stress

EXPECTED OUTCOMES FOR THE CLIENT WITH *INEFFECTIVE COPING*

The client whose coping and problem-solving abilities interfere with life will need assistance with setting realistic outcomes. Basic expected outcomes for the client with *Ineffective coping* include that the client will do the following:

- Demonstrate effective coping behaviors as evidenced by identifying the stressor, identifying usual coping behaviors, discussing coping alternatives, and choosing and using a coping strategy in an actual situation
- Effectively solve a problem, as evidenced by identifying the problem, discussing the steps of the problem-solving process, applying the problem-solving process to the problem in discussion, and implementing the problem-solving process
- Return to a previous level of functioning, as evidenced by maintenance of an adequate balance of rest and sleep, achievement of an appropriate level of social interaction and daily activities, and development of problem-solving techniques to decrease the effects of stress

EXPECTED OUTCOMES FOR THE CLIENT WITH *INEFFECTIVE DENIAL*

Denial can be a useful coping mechanism for defending against a stressful event. Rather than setting a goal of eliminating denial, help the client to increase stress tolerance and to use healthy coping skills. Expected outcomes for a client with *Ineffective denial* may include that the client will do the following:

- Demonstrate a low-to-moderate anxiety level, as evidenced by reduced signs and symptoms, resulting from relaxation techniques
- Receive the facts of the illness in a positive manner and use that information in a way that allows compliance with the health care regimen to achieve the full health potential

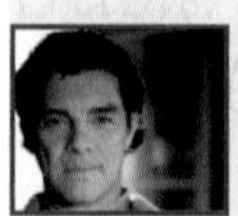

Mr. Osceola will not look at his leg while you rapidly change the dressing. You note that the amputation incision is coming open in the center and producing large amounts of foul, purulent drainage from the opening. The skin is red and edematous around the incision. You place a new dressing on the leg and ask Mr. Osceola if he knows that his leg is infected. Can you write an expected outcome that would indicate Mr. Osceola is making progress toward acceptance of the seriousness of his condition?

INTERVENTION

Effective nursing actions are based on an understanding of the concepts of stress and coping behaviors. Interventions are focused on increasing coping skills, preventing a crisis, intervening in crisis, and teaching stress management techniques to effectively deal with stressors.

INTERVENTIONS TO INCREASE COPING SKILLS

Therapeutic Relationship. Interventions to increase coping skills require establishing a therapeutic relationship and setting mutual goals with the client.

You and the client collaborate on the following:

- Analyzing and defining the problem (the situation and coping behaviors)
- Defining goals
- Identifying the interventions that can be implemented to solve the problem or decrease the severity of symptoms

You can help the client cope more effectively by using social supports, protecting a vulnerable self, practicing adaptive thinking, increasing receptivity, and learning new information.

Enhancing Social Supports. Positive support, given with unconditional positive regard, provided by a client's social circle is important for effective coping. Encourage and enlist the involvement of family and significant others to help the client tolerate the stressful event. Teach or role-model effective support.

If the client has little or no social support, contact appropriate support groups of the client's choosing, such as clergy, or social services to aid the client with further coping strategies. You, as the nurse, can also enhance social support by listening and using therapeutic communication, teaching techniques, and supportive behaviors. You can also provide support to the client by ensuring access to telephones, by encouraging expansion of social and personal contacts, and by helping significant others gain access to special visitations during critical care or prolonged hospitalizations.

Protecting a Vulnerable Self. Because defense mechanisms may initially allow clients to protect or defend themselves to reduce stress or anxiety, you should avoid breaking through their defenses unless you first teach an alternative way to cope. You can use cognitive techniques to reframe the stressor in more acceptable terms, help clients identify their strengths, or introduce information about the stressor in small, manageable amounts. When clients feel safe and anxiety is controlled, you may be able to help them recognize the negative effects of defensive behavior.

> ***Action Alert!*** Avoid confronting a client in denial unless you have evidence that the client can cope with the loss of this defense mechanism.

Practicing Adaptive Thinking. Cognitive therapy refers to methods of treatment that help a person change attitudes, perceptions, and patterns of thinking from irrational to realistic thoughts about the self and situations. Here are two techniques.

Self-Suggestion. To use suggestion for stress reduction, start by obtaining data on sources of the client's stress. Then agree on an individualized stress reduction self-suggestion. Help the client to a relaxed state. Then repeat or ask the client to repeat the stress reduction self-suggestion.

Once the stressful situation has been identified, you and the client decide which portion of the situation to focus on and how the suggestions can be worded most effectively for that client. For example, in a situation in which a client becomes highly stressed while talking with a physician, the client may be taught to self-suggest with the statement "I can stay calm when talking with my doctor."

Coping Thoughts. This approach is based on cognitive psychology theory, which holds that thoughts rule feelings. The way the future or present is imagined intensifies or decreases the feelings experienced. For example, being late for an assignment can result in stress, or it may result in a calm, problem-focused response. Positively interpreting lateness will most likely lead to feelings of calmness. Negatively interpreting the event can bring knots to the stomach, an increased heart rate, and rapid respirations.

When working to reverse negative thoughts, coping statements can be used to reduce stress at various points in the stressful situation. For example, when anticipating the situation, you could say (or teach the client to say), "I'm going to be all right. I won't let this upset me." As the situation begins, you could say, "I'll take this step by step. I'm handling this right now." And when the situation ends, you could say, "I got through this, and I did well. I'm able to handle this situation."

Inner Dialogue. Inner dialogue may be of help to clients who are unable to verbalize their thoughts and feelings directly. People who use self-blame or guilt may also find help through inner dialogue. It is a structured way of providing positive direction without focusing on self-destructive feelings. Clients who want to solve a work-related problem can turn to their inner "work" advisers.

Inner dialogue is based on the idea that everyone has intuitive wisdom. Before using the inner adviser, clients must prepare. Have the client ask the following:

- If I had an inner adviser, what would he, she, or it look like?
- What characteristics would my inner adviser have that would be helpful to me?
- What is the best way to communicate with my inner adviser?
- What are my usual body symptoms that could be giving me messages about imbalances in my body or mind?
- In what ways have I been stressing myself lately?

The answers to these questions provide valuable clues to help clients create a dialogue with themselves to become receptive to their own intuitive wisdom.

> ***Action Alert!*** Use mutual goal setting to explore interventions that are consistent with the client's values and beliefs.

Gaining Control Through Knowledge. A common source of anxiety and stress is the inability to control a situation; this often accompanies a serious illness. Knowledge is power, and although it may not change the situation, it can increase the sense of control. Fear of the unknown is a major contributor to stress. Provide information to help the client and family feel a sense of control. However, you must assess the client's readiness to receive information.

INTERVENTIONS TO PREVENT A CRISIS

Preventing a crisis is always preferable to intervening in a crisis that already exists. To help prevent a crisis, make sure that the client's basic needs are met before you leave the unit or the client's home or the client leaves the clinic. If you are working in an institutional setting, communicate clearly to staff regarding client's additional unmet needs before you leave for the day. If appropriate, before discharging a client, make a referral to a home health care agency after consulting with client about any anticipated unmet needs.

Anticipate situations that could precipitate a crisis. Tell clients you are available to talk. For example, you can talk with your clients before their surgery, and give them an opportunity to discuss their thoughts, feelings, and expected body or life changes. Prepare them for expected changes. Refer them to appropriate support groups for pertinent life changes. They may benefit from a new-parent group, a group of new retirees, an ostomy group, or a group for newly diagnosed diabetics.

In addition, guided imagery, using your imagination to go to an imaginary place, situation, or event that is considered relaxing, has been shown to be helpful for presurgical clients (Box 47-4).

INTERVENTIONS DURING CRISIS

Realize that your clients in crisis are probably already overloaded with decisions, thoughts, and feelings. Use the following interventions to help them navigate the crisis successfully:

- As needed, orient clients to who you are and where they are.
- Use a calm, slow tone of voice, attentive body posture, and eye contact.
- Use short phrases to reduce sensory input.

BOX 47-4 *Stress Management Skills*

BIOFEEDBACK

Biofeedback is a technique of physiological self-control using instruments that measure bodily processes such as skin temperature, heart rate, muscle electrical activity, galvanic skin response, and sometimes brain waves. Breathing, progressive muscle relaxation, a sense of "mindfulness," and an alert yet passive "letting go" attitude are all elements of biofeedback. The client is taught the techniques and encouraged to practice them regularly. It has been widely used in pain programs, by physical therapists, with clients who have respiratory conditions, and by many psychotherapists.

GUIDED IMAGERY

Guided imagery is a powerful intervention. Clients simply use their imagination to go to an imaginary place, situation, or event that they consider relaxing. The type of conditions that respond well to visualization include those aggravated by stress, pain, anxiety associated with medical procedures, sleep disturbance, body or self-imagine disturbance (see illustration).

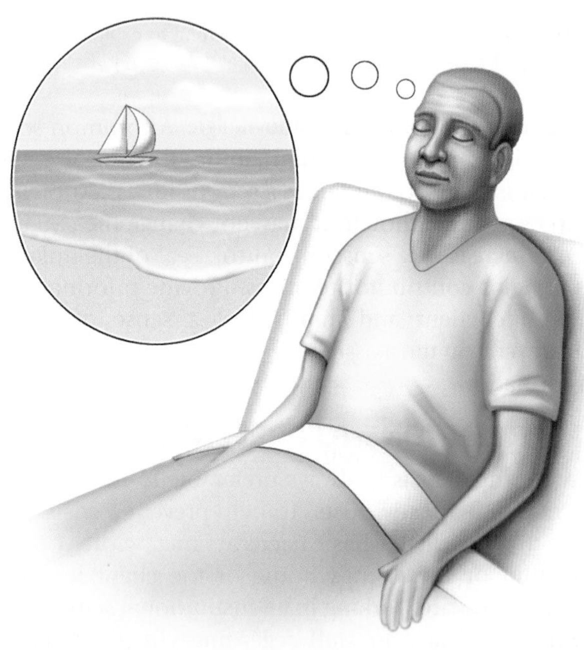

MASSAGE

Nurses or massage therapists manipulate muscle and connective tissue to enhance function of those tissues and promote relaxation and well-being.

MEDITATION/RELIGION

Meditation is an effective way to calm the body and mind. The practice of meditation is used to find a sense of oneness with self, with other people, and with the universe or a god. The therapeutic benefits of meditation include relaxation, stress relief, improved functioning of the immune system, and improved mental health. Although meditation may sound like an esoteric practice, it is a part of many religions. To many people, prayer, or religious contemplation, is a form of meditation.

Studies have shown better clinical outcomes for clients who practice their religious faith. You can encourage your clients to practice their own religious beliefs while in the hospital.

MUSIC

Music has been proven effective in producing relaxation and desired changes in emotions, behavior, and physiology. It can be useful to reduce stress and anxiety, for example, in clients with cancer, surgical clients, and newborn infants in the nursery. Noise levels in hospitals should be less that 45 dB during the day and less than 35 dB at night.

PROGRESSIVE MUSCLE RELAXATION

Progressive muscle relaxation is a process of alternately tensing and relaxing muscle groups to promote awareness of subtle degrees of tension. It reduces anxiety and allows clients to experience a heightened sense of comfort. This technique can be easily taught by nurses at the bedside and reinforced with taped instructions (see Box 42-6, in Chapter 42).

SLEEP

Promoting rest and sleep is an important aspect of care when a client is admitted to the hospital. Disturbance in the sleep cycle is linked to increased intrusive thoughts, avoidance behavior during stressful situations, and a lower number of circulating natural killer cells (see Chapter 36).

RELAXATION

Relaxation comes in many forms, and people do many things to relax. A very important form of relaxation involves doing very little, or even "nothing." This is very difficult for many people. Relaxation of the body facilitates the creation of positive internal images by way of inner communication involving all senses, which in turn signal the muscles to relax and promote better health. It can be beneficial for decreasing anxiety, easing muscle tension, decreasing fatigue, promoting sleep and rest, and reducing pain.

THERAPEUTIC TOUCH

Therapeutic touch is derived from an ancient technique called laying-on of hands. It is based on the premise that it is the healing force of the nurse that affects the client's recovery. Healing is promoted when the body's energies are in balance, and, by passing their hands over the client, nurses can identify energy imbalances.

- Avoid talking about the future; instead, stay with what the client is experiencing at the moment.
- Point out any movement toward dealing with the crisis: "You're sounding calmer now."

As the client's anxiety level declines (speech slows, for example, or pacing stops), begin to focus on problem solving. Use such phrases as, "If I hear you right, the problem is that. . . ." Identify the client's strengths as you observe them, and stress their importance in helping the client get through this crisis.

Once the problem is identified, locate resources to help with the crisis. For example, a possible resource might be a referral to a clinical specialist in psychiatric or mental health nursing. Another resource might be a friend who could bridge the gap between a hospital stay and going home by providing companionship for the discharged client.

Tell a hospitalized suicidal client that you must share this information with other staff involved in the client's care, so they can help keep him or her safe. Strictly follow hospital protocol for suicidal clients. This may entail the client being placed on one-on-one observation, evaluated by a mental health professional, or transferred to a psychiatric unit for safety. On discharge make sure the client has the 24-hour crisis phone number and agrees to call that number, another health care professional or the hospital unit, if appropriate, at specific times until the crisis passes.

> ***Action Alert!*** If the client says, "I wish I were dead" or other expressions of suicidal and homicidal thoughts, feelings, or actions, immediately inform the nurse in charge for prompt evaluation.

INTERVENTIONS TO HELP EFFECTIVELY MANAGE STRESSORS

Stress is a component of our daily life. Each individual responds to stress differently, and thus different interventions work for different individuals. Our body is affected by various physiological changes during stressful situations. These changes could be healthy or detrimental to health. Physiological changes that are detrimental to health can sometimes be managed by a relaxation technique. The achievement of relaxation produces diminished muscle tension, slowed respiratory rate, decreased blood pressure, slowed metabolic rate, dilation of peripheral vessels, and constriction of pupils. Level of consciousness moves to beta activity (associated with increased creativity, memory, and ability to concentrate), ultimately realizing adaptive functioning. Techniques that may help an individual deal with stress include focusing, reconstructing, compensating, and using various stress management techniques.

Focusing. Focusing involves sensing inwardly, in your body, the way it feels about the situations in your life. Ask clients to focus on recognizing their body's signals that stress is interfering with comfort. To help clients with focusing, ask, "Where do you feel the stress in your body?" Examples are an uneasy feeling in the pit of their stomach that tells them that something is not right or the heaviness in their heart after the doctor leaves their bedside. Ask them to make a list of things that are bothering them today. After they complete the list, ask, "What is keeping you from feeling okay today?" Help a client develop affirmations, such as "This day is getting better and better," or in collaboration with the clients figure out what helps them to enhance their comfort.

Reconstructing. Clients can enhance resilience by reconstructing stressful situations in a way that puts the experience in perspective. Help them reconstruct a stressful situation by asking them to think about a recent episode of distress. Then have them write down three things that could have happened to make it turn out better. Finally, ask the clients to write down three ways it could have gotten worse. This exercise increases their ability to put the situation in perspective—a useful technique for reducing stress.

Compensating. Compensating through self-improvement will lower a client's stress level. It works most effectively with stressors that cannot be avoided, such as illness, impending divorce, or the loss of a loved one. The feeling of loss of control that results from this kind of event can be balanced by taking on a new challenge, such as learning to sew, teaching someone a skill, or helping someone else. These efforts can reassure clients that they can cope with life.

Stress Management Skills. Client teaching is one of your most important nursing interventions. Knowledge of various stress management techniques will help you provide a more comprehensive and holistic approach in caring for your clients. They can be used in combination with prescribed medical treatments. See Box 47-4 for various stress management skills you can teach your clients.

You may also recommend that your clients lead healthy lifestyles, including good nutrition, adequate sleep and exercise, and limiting alcohol or other drug use. Several interventions can be used simultaneously to enhance stress reduction and coping (Box 47-5).

EVALUATION

Maintaining the effectiveness of a client's coping abilities is an ongoing process that includes client input. Evaluation of the expected outcomes will let you know if your interventions and nursing care were effective. If stressors were not identified, stress was not reduced, and new coping behaviors were not effective, then the overall goals were not met. Reassess, and adjust the care plan to meet the client's needs.

BOX 47-5

Considering the Alternatives

Alternative Therapies for Stress Tolerance and Coping

Transcendental Meditation

Advantages

Can improve blood pressure and insulin resistance in clients who have stable coronary heart disease (Paul-Labrador, Polk, & Dwyer, 2006)

Requires no equipment, no special location, and no physical exertion

May modulate the physiological response to stress

Disadvantages

Requires training and continued practice by client

May be perceived as conflicting with religion

More applicable to long-term stress than crisis situations

Art Therapy

Advantages

Reduces stress, decreases anxiety, and increases positive emotions (Walsh, Martin, & Schmidt, 2004)

Psychologically noninvasive (client can choose to not reveal perceived stressors)

May appeal to people who do not want to take medication or supplements

Disadvantages

Cost of supplies (paper, markers, fabric, paint, etc.)

Time to create the art

Clients may resist participation if they do not perceive themselves as artistic

Multivitamin With Calcium, Magnesium, and Zinc

Advantages

Reduces anxiety and perceived stress (Carroll, Ring, Suter, & Willemsen, 2000)

Requires less time than other stress coping methods

Easy administration and fewer side effects than medication

Disadvantages

May interact with medications

Cost of supplement

Clients may think what they eat is not important as long as they take the supplement

Carroll, D., Ring, C., Suter, M., & Willemsen, G. (2000). The effects of an oral multivitamin combination with calcium, magnesium, and zinc on psychological well-being in healthy young male volunteers: A double-blind placebo-controlled trial. *Psychopharmacology, 150*(2), 220-225.

Paul-Labrador, M., Polk, D., & Dwyer, J. H. (2006). Effects of a randomized controlled trial of transcendental meditation on components of the metabolic syndrome in subjects with coronary heart disease. *Archives of Internal Medicine, 166*(11), 1218-1224.

Walsh, S. M., Martin, S. C., & Schmidt, L. A. (2004). Testing the efficacy of a creative-arts intervention with family caregivers of patients with cancer. *Journal of Nursing Scholarship, 36*(3), 214-219.

The home health care nurse who worked with Mr. Osceola knew that she would need to help him integrate his cultural beliefs and practices with biomedical health care or his life would be threatened from a serious osteomyelitis. To evaluate the diagnosis of *Ineffective coping,* she might write a nursing note like the one below.

SAMPLE DOCUMENTATION NOTE FOR MR. OSCEOLA

Shaman accompanied nurse to visit Mr. Osceola. Removed alcohol from his home and performed a ceremony with Mr. Osceola and gave him an amulet to wear around his neck. Secured Mr. Osceola's agreement to allow the nurse to visit daily, dress the wound, and administer insulin and an antibiotic.

▼ KEY PRINCIPLES

- Stress can be physiological, psychosocial, cultural, developmental, or situational.
- Stress, stressors, and adaptation interact in a highly individualized way to give a total mind, body, and spirit effect.
- Homeostasis is a healthy, relatively balanced state that is maintained by physiological balancers, coping behaviors, defense mechanisms, and resilience.
- Psychoneuroimmunology refers to the interface between the brain and immunology. The evidence for the effects of stress on immune competence is compelling.
- Coping is situation specific and a major component in the relationship between stress and health. It can be adaptive or maladaptive.
- Anxiety is a common reaction to stress in both clients and nurses. At higher levels, anxiety may precipitate a crisis.
- Illness can be thought of as an imbalance that occurs when the body cannot adapt to complex physical and emotional stressors in the environment.
- Crises are either developmental or situational and upset the balanced or stable state.
- Balance is restored through either solving the problem or adapting to the lack of a solution.
- Resilience is the process of identifying or developing resources and strengths to flexibly manage stressors to gain a positive outcome, a sense of confidence, mastery, and self-esteem.
- Techniques that may help an individual deal with stress include focusing, reconstructing, compensating, and various stress management techniques.

■ REVIEW QUESTIONS

1. The nurse knows that a developmental crisis occurs when the client:

1. Uses mental processes to reduce her stress
2. Experiences a natural disaster
3. Is unable to complete the tasks for a particular developmental level
4. Is uneasy about her job interview

2. The client who behaves in ways that are appropriate for an earlier developmental period is using the defense mechanism:
1. Identification
2. Suppression
3. Regression
4. Projection

3. The nurse could use all of the following techniques to help a client reduce stress **except**:
1. Focusing
2. Compensating
3. Exercising
4. Reconstructing

4. The first step the nurse would do to assist a client in working through the stress of having a leg amputated and its consequences is:
1. Confront the client's denial
2. Refer the client to a psychiatrist
3. Establish a therapeutic relationship
4. Help the client identify past coping strategies

5. When the nurse had clients use their imagination to go to an imaginary place that they consider relaxing during a painful procedure the nurse was having the clients use:
1. Biofeedback
2. Imagery
3. Mediation
4. Progressive muscle relaxation

Bibliography

Ackley, B. J., & Ladwig, G. D. (2006). *Nursing diagnosis handbook: A guide to planning care* (7th ed.). St. Louis, MO: Mosby.

*American Psychiatric Association. (2000). *Diagnostic and statistical manual of mental disorders* (4th ed., Text Revision). Washington, DC: Author.

Anselmo, J. (2005). Relaxation: The first step to restore, renew, and self-heal. In B. M. Dossey, L. Keegan, & C. Guzzetta (Eds.), *Holistic nursing: A handbook for practice* (4th ed., pp. 521-560). Boston: Jones and Bartlett.

Cunningham, M. F., Hanson-Heath, C., & Agre, P. (2003). A perioperative nurse liaison program: CNS interventions for cancer patients and their families. *Journal of Nursing Care Quality, 18*(1), 16-21.

Johnson, M., Bulechek, G., Butcher, H., Dochterman, J. M., Maas, M., Moorhead, S., et al. (Eds.). (2006). *NANDA, NOC, and NIC linkages: Nursing diagnoses, outcomes, & interventions.* St. Louis, MO: Mosby.

NANDA International. (2005). *Nursing diagnoses: Definitions and classification, 2005-2006* (6th ed.). Philadelphia: Author.

O'Brien, B. L., Anslow, R. M., Begay, W., Pereira, B. A., & Sullivan, M. P. (2002). Twenty-first century rural nursing: Navajo traditional and Western medicine. *Nursing Administration Quarterly, 26*(5), 47-57.

*Selye, H. (1956). *The stress of life.* New York: McGraw-Hill.

Stuart, G. W., & Laraia, M. T. (2005). *Principles and practice of psychiatric nursing* (8th ed.). St. Louis, MO: Mosby.

Swanson, E. (2006). *NANDA, NOC and NIC linkages: Nursing diagnoses, outcomes, & interventions* (2nd ed.). St. Louis, MO: Mosby.

Thobaben, M. (2004). Alternative approaches to mental health care. *Home Health Care Management & Practice, 16*(6), 528-533.

Thobaben, M., Fossett, B., & Nadler-Moodie, M. (2004). Nursing management of the patient who is anxious. In *Psychiatric principles and applications for general patient care* (4th ed.). Brockton, MA: Western Schools.

Thobaben, M. (2005). Defense mechanisms and defense levels. *Home Health Care Management & Practice, 17*(4), 330-332.

Tyrrell, M. (2005). School phobia. *Journal of School Nursing, 21*(3), 147-151.

White, K. S., & Farrell, A. D. (2006). Anxiety and psychosocial stress as predictors of headache and abdominal pain in urban early adolescents. *Journal of Pediatric Psychology, 31*(6), 582-596.

*Asterisk indicates a classic or definitive work on this subject.

Chapter 48

Supporting Family Coping

Media Resources

- Evolve Website http://evolve.elsevier.com/Harkreader/
- Companion CD

Learning Objectives

After studying this chapter, you should be able to do the following:

- Describe the concepts of family, family function, family roles and family coping
- Describe the role of family member as caregiver
- Discuss a variety of factors affecting an individual family member's ability to provide care
- Assess the family, especially noting major stressors that may interfere with healthy coping, place the client at risk, or both, and clients experiencing or at *Risk for caregiver role strain*
- Diagnose family problems that respond to nursing care and differentiate among the variety of diagnoses that may be appropriate for clients who are caregivers
- Plan for goal-directed interventions to prevent or correct family problems identified by nursing diagnoses
- Evaluate outcomes that describe progress toward or resolution of family problems, including those experiencing *Caregiver role strain*

Key Terms

caregiver
caregiver burden
caregiver burnout
caregiver stress
caring
closed system
coping patterns
dysfunctional families
extended family
family
family-centered nursing
family dynamics
intergenerational family
nuclear family
objective caregiver burden
open system
role conflict
role stress
single-parent family
subjective caregiver burden
system

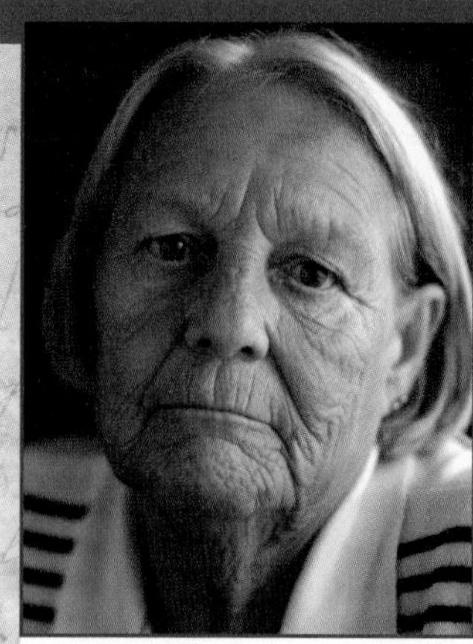

Mrs. LaVerne Roddy, age 78, was married to Laurence for 60 years. After his death 2 years ago, LaVerne felt overwhelmed by her transition to widowhood. She lost weight, had difficulty sleeping, and became uncharacteristically forgetful, anxious, and angry. She stopped attending church regularly, doing her beloved yard work, socializing with family and friends, and going to the senior center.

At first, her family attributed this change of behavior to her grief over the loss of her husband. As time passed, they became increasingly concerned about her and had Mrs. Roddy evaluated by the nurse practitioner, her primary care provider. After an extensive work-up, the nurse practitioner informed the family that Mrs. Roddy had primary degenerative dementia of the Alzheimer type.

The nurse gave the family a referral for a home evaluation. The home health care nurse performed a functional assessment of Mrs. Roddy and established a plan of care. Sadly, the client failed to respond to the nursing interventions and progressively declined from independence to total dependence. The family declined to place her in a skilled nursing facility because they had a close and loving relationship with Mrs. Roddy, as well as cultural and spiritual beliefs about caring for their parent. However, they were at *Risk for caregiver role strain* (see key nursing diagnoses box) because of the multiplicity of Mrs. Roddy's problems.

KEY NURSING DIAGNOSES FOR FAMILY COPING

Caregiver role strain: Difficulty in performing the caregiver role

Risk for caregiver role strain: A caregiver is vulnerable for felt difficulty in performing the family caregiver role

Readiness for enhanced family coping: Effective managing of adaptive tasks by family member involved with the client's health challenge, who now is exhibiting desire and readiness for enhanced health and growth in regard to self and in relation to the client

Compromised family coping: A usually supportive primary person (family member or close friend) is providing insufficient, ineffective, or compromised support, comfort, assistance, or encouragement that may be needed by the client to manage or master adaptive tasks related to his or her health challenge

Disabled family coping: Behavior of significant person (family member or other primary person) that disables his or her capacities and the client's capacities to effectively address tasks essential to either person's adaptation to the health challenge

Impaired parenting: Inability of the primary caretaker to create, maintain, or regain an environment that promotes the optimum growth and development of the child

CONCEPTS OF FAMILY

Family-centered nursing is health care that focuses on the health of the family as a unit and on the maintenance and improvement in the health and growth of each person in that unit. The recipient of care is the family itself. This nursing care focuses on the family's response to actual or potential health problems or to life processes that can be treated by nursing care. It involves intervening to help the family manage the impact of stressors on the family. You will have opportunities to assess families for threats to healthy family coping when either an individual or the family interacts with the health care delivery system. Recognition of various types of families and their strengths and weaknesses underlies family assessment.

THEORETICAL APPROACHES TO FAMILY

The application of nursing theories offers a conceptual approach to family assessment.

Developmental Theories. Understanding a family from a developmental perspective is assessing family development throughout families' generational life cycles. Knowing individual and family developmental tasks, you can determine the family unit's health by assessing the family's successful mastery of appropriate tasks while observing whether individual family members' actions are appropriate to their developmental level (Table 48-1).

Family Systems Theory. The study of the family can be approached as the study of a system (family) with subsystems (individual members) interacting with each other. A **system** is a set of integrated, interacting parts that function as a whole, with structure and patterns of function that accomplish the work of the whole. As the system tries to maintain balance or equilibrium, its boundaries filter and regulate what passes through. An **open system** exchanges matter, energy, and information with other systems and with the environment. A **closed system** is a set of integrated interacting parts that function as a whole and do not interact with other systems or the environment.

Table 48-1 Family Developmental Tasks by Developmental Stage and Age

FAMILY STAGE	AGE OF CHILDREN	FAMILY TASKS
The family during pregnancy	Fetal development	• Maintaining health of fetus • Allocating resources • Dividing labor • Transition of identity into parenthood • Socialization order • Maintaining motivation and morale
The family with a neonate	Newborn	• Maintaining control over the childbirth events • Communicating effectively with each other and significant others • Maintaining satisfying relations with each other and significant others • Resolving the birthing experience
The family with an infant	Oldest child 6 weeks to 1 year	• Meeting physical and emotional needs of the infant • Assigning roles • Incorporating the infant into the family • Reallocating resources • Promoting physical and emotional development • Adapting lifestyle to the changing infant • Incorporating new family structure into society • Maintaining interpersonal relationship • Establishing goals, priorities, and values
The family with a toddler or preschooler	1 to 5 years	• Initiating and maintaining a home • Maintaining physical growth and well-being (air, food, safety)
The family with a school-age child	6 to 12 years	• Meeting the physical needs of the family • Expanding family communications and activities • Maintaining marital satisfactions • Socialization and education of the children • Developing the potential of all individual family members • Communicating effectively with all family members
The family with an adolescent	13 to 19 years	• Allowing and providing for individual differences and needs • Working out a system of financial and family responsibility • Maintaining open communication among family members • Widening the horizons of adolescents and their parents • Maintaining family ethnical and moral standards
The family during the child's transition to adulthood	20 to 44 years	• Continuance of physical care • Redefining need-response pattern • Supporting maturation of the child • Allocating resources • Maintaining family relationships • Establishing priorities and maintaining goals • Evaluating and maintaining socioeconomic security for the future • Evaluating and maintaining family accomplishments • Changing and maintaining family relationships
The family in senescence	45 to 75 years	• Maintaining socioeconomic security to death • Reviewing family accomplishments • Changing and maintaining family relationships • Children planning for or assuming care of parents

The family is a set of interacting elements—that is, the individual members, who interact to create the family unit. The relationships are structured for the division of labor and for meeting the needs of the family. The family has boundaries that define who are family members and control access or interaction with the outside world. These boundaries protect the family as a unit, but they may also prevent entry of sources of support and nurturance. The healthy family is an open system with complex interactions both within the family and in the external world. It controls its boundaries through its values, beliefs, attitudes, and rules. It is self-regulating and can adjust the family unit as the needs of its members change so that harmony and balance exist. When the open family system loses its balance, outside help can assist in its stabilization. The closed family system excludes others, functions in isolation, and is the pathological model.

When you assess the family as a system, you observe whether the system is working and whether the subsystems are functioning. In addition, you observe whether the system is open (that is, available for input) or closed (that is, having limited outside support or input).

Interactional Theory. Interactional theory emphasizes the internal dynamics of family life or how the individual members interact with one another and with the family as a whole. **Family dynamics** is the ever-changing pattern of interaction among family members; it is the forces at work within the family that create patterns of behavior. Thus, interactionalists would examine family life in terms of how power is assigned, how children are disciplined and by whom, who is assigned the caretaking role, or whether communication is direct or indirect. They might describe the family by describing roles, the decision-making process, conflict, and reaction to stress.

In a well-functioning family, the interactional dynamics maintain a state of equilibrium—that is, adjustments are continually made to keep the needs of the members balanced. Rigidity, suppression, or lack of spontaneity, especially in a family member who is not interacting, throws the family into disequilibrium. Interactionalists view the family as being relatively closed to outside systems, and they emphasize analysis of the internal aspects of family dynamics.

FAMILY STRUCTURE AND FUNCTION

Family Structure. Family structure is how the family is organized. It includes the individuals that compose the family, their relationships, and the interactions between family members and with other social systems.

A **family** is two or more people united by a common goal to create a physical, cultural, spiritual, and nurturing bond that will promote the physical, mental, spiritual, and social development of each of its members, while maintaining cohesiveness as a unit. It is the basic social unit of society and has needs as a unit. It can be forged by blood (genetics), law (marriage or adoption), or spirit.

Nuclear Family. The **nuclear family** is composed of a husband, a wife, and their child or children living in a common household with one or both spouses gainfully employed. This can include first marriage families, blended or stepparent families, and adoptive families. A binuclear family refers to the postdivorced family in which the children are part of two nuclear families with varying degrees of cooperation (i.e., co-parenting and joint custody) and time spent in each household.

Intergenerational Family. An **intergenerational family** includes more than one generation of a family living together in one residence or within a small geographical area. This type of family exists because of cultural values, the family's financial status, safety concerns, or because older parents or other disabled family members cannot care for themselves physically, financially, or emotionally. Multiple generations often enrich family life (Figure 48-1).

Extended Family. The **extended family** unit includes the nuclear family as well as other relatives such as aunts, uncles, cousins, and grandparents who are committed to maintaining family ties. They may live in the same household, in close proximity, or in geographically different places. The defining characteristic is identification as a family unit and maintaining an interrelatedness that is mutually supportive, such as caring for older adult members by younger members and caring for the young by older family members.

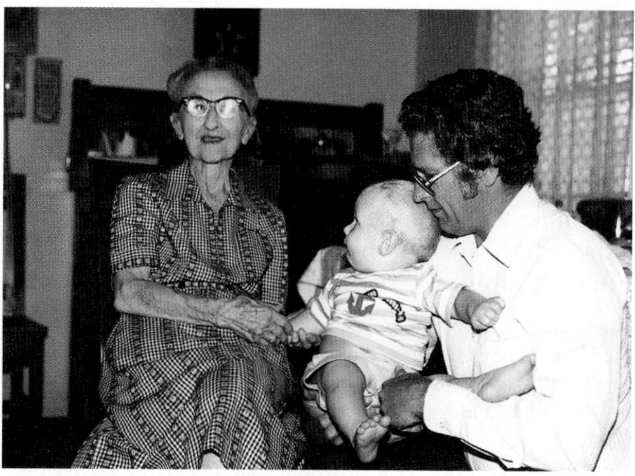

FIGURE 48-1 Multiple generations enrich family life.

Single-Parent Family. **Single-parent families** are households in which the children live with one parent, usually because of divorce, out-of-wedlock birth, or the death of a spouse. Without a partner, single-parent families can find it harder to manage as a family unit because more energy may be required to meet basic needs. When parents feel powerless to protect and provide for their families, they may experience low self-esteem, frustration, resignation, or fatalism, which may lead them to escape the resulting pain with alcohol, drugs, abusiveness, abandonment, or suicide. Adolescent single parents have been found to be at increased risk for a variety of social, psychological, and physiological problems, including poverty, domestic violence, and low educational attainment. Single-parent families are not homogeneous but are diverse in terms of resources, and each family has its own set of problems and strengths.

Action Alert! Treat every single-parent family as unique. Identify the strengths and weaknesses of each single-parent family to gain a better understanding of the family's needs. Keep in mind that single-parent families can be functional, healthy family units.

Nontraditional Families. There are many nontraditional family structures. A heterosexual cohabiting family is an unmarried couple living together with or without children. A communal family is a household of more than one monogamous couple with children, each of which shares resources and socializes the children as a group activity. A lesbian or gay family includes either a female or a male couple living together with or without children. A foster family is a household of a single parent or two parents with foster children and may include the parents' own children. Children are placed in foster homes when their parents are unable to care for them or are unfit.

The profile of the American family is changing. There are more unmarried couples living together, opposite-sex couples and same-sex couples with children present in the home. There is no right or wrong or improper form of family.

> ***Action Alert!*** You will not be able to deliver effective family nursing care if you believe your own family structure is the only "correct" one.

Family Functions. The family's organization and functioning are based on a mixture of societal and cultural behaviors and rituals. Families function to satisfy both the needs of individuals within the family and the needs of the family as a social unit. The primary functions include the following:

- *Affective function* needs are met by providing psychosocial protection and support of the family members. Families confer feelings of acceptance and value on their members through love, intimacy, nurturing, acceptance, caring, sharing, and support (Figure 48-2).
- The *economic functions* of the family include having sufficient resources and allocating these resources to provide food, clothes, shelter, recreation, education, and quality of life.
- The *health care function* is to provide for nutrition, mental health, immunizations, and physical well-being.
- *Reproductive functions* are to maintain family continuity over the generations and to achieve societal survival.
- The *socialization and social placement function* includes socialization of children by helping them become productive members of their society, as well as the conferring of status on family members (Friedman, Bowman, & Jones, 2003).

FAMILY ROLES

In families, roles are structured for the division of labor and the distribution of power (Figure 48-3). Family power is the ability of individual members to change the behavior of other family members. Power may be formally assigned by designating one person as head of the household. A woman may assign her husband the role of repairman by openly stating that she does not have the skill to do home repairs. Power can be destructive, such as a husband maintaining control over the finances, or mutually shared among family members to meet both common and individual needs.

CAREGIVING ROLE

Although caregivers can be both professional and nonprofessional, the focus of this chapter is on nonprofessional caregivers who have family or personal ties to clients who receive the care. The family caregiver role is not new. Caregiving is a role that is inherent in family life, but individual family members and diverse family units define it differently. Before health care facilities existed, families routinely cared for their ill members themselves or hired help if they were financially able. Lack of adequate health insurance and changes in health care delivery, such as shorter hospital stays and increased technological advances, have led to the increased use of family caregivers and home health care.

A **caregiver** is one who provides care to a dependent or partially dependent family member or friend. **Caring** is a behavior of having regard for, cherishing, protecting, being responsible for, or attending to needs of others; it is universally observed in human beings and influenced by society, culture, values, and sex. When we care, we consider others' points of view, their objective needs, and what they expect of us. Our attention, our mental engrossment, is not on ourselves but on the recipient of care. "Caring for" includes those actions and behaviors that are associated with "doing for" the receiver of care.

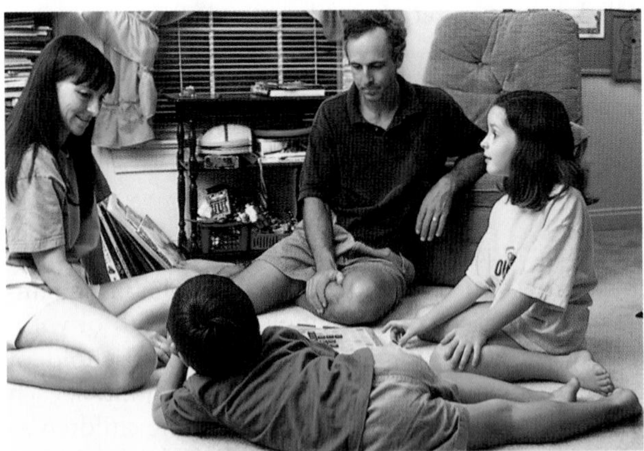

FIGURE 48-2 Families confer feelings of acceptance and value on their members by the development of love, intimacy, nurturing, acceptance, caring, sharing, and support.

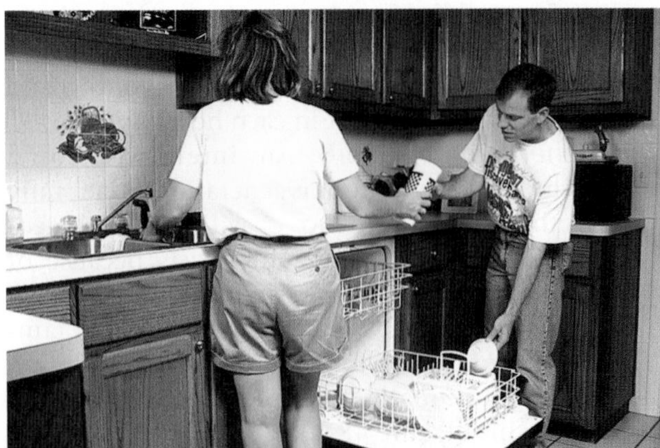

FIGURE 48-3 Family roles are structured for the division of labor and the distribution of power.

Caring "about" involves positive and unconditional regard for the recipient of care. Thus caregiving can be the direct meeting of physical or emotional needs, practical supportive acts, a state of empathy, or a warm feeling with no action involved.

Dysfunctional families either cannot meet the needs of the families or function in a way that is harmful to their members. Although all families function ineffectively at times, the dysfunctional family is usually in pain and consistently functions at the expense of one or more family members. Dysfunctional families have ineffective communications and living patterns, marginal health practices, strained or poor coping skills, and ineffective child-rearing practices. Indicators of ineffective family coping include family members who deny or trivialize problems, detach themselves, or refuse to offer any help. When there is tension, the family may sit apart and not make eye contact. They may uneasily watch each other's movements and give very cautious responses to avoid (or to prompt) conflict.

Dysfunctional families are not necessarily abusive; however, family violence can occur in dysfunctional families. It is an intentional or negligent act by a family member that causes harm or a serious risk of harm to another member, including children, spouses, and older adults. Child abuse is a serious and growing problem. Abuse of older adults, similar to other forms of family violence, affects men and women and families from all ethnic backgrounds and social status. According to the National Center on Elder Abuse (2005), abuse may be the following:

- *Physical abuse*—Inflicting, or threatening to inflict, physical pain or injury or depriving a vulnerable family member a basic need
- *Emotional abuse*—Inflicting mental pain, anguish, or distress on a family member through verbal or nonverbal acts
- *Sexual abuse*—Nonconsensual sexual contact of any kind
- *Exploitation*—Illegal taking, misuse, or concealment of funds, property, or assets of a vulnerable family member
- *Neglect*—Refusal or failure by caregivers to provide food, shelter, health care, or protection for a vulnerable family member
- *Abandonment*—The desertion of a vulnerable family by a family member who has assumed the responsibility for care or custody of that person

FACTORS AFFECTING FAMILY COPING

Many factors affect the family's ability to cope, including the characteristics of the family, socioeconomic factors, and psychological factors. The family members' culture, religious values, social values, communication patterns, support for each other, and communities must be considered.

RISK FACTORS ACROSS THE LIFE SPAN

Family coping is the family unit's method of managing the stressors of family life through each developmental stage and change in family circumstance. The ability to cope is affected by characteristics of the family.

Developmental Stage. As a family progresses through the developmental stages, from forming a marriage to launching the youngest child into the adult world, the family makes adjustments, learns new coping strategies, and uses transitional crises as a means of family growth. Positive predictors of successful transition from one stage to the next include successful completion of the last developmental stage, a history of effective family support for family members in transition, willingness to redefine family roles and responsibilities, and a history of successes, individually and as a family.

Situational Stressors. Families are exposed to multiple situational stressors. Any relationship can be a stressor, and when an additional component is added, such as divorce or an out-of-wedlock conception, it can cause a loss of equilibrium for the members of a family. Other stressors include work and family conflicts, financial and job-related stress, and the struggle to care for older parents. Family stress is the tension or strain produced as the family's response to any outside force—or stressor—that affects the family. The response to stressors creates a situation in which normal family processes, employed to attain goals and maintain status quo, are in disequilibrium. Stressors can be a threat or a challenge, depending on how the family perceives them and the duration of the presence of the stressors.

Coping Patterns. **Coping patterns** are the specific protective behaviors used by an individual or a family to respond to stressful situations. These patterns produce varying degrees of success.

Effective Coping. Healthy families have resources for successfully managing stress. Stress that is perceived as an opportunity or a challenge is often a positive experience for the family. Through good problem-solving skills, the family develops its coping skills. When one family member becomes ill and the other family members must provide the care, the family can grow. The family can feel good about the way they handled the stressor, which can enhance their collective self-esteem. Effective management of stressors is a family strength.

Examples of strategies used by families who have effective coping skills include the following:

- Discussing problems and concerns among family members
- Demonstrating human emotional responses, such as crying or laughing
- Confronting stressors realistically
- Seeking professional guidance if necessary

Healthy families can reappraise and reorder priorities in work and private life on the basis of family values. They work off stress and anger by doing meaningful tasks and using stress-reducing mechanisms such as prayer and meditation, yoga, deep-breathing exercises, relaxation tapes, imagery, or biofeedback.

Ineffective and Dysfunctional Coping. Unhealthy families lack resources for managing stress. Stress perceived by the family as a danger or a threat that could overwhelm their coping skills is negative stress. The number of stressors, the critical importance of the stressor, or the overwhelming threat of the stressor can cause the family to feel overwhelmed.

Ineffective coping is the use of defense mechanisms, communication, problem identification, and decision making by one or more family members that results in maladaptive behavior or negative consequences. Ineffective coping skills, such as the use of drugs, blur the reality of the situation until problems become overwhelming. Failure to satisfactorily resolve a stressor contributes to lowered self-esteem and increases the use of maladaptive coping skills in future stressful situations. When caregivers and families are under stress, both cognitive and noncognitive processes direct their coping behavior. If their usual coping patterns are ineffective because of a crisis, the family can become vulnerable to damaging stress.

Action Alert! Assess families involved in caregiving for how well they are coping.

CULTURAL AND LIFESTYLE FACTORS

Cultural. Cultural expectations may also place caregivers at risk for *Caregiver role strain.* Conflicts may exist between what is expected from one's culture and what can actually be accomplished. In some cultures, women are expected to care for dependent relatives. Such cultural practices may have been conceived during an era when women were expected to remain at home and were not part of the workforce. Today, such expectations may not be feasible. When working women try to assume all expected roles, *Caregiver role strain* may occur. You must be culturally sensitive when developing nursing interventions to prevent *Caregiver role strain* and care recipient stress. Box 48-1 illustrates the importance of culture for the Roddy family.

Lifestyle. Meeting the needs of dependent family members is emotionally taxing for caregivers. Family dynamics suffer when interactions and relationships stop working efficiently to accomplish the family's functions and tasks. The stress created by caring for a dependent family member causes new roles to emerge. Multiple roles can create role stress and role conflict, thus compromising family functions. **Role stress** is an emotion that occurs when a person has difficulty meeting the demands of a role. It can occur when competing demands interfere, when the family structure is rigid, or when role expectations are unrealistic. **Role conflict** is incompatible expectations for behavior within a role, between two or more roles, or when a role is incongruent with a person's beliefs and values. Role conflict can be manifested as interrole conflict, in which competing roles are in conflict. Intersender role conflict occurs when two people have different expectations of how the role will be performed. Personal role conflict is an inner conflict between values held internally and opposing external values that the role demands.

Caregiver stress refers to the caregiver's reaction to physical, emotional, sociocultural, financial, and environmental stressors brought on by the caregiving experience. In many cases, caregivers enter their roles with ambivalent feelings. Love for family members and the satisfaction derived from helping coexist with feelings of resentment about their loss of privacy and frustration at believing they have no control over what happens. Caregiver stressors can originate from intrafamily, interfamily, or extrafamily sources. One common intrafamily (within a family/member) stressor is a lack of time for oneself. Research has shown that many caregivers have no leisure time and receive inconsistent or no help from family or friends. Another intrafamily stressor results

BOX 48-1 *Cross-Cultural Care*

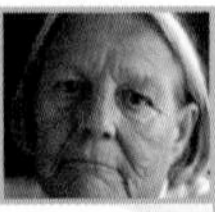

Caring for an Irish American Catholic

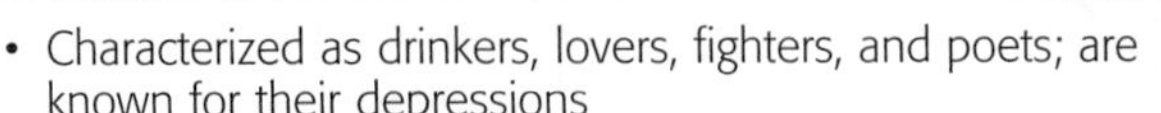

If you ask Mrs. Roddy's daughter about her family, she will tell you she is Irish and proud of it. She remembers her grandmother telling stories about her family building this country by working on the railroads. However, she has no ties to an Irish community or to any family in Ireland. Although each client is unique, many Irish Americans tend to share certain characteristics:

- Feel family loyalty and provide support to extended family
- Many are Catholic; may also be Protestant
- Outgoing, friendly manner; may exhibit stoicism
- Characterized as drinkers, lovers, fighters, and poets; are known for their depressions
- Proud of doing hard work and hard play
- If Catholic, may avoid birth control and abortion
- May desire visits from a priest and the Sacrament of the Sick if dying
- Prefer that a dying newborn be baptized, even by a nurse, to aid the infant's entrance to heaven

from feelings about lack of appreciation for one's efforts. Caregiver surveys indicate that many caregivers feel taken for granted and unappreciated. An example of an interfamily (between family members) stressor is when a caregiver has feelings of unrelenting stress from caring for a dependent member of the extended family. An example of an extrafamily (from outside the family) stressor is when a caregiver quits work to care for a family member and then experiences a financial hardship.

The financial cost associated with caregiving can cause many families to experience financial difficulties. Financial setbacks are especially prevalent in families whose members have to leave the workforce to care for a dependent family member. These families are placed at risk for *Caregiver role strain* due to financial instability.

When caregivers have an inadequate social support system, they are more likely to experience *Caregiver role strain*. The caregiver's social support system may include relatives, friends, and others who will help in caring for the dependent family member. Support can include financial, emotional, or daily caregiving assistance. Box 48-2 describes a caregiver's perspective of the importance of support.

Caregivers who are under stress suffer physical and emotional disabilities that interfere with their caregiver capabilities. Because of this, you should educate caregivers about the dangers of stress and offer them self-help strategies to eliminate it or reduce its effects.

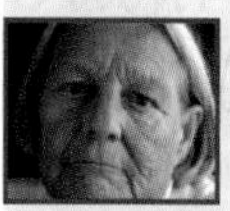

What role stressors and conflicts can you imagine are present in the Roddy family?

Action Alert! Offer caregivers self-help strategies to reduce the detrimental effects of caregiver stress.

Caregiver Burden. **Caregiver burden** refers to strain or load borne by a family member who cares for an older adult, chronically ill, or disabled family member. It is a multidimensional response to physical, psychological, emotional, social, and financial stressors associated with the caregiving experience. **Subjective caregiver burden** refers to the caregiver's personal appraisal of a caregiving situation and the extent to which the person perceives it to be a burden. The caregiver's perception of the burden, rather than the perception of other family members or

BOX 48-2 *A Caregiver's Perspective*

"It Helps—and Hurts—to Remember Who They Were"

Not long after my wife of 42 years retired from her job at the district court, she began to show what I thought were signs of depression. We were leaving our 10-room house, now emptied of seven children, for a smaller, cozier place, and she was having difficulty packing. She was more quiet and forgetful, just seemed to be losing her zip. She also misplaced things. I found a bank book in her raincoat pocket, a plastic bag with several of her rings in the pocket of a jacket she seldom wore. Seven years later, I'm still trying to find her engagement ring.

Before her annual physical, I tipped off the internist about her symptoms. He referred us to a neurologist, who ordered an extensive series of tests. Ruling out any physiological problem left only one possibility: Alzheimer's.

I immediately joined the Alzheimer's Association, got a medical ID bracelet for my wife, contacted social service agencies, and talked with my colleagues at the Visiting Nurses Association. They told me to start looking at rest homes immediately, which I did. Before long, I applied at a facility that offered both day care and full-time care. Good advice; there's a long waiting list now.

One day my wife slipped out of the house and then couldn't find her way back. Because of her work at the courthouse, the police knew her and brought her home. That's when I had alarms installed on the doors.

I hired a companion for her who claimed to have cared for a grandmother with Alzheimer's; she didn't work out for us, however. Then I hired a neighbor who had worked in a day care facility for Alzheimer's clients. That worked until the neighbor said my wife needed to be in full-time day care. A good solution, temporarily. She adjusted very well to the structured routine and simple exercises.

Then rages began at home. She would throw things and strike out at me, although at 4 feet 11 inches tall, she wasn't much of a threat to my 6-foot, 200-pound frame. In addition, she would be up, prowling the house in the middle of the night. When the final stages of incontinence began, my macho "I can take care of anything" attitude crumbled. I knew she needed more care than I could provide.

Six years after the diagnosis, she became a resident at the same place where she had been in day care. It was an easy transition. The experts say Alzheimer's clients do not suffer physical pain, but every family suffers. Depression and guilt are common. What makes the biggest difference for the caregiver is support—or lack of it—from family and friends. We are blessed with wonderful kids—six daughters and a son. The ones who live nearby visit her often. They pay to have my house cleaned and keep my freezer stocked with food. They call often.

People find it hard to visit Alzheimer's clients—even family members. As soon as my wife went into the rest home, I called her three closest friends. Not one has gone to see her.

She gets wonderful care. The place is mostly staffed with RNs. But regardless of how good the care is, you need to be there every day to keep an eye on the little things. Massachusetts has a good system for monitoring all convalescent homes. When I asked the Department of Public Health for the report on my wife's facility, they sent an eight-page review. Out of a possible score of 80, the place rated 79.

Outside each resident's room, there's a brief biography of that person. You find people from all walks of life: a federal district court judge, a nun who taught French, a nun who ran a convalescent home, an attorney, the owner of a bus company, a Ph.D. educator, a hospital chaplain, and a former football player. It helps—and hurts—to remember who they were.

health care providers, determines the impact on his or her life. **Objective caregiver burden** refers to the visible, tangible costs to the caregiver as measured in required behaviors or disruptions. Caregivers may experience a greater burden when they also hold a job. Financial losses occur when they are forced to reduce work hours or quit working so they can care for a family member.

The caregiving responsibility is not always assumed by choice but because of a blend of responsibility, desire, and family or sociocultural expectations. Some burdens cannot be measured. For example, when the caregiver and the care receiver have a history of incompatibility, they may find it difficult to care *about* each other. The stress from such a relationship can lead to *Caregiver role strain*. The greatest needs for these caregivers may be emotional support and respite care.

Caregiver Burnout. **Caregiver burnout** is a depletion of physical and mental energy caused by providing care for a chronically ill person over a long period. The more complicated the treatment program or needs of the receiver, the greater the risk for caregiver burnout. Caregiver behaviors that suggest burnout include ongoing and constant fatigue, decreasing interest in work and work production, withdrawal from social contacts, increasing fear of death, increasing use of stimulants or alcohol, sleep disturbances, a change in eating patterns, and feelings of helplessness and depression.

Family caregivers who experience burnout are generally involved in unrelenting daily care of family members as opposed to several hours per day for a few days a week. They may feel unable to divorce themselves from the caregiving situation because of family, cultural, personal, or financial reasons.

It is important for you to intervene before burnout occurs in family caregivers. Helping caregivers recognize unrealistic expectations of themselves and the need for respite care are essential nursing interventions.

> ***Action Alert!*** Support caregivers with problem-solving and decision-making activities when they experience emotional upheavals.

Caregiver Role Strain. Caregivers are at increased *risk for caregiver role strain* when they have trouble performing the caregiver role (NANDA International [NANDA-I], 2005). This strain is associated with the burden and responsibilities involved in the care of dependent family members. It can result from the developmental level of the caregiver (too young to provide the care), the living environment (inadequate space), situational stressors (financial problems), or a need for extensive care (family member has Alzheimer's disease).

Caregiver role strain can also occur when there are unresolved conflicts between the caregiver and care recipient or when there is resentment, anger, or guilt about taking on the role of caregiver. For example, the wife of an older brain-impaired care recipient may resent being in the caregiver role because of an earlier history of abuse from her husband. The burden of this arrangement may be especially trying and energy depleting for her. *Caregiver role strain* can also occur when caregivers neglect their own health or let existing conditions worsen.

Caregiver role strain may be minimized when the recipient and the caregiver predetermine how and by whom the care will be provided. The caregiver agrees to accept the role and makes preparations.

> ***Action Alert!*** Be knowledgeable about and alert to the cues that indicate family *Caregiver role strain.*

Most caregivers experience some type of psychological distress while they perform caregiver duties, but their coping patterns and the quality and quantity of support provided by their social network can minimize their stress. The more serious and demanding the care is, the greater the likelihood the caregiver will experience psychological problems, including becoming clinically depressed.

ASSESSMENT

GENERAL ASSESSMENT OF FAMILIES

Applying the philosophy of family-centered nursing, individual problems are also family problems. Your assessment identifies the strengths and weaknesses and the coping abilities of both individual and family.

During your first visit with the family, you need to begin establishing a trusting relationship. You do this by being honest, nonthreatening, and caring with them. You will need to develop a systematized method for family assessment that includes the information you need but does not subject the family to unnecessary intrusion. You will need to be able to distinguish healthy family behavior from dysfunctional behavior.

> ***Action Alert!*** Reflect on your own values to prepare for a family home visit. What are your thoughts about the family? Do you possess any biases or prejudices that would prevent you from giving good nursing care?

Demographic Data. The assessment begins with verifying the information on the referral sheet and obtaining family data. You will want to determine the family members, including their age, sex, developmental stage, and roles. You can obtain additional cues regarding the family's state of health.

Family Dynamics. Observe the patterns of relating to one another. One of your challenges will be to determine whether the family works well together. When assessing the family, obtain information through what they say and through your observations of body gestures, vocal tones, facial expressions, word selection, and congruent messages. Your family assessment will determine whether the family is functional or dysfunctional.

Action Alert! Pay attention to your instincts. Tension and hostility can be felt. Think about situations you have experienced. When there was tension in the air, could you almost feel it?

Family Strengths. A healthy family will show genuine interest in learning to help the client. Their relationships are caring with a sense of togetherness and with a willingness to help in managing a problem. You will make observations of the family's adaptive ability, communication patterns, ability to function as a system, physical needs, ability to protect their members, health promotion activities, and community support. Table 48-2 suggests questions that might be asked in each of these areas.

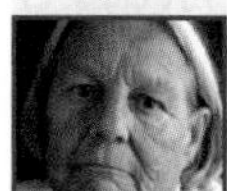

Review the list of questions in Table 48-2. What data would you gather for the Roddys? How would you gather these data?

Family Roles. Find out who the primary caregiver is and what the role expectations of other family members are. In most settings, caregivers are not considered clients, so their specific needs may go unmet. However, to ensure that the needs of clients are met, you need to assess the needs of the caregivers as well. Ask questions about their perceptions of the caregiving process: ask about their understanding of their responsibilities as caregivers, their expectations (and their family's expectations) of the caregiving duties, their relationship with the care receiver, and their other responsibilities, such as work and child care. Several caregiver assessment tools are available to help you collect these data. Some assess the caregiver's physical and mental health, and others assess family dynamics, perceptions of caregiving, the adequacy of social support systems, and cultural expectations.

Family Stressors. Although you might not ask a list of specific questions about family stressors, if you listen and allow the family to express themselves, you will often discover stressors not directly related to the caregiving situation.

Table 48-2 Family Assessment Criteria

CRITERIA	ASSESSMENT QUESTIONS
Physical needs	• Is the family shelter adequate? • Does the family shelter provide the basic essentials that will allow proper food consumption, such as an operating refrigerator and stove? • Is there an adequate water supply, and is the water that flows from the faucet safe to drink? • Is the home warm and cool enough? • How is the home heated? • Is there money for fuel? • Is there a working toilet and a bathtub or shower where adequate hygiene measures can be carried out? • Is there enough money for soap? • Are there beds where each family member can be assured of a restful sleep? • Can the family shelter offer room for activity, such as a television, a room where children can play, and toys? • Is there adequate food in the refrigerator or cupboard? • If the family qualifies for food stamps or extra food, like a bag of wheat or flour, can someone prepare an adequate meal? • Are there proper cooking and eating utensils? • Are bathroom facilities easily accessible for the recovering client? • How many stairs must the client climb to get into the home? • Is the home clean, well ventilated, and well kept, or is it dirty, unkempt, and lacking such essentials as a flushing toilet or hot water?
Protection	• If the family is fearful, what is the source of the fear? Is it outside, as in a dangerous neighborhood? Or is it inside, as in an abusive parent or mate? • What options are available for the fearful? • Is there a social worker in the picture? Collaborative work is sometimes essential when dealing with families that have multiple problems. • Are adults allowed to smoke where there are children? • Are safety belts and child seats used appropriately? • Are dangerous chemicals, medications, and matches safely stored out of reach of children?
Health promotion	• Do family members smoke, drink to excess, or use illegal drugs? • Do family members exercise, wear safety belts when driving, and wear helmets when bike riding? • Do family members eat well-balanced meals (ask for a sample daily menu), see a dentist, and get proper amounts of sleep? • When someone is ill, does the family have all the integrity and resources, physically, mentally, emotionally, and economically, to intelligently handle the stressors inherent in sickness and the individual autonomy to meet their own needs?

Continued

Table 48-2 Family Assessment Criteria—cont'd

CRITERIA	ASSESSMENT QUESTIONS
Communication	• Do family members feel understood by each other? • What is their communication network like? Can you observe basic communication errors? • Do all family members feel safe and important enough to share their feelings and opinions? Have they had a lot of practice? Do they do it well or superficially? • How well does the family listen? How well do they receive the messages sent? • Are messages sent in an intimidating, manipulative way, or are they "I think . . . " or "I feel . . . " statements? • Do family members assume they understand, or is there valuable feedback? • Does the family share, or do they have secrets? Is not sharing a power move or a destructive habit—a way to avoid conflict? • How does the family react to transmitted messages? Do they respect the feelings of the sender? Do they react inappropriately emotionally? Do they ask questions to get more information? • Do they value messages and apply them appropriately?
Family as a system	• Does the family interact with the community? • Does the family accept public assistance if it is needed? • Are the subsystems of the family (each family member) able to reach his or her own potential, or are they stifled in a closed system? • If there is a disrupting force, what mechanisms do they have to reach equilibrium?
Community support	• Is the community air quality within acceptable limits for pollution? Is the water safe to drink? Is there adequate garbage collection? Are police visible? • Is transportation available, or are stores close by to get essentials? • What does this community offer in shared values and ethnicity to your client? Are there places to worship, hospitals, and other support systems that help in a crisis? • How is the fire station and ambulance service? How far away are they? • Is there a newspaper to support the community's communication system? • Are there cultural offerings in which the entire family can participate and enjoy? • Are there parks and playgrounds? • Are there organized sports and places children can go to after school, such as a YMCA, a Boy's Club, or the Girl Scouts? Is there a good school system, with an active parent–teacher association? • Can students walk safely or ride a short distance to school? Is public transportation available? • What services are available for the old and infirm? • Does the community offer intellectual stimulation with theater, plays, and museums? Is it a friendly town where children can run and play? Is it safe? • Will this community support your client and the family?
Adaptive abilities	• Who is identified as the client? • Do all family members have their physical, mental, emotional, socioeconomic, and spiritual needs met within the context of the family? • Is a stressor seen by the family as an opportunity to grow, or does it throw a family's functional ability into disequilibrium? • Can the family help itself when out of balance? • Can family members accept help when their needs overwhelm their resources? • Are family members flexible in adapting or adopting roles? • Does the family communicate effectively? • How does the client like being cared for at home?

Use of Formal and Informal Support Systems. Determine the family's knowledge of community resources, such as adult day care, nursing home, and rehabilitation facilities. Ask if there are friends or extended family who can be called on for help. If caregiving became difficult, would the family consider a long-term care facility?

FOCUSED ASSESSMENT FOR *READINESS FOR ENHANCED FAMILY COPING*

Readiness for enhanced family coping is a wellness nursing diagnosis that allows you to be a family advocate, a teacher, an observer, and a tender of the sick. Families whose members are effectively managing adaptation to the health challenges of their members but are asking for help to do better are given this diagnosis. It reflects families who demonstrate readiness for enhanced health and growth for themselves and the client.

Defining Characteristics. The family with potential for growth is recognized by health-promoting behaviors. They may ask questions about health care, ask about resources for knowledge, or ask for assistance in other ways. When the family's needs are sufficiently gratified and adaptive tasks effectively addressed to enable goals of self-actualization to surface, the family has the potential for growth.

This wellness diagnosis is used when families indicate that they wish to retake control of a situation or when they show a willingness to be taught ways of seeking a higher level of wellness. These families have achieved appropriate developmental tasks and have adequate support systems to achieve further personal and family growth. Healthy families effectively manage to adapt to health challenges of their family members.

Related Factors. Because this diagnosis implies that the family is seeking a higher level of wellness, the family will generally express the related factors in the form of a request for service. Some related factors may include expressing a need for knowledge of treatments, services, or prognosis or expressing a need for contacting a support network or service provider.

FOCUSED ASSESSMENT FOR *COMPROMISED FAMILY COPING*

The diagnosis of *Compromised family coping* indicates that an untoward event or a crisis has occurred to alter the family's ability to function or support individuals within the family in a helpful manner. It can occur in reasonably functional families who have never had a major crisis or in dysfunctional families whose support systems are under pressure and who are unable to meet a health challenge.

Defining Characteristics. Defining characteristics for *Compromised family coping* include both objective and subjective elements. The family may not recognize that their coping is compromised. However, this family is usually trying to meet the needs of its members but feels the efforts are not adequate.

The following are examples of cues to compromised coping from clients or family members:

- Clients express concerns about family members' response to the health problem or with personal reactions (such as fear, anticipatory grief, guilt, anxiety) to their illness, disability, or other situational or developmental crises.
- Family members may be overly protective of the client, investing all energy into being sure that their needs are met while other family members may be neglected.
- Family members express concern about an inadequate understanding or knowledge base, which interferes with effective assistive or supportive behavior (NANDA-I, 2005).

Related Factors. Related factors for *Compromised family coping* include temporary preoccupation by a family member who is trying to manage emotional conflicts and personal suffering and is unable to perceive or act effectively in regard to the client's needs. The family may experience temporary disorganization and role changes. There may be prolonged disease or disability progression that exhausts the supportive capacity of family members. There may other situational or developmental crises or situations the family members may be facing (NANDA-I, 2005).

FOCUSED ASSESSMENT FOR *DISABLED FAMILY COPING*

Disabled family coping is a diagnosis that indicates that the destructive behavior of a family member has disrupted the family's ability to function. The nurse needs to make a decision about the safety of the client and the family. Family members often have significant physical, cognitive, or psychological problems, such as psychiatric disorders, illegal drug use, rebellion against authority, abusive relationships, or geographical or social isolation.

Defining Characteristics. When a crisis has totally broken down or disabled the family's coping abilities, the signs of family dysfunction are more dramatic. The client's or family's needs may not be being met. The family members in the caregiving role may behave with intolerance, aggression, or hostility toward the client, providing care in a harsh manner. In other cases, the client's needs may be disregarded to the point of negligence or even abandonment. The family caregivers may be neglecting other family members or themselves and may develop illnesses or complain of symptoms. They may make decisions that are detrimental to the family's economic or social well-being (NANDA-I, 2005).

Related Factors. Related factors for *Disabled family coping* include families who have relationship problems or unresolved family issues, such as chronically unexpressed feelings of guilt, anxiety, or hostility. Other related factors include families who have ineffective or destructive family communication or coping styles that differ or conflict among family members (NANDA-I, 2005).

FOCUSED ASSESSMENT FOR *CAREGIVER ROLE STRAIN*

Defining Characteristics. Defining characteristics for the diagnosis *Caregiver role strain* includes caregivers' having difficulty in performing required caregiving tasks, concerns about future caregiving responsibilities, including the possible need to institutionalize an ill family member, and apprehension about a family member's future health status and their own (NANDA-I, 2005).

> ***Action Alert!*** When caregivers experience stress-related or opportunistic illnesses (such as hypertension, gastrointestinal upset, headaches, or colds) it may indicate that they are experiencing *Caregiver role strain.*

Related Factors. Factors that contribute to the caregiver's effectiveness in performing the unrelenting or complex care requirements of the care receiver may be classified as psychosocial, developmental, and situational. Refer to Table 48-3 for examples of each factor.

FOCUSED ASSESSMENT FOR *IMPAIRED PARENTING*

Impaired parenting occurs when parents either have inadequate parenting skills or experience crises that have interfered with their adjustment to parenting.

Defining Characteristics. Defining characteristics for *Impaired parenting* include those for the infant or child and those for the parent. Characteristics that apply to the infant or child include physical problems, such as

Table 48-3 Factors Affecting Caregiver Effectiveness

CATEGORY	EXAMPLES OF INFLUENTIAL FACTORS
Developmental	• Caregiver developmentally not ready for caregiver role, as when a young adult must care for a middle-age parent • Developmental delay of the receiver or caregiver • Family's stage of development conflicts with caregiving requirements, as when a newly married couple must care for a sick sibling rather than preparing for child rearing
Psychosocial	• Psychosocial or cognitive problems in the receiver of care • Marginal coping patterns in caregiver • History of poor relationship between caregiver and care receiver • Caregiver is spouse • Care receiver exhibits bizarre behavior • Relationship of caregiver to receiver (spouse, sibling, parent, child, friend, other relative, acquaintance) • Family coping patterns • Spiritual, religious, or cultural beliefs • Financial risk borne by caregiver
Situational	• Abuse or violence in the family • Situational stressors such as loss, disaster, crisis, poverty or major life events such as birth, hospitalization, leaving home, returning home, marriage, divorce, employment, retirement, or death • Poor family dynamics before caregiving began • Duration of caregiving required • Inadequate physical environment for providing care (housing, transportation, community services, equipment) • Family or caregiver isolation • Lack of respite and recreation for caregiver • Inexperience with caregiving • Caregiver's competing role commitments • Complexity and amount of caregiving tasks required
Physiological	• Severity of the recipient's illness • Addiction or codependency • Premature birth or congenital defect • Discharge from health care facility with significant home health care needs • Impaired caregiver health • Unpredictable course of illness or unstable caregiver health

frequent illnesses, failure to thrive, or accidents; cognitive problems, such as poor academic performance; psychological problems, such as behavioral disorders; and social problems, such as lack of social competence, running away, and evidence of physical and psychological trauma or abuse (NANDA-I, 2005).

Characteristics that apply to the parent include the following: child neglect, abuse, or abandonment; verbalization of inability to control the child or inability to meet the child's needs; negative statements about the child; and deficient or poor parent-child interaction (NANDA-I, 2005).

Related Factors. In general, factors related to *Impaired parenting* are contained in five main categories:

- *Social:* lack of access to resources, social isolation, job problems, marital conflict, lack of social support, poor coping and problem-solving skills, and problems with being or acting as a parent
- *Knowledge:* inadequate knowledge of child health and parenting skills, unrealistic expectations, and inability to recognize an infant's cues
- *Physiological:* physical illness
- *Infant or child:* premature birth, illness, prolonged separation from parent, difficult temperament or "wrong" gender, unwanted pregnancy, and physical or developmental abnormality
- *Psychological:* a history of substance abuse, disability, depression, difficult labor and delivery, adolescent parent, and poor prenatal care (NANDA-I, 2005)

DIAGNOSIS

The key to determining accurate nursing diagnoses is to obtain all relevant information, verify it, and then cluster it appropriately. You may need to use a wide variety of nursing diagnoses (Table 48-4). You would use the diagnosis of *Caregiver role strain* when your data indicate that family caregivers feel or exhibit difficulty in performing their family caregiver roles. The diagnosis *Risk for caregiver role strain* is used when family caregivers are vulnerable for felt difficulty in performing their family caregiver roles (NANDA-I, 2005).

PLANNING

EXPECTED OUTCOMES FOR THE FAMILY WITH *READINESS FOR ENHANCED FAMILY COPING*

As a nurse, you should always plan with the family, not for the family. You need to reinforce the family's efforts and help them anticipate what they may need. The

Table 48-4 Clustering Data to Make a Nursing Diagnosis

Family Coping Problems

DATA CLUSTER	DIAGNOSIS
Martha has three children, ages 3, 5, and 9. The 3-year-old has been diagnosed with cystic fibrosis. Martha has been a devoted mother, enjoying creating fun activities for the children and being a Girl Scout leader. Currently she is focusing her attention on the youngest child. The 9-year-old is expected to feed and dress the 5-year-old.	*Impaired parenting* related to overwhelming care needs of child with cystic fibrosis
Mitch Reeves is a 55-year-old man who has had quadruple coronary artery bypass grafting and has residual heart failure. He is on extended medical leave. His wife is planning to build a new, larger house and expects him to be able to negotiate with the builders. She has previously been a realistic and thoughtful homemaker.	*Disabled family coping* related to wife's denial of possible long-term effects from open heart surgery
Rebecca, age 75, has been living with her mother, age 95, and providing financial and emotional support. The relationship has been mutually satisfying and beneficial to both Rebecca and her mother. Her mother had been healthy and active until she recently fractured her ankle. Rebecca tells the nurse that she does not know how to manage her mother's care. Rebecca's diabetes is out of control, and she is learning to give herself insulin.	*Compromised family coping* related to recent injury confounding the care situation
Mary Elizabeth has a 7-year-old child diagnosed with attention-deficit/hyperactivity disorder. She has just been accepted into a community college semiconductor technology program. She needs the training to obtain a better job because she is recently divorced.	*Risk for impaired parenting* related to multiple stressors
John is 35 years old. His wife recently died from cancer. He has two children, ages 6 and 10. John has been working long hours in an effort to manage his grief. He often comes home after his own mother has put the children to bed. On weekends he spends time on household chores. The 6-year-old has started wetting the bed again, and the 10-year-old is acting out in school. John says he cannot deal with any problems, that his mother will have to handle it.	*Interrupted family processes* related to situational crisis of wife's death
Linda has a 4-year-old child. She is a single mother and works at a minimum-wage job. She attends college. She is currently in the hospital with a ruptured appendix. She tells the nurse that she is unable to be an adequate mother to her child.	*Parental role conflict* related to crisis precipitated by acute illness

specific outcomes will reflect the family's expressed needs.

EXPECTED OUTCOMES FOR THE FAMILY WITH *COMPROMISED FAMILY COPING*

Goals can include that the family members will be able to do the following:

- Identify their strengths and weaknesses
- Realistically appraise the changes that the health situation will mean for them and share thoughts and feelings about it
- Be able to plan together and prioritize the needs of each family member
- Take effective action to manage and adapt to the new family situation

EXPECTED OUTCOMES FOR THE FAMILY WITH *DISABLED FAMILY COPING*

If the family meets the criteria for *Disabled family coping,* they are dysfunctional. The focus of your care may need to shift to providing protection for vulnerable family members and getting the family to professional care providers. The following outcomes are in addition to the ones previously listed:

- The client will be protected from abuse, mistreatment, neglect, or abandonment.
- Family members will have a realistic understanding of the needs of the client and provide care that is safe and effective.

BOX 48-3 *Older Adults*

Factors Affecting Older Adults' Caregivers

Lack of time
Emotions, such as anxiety, guilt, depression, worry
Decreased social contacts
Loss of other relationships
Increased expenses
Family conflicts
Fatigue

- Family members will identify their developmental and situational needs and discuss appropriate means to achieve them, including using social support systems and/or professional counseling.

EXPECTED OUTCOMES FOR *CAREGIVER ROLE STRAIN*

The outcomes for *Caregiver role strain* includes your being empathic to families and being able to listen to them without giving advice. The family members will share their frustrations about their caregiver roles and identify plans to improve their daily life, including identifying their support systems (Box 48-3).

The plan of care that the family is given on discharge from an acute care setting is reevaluated in the home setting and revised as needed to meet the needs of the family.

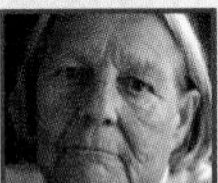

Mrs. Roddy developed a urinary tract infection and needed to be hospitalized. While there, she developed acute respiratory failure and required mechanical ventilation. Attempts to wean her from the ventilator failed, and the family faced the decision of whether to bring her home or admit her to a long-term care facility. What factors did the family need to consider in deciding whether to care for Mrs. Roddy at home?

EXPECTED OUTCOMES FOR *IMPAIRED PARENTING*

The following are examples of goals for *Impaired parenting* that is involved with a parent-child role conflict:

- The parents will gain an understanding of their nurturing role during a specific illness.
- The parents will be able to discuss the balance needed between work and personal responsibilities while being a support to each other and to other family members.
- The parents will be able to identify what they need for support, both internally and externally, to function as a family.

INTERVENTION

INTERVENTIONS TO ESTABLISH A NURSE-FAMILY RELATIONSHIP

Nursing interventions used to establish a nurse-family relationship include establishing trust, active listening, overcoming family resistance, and reinforcing family strengths. You need to develop a working relationship with all family members that is based on trust. Establishing trust in a closed family system is a slow process. A full explanation of your role and the services the agency offers should be given at the level of the family's understanding.

You will need to use active listening skills to understand the problem(s) from the family's perspective. This involves hearing what the family is saying and using your communication skills to help family members express and explore their thoughts and feelings without pressing for information if a person is reluctant to tell. The initial meeting with a family is used to establish that you are an informed resource who will honor the family's confidences and respect the family's members. You can begin by offering nonthreatening general information regarding parenting, developmental stages, relationships, or caregiving as appropriate to the family's needs. You will use your communication skills, such as reflection, to make sure you understand what each family member is expressing.

When behavior patterns are well established, resistance to outside help and to change is a normal reaction. Resistance can be overcome by having the family assume control through the process of mutual goal setting. You must know how to sensitively approach the family. Your level of understanding of their power structure and their cultural influences could garner support or promote family resistance. Give a description of your nursing interventions and what will most likely happen if the interventions are successful or what will continue to happen if they fail. Provide support and praise for the family strengths as developmental or situational stressors are managed. Reinforcing family strengths will help the family grow and change (Figure 48-4).

INTERVENTIONS TO PROMOTE FAMILY PROBLEM SOLVING

Nursing interventions to help families with problem solving are helping them to define their problem(s), acknowledging their feelings, and exploring their coping skills. You can help them limit the scope of their problem(s) and explore solutions. You can help the family identify the areas of family coping that keep them vulnerable and discuss ways to strengthen their defenses. You can help them by attempting to identify their underlying feelings that may be keeping them from working out a solution.

The family may want to start by discussing how they interacted before the current situation (family illness, birth of a baby) arose; this may help them see and understand the negative interactions they have been using with each other. When a family is faced with a problem that is long term or extensive, seeing the problem in its entirety can be overwhelming. Stay in the "now," and keep the family in reality. Offer information related to a specific problem. By the time the family members have worked together to identify their problems and have defined the source of the problems, many ideas for solutions have probably been offered. Plans to implement these proposed solutions should be made. You should support any family strengths the family may have identified.

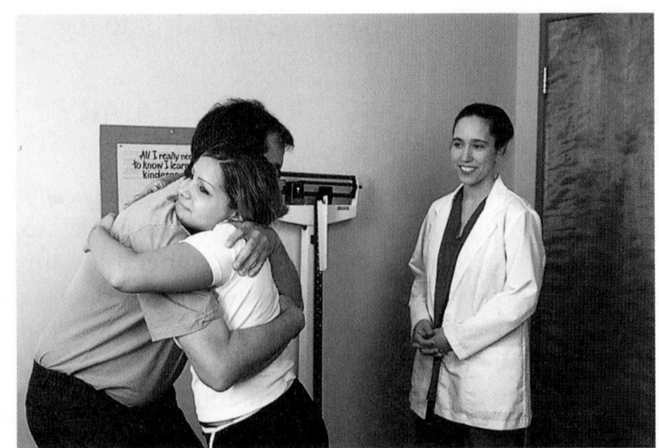

FIGURE 48-4 Reinforcing family strengths will help the family grow and change.

INTERVENTIONS TO CHANGE FAMILY BEHAVIORS

Interventions to change family behaviors include role modeling effective behaviors, providing education, and identifying destructive behaviors, which is an advanced nursing skill. Role modeling is an effective method of teaching caregiving skills. This is a particularly effective intervention for parents of infants and young children (Figure 48-5) and families caring for members who are sick. When you have developed a trusting relationship with the family, they will allow you to function as a role model. When this occurs, you will be able to gain better insight into the family's stressors.

A key to providing effective education for clients is identifying their readiness to learn. Information provided when the family is stressed or not focused may not be remembered or may be rejected. The topics are based on the identified family problems and the family's need for knowledge to understand their problems, to identify solutions, and to implement needed changes to accomplish their goals.

INTERVENTIONS TO PREVENT *CAREGIVER ROLE STRAIN*

Providing Empathy. Assessment data may reveal that the caregivers need to vent or be praised for doing a good job. Performing the tasks of a caregiver can be a lonely, isolating experience that can prompt feelings that no one understands the difficulties and demands of the job. When visiting a caregiver, allow time to share feelings. Convey admiration for positive behaviors that you observe, such as devotion, love, a little job well done, or the client's sense of satisfaction and involvement in family life. Listen to the caregiver's feelings, communicate understanding, and promote a sense of competency not just once but as often as is needed to achieve positive results. Encourage the family, and support them in their decision making.

Help caregivers appreciate the task they have undertaken by giving information about the difficulties of caregiving responsibilities. Educate caregivers about self-care activities that can be used to alleviate *Caregiver role strain* (Box 48-4).

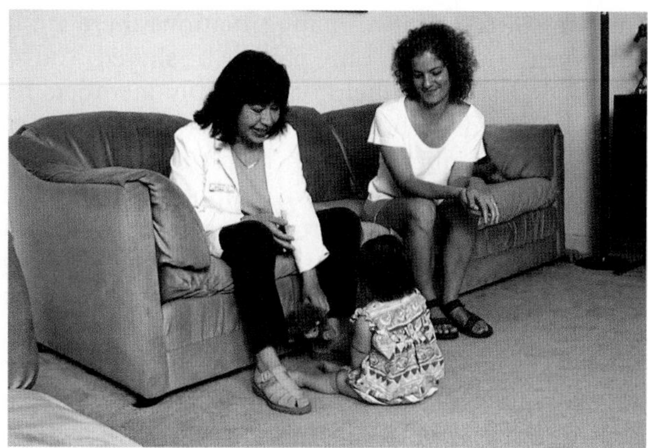

FIGURE 48-5 Role modeling is an effective method of teaching caregiving skills.

Promoting Realistic Appraisal. Caregivers may have unrealistic goals and objectives for the caregiving situation. You can help a caregiver assess the reality of the length of time care will be needed, how much recovery is possible, how much cooperation or self-help can be expected from the family member, and what elements of care are essential. The caregiver may be in denial or uninformed about the demands of the situation.

Help family caregivers be realistic. Many caregivers are not aware of the responsibilities involved in the day-to-day care of a dependent family member. Asking them to describe a typical day and how they will maintain their present schedules and caregiver responsibilities will help them understand that their caregiver responsibilities are in some cases overwhelming. Caregivers should make plans for maintaining physical and emotional health and relationships with family and friends. You can help the caregiver develop a plan for scheduling needed respite time. The caregiver needs to have "me" time to unwind from the pressures of the caregiving role and to maintain good health.

Using Resources. *Caregiver role strain* often stems from a lack of knowledge about available resources or unwillingness to accept assistance. Many caregivers try to take care of their family members alone or with a few family members. They are unaware of the resources available to them in the community or how to request help from others. You can provide family members with information about community resources and their health insurance and/or Medicare or Medicaid benefits. Volunteers can be called to sit with family members while the caregiver goes to the grocery store, has lunch with friends, or otherwise takes a break from their caregiving role.

Some caregivers decline help because they associate asking for help with begging or not being able to manage their own affairs. Statements such as "I never depend on anyone to help me" or "We aren't destitute" demand investigation. Make sure that caregivers understand the relationship between overextending themselves as caregiver and the high probability that they will suffer the ill effects of excessive stress. Encourage them to take care of themselves so they can continue to effectively take care of their loved one.

If you can, talk to family members privately—that is, not in front of the caregiver. Interesting facts may surface during this discussion. For example, other family members may not be aware that the primary caregiver is at risk for *Caregiver role stain.* Sometimes, when family members become aware of the difficulties the primary caregiver is experiencing, they are willing to provide help with caregiving. For family members who cannot provide direct care, providing emotional support to the

BOX 48-4 *Teaching Strategies for Reducing Caregiver Role Strain*

ESTABLISH PARTNERSHIPS IN YOUR FAMILY MEMBER'S CARE

- Establish good relationships with health care providers. They can make sure your family member receives good health care, and they can provide information about the person's medical condition, what to expect in the future, and available community resources.
- Contact a professional with whom you feel comfortable talking about the frustrations of providing care. Clergy, social workers, psychologists, and psychiatric nurses are trained to provide counseling on caregiving issues.
- Join a caregiver support group. This is another good place to share your frustrations and obtain help in managing your stress, locating resources, reducing feelings of isolation, and obtaining support.
- If you have an employee assistance program at work, use it to obtain help with feelings about your caregiver role and to learn about community resources that can help to alleviate your stress.
- Involve your family from the beginning by sharing your concerns with them and dividing up, when possible, the caregiving responsibilities.
- Take time to consider how you might take better care of yourself.

TAKE CARE OF YOURSELF

- Set realistic goals. Trying to balance caregiving with time for yourself, work, and other obligations is difficult. Determine your priorities, and turn to others for help with your caregiving responsibilities.
- Carve time out for yourself, even an hour a day. Do something you enjoy, such as reading a book or going to lunch with a friend. Do not give up your favorite pastimes or withdraw from your friends.
- Accept your feelings. Recognize that you may be grieving. Talk about your feelings with a family member, close friend, or counselor.
- Recognize signs of stress. Are you feeling irritable, helpless, hopeless? Do minor things upset you or make you cry? Are you having trouble sleeping, gaining or losing weight, or feeling exhausted all the time? Are you getting ill more often than you used to? Use a support group, get counseling, and use respite care.
- Get some exercise each day. Take a walk, take stairs instead of an elevator, walk when you are on the phone, put energy into housework, mow the lawn, and so on.
- Recognize your limits. Maybe you will not be able to continue to provide care until the care recipient dies. Learn to continue to "let go" from the start, and share your caregiver burdens with other family members or professional caregivers.

Modified from National Family Caregivers Association. (2005). *Tips & guides*. Retrieved November 11, 2005, from http://www.thefamilycaregiver.org/ed/tips.cfm.

primary care provider with visits or phone calls may help to reduce caregiver role strain.

Providing Direct Assistance. You may need to intervene to help caregivers obtain information and support. First, determine the care that is being provided by caregivers. Typically, caregivers provide services as personal care, medical treatments, meals, housekeeping, and managing finances. Help caregivers identify both professional and volunteer (family, friends, neighbors, church) resources. Advise caregivers if they ask for help from family and friends, they may feel good they are providing a "little help."

When a family member can no longer remain safely in the home, you will need to help the family and client identify alternative residential options, such as assisted living facilities. This type of residence provides people with a feeling of independence while providing them with a safe and supervised environment that includes regular meals, reminders to take needed medication, and immediate help if an emergency should arise.

For family members who are too frail or sick to live in assisted living facilities, a skilled nursing facility (nursing home) may be considered. You can help families and clients with this difficult decision by suggesting they evaluate the available nursing homes in terms of the quality of life and type of care they offer their residents and their safety records. The Medicare Internet website has information about the Medicaid- and Medicare-certified nursing homes in the United States. It includes information on payment and patient rights and a nursing home checklist that will help families evaluate the nursing homes that they visit (U.S. Department of Health and Human Services, 2005).

Discuss the advantages and disadvantages of each out-of-home option, but allow decision making to remain with the family members. Support their decisions to help minimize the guilt feelings they may experience when the ill family member needs to be placed in a facility.

INTERVENTIONS TO PREVENT *RISK FOR CAREGIVER ROLE STRAIN*

Engaging Assistance From Family and Friends. When possible and with the permission of the caregiver, engage other family members in the appraisal of the caregiver's situation. Allow each member the opportunity to share their frustration and concerns about the changes in family function created by the need for caregiving. Stress that in many situations there are no problems to be solved, only pain to be shared. You are in a good position to help other family members recognize the needs of both the caregiver and the dependent family member. You can help them identify the kinds of support they can give. Emphasize the importance of emotional support—that is, regular phone calls, cards, letters, and visits. Discuss the need to give caregivers "permission" to enjoy themselves (respite care, vacations, and day trips).

If caregivers have access to the Internet, you can encourage its use as a support system. It can give them easy access to resources that meet their needs, such as information about their family member's health problems. It can provide them with Internet caregiver support groups.

And it can serve as a diversionary intervention for caregivers unable to leave the home at regular intervals.

Encouraging Social Support and Advocacy. Encourage caregivers to use a social support system to help manage their emotional needs. Support groups can help caregivers appraise the reality of their situations and provide them with information about methods of care and resources. You can link caregivers with social support resources.

Many caregiver advocacy groups are recruiting members who will speak out and demand an improvement in the quality and quantity of caregiving services at the local, state, and federal levels. The opportunity to join with other caregivers advocates can be a satisfying social outlet for some caregivers.

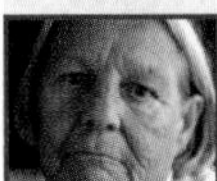

Mrs. Roddy's family attended a discharge planning conference in which the discharge team discussed her deteriorating condition and the health care options available for the family. Because Mrs. Roddy had expressed a desire to remain in her home and had not wanted to go to a nursing home, the family decided to try home health care. After the family caregivers were instructed in the care of a ventilator-dependent client and declared competent caregivers, Mrs. Roddy was discharged home with a tracheostomy, gastrostomy tube feedings, Foley catheter, heparin lock, and therapeutic bed. A home health care nurse collaborated with the family and the home health care team. What interventions on the part of the home health care nurse might help to prevent *Caregiver role strain?*

EVALUATION

Periodically reassess the family for changes in the health care situation and for the development of new stressors. The family is evaluated in relationship to each nursing intervention. If the goals are realistic and comprehensive, the client should be receiving effective care without disrupting the needs of the entire family.

Include assessment of factors that have an impact on the outcomes of the nursing process, such as the compliance of the client and family, the quality of the care given, the consistency of the support systems, and a realistic time frame for reaching the goals. When the goals are not met, you need to reevaluate every step of the nursing process. Remember that a family unit is a dynamic unit; the situation may have changed in such a way that the plan cannot be carried out effectively. Did everyone do his or her job? Did the interventions achieve what you and the family expected and wanted?

If the family has been involved in the process, they will be willing to reassess and continue. In collaboration with the family caregivers, evaluate progress toward preventing or reducing *Caregiver role strain.* Did you successfully reduce the caregivers' apprehension about their ability to provide care? Did the caregivers receive the type of help they needed to take care of themselves? Point out the family successes, and identify the areas where more work is needed. Families will respond, especially when they can see that their efforts have been recognized and appreciated.

Caregiver role strain can have a strong detrimental influence on caregivers and their families. Successful nursing care can prevent caregiver burnout and the physical and emotional disorders associated with it. Your care can make a tremendous difference in the lives of caregiving families.

When Mrs. Roddy is discharged from the hospital, the nurse writes the following discharge note.

Sample Documentation Note for Mrs. Roddy

Discharged on a mechanical ventilator to tracheostomy, gastrostomy tube with continuous feedings, Foley catheter, and saline lock intravenous access. Family has practiced caring for the tracheostomy site, suctioning, and managing the ventilator. Respiratory therapist will accompany the client home and make sure the ventilator is functioning properly. Family has practiced tube-feeding technique and has been instructed in skin care, Foley care, and saline lock care. Home health care nurse will visit tomorrow to review care and the family's plan for care.

▼ KEY PRINCIPLES

- The family as a client is the essence of family-centered nursing care.
- Family nursing care is based on the family response to actual or potential health problems.
- Knowing individual and family developmental tasks, nurses can determine the family unit's health by assessing the family's successful mastery of appropriate tasks while also observing whether individual family members' actions are appropriate to their developmental level.
- The healthy family is an open system with complex interactions both within the family and with the external world.
- The interactionalist would describe the family by describing roles, the decision-making process, communication, conflict, and reaction to stress.
- Family roles are structured for the division of labor and the distribution of power.
- Family function can be compromised by role stress and role conflict.
- Stressors can be a threat or a challenge. It depends on how the family perceives them.
- Healthy families have resources for managing stress.
- Caregivers are at risk for role strain from the burden, responsibilities, and stress associated with caregiving.
- Caregivers are not clients of the health care system; as such, their specific needs may go unmet.
- *Ineffective coping* can be caused by the number of stressors and the critical importance of, or the overwhelming threat of, the particular stressor.
- The key to determining accurate nursing diagnoses is obtaining all relevant information, verifying it, and then clustering it appropriately.
- The *Readiness for enhanced family coping* diagnosis is a wellness nursing diagnosis that is observed in families whose members are effectively managing adaptation to a health challenge of one of its members.
- Nurses need to be alert to the unmet needs of caregivers as well as of care recipients.

Continued

- The diagnosis *Caregiver role strain* is used when family caregivers feel or exhibit difficulty in performing their family caregiver roles.
- The diagnosis *Risk for caregiver role strain* is used when family caregivers are vulnerable for felt difficulty in performing their family caregiver roles.
- A healthy family is one whose members are genuinely interested in what the nurse has to say and are willing to help the client.
- Interventions to establish a nurse-family relationship are establishing trust, listening actively, overcoming resistance, and reinforcing family strengths.
- Interventions for problem solving are defining the problem, acknowledging feelings, exploring coping skills, limiting the scope, and exploring solutions to problems.
- Interventions to change behaviors are role modeling effective behaviors, providing education, and identifying destructive behaviors.
- Interventions include helping caregivers identify when they need to examine other options, such as respite care, nursing home placement, or hospice care.

REVIEW QUESTIONS

1. The family is composed of the husband and his child from a previous marriage and his wife, whose children stay with them during the summer. The nurse knows this is an example of a(an):

1. Intergenerational family
2. Binuclear family
3. Extended family
4. Nuclear family

2. The nurse knows that providing psychosocial protection and support of the family members is an example of which type of family function?

1. Affective
2. Economic
3. Health care
4. Socialization

3. The nurse knows healthy families may use which of the following strategies to manage stress?

1. Keeping their concerns about the family member's care within the family.
2. Controlling all emotions when the nurse is making a home visit.
3. Discussing problems among members.
4. Not recognizing their problems

4. The wife of an older client who is brain impaired resents being in the caregiver role because of an earlier history of abuse from her husband. The burden of this arrangement may be especially trying and energy depleting for her. The most appropriate nursing diagnosis is:

1. *Risk for caregiver role strain*
2. *Readiness for enhanced family coping*
3. *Caregiver role strain*
4. *Disabled family coping*

5. Which nursing intervention would be the most appropriate in assisting a family caregiver with preventing role strain?

1. Discussing the caregiver's situation with other family members
2. Suggesting placement for the family member in a skilled nursing facility
3. Reassuring the caregiver that caregiving will get easier
4. Referring the family caregiver to other resources

Bibliography

Black, C., & Ford-Gilboe, M. (2004). Adolescent mothers: Resilience, family health work and health-promoting practices. *Journal of Advanced Nursing, 48*(4), 351-360.

Family Caregiver Alliance. (2005). *Fact sheet: Selected caregiver statistics*. Retrieved October 28, 2005, from http://www.caregiver.org/caregiver/jsp/content_node.jsp?nodeid=439.

Feinberg, L. F., Newman, S. L., Gray, L., & Kolb, K. N. (2004). *The state of the states in family caregiver support: A 50 state study*. San Francisco, CA: Family Caregiver Alliance.

Friedman, M. M., Bowman, V. R., & Jones, E. (2003). *Family nursing: Research, theory, and practice.* Upper Saddle River, NJ: Prentice Hall.

Hanson, S. M. H., Gedaly-Duff, V., & Kaakinen, J. R. (2005). *Family health care nursing: Theory, practice & research* (3rd ed.). Philadelphia: F. A. Davis.

Johnson, M., Bulechek, G., Butcher, H., Dochterman, J. M., Maas, M., Moorhead, S., et al. (Eds.). (2006). *NANDA, NOC, and NIC linkages: Nursing diagnoses, outcomes, & interventions.* St. Louis, MO: Mosby.

Ladwig, G. B., & Ackley, B. J. (2006). *Mosby's guide to nursing diagnosis*. St. Louis, MO: Mosby.

NANDA International. (2005). *Nursing diagnoses: Definitions and classification, 2005-2006* (6th ed.). Philadelphia: Author.

National Alliance for Care-giving. (2004). *About family caregiving 101*. Retrieved November 10, 2005, from http://www.familycaregiving101.org/about/.

National Center on Elder Abuse. (2005). *Frequently asked questions: What is elder abuse*. Retrieved November 11, 2005, from http://www.elderabusecenter.org/default.cfm?p=faqs.cfm.

National Family Caregivers Association. (2005). *Tips & guides*. Retrieved November 11, 2005, from http://www.thefamilycaregiver.org/ed/tips.cfm.

National Family Caregivers Association. (2005). *Who are America's family caregivers?* Retrieved November 8, 2005, from http://www.thefamilycaregiver.org/who/.

Thobaben, M. (2006). Family caregiving in home health. *Home Health Care Management & Practice, 18*(3), 250-252.

Thobaben, M., & Duncan, R. (2003). Domestic elder abuse by health care providers. *Home Health Care Management & Practice, 15*(2), 168-169.

U.S. Department of Health & Human Services, Centers for Medicare & Medicaid Services, Medicare. (2005). *Nursing homes*. Retrieved November 13, 2005, from http://www.medicare.gov/Nursing/Overview.asp.

Chapter 49

SUPPORTING SPIRITUALITY

Media Resources

- Evolve Website http://evolve.elsevier.com/Harkreader/
- Companion CD

Learning Objectives

After studying this chapter, you will be able to do the following:

- Relate the concepts of spirituality, religion, and faith to the concept of providing spiritual care in nursing
- Discuss the factors affecting a client's spiritual and religious needs
- Assess a client for spiritual well-being
- Write nursing diagnoses for clients with spiritual distress or impaired religiosity
- Plan individualized care for clients experiencing spiritual distress or impaired religiosity
- Evaluate interventions for relieving spiritual distress or impaired religiosity
- Discuss nursing care for enhancing spiritual well-being or religiosity

Key Terms

agnostic
atheist
faith
hope
monotheism
polytheism
religion
religiosity
spiritual distress
spiritual health
spiritual well-being
spirituality

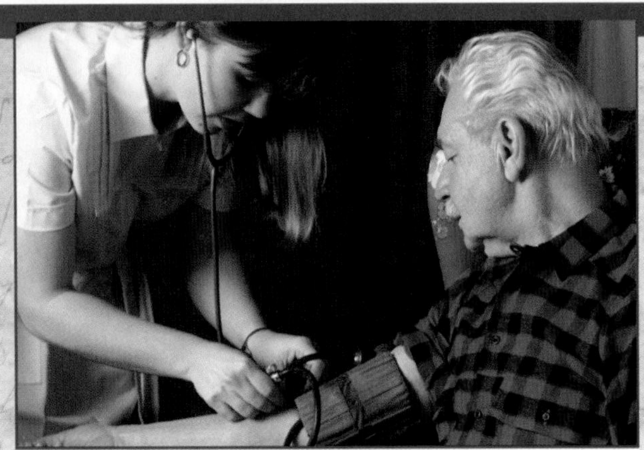

Mr. Guevara is a 56-year-old master electrician who has just returned home from the hospital after a radical prostatectomy (removal of prostate gland) for invasive carcinoma 4 days ago. His suprapubic wound has a 3-cm opening that requires daily wound care. You make plans to assist Mr. Guevara in managing his wound care and supporting his recovery from surgery. You discover that Mr. Guevara has spiritual and religious needs in addition to his obvious physical and psychological needs. You consider the nursing diagnoses that apply to spirituality (see key nursing diagnoses box).

KEY NURSING DIAGNOSES FOR SPIRITUALITY

Readiness for enhanced spiritual well-being: Ability to experience and integrate meaning and purpose in life through connectedness with self, others, art, music, literature, nature, or a power greater than oneself

Risk for spiritual distress: At risk for impaired ability to experience and integrate meaning and purpose in life through the individual's connectedness with self, others, art, music, literature, nature, and/or a power greater than oneself

Spiritual distress: Impaired ability to experience and integrate meaning and purpose in life through connectedness with self, others, art, music, literature, nature, or a power greater than oneself

Readiness for enhanced religiosity: Ability to increase reliance on religious beliefs and/or participate in rituals of a particular faith tradition

Risk for impaired religiosity: At risk for impaired ability to exercise reliance on religious beliefs and/or participate in rituals of a particular faith tradition

Impaired religiosity: Impaired ability to exercise reliance on beliefs and/or participate in rituals of a particular faith tradition

CONCEPTS OF SPIRITUALITY

SPIRITUALITY

Spirituality is an abstract and elusive term defined in the dictionary as an attachment to the values of the spirit. The human spirit is described as the immaterial aspect of a person, which never dies. Spirituality then is the core of a person that interprets and unifies the whole being: the physical, emotional, social, cognitive, and spiritual dimensions. One's spirituality serves to shape and give meaning to life and to what one can be.

From an analysis of the literature, **spirituality** is defined as the experiences and expressions of one's spirit in a unique and dynamic process reflecting faith in God or a supreme being; connectedness with oneself, others, nature, or God; and integration of the dimensions of mind, body, and spirit (Meraviglia, 2004). Table 49-1 lists characteristics of spirituality (Meraviglia, 1998).

Spirituality is seen in everything one is, one knows, and one does. It involves not only being but knowing and doing, encompassing a person's sense of meaning and purpose in life as well as religious beliefs or practices, such as prayer (Figure 49-1). However, this idea of personal spirituality transcends any structured religion.

Spirituality is a sense of connectedness with oneself, others, nature, or God that has both vertical and horizontal dimensions. The vertical dimension represents one's relationship with God or a supreme being. The experience of God as a transcending (yet personal) being is included in this dimension. The horizontal dimension of spirituality encompasses one's relationships with self, others, and nature, and one's supreme values and beliefs, such as hope and love. Pargament (1997) states that spirituality toward God (the vertical dimension) is the primary focus of our spirit, and the remaining forms of connectedness (the horizontal dimension) stem from this focal point.

RELIGION

Religion is a belief system about God or a supreme being, including rituals and traditions. Religion can also mean a social institution in which people participate together, rather than an individual's solitary search for meaning in life. **Religiosity** is a person's reliance on religious beliefs or participation in rituals of a particular faith tradition.

Typically, religion includes a personal commitment to God with worshipful devotion and conduct. Religious practices are conducted in accordance with divine commands, especially as found in sacred writings or declared by authoritative teachers. Religion can therefore be viewed as a service to God, organized within a specified set of beliefs and practices.

Table 49-1 Characteristics of Spirituality

CHARACTERISTIC	ELEMENTS
General	• Connectedness to all things • Unity or wholeness permeating all of life and manifested through becoming and connecting; cannot occur in isolation
Being (important relationships and sense of connection with oneself)	• Going inward • Being in touch with self • Sense of communion with others, God, and the world • Being open to new things • Feeling of inner synchrony and harmony
Knowing (what and how one knows)	• Evolving understanding of the processes and events of life • Receptive openness to life • Active seeking and discovering • Trusting in one's own experiences
Doing (what one does and how one acts)	• Connection with something bigger than the self • Activities such as prayer, going to church, meditation, rituals • Being with others, assisting friends, raising children, caring for parents • With the earth, gardening, recycling, composting

Information from Meraviglia, M. G. (1998). Critical analysis of spirituality and its empirical indicators: Prayer and meaning in life. *Journal of Holistic Nursing, 17*(1), 18-33.

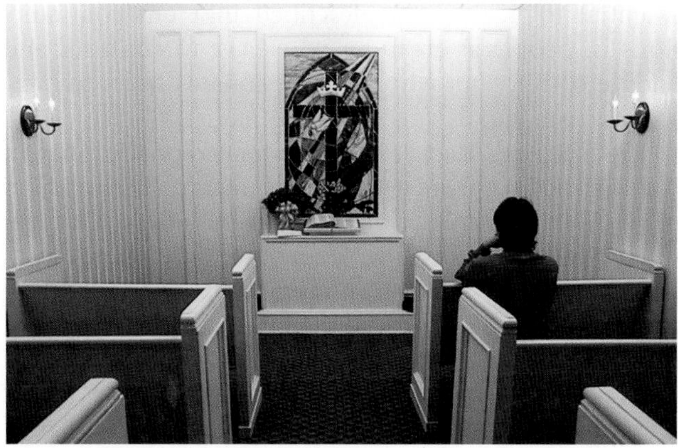

FIGURE 49-1 Spirituality encompasses a person's sense of meaning and purpose in life, in addition to religious beliefs or behaviors, such as prayer.

Spiritual and religious expressions are not necessarily synonymous. A person can be spiritual without being religious and religious without being spiritual. Spirituality has to do with experience; religion has to do with the conceptualization of that experience. Spirituality focuses on what happens in the heart, whereas religion tries to capture and explain that experience.

Many religions of the world are based on a belief in a singular God. **Monotheism** is the belief in the existence of one God who created and rules the universe. Other faiths, such as Native American beliefs, perceive many spirits in the world. **Polytheism** is the belief in more than one god. Still other faiths, such as Hinduism, see many gods coexisting but all as manifestations of the one Absolute God.

FAITH

Faith is belief in or commitment to something or someone greater than oneself that helps a person realize his or her purpose. By definition, faith is belief without proof. Each person chooses what to believe. Faith is universal, a part of living, a part of acting, and a part of self-understanding (Fowler & Keen, 1985).

Faith is further described as relating the boundaries and depths of experience to a source, center, and standard of values in life, which includes the total being. The content of a person's faith, the person's values, beliefs, symbols, and rituals, are important in influencing the person's behavior and shaping his or her personality. Although faith is always an inner knowing and belief in a supreme being, it includes a social or interpersonal dimension, which is reflected through relationships with friends, family, and neighbors.

An **atheist** is a person who has no faith in God or a supreme being and denies the possibility of God's existence. Atheists find meaning in life through their relationships, work, or secular humanism, which is a set of beliefs about the world without the notion of God. Some people do not believe in God and also feel no need to find an alternative set of principles.

An **agnostic** is a person who is undecided about the existence of God or a supreme being. Because God is not provable, agnostics believe silence on the issue is a wise position. Some agnostics argue that there is not an ultimate meaning in life, only the meaning that individuals invest in life. All such decisions are a matter of choice and faith.

SPIRITUALITY AND HEALTH

The human-environment connection is a mutual process in which people exist in open relationship with God or a supreme being and thus become more than just the sum of their parts. This concept of a person expands the traditional definition of health. Holistic health is the understanding that health includes the whole person: the physical, emotional, cognitive, social, and spiritual dimensions.

Personal spiritual experiences can enhance feelings of compassion, peace of mind, and connection. These feelings represent a balance between inner and outer aspects of human experience. Beliefs about spirituality, life after death, and meaning in life are important aspects of health and wellness. For example, Dalmida (2006) found that spirituality was an effective resource to enhance the psychological well-being and health-related quality of life in women who are human immunodeficiency virus (HIV) positive.

Taylor (2002) described the spiritual needs of clients as the need to experience God's presence, have the opportunity to pray, gain a sense of purpose and meaning in life, feel peaceful, and resolve bitter feelings. Additional spiritual needs during a terminal illness include the need to confess and be forgiven, to be loved and love others, to maintain an attitude of hope, and to accept and prepare for death.

The spirit integrates one's personality and provides some sense of direction and order to live by. In addition, one's spirituality stimulates a sense of selflessness and a willingness to do more for others than for oneself. **Spiritual well-being** is the process of being and becoming by reflecting one's spiritual experiences. Spiritual well-being represents the totality of a person's inner resources, the wholeness of spirit and unifying dimension, a process of transcendence, and perception of life as having meaning (Ellison & Paloutzion, 1983). Spiritual well-being includes the following:

- Concern for others and self
- Sense of meaning and enjoyment in life
- Commitment to purposes greater than the self
- Sense of connectedness
- Means for moving through debilitating guilt, anger, or anxiety
- Life-affirming relationships or interconnectedness with God or a supreme being, self, community, and environment

Spiritual well-being is closely related to hope. **Hope** is an interpersonal process created through trust and nurtured by trusting relationships with others, including God. Hope is the belief, expectation, or trust that things will be better in the future. Hope is necessary for people to survive illness or difficult times.

Spiritual health refers to a state of wholeness of the spiritual dimension. It includes the following:

- Sense of personal fulfillment
- Sense of peace with the self and the world
- Sense of fulfillment in life and interaction with self and others
- Ability to discover and articulate a basic purpose in life
- Ability to experience love, joy, peace, and fulfillment
- Ability to live in wholeness consistent with the values of community and self

Spiritual distress is an impaired ability to experience and integrate meaning and purpose in life through connection with self and others, which causes anguish of the human spirit. Relieving spiritual distress in clients is an important factor for optimizing holistic health and healing (NANDA International [NANDA-I], 2007).

SPIRITUALITY IN NURSING

Nursing recognizes the spiritual aspect of human nature as an integral component of a person's sense of wellness. Facilitating spiritual well-being is one approach to attaining and maintaining holistic health. Nursing theorists have long recognized the importance of spirituality.

Travelbee (1971) underscored the significance of spiritual values by emphasizing the importance of finding meaning in illness, thus suggesting that spirituality is essential to health. She described inherent contradictions in people as creatures who have to confront and endure conflict but who have the innate ability to transcend the material aspects of their nature.

Paterson and Zderad (1988) elaborated on the inherent contradictions that are part of being human. By emphasizing the conflict between the spiritual and material dimensions of the self, this theory supports the dimension of assisting clients with confronting spiritual dilemmas.

Watson (1985) incorporated the abstract spiritual concepts of soul, spirit, and transcendence to explain the nature of a person and the goals of nursing. For Watson, one's spirituality is a developmental phenomenon growing and changing through life experiences. Maintaining faith, hope, and altruistic values enhances this developmental process.

Newman (1986) characterized spiritual growth as movement toward a state of absolute consciousness in which the spatial-temporal self is transcended. In this state, the person is aware of a unity that includes but is greater than the self, and there is an experience of unconditional love. As development of the physical self becomes more restricted with aging, former methods of coping no longer work. Transcendence offers an alternative to the spiritual impasse that older adults or the severely ill may experience: an awareness that extends beyond the physical self. Spirituality is integral to the health process at all ages but particularly in later life.

Roy (1988) stated that one assumption about the healing process is the premise that human nature is rooted in connectedness to the absolute truth of the creator. Although not stated in Roy's original theory, implicit in her work is that healing involves a relationship with God.

Most nurses strive to give holistic care, but research has shown that nurses commonly avoid addressing spirituality. Fewer than 36% of nurses reported giving frequent spiritual support to their clients (Vance, 2001). Barriers to giving spiritual care are cited as insufficient time, lack of education, privacy of client, and lack of confidence. Interestingly, nurses who reported more spiritual well-being provided more spiritual care to their clients yet still identified the same barriers.

OVERVIEW OF MAJOR RELIGIONS

Health care includes clients who practice a diversity of religions. If the client states a faith, you should know resources for obtaining more information about that faith, especially the most common religions (Table 49-2). All religions fulfill the purpose of describing and explaining spiritual experiences. You need to be aware of the particular beliefs and practices of each religion to assess and care for the spiritual needs of your clients.

Christianity. The central figure in Christianity is Jesus of Nazareth. Jesus is considered the Christ, the Savior who was foretold and expected by the Jewish people. Christianity is one of the largest world religions, with the predominant groups being the Roman Catholic Church, the Protestant churches, and the Eastern Orthodox Church.

Christianity's primary beliefs include the following:

- Focus on Jesus Christ as the son of God
- Trinitarian God (Father, Son, and Holy Spirit)
- Redemption of people from sin through the death and resurrection of Jesus
- Holy Spirit of God given to all believers
- Revelation of God's truth in the Bible
- Final judgment by God at the end of one's life

Each group within Christianity has unique beliefs and practices. The Roman Catholic Church relies on scripture and tradition for its beliefs and practices. Members must attend church services regularly and participate in the sacraments of the faith, which include baptism, confirmation, communion, confession, and sacrament of the sick. The Eastern Orthodox Church is similar in terms of the worship service, but leadership is provided by the patriarchs instead of the pope, priests can marry instead of remaining celibate, and members do not say rosary prayers.

The Protestant churches have many denominations with a variety of different beliefs. Primarily, Protestant churches rely on the Bible instead of tradition as the basis for beliefs and practices. Another unique belief of Protestant Christians is the forgiveness of all believers' sins through faith in Jesus Christ, with good deeds not contributing to salvation.

To provide appropriate spiritual care, identify the specific beliefs and practices of Christian clients. Based on this individualized assessment, you can determine the spiritual needs of the client and establish effective interventions to meet those needs. With Christian clients, you should be sensitive to their need for quiet prayer time. Roman Catholics and Eastern Orthodox Christians may desire a priest to administer communion and sacrament of the sick (anointing for healing). They may want pictures of saints or angels in the room for spiritual and emotional comfort. Protestants may want to talk about life and illness openly in regard to their personal relationship with Jesus.

Judaism. As with most major religions, Judaism represents a religion and a way of life that influence the community of believers through conduct and culture. Judaism began well over 4000 years ago when God, the creator of the universe, called Abraham into a covenant relationship. The covenant extends to all of Abraham's descendants, making them a kingdom of priests and a holy nation.

The fundamental teachings of Judaism are grouped around the concept of monotheism. Central to the religion is the belief that people are at the core of God's

Table 49-2 Ten Largest Religions in the United States (Self-Identification, 2001)

RELIGION	ESTIMATED NUMBER OF ADULTS	ESTIMATED PERCENTAGE OF TOTAL ADULTS
Protestant	108,633,000	52.5%
Roman Catholic	50,873,000	24.1%
No religion	27,539,000	13.2%
Judaism	2,831,000	1.3%
Islam	1,104,000	0.5%
Buddhism	1,082,000	0.5%
Agnostic	991,000	0.5%
Atheist	902,000	0.4%
Hinduism	766,000	0.4%
Unitarian Universalist	629,000	0.3%

From Adherents.com. Retrieved October 29, 2005, from http://www.adherents.com/rel_USA.html#religions.

creation. Judaism also teaches that people are basically good because they are made in God's image. God is seen as just, merciful, and compassionate. The Jewish people are called to be like God and to worship God through their lives. The Torah (sacred writings of the Law) and the Talmud (Oral Law) are viewed as divine revelations on the rules for living and the experiences of others with God.

There are several Jewish sects, and they adopt different religious practices that you need to be aware of in providing spiritual care. Orthodox Jews comply with the traditional beliefs and practices of Judaism. They strictly follow the Torah and Talmud, which include practices of daily worship, dietary regulations (no pork or shellfish, and foods are to be prepared in a kosher, or proper, manner), traditional prayers in Hebrew, study of the Torah, special clothing and head covering, and observance of the Sabbath (Saturday as a holy day). Conservative Jews follow the traditional practices of Orthodox Judaism with some modifications. They adhere to most of the dietary regulations and the Sabbath. Conservative Judaism provides a middle ground to the liberal Reform Judaism that abandoned the traditional practices for modernization. Reformed Jews believe in the one true God and practice the ethical principles of Judaism but have removed the lifestyle restrictions of Orthodox Judaism.

In caring for a Jewish client, you will need to determine the specific beliefs and practices embraced by the person. Providing privacy for daily prayers is very important for many Jewish clients, as is the need to keep the Sabbath by refraining from physical and recreational activities. Knowledge of the client's dietary restrictions and the need for kosher food items is imperative in providing for health and spiritual care.

Islam. The religion of Islam began with Muhammad during the 600s in Arabia. He began to have visions and revelations while meditating in the caves around Mecca in which the angel Gabriel delivered messages from God, known as Allah, about God's greatness and human beings' sinful nature. Allah is viewed as the only God, who created the universe and sustains its inhabitants. Muhammad is considered the last prophet of God in a long line of prophets, which include Abraham, Isaiah, and Jesus (from Judaism and Christianity).

The revelations from Allah were written down and form the sacred book of the Qur'an for the Muslims. Most of the book includes the Islamic laws concerning the spiritual life of daily prayers, fasting, pilgrimage to Mecca, giving, and attaining salvation; and social laws on inheritance, crime, personal conduct, and marriage. The Qur'an includes stories from the Hebrew Bible about Adam and Eve, Abraham, and Joseph.

Muhammad and his successors conquered vast territories and imposed the religious and governmental laws of Islam on the people. The religion spread very rapidly into the Middle East, India, Europe, and Africa. There are currently two main sects of Islam, which are the traditionalist Sunni (the largest group) and the Shi'ite. The predominant difference between the sects is that the Sunni have combined regional customs with the Qur'an Law. There are four subgroups of Sunni in the Islam community (Sunnite, 2006).

Islamic religious practices include the Five Pillars of Islam, which the believer is to practice faithfully. The Five Pillars include the following:

- Recite the creed, "There is no God but Allah, and Muhammad is the messenger of Allah."
- Observe the five prayer times each day.
- Give at least 2.5% of one's income to help the poor.
- Fast during the day in the month of Ramadan.
- Go once during one's lifetime on a pilgrimage to Mecca.

The Law or Shari'ah describes the way of life for Muslims, including beliefs and practices.

The Islamic religion has special implications for you in caring for a Muslim client. You must be aware of the spiritual need for daily prayer time at sunrise, noon, midafternoon, sunset, and bedtime. Muslims must wash before each prayer time even if they are sick. They are forbidden to eat pork and drink alcohol. Muslim women are required to cover all of the body and maintain modesty in all situations.

Buddhism. Buddhism originated with the teachings of Buddha Gautama in approximately 550 BC in India. Gautama followed the early beliefs of Hinduism to find enlightenment. After a long period of spiritual growth, he began to teach the people about his experiences and his transformation to Buddha. Central to Buddhism are the Four Noble Truths, which include the following:

- Life is suffering.
- Suffering is a result of one's desires for pleasure, power, and existence.
- To stop suffering, one must stop desiring.
- The way to stop desiring, and thus suffering, is to follow the Eightfold Path. It includes right views, right intention, right speech, right action, right livelihood, right effort, right awareness, and right concentration.

Through this process, one experiences a state of release known as Nirvana. To Buddha, there was no encounter with the self or godhead as in Hinduism. When he died, Buddha is believed to have entered a final state of Nirvana.

Over the years, several traditions of Buddhism have arisen. The Theravada tradition emphasizes the composite nature of all things and the absence of gods to help. This tradition has spread throughout Southeast Asia. The Mahayana tradition stresses an expanded understanding of the universe with celestial beings and a godhead. This tradition is the predominant type of Buddhism throughout East Asia, including China, Korea, and Japan. The Tantrayana sect of Buddhism is the major type in Tibet and Mongolia. This tradition describes a visualized god and uses tantric rituals to experience Nirvana, such as sacred gestures and sounds (Britannica Online, 2005).

Because of the various sects of Buddhism with differing beliefs, they cannot be assessed as a group when providing spiritual care. You need to assess the specific beliefs the Buddhist holds and then consider those beliefs and practices when caring for the client's spiritual needs.

Buddhists use yoga meditation as a religious practice to attain peace. The concept of balance is important to Buddhists. They stress the middle path in life, emphasizing self-control and discipline. The Chinese believe that yin, the shady side of the mountain, and yang, the sunny side, demonstrate this idea of balance. Along with this understanding of life is the notion of the dynamic flow of the energy in the universe. There is also a feeling of unity with all of the people and things in the world. Buddhists want to be aware of the unity but remain nonattached (Eliade & Couliano, 2000).

Hinduism. Hinduism is a complex belief system from India dating back 3000 years. In this religion, the person is seen as being on a spiritual journey to discover the self or consciousness. The self is considered to be absolute truth. The true nature of the self is connected with the supreme consciousness of the cosmos known as Brahma. Brahma, then, is the source of all existence, literally the godhead of creation. Hindus worship many gods, such as Vishnu and Shiva, which are believed to be the embodiment of the godhead.

A key concept in Hinduism is Maya. Maya refers to the world that appears to us, the material objects around us. It represents an illusion of time and space. For Hindus, Maya impedes an awareness of the self by keeping one's focus on the things of the world.

Rebirth is another belief central to Hinduism. When anyone dies, he or she is reborn as another creature on the basis of deeds in a previous existence. When a person performs perfect deeds, attains perfection, knowledge, or is extremely ascetic, the person will earn salvation from the process of rebirth.

Hinduism has many religious practices for the spiritual journey of finding the self. Yoga is one such practice, helping people integrate mind, body, and spirit so that they can encounter the self and attain perfect knowledge. Within yoga there are steps for achieving integration, such as physical posturing, breathing control, concentration, meditation, and enlightenment. Yoga is also practiced by people of other religions.

The rituals of worship facilitate the spiritual journey. Worship is primarily done individually by meditating to encounter the self. Believers also gather in temples to chant prayers or scripture (Figure 49-2).

Hinduism is not just a religion but represents both a lifestyle and a social structure for its followers. Because of this, the beliefs have implications for spiritual care.

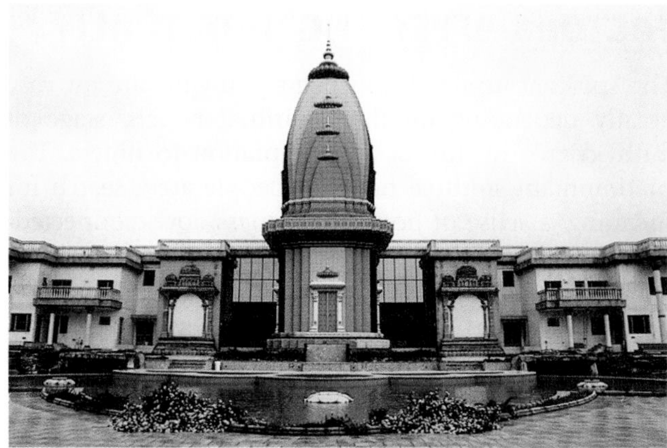

FIGURE 49-2 In Hinduism, believers gather in Hindu temples to chant prayers or scripture.

The law of karma is an example of Hinduism's influence on the lifestyle by the understanding of personal health and well-being. Karma is the belief that for every action there is a corresponding reaction. For Hindus, karma is central to health, and all thoughts and actions have effects on the body and mind. Personal harmony is maintained by following this law of nature. Physical illness is explained by previous actions, even actions in another life (Eliade & Couliano, 2000).

Native American Religion. The Native American people, also known as American Indians, are separated by over 500 languages but share similar religious beliefs. The people worship many gods and the objects that surround them, such as the Sun and Moon. They worship a sacred power represented in mythological beings. Many Native Americans believe in good and evil forces, which are manifested through spirits.

Most tribes have a shaman or medicine man on whom they rely for spiritual knowledge. The shaman performs special rituals to ensure tribal survival and prosperity. The Native American people worship the land and hold tribal grave sites as sacred.

The Native American Church is the most widespread religious group today among Native Americans. This religion is also known as Peyotism for its use of the hallucinogenic substance, peyote. The beliefs of the religion combine ideas from Christianity and traditional Indian beliefs, such as the belief in one God, known as the Great Spirit, and belief in the Peyote Spirit, which is similar to Jesus. Peyote is eaten to enhance communication with God and to receive spiritual power (Britannica Online, 2005).

An understanding of the general spiritual beliefs of Native Americans will help you care for their spiritual needs. You need to assess each client's personal beliefs to provide care unique to that person. Always maintaining an unbiased attitude to unique spiritual beliefs will allow you to care for all clients.

FACTORS AFFECTING SPIRITUALITY

The spiritual needs of the clients you will care for vary greatly depending on their spiritual beliefs, stage of faith, degree of illness, and adaptation to illness. The predominant spiritual needs of people are a search for meaning, a sense of hope, forgiveness, love, connectedness, and a sense of purpose. Many factors can affect spiritual needs, including life span, physiological, and cultural and lifestyle factors.

FACTORS ACROSS THE LIFE SPAN

Children. Meeting the spiritual needs of children is usually concerned with teaching children and helping them apply religious principles in their daily lives. Children do not have a spiritual crisis in the same sense as adults. The defining characteristics of *Spiritual distress* do not fit children. Children sometimes feel a sense of confusion about God when prayers do not seem to be answered. For example, the child may pray for a parent with cancer to get well, but the parent may die anyway. However, children who are victims of abuse or other difficult family situations and who appear to be hurting at their inner core could be described as being in spiritual distress. You can do much to help meet the spiritual needs of these and all children (Figure 49-3).

Adolescents and Young Adults. Adolescence is a time of questioning the meaning of life and the religious teachings that have been a part of childhood. Some degree of spiritual distress is a normal part of adolescence. The adolescent needs someone who will listen without judging or offering advice while they explore questions of their faith. Spiritual distress is closely related to depression and suicide, both of which have a high incidence in adolescence.

Young adults often separate themselves from family, culture, and religion when they leave home for college or after getting a job. When the young adult is a long way from home, it is easy to stop the religious practices that have been a part of childhood. But when a crisis occurs, they need to be in touch with a source of spiritual strength. Young adulthood is a time of seeking to be in touch with the spiritual self and exploring alternative forms of spiritual guidance such as astrology, alternate religions, and New Age methods.

Middle Adults. The American dream has led many people to pursue financial success, an appealing appearance, and social recognition as the path to a full and satisfying life. However, these extrinsic signs of success are not necessarily associated with happiness. Close interpersonal relationships are more important to personal satisfaction and sense of success. Adults during their middle age years often reevaluate their life priorities and develop other aspects of their life. During midlife, success-driven adults may shift their emphasis to friends and family.

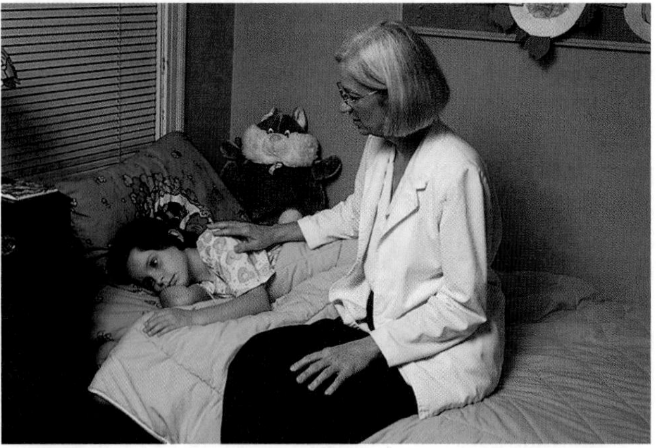

FIGURE 49-3 Nurses can have an important role in meeting the spiritual needs of children who are sick or suffering from spiritual distress.

Spirituality becomes more important as middle-age adults discover discontent with their lives. The uneasiness or dissatisfaction with life can be a significant impetus for exploring spiritual beliefs. For many middle-age adults, this time in life is for connecting with the values and beliefs from their childhood. For others the transition of middle age is a time for expanding and refining spiritual ideas. The opportunity to explore spirituality can provide adults with a foundation for healthier living as old age approaches.

Older Adults. Religion and spirituality become increasingly more important as a person ages. In fact, religion is the key to life satisfaction for many older adults. A sense of the encompassing love of God is basic to the emotional security and spiritual foundation for older adults at the end of life.

Older adults have an enhanced reasoning ability to transcend the immediate and derive meaning from conflict. They are more than problem solvers; they are problem transformers. Older adults are often more concerned with the Why of a situation than with the What or the How. There is transcendence of preoccupation with the physical self and increased awareness of the spiritual self. As an individual grows older, there is less emotional investment in externals and more attention to the inner self and perception and organization of life and its events.

It is important for older adults to be respected as spiritual beings because of their spiritual perception of themselves. Older adults become concerned about the meaning of their past. The way an older adult remembers the past, lives in the present, and anticipates the future often reflects spiritual views. Older adults need the following:

- Sense of worth despite physical decline
- Sense of trust in self and trust in God or a supreme being
- Sense of forgiveness toward self and others
- Affirmation of the meaning of the life they have lived

Table 49-3 Characteristics of Spiritual Well-Being in the Older Adult: Relationships and Time

CHARACTERISTIC	ELEMENTS
RELATIONSHIPS	
An ultimate other	• Believes in a supreme being • Trusts in God • Communicates with God through prayer • Participates in religious practices
The nature of others	• Accepts or tolerates differences with others • Expresses mutual love and concern • Expresses mutual forgiveness • Accepts and gives help • Appreciates nature
Self	• Accepts self and situations in life • Values inner self • Values self-determination • Has a positive attitude • Expresses life satisfaction
TIME	
Past	• Recognizes parental and other influences • Expresses sociocultural ties with past situations and outcomes • Describes ties with a formal belief system • Describes past religious practices and rituals • Expresses growth and change over time
Present	• Lives up to potential • Expresses congruency between values and practice • Open to growth and change • Participates in communal prayers or rituals • Finds meaning and purpose in life
Future	• Sets goals • Hopes in ultimate integration • Hopes in afterlife • Searches for meaning and purpose in life

- Transcendence of losses to enable the person to live more fully in the present
- Love and care for the self as well as others

Table 49-3 lists characteristics of spiritual well-being in the older adult. In older adults, feelings such as happiness, usefulness, and life satisfaction are positively correlated with religious participation and other forms of spirituality. Furthermore, spirituality is the predominant coping strategy used by older adults to enhance well-being. Spiritual or religious beliefs help to transcend the negative stereotypes of aging and maintain or gain a sense of meaning and autonomy in society. However, spiritual expression tends to change in later life. Participation in organized religious practices diminishes and more personal forms of spiritual expression increase.

PHYSIOLOGICAL FACTORS

Many illnesses are perceived as a threat to a sense of well-being, which can initiate a spiritual conflict. Diseases that are life threatening or chronic are especially capable of stimulating such a crisis. For example, when a person is initially diagnosed with cancer, doubts and fears may arise about the future. The meaning and purpose of the disease may also be questioned.

Pain can present a challenge to spiritual beliefs. The presence of extensive or uncontrollable pain has long been understood to initiate spiritual as well as mental pain. For example, a client who experiences an automobile accident with serious physical injury may call into question beliefs in a God who caused such discomfort. Pain can also prevent a client's usual involvement in religious activities.

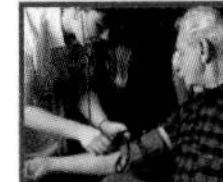

When Mr. Guevara returns home from the hospital after his surgery, you are assigned to conduct an admission assessment. What types of questions will you ask to assess Mr. Guevara's spirituality? Do you expect his diagnosis of prostate cancer will affect his sense of spiritual well-being? Are Mr. Guevara's religious practices important in his recovery from surgery?

CULTURAL AND LIFESTYLE FACTORS

Culture and Religion. The broader culture and subculture to which a client belongs can influence spiritual needs and preferences (Box 49-1). The beliefs and religious practices of the cultural group will determine what type of spirituality is most appropriate. As pointed out in the overview of world religions, all religious beliefs and practices are bound to the culture and guide the group's lifestyle.

The philosophical views of the culture toward God or a supreme being, sin, salvation, forgiveness, health, and the future affect how clients respond to changes in their health. For example, a client from India, raised as a dedicated Hindu, would express a fatalistic belief in the future and a lack of control over future events. A Jewish client from America might appear more optimistic about the future because the client believes he or she can cry out for God's mercy.

The leadership pattern of the culture may affect clients' spiritual needs as well. People tend to follow the advice of their leaders. You need to be aware of the potential influence of leadership patterns when assessing your clients' spiritual needs.

Psychosocial Factors. Various psychological and social factors can influence spiritual needs. Socially, a support system and social roles can influence spiritual responses to illness. Psychologically, a personality type, outlook on life, coping style, and meaning ascribed to life affect spirituality. Keep in mind that clients may adhere to many different ways of thinking about personalities and how they relate to health.

A client's general outlook on life stems from his or her personality. Both of these psychological factors influence the client's coping ability in times of distress or illness. Coping styles that might interfere with effective

BOX 49-1 *Cross-Cultural Care*

Caring for a Mexican American Client

Jesse Guevara, the client whose story we've been following throughout the chapter, is of Mexican descent. His family immigrated to Arizona in the early 1900s and settled near Tucson. Although each person is unique, Mexican Americans have a tendency to value the following:

- Traditional values of family roles, including men heading the family and women taking care of the family
- Working hard, even under difficult situations, to support the family
- Providing direct help to family and extended family members
- Following the rules
- Stoicism; not complaining about discomfort
- Putting the needs of other family members before their own
- Denying the severity of health-related issues

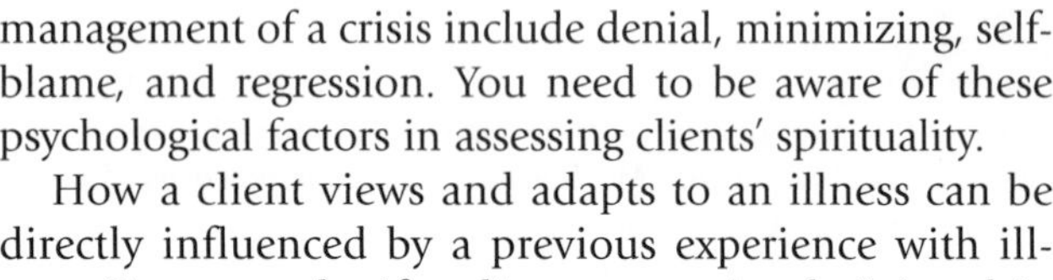

management of a crisis include denial, minimizing, self-blame, and regression. You need to be aware of these psychological factors in assessing clients' spirituality.

How a client views and adapts to an illness can be directly influenced by a previous experience with illness. For example, if a client was seriously injured in an automobile accident and experienced spiritual growth during that time, the thought of a critical illness might not pose such a threat to the client's sense of spiritual well-being.

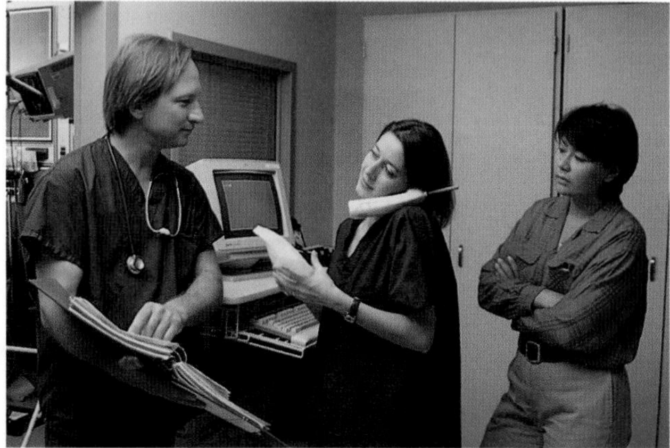

FIGURE 49-4 Nurses are sometimes so busy with the hectic pace of health care that they do not take the time to care for the spiritual needs of clients.

ASSESSMENT

Because nursing focuses on the whole person, you are responsible for supporting the client's spirit as a tool for healing. Clients who feel hopeless are more likely to die, even when there is insufficient disease to justify the death. Those who are joyful are more likely to live even in the face of overwhelming illness. We begin the nursing process portion of this chapter with assessment of spiritual needs.

GENERAL ASSESSMENT OF SPIRITUALITY

Information about the client's spiritual condition is obtained from observation of behaviors and interactions with the client. Major factors that interfere with the spiritual assessment are time constraints and severity of illness. Nurses are frequently too busy with the hectic pace of health care to conduct a thorough assessment of spiritual needs (Figure 49-4).

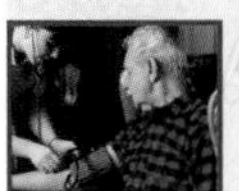

During your assessment of Mr. Guevara, you discover that he used to attend a nondenominational Christian church but stopped 12 years ago when he got a divorce. He and his present wife do not practice "all that church stuff." He says his wife is an agnostic. What can you ask Mr. Guevara to find out more about his spiritual beliefs? Do you think Mrs. Guevara's disbelief has influenced Mr. Guevara's spiritual beliefs or practices?

Health History. The health history in most settings asks if the client has a religious preference. To gain more than this limited amount of information, you need to ask additional questions about spiritual beliefs and practices.

Specific objective data can be sought; ask openly about current religious practices and whether the client would like to visit the chapel or have a cleric, rabbi, or other religious leader visit. Sometimes, just asking, "How can I help you?" is sufficient. These are acceptable, nonthreatening questions. You can also ask about the appropriate care for any religious item to prevent its loss and yet have it readily available for the client.

You can encourage clients to express their thoughts and feelings. You can listen to the stories they tell to identify the role of spirituality in their life and health. Box 49-2 offers an example of one client's story. You can determine how clients perceive their lives and relationships with self, others, and God.

In summary, then, you must use cues to formulate open-ended, nonjudgmental questions and statements that facilitate the development of a trusting nurse-client relationship in which spiritual needs, such as those of purpose, love, belonging, and self-worth, can be examined and appropriate interventions planned.

BOX 49-2 *A Patient's Perspective*

"I Walk by Faith, Not Just by What I See"

In 1956, people had begun to think of polio as history. I was 4 years old and had been given two out of three doses of the Salk vaccine, so no one thought I could have polio. But they were wrong. I don't remember much about the early months in the hospital, but my parents said it was touch-and-go for a while. I do remember the rehabilitation, however. My mother had me doing intensive exercises with sandbags, mostly to strengthen my right leg.

Those exercises paid off. I recovered full use of my legs and was able to play sports, so we thought it was just a "mild" case. I was an active, happy kid, successful in school, went to college, married right after graduation, and went East with my wife to enter seminary.

During a general examination in late 1994, the doctor said my blood pressure was too high and told me to lose weight, so I started working out. That's when the unexplained falling started. When I fell and broke my finger the following spring, I thought I had slipped on the steps but then realized that my legs felt weak, especially the right leg. The doctor did some manual strength tests and referred me to a neurologist. More tests followed. By July 1995 the diagnosis of post-polio syndrome came as no surprise. The strength was (and is) deteriorating in both legs, but it's more acute in the left leg because of all those years favoring the right leg.

Unlike many people with postpolio syndrome, I'm not in pain. But the weakness in my legs and the crushing fatigue (the most common symptom) have imposed limits I feel I'm too young to accept at age 46. My running days are over, so tennis is gone. I have trouble going down steps or even a slope because my quadriceps muscles are shot. Last winter, I decided it was time to wear a brace on my right knee. Now that summer is here and I sometimes wear shorts, I've begun to experience what it means to be visibly imperfect. People treat you differently. They don't know what to do or say. I realize how easily we categorize someone as handicapped—not quite a person—how wrong it is to define a person in terms of an affliction, and how important it is to recognize there's lots more to a person than meets the eye.

The fatigue is more than physical. It's also brain fatigue that renders you incapable of doing anything. It has affected the quality and quantity of my work. And I have a terrible time sleeping (also a common problem), so I'm working with a sleep disorder clinic. To conserve my flagging energy, I'm talking with the other two pastors in the church about reducing my workload.

One of the biggest challenges of this condition is the uncertainty, the unpredictability of the problem. No one knows whether the deterioration will continue, perhaps to paralysis, or whether it will abate at some point. The progression is different in every person affected. Thinking too far ahead discourages me, so I just try to focus on today. My wife and family give me enormous support and a fair amount of laughter. My parents offer tremendous encouragement.

I feel blessed that I can get around, that I'm not crippled. This is just one thing in my life. It's real—and the most pressing thing I have to face—but it's just one thing. I'm laboring not to let this condition define me. This affliction has caused me to stop and think about what I'm doing with my life—what's most important. I'm starting to get a clearer picture. But meanwhile, I walk by faith, not just by what I see. That's the heart of Christian life.

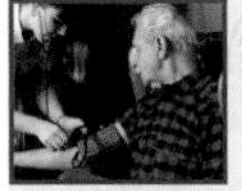

After talking more with Mr. Guevara, you learn that he has begun to pray after learning about his cancer. He also tells you that he has been thinking about going to church when he can drive again. What can you say to encourage Mr. Guevara in pursuing the fulfillment of his spiritual needs? Would you offer to provide him spiritual care?

Assessment Tools. Caring for spiritual needs is central to holistic nursing care and to healing. The spiritual nature of a person cannot be directly observed or measured. Yet, in the company of someone profoundly depressed, the void created by lack of spiritual connections has an infectious, damping effect on your own spirit. Likewise, the high-spirited, ebullient individual who bubbles over with life and enthusiasm is easily recognized. If you are to give holistic care to your clients, you must know how to assess their spiritual needs.

Thoroughly assessing spiritual needs is difficult because spiritual dimension is abstract and elusive. Because of the pluralism of ideologies, philosophies, and creeds, discrepancies may occur between your beliefs and those of the client. Your own beliefs may interfere with identifying subtle cues to the client's spiritual needs. The confusion between religion and spirituality can also complicate the assessment.

The most widely known assessment tool in nursing consists of a series of questions addressing personal beliefs (Stoll, 1979). The tool is a challenging instrument requiring extensive time and thought to complete. It provides you with significant information about the client's spirituality, enabling you to plan spiritual nursing care. Box 49-3 gives guidelines for spiritual assessment.

To appraise a client's spiritual needs, ask questions such as the following:

- Is God important to you right now? Has God been important in the past?
- Are your religious practices meaningful for you now? In the past?
- Have you found your prayers to be helpful now? In the past?
- Has your current illness affected your spiritual experiences?

The format of these questions provides you with an efficient and effective means for assessing the clients' current spiritual needs in comparison to their previous

BOX 49-3 *Guidelines for Spiritual Assessment*

To Determine Client's Beliefs, Values, and Concept of God or Divine Being
- Is religion or God significant to you? If yes, can you describe how?
- Is prayer helpful to you? What happens when you pray?
- Does a God or deity function in your personal life? If yes, can you describe how?
- How would you describe your God or what you worship?

To Determine Client's Sources of Hope and Strength
- Who is the most important person to you?
- To whom do you turn when you need help? Are they available?
- In what ways do they help?
- What is your source of strength and hope?
- What helps you the most when you feel afraid or need special hope?

To Determine Client's Religious Practices
- Do you feel your faith (or your religion) is helpful to you? If yes, would you tell me how?
- Are there any religious practices that are important to you?
- Has being sick made any difference in your practice of praying?
- Has being sick made any difference in your religious practices?
- What religious books or symbols are helpful to you?

To Determine Client's Perception of Relationship Between Spiritual Beliefs and Health
- What has bothered you most about being sick (or what is happening to you)?
- What do you think caused this to happen to you?
- Has being sick (or what has happened to you) made any difference in your feelings about God or the practice of your faith?
- Is there anything that is especially frightening or meaningful to you?

Data from Stoll, R. I. (1979). Guidelines for spiritual assessment. *American Journal of Nursing, 79*(9), 1574-1577.

spiritual experiences. In this way you are prepared to address specific needs.

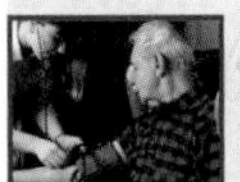

As you finish providing wound care, Mr. Guevara begins to tell you his concerns about dying from cancer. What can you say in response to his fears of dying? How will your own spiritual beliefs about life and death affect your care of Mr. Guevara? What are the defining characteristics Mr. Guevara is exhibiting? What nursing diagnosis do you think is most appropriate?

FOCUSED ASSESSMENT FOR *SPIRITUAL DISTRESS*

Spiritual distress is an impaired ability to experience and integrate meaning in life through connections. The client expresses this distress both verbally and behaviorally. Sometimes it is a direct expression of loss of faith, anger at God, or questioning the meaning of life and death. *Spiritual distress* includes the spiritual needs for forgiveness, love, hope, trust, and meaning and purpose in life. Often the subject arises when the client cannot sleep, is crying, or has other obvious signs of distress. Misdirected anger or hostility may occur secondary to spiritual distress.

Factors related to *Spiritual distress* include the following:
- Challenged belief and value system (e.g., due to moral or ethical implications of therapy or to intense suffering)
- Separation from religious or cultural ties

Clients who are experiencing a crisis are susceptible to spiritual distress. Some treatment factors can cause spiritual distress. Depending on the client's religious faith, abortion, blood transfusions, amputation, or even being socially isolated can create spiritual conflict.

Risk for spiritual distress can be precipitated by loneliness, fear of the unknown, guilt or expressions of regret, anger toward God or a supreme being, loss of hope, and a change in relationships, values, and beliefs. Any client verbalizing such feelings is at high risk for spiritual distress. Risk factors for spiritual distress also include anxiety, blocks to self-love, inability to forgive, stress, substance abuse, and disasters.

FOCUSED ASSESSMENT FOR *READINESS FOR ENHANCED SPIRITUAL WELL-BEING*

By its nature, this nursing diagnosis has defining characteristics but no risk factors. These include the following:
- Inner strengths, such as self-consciousness, awareness, transcendence, or a unifying or sacred force
- Unfolding mystery, which is a person's experience about the purpose, meaning, uncertainty, and mystery of life
- Connections with self, others, the environment, and God or a supreme being

FOCUSED ASSESSMENT FOR *IMPAIRED RELIGIOSITY*

Impaired religiosity is an alteration in the ability to exercise reliance on religious beliefs and rituals. The client may be having difficulty with maintaining all required religious practices or rituals, dietary regulations, or observations. Other characteristics of impaired religiosity include emotional distress because of separation from religious community or concerns about religious beliefs and practices.

Physical illness, ineffective coping, personal crisis, anxiety, or fear can be factors related to the development of *Impaired religiosity*. Other related factors include barriers to participation in religious practices, spiritual crises or suffering, life transitions, impaired social integration or life-threatening conditions.

Risk for development of *Impaired religiosity* can be related to similar client concerns, especially hospitalization, ineffective coping with illness or personal crises, depression, and social isolation from religious community.

FOCUSED ASSESSMENT FOR *READINESS FOR ENHANCED RELIGIOSITY*

This nursing diagnosis has defining characteristics but no risk factors. The characteristics of *Readiness for enhanced religiosity* include the following:

- Acknowledges need for participation in religious ceremonies, rituals, or services
- Asks for clergy, rabbi, or religious leader
- Expresses need for forgiveness or reconciliation with others

DIAGNOSIS

Spiritual needs can be confused with psychological or social needs, thus leading to the wrong diagnosis and plan of care. By focusing on the defining characteristics, you can determine which diagnosis is most appropriate for the client's needs. For the spiritual nursing diagnoses, the major issues are the client's relationship to God or a supreme being, beliefs and values, and search for meaning and purpose in life.

RELATED NURSING DIAGNOSES

Spiritual distress or impaired religiosity may not be the most obvious presenting need. However, many nursing diagnoses can have an element of spiritual distress. You need to differentiate *Spiritual distress* or *Impaired religiosity* from related nursing diagnoses, such as *Ineffective coping, Hopelessness,* and *Complicated grieving.*

- *Ineffective coping:* A nursing diagnosis frequently confused with spiritual needs is *Ineffective coping,* which is the impairment of adaptive behaviors and problem-solving abilities in meeting life's demands and roles (see Chapter 47). The defining characteristics of *Ineffective coping* are that the client is not dealing with life events appropriately. If the client exhibits increased anxiety, unhappiness, pessimism, nonperformance of activities of daily living, or drug abuse, then the client's primary diagnosis should be *Ineffective coping.*
- *Hopelessness:* Occasionally you must decide whether the diagnosis of *Hopelessness* or that of *Spiritual distress* or *Impaired religiosity* is more appropriate for a client's needs. Hopelessness is a state in which the person sees limited or no alternatives or personal choices available and is unable to mobilize energy. The characteristics are behavioral and include passivity, slow response, decreased affect, and despondency. Spiritual distress, with a loss of belief in God or a supreme being, may be a related factor for feelings of hopelessness. By conducting a thorough assessment of the spiritual domain, you can distinguish between *Spiritual distress, Impaired religiosity,* and *Hopelessness.*
- *Complicated grieving:* To differentiate between *Complicated grieving, Impaired religiosity,* and *Spiritual distress,* you need to conduct a complete assessment of the psychological and spiritual dimensions. Complicated grieving is a process of maladaptive and excessive emotional responses after experiencing a significant loss. It can lead to spiritual distress with questions revolving around the meaning of life and death. The defining characteristics of *Complicated grieving* are different from those of *Impaired religiosity* or *Spiritual distress.* These behaviors include alterations in lifestyle, such as eating, sleeping, activity, physical symptoms of fear and anxiety, and distorted emotional reactions, such as anger, denial, and low self-esteem.

In finalizing a diagnosis, keep in mind that you may tend to feel comfortable with cues that support your diagnosis and overlook or deny those that do not. Self-knowledge is crucial when trying to understand a client and cluster data to arrive at appropriate diagnoses (Table 49-4). Therefore be aware of and open to your own spiritual biases and beliefs. In addition to *promoting* positive spirituality, you must *possess* positive spirituality.

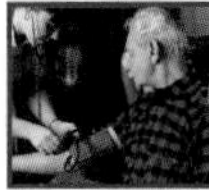

During your next visit, you talk with Mr. Guevara about the nursing diagnoses *Spiritual distress* and *Impaired religiosity* and your tentative plans for spiritual care. Mr. Guevara is very pleased you will be helping him with his spiritual needs, but Mrs. Guevara expresses her disagreement with the plans. What will you say to the couple, because their needs are quite different?

PLANNING

You need to plan your nursing care of clients who have spiritual distress or impaired religiosity by establishing expected outcomes in conjunction with the client. Given the complex nature of the spiritual domain, a specific target date for achieving expected outcomes might be unrealistic.

The overall expected outcome for the client with *Spiritual distress* is that the client will develop an inner spiritual peace and a sense of spiritual well-being. Additional outcomes are based on individual needs. An expected outcome for a client who expresses questions about the meaning of life or suffering would be that the client will experience a greater sense of meaning, purpose, and hope in living with an illness. For a client expressing inner conflict about beliefs, an outcome would be that the client will have a clearer understanding of personal beliefs and values. When clients talk about a conflict in their relationship with

Table 49-4 Clustering Data to Make a Nursing Diagnosis

Spiritual Problems

DATA CLUSTER	DIAGNOSIS
A young African American woman who recently lost her infant expresses disbelief in God, confusion about her former beliefs, and guilt about the child's death.	*Spiritual distress* related to loss of child, sense of guilt, and conflict about beliefs
A Native American man is talking about suicide after losing his wife and son in an automobile accident. He has been treated for bipolar disease for 10 years, has resumed drinking since their deaths, and is angry with God for taking them.	*Ineffective coping* related to loss of loved one, psychiatric disorder, and drinking problem
An older adult immigrant from Vietnam is diagnosed with ovarian cancer that has metastasized. She understands her condition and expresses a readiness for death.	*Readiness for enhanced spiritual well-being* related to terminal cancer
A recently retired man suffers a massive stroke with complete left hemiparesis. He talks about his lack of spiritual beliefs, sense of things being unreal, feelings of anger, and denial about lost health.	*Complicated grieving* related to multiple losses, including employment, career, health, and physical independence
A 13-year-old girl is being evaluated for sexual abuse by her stepfather. She talks about her anger at God, recent nightmares, and meaning of her life.	*Spiritual distress* related to sexual abuse and confusion with meaning in life
A Philippine woman had a ruptured ectopic pregnancy. She expresses concern that not receiving communion while hospitalized and being allowed nothing by mouth (NPO) will keep her from healing	*Impaired religiosity* related to surgical procedure, hospitalization, loss of baby, and inability to receive communion
An adolescent boy survives a motorcycle accident with only a fractured right leg. He expresses interest in knowing more about God.	*Readiness for enhanced religiosity* related to accident and new appreciation of life

God or anger at God for their poor health, then an appropriate outcome would be that they will develop meaningful relations with God or a supreme being, themselves, and others.

There are four goals for you in helping a client confront spiritual distress. First, you may help the client create, maintain, or renew relationships. As people review their lives, they may experience guilt as they consider unfulfilled expectations for themselves or acts of omission or commission toward themselves or others. To relieve this spiritual pain, there must be a sense of forgiveness. Persons of all belief systems should be assisted in resolving human differences and renewing relationships whenever these are recognized as sources of spiritual pain. Second, everyone has a need for love expressed through relationships and seen in words and acts of kindness. This positive regard or love must be unconditional even for those who are unpleasant or apparently unresponsive to the family's efforts or to yours.

Third, you can help clients search for meaning. However helpful you wish to be, though, in the final analysis they themselves must create personal meaning. You can engage in supportive actions, such as being with and listening to a client, even when the final outcome is submission to suffering and death. Last, there is always the need for hope, which suggests the possibility of future good. Hope can simply be for freedom from pain or for the ability to perform certain tasks. Even a dying person can hope for a reunion with deceased loved ones, union with God, or at least a superior alternative to the current painful situation. Those who do not believe in an afterlife may believe in the transfer of physical energy, being remembered by others, or leaving a legacy to their children or community. You can help the client see hope in each remaining moment and the chance to make a positive difference while such moments continue.

Outcomes for *Readiness for enhanced spiritual well-being* might be that the client experiences a heightened sense of connectedness. The connectedness may be with self, others, God or a supreme being, or the environment.

The overall expected outcome for the client with *Impaired religiosity* is that the client will strength his or her reliance on religious beliefs and practices. Additional outcomes are based on individual needs. An expected outcome for a client who expresses emotional distress because of separation from the religious group would be that the client will experience connection with his or her religious community through visits and telephone calls while in the hospital. For a client demonstrating difficulty adhering to religious rituals or conflict with customs and healthy lifestyle, an outcome statement would be the client will demonstrates balance between religious practices and a healthy lifestyle. When a client questions his or her religious beliefs or customs, then an appropriate outcome would be that the client will express satisfaction with his or her religious beliefs and practices.

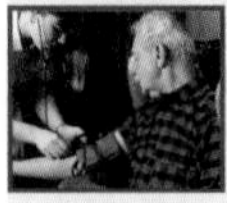

You provide spiritual care for Mr. Guevara on each subsequent home visit. What spiritual interventions are most appropriate for Mr. Guevara? What spiritual interventions are available for Mrs. Guevara?

INTERVENTION

INTERVENTIONS TO RELIEVE *SPIRITUAL DISTRESS*

Thinking about meaning should not be perceived as a problem. *Spiritual distress* can be an opportunity for growth and change. Spiritual distress is not a pathological condition but is part of experiencing the meaning and fullness of life. Recognizing that all persons face crises at times throughout life allows you to care for clients who are struggling to both understand and shape the meaning of life. Even a beginning nurse can implement initial interventions.

Communicating Effectively. Communicating effectively about spiritual needs requires sensitivity, concern, empathy, a willingness to listen, and a nonjudgmental attitude. It also requires communication that is direct, specific, and clear. For example, if a client asks if he is going to die, you can refocus the question onto the client's fear of dying. On the other hand, simply listening to the client can be healing. A client experiencing spiritual distress does not require answers but needs someone who will listen and hear with empathy. Listening with nonjudgmental regard is the single most therapeutic action you can take.

If listening to clients debating the meaning of life makes you anxious, you will need to examine your own beliefs so that you are more comfortable with them and capable of listening without feeling anxious or defensive. It is important to acknowledge the client's true feelings, even when they are negative. Any person with an illness may suddenly be faced with doubts and fears about being dependent on others or dying. Common responses include grief over loss, unbearable anxiety, and anger at God. Dwelling on such feelings may cause considerable spiritual distress. You can help a great deal by just acknowledging how terrible such feelings and fears can be. Be sure to stress that grappling with strong feelings, such as anger, fear, or despair, is normal when facing severe illness or hospitalization. Finally, continue to comfort the client with your physical presence, which demonstrates your availability and caring.

Active Listening. Using yourself therapeutically by active listening requires connection with each client. Active listening includes many caring behaviors, such as taking time, touching, hearing what is said, being present and available, giving "good" nursing care and extra attention, and being understanding and accepting. Perhaps most important is that clients perceive these caring behaviors even in the midst of routine nursing activities.

It is very easy to avoid having to use yourself therapeutically. You can do this by giving pain or sleep medication, making it clear that you are too busy to talk, ignoring nonverbal cues, or refusing to hear the true message of what a client is saying. Even prayer can be misused if rote recitations are used to respond to hard questions or as a means of closing the discussion rather than dealing with feelings or issues.

It is also easy for your own feelings to interfere with your ability to listen. Feelings of isolation, fear, guilt, anger, grief, or being overwhelmed may require you to temporarily leave the situation until you can address your personal feelings. You cannot expect to always be able to listen to deep emotions. Time out is acceptable so that you will be able to continue giving quality care at a later time.

Lack of spiritual care is often attributed to time constraints. However, spiritual care typically is not time consuming, nor does it require extensive knowledge of different religions and philosophies. Brief comments about a supreme being's care, an encouraging word or touch, and visits of 5 to 10 minutes are all forms of spiritual care and active listening. Spiritual care is viewed by clients as a reciprocal relationship.

Being Present With the Client. Presencing with clients on their journey can be a valuable method of support, both for them and for you. You can view just being with clients as presencing. Thus you can have a vital role even when you are unable to alter what is happening to the client physically.

Presencing is an important aspect of the caregiver's role. Being with the client requires you to enter into the reality of suffering to develop a sense of communion with the sufferer. You offer quiet sharing of your presence and help the person bear the burden of suffering. Presencing involves both your presence and comfort of the client.

Promoting a Spiritual Environment. Minor alterations in the hospital environment can bring the client tremendous spiritual comfort. Encourage family or friends to bring in inspirational art, such as paintings or prints. For example, paintings or photographs depicting a spiritual leader can be a source of comfort. Personal religious objects such as prayer beads, statues, and incense also may relieve spiritual distress, as do many sacred texts such as the Bible, the Qur'an, a book of prayers, or sacred poetry. Music can be used therapeutically. In addition to suggesting religious television or radio programs, encourage family and friends to bring the client CDs or tapes of chants, hymns, or other inspirational music.

The internal environment may also be manipulated. For example, you can teach the client to use meditation, relaxation, and guided imagery. Meditation is an act of surrender, of letting go of usual preoccupations. Besides having positive psychological and physiological effects, it is a means by which the client can sense and experience directly or know intuitively what the conscious mind may deny or avoid. Many hospitals have relaxation or guided-imagery audiotapes or videotapes, with images such as a flickering fire or waves on a beach.

Helping the Client Maintain Relationships. Illness commonly causes isolation. The loss of ongoing contact with family, friends, and worshipers at church or other spiritual centers is often acutely felt. Being cut off from others is a form of suffering. Clients who identify themselves in relation to their faith community may be particularly vulnerable to a sense of spiritual isolation. You can help relieve the client's spiritual distress by recommending that family members contact the client's spiritual community and arrange for visits, phone calls, or gifts of cards or flowers as appropriate.

Helping the Client Explore Meaning. While giving routine care, you can also help clients explore their thoughts about the meaning of illness, suffering, or life. Simple questions can help the client focus on meaning, as can the therapeutic techniques of reminiscence, visualization, life-review processes, and contemplation of literature.

Both you and the client may recognize the importance of illness in growth. Through pain, the person is alerted to be quiet, to allow the process to ferment, and to be inspired by the quiet. In aloneness, the person discovers the need for the presence and touch of another. Because most humans are ambivalent and somewhat unsure about the meaning of life, the client may need a supportive listener to encourage exploration of the meaning of this experience. It is often not the experience itself but its meaning that is important. Your reflective listening can allow your clients to explore their beliefs and feelings.

An intervention you can use to help clients find meaning is the use of *reminiscence.* Through reminiscence, clients can examine their life experiences to discover new meanings or reconnect to forgotten moments that represent significant meaning. Finding meaning through reminiscence helps clients maintain ego integrity.

Another method for exploring meaning is to encourage clients to engage in a *life review.* The immediate result can be an autobiography to be given to family members or stories of childhood events to be given to children or grandchildren, but the most important outcome is the clients' increased understanding of their own lives. Such an understanding may help them accept current circumstances, regardless of the expected long-term outcome.

You can also help clients explore meaning through literature, including myth, metaphor, biographies, poetry, and song lyrics. When clients come to the end of one stage in life and the beginning of a new one, as occurs with traumatic injury or debilitating illness, they may experience tremendous anxiety, pain, and turmoil. Myths deal with the thresholds of such passages and function to bring the person into harmony with destiny. You can offer to read such literature aloud or to leave books at the bedside for the client to read.

Stories that use subtle metaphors allow a truth to be shared without the glare of reality. Using metaphor in the search for truth, meaning, and significance allows clients to confront issues of self-identity gently and helps them to see the universality of their suffering. Biographies are less subtle but equally revealing and inspiring. Some clients find poetry and songs a source of understanding when they reveal the insights of others whose sufferings were similar to their own.

Transcending the present situation and perceiving higher meaning and purpose may require that you share personal past situations of suffering and ways that you have discovered meaning and purpose. Examining meaning and purpose in life through inward reflection is advocated for you to be able to help clients articulate their inward struggles.

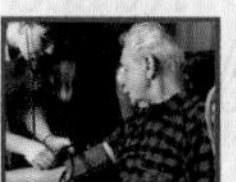

After 6 weeks, Mr. Guevara's suprapubic wound has healed, and he will be discharged from home health care. He tells you that he will need radiation therapy for the treatment of metastatic cancer. He appears quite distressed about the change in his condition and voices doubts about God's care of him. What plans can you make for Mr. Guevara's spiritual needs after his discharge from your care?

INTERVENTIONS TO ENHANCE SPIRITUAL WELL-BEING

Encouraging Hope. Hope is the means by which a person maintains integrity while in the midst of illness and disease. Hope assists a client in coping with health problems and has been found predictive of favorable outcomes.

Bays (2001) studied hope in older adults who had had a stroke. Bays found that the patterns of hope included positive and active participation, forward-moving process, inner strength, faith in God, comparisons with others, and realistic possibilities of the future. Factors associated with having hope were the person's connections with family and their awareness of their spiritual dimension.

Especially when the clients are older adults, you may have to help them confront the possibility of death and yet have hope. One approach is to encourage them to be aware of nature's cycle. Suggest that they take the time to watch the changes in the sky, the rising and setting of the sun, the falling of leaves, and the beginning of new growth. Watching the daily and seasonal changes can help put into perspective the cycle of life and death, dying and rebirth, year after year. Humankind is part of the cycle of life and death, too.

You can teach clients *reality surveillance.* By reconstructing past events and reasoning about them, the client searches for clues that hope is feasible. They may need help in devising and revising goals, such as small steps in physical progress or defining tasks to be done or relationships that need renewal. Small goals can be set to help make each day more positive. For example, humanity's unlimited potential for *becoming* provides a continuous reason to hope. Thus clients can hope to be the best person possible today. Or they can look forward to a specific event, such as a wedding or family reunion. If there is reason to believe they may not be able physically to participate in the event, clients can personally dictate an audiotape or write a letter to those who will be present to express love and good wishes. You can encourage expression using symbolic imagery in art, music, poetry, or stories.

Hope refers to the belief that whatever the outcome of a specific illness, everything will be all right. Such hope can be fostered when you share stories about people who have overcome great difficulties or personal events of overcoming troubles. Self-disclosure can help clients feel that they know the caregiver much better. Consequently, clients can feel that they can transcend the present situation to a hoped-for better future.

Many books are available that may give hope and joy to clients, even those who are dying. Such books are often very uplifting and optimistic because they demonstrate continued growth and development, love, and enjoyment of life until the end. Regardless of the specific illness or disease, there are probably books written by people suffering the same problem, which helps confirm that the client is not alone in suffering. Such books may also give hints as to coping mechanisms that proved helpful to others.

Helping the Client Interpret Crises as Spiritual Growth. Physical illness can be a crisis that forces clients to seek meaning in the chaos they are feeling. It may prompt clients to try to resolve interpersonal problems, their relationship with God, or feelings of failure from not having achieved certain life goals. Your first duty in such situations is to help clients achieve clarity about the problem.

Smucker (1996) described three stages of spirituality from her study of people experiencing some type of crisis. The first stage is "breaking the web of life." It happens when an event occurs unexpectedly. Feelings during this stage range from anxiety to fearfulness. Clients may express concern as they try to make sense of the circumstances. With the passage of time and with personal effort, the second stage begins.

Smucker calls the second stage "rebuilding the web of life." During this stage of spiritual crisis, people focus on the return of stability to their life. They became aware of the changes that have occurred in their life and choose to find meaning in these events. Many people feel their faith deepen and become more real during this time.

The third stage is known as "wondering." In this stage, people describe awe at the mysteries of life as they realize that they have not found answers. Rather than being frustrated at the limits of human knowing, however, they conclude that the ways of God are unfathomable. Believing in a higher being helps them to live even without rational answers.

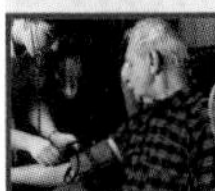

Mr. Guevara has undergone 4 weeks of radiation therapy to his pelvis. It causes diarrhea and skin breakdown near his anus. You are reinstated to provide wound care and pain management. How does spiritual distress and suffering affect the management of pain? Why would you want to differentiate between spiritual, emotional, and physical pain and suffering?

Helping the Client Deal With Suffering. You can help clients interpret the causes of suffering and determine what the appropriate responses might be. Pain is a physical response to injury and is easy to alleviate by comfort measures and medical treatment, such as drugs or surgery. It is much harder to reduce suffering, which is the client's personal interpretation of the pain.

To effectively intervene with a suffering client, you need to understand the meaning of suffering. Different religions emphasize different meanings for suffering, but it is most commonly perceived as punishment, mystery, or redemption. Punishment is often the first thought. Many clients ask, "What did I do to deserve this?" Most of us realize that some lifestyle behaviors can lead directly to illness, and many people believe that strong faith can lead to healing. Therefore clients may blame themselves for their bad habits or not having sufficient faith to achieve healing. Assess for self-blame from the client or the client's family, and reassure them that they are not responsible.

Some religions place suffering in the realm of mystery. According to these traditions, the meaning of illness is not really understandable. The question is not "Why me?" but "Why not me?" Other ancient traditions suggest that suffering is instructive, that a person will learn by suffering, and that suffering will bring about a reordering of personal values that leads to redemption. Many recent theorists propose that some illnesses may be chosen by the soul for an important spiritual purpose, such as to advance the sufferer's spiritual development.

You can help your clients identify and explore their own interpretation of suffering. By being present with clients you can allow them to verbalize their concerns about the meaning of their suffering. Listening and clarifying the interpretations of suffering can help clients deal with it. Also, you can encourage clients to find some positive aspects to their suffering. As they discuss it with you and their family and friends, clients will feel some release from the extreme burden of the suffering.

INTERVENTIONS TO RELIEVE *IMPAIRED RELIGIOSITY*

Encouraging the Client's Participation in Religious Practices. There are varying levels of commitment to religion. Some people follow the rituals of their religion very closely; others accept the beliefs but feel that certain rituals are outdated. A discussion of religious practices with the client will help you provide appropriate care.

Rituals and religious practices can sustain the client. Rituals bring a sense of unity, providing identification with the past and hope for the future. Healing rituals are a part of the practice of most forms of religion. Many clerics are willing to have a healing service in the hospital, either at the bedside or in the chapel, with both client and family present. You may help the client engage in a ritual or celebrate a holy day by contacting the spiritual advisor, discussing the ritual with other members of the health care team, and planning the day's activities around the planned ritual.

Other religious interventions may be planned according to the client's religious preference. Many books are available that give the implications of typical nursing interventions for persons of various faiths. For example, in relation to cleanliness, Jewish men wash their hands before daily prayers and before and after meals. To support the practice, you may offer to supply a warm, wet washcloth before and after prayers and meals.

Providing Access to Spiritual Leaders. It is your responsibility to make sure that clients receive care by being supportive and helpful, but you do not always have to personally give care. If you feel unable to be supportive, call another nurse who is more comfortable with spiritual issues, or ask the clients if they would like to speak with a member of the pastoral care staff or another spiritual advisor (Figure 49-5).

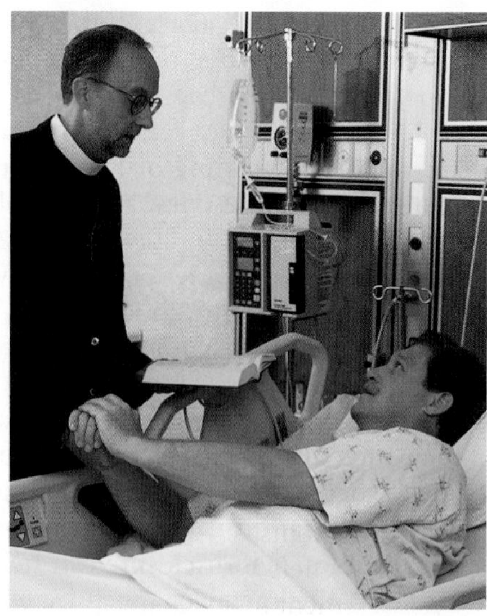

FIGURE 49-5 If you feel unable to meet the spiritual needs of clients, you can ask the client if he would like to speak with a member of the pastoral care staff or another spiritual advisor.

When illness requires clients to engage in behaviors that they usually avoid, it is often helpful to have a spiritual leader discuss the spiritual restrictions in relation to therapeutic requirements. For example, clients can be excused from a spiritual fast if food is needed for healing. Having a spiritual leader describe the exemption with clients after you explain the purpose of the therapy is often helpful.

Even for those who do not consider themselves religious, when a clergy member or chaplain appears, the client's imagination and memories of their spiritual tradition and heritage may be triggered and a therapeutic interaction may result. In many hospitals in the United States, a visit by a Christian minister is routine. Be aware that such a visit may not be welcomed by clients of a different faith. Ask such clients if they would like you to contact their own spiritual advisor. In any case, it is always acceptable to simply ask if a visit with a cleric would be helpful or if the client would like to visit the hospital chapel.

The chapel itself can be very helpful. Quiet time alone in a pew can sometimes help a client pray with a better sense that God is listening. Religious symbols are often therapeutic. Clients imaging God, a supreme being, or just love surrounding them will often feel better even when nothing else can be done. The feeling of being alone is reduced in such a setting.

Any request by a client for a spiritual counselor should be honored. Especially in emergency cases, clergy must be called. Most religious leaders know how to support the client without interfering in medical interventions, even in such acute care settings as the operating room or emergency department.

Religious leaders of most faiths wear specific clothing and are often addressed by a specific title to indicate their religious position. To demonstrate your respect and support for the client's faith, determine the proper title for religious leaders of that faith and call the leader by that title.

INTERVENTIONS TO ENHANCE *RELIGIOSITY*

Assist Clients With the Observance of Religious Practices. Many clients use placing one's faith and trust in God and obtaining strength from God as effective coping strategies for dealing with health crises. Another helpful religious practice is the use of prayer. Prayer has been called the raising of the mind and heart to God. For many clients, it is a source of strength as well as a cry for understanding, for the power to endure, and for the wisdom to grow. Praying for help and healing is an action accepted in almost all cultures, although the objectives of such prayers may differ.

You can offer to say a prayer personally, to be present while the client prays, or to request that a minister, priest, or rabbi be present to share in the prayer. Many clients have favorite texts from sacred writings that they recite as a prayer when words otherwise fail. When clients are very ill or weak, or have impaired vision, you may offer to read their favorite prayers aloud for them.

Identify Clients at Risk for Excessive Dependence on Religious Beliefs. As a nurse providing spiritual care to your clients you need to be aware of religious beliefs that have the potential of being harmful for ill clients. For instance, Jehovah's Witnesses refuse to have blood products, and Christian Scientists frequently oppose the use of medications for healing. In addition, there are religious beliefs that cause psychological harm. An example of this type of religious belief is the idea that disease is a result of sin and must be accepted as God's punishment and seeking medical care shows lack of faith or rebellion (Taylor, 2002).

After identifying clients at risk for excessive dependence on religious beliefs you need to conduct a thorough spiritual assessment to determine how their beliefs will guide their behaviors. You can ask clients what they think God will gain from watching them suffer or how this belief compares to the image of a loving God. It might be necessary for you to contact their spiritual leader to consult on the meaning and application of the potentially harmful religious belief.

When you are working with a client with religious beliefs different from your own, remember to always consider your own personal biases. It may be possible that you are having the spiritual crisis concerning the opposing religious beliefs instead of your client.

EVALUATION

To evaluate the plan of care, determine if the outcomes have been achieved (Box 49-4). Spiritual health, a sense of spiritual well-being, and enhanced religiosity constitute processes that span an entire lifetime. It is appropriate for you to evaluate the expected outcomes for evidence of individual improvement.

A sample documentation note for Mr. Guevara might look like the one below.

Sample Documentation Note for Mr. Guevara

Client openly discusses a sense of meaning in life with cancer. Able and willing to discuss previous and potential religious beliefs and spiritual experiences. Reports that he is beginning to accept life with cancer and reports great satisfaction from his prayers. Verbalizes that he is pleased the pastor came to visit and plans to start attending church services when he is able to drive.

When clients have been successful in confronting spiritual distress, you can expect them to continue in their relationship with their God and engage in spiritual practices not detrimental to their health. Rather than expressing negative feelings of fear, guilt, or anxiety, they will express feelings of peace and wholeness. Last, clients may verbalize hope, trust, and satisfaction with their spiritual condition; life will have meaning and purpose.

If your interventions are successful, clients will show signs of improving spiritual health and well-being. Spiritual well-being requires a relationship with self, others, the environment, and God or a supreme being. The person looks simultaneously to the past, lives in the present, and hopes for the future. Characteristics of spiritual well-being include the following:

- Sense of inner peace
- Compassion for others
- Reverence for life
- Gratitude
- Appreciation of both unity and diversity
- Humor
- Wisdom
- Generosity
- Ability to transcend the self
- Capacity for unconditional love

BOX 49-4 *Nursing Care Plan*

A Client With Spiritual Distress

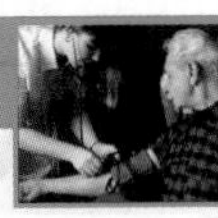

Initial Data

Mr. Guevara is a 56-year-old master electrician who has just returned home from the hospital after a radical prostatectomy for invasive carcinoma 4 days ago. His suprapubic wound has a 3-cm opening that requires daily wound care.

Nursing Assessment

As the nurse, you make plans to assist Mr. Guevara in managing his wound care and supporting his recovery from surgery. You discover that Mr. Guevara has spiritual needs in addition to the obvious physical and psychological needs. During your assessment you also find out that he used to attend a nondenominational Christian church but stopped 12 years ago when he got a divorce. He and his present wife do not practice "all that church stuff." He says his wife is an agnostic. After talking more with Mr. Guevara, he tells you he has begun to pray again since learning about his cancer. Mr. Guevara also tells you he has been thinking about going to church when he can drive again. As you finish providing wound care, Mr. Guevara begins to tell you about his concerns about dying from the cancer.

Continued

BOX 49-4

Nursing Care Plan—cont'd

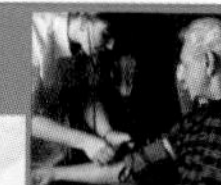

A Client With Spiritual Distress—cont'd

NANDA-I Nursing Diagnosis	NOC Expected Outcomes With Indicators	NIC Interventions With Selected Activities	Evaluation Data
Spiritual Distress **Related Factors:**	***Spiritual Well-Being***	***Spiritual Growth Facilitation***	***After 2 Weeks***
• Conflict about spiritual beliefs	• Client will experience a greater sense of meaning in living with cancer.	• Listen to client's concerns and feelings. Provide time to be with client.	• Client discusses his sense of meaning of living with cancer.
• Concern about relationship with God	• Client will have a sense of belonging.	• Encourage client to contact church of interest to have home visit with clergy. Encourage visits from spiritual counselor.	• Client calls a nearby church, and minister comes to visit him.
• Diagnosis of prostate cancer	• Client will have a clearer understanding of personal beliefs.	• Allow client to verbalize previous beliefs and spiritual experience.	• Client talks about previous and potential spiritual beliefs and experiences.
	• Client will establish meaningful relationship with himself, God, and others.	• Provide opportunity for client to explore new spiritual beliefs.	
		• Encourage client to take responsibility for own life.	• Client begins to accept life with cancer.
		• Encourage client to pray.	• Client reports great satisfaction from his prayers.
		• Encourage client to contact spiritual family members and friends during recovery.	• Client contacts former friend with strong spiritual beliefs.

Critical Thinking Questions

1. Do you expect Mr. Guevara's diagnosis of prostate cancer will affect his sense of spiritual well-being?
2. Do you think Mrs. Guevara's disbelief has influenced Mr. Guevara's spiritual beliefs and practices?
3. What can you say to encourage Mr. Guevara in pursuing the fulfillment of his spiritual needs?
4. How will your own spiritual beliefs about life and death affect your care of Mr. Guevara?

Nursing outcome and intervention labels from Ackley, B. J., & Ladwig, G. B. (2006). *Nursing diagnosis handbook: A guide to planning care* (7th ed.). St. Louis, MO: Mosby.

Clients have reported that being ill made them receptive to spiritual care. Health care providers who spend brief moments with clients and give spiritual care are remembered months and years later as a spiritual caregiver. The clients described these caregivers as full of love, accepting, and spiritually focused. Clients said that spiritual care was important to their coping with their illness and to their recovery. Some felt it brought them through the experience.

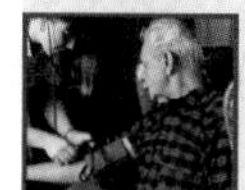

Mrs. Guevara calls to tell you Mr. Guevara has been admitted to the hospital for management of his pain. She expresses her fear of his dying. How can you provide emotional support while being sensitive to Mrs. Guevara's spiritual beliefs? Will this cause you any distress?

▼ KEY PRINCIPLES

- Spirituality is the experiences and expressions of one's spirit in a unique and dynamic process reflecting faith in God or a supreme being; connectedness with oneself, others, nature, or God; and integration of the dimensions of mind, body, and spirit.
- Religion is a belief system, including rituals and traditions. It is also a social institution in which people participate to search for meaning in life.
- Faith is belief in or commitment to something or someone; it helps a person realize purpose and meaning in life.
- Spiritual health enables and motivates us to search for meaning and purpose in life, to seek the supernatural or some meaning that transcends us.

- Spiritual well-being represents the totality of a person's inner resources, the wholeness of spirit and unifying dimension, a process of transcendence, and the perception of life as having meaning.
- Nursing care of a client's spiritual needs should always be based on respect for the person and his or her personal beliefs.
- Barriers to spiritual nursing care include lack of preparation, objective empathy, lack of time, confusion of spiritual needs with psychosocial needs, materialism, empiricism, and lack of personal spiritual beliefs.
- The major religions of North America include Christianity, Judaism, Islam, Buddhism, Hinduism, and Native American.
- Life span, physiological, and cultural and lifestyle factors affect individual spiritual needs.
- On the basis of a thorough assessment, you can plan spiritual care for clients with the nursing diagnoses *Spiritual distress, Risk for spiritual distress, Readiness for enhanced spiritual well-being, Impaired religiosity, Risk for impaired religiosity,* and *Readiness for enhanced religiosity.*
- *Spiritual distress* is an impaired ability to experience and integrate meaning and purpose in life through connectedness with self, others, art, music, literature, nature, or a power greater than oneself.
- *Impaired religiosity* is an impaired ability to exercise reliance on beliefs and/or participate in rituals of a particular faith tradition.
- Interventions to relieve spiritual distress include communicating effectively, active listening, being present with the client, promoting a spiritual environment, helping the client maintain relationships, and helping the client explore meaning.
- Interventions to enhance spiritual well-being are encouraging hope, helping the client interpret crisis as spiritual growth, and helping the client deal with suffering.
- Interventions to relieve impaired religiosity include encouraging the client's participation in religious practices and providing access to spiritual leaders.
- Interventions to enhance religiosity are assisting the client in the observance of religious practices and identifying clients at risk for excessive dependence on religious beliefs.
- Evaluation of the nursing process is based on an appraisal of the expected outcomes specified for and with the client.

REVIEW QUESTIONS

1. The nurse finds a hospitalized 48-year-old woman newly diagnosed with colon cancer crying quietly in her room. The nurse learns by talking with the client that the client is actually quite angry and "cannot understand why God would let this happen." Which of the following nursing diagnoses would be most appropriate for the nurse to use in planning care?

1. *Ineffective coping*
2. *Impaired religiosity*
3. *Spiritual distress*
4. *Readiness for enhanced spiritual well-being*

2. A client asks a family member to bring in a Bible and prayer beads from home. The nurse interprets this request as an expression of which of the following?

1. Faith
2. Religiosity
3. Spirituality
4. Prayer

3. The nurse is assigned to the care of a male client involved in an automobile accident that resulted in leg amputation and subsequent phantom pain. The nurse would formulate which of the following as the most appropriate goal for the nursing diagnosis of *Spiritual distress* after hearing the client question how he can have a meaningful life with this pain and disability?

1. Reports becoming resigned to the fact that pain and suffering will someday have meaning in his life
2. Develops a meaningful relationship with God, himself, and other significant people in his life
3. Expresses a greater sense of meaning, purpose and hope in living with a chronic health problem
4. States a clearer understanding of his personal beliefs and values

4. A client with spiritual distress who will soon undergo a kidney transplant says to the nurse, "I'm afraid that I will die after this operation. Even if I don't, I'll probably just be a bigger burden than when I was on dialysis." Which of the following is the best response by the nurse?

1. "Hopefully your past belief in God will carry you through this. Do you think you can regain your faith?"
2. "The success rate for this surgery is high, and the burden on your family will probably be reduced because you won't need dialysis anymore."
3. "Your family does not think of you as a burden, and I do not know of anyone who has died after kidney transplant."
4. "It must be very difficult to have such feelings, even though they are very common for people who undergo major surgery."

5. The nurse is using reminiscence as a therapeutic intervention when working with a client who has spiritual distress. Which strategy is this nurse using?

1. Being present with the client
2. Helping the client explore meaning
3. Promoting a spiritual environment
4. Helping the client maintain relationships

Bibliography

Ackley, B. J., & Ladwig, G. B. (2006). *Nursing diagnosis handbook: A guide to planning care* (7th ed.). St. Louis, MO: Mosby.

Bays, C. (2001). Older adults' description of hope after a stroke. *Rehabilitation Nursing, 26*(1), 18-20, 23-27.

Britannica Online. (2006). *Britannica encyclopedia.* Chicago: Britannica.

Dalmida, S. (2006). Spirituality, mental health, physical health, and health-related quality of life among women with HIV/AIDS: Integrating spirituality into mental health care. *Issues in Mental Health Nursing, 27*(2), 185-198.

*Eliade, M., & Couliano, I. (2000). *The HarperCollins concise guide to world religions.* San Francisco: HarperCollins.

*Ellison, C., & Paloutzion, R. (1983). Spiritual well-being: Conceptualization measurement. *Journal of Psychology and Theology, 11*(4), 330-340.

*Fowler, J., & Keen, S. (1985). *Life maps: Conversations on the journey of faith.* Waco, TX: Word Books.

Gaskamp C, Sutter R, Meraviglia M, Adams S, Titler MG. (2006). Evidence-based guideline: Promoting spirituality in the older adult. *Journal of Gerontological Nursing, 32*(11), 8-13.

Gaskamp, C., Sutter, R., & Meraviglia, M. (2004). *Promoting spirituality in older adults, evidence-based protocol* Gerontological Nursing Interventions Research Center, The University of Iowa, College of Nursing.

Hermann, C. (2006). Development and testing of the spiritual needs inventory for patients near the end of life. *Oncology Nursing Forum, 33*(4), 737-744.

*Hungelmann, J., Kenkel-Rossi, E., Klassen, L., & Stollenwerk, R. (1985). Spiritual well-being in older adults: Harmonious interconnectedness. *Journal of Religion and Health, 24*(2), 147-153.

*Meraviglia, M. (1998). Critical analysis of spirituality and its empirical indicators: Prayer and meaning in life. *Journal of Holistic Nursing, 17*(1), 18-33.

Meraviglia, M. (2004). Spirituality in people with lung cancer. *Oncology Nursing Forum, 31*(1), 89-94.

Meraviglia, M. (2006). Effects of spirituality in breast cancer survivors. *Oncology Nursing Forum, 33*(1), E1-7.

NANDA International. (2007). *Nursing diagnoses: Definitions and classification, 2006-2007* (7th ed.). Philadelphia: Author.

*Newman, M. A. (1986). *Health as expanding consciousness.* St. Louis, MO: Mosby.

*Pargament, K. I. (1997). *The psychology of religion and coping: Theory, research, practice.* New York: Guilford Press.

*Paterson, J. G., & Zderad, L. T. (1988). *Humanistic nursing.* New York: National League for Nursing.

*Roy, C. (1988). An explication of the philosophical assumptions of the Roy adaptation model. *Nursing Science Quarterly, 1*(1), 26-34.

Skala, K., & McCoy, P. (2006). Spiritual assessment of patients with cancer: The moral authority, vocational, aesthetic, social, and transcendent model. *Oncology Nursing Forum, 33*(4), 745-751.

Smucker, C. (1996). A phenomenological description of the experience of spiritual distress. *Nursing Diagnosis, 72*(2), 81-89.

*Stoll, R. I. (1979). Guidelines for spiritual assessment. *American Journal of Nursing, 79*(9), 1574-1577.

Tanyi, R. (2006). Spirituality and family nursing: Spiritual assessment and interventions for families. *Journal of Advanced Nursing, 53*(3), 287-294.

*Taylor, E. J. (2002). *Spiritual care: Nursing theory, research, and practice.* Upper Saddle River, NJ: Prentice Hall.

Taylor, E. J. (2006). Prevalence and associated factors of spiritual needs among patients with cancer and family caregivers. *Oncology Nursing Forum, 33*(4), 729-735.

*Travelbee, J. (1971). *Interpersonal aspects of nursing* (2nd ed.). Philadelphia: Davis.

*Vance, D. L. (2001). Nurses' attitudes towards spirituality and patient care. *Medsurg Nursing, 10*(5), 264-278.

*Watson, J. (1985). *Human science and human care* (p. 46). Norwalk, CT: Appleton-Century-Crofts.

Chapter 50

THE SURGICAL CLIENT

Media Resources

- evolve Evolve Website http://evolve.elsevier.com/Harkreader/
- 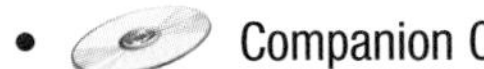 Companion CD

Learning Objectives

After studying this chapter, you should be able to do the following:

- Describe the surgical experience using the perioperative phases as a framework
- Identify factors that may affect the surgical outcome of a perioperative client
- Conduct a preoperative nursing history and physical assessment to identify client strengths and factors that increase risks for perioperative complications
- Describe the nursing role in the psychological and educational preparation of the surgical client
- Differentiate between general, regional, and local anesthesia
- Discuss the role of the perioperative nurse when managing the intraoperative care of the surgical client
- Identify priority intraoperative nursing diagnoses
- Design an intraoperative nursing care plan
- List factors that may affect a postoperative client in the immediate recovery period
- Explain the nursing management of potential complications the client faces postoperatively

Key Terms

ambulatory surgery
anesthesia
anesthesiologist
certified registered nurse anesthetist (CRNA)
circulating nurse
general anesthesia
intraoperative phase
local anesthesia
malignant hyperthermia (MH)
perioperative
perioperative nursing
postanesthesia care unit (PACU)
postoperative phase
preoperative phase
regional anesthesia
registered nurse first assistant (RNFA)
scrub nurse

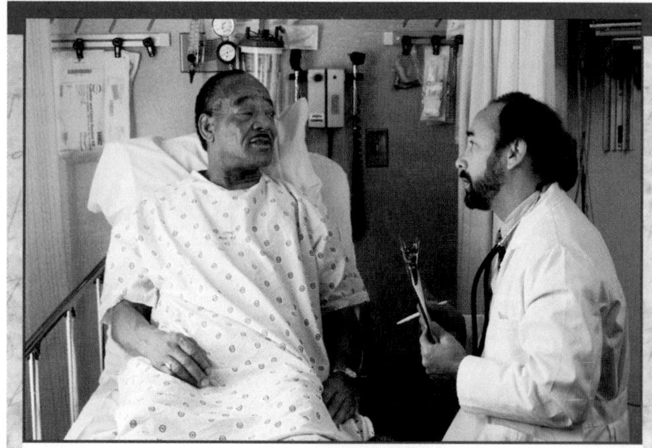

Berris Warren, an alert, oriented, 61-year-old Afro-Caribbean man, has prostate cancer. His cancer was diagnosed by his primary physician in Jamaica 1 month ago, after repeated episodes of inability to urinate. He admitted having urinary difficulty for about 9 months. His daughter, a pediatric nurse practitioner, assisted him in getting a second opinion from a urologist in Atlanta, Georgia, where she and her family live. The cancer was confirmed, and Mr. Warren was scheduled for a prostatectomy in 2 weeks. His surgical experience has begun.

CONCEPTS OF THE SURGICAL EXPERIENCE

Surgery is an invasive medical procedure performed on all parts of the human body to diagnose or treat illnesses, correct deformities and defects, repair injuries, and cure certain diseases. Clients who require surgery enter the health care setting in a wide variety of situations—for example, clients awaiting planned surgery may feel relatively healthy, whereas those facing emergency surgery for a traumatic injury may be in much distress. Surgical clients may be any age and at any point on the health-illness continuum.

Nurses assume important and active roles in caring for the client before, during, and after surgery. The combination of collaborative and independent nursing care prevents complications and promotes optimal outcomes for the surgical client. The nursing process is used during each phase of the client's surgical experience to promote the recovery of health, prevent further injury or illness, and facilitate coping.

SETTINGS

In the past, the client was admitted to the hospital the day before a scheduled surgery for completion of preoperative assessments and laboratory testing. Surgery was usually performed in a hospital operating room (OR) and involved several days of recovery in the hospital. For some procedures, this is still the case. However, because of cost containment measures and technological advances, many surgical clients are admitted on the day of surgery or are not admitted to a hospital at all. Increasingly, surgical procedures are being performed in emergency departments, doctor's offices, free-standing surgery clinics, mobile surgical units, and outpatient surgical units in hospitals. **Ambulatory surgery** is same-day or outpatient surgery that can be performed with general or local anesthesia, usually takes less than 2 hours, and requires less than a 3-hour stay in a recovery area.

Ambulatory surgery has steadily increased over the last decade. Smaller, less invasive incisions, reduced cost, and decreased length of stay in the health care system are some of the reasons clients and physicians alike prefer ambulatory surgery. In some cases, ambulatory surgery has been mandated by third-party payers—private insurance companies, government insurers (Medicare and Medicaid), and health management organizations.

CLASSIFICATION OF SURGICAL PROCEDURES

Surgical procedures are classified according to the client's admission status, urgency, degree of risk, and purpose (Table 50-1). Classifications for a given procedure may overlap. An elective procedure may be ambulatory and diagnostic, or the same procedure may be performed for different reasons on a hospitalized client.

Surgical procedures may also combine several classifications (such as a client who has sustained multiple traumatic injuries in an automobile accident and may require major, reconstructive, and emergency surgery). It is important to remember that regardless of the defined degree of risk, any surgical procedure imposes physical and psychological stress and seldom is considered minor by the client. The classification system indicates the type of nursing care a client might require.

Perioperative Phases. All clients progress through the surgical experience in three phases. The word **perioperative** (with the Greek prefix *peri,* meaning "around") is used to describe the preoperative, intraoperative, and postoperative phases of the surgical experience. **Perioperative nursing** is a specialized area of practice that provides continuity of nursing care for the surgical client throughout the surgical process. Historically, the term *operating room nursing* was used to describe the surgical care of clients. However, with the advent of technology, multiple surgical settings, and managed care, the surgical care of the client is no longer based just in the operating room.

In some facilities, the same perioperative nurse assesses a client's health status preoperatively, identifies specific client needs, teaches and counsels, attends to the client's needs intraoperatively in the OR, and then follows the client's recovery postoperatively. In other institutions, different nurses care for the surgical client during each

Table 50-1 Classification of Surgical Procedures

TYPE	DESCRIPTION	EXAMPLES
ADMISSION STATUS		
Ambulatory (outpatient)	Client enters setting, has surgical procedure, and is discharged on the same day	• Breast biopsy • Cataract extraction • Hemorrhoidectomy • Scar revision
Same-day admit	Client enters hospital and undergoes surgery on the same day and remains for convalescence	• Carotid endarterectomy • Cholecystectomy • Mastectomy • Vaginal hysterectomy
Inpatient	Client is admitted to hospital, undergoes surgery, and remains in hospital for convalescence	• Amputation • Heart transplant • Laryngectomy • Resection of aortic aneurysm
URGENCY		
Elective	Delay of surgery has no ill effects; surgery is performed on basis of client's preference	• Breast reconstruction • Hernia repair • Joint bunionectomy • Tonsillectomy
Urgent	Necessary for client's health and may prevent further damage; usually done within 24-48 hours	• Amputation • Colon resection for obstruction • Coronary artery bypass
Emergency	Performed as soon as possible to save client's life or to preserve a body part or organ	• Control of hemorrhage • Repair perforated ulcer • Tracheostomy
DEGREE OF RISK		
Major (elective, urgent, or emergent)	To improve or maintain health, to restore function, or to preserve life; includes opening the abdomen, thorax, or cranium	• Exploratory laparotomy • Nephrectomy • Traumatic injury repair
Minor (usually elective)	Restores function or corrects deformities, such as lesions	• Arthroscopy • Cataract extraction • Dilatation and curettage • Removal of warts • Tooth extraction
PURPOSE		
Diagnostic	Surgical exploration to assist in making a diagnosis (may involve biopsy)	• Breast biopsy • Bronchoscopy • Exploratory laparotomy • Skin biopsy
Ablative	Removal or excision of diseased body part or organ	• Amputation • Appendectomy • Colon resection • Thyroidectomy
Palliative	Reduces intensity of disease or illness symptoms but is not intended to be curative	• Arthroscopy • Colostomy • Debulking of malignant tumor • Nerve root resection
Constructive	Restores function in congenital anomalies	• Cleft palate repair • Closure of atrial-septal heart defect
Reconstructive	Restores function or appearance to traumatized tissue	• Breast reconstruction • Internal fixation of fracture • Scar revision • Skin graft
Transplant	Replaces malfunctioning organs	• Cornea • Heart • Joints • Kidney

phase of the surgical experience. Provision of safe, consistent, and effective nursing care during each phase of surgery is a major responsibility.

Preoperative Phase. The **preoperative phase** begins when the decision for surgical intervention is made. The range of nursing activities includes, but is not limited to, preoperative assessment of the client's physical, psychological, and social states; the assessment of preoperative and postoperative educational needs; the planning of nursing care and education that is required to prepare the client for surgery; and the implementation and evaluation of nursing interventions. This phase ends when the client is safely transported into the OR for the surgical procedure.

Intraoperative Phase. The **intraoperative phase** begins with the client's entry into the OR and ends when the client is transferred to the recovery room or to another area such as the intensive care unit, where attention is given in the immediate postoperative period. During this phase, focus is on the continuing assessment and diagnosis of the client's physiological and psychological responses and the implementation and evaluation of interventions to promote safety and privacy, as well as prevent wound infection and promote healing.

Safe and effective intraoperative care requires a team effort (Figure 50-1). Each member of the surgical team brings unique skills that must be coordinated to achieve desired client outcomes. Team members are categorized as sterile or nonsterile in relation to the sterile surgical field.

Sterile team members are those who scrub their hands and arms, don sterile attire, use sterile instruments and supplies, and work in the sterile surgical field. Members of the sterile surgical team include the surgeon; physician's assistants and registered nurse first assistants; and the scrub person, who may be a registered nurse, a licensed vocational or practical nurse, or a surgical technician.

The **registered nurse first assistant (RNFA)** is an expanded nursing role, requiring additional education, in which the perioperative nurse works as a first assistant during the surgical procedure. The RNFA is a perioperative role that is gaining legislative acceptance as a way to serve the public's health care needs in a cost-effective manner. The RNFA replaces an assisting surgeon and therefore is more cost effective when viewed by insurance reimbursement guidelines. The RNFA may perform the following functions during the surgical procedure: handling tissue and organs with instruments, providing exposure of surgical site, suturing tissue, and providing hemostasis. These functions are independent of the scrub nurse role, because the RNFA does not concurrently function as the scrub person. The RNFA may also be involved in preoperative and postoperative care of the client.

The **scrub nurse** is a nurse whose special qualifications include knowledge of aseptic technique, instruments and equipment, anatomy and physiology, surgical procedures, and, most importantly, promotion of client safety. This knowledge helps the scrub nurse anticipate the needs of the surgical team and thus reduces the duration of anesthesia time for the client. The scrub nurse sets up and maintains the sterile field; hands supplies and instruments to the surgeon and assistants; keeps an accurate count of instruments, sponges, and sharps; monitors aseptic technique; and uses the nursing process to ensure client safety. When the scrub role is performed by someone other than the nurse, that person is in a delegated technical role and under the supervision of a perioperative registered nurse. These technically trained unlicensed assistive personnel are called operating room technicians or surgical technicians.

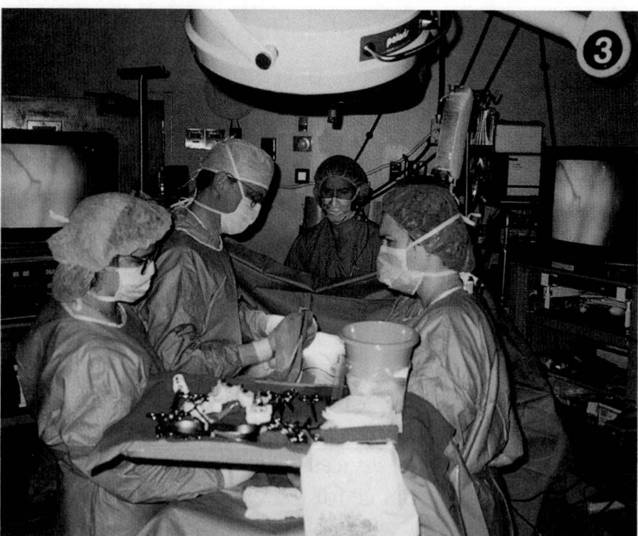

FIGURE 50-1 Safe, effective intraoperative care requires a team effort.

Members of the nonsterile surgical team have responsibilities outside the sterile field and do not wear sterile attire. The nonsterile team members include, but are not limited to, the anesthesiologist, the nurse anesthetist, and the circulating nurse. The **circulating nurse,** or circulator, who must be a registered nurse, helps meet the individual needs of the client during all three phases of the surgical experience. The circulating nurse coordinates the care of the client, is the client's advocate, and manages activities outside the sterile field. The nursing process is the framework used to meet client needs and achieve the desired overall outcomes. The circulating nurse does the following:

- Provides emotional support to the client before induction of anesthesia
- Performs preoperative and ongoing client assessment
- Directs and assists with proper positioning of the client
- Ensures correct sponge, sharps, and instrument counts
- Performs the surgical skin preparation
- Creates and maintains a safe environment

- Implements and enforces policies and procedures to ensure client safety
- Administers medications and solutions to the sterile field
- Manages catheters, tubes, drains, and specimens
- Protects the client's privacy and dignity
- Documents client assessment data and care needs, with outcomes
- Communicates relevant information to other team members and to the client's family

Other members of the nonsterile surgical team are radiology and laboratory technicians, perfusionists, staff development educators, pathologists, nurse's aides, and personnel from materials management, environmental services, and central services. All participate in ensuring a safe surgical experience for the client. However, it is the perioperative nurse who coordinates the contributions of each surgical team member.

Postoperative Phase. The **postoperative phase** can be divided into two segments of care: the immediate and the ongoing postoperative periods. In the immediate postoperative period, there is an evaluative assessment by the perioperative nurse and the client is admitted to the postanesthesia care unit. The **postanesthesia care unit (PACU),** previously known as the recovery room or postanesthesia room, is an area where clients remain until they regain consciousness from the effects of anesthesia. Most clients who have received general anesthesia, major regional anesthesia, or monitored local anesthesia are transferred to a PACU. The perioperative nurse in some cases may actually provide care for the client in the PACU; however, it is more common for the perioperative nurse to give a transfer-of-care report to a postanesthesia nurse. The PACU nurse is skilled in the care of clients immediately after surgery and has in-depth knowledge of anesthetics, pain management, and surgical procedures.

Nursing care in the PACU involves immediate assessment of changes in the physical and psychological status of the client, along with appropriate planning and implementation of care, such as frequent monitoring of airway patency, vital signs, and neurological status; providing intravenous fluids and blood; accurately assessing output from all drains; and providing a thorough transfer report of the client's status to the nurse receiving the client on the unit and to the client's family and friends.

After transfer to the surgical unit or ambulatory recovery area, the client is in the ongoing phase of postoperative care. This period includes all care given during the course of surgical convalescence until the time of discharge, and it continues with assisted care or self-care at home.

Discharge planning, which includes teaching and referral, is also part of the ongoing care throughout the client's surgical experience. The client and family are prepared to assume any care that may be needed after discharge. If needed, community resources are used. A community or home health care nurse is a valuable resource for the client with needs after discharge.

ANESTHESIA

Anesthesia is the partial or complete loss of sensation with or without a loss of consciousness that results from administration of an anesthetic agent. Anesthetics are given by an **anesthesiologist,** a medical physician who specializes in anesthesiology, or by specifically trained physician's assistants. Another anesthesia provider, the **certified registered nurse anesthetist (CRNA)** is an advanced practice registered nurse who has been specifically educated in the administration of anesthetic agents.

The role of the perioperative nurse in anesthesia management begins with the preoperative assessment and ends when the client recovers from the effects of anesthesia. An understanding of the following concepts enhances the perioperative nurse's ability to collaborate with anesthesia providers: anesthesia risk classifications, choice of anesthetic agents, client positioning principles, induction and intubation techniques, levels of general anesthesia, malignant hyperthermia, and client monitoring parameters during local and regional anesthesia procedures. These concepts are discussed further throughout this chapter. As the client's advocate, perioperative nurses also maintain a quiet environment once the client has entered the operating room and provide emotional support to help reduce client anxiety.

The anesthesiologist considers multiple factors when selecting anesthetic techniques and agents. Before surgery, the anesthesiologist evaluates the physical condition and age of the client; the presence of coexisting diseases; the type, site, and duration of the operation; the client's preference; and the surgeon's preference. The American Society of Anesthesiologists (ASA) has developed a classification system to identify risk factors on the basis of the client's health status (Table 50-2). As part of the preoperative evaluation, the anesthesiologist places the client in a class according to physical status. For example, a traumatically injured client with severe head and neck injuries who was evaluated by the neurosurgeon before surgery would be given a classification of P5. This identifies a client who is not expected to survive 24 hours and is an extreme risk for anesthesia.

Preoperative medications may be ordered by the anesthesiologist or surgeon to reduce preoperative anxiety, minimize secretions in the respiratory tract, decrease acidity and production of gastric secretions, relieve pain, and decrease metabolism so that less anesthetic agent is necessary. Medications are selected on the basis of the preoperative assessment findings and the demands of the intended surgical procedure.

Table 50-2 ASA Physical Status Classification System

P1	Normal healthy client
P2	Client with mild systemic disease
P3	Client with severe systemic disease
P4	Client with severe systemic disease that is a constant threat to life
P5	Moribund client who is not expected to survive without the operation
P6	Declared brain-dead client whose organs are being removed for donor purposes

From American Society of Anesthesiologists. Retrieved December 12, 2005, from www.asahq.org/clinical/physicalstatus.html.

Anesthesia is used to produce a loss of sensation with or without the loss of consciousness, and it also provides analgesia, reflex loss, and muscle relaxation during a surgical procedure. Therefore the goal of anesthesia is the elimination of pain and awareness at a level of anesthesia that is safe for the client. One of three types of anesthesia is used during surgical procedures: general, regional, or local.

General Anesthesia. **General anesthesia** is produced by inhalation or by injection of anesthetic drugs into the bloodstream, or a combination of both, and causes the client to lose all sensation and consciousness. The client also experiences amnesia of surgical events. General anesthesia is accomplished in four phases: preinduction, induction, maintenance, and reversal.

The *preinduction phase* begins as soon as the client is brought into the operating room. Monitoring devices are applied to the client, with a brief explanation of each device. Methods for intraoperative monitoring include the following:

- Electrocardiogram (ECG) continuously displayed
- Arterial blood pressure and heart rate determined, evaluated, and documented as baseline data
- Pulse oximetry
- Body temperature readings
- Respirometer and inspiratory pressure readings
- End-tidal CO_2 analysis

The use of additional invasive monitors or special monitoring equipment, if deemed necessary, is based on the cardiovascular and pulmonary status of the client, the surgical procedure, and the chance of significant physiological changes.

The *induction phase* begins with the introduction of anesthetic agents and ends with endotracheal intubation and stabilization of the client. Induction involves putting the client safely to sleep. A patent airway and adequate ventilation must be ensured at all times.

The *maintenance phase* starts when stabilization is accomplished. During this period, the client is positioned for the procedure, the skin is prepared, and the surgery is performed. The anesthesiologist or CRNA maintains the proper depth of anesthesia while constantly monitoring physiological parameters such as vital signs and oxygen and carbon dioxide levels.

The final phase of anesthesia is the *reversal phase*. As the anesthetic agents are withdrawn or the effects are reversed pharmacologically, the client begins to awaken. The endotracheal tube is removed once the client is able to reestablish voluntary breathing of sufficient volume. It is critical to ensure airway patency in this period, because extubation may cause bronchospasm or laryngospasm. Other potential problems during this phase include vomiting with risk for aspiration, slow spontaneous respirations, and uncontrolled reflex movements or shivering.

General anesthesia has both advantages and disadvantages. One advantage is that it can be used for clients of any age and for any surgical procedure, and it leaves the client unaware of the physical trauma. Also, rapid excretion of the anesthetic agent and prompt reversal of its effects are considered advantageous.

Disadvantages of general anesthesia include risks associated with circulatory and respiratory depression. Clients with serious respiratory or circulatory diseases, such as emphysema or congestive heart failure, are at a high risk for complications during and after surgery.

Regional Anesthesia. When general anesthesia is contraindicated or not a desirable choice, regional anesthesia may be used. **Regional anesthesia** is a type of anesthesia in which medication is instilled into or around the nerves to block the transmission of nerve impulses in a particular area or region. Regional anesthesia produces analgesia and reduced reflexes. There are several techniques for regional anesthesia, and the choice depends on the type and length of surgery, the preferences of the anesthesiologist and surgeon, and, if possible, the preference of the client. Regional anesthesia techniques require the skill of an anesthesiologist and may be used for complex procedures.

When receiving regional anesthesia, the client is awake during the procedure but does not perceive pain. Regional anesthesia is often supplemented with sedatives and narcotics for one or more of the following purposes: to decrease anxiety, to decrease awareness of the surroundings, and to provide additional analgesia. A screen is usually used to restrict the client's view of the surgical area and to protect the sterile field. Regional anesthesia may be classified further as follows.

Nerve Block Anesthesia. Nerve block anesthesia involves injection of the anesthetic agent into and around a nerve group or nerve trunk to produce a lack of sensation over a specific body area. Major blocks involve multiple nerves, such as the brachial plexus or an axillary nerve block that would anesthetize the arm.

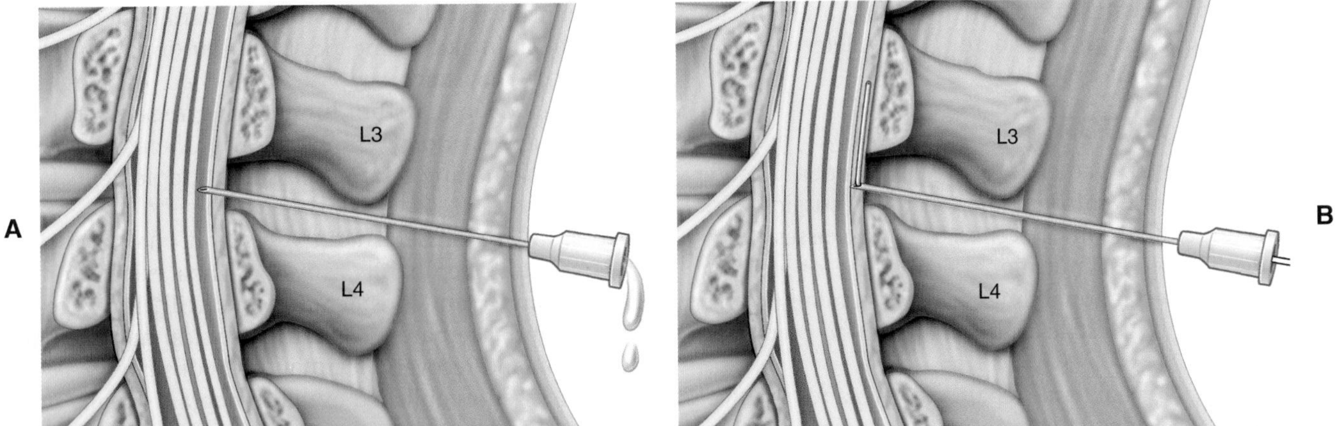

FIGURE 50-2 Placement of needle for spinal anesthesia **(A)** and catheter for epidural anesthesia **(B)**.

Minor blocks involve a single nerve (a facial nerve, for example).

Bier Block Anesthesia. Intravenous block anesthesia, otherwise known as Bier block anesthesia, is used most often for procedures involving the arm, wrist, and hand. An occlusion tourniquet is put on the extremity to prevent absorption of the injected intravenous drug beyond the involved extremity.

Spinal Anesthesia. Spinal anesthesia is also known as a subarachnoid block. Surgeries of the lower abdomen, perineum, and lower extremities are likely candidates for this type of regional anesthesia. It requires a lumbar puncture through one of the interspaces between the second lumbar disk (L2) and the sacrum (S1), such as at the L3-4 interspace (Figure 50-2, *A*). Cerebrospinal fluid (CSF) dripping from the needle cannula confirms correct placement before injection of the anesthetic. With spinal anesthesia, continued leakage of CSF from the needle insertion site may cause decreased CSF pressure and result in postoperative headaches. Bed rest with restrictions on elevating the head of the bed, maintaining hydration, and applying pressure to the puncture site combat this common side effect.

Epidural Anesthesia. Epidural anesthesia occurs when local anesthetic agents are injected into the epidural space, which is located outside the dura mater of the spinal cord. This type of anesthesia is used frequently for surgeries involving the abdomen and lower extremities. Advantages of epidural anesthesia are reduced risk for headaches or hypotensive reactions (Figure 50-2, *B*).

Local Anesthesia. **Local anesthesia** is any agent that induces a temporary loss of feeling as a result of the inhibition of nerve endings in a specific part of the body. Topical application and local (or extravascular) infiltration are the usual routes of local anesthesia techniques.

Topical surface anesthesia is applied to the mucous membranes or skin to block nerve impulses at that site. *Local nerve infiltration* is achieved by the injection of an agent around a local nerve to depress nerve sensation over a limited area of the body. This technique is used during minor surgical procedures such as skin and muscle biopsies, removal of superficial cysts, and suturing of small wounds.

The Association of periOperative Registered Nurses (AORN) *Standards, Recommended Practices, and Guidelines* (2005) for perioperative nurses has documents that are applicable to situations in which the perioperative nurse cares for a client receiving local anesthesia with or without sedation or analgesia in the absence of anesthesia professionals. The perioperative nurse is then responsible for monitoring the client and for the administration of supplemental medications to sedate the client during the procedure.

INFORMED CONSENT

Before surgery, the surgeon is required to ask the client to sign a legal document stating the client's informed consent to have the operative procedure performed. Informed consent implies that the client has agreed to allow something to happen, such as surgery, on the basis of a full disclosure of facts needed to make an intelligent decision. This document serves to legally protect the client, nurse, physician, and health care facility. Chapter 2 discusses informed consent in detail.

> ***Action Alert!*** Notify the surgeon immediately if a client is unsure about the nature of the surgical procedure that is about to be performed. Act as a client advocate, and do not allow the surgery to proceed if the client may not have been informed adequately.

FACTORS AFFECTING SURGICAL OUTCOME

To determine the level of surgical risk, screening the client for factors affecting surgical outcome may help prevent perioperative complications. Lifestyle habits, cultural and religious practices, developmental stage, socioeconomic status, psychological state, and physiological factors are all considered when determining a client's surgical outcome.

LIFESTYLE FACTORS

A nursing history gathered about the client's lifestyle provides valuable information regarding surgical risk and postoperative convalescence. The areas assessed related to lifestyle are nutritional status; use of alcohol, tobacco, and recreational drugs; activities of daily living; and occupation. Lifestyle factors are critical to predicting recovery.

Nutrition. Normal tissue repair and resistance to infection depend on adequate nutrition. Surgery increases the body's need for nutrients. Both malnutrition and obesity increase surgical risk. Nutritional deficiencies of protein and vitamins A, C, and B complex are particularly significant because each of these substances is essential for wound healing. A malnourished client is prone to fluid and electrolyte imbalances, reduced energy stores, improper wound healing, and infection after surgery. Both obese and underweight clients are at risk for intraoperatively acquired pressure ulcers at pressure points because of positioning required for surgery. Elective surgeries may be postponed until the client loses or gains weight and other nutritional deficiencies are corrected. Chapters 24 and 25, respectively, cover the promotion and restoration of nutritional status.

The obese client also has other possible complications to consider. Obese clients usually have reduced ventilatory and cardiac function, and positions required for surgery may limit ventilation further. Inhalation anesthesia is absorbed and stored by adipose tissue and then released postoperatively. Therefore the obese client requires more anesthetic during surgery and recovers more slowly from its effects. Fatty tissue is also more difficult to suture and has less resistance to infection, which may lead to the postoperative complications of delayed wound healing, wound infection, and dehiscence of the wound.

Specifically ask clients about their vitamin, herbal, or supplement intake. Some popular nutritional supplements that may have a detrimental effect on surgical clients include, but are not limited to, garlic, vitamin E, and eicosapentaenoic acid (fish oil). Clients may be asked to stop taking certain herbs and supplements before surgery.

Activity and Exercise. The quantity and quality of clients' rest and sleep habits as well as their exercise program are important considerations in facilitating recovery. Rest and sleep are essential to physical and mental restoration and recovery from the stress of surgery. A client with a well-established exercise program usually has improved body systems function, which decreases the risks of surgery. Information gained during a preoperative nursing history allows individualizing interventions to promote rest, sleep, and exercise.

Substance Abuse. Ask the client about possible drug use, abuse, and addiction. The categories of agents most likely to be abused include tobacco, alcohol, opioids, marijuana, and cocaine. Encourage the client to answer truthfully, and ask the questions in a nonjudgmental, matter-of-fact manner. Most clients, when informed of the potential interactions of these drugs and anesthetic medications, will respond truthfully about their drug use. Clients whose alcohol intake is habitual and in large amounts usually require larger doses of anesthesia and postoperative analgesics for sedation and pain relief. Clients who smoke are at higher risk for respiratory complications after surgery. The potential for postoperative complications is increased for clients who use, abuse, or are addicted to recreational drugs, alcohol, or tobacco.

CULTURAL AND RELIGIOUS FACTORS

Cultural influences also affect the client's responses to and perceptions of a surgical experience (Box 50-1). Chapter 3 goes into depth about the cultural context of nursing practice. Nurses frequently care for clients whose cultural beliefs are different from their own. In educating clients, ignorance of cultural differences can pose serious

BOX 50-1 *Cross-Cultural Care*

Caring for an Afro-Caribbean Client

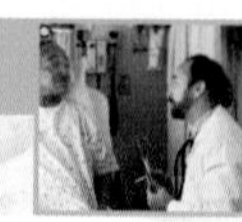

Berris Warren, the client we have been reading about in this chapter, is from Jamaica and of African descent. He was born in a small village outside of Kingston, Jamaica. His family has been on the island since the seventeenth century. They were some of the first slaves brought from Africa by the Spanish. Growing sugar cane and bananas has been a part of his life as long as he can remember. Although each client is unique, many Afro-Caribbeans hold the following values:

- Religion and spirituality
- Music
- Humor
- Extended family (especially in rural communities)
- A collective or communal view of society
- Community responsibility for children
- Playing down achievements to avoid standing out
- Enjoying life and finding immediate gratification
- Respecting others by looking away and covering one's mouth when laughing

problems; if you alienate them, you run the risk of your teaching being ignored. Awareness of cultural background (language spoken, foods eaten, family interactions and participation, personal space, and health beliefs and practices) may be required to effect nursing interventions.

If you know what meaning religion holds for the client, you can identify a possible source of support. Support the client's spiritual needs through acceptance, participation in prayer, or referral to clergy or chaplain. Faith in a higher being provides support and helps to reduce fears.

DEVELOPMENTAL FACTORS

Infants and older adults are greater surgical risks than children and young to middle-age adults. The neonate has a lower total blood volume, which makes a small blood loss a serious situation because of the risk for dehydration. The infant also has difficulty maintaining a stable body temperature during surgery because the shivering reflex is not well developed, making potential hypothermia more likely.

With an increasingly older population undergoing surgical procedures, assessment of physiological changes is critical to providing safe holistic care to older clients. Geriatric clients are at additional risk from surgery because of impaired circulation from limited cardiac function and arteriosclerotic disease. Careful assessment and special attention to risk factors that threaten impending ventilatory, renal, metabolic, infectious, or thromboembolic complications are imperative for the prevention of postoperative complications in this population. Physiological changes related to aging decrease the older client's ability to respond to surgical stressors; they may also alter the response to medications given perioperatively and prolong or alter the healing process (Table 50-3). Energy reserves are usually limited, and hydration and nutritional status may be poor. The most critical aspect affecting perioperative care is the decreased homeostatic capacity in the older adult client.

SOCIOECONOMIC FACTORS

Economic factors influence both the immediate surgical intervention and the follow-up care. Make appropriate referrals to social workers early in the preoperative phase so that discharge planning can be initiated. Most surgical procedures require that the client not return to work right away, and some necessitate a change in the client's occupation. Assess the client's work history to anticipate the effects surgery may have in this area, and individualize teaching plans and referrals.

PHYSIOLOGICAL FACTORS

The client's medical history serves as a framework of care to be provided by the nurse, the anesthesia provider, and the surgeon. Physiological factors that may affect surgical outcome include illnesses, medications, and previous surgery.

Illnesses. Preexisting illnesses can influence the client's ability to tolerate anesthesia and surgery and to reach a full recovery (Table 50-4). A review of the medical history will alert you to past hospitalizations and client outcomes. Pathological changes associated with past and present illnesses increase surgical risk and the

Table 50-3 How Physiological Changes of Aging Increase Surgical Risk

BODY SYSTEM	CHANGES	RISK
Pulmonary	• Reduced range of movement in diaphragm • Lung tissue stiffened • Air spaces enlarged	• Reduced vital capacity • Diminished cough reflex • Decreased oxygenation of blood
Cardiovascular	• Degenerative changes in heart • Rigidity of arterial walls • Reduced innervation of heart • Arterial walls thickened	• Reduced cardiac reserve • Predisposes to hemorrhage and rise in blood pressure • Predisposes to thrombus formation
Renal	• Reduced bladder capacity • Reduced blood flow to kidneys	• Postoperative urine retention due to larger amount of urine that stays in bladder after voiding • Increases danger of shock when blood loss occurs
Neurological	• Decreased reaction time • Sensory losses • Increased pain tolerance	• Confusion following anesthesia • Less able to respond to early warning signs of postoperative complications
Metabolic	• Lower basal metabolic rate • Reduced number of red blood cells • Change in total amounts of potassium and water volume	• Reduces total oxygen consumption • Reduces ability to carry oxygen to tissues • Predisposes to fluid and electrolyte imbalances
Integumentary	• Decreased vascularity and turgor of skin	• Predisposes to pressure ulcers
Gastrointestinal	• Decreased motility of gastrointestinal tract	• Predisposes to constipation • Raises the risk of paralytic ileus

Table 50-4 Medical Conditions That Increase Surgical Risk

MEDICAL CONDITION	ASSOCIATED RISK
Respiratory disorders, such as asthma, bronchitis, and emphysema	• Hypoventilation and spasms of bronchus or larynx • Respiratory depression from general anesthesia • Reduced ability to compensate for acid-base imbalances
Cardiovascular disorders, such as congestive heart failure or recent myocardial infarction	• Increased demands on myocardium (from stress of surgery) to maintain cardiac output • Increased risk of myocardial infarction • Increased risk of hemorrhage, shock, hypotension, thrombophlebitis, stroke, and fluid volume overload
Diabetes mellitus	• Increased susceptibility to infection • Delayed wound healing from altered glucose metabolism and circulatory impairment • Increased risk for fluctuating blood glucose levels, possibly leading to life-threatening hypoglycemia or ketoacidosis
Renal and liver disease	• Altered metabolism and elimination of drugs administered during surgery • Poor tolerance for general anesthesia
Malnutrition	• Increased risk for fluid, electrolyte, and acid-base imbalances • Predisposed to hemorrhage and delayed wound healing • Increased risk of organ failure and shock because client's metabolic reserves may not be sufficient to allow the body to respond to the physical stress of surgery • Poor wound healing and infection from increased metabolic demands of surgery
Obesity	• Delayed wound healing • Infection and wound dehiscence • Pneumonia and atelectasis • Thrombophlebitis • Arrhythmias and heart failure
Alcoholism	• Probable malnourishment and possible delirium tremens (withdrawal symptoms) • Increased risk of infection and physical injury • Possible need for increased dose of general anesthesia • Liver damage may predispose to hemorrhage
Nicotine abuse	• Respiratory complications, such as atelectasis, pneumonia, and bronchitis, from increased secretions and decreased ability to expectorate

potential for postoperative complications. Clients planning for ambulatory surgery should also be assessed for major medical problems that may raise their risk for complications. If the client is at increased risk, surgery as an outpatient may not be possible.

Although the presence of an acute infection usually results in the cancellation of elective surgery, clients with active chronic infections such as acquired immunodeficiency syndrome and tuberculosis may still have surgery. When preparing the client for surgery, remember that standard universal precautions need to be taken with every client.

Medications. Review of the client's current medication regimen is essential. Polypharmacy (the concurrent use of multiple medications) occurs in all age-groups but is more common with older adults. Studies have shown that clients age 65 and over use more medications because these clients often present with multiple disease states, such as diabetes, hypertension, congestive heart failure, and chronic renal failure (Kutchta & Golembiewski, 2004). The use of multiple medications predisposes clients to adverse drug reactions and interactions with other medications in the perioperative setting.

A number of pharmacological categories are used routinely during the client's surgical experience. These include anesthesia agents, antimicrobials, anticoagulants, hemostatic agents, oxytocics, steroids, diagnostic imaging dyes, diuretics, central nervous system agents, and emergency protocol medications. Large numbers of medications increase the chance of interactions.

It is also common for clients to use herbal remedies as alternative or complementary medicines. Ask clients about their use of herbal remedies, either as dietary supplements (discussed previously under Nutrition) or as medicines (MacKichan & Ruthman, 2004). Unless specifically asked, some clients may not consider their natural remedies as medicines. Even though herbs are natural products, they act like medications and may interact or potentiate other medications or interfere with surgical procedures (Table 50-5).

Some medications may be canceled when a client goes to surgery. However, it is important to know the purposes and actions of drugs, because specific medications may be given to clients with diseases such as diabetes. The anesthesiologist, in collaboration with the client's physician and surgeon, will determine whether these medications should be taken the day of surgery and whether they should be taken postoperatively (Table 50-6).

Remember to assess for allergies to drugs that may be given during any phase of the surgical experience.

Table 50-5 Preoperative Considerations for Commonly Ingested Herbs

HERB	COMMON USES	PREOPERATIVE CONSIDERATIONS
Ginseng	• Stress • Gastric disturbances	• Has anticoagulation factors. • Causes hypoglycemia and edema. • May cause hypertension or tachycardia. • Discontinue before surgery.
Ginger	• Motion sickness • Cough • Menstrual cramps • Intestinal gas	• Risk of prolonged clotting times. • Preoperative assessment should include clotting studies. • Discontinue before surgery.
St. John's wort	• Antidepressant • Antiviral properties • Antiinflammatory action	• Should not be used with other psychoactive drugs, monoamine oxidase inhibitors, or serotonin reuptake inhibitors. • Discontinue before surgery because of possible drug interactions.
Echinacea	• Antibacterial and antiviral properties	• May cause allergic reactions. • Decreases effectiveness of immunosuppressants. • May cause immunosuppression.

Table 50-6 Medications That May Influence the Intraoperative Course

MEDICATION TYPE	INTRAOPERATIVE EFFECTS
Anticoagulants	• Alter normal clotting factors and thereby increase risk of hemorrhage
Antihypertensives	• Interact with anesthetics to cause bradycardia, hypotension, and impaired circulation
Antiarrhythmics	• Can reduce cardiac contractility and impair conduction during anesthesia
Anticonvulsants	• Certain anticonvulsants (phenytoin and phenobarbital, for example) can alter metabolism of anesthetic agents after long-term use
Corticosteroids	• With prolonged use, cause atrophy of adrenal glands, which decreases body's ability to withstand stress
Insulin	• Diabetic client's need for insulin preoperatively is reduced because of fasting (NPO) status
Diuretics	• Potentiate electrolyte and fluid imbalances
Antidepressants	• Increase the hypotensive effects of anesthesia
Antibiotics	• Potentiate the action of anesthetic drugs

Ask the client to tell you what exactly happened when they took a drug reported as an allergen. It is also important to inquire about nondrug allergies, including allergies to foods, chemicals, pollen, antiseptics used to prepare the skin for surgery, and latex rubber products. The client with a history of allergic responsiveness has a greater potential for demonstrating hypersensitivity reactions to anesthesia agents. Many facilities require that the client receive an allergy identification band to be worn before going to surgery. Flag the front of the client's chart to alert all health care providers to the client's allergy status.

Previous Surgery. A past experience with surgery can indicate physical and psychological responses to the planned surgery and can alert the nurse to special needs and possible risk factors. Complications such as anaphylaxis (an allergic reaction) during previous surgery signal the need for preventive measures for the upcoming procedure. Complications such as thrombophlebitis or pneumonia after a prior surgery indicate needed preoperative teaching and careful postoperative monitoring. Reports of severe anxiety before previous surgery may indicate the need for additional emotional support and teaching.

PSYCHOLOGICAL FACTORS

Client perceptions of the upcoming surgery, individual coping patterns, perceived body image, and sexuality issues all affect the surgical client psychologically. Understanding more about the client's psychological factors may influence the surgical outcome beneficially.

Perceptions of the Surgical Procedure. A well-informed client knows what to expect and in general accepts and copes more effectively with surgery and recovery. Misconceptions about the surgical outcome or the actual perioperative process can cause undue stress and fear. Because people respond on the basis of their perceptions, it is important to find out exactly how the surgery is perceived. Identify the client's perceptions of the procedure to better plan for teaching and emotional preparation measures.

A client's perceptions of and reactions to the surgical experience are influenced by sociocultural factors, including family health beliefs and practices, economic factors, and cultural background. Assessing the social situation of the client and family is particularly important if you are incorporating the family as part of the client's plan of care during the perioperative period. A client who has been brought up in a family that believes surgery is the last option in treating an illness may refuse to have surgery or may be convinced that death will result. The resulting anxiety may be manifested in physical symptoms, such as circulatory changes, palpitations, and nausea that may make this particular client even more susceptible to surgical risk. Reactions to teaching, physical care, and pain are also influenced by family values (Majasaari, Sarajarvi, Koskinen, Autere, & Paavilainen, 2005).

Coping Patterns and Support Systems. Surgery is a significant and stressful event in the life of the client and family. The client is concerned about the surgery and whether it will improve health. Hospitalization and the convalescent period may be lengthy and costly. Clients often feel they have very little control over their situation. Determine the client's coping patterns, support systems, and sociocultural needs to better understand the impact surgery has on a client's and family's emotional health.

Determine whether family members can provide support. The effect of others on the client's level of anxiety needs to be determined. Encourage significant others to be part of the surgical experience if they are able to provide support before and after surgery.

Body Image. Surgery can leave permanent disfigurement or alteration in body function. Concern over mutilation or loss of a body part compounds a client's fears. Removal of certain body parts may affect the client's feelings about appearing feminine, masculine, or even as a whole person. The client's perceptions about alterations of the body from surgery are an important assessment consideration.

Sexuality. The physical and psychological aspect of a client's sexuality is often affected by surgery. Excision of a breast, a colostomy, or removal of the prostate gland may affect a client's sexuality. Even minor surgeries such as a hernia repair or a cervical biopsy force clients to temporarily refrain from sexual intercourse. Encourage clients to express sexuality concerns. The client facing even temporary sexual dysfunction requires support. Include the client's sexual partner in discussions about sexuality to provide the couple a shared understanding on how to cope with sexual function limitations. Chapter 46 provides more information on sexuality.

PREOPERATIVE PHASE

After the client decides to have surgery, preoperative preparation begins, and assessment is the first step. Analysis of assessment data allows determination of risk factors, prevention measures needed, particular nursing interventions, and probable surgical outcome.

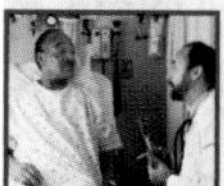

Mr. Warren, accompanied by his wife and daughter, is at the hospital completing his diagnostic testing and preoperative teaching. This is his first surgery and hospitalization. He received only minimal preoperative education from the urologist. Mr. Warren is asking the perioperative nurse many questions about the upcoming surgical events. On the basis of this information, which nursing diagnoses for the preoperative phase (see key nursing diagnoses box) might the nurse want to consider to help Mr. Warren and his family cope with the rapidly approaching surgery?

KEY NURSING DIAGNOSES FOR PREOPERATIVE PHASE

Anxiety: A vague uneasy feeling of discomfort or dread accompanied by an autonomic response (the source often nonspecific or unknown to the individual); a feeling of apprehension caused by anticipation of danger. It is an alerting signal that warns of impending danger and enables the individual to take measures to deal with threat

Grieving: A normal, complex process that includes emotional, physical, spiritual, social, and intellectual responses and behaviors by which individuals, families, and communities incorporate an actual, anticipated, or perceived loss into their daily lives

Risk for latex allergy response: At risk for an allergic response to natural latex rubber products

Deficient knowledge: Absence or deficiency of cognitive information related to a specific topic

ASSESSMENT

The importance of preoperative assessment cannot be overemphasized. It is an interdisciplinary activity, and responsibility for the assessment extends to all members of the health care team. Analysis of the preoperative assessment information is used to prepare the client physically and mentally for surgery and to communicate pertinent information to other surgical team members. Preoperative data are also used through the intraoperative and postoperative phases.

GENERAL ASSESSMENT OF THE PREOPERATIVE CLIENT

Approach assessment of the preoperative client in a holistic manner by gathering information about the physiological, psychological, spiritual, and social needs of the client and family or significant others. From these baseline data, identify surgical risk factors, physical and psychological support needs, and teaching needs, and determine the priority of nursing care. Assessment of the preoperative client is done by taking a nursing history and health history, performing a physical examination, and analyzing laboratory data. This initial client database demonstrates the holistic assessment approach needed to determine care priority of the surgical client.

Health History

Nursing History. When taking a history, you are screening the preoperative client for risks that may cause

Table 50-7 Preoperative Physical Assessment

SYSTEM	ASSESSMENT	PURPOSE
General survey	• Height	• Determination of nutritional status
	• Weight	• Baseline data for preoperative and postoperative phases
	• Vital signs	• Indication of underlying imbalances or infection
	• General	• Reflects energy levels and physical and emotional status
Integumentary	• Skin turgor	• Evidence of hydration
	• Bony prominences	• Indication of potential for injury or pressure ulcers
	• Mucous membranes	• Indication of hydration and oxygenation
Respiratory	• Breathing rate, depth, and rhythm; adventitious sounds; diameter and shape of thorax	• Abnormalities may indicate a preexisting condition that could raise the risk of respiratory trouble during surgery or of atelectasis or pneumonia after surgery
Cardiovascular	• Peripheral pulses and apical pulse, rate, rhythm, character	• Baseline data for intraoperative and postoperative phases of care
	• Presence of edema or other abnormal finding	• Abnormal findings indicate possible complications, such as thrombophlebitis, emboli, or arrhythmias
Neurological	• Level of consciousness and level of motor and sensory function	• Provides baseline data for postoperative assessments and identifies limitations to activity
Abdomen	• Size, shape, bowel sounds, and last bowel movement	• Provides baseline data for postoperative assessments

complications during the perioperative period. The nursing history is an assessment of risk factors and strengths in the client's physical and psychosocial status. Other sources of information are the client's family or significant others. Data that are significant to the surgical experience include the health history, medication and nutritional supplement usage, lifestyle, coping patterns and support systems, and client perceptions of self and of the surgical procedure.

The nursing history interview is often a time when cues from verbal and nonverbal communication may be used to identify fears and concerns related to the client's perception of the surgery and to plan interventions to provide the information and emotional support necessary for successful recovery from surgery. Therapeutic communication skills are essential in establishing a trusting nurse-client relationship necessary to identify and resolve fears. Reduction of fear is of major importance in preoperative preparation, because emotional stress added to the physical stress of surgery increases surgical risk.

Surgical Health History. A health history is taken by the surgeon to determine pathological conditions and to provide a basis for planning surgical care. The collection of data about the client before surgery is probably completed in the surgeon's office. If a client has chronic medical problems (cardiac, pulmonary, renal), a medical physician, possibly a specialist, may also be consulted to provide medical clearance for the client before surgery. This clearance usually involves further diagnostic testing to determine the level of surgical risk related to the chronic status. The term *medical clearance* implies that the client is rated as a low surgical risk.

Physical Examination. Clients should be in optimal physical condition before surgery. A thorough examination of all body systems should be performed to assess the client's status (Table 50-7). Collect physiological data preoperatively to obtain baseline data for comparison during the intraoperative and postoperative phases of care and to identify potential problems that may require preventive nursing interventions before, during, and after surgery.

BOX 50-2 *Commonly Ordered Preoperative Tests*

- Blood studies
  - Red blood cell count
  - Hematocrit
  - Hemoglobin
  - White blood cell count with differential
  - Prothrombin or partial thromboplastin time
  - Type and crossmatch
  - Creatinine
  - Blood urea nitrogen
  - Electrolytes
  - Human chorionic gonadotropin (pregnancy test)
  - Fasting glucose level
- Urinalysis
- Chest radiograph
- Electrocardiogram

Diagnostic Tests. Clients may undergo preoperative preparation several days before surgery or immediately before surgery if the procedure is done on an emergency basis. Usually, preadmission testing is done in the hospital, the physician's office, or an outpatient laboratory. Many facilities have written protocols for preoperative tests. The surgeon orders preoperative radiological and other laboratory tests (Box 50-2).

Abnormalities may warrant treatment before the client has surgery. Check the physician's orders carefully, and see that they are carried out to ensure that the results are obtained before surgery. In many institutions, the nurse screens the test results for abnormalities and informs the surgeon and anesthesiologist as appropriate. The window of time for laboratory and diagnostic testing acceptability before surgery is determined by each institution.

With the testing completed, the client anticipating a scheduled surgery usually enters the hospital the day surgery is performed. The traditional preoperative routine, with the client entering the hospital the day before surgery, is not usually done now unless the client has special therapy or testing needs. Regardless of the method of entry into the setting, you must be able to properly prepare the client for surgery.

FOCUSED ASSESSMENT FOR *ANXIETY*

Anxiety, which is present in most surgical clients to a certain degree, is a state in which a person experiences generalized feelings of unease and apprehension that are triggered by an actual or a perceived threat. Anxiety interferes with the client's ability to concentrate, recall information, and process new information. Assessment that focuses on identification of the nursing diagnosis *Anxiety* as soon as the client consents to surgery provides an opportunity to work with the client and family members in developing a plan of care that addresses anxiety management.

Identify anxiety in a client by looking for its objective signs and listening for its subjective cues (see Chapter 42). Encourage the client to be open in expressing and communicating thoughts and feelings. Ask clients about past hospital experiences that frightened them or that cause them to have concern about their current surgery.

FOCUSED ASSESSMENT FOR *GRIEVING*

The nursing diagnosis *Grieving* is the expectation by the client that he or she will experience a disruption in familiar patterns concerning other people, possessions, job, status, home, and parts and processes of the body after surgery (see Chapter 45).

Focus the preoperative assessment to determine the sequence of subjective states in which there is the expectation of, or actual, loss of life, bodily function, or activity. Discussing with the client the type of loss expected, feelings about control of the situation, and usual patterns of coping with loss leads to individualizing the plan of care for the client.

FOCUSED ASSESSMENT FOR *RISK FOR LATEX ALLERGY RESPONSE*

Focused assessment of risk factors will help you identify clients who need the nursing diagnosis *Risk for latex allergy response.* In assessing the client's past experience, identify those at risk for a systemic reaction; for example, clients may relate stories of complicated anesthesia events, hives from blowing up a balloon, or severe swelling of the labia with a urinary catheterization.

With the advent of universal precautions (now called standard precautions) in the late 1980s, the use of latex gloves dramatically increased, and latex allergies became much more common. Basically, every health care worker wears gloves. Most gloves are powdered to facilitate donning. The powder adsorbs protein allergens from latex gloves and deposits them on skin and into surgical wounds; it also aerosolizes the protein allergens. Aerosolized latex allergens are carried in ventilation systems, causing need for further prevention measures.

Latex allergy is classified into three categories: irritant reaction, and types IV and I allergic reactions. The irritant reaction, which is most commonly seen, is actually a nonallergic reaction. The type IV allergic reaction to latex is a cell-mediated response to the chemical irritants found in latex products. The true latex allergy is the type I allergic reaction, and it occurs shortly after exposure to the proteins in latex rubber. The type I reaction is an IgE-mediated systemic reaction that occurs when latex proteins are touched, inhaled, or ingested.

Factors influencing the diagnosis *Risk for latex allergy response* are the person's susceptibility and the route, duration, and frequency of latex exposure (AORN, 2005). Risk factors for latex allergy response include the following:

- History of anaphylactic reaction of unknown etiology during a medical or surgical procedure
- Multiple surgical procedures (especially from infancy)
- Food allergies (specifically kiwi, bananas, avocados, chestnuts)
- A job with daily exposure to latex (medical, nursing, food handlers, tire manufacturers)
- Conditions needing continual or intermittent catheterization
- History of reactions to latex (balloons, condoms, gloves)
- Allergy to poinsettia plant
- History of allergies and asthma

FOCUSED ASSESSMENT FOR *DEFICIENT KNOWLEDGE*

The nursing diagnosis *Deficient knowledge* means the client or family is demonstrating an inability to learn and comprehend information about the surgical experience or an inability to perform skills as needed to improve the client's level of wellness. Deficient knowledge of perioperative activities related to a lack of exposure is a common nursing diagnosis during the preoperative phase of care and may continue throughout the client's surgical experience.

Identify the client's learning needs, and you can individualize the plan of care by determining related factors. At times, *Deficient knowledge* may be related to psychosociological barriers, such as denial of a health situation, the impending surgery, or both (see Chapter 13). Knowledge deficits often exist simply because it is the client's first surgical experience (Figure 50-3). The client may have received inaccurate information or have difficulty understanding because of the mode of presentation (e.g., when talking faster than the client can follow).

DIAGNOSIS

Cluster preoperative assessment data to identify nursing diagnoses and related factors for the client and family (Table 50-8). Diagnosis gives direction for specific care interventions provided during the surgical experience. Preoperative nursing care includes the physical and psychological care given before a surgical procedure to promote comfort and prevent complications during or following surgery. To effectively manage the care of a surgical client, preventive care is essential. The nature and type of surgery, as well as the client's health status, affect the choice of nursing diagnoses.

In the preoperative phase, the client may experience emotional distress that can affect the surgical experience in numerous ways. Risk factors may be present without the client's presenting signs and symptoms. Many preoperative nursing diagnoses reflect assessment of potential risk and are made to allow interventions that will meet client needs during the intraoperative and postoperative phases. Nursing care throughout the perioperative period must be consistent and documented, because the preoperative nursing diagnoses are the basis for consistent holistic care from admission through recovery. Preventive care is essential to manage the surgical client effectively. The nature and type of surgery, as well as the client's health status, suggest defining characteristics for many diagnoses.

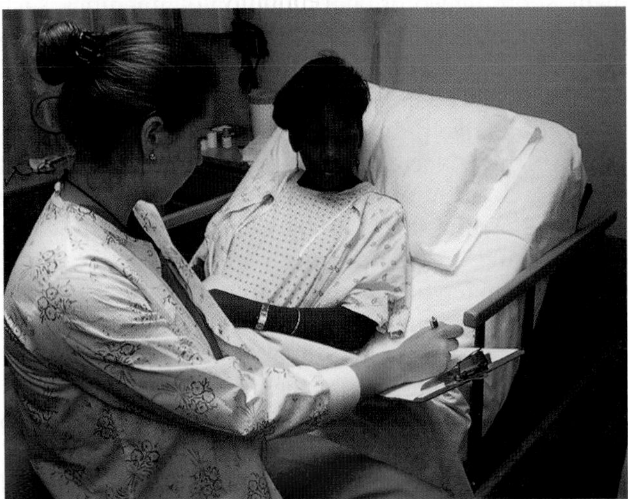

FIGURE 50-3 Often, knowledge deficits occur when the client is undergoing her first surgical experience.

PLANNING

The planning process includes setting priorities, establishing client goals or expected outcomes, and selecting nursing interventions for care of the surgical client. The focus of perioperative nursing is to minimize the client's risks before and during surgery to maximize the potential for positive outcomes during postoperative recovery. However, the primary goal of the preoperative phase is that the client be psychologically and physically prepared for surgery.

EXPECTED OUTCOMES FOR THE CLIENT WITH *ANXIETY*

The overall expected outcome for preoperative clients experiencing anxiety is that they will demonstrate, both verbally and behaviorally, a decrease in anxiety. The client may verbalize the experience of anxiety, describe past coping methods that were successful, exhibit a reduction in physical symptoms of anxiety, interact with others in a focused manner, or choose a decisive course of action from a list of alternatives.

Because *Anxiety* may be present throughout the entire perioperative period, the expected outcomes that the client attains may be new methods of coping with stress and controlling anxiety. Some examples of outcome criteria include identifying sources of anxiety, describing

Table 50-8 Clustering Data to Make a Nursing Diagnosis

Perioperative Problems

DATA CLUSTER	DIAGNOSIS
A 26-year-old registered nurse in the outpatient clinic for a cervical cone biopsy is discussing preoperative data with the admitting nurse. She reports a recent rash on her hands and swelling of her eyelids at the end of each day at work, and she is allergic to bananas.	*Risk for latex allergy response* related to history of recent sensitivity to latex items and history of allergies
A 71-year-old librarian diagnosed with breast cancer weighs 88 pounds and is 5 feet 3 inches in height. She is scheduled for mastectomy this morning.	*Risk for perioperative-positioning injury* related to emaciated state
Client says, "I can't go home! I'm so sick and need extra help." Client refuses to get out of bed and complete morning care. Abdominal incision is healing without complications.	*Delayed surgical recovery* related to perception of needing more time to recover in the hospital setting

symptoms of increasing anxiety, verbalizing long-term coping strategies (exercise, meditation, relaxation techniques), and discussing methods to enlarge, or make better use of, an existing support system.

EXPECTED OUTCOMES FOR THE CLIENT WITH *GRIEVING*

The outcome expected for *Grieving* is that the client will adjust or adapt to the expected loss and reinvest energy and activities in living a productive and meaningful life. This would be a progressive movement through stages of grief toward resolution and adaptation to the diagnoses, treatment regimen, and possible surgical outcome.

EXPECTED OUTCOMES FOR THE CLIENT WITH *RISK FOR LATEX ALLERGY RESPONSE*

The outcome for clients with the nursing diagnosis *Risk for latex allergy response* is that they will not experience a latex allergy response. This outcome includes all classifications of latex allergy: irritant reaction and types IV and I reactions.

EXPECTED OUTCOMES FOR THE CLIENT WITH *DEFICIENT KNOWLEDGE*

The expected outcome for clients with the nursing diagnosis *Deficient knowledge* is that they verbalize adequate knowledge and understanding of expected preoperative procedures and care, intraoperative routines, and procedures to be performed postoperatively to prevent complications. Teaching is continued and reinforced throughout the entire surgical experience (see Chapter 13).

For the surgical client, outcomes for the preoperative phase include communication of a lack of knowledge and desire to know, setting of realistic learning goals, and expression of new knowledge and decreased anxiety related to fear of unknowns, misconceptions, or misinformation.

Outcomes for the intraoperative phase include description of the surgical procedure and its purpose in general terms, identification of routine monitoring to be done intraoperatively, and verbalization of events and sensations expected in the OR.

Outcomes for the postoperative phase include the following:

- Accurate demonstration of desired postoperative skills (use of incentive spirometer and turning-coughing-deep-breathing [TCDB] exercises)
- Verbalization of expectations and understanding of usual postoperative pain control and comfort measures (patient-controlled analgesia pump usage and splinting the incision) by applying pressure during movement
- Discussion of signs and symptoms of wound infection
- Verbalization of lifestyle modifications needed to follow the prescribed postoperative regimen.

INTERVENTION

The perioperative nurse performs nursing interventions according to the priorities established by the nursing diagnoses. The focus of preoperative intervention is to assist the client with both psychological and physical preparation for surgery and postoperative recovery. Many of these interventions are continued throughout the client's surgical experience.

INTERVENTIONS TO REDUCE ANXIETY

Because most clients experience some form of anxiety when confronted with surgery, help them identify the source of their anxiety and suggest strategies for managing it. Interventions should focus on providing information about the impending surgery, clarifying misinformation the client may have, teaching the client relaxation techniques, helping the client explore the source of anxiety, and communicating the client's psychosocial status to the other health care team members. Include interventions that provide support to the client, particularly during the period immediately before surgery. Gentle physical contact, a quiet and unhurried environment, soothing words, and provision of amenities, such as a warm blanket and headphones for listening to music, help the client deal with anxiety.

Anxiety level will influence how you prepare the client preoperatively. One purpose of preoperative teaching is to help decrease the anxiety that might result from a lack of information about the surgery. Because of short hospital stays, discharge teaching must be initiated during the preoperative period. Be aware of the effects of anxiety on learning, and allow time for repetition, reinforcement, and verification of the client's understanding.

Preoperative information helpful to most clients relates to preoperative tests and activities, events related to the surgery itself, and what will happen in the postoperative phase of surgery. Clients are less anxious and participate more readily if they know the reasons for perioperative activities. Allowing clients to participate in decision making concerning their care when that is a realistic option helps them maintain some control over the perioperative events.

Teach clients activities that help decrease anxiety and gain a sense of control. The most common approaches include relaxation exercises, music therapy, and guided imagery. Use therapeutic communication skills and techniques to establish a supportive and trusting nurse-client relationship and to facilitate psychological safety and security. Listen carefully, give the client time to talk, and watch for clues of disabling anxiety. Provide an empathetic, private environment for the client to cry and express anger. The client may also be provided preferred music or a familiar personal object to soothe anxiety.

INTERVENTIONS TO PROMOTE FUNCTIONAL GRIEVING

When a client is confronted with surgery and a perceived loss, grieving on a functional level is necessary, as well as physically and emotionally healthy. On the other hand, dysfunctional grieving has a negative impact on the well-being of the client and can lead to physical and psychological imbalance.

Identify *Grieving*, and help clients move along the grief continuum to a point where they are able to deal with the stressors of surgery. Assist them in identifying the grief and understanding that grieving is common. Discuss the stages of grieving with the clients, and provide encouragement to set goals in response to the expected loss. This enhances their understanding of the normalcy of grief and their ability to cope.

If defining characteristics of *Grieving* are present, document and communicate the findings to the appropriate members of the health care team, such as psychologists, pastoral services, and social workers. Encourage the client to seek help from these resources. Listen and show empathy if the client exhibits behaviors such as crying, anger, or sorrow. Show concern, understanding, and support. If not contraindicated because of the client's cultural practices, establish body contact with the client by touching the hand or shoulder, and explain that feelings of loss are normal.

INTERVENTIONS TO PREVENT LATEX ALLERGY RESPONSE

To provide a latex-safe environment for susceptible clients, all surgical clients should be screened for the *Risk for latex allergy response* before admission. Identification of clients at risk is the initial step in providing prevention.

When a client with a suspected or known latex allergy is scheduled for surgery, all potential risk areas (latex use) are avoided and the client is admitted directly to the OR as the first case of the day if possible. Many facilities have converted isolation rooms into latex-safe environments for care of the perioperative client with latex allergy. Ensure that everyone on the health care team is aware that a client is, or may be, latex allergic. Place a medical alert band or allergy band around the client's wrist, and clearly flag the chart about the latex reaction status. Remove all natural rubber latex products from a known or suspected latex-allergic client's care area. Use latex-free pharmaceutical measures to prepare the client's medications. Have a crash cart standing by stocked with latex-free equipment, supplies, and drugs for treating anaphylaxis. As ordered, give prophylactic treatment with glucocorticoid steroids and antihistamines to latex-allergic clients preoperatively. Box 50-3 lists interventions for the perioperative care of clients with *Risk for latex allergy response.*

The risk for the health care worker's becoming sensitized to latex ranges from 10% to 17% (AORN, 2005). You need to know about the risks of latex to protect clients, latex-sensitive colleagues, and yourself. Wash, rinse, and dry hands thoroughly after removing gloves or between glove changes. Never wear oil-based lotions with latex gloves. Oil breaks down latex, damages the glove as a barrier, and releases additional allergens. Non–oil-based products are compatible with latex.

INTERVENTIONS TO INCREASE CLIENT KNOWLEDGE

Assess the client's level of understanding and willingness to learn to determine the level of knowledge deficit before implementing preoperative teaching. Minimally, knowledge concerning surgical routines, nothing-by-mouth (NPO) requirements, TCDB exercises, wound site splinting, postoperative pain management, postoperative leg exercise, and discharge instructions should be identified. Go over written material with the client. Validate comprehension of the information by asking questions and requesting return demonstrations. Remember that anxiety can interfere with comprehension.

Teaching postoperative activities is done in the preoperative phase and is the nurse's responsibility. Clients and families need to know about the surgical events and sensations, how to manage pain, and how to perform the physical activities necessary to decrease postoperative complications and facilitate recovery. The teaching-and-learning process should be individualized to meet both specific and common needs of surgical clients.

The timing of teaching is a significant consideration; teaching that is done too far in advance of surgery or when the client is highly anxious will be less effective.

BOX 50-3 *Responding to a Client's Risk for Latex Allergy*

LATEX-ALERT CLIENT (HIGH RISK FOR ALLERGIC RESPONSE)
- No premedications are required.
- No special pharmaceutical protocols are required.
- Use nonlatex gloves.
- Use latex-safe supplies.
- Keep a latex-safe supply cart available in client's area.

LATEX-ALLERGY CLIENT (SUSPECTED OR KNOWN ALLERGIC RESPONSE)
- Administer prophylactic treatment with steroids and antihistamines preoperatively.
- Prepare a latex-safe environment, include latex-safe supply cart and crash cart.
- Apply cloth barrier to client's arm under a blood pressure cuff.
- Use medications from glass ampules.
- Do not puncture rubber stoppers with needles.
- Wear synthetic gloves.
- Use latex-free syringes.
- Use latex-safe (polyvinyl chloride) intravenous (IV) tubing.
- Do not use latex preparation on IV bags.

Many facilities provide preoperative teaching sessions before admission so that the client is prepared for surgery. Whether done before or after admission, a preoperative teaching checklist gives nurses organized and comprehensive guidelines for instruction. Check at your clinical facility to see an example of teaching items found on a preoperative checklist.

TEACHING THE CLIENT ABOUT SURGICAL EVENTS AND SENSATIONS

Clients and their families need to know when surgery is scheduled, the approximate length of surgery, the time spent in the recovery room, and what will be done before, during, and after surgery. An explanation of surgical events includes a description of the various members of the perioperative health care team. Preparatory information helps clients and their families anticipate the steps of a procedure and form a realistic mental picture of the surgical experience. When events occur as predicted, the client is better able to cope.

Clients also need to know about sensations typically experienced before, during, and after surgery. Informing the client about sensations in the OR will reduce anxiety before the client is anesthetized. Sensations will differ depending on the type of surgery, but teaching should include descriptions of the following:

- Feelings experienced from preoperative medications, such as drowsiness and a dry mouth
- Sights and sensations (bright lights, cold temperatures) that are common in the OR
- Information about the numerous monitoring devices that will be placed on the client before anesthetization, such as a blood pressure cuff, pulse oximeter, and ECG pads
- Sensations that normally occur after surgery and anesthesia, such as a sore throat from an endotracheal tube, blurred vision from ophthalmic ointment, incisional pain, and tightness of the dressings

TEACHING THE CLIENT ABOUT PAIN MANAGEMENT

Pain is an expected and normal part of the surgical experience and an area of great concern for the client and family (see Chapter 37). Inform clients that pain medicine will be available to assist with pain management postoperatively. Encourage them to use the pain medication as often as needed to achieve an optimal activity level postoperatively. Surgical clients may avoid taking pain medications for fear of becoming addicted. They should be informed that most drug dosages and the required intervals between them are not sufficient to cause dependence.

Pain medications allow clients to manage pain and raise their ability to carry out activities and exercises necessary to recovery. Explore with the client effective coping mechanisms used to manage pain, such as medications, position changes, back rubs, wound splinting, relaxation, biofeedback, and warm moist or dry heat applied to the painful site. Introduce the client to the technique of rating pain on a scale of 0 (no pain) to 10 (worst possible pain) to allow the nurse and client better communication and evaluation of pain management.

If intramuscular or oral analgesics will be used, the client needs to know the schedule for these drugs. Pain medications usually are ordered on an as-needed (prn) basis, with a time restriction between doses (such as every 3 to 4 hours). Pain medications are usually given parenterally for the first few days and as long as a client is NPO; with food intake and decreasing pain levels, oral pain medications are then administered.

Patient-controlled analgesia (PCA) is commonly used and provides the client with control over pain. The PCA medications may be either intravenous or via epidural catheter. Instruct the client in how to operate the PCA pump and the importance of self-administering medication as soon as pain becomes noticeable and before any activity. If the client or nurse waits until the postoperative pain is at an excruciating level, the analgesic may not provide relief. The time intervals between doses and the amount of medication that can be used within a given period are programmed into the device. You are responsible for assessing the effectiveness of the pain relief. Alternate methods of pain control are also encouraged for use with PCA for better relief of pain after surgery (Figure 50-4).

TEACHING THE CLIENT ABOUT POSTOPERATIVE PHYSICAL EXERCISES

Given a rationale for postoperative activities and procedures, clients are better prepared to participate in their own care. Every preoperative teaching program should in-

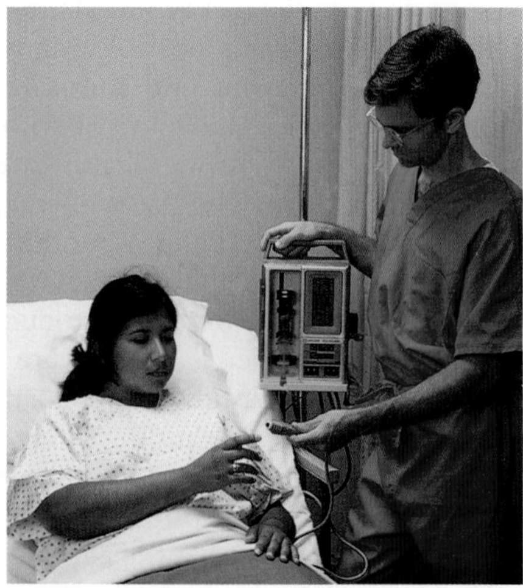

FIGURE 50-4 Teach the client how to operate the PCA pump, stressing the importance of self-administering pain medication as soon as pain becomes noticeable.

clude explanations and demonstrations of postoperative exercises designed to prevent postoperative complications. The most common causes of postoperative complications are pulmonary and cardiovascular alterations, including atelectasis, pneumonia, thrombophlebitis, and emboli.

Physical activities to decrease the potential for complications are taught in the preoperative phase. The client should be able to verbalize and demonstrate the activities before surgery.

Turning Exercises. Turning in bed improves venous return and respiratory function and increases gastrointestinal peristalsis. Incisional pain makes moving and turning in bed difficult, and this activity should be practiced before surgery. The client should turn from side to side at least every 2 hours.

Coughing. Coughing facilitates removal of retained mucus from the respiratory airways and is usually taught in conjunction with the deep-breathing exercise. A deep cough is more beneficial than merely clearing the throat. The client must anticipate incisional discomfort and understand the importance of coughing. Splinting an incision minimizes pain during coughing exercises (Figure 50-5). Advise the client to perform exercises during the period when pain medication has reached its peak effectiveness.

Deep Breathing. While the client is under general anesthesia, the cough reflex is suppressed, mucus accumulates in the tracheobronchial passages, and the lungs do not fully ventilate. After the surgical procedure, respirations are often less effective because of the anesthesia, pain medications, and pain from the incision. As a result, alveoli do not inflate and may collapse and secretions are retained, increasing the potential for atelectasis and pneumonia.

Diaphragmatic breathing improves lung expansion and oxygen delivery without using excess energy. The client learns to use the diaphragm during deep-breathing exercises, and eventually the client's lung volume improves.

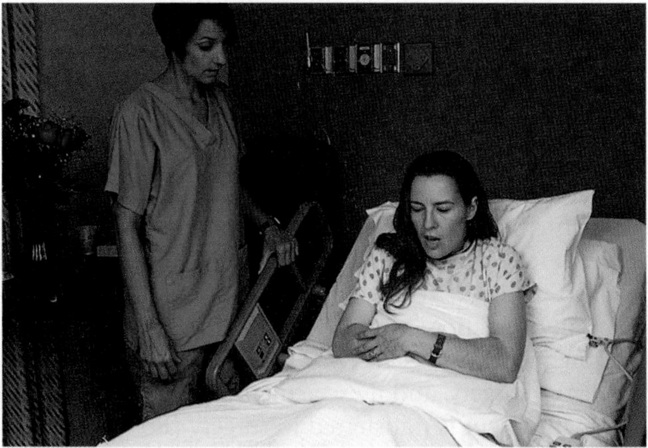

FIGURE 50-5 Preoperatively, teach the client to splint her incision to minimize pain during coughing.

To facilitate deep breathing, the physician often orders an incentive spirometer for the client's use. Incentive spirometry encourages forced inspiration and helps reinflate collapsed alveoli and remove secretions. The therapy is effective in preventing postoperative atelectasis. Chapter 34 discusses respiratory function in depth.

Leg Exercises. During surgery, venous blood return from the legs slows; some surgical positions may also decrease venous return. Postoperative bed rest potentiates this decreased venous blood return, and venous stasis occurs. With circulatory stasis of the legs, thrombophlebitis and resultant emboli are potential complications. Leg exercises increase venous return through flexion and contraction of the quadriceps and gastrocnemius muscles.

Leg exercises should be encouraged 10 to 12 times every 1 to 2 hours. You should assist the client in doing these exercises for the first 24 to 48 hours after surgery and as necessary thereafter, depending on risk factors and the client's status. Crossed legs, pillows behind the knees, and elevation of the bed's knee section must be avoided. Leg exercises must be individualized to client needs, physical condition, physician preference, and hospital protocol.

Some surgeons routinely order elastic stockings or mechanical sequential compression devices to stimulate and enhance venous return when leg muscles contract. These aids are useless if the legs are not exercised and may actually impair circulation if the legs remain inactive or the stockings or devices are inappropriately sized or applied.

TEACHING THE CLIENT ABOUT PREOPERATIVE PHYSICAL PREPARATION

The physical preparation of the preoperative client depends on the client's health status, type of surgical procedure, and physician's orders. You, as the nurse, are responsible for the preparation and safety of the client on the day of surgery in the areas of nutrition and fluid balance, skin preparation, elimination, and rest and sleep. Independent as well as interdependent nursing interventions will be needed to prepare the client physically for surgery.

Maintaining Nutrition and Fluid Balance. Clients need to be well nourished and hydrated before surgery to counteract intraoperative fluid and electrolyte loss and to promote healing postoperatively. Preoperative assessment data provide the information for individualizing interventions regarding the need for preoperative supplemental nutrition, fluids, or electrolytes. If the client's laboratory results show a hemoglobin level of less than 10 g/100 mL and hematocrit less than 30%, blood may be ordered by the physician to be given preoperatively to maintain volume and increase oxygenation of tissues during surgery.

The diet ordered for the preoperative client will depend on the type of procedure and the choice of anesthesia. Clients having general anesthesia or major regional anesthesia are placed on NPO status up to 8 hours before the surgery. Approximately 6 hours of fasting leaves the client's gastrointestinal tract relatively empty of food, so the risks for vomiting or aspirating emesis during surgery are minimized greatly by the NPO status. The risk for aspiration of gastric fluids still remains. You should explain the rationale for being NPO, remove all food and fluids from the bedside, and place a sign above the bed to notify others of the restriction. The client who is at home the night before surgery must also understand the importance of not taking food or fluids and be willing to follow these restrictions. Notify the surgeon and the anesthesiologist if the client eats or drinks during this fasting period.

It is common practice to give antacids (to raise gastric fluid pH) or histamine blockers (to decrease gastric acid production) to high-risk clients, such as those with obesity, pregnancy, traumatic injury, intestinal obstruction, hiatal hernia, or active gastrointestinal bleeding, on the morning of surgery. This is a measure to prevent damage to tracheobronchial mucosa if aspiration occurs. In some situations, the client is allowed to take oral medications, either preoperative or maintenance, with sips of water while on preoperative NPO status.

Preparing the Skin. An alteration in skin integrity, such as a surgical incision, provides a potential site for infection. Surgical site infections are the second most common type of nosocomial infection and account for close to one third of all hospital-acquired infections. Surgical site infection is a risk for all perioperative clients and is considered during each phase of the surgical experience.

Without proper skin preparation, the risk for the development of a postoperative skin infection increases. Bathing the evening before surgery with an antimicrobial or bacteriostatic soap, with particular attention to the proposed surgical site, is believed to reduce the incidence of postoperative wound infections. If the surgery involves the head, neck, or upper chest area, the client may be required to shampoo the hair (AORN, 2005; Mangram, Horan, Pearson, Silver, & Jarvis, 1999).

The incisional site is usually shaved before surgery because hair is a reservoir for bacteria. Hair clippers or depilatory creams may be used to remove hair. Shaving the skin with a razor is not recommended because the microscopic injury that regularly accompanies razor shaving has been found to raise the potential for surgical site infection (Seropian & Reynolds, 1971). Each agency or facility should have policies and protocols regarding the timing, method, and people responsible for the preoperative skin preparation of surgical clients (AORN, 2005; Mangram et al., 1999).

Preparing the Bowel and Bladder. Use assessment data to establish the preoperative baseline related to the client's elimination pattern, and determine the need for an order for further bowel elimination. If the client has not had a bowel movement for several days or has had barium diagnostic testing, an enema helps prevent postoperative constipation. Bowel surgery, such as a colon resection, often necessitates a preoperative bowel evacuation to empty the bowel of feces, because an empty bowel prevents contamination of the surgical area during surgery. Manipulation of the bowel during abdominal surgery results in absence of peristalsis for up to 24 hours and sometimes longer. Enemas and cathartics cleanse the gastrointestinal tract to prevent incontinence and contamination during surgery.

The bladder is usually not prepared until immediately before surgery. Instruct the client to void just before transferring to the holding room. If the client has to void after receiving preoperative sedative medications, a bedpan or urinal is provided to prevent injury from falls. An empty bladder minimizes incontinence during surgery. Indwelling urinary catheters increase the risk for urinary tract infections and are not routinely inserted for all surgical procedures. However, a catheter may be placed for clients undergoing intestinal, gastrointestinal, obstetrical, and gynecological surgery. It is important for the bladder to remain empty and decreased in size during these procedures to avoid its being injured when the surgeon is working in the pelvic region. Indwelling catheters, if ordered, are usually inserted in the OR immediately after the client has been anesthetized.

Promoting Rest and Sleep. Rest and sleep are important for reducing stress before surgery and are essential for normal healing and recovery after surgery. Promote rest and sleep in the preoperative phase by assisting the client in meeting psychological needs, by providing a quiet environment, and by keeping to the client's usual bedtime routine as much as possible. Frequently the physician orders a sedative-hypnotic or antianxiety agent to be taken the night before surgery. An advantage to ambulatory or same-day surgery is that the client is able to sleep at home the night before surgery and will probably sleep better in the familiar environment.

Ensuring Physical Readiness. The day of surgery preparation varies greatly depending on whether the client is admitted to a facility or presents as an ambulatory surgical client. For clients previously admitted to the hospital, you will provide their physical readiness for surgery. For clients with ambulatory status, they or a family member will share in the preoperative preparation activities. Immediately before surgery, you are responsible for the final preparation of the client, as well as for determining that all orders have been carried out and the medical record is complete and ready to accompany the client to the OR.

A preoperative checklist outlines the responsibilities on the day of surgery, and these activities must be completed before the client is transferred to surgery (Box 50-4). This list helps to ensure that no preoperative detail has been omitted that may affect the client's intraoperative and recovery periods. It is especially important to determine that all preoperative orders and procedures have been completed and that documentation is complete before any preoperative medications are given to the client. Verify the presence of a signed informed consent for surgery, laboratory data, history and physical examination report, baseline vital signs, and completed nurse's notes.

Prosthetic devices of any type may be damaged or lost during surgery. Therefore the client must remove all removable prosthetics, including partial and complete dentures and artificial eyes and limbs. If the client has a brace, check with the surgeon to determine whether the brace should remain on the client during surgery.

In some agencies, nurses inventory all removable client devices and secure them. It is common for family members to keep the items, or you may secure the devices at the client's bedside or in the facility's safe. Refer to institutional policies.

Removing dentures can be embarrassing for the client; therefore, if dentures are to be removed before surgery, privacy should be offered. Document and inform surgical team members of the client's feelings about removal and of denture location. Dentures are placed into a container labeled with client's name for safekeeping after removal. In some instances, dentures are left in place until after the first stages of anesthesia. Having well-fitted dentures in place can provide a better seal for ventilation before intubation in the OR.

Anything in or around the eye may irritate or injure the eye during surgery; therefore contact lenses, false eyelashes, and eye makeup must be removed. Glasses and hearing aids are also removed; for the severely hearing impaired, this should not be done until immediately after induction of anesthesia. Allowing the client to be able to see and hear with the use of these aids facilitates communication and raises the client's sense of control in the preoperative setting.

EVALUATION

Evaluate preoperative outcomes before the client goes to surgery (Box 50-5). Evaluation of several outcomes continues into the postoperative period. Frequently, there is limited time for evaluation, because the client's surgery may be emergent, or tests are barely completed by the time the client is sent to surgery. The plan of care for a preoperative client is effective and the outcomes are met if the client is physically and emotionally prepared for surgery.

BOX 50-4 *Examples of Items on a Preoperative Checklist*

DAY BEFORE SURGERY

Check the items that are completed, and document why if not complete.

- Consent forms: admission, general, surgical, anesthesia, blood
- Allergies: medications, foods, environmental, latex
- History and physical on chart or dictated
- Admission database in chart
- Preanesthesia evaluation completed
- Old chart obtained
- Laboratory work completed and results in chart
- Blood ordered: type and screen, type and crossmatch, number of units, autologous, directed donor
- ECG results in chart
- X-ray film results in chart or films with chart
- Surgeon notification if abnormal laboratory work
- Advance directives
- Addressograph plate on chart

DAY OF SURGERY

Check the items that are completed, and document why if not complete.

- NPO since ______________
- Voided/catheter emptied
- Shave/skin preparation (nail polish, makeup, hairpins removed)
- Antiembolism stockings/sequential compression device
- Dentures, contacts/glasses, prostheses, jewelry removed; hearing aid left in place
- Preoperative teaching completed and documented
- IV started and infusing
- Preoperative medications administered and documented

ECG, Electrocardiogram; *NPO*, nothing by mouth; *IV*, intravenous.

BOX 50-5 *Nursing Care Plan*

A Preoperative Client

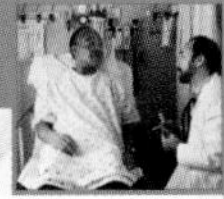

Preoperative Data

Mr. Warren is scheduled for surgery in 5 days. He is in the preadmissions office of the hospital's admitting area. The preoperative nurse is gathering assessment data and assisting Mr. Warren with preoperative preparation. He has many questions about the intraoperative and postoperative events of his surgical experience. Mr. Warren states that his doctor told him the reasons for the surgery and the outcome probabilities. He knows what the doctor is going to do and why but is unsure of the rest of the process. Mr. Warren's daughter acts as translator periodically because of his heavy Jamaican patois.

Continued

BOX 50-5

Nursing Care Plan—cont'd

A Preoperative Client—cont'd

Physician's Orders

Admit morning of scheduled surgery
Surgical procedure: nerve-sparing radical retropubic prostatectomy
Admitting diagnosis: prostate cancer
Routine preoperative labs: CBC with differential, chest x-ray, ECG, prothrombin and partial thromboplastin time, type and crossmatch with 4 units specify available, creatinine, blood urea nitrogen, electrolytes
Attach last week's ultrasonography report, biopsy results, urology studies, and office labs
NPO
Finger stick glucose testing at 7:30 AM
Pentobarbital 100 mg IM on call to OR
Start IV 1000 ml D_5 lactated Ringer's at 100 mL/hr
To OR with thigh-high antiembolism stockings and sequential compression stockings

Nursing Assessment

61-year-old Jamaican man diagnosed with prostate cancer. Awake, alert, and oriented ×3 and to situation. History of arthritis and recently diagnosed with diabetes. Says he takes no medications for diabetes. Takes occasional aspirin for arthritis pain—"Only when it flares up." No complaints of arthritis pain at present. Reports last aspirin dose 2 weeks ago. Takes no vitamins or dietary supplements. However, does take some herbals: sarsaparilla tea for arthritis and corn silk tea for bladder problems. Denies ingestion of herbs over last 2 weeks. Anesthetist informed of herbal usage. Temperature 98.4° F, pulse 84, respirations 20, BP 138/88 sitting. Skin intact, warm, and dry with pink, moist oral mucosa. Lungs clear bilaterally. Heart sounds regular in rate and rhythm. Abdomen soft, nondistended, with normoactive bowel sounds auscultated. No complaints of pain, only comments about slow flow of urine, difficulty in starting stream, and occasional burning with urination. Reports recent notice of vague heavy feeling in his back. Asking multiple questions about perioperative course of events. Wife and daughter in attendance. Daughter translates some of her father's phrases for clarity. Scheduled for prostatectomy in 5 days. This is client's first surgical experience.

NANDA-I Nursing Diagnosis	NOC Expected Outcomes With Indicators	NIC Interventions With Selected Activities	Evaluation Data
Deficient Knowledge	***Knowledge: Treatment***	***Teaching***	
Related Factors: • Lack of exposure • First surgical experience • Lack of knowledge	• Will describe four events that occur in holding area and OR.	• Provide teaching booklets "Prostate Surgery and You" and "The Surgical Experience.	• Handed booklets to daughter and asked for verbalization about the areas and the events. Discussed perioperative course of events.
	• Will describe routine postoperative nursing care events.	• Explain events that will occur in holding area (e.g., shave prep, monitoring vital signs) and in OR (e.g., cold, OR bed, anesthesia).	• Listened intently and looked at daughter frequently. Held wife's hand. Asked questions during and at end of the explanation.
	• Will demonstrate postoperative exercises, splinting, and use of patient-controlled analgesia (PCA) pump.	• Explain and demonstrate common activities that occur postoperatively in the PACU and on the surgical unit (monitoring, catheter care, activity, diet, pain control, sequential compression stockings).	• Client asked questions regarding catheter and compression stockings. Stated he understood.
		• Demonstrate turning-coughing-deep-breathing (TCDB) exercises, splinting incision, and PCA pump usage.	• Daughter emphasized the PCA usage to her father. Client return demonstrated all activities properly.

Critical Thinking Questions

1. Why do you think Mr. Warren handed the booklets about his surgery and surgical experience to his daughter? How would you determine the usefulness of the booklets to Mr. Warren?
2. Mr. Warren is from Jamaica and plans to recuperate at his daughter's home in Atlanta after discharge from the hospital. What other teaching may be needed related to home health care?
3. Prostatectomy can sometimes cause impotence. How would you approach discussion about postoperative sexual activities and coping with possible sexual dysfunction?

Nursing outcome and intervention labels from Johnson, M., Bulechek, G., Butcher, H., Dochterman, J. M., Maas, M., Moorhead, S., et al. (Eds.). (2006). *NANDA, NOC, and NIC linkages: Nursing diagnoses, outcomes, & interventions.* St. Louis, MO: Mosby.

INTRAOPERATIVE PHASE

The intraoperative phase of the surgical experience begins when clients enter the OR and ends when they are transferred to a recovery area. The perioperative nurse is the client's advocate during surgery. Knowledge of the client gained through assessment provides information necessary to provide care specifically for that client. You, the perioperative nurse, compensate for the client's inability to provide self-care by devising a nursing care plan to protect the client during surgery.

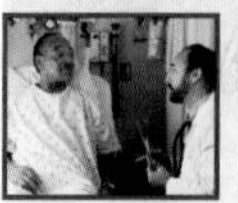

The holding area is busy with numerous clients and health care personnel talking and doing various activities of preparation. Mr. Warren has spoken with the surgeon and has been thoroughly assessed by anesthesia personnel and the circulator. His lower abdominal incision site has been shaved. Intravenous (IV) fluids are infusing, and the CRNA just gave another medication through the line. Mr. Warren is very drowsy but is holding his wife's hand very tightly. His daughter is rubbing his forehead. The circulating nurse arrives at his side and announces it is time to go for his procedure. His family kiss him, and he is taken to the OR suite prepared for him by the CRNA and the circulator.

During his assessment, the circulator determines that *Risk for perioperative positioning injury* is an important nursing diagnosis for Mr. Warren. Why might that be an appropriate diagnosis, given Mr. Warren's health history? What other nursing diagnoses (see key nursing diagnoses box) might be appropriate?

KEY NURSING DIAGNOSES FOR INTRAOPERATIVE PHASE

Risk for infection: At risk for being invaded by pathogenic organisms
Risk for perioperative positioning injury: At risk for inadvertent anatomical and physical changes as a result of posture or equipment used during an invasive/surgical procedure
Risk for injury: At risk for injury as a result of environmental conditions interacting with the individual's adaptive and defensive resources
Risk for imbalanced body temperature: At risk for failure to maintain body temperature within normal range

ASSESSMENT

The focus of nursing care during this phase is to ensure client privacy and safety. Maintaining a safe environment includes protecting the client from injury, infection, and complications arising from anesthesia and the surgery itself.

The holding area, a unit usually connected to the OR suites, is where the surgical team further prepares the client for surgery. The circulator is usually the first member of the surgical team encountered by the client. Assessment activities and certain interventions are conducted in the holding area before the client is taken to the OR suite.

GENERAL ASSESSMENT OF THE INTRAOPERATIVE CLIENT

Assessment data are obtained from a combination of chart review, client and family interviews, observations, and physical and psychosocial assessments. Intraoperative assessment of the client begins with verification and analysis of preoperative data to determine priority of care. A nursing history and brief physical examination are usually completed immediately before the surgery.

Health History. While the client is in the holding area, establish baseline assessment data for intraoperative and postoperative care. The assessment data provided by the client and data from the nursing units (outpatient and inpatient) are important. The preoperative assessment information, preoperative checklist, type of surgery scheduled, and immediate client needs influence the intraoperative plan of care. You may also carry out immediate preoperative care, possibly including skin preparation, starting intravenous fluids, and giving medications.

Chart assessment and identification of the surgical client requirements vary with each facility, client condition, and specific surgical procedures. This assessment activity is a final validation of medical record contents and identification of the client and surgical site. The following is usually included in this validation process:

- Identification of the client
- Identification of the surgical site
- History and physical examination report
- Operative consent form
- Preoperative medications
- Last intake of food and fluids
- Urinalysis
- Pregnancy status
- Complete blood count and electrolyte values
- Chest radiograph and electrocardiogram
- Verification of medications given preoperatively (sedatives, antibiotics, eye drops)
- Values or beliefs that may require intraoperative care adjustments
- Communication impairments
- Location of valuables and prostheses
- Location of family and significant others

Physical Examination. Physical assessment data important to intraoperative nursing care include vital signs, height, weight, age, allergic reactions, condition of skin, skeletal and muscle impairments, sensory or perceptual difficulties, level of consciousness, and any source of pain. Baseline vital signs are important data when anesthetics and other drugs are administered.

The surgical team is guided by the height and weight of the client for dosages of anesthetic drugs and even for the width and length of the operating table. Age can indicate special needs for clients, such as warming units or lights for neonates or special padding for the frail skin of older clients. Allergic reactions can be avoided with measures as simple as a change in the solution used to prepare the skin or as extensive as providing a latex-safe environment for latex-allergic clients. The condition and cleanliness of the skin determine the amount and type of intraoperative skin preparation and will alert the surgical team to the potential for infection or skin integrity breakdown. Knowledge of skeletal and muscle impairments helps prevent positional injuries. Vision or hearing impairments may lead you to adapt communication techniques to meet individual client needs. Increased safety measures may be necessary when a client presents with an altered mental status or decreased level of consciousness. Identify and communicate sources of pain to others in the surgical team to prevent unnecessary discomfort for the client.

Once clients have been properly identified and thoroughly assessed, discuss with them the next steps using some details and basic information about the operating room itself. Fear of the unknown, fear of losing control, and misconceptions can increase their anxiety. Transport them from the holding area into the operating room prepared specifically for their surgical procedure. The clients are usually still awake and will see several people in complete surgical attire, which includes masks, protective eyewear, gowns, and sterile gloves. There are rows of shiny, silver instruments on tables, and the room is cold. Provide emotional and physical support to the client by providing reassurance, further explanations, warm blankets, and a caring touch on the hand or shoulder. Depending on the type of procedure, assist the client to the operating bed and place a safety strap across the client's thighs. The surgical procedure will begin after induction of anesthesia and positioning of the client. As the circulating nurse, assist the anesthesia provider with the induction of anesthesia and intubation. Stand by the client and offer reassurance while at the bedside (Figure 50-6). Fear of never awakening and fear of the unknown are uppermost in the client's mind at this time. Your presence will reduce anxiety and provide emotional support during induction. Remain as the client's advocate throughout this intraoperative stage of care through continued assessment and intervention as needed by the client's physical and emotional status.

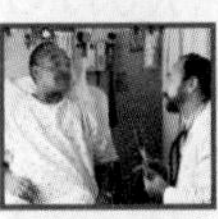

Mr. Warren is transported to the OR via stretcher. He is assisted to the OR bed. What steps should the nurse take to ensure client safety and warmth?

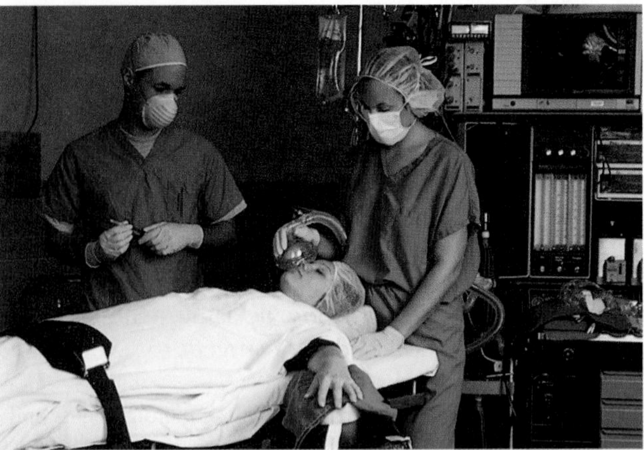

FIGURE 50-6 During induction of anesthesia, stand by the client and provide reassurance.

FOCUSED ASSESSMENT FOR *RISK FOR INFECTION*

The skin, which is the body's first line of defense, is violated by a surgical incision. Although the incision is aseptically created and controlled, the risk for wound infection is increased by the presence of a portal of entry for pathogenic microorganisms. Assess for other factors that may indicate a higher chance for postoperative infection.

The intraoperative nursing diagnosis *Risk for infection* is defined as the accentuated risk for invasion of a surgical wound by pathogenic organisms from either exogenous or endogenous sources. Exogenous infection is acquired from organisms outside the client's body. Endogenous infections come from the large number of microorganisms found in and on the client's body.

Besides the skin incision, other risk factors that can influence a client's risk for wound infection include malnutrition, obesity, extremes of age, inadequate tissue perfusion (large blood loss), history of exposure to infectious diseases and inadequate secondary defenses (immunosuppression, reduced hemoglobin concentration, leukopenia), substance abuse, wound classification (contaminated or infected), and a break in surgical aseptic technique.

FOCUSED ASSESSMENT FOR *RISK FOR PERIOPERATIVE POSITIONING INJURY*

Positioning of the client for surgery is one of the most important aspects of perioperative nursing. Surgical positioning is securing the client's body into a place that allows optimal exposure of the surgical site together with the least compromise to physiological function and the least mechanical stress. The client is particularly vulnerable to positioning injury when the procedure is performed under general anesthesia. Physiological, musculoskeletal, and integumentary systems can be severely compromised at a time when the client is unable to alert you to a problem.

When the client is at risk for injury as a result of the environmental conditions found in the perioperative setting, the nursing diagnosis of *Risk for perioperative positioning injury* is made. During surgery, the risks of impaired gas exchange, neuromuscular impingement, vascular compromise, and tissue injury are accentuated for all clients because of surgical positioning.

Assessment relative to positioning includes gathering data about the scheduled procedure, age, height, weight, activity level, muscle tone, nutritional status, skin condition, and cardiopulmonary status. Assess skin status of clients of all ages with particular attention to the very young and the very old. Assess medical history, preexisting mobility, and range of motion. Principles of client positioning are grounded in knowledge of anatomy and physiology, range of motion, and vulnerable points and positions.

Risk Factors. The degree of risk for positioning injury depends on whether the client receives general or regional anesthesia, on the type and length of procedure, on the required position, and on the client's overall condition at the time of surgery. Anesthetic agents and muscle relaxants depress the pain and pressure receptors and cause muscle relaxation and loss of tone. The normal defense mechanisms cannot guard against joint damage and muscle stretch and strain. When an anesthetized client is in an exaggerated position, injury may occur. Evidence of hyperextension injury can range from mild postoperative discomfort to dislocation.

During surgery, clients are immobile and cannot reposition themselves to relieve discomfort from prolonged pressure. The period of immobility is even longer than the length of the surgical procedure, given that prolonged pressure begins with sedation and includes the time the client is in the preoperative area, the surgery, and the immediate recovery period. Therefore surgery is one of the few times when a client who is not normally at risk for pressure ulcers is at high risk (see Chapter 32). Anesthetic agents also disrupt normal vasodilation and constriction, decreasing perfusion to the bony prominences.

Administration of anesthetics also results in nervous system depression. As a client advocate, you must be aware that when nervous system depression takes place, the body's compensatory actions are no longer functioning. Failure to recognize and relieve pressure to peripheral nerves may result in minor sensory motor loss to permanent paralysis.

Figure 50-7 illustrates some common perioperative positions and the padding provided to relieve pressure in each position. Extreme positions such as Trendelenburg's, in which the head and upper body are lower than the feet, affect circulation and oxygen–carbon dioxide exchange. Positions can also decrease compliance of the lungs and the ability of the thoracic cage to expand, with hypoventilation resulting.

FOCUSED ASSESSMENT FOR *RISK FOR INJURY*

Besides perioperative-positioning injury, the possibility of injury to the client during the intraoperative phase of the surgical experience may be related to retained foreign objects or electrical or burn hazards. The OR is one of the most technically driven areas in a health care facility and contains sophisticated and potentially hazardous equipment.

The diagnosis *Risk for injury* is defined as a state in which a person is at risk for injury as a result of environmental conditions interacting with the client's adaptive and defensive resources. The use of sponges, sharps, instruments, and electrical devices, inherent to the OR environment, constitutes environmental risk.

Extraneous objects such as sponges, sharps (needles, blades), and instruments left inadvertently in the client during surgery can result in postoperative pain, infection, obstruction, extended hospital stay or readmittance, additional surgery and cost, and delayed surgical recovery. One way to reduce the potential for retained foreign objects is by surgical counts.

The AORN (2005) has recommended counting sponges, sharps, and instruments for all surgical procedures and has advised that counts be documented and that counting be enforced through institution policy and procedure. The need to bypass surgical counts exists only in extreme emergency situations and should be documented as such.

Electrocautery as a means of controlling bleeding is practiced routinely in most of the surgical cases today. Radiofrequency electrical current is passed through the body with a hand-held active electrode for the purpose of cutting tissue or coagulating bleeding tissues (commonly called Bovie or cautery). The amount of power and the type of current (cut, coagulate, or a combination) are regulated by controls on the electrocautery unit and the electrode. A grounding pad, or dispersive pad, is provided to complete the electrical circuit through the body and back to the generator or the electrosurgical unit. Injuries can occur at the dispersive site, at the active electrode, or elsewhere, such as ECG electrode sites or a body part touching metal.

Lasers provide another method for hemostasis during surgery. Lasers deliver high-beam energy directly onto tissues. The water in cells evaporates so quickly that the cell actually explodes and vaporizes. This thermal effect cuts, cauterizes, and sterilizes tissue. Laser use during surgery is the responsibility of the entire surgical team. Lasers can cause thermal reactions that can lead to fire, skin burns, and optical damage by either direct or scattered radiation. Specific laser safety precautions must be followed to prevent injury.

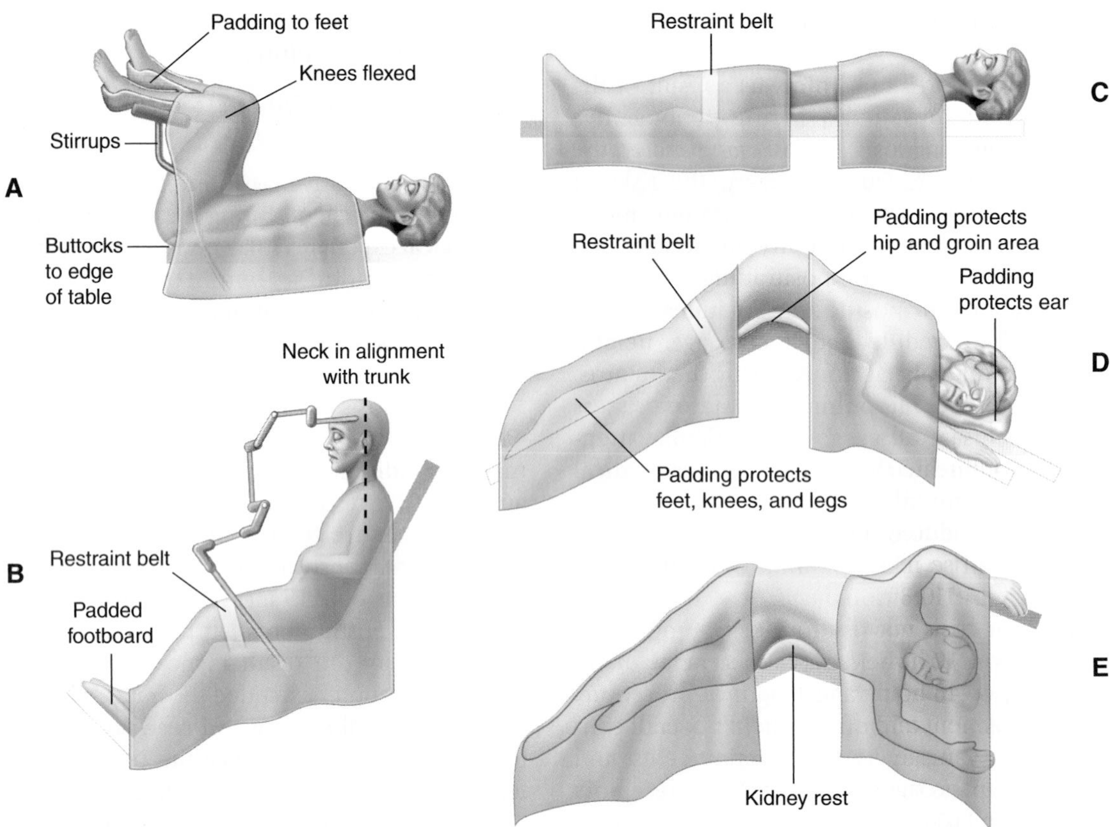

FIGURE 50-7 Common perioperative positions and the padding provided to relieve pressure in each position. **A,** Lithotomy position, used for vaginal and perineal procedures. **B,** Sitting position, used for neurological procedures. **C,** Supine position (the most common position). Potential pressure points are the occiput, scapula, olecranon, thoracic vertebrae, sacrum, coccyx, and calcaneus. **D,** Jackknife position, used for gluteal and anorectal surgeries. **E,** Lateral kidney position, used for procedures requiring a retroperitoneal approach.

FOCUSED ASSESSMENT FOR *RISK FOR IMBALANCED BODY TEMPERATURE*

All intraoperative clients are at risk for alteration in body temperature regulation—the state in which a person is at risk for failure to maintain body temperature within the normal range. Hypothermia is the most common alteration and is described as a core body temperature below 97° F (36.1° C). Hyperthermia, seen when an individual's body temperature is elevated above 99° F (37.2° C), is not as commonly seen in the intraoperative setting but can be a serious problem when it occurs.

Perioperative temperature management is important because it has tremendous effects on surgical client outcomes. Normally, the human body, by a combination of behavioral and physiological responses, can maintain a steady internal (core) body temperature close to (37° C) 98.6° F (37° C) despite large external temperature changes. When a surgical client undergoes general or major regional anesthesia (e.g., epidural anesthesia) for periods longer than 1 hour, hypothermia is expected because anesthesia disrupts the behavioral and physiological mechanisms of thermoregulation. Other factors that place clients at risk for the development of hypothermia include the following:

- Complaints of feeling cold
- Cold operating room environment
- Major fluid or blood loss
- Infusion of cold fluids/blood
- Large volume of irrigation
- Exposure of large body cavity
- Client's age (pediatric or geriatric)
- Client's physical status/preexisting conditions

Any level of hypothermia can cause serious complications. Even mild hypothermia (temperature <96.8° F [36° C]) has been associated with adverse effects on body systems and functions. The more *at risk* the client and the more significant the hypothermia, the greater the likelihood of adverse outcomes. Intraoperatively induced hypothermia causes postoperative complications that lengthen time spent in the PACU and potentially lengthen hospital stays. Complications include postoperative vasoconstriction and shivering, with increased postoperative pain, impaired wound healing, increased clotting time resulting in postoperative bleeding, decreased drug metabolism and clearance, and increased cardiac output.

Signs that indicate hypothermia include reduction in body temperature below the normal range, pallor, cool skin, cyanotic nail beds, piloerection (goose bumps), slow capillary refill, tachycardia, and hypertension. Assess the client for malnutrition, extremes of age, chronic illness, or trauma, because these conditions further increase the risk for hypothermia (AORN, 2005; American Society of PeriAnesthesia Nurses [ASPAN], 2001).

Anesthetic agents may also trigger a hyperthermic response known as malignant hyperthermia. **Malignant hyperthermia (MH)** is a rare, autosomal dominant, inherited syndrome that causes rigidity of the skeletal muscles and is life threatening. It is triggered by anesthetic inhalation agents and neuromuscular blocking medications used to induce general anesthesia. It is characterized by a rapid rise in temperature, with temperatures rising as high as 110.8° F (43.3° C).

The syndrome or crisis may develop during induction of anesthesia or up to 12 hours after receiving anesthesia, and it may recur up to 48 hours after treatment. A delay in recognition and treatment can result in sudden death from cardiac arrest, brain damage, body system failure, or disseminated intravascular coagulation (AORN, 2005).

Action Alert! Bring the MH cart right away if the client develops malignant hyperthermia. Immediately assist with termination of anesthesia and surgery. Assist the anesthesia provider by preparing drugs from the MH cart. Dantrolene sodium, a skeletal muscle relaxant, is the primary drug given during the crisis. Prepare to begin active cooling. Use iced saline to lavage any open body cavities, and cool the body further with cooling blankets and ice packs at the groin, neck, axillae, and head.

DIAGNOSIS

Nursing diagnoses from the preoperative phase are reviewed after the intraoperative assessment and modified to individualize the care plan for the client in the operating room. Additional diagnoses are added to provide direction for the intraoperative and postoperative care of the client. Possible diagnoses are related to the incision, the OR environment, the effects of anesthesia, and the provision of client comfort, safety, and support during the intraoperative period.

PLANNING

The overall focus of intraoperative planning is the safety of the client. During the planning of care, the environment, equipment, and supply needs are prioritized according to the availability of assessment data. Procedural basics for the surgical team's care of the client can be anticipated on the basis of the client's age, scheduled procedure, and surgeon's preferences of instrumentation and supplies. Once the client is assessed, an individualized plan of care is made.

EXPECTED OUTCOMES FOR THE CLIENT WITH *RISK FOR INFECTION*

The expected outcome for the diagnosis *Risk for infection* is that the client remain free from surgical site infection. Surgical asepsis will be maintained during the client's surgical procedure. The client's temperature will remain below 100.8° F (38.2° C), with other vital signs and laboratory values remaining within normal limits. The incision site will be free of erythema, induration, undue tenderness, and purulent drainage. The edges of the incision maintain approximation, and dehiscence of the wound will not occur.

EXPECTED OUTCOMES FOR THE CLIENT WITH *RISK FOR PERIOPERATIVE POSITIONING INJURY*

The outcome for *Risk for perioperative positioning injury* is for the client to remain free from injury related to positioning during surgery. This includes the following outcome criteria:

- Effective breathing patterns with no restrictions to ventilation
- Adequate cardiac output with no significant episodes of hypertension or hypotension
- Surgical positioning that facilitates adequate gas exchange and maintains adequate ventilation/perfusion ratio
- Skin integrity maintained to avoid physical breakdown
- No evidence of neurological, musculoskeletal, or vascular compromise, including numbness, tingling, weakness, or pain of positioned limbs that was not present preoperatively
- No alteration in tissue perfusion, such as reddened, ulcerated, edematous, or excoriated skin areas

EXPECTED OUTCOMES FOR THE CLIENT WITH *RISK FOR INJURY*

The outcome for the client with the diagnosis *Risk for injury* is for the client to remain free from injury related to retained foreign objects or electrical or burn hazards. The client will not have any retained sponges, instruments, or sharps following wound closure—unless such placement was deliberate and recorded. The client will be free from injury related to the use of electrical equipment as evidenced by absence of skin lesions, burns, neuromuscular damage, and signs of electrical shock.

EXPECTED OUTCOMES FOR THE CLIENT WITH *RISK FOR IMBALANCED BODY TEMPERATURE*

The expected outcome for clients with *Risk for imbalanced body temperature* is that they maintain core body temperature ranging from 97.3° F (36.3° C) to 98.8° F (37.1° C) during perioperative care. They also show no complications associated with hypothermia, such as soft tissue injury, dehydration, or hypovolemic shock when rewarmed. Any genetic disposition for malignant hyperthermia is known, and there is no diaphoresis, shivering, or tachycardia. Adequate oxygen is delivered to tissues.

INTERVENTION

The AORN *Standards, Recommended Practices, and Guidelines* (2005) provide specific guidelines for perioperative nurses to ensure positive outcomes for surgical clients. These guidelines include recommendations for instrument and supply sterilization, use of aseptic technique principles to create a sterile field, prevention of physical injury, and adequate skin preparation of the surgical client. Follow these standards, recommended practices, and specific hospital policies during perioperative nursing intervention. Interventions for the aforementioned nursing diagnoses are based on the AORN *Standards, Recommended Practices, and Guidelines.*

INTERVENTIONS TO PREVENT INFECTION

Decrease risk for wound infection by using sterile technique and following recommended practices and your facility's policies. Interventions that reduce the potential for developing surgical site infections include maintaining a sterile field (see Chapter 22) and monitoring and controlling the client's environment. Initiate corrective measures when a break in technique occurs, because contamination of the sterile field may lead to wound contamination and subsequent infection.

Classify the surgical wound according to the degree of contamination of the wound and surrounding tissue (Table 50-9). Classification helps to assess the risk for wound infection from an endogenous source and determine the need for antibiotic therapy.

Administer antibiotics as ordered because intraoperative administration of antibiotics can reduce the incidence of wound infection and lessen its severity. The presence of pathogenic microorganisms is verified by obtaining intraoperative aerobic and anaerobic cultures for laboratory analysis.

Timeliness and preparedness of the surgical team can decrease operative time, thus reducing the amount of time a client has an open surgical wound. Also, it is important to ensure that all surgical team members wear appropriate operating room attire, because the human body is a major source of microbial contamination. Maintain an operating room temperature of 68.8° to 75.8° F (20.4° to 24.3° C) and a relative humidity at 50% ± 10%, unless contraindicated, because cooler air temperatures and lower humidity inhibit microbial growth.

The surgical skin preparation is intended to prevent introduction of exogenous microbes into the incision site and should incorporate aseptic technique. Intraoperative routines for skin preparation should also comply with institutional protocol. The AORN (2005) recommended practices for skin preparation of clients may be used as the basis for a generic plan of care for operative site preparation before the incision is made. An ideal skin preparation agent should be easy to apply, dry quickly, and deliver broad-spectrum antimicrobial protection for the duration of the surgery. The choice of antimicrobial agent and skin preparation technique may vary from institution to institution.

Assess and document the condition of the client's skin before beginning the skin preparation. Allergies, especially to chemicals, should be documented. Maintain the client's privacy by exposing only the area to be prepared. Don sterile gloves. The area of the "prep" should be wide enough to include the surgical site and a substantial area surrounding it. The center of the sterile field is the surgical incision site. Start the preparation at the incision site, moving outward in continually expanding circles away from the surgical site and not returning to the original site with the sponge. Time, area, solutions used, and skin condition are charted. After preparation of the skin, sterile members of the surgical team drape the area intended for incision. Only the site to be incised is left exposed.

The perioperative nursing documentation provides necessary data for further intervention to prevent postoperative infection. Documentation includes the operative procedure; type of anesthesia; surgical times; wound classification; antibiotics given; presence of packing, drains, indwelling catheters, and other invasive devices; implants and tissue or organ transplants; type of dress-

Table 50-9 Surgical Wound Classifications

TYPE OF WOUND	DEFINITION
Clean	• No break in aseptic technique • Gastrointestinal, genitourinary, or respiratory tract not entered • No inflammation present
Clean-contaminated	• Minor break in aseptic technique • Gastrointestinal, genitourinary, or respiratory tract entered without spillage
Contaminated	• Major break in aseptic technique • Gross spillage from gastrointestinal tract or infected biliary or genitourinary tract
Dirty-infected	• Acute inflammation present • Traumatic wound with devitalized tissue or foreign body • Fecal contamination with delayed treatment • Established infection before surgery

ing applied; estimated blood loss; and evaluation of each expected outcome.

INTERVENTIONS TO PREVENT PERIOPERATIVE POSITIONING INJURY

Positioning the client for surgery is a shared responsibility. The surgeon, perioperative nurse, and anesthesia provider all communicate to determine positioning needs. Positioning usually follows induction of general anesthesia; when an alternative anesthetic technique (such as regional or local) is used, the anesthesia provider indicates the time for positioning of the client to protect the integrity of the airway. Positioning should provide physiological alignment for all points while at the same time providing protection from the sequelae of pressure, abrasion, prolonged stretching or compression of nerves, and other injuries. When positioning the client for surgery, pay particular attention to the following goals:

- Provide adequate thoracic excursion.
- Provide correct body alignment.
- Prevent pressure on bony prominences, skin, and eyes.
- Prevent occlusion of arteries and veins.
- Avoid stretching and compression of nerve tissue.
- Avoid unnecessary exposure of the client's body.
- Make allowance for previously assessed aches, pains, or deformities.

Provide adequate padding, positional devices, and support for the client during positioning for surgery. Possible pressure areas and bony prominences are given special attention and may be given extra padding to prevent complications. There are numerous positions in which the client may be placed. The supine position is the most common position used. The lithotomy position is used for pelvic and perineal surgeries. The prone position provides access for back surgeries (laminectomy). Other positions include Trendelenburg's, lateral, kidney, jackknife, and sitting.

Attachments and padding are used to keep extremities within the client's anatomical range of motion. The position of extremities and positioning devices should be rechecked during longer procedures to ensure no displacement has occurred. Monitor and document the circulation to all four extremities. During long surgical procedures, intervene with changes in the client's position at least every 2 hours to increase circulation and relieve pressure at pressure areas to prevent circulatory compromise and intraoperatively acquired pressure ulcers.

> ***Action Alert!*** Protect all bony prominences and pressure areas carefully. You have a key role in recognizing and preventing intraoperatively acquired pressure ulcers. Pressure ulcers that develop in the OR typically develop 1 to 3 days postoperatively. The damage from intraoperative pressure originates deep within the tissues at the bone and not on the skin surface as other pressure ulcers do.

INTERVENTIONS TO PREVENT INJURY

Count sponges, sharps, and instruments according to institutional protocol. Perform counts at change of shift or during any personnel relief. Only x-ray–detectable sponges are used in the wound. Items deliberately left in the body are documented, such as nasal packing. When an incorrect count occurs, inform the surgeon and recount. Enlist all surgical team members to assist in locating the missing item. Common policy is that if a count remains incorrect after search, an incident report is filed, and a radiograph is taken. If the radiograph reveals the retained object, appropriate measures are taken to retrieve it, and surgery is completed. Document counts, any corrective action, and results of subsequent counts.

During the preparation for the procedure, check all electrical equipment and alarms for proper working order. Before and after electrosurgical unit use, assess the client's skin integrity, especially at positional pressure points and under the dispersive pad. If the client is repositioned at all during the procedure, reconfirm the integrity of the dispersive pad placement. Position the client free from contact with metal surfaces. After surgery, remove the dispersive pad slowly to prevent denuding of the skin. Check the client for incidental burns with particular attention given to ECG electrode sites.

The perioperative nurse ensures that only qualified personnel operate the laser, provides a safe and properly functioning laser unit, monitors the use of protective devices, and protects the client and surgical team from laser injury. Cover the eyes of the client appropriately, and follow all precautions for the use of lasers.

INTERVENTIONS FOR IMBALANCED BODY TEMPERATURE

The most common body temperature alteration seen in the OR is hypothermia. The cool OR environment, the client's inactivity and lack of clothing, extensive and invasive surgical procedures, and decreased metabolic rate from drugs all lower the client's body temperature. There are several intraoperative interventions to preserve or even increase the client's temperature, including warmed cotton blankets, thermal drapes, fluid warmers, water mattresses, and forced-air warming systems. Place warm coverings on the client's body, extremities, and head. Use warm saline irrigation to decrease the amount of body core temperature loss. Continuous temperature monitoring is important. If large volumes of intravenous fluids are given, provide a fluid-warming unit.

EVALUATION

Upon closure of the wound and placement of a sterile dressing, perform a postoperative evaluation of the client (Box 50-6). Document specific evaluative findings on the intraoperative record. Evaluation data will continue to be gathered postoperatively because some complications (e.g., wound infection) may occur days after the procedure.

BOX 50-6

Nursing Care Plan

An Intraoperative Client

Intraoperative Data

Mr. Warren is transported via stretcher to his OR suite. He notices how cool it is and comments on all the equipment and masked people he sees. The circulator reminds him that his room was specially prepared for him and that she will be with him from start to finish. They reach OR #14 and go through the double doors. The nurse and anesthesia personnel help Mr. Warren move safely over to the OR bed. A safety strap is applied and warm blankets are placed over him. He states that he puts himself in God's hands and holds the circulator's hand tightly. Mr. Warren breathes deeply from the oxygen mask that is placed over his mouth and nose.

Physician's Orders

Insert 22 Fr. Foley cath to drainage

Use prostatectomy procedure card for routine orders and particulars for this surgeon

Nursing Assessment

Mr. Warren, a 61-year-old Afro-Caribbean man, was admitted this AM for nerve-sparing radical retropubic prostatectomy with admitting diagnosis of prostate cancer. Prostate ultrasound, biopsy, and urology reports in chart. Other lab results within normal limits. 4 units O-negative blood available. Height: 5′10″ Weight: 220. History of arthritis and recently diagnosed with diabetes. Glucose test reading: 148 at 7:30 AM. Reports on no medications with occasional aspirin usage. Last aspirin usage 2 weeks ago. Ambulatory with full range of motion to extremities. Finger joints slightly enlarged with minimal decrease in range of motion. No complaints of joint pain, just stiffness reported. States recent "heavy feeling in my lower back." NPO since last night. IV infusing left forearm. Voided "best I could" before leaving preop admitting area. TED hose and sequential stockings on client, who states "keeping me warm." Skin intact, dry, and slightly cool to touch. Provided warm blankets and OR cap for head. Peripheral pulses palpable and equal. Wife and daughter at side of stretcher before transfer to OR. To OR #14 via stretcher.

NANDA-I Nursing Diagnosis	NOC Expected Outcomes With Indicators	NIC Interventions With Selected Activities	Evaluation Data
Risk for Perioperative-Positioning Injury			
Related Factors: • 61 years old • General anesthesia • History of arthritis • Diabetes	• Will remain free from injury related to positioning during surgery.	• Assess mobility and range of motion (ROM), skin integrity, and neurovascular status before positioning.	• Decreased joint movement in hands and feet. Shoulder and hip ROM full, but client complains of feeling stiff—arthritis. Reports recent lower back discomfort. Diabetic. Skin integrity intact.
		• Reassess mobility and ROM, skin integrity, and neurovascular status 24 hours postoperatively.	• Client expressed no complaints of pain, numbness, or change in ROM. Able to raise arms above head. No pressure point signs of breakdown. Will reassess in 48 hours.
	• Maintain skin integrity with no physical breakdown.	• Use special high-risk positioning aids for extra support and padding during care.	• Placed gel pads at occiput and sacrum, foam protectors to heels and elbows, and pillow under knees. No signs of redness or excoriation noted postprocedure. Will reevaluate in 72 hours.
	• No evidence of neurological, musculoskeletal, or vascular compromise.	• Compare preop assessment data to postop assessment data 24 hours after surgery.	• Peripheral pulses remained intact and same during perioperative course. No numbness, tingling, or pain reported. No signs of skin breakdown. Will reevaluate in 48 hours.

Critical Thinking Questions

1. Why do you think the antiembolism stockings and the sequential compression device are in place during the surgical procedure? Does the length of the procedure make a difference to the client's circulation? Why or why not?
2. The nurse took extra precautions with the client when positioning. Why would you consider Mr. Warren to be at risk for positioning injury?
3. Once the client is in final position, the perioperative nurse should do an overall check to ensure that positioning will not cause injury. Describe at least four factors that the perioperative nurse should assess.

Nursing outcome and intervention labels from Johnson, M., Bulechek, G., Butcher, H., Dochterman, J. M., Maas, M., Moorhead, S., et al. (Eds.). (2006). *NANDA, NOC, and NIC linkages: Nursing diagnoses, outcomes, & interventions.* St. Louis, MO: Mosby.

Intraoperative care of the client focuses on risk management and prevention of injury related to anesthesia, positioning and equipment, environment, and the actual surgical procedure itself. The intraoperative nurse's notes are the documentation of client care in the OR.

The plan of care for an intraoperative client is effective and outcomes are met if the client is physically safe and complications are prevented. However, responsibility to the client does not end for the perioperative nurse in the OR with the application of a sterile dressing. Perioperative nursing care continues during the postoperative phase.

POSTOPERATIVE PHASE

The immediate postoperative phase of nursing care begins as soon as the surgical procedure is concluded. The postoperative course involves both the immediate postoperative period and the ongoing postoperative convalescence. For an ambulatory client, the immediate postoperative period lasts only 1 to 2 hours and convalescence will occur at home. For a hospitalized client, the immediate postoperative period may last several hours, with convalescence taking 1 or more days in the hospital setting, depending on the extent of surgery and the client's response. Further recovery will then take place at home or perhaps in an extended care facility.

ASSESSMENT

Assessment of postoperative clients includes the critical variables that affect recovery and convalescence. Knowledge of preoperative condition, anesthesia type, length of operation, amount of blood loss, intake and output, and the organ system involved in the surgery will help direct the plan of care for the postoperative client. You must be skilled at recognizing change in the client's status, because any variation from normal may signal the onset of complications. Therefore assessment is the key in prevention of postoperative complications.

GENERAL ASSESSMENT OF THE IMMEDIATE POSTOPERATIVE CLIENT

While applying humidified oxygen and various monitoring devices (such as a cardiac monitor, pulse oximeter, or blood pressure cuff), perform a rapid initial assessment of the client's airway, breathing, and circulatory adequacy immediately upon receiving the client in the PACU. The anesthesia provider gives a report to the PACU nurse about the client's surgical status. The American Society of PeriAnesthesia Nurses (2004) recommends that a comprehensive report from anesthesia providers include the following:

- Relevant preoperative status (vital signs, laboratory values, allergies)
- Anesthesia technique used during the procedure
- Type of surgical procedure performed
- Anesthetic agents used
- Length of time anesthesia was administered
- Time that reversal agents were given
- Estimated blood loss and replacement fluids given

The circulating nurse corroborates previously reported data about the preoperative status of the client and includes information about the presence of tubes, drains, and catheters; wound status; any surgical complications; and the types of communication with the client's family members. During this report, the client is continuously monitored.

After reviewing events occurring in the OR, assess the client's status on a continual basis and initiate interventions immediately as needed. The PACU nursing care plans are designed to do the following:

- Determine the client's physiological status at the time of admission to the PACU
- Reevaluate the client so that physiological trends become apparent
- Establish the client's baseline parameters
- Assess the ongoing status of the surgical site
- Assess recovery from anesthesia
- Compare current client status with discharge criteria

Care of the immediate postanesthesia client usually occurs over a 1- to 3-hour period. Assisting the client to a safe physiological level of function after anesthesia is the main objective, with basic care prioritized in relation to the client's airway, breathing, and circulation. Common postoperative problems in the immediate recovery stage include airway compromise, respiratory insufficiency, cardiac compromise, neurological compromise, hypothermia, pain, and nausea and vomiting.

Action Alert! Hyperextend the client's head, and begin positive-pressure ventilation when laryngospasm occurs. Laryngospasm requires immediate response and intervention. Laryngospasm is a respiratory emergency caused by reflex contractions of the pharyngeal muscles, which cause spasms of the vocal cords and prevent the client from a positive-pressure inspiration. Signs and symptoms include dyspnea, hypoxia, hypoventilation, absence of breath sounds, and hypercarbia. Medications used in the treatment of laryngospasm include lidocaine, steroids, and atropine. Endotracheal intubation is required if the laryngospasm persists or if hypoxia cannot be corrected.

The client may be discharged from the PACU to an inpatient unit, intensive care unit, ambulatory care unit, or home. The choice of the site will be based on client acuity, access to follow-up care, and the potential for postoperative complications. Clients are ready for discharge from the PACU when they have demonstrated recovery from the effects of anesthesia; have a patent airway, stable vital signs, and minimal wound or other drainage; have returned to preoperative level of consciousness; have adequate urinary output; and have no unresolved acute problems. Following evaluation and documentation of the client's condition, the client is discharged according to written protocols and discharge criteria. Often a numerical scoring system is used to reflect the client's readiness for discharge.

ONGOING GENERAL ASSESSMENT OF THE POSTOPERATIVE CLIENT

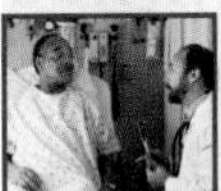

Mr. Warren is transferred by nurses from the stretcher to his bed in a semiprivate room. He spent 2 hours in the PACU before transfer. He remains drowsy but responds appropriately to questions and simple commands. Mr. Warren hums, sings, and dozes. Vital signs remain stable. His abdominal dressing is dry and intact, with a Jackson-Pratt drain on the right side collecting bright red bloody drainage. He has a Foley catheter in traction, and it is patent with pink to red urine draining. No clots in the tubing are noted. IV fluids are infusing, and PCA is in use. The client is not complaining of pain upon transfer. What immediate postoperative teaching about PCA would be appropriate for Mr. Warren? What nursing diagnoses might be appropriate for Mr. Warren in the immediate postoperative phase?

The client is received in the unit room and safely transferred to a bed by the PACU nurse and the unit nurse. Report is given about the client's surgical and PACU course with a review of the PACU record and clarification of physician orders. The unit nurse completes a set of immediate vital signs for comparison to postanesthesia findings before the PACU nurse leaves the room. Minor vital sign changes normally occur after transporting a client.

Your first assessment of the client's general condition includes respiratory and cardiovascular status, level of consciousness, condition of dressings and drains, intravenous fluid status, skin integrity, and comfort level. Institutional protocol for assessment routines should be followed. Common time frames for continuing postoperative assessment activities are every 15 minutes the first hour, every 30 minutes for 2 hours, every hour for 4 hours, and then every 4 hours as needed. Assessments may be more frequent if the client's condition requires. The initial findings are used as a baseline for identifying any postoperative changes.

After you complete the first assessment of the client and determine stability, allow the family to visit. Explain the purpose of the frequent postoperative procedures. Inform the family of the client's condition and that the client may fall in and out of sleep (common after general anesthesia) for most of the day. The family is also instructed and enlisted to maintain safety for the client, such as keeping the side rails up, the call bell in reach, and the bed in its lowest position.

A number of potential complications may occur during the postoperative phase on the surgical unit, as described in the preoperative and intraoperative sections of this chapter. Nursing management activities are also based on an awareness of potential complications of surgery in general, as well as complications specific to the client's surgical procedure itself.

KEY NURSING DIAGNOSES FOR POSTOPERATIVE PHASE

Ineffective airway clearance: Inability to clear secretions or obstruction from the respiratory tract to maintain a clear airway

Ineffective tissue perfusion (specify renal, cerebral, cardiopulmonary, gastrointestinal, peripheral): Decrease in oxygen resulting in failure to nourish tissues at the capillary level

Acute pain: An unpleasant sensory and emotional experience arising from actual or potential tissue damage or described in terms of such damage (International Association for the Study of Pain); sudden or slow onset of any intensity from mild to severe with an anticipated or predictable end and a duration of less than 6 months

Impaired urinary elimination: Disturbance in urine elimination

Nausea: An unpleasant, wavelike sensation in the back of the throat or epigastrium or throughout the abdomen that may or may not lead to vomiting

Risk for constipation: At risk for a decrease in normal frequency of defecation accompanied by difficult or incomplete passage of stool and/or passage of excessively hard, dry stool

Disturbed body image: Confusion in mental picture of one's physical self

Delayed surgical recovery: An extension of the number of postoperative days required for individuals to initiate and perform on their own behalf activities that maintain life, health, and well-being

FOCUSED ASSESSMENT FOR *INEFFECTIVE AIRWAY CLEARANCE*

Assess the patency of the airway, respiratory rate, patterns of respiratory work, and breath sounds to identify potential alterations in respiratory function (see Chapter 34). Results should be compared to the client's preoperative status.

Assess the intensity of breath sounds and for the presence of adventitious breath sounds. Monitor for the client's use of accessory muscles. Note the amount and quality of secretions, because these will indicate the presence of respiratory infection and hydration of the mucociliary blanket.

The postoperative client is at particular risk for *Ineffective airway clearance.* A common cause of ineffective airway clearance is airway obstruction due to relaxation of the tongue on the posterior pharyngeal wall.

Residual effects of anesthetic drugs and muscle relaxants affect muscle control over the tongue and jaw and may decrease cough and gag reflexes.

Postoperative immobility or even the expected decreased mobility can cause clients to take shallow breaths. Many postoperative clients, especially those who have had major abdominal or thoracic surgery, have a tendency to take shallow breaths and to avoid coughing because of the pain it causes. The postoperative development of atelectasis and pneumonia is directly related to hypoventilation, constant recumbent position, ineffective coughing, and smoking. Without medical and nursing intervention, atelectasis can progress to pneumonia when microorganisms grow in the stagnant mucus and an infection develops. Other related factors include airway spasm; presence of artificial airway; excessive secretions; coexisting respiratory disease; tracheobronchial irritation (endotracheal intubation and anesthetic agents); obesity; flow of blood, vomitus, or secretions into airway; and alteration in level of consciousness caused by continued sedation.

FOCUSED ASSESSMENT FOR *INEFFECTIVE TISSUE PERFUSION*

General assessment activities of tissue perfusion include monitoring of the client's blood pressure, heart rate, pulses, and skin temperature and color (see Chapter 35). Results should be compared with the client's preoperative baseline status. Review the chart for information about the surgical procedure performed and equipment used for positioning during the surgery, because these factors are involved in the postoperative client's risk for altered tissue perfusion. Assess the client for postoperative dehydration due to inadequate fluid replacement, intraoperative blood loss, and postoperative bleeding, vomiting, or wound drainage. Fluid volume deficit leads to decreases in cardiac output and tissue perfusion.

Blood clots may form in the leg veins as a result of inactivity, pressure, and body position, all of which lead to stasis and decreased tissue perfusion. Because it may lead to pulmonary embolism, deep vein thrombosis is a potentially life-threatening complication. Deep vein thrombosis is seen more commonly in the older client, the obese client, and the immobilized client.

Fainting or syncope in the postoperative client may indicate decreased cardiac output, fluid deficits, or defects in cerebral tissue perfusion. Syncope develops when the postoperative client sits up rapidly or during the first ambulation attempts.

Clients with previous history of atherosclerosis, malnutrition, obesity, and cigarette smoking are commonly seen with perfusion problems. Inadequate exchange problems that occur with hypothermia, hypoventilation, and immobility can alter tissue perfusion. Anesthetic agents and other medications are related to perfusion compromise because of vasodilation and vasoconstriction properties. Hypovolemia due to hemorrhage or dehydration can cause life-threatening perfusion alterations.

FOCUSED ASSESSMENT FOR *ACUTE PAIN*

Postoperative pain is caused by injured nerve fibers in incised or traumatized tissue. Assessment of pain is ongoing throughout the postoperative phase and often begins as the client returns to consciousness in the PACU. A surgical client's pain increases as the effects of anesthesia wear off.

The most important information in pain assessment is the client's report (see Chapter 37). Although observation of a client's behavioral symptoms provides objective information, it cannot be considered conclusive evidence for the identification of pain. Assess and reassess pain frequently during the postoperative period. Determine the frequency of assessment on the basis of complaints of pain, severity, and operation performed. Increase the frequency of your assessments if pain is poorly controlled or if interventions change.

Observe for indications of pain such as restlessness or grimacing. Question the client about the characteristics and degree of pain. Note the onset, site, duration, intensity, associated aggravating and alleviating factors, and the client's description of the pain. Ask the client to rate the pain using a pain scale. Pain assessment begins in the PACU and continues during postoperative convalescence.

The incision may be only one source of pain. Surgical manipulation, presence of irritating drainage tubes, tight dressings or casts, and the muscular strains from positioning on the OR table are all factors that may make the client express high levels of pain. Severity of pain may be related to the type of surgical procedure performed. Severity of pain is also associated with the type of anesthetic agent used. Clients who received regional anesthesia may not experience pain in the PACU but will do so later.

FOCUSED ASSESSMENT FOR *IMPAIRED URINARY ELIMINATION*

Assessment of intake and output should include all potential sources. Observe color, clarity, and odor of urine. Assess for signs of dehydration. Assess the bladder by palpating the lower abdomen to ascertain distention, especially for clients who have received spinal or epidural anesthesia or undergone urinary tract instrumentation (Figure 50-8).

Urinary elimination can be altered by anesthesia, manipulation of pelvic structures during surgery, inactivity and a recumbent position, and altered food and fluid intake during the perioperative period (see Chapter 30). Urinary retention and urinary tract infections are common postoperative complications.

FOCUSED ASSESSMENT FOR *NAUSEA*

Nausea is an unpleasant, wavelike sensation in the back of the throat, in the epigastrium, or throughout the abdomen that may or may not lead to vomiting. Nausea is a postoperative problem that affects a large number of clients. It may begin in the PACU and continue for several days postoperatively.

Assess the client carefully to differentiate between nausea that is narcotic induced and nausea caused by improper gastric emptying. Assess the abdomen visually for distention. Assess the client's ability to tolerate diet, and determine whether the client is vomiting. Look for possible complications from vomiting, which include fluid and electrolyte imbalances, increased pain, and aspiration.

Postoperative nausea can be caused by multiple factors. Anesthesia agents and opiate narcotics can stimulate chemoreceptors in the inner ear and the vomiting center in the brain. Many anesthetics are retained in fat cells, so the obese client may be more prone to nausea and vomiting. Clients with a history of motion sickness are likely candidates for postoperative nausea and vomiting. If a client reports nausea after a previous surgery, he or she will very likely be nauseated after this surgery.

Manipulation of the intestines during abdominal surgery decreases bowel activity postoperatively. Inactivity postoperatively maintains a sluggish bowel. If sufficient bowel peristalsis does not occur, gastric juices, liquids, and any food taken are unable to leave the stomach through the bowel, so they are regurgitated or vomited. Fluid volume deficit and electrolyte imbalances may also cause nausea and vomiting.

FOCUSED ASSESSMENT FOR *RISK FOR CONSTIPATION*

Frequently, bowel elimination is altered after abdominal or pelvic surgery and sometimes after other surgical procedures as well. Return to normal gastrointestinal function may be delayed by general anesthesia, narcotic analgesia, decreased mobility, or altered fluid and food intake during the perioperative period. *Risk for constipation* is commonly present in the postoperative client (see Chapter 29).

The essential assessment for postoperative gastrointestinal function is the auscultation of the abdomen to determine the presence, frequency, and characteristics of the client's bowel sounds. Bowel sounds are diminished or frequently absent in the immediate postoperative period when peristalsis is decreased.

Motility of the large intestine may be reduced for 3 to 5 days, although small intestine motility normally resumes within 24 hours. Swallowed air and gastrointestinal secretions may accumulate in the colon, producing flatulence and gas pains. A distended abdomen with absent or high-pitched bowel sounds may indicate paralytic ileus, which is an absence of peristalsis with resultant intestinal obstruction.

Action Alert! Assess bowel sounds carefully. The intestinal obstruction and abdominal distention of paralytic ileus is painful, and the client faces possible surgical intervention to release the obstruction. Paralytic ileus is first treated nonsurgically by bowel decompression, which is the insertion of a nasogastric tube with intermittent to constant low suction.

FOCUSED ASSESSMENT FOR *DISTURBED BODY IMAGE*

Assessment of the client's and family's perception of the surgery and its altering effects is important. Be alert for signs of postoperative anxiety and depression. These responses may develop in any client as part of the grief response to a loss of a body part or organ or as a disturbance in body image. Clients may show revulsion toward their appearance, such as refusing to look at an incision.

If surgery led to an impairment of a body function, the client's role within the family may change significantly. The fear of not being able to return to a functional role in the family may cause the client to avoid participating in the plan of care, even for discharge to home. The family plays a crucial role in the efforts to improve the client's self-concept (see Chapter 41).

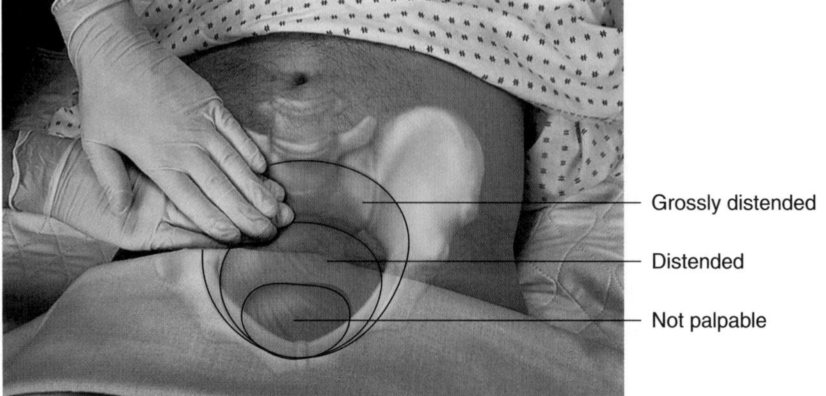

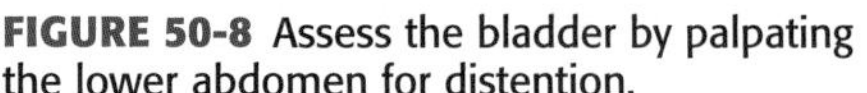
FIGURE 50-8 Assess the bladder by palpating the lower abdomen for distention.

FOCUSED ASSESSMENT FOR *DELAYED SURGICAL RECOVERY*

When clients extend the number of postoperative days usually required to perform the activities that maintain their life, health, and well-being, the nursing diagnosis of *Delayed surgical recovery* is made. Failure of the client to become actively involved in recovery adds to the risk for delayed healing and increases the incidence of complications.

The diagnostic cues of *Delayed surgical recovery* are evidence of interrupted healing, continued spiking fever, loss of appetite with or without nausea, requiring moderate to full assistance to complete self-care, reports of pain at high levels, and postponement of returning to employment or work activities.

The stress of inadequate nutrition, impaired circulation, and metabolic alterations raises the risk for delayed healing during the postoperative period. The physical stresses to the wound during coughing, vomiting, distention, and general movement of body parts are also key factors specific to delayed recovery. The general related factors of *Delayed surgical recovery* are lack of knowledge, depression, malnutrition, and postoperative complications, such as paralytic ileus, pneumonia, thrombophlebitis, and wound infection.

Evaluate the client's general condition, chronic disease processes, and laboratory test results. The incidence of wound sepsis is higher in clients who are older, immunosuppressed, or malnourished or have had a lengthy surgical procedure (longer than 3 hours) or a prolonged hospital stay. Monitor vital signs because elevated temperatures can occur at any time postoperatively and may mean different things. Transient low-grade fever is considered normal. If inflamed tissue was excised during the operation, you should expect a constant elevated temperature for 3 to 5 days postoperatively. Gradually, the temperature will return to normal. A temperature that is intermittently high, called a spiking temperature, may mean something more serious. Determining the source of the fever is crucial. Spiking temperatures during the first 2 postoperative days are usually pulmonary in origin. Auscultate lung sounds for adventitious noise or decreased sounds, and encourage coughing and deep-breathing exercises. From the fourth to seventh day, suspect wound complications if temperatures are spiking. Thrombophlebitis can cause a fever from the sixth to the tenth day.

Ongoing assessment of the client's surgical site also identifies early signs and symptoms of wound infection. Evidence of a wound infection is usually not apparent before the third to fifth postoperative day. Local manifestations are redness, swelling, increasing pain, or tenderness at the site. Systemic signs are fever and leukocytosis.

Assessment of the surgical wound requires knowledge of the type of wound, the specific surgical procedure, and basic knowledge of wound healing principles. Assess for wound pain. When incisional pain is accompanied by an increased or purulent drainage, it usually indicates delayed healing or presence of infection. Incisional pain is usually most severe for the first 3 days and then it should progressively diminish. Assess the amount, color, odor, and consistency of wound drainage from the wound, on the dressings, and in drainage reservoirs.

Use the database completed preoperatively to assess the client's needs related to learning abilities and support resources. The client may be sent home with continued need for special supplies, equipment, assistance with activities of daily living, special medications, or dressing changes. Assess for the particular needs and determine the teaching and referrals needed for continued care.

DIAGNOSIS

Determine the status of identified preoperative and intraoperative problems, and cluster new assessment data to identify additional postoperative diagnoses. The focus of postoperative nursing care is again prevention of complications. Previously diagnosed problems, such as *Deficient knowledge* and *Risk for infection,* usually continue as postoperative nursing diagnoses.

PLANNING

Care of the postoperative client is planned to maximize the potential for positive recovery outcomes.

EXPECTED OUTCOMES FOR THE CLIENT WITH *INEFFECTIVE AIRWAY CLEARANCE*

The overall expected outcome for *Ineffective airway clearance* is for the client's airway to remain patent. The client will show no signs of pulmonary compromise, and adventitious breath sounds are absent upon auscultation (Figure 50-9). Oxygen level is in the normal range, arterial blood gas levels remain at baseline, and ventilation is adequate.

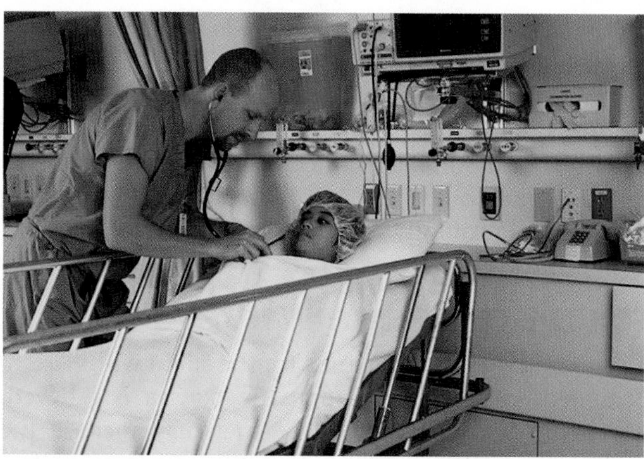

FIGURE 50-9 Expected outcomes for the postoperative client with ineffective airway clearance include the absence of adventitious breath sounds on auscultation.

The client will experience no alterations in respiratory function as evidenced by the following criteria:

- Alert, oriented, and displays no agitation or somnolence
- Shows no signs of aspiration
- Respiratory rate stays within 5 of baseline rate
- Auscultation reveals no adventitious breath sounds
- Coughs effectively and expectorates normal sputum

EXPECTED OUTCOMES FOR THE CLIENT WITH *INEFFECTIVE TISSUE PERFUSION*

The expected outcome for the client with *Ineffective tissue perfusion* is to return tissue perfusion and cellular oxygenation to, or maintain them within, normal parameters as evidenced by the following:

- All pulses palpable
- Extremities warm with normal color
- No complaints of pain or tingling to limbs
- Vital signs normal for client
- Bowel sounds present
- 1500 to 3000 mL output daily, or equivalent to intake
- Alert with recent memory normal
- Hemoglobin 15.5 ±1.1 g/100 mL in men and 13.7 ± 1.0 g/100 mL in women
- Partial thromboplastin time 25 to 39 seconds
- Arterial blood gases within normal limits

EXPECTED OUTCOMES FOR THE CLIENT WITH *ACUTE PAIN*

The overall expected outcome for *Acute pain* is that the client will verbalize that pain is relieved or adequately controlled. Specific criteria include that the location and nature of the pain are described, factors that worsen or relieve the pain are identified, and the client describes and carries out appropriate interventions for pain relief.

EXPECTED OUTCOMES FOR THE CLIENT WITH *IMPAIRED URINARY ELIMINATION*

The client with *Impaired urinary elimination* will have the expected outcome that the bladder will not be palpable after voiding. The following criteria will also be met: voiding occurs in 150- to 400-mL amounts; absence of dribbling or dysuria is reported; postvoid residual is less than or equal to 100 mL; and difficulties with urinating are reported promptly.

EXPECTED OUTCOMES FOR THE CLIENT WITH *NAUSEA*

The overall expected outcome for the client with *Nausea* is that the client reports that the nausea is relieved. Further outcome criteria to be met may include the ability to take fluids and food, identification of the factors that worsen or alleviate nausea, and vomiting does not occur.

EXPECTED OUTCOMES FOR THE CLIENT WITH *RISK FOR CONSTIPATION*

The expected outcome for the client at *Risk for constipation* is that the client's bowel schedule returns to normal patterns. Further goals to be met include the evacuation of soft, formed stool without undue straining, drinking 2000 to 3000 mL of fluid daily, and describing normal bowel function and how fluids, diet, and exercise affect function.

EXPECTED OUTCOMES FOR THE CLIENT WITH *DISTURBED BODY IMAGE*

The overall expected outcome is that the client will use adaptive behaviors in response to alterations in psychosocial function. Specific goals may include the client's expressing comfort with the new body image, verbalizing ways to cope with the alteration, demonstrating ways to enhance relaxation and stress reduction, and discussing feelings, and coping effectiveness as a family unit.

EXPECTED OUTCOMES FOR THE CLIENT WITH *DELAYED SURGICAL RECOVERY*

The overall expected outcome for the client with *Delayed surgical recovery* is that the client will return to a functional state of health within the limits imposed by surgery. The client will contribute to the recovery process by actively participating in planning for discharge, performing activities related to postoperative care, and progressively demonstrating self-care activities.

INTERVENTION

Dramatic and life-threatening changes can occur in the early postoperative phase. Prevention of complications is inherent in postoperative care, and prompt recognition and immediate intervention are imperative for the continued well-being and recovery of the client.

INTERVENTIONS TO MAINTAIN THE AIRWAY

Determine the cause of a compromised airway, and initiate corrective action. Perform endotracheal suctioning when secretions are present. Endotracheal suctioning should be done only when a real need for it exists, because it may traumatize the airway. Note stridor, a change in skin color, and any change in mental alertness.

Action Alert! Determine the cause of the ineffective airway, and correct the problem immediately. The first step is recognition; the second is an open airway. The client's tongue may be relaxed because of anesthesia, narcotics, or muscle relaxants. Or it may become edematous because of an allergic reaction or surgical manipulation. Blood or secretions may be compromising the airway as well.

If the client is nauseated or still stuporous, place the client on one side so that secretions or vomit can flow out of the mouth. If level of consciousness and conditions allow, position the client with the head slightly elevated. This position promotes chest expansion and better ventilation. Administer oxygen as needed and as warranted. Some clients, such as compromised trauma clients, may remain on the mechanical ventilator postoperatively. Mechanically ventilated clients will require critical care by specially educated nurses.

Monitor vital signs, because changes from baseline may indicate increased respiratory and cardiac work related to increased airway resistance, hypoxemia, or the presence of respiratory infection. Monitor arterial oxygen tension (PaO_2) and hemoglobin saturation via pulse oximetry. Stimulate the client, and ask him or her to take deep breaths.

TCDB exercises help the client prevent alveolar collapse and move secretions to large airway passages for easier expectoration. Splinting the incision with a pillow or rolled blanket provides support to the incision and facilitates a deeper cough with expectoration of secretions. Adequate and frequent pain medications should be given because incisional pain is often the greatest deterrent to client participation in ambulation and TCDB exercises. Provide emotional support during these exercises by maintaining contact through touch and communication.

Instruct the client to use the incentive spirometer for maximum inspiration. Encourage early ambulation to increase chest wall expansion and stimulate respiratory rate and circulation. Educate the client about the essential need to maintain hydration, parenteral or oral, to keep secretions thin and loose. Provide oral hygiene frequently for the client to maintain integrity of mucous membranes.

INTERVENTIONS TO PROMOTE TISSUE PERFUSION

Promotion of tissue perfusion is accomplished with simple interventions for the most part. Monitor the client's blood pressure, heart rate, pulses, and skin temperature and color. Compare findings with the preoperative baseline status of the surgical client. Facilitate venous return from the lower extremities by helping the client with leg exercises and ambulation.

Some surgeons prescribe elastic antiembolism stockings or sequential compression devices to stimulate venous return in the legs. Sequential compression devices used with antiembolism stockings are especially effective in reducing deep vein thrombosis in general surgical high-risk clients.

Action Alert! Assess for complaints of swelling, inflammation, aching, or pain in the calf with walking or with dorsiflexion of the foot. These complaints are symptoms of thrombophlebitis.

Promote cerebral perfusion and prevention of syncope by making changes slowly in the client's position. Progression to ambulation can be achieved by first raising the head of the bed, assisting the client to a sitting position on the bedside with legs dangling, and then assisting to a standing position by the bed. If the client voices no complaints and no change in vital signs occurs, start ambulation. If faintness occurs, help the client to a sitting position and then to lie down. Many times the physician will order that the client stand at the bedside the evening of surgery, with ambulation beginning the first postoperative day. Progressive increases in levels of activity promote tissue perfusion, and the client will usually feel less faint with each activity (Figure 50-10).

INTERVENTIONS TO REDUCE OR ALLEVIATE PAIN

Pain is expected after surgery. Nevertheless, the client should receive substantial relief from and control of this pain. Managing acute postoperative pain is an important nursing intervention before, during, and after surgery. Excellent pain control techniques not only can lead to improved client outcomes but also can reduce the cost of care because of a more rapid recovery period. Successful pain management involves the cooperative efforts of the client, physician, and nurse, and it begins with preoperative education (see Chapter 37).

Interventions for pain include pharmacological and behavioral actions. The most rapid relief from pain is provided through intravenous narcotics; more sustained relief may be through the use of epidurals, PCA, or regional anesthesia techniques. Many clients achieve adequate pain relief through intramuscular or oral administration of analgesic medications. Documentation of the medication's effectiveness is important.

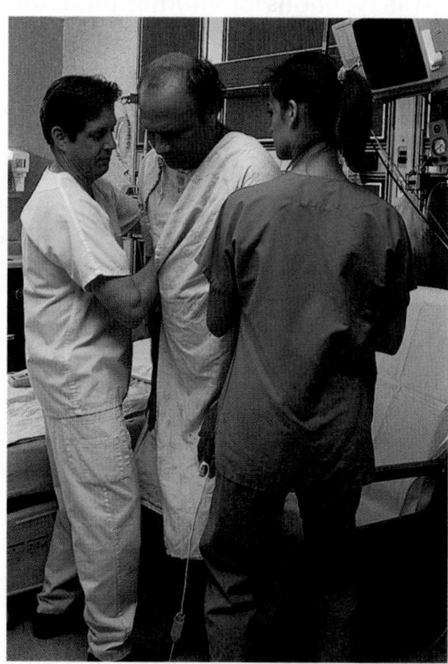

FIGURE 50-10 Progressive increases in levels of postoperative activity promote tissue perfusion.

Various nonpharmacological approaches to pain management are used alone or in conjunction with drug therapy to control acute postoperative pain. Relaxation, distraction, massage, acupuncture, and therapeutic touch are several approaches to pain management. Transcutaneous electrical nerve stimulation (TENS) has also been successful in decreasing postoperative pain for many clients.

INTERVENTIONS TO PROMOTE URINARY ELIMINATION

The urine of the postoperative client should be examined for both quantity and quality, with the urine color, amount, consistency, and odor noted. Indwelling urinary catheters should be assessed for patency, and urine output should be at least 0.5 mL/kg/hr. Urine output is one of the most valuable clinical indicators of renal perfusion. A drop in renal arterial pressure and flow produces renal arterial vasoconstriction and results in decreased glomerular filtration and decreased urine output. Normal urine flow is a minimum of 50 mL/hr for an adult. If no voiding occurs within 6 to 8 hours after surgery, the lower abdomen should be inspected and the bladder palpated and percussed for distention.

Low urine output (800 to 1500 mL) in the first 24 hours postoperatively may be expected, regardless of fluid intake, because of the physiological stress of surgery, preoperative fluid restriction, and loss of fluids during surgery. The inability to urinate, with urinary retention, may occur postoperatively as a result of the recumbent position or of the effects of anesthesia and narcotics, inactivity, nervous tension, or surgical manipulation in the pelvic region. Incisional pain may alter perceptions and interfere with the client's awareness of the less intense sensation arising as the bladder fills with urine.

Nursing interventions promoting the return of normal urinary elimination include the following:

- Monitor intake and output balance.
- Assist with a normal position to void (sitting for women and standing for men).
- Provide reassurance regarding ability to void, and use the techniques to assist in voiding (such as running water or pouring warm water over the perineum).
- Maintain ordered rate of intravenous fluids.
- Encourage oral fluids, when ordered.
- Provide privacy when the client is using a bedpan, commode, or bathroom.
- Assess for bladder distention if the client has not urinated within 6 hours after surgery or if client voids in amounts less than 100 mL.
- Insert a straight or indwelling catheter as ordered.

INTERVENTIONS TO REDUCE OR ALLEVIATE NAUSEA

Determine the onset, duration, and frequency of nausea symptoms. Is it associated with anesthesia agents or narcotic pain medications? Administer appropriate medications. If the client is actively vomiting, choose a route other than by mouth for drug administration.

Ask the client what he or she usually does when nauseated. Provide a cool cloth for the neck or forehead. Place an emesis basin and call bell within reach, turn off lights, and allow the client to rest quietly. Attempt to rid the room of strong odors or food smells.

Auscultate for gurgling and rumbling sounds in all four quadrants to indicate return of peristalsis. Ask clients whether they have passed flatus, because both bowel sounds and active flatus indicate active peristalsis.

If the client is unable to take fluids by mouth or is actively vomiting, monitor hydration status and intravenous infusions carefully. Keep an accurate intake and output record. Monitor heart rate, blood pressure, and laboratory findings such as electrolytes and hematocrit for signs of fluid volume deficit. Electrolyte imbalances can also be the cause of nausea with vomiting.

INTERVENTIONS TO PREVENT CONSTIPATION

Preventing constipation is preferable to treating it. Interview the client about the presence or absence of the following subjective symptoms that may indicate return of gastrointestinal motility or postoperative ileus:

- Abdominal pain
- Flatus within previous 8 hours
- Bowel movement in previous 12 to 24 hours
- Nausea, vomiting, or both
- Feeling bloated
- Return of appetite
- Abdominal cramps

Assess for the return of peristalsis by inspecting the abdomen for presence or absence of distention. Auscultate bowel sounds every 8 hours until the client experiences the first flatus and bowel movement, then twice daily, and as needed until discharge. Palpate the client's abdomen in a systematic fashion, taking precautions not to cause discomfort. Palpation includes assessment of presence or absence of abdominal firmness and tenderness. Encourage and assist with early ambulation if it is not contraindicated. Unless there is a medical condition to restrict fluids (such as renal failure), facilitate daily fluid intake of 2500 to 3000 mL by offering fluids of the client's choice and placing a ready supply at the bedside. Encourage the intake of high-fiber foods unless contraindicated by diet restrictions. Maintain privacy at all times when clients use the bathroom, bedpan, or commode. Assist the client with a more normal position for defecation on a bedpan by raising the head of the bed if not contraindicated. Discourage the use of irritant or stimulant type of laxatives because they irritate the entire bowel. Administer glycerin suppositories or mineral oil enemas as ordered for constipation.

INTERVENTIONS TO PROMOTE REALISTIC BODY IMAGE

To facilitate coping and to promote a realistic body image, provide the client with privacy and accept each client as an individual. Identify through verbal and nonverbal cues those who may be at risk for inability to cope with a body alteration, and offer opportunities for clients and families to verbalize their feelings about the change. Encourage the client to be part of decision making throughout the postoperative experience, and provide honest information to the client and family about all aspects of care. Collaborate with other members of the health care team, and provide referrals to meet psychosocial needs as necessary.

INTERVENTIONS TO PROMOTE SURGICAL RECOVERY

You have an important role in the recovery of the postoperative client. You are usually the first to recognize postoperative problems. Frequent assessment enables you to detect postoperative complications, initiate treatment or referrals, and promote surgical recovery.

The most significant general nursing measure to prevent postoperative complications is early ambulation. It has been nearly 50 years since it was first advocated, and the value of early ambulation is still just as significant. The exercise associated with walking increases muscle tone, improves gastrointestinal and urinary tract function, stimulates circulation, and maintains normal respiratory function.

Nursing care of surgical wounds is directed at preventing and monitoring for wound complications, and it includes the following:

- Maintain aseptic technique in dressing changes and care of drains and tubes.
- Use medical asepsis (hand hygiene protocols).
- Maintain nutritional status; encourage diet selection high in carbohydrates, proteins, calories, and vitamins.
- Maintain hydration.
- Assess the wound for approximation of wound edges, color of the wound and surrounding area, drains or tubes, condition of sutures or staples, and signs of dehiscence or evisceration.

Action Alert! Have the client lie down; cover the wound with a sterile saline dressing, and call the surgeon immediately if dehiscence and evisceration occur. Clients who are obese have a greater risk for wound dehiscence and evisceration.

As the client enters the discharge period of postoperative care to recuperate outside the hospital setting, provide individualized information and support to aid the client in meeting self-care needs (Figure 50-11). Postoperatively, the client will be able to perform many self-care activities and will be encouraged to do those activities and more. Raise the client's confidence and involvement in the recovery process by encouraging preoperative participation in care planning for the eventual discharge from the hospital. All teaching activities should be accompanied by written information and guidelines for the client to refer to while at home. This is important when a large amount of detailed information is presented, such as a wound dressing change.

Because the hospital stay is often very brief, you must make an organized, coordinated effort to educate the client and family members. Specifics and teaching needs may vary, but the most common needs include the following:

- Care of wound site and any dressings
- Signs and symptoms of a wound infection, and when to call the physician
- Symptoms to be reported that may occur in other parts of the body
- Medications and why, when, and how to take them
- Activities allowed and restricted (such as driving, sexual intercourse, returning to work) and when various activities may be resumed
- When and where to return for follow-up care (provide phone number if needed)
- Specific questions and concerns on an individual basis

The client must be accompanied by a responsible adult at discharge. Written and verbal instructions, prescriptions, and immediate supplies are given to the client. Include copies of signed (by client or designee) discharge instructions in the legal medical record. A follow-up evaluation of the client's status may be made by telephone several days later, and any specific concerns are addressed at that time.

A client with *Delayed surgical recovery* may need to be transferred to a long-term or extended-care facility or have home health care nursing visits. Collaboration and further education of the client and the family will be needed before the client's leaving the hospital. Assessment of and planning for special needs and supplies should be reflected in the transfer or discharge documentation. Continued care and evaluation of recovery will continue until the client returns to an optimal level of health.

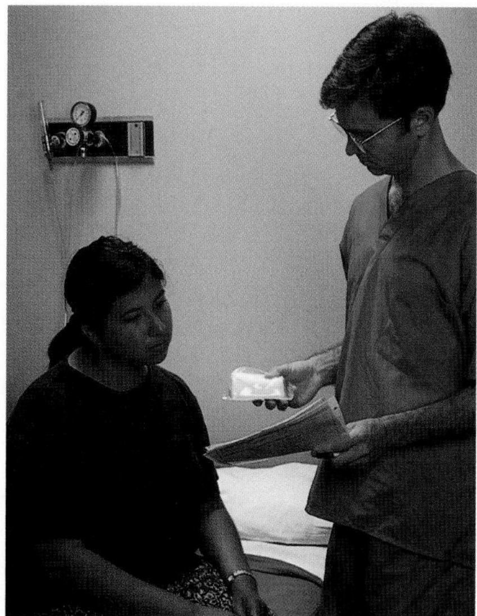

FIGURE 50-11 In preparing for discharge, provide individualized information and support for the postoperative client.

EVALUATION

Evaluate the postoperative client thoroughly (Box 50-7). Keep in mind, however, that postoperative evaluation of outcomes is not always readily apparent. The client's stay is usually short, and access to the client for outcome evaluation is sometimes difficult. Approach evaluation of care collaboratively, because nursing care provided intraoperatively related to a preoperative diagnosis may not have progressed to the evaluation stage until the client is preparing for postoperative discharge.

BOX 50-7 *Nursing Care Plan*

A Postoperative Client

Postoperative Data

Mr. Warren arrived on the GU unit at 2:30 PM on the day of his surgery. The transfer from PACU went smoothly, and the client was stable. At 4:00 AM, Mr. Warren was having dry heaves and complaining of the worst "sickness in my belly and brain" that he has ever experienced. The nurse works with the client to determine the cause of the nausea.

Physician's Orders

Vital signs q30 minutes ×4, q1h ×4, q2h ×2, then q4h
NPO until awake, then clear liquid diet as tolerated
Nothing per rectum
Maintain Foley traction, do not manipulate catheter. Strict intake and output.
No irrigation of Foley—if low output or clots, call physician stat
D_5 1/2 NS 1000 mL at 125 mL/hr alternate with D_5 LR at 125 mL/hr
Drain Jackson-Pratt drain q4h and record
CBC and platelet count, electrolytes, blood urea nitrogen, and creatinine on 3rd postop day
Kefzol 1 g q8h for 5 days
PCA orders and pain control per anesthesia department
Phenergan 50 mg IM q4h prn nausea
Antiembolism stockings with sequential compression device—until ambulating in halls

Nursing Assessment

Client complaining of severe nausea and presenting with dry heaves. Emesis basin at bedside. Placed cool cloth on forehead. Skin cool, clammy, and ashen in color. BP 108/70, pulse 88, respirations 26, and axillary temperature 97.2° F. Bowel sounds hypoactive ×4 quadrants with abdomen softly distended. Lower abdominal dressing bulky, dry, and intact. Jackson-Pratt drain to right of dressing with sanguineous drainage. Foley catheter traction intact and draining pink urine with occasional small bloody clots. IV fluids infusing left forearm without redness, edema, or pain, PCA intact with client using button q30 minutes to q1 hour. Reports lower abdominal incision pain at 4 on scale of 0 to 10. Sequential hose over TED hose in progress. Daughter at bedside.

NANDA-I Nursing Diagnosis	NOC Expected Outcomes With Indicators	NIC Interventions With Selected Activities	Evaluation Data
Nausea **Related Factor:** • Postsurgical anesthesia	***Comfort Level***		
	• Identify factors that worsen or alleviate nausea.	• Ask client to identify what makes the nausea worse and what makes it better.	• Client says "Lord have mercy—it's bad" while lying very still. States never had motion sickness problems in past. PCA morphine in progress.
		• Administer antiemetic medications.	• Phenergan 50 mg IM given with marked decrease in nausea. Able to sit on side of bed and do TCDB exercises 40 minutes after administration of antiemetic.
		• Consult physician for a change in pain medication.	• Called physician and requested change to Dilaudid for client. Received orders to change IV medication in PCA pump to Dilaudid (noted to cause less nausea) for pain relief. Changed PCA pump to Dilaudid at 8 AM.
	Hydration		
	• Has no vomiting.	• Provide cool cloth for neck, forehead, or both.	• Client has not vomited, just had dry heaves. Comfort measures were welcomed.
		• Place emesis basin and call bell within reach.	• Emesis basin and call light are both within client's reach.
		• If vomiting, monitor hydration status and continue IV infusions.	• Not vomiting, but while nauseated, continued IV infusions and monitored hydration status.

BOX 50-7
Nursing Care Plan—cont'd
A Postoperative Client—cont'd

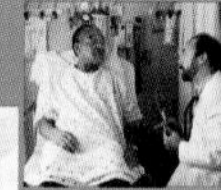

NANDA-I Nursing Diagnosis	NOC Expected Outcomes With Indicators	NIC Interventions With Selected Activities	Evaluation Data
	Nutritional Status		
	• Able to take fluids and food.	• Offer only cool clear liquids, and progress as client tolerates.	• First day postop orders for clear liquids only. Took sips on 7-3 shift and progressed to 600 mL intake on 3-11 shift.
	Symptom Severity		
	• Reports the nausea is relieved.	• Assess complaint of nausea for onset, duration, and frequency as needed.	• Complained of severe nausea at 4:00 AM and moderate nausea at 9:00 AM. After giving antiemetic ×2 and changing PCA medication at 8:00 AM, client reported relief of nausea.

Critical Thinking Questions

1. What do you think may be causing Mr. Warren's nausea? What other nursing measures besides those mentioned here may help the client with his nausea?
2. If Mr. Warren began vomiting, it would affect his hydration status. How do you assess for hydration status? Would dehydration cause additional problems because of his particular type of surgery?
3. The dry heaves Mr. Warren is experiencing can cause abdominal incision pain because of the abdominal muscle use during retching. How could you assist the client with supporting the abdominal incision during this type of situation?

Nursing outcome and intervention labels from Johnson, M., Bulechek, G., Butcher, H., Dochterman, J. M., Maas, M., Moorhead, S., et al. (Eds.). (2006). *NANDA, NOC, and NIC linkages: Nursing diagnoses, outcomes, & interventions.* St. Louis, MO: Mosby.

In the evaluation of *Risk for infection* or *Delayed surgical recovery,* you may need to call the client at home and ask specific questions, or perhaps you will evaluate the outcomes in collaboration with the surgeon's office after the client's first postoperative office visit. Documentation of postoperative evaluation of outcomes is placed in the client's chart.

▼ KEY PRINCIPLES

- Clients confronted with impending surgery face both psychological and physiological stressors.
- The anticipation of surgery may cause anxiety for many clients, who associate surgery with pain, possible disfigurement, loss of independence, and even death.
- Previous illnesses, chronic diseases, and past surgeries influence the ability of the client to tolerate surgery.
- The geriatric client is at higher surgical risk because of declining physiological status.
- The time before, during, and after surgery is called the perioperative period; it is divided into preoperative, intraoperative, and postoperative phases.
- Preoperative assessment data gathered about the surgical client provide an important baseline with which to compare intraoperative and postoperative assessment data.
- Nursing diagnoses of the surgical client may have implications for nursing care during one or all phases of perioperative care.
- Primary responsibility for informed consent rests with the surgeon. However, verification of informed status is an advocacy responsibility of the nurse.
- Structured and timely preoperative teaching positively influences the recovery of surgical clients.
- A major focus of perioperative nursing care during the intraoperative phase is maintenance of client safety through advocacy and prevention of complications.
- Immediate postoperative nursing care in the PACU focuses on prevention of complications from anesthesia and surgery.
- Ongoing postoperative care of the surgical client is planned to facilitate recovery from surgery and to teach the client how to cope with alterations.
- Evaluation of all perioperative care is at times difficult, because the client may be discharged from your care before the outcome is ready for evaluation.

■ REVIEW QUESTIONS

1. The nurse understands older adult clients undergoing surgery are at increased risk because:

1. These clients are predisposed to constipation due to increased motility of the gastrointestinal tract
2. Impaired circulation and decreased cardiac reserve may predispose these clients to hemorrhage and increased blood pressure

Continued

3. These clients are prone to hyperthermia due to an increased metabolic rate and decreased adipose and muscle mass
4. These clients usually have higher basal metabolic rates that decreases total oxygen consumption

2. The nurse is caring for a client who is 7 hours postoperative and has not voided, despite repeated attempts. The client complains of feeling the urge to void, and the bladder is palpable. The nurse intervenes by:

1. Restricting fluid intake until the client is able to void
2. Administering analgesic medication as ordered to promote relaxation
3. Inserting an indwelling urinary catheter as ordered to hasten the return of bladder tone
4. Performing straight urinary catheterization as ordered to relieve bladder distention

3. The nurse is doing preoperative teaching for a client who is to undergo a hysterectomy. The client voices concern about postoperative pain. The nurse responds by saying:

1. "You should expect very little discomfort after surgery, but there is pain medicine available."
2. "Some discomfort is to be expected after surgery, but you don't want to get addicted to pain killers."
3. "Try not to worry about it. The nurses will take good care of you."
4. "Medications will be available to relieve your pain. Please request your medicine when needed."

4. The postoperative abdominal surgery client complains that he felt something "give way" in his incision. Upon assessing the wound the nurse notes a large amount of serosanguineous drainage, wound edges are *not* approximated, and intestines are protruding from the wound. The nurse immediately:

1. Covers protruding internal organs with sterile gauze moistened with sterile saline
2. Encourages the client to turn, cough, and deep breathe while splinting the opening
3. Paints the open wound with an antimicrobial solution to prevent infection
4. Reinserts the organs and applies a pressure dressing to prevent further organ protrusion

5. On admission of a client to the PACU from surgery, the nurse places the HIGHEST priority on assessing the:

1. Client's level of consciousness
2. Condition of the surgical site
3. Adequacy of airway and breathing
4. Status of fluid and electrolyte balance

Bibliography

*Agency for Health Care Policy and Research. (1992). *Clinical practice guideline: Acute pain management—Operative or medical procedures and trauma.* Rockville, MD: U.S. Dept. of Health and Human Services.

Alleyne, M. (1996). *Africa: Roots of Jamaican culture.* Chicago: Research Associates School Times.

*American Nurses Association. (1996). *Latex allergy: Protect yourself—protect your patients* [Brochure]. Washington, DC: Author.

*American Nurses Association. (1997). *Position statement: Latex allergy.* Washington, DC: Author.

American Society of Anesthesiologists. (2004). Practice guidelines for acute pain management in the perioperative setting. *Anesthesiology, 100*(6), 1573-1581.

*American Society of PeriAnesthesia Nurses. (2001). Clinical guideline for the prevention of unplanned perioperative hypothermia. *Journal of PeriAnesthesia Nursing, 16*(5), 303-314.

American Society of PeriAnesthesia Nurses. (2004). *ASPAN: Standards for perianesthesia nursing practice.* Cherry Hill, NJ: Author.

Association of periOperative Registered Nurses. (2002). *Perioperative Nursing Data Set: The perioperative nursing vocabulary.* (2nd ed.). Denver, CO: Author.

Association of periOperative Registered Nurses. (2005). *AORN standards, recommended practices, and guidelines with official AORN statements.* Denver, CO: Author.

Johnson, M., Bulechek, G., Butcher, H., Dochterman, J. M., Maas, M., Moorhead, S., et al. (Eds.). (2006). *NANDA, NOC, and NIC linkages: Nursing diagnoses, outcomes, & interventions.* St. Louis, MO: Mosby.

Joint Commission on Accreditation of Healthcare Organizations. (2003). *Improving the quality of pain management through measurement and action.* Oakbrook Terrace, IL: Joint Commission Resources.

Kuchta, A., & Golembiewski, J. (2004). Medication use in the elderly patient: Focus on the perioperative/perianesthesia setting. *Journal of PeriAnesthesia Nursing, 19*(6), 415-427.

MacKichan, C., & Ruthman, J. (2004). Herbal product use and perioperative patients. *AORN Journal, 79*(5), 948-959.

Madsen, D., Sebolt, T., Cullen, L., Folkedahl, B., Mueller, T., Richardson, C., & Titler, M. (2005). Listening to bowel sounds: An evidence-based practice project. *American Journal of Nursing, 105*(12), 40-49.

Majasaari, H., Sarajarvi, A., Koskinen, H., Autere, S., & Paavilainen, E. (2005). Patients' perceptions of emotional support and information provided to family members. *AORN Journal, 81*(5), 1030-1039.

*Mangram, A. J., Horan, T. C., Pearson, M. L., Silver, L. C., Jarvis, W. R. (1999). Hospital Infection Control Practices Advisory Committee: Guideline for prevention of surgical site infection, 1999. *Infection Control and Hospital Epidemiology, 20*(4), 250-278.

Mews, P. A. (2000). Establishing and maintaining a sterile field. In M. L. Phippen & M. P. Well (Eds.), *Patient care during operative and invasive procedures* (pp. 78-79). Philadelphia: Saunders.

Miaskowski, C. (2005). Patient-controlled modalities for acute postoperative pain management. *Journal of PeriAnesthesia Nursing, 20*(4), 255-267.

*Porter, J., & Jick, H. (1980). Addiction rare in patients treated with narcotics. *New England Journal of Medicine, 302*(2), 123.

Rothrock, J. C. (2003). *Alexander's care of the client in surgery* (12th ed.). St. Louis, MO: Mosby.

*Seropian, R., & Reynolds, B. M. (1971). Wound infections after preoperative depilatory versus razor preparation. *The American Journal of Surgery, 121*(3), 251-254.

*Sessler, D. I. (1993). Perianesthetic thermoregulation and heat balance in humans. *The FASEB Journal, 7*(8), 638-644.

Ulmer, B. C. (2002) Use of electrosurgery in the perioperative setting. *Plastic Surgical Nursing, 22*(4), 173-178.

Wagner, V. D. (2003) Impact of perioperative normothermia management on patient safety. *Surgical Services Management, 9*(4), 38-43.

*Asterisk indicates a classic or definitive work on this subject.

Review Questions Answers

Chapter 1
1. 3
2. 1
3. 2
4. 1
5. 2

Chapter 2
1. 1, 2
2. 2
3. 4
4. 1, 3, 5
5. 1

Chapter 3
1. 2
2. 3
3. 1
4. 1
5. 2

Chapter 4
1. 1
2. 2
3. 1
4. 3
5. 1

Chapter 5
1. 1
2. 3
3. 2
4. 3
5. 2

Chapter 6
1. 3
2. 1
3. 2
4. 1
5. 2

Chapter 7
1. 3
2. 1
3. 2
4. 4
5. 2

Chapter 8
1. 3
2. 1
3. 2
4. 3
5. 4
6. 2
7. 2

Chapter 9
1. 3
2. 2
3. 1
4. 2
5. 2

Chapter 10
1. 2
2. 4
3. 2
4. 1
5. 2

Chapter 11
1. 2
2. 4
3. 3
4. 1
5. 4

Chapter 12
1. 1
2. 3
3. 4
4. 3
5. 2

Chapter 13
1. 4
2. 2
3. 3
4. 4
5. 3

Chapter 14
1. 2
2. 2
3. 2
4. 2
5. 2

Chapter 15
1. 4
2. 2
3. 3
4. 4
5. 1

Chapter 16
1. 3
2. 1
3. 1
4. 2
5. 2

Chapter 17
1. 2
2. 1
3. 3
4. 3
5. 4

Chapter 18
1. 1
2. 2, 3
3. 2
4. 1
5. 2

Chapter 19
1. 2
2. 2
3. 1
4. 1
5. 4

Chapter 20
1. 1
2. 4
3. 2
4. 3
5. 2

Chapter 21
1. 4
2. 4
3. 3
4. 1
5. 4

Chapter 22
1. 3
2. 1
3. 4
4. 3
5. 4

Chapter 23
1. 3
2. 1
3. 1
4. 3
5. 3

Chapter 24
1. 3
2. 1
3. 4
4. 3
5. 4

Chapter 25
1. 3
2. 4
3. 2
4. 2
5. 1

Chapter 26
1. 2
2. 4
3. 2
4. 3
5. 2

Chapter 27
1. 3
2. 2
3. 4
4. 1
5. 2

Chapter 28
1. 1
2. 4
3. 2
4. 3
5. 2

Chapter 29
1. 1
2. 4
3. 2
4. 2
5. 2

Chapter 30
1. 2
2. 4
3. 2
4. 2
5. 2

Chapter 31
1. 3
2. 4
3. 1
4. 2
5. 4

Chapter 32
1. 2
2. 4
3. 1
4. 4
5. 2

Chapter 33
1. 1
2. 3
3. 1
4. 2
5. 2

Chapter 34
1. 2, 3, 4, 5, 6
2. 1
3. 2
4. 3
5. 3
6. 1

Chapter 35
1. 3
2. 2
3. 1
4. 1
5. 3

Chapter 36
1. 4
2. 1
3. 2
4. 3
5. 1

Chapter 37
1. 2
2. 4
3. 1
4. 2
5. 4

Chapter 38
1. 2
2. 4
3. 1
4. 2
5. 4

Chapter 39
1. 2
2. 4
3. 1
4. 2
5. 4

Chapter 40
1. 1
2. 2
3. 2
4. 4
5. 1

Chapter 41
1. 2
2. 2
3. 3
4. 2
5. 4

Chapter 42
1. 1
2. 4
3. 1
4. 1
5. 3

Chapter 43
1. 1
2. 3
3. 4
4. 4
5. 2

Chapter 44
1. 3
2. 3
3. 4
4. 4
5. 3

Chapter 45
1. 4
2. 3
3. 2
4. 1
5. 1

Chapter 46
1. 2
2. 3
3. 3
4. 3
5. 2

Chapter 47
1. 3
2. 3
3. 3
4. 3
5. 2

Chapter 48
1. 2
2. 1
3. 3
4. 3
5. 4

Chapter 49
1. 3
2. 2
3. 3
4. 4
5. 2

Chapter 50
1. 2
2. 4
3. 4
4. 1
5. 3

Review Questions Answers Rationales

Chapter 1

1. The correct answer is 3. The term *client* refers to a person who participates actively in his or her own care along with health care providers.
2. The correct answer is 1. Nursing informatics is a new area for nursing influenced by advancements in computer technology.
3. The correct answer is 2. HIPAA has positively affected clients' rights to privacy and confidentiality of health information.
4. The correct answer is 1. A nurse who attends a 2-year program should expect to receive an associate's degree in nursing.
5. The correct answer is 2. The professional organization for nurses in the United States is the American Nurses Association.

Chapter 2

1. The correct answer is 1, 2. Answers 3 and 4 are legal requirements.
2. The correct answer is 2. The nurse is attempting to hold him against his will; therefore false imprisonment is the most likely charge. However, assault and battery is also possible.
3. The correct answer is 4. Even though the nurse was not assigned to the client, she had a duty to the client. However, no harm resulted; thus there was no damage.
4. The correct answer is 1, 3, 5. A nurse practice act is a legal guide for practice. Generally a nursing license is only valid in the state that issues the license.
5. The correct answer is 1. Most nurses are at-will employees; only 17% are members of a collective bargaining unit. Litigation can be brought against you as well as your employer. Check your nurse practice act for your obligation to report substandard nursing practice.

Chapter 3

1. The correct answer is 2. It is important to clarify one's own values before caring for clients of different cultures recognition.
2. The correct answer is 3. The goal of humanistic care is to gain full understanding of human beings and their humanity.
3. The correct answer is 1. Awareness, sensitivity, respect, and the are attributes of culturally competent practitioners.
4. The correct answer is 1, Madeline Leininger.
5. The correct answer is 2. Communication, space, social organization, time, environmental control, and biological variation are the phenomena described in Giger and Davidhizar's model.

Chapter 4

1. The correct answer is 1. Health promotion is a means to modifying a client's knowledge, attitudes, and skills to adopt behaviors leading to a healthier lifestyle, thus achieving a higher level of wellness.
2. The correct answer is 2. This would be out of the scope of practice for 1 and 3. The physician's assistant could do it, but the nurse is likely to have more experience with home wound management.
3. The correct answer is 1. This client can remain at home and go to an outpatient clinic for infusions.
4. The correct answer is 3. With the retrospective system, payment is determined after the provision of care and is based completely on the costs incurred by the facility.
5. The correct answer is 1. This data is the only information that tells us how many people utilize the available services. The other information is related to quality of care.

Chapter 5

1. The correct answer is 1. The received view measures well-being against established norms.
2. The correct answer is 3. Nightingale's theory focuses on manipulation of the environment to provide the best client outcomes.
3. The correct answer is 2. Eriksson is the author of the theory of caring science.
4. The correct answer is 3. Considering possible outcomes based on actions taken is the goal of critical thinking.
5. The correct answer is 2. The T.H.I.N.K. model was developed by nurse educators.

Chapter 6

1. The correct answer is 3. You need to analyze the symptom of pain.
2. The correct answer is 1. This client needs continuous assessment to determine that his condition is stable in this critical period.
3. The correct answer is 2. You have reason to believe that the client may not be a totally reliable source. Examining the abdomen may give some information but not enough to diagnose constipation.
4. The correct answer is 1. This prepares the client for the end of the interview. Your last question should always be, "Do you have any questions?"
5. The correct answer is 2. The nutritional–metabolic pattern includes the client's dietary habits in relation to metabolic need. Diabetes is managed by diet and medication to regulate blood glucose level.

Chapter 7

1. The correct answer is 3. Comparing a current temperature reading to previous readings helps the nurse to determine whether the current reading is a change from a previous state and thereby interpret the measurement most accurately.
2. The correct answer is 1. The nurse should measure an apical pulse instead of a radial pulse on any client who is receiving medication that could affect the heart rate, such as digitalis and beta-adrenergic blockers.
3. The correct answer is 2. Because the reading is within normal parameters for an adult, the nurse should chart the finding in the medical record.
4. The correct answer is 4. Factors such as lung disease and decreased circulation (from disease or cool temperatures) can lower the oxygen saturation. For this reason, it would be important to measure it for this client.
5. The correct answer is 2. To measure orthostatic blood pressure, take measurements when the client is lying, sitting, and finally standing. Wait approximately 2 minutes between each reading.

Chapter 8

1. The correct answer is 3. Distal means away from the point of origin of the arm.
2. The correct answer is 1. The client who was in a motor vehicle accident may have sustained a head injury.
3. The correct answer is 2. To test peripheral vision, the client looks straight ahead and you determine at what point the client can see an object in the peripheral vision.
4. The correct answer is 3. The client should continue to hear the vibration of the tuning fork after it is removed from the mastoid bone for the same number of seconds as it was heard on the mastoid bone.
5. The correct answer is 4. Lymph nodes are generally not palpable but are within normal limits if smooth, firm, less than 1 cm in diameter, mobile, and nontender.
6. The correct answer is 2. There is very little access to the lower lobes on the anterior surface.
7. The correct answer is 2. A bruit is a swishing sound produced by blood flow through a narrowed vessel.

Chapter 9

1. The correct answer is 3. A nursing diagnosis is the client's response to illness or health needs.
2. The correct answer is 2. The client is at the center of nursing care; therefore 2 is the best answer.
3. The correct answer is 1. This is an actual diagnosis. The client clearly needs help with bathing and other personal care.
4. The correct answer is 2. The intervention with the goal of mobility is to teach him to walk with crutches. The goal comes from the label, and the interventions come from the related factor.
5. The correct answer is 2. Answer 2 directs you to teaching in all three areas listed. Answer 1 only covers one area of teaching; answer 3 has no evidence to substantiate the diagnosis. Answer 4 would be contrary to medical orders.

Chapter 10

1. The correct answer is 2. "Demonstrate" is measurable. The nurse can observe the actual behavior and whether correct technique is used. Choice 1 and choice 4 are incorrect. The verbs (understand, know) used in these choices are not measurable. Choice 3 is incorrect—this statement is vague and is not measurable.
2. The correct answer is 4. The nurse can always help clients understand about medications and does not require a physician's order. Choices 1, 2, and 3 are incorrect. Choice 1 is a direct but physician-initiated intervention. Choice 2 is an indirect intervention. Choice 3 is an indirect intervention.
3. The correct answer is 2. The nurse should evaluate the client's responses to the intervention provided. Choice 2 is correct because the nurse knows the oral analgesic medication should work in 30 minutes and asks the client to evaluate the pain severity with the scale. Choices 1, 3, and 4 are incorrect. Choice 1 hints that the client is "pretty comfortable," and some clients may reply "yes" even though they have some degree of pain. Choice 3 assumes both PCA pump and oral medication work. The client's responses to the intervention of oral medication are not elicited. Choice 4 asks a general question and hints that oral medication is "better." The client is asked to compare the PCA pump with oral medication, and the client is not asked to describe the effects of oral medication on pain relief.
4. The correct answer is 1. Data (states that music helps him to relax and feel less pain; took a 90-minute nap; listened to a CD) indicate that his pain was reduced, which met the outcome criteria. Choices 2 and 3 are incorrect—there are no data to support that outcome criteria are not met or are partially met. Choice 4 is incorrect—data indicate the evaluation of the outcomes.
5. The correct answer is 2. The nurse needs specific data to evaluate whether outcomes are met or partially met and needs to involve the client when possible. Choice 1 is incorrect—it indicates that the nurse lacks specific understanding of the client's plan of care. Choice 3 is incorrect—it is very important for the nurse to evaluate the plan of care and revise the plan of care based on the client's responses so that individualized nursing care can be provided. Choice 4 is incorrect—the client should always be involved whenever possible in planning and evaluating care.

Chapter 11

1. The correct answer is 2. The Joint Commission on Accreditation of Healthcare Organizations has standards for documentation on client medical records.
2. The correct answer is 4. This situation requires an incident report because it represents a variance in the expected operations of the unit. Client belongings should not be lost, and the hospital may be liable to replace them.
3. The correct answer is 3. It is appropriate to document the finding as a late entry.
4. The correct answer is 1. Drawing a single line through an error and writing "void" is a correct method of correcting an error.
5. The correct answer is 4. The intake and output record is used to document fluids the client drinks or receives by other means and to record output by the client.

Chapter 12

1. The correct answer is 1. During the orientation phase of a therapeutic relationship, the nurse and client initiative an agreement that forms their working relationship and the basis for the work the nurse and the client will do together.
2. The correct answer is 3. The person to whom a message is aimed is the decoder (receiver) element of a model for communication process.
3. The correct answer is 4. Paralanguage refers to nonverbal components of spoken language. These components give speech its rhythm and humanness and include stress, accent, pitch, pause, intonation, rate, volume, and quality.
4. The correct answer is 3. When the nurse is using the therapeutic communication technique, focusing, the nurse selects one topic for exploration from among several possible topics presented by the client.
5. The correct answer is 2. When the nurse parrots, the nurse mechanically repeats the client's words without evaluating what has been said and without helping the client to think things through.

Chapter 13

1. The correct answer is 4. Assessment is the first step of the nursing process and the first step of the teaching-learning process.
2. The correct answer is 2. Verbalization that a client has no knowledge, incomplete knowledge, or incorrect knowledge is a defining characteristic for the nursing diagnosis *Deficient knowledge,* which is the most common nursing diagnosis related to client teaching.
3. The correct answer is 3. This is the best learning objective because it contains the performance (ambulates 25 feet with walker), the condition (by end of shift), and the criterion (independently).
4. The correct answer is 1. Two disadvantages of group teaching that make individual instruction preferred are the lack of ability to pace your teaching to individual learning rates and the possibility that some clients will be too intimidated to ask questions in front of the group.
5. The correct answer is 3. Because the client learned a new skill, the most effective evaluation is to see a return demonstration of the skill.

Chapter 14

1. The correct answer is 2. This service meets the needs of the community for access to care. Although the remaining services may be in keeping with the concept of a community hospital, each one limits access and therefore is in conflict with the concept of optimal access.
2. The correct answer is 2. The charge nurse is empowering the staff nurses to make decisions about documentation.
3. The correct answer is 2. Choice 2 is the only evaluation to determine the methods of care while the nurses are performing the care.
4. The correct answer is 2. Choice 2 is primary nursing. Although the charge nurse might be identified as the client's nurse, it is not likely that the client will have much contact with this nurse who is responsible for the whole unit.
5. The correct answer is 2. The goal of the health care team is optimal benefit to the client. The remaining answers are relevant to how the team functions, but the goal is client oriented.

Chapter 15

1. The correct answer is 4. A research problem is an observation, situation, occurrence, or even a hunch that an investigator chooses to research.
2. The correct answer is 2. Because of the double-blind method used in studies that are experimental in nature, the participant in a research study is not aware of whether he or she is assigned to a control or experimental group.
3. The correct answer is 3. Validity is the ability of an instrument to measure what it is designed to measure.
4. The correct answer is 4. The Hawthorne effect occurs when student subjects act in a way that is different than they usually act.
5. The correct answer is 1. Level 1 evidence is obtained from a systematic review of all relevant randomized controlled trials (RCTs).

Chapter 16

1. The correct answer is 3. This is correct motor ability at this age.
2. The correct answer is 1. This is correct growth for age.
3. The correct answer is 1. Further examination is appropriate for this age if there is difficulty kicking a ball.
4. The correct answer is 2. This is the correct crisis for a school-age child.
5. The correct answer is 2. This is a demonstration of a fine motor skill.

Chapter 17

1. The correct answer is 2. Self-image in relationship to peers is the most important task for an adolescent.
2. The correct answer is 1. Dental maturity is evident in the mid 20s.
3. The correct answer is 3. Development of hypertension is one of the major risks associated with obesity. Being overweight also increases the risk of coronary artery disease and diabetes.
4. The correct answer is 3. Uninsured clients may die from lack of health care insurance. They avoid spending money because they know the high price of health care.
5. The correct answer is 4. Obesity in childhood has increased the risks of diabetes, hypertension, and coronary artery disease in children as we previously had seen only in adults because of the lifestyle choices of today's children.

Chapter 18

1. The correct answer is 1. This older adult woman is creating a new life structure by making use of her retirement years by doing volunteer work. The remaining answers would be more relevant to Erikson's stages of psychosocial development.
2. The correct answer is 2, 3. Depression may occur, but not for this reason. AIDS is a growing problem in older adults because people are living longer with AIDS, but it would not yet be part of routine screening. Cancer and heart disease are among the leading causes of death.
3. The correct answer is 2. Older adults do not lose intelligence but do learn more slowly. The book might work for some elders, but a whole book is likely to contain information that is not necessarily relevant or need-to-know information.
4. The correct answer is 1. Assisted living would provide meals and socialization; many assisted living environments also offer medication monitoring and assistance

with bathing for an additional fee. The community-based day care would provide the socialization but not assistance with bathing and medications. Home health care might meet her physical needs but would not provide socialization. Nursing home care is a higher level of care.
5. The correct answer is 2. The data given suggest that she is fully able to participate in a rehabilitation program.

Chapter 19
1. The correct answer is 2. An optimal state of well-being is a choice, achieved through active pursuit of good health.
2. The correct answer is 2. The remaining three answers identify populations that are at risk. The action is designed to reduce a specific risk.
3. The correct answer is 1. Tertiary prevention is reducing the effects of a disease or illness that has occurred. It also includes preventing complication or deterioration.
4. The correct answer is 1. This man is strictly defining health as the absence of disease.
5. The correct answer is 4. We have no information to decide her health is poor; what we know is she plans to improve her health. However, her environment is unfavorable.

Chapter 20
1. The correct answer is 1. In the precontemplation stage, the person does not intend to change a high-risk behavior in the foreseeable future (the next 6 months); however, the person may agree to make changes under pressure from family and friends. These changes are usually minimal and last only as long as pressure continues to be applied.
2. The correct answer is 4. Perceived barriers refers to perceived negative aspects of a health action or the perceived impediments to undertaking the recommended behaviors. In this case, the client is expressing that it will be difficult to make dietary changes that have been long-standing.
3. The correct answer is 2. The value-expectancy theory suggests that behavior is rational and economical. Furthermore, people will not invest in a goal if they perceive that the goal is impossible to achieve. This is why, for some people, achieving small steps is more successful than attempting major change, in this case, a more manageable exercise program.
4. The correct answer is 3. *Health-seeking behaviors* is appropriate when a person is in a state of wellness but is seeking ways to achieve a higher level of wellness. This nursing diagnosis applies to this client.
5. The correct answer is 2. Support groups provide a means of social support to clients and may be very effective in helping clients achieve and maintain health goals.

Chapter 21
1. The correct answer is 4. In the excretion phase, medications are eliminated from the body. Because the kidneys are a prime organ of excretion, it is likely that medication dosages will need to be reduced for several ordered medications.
2. The correct answer is 4. The physician who wrote the original order should be contacted to clarify what the order was intended to convey.
3. The correct answer is 3. The next action should be one that obtains additional information on the herbs used, amounts and type of preparation, and frequency of use. Once this information is known, the list can be compared to medications ordered for the client to determine contraindications or increased risk of adverse effects.
4. The correct answer is 4. If the dose is 6 mg and each tablet has 2 mg, then 3 tablets are needed to administer the correct dose.
5. The correct answer is 4. The client described in the question is overweight and will have an increased amount of subcutaneous tissue to penetrate before reaching muscle tissue. For this reason, a $1\frac{1}{2}$-inch needle would be a better choice than a 1-inch needle.

Chapter 22
1. The correct answer is 3. When a client can transmit an infection by respiratory secretions or droplets, then the client needs to be placed on droplet precautions.
2. The correct answer is 1. The nurse would put on the gown first.
3. The correct answer is 4. Because corticosteroids and diabetes delay healing, this client is at increased risk for ineffective protection.
4. The correct answer is 3. Malaise is one of a cluster of symptoms that may be noted when a client develops a systemic infection.
5. The correct answer is 4. The flap that is toward the nurse is opened last.

Chapter 23
1. The correct answer is 3. Clients are often injured from a fall when attempting to climb over the side rails. Two side rails up serves as a reminder to call for help without creating a barrier of four side rails, which may actually increase the risk for injury.
2. The correct answer is 1. This client has the most risk factors.
3. The correct answer is 1. Your objective is to immediately get unsafe equipment out of the room.
4. The correct answer is 3. The first step in RACE is to rescue the client.
5. The correct answer is 3. Because she could do serious damage to herself, an immediate solution to the problem is required. Follow up with a call to the physician for a restraint order. Reevaluate the need for restraints frequently, and consider other solutions.

Chapter 24
1. The correct answer is 3. Vitamin A is a fat-soluble vitamin, which is stored by the body. For this reason, it is important not to take excessive supplements to avoid toxicity.
2. The correct answer is 1. The most popular and easiest method for obtaining data about dietary intake is the 24-hour recall. The client is asked to recall everything eaten the previous day or within the last 24 hours.
3. The correct answer is 4. The normal body mass index is 18.5 to 24.9. This client should be further evaluated for overweight status.
4. The correct answer is 3. Two minerals of special concern include iron in girls from the time they begin menstruation and calcium in both boys and girls for bone growth and optimal bone mass. Adequate calcium remains one of the best protectors against age-related bone loss and fractures.
5. The correct answer is 4. Eggs belong to the meat and beans food group.

Chapter 25

1. The correct answer is 3. Eating disorders affect adolescent girls with greater frequency than boys. However, girls and boys who compete in sports requiring low body fat, such as track, dance, rowing, gymnastics, or wrestling, are more at risk for eating disorders in the unspecified category.
2. The correct answer is 4. Because of greatly restricted voluntary intake of calories and nutrients, the client with anorexia nervosa is likely to have the nursing diagnosis *Imbalanced nutrition: less than body requirements.*
3. The correct answer is 2. Salt intake can worsen high blood pressure (hypertension) and possibly aggravate other cardiac conditions in which the client is at risk for fluid overload, such as heart failure.
4. The correct answer is 2. To reduce the risk of aspiration, the head of bed should be elevated to at least 30 degrees.
5. The correct answer is 1. Infection is a serious complication of TPN therapy, because the increased dextrose load provides an excellent medium for bacterial growth. Fever is a sign of infection, whereas the other vital signs do not reflect this risk.

Chapter 26

1. The correct answer is 2. Abnormal potassium levels can lead to cardiac dysrhythmias. The normal reference range for serum potassium is 3.5 to 5.0 mEq/L.
2. The correct answer is 4. Weight is a reliable indicator of fluid status. One kilogram of weight (2.2 pounds) is equal to 1000 mL of fluid.
3. The correct answer is 2. The low pH and high CO_2 indicate that the client has a respiratory acidosis.
4. The correct answer is 3. A preliminary action for nursing procedures is to explain the procedure to the client.
5. The correct answer is 2. The flow rate of an intravenous infusion should be checked once per hour.

Chapter 27

1. The correct answer is 3. Redness, warmth, and heat after the third to fourth postoperative day are signs of infection.
2. The correct answer is 2. Infection in chronic wounds include the classic manifestations of pain, erythema, swelling, and purulent drainage, as well as delayed wound healing, friable granulation tissue, discoloration of granulation tissue, foul odor, and serous drainage accompanied by inflammation.
3. The correct answer is 4. A nurse is unable to stage ulcers with necrotic tissue because he or she is unable to detect the depth of the wound until the necrotic tissue is removed.
4. The correct answer is 1. The bacteria may not be present in all parts of the wound; therefore you should cover the entire wound bed.
5. The correct answer is 2. Vacuum-assisted wound therapy is used for a large wound with a large amount of drainage.

Chapter 28

1. The correct answer is 1. During the initiation phase of fever, pyrogens act on the hypothalamus to reset the temperature set-point to higher than body temperature. The client will feel cold and may have chills.
2. The correct answer is 4. Any hospitalized client is at risk for fever caused by infection. However, immunosuppressed people are at particular risk. The client who had gallbladder surgery is not immunosuppressed, whereas the other clients are. Examples of causes of immunosuppression include neoplasms (cancer), infection with human immunodeficiency virus, and medications received after an organ transplant.
3. The correct answer is 2. Expected outcomes for the client with hypothermia include return of body temperature to normal and absence of complications. Because the area involved suffered damage such as necrosis, the goal of care for minimal to no tissue necrosis was not fully met.
4. The correct answer is 3. The nurse would expect to implement the use of a cooling blanket with an appropriate physician order and only if the temperature spikes to a high level despite treatment with other measures.
5. The correct answer is 2. The temperature of clients at risk for infection should be measured every 4 hours. It is unnecessary to monitor the temperature more frequently because the client does not actually have a fever. If temperature is monitored less frequently than every 4 hours, a febrile episode may occur between temperature measurements.

Chapter 29

1. The correct answer is 1. GoLYTELY is a large volume of a fluid and electrolyte solution; therefore it is less likely to deplete the body's fluids and electrolytes.
2. The correct answer is 4. Fluid loss can result in dehydration, which would be the most serious consequence of diarrhea.
3. The correct answer is 2. Frequent passage of small, liquid stool is characteristic of fecal impaction.
4. The correct answer is 2. An oil retention enema will lubricate a hard mass of stool.
5. The correct answer is 2. Answer 2 has the most fiber; fiber in the diet assists peristalsis.

Chapter 30

1. The correct answer is 2. Age alone is insufficient as a cause of urinary incontinence. You should provide adequate fluids and help her to a bedside commode or bathroom at frequent intervals.
2. The correct answer is 4. Standing is the most natural position for most men to urinate.
3. The correct answer is 2. The Kegel exercises are a simple, noninvasive method of controlling stress incontinence.
4. The correct answer is 2. Foley catheters should not be used solely for the purpose of managing incontinence because of the infection rate.
5. The correct answer is 2. Dependent coils will collect urine, which could grow bacteria, which can migrate up the tubing.

Chapter 31

1. The correct answer is 3. The sebaceous glands secrete an oily substance called sebum, which helps to keep the skin soft and supple and inhibits the growth of certain bacteria on the skin.
2. The correct answer is 4. Gingivitis is an inflammation of the gums usually manifested by the primary symptom of bleeding of the gums.
3. The correct answer is 1. Giving a complete bed bath is giving the complete bath without any assistance from the client.
4. The correct answer is 2. A surgical bed is made for the client who is returning from the operating room on a stretcher. It is an *open bed* and the sheets are fanfolded to one side of the bed to receive the client from a stretcher.
5. The correct answer is 4. A sitz bath is given to decrease pain and inflammation for pain relief from hemorrhoids.

Chapter 32

1. The correct answer is 2. Scoliosis, which is a lateral deviation of the spine, is typically diagnosed in preadolescent and adolescent children.
2. The correct answer is 4. The standard walker is used for clients who can bear partial weight, and it must be picked up to be used correctly. Therefore the upper body strength must be adequate.
3. The correct answer is 1. This step is done first.
4. The correct answer is 4. The transfer belt allows the nurse to guide the client, and it offers support during the transfer.
5. The correct answer is 2. Before teaching a client to ambulate with crutches, the nurse should check the distance between the axilla and the top of the crutch. It should be at least three finger widths, or 1 to 2 inches (2.5 to 5 cm). If the crutches are not the correct length, the client could sustain axillary nerve damage.

Chapter 33

1. The correct answer is 1. The suddenness of the symptoms make you suspect pulmonary embolism; symptoms of pneumonia would not develop as rapidly.
2. The correct answer is 3. If you move her up too far and she slides down in bed when you raise her head, a shearing force may be created.
3. The correct answer is 1. The combination of antiembolism stockings and passive leg exercises prevents venous stasis.
4. The correct answer is 2. The client should move slowly, allowing time for the circulation to adjust to the position change. Good fluid balance may help in conjunction with moving slowly.
5. The correct answer is 2. She should be able to assist you with turning her. This time would not be appropriate for teaching her to turn herself.

Chapter 34

1. The correct answer is 2, 3, 4, 5, 6. You are assessing her for her respiratory status but also considering that oxygen deficit can affect all body system. More pertinent than S_1 and S_2 heart sounds is whether or not she has an irregular heart rhythm. Pedal pulses are generally assessed to determine arterial occlusive disease.
2. The correct answer is 1. Wheezes indicates narrowed airways, which causes airway resistance.
3. The correct answer is 2. Standing erect is the only position that does not limit expansion of the chest.
4. The correct answer is 3. Dyspnea is a subjective complaint of difficult breathing. Each of the other answers could be an indication that the client may be having a problem with breathing, but you need to verify it with the client.
5. The correct answer is 3. There are earlier signs of hypoxemia present. The student may have mistaken unconsciousness for sleeping. She should have aroused the client, had her take deep breaths, measured her oxygen saturation with the pulse oximeter, and called the staff nurse to the bedside.
6. The correct answer is 1. A face mask provides 40% oxygen at 6 LPM to 65% oxygen at 12 LPM. A nasal cannula provides up to 40% oxygen at 6 LPM but is highly irritating to the nose. At higher liter flows a face mask should be used.

Chapter 35

1. The correct answer is 3. You need to check the pulses to determine that a blood clot has not formed in the artery and observe the site for bleeding.
2. The correct answer is 2. The other menus have at least one item that is high in fat.
3. The correct answer is 1. This tachycardia would decrease cardiac output. All of the data in answer 1 are consistent with decreased cardiac output.
4. The correct answer is 1. Coumadin is an anticoagulant, and his INR is at the upper range. It will not affect his blood pressure, it is unaffected by sodium, and the prescription is often continued for life.
5. The correct answer is 3. Because he has attacks infrequently, a prn medication may be sufficient.

Chapter 36

1. The correct answer is 4. Rapid eye movement (REM) sleep is the stage of sleep characterized by rapid saccadic movement of the eyes. During this stage, the activity of the brain's neurons is quite similar to that during waking hours. Most of the vividly recalled dreams occur during REM sleep.
2. The correct answer is 1. Decreasing liquids 2 to 4 hours before bedtime can help decrease the need to void during the night.
3. The correct answer is 2. Narcolepsy is characterized by abnormal sleep tendencies as well as by pathological REM sleep, manifested as excessive daytime sleepiness, disturbed nighttime sleep, cataplexy, sleep paralysis, and hypnagogic hallucinations.
4. The correct answer is 3. Developing a bedtime routine helps establish good sleep habits.
5. The correct answer is 1. Infants sleep an average of 16 to 17 hours a day. However, they often alternate between REM sleep and wakefulness, skipping stages 1 through 4 of NREM. This phenomenon shortens the duration of each sleep period. Their sleep cycle is also shorter, lasting about 40 to 50 minutes instead of 90.

Chapter 37

1. The correct answer is 2. The rating scale is used to assess the intensity of pain, with 0 being no pain and 10 being the most severe.
2. The correct answer is 4. Because arthritis is a chronic condition, this client is most likely to be at risk for chronic pain.
3. The correct answer is 1. It is true that children will not always tell you when they are in pain, so it is important to diligently assess for pain in children.
4. The correct answer is 2. Opioid analgesics are metabolized by the liver and are excreted by the kidneys; therefore they may be contraindicated in certain instances of hepatic or renal dysfunction.
5. The correct answer is 4. Clients who are the best candidates for PCA are those who are alert and have the cognitive ability to use the device.

Chapter 38

1. The correct answer is 2. Furosemide (a diuretic) and aminoglycosides (antibiotics), among others, can cause ototoxicity.
2. The correct answer is 4. A Snellen eye chart is used to measure both near and distance vision.
3. The correct answer is 1. Facing the client while speaking enables the client to read the lips as well as listen to a communication.
4. The correct answer is 2. Directing the fluid toward the posterior wall of the ear canal prevents accidental damage to the tympanic membrane.
5. The correct answer is 4. Bright lights can cause glare and further impair vision for a client who is already visually impaired.

Chapter 39

1. The correct answer is 2. This is a true statement. Communication is vital to human interactions beginning with the first interactions between a mother and an infant and continuing throughout the life span.
2. The correct answer is 4. Wernicke's area is located in the brain and is responsible for comprehension of speech and is not considered a component of the anatomy of sound production.
3. The correct answer is 1. These are lifestyle factors that affect verbal communication.
4. The correct answer is 2. The diagnosis of *Impaired verbal communication* is the problem clients with expressive (Broca's) aphasia have because they have difficulty with verbally expressing their needs.
5. The correct answer is 4. Alternative communication methods help ensure that the client can communicate needs to the nurse, which reduces the frustration of not being able to vocalize them.

Chapter 40

1. The correct answer is 1. It is difficult for a person with chronic confusion to learn; however, with time, patience, and repetition, new learning can take place, at least in some cases.
2. The correct answer is 2. Although she does have chronic confusion, you should look for causes of acute confusion before concluding her symptoms are chronic. Oxygen deficit is the first thing you should suspect.
3. The correct answer is 2. Seeing her dead husband is likely a hallucination.
4. The correct answer is 4. The information she can give is generally enough to determine that she is oriented but is insufficient to determine the absence of confusion.
5. The correct answer is 1. The best way to avoid catastrophic events is to recognize triggers to these events and avoid the triggers.

Chapter 41

1 The correct answer is 2. The client is making a statement about her view of herself.
2. The correct answer is 2. Learning to be independent in the use of a toilet is learning autonomy.
3. The correct answer is 3. Having self-esteem is often built on positive relationships with others.
4. The correct answer is 2. Each person will have his or her own time frame for adjustment. The nurse should allow time to experience the impact of the event and for the meaning of the event to come into conscious awareness.
5. The correct answer is 4. The client must be involved in developing goals and outcomes; otherwise the client is unlikely to work toward goal attainment.

Chapter 42

1. The correct answer is 1. Hyperventilation is a physical symptom of stress.
2. The correct answer is 4. Learning to identify situations that trigger anxiety will help the client deal with the anxiety.
3. The correct answer is 1. These are the divisions of the autonomic nervous system.
4. The correct answer is 1. These are symptoms of mild anxiety.
5. The correct answer is 3. Anxiety does not directly affect the client's financial status.

Chapter 43

1. The correct answer is 1. A population is a group of people who share common characteristics.
2. The correct answer is 3. Vulnerable populations are those with limited resources and social support.
3. The correct answer is 4. Individuals 85 years old or older are at greatest risk for suicide.
4. The correct answer is 4. These factors are demographic data.
5. The correct answer is 2. Although communication is a part of the empowerment process, empowerment is not achieved through communication alone.

Chapter 44

1. The correct answer is 3. The social worker is the team member who knows the most about medical insurance coverage. The other team members listed are not considered the experts in this area, and this is not the focus of their job
2. The correct answer is 3. This is the only answer that combines all of the components of an interdisciplinary team goal: it is measurable, time-limited, and realistic, and it involves several team members. Each of the other choices leaves out an essential component.
3. The correct answer is 4. All or any of the answers may be correct, depending on the multiple factors that affect rehabilitation and recovery, as discussed in this chapter.
4. The correct answer is 4. Swallowing problems is the only answer that does not directly relate to defining characteristics of *Ineffective role performance.* All of the other choices are appropriate.
5. The correct answer is 3. The FIM scale is the most widely used and reliable scale for measuring functional independence. The Barthel and Katz are fine instruments but not as comprehensive or widely tested as the FIM. The Kenny self-care scale is fictitious.

Chapter 45

1. The correct answer is 4. Reflection is the middle phase in which the person is attempting to achieve stability and control while reconciling the loss. Answer 1 is the first stage; answer 3 is the last stage; answer 2 often happens in the last stage.
2. The correct answer is 3. Disenfranchised grief lacks social acknowledgment, validation, and support for the bereaved.
3. The correct answer is 2. She is experiencing a normal feeling that her father is there.
4. The correct answer is 1. Reduced peripheral circulation could reduce the absorption of intramuscular medications.
5. The correct answer is 1. Secretion accumulation in the lungs is sometimes called "death rattle."

Chapter 46

1. The correct answer is 2. A nurse with awareness of his or her feelings, thoughts, and personal biases concerning sexual matters is best able to assist clients with sexual disorders.
2. The correct answer is 3. The most important knowledge a nurse can have is to understand his or her own personal views before working with clients with sexual dysfunctions.
3. The correct answer is 3. Securing quiet family time and being honest with children will help them feel secure. Using calm and easy language will help them.
4. The correct answer is 3. This answer would create unnecessary fear and is not true. Although death may occur during

sex, it is uncommon and not necessarily related to a prior heart attack.

5. The correct answer is 2. The accepted term is *sexual partner.* You may also use such words as *significant other* or *your partner.*

Chapter 47

1. The correct answer is 3. A developmental crisis occurs when a person is unable to complete the tasks for a particular developmental level.
2. The correct answer is 3. Regression is behaving in ways that were appropriate at earlier developmental periods.
3. The correct answer is 3. Exercise is not a long-term solution against stressors.
4. The correct answer is 3. Interventions to increase coping skills require establishing a therapeutic relationship and setting mutual goals with the client.
5. The correct answer is 2. Imagery is using your imagination to go to an imaginary place, situation, or event that is relaxing.

Chapter 48

1. The correct answer is 2. A binuclear family refers to the postdivorced family in which the children are part of two nuclear families with varying degrees of cooperation (i.e., co-parenting and joint custody) and time spent in each household.
2. The correct answer is 1. Affective function needs are met by providing psychosocial protection and support of the family members.
3. The correct answer is 3. An effective coping skill is when families discuss their problems.
4. The correct answer is 3. *Caregiver role strain* can occur when there are unresolved conflicts between the caregiver and care recipient or when there is resentment, anger, or guilt about taking on the role of caregiver.
5. The correct answer is 4. The role of the nurse is to assist the family caregiver with other available options or to obtain an order for a social service referral.

Chapter 49

1. The correct answer is 3. *Spiritual distress* is an impaired ability to experience and integrate meaning in life through connections. The client expresses this distress both verbally and behaviorally. Sometimes it is a direct expression of loss of faith, anger at God, or questioning the meaning of life and death. Often the subject arises when the client cannot sleep, is crying, or has other obvious signs of distress.
2. The correct answer is 2. Religiosity represents a person's dependence on and involvement in religious practices and behaviors.
3. The correct answer is 3. An expected outcome for a client who expresses questions about the meaning of life or suffering would be that the client will experience a greater sense of meaning, purpose, and hope in living with an illness.
4. The correct answer is 4. Any person with an illness may suddenly be faced with doubts and fears about being dependent on others or dying. Dwelling on such feelings may cause considerable spiritual distress. It is very helpful to acknowledge how terrible such feelings and fears can be. Be sure to stress that grappling with strong feelings, such as anger, fear, or despair, is normal when facing severe illness or hospitalization.
5. The correct answer is 2. An intervention you can use to help clients find meaning is the use of reminiscence. Through reminiscence, clients can examine their life experiences to discover new meanings or reconnect to forgotten moments that represent significant meaning.

Chapter 50

1. The correct answer is 2. Impaired circulation and decreased renal function may delay recovery from anesthesia.
2. The correct answer is 4. Inserting a straight urinary catheter will immediately relieve bladder distention and discomfort.
3. The correct answer is 4. Pain medications allow clients to manage pain and raise their ability to carry out activities necessary for recovery.
4. The correct answer is 1. Protection of the internal organs from infection is a priority, and a sterile saline dressing will also prevent the dressing from sticking to the organs.
5. The correct answer is 3. The priority assessment is always the client's airway and breathing status.

Appendix A ANA Standards of Nursing Practice and Professional Performance

STANDARD 1. ASSESSMENT

THE REGISTERED NURSE COLLECTS COMPREHENSIVE DATA PERTINENT TO THE PATIENT'S HEALTH OR THE SITUATION.

Measurement Criteria

The registered nurse:

Collects data in a systematic and ongoing process.

Involves the patient, family, other healthcare providers, and environment, as appropriate, in holistic data collection.

Prioritizes data collection activities based on the patient's immediate condition, or anticipated needs of the patient or situation.

Uses appropriate evidence-based assessment techniques and instruments in collecting pertinent data.

Uses analytical models and problem-solving tools.

Synthesizes available data, information, and knowledge relevant to the situation to identify patterns and variances.

Documents relevant data in a retrievable format.

STANDARD 2. DIAGNOSIS

THE REGISTERED NURSE ANALYZES THE ASSESSMENT DATA TO DETERMINE THE DIAGNOSES OR ISSUES.

Measurement Criteria

The registered nurse:

Derives the diagnoses or issues based on assessment data.

Validates the diagnoses or issues with the patient, family, and other healthcare providers when possible and appropriate.

Documents diagnoses or issues in a manner that facilitates the determination of the expected outcomes and plan.

STANDARD 3. OUTCOMES IDENTIFICATION

THE REGISTERED NURSE IDENTIFIES EXPECTED OUTCOMES FOR A PLAN INDIVIDUALIZED TO THE PATIENT OR THE SITUATION.

Measurement Criteria

The registered nurse:

Involves the patient, family, and other healthcare providers in formulating expected outcomes when possible and appropriate.

Derives culturally appropriate expected outcomes from the diagnoses.

Considers associated risks, benefits, costs, current scientific evidence, and clinical expertise when formulating expected outcomes.

Defines expected outcomes in terms of the patient, patient values, ethical considerations, environment, or situation with such consideration as associated risks, benefits and costs, and current scientific evidence.

Includes a time estimate for attainment of expected outcomes. Develops expected outcomes that provide direction for continuity of care.

Modifies expected outcomes based on changes in the status of the patient or evaluation of the situation.

Documents expected outcomes as measurable goals.

STANDARD 4. PLANNING

THE REGISTERED NURSE DEVELOPS A PLAN THAT PRESCRIBES STRATEGIES AND ALTERNATIVES TO ATTAIN EXPECTED OUTCOMES.

Measurement Criteria

The registered nurse:

- Develops an individualized plan considering patient characteristics or the situation (e.g., age and culturally appropriate, environmentally sensitive).
- Develops the plan in conjunction with the patient, family, and others, as appropriate.
- Includes strategies within the plan that address each of the identified diagnoses or issues, which may include strategies for promotion and restoration of health and prevention of illness, injury, and disease.
- Provides for continuity within the plan.
- Incorporates an implementation pathway or timeline within the plan.
- Establishes the plan priorities with the patient, family, and others as appropriate.
- Utilizes the plan to provide direction to other members of the healthcare team.
- Defines the plan to reflect current statutes, rules and regulations, and standards.
- Integrates current trends and research affecting care in the planning process.
- Considers the economic impact of the plan.
- Uses standardized language or recognized terminology to document the plan.

STANDARD 5. IMPLEMENTATION

THE REGISTERED NURSE IMPLEMENTS THE IDENTIFIED PLAN.

Measurement Criteria

The registered nurse:

- Implements the plan in a safe and timely manner.
- Documents implementation and any modifications, including changes to or omissions of the identified plan.
- Utilizes evidence-based interventions and treatments specific to the diagnosis or problem.
- Utilizes community resources and systems to implement the plan.
- Collaborates with nursing colleagues and others to implement the plan.

STANDARD 5A: COORDINATION OF CARE

THE REGISTERED NURSE COORDINATES CARE DELIVERY.

Measurement Criteria

The registered nurse:

- Coordinates implementation of the plan.
- Documents the coordination of the care.

STANDARD 5B: HEALTH TEACHING AND HEALTH PROMOTION

THE REGISTERED NURSE EMPLOYS STRATEGIES TO PROMOTE HEALTH AND A SAFE ENVIRONMENT.

Measurement Criteria

The registered nurse:

- Provides health teaching that addresses such topics as healthy lifestyles, risk-reducing behaviors, developmental needs, activities of daily living, and preventive self-care.
- Uses health promotion and health teaching methods appropriate to the situation and the patient's developmental level, learning needs, readiness, ability to learn, language preference, and culture.
- Seeks opportunities for feedback and evaluation of the effectiveness of the strategies used.

STANDARD 5C: CONSULTATION

THE ADVANCED PRACTICE REGISTERED NURSE AND THE NURSING ROLE SPECIALIST PROVIDE CONSULTATION TO INFLUENCE THE IDENTIFIED PLAN, ENHANCE THE ABILITIES OF OTHERS AND EFFECT CHANGE.

Measurement Criteria for the Advanced Practice Registered Nurse

The advanced practice registered nurse:

- Synthesizes clinical data, theoretical frameworks, and evidence when providing consultation.
- Facilitates the effectiveness of a consultation by involving the patient in decision-making and negotiating role responsibilities.
- Communicates consultation recommendations that facilitate change.

Measurement Criteria for the Nursing Role Specialty

The registered nurse in a nursing role specialty:

- Synthesizes data, information, theoretical frameworks and evidence when providing consultation.
- Facilitates the effectiveness of a consultation by involving the stakeholders in the decision-making process.
- Communicates consultation recommendations that influence the identified plan, facilitate understanding by involved stakeholders, enhance the work of others, and effect change.

STANDARD 5D: PRESCRIPTIVE AUTHORITY AND TREATMENT

THE ADVANCED PRACTICE REGISTERED NURSE USES PRESCRIPTIVE AUTHORITY, PROCEDURES, REFERRALS, TREATMENTS, AND THERAPIES IN ACCORDANCE WITH STATE AND FEDERAL LAWS AND REGULATIONS.

Measurement Criteria for the Advanced Practice Registered Nurse

The advanced practice registered nurse:

Prescribes evidence-based treatments, therapies, and procedures considering the patient's comprehensive healthcare needs.
Prescribes pharmacologic agents based on a current knowledge of pharmacology and physiology.
Prescribes specific pharmacological agents and/or treatments based on clinical indicators, the patient's status and needs, and the results of diagnostic and laboratory tests.
Evaluates therapeutic and potential adverse effects of pharmacological and non-pharmacological treatments.
Provides patients with information about intended effects and potential adverse effects of proposed prescriptive therapies.
Provides information about costs, alternative treatments and procedures, as appropriate.

STANDARD 6. EVALUATION

THE REGISTERED NURSE EVALUATES PROGRESS TOWARDS ATTAINMENT OF OUTCOMES.

Measurement Criteria

The registered nurse:

Conducts a systematic, ongoing, and criterion-based evaluation of the outcomes in relation to the structures and processes prescribed by the plan and the indicated timeline.
Includes the patient and others involved in the care or situation in the evaluative process.
Evaluates the effectiveness of the planned strategies in relation to patient responses and the attainment of the expected outcomes.
Documents the results of the evaluation.
Uses ongoing assessment data to revise the diagnoses, outcomes, the plan, and the implementation as needed.
Disseminates the results to the patient and others involved in the care or situation, as appropriate, in accordance with state and federal laws and regulations.

ANA STANDARDS OF PROFESSIONAL PERFORMANCE

STANDARD 7. QUALITY OF PRACTICE

THE REGISTERED NURSE SYSTEMATICALLY ENHANCES THE QUALITY AND EFFECTIVENESS OF NURSING PRACTICE.

Measurement Criteria

The registered nurse:

Demonstrates quality by documenting the application of the nursing process in a responsible, accountable, and ethical manner.
Uses the results of quality improvement activities to initiate changes in nursing practice and in the healthcare delivery system.
Uses creativity and innovation in nursing practice to improve care delivery.
Incorporates new knowledge to initiate changes in nursing practice if desired outcomes are not achieved.
Participates in quality improvement activities. Such activities may include:
Identifying aspects of practice important for quality monitoring.
Using indicators developed to monitor quality and effectiveness of nursing practice.
Collecting data to monitor quality and effectiveness of nursing practice.
Analyzing quality data to identify opportunities for improving nursing practice.
Formulating recommendations to improve nursing practice or outcomes.
Implementing activities to enhance the quality of nursing practice.
Developing, implementing, and evaluating policies, procedures and/or guidelines to improve the quality of practice.
Participating on interdisciplinary teams to evaluate clinical care or health services.
Participating in efforts to minimize costs and unnecessary duplication.
Analyzing factors related to safety, satisfaction, effectiveness, and cost/benefit options.
Analyzing organizational systems for barriers
Implementing processes to remove or decrease barriers within organizational systems.

STANDARD 8. EDUCATION

THE REGISTERED NURSE ATTAINS KNOWLEDGE AND COMPETENCY THAT REFLECTS CURRENT NURSING PRACTICE.

Measurement Criteria

The registered nurse:

Participates in ongoing educational activities related to appropriate knowledge bases and professional issues.

Demonstrates a commitment to lifelong learning through self-reflection and inquiry to identify learning needs.
Seeks experiences that reflect current practice in order to maintain skills and competence in clinical practice or role performance.
Acquires knowledge and skills appropriate to the specialty area, practice setting, role, or situation.
Maintains professional records that provide evidence of competency and lifelong learning.
Seeks experiences and formal and independent learning activities to maintain and develop clinical and professional skills and knowledge.

STANDARD 9. PROFESSIONAL PRACTICE EVALUATION

THE REGISTERED NURSE EVALUATES ONE'S OWN NURSING PRACTICE IN RELATION TO PROFESSIONAL PRACTICE STANDARDS AND GUIDELINES, RELEVANT STATUTES, RULES, AND REGULATIONS.

Measurement Criteria

The registered nurse's practice reflects the application of knowledge of current practice standards, guidelines, statutes, rules, and regulations.

The registered nurse:

Provides age-appropriate care in a culturally and ethnically sensitive manner.
Engages in self-evaluation of practice on a regular basis, identifying areas of strength as well as areas in which professional development would be beneficial.
Obtains informal feedback regarding one's own practice from patients, peers, professional colleagues, and others.
Participates in systematic peer review as appropriate.
Takes action to achieve goals identified during the evaluation process.
Provides rationales for practice beliefs, decisions, and actions as part of the informal and formal evaluation processes.

STANDARD 10. COLLEGIALITY

THE REGISTERED NURSE INTERACTS WITH AND CONTRIBUTES TO THE PROFESSIONAL DEVELOPMENT OF PEERS AND COLLEAGUES.

Measurement Criteria

The registered nurse:

Shares knowledge and skills with peers and colleagues as evidenced by such activities as patient care conferences or presentations at formal or informal meetings.
Provides peers with feedback regarding their practice and/or role performance.
Interacts with peers and colleagues to enhance one's own professional nursing practice and/or role performance.
Maintains compassionate and caring relationships with peers and colleagues.
Contributes to an environment that is conducive to the education of healthcare professionals.
Contributes to a supportive and healthy work environment.

STANDARD 11. COLLABORATION

THE REGISTERED NURSE COLLABORATES WITH PATIENT, FAMILY, AND OTHERS IN THE CONDUCT OF NURSING PRACTICE.

Measurement Criteria

The registered nurse:

Communicates with patient, family, and healthcare providers regarding patient care and the nurse's role in the provision of that care.
Collaborates in creating a documented plan focused on outcomes and decisions related to care and delivery of services that indicates communication with patients, families, and others.
Partners with others to effect change and generate positive outcomes through knowledge of the patient or situation.
Documents referrals, including provisions for continuity of care.

STANDARD 12. ETHICS

THE REGISTERED NURSE INTEGRATES ETHICAL PROVISIONS IN ALL AREAS OF PRACTICE.

Measurement Criteria

The registered nurse:

Uses the Code of Ethics for Nurses With Interpretive Statements (ANA, 2001) to guide practice.
Delivers care in a manner that preserves and protects patient autonomy, dignity, and rights.
Maintains patient confidentiality within legal and regulatory parameters.
Serves as a patient advocate assisting patients in developing skills for self advocacy.
Maintains a therapeutic and professional patient-nurse relationship with appropriate professional role boundaries.
Demonstrates a commitment to practicing self-care, managing stress, and connecting with self and others.
Contributes to resolving ethical issues of patients, colleagues, or systems as evidenced in such activities as participating on ethics committees.
Reports illegal, incompetent, or impaired practices.

STANDARD 13. RESEARCH

THE REGISTERED NURSE INTEGRATES RESEARCH FINDINGS INTO PRACTICE.

Measurement Criteria

The registered nurse:

Utilizes the best available evidence, including research findings, to guide practice decisions.

Actively participates in research activities at various levels appropriate to the nurse's level of education and position. Such activities may include:

Identifying clinical problems specific to nursing research (patient care and nursing practice).

Participating in data collection (surveys, pilot projects, formal studies).

Participating in a formal committee or program.

Sharing research activities and/or findings with peers and others.

Conducting research.

Critically analyzing and interpreting research for application to practice.

Using research findings in the development of policies, procedures, and standards of practice in patient care.

Incorporating research as a basis for learning.

STANDARD 14. RESOURCE UTILIZATION

THE REGISTERED NURSE CONSIDERS FACTORS RELATED TO SAFETY, EFFECTIVENESS, COST, AND IMPACT ON PRACTICE IN THE PLANNING AND DELIVERY OF NURSING SERVICES.

Measurement Criteria

The registered nurse:

Evaluates factors such as safety, effectiveness, availability, cost and benefits, efficiencies, and impact on practice, when choosing practice options that would result in the same expected outcome.

Assists the patient and family in identifying and securing appropriate and available services to address health-related needs.

Assigns or delegates tasks, based on the needs and condition of the patient, potential for harm, stability of the patient's condition, complexity of the task, and predictability of the outcome.

Assists the patient and family in becoming informed consumers about the options, costs, risks, and benefits of treatment and care.

STANDARD 15: LEADERSHIP

THE REGISTERED NURSE PROVIDES LEADERSHIP IN THE PROFESSIONAL PRACTICE SETTING AND THE PROFESSION.

Measurement Criteria

The registered nurse:

Engages in teamwork as a team player and a team builder.

Works to create and maintain healthy work environments in local, regional, national, or international communities.

Displays the ability to define a clear vision, the associated goals, and a plan to implement and measure progress.

Demonstrates a commitment to continuous, lifelong learning for self and others.

Teaches others to succeed by mentoring and other strategies.

Exhibits creativity and flexibility through times of change.

Demonstrates energy, excitement, and a passion for quality work.

Willingly accepts mistakes by self and others, thereby creating a culture in which risk-taking is not only safe, but expected.

Inspires loyalty through valuing of people as the most precious asset in an organization.

Directs the coordination of care across settings and among caregivers, including oversight of licensed and unlicensed personnel in any assigned or delegated tasks.

Serves in key roles in the work setting by participating on committees, councils, and administrative teams.

Promotes advancement of the profession through participation in professional organizations.

Appendix B

Abbreviations Used in Documentation

a	of each
Abn	abnormal
ADA	American Diabetes Association, American Dietetic Association
ADLs	activities of daily living
ad lib	as desired
AKA	above-knee amputation
AM	before noon (morning)
AMA	against medical advice
amt.	amount
ax	axillary
B; bil.	bilateral
bid	twice a day
BP; B/P	blood pressure
BR	bed rest
BRP	bathroom privileges
bs; BS	breath sounds
BS	bedside
BSC	bedside commode
c̄	with
cath	catheter or catheterization
CBB	complete bed bath
CBR	complete bed rest
CC	chief complaint
c/o	complains of
DOA	dead on arrival or date of admission
DOB	date of birth
DTR	deep tendon reflexes
Dx.	diagnosis
EBL	estimated blood loss
e.g.	for example
ENT	ear, nose, throat
EOM	extraocular movement
etiol.	etiology
ETOH	alcohol
fx	fracture
GI	gastrointestinal
GU	genitourinary
gyn	gynecology
h; hr	hour
H/A	headache
HEENT	head, eyes, ears, nose, throat
HL	heparin lock
H_2O	water
H_2O_2	hydrogen peroxide
HOB	head of bed
hosp.	hospital
H&P	history and physical
ht.	height
Hx.	history
ICU	intensive care unit
I&D	incise and drain
I&O	intake and output
IV	intravenous
IVF	intravenous fluids
IVPB	intravenous piggyback
JCAHO	Joint Commission on Accreditation of Healthcare Organizations
KVO; TKO	keep vein open; to keep open
L	liter
L; lt.	left
lb; #	pound
LLE	left lower extremity
LLL	left lower lobe
LLQ	left lower quadrant
LMP	last menstrual period
LOC	level of consciousness
maew	moves all extremities well
MD	medical doctor
NG; N/G	nasogastric
NKA	no known allergies
noct.	nighttime
NPO	nothing by mouth
N&V	nausea and vomiting
NVD	normal vaginal delivery
o; os	orally; by mouth
O_2	oxygen
OOB	out of bed (up and about)
OP	outpatient
OR	operating room
OT	occupational therapy
OTC	over the counter
p̄	after
pc	after meals
PEARL	pupils equal and reactive to light
per	by
PERRL	pupils equal, round, reactive to light
PERRLA	pupils equal, round, reactive to light with accommodation
PM	after noon
PMH	previous medical history
PND	paroxysmal nocturnal dyspnea
PO	by mouth
POD	postoperative day

postop.	postoperative
PP	postpartum
prep	prepare for
prn	as needed
pt.	patient
PT	physical therapy
q	every
qh	every hour
qid	four times a day
qs	sufficient quantity
RLE	right lower extremity
RLL	right lower lobe
RLQ	right lower quadrant
ROM	range of motion
R; rt.	right
R/T	related to
RTO	return to office
RUQ	right upper quadrant
Rx	prescription, treatment
$\bar{s}$	without
S/P	status post
SR	side rail
S/S	signs and symptoms
surg.	surgery
sym	symmetrical
TBA	to be absorbed
temp.	temperature
tid	three times a day
TLC	tender loving care
t.o.	telephone order
TPR	temperature, pulse, and respiration
tx.	treatment
UO	urinary output
V.O.; v.o.	verbal order
vol.	volume
VS	vital signs
W/C	wheelchair
WD	warm and dry
WD/WN	well developed, well nourished
WNL	within normal limits
wt.	weight, weigh
y/o	years old

Appendix C

Quick Guide to Medical Terminology

GENERAL GUIDELINES FOR USING TERMS

1. Divide the words into component parts.
   a. Root: foundation of the term
   b. Suffix: word ending
   c. Prefix: word beginning
   d. Combining vowel: often the letter "o" links the components
2. Interpret the word.
   a. Start with the suffix, then read the beginning and middle.
3. Spelling: Drop the combining vowel before a suffix beginning with a vowel, but keep it when it occurs between two root words.
4. Pronounce the word.
   a. Pronounce one component at a time. The following hints may help:
      i. Pronounce "-es" at the end of a word as a separate syllable, "-eez" (example: nares).
      ii. Pronounce "-i" (when it forms a plural at the end of a word) as "eye."
      iii. Pronounce "pn" as an "n" (example: pneumothorax).
      iv. The "ch" is often pronounced as a "k" (example: chronic, chromic).
   b. Decide which syllable to emphasize.
      i. Use a dictionary.
      ii. Often the emphasis comes in the second syllable for three-syllable words, and in the third syllable for four-or-more syllable words.
      iii. As you become more facile with medical terminology, the proper placing of the accent will become more natural.

KEY PREFIXES

DESCRIBING TIME AND PLACE

ante-	before
anti-	against
circum-	around
contra-	opposite, against
dorso-, dorsi-	back
endo-	within
epi-	on, over, upon
extra-	outside of
gen-	beginning, origin
hypo-	below, under
inter-	between parts
intra-	within a part
juxta-	near
medi-	middle
noct-	night
para-	beside, beyond
peri-	around
post-	after
pre-	before
sub-	beneath
supra-	above

RELATED TO TYPE

a-, an-	without, absent
ankyl-	crooked, bent, fused, stiff
auto-	self
bio-	life
brady-	slow
eu-	good, true, normal
glyco-, gluco-	sugar, sweet
hetero-	other, different
homo-	same
hydro-	water
iso-	same, equal
mal-	bad
neo-	new, new and different
non-	not
normo-	normal
ortho-	straight, erect, correct, normal
oxy-	sharp, acute
path-	disease, suffering
pseudo-	false
sclero-	hard
tachy-	fast
toxic-	poisonous
xero-	dry

DESCRIBING DIRECTION

ab-	away from
ad-	toward, to
de-	away, not, down
dextro-	right
e-	out
ex-	away from, out completely
par-	aside, beyond, apart, from, against
re-	back, again
retro-	backward, behind
sinister(o)-	left

DESCRIBING NUMBER OR QUANTITY

ambi-, amphi-	both
bi-	two
centi-	100
deca-	10
di-, dis-	twice, doubly
diplo-	double
hemi-	half
holo-	whole, all
milli-	1000
mono-	one
multi-	many
nulli-	none
pan-	all
poly-	many
quadr(i)-	four
semi-	half
tetra-	four
tri-	three
uni-	one

DESCRIBING SIZE AND AMOUNT

brachy-	short
brevi-	short, slow
macro-, mega-	large
micro-	small
olig(o)-	little, small scanty, deficient

DENOTING COLOR

alba-	white
chloro-	green
cirrh-	yellow
cyano-	blue
erythro-	red
leuko-	white
lute-	yellow
nigro-	black
rube-	red
xantho-	yellow

MISCELLANEOUS

pyo-	pus
pyro-	fever, heat

KEY SUFFIXES

NOUN SUFFIXES

-ance	quality or act of
-cide	killer
-ectasia, -ectasis	dilation or expansion of
-form	shape
-gen	production of
-ician, -ist	one charged with or skilled in
-meter	measure
-ology	study of
-phylaxis	protection
-poiesis	production of, formation of
-stenia	strength

ADJECTIVAL SUFFIXES

-ac	pertaining to
-ad	toward, in the direction of
-al	pertaining to
-ary	that which is, pertaining to
-fugal	driving or traveling away from
-ic	pertaining to
-trophic	related to nutrition, growth, development
-tropic	turning toward, or changing

DENOTING A STATE OR CONDITION

-algia	pain
-atresia	abnormal closure
-cele	swelling, tumor
-cyst	bladderlike sac
-dynia	pain
-ema	swelling, distention
-emia	in the blood
-esthesia	feeling, nervous sensation
-ia, -iasis	a diseased condition
-ism	a condition of
-itis	inflammation
-kinesia	movement
-lepsy	seizure
-lexia	words, speech
-malacia	softening
-oma	tumor
-paresis	slight paralysis
-pathy	suffering, disease
-penia	deficiency, lack
-phagia	swallowing
-phasia	speech
-philia	love of
-phobia	fear of
-plegia	paralysis
-praxia	action
-ptosis	dropping, or downward displacement
-rrhage, -rrhagia	bursting forth
-rrhea	flow, discharge
-stasis	state of being at a standstill
-sthenia	strength
-tonia	stretching, putting under tension
-vert	turn

RELATED TO A SURGICAL OR DIAGNOSTIC PROCEDURE

-centesis	puncture of a cavity
-cis	cut
-desis	binding, fusion
-ectomy	excision, cutting out
-gram, -graphy	act or method of recording
-lysis	setting free, dissolution
-ostomy	creation of a mouth or opening
-otomy	cutting into
-pexy	fixation
-plasty	molding or shaping
-scope, -scopy	looking at, examining
-sect	cut
-tome	instrument for cutting
-tripsy	rubbing or crushing

RELATED TO CHEMICAL COMPOUNDS

-ase	enzyme
-ol	oil, or alcohol
-ose	carbohydrate
-yl	matter, substance, a radical

MISCELLANEOUS

-sepsis	infection
-septemia	infection in the blood

KEY SUFFIXES/PREFIXES BY BODY SYSTEM

CARDIOVASCULAR/RESPIRATORY/BLOOD

COMBINING FORM	RELATED STRUCTURE	EXAMPLE	DEFINITION OF EXAMPLE
adenoido-	adenoids	adenoidectomy	cutting out of the adenoids
alveolo-	air sac, alveolus	alveolar	pertaining to the alveoli
angio-	vessel	angiogram	radiographic recording of blood vessels
aorto-	aorta	aortogram	radiographic recording of the aorta
artero-, arterio-	artery	arteriosclerosis	a condition of hardened arteries
athero-	yellowish plaque	atherosclerosis	a condition of yellow plaque in arteries
atrio-	atrium (hall or entryway)	atriomegaly	enlargement of the smaller chambers of the heart (which give entry into the ventricles)
baso-	base (alkaline)	basophils	cells that attract alkaline stain
brachio-	arm	brachial artery	the main artery in the arm
bronchiolo-	bronchiole	bronchiolitis	inflammation of the bronchioles
broncho-, bronchio-	bronchus	bronchoscope	an instrument to view the bronchus
capno-	carbon dioxide	hypercapnia	a condition of high carbon dioxide
chromo-	color	chromophobic cells	cells that do not stain with acid or alkaline dye
corono-	crown	coronary arteries	the arteries that go around the surface of the heart
cyto-	cell	cytology	study of cells
eosino-	red, rosy	eosinophils	cells that stain with red acidic xanthene dye (eosin)
epiglotto-	epiglottis	epiglottoplasty	reconstructive surgery of the lidlike cartilaginous structure over the entrance to the windpipe; glottis is from Greek, "mouth of the windpipe"
granulo-	granules	granulocytes	cells with a granular appearance (basophils, eosinophils, and neutrophils)
hemo-	blood	hemolysis	destruction of red blood cells
hemoglobino-	hemoglobin	hemoglobinemia	free hemoglobin in the blood plasma
laryngo-	larynx	laryngospasm	muscular spasm of the larynx
leuko-	white	leukocyte	white blood cell
lobo-	lobe	lobectomy	cutting out of a lobe
mediastino-	mediastinum	mediastinotomy	cutting into the mediastinum
mono-	one	monocyte	a cell with one nucleus
myelo-	bone marrow	myelopoiesis	formation of bone marrow
neutro-	neutral (neither acid nor alkaline)	neutrophils	blood cells that take neither acid nor alkaline stain
oxy-	oxygen	oximeter	device to measure oxygen
pectoro-	thorax, chest	pectoral	pertaining to the chest
pericardio-	around heart	pericardial	around the heart
phago-	eat, swallow	dysphagia	difficulty swallowing
pharyngo-	pharynx	pharyngeal	pertaining to the pharynx
phlebo-	vein	phlebotomy	cutting into a vein
phono-	voice	phonogram	recording of a voice
phreno-	diaphragm	phrenic nerve	a nerve supplying the diaphragm
pleuro-	lung	pleuritis	inflammation of the lung
pneumo-, pneumono-	air, lung	pneumonia	a condition of the lungs
sidero-	iron	hemosiderin	an iron-rich pigment produced by hemolysis
sphygmo-	pulse	sphygmomanometer	a thin (manos) tube to measure the pressure of the pulse (blood pressure)
spiro-	breathing	spirograph	a record of breathing
stetho-	chest	stethoscope	a scope used on the chest
telo-	complete	atelectasis of lung	absence of complete expansion (ektasis)
thoraco-	chest	thoracentesis	puncture of the chest
thrombo-	clot	thrombocytopenia	diminished clot-forming cells (platelets)
tracheo-	trachea	tracheobronchoscopy	visually examining the trachea and bronchus
valvulo-	valve	valvuloplasty	a repair of a valve
vasculo-	vessel	vasculitis	inflammation of vessels
vaso-	vessel	vasodilation	expansion or dilation of a vessel
veno-	vein	venogram	a recording of veins
ventriculo-	ventricle	ventricular rhythm	a heart rhythm originating in (pertaining to) the ventricles

DIGESTIVE SYSTEM

COMBINING FORM	RELATED STRUCTURE	EXAMPLE	DEFINITION OF EXAMPLE
ascites	literally means bag	acetic	refers to an abnormal accumulation of fluid in the peritoneal cavity
bucco-	cheek	buccogingival	pertaining to the cheeks and gums
chole-	bile	choleic	pertaining to bile
cholecysto-	the sac that stores bile (gallbladder)	cholecystectomy	cutting out the gallbladder
choledocho-	common bile duct	choledochoplasty	repair of the common bile duct
colo-	colon	colostomy	making a new opening into the colon
-emesis	vomiting	hematemesis	vomiting with blood
gingivo-	gums	gingivitis	inflammation of the gums
glosso-	tongue	glossopharyngeal	pertaining to the tongue and pharynx
hepato-	liver	hepatotoxicity	a state of being toxic to the liver
		hepatomegaly	enlargement of the liver
ileo-	small intestine	ileostomy	a new opening into the small intestine
jejuno-	jejunum	jejunostomy	a new opening into the jejunum
litho-	stone	cholelithiasis	a condition of stones in the gallbladder
naso-	nose	nasogastric tube	a tube passed through the nose to the stomach
-orexia	appetite	anorexia	lack of appetite
palato-	palate	palatopharyngo-plasty	a surgical repair of the palate and pharynx
pancreato-	pancreas	pancreatitis	inflammation of the pancreas
para	past, beyond	paracentesis	a puncture through the skin into (usually the peritoneal cavity)
-pepsia	digestion	dyspepsia	difficulty with digestion
peritoneo-	peritoneum	peritoneal	pertaining to the peritoneum
-phagia	swallowing	dysphagia	difficult swallowing
procto-	anus or rectum	proctoscopy	using a scope to view the anus and rectum
pyloro-	pyloric valve	pyloric stenosis	a condition of narrowing of the pyloric valve
-rhea	flowing through or out	diarrhea	a flow out of; usually refers to excessive flow of stool
rhino-	nose	rhinoplasty	a surgical repair of the nose
sigmoido-	sigmoid colon	sigmoidoscopy	using a scope to look at the sigmoid colon
-spasm	sudden, involuntary contraction of muscles	esophagospasm	sudden, involuntary muscle contraction in the esophagus
steato-	fatty	steatorrhea	an abnormal amount of fat in the stool
stomato-	mouth	stomatopathy	disease of the mouth

FEMALE REPRODUCTIVE SYSTEM

COMBINING FORM	RELATED STRUCTURE	EXAMPLE	DEFINITION OF EXAMPLE
amnio-	amnion	amniocentesis	puncture of the amnion
cervio-	cervix, neck	cervicitis	inflammation of the cervix
chorio-	chorion	choriotrophic	pertaining to growth of the chorion
colpo-	vagina	colposcopy	use of an instrument to view the vagina
culdo-	cul-de-sac	culdocentesis	puncture of the cul-de-sac of the vagina
episio-	vulva	episiotomy	cutting of the vulva
galacto-	milk	galactorrhea	the flow of milk
gyneco-	woman, female	gynecomastia	a condition of having female breasts
hystero-	uterus, womb	hysterectomy	cutting out of the uterus
lacto-	milk	lactogenesis	production of milk
mammo-	breast	mammoplasty	repair or reconstruction of the breast
masto-	breast	mastitis	inflammation of the breast
meno-	menses, menstruation	dysmenorrhea	difficulty with flow of menses
oo-	egg	oophorectomy	removal of the ovaries
oophor-	to bear eggs (ovaries)	oophorsalpingectomy	removal of the ovaries and fallopian tubes
ovulo-	egg	anovulatory	state of not producing eggs
utero-	uterus, womb	uterine myomectomy	cutting out of muscle of the uterus
vagino-	vagina	vaginal repair	a surgical repair pertaining to the vagina
vulvo-	vulva	vulvectomy	removal of the vulva

MALE REPRODUCTIVE SYSTEM

COMBINING FORM	RELATED STRUCTURE	EXAMPLE	DEFINITION OF EXAMPLE
andro-	male	androgen	production of a man (male hormone)
balano-	glans penis	balanitis	inflammation of glans penis
cryo-	cold	cryosurgery	surgery using cold to cut or destroy
crypto-	hidden	cryptorchism	hidden (undescended) testes
epididymo-	epididymis	epididymitis	inflammation of the epididymis
orcho-, orchio-, orchido-	testis, testicle	orchitis	inflammation of the testis
prostato-	prostate gland	prostatectomy	cutting out of the prostate gland
semini-	semen, seed	seminal vesicles	saclike structures containing sperm
spermo, spermato-	spermatozoa, semen	oligospermia	scanty number of sperm
testo-	testis, testicle	testicular	referring to the testes
varico-	varicose veins	varicocele	collection of varicose (swollen, twisted) veins above the testes
vaso-	vessel, duct	vasectomy	cutting of ducts (vas deferens)

NERVOUS SYSTEM

COMBINING FORM	RELATED STRUCTURE	EXAMPLE	DEFINITION OF EXAMPLE
cerebello-	cerebellum	cerebellar	pertaining to the cerebellum
cerebro-	cerebrum	cerebrospinal fluid	fluid that bathes the cerebrum and spinal column
duro-	dura mater	subdural hematoma	a tumor (pool) of blood below the dura mater
encephalo-	brain	encephalopathy	disease of the brain
glio-	glue	glial	pertaining to stromal or connective tissue
meningo-	membranes, meninges	meningitis	inflammation of the meninges
myelo-	spinal cord	myelogram	x-ray film of spinal cord
neuro	nerve	neuroma	a tumor of a nerve
ponto-	pons	pontine	pertaining to the pons
radiculo-	nerve root (of spinal nerves)	radiculopathy	disease of the spinal nerve roots
thalamo-	thalamus	thalamic	pertaining to the thalamus
theco-	sheath (refers to the meninges)	intrathecal	within the subarachnoid space
vago-	vagus (cranial nerve X)	vagal	pertaining to the vagus nerve

IMMUNE SYSTEM

COMBINING FORM	RELATED STRUCTURE	EXAMPLE	DEFINITION OF EXAMPLE
immuno-	protection	immunosuppression	a state of low protection
lympho-	lymph	lymphoma	tumor of lymph tissue
lymphadeno-	lymph node	lymphadenopathy	disease of lymph nodes
spleno-	spleen	splenomegaly	enlarged spleen
thymo-	thymus	thymectomy	cutting out of the thymus gland
toxo-	poison	toxicology	study of toxins

MUSCULOSKELETAL SYSTEM

COMBINING FORM	RELATED STRUCTURE	EXAMPLE	DEFINITION OF EXAMPLE
calco-	calcium	hypercalcemia	excess calcium in the blood
kypho-	hump	kyphosis	a condition of being humpbacked (excess outward curve of the cervical spine)
lordo-	curve, swayback	lordosis	a condition of excess inward curvature of the lower back
lumbo-	loins, lower back	lumbodynia	pain in the lower back
ortho-	straight	orthopedics	literally, straight child; has come to mean a branch of medicine dealing with the musculoskeletal system
osteo-	bone	osteomyelitis	an infection of the bone and bone marrow
scolio-	crooked, bent	scoliosis	a condition of having a crooked spine
spondylo-	vertebra	spondylitis	inflammation of the vertebrae

SKIN (INTEGUMENTARY) SYSTEM

COMBINING FORM	RELATED STRUCTURE	EXAMPLE	DEFINITION OF EXAMPLE
adipo-	fat	adipose tissue	fat tissue
causo-	burn, burning	causalgia	a painful sensation of burning
cutaneo-	skin	subcutaneous	under the skin
dermo-, dermato-	skin	dermabrasion	scraping away the skin
diaphoro-	profuse sweating	diaphoresis	a state of profuse sweating
erythemo-	redness	erythema	redness
hidro-	sweat	anhidrosis	a state of the absence of sweat
ichthyo-	scaly, dry	ichthyosis	dry, scaly skin
kerato-	hard, horny tissue	keratosis	a state of hard, horny tissue (usually the skin)
lipo-	fat	lipoma	a fatty tumor
myco-	fungus	dermatomycosis	a condition of fungus growth on the skin
onycho-	nail	onychophagia	biting the nails
pilo-	hair	pilosebaceous cyst	a fluid-filled sac formed by a hair follicle and its gland that produces sebum
sebo-	sebum	seborrhea	excess flow of sebum (causes dandruff)
squamo-	scalelike	squamous epithelium	flat, scalelike skin cells
tricho-	hair	trichomycosis	a condition of fungus of the hair
unguo-	nail	subungual	a state of being under the nail

URINARY SYSTEM

COMBINING FORM	RELATED STRUCTURE	EXAMPLE	DEFINITION OF EXAMPLE
albumino-	albumin	albuminuria	albumin in the urine
azoto-	nitrogen	azotemia	excess nitrogenous products in the blood
calico-, calio-	calyx or calix	caliceal	pertaining to the calyx of the kidney
dipso-	thirst	polydipsia	excess thirst
glomerulo-	glomerulus	glomerulonephritis	an inflammation of the glomerulus of the kidney
keto-	ketones	ketoacidosis	a condition of excess ketone acids
litho-	stones	lithiasis	a condition of having stones
meato-	mouth or opening	meatorrhaphy	suturing of the meatus
nephro-	kidney	paranephrotic abscess	an abscess close to but on the outside of the kidney
nocti-	night	nocturia	urinating at night
oligo-	scanty	oliguria	a scanty amount of urine
-poietin	substance that forms	erythropoietin	a substance that forms erythrocytes
pyelo-	pelvis of kidney	trigonitis	nflammation of the trigone
reno-	kidney	pananephrotic abscess	an x-ray film of the kidney
trigono-	trigone muscle	trigonitis	inflammation of the trigone
uretero-	ureter	ureterovesicular valve	a valve between the ureter and the bladder
-uria	urine	pyuria	pus in the urine
urino-	urine	urinary	pertaining to urine
uro-	urine	urometer	an instrument to measure urine
vesico-	vessel; refers to bladder	vesicoureteral	pertaining to the jun ction between the bladder and ureter

SENSORY SYSTEM

Eye

COMBINING FORM	RELATED STRUCTURE	EXAMPLE	DEFINITION OF EXAMPLE
amblyo-	dull, dim	amblyopia	dull or dim vision (eyes)
aqueo-	water	aqueous humor	a watery body substance in the posterior chamber of the eye
blepharo-	eyelid	blepharitis	inflammation of eyelid
conjunctivo-	conjunctiva	conjunctivitis	inflammation of conjunctiva
corneo-	cornea	corneal	pertaining to the cornea
coro-	pupil	corectasis	dilatation of the pupil
cyclo-	ciliary body or muscle of the eye	cycloplegia	paralysis of the ciliary body
dacryo-	tears, tear duct	dacryocyst	cysts of tear ducts
diplo-	double	diplopia	double vision
glauco-	gray	glaucoma	mass or collection of fluid (aqueous humor) producing a dull gray-green gleam in advanced cases
iro-, irido-	iris	iritis	inflammation of the iris
kerato-	cornea	keratitis	inflammation of the cornea
lacrimo-	tears	lacrimal ducts	the ducts that produce tears
mio-	small, less	miosis	nearsightedness (associated with constriction of pupils)
mydro-	widen, enlarge	mydriasis	farsightedness (associated with widening of pupils)
oculo-	eye	intraocular	inside the eye
ophthalmo-	eye	ophthalmologist	a person who studies the eye (a medical doctor who treats disorders of the eye)
opto-, optico-	eye, vision	optical	pertaining to vision
palpebro-	eyelid	palpebral	pertaining to the eyelid
phaco-, phako-	lens of the eye	aphakia	result of extraction of a cataract
presbyo-	old age	presbyopia	visual changes that occur with old age
pupillo-	pupil	pupillary	pertaining to the pupil
retino-	retina	retinopathy	disease of the retina
sclero-	sclera (white of the eye)	sclerostomy	opening into sclera
uveo-	uvea (vascular layer)	uveitis	inflammation of the iris, ciliary body, and choroids
vitreo-	glassy	vitreous humor	watery, transparent (hence glassy) body substance in the anterior chamber of the eye

Ear

COMBINING FORM	RELATED STRUCTURE	EXAMPLE	DEFINITION OF EXAMPLE
acouso-	hearing	acoustic	pertaining to hearing
audio-	sense of hearing	audiometry	measurement of hearing
auro-	ear	aural	pertaining to the ear
cochleo-	cochlea	cochlear	pertaining to the cochlea
mastoido-	mastoid process	mastoiditis	inflammation of the mastoid
myringo-	eardrum	myringotomy	cutting into the eardrum
ossiculo-	ossicle	ossiculoplasty	repair of the ossicle
oto-	ear	ototoxic	toxic to the ear
salpingo-	eustachian tube, auditory tube	salpingopharyngeal drainage	drainage from the eustachian tube into the back of the oral cavity
stapedo-	stapes	stapedectomy	removal of the third bone of the middle ear
tympano-	eardrum, tympanic membrane	tympanoplasty	repair of the eardrum
vestibulo-	vestibule	vestibular neuronitis	an inflammation of the nerves of the vestibule resulting in dizziness

Appendix D HIPAA Privacy Act: Fact Sheet—Protecting the Privacy of Patients' Health Information

OVERVIEW

The first-ever federal privacy standards to protect patients' medical records and other health information provided to health plans, doctors, hospitals, and other health care providers took effect on April 14, 2003. Developed by the Department of Health and Human Services (HHS), these new standards provide patients with access to their medical records and more control over how their personal health information is used and disclosed. They represent a uniform, federal floor of privacy protections for consumers across the country. State laws providing additional protections to consumers are not affected by this new rule.

Congress called on HHS to issue patient privacy protections as part of the Health Insurance Portability and Accountability Act of 1996 (HIPAA). HIPAA included provisions designed to encourage electronic transactions and also required new safeguards to protect the security and confidentiality of health information. The final regulation covers health plans, health care clearinghouses, and those health care providers who conduct certain financial and administrative transactions (e.g., enrollment, billing, and eligibility verification) electronically. Most health insurers, pharmacies, doctors, and other health care providers were required to comply with these federal standards beginning April 14, 2003. HHS has conducted extensive outreach and provided guidance and technical assistance to these providers and businesses to make it as easy as possible for them to implement the new privacy protections. These efforts include answers to hundreds of common questions about the rule, as well as explanations and descriptions about key elements of the rule. These materials are available at http://www.hhs.gov/ocr/hipaa.

PATIENT PROTECTIONS

The new privacy regulations ensure a national floor of privacy protections for patients by limiting the ways that health plans, pharmacies, hospitals, and other covered entities can use patients' personal medical information. The regulations protect medical records and other individually identifiable health information, whether it is on paper, in computers, or communicated orally. Key provisions of these new standards include the following:

- **Access to Medical Records.** Patients generally should be able to see and obtain copies of their medical records and request corrections if they identify errors. Health plans, doctors, hospitals, clinics, nursing homes, and other covered entities generally should provide access to these records within 30 days and may charge patients for the cost of copying and sending the records.
- **Notice of Privacy Practices.** Covered health plans, doctors, and other health care providers must provide a notice to patients about how they may use personal medical information and their rights under the new privacy regulation. Doctors, hospitals, and other direct-care providers generally will provide the notice on the patient's first visit following the April 14, 2003, compliance date and upon request. Patients generally will be asked to sign, initial, or otherwise acknowledge that they received this notice. Health plans generally must mail the notice to their enrollees by April 14 and again if the notice changes significantly. Patients also may ask covered entities to restrict the use or disclosure of their information beyond the practices included in the notice, but the covered entities would not have to agree to the changes.
- **Limits on Use of Personal Medical Information.** The privacy rule sets limits on how health plans and covered providers may use individually identifiable health information. To promote the best quality care for patients, the rule does not restrict the ability of doctors, nurses, and other providers to share information needed to treat their patients. In other situations, though, personal health information generally may not be used for purposes not related to health care, and covered entities may use or share only the minimum amount of protected information needed for a particular purpose. In addition, patients would have to sign a specific authorization before a covered entity could release their medical information to a life insurer, a bank, a marketing firm, or another outside business for purposes not related to their health care.
- **Prohibition on Marketing.** The final privacy rule sets new restrictions and limits on the use of patient information for marketing purposes. Pharmacies, health plans, and other covered entities must first obtain an individual's specific authorization before disclosing their patient information for marketing. At the same time, the rule permits doctors and other covered entities to communicate freely with patients about treatment options and other health-related information, including disease-management programs.

- **Stronger State Laws.** The new federal privacy standards do not affect state laws that provide additional privacy protections for patients. The confidentiality protections are cumulative; the privacy rule will set a national "floor" of privacy standards that protects all Americans, and any state law providing additional protections would continue to apply. When a state law requires a certain disclosure—such as reporting an infectious disease outbreak to the public health authorities—the federal privacy regulations would not preempt the state law.
- **Confidential Communications.** Under the privacy rule, patients can request that their doctors, health plans, and other covered entities take reasonable steps to ensure that their communications with the patient are confidential. For example, a patient could ask a doctor to call his or her office rather than home, and the doctor's office should comply with that request if it can be reasonably accommodated.
- **Complaints.** Consumers may file a formal complaint regarding the privacy practices of a covered health plan or provider. Such complaints can be made directly to the covered provider or health plan or to HHS' Office for Civil Rights (OCR), which is charged with investigating complaints and enforcing the privacy regulation. Information about filing complaints should be included in each covered entity's notice of privacy practices. Consumers can find out more information about filing a complaint at http://www.hhs.gov/ocr/hipaa or by calling (866) 627-7748.

HEALTH PLANS AND PROVIDERS

The privacy rule requires health plans, pharmacies, doctors, and other covered entities to establish policies and procedures to protect the confidentiality of protected health information about their patients. These requirements are flexible and scalable to allow different covered entities to implement them as appropriate for their businesses or practices. Covered entities must provide all the protections for patients cited above, such as providing a notice of their privacy practices and limiting the use and disclosure of information as required under the rule. In addition, covered entities must take some additional steps to protect patient privacy:

- **Written Privacy Procedures.** The rule requires covered entities to have written privacy procedures, including a description of staff that has access to protected information, how it will be used, and when it may be disclosed. Covered entities generally must take steps to ensure that any business associates who have access to protected information agree to the same limitations on the use and disclosure of that information.
- **Employee Training and Privacy Officer.** Covered entities must train their employees in their privacy procedures and must designate an individual to be responsible for ensuring the procedures are followed.
  If covered entities learn an employee failed to follow these procedures, they must take appropriate disciplinary action.
- **Public Responsibilities.** In limited circumstances, the final rule permits—but does not require—covered entities to continue certain existing disclosures of health information for specific public responsibilities. These permitted disclosures include: emergency circumstances; identification of the body of a deceased person or the cause of death; public health needs; research that involves limited data or has been independently approved by an Institutional Review Board or privacy board; oversight of the health care system; judicial and administrative proceedings; limited law enforcement activities; and activities related to national defense and security. The privacy rule generally establishes new safeguards and limits on these disclosures. Where no other law requires disclosures in these situations, covered entities may continue to use their professional judgment to decide whether to make such disclosures based on their own policies and ethical principles.
- **Equivalent Requirements for Government.** The provisions of the final rule generally apply equally to private sector and public sector covered entities. For example, private hospitals and government-run hospitals covered by the rule have to comply with the full range of requirements.

INFORMATION FOR NURSES AND NURSING STUDENTS

1. The right to privacy has a basis in the Constitution of the United States.
2. Laws requiring the protection of health privacy in the United States have been enacted primarily by the states. State laws (like those covering HIV testing or mental health) giving privacy protections continue to apply.
3. The HIPAA statute establishes the first federal, comprehensive protection of health information ensuring a basic level of privacy of health information. Some of the topics HIPAA addresses include accountability of medical records, type of medical information protected, and disclosure requirements.
4. Neither HIPAA nor any of the state laws appear to offer individuals the absolute right to restrict disclosure of their health information. HIPAA permits disclosure of health information without individual authorization for public health, emergencies, national defense, and other limited situations.
5. Privacy protection guidance is also found in the professional codes of conduct developed by organizations such as the American Medical Association, American Nurses Association, the American Hospital Association, the American Psychiatric Association, and the American Dental Association. The opinions and interpretation of the codes guide the professional standards and practice for their members. The codes do not have the force of law, but providers often recognize them as binding rules.
6. The HIPAA rules identify the health care providers, health plans, pharmacies, and other entities required to comply with the rules. Generally, health-related entities that conduct certain financial and administrative transactions are covered. All medical records and other individually identifiable health information communicated by any means, that is paper, oral, or electronically, are controlled by HIPAA rules.
7. For the purposes of treatment, providers of health care are allowed access to the full medical record. However, patient consent is required prior to releasing any medical information for payments, other treatment, health care operations or other nonroutine uses of the information. Disclosures of information must be limited to the minimum amount of information necessary for the purpose of the disclosure.

From HIPAA privacy act fact sheet. Released April 14, 2003. United States Department of Health & Human Services, www.hhs.gov/news/facts/privacy.html.

8. Duties of nurses and nursing students regarding the right to privacy associated with protected health information are essentially the same as before the implementation of HIPAA. These include the duty to:
   a. Know how your health care agency implements HIPAA requirements for disclosure of protected medical information. A form signed by the patient may be required.
   b. Understand patients' rights under HIPAA and how your agency assures these rights.
   c. Keep all information about the patient confidential except to disclose information for purposes of the patient's treatment or education.
   d. Check for authorization to release health-related information about your patient prior to giving information to insurance companies, patient's employer, friends or family members, or anyone else not involved in direct care.
   e. Remove any identifying information from personal notes or assignments for educational purposes, and never leave notes about the patient accessible to others. Any student assignments related to clients must be maintained in a secure and confidential manner—even if the data is de-identified. This means that assignments, logs, and care plans cannot be left unattended at school, at home, in your car, or on your computer.
   f. Never copy the patient's medical record.
   g. When discussing the patient's health care information for educational purposes, be sure the environment is private.
   h. When it is necessary to fax patient information for purposes of treatment, a cover sheet should be used and you should know there are security measures at the site of the receiving fax machine. In general, students should not fax client information at any time.
   i. Remember that violations of HIPAA privacy standards can result in penalties.

From United States Department of Health and Human Services Office of Civil Rights—HIPAA. Medical privacy—national standards to protect the privacy of personal health information, www.hhs.gov/ocr/hipaa. Last revised April 14, 2003.

GLOSSARY

abrasion a mechanical injury resulting from scraping away of skin or mucous membrane (Chapter 27) [audio]
abstract (concepts) conceived apart from concrete reality; those concepts that are not observable, such as caring and hope (Chapter 5)
abstract (research) a short summary that contains brief information about the purpose of the study, the number of subjects, the methodology used to select subjects, the type of study being conducted, and the major results from the study (Chapter 15)
access a complex construct representing the personal use of health care services and the structures or processes that facilitate or impede that use (Chapter 4)
accommodation the adjustment of the eye for seeing objects at various distances (Chapter 8)
accountability the obligation, conferred by virtue of one's position, to provide an accounting or rationale for personal actions or the actions of others (Chapter 14)
accreditation a process that monitors an educational program's ability to meet predetermined standards for student outcomes (Chapter 2)
acting-out behaviors inappropriate or unexpected client behaviors that communicate a message about the client's true or subconscious feelings and concerns (Chapter 12)
action stage the stage of change in which the person changes risky behaviors and the context of the behavior (environment, experience) and makes significant efforts to reach goals (Chapter 20)
active listening participation in a conversation with a client in which the nurse attends to what the client says and has a part in helping the client clarify, elaborate, and give additional pertinent information (Chapters 6 and 12)
active processing a systematic series of mental actions to analyze and interpret information about a client (Chapter 6)
active transport an active process by which molecules move from an area of lower concentration to an area of higher concentration with an expenditure of energy (Chapter 26)
activities of daily living (ADLs) the basic activities usually performed in the course of a normal day in a person's life, such as eating, toileting, dressing, bathing, or brushing the teeth (Chapter 44)
acute pain short-term, self-limited pain with a probable duration of less than 6 months; expected to resolve when the tissue heals (Chapter 37)
adaptation the change that occurs as a result of assimilation and accommodation; also called coping behavior (Chapter 42); a process through which individuals accommodate to changes in the internal or external environment to preserve functioning and pursue goals (Chapter 47)
adaptive coping a process that fosters problem solving, growth and development, and the ability to perceive reality and respond in a way that supports emotional and physical well-being (Chapter 47)
adjuvant analgesic any medication that may increase analgesic efficacy, thus allowing for a smaller opioid dosage (Chapter 37) [audio]
administrative law the rules and regulations delineating the methods or actions that conform to enacted law (e.g., statutory law) and provide the detail necessary to implement them (Chapter 2)
admit note the opening nurse's note acknowledging the arrival of a new client (Chapter 11)
adolescence the period of transition between childhood and adulthood (Chapter 17)
advance directive a written document that provides direction for health care when a person is unable to make his or her own treatment choices (Chapter 2)
adverse effect serious medication effect that may or may not be expected and is potentially dangerous to the client (Chapter 21)
affect the observable expression of feelings or emotions (Chapter 40)
affective learning domain the learning domain that relates to ethics or principles that guide moral behavior and to reasoning that determines right behavior (Chapter 13)
afterload the final determinant of stroke volume, defined as the pressure against which the left ventricle pumps (aortic systolic pressure); higher aortic pressure forces the heart to work harder, and less blood is ejected from the ventricles with each contraction (Chapter 35)
ageism a stereotyping, prejudice, or discrimination against people, especially older adults, based on their age (Chapter 18)
agnosia the failure to recognize or identify objects despite an intact sensory ability (Chapter 40) [audio]
agnostic a person who is undecided about the existence of God or a higher power (Chapter 49)
agonist analgesic an opioid that stimulates activity at an opioid receptor site to produce analgesia (Chapter 37) [audio]
alopecia loss of hair, and baldness (Chapter 31)
ambulatory surgery same-day or outpatient surgery that can be performed with general or local anesthesia, usually taking less than 2 hours and requiring less than a 3-hour stay in a recovery area (Chapter 50)
amino acids compounds composed of carbon, hydrogen, oxygen, and an amino group, and classified as essential or nonessential depending on whether the body can manufacture them from other sources (Chapter 24)
analgesia reduction of the perception or experience of pain (Chapter 37)
anaphylaxis a severe allergic reaction that requires immediate intervention to prevent possible death (Chapter 21) [audio]
androgyny an anthropological term meaning that a person may display both male and female characteristics and may relate to both a male and a female gender identity and role (Chapter 46) [audio]
anesthesia partial or complete loss of sensation, with or without loss of consciousness, as a result of being given an anesthetic agent (Chapter 50) [audio]
anesthesiologist a medical physician who specializes in anesthesiology and provides anesthesia for surgical clients (Chapter 50) [audio]
anger a strong feeling of displeasure and belligerence aroused by a real or supposed wrong; occurs in grief as the denial and disbelief are replaced with the growing awareness of the reality of a loss (Chapter 45)
anion a negatively charged ion, such as chloride, bicarbonate, phosphate, sulfate, or proteinate (Chapter 26)
anorexia lack of appetite (Chapter 25) [audio]
antagonist a drug, such as naloxone, that blocks activity at *mu* and *kappa* receptors by displacing opioid analgesics currently attached to them (Chapter 37) [audio]
antagonistic effect an effect that occurs when one drug reduces or negates the effect of another, which may be accidental or purposeful (Chapter 21)
anthropometric measurements measurements of physical characteristics of the body (such as height and weight), as well as the amount of muscle or fat tissue in the body (Chapter 24) [audio]
antibacterial kills off bacteria (Chapter 22)
antibiotic a drug that kills bacteria (Chapter 22) [audio]
antibody a circulating protein that recognizes and destroys foreign invaders, or antigens (Chapter 22) [audio]

anticipatory grief intellectual and emotional responses and behaviors by which individuals, families, and communities attempt to work through the process of modifying self-concept on the basis of the perception of potential loss (Chapter 45)

antidiuretic hormone (ADH) substance produced by the hypothalamus and secreted by the posterior pituitary gland that causes the kidneys to retain water (Chapter 35) [audio]

antimicrobial having the ability to limit the spread of microorganisms (Chapter 22) [audio]

anuria the absence of urine (Chapter 30) [audio]

anxiety a diffuse, highly uncomfortable, sometimes vague sense of apprehension or dread accompanied by one or more physical sensations (Chapters 42 and 47)

anxiety disorders serious medical illnesses that fill clients' lives with overwhelming anxiety and fear; unlike the brief anxiety caused by a stressful event, anxiety disorders are chronic, relentless, and can grow progressively worse if not treated (Chapter 42)

anxiolytics antianxiety medications that act on the central nervous system to disrupt the feelings of anxiety and associated symptoms such as muscle tension and restlessness (Chapter 42)

aphasia a language disorder resulting from brain damage or disease to speech centers in the brain resulting in a variety of difficulties in formulating, expressing, and understanding language (Chapter 39) [audio]

apical pulse the heart rate counted at the apex of the heart on the anterior chest (Chapter 7) [audio]

APIE (PIE) charting a method of charting that evolved from the problem-oriented type of medical record and that is designed to allow documentation using the nursing process; the acronym standing for assessment, problem identification, interventions, and evaluation (Chapter 11)

apraxia the inability to carry out motor activities despite the functional ability to perform them (Chapter 40) [audio]

arousal erotic excitement that precedes sexual response and occurs in the presence of physically and emotionally pleasurable stimuli (Chapter 46)

articulation the process of molding sounds into enunciated words and phrases (Chapter 39)

asphyxiation an interruption in breathing from a severe lack of oxygen (asphyxia) because there is either no source of air, an inadequate supply of oxygen in the air, or inadequate inhalation (Chapter 23)

aspiration the inspiration of foreign material into the airway (Chapter 23)

assault an attempt or threat to touch another person unjustly (Chapter 2)

assessment the process of gathering data about the client's health status to identify the concerns and needs that can be treated or managed by nursing care (Chapter 6)

atheist a person who believes there is no God or higher power (Chapter 49)

atherosclerosis pathological condition in which fat and plaque are deposited on the intimal surface of arteries (Chapter 35) [audio]

atrophy decrease in the size or physiological activity of a normally developed tissue or organ as a result of inactivity or diminished function (Chapter 33) [audio]

attachment development of strong ties of affection of an infant with a significant other (mother, father, sibling, caretaker) (Chapter 16)

attending behaviors nursing behaviors that show that you are paying attention to and listening to what the client is saying (Chapter 12)

attention the ability to focus on an object or activity (Chapter 40)

atypical analgesic a drug not primarily indicated for managing pain but used to treat specific types of pain, such as an anticonvulsant to treat neuropathic pain (Chapter 37)

auditory pertaining to the sensation of hearing (Chapter 38)

auscultation the process of listening to sounds generated within the body (Chapter 8)

auscultatory gap absence of a second Korotkoff sound, a common finding in hypertension (Chapter 7)

authority the ability or legitimate power to make decisions, implement strategies, and elicit work (Chapter 14)

autonomy an individual's ability to independently make decisions and take action using critical thinking skills, a body of knowledge, and own expertise as a member of a profession (Chapters 1 and 2)

awareness the state of being awake and alert enough to react to stimuli; also known as consciousness (Chapter 40)

bacterium a single-celled organism that can reproduce outside of cells (Chapter 22)

bacteriuria the presence of bacteria in the urine (Chapter 30)

baroreceptors specialized cells located in the aorta and carotid arteries that detect pressure changes in the vascular system (Chapter 35)

basal metabolic rate the amount of energy needed to maintain essential basic body functions, expressed as calories per hour per square meter of body surface (Chapter 7)

battery the actual willful touching of another person that may or may not cause harm (Chapter 2)

bed rest a prescribed or self-imposed restriction to bed for therapeutic reasons (Chapter 33)

beneficence the promotion of good by the performance of actions that benefit others (Chapter 2)

Benner's stages of skill acquisition application of the Dreyfus model of skill acquisition to nursing practice through five levels of proficiency in acquiring and developing skill in decision making (Chapter 5)

bereavement the experience of a loss; usually applies to the loss by death of an immediate family member (Chapter 45)

bioavailability the amount of an administered drug that is available for activity in the target tissue (Chapter 21)

biographical data information that identifies and describes a person, such as name, address, age, sex, religious affiliation, race, and occupation (Chapter 6)

biotransformation the process of inactivating and breaking down a drug, also called drug metabolism (Chapter 21)

bisexual sexual orientation in which one may be sexually attracted to members of either sex (Chapter 46)

body image a person's perception of his or her body; the physical dimension of self-concept, or how a person perceives and evaluates appearance and function of self (Chapter 41)

body language nonverbal communication behaviors that are accomplished by the movement of the body or body parts, by the presentation of ourselves to the world, and by the use of our personal space (Chapter 12)

bowel incontinence inability to voluntarily control the passage of feces and gas (Chapter 29)

bradycardia an abnormally slow heart rate, usually below 60 beats per minute (Chapters 7 and 35) [audio]

bradypnea a respiratory rate below 12 breaths per minute for an adult (Chapter 7) [audio]

breakthrough pain intermittent episodes of pain that occur despite continued use of an analgesic (Chapter 37)

Broca's area the center of motor speech control, located in the frontal lobe of the brain and responsible for controlling muscles of the mouth, tongue, and larynx, which produce speech (Chapter 39)

bronchial breath sounds normal sounds heard with a stethoscope over the main airways, including trachea and sternum; inspiration longer than expiration (Chapter 8)

bronchospasm spasm of the smooth muscle of the bronchi and/or the bronchioles that results in decreased airway diameter (Chapter 34) [audio]

bronchovesicular breath sounds normal breath sounds that occur between sounds of the bronchial tubes and those of the alveoli, or a combination of the two sounds; expiration and inspiration of equal duration, sounding like blowing through a hollow tube (Chapter 8) [audio]

bruxism characterized by violent, repetitive grinding of the teeth that occurs during the lighter stages of sleep or during partial arousals (Chapter 36) [audio]

burn injury caused by excessive exposure to heat, electricity, chemicals, gases, radioactivity, or thermal agents (Chapter 23)

calorie a measure of the energy content of food, also called a kilocalorie (Chapter 24)

capitation payment system a form of payment for health care services agreed on between the purchaser of care and the provider, with the provider receiving a flat fee to provide a defined level of care whether the enrollee receives the care or not (Chapter 4)

carbohydrate a simple or complex compound composed of carbon, oxygen, and hydrogen (Chapter 24)

cardiac output the amount of blood pumped by the ventricles of the heart per minute (Chapter 35)
cardinal signs and symptoms data of greatest significance in diagnosing a particular illness, disease, or health problem (Chapter 6)
care map *see* clinical pathway
care plan conference the action of a group (health care team) conferring or consulting together to plan care for the client (Chapter 10)
caregiver one who provides care to a dependent or partially dependent family member or friend (Chapter 48)
caregiver burden unrelenting physical, psychological, social, or financial problems that occur when a caregiver provides for the health needs of an impaired family member or friend (Chapter 48)
caregiver burnout depletion of physical and mental energy caused by providing care for a chronically ill person over a long period of time (Chapter 48)
caregiver stress the caregiver's reaction to physical, emotional, sociocultural, financial, and environmental stressors brought on by the caregiving experience (Chapter 48)
caries decalcification of the tooth enamel leading to continued destruction of the enamel and dentin with resulting cavitation of the tooth (Chapter 31)
caring a behavior of having regard for, cherishing, protecting, being responsible for, or attending to needs of others; universally observed in human beings and influenced by society, culture, values, and sex (Chapters 5 and 48)
case management a care delivery system that focuses on the management of client care across an episode of illness (Chapter 10)
catabolism production of glucose from the breakdown of muscle and lean body mass (Chapter 25)
cathartic a medication, stronger than a laxative, used to induce emptying of the bowel (Chapter 29)
cation a positively charged ion, such as sodium, potassium, calcium, magnesium, or hydrogen (Chapter 26)
cephalocaudal from head toward feet; in neuromuscular growth and development, the normal pattern (Chapter 16) [audio]
certification a voluntary process by which a nurse can be granted recognition for meeting certain criteria established by a nongovernmental association (Chapter 2)
certified registered nurse anesthetist (CRNA) an advanced practice registered nurse who has been specifically educated in the administration of anesthetic agents and provides anesthesia for clients under an anesthesiologist's supervision (Chapter 50)
cerumen waxy secretion of the glands of the external acoustic meatus; commonly known as earwax (Chapter 31) [audio]
change-of-shift report oral report given at the end of a shift to the next nurse who will assume responsibility for care of the client (Chapter 14)
charting by exception a method of charting that provides documentation in progress notes only if data are significant or abnormal (Chapter 11)
chemical name the name that precisely describes the chemical and molecular structure of a medication (Chapter 21)
chest percussion use of cupped hands to rhythmically clap on the chest wall over various segments of the lungs to mobilize secretions (Chapter 34)
chest physiotherapy an approach to mobilizing and draining secretions from gravity-dependent areas of the lung that uses a combination of postural drainage, chest percussion, and vibration (Chapter 34)
chief complaint the problem that caused the client to seek health services, call the doctor, or request a visit with a nurse, in the client's own words (Chapter 6)
choking an internal obstruction of the airway by a foreign body, such as food (Chapter 23)
chronic illness all impairments or deviations from normal that fit one or more of the following descriptions: are permanent, leave residual disability, are caused by a nonreversible pathological condition, require special training of the client for rehabilitation, or can be expected to require a long period of supervision, observation, or care (Chapter 44)
chronic pain long-term, constant, or recurring pain with a duration of more than 6 months and without an anticipated or predictable end (Chapter 37)
chronicity a broad term that encompasses chronic illnesses as well as disease or congenital defects that permanently alter a person's previous health status (Chapter 44)
circadian rhythm a biorhythmic pattern that is regularly repeated at 24-hour intervals (Chapter 36)
circulating nurse a registered nurse (also called a circulator) who helps clients meet individual needs during all three phases of the surgical experience, coordinates the client's care, acts as the client's advocate, and manages activities outside the sterile field (Chapter 50)
civil law regulates disputes between individuals or between individuals and groups (Chapter 2)
claudication cramplike pains in the calves caused by poor circulation of the blood to the leg muscles (Chapter 35) [audio]
client an individual who participates with health care providers in planning and implementing own health care (Chapter 1)
clinical judgment a conclusion or an opinion about a problem or situation that requires nursing care; may determine the cause of the problem, distinguish between similar problems, or discriminate between two or more courses of action (Chapters 5 and 9)
clinical pathway a standardized multidisciplinary care plan that projects the expected course of the client's treatment and progress over the hospital stay (Chapters 10 and 11)
closed question question that calls for a specific response from the client (Chapter 6)
closed system a set of integrated, interacting parts that function as a whole and do not interact with other systems or the environment (Chapter 48)
code status the specific orders for a client related to whether to begin resuscitative actions, defining the extent of those actions, at the time of a cardiac or respiratory arrest (Chapter 45)
cognition the process of knowing and interacting with the world, also known as thought (Chapter 40)
cognitive learning domain the learning domain that encompasses knowledge, comprehension, and critical thinking skills (Chapter 13)
collaboration the act of two or more health care professionals working cooperatively to achieve a common goal, with equal value given to each person's opinion (Chapter 10)
collaborative problem a clinical problem that cannot be solved by the nurse alone (or by the nursing staff) but that requires treatments or medications that the nurse is not able to do or not licensed to order (Chapter 9)
colloid a macromolecule, such as a protein, that is too large to pass through a cell membrane and that does not readily dissolve into a solution (Chapter 26) [audio]
colloid osmotic pressure osmotic pressure exerted by large molecules, such as protein (Chapter 26)
colostomy a surgical procedure involving the creation of an opening between the colon and the abdominal wall (Chapter 29)
common law standards and rules applicable to our interactions with one another that are recognized, affirmed, and enforced through judicial decisions (Chapter 2)
communication a complex process in which information is exchanged between two or more individuals, called senders and receivers (Chapters 12 and 39)
community a geographical location, or an aggregate or population of individuals who have one or more personal or environmental characteristics in common (Chapter 43)
community forum an open meeting where members of a community or group may come to share opinions and concerns about a particular issue (Chapter 43)
community health nursing nursing that promotes and preserves the health of populations by (1) understanding and applying concepts of public health and community, (2) working with community organizations to assist in community development, (3) providing generalist care to selected individuals, families, and groups, and (4) providing health promotion, health maintenance, health education, and coordination of care (Chapter 43)
community reintegration the return and acceptance of a disabled person as a participating member of the community (Chapter 44)
complicated grief a disorder that occurs after the death of a significant other, in which the experience of distress accompanying bereavement fails to follow normative expectations and manifests in functional impairment (Chapter 45)
computerized care plan a care plan generated by a computer program with inputs from an operator (Chapter 10)

computerized provider order entry (CPOE) electronic documentation of orders by health care providers directly into a clinical information system

concept an idea, thought, or notion conceived in the mind (Chapter 5)

concrete operations stage of cognitive development at which children begin to project the self into other people's situations and realize that their own way of thinking is not the only way (Chapter 16)

concurrent audit an evaluation method to inspect the nursing staff's compliance with predetermined standards and criteria while the nurses are providing care (Chapter 14)

confidentiality the client's right to privacy in the health care delivery system; includes the nurse's ethical obligation to maintain client confidentiality (Chapter 2)

confusion the state in which the individual experiences or is at risk of experiencing a disturbance in cognition, altered memory, and orientation of an undetermined origin or onset (Chapter 40)

consciousness the state of being awake and alert enough to react to stimuli, also known as awareness (Chapter 40)

conservation in the context of developmental theory, a child's ability to understand that changing the shape of a substance does not change its quality (Chapter 16)

constipation a condition in which feces are abnormally hard and dry and evacuation is abnormally infrequent (Chapter 29)

constitutional delay of puberty an absence of early signs of puberty, such as Tanner stage II breasts by age 13 for girls or Tanner stage II genitalia by age 14 for boys (Chapter 17)

consultation the act of two or more health care professionals (one of whom is an expert or specialist solicited to offer an opinion) deliberating for the purpose of making decisions (Chapter 10)

contemplation stage the stage of change in which the individual intends to change within the next 6 months (Chapter 20)

context the condition within which a communication occurs (Chapter 12)

continuing education informal courses that assist professional nurses in developing and maintaining clinical expertise and knowledge that promotes the quality of nursing care (Chapter 1)

continuous quality improvement (CQI) a systematic ongoing approach to the methods of controlling and improving quality of health care from the perspective of both professionals and clients (Chapter 14)

contract an agreement between two or more individuals creating certain rights and obligations in exchange for goods or services (Chapter 2)

contracture an abnormal condition of joint flexion resulting from shortening of muscle fibers and associated connective tissue, with resistance to stretching and eventually to flexion and, finally, to permanent fixation (Chapter 33)

controlled substance a drug that affects the mind or behavior, may be habit forming, and has a high potential for abuse, including narcotics, barbiturates, and illegal drugs (Chapter 21)

coping the ability to deal with dangerous, threatening, or challenging situations (Chapter 47)

coping patterns specific protective behaviors used by an individual or family to respond to stressful situations (Chapter 48)

cough a sudden audible, forceful expulsion of air from the lungs, usually an involuntary, reflexive action in response to an irritant (Chapter 34)

counseling a method of communication that actively involves the client in the recognition of personal risk factors and management of necessary behavior changes (Chapter 20)

credentialing methods by which the nursing profession attempts to ensure and maintain the competency of its practitioners (Chapter 2)

criminal law definition of specific behaviors determined to be inappropriate in the orderly functioning of society (Chapter 2)

crisis an upset in a balanced or stable state for which the usual methods of adaptation and coping are not sufficient (Chapter 47)

critical pathway *see* clinical pathway

critical periods times when a person has an increased vulnerability to physical, chemical, psychological, or environmental influences (Chapter 16)

critical thinking purposeful, self-regulatory judgment that gives reasoned and reflective consideration to evidence, contexts, conceptualizations, methods, and criteria (Chapter 5)

cue an indicator of the presence or existence of a problem or condition that represents a client's underlying health status (Chapters 6 and 9)

cultural competence having enough knowledge of cultural groups that are different from your own to be able to interact with a member of a group in a manner that makes the person feel respected and understood (Chapter 3)

culture a patterned behavioral response developed over time as a consequence of imprinting the mind through social and religious structures and intellectual and artistic manifestations (Chapter 3)

cyanosis a state of blue color to the skin that results from the concentration of deoxygenated hemoglobin close to the surface of the skin (Chapter 34)

data pieces of subjective or objective information about the client or the signs and symptoms of disease (Chapter 6); information that a researcher is interested in collecting (Chapter 15)

data collection the process by which the researcher acquires subjects and collects the information necessary to answer the research question (Chapter 15)

database all of the information that has been collected about the client and recorded in the health record as a baseline for the initial plan of care (Chapter 6)

débridement the removal of dirt, foreign matter, and dead or devitalized tissue from a wound (Chapter 27) [audio]

decision making choosing between two or more options as a means to achieve a desired result (Chapter 5)

decoder (receiver) the person to whom a message is aimed (Chapter 12)

deep vein thrombosis (DVT) the condition caused when a blood clot (thrombus) develops in the lumen of a deep leg vein, such as the tibial, popliteal, femoral, or iliac vein (Chapter 33) [audio]

defamation either a false communication or a careless disregard for the truth that results in damage to someone's reputation (Chapter 2)

defendant the person against whom a lawsuit is filed (Chapter 2)

defense mechanism method used to protect oneself from stress and maintain psychological homeostasis (Chapter 47)

defining characteristic descriptor of a client's behavior that determines whether a nursing diagnosis is present and whether a particular diagnosis is appropriate or accurate (Chapter 9)

deglutition the reflex passage of food, fluids, or both from the mouth to the stomach, also known as swallowing (Chapter 25) [audio]

dehiscence partial or total separation of the edges of a wound (Chapter 27) [audio]

delegation assigning responsibility for certain tasks to other people, thereby allowing the nurse to concentrate on aspects of care that require the skill of a registered nurse (Chapter 14)

delirium a disturbance in consciousness and a change in cognition that develops over a short period of time (Chapter 40) [audio]

delusions false personal beliefs (Chapter 40)

dementia multiple cognitive deficits that include impairment of memory and judgment resulting in a progressive decline in intellectual functioning, synonymous with chronic confusion (Chapter 40) [audio]

demographic data factual information that can be counted to describe populations of clients (Chapter 6)

denial an attempt by the mind to alter a person's perception of reality by refusing to believe, recognize, or acknowledge an event such as death or catastrophic illness (Chapter 45)

dentures a complement of teeth, either natural or artificial; the term ordinarily used to designate an artificial replacement for the natural teeth (Chapter 31)

dependent variable the variable hypothesized to change with treatment and thus to have been caused by an independent variable (Chapter 15)

descriptor axis 6 of the NANDA-I taxonomy; a judgment that modifies, limits, or specifies the meaning of a nursing diagnosis, such as *decreased, deficient, excessive,* or *readiness* (Chapter 9)

development a progression of behavioral changes that involve the acquisition of appropriate cognitive, linguistic, and psychosocial skills (Chapter 16)

developmental crisis occurs when a person is unable to complete the tasks of a developmental level (Chapter 47)

diagnosis-related groups (DRGs) a system of classification or grouping of clients

according to medical diagnosis for the purpose of paying hospitalization costs (Chapter 4)
diagnostic label a concise term or phrase that represents a pattern of related signs and symptoms; also known as a nursing diagnosis (Chapter 9)
diagnostic reasoning the process of clustering assessment data into meaningful sets and generating hypotheses about the client's human responses (Chapters 5 and 9)
diaphragmatic (abdominal) breathing breathing in which the majority of ventilatory work is accomplished by the diaphragm and abdominal muscles; deliberate use of the diaphragm and abdominal muscles to control breathing (Chapter 34)
diarrhea rapid movement of fecal matter through the intestine, resulting in poor adsorption of water, nutrients, and electrolytes and producing abnormally frequent evacuation of watery stools (Chapter 29) [audio]
diastole relaxation of the ventricles of the heart (Chapter 35) [audio]
diastolic blood pressure the constant pressure in the arteries during myocardial relaxation (Chapter 7) [audio]
differential cell count a breakdown of the number of white cells into their different types (Chapter 22)
differential diagnosis the process of deciding among several possible diagnoses to most accurately describe the client's problem (Chapter 9)
differentiated development a normal pattern of development, which becomes increasingly differentiated over time, starting with a generalized response and progressing to a skilled specific response (Chapter 16)
diffusion a passive process by which molecules move through a cell membrane from an area of higher concentration to an area of lower concentration without the expenditure of energy (Chapter 26)
disaccharide a molecule that forms when two monosaccharides condense (join together) to form a double sugar (Chapter 24) [audio]
discharge note a nursing note that reflects the circumstances around the release of a client from a facility (Chapter 11)
discharge planning preparation for moving a client from one level of care to another within or outside of the current health care agency (Chapter 10)
disease a specific disorder characterized by a recognizable set of signs and symptoms, attributable to heredity, infection, diet, or environment (Chapter 19)
disenfranchised grief grief that lacks social acknowledgment, validation, and support for the bereaved (Chapter 45)
disuse the condition that occurs when organs or body parts are no longer used (Chapter 33)
diuresis increased secretion of urine (Chapter 30)
diversity differences in modes or patterns of care between cultures, including specific patterns of care within cultural groups (Chapter 3)
documentation the recording of information relevant to assessment, planning, implementation, and client response; a legal record that is permanent and retrievable for future purposes (Chapter 11)
durable power of attorney for health care a document that designates a person to make decisions about the client's medical treatment in the event that the client becomes unable to do so, also called a proxy directive (Chapter 2)
dysarthria impaired articulation of speech (Chapter 39) [audio]
dysfunctional families families that cannot meet the needs of their members, often consistently functioning at the expense of one or more members (Chapter 48)
dysfunctional grief extended, unsuccessful use of intellectual and emotional responses by which individuals, families, and communities attempt to work through the process of modifying self-concept on the basis of the perception of potential loss (Chapter 45)
dysphagia difficulty in swallowing (Chapters 25 and 39) [audio]
dysphonia difficulty in producing vocal sounds (Chapter 39) [audio]
dyspnea the subjective sensation of difficulty in breathing (Chapter 34) [audio]
dysrhythmia abnormalities of heart rate or rhythm (Chapter 35) [audio]
dyssomnias primary sleep disorders initiating or maintaining sleep or excessive sleep (Chapter 36) [audio]
dysuria difficult or painful urination (Chapter 30) [audio]
ecchymosis a hemorrhagic infiltration of the skin producing a bluish discoloration that changes to yellow as the blood cells are broken and reabsorbed; a bruise (Chapter 8)
edema abnormal accumulation of fluid in the interstitial spaces of tissues; commonly known as swelling (Chapter 35)
egocentrism the tendency to spend so much time thinking about and focusing on one's own thoughts and changes in one's own body that one comes to believe that others are focused on them as well (Chapter 17)
electrolyte a substance that, when placed in water or another solvent, separates into electrically charged particles (ions) (Chapter 26)
electronic health record (EHR) a computerized account of a client's health information across several episodes of care and different facilities (Chapter 11)
electronic medical record (EMR) a computerized account of a client's admission or care episode within a health care facility (Chapter 11)
electronic medication administration record (eMAR) a computerized version of a medication administration record (Chapter 11)
emic dimension a person's or social group's subjective perception and experiences related to health (Chapter 20)
empathy accurate perception of the client's feelings (Chapter 12)
empirical based on observation or experience (Chapter 5)
encoder (sender) the person who initiates a transaction to exchange information, convey thoughts and feelings, or engage another (Chapter 12)
endorphin an internally secreted, opioid-like substance released by a signal from the cerebral cortex that attaches to opioid receptors and blocks transmission of the pain signal (Chapter 37) [audio]
endotracheal tube a catheter passed through the nose or mouth into the trachea for the purpose of establishing an airway (Chapter 34) [audio]
enteral nutrition provision of nutrition through a tube in the gastrointestinal tract (Chapter 25) [audio]
enuresis recurrent involuntary urination that occurs during sleep (Chapter 30) [audio]
environmental resources a domain for describing vulnerable populations; includes access to health care and quality of health care (Chapter 43)
epidemiology study of the cause and distribution of disease, disability, and death among groups of people (Chapter 43)
epidural analgesia pain relief provided by placing a catheter between the spinal vertebra and the dura mater to allow the diffusion of an analgesic drug across the dura mater into the cerebrospinal fluid (Chapter 37) [audio]
epithelialization movement of epithelial cells to the wound bed (Chapter 27) [audio]
equianalgesia the dosages of different drugs, or of the same drug by different routes, that provide the same amount of pain relief (Chapter 37) [audio]
eschar thick, leathery, necrotic, devitalized tissue (Chapter 27) [audio]
ethics the branch of philosophy that systematically examines behavior to determine what constitutes good, bad, right, and wrong in human behavior and provides guidance for action (Chapter 2)
ethnic describing a group of people of the same race or national origin who are distinctive on the basis of traditions of religion, language, or appearance from the larger cultural system in which they live (Chapter 3)
ethnicity qualities that reflect the characteristics a group may share in some combination (Chapter 3)
ethnocentrism the belief that one's own ethnic beliefs, customs, and attitudes are correct and thus superior (Chapter 3)
etic dimension the objective interpretation of health by a scientifically trained practitioner (Chapter 20)
etiology the cause of a disease (Chapter 19)
eupnea easy, quiet respiration with a rate of 12 to 20 breaths per minute in an adult at rest (Chapter 7) [audio]
evaluation a systematic and ongoing process of examining whether expected outcomes have been achieved and whether nursing care has been effective (Chapter 10)
evidence-based practice a conscientious integration of the best research evidence into clinical practice and decisions about client care (Chapter 15)
evisceration protrusion of internal organs through an incision (Chapter 27) [audio]
exclusive provider organization (EPO) a type of group health care practice in which enrollees are restricted to the list

of preferred providers of health care (the exclusive providers) (Chapter 4)

excoriation an injury to the epidermis caused by abrasion, scratching, a burn, or chemicals (such as sweat, wound drainage, feces, or urine) coming in contact with skin (Chapter 33) [audio]

executive function a constellation of cognitive abilities that include the ability to plan, organize, and sequence tasks and manage multiple tasks simultaneously; includes self-monitoring and self-correcting behaviors (Chapter 40)

expected outcome desired result from nursing care expressed in terms of measurable client behaviors (Chapter 10)

experimental research a study in which the researcher manipulates a treatment or intervention, randomly assigns subjects to either a control or an experimental group, and has control over the research situation (Chapter 15)

extended family family unit that includes the nuclear family and other relatives, such as aunts, uncles, cousins, and grandparents, who are committed to maintaining family ties (Chapter 48)

exudate fluid and cells that have escaped from blood vessels during the inflammatory response and are left in surrounding tissues (Chapter 27) [audio]

faith belief in or commitment to something or someone that helps a person realize purpose without proof of its existence (Chapter 49)

false imprisonment the restraining, with or without force, of another person against his or her wishes (Chapter 2)

family two or more people united by a common goal to create a physical, cultural, spiritual, and nurturing bond that will promote the physical, mental, spiritual, and social development of each of its members while maintaining cohesiveness as a unit (Chapter 48)

family-centered nursing health care that focuses on the health of the family as a unit, as well as the maintenance and improvement in the health and growth of each person in that unit (Chapter 48)

family dynamics the ever-changing pattern of interaction among family members; the forces at work within the family that create patterns of behavior (Chapter 48)

fear an intense feeling of dread related to an identifiable source of threat that the person can verify as real (Chapter 42)

fecal impaction a collection of puttylike or hardened feces in the rectum or sigmoid colon that prevents the passage of normal stool and becomes more and more hardened as the colon continues to absorb water from it (Chapter 29) [audio]

feces body waste discharged from the intestine, also called stool, excreta, or excrement (Chapter 29) [audio]

feedback the process by which effectiveness of communication is determined (Chapter 12)

fever a regulated rise in temperature that is mediated by a rise in temperature set-point (Chapter 28)

fiber the structure of which plants are composed, including cellulose, hemicellulose, pectins, gums, and mucilages (Chapter 24)

fidelity an ethical principle having to do with honoring agreements and keeping promises (Chapter 2)

filtration the passage of water and certain smaller particles through a semipermeable membrane assisted by hydrostatic or capillary pressure (Chapter 26)

first pass effect partial metabolism of opioid analgesics by the liver before they reach the systemic circulation, thereby resulting in a decrease in opioid availability (and thus requiring an increased dosage) (Chapter 37)

fistula an abnormal passage between two internal organs or between internal organs and the external skin surface (Chapter 27) [audio]

flaccid the state of being weak, soft, and flabby, lacking normal muscle tone, or having no ability to contract (Chapter 32)

flatulence the presence of abnormal amounts of gas in the gastrointestinal tract, causing abdominal distention and discomfort (Chapter 29) [audio]

flatus the air and gas that accumulate in the gastrointestinal tract from swallowing air and from digestion and that passes through the anus (Chapter 29)

flow sheet a form used to document data that can be more easily followed in graphic or tabular form (Chapter 11)

focus charting a method of charting that addresses client problems or needs and includes a column that summarizes the focus of the entry (Chapter 11)

focus group method of data collection in which 6 to 12 people from a group or aggregate are brought together for discussion, guided when necessary by a skilled, nonjudgmental leader (Chapter 43)

footdrop a contracture deformity in which the muscles of the anterior foot are lengthened and the muscles of plantar flexion along with the Achilles tendon are shortened, resulting in plantar flexion of the foot (Chapter 33)

formal operations abstract reasoning (Chapter 17)

for-profit a business operating for the purpose of making a profit (Chapter 14)

fraud the false representation of some fact, with the intention that it will be acted on by another person (Chapter 2)

friction injury injury in which the epidermal layer of skin is rubbed off, possibly from a restraint, a dressing, bed linens, or a tube (Chapter 33)

functional health patterns the positive and negative behaviors a person uses to interact with the environment and maintain health (Chapter 6)

functional urinary incontinence an unpredictable, involuntary passage of urine in the presence of normal bladder and urethral function; sometimes occurring without cognitive awareness of the need to void (Chapter 30)

functional limitations difficulties that people with physical challenges face in performing activities of daily living (Chapter 44)

gate control theory theory about an alteration in the transmission of the ascending pain signal by a spinal gating mechanism located in the dorsal horn; the pain signal may be inhibited or facilitated by multiple variables (Chapter 37)

gender a person's sex, either male or female (Chapter 46)

gender identity the internal belief or sense that one is male or female (Chapter 46)

gender role the outward appearance, behaviors, attitudes, and feelings deemed culturally appropriate for males or females (Chapter 46)

general anesthesia loss of all sensation, consciousness, and memory of the surgical event as a result of inhaling an anesthetic drug, having it injected into the bloodstream, or both (Chapter 50)

generic name the name (also called a nonproprietary name) assigned to a drug by the United States Adopted Names Council when the drug is first manufactured (Chapter 21)

geriatric nursing branch of nursing that deals with the problems and diseases of old age and aging people (Chapter 18)

gerontology the comprehensive study of aging and the problems of older adults (Chapter 18)

gingivitis inflammation of the gums, usually manifested by the primary symptom of bleeding of the gums (Chapter 31) [audio]

glycogen the form in which carbohydrates are stored in the muscle tissue of humans and animals (Chapter 24) [audio]

goals broad, general statements about the desired results of nursing care; should be measurable through the delineation of expected outcomes (Chapter 10)

Gram stain a microscopic test used to identify a culture sent to the laboratory (Chapter 22)

granulation tissue any soft pink fleshy projections that form during the healing process in a wound that does not heal by primary intention; it consists of capillaries surrounded by fibrous collagen (Chapter 27)

grief a normal, complex process that includes emotional, physical, spiritual, social, and intellectual responses and behaviors by which individuals, families, and communities incorporate an actual, anticipated, or perceived loss into their daily lives (Chapter 45)

grief attack unexpected, involuntary resurgence of acute grief-related emotions and behaviors triggered by routine events, sometimes accompanied by uncontrollable crying or emotional display (Chapter 45)

grief work efforts (necessary to complete the normal grieving and mourning process) by a grieving person to acknowledge the physical and psychological pain of bereavement and to integrate the loss into the future (Chapter 45)

growth the physiological development of a living being and the quantitative (measurable) change seen in the body (Chapter 16)

guaiac a reagent used for detecting occult blood in the stool (Chapter 29)

gustatory pertaining to the sensation of taste (Chapter 38)

gynecomastia a benign increase in breast tissue associated with puberty in boys (Chapter 17)

hallucinations sensory reactions in the absence of real stimuli (Chapter 40)

health not just the absence of disease but the maximization of one's potential within the limitations that an individual might possess, including the entire individual's makeup: physical, social, spiritual, and psychological (Chapter 1)

health goals broad outline of what needs to be done to achieve health for individuals, families, or communities (Chapter 19)

health maintenance organization (HMO) a type of group health care practice that provides basic and supplemental health maintenance and treatment services to voluntary enrollees who prepay a fixed periodic fee set without regard to the amount or kind of services received (Chapter 4)

health perception the knowledge and experience of one's state of wellness and well-being (Chapter 19)

health promotion the advancement of health through the encouragement of activities that enhance the wellness of individuals, families, or communities (Chapters 4 and 19)

health status the third domain of the vulnerable populations conceptual model; it includes age- and gender-specific morbidity and mortality (Chapter 43)

health within illness a state that can expand human potential by providing an opportunity for personal growth and well-being despite having an illness (Chapter 19)

health-illness continuum a range that extends from high-level wellness (an optimal state of mental and physical well-being), to a neutral state in which the person cannot be considered either healthy or ill, to illness and premature death (Chapter 19)

heat exhaustion a rise in body temperature that is usually related to inadequate fluid and electrolyte replacement during physical activity (Chapter 28)

heat stroke an elevation of body temperature that is usually above 40.6° C (105° F) with altered central nervous system function (Chapter 28)

hematoma an accumulation of bloody fluid beneath tissue (Chapter 27) [audio]

hematuria the presence of blood in the urine (Chapter 30) [audio]

hemiparesis a numbness or other abnormal or impaired sensation experienced on only one side of the body and limiting activities of daily living (Chapter 32) [audio]

hemiplegia paralysis of one side of the body (Chapter 32) [audio]

hemoptysis coughing and spitting up blood as a result of bleeding from any part of the lower respiratory tract (Chapter 34) [audio]

hemorrhage bleeding from a wound bed or site (Chapter 27)

heterosexual sexual orientation in which one is sexually attracted to members of the opposite sex (Chapter 46)

holistic care an approach to client management that includes the individual's physical, social, spiritual, and psychological needs (Chapter 1)

homeostasis a state of internal stability of our physiology and our emotions (Chapters 42 and 47)

homophobia a fear of becoming homosexual through contact with lesbians or gay men or through having close or intimate feelings toward someone of the same sex (both myths) (Chapter 46)

homosexual sexual orientation in which one is sexually attracted to members of the same sex (Chapter 46)

hope an interpersonal process created through trust and nurtured by a trusting relationship with others, including God (Chapter 49)

hospice a cluster of special services that address the special needs of dying persons and their families (Chapter 45)

human capital a dimension of the resource availability domain of the vulnerable populations conceptual model that includes income, jobs, education, and housing (Chapter 43)

humanistic care understanding and knowing a client in as natural or human a way as possible while helping or guiding the client to achieve certain goals, make improvements, reduce discomforts, or face disability or death (Chapter 3)

hydrostatic pressure pressure exerted by the fluid within a compartment that results from the weight of the fluid (Chapter 26)

hypercapnia high carbon dioxide level in the blood, usually resulting from failure of the lungs to remove this gas (Chapter 34) [audio]

hypersensitivity reaction a mild allergic reaction to a drug (Chapter 21)

hyperthermia an elevation in body temperature related to an imbalance between heat gain and heat loss (Chapter 28)

hypertonic having an osmotic pressure greater than that of the solution to which it is being compared (Chapter 26)

hyperventilation increase in the rate and depth of breathing, clinically defined as a partial pressure of carbon dioxide ($PaCO_2$) less than 35 mm Hg; also known as hyperpnea (Chapter 34)

hypnotic a drug that acts on the central nervous system to shorten sleep onset, reduce nighttime wakefulness, or decrease anxiety when insomnia is associated with increased anxiety (Chapter 36) [audio]

hypomotility decreased peristalsis resulting from lack of stimulation of the gastrocolic reflex (Chapter 33) [audio]

hypostatic pneumonia inflammation of the lungs caused by stasis of secretions, which become a medium for bacterial growth (Chapter 33)

hypothermia a state in which body temperature is reduced below normal (Chapter 28) [audio]

hypothesis a tentative prediction of the relationship between two or more variables being studied (Chapter 15)

hypotonic having an osmotic pressure less than that of plasma (more water, less solute) (Chapter 26)

hypoventilation decrease in the rate and depth of breathing, clinically defined as $PaCO_2$ greater than 45 mm Hg (Chapter 34)

hypoxemia deficient oxygenation of the blood (Chapter 34) [audio]

hypoxia deficient oxygenation of body tissues (Chapter 34) [audio]

iatrogenic infection an infection acquired as the direct result of a medical, nursing, or other treatment (Chapter 22) [audio]

idiosyncratic response an unexplained and unpredictable response to a medication (Chapter 21)

ileostomy a surgical procedure involving the creation of an opening between the ileum and the abdominal wall (Chapter 29)

illness a personal experience of feeling unhealthy; involves changes in a person's state of well-being and social function (Chapter 19)

illness prevention the use of immunizations or medications or other methods that avert disease or detect disease in the earliest, most treatable stages (Chapter 4)

immobility the inability to move the whole body or a body part (Chapter 33)

immunization medication administered to activate an immune response before exposure to the disease agent (Chapter 22)

immunocompromised a state of not having an intact immune system (Chapter 22)

immunosuppression use of medications to suppress the body's immune system (Chapter 22) [audio]

inactivity lack of performing or being of use; usually related to an individual who is not active but sedentary or inert (Chapter 33)

incentive spirometer a device that provides a visual goal for and measurement of inspiration, thus encouraging the client to execute and sustain maximal inspiration (Chapter 34)

independent variable the variable that should stay constant during a study, although it influences or even causes a change in another variable (Chapter 15)

individualized care plan a plan written specifically for each client who enters a health care facility and developed from the admission history, physical and functional assessments, and problems anticipated from the physician's treatment plan (Chapter 10)

infection clinical syndrome caused by the invasion and multiplication of pathogens (Chapter 22) [audio]

infection control measures used to prevent or control the spread of an infection (Chapter 22)

inference the process of attaching meaning to data or reaching a conclusion about data; based on a premise that supports or helps support a conclusion (Chapter 6)

inflammatory response a localized reaction to injury that is activated when there is tissue damage (Chapter 22) [audio]

informed consent the legal right of a client to receive adequate and accurate information about his or her medical condition and treatment (Chapter 2), or of a potential research participant to receive sufficient information about a research project to enable him or her to consent voluntarily to participate or decline to participate (Chapter 15)

injury trauma or damage to some part of the body (Chapter 23)

inotropic agent a medication that increases the contractility of the heart muscle, thereby increasing cardiac output (Chapter 35) [audio]
insomnia characterized by difficulty initiating or maintaining sleep, sleeping too lightly, easily disrupted sleep with many spontaneous arousals, or early-morning awakenings and the subjective sense that sleep quality is poor and inadequate (Chapter 36)
inspection the systematic visual examination of the client (Chapter 8)
institutional review board (IRB) a committee whose duties include making sure that proposed research meets the federal requirements for ethical research (Chapter 15)
instrumental activities of daily living (IADLs) food preparation, housekeeping, laundry, transportation, using the telephone, shopping, and handling finances (Chapter 45)
instruments the tools a researcher uses to conduct a study (Chapter 15)
interdisciplinary team a group of people working together with the client to achieve mutually established rehabilitation goals for recovery or adaptation; an array of doctors, nurses, physical and occupational therapists, social workers, psychologists, and nutritionists make up the team (Chapter 44)
interface pressure pressure created in tissues that are compressed between the bones and a support surface by the weight of the body (Chapter 33)
intergenerational family a family with more than one generation living together in one residence or within a small geographical area (Chapter 48)
interval or progress note a nursing note that is entered at various times during a shift and reflects any aspect of change in the client's condition, or anything affecting the client such as tests, stat or prn medications, and procedures (Chapter 11)
interview a planned series of questions designed to elicit information for a particular purpose (Chapter 6)
intradermal route (ID) injection into the dermal layer of the skin (the dermis) (Chapter 21) [audio]
intramuscular route (IM) injection into muscle tissue (Chapter 21) [audio]
intraoperative phase surgical phase that starts with the client's entry into the operating room and ends when the client is transferred to the recovery room or other area to receive immediate postsurgical attention (Chapter 50) [audio]
intrathecal analgesia pain relief provided by placing a catheter in the subarachnoid space between the dura mater and the spinal cord to allow immediate drug diffusion into the cerebrospinal fluid (Chapter 37) [audio]
intravenous route (IV) injection into a vein (Chapter 21) [audio]
intuition an ability to understand the whole without having to systematically examine the parts (Chapter 6)
invasion of privacy occurs when the client's private affairs are unreasonably intruded upon by the nurse (Chapter 2)
ischemia decreased supply of oxygenated blood to tissues (Chapter 35)
isolation identification of a client who has an infection and implementation of precautions to prevent the spread of that infection (Chapter 22)
isometric exercise a form of active exercise that increases muscle tension by applying pressure against stable resistance, where there is no joint movement and the length of the muscle remains unchanged, but the tone and strength are maintained or increased (Chapter 32)
isotonic having an osmotic pressure equal to that of the solution to which it is being compared (Chapters 26 and 32)
isotonic exercise a form of active exercise in which the muscle contracts and moves with little change in resistance (Chapter 32)
judgment the ability to make rational decisions (Chapter 40)
justice an ethical principle based on moral rightness, fairness, or equity (Chapter 2)
Kegel exercises exercises performed to strengthen the pelvic and vaginal muscles to help control stress incontinence in women (Chapter 30)
key informant a community leader, professional, politician, or business person who has knowledge of the needs of the community and who can act as a useful source of data and a supporter of new programs (Chapter 43)
kinesthetic pertaining to the sensation of position (Chapter 38)
Korotkoff's sounds five distinct sounds heard while measuring blood pressure (Chapter 7)
kyphosis an abnormal condition of the vertebral column characterized by increased convexity in the thoracic spine when viewed from the side (Chapter 32)
language a set of words having meanings that are comprehensible within a group (Chapter 12)
law a body of rules of action or conduct prescribed by a controlling authority, which is the government (Chapter 2)
laxative a medication, less potent than a cathartic, used to induce emptying of the bowel (Chapter 29)
leadership a means of shaping the future through influencing others to change direction in thinking or acting; leadership differs from management in that it empowers the followers with a vision and the desire to achieve high goals (Chapter 14)
leading question a question that suggests a possible response (Chapter 6)
learning the acquisition of knowledge, behavior, or skill through experience, practice, study, or instruction (Chapter 13)
learning contract an agreement in which each party (nurse and client) agrees to contribute certain things; the nurse provides information, and the client agrees to use that information (Chapter 13)
learning objective a statement that describes the intended results of learning rather than the process of instruction (Chapter 13)
lesion a wound, injury, or pathological change in the body (Chapter 8)
liability the legal obligation or responsibility to provide care to a client that meets the accepted standards of care (Chapter 2)
libido the conscious or unconscious sex drive; desire for pleasure or satisfaction (Chapter 46) [audio]
license the granting, by a constituted authority, of formal permission to practice a particular profession (Chapter 2)
licensed vocational nurse (LVN)/ licensed practical nurse (LPN) a licensed nurse who has a defined set of technical skills and works under the direction of the professional registered nurse (Chapter 1)
lifestyle a behavior or group of behaviors, chosen by the person, that may have either a positive or a negative influence on health (Chapter 20)
living will document that provides written instructions about when life-sustaining treatment should be terminated (Chapter 2)
loading dose an initial medication dose that exceeds the maintenance or therapeutic dose (Chapter 21)
local anesthesia a temporary loss of feeling in an area of the body caused by the inhibition of nerve endings after being given a certain type of anesthetic drugs, usually by topical application or local (or extravascular) infiltration (Chapter 50)
long-term goal a goal that reflects an expectation that resolution of the nursing diagnosis will take place in small, measurable steps but may take weeks or months; may be ongoing in the rehabilitative or long-term care setting (Chapter 10)
loss the removal, change, or reduction in value of something valued or held dear, and the feelings that result (Chapter 45)
maceration a softening of the epidermis caused by prolonged contact with moisture, such as a wet sheet or diaper (Chapters 27 and 33) [audio]
maintenance stage the stage of change that takes place during the 6 months after the person changes the high-risk behavior (Chapter 20)
maladaptive coping methods or efforts directed toward management of dangerous, threatening, or challenging situations and producing feelings and behaviors that decrease the quality of life and lead to unhealthy outcomes (Chapter 47)
malaise a feeling of indisposition (Chapter 28)
malignant hyperthermia (MH) a rare, life-threatening, autosomal-dominant inherited syndrome that rapidly causes a very high temperature after anesthetic inhalation agents and neuromuscular blocking medications are given to induce general anesthesia (Chapter 50) [audio]
malnutrition a disorder characterized by insufficient or excessive nourishment of body tissue caused by improper diet or impaired absorption or metabolism of nutrients (Chapter 25)
malpractice acts of negligence by a professional person as compared to the actions of another professional person in similar circumstances (Chapter 2)

managed care a system that combines the functions of health insurance and the actual delivery of care in a way that controls utilization and cost of services by limiting unnecessary treatment (Chapter 4)
management implementation of strategies that promote effective and efficient use of resources (human, technological, supplies, time) to achieve organizational goals (Chapter 14)
Medicaid a welfare program, supported jointly by federal and state governments, providing partial health care services for indigent people (Chapter 4)
medical asepsis practices to reduce the numbers of pathogenic microorganisms in a person's environment (Chapter 22)
medical model a philosophy of health care delivery in which identification and treatment of an illness or disease is the focus of care (Chapter 4)
Medicare a federally funded national health insurance program in the United States for people over 65 years of age (Chapter 4)
memory the retention or storage of information learned about the world (Chapter 40)
menarche the time of the first menstrual period (Chapter 17) [audio]
menopause the second stage in the female climacteric, during which hormone production is reduced, the ovaries stop producing eggs, and menstruation ceases (Chapter 18)
message the content a sender wishes another person (the receiver) to receive in the process of communication (Chapter 12)
metabolic acidosis a pathological condition caused by an increase in noncarbonic acids, a decrease in bicarbonate in the extracellular fluid, or both (Chapter 26)
metabolic alkalosis a pathological condition caused by an increase in bicarbonate, a decrease in acid in the extracellular fluid, or both (Chapter 26) [audio]
metabolism the process by which energy from nutrients is used by the cells or stored for later use (Chapter 24) [audio]
micturition the process of emptying the bladder (Chapter 30) [audio]
middle adulthood the period of time between age 35 and age 64 (Chapter 18)
midlife crisis a stressful life period during middle adulthood, precipitated by the review and reevaluation of one's past, including goals, priorities, and life accomplishment, during which the person experiences inner turmoil, self-doubt, and major restructuring of personality (Chapter 18)
milliequivalent one thousandth of a chemical equivalent; the measurement used to express the chemical activity or combining power of an ion (Chapter 26) [audio]
milliosmole the amount of dissolved particles needed to produce a unit of force (Chapter 26)
minerals inorganic elements, present in small amounts in virtually all body fluids and tissues (Chapter 24)
minimum data set the least amount of information to be collected on every client entering an institution or being admitted to a particular service within an institution (Chapter 6)
mixed agonist-antagonist analgesic analgesic that attaches to both the *kappa* and *mu* opioid receptor sites, simultaneously providing analgesia at the *kappa* site and blocking activity at the *mu* site if given after the client receives a morphinelike drug (Chapter 37) [audio]
modulation an internal or external restraining of the nociceptive process that inhibits transmission of the pain signal at any place along the transmission pathway (Chapter 37)
monosaccharide a six-carbon sugar (a carbohydrate subunit), such as glucose, fructose, or galactose (Chapter 24) [audio]
monotheism belief in the existence of one God who created and rules the universe (Chapter 49)
morals standards of conduct that represent the ideal in human behavior that would be put forward by all rational persons as a guide to our relationships to others (Chapter 2)
mourning social and cultural acts used by a bereaved person to express thoughts and feelings of sorrow (Chapter 45)
multicultural society a society composed of more than one culture or subculture (Chapter 3)
multiple sleep latency test a direct, objective measure of sleepiness used to evaluate excessive somnolence and daytime sleepiness (Chapter 36)
narcolepsy characterized by abnormal sleep tendencies as well as by pathological REM sleep, manifested as excessive daytime sleepiness, sudden daytime sleep attacks usually last 20 to 30 minutes, disturbed nighttime sleep, cataplexy, sleep paralysis, and hypnagogic hallucinations (Chapter 36)
narrative charting a method of charting that provides information in the form of statements that describe events surrounding client care (Chapter 11)
National Council Licensure Examination for Registered Nurses (NCLEX-RN) successful passage required for licensure as a registered nurse (Chapter 1)
necrosis localized death of tissues caused by disease, oxygen deficit, or injury (Chapter 35)
negligence an act of omission or commission by a lay person resulting in harm or injury (Chapter 2)
neologism the creation of words that are meaningless to the listener; a common language problem of the aphasic client (Chapter 39) [audio]
neuropathic pain transmission of a pain signal from the site of injury to the higher brain centers via a nervous system that has been damaged in some way (Chapter 37) [audio]
neurotransmitter A chemical messenger released from the synaptic terminal of a neuron at a chemical synapse that diffuses across the synaptic cleft and binds to and stimulates the postsynaptic membrane (Chapter 40)
nightmare disorder the repeated occurrence of frightening dreams that lead to awakenings from sleep that occurs primarily during rapid eye movement (REM) sleep and may occur every 90 to 110 minutes (Chapter 36)
nociception transmission of a pain signal from a site of tissue damage to areas of the brain where perception occurs (Chapter 37) [audio]
nociceptive pain pain transmitted from a site of injury to the higher brain centers via an intact nervous system (Chapter 37)
nociceptor primary afferent fiber that initiates the pain experience when stimulated by tissue damage (Chapter 37)
nocturia nighttime urination (Chapter 30) [audio]
nocturnal emission a discharge of semen during sleep (Chapter 17)
nocturnal enuresis bed-wetting; repeated urination during nighttime sleep that disrupts the sleep cycle (Chapter 36)
nonelectrolyte a substance, such as glucose, that does not ionize and thus does not carry an electrical charge (Chapter 26)
nonexperimental research a type of study in which the researcher collects data without the introduction of a treatment or intervention (Chapter 15)
nonmaleficence the concept that no harm is done by the practitioner (Chapter 2)
nonopioid analgesic a drug that provides analgesia at the peripheral level by a mechanism other than those that occur at the opioid receptor sites (Chapter 37)
nonprofit in the context of medicine, referring to an institution that does not make a profit (Chapter 14)
non–rapid eye movement (NREM) sleep a sleeping period without rapid eye movement (REM) (Chapter 36)
nonverbal communication a set of behaviors that conveys messages either without words or by supplementing verbal communication (Chapter 12)
normal grief a response to bereavement, separation, or loss that includes emotional, physical, cognitive, and behavioral responses within an expected range for any person with such an experience, but retaining uniqueness for each individual (Chapter 45)
nosocomial infection an infection that is acquired from a reservoir in the hospital (Chapter 22) [audio]
not-for-profit refers to institutions whose purpose is not to make a profit but to reinvest it into services provided (Chapter 14)
nuclear family husband, wife, and offspring living in a common household, usually with one or both partners gainfully employed (Chapter 48)
nurse manager a nurse responsible for managing the operation and expenses of a health care organization that employs nurses as the means to produce health (Chapter 14)
nurse-initiated intervention any treatment initiated by the nurse in response to a nursing diagnosis; an autonomous action based on scientific rationale that is executed to benefit the client in a predicted way related to the nursing diagnosis and projected outcome (Chapter 10)

nursing an accountable discipline guided by science, theory, a code of ethics, and the art of using care and comfort to treat human responses to health and illness (Chapter 1)
nursing care plan (NCP) a guide for client care that identifies client problems in need of nursing care (specified by nursing diagnoses), predicts outcomes that are sensitive to nursing care, and lists interventions that will result in the expected outcomes (Chapter 10)
nursing diagnosis a clinical judgment about individual, family, or community responses to actual or potential health problems or life processes (Chapter 9)
nursing history a narrative of the client's past health and health practices that focuses on information needed to plan nursing care (whereas a medical history focuses on illness and the treatment of disease) (Chapter 6)
nursing intervention any treatment, based on clinical judgment and knowledge, that a nurse performs to enhance client outcomes (Chapter 10)
Nursing Interventions Classification (NIC) a system of standardized language appropriate for computerized client information systems to describe the component of client care that is nursing practice (developed at the University of Iowa) (Chapter 10)
Nursing Outcomes Classification (NOC) a system of standardized language for measuring the effects of nursing care using indicators sensitive to nursing intervention (Iowa Outcomes Project) (Chapter 10)
nursing process a clinical decision-making framework that includes critical thinking, diagnostic reasoning, and clinical judgment; composed of five interwoven phases: assessment, diagnosis, planning, intervention, and evaluation (Chapter 5)
nursing-sensitive client outcome a client result that can be achieved by nursing intervention (Chapter 10)
nutrient a biochemical substance used by the body for growth, maintenance, and repair (Chapter 24)
nutrition the science of food and nutrients and of the processes by which an organism takes them in and uses them for energy to grow, maintain function, and renew itself (Chapter 24)
nutritional status the condition of the body resulting from its use of the essential nutrients available to it (Chapter 24)
object permanence the awareness that unseen objects do not disappear, evidenced by the infant searching for an object that has been moved out of sight (Chapter 16)
objective caregiver burden the visible, tangible cost to the caregiver as measured in required behaviors or disruptions (Chapter 48)
objective data characteristics about the client that are directly observable (Chapter 6)
obstructive sleep apnea (OSA) a sleep disorder manifested by periodic cessation of airflow at the nose and mouth during inspiration and that arouses the person from sleep (Chapter 36) [audio]
occult blood an amount of blood too small to be seen without a microscope (Chapter 29)
official name the name assigned by the Food and Drug Administration (often the same as the generic name) after a drug is approved (Chapter 21)
older adult any person over age 65 (Chapter 18)
olfactory pertaining to the sensation of smell (Chapter 38)
oliguria a diminished, scanty amount of urine (Chapter 30) [audio]
open system a system that exchanges matter, energy, and information with other systems and with the environment (Chapter 48)
open-ended question a question that allows the client freedom in the manner of response (Chapter 6)
operational definition the meaning of a concept precisely as it is being used in a study, defined in a manner that specifies how concepts will be measured (Chapter 15)
ophthalmoscope an instrument used to visualize the retina, including the optic disc, macula, and retinal blood vessels, through the pupil (Chapter 8) [audio]
opinion survey a method of data collection performed through telephone interviews, mailed questionnaires, door-to-door interviews, or at clinic sites (Chapter 43)
opioid analgesic any morphinelike drug that attaches to the opioid receptors and produces analgesia by blocking substance P, a powerful neurotransmitter of the pain signal (Chapter 37) [audio]
opioid naive having had no or minimal previous exposure to opioid analgesics (Chapter 37)
opioid receptor the portion of a nerve cell to which an opioid or opioid-like substance can bind (Chapter 37)
orgasm sexual tension evidenced by muscular spasm and engorgement of blood vessels reaching maximum intensity; a highly pleasurable and totally involuntary response (Chapter 46)
orientation awareness of person, place, and time (Chapter 40)
orientation phase a phase of the interview process in which there is a brief exchange to establish the purpose, the procedure, and the nurse's role (Chapter 6)
orthostatic hypotension blood pressure variation in which blood pressure drops by 20 mm Hg or more with position changes; a temporary condition of low blood pressure caused by the failure of compensatory mechanisms to regulate pressure as the person moves from a lying to a sitting or standing position (also called **orthostatic intolerance**) (Chapters 7 and 33) [audio]
osmolality the number of milliosmoles per kilogram of water (Chapter 26) [audio]
osmolarity the number of milliosmoles per liter of solution (Chapter 26) [audio]
osmosis the movement of water through a semipermeable membrane from an area of lower concentration of particles to an area of higher concentration of particles (Chapter 26) [audio]
osteoporosis a condition in which there is a decreased mass per unit volume of normally mineralized bone, primarily from a loss of calcium, that makes bones brittle and porous (Chapter 33) [audio]
ostomy a surgical procedure that creates an opening through the abdomen into the intestine to allow fecal matter to exit the intestine from a site other than the anus (Chapter 29) [audio]
otoscope a hand-held instrument used to examine the external ear, the eardrum, and, through the eardrum, the ossicles of the middle ear (Chapter 8) [audio]
ototoxic capable of damaging cranial nerve VIII or the organs of hearing and balance (Chapter 38)
oxygen saturation the percent of saturation of the client's arterial blood with oxygen, usually 95% to 100%; also abbreviated as SaO_2 (Chapter 7)
pain an unpleasant sensory and emotional experience associated with actual and potential tissue damage, described in terms of such damage (Chapter 37)
pain behavior anything a person says or does that implies the presence of pain (Chapter 37)
palliative care the control of pain, symptoms, and distress for clients whose disease is not responsive to curative treatment (Chapter 45)
palpation a form of touch or feeling with the hand to obtain information about temperature, moisture, texture, consistency, size, shape, position, and movement (Chapter 8)
panic profound terror experienced with an intense urge to escape or fight; accompanied by disintegration of personality organization and inability to control thoughts and actions (Chapter 42)
paralanguage the nonverbal components of spoken language, which give speech its rhythm and humanness and include stress, accent, pitch, pause, intonation, rate, volume, and quality (Chapter 12)
paralytic ileus a temporary stoppage of peristalsis caused by direct handling of the bowel during surgery (Chapter 29) [audio]
paraparesis a numbness or other abnormal or impaired sensation in the legs and trunk (Chapter 32) [audio]
paraphasia a word substitution problem in the aphasic client who speaks fluently (Chapter 39) [audio]
paraplegia paralysis characterized by motor or sensory loss in the legs and trunk (Chapter 32) [audio]
parasomnias difficulties with abnormal movements and behaviors that occur during sleep rather than difficulties with sleep itself; examples include nightmare disorder, sleep terror disorder and sleepwalking disorder (Chapter 36)
parenteral nutrition provision of total nutrition through a central or peripheral intravenous catheter (Chapter 25)
parenteral route a route for medication administration that is outside the gastrointestinal tract (Chapter 21) [audio]
parish nurse a registered nurse who is employed by (or volunteers at) a religious or health care organization for the purpose of providing nursing care to members of a church congregation (Chapter 43)

participant observation a method of community assessment that examines formal and informal social systems at work, in which the researcher shares in the life activities of the group while observing and collecting data (Chapter 43)

pathogen a disease-producing microorganism (Chapter 22) [audio]

patient-controlled analgesia (PCA) a drug delivery approach that employs an external infusion pump to deliver an opioid dose on a "client demand" basis (Chapter 37)

peer review the evaluation of the performance of one staff member by another staff member, on the same level in the hierarchy of the organization or similar in qualifications, to judge the quality of care provided or other measures of professional/job performance (Chapter 14)

perceived barriers negative perceptions and beliefs about aspects of a health action, or viewed impediments to undertaking the recommended behaviors (Chapter 20)

perceived benefits positive perceptions and beliefs about the effectiveness of the recommended actions in preventing the health threat (Chapter 20)

perceived severity perceived seriousness of contracting an illness or leaving it untreated (Chapter 20)

perceived susceptibility subjective perception of the risk of contracting a health condition (Chapter 20)

perception conscious mental recognition or registration of a sensory stimulus, as, for example when a person smells a sweet fragrance and gets the mental image of a cherry (Chapter 38)

percussion the use of short, sharp strikes to the body surface to produce palpable vibrations and characteristic sounds (Chapter 8)

performance appraisal an organized and uniform method of evaluation of a nurse's job contribution, quality of work, and potential for advancement, made by the nurse's supervisor (Chapter 14)

perineum the pelvic floor and associated structures of the pelvic outlet, bounded anteriorly by the symphysis pubis, laterally by the ischial tuberosities, and posteriorly by the coccyx (Chapter 31) [audio]

perioperative the preoperative, intraoperative, and postoperative phases of the surgical experience (Chapter 50) [audio]

perioperative nursing a specialized area of practice that describes the provision of care for the surgical client throughout the continuum of care (Chapter 50)

peripheral vascular resistance the impediment to blood flow in a vessel created by the diameter of the vessel and the viscosity of the blood (Chapter 7) [audio]

peristalsis rhythmic smooth-muscle contractions of the intestinal wall that propel the intestinal contents forward toward the anus (Chapter 29) [audio]

personal identity the organizing principle of the personality that accounts for the unity, continuity, consistency, and uniqueness of an individual (Chapter 41)

personal space a private zone around our body that we believe is an extension of ourselves and belongs to us (Chapter 12)

pharmacokinetics the activity of a drug from the time it enters the body until it leaves (Chapter 21) [audio]

phonation the production of sound by the vibration of the vocal cords (Chapter 39)

physical dependence an involuntary physiological phenomenon that occurs after repeated exposure to an opioid analgesic that causes withdrawal symptoms if the opioid is abruptly withdrawn or an opioid antagonist is administered (Chapter 37)

physician-initiated intervention a treatment initiated by a physician in response to a medical diagnosis but carried out by a nurse in response to a physician's order (Chapter 10)

plaintiff the party bringing a lawsuit that alleges certain facts and outcomes (Chapter 2)

plaque a soft, thin film of food debris, mucin, and dead epithelial cells that is deposited on the teeth and provides a medium for the growth of bacteria (Chapter 31)

point of maximal impulse (PMI) the point on the chest wall where the apex of the heart is closest and the heartbeat can be felt (Chapter 8)

poisoning an adverse condition or physical state resulting from the administration of a toxic substance (Chapter 23)

policy a set of rules and regulations that govern nursing practice and nursing care; guidelines that are often more general than in a protocol or procedure in order to apply in multiple situations (Chapter 14)

polysaccharide a group of monosaccharides joined together in a chain; can be converted back to monosaccharides by acid hydrolysis (Chapter 24) [audio]

polysomnography the continuous measurement and recording of physiological activity during sleep using electroencephalogram, electrooculogram, electrocardiogram, and electromyogram tracings to monitor brain activity, eye movements, heart rate and rhythm, and muscle movements (Chapter 36) [audio]

polytheism belief in more than one god (Chapter 49)

polyuria a large amount of urine, usually associated with diabetes mellitus or diabetes insipidus (Chapter 30) [audio]

population a group of individuals who share common characteristics (Chapter 43)

population health the consideration of health problems encountered as a result of being a part of a group, and the focus on interventions for a population rather than for an individual (Chapter 19)

postanesthesia care unit (PACU) a nursing care unit where clients remain until they regain consciousness from the effects of anesthesia (previously known as the recovery room or postanesthesia unit) (Chapter 50)

postoperative phase period following an operation, which can be divided into two segments of care: the immediate postoperative period (including an evaluative assessment by the perioperative nurse and admittance to the postanesthesia care unit) and the ongoing postoperative period (including all care given during the course of surgical convalescence to the time of discharge, and continuing with assisted care or self-care at home) (Chapter 50)

postural drainage a technique in which the client assumes one or more positions that will facilitate the drainage of secretions from the bronchial airways (Chapter 34)

PQRST model a model for the assessment of pain: P stands for provoking incident; Q stands for quality; R stands for region, radiation, or relieving factors; S stands for severity; and T stands for timing (Chapter 32)

precontemplation stage the first stage in the change process, in which a person does not intend to change a high-risk behavior in the foreseeable future (the next 6 months), primarily because of a lack of awareness of the long-term consequences of the behavior (Chapter 20)

precordium the area on the anterior chest overlying the heart and great vessels (Chapter 8)

preferred provider organization (PPO) an organization of physicians, hospitals, and pharmacists whose members discount their health care services to subscriber clients; may be organized by a group of physicians, an outside entrepreneur, an insurance company, or a company with a self-insurance plan (Chapter 4)

preload the amount of blood in the left ventricle immediately before contraction; the main force that stretches cardiac muscle fibers (Chapter 35)

preoperative phase phase that begins with the decision for surgical intervention and ends when the client is safely transported into the operating room for a surgical procedure (Chapter 50)

preparation stage the third stage in the change process, in which a person intends to take action in the very near future, usually within the next month (Chapter 20)

presbycusis a sensorineural hearing loss of high-frequency tones that occurs in older adults and may lead to a loss of all hearing frequencies (Chapter 38) [audio]

presbyopia loss of near vision in older people that results from reduced elasticity in the lens and weakened ciliary muscles (Chapter 38) [audio]

prescription an order for a medication that contains the client's name, medication name, dose, route, frequency, amount of the medication to be dispensed, number of refills allowed (if any), and the physician's signature (Chapter 21)

pressure ulcer any lesion caused by ischemia from unrelieved pressure that leads to damage of the skin and underlying tissues (Chapter 27 and 33)

preventive health care the recognition of the risk of disease and actions taken to reduce that risk (Chapter 19)

primary health care all care necessary to people's lives and health, including health education, nutrition, sanitation, maternal and child health care, immunizations, prevention, and control of endemic disease (Chapter 19)

primary hypersomnia excessive sleepiness that is severe enough to cause clinically significant distress or impairment in occupational, social, and/or other areas of functioning that lasts at least 1 month as evidenced either by prolonged sleep episodes or by daytime sleep that occurs almost daily (Chapter 36)

primary lesion the first lesion to appear on the skin in response to a causative agent; usually has a recognizable structure (Chapter 27)

primary nursing a method of client assignments that gives the client a nurse who is at the bedside and responsible for the client's care over a 24-hour period (Chapter 14)

primary prevention actions that are considered true prevention because they precede disease or dysfunction and are applied to clients considered physically and emotionally healthy to protect them from health problems (Chapter 19)

problem solving defining a problem, selecting information pertinent to its conclusion (recognizing stated and unstated assumptions), formulating alternative solutions, drawing a conclusion, and judging the validity of the conclusion (Chapter 5)

problem-oriented medical records a form of documentation originally designed to organize information according to identified client problems, with all members of the health care team documenting information sequentially (Chapter 11)

procedural law establishes the manner of proceeding used to enforce a specific legal right or obtain redress (Chapter 2)

procedure a detailed description of a specific method of performing nursing care (Chapter 14)

profession a group of specialized individuals that supports, promotes, and maintains the practice of a specific skilled role through legal and public means; the role requires advanced education and training to perform (Chapter 1)

professional misconduct a violation of the nurse practice act that can result in disciplinary action against a nurse (Chapter 2)

proprioception sensation pertaining to stimuli originating from within the body regarding spatial position and muscular activity or to the sensory receptors that they activate (Chapter 32) [audio]

prospective payment system (PPS) a payment system in which the amount to be paid for a specific service is predetermined (Chapter 4)

protein a compound containing polymers of amino acids linked together in a chain by polypeptide bonds (Chapter 24)

protocol rules for action that contains detailed guidelines for nursing care for clients with specific conditions (Chapter 14)

proximodistal a normal pattern of skill development, which moves from the midline of the body outward (Chapter 16)

pseudoaddiction a syndrome of abnormal behavior that develops as a direct consequence of inadequate pain management (Chapter 37)

pseudodementia depression that is misinterpreted as dementia (Chapter 40)

psychological dependence (addiction) a chronic disorder demonstrated by overwhelming involvement with obtaining and using a drug for its mind-altering effects (Chapter 37)

psychomotor learning domain the learning domain concerned with physical and motor skills (Chapter 13)

psychoneuroimmunology the study of the interface between the brain and immunology (Chapter 47)

psychosocial adaptation the process by which a person adjusts, copes, or responds to the functional, psychological, and social changes that occur with the onset and experience of living with a physical/mental limitation or chronic illness (Chapter 44)

public health nursing the practice of promoting and protecting the health of populations through nursing activities to improve the quality of life (including its physical, mental, and social aspects), to prevent disease, and to control communicable disease consistent with available knowledge and resources using knowledge from nursing, social science, and public health science (Chapter 43)

public law regulates the relationship of individuals to government agencies and may be administrative, constitutional, or statutory (Chapter 2)

pulmonary embolus a condition that results when a piece of a deep vein thrombus breaks free, floats in the blood stream to the pulmonary circulation, and lodges in a pulmonary blood vessel (Chapter 33) [audio]

pulse deficit the condition of the apical pulse rate exceeding the radial pulse rate (Chapter 7)

pulse oximeter a device for measuring the oxygen saturation of functional hemoglobin in the blood (Chapter 7) [audio]

pulse oximetry measuring oxygen saturation of functional hemoglobin in the blood (Chapter 34)

pulse pressure the amount of pressure that produces the palpable pulse (the difference between systolic and diastolic blood pressures) (Chapter 7)

pursed-lip breathing a technique of mouth breathing that creates slight resistance to exhalation by contracting the lips to reduce the size of the opening, thus maintaining an even reduction of intrathoracic pressure during exhalation (Chapter 34)

pyrogen an agent that causes or stimulates a fever (Chapter 28)

quadriparesis a numbness or other abnormal or impaired sensation in all four limbs and the trunk (Chapter 32) [audio]

quadriplegia an abnormal condition characterized by paralysis of the arms, legs, and trunk below the level of an associated injury to the spinal cord (Chapter 32) [audio]

qualitative research a type of study that uses ideas analyzed as words (as opposed to numbers) (Chapter 15)

quality assurance a process of evaluating the outcome of care measured against predetermined standards and implementing methods of improvement (Chapter 14)

quantitative research a type of study that uses variables analyzed as numbers (as opposed to words) (Chapter 15)

quarantine the process of isolating people infected by a communicable disease to prevent its spread to large numbers of other people (Chapter 22)

quasi-experimental research a type of study in which the researcher manipulates a treatment or intervention but is unable to randomize subjects into groups or lacks a control group (Chapter 15)

range-of-motion exercises any body action (active or passive) involving the muscles, joints, and natural directional movements, such as abduction, extension, flexion, pronation, and rotation (Chapter 32)

rapid eye movement (REM) sleep the stage of sleep characterized by eyes jerking rapidly in various directions (Chapter 36)

recommended dietary allowance (RDA) the level of a nutrient that is adequate to meet the needs of almost all healthy people, as determined by the Food and Nutrition Board of the National Research Council (Chapter 24)

referral a process designed to provide the client with access to health care and supportive services that are not available from the sending institution (Chapter 20)

referred pain pain experienced at a site distant from the injured tissue (Chapter 37)

reflex urinary incontinence unexpected voiding without awareness of the need to void, specific to the client with a spinal cord injury (Chapter 30)

regional anesthesia a type of anesthesia that produces analgesia, relaxation, and reduced reflexes after medication is instilled into or around the nerves to block the transmission of nerve impulses (Chapter 50)

registered nurse a licensed, professional individual who practices under state guidelines to provide care in a safe and effective manner in various health care settings in a variety of roles (Chapter 1)

registered nurse first assistant (RNFA) an expanded nursing role, requiring additional education, in which the perioperative nurse works as a first assistant during the surgical procedure (Chapter 50)

registration a process by which an applicant provides specific information to the state agency administering the nursing registration process (Chapter 2)

rehabilitation the process of adaptation, or recovery, through which an individual suffering from a disabling condition, whether temporary or irreversible, participates to regain, or attempt to regain, maximum function, independence, and restoration (Chapters 4 and 44)

rehabilitation nursing a specialty in which nurses with expert knowledge in the care of clients and families affected by chronic illness or disability assist them with goal attainment, prevention of complications, promotion of self-care, and reintegration into the community (Chapter 44)

related factors factors that appear to be related to a nursing diagnosis and help define how the problem should be managed (Chapter 9)

relative risk the second domain of the vulnerable populations conceptual model; defined as the ratio of the risk of poor health among populations who do *not* receive resources and *are* exposed to risk factors, to the risk in those populations who *do* receive resources and are *not* exposed to these risk factors (Chapter 43)

religion a belief system that includes dogma, rituals, and traditions, and also a social institution in which people participate together rather than alone (Chapter 49)

religiosity a person's dependence on and involvement in religious practices and behaviors (Chapter 49)

renal calculi stones formed in the kidney when the excretion rate of calcium or other minerals is high, as when osteoclastic activity releases calcium from the bones during immobility (Chapter 33) [audio]

rescue dose administration of as-needed doses of an immediate-release analgesic in response to breakthrough pain and in addition to the scheduled analgesic dosage (Chapter 37)

research design a researcher's strategy for testing a hypothesis (Chapter 15)

research problem an observation, situation, occurrence, or even a hunch that an investigator chooses to research (Chapter 15)

residual urine the amount of urine remaining in the bladder after voiding (Chapter 30)

resilience the ability to identify or develop resources and strengths and to flexibly manage stressors to gain a positive outcome, a sense of confidence, mastery, and self-esteem (Chapter 47)

resonance the forced vibration of a structure that is related to a source of sound and results in changes in the quality of the sound (Chapter 39)

resource availability the first domain of the vulnerable populations conceptual model, involving the availability of socioeconomic and environmental resources (Chapter 43)

respiration the exchange of oxygen and carbon dioxide between the atmosphere and the cells of the body; also, a series of metabolic activities by which living cells break down carbohydrates, amino acids, and fats to produce energy in the form of adenosine triphosphate (ATP) (Chapter 34)

respiratory acidosis a state of having a pH of the blood that is less than normal (below 7.35) from respiratory causes; a result of the retention of carbon dioxide (CO_2), which is an acid, and a resultant decrease in pH (Chapter 26) [audio]

respiratory alkalosis a state of having a pH of the blood that is greater than normal (above 7.45) from respiratory causes; a result of rapid or excess elimination of CO_2, resulting in a increase in pH with a decrease in the partial pressure of CO_2 ($PaCO_2$) (Chapter 26)

respiratory excursion the degree to which the chest wall expands with inhalation; a measure of the ability of the lungs to expand (Chapter 8)

responsibility having the duty to act or direct the actions of others to achieve a goal (Chapter 14)

rest a state of being physically and mentally relaxed and free from anxiety while being awake and alert (Chapter 36)

restless legs syndrome a familial sleep disorder characterized by intense, abnormal, lower extremity sensations and irresistible leg movements that delay sleep onset (Chapter 36)

restraint a device (usually a wristlet, anklet, or other type of strap) intended for medical purposes that limits movement to the extent necessary for treatment, examination, or protection of the client (Chapter 23)

reticular activating system portion of the midbrain and thalamus that keeps the brain aroused and controls the sleep-wake cycle, level of consciousness, the ability to direct attention to specific tasks, and the perception of sensory input that might alter behavior (Chapter 38) [audio]

retirement the permanent withdrawal from one's job (Chapter 18)

retrospective audit a method of reviewing or evaluation by inspecting the medical record for documentation of compliance with standards, characterized by being an after-the-fact review of care that has been provided (Chapter 14)

retrospective payment system a payment system in which the amount of insurance paid was based on the service received (Chapter 4)

risk factors factors in the internal or external environment that increase the vulnerability of a person, family, or community to an unhealthful state or event (Chapter 9)

"risk for" nursing diagnosis a nursing diagnosis that describes human responses that *may* develop in a vulnerable person, family, or community (Chapter 9)

risk management a process of identifying, evaluating, and reducing or financing the cost of predictable losses, including loss from litigation (Chapter 14)

role a homogeneous set of behaviors, attitudes, beliefs, principles, and values that are normatively defined and expected of a person in a given social position or status in a group (Chapter 41)

role conflict incompatible expectations for behavior within a role, between two or more roles, or when a role is incongruent with a person's beliefs and values (Chapter 48)

role performance the roles a person assumes or is given, including the actions, thoughts, and feelings associated with those roles, as defined in terms of relationship to others (Chapter 41)

role stress emotion that occurs when a person has difficulty meeting the demands of a role (Chapter 48)

sampling the process of selecting subjects from the population being studied (Chapter 15)

sandwich generation middle-age adults caught between the needs of adjacent generations, caring for ill or frail parents while handling the competing demands of children and employment (Chapter 18)

scrub nurse a licensed or registered nurse with special qualifications that include knowledge of aseptic technique, instruments, and equipment; anatomy and physiology; surgical procedures; and, most importantly, promotion of client safety (Chapter 50)

searching in the context of the grief reaction, conscious and unconscious efforts by the bereaved to negate the reality of the loss through finding the deceased alive and well (Chapter 45)

secondary lesion a change in a primary lesion in the epidermal layer caused by any of several factors, including scratching, rubbing, medications, and the client's medical condition or disease process (Chapter 27)

secondary prevention actions that focus on the early diagnosis and prompt treatment of people with health problems or illnesses who are at risk for developing complications or worsening conditions (Chapter 19)

selective attention the act of consciously choosing when and to whom a person will give attention, and when to allow thoughts and feelings to enter the conscious mind (Chapter 45)

self-concept a relatively enduring set of attitudes and beliefs about both the physical self and the psychological self (Chapter 41)

self-efficacy the conviction that one can successfully execute a behavior required to produce desired outcomes (Chapter 20)

self-esteem one's evaluation of self; based on perceptions of how one is viewed by others as well as on the view of oneself (Chapter 41)

sensation the reception of stimulation through receptors of the nervous system (Chapter 38)

sense of presence nonthreatening, comforting perception by the bereaved of the presence of the deceased through one or more of the senses or in dreams, fortuitous events, or conversations (Chapter 45)

sensory channel the means by which a message is sent; primarily sensory: visual, auditory, and kinesthetic (Chapter 12)

sensory deprivation inadequate reception or perception of environmental stimuli (Chapter 38)

sensory overload excessive environmental stimuli, or stimulus beyond the person's ability to absorb or comprehend (Chapter 38)

sensory stimulation the activation and exhilaration of the senses (Chapter 16)

septicemia infection in the bloodstream (Chapter 22) [audio]

set-point the temperature that thermoregulatory mechanisms attempt to maintain (Chapter 28)

sexual desire a wish to participate in sexual intimacy that is activated by thoughts, fantasies, emotions, and psychological wants and needs (Chapter 46)

sexual dysfunction a change or disruption in sexual health or function that the affected person views as unrewarding or inadequate (Chapter 46)

sexual identity a perception of self as male or female (Chapter 46)

sexual orientation description of a person's sexual attraction and feelings of erotic potential toward a partner or toward members of either sex (heterosexual, homosexual, or bisexual) (Chapter 46)
sexual patterns a person's chosen expressions of sexuality (Chapter 46)
sexual response cycle phases of response in relation to sexual stimuli (Chapter 46)
sexuality the state or quality of being sexual, including the collective characteristics that distinguish male and female (Chapter 46)
shear a mechanical force that acts on an area of skin in a direction parallel to the body's surface (Chapter 33)
short-term goal a resolution of the nursing diagnosis that can be accomplished in an hour, a day, or a week; sometimes an intermediary goal that shows progress toward the longer-term goal (Chapter 10)
side effect an unintended or unplanned effect of a medication; often not dangerous (Chapter 21)
signs characteristics of disease or dysfunction that can be observed directly as objective data (Chapter 6)
single-parent family a household where children live with one parent (Chapter 48)
situational crisis a hazardous situation that is not easily anticipated and for which a person is inadequately prepared (Chapter 47)
sleep a state marked by reduced consciousness, diminished activity of the skeletal muscles, and depressed metabolism (Chapter 36)
sleep deprivation a state resulting when an individual does not get enough sleep (Chapter 36)
sleep terrors a parasomnia (also known as night terrors) that occurs during slow-wave sleep and is characterized by arousal, agitation, and signs of sympathetic nervous system activity, such as dilated pupils, increased sweating, tachypnea, and tachycardia (Chapter 36)
sleep terrors disorder the repeated occurrence of sleep terrors, abrupt awakenings from sleep usually beginning with a panicky scream or cry (Chapter 36)
sleepwalking disorder a slow-wave sleep parasomnia associated with stereotypical "sleepwalking" behaviors (Chapter 36)
slough necrotic tissue that is moist, stringy and yellow in color; it must be cleansed and removed to allow the wound to heal (Chapter 27)
SOAP charting a method of charting used to record progress notes with problem-oriented medical records; mnemonic stands for subjective data, objective data, assessment, and plan (Chapter 11)
social integration a dimension of the resource availability domain of the vulnerable populations conceptual model; refers to having a harmonious relationship with the society in which the person participates as a full member (Chapter 43)
social status a dimension of the resource availability domain of the vulnerable populations conceptual model; refers to the position of an individual in relation to others in the society as reflected in power to control the political process and the distribution of resources (Chapter 43)
social support the subjective feeling of belonging, or being accepted, loved, esteemed, valued, and needed for oneself, not for what one can do for others (Chapter 20)
somatic pain well-localized pain, usually from bone or spinal metastases or from injury to cutaneous or deep tissues (Chapter 37)
spastic describes muscle contractions caused by reflex activity rather than by central nervous system control (Chapter 32)
spiritual distress a disruption that pervades a person's being and that integrates and transcends one's biological and social nature, resulting in distress of the human spirit (Chapter 49)
spiritual health a state of wholeness of the spiritual dimension (Chapter 49)
spiritual well-being a process of being and becoming that surrounds the totality of a person's inner resources, the wholeness of spirit and unifying dimension, a process of transcendence, and the perception of life as having meaning (Chapter 49)
spirituality a process and sacred journey, an essence or life principle of a person, the experience of the radical truth of things, and a belief that relates a person to the world and gives meaning to existence (Chapter 49)
sputum mucus secreted from the lungs, bronchi, and trachea; may include epithelial cells, bacteria, and debris (Chapter 34)
standard precautions a set of actions, including hand hygiene and the use of barrier precautions, designed to reduce transmission of infectious organisms (Chapter 22)
standardized care plans plans that provide the usual nursing management for a nursing problem or a medical/surgical condition; typically written by a group of nurses who use their collective expertise to produce a plan to direct nursing care for clients with specific medical diagnoses (such as myocardial infraction) or nursing diagnoses (such as *Pain* or *Anxiety*) (Chapter 10)
standards of nursing practice a set of nursing actions that are generally agreed on by nurses as constituting safe and effective client care (Chapter 1)
standards of practice standards that describe a "competent level of nursing care as demonstrated by the critical thinking model known as the nursing process" (ANA, 2004) (Chapters 10 and 14)
standards of professional performance "authoritative statements that describe a competent level of behavior in the professional role, including activities related to quality of care, performance appraisal, education, collegiality, ethics, collaboration, research, and resource utilization" (ANA, 2004) (Chapter 14)
starch the form in which plants store glucose (Chapter 24)
statutory law law enacted by the state or federal legislative branch of government (Chapter 2)
steatorrhea gray stool mixed with observable fat and mucus and caused by malabsorption of fat (Chapter 29) [audio]
stereotyping the assumption that an attribute present in some members of a group is present in all members of a group (Chapter 3)
stoma a surgically created opening between the abdominal wall and intestine through which fecal material passes (Chapter 29)
strangulation constriction of the airway from an external cause (Chapter 23)
stress a physiological response produced by the normal wear and tear of bodily processes and external and internal demands (Chapter 47)
stress urinary incontinence the reported or observed dribbling of urine with increased abdominal pressure (Chapter 30)
stressor a cause of stress, such as extreme hot or cold, an argument, a virus, an examination, cigarette smoke, a death, or any of the countless demands of the environment (Chapter 47)
stroke volume amount of blood ejected from the heart with each contraction (Chapter 35)
subcutaneous (subcut) route injection of medication into subcutaneous tissue (which lies directly underneath the dermis) (Chapter 21)
subjective caregiver burden a caregiver's personal appraisal of a caregiving situation and the extent to which the caregiver perceives it to be a burden (Chapter 48)
subjective data information that is provided by the client and cannot be directly observed (Chapter 6)
substantive law the part of law that stipulates one's rights and duties, in contrast to procedural law, which guides the enforcement of rights (Chapter 2)
suffering an unpleasant emotional response to pain (Chapters 36 and 37)
sundowning the nocturnal exacerbation of disruptive behaviors and agitation associated with clients who have dementia (also called the **sundown syndrome**) (Chapters 36 and 40)
supportive care the medical, nursing, psychological, and social services that together help a client manage chronic illness, disability, or terminal illness when rehabilitation or restoration is not a realistic goal; also, the care that maintains physiological processes until the body can heal or definitive therapy can take effect (Chapter 4)
surgical asepsis the protection of the client against infection before, during, and after surgery using sterile technique (Chapter 22) [audio]
symbolic play pretend or imaginative play that enables the preschooler to recreate experiences and to try out roles (Chapter 16)
symptoms subjective information that is indicative of disease as perceived by the client (Chapter 6)
synergistic effect the result of one drug enhancing or increasing the effect of another drug; may be accidental or purposeful (Chapter 21)

synovium the inner layer of the articular capsule surrounding a freely movable joint that is loosely attached to the external fibrous capsule and secretes a thick fluid to lubricate the joint and absorb shock (Chapter 32)

system a set of integrated, interacting parts that function as a whole, with structure and patterns of function that accomplish the work of the whole (Chapter 48)

systole contraction of the ventricles of the heart (Chapter 35)

systolic blood pressure the maximum force of blood in the arteries during myocardial contraction (Chapter 7)

tachycardia an abnormally fast heart rate, usually above 100 beats per minute (Chapters 7 and 35) [audio]

tachypnea a respiratory rate above 20 breaths per minute for an adult (Chapter 7) [audio]

tactile pertaining to the sensation of touch (Chapter 38)

tactile fremitus a vibration in the chest wall that is felt on the thorax while the client is speaking (Chapter 8)

target organ the type of body tissue affected by a medication (Chapter 21)

tartar a yellowish film of calcium phosphate, carbonate, food particles, and other organic matter deposited on the teeth by saliva (Chapter 31)

taxonomy a system of naming and classification of phenomena (Chapter 9)

teaching a set of planned activities performed to influence knowledge, behavior, or skill (Chapter 13)

teaching plan an organized, individualized, written presentation of what the client must learn and how the instructions and information needed will be provided (Chapter 13)

team nursing a work group organization in which a group of clients are assigned to a team (including registered nurses, vocational or practical nurses, student nurses, and nursing assistants) who work together and share responsibility for the care of these clients (Chapter 14)

telegraphic speech telegram-like speech that lacks grammatical elements, such as articles, prepositions, and conjunctions (Chapter 39)

teratogenic potential the possibility that a medication will harm a developing fetus (Chapter 21) [audio]

termination in the context of an interview or a nurse-client relationship, the last phase; marked by ensuring that the expectations are met and that client satisfaction is present (Chapter 6)

termination stage in the context of behavior change, the stage in which the person is no longer tempted to engage in the old behavior (Chapter 20)

tertiary prevention actions taken when a defect or disability is permanent and irreversible; intended to minimize the effects of the disease or disability by interventions directed at preventing complications and deterioration (Chapter 19)

thanatology the discipline of study and research that deals with death and death-related topics (Chapter 45)

theoretical framework a logical but abstract structure that suggests the relationship among the variables in a research study (Chapter 15)

theory a group of propositions used to describe, explain, or predict a phenomenon (Chapter 5)

therapeutic effect the intended effect or action of a medication (Chapter 21)

therapeutic rapport a special bond that exists between a nurse and a client who have established a sense of trust and a mutual understanding of what will occur in their relationship (Chapter 12)

therapeutic relationship a helping relationship in which nurses are helpers and clients are those seeking help; personal, client-focused, and aimed at realizing mutually determined goals (Chapter 12)

thermogenesis the generation of heat from the chemical reactions that take place in cellular activity (Chapter 7) [audio]

thermolysis the processes through which heat is dispersed from the body through radiation, conduction, convection, and evaporation (Chapter 7) [audio]

T.H.I.N.K. model a critical thinking model that incorporates five modes of thinking: total recall, habits, inquiry, new ideas and creativity, and knowing how you think (Chapter 5)

third spacing the movement of fluid into an area that makes it physiologically unavailable, such as the peritoneal space (ascites), the pericardial space (pericardial effusion), the pleural space (pleural effusion), or the vesicles produced by a burn wound (Chapter 26)

tidal volume the volume of air that flows in and out of the lungs with quiet, easy respiration (Chapter 7)

tolerance an involuntary physiological phenomenon that occurs after repeated exposure to an opioid analgesic in which pain relief decreases despite a stable or escalating opioid dosage (Chapter 37)

topical route method of administering a medication directly to a body site, such as the skin, eyes, ears, nose, throat, vagina, or rectum (Chapter 21)

tort a civil wrong committed by one person against another person or his or her property; can be intentional or unintentional (Chapter 2)

total client care the provision of comprehensive care to a small group of clients by one nurse, avoiding the fragmentation of care into a series of seemingly unrelated tasks (Chapter 14)

total urinary incontinence inability to control urination, usually in immobile, cognitively impaired persons; results in undergarments or bed being almost continually wet (Chapter 30)

toxic effect a harmful result caused by an accumulation of a medication in the body (Chapter 21)

transactional leadership leadership that seeks to motivate others through a cost-benefit, economic exchange in which followers' material and psychic needs are met in return for services rendered by the follower (Chapter 14)

transcultural nursing culturally competent nursing care focused on differences between and similarities among cultures with respect to caring, health, and illness and based on the client's cultural values, beliefs, and practices (Chapter 3)

transfer note a nursing note that reflects the movement of a client from one location to another, either within the agency or to another agency (Chapter 11)

transformational leadership leadership that seeks to motivate others by inspiration, arousing and satisfying higher needs, thus engaging the full person of the follower and stimulating intellectual growth; considers individual needs for support, encouragement, and developmental experiences (Chapter 14)

trauma a physical injury or wound caused by a forceful, disruptive, or violent action (Chapter 23)

triglyceride a molecule composed of three fatty acids and a glycol unit; the chief form of fat in the diet and the main form of fat transport in the blood (Chapter 24) [audio]

trochanter roll the roll of a sheet placed under a client's hip to prevent external rotation of the trochanter (hip joint) in the supine position (Chapter 33) [audio]

turgor a reflection of the skin's elasticity, measured as the time it takes for the skin to return to normal after being pinched lightly between the thumb and forefinger (Chapter 8)

unconditional positive regard respect for the client that is not dependent on the client's behavior (Chapter 12)

universality a common mode or value of caring or a prevailing pattern of care across cultures (Chapter 3)

unlicensed assistive personnel (UAP) an unlicensed individual who is trained to function in an assistive or supportive role to the licensed nurse in the provision of direct client care or activities peripherally related to the provision of care that have been delegated by the nurse (Chapter 4)

urge urinary incontinence the reported or observed sudden desire to urinate and immediate seeking of toileting facilities (Chapter 30)

urinalysis a physical, chemical, and microscopic examination of the urine (Chapter 30) [audio]

urinary frequency urination that occurs at shorter-than-usual intervals without an increase in daily urine output (Chapter 30)

urinary hesitancy a delay in starting the urine stream, commonly with a decreased force of the stream (Chapter 30)

urinary incontinence involuntary passage of urine (Chapter 30)

urinary retention the inability to pass all or part of the urine that has accumulated in the bladder (Chapter 30)

urinary urgency a sudden, forceful urge to urinate (Chapter 30)
urination the common term for the act of micturition (Chapter 30) [audio]
validation substantiating or confirming the accuracy of the information against another source or by another method (Chapter 6)
Valsalva maneuver holding the breath and creating forced expiratory effort against a closed glottis while tightening muscles to perform work (Chapter 33)
values ideals, beliefs, and patterns of behavior that are prized and chosen by a person, group, or society (Chapter 2)
values clarification a process that allows us to identify our personal values and develop self-awareness (Chapter 2)
ventilation the process of exchanging air between the ambient air and the lungs; *pulmonary ventilation* (the total exchange of air) and *alveolar ventilation* (the effective ventilation of the alveoli) (Chapter 34)
veracity an ethical principle concerning adherence to the truth, thus requiring consistent, continual truth telling (Chapter 2)
verbal communication the use of words to convey messages (Chapter 12)
vesicular breath sounds the normal rustling and swishing breath sounds heard with a stethoscope over the lung periphery; characteristically higher pitched during inspiration and falling rapidly during expiration (inspiration longer than expiration) (Chapter 8) [audio]
vibration a technique of chest physiotherapy whereby the chest wall is set in motion by oscillating movements of the hands or a vibrator for the purpose of mobilizing secretions (Chapter 34)
virulence the power of an organism to cause disease; influenced by invasiveness (ability to adhere to mucosal cells, invade host tissue, and multiply and spread within the host) and toxigenicity (ability to produce substances that can damage the host) (Chapter 22)
virus a microorganism much smaller than a bacterium that can replicate only inside a host cell (Chapter 22)
visceral pain poorly localized pain that results from nociceptor activation by stretching, distention, or contraction of smooth muscle walls; ischemia of the visceral wall; irritation or inflammation; or torsion or traction on mesenteric attachment organs (Chapter 37) [audio]
viscosity the relative ability of a fluid to flow (Chapter 35)
visual pertaining to the sensation of sight (Chapter 38)
vitamin an organic substance found in food that serves as a coenzyme in enzymatic reactions (Chapter 24)
void a term synonymous with micturition and urination that is used most often in clinical settings (Chapter 30)
vulnerability a feeling or experience of helplessness, lack of control, and inadequate resources for defense when faced with threat or danger (Chapter 42)
vulnerable population a subgroup of a larger population that has an increased risk of health problems because of exposure or coexisting health or nonhealth problems (Chapter 43)
well-being a subjective perception of a good and satisfactory existence in which the individual has a positive experience of personal abilities, harmony, and vitality (Chapter 19)
wellness a state of optimal health or optimal physical and social functioning (Chapter 19)
wellness nursing diagnosis the desire in an individual, family, or community to move toward a quality, or higher state, of being healthy, usually involving deliberate action (Chapter 9)
Wernicke's area the portion of the brain that helps control the content of speech and affects auditory and visual comprehension (Chapter 39)
windshield survey a method of data collection in which the researcher or surveyor drives through a neighborhood to conduct a general assessment of that neighborhood through observation (Chapter 43)
working phase a phase of the interview process in which the client and the nurse work together to review the client's health history and establish potential and actual problems that will be addressed in the care plan (Chapter 6)
wound a disruption of the normal anatomical structure and function that results from pathological processes that arise internally or externally to the involved organ(s) (Chapter 27)
wrist drop a contracture of the wrist in the flexed position (Chapter 33)
young adulthood the period of time between ages 20 and 35 (Chapter 17)
zeitgeber environmental trigger or synchronizer that adjusts the human body's internal clock to a 24-hour solar day; may be physical (sunlight) or social (meals) (Chapter 36)

INDEX

NOTE: Page numbers followed by f indicate figures; those followed by t indicate tables; and those followed by b indicate boxed material.

Clustering Data to Make a Nursing Diagnosis

Cross-Cultural Care

Evidence-Based Practice

Key Nursing Diagnoses